Success in the Classroom, in Clinicals, and on the NCLEX-RN®

Classroom

- Detailed lecture notes organized by learning outcome
- Suggestions for classroom activities
- Guide to relevant additional resources
- Comprehensive PowerPoint™ presentations integrating lecture, and images
- Online course management systems complete with instructor tools and student activities

Clinical

- Suggestions for Clinical Activities and other clinical resources organized by learning outcome

Real Nursing Simulations Facilitator's Guide: Institutional Edition

- 25 simulation scenarios that span the nursing curriculum
- Consistent format includes learning objectives, case flow, instructions for set up, student debriefing questions and more!
- Companion online course cartridge with student exercises, activities, videos, skill checklists, and reflective questions also available for adoption

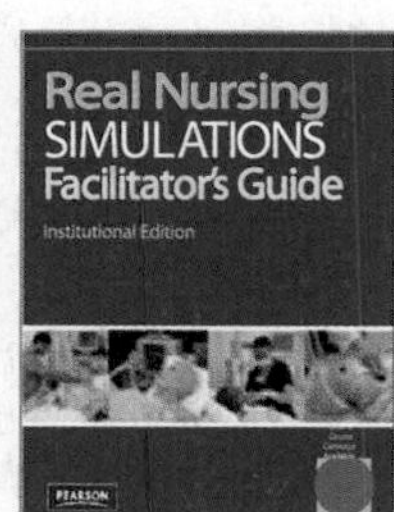

NCLEX-RN®

- Test Item Files with NCLEX®-style questions and complete rationales for correct and incorrect answers mapped to learning outcomes. *available in TestGen, Par Test, and MS Word*

Instructor Resources

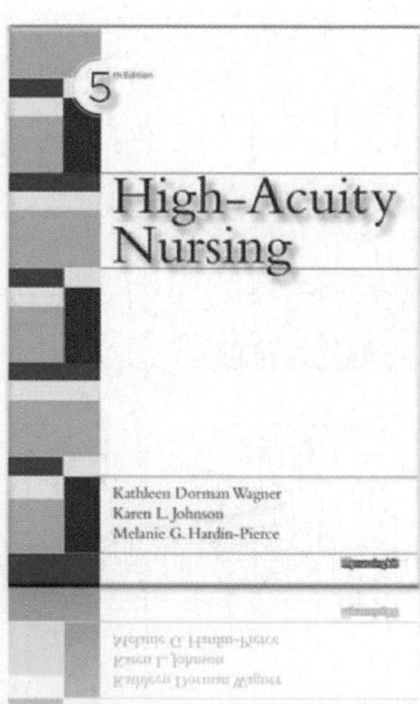

More *information and instructor resources*
visit **www.mynursingkit.com**

HIGH-ACUITY NURSING

HIGH-ACUITY NURSING

FIFTH EDITION

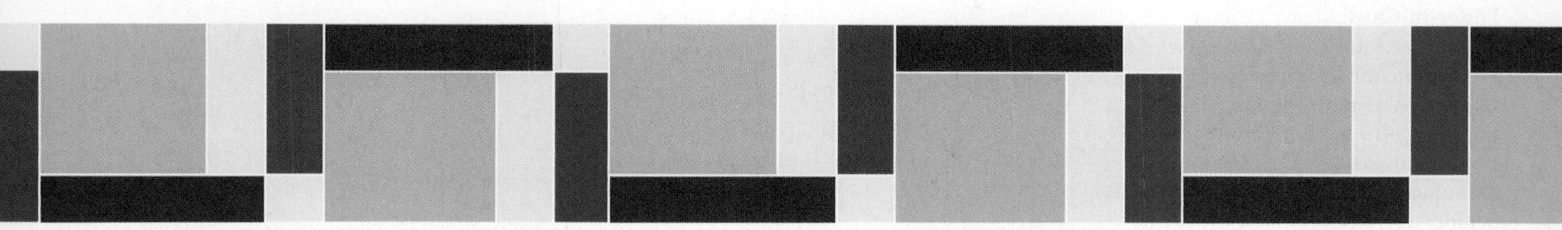

Kathleen Dorman Wagner, EdD, MSN, RN
University of Kentucky College of Nursing
Lexington, Kentucky

Karen L. Johnson, PhD, RN
University of Maryland School of Nursing
University of Maryland Medical Center
Baltimore, Maryland

Melanie G. Hardin-Pierce, DNP, RN, ACNP-BC
University of Kentucky College of Nursing
Central Baptist Hospital
Lexington, Kentucky

Pearson
Boston Columbus Indianapolis New York San Francisco Upper Saddle River
Amsterdam Cape Town Dubai London Madrid Milan Munich Paris Montreal Toronto
Delhi Mexico City Sao Paulo Sydney Hong Kong Seoul Singapore Taipei Tokyo

Library of Congress Cataloging-in-Publication Data
Wagner, Kathleen Dorman.
High-acuity nursing / Kathleen Dorman Wagner, Karen L. Johnson, Melanie G. Hardin-Pierce. — 5th ed.
p.; cm.
Includes bibliographical references and index.
ISBN-13: 978-0-13-504926-6
ISBN-10: 0-13-504926-1
1. Intensive care nursing. I. Johnson, Karen L., (date)– II. Hardin-Pierce, Melanie G. III. Title.
[DNLM: 1. Critical Care—methods. 2. Critical Illness—nursing. 3. Nursing Process. WY 154 W133h 2010]
RT120.I5K53 2010
616.02'8—dc22

2009017700

Publisher: Julie Levin Alexander
Publisher's Assistant: Regina Bruno
Editor-in-Chief: Maura Connor
Executive Acquisitions Editor: Pamela Fuller
Development Editor: Jennifer Blackwell
Editorial Assistant: Jennifer Aranda/Lisa Pierce
Managing Production Editor: Patrick Walsh
Production Liaison: Cathy O'Connell
Manufacturing Manager: Ilene Sanford
Senior Art Director: Maria Guglielmo
Art Director: Chris Weigand
Director of Marketing: Karen Allman
Marketing Specialist: Michael Sirinides
Marketing Assistant: Crystal Gonzalez
Digital Media Product Manager: Travis Moses-Westphal
Media Project Manager: Rachel Collett
Manager, Rights and Permissions: Zina Arabia
Manager, Visual Research: Beth Brenzel
Image Permission Coordinator: Richard Rodrigues
Full-Service Project Management: Elm Street Publishing Services
Composition: Integra Software Services Pvt. Ltd.
Printer/Binder: Courier/Kendallville
Cover Printer: Lehigh-Phoenix/Hagerstown

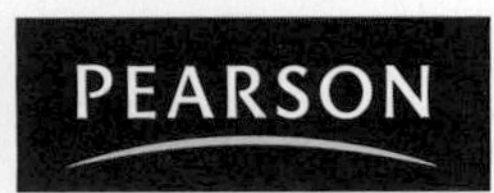

www.pearsonhighered.com

10 9 8 7 6 5 4
ISBN-10: 0-13-504926-1
ISBN-13: 978-0-13-504926-6

About the Authors

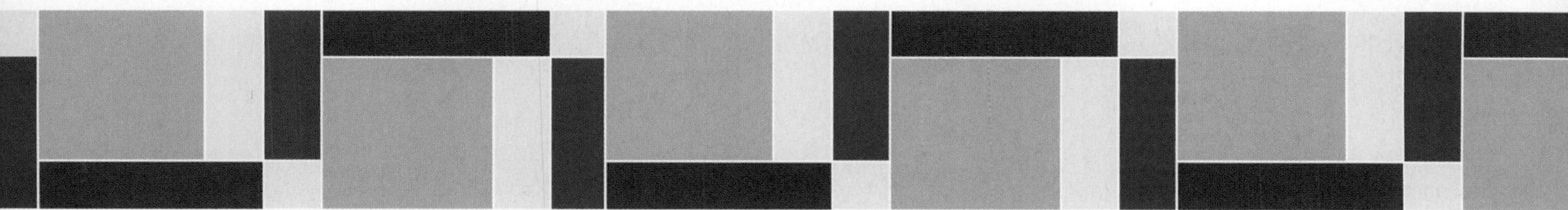

Kathleen Wagner, EdD, MSN, RN, is a lecturer in the undergraduate program in the College of Nursing at the University of Kentucky. As a nurse educator, she teaches pathopharmacology and high-acuity nursing. She is also the educational consultant for the undergraduate program at the University of Kentucky. She has a doctorate in instructional systems design with a focus on learning transfer and case method instruction.

Karen Johnson, PhD, RN, is an associate professor at the University of Maryland School of Nursing and director of nursing, research & evidence-based practice at the University of Maryland Medical Center.

Melanie Hardin-Pierce, DNP, RN, ACNP-BC, is an assistant professor in the University of Kentucky College of Nursing, where she teaches in both the undergraduate and graduate programs. She earned her Doctor of Nursing Practice degree at the University of Kentucky studying oral health in mechanically ventilated patients. She is a board-certified acute-care nurse practitioner who practices as a critical care intensivist in Central Baptist Hospital, Lexington. She is the primary investigator in funded research that examines inflammation, cardiovascular function, and weaning outcomes in mechanically ventilated adults.

Thank You

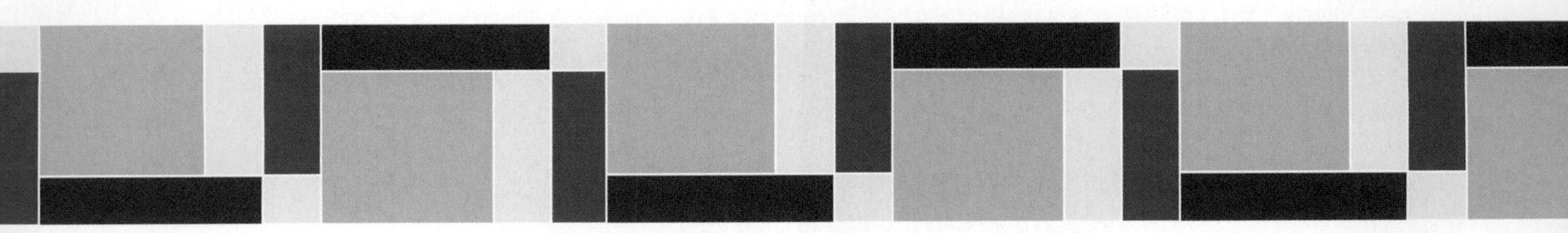

We extend a heartfelt thanks to our contributors and reviewers, who gave their time, effort, and expertise so tirelessly to the development and writing of this new edition of our book.

Contributors

Tonya L. Appleby, MSN, RN, ACNP-BC
University of Maryland School of Nursing
Baltimore, Maryland

Jill Arzouman, MS, RN, ACNS, BC
University Medical Center
Tucson, Arizona

Beth Augustyn, MSN, RN, ACNP, CCRN
Chest Medicine Consultants
Chicago, Illinois

Susan Bohnenkamp, MS, APRN-BC, CNS, CCM
University Medical Center
Tucson, Arizona

Zara R. Brenner, MS, RN-BC, ACNS-BC
The College at Brockport
Brockport, New York
Rochester General Hospital
Rochester, New York

Lacey Troutman Buckler, MSN, RN, ACNP-BC
University of Kentucky Gill Heart Institute
Lexington, Kentucky

Joan Davenport, PhD, RN, CCRN
University of Maryland School of Nursing
Baltimore, Maryland

Theresa M. Glessner, MSN, RN, ACNP-BC, NEA-BC, CCRN
Cardiothoracic Service
Rochester General Hospital
Rochester, New York

Kiersten Henry, MS, APRN-BC, ACNP, CCNS, CCRN-CMC, TTS
Montgomery General Hospital
Olney, Maryland

Donna Jarzyna, MS, RN-C, CNS-BC
University Medical Center
Tucson, Arizona

Julia King, MSN, RN, CCNS, ACNP-BC
United States Navy
Portsmouth Naval Medical Center
Portsmouth, Virginia

Maureen E. Krenzer, MS, RN, NP, ACNS-BC
Rochester General Hospital
Rochester, New York
Wegmans School of Nursing at St. John Fisher College
Rochester, New York

Kristine Hart L'Ecuyer, MSN, RN, CCNS
Saint Louis University School of Nursing
St. Louis, Missouri

Helen M. Lach, PhD, RN, GCNS-BC
Saint Louis University School of Nursing
St. Louis, Missouri

Virginia LeBaron, MS, ACNP-BC, AOCN, ACHPN
University Medical Center,
Tucson, Arizona

Nancy Munro, RN, MN, CCRN, ACNP
National Institutes of Health
Bethesda, Maryland

Angela C. Muzzy, MSN, RN, CCRN
University Medical Center
Tucson, Arizona

Grace Nolde-Lopez, MS, RN, CWOCN, CRRN, ANP-BC
CNS Medical Group
Englewood, Colorado

Gail Priestley, MSN, RN, APRN–BC, CCRN, CNS
University Medical Center
Tucson, Arizona

Clifford C. Pyne, MS, RN, ACNP-BC
Peninsula Cancer Institute
Newport News, Virginia
Chesapeake Free Clinic
Chesapeake, Virginia

Valerie Sabol, MSN, RN, CCRN, ACNP-BC
University of Maryland School of Nursing
Baltimore, Maryland

Kara Adams Snyder, MS, RN, CCRN, CCNS
University Medical Center
Tucson, Arizona

Diana Thacker, MSN, RN, CPTC
Kentucky Organ Donor Affiliates
Lexington, Kentucky

Paul Thurman, MS, RN, ACNP, CCNS, CCRN, CNRN
R. Adams Cowley Shock Trauma Center, University of Maryland Medical Center
Baltimore, Maryland

Vicky L. Turner, MSN, RN, ACNP-BC, CCRN
University of Kentucky Hospital
Lexington, Kentucky

Supplement Contributors

Josephine Lister Hendrix, MSN, FNP-C
Instructor, Health Occupations
Northwestern Michigan College
Traverse City, Michigan

Laura A. Schmidt, MSN, FNP-BC
Director, Allied Health
Northwestern Michigan College
Traverse City, Michigan

Betsy Swinny, MSN, RN, CCRN
Faculty II
BHS School of Health Professions
San Antonio, Texas.

4th Edition Contributor Acknowledgments

Adam DaDeppo
Dayna Gary
Conrad Gordon
Kathy Hausman
Jane Lacovara
Catherine McDonald
Ted Rigney
Allison Steele
Amy Tarbay
Michelle Willis

Reviewers

Andrea Dodge Ackermann, PhD, RN, CCRN
Mount Saint Mary College
Newburgh, New York

Melanie Akers, MSN, RN, BC
Marshall University
College of Health Professions
Huntington, West Virginia

Beverly Anderson, MSN, RN
Salt Lake Community College
West Jordon, Utah

Jeane Asel, MS, RN, APRN-BC, CCRN
Texas Woman's University
Dallas, Texas

Donna Garbacz Bader, MSN, RNC, CFN, D-ABMDI
Assistant Professor
BryanLGH College of Health Sciences
Lincoln, Nebraska

Angela Balistrieri, MSN, RN, CCRN
Mercy Hospital School of Nursing
Pittsburgh, Pennsylvania

Cheryl L. Bausler, PhD, RN
University of Missouri
Sinclair School of Nursing
Columbia, Missouri

Michele L. Beatty, MSN, RN
Southern Illinois University Edwardsville
Edwardsville, Illinois

Alice Blazeck, DNSc, RN
University of Pittsburgh
School of Nursing
Pittsburgh, Pennsylvania

Marylee Bressie, MSN, RN, CCRN, CCNS, CEN
Spring Hill College
Mobile, Alabama

Ann H. Crawford, PhD, RN, CNS
University of Mary Hardin-Baylor
Belton, Texas

David G. Curry, PhD, APRN
SUNY Plattsburgh
Plattsburgh, New York

Kelly Dempsey, MSN, RNC
Indiana University East
Richmond, Indiana

M. Joyce Dienger, PhD, RN
University of Cincinnati
College of Nursing
Cincinnati, Ohio

Linda Dune, PhD, RN, CCRN, CEN, Dipl ABT
University of Houston-Victoria
School of Nursing
Sugar Land, Texas

C. Suzanne Gosse, PhD, RN
Indiana State University
College of Nursing, Health and Human Services
Terre Haute, Indiana

Sheila Grossman, PhD, FNP-BC
Fairfield University School of Nursing
Fairfield, Connecticut

Karla Hanson, MS, RN
South Dakota State University
Brookings, South Dakota

Margaret Harvey, PhD, ACNP-BC
UT Health Science Center
Memphis, Tennessee

Stacey J. Jones, MSN, CRNP
Troy University School of Nursing
Troy, Alabama

Joan E. King, PhD, ACNP-BC, ANP-BC
Program Director for the Acute Care Nurse Practitioner Program
Vanderbilt University
School of Nursing
Nashville, Tennessee

Karen S. March, PhD, RN, CCRN, ACNS-BC
York College of Pennsylvania
York, Pennsylvania

Diane Mulbrook, MA, RN
Mount Mercy College
Cedar Rapids, Iowa

David G. Parkhurst, MSN, RN, FNP, APRN-BC
Sonoma State University
School of Nursing
Rohnert Park, California

Marian Pezdek, MS, RN
Joliet Junior College
Joliet, Illinois

Carrie L. Pucino, MS, RN, CCRN
York College of Pennsylvania
York, Pennsylvania

Gail Rattigan, MSN, R.N., FNP-BC
Nevada State College
Henderson, Nevada

Maria A. Revell, DSN, RN, COI
Middle Tennessee State University
School of Nursing
Murfreesboro, Tennessee

Vanessa Sammons, MSN, APRN, BC, CNE
Morehead State University
Morehead, Kentucky

Laura A. Schmidt, MSN, FNP-BC
Director, Allied Health
Northwestern Michigan College
Traverse City, Michigan

Margi J. Schultz, PhD, RN
GateWay Community College
Phoenix, Arizona

Deborah Jane Schwytzer, MSN, RN, CEN
University of Cincinnati
College of Nursing
Cincinnati, Ohio

Susan B. Sepples, PhD, MS, CCRN
University of Southern Maine
Portland, Maine

Nita Slater, MSN, RN
University of Arizona
College of Nursing
Tucson, Arizona

Scott Suttles, BSN, RN, CCRN-CSC, NREMT-P
Morehead State University
Morehead, Kentucky

Laura B. Sutton, PhD, ACNS-BC
University of Florida
College of Nursing
Gainesville, Florida

Jeanine M. Karle Swails, MSN, RN, CNRN
University of Cincinnati
College of Nursing
Cincinnati, Ohio

Rita Trivette, MSN, CNN
Milligan College
Milligan College, Tennessee

Judy Walloch, EdD, RN, CNE
Graham Hospital School of Nursing
Canton, Illinois

Shirley Kay Woolf, MSN, MA, RN, CCRN, CNE
Indiana University
School of Nursing
Indianapolis, Indiana

Kathleen Zellner, PhD, MSN, RN
Bellin College of Nursing
Green Bay, Wisconsin

Preface

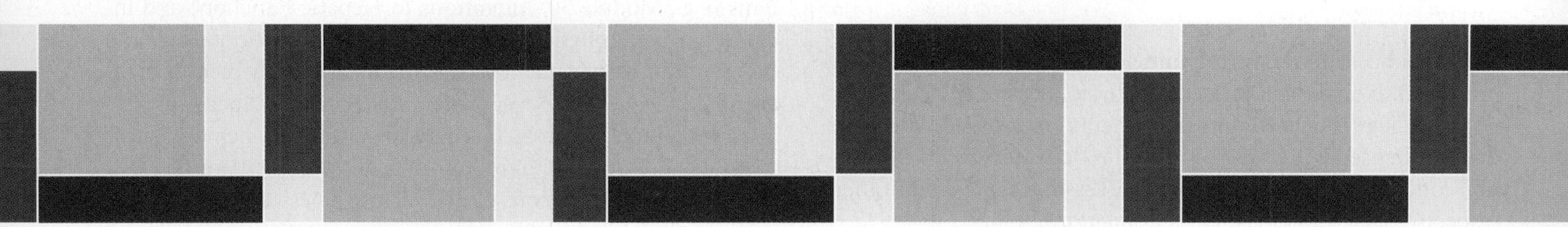

When the first edition of *High-Acuity Nursing* was published in 1992, the term *high-acuity* was largely confined to leveling patient acuity for determining hospital staffing needs rather than being applied to nursing education. Today, there is a growing trend toward offering a high-acuity nursing course as part of the required undergraduate nursing curriculum. This, we believe, reflects the changing nature of the acute-care adult patient population and the need to adequately prepare new nurses to meet these rapidly changing needs.

The term *high-acuity* refers to a level of patient problems beyond uncomplicated acute illness on a health–illness continuum. Today, high-acuity patients are increasingly found outside of critical-care units or even acute-care institutions. The patient population is older and faces an increased number of health issues upon entering the health-care system. Hospitalized patients are being discharged earlier, often in a poorer state of health. In the home-health setting, nurses provide care to patients with mechanical ventilators, central intravenous (IV) lines, IV antibiotic therapy, and complicated injuries. Whereas critical-care units are considered specialty areas within the hospital walls, much of the knowledge required to work within those specialties is generalist in nature. It is this generalist knowledge base that is needed by all nurses who work with patients experiencing complex care problems to assure competent and safe nursing practice.

Purpose of the Text

The *High-Acuity Nursing* text delivers critical information using learner-focused, active learning principles, with concise language and a user-friendly format. The book's design breaks down complex information into small, discrete chunks for easy understanding. Self-testing is provided throughout the text, using Pretests, short section quizzes, and Posttests. All answers to the section review quizzes are provided to give learners immediate feedback on their command of section content before proceeding to the next module section.

The self-study modules in this book focus on the relationship between pathophysiology and the nursing process with the following goals in mind

1. To revisit and translate critical pathophysiological concepts pertaining to the high-acuity adult patient in a clinically applicable manner.
2. To examine the interrelationships among physiological concepts.
3. To enhance clinical decision-making skills.
4. To provide immediate feedback to the learner regarding assimilation of concepts and principles.
5. To provide self-paced learning.

Ultimately, the goal is for the learner to be able to approach patient care conceptually, so that care is provided with a strong underlying understanding of its rationale.

This book is appropriate for use in multiple educational settings, including undergraduate nursing students, novice nurses, novice critical-care nurses, and home-health nurses. It also serves as a review book for the experienced nurse wanting updated information about high-acuity nursing for continuing education purposes. Hospital staff development departments will find it useful as supplemental or required reading for nursing staff, or high-acuity/critical care classes.

Organization of the Text

The book consists of ten parts: Special Topics, Hematologic (Cellular Function), Pulmonary Gas Exchange, Cardiac Output, Tissue Perfusion, Neurologic, Fluid and Electrolyte Balance, Metabolic: Regulation of Internal Environment, Metabolic: Nutrition, and Tissue Integrity. Part One: Special Topics is composed of four introductory chapters (called modules) with topics that apply across high-acuity problems, including an introduction to high-acuity nursing and care of high-acuity patients, acute pain management, and important considerations when caring for the high-acuity older adult. Parts 2 through 10 present topics that represent the more common complex problems, assessments, and treatments associated with high-acuity adult patients. All modules contain Module Objectives, Pretest, Section Review Questions, and Posttest. Each module is divided into small sections that cover one facet of the module's topic (e.g., pathophysiology or nursing management), and each section ends with a short self-assessment review quiz. Key words are bolded throughout the modules to indicate glossary terms defined in the textbook's Glossary. Parts 2 through 10 of the book are composed of two different types of modules, including *Determinants and Assessment* modules and *Alterations* modules.

Determinants and Assessment Modules

Each part begins with an overview of normal concepts that provides a solid foundation for understanding the diseases being presented. Normal anatomy and physiology are reviewed and relevant diagnostic tests and assessments are profiled. The more disease-focused (Alterations) modules draw heavily on the normal concepts, diagnostic tests, and assessments covered in their respective *Determinants and Assessment* module.

Alterations Modules

Following each *Determinants and Assessment* module is a series of organ- or concept-specific modules that focus on a single topic area. The majority of *Alterations* modules are based on body systems (e.g., Module 30, Alterations in Hepatic Function) and include the pathophysiology, assessments, diagnostic testing, and collaborative management of disorders commonly seen in high-acuity adult patients. Several *Alterations* modules focus on supportive therapies, such as mechanical ventilation, hemodynamic monitoring, ECG rhythm monitoring, and complex wound management; or complications of high-acuity illness, such as multiple organ dysfunction syndrome or sensory motor complications of acute illness. The pathophysiologic basis of disease is emphasized in this textbook with the belief that strong foundational knowledge about the basis of disease improves learner understanding of the associated disease manifestations and rationales for treatment.

New to This Edition

The fifth edition has undergone major revamping of content to address concerns specific to the high-acuity population. We are extremely excited to have upgraded the textbook to full color with this edition. The book parts have been reorganized and expanded to improve the module organization.

- A new book part, Hematologic, has been added to better describe the many blood cell-related disorders and considerations that significantly impact this patient population.
- All modules have been updated and substantially reorganized, with normal concepts being moved into the *Determinants and Assessment* modules. This allows the *Alterations* modules to focus on related disease states.
- The glossaries and abbreviations that were previously located at the beginning of each module are now located in a formal Glossary in the back of the book to reduce definition redundancy.
- Nursing management of the high-acuity patient has been significantly increased throughout the book, as has pharmacotherapy, to include two new sets of special elements, NURSING CARE and RELATED PHARMACOTHERAPY boxes.
- Test items have been revised to reflect the changes in content and Posttest answers now include rationales.
- Research has been integrated throughout the content and *Emerging Evidence* boxes are included in the modules to emphasize the importance of evidence-based practice.
- A new module focusing on the older high-acuity patient has been added to reflect the high percentage of elderly patients who require high-acuity nursing care.
- The organ transplant module has been expanded to include hematopoietic stem cell transplantation.
- The ECG rhythm interpretation chapter has been expanded to include more rhythm interpretation exercises.
- A new module, Sensory Motor Complications of Acute Illness, addresses a variety of neurological alterations that are commonly noted in the high-acuity patient population, such as altered mentation and consciousness, neuromuscular weakness syndromes, and common seizure-related complications.
- The nursing management modules found in the previous editions of the book have been moved to the book's online platform as Web-based exercises.
- A summary section has been added to each module and is found on MyNursingKit. Important points are identified and emphasized, enhancing learner review of the material.
- Each module also has a new online Critical Thinking Checkpoint exercise that includes a case scenario and higher-level (critical thinking) short-answer questions that pertain to a major concept in the module, and exemplar answers are provided. The *Critical Thinking Checkpoint* exercises are found in MyNursingKit. The answers to the Pretests and Posttests will be found on MyNursingKit as well.

Summary

This text is a series of reality-based modules that focus on concepts frequently encountered in high-acuity patients. It is not designed as a comprehensive review of pathophysiology or medical-surgical nursing. The book's format reduces learner feelings of being overwhelmed by complex information. Learners are more apt to feel in command of the concepts, giving them the confidence to proceed to the more complex concepts. The fifth edition of *High-Acuity Nursing* has maintained the overall look and feel of the previous editions, with some valuable changes. Although the fifth edition has been reorganized, we have not compromised our interactive approach. The ultimate goal of this book continues to be to enhance the preparation of nurses for practice in today's health care settings.

Kathleen Dorman Wagner
Karen L. Johnson
Melanie G. Hardin-Pierce

Acknowledgments

I would like to once again acknowledge our dear friend, mentor, and colleague, Dr. Pamela Kidd, who co-edited the first three editions of *High-Acuity Nursing.* Without her quiet leadership and competence, creativity and support, this unique textbook would not exist. My heartfelt thanks go out to my friend and colleague, Dr. Karen Johnson, for her continued support in bringing this fifth edition into fruition. I would also like to thank our newest editor, Dr. Melanie Hardin-Pierce, for her willingness to take on the editorial task with so many other commitments on her plate. Editing and contributing to a textbook is not for the faint of heart! To Don, Becky, Debby, Tom and now our little Zoe —my family, my joy.

–KDW

Twenty years ago our colleague, Dr. Pamela Kidd, came up with the idea for this unique textbook. We honor her memory by striving for excellence with each new edition. Thank you, my dear friend Dr. Kathy Wagner, for your leadership, organization, and amazing creativity on this edition. To Dr. Melanie Hardin-Pierce, thank you for joining us; we could not have done this edition without you. A soul-full and heartfelt thank-you to my husband Steve for his everlasting love and support throughout my career. Without you, everything else is meaningless. Nineteen years ago, I wrote the shock module while in labor with my son Christopher. To Christopher, now in college, I am so proud of you! Thank you for your humor and love. To Amy, I am so proud of the beautiful, intelligent young lady you have become. Thank you for sacrificing countless evenings and weekends as I worked on "the book." Now, let's go shopping!

–KLJ

I want to thank my friend and mentor, Dr. Kathleen Wagner, for her guidance and support on this revision. Her competent leadership, patience, and sense of humor gave me hope and made this revision work possible for us all. She bailed me out of some difficult situations, for which I am eternally grateful. My appreciation also goes to Dr. Karen Johnson, the reviewers, contributors, the PH staff, and to the enduring legacy of Dr. Pamela Kidd, all of whom made this text and revision possible. It is indeed an honor and a privilege to be a part of this team. This acknowledgment would not be complete without honoring my husband Mike and daughters Chelsea and Haley, who offered me support, cooked my meals, and tolerated all of my "book clutter" this past year while encouraging me along the way. They are priceless, and I love them.

–MHP

Contents

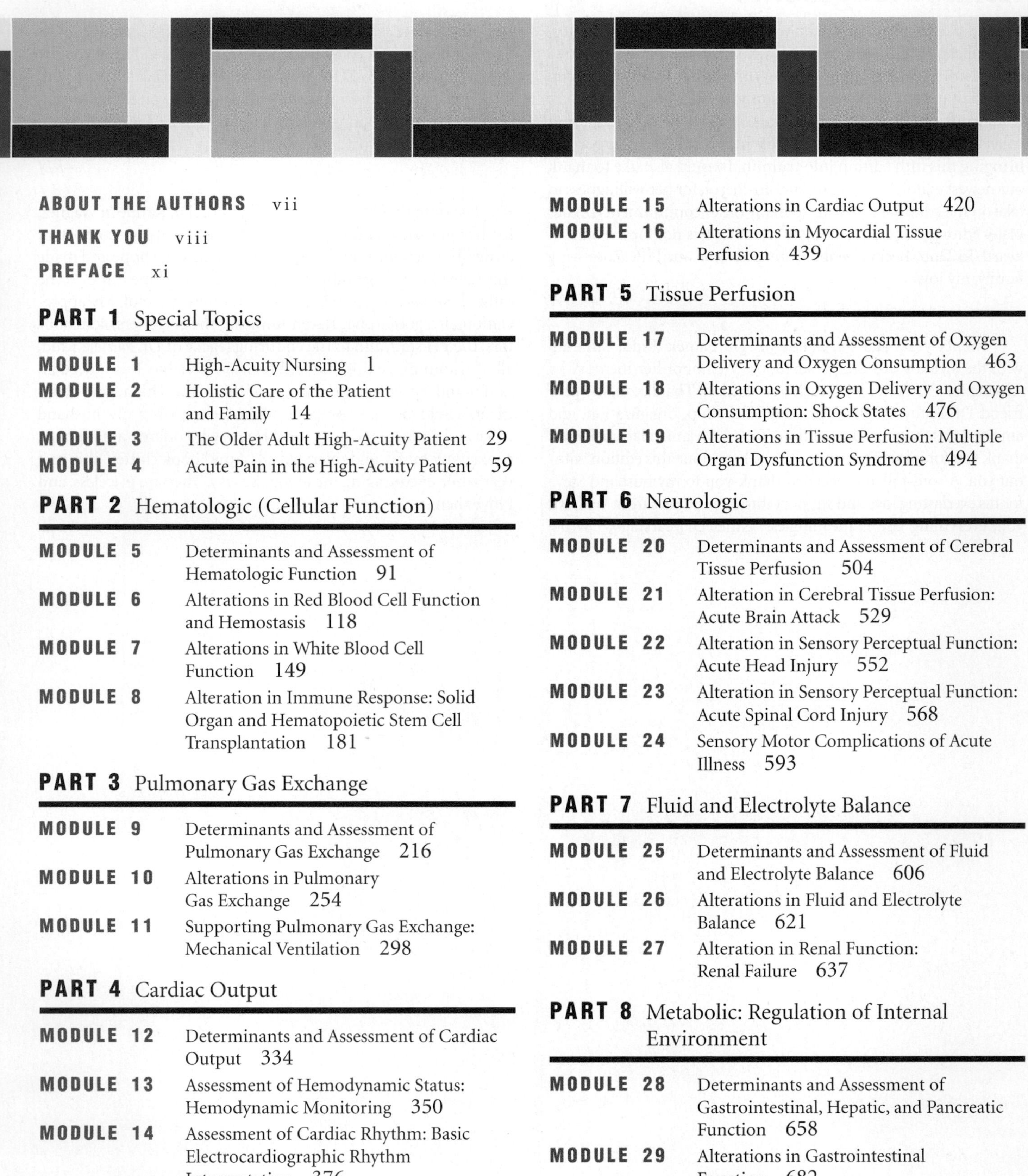

HIGH-ACUITY NURSING

MODULE

1 High-Acuity Nursing

Jill Arzouman

OBJECTIVES

Following completion of this module, the learner will be able to

1. Discuss the various health care environments in which high-acuity patients receive care.
2. Identify the need for resource allocation and staffing strategies for high-acuity patients.
3. Examine the use of technology in high-acuity environments.
4. Identify the components of a healthy work environment.
5. Discuss the importance of patient safety in the high-acuity environment.

This module is written at a core knowledge level for individuals who provide nursing care for high-acuity patients, regardless of the practice setting. The focus of the module is on the environment in which high-acuity nursing care is given. The module consists of five sections. Section One discusses the environments in which high-acuity patients are placed to receive care. Section Two addresses staffing strategies and resource allocation. The use of technology in the high-acuity environment is discussed in Section Three. Section Four addresses the components of a healthy work environment. Section Five examines patient safety in the high-acuity environment. All Section Reviews include answers. It is suggested that the learner review those concepts answered incorrectly in the review questions before proceeding to the next section.

PRETEST

1. Which of the following has been shown to reduce mortality and life-threatening complications in hospitalized patients?
   A. constant surveillance of patients by nurses
   B. admission to the ICU
   C. treatment by a good physician
   D. admission to a university hospital
2. An intermediate-care unit serves as a place for the monitoring and care of patients
   A. with moderate or potentially severe physiologic instability
   B. who require technical support
   C. who do not require life-sustaining support
   D. all of the above
3. Intensive care units were first developed in the year
   A. 1900
   B. 1945
   C. 1960
   D. 1980
4. Which of the following professional organizations has mandated that the safest nurse-to-patient ratio in high-acuity settings is 1:4?
   A. American Association of Critical Care Nurses
   B. Academy of Medical Surgical Nurses
   C. Society of Critical Care Medicine
   D. none of the above
5. Hospitals that achieve Magnet Accreditation
   A. recruit and attract unlicensed assistive personnel
   B. recruit and retain registered nurses
   C. give nurses higher salaries
   D. can attract nurses, but have difficulty retaining nurses
6. Which of the following play an important role in determining allocation and utilization of ICU resources?
   A. physicians and nurses
   B. patient wishes
   C. families
   D. all of the above
7. Technology causes difficulties when
   A. the machine becomes the primary focus instead of the patient
   B. the machines leave little surface area for physical contact
   C. the machines create fear in the patient and family
   D. all of the above
8. It is essential that the nurse validate technologic data with
   A. the critical care provider
   B. other technologic data

C. nursing assessment data
D. none of the above

9. Stress is a major component of
   A. working in high-acuity settings
   B. burnout
   C. compassion fatigue
   D. depression
10. Which of the following are symptoms of nurse burnout?
   A. cigarette smoking
   B. chronic fatigue
   C. hostility and negativism
   D. all of the above
11. Which of the following can be used positively to cope with burnout and stress?
   A. critical incident stress debriefing
   B. alcohol
   C. change in career
   D. withdrawal
12. A healthy work environment is characterized by
   A. frequent social gatherings
   B. potluck luncheons
   C. nurses being recognized and valued as partners in policy making
   D. low rate of absenteeism
13. High levels of team work in high-acuity settings results in
   A. frequent visits of past patients
   B. decreased length of stay and decreased mortality
   C. increased length of stay and increased mortality
   D. higher use of precious resources
14. Which of the following jeopardize patient safety?
   A. nursing shortage
   B. overtime hours
   C. excessive documentation
   D. all of the above

Pretest answers are found on MyNursingKit.

SECTION ONE: High-Acuity Environment

At the completion of this section, the learner will be able to discuss the various health care environments in which high-acuity patients receive care.

The nurse caring for the high-acuity patient must be able to analyze clinical situations, make decisions based on this analysis, and rapidly intervene to ensure optimal patient outcomes. It is required that the nurse be comfortable with uncertainty and patient instability. The nurse is instrumental in treating patients' health problems as well as their reactions to the health care environment. The nurse is the only member of the health care team who remains at the bedside and, as a result, is frequently the one who coordinates patient care.

The nurse is often the first member of the health care team to detect early signs of an impending complication. Constant surveillance by the nurse involves assessing and monitoring the patient for signs of subtle changes over time. Many times, subtle changes in a patient's condition are clues of a possible impending complication. Prevention of complications in the patient is one of the primary goals of the acute care nurse. Evidence suggests that constant surveillance of patients by nurses reduces mortality and life-threatening complications in the hospitalized patient (Clarke & Aiken, 2006).

Intensive care units (ICUs) were first developed in the early 1960s. There were multiple reasons for their development, including (1) the implementation of cardiopulmonary resuscitation (CPR) so that people might survive sudden death events; (2) better understanding of the treatment of hypovolemic shock related to recent war experiences; (3) the implementation of emergency medical services, resulting in improved transport systems; (4) the development of technologic inventions that required close observation for effective use (electrocardiographic monitoring); and (5) the initiation of renal transplant surgery. The first ICUs were recovery rooms. Patients admitted were still anesthetized. Problems resulted, however, when the volume of surgical procedures increased, and recovery rooms quickly became full. The patient who required extra equipment and prolonged observation was placed in the newly created ICU.

Although high-acuity patients are viewed historically as being in an acute care unit, because of the shortage of acute care beds this is no longer true. This shortage of beds combined with skyrocketing costs for health care requires practitioners to make decisions about where in the hospital high-acuity patients are placed so that they receive the most efficient and cost-effective care. This may mean the patient is placed in an ICU, an **intermediate-care unit (IMC),** or in a medical–surgical acute care unit. These triage decisions require a systematic approach so that optimal outcomes and controlled costs are achieved.

The use of intermediate–care or step-down units may provide an efficient distribution of resources for the patient whose acute illness requires less monitoring equipment and staffing than an ICU (American College of Critical Care Medicine [ACCM], 1998). The intermediate-care unit serves as a place for the monitoring and care of patients with moderate or potentially severe physiologic instability who require technical support but not necessarily artificial life support; it is reserved for those patients requiring less-than-standard intensive care but more than that which is available from ward care (ACCM, 1998). Guidelines for the admission and discharge for adult intermediate-care units are available (ACCM, 1998).

TABLE 1–1 Prioritization of Admission, Discharge, and Triage of Acutely Ill Patients in an ICU

PRIORITY FOR ICU PLACEMENT	DESCRIPTION OF PATIENT CHARACTERISTICS
Priority 1	Acutely ill, unstable, and requires intensive treatment and monitoring that cannot be provided outside of the ICU (mechanical ventilation, continuous vasoactive drug infusions). There are no limits on the extent of intended interventions. Examples of these patients may include postoperative or acute respiratory failure patients requiring mechanical ventilator support, and shock or hemodynamically unstable patients receiving invasive monitoring and/or vasoactive drugs.
Priority 2	Requires intensive monitoring, may potentially need immediate intervention. There are no limits on the extent of intended interventions. Examples include patients with chronic comorbid conditions who develop acute severe medical or surgical illness.
Priority 3	Critically ill and unstable with a reduced likelihood of recovery because of underlying disease or nature of the acute illness. May receive intensive treatment to relieve acute illness; however, limits on therapeutic efforts may be set, such as no intubation or cardiopulmonary resuscitation. Examples include patients with metastatic malignancy complicated by infection, cardiac tamponade, or airway obstruction.
Priority 4	Generally not appropriate for ICU admission. Admission should be made on an individual basis, under unusual circumstances, and at the discretion of the ICU director. Examples include patients with peripheral vascular surgery, stable diabetic ketoacidosis, conscious drug overdose, and patients with terminal and irreversible illness facing immediate death.

Data from Task Force of the American College of Critical Care Medicine, Society of Critical Care Medicine. (1999). Guidelines for intensive care unit admission, discharge, and triage. *Critical Care Medicine, 27*(3), 635.

The Society of Critical Care Medicine (SCCM) recommends using a prioritization model to help make decisions about appropriate admission, discharge, and triage of acutely ill patients in an ICU (ACCM, 1999). The model defines which patients may benefit most from receiving care in an ICU. This prioritization model is summarized in Table 1–1. Priority 1 includes the most critically ill and Priority 4 includes those who are generally not appropriate candidates for ICU admission.

ICUs vary from hospital to hospital in terms of the services provided, the personnel, and their level of expertise. Large medical centers frequently have multiple ICUs defined by specialty area (neurosurgical ICU, trauma ICU). Small hospitals may have only one ICU designed to care for a variety of patients with medical or surgical disease processes. Although the types and varieties of ICUs may differ from one hospital to the next, all ICUs have the responsibility of providing services and personnel to ensure optimal care. The American College of Critical Care Medicine has identified three levels of ICUs as determined by resources available to the hospital (Haupt et al., 2003). These levels are summarized in Table 1–2.

When a patient requires more comprehensive or specialized care, a decision must be made to transfer the acutely ill patient to a higher level of ICU care where additional personnel and resources are available. Transporting a patient from one area of the hospital to another or from one hospital to another includes risk. The decision to transport a patient must include an assessment of the risk-to-benefit ratio. Guidelines for the transfer of critically ill patients are available to help make these important decisions (Warren, 2004). According to these guidelines, hospitals should have policies and procedures that address pre-transport coordination and communication, personnel who must accompany the patient, equipment to accompany the patient, and the monitoring that will be required during the transport. It is recommended that clinicians use an algorithm (Fig. 1–1) in the decision-making process of transferring acutely ill patients to a higher level of care.

TABLE 1–2 ACCM's (2003) Definitions of ICU Levels of Care

ICU LEVEL	DESCRIPTION OF SERVICES, PERSONNEL
Level I	Hospitals with ICUs that provide comprehensive care for patients with a wide range of disorders. Sophisticated equipment is available. Units are staffed with specialized nurses and HCPs with critical care training. Comprehensive support services are available and include pharmacy, respiratory therapy, nutritional support, social services, and pastoral care. These units may be located within an academic teaching hospital or may be community based.
Level II	Hospitals with ICUs that have the capability of providing comprehensive care to most critically ill patients but not to specific patient populations (neurosurgical, cardiothoracic, trauma).
Level III	Hospitals with ICUs that have the ability to provide initial stabilization of critically ill patients but are limited in ability to provide comprehensive care for all patients. Able to care for ICU patients requiring routine care and monitoring.

Data from *ACCM (2003).*

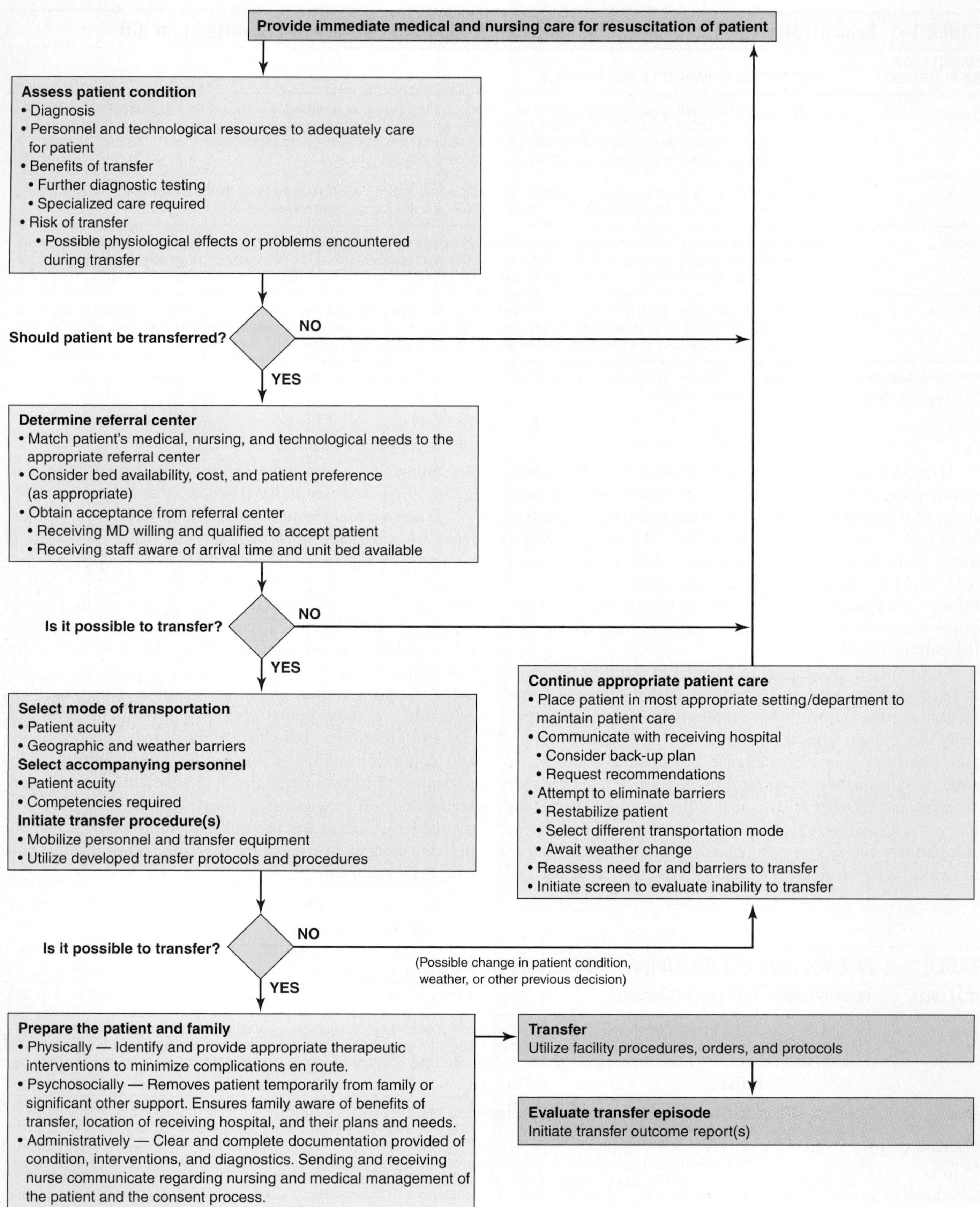

Figure 1–1 ■ Decision-making tree: transferring to a higher level of care. *(American College of Critical Medicine. (1993). Guidelines for the transfer of critically ill patients. Critical Care Medicine, 21, 934.* Used with Permission.*)*

SECTION ONE REVIEW

1. Intermediate-care units
   A. are outdated and should not be used
   B. are labor intensive and are not cost effective
   C. provide an efficient distribution of resources
   D. are reserved for patients with life-threatening illnesses
2. Which of the following priority levels means that the patient is acutely ill and unstable and requires intensive treatment and monitoring that cannot be provided outside the ICU?
   A. Priority 1
   B. Priority 2
   C. Priority 3
   D. Priority 4
3. Which of the following has been shown to reduce mortality and life-threatening complications in the hospitalized patient?
   A. a nurse patient ratio of 1:2
   B. constant surveillance of patients by nurses
   C. high technology ICUs
   D. IMC's
4. A hospital with an ICU that has the capability of providing comprehensive care to most critically ill patients but not to trauma patients meets criteria for Level ___ICU.
   A. I
   B. II
   C. III
   D. IV
5. Policies and procedures for the transfer of critically ill patients should address
   A. personnel who accompany the patient.
   B. equipment that should accompany the patient.
   C. monitoring that is required during transport.
   D. all of the above.

Answers: 1. C, 2. A, 3. B, 4. B, 5. D.

SECTION TWO: Resource Allocation

At the completion of this section, the learner will be able to identify the need for staffing strategies and resource allocation for high-acuity patients.

Nursing Staffing

Nurses willing to work with acutely ill patients are a precious commodity. Decreased third-party reimbursement and managed care encourage shorter hospital lengths of stay. As a cost-reducing measure, hospitals reduced professional nursing staff positions. In the late 1990s, hospital restructuring and reengineering forced bedside nurses to embrace new concepts such as role redesign, work transformation, and patient-centered care (Boston-Fleischhauer, 2008). Hospital employees, including nurses, were required to cross-train and "float" to care for patients outside their specialty areas. Unlicensed assistive personnel (UAP) were trained and supervised by nurses to complete patient care tasks. All these changes led to decreased job satisfaction and nurses leaving practice in high-acuity areas. Other factors have contributed to the shortage of nurses. The registered nurse (RN) workforce is rapidly aging and fewer young people are choosing nursing as a career. In addition, as the population continues to age, more patients will require high-acuity care. The nursing shortage issues are multifaceted and will continue to require comprehensive solutions. This may include federal funding for nursing education, changes in state regulations related to staffing standards, and increased public awareness (AACN, 2001).

A decrease in the number of professional nurses forced hospitals to increase nurse–patient ratios. The result: One nurse cares for more patients. What is the appropriate nurse–patient ratio in high-acuity settings? The Academy of Medical Surgical Nurses (AMSN) is not in favor of establishing predetermined ratios. Rather, the needs of the patient and skill mix of the nursing staff must be considered when making decisions about staffing patterns. Adequate resources must be available to evaluate the patient/family response to treatment, education, and pharmacological interventions (AMSN, 2000). The position of the American Association of Critical Care Nurses (AACN) is consistent with that of AMSN. Staffing is both a process and an outcome. Optimal care is provided when the patient's needs are matched with the caregiver's competencies. The first principle of staffing should be to provide safe and effective patient care. The patient's acuity level and required intensity of their nursing care requirements should determine the nurse–patient ratio (AACN, 2003).

The reduction in professional nursing staff encouraged an upgrade of nursing assistant skills. The AMSN supports the use of UAP to enable the professional nurse to provide nursing care (AMSN, 1998). When UAP provide direct patient care, they are accountable to, and work under, the direct supervision of the professional nurse. The registered nurse must use leadership skills to safely and legally delegate tasks to the UAP.

One potential solution to the nursing shortage has been the Magnet Recognition Program®. This concept, originally developed in the 1980s by the American Nurses Credentialing Center, awards hospitals a **Magnet designation** if they are able to create working environments that are successful in recruiting and retaining professional nurses. In effect, these environments act like magnets to attract nurses. Hospitals that achieve "Magnet status" have practice models that promote professional nursing. Nurses who work at Magnet hospitals are more involved in decision making, report better relations with physicians,

Emerging Evidence

- In a study of 232,342 surgical patients in 168 hospitals, investigators found that surgical mortality rates were more than 60% higher in the poorly staffed hospitals with the poorest patient care environments than in hospitals with better care environments (best staffing ratios, most highly educated nurses). The study also included data from 10,184 nurses. Analyses revealed three factors that improve nurse retention and patient outcomes: improved RN staffing, moving to a more educated workforce, and improving the care environment. Hospitals with even some of the Magnet hospital features (investments in staff development, quality management, frontline manager supervisor ability, and good relationships with physicians) were associated with better nurse and patient outcomes *(Aiken, Clarke, Sloane et al., 2008).*
- In a study involving 16 unit managers, 1,137 patients, and 296 observations from RNs over time, investigators found that as nurse-to-patient ratios climbed higher, nurses reported lower perceptions of quality of care and work environment on the unit, lower perceptions of unit leadership, and higher job stress. Patients in units with a higher proportion of RNs reported higher levels of independence in activities of daily living and patients reported higher ratings of their self-care ability on units with more experienced RNs *(Hall, Doran, Pink, 2008).*

and have higher nurse–patient ratios. Hospitals with Magnet status report their patients have shorter ICU stays and shorter hospital stays. The Magnet hospital program has been successful over time but it can be improved. Further studies are needed to evaluate the effects of Magnet hospital status on patient outcomes and to update and identify the essential components of magnetism (Kramer & Schmalenberg, 2005).

Decreasing Resources – Increasing Care Needs

Decisions about allocation of resources must be made when there is a need to place patients in acute care areas (specifically in ICU or step-down), but there are no beds available. Who is in need of the greatest health care resources when they are acutely ill? The priority levels depicted in Table 1–1 were developed to assist clinicians in making these tough decisions about admission, discharge, and triage in high–acuity care areas. Some could argue that ICU resources should be used for patients who will have the greatest probability of benefiting or have a higher quality of life. If resource allocation were based on these principles, the actual precipitating event that created the need for resources would be irrelevant. Therefore, oncology patients, trauma patients, the young, and the old would be considered equally. Futility of treatment and informed refusal by the patient may be acceptable reasons for health care providers (HCPs) to limit treatment. Although these issues occur daily in the care of high-acuity patients, they also occur in a larger context of society that includes ethical, economic, and legal considerations (Simone, 2007).

Oncology patients are often stereotyped as not being candidates for aggressive treatment. However, they frequently become acutely ill from therapeutic interventions. Should these patients be denied access to resources when their conditions are induced? During a patient's final hours, high-acuity care may be deemed appropriate because intensive efforts may be required to ensure suffering is minimized during and after removal from life support. Often there is no reliable timetable for when a patient progresses from being very ill to actually dying (Wingate & Wiegand, 2008).

Age has been used to justify the withholding of resources from the elderly. Extended care in the ICU has been questioned because of this patient population's high mortality rate. However, some studies of healthy elderly patients have shown that they often fare as well as younger patients. Elderly patients with minimal comorbidities appear to have similar health benefits following coronary artery bypass surgery when compared with younger patients. The severity of illness episode, admitting diagnosis, and the patient's previous health status contribute to patient outcomes. A high-acuity patient admitted to the hospital with a preexisting chronic medical condition may pose a greater risk of dying when compared to a patient who is not chronically ill.

It is difficult to predict who will benefit from care in high-acuity areas. Severity of illness scales and probability models were developed for this purpose. The Injury Severity Scale, New Injury Severity Scale, Acute Physiologic and Chronic Health Care Evaluation, and Trauma Registry Abbreviated Injury Scale are examples of severity of illness scales used in hospitals (Moore, 2008). However, the exclusive use of such indices has not been a completely accurate predictor of outcomes. Other factors must be taken into account. For example, the functional capacity of the patient prior to illness has been associated with outcomes as well as age and physiologic status (Moore, 2008). Mortality is usually the outcome studied in high-acuity care. Outcomes may also include patient comfort, quality of life, functional status, and other variables in addition to living and dying. While the use of severity of illness scales is important to compare patient populations for research and resource allocation (Moore, 2008), patients and their families consider multiple outcomes when deciding whether to withdraw life support.

Making decisions about allocation of resources is a real, but unspecified, aspect of the nursing role with high-acuity patients. These decisions force health care providers to make comparisons based on personal beliefs. Technology alone cannot provide information about who may live and die. Families play an important role in resource utilization. Family involvement in these decisions may ultimately decrease the use of technological resources and increase comfort measures during the last hours before death. Goals for care must be discussed with the patient and family allowing ample time for meaningful discussion (Wingate & Wiegand, 2008). Patients who die in high-acuity areas consume significant resources. The value of end-of-life care is subjective and cost alone cannot be used to justify the use of health care resources (Simone, 2007). Each patient situation is different.

SECTION TWO REVIEW

1. Unlicensed assistive personnel (UAP) may
   A. not work in high-acuity environments
   B. work independently as long as they notify the RN at the end of their shifts
   C. perform only those tasks delegated to them by a professional nurse
   D. obtain a patient health history
2. Hospitals that achieve the designation of Magnet status
   A. use UAP to deliver most nursing care
   B. have practice models that promote professional nursing
   C. indicate the hospital that has low nurse–patient ratios
   D. are not desirable places to work for professional nurses
3. Some argue that ICU resources should be used for patients with
   A. cancer
   B. advanced age
   C. DNR orders
   D. the greatest possibility of benefiting
4. What is the appropriate nurse-patient ratio in a high-acuity setting?
   A. 1 nurse to 2 patients
   B. 1 nurse to 4 patients
   C. 1 nurse to 6 patients
   D. The patient's acuity and required intensity determines the nurse–patient ratio
5. What is the timeline for when a patient progresses from being very ill to actually dying?
   A. there is no reliable timeline
   B. usually minutes
   C. 12 hours
   D. 24 hours

Answers: 1. C, 2. B, 3. D, 4. D, 5. A

SECTION THREE: Use of Technology in High-Acuity Environments

At the completion of this section, the learner will be able to examine and discuss the use of technology in the high-acuity environment.

In medical, business, academic, and many other work environments, technology influences how we communicate, document, evaluate, and conduct business—whether that business is making a product or taking care of patients. A major advantage of having technology available in the ICU environment is that the patient's status can be monitored continuously, using sensitive physiologic indicators of changing status. In the unstable patient, the ability to assess a possible problem before it becomes a full-blown complication may make the difference between life and death for that patient. Technology is also a useful tool that can assist high-acuity nurses and other health care professionals in making critical decisions. Although decision making is viewed as somewhat artful and intuitive, computers use a scientific, programmed approach based on a massive database and algorithmic decision-making trees. Computer software programs are available to help diagnose patient conditions. Furthermore, handheld computer devices, such as the personal digital assistant (PDA), can provide quick bedside access to drug and diagnostic information (Farrell & Rose, 2008).

While technology has provided the nurse with many advantages and improved patient outcomes, it has also given rise to some important issues. Nurses who care for acutely ill patients must be able to use technology in the caring process and still recognize its limits.

Patient Depersonalization

A major criticism of nurses who work with high-acuity patients is that they are too technologically oriented. The focus of nursing care in high-acuity patient care units is on monitoring patients for subtle physiologic changes. This monitoring requires the nurse to use multiple technologies. The patient interfaces with members of the health care team and medical equipment in the diagnosis and management of the patient's disease process. Difficulties arise when machines, rather than individual patient needs, become the focus of care of the high-acuity patient. Technology must be used to enhance care, not take the place of a nurse's personal knowledge, observation skills, and senses.

Technical devices present mechanical impediments to touching the patient. Little surface area may be available for physical contact and this may lead to a feeling of depersonalization. Technology may evoke fear in patients and contribute to their anxiety about their recovery process.

Overload and Overreliance Issues

Having responsibility for multiple pieces of equipment can increase the nurse's stress level. Because of the massive amount of patient data available, nurses may be reaching a saturation point in data processing. Technology can be so intriguing that its primary purpose—to support the well-being of the patient—is lost. Technology may create demands where no demands existed before, such as that which occurs with the fragmentation of patients into subpopulations (e.g., bone marrow transplant unit, cardiac surgery unit). Each subpopulation has its own special staff competing for hospital resources. Machines compete with the patient for nursing surveillance. It is possible that nurses become so dependent on monitoring devices that they completely trust the equipment, even when the data conflict with their own clinical assessments.

Finding a Balance

The skilled nurse who practices in a high-acuity setting must be able to bridge the gap between complex technology and the art of caring. When new technologies are introduced at the bedside, it is commonplace for the nurse to focus initially on the technology because of the need to gain proficiency in the use of this technology to support patient care. It is important for the nurse to be given the opportunity to become familiar with a technology before its use in patient care fosters proficiency; thus, appropriate training in use of high-tech equipment is crucial. A high degree of comfort with technology prevents it from becoming the focus of care. Nurses are at risk for becoming overly dependent on technology for clinical decision making, making it essential that the nurse validate the technologic data with nursing assessment data. The health care practitioner, not the technology, is ultimately responsible for clinical decisions. The element of human touch must never be removed from the bedside (Catalano & Fickenscher, 2007).

SECTION THREE REVIEW

1. Inherent hazards to the use of technology include
   A. fragmentation of patients into subpopulations
   B. increasing the nurse's stress level
   C. allowing greater time for patient contact
   D. A and B
2. Technical devices
   A. present mechanical impediments to touching
   B. lead to a feeling of depersonalization
   C. may evoke fear in patients
   D. all of the above
3. The focus of care of the high-acuity patient should always be on the
   A. bedside machines
   B. individual patient needs
   C. alarms on the machines
   D. the nurse's needs
4. It is essential that the nurse validate the technologic data with
   A. nursing assessment data
   B. the HCP
   C. other technologic data
   D. another nurse
5. What could nurses use to provide quick access to drug information?
   A. the internet
   B. a textbook
   C. PDA
   D. ask another nurse

Answers: 1. D, 2. D, 3. B, 4. A, 5. C

SECTION FOUR: Healthy Work Environment

At the completion of this section, the learner will be able to identify the components of a healthy work environment in high-acuity settings.

Stressors and Satisfying Factors

The term **burnout** has been used to describe feelings of personal and professional frustrations, job dissatisfaction, job insecurities, and emotional and physical exertion (Katz et al., 2005). It is a syndrome of emotional exhaustion, depersonalization, and reduced personal accomplishments that occur among individuals who work with people on a daily basis (Katz et al., 2005). When asked to describe burnout, nurses invariably talk about being overworked, frustrated, emotionally detached, and less productive at home (Espeland, 2007). Nurses work in demanding situations over long periods of time. The quest to provide high-quality patient care in a work environment that has decreasing resources and increasing responsibilities creates conflict. This conflict creates feelings of personal and professional frustrations and results in burnout (Davies, 2008). Symptoms indicative of burnout are summarized in Table 1–3.

Patients' conditions change rapidly in high-acuity units and this may be a source of burnout for nurses who work in these areas because it requires philosophical flexibility. A patient with a poor prognosis may have a prolonged stay that involves the use of multiple technologies. Then in the middle of a shift, a decision is made to cease these efforts. The patient may improve, requiring reevaluation and escalation of care. Conversely, a patient is declared dead by brain death criteria, and immediately thereafter may become an organ donor. This requires the nurse to shift from caring for a patient, to caring for organs for another patient. It is also quite common to have a patient die and, within minutes after death, the nurse is told there is a new patient waiting to come into that very same bed. The nurse is required to grieve or mourn a death and then minutes later reinvest energy in a new patient. A significant degree of uncertainty is confronted on a daily basis. A broad-based end-of-life care curriculum may be instrumental in assisting the high-acuity nurse to cope with the daily stress of changing patient conditions.

Stress is a major component of burnout. A current reason for stress and subsequent burnout by nurses is the nursing shortage, long working hours, and loss of concentration (Davies, 2008). Other sources of stress include giving emotional support during patient suffering, feelings of powerlessness in a physician controlled environment and dealing on a daily basis with pain and traumatic loss (Katz et al., 2005).

TABLE 1–3 Symptoms of Burnout

Behavioral	
Withdrawal Risk taking and impulsiveness Ambivalence Decreased productivity	Contemplating career change Increased use of caffeine, alcohol, and nicotine
Physiologic	
Chronic fatigue Frequent minor ailments Sleep changes	Appetite change Sexual difficulty
Psychological	
Attempt to blame others Stereotype patients Nightmares	Depression Hostility and negativism Loss of tolerance
Cognitive	
Decreased ability to make decisions Poor judgment	Lack of initiative Forgetfulness

Coping with Stress and Burnout

The social environment of the nursing unit plays a role in nurses' perceived levels of stress. Stress can be labeled as either "good" or "bad" (Davies, 2008). A positive social climate, characterized by strong managerial support and cohesiveness among the staff, serves as a buffer for the negative effects of stress. Environmental uncertainty, as measured by the number of admissions, discharges, and transfers in the high-acuity area, can result in emotional exhaustion. Nurses must enhance self-awareness of personal sources of tension. Once these sources of tension are identified, strategies for alleviating stressors can be developed.

Establishing critical incident stress debriefings (CISDs) may facilitate coping with specific situations. These are structured group discussions, usually occurring within several days post-crisis, designed to address symptoms of stress, assess the need for follow up, and provide a sense of closure. These sessions are a formal way of managing stress before it becomes debilitating or fosters burnout. Another strategy to prevent burnout is to assist nurses during orientation in formulating clear ideas of their professional roles and responsibilities within the high-acuity environment. Offering new nurses the opportunity to meet in small groups provides a safe, confidential environment to share experiences. Promoting a sense of community can also provide the ability to share stresses and joys, and to seek feedback for continuing performance improvement (Halfer, 2007).

Healthy Work Environment

In 2001 AACN made a commitment to promote healthy work environments that support quality patient care and high levels of nurse satisfaction. Six standards were identified which are critical to create and sustain a **healthy work environment** (AACN, 2005). These standards are listed in Table 1–4. AACN believes that the implementation of these standards will be an important step in meeting the commitment for a healthy work environment. This will, in turn, lead to improved patient safety, enhanced recruitment and retention, and positive patient outcomes (AACN, 2005).

Organizations can implement strategies to improve the working environment but it is the nurse who must validate the effectiveness. High-acuity nurses are the gatekeepers of patient safety. Structures, processes, and outcomes are required for quality care—that is, having the "right things in place" to do the "right things" so that the "right outcomes" will happen. A healthy and productive work environment allows the nurse to give excellent care to patients while achieving job satisfaction (Kramer & Schmalenberg, 2008).

TABLE 1–4 AACN Standards for Healthy Work Environments

STANDARD	DEFINITION
Skilled Communication	Nurses must be as proficient in communication skills as they are in clinical skills.
True Collaboration	Nurses must be relentless in pursuing and fostering true collaboration.
Effective Decision Making	Nurses must be valued and committed partners in making policy, directing and evaluating clinical care and leading organizational operations.
Appropriate Staffing	Staffing must ensure the effective match between patient needs and nurse competencies.
Meaningful Recognition	Nurses must be recognized and recognize others for the value each brings to the work of the organization.
Authentic Leadership	Nurse leaders must fully embrace the imperative of a healthy work environment, authentically live it, and engage others in its achievement.

Data from AACN (2005). Standards for establishing and sustaining healthy work environments: A journey to excellence. *American Journal of Critical Care, 14*, 187–197.

SECTION FOUR REVIEW

1. The term *burnout* describes feelings of
   A. personal and professional frustrations
   B. job dissatisfaction
   C. physical and emotional exertion
   D. all of the above
2. Risk taking, impulsiveness, decreased productivity, and increased use of caffeine and alcohol are behavioral symptoms of
   A. compassion fatigue
   B. job satisfaction
   C. burnout
   D. hardiness
3. Components of a healthy work environment include which of the following? (choose all that apply)
   A. true collaboration
   B. appropriate staffing
   C. authentic leadership
   D. individual priorities
4. Which of the following can help buffer the negative effects of stress? (choose all that apply)
   A. environmental uncertainty
   B. positive social climate
   C. managerial support
   D. cohesiveness among staff
5. CISDs can be used to (choose all that apply)
   A. assess high-acuity patients
   B. help families cope with stress
   C. address staff symptoms of stress
   D. provide staff with a sense of closure

Answers: 1. D, 2. C, 3. (A, B, C), 4. (B, C, D), 5. (C, D)

SECTION FIVE: Ensuring Patient Safety in High-Acuity Environments

At the completion of this section, the learner will be able to discuss the importance of patient safety in the high-acuity environment.

The Culture

Patient safety and healthy work environments are closely linked. For many years industry has examined work culture and its effect on job performance and outcomes. Only recently has this been examined in health care. Reports from the Institute of Medicine highlighted unsafe patient conditions and were instrumental in launching patient safety initiatives (Huang et al., 2007). Research has shown a correlation between working conditions, teamwork, and patient outcomes. High levels of teamwork result in decreased length of stay and decreased mortality (Huang et al., 2007).

Health care errors have become recognized as a public health problem. Failure to disclose errors was part of the socialization process for many years. Now, errors are publicly reported in the media and on the Internet. While some argue that health care professionals are human and apt to make mistakes, others feel that any medical mistake is unacceptable. For many years the fear of making mistakes was linked to a culture of blame. A nurse experienced reprimands from non-supportive administrators and loss of respect from colleagues when reporting an error (Wolf, 2007). The gradual shift to a culture of caring and support has been shown to increase error reporting and lead to systems improvement (Simpson, 2005).

Patient Safety

The Joint Commission (TJC) is an accrediting organization committed to improving patient safety. TJC's mission is to continuously improve the safety and quality of care provided to the public through the provision of health care accreditation that supports process improvement in health care organizations. The TJC established "National Patient Safety Goals" for acute care hospitals (TJC, 2009). These goals are summarized in Table 1–5.

TABLE 1–5 National Patient Safety Goals for Acute-Care Hospitals

- Improve the accuracy of patient identification
- Improve the effectiveness of communication among caregivers
- Improve the safety of using medications
- Reduce the risk of health care associated infections
- Accurately and completely reconcile medications across the continuum of care
- Reduce the risk of patient harm resulting from falls
- Encourage patients' active involvement in their own care as a patient safety strategy
- Improve recognition and response to changes in patient condition

Data from TJC *(2009)*.

To improve the accuracy of patient identification, the nurse should use at least two patient identifiers when providing care, treatment, and services. For example, a two-person verification process should be used before initiating a blood or blood component product. Effectiveness of communication among caregivers should be improved. One way to accomplish this safety goal is to use a "read-back" process. For example, when reporting critical laboratory test results, the person giving the test result should verify the test result by having the person receiving the information record and read back the test results. To improve the safety of using medications, The Joint Commission recommends that all medication labels are verified both verbally and visually by two people whenever the person preparing the medication is not the person who will be administering it. To reduce the risk of health care associated infections, hospitals must implement evidence-based guidelines to prevent central-line associated blood stream infections. This includes annual education for health care workers who are involved with caring for patients with central-lines to have education about infections and the importance of prevention. Medication reconciliation across the continuum of care should be done accurately and completely. For example, when a patient is transferred from the ICU to a high-acuity unit, the ICU nurse informs the high-acuity nurse about the up-to-date reconciled medication list and documents the communication. To reduce the risk of patient harm resulting from falls, hospitals must implement a fall reduction program. Staff should received education and training for this program.

As another safety strategy, patients should be encouraged to actively participate in their own care. The patient and family should be educated on available reporting methods for concerns related to care, treatment, services, and patient safety issues. The Joint Commission requires hospitals to improve recognition and response to changes in patient condition. This means that hospitals must have a method that enables health care staff members to directly request additional assistance from a specially trained individual when the patient's condition appears to be worsening. The Joint Commission requires adherence to a Universal Protocol. For example, a time-out process must be performed prior to starting a procedure, such as the bedside insertion of a percutaneous tracheostomy. The purpose of this time-out is to conduct a formal assessment that the correct patient, site, positioning, and procedure are identified, that all relevant documents (such as a consent), and necessary equipment are available. The completed components must be clearly documented.

For a hospital to receive The Joint Commission accreditation, the organization must demonstrate and provide evidence that it is meeting these safety goals. High-acuity nurses must actively participate in ensuring these goals are met.

Technology and Patient Safety

Technology has been introduced to prevent errors. One example is the implementation of computerized provider order entry (CPOE) systems. These systems block incorrect medication orders; warn against drug interactions, allergies and overdoses; provide current, accurate drug information; and alert to sound-alike drug names (Wolf, 2007). Many hospitals have implemented CPOE and benefited from cost savings and error reduction (Kaushal, et al., 2006).

Manufactured devices may be a source of potential errors. Devices are carefully engineered to be fail-safe; however, adverse incidents do happen. The nurse must be competent in using the equipment. It is the responsibility of the nurse to report medical device failure when it occurs and remove the item from service (Wolf, 2007).

Barcode point of care (BPOC) is another technology recently introduced to prevent errors. This system allows nurses to scan their badges as well as patient wristbands to access medication profiles. The nurse is then able to obtain the right medication, for the right patient, in the right dose, at the right time, and via the correct route (Topps, et al., 2005).

The use of personal digital assistants (PDAs) has helped to improve practice and decrease errors. Nurses have found these devices essential for checking medications, calculating doses, and accessing reference material (Taylor, 2005). While these systems have been effective in reducing errors, they are not infallible. The human component cannot be discounted.

Other Factors Contributing to Patient Safety

Patients trust their care to nurses who must deal with workforce shortages and ever-changing therapies and technologies. AACN's position (2003) is that the nursing shortage, overtime hours and excessive documentation jeopardize patient safety. A strong educational foundation and solid orientation will allow for the high-acuity nurse to provide more efficient, safer care (AACN, 2003). The Institute of Medicine has suggested performance standards for health care professionals that focus on patient safety. AACN (2003) believes that specialty certification addresses this need. Hospitals that create a culture of respect and professionalism are more likely to have experienced, certified nurses in an environment where safety is valued. Research continues to indicate that adequate staffing, well-educated nurses, positive physician-nurse relationships, and responsible management are the keys to decreasing errors (Clarke & Aiken, 2006).

SECTION FIVE REVIEW

1. The current patient safety and healthy work environment cultures in the high-acuity environment promote
   - **A.** an increase in error reporting and systems improvement
   - **B.** a decrease in error reporting
   - **C.** a culture of blame
   - **D.** the failure to publicly disclose medical errors
2. Which of the following contribute to medical errors? (choose all that apply)
   - **A.** staffing ratios
   - **B.** overtime
   - **C.** excessive documentation
   - **D.** specialty certification
3. Which of the following technologies reduce errors? (choose all that apply)
   - **A.** ANCC
   - **B.** BPOC
   - **C.** PDA
   - **D.** CPOE
4. Which of the following must be done to ensure patient safety before administering a blood product?
   - **A.** One person should verify correct transfusion.
   - **B.** Two people should verify correct transfusion and correct patient.
   - **C.** Confirm the order with the HCP.
   - **D.** Insert a 22-gauge IV catheter.
5. What should be done to ensure patient safety when the nurse preparing a medication is not the same nurse who administers the medication? (choose all that apply)
   - **A.** This should never be done.
   - **B.** Confirm the order with the HCP.
   - **C.** Labels should be verbally verified by the two nurses.
   - **D.** Labels should be visually verified by the two nurses.

Answers: 1. A, 2. (A, B, C), 3. (B, C, D), 4. B, 5. (C, D)

POSTTEST

1. The ICU nurse received a report from the medical-surgical unit. They are requesting a transfer of a patient to the ICU. This patient is in acute respiratory failure and requires mechanical ventilation. He has profound hypotension and will require vasoactive drugs to help manage his blood pressure. Based on the SCCM prioritization model, what is this patient's priority for ICU placement?
   - **A.** Priority 1
   - **B.** Priority 2
   - **C.** Priority 3
   - **D.** Priority 4
2. A nurse is interviewing for a position in a local community hospital. The nurse recruiter states the ICU is a Level III ICU. Which of the following statements describes the resources available at this hospital to care for critically ill patients?
   - **A.** Units are staffed with specialized equipment, specialty trained nurses, and HCPs and can provide comprehensive care for patients with a wide range of disorders.
   - **B.** The ICU has the capability of providing comprehensive care for patients with a wide range of disorders.
   - **C.** The unit has the ability to provide initial stabilization of patients but is limited in the ability to provide comprehensive care for all patients.
   - **D.** Sophisticated equipment is available and the hospital is most likely an academic institution.

3. A patient is admitted to the IMC. His wife states that she heard on the news that IMCs with a nurse-to-patient ratio of 1:4 provide the best care. Which statement by the nurse is the best response?
   - **A.** That is correct, but that is not how this unit is staffed.
   - **B.** Many professional organizations, as does our hospital, disagree with using a specific ratio of nurses to patients. We match the individual patient's needs with nursing care requirements.
   - **C.** There is just no way to provide the resources to evaluate every patient and family response to treatments.
   - **D.** A 1:4 ratio is unsafe. Please write a letter to your legislator and tell them we need help.
4. Mr. B. is a patient in the IMC. After 3 days of being on the unit, he asks the nurse "What is the difference between an RN and a UAP? I don't understand. It seems to me like you do the same things." Which statement by the nurse would be the best response?
   - **A.** There is really not much difference, except in pay.
   - **B.** We have different educational backgrounds.
   - **C.** They were hired to help with the nursing shortage.
   - **D.** They are trained and supervised by nurses to complete specific care tasks.
5. The nurse is most concerned if which of the following signs and symptoms are observed in a patient with a history of asthma?
   - **A.** The pulse oximeter alarms at 80 percent.
   - **B.** The patient states he "can't get all of his air out."
   - **C.** The infusion alarm says "infusion complete."
   - **D.** A and B are correct.
6. The focus of nursing care for high-acuity patients is on monitoring
   - **A.** devices, machines, technical equipment
   - **B.** alarms that indicate patient changes
   - **C.** monitoring patients for subtle physiologic changes
   - **D.** massive amounts of patient data
7. A co-worker has become increasingly withdrawn from unit social activities. He is often late for work and is ambivalent about warnings from the nurse manager. He has become very hostile and negative about any proposed changes in the unit. The nurse should recognize that the co-worker is exhibiting symptoms of which condition?
   - **A.** burnout
   - **B.** stress
   - **C.** job dissatisfaction
   - **D.** conflict
8. A high-acuity nursing unit has an "Operations Council." The members include the unit's medical director, nurse manager, staff nurses, UAP, respiratory therapists, and a nutritionist. The Council initiates policies and procedures and evaluates clinical care on the unit. These activities reflect which of the following AACN standards for a healthy work environment?
   - **A.** meaningful recognition
   - **B.** effective decision making
   - **C.** authentic leadership
   - **D.** appropriate staffing
9. The hospital is planning to implement a CPOE system. A co-worker sees no benefits from implementing this technology. Which statement by the nurse is the best response to this co-worker's concerns?
   - **A.** You are right. These systems have been shown to cause medication errors.
   - **B.** You are right. These systems have been shown to cause drug interactions.
   - **C.** Actually, hospitals that have implemented CPOE have benefited from error reduction.
   - **D.** Actually, these systems reduce medication errors but have been found to be way too expensive.
10. The high-acuity unit's Operations Council is seeking suggestions for the use of technology to prevent errors on the unit. What statement by the nurse is the best response to this request?
   - **A.** Barcode point-of-care has been shown to reduce medication errors.
   - **B.** PDAs have been shown to increase errors.
   - **C.** We need more infusion pumps as they are fail-safe.
   - **D.** All technology is fail-safe.

Posttest answers with rationale are found on MyNursingKit.

PEARSON

EXPLORE mynursingkit™

MyNursingKit is your one stop for online chapter review materials and resources. Prepare for success with additional NCLEX®-style practice questions, interactive assignments and activities, web links, animations and videos, and more!

Register your access code from the front of your book at **www.mynursingkit.com.**

REFERENCES

AMSN (Academy of Medical Surgical Nurses). (2000). Position statement: Staffing standards for patient care. Available at: http://www.medsurgnurse.org. Accessed April 16, 2008.

AMSN (Academy of Medical Surgical Nurses). (1998). Position statement: Unlicensed assistive personnel. Available at: http://www.medsurgnurse.org. Accessed April 16, 2008.

Aiken L. H., Clarke S. P., Sloane D. M., et al. (2008). Effects of hospital care environment on patient mortality and nurse outcomes. *Journal of Nursing Administration 38(5)*, 223–229.

AACN (American Association of Critical Care Nurses). (2005). AACN Standards for establishing and sustaining healthy work environments: a journey to excellence. *American Journal of Critical Care*, 14, 187–197.

AACN (American Association of Critical Care Nurses), American College of Chest Physicians, American Thoracic Society, Society of Critical Care Medicine. (2001). Critical care workforce partnership position statement: The aging of the U.S. population and increased need for critical care. Available at: http://www.aacn.org. Accessed April 10, 2008.

AACN (American Association of Critical Care Nurses). (2003). Written statement to the institute of medicine committee on work environment for nurses and patient safety. Available at: http://www.aacn.org. Accessed April 10, 2008.

ACCM (American College of Critical Care Medicine). (1993). Guidelines for the transfer of critically ill patients. *Critical Care Medicine, 21*, 931–937.

ACCM (American College of Critical Care Medicine). (1998). Guidelines on admission and discharge for adult intermediate care units. *Critical Care Medicine, 26(3)*: 608.

ACCM (American College of Critical Care Medicine). (1999). Guidelines for intensive care unit admission, discharge, and triage. *Critical Care Medicine, 27(3)*, 633–638.

Boston-Fleischhauer, C. (2008). Enhancing healthcare process redesign with human factors engineering and reliability science, Part 1: Setting the context. *Journal of Nursing Administration, 38(1)*, 27–32.

Catalano, K. & Fickenscher, K. (2007). Emerging Technologies in the OR and their effect on perioperative professionals. *AORN*, 86(6), 958–960, 962–969.

Clarke, S., & Aiken, L. (2006) More nursing, fewer deaths. *Quality and Safety in Healthcare, 15*, 2–3.

Davies, W. (2008). Mindful meditation: healing burnout in critical care nursing. *Holistic Nursing Practice. 22(1)*, 32–36.

Espeland, K. (2006). Overcoming burnout: how to revitalize your career. *Journal of Continuing Education in Nursing, 37*, 179–180.

Farrell, M. & Rose, L. (2008). Use of mobile handheld computers in nursing education. *Journal of Nursing Education. 47(1)*, 13–19.

Halfer, D. (2007). A magnetic strategy for new graduate nurses. *Nursing Economics*, 25(1), 6–11.

Hall, L. M., Doran D., & Pink, L. (2008). Outcomes of interventions to improve hospital nursing work environments. *Journal of Nursing Administration 38(1)*, 40–46.

Haupt, M. T., Bekes, C. E., Carl, L. C., et al. (2003). Guidelines on critical care services and personnel: recommendations based on a system of categorization of resources: three levels of care. *Critical Care Medicine, 3(11)*, 2677–2683.

Huang, D., Clermont, G., & Sexton, J., et al. (2007). Perceptions of a safety culture vary across intensive care units of a single institution. *Critical Care Medicine, 35(1)*, 165–176.

Katz, J., Wiley, S., & Capuano, T., et al. (2005). The effects of mindfulness based stress reduction on nurse stress and burnout. Part 2. a quantitative and qualitative study. *Holistic Nursing Practice*, 19, 26–32.

Kaushal, R., Franz, C., Glaser, J., et al. (2006). Return on investment for a computerized physician order-entry system. *Journal of the American Medical Informatics Association, 13(3)*, 261–266.

Kramer, M. & Schmalenberg, C. (2005). Best quality patient care: a historical perspective on magnet hospitals. *Nursing Administration, 29(3)*, 275–287.

Kramer, M. & Schmalenberg, C. (2008). Confirmation of a healthy work environment. *Critical Care Nurse*, 28(2), 56–63.

Moore, L., Lavoie, A., LeSage, N., et al. (2008). Consensus or data – derived anatomic injury severity scoring. *The Journal of Trauma, Injury, Infection and Critical Care, 64(2)*, 420–426.

Simone, J. (2007). Ethics and medical economics: rationing care. *Oncology Times, 29(6)*, 2, 4–5.

Simpson, R. (2005). Patient and nurse safety: how information technology makes a difference. *Nursing Administration Quarterly, 29(1)*, 97–101.

Topps, C., Lopez, L., Messmer, P., et al. (2005). Perceptions of pediatric nurses toward bar-code point of care medication administration. *Nursing Administration Quarterly, 29(1)*, 102–107.

TJC (The Joint Commission). (2009). National Patient Safety Goals. http://www.jointcommission.org/PatientSafety/NationalPatientSafetyGoals.09_hap_npsgs.htm.

Warren, J., Fromm, R. E. Jr., Orr, R. A., et al. (2004). Guidelines for the inter- and intrahospital transport of critically ill patients. Critical Care Med 32(1): 256–262.

Wingate, S. & Wiegand, D. (2008). End-of life care in critical care for patients with heart failure. *Critical Care Nurse, 28(2)*, 84–95.

Wolf, Z. (2007). Pursuing safe medication use and the promise of technology. *MEDSURG Nursing, 16(2)*, 92–100.

MODULE

2 Holistic Care of the Patient and Family

Jill Arzouman

OBJECTIVES Following completion of this module, the learner will be able to

1. Discuss stages of illness a high-acuity patient may experience.
2. Identify ways the nurse can help high-acuity patients cope with an illness and/or injury event.
3. Describe the principles of patient- and family-centered care in the high-acuity environment as it relates to educational needs of visitation and policies.
4. Discuss the importance of awareness of cultural diversity when caring for high-acuity patients.
5. Examine the role of palliative care in the high-acuity environment.
6. Identify environmental stressors, their impact on high-acuity patients, and strategies to alleviate those stressors.
7. Examine personal values as they relate to the nurse's role in working with high-acuity patients.
8. Discuss end-of-life issues to be considered in caring for high-acuity patients.

This module focuses on the role nurses play in providing holistic care for the patient and family in the high-acuity environment. The module is divided into six sections. Sections One and Two address the stages of acute illness and strategies that can be used to help patients to cope with acute illness. Section Three examines the principles of family-centered care as well as educational needs of the patient and family. Cultural diversity is addressed in Section Four. The role of palliative care for the high-acuity patient is discussed in Section Five along with environmental stressors and their impact on the high-acuity patient. Section Six focuses on end-of-life care and assessment of sources of conflict. Each section includes a set of review questions to help the learner evaluate his or her understanding of the section's content before moving on to the next section. All Section Reviews include answers. It is suggested that the learner review those concepts answered incorrectly in the review questions before proceeding to the next section.

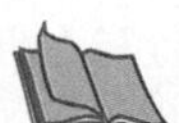

PRETEST

1. During the resolution stage of illness, the high-acuity nurse should design interventions that
   A. assist with patient problem solving
   B. provide accurate information
   C. promote self-care and independence
   D. do not stress reality
2. Family is defined as
   A. however the patient wishes to define it
   B. a blood relative
   C. a spouse, child, and parents
   D. legally authorized representative
3. The use of massage therapy is contraindicated in which of the following?(choose all that apply)
   A. burns
   B. during dressing changes
   C. bruises
   D. phlebitis
4. Patients who use complementary and alternative therapies (CAT)
   A. do not always relay this information to their health care providers
   B. are normally stressed individuals
   C. are decreasing in numbers
   D. have up-to-date information
5. Which of the following can inhibit learning in high-acuity patients?
   A. Hypoxemia
   B. Hyperglycemia
   C. Nitroglycerine
   D. Dopamine
6. Advantages to having families at the bedside during CPR include
   A. the ability to calm the patient
   B. removal of doubt as to what is happening to the patient

C. the ability to see that more could have been done for the patient
D. a healthy increase in anxiety and fear

7. Cultural competence is defined as
A. having knowledge about various cultural beliefs
B. lack of prejudice for other ethnic groups
C. awareness of one's own thoughts and feelings without letting it influence caring for patients with different backgrounds
D. human biological variation

8. Sources of diversity may include
A. race
B. ethnicity
C. sexual orientation
D. all of the above

9. The goal of palliative care is to
A. promote peaceful death
B. improve the quality of care
C. institute DNR orders
D. withdraw life support

10. A patient may be referred to palliative care for
A. uncontrollable level of pain
B. transfer between ICU settings with evidence of progress
C. infrequent emergency room visits
D. IMC setting with documented progress

11. The Patient Self Determination Act (1990) requires that all patients be given information about their right to formulate advanced directives for (choose all that apply)
A. treatment directives
B. appointment directives
C. pain medication
D. natural death

12. Barriers to end-of-life care in the high-acuity environment include (choose all that apply)
A. nursing time constraints
B. communication challenges
C. inadequate staffing patterns
D. non-communicative patients

Pretest answers are found on MyNursingKit.

SECTION ONE: Stages of Acute Illness

At the completion of this section, the learner will be able to discuss the stages of illness a high-acuity patient may experience.

High-acuity illness produces a loss of self-image and impacts self-esteem. The patient may need to adapt to loss of health, loss of limb, disfigurement, or a necessary change in lifestyle. Change may precipitate grieving. According to Suchman (1965), high-acuity patients may respond to these losses by experiencing certain predictable phases. Table 2–1 summarizes Suchman's stages of illness, manifestations, and nursing interventions appropriate for each stage. The first stage is shock and disbelief because the diagnosis does not have an emotional meaning. The patient may be uncooperative because he is projecting difficulties onto hospital procedures, equipment, and personnel. In this stage, a patient may worry more about the equipment being used than about the diagnosis because the diagnosis may be a threat to life. The denial stage can have positive effects. It may protect the patient against the emotional impact of the illness and conserve energy by removing worry. The nurse should function as a noncritical listener.

The awareness stage is characterized by an attempt to regain control. Patients may express guilt about the illness or injury as a gesture of assuming responsibility for events over which they may or may not have actual control. The patient may be demanding or exhibit signs of withdrawal. Both signs are indicative of anger toward self or others. The nurse should not argue with the patient. Consistent, dependable nursing care should be provided.

During the next stage, restitution, the patient may verbalize fears about the future. New behaviors are initiated that reflect new limitations. The patient may feel sad and have frequent crying episodes. Relationships with family and friends may be reorganized. The nurse can assist by building communication to assist with problem solving. Resolution, the final stage, involves identity

TABLE 2–1 Suchman's Stages of Illness

STAGE	DEFINITION	MANIFESTATIONS	INTERVENTIONS
Shock and disbelief	Diagnosis does not have an emotional meaning	Patient may be uncooperative or worry excessively	Provide accurate information when asked
Denial	Patient rejects diagnosis	Patient may act like nothing is wrong	Nurse is noncritical; clarify statements but do not stress reality
Awareness	Attempt to regain control	Demanding and angry or quiet and withdrawn	Provide consistent nursing care; do not argue with patient
Restitution	Diagnosis is accepted	Sadness and crying; attempt to improve relationships with family and friends	Assist patient with problem solving
Resolution	Patient's identity is changed	Patient may openly participate in care	Promote self-care and independence

change. The patient may begin to think of the illness as a growing experience. Limitations are accepted as consequences and not as defects.

These stages are not fixed but reflect a dynamic process of adjusting to an acute situation. The patient may regress to an earlier stage during periods of heightened anxiety. One aim in caring for the high-acuity patient is to foster a feeling of security. A patient may feel vulnerable because of physiological changes, such as paralysis. Changes in patient care routines can increase patient anxiety, even when these changes mean the patient is getting better. Examples include removing cardiac electrodes, weaning from mechanical ventilation, reducing pain medication, and increasing mobility.

The high-acuity patient cannot be considered in isolation of family members. The family is defined according to however the patient wishes to define family. The high-acuity nursing unit has evolved from a restrictive environment into a more inclusive environment for families. This change is the result of an increasing body of research that demonstrates positive outcomes when family members actively participate in the recovery process of their loved one. Because of this important role, the nurse must identify and meet family needs so that they can fully participate in the care of the patient.

Nursing research has demonstrated that families frequently need information, comfort, support, assurance, and accessibility (Counsell & Guin, 2002). Families want frequent communication about the patient's condition. They want to know why particular interventions are initiated. They experience high levels of emotional distress and need to be reassured frequently and honestly that the patient is receiving the best care possible. Communication must be open, honest, direct, frequent, and ongoing (Auerbach et al., 2005). A frequent meeting with the family assures healthy coping mechanisms and helps the nurse to develop a family-centered plan of care.

SECTION ONE REVIEW

1. A patient was involved in a motor vehicle crash and sustained multiple lower extremity fractures. He will need additional surgery and prolonged physical therapy. The nurse finds Mr. Abe drawing plans for remodeling his porch to accommodate a wheelchair. This behavior reflects which stage of illness?
   A. denial
   B. awareness
   C. restitution
   D. resolution
2. When interacting with a patient in denial, the nurse should
   A. reinforce reality
   B. function as a noncritical listener
   C. explain the current treatment plan
   D. help the patient to recall the injury event
3. An appropriate nursing intervention for a patient experiencing high anxiety is
   A. active listening
   B. providing accurate information
   C. exhibiting empathy
   D. acknowledging loss
4. Which of the following changes can induce anxiety in the high-acuity patient? (choose all that apply)
   A. weaning from mechanical ventilation
   B. reducing pain medication
   C. increasing mobility
   D. family visitation
5. A patient was just admitted to the high-acuity unit. The family has just arrived and wants to speak with the patient's nurse. Which of the following may be their most important need at this time?
   A. information
   B. sleeping
   C. food
   D. relaxation exercises

Answers: 1. D, 2. B, 3. B, 4. (A, B, C), 5. A

SECTION TWO: Coping with Acute Illness

At the completion of this section, the learner will be able to identify ways the nurse can help high-acuity patients cope with an illness or injury event.

There is an increasing body of research on the importance of the search for meaning in life-changing events. **Spirituality,** a sense of faith and transcendence, and a sorting-out of old life views are frequently part of the experience of the patient and family during acute illness or injury. Questions such as "Why me?" "Why this?" and "Why now?" become part of the patient's and family's quest for meaning. The nurse can provide a sounding board for such questions and act as a nonjudgmental listener as patients and families sort out their answers.

Various strategies can be used to help patients cope with the psychological and physical stressors of an acute illness. **Complementary and alternative therapies** (CAT) may be beneficial to the high-acuity patient as a way of reducing stress. CAT may be used in lieu of, or as a complement to, standard medical treatment. It is important to remember that all patients are in need of healing, even if they cannot be cured. The decision to use CAT must be an informed decision. Some patients, because of personal feelings or cultural differences, may not be comfortable with massage or touch therapy. In this situation, the CAT will actually add stress and may inhibit relaxation. Many patients who are using CAT do not tell their health care provider. As the numbers of patients using CAT increases, so does the risk for side effects. A patient may experience interactions from allopathic medications or adverse effects from overuse. The high-acuity nurse must be knowledgeable about CAT to provide correct information to patients (Tracy, Lindquist et al., 2005).

Aromatherapy is the use of oils to reduce stress and anxiety. Aromatic plant oils such as hiba, lavender, jasmine, and others have been shown in small, limited studies to reduce stress and anxiety in acutely ill patients. These oils may be inhaled or used as an enhancement to massage therapy. When inhaled, the oils travel through the olfactory bulb to the limbic system for processing. When used with massage, oils are absorbed through the skin into the bloodstream (Halm, 2008). Aromatherapy is recognized by many state boards of nursing as a component of holistic nursing. Research on the therapeutic effects of essential oils is limited and must be expanded. Aromatherapy and touch therapy will continue to play an essential role in promoting comfort and relaxation in patients.

Humor has been recognized for years as a way of relieving stress. Unlike aromatherapy, which is easy to apply, humor may be tricky to deliver by the high-acuity nurse. However, a skilled nurse may use humor as one complementary and alternative therapy. Humor may be effective in reducing pain, showing the human side of the health care team and helping the patient and family cope. When used effectively humor strengthens the bond between the patient, family, and nurse. Some patients may not be accepting of humor when facing a serious illness and this makes humor a risky strategy (Penson, Partridge et al., 2005).

Massage is manipulation of soft tissues of the body using hands. Massage and therapeutic touch may help patients relax, reduce anxiety, and promote sleep. In addition, these therapies are designed to have a positive effect on vascular, muscular, and nervous systems. The use of massage therapy to relieve pain is widespread as an acceptable intervention. The high-acuity nurse may use massage therapy to treat all components of pain, which includes physical, spiritual, emotional, and social domains (Liu & Tonks, 2008). Contradictions to massage therapy as summarized by Ernest et al. (2006) are listed in Table 2–2.

Guided imagery is a CAT that uses the patient's past positive experiences to promote a vision or fantasy that encourages relaxation. In imagery, the patient focuses on positive thoughts and experiences and blocks out negative thoughts. Nurses can guide patients through imagery by asking them to place themselves in environments where they remember feeling relaxed. Many people recall the beach or ocean as having a calming effect. An example of imagery is the thought of lying on a beach on a deserted island, listening to the pounding of the surf on the shore, watching the graceful sway of the palm trees, and feeling the cool breezes, while at the same time feeling the warmth of the sun on the skin. Imagery provides an opportunity for the patient to take a vacation or temporary mental escape from the day-to-day realities of the high-acuity environment. Imagery is a CAT that may be beneficial for patients experiencing extensive and painful dressing changes, anxiety, depression, mood disturbance, or pain (Deng et al., 2007). The following case study demonstrates the use of imagery. The case study is referred to again in Section Three.

TABLE 2–2 Contraindications to Massage Therapy

Advanced osteoporosis
Bone fractures
Burns
Deep vein thrombosis
Eczema
Phlebitis
Skin infections

A 79-year-old man had an exploratory laparotomy for a perforated duodenal ulcer. He has a history of chronic airflow limitation and takes daily prednisolone. His wound is healing by secondary intention and he experiences significant pain during his dressing changes.

The nurse prepares the environment by dimming lights and decreasing noise. He places a sign outside the patient's room indicating that an imagery session is in progress. The nurse promotes relaxation by encouraging the patient to imagine that each muscle is going limp starting at the top of his head. He describes it as a heavy, good feeling. The nurse tells the patient to concentrate on each body section separately (neck, shoulders, and so on). The patient closes his eyes and concentrates on his body.

Nurse: "As the old dressing is removed, your new tissue is getting fresh nutrients because dead skin and bacteria are being removed along with the gauze. Imagine a tiny skin cell with hands that reach out to join another skin cell to make a firm chain. Although you are a little uncomfortable, you want the dressing to be removed because the new skin cells cannot grow underneath the debris from the old cells. As the new cells get nutrients, there is less drainage and less discomfort. Now, imagine that the skin is completely together just like it was before surgery. There is no need for more dressing changes. Each time your dressing is changed, concentrate on this image of the skin cells joining hands to make a firm chain that is completely together and healed. Imagine the cells getting fresh air and food that make them strong."

The goal of this imagery session was to describe positive aspects of the dressing change, in order to replace the patient's fear with a positive image of healing.

In addition to the therapies discussed above, the high-acuity patient may pursue other CATs, such as meditation, yoga, tai chi, hypnosis, relaxation techniques, or music therapy. Manipulation of energy fields and acupuncture, diet, and dietary supplements have also gained popularity. The high-acuity nurse must be able to provide evidence-based practice to guide the patient to receive benefit from CAT while avoiding harm (Deng, 2007).

SECTION TWO REVIEW

1. Complementary and alternative therapies may be used (choose all that apply)
   - **A.** in lieu of standard medical treatment
   - **B.** as a complement to standard medical treatment
   - **C.** only with a physician's order
   - **D.** in limited situations

2. Humor is
   - **A.** not a way to relieve stress
   - **B.** a CAT that can be used with high-acuity patients
   - **C.** ineffective in reducing pain
   - **D.** interferes with the bond between patient and nurse

(*continued*)

(continued)

3. Aromatherapy (choose all that apply)
   A. is the use of oils to reduce stress and anxiety
   B. includes plant oils that may be applied topically
   C. may be used to enhance massage therapy
   D. cannot be used with high-acuity patients
4. Contraindications to massage therapy include (choose all that apply)
   A. advanced osteoporosis
   B. bone fractures
   C. burns
   D. deep vein thrombosis
5. Guided imagery may be a useful strategy for patients with (choose all that apply)
   A. anxiety
   B. depression
   C. pain
   D. hypotension

Answers: 1. (A, B), 2. B, 3. (A, B, C), 4. (A, B, C, D), 5. (A, B, C)

SECTION THREE: Patient- and Family-Centered Care

At the completion of this section, the learner will be able to describe the principles of patient- and family-centered care in the high-acuity environment as it relates to educational needs and visitation policies.

Educational Needs of Patients and Families

High-acuity patients have a right to know and understand what procedures are being done to and for them. Initially, when teaching high-acuity patients, the goal is to decrease stress and promote comfort rather than to increase knowledge. The patient and family may not recall what the nurse said ten minutes later, but the patient's blood pressure may be decreased or the pain lessened. As adult learners, high-acuity patients focus on learning in order to solve problems. Thus, the nurse must assess what the patient considers to be problematic in order to make learning meaningful. Basic questions about what the patient and family want to know will assist the nurse in focusing content. It is also helpful to identify what the patient already knows. An interpersonal relationship allows for the patient to trust the abilities and knowledge of the nurse. For the high-acuity patient to learn, he or she must feel secure.

Several factors inhibit learning in high-acuity patients. Patients may be fatigued because of hypoxemia, anemia, and hypermetabolism. Barriers to communication, such as endotracheal tubes, many hourly procedures, and diagnostic tests interfere with teaching and learning. Pain diminishes a person's ability to concentrate; drugs may depress the central nervous system and affect memory. The nurse should assess the patient for the presence of these factors. Physiologic needs take precedence over the need to know and the need to understand. Once the patient's condition has stabilized, however, the patient may be able to concentrate on learning. Educational needs of both patients and families, according to Palazzo (2001), are summarized in Table 2–3. It is important for the nurse to incorporate adult learning theory in high-acuity areas.

The patient, discussed in Section Two, is improving. His arterial blood gases (ABGs) have improved, and he is being weaned from mechanical ventilation. The nurse has been teaching him about his wound care, explaining that he is at an increased risk of a wound infection because he is also receiving corticosteroids. Up to this point, the patient has been eager to learn and has asked questions using a writing board; however, this morning he appears anxious.

Before teaching the patient, the nurse assesses the cause of his anxiety. Is it related to hypoxemia secondary to being weaned from mechanical ventilation? The nurse draws blood for an ABG, and the results are within normal limits. The patient's anxiety may be related to the fear of not being able to breathe without the ventilator. On questioning, the patient admits he is frightened about leaving the ICU and moving to another unit. The nurse explains to the patient that he will be assessed regularly to determine his ability to remain off the ventilator. Next,

TABLE 2–3 Educational Needs of Patients and Families

EDUCATIONAL NEEDS	NURSING CONSIDERATIONS
Current information about patient progress	Both families and patients need daily information on progress towards recovery. Trends in vital signs, results of laboratory tests, and wound healing are physiological indicators that the nurse may discuss with the patient. In general, the high-acuity environment encourages a highly motivated learner.
Informed decision making	Most adults are self-directed and want to make informed decisions themselves, not to have decisions made by someone else.
Acknowledgment of past	The adult learner has a lifetime of experiences that influence their values and opinions, and shape their decisions.
Optimal learning environment	Using the right time and environment is conducive to the learning process. Transforming the high-acuity environment into a learning environment will enhance the learning process and improve retention. Presenting the information at the appropriate time is important.
Orientation to routines and care	Teaching patients and families procedures that will improve their daily life is productive. Teaching patients and families to perform complementary and alternative therapies to relieve pain, reduce stress, and induce sleep may be beneficial to all.
Motivation	Adults are motivated to learn something new when it will have a direct effect on their daily lives.

he explains when he will be transferred to a lower-acuity unit and how he will continue to be monitored.

The transfer to a less acute unit may precipitate **transfer anxiety** in the patient or family. Transfer anxiety has been defined as anxiety experienced by the individual who moves from a familiar, somewhat secure environment, to an environment that is unfamiliar (Roberts, 1976). Although discharge from the ICU is a positive step in terms of physical recovery, many patients experience high levels of anxiety with the transfer from the ICU to another high-acuity unit (Chaboyer 2005; Chaboyer, 2007). There are several strategies that can be used to decrease transfer anxiety. A structured transfer plan is often helpful. The transfer plan should include strategies to encourage patient and family questions as well as their active involvement in the transfer plan. Optimally, it is best to transfer the patient during the daytime, although this is not always possible. The patient and family should receive information about unit routines and any new equipment. The patient and family should be introduced to the receiving nurse before the transfer.

Visitation Policies

There has been considerable debate about the effectiveness of open visitation policies in the ICU's. Some feel while open visitation may be psychologically supportive, it comes with harmful physiological consequences, interferes with time nurses need to spend caring for patients, and therefore leads to delays in care (Marco, 2006). Many ICUs in the United States continue to have restrictive visiting policies (Lee, Friedenberg, Mukpo et al., 2007). However, the emphasis on family- and relationship-based care has changed restrictions on ICU visiting hours (Kleinpell, 2008). Research continues to demonstrate that most patients and their family members prefer open visitation policies (Quinio, Savry, Deghelt et al., 2002; Garrouste-Orgeas, Philippart, & Timsit, 2008). Furthermore, research has shown that patients who have unrestricted visiting hours have less risk of cardiovascular complications, decreased mortality, and experience less stress and less anxiety (Fumagalli, Boncinelli, Lo Nostro et al., 2006). Clinical practice guidelines provide support for family visitation in the ICU (Davidson, Powers, Hedayat et al., 2007).

Finding a balance between patient, family, and staff needs is a priority (Farrell, Joseph, & Schwartz-Barcott, 2005). Observing patient–family interactions can provide information about the nature of the patient–family relationship and clues to family needs. The more acutely ill the patient, the more urgent it becomes for family members to be at the bedside to participate in decisions about the plan of care.

Children are often restricted from visiting adult inpatient units because adults often believe they will be overwhelmed and unable to cope or understand. Hospital policies often prevent children from entering high-acuity units because of the risk of infection. Acute illness is a source of stress and disruption for the entire family, especially children. That said, visiting may reassure the child that the family member is alive and has not left them permanently. In the instances where the high-acuity patient may not survive, the opportunity to "say goodbye" is very important. The nurse must use age-appropriate language when discussing illness with children. This allows for the planning of specific nursing interventions to best meet the needs of the child (Ihlenfeld, 2006).

TABLE 2–4 Advantages of Family Presence During CPR

- The ability of the family to grasp the seriousness of the patient's illness
- Family members see firsthand that everything was done for the patient
- Families move more positively through the grieving process
- Removal of doubt by families about what is happening to the patient
- Families experience less anxiety and fear
- Provision of a sense of closure for families who lose a loved one
- Facilitation of the grieving process by families who lose a loved one

Historically, family members have been restricted from visiting during invasive procedures and cardiopulmonary resuscitation (CPR). Reasons for these restrictions included fear that the family might lose control, unpleasantness of what families will see, insufficient room at the bedside, and increased risk of litigation. Many hospitals do not have written policies for family presence during CPR, yet it appears that most nurses believe families should be present. Advantages of having the family present, as summarized by Twibell (2008), are listed in Table 2–4.

Families may need guidance regarding how to visit with the patient. The nurse may discuss with the family what the patient looks like prior to the family visit. It is helpful for the family to know that they should speak to the patient in a normal tone of voice, to be comfortable simply being with the patient and not speaking at all, and to ask questions away from the bedside. Flexible visitation can be established when nurses are consistent and communicate effectively with visitors. A contract between the nursing staff and family members may be effective. Other resources can be helpful in dealing with visitors such as pastoral care, patient relations staff, social services, local support groups, physicians, and hospital administration. Staff must be prepared to set limits to visitation. Written hospital policies should include guidelines that define acceptable behavior and include a zero-tolerance policy that addresses unacceptable behavior, such as drug/alcohol usage, physical or verbal abuse, or the presence of weapons.

Patient- and family-centered care, a concept embraced by an increasing number of hospitals, is a care delivery model that is patient/family-focused. In this care delivery model, family members are not kept away from the bedside of the acutely ill patient. Instead, they are welcomed and encouraged to be present and active in care. Although the nurse is instrumental in making family-centered care a core value in the high-acuity area, all members of the multidisciplinary team play a role in ensuring the families' needs are met. The essential components of patient- and family-centered care, according to Carmen (2008) are summarized in Table 2–5.

TABLE 2–5 Components of Patient- and Family-Centered Care

- Open visitation – families are not considered "visitors"
- Inclusion in policy decision making – families serve on hospital committees
- Inclusion in patient care decision making – families "round" with the health care team
- Education of families about health care information
- Including families in designing comfortable spaces – families are facility advisors

SECTION THREE REVIEW

1. The initial goal when teaching high-acuity patients is to (choose all that apply)
   A. decrease stress
   B. promote comfort
   C. increase knowledge
   D. establish a trusting relationship
2. Which of the following factors may inhibit learning in high-acuity patients? (choose all that apply)
   A. fatigue
   B. educational level
   C. pain
   D. socioeconomic status
3. Which of the following strategies should the nurse use to reduce transfer anxiety?
   A. Introduce the patient and family to the receiving nurse before the transfer occurs.
   B. Transfer the patient during the night while they are sleeping.
   C. Do not include the family in the transfer until it's over.
   D. Inform the patient they will not receive as much nursing care in the lower acuity unit.
4. Patients who have unrestricted visiting hours may experience
   A. fatigue
   B. depression
   C. decreased cardiovascular complications
   D. increased anxiety
5. Family presence during CPR contributes to
   A. family members seeing firsthand that everything was done
   B. family members having more difficulty moving through the grieving process
   C. increased fear and anxiety
   D. inability to promote a sense of closure

Answers: 1. (A, B), 2. (A, C), 3. A, 4. C, 5. A

SECTION FOUR: Cultural Diversity

At the completion of this section, the learner will be able to discuss the importance of the awareness of cultural diversity when caring for high-acuity patients.

Cultural Competence

Cultural competence is defined as an awareness of one's own thoughts and feelings without letting them influence caring for patients with different backgrounds. With this self-awareness comes knowledge, understanding, respect, and acceptance for the patient's culture (Flowers, 2004). The American Nurses Association (ANA) has recognized the need for nurses to provide culturally competent care. The ANA Code for Nurses (2001a) states that nurses should "practice with compassion and respect for the inherent dignity, worth and uniqueness of every individual." Nurses who are culturally competent are sensitive to the culture, race, gender, sexual orientation, social class, and economic status of their patients. Cultural competence is more than just knowledge of another ethnic group. It includes effective communication, cultural assessment, interpretation and, lastly, intervention (Lipson, Dibble, & Minarik, 2001). High-acuity environments are stressful for patients and their families. It is essential that the nurse provide culturally competent care. The patient's perceived level of stress will be decreased if awareness of cultural beliefs is incorporated into the nursing interventions (Flowers, 2004).

Cultural Assessment

The high-acuity environment is not always the most conducive environment for a thorough cultural assessment. However, the nurse cannot provide excellent care without knowledge of the patient's cultural background. Questions that may be asked or observed to better understand a patient's culture, as suggested by Lipson and colleagues (2001) are listed in Table 2–6.

Effective communication may be hindered by language differences. When family members serve as interpreters, the complete message may not be transmitted due to lack of medical vocabulary or family role conflicts. The family member may transmit the information with his or her own perceptions.

TABLE 2–6 Cultural Assessment – Questions to Ask or Observe

1. Where was the patient born? Is he/she an immigrant? How long has he/she lived in this country?
2. What is the patient's ethnic affiliation?
3. Who makes up the patient's support system? Does the patient live in an ethnic community?
4. What is the primary (or secondary) language? What language does the patient/family prefer to speak/write?
5. How does the patient communicate nonverbally?
6. What is the patient's religious preference? Does it play an important role in his/her life?
7. Does the patient have food preferences or prohibitions?
8. What is the patient's economic status?
9. Does the patient have specific health/illness practices or beliefs?
10. Does the patient/family have specific customs or beliefs related to illness, birth, or death?

Certain details may be eliminated due to embarrassment. When working with an interpreter, the high-acuity nurse must exhibit patience. Speaking in short units of speech and using simple language may convey the information more effectively. Observe the patient for nonverbal cues.

Other Sources of Diversity

In addition to assessing a patient's cultural background, other sources of diversity must be considered. Immigrants and refugees may have specific health beliefs and practices. It is important to determine why these patients left their country and what drew them to the United States. Racial and ethnic considerations must be taken into account. **Race** refers to human biological variation while **ethnicity** refers to a set of social, cultural, and political beliefs held by a group of individuals. Socioeconomic status (income, education, and occupation) may have a strong influence on health care beliefs and access to the health care system. Sexual orientation should be taken into account. The nurse must collect these important data and communicate in a nonjudgmental manner.

Developing Cultural Competence

How, then, does a high-acuity nurse develop cultural competence? One model proposed by Rust et al. (2006) suggested a core set of skills defined by the mnemonic CRASH (Table 2–7). In considering culture, the high-acuity nurse must assess individual patient characteristics such as national origin, faith, and education. Accounting for individual characteristics helps to prevent stereotyping. Conveying respect for the patient's unique health/illness beliefs is essential for developing cultural competence. Assessing and affirming differences is crucial as it relates to language preferences. Educational material must be presented in a language and at a level of understanding that meets the needs of the patient. Sensitivity is addressed during the initial assessment of health practices, health beliefs, dietary preferences, and home remedies. Providing care with humility requires looking at the patient's culture without judgment (Broome & McGuiness, 2007).

TABLE 2–7 Using CRASH to Develop Cultural Competence

C	consider **C**ulture
R	show **R**espect
A	**A**ssess and **A**ffirm differences
S	**S**how **S**ensitivity and **S**elf-awareness
H	provide care with **H**umility

SECTION FOUR REVIEW

1. Cultural diversity
   - **A.** plays no role in the care of the high-acuity patient
   - **B.** plays an important role in the care of the high-acuity patient
   - **C.** is comprised of four components
   - **D.** is comprised of six components
2. Which of the following is not a source of cultural diversity?
   - **A.** age
   - **B.** socioeconomic status
   - **C.** sexual orientation
   - **D.** disabilities
3. Effective communication is enhanced by
   - **A.** disregarding nonverbal cues
   - **B.** incorporating medical vocabulary
   - **C.** avoiding eye contact
   - **D.** speaking in small units of speech
4. Which of the following is a term that describes a set of social, cultural, and political beliefs held by a group of individuals?
   - **A.** race
   - **B.** socioeconomic status
   - **C.** ethnicity
   - **D.** sexual orientation
5. Which of the following skills by the nurse demonstrates cultural competence? (choose all that apply)
   - **A.** show respect
   - **B.** assess and affirm differences
   - **C.** show sensitivity
   - **D.** provide care with humility

Answers: 1. B, 2. A, 3. D, 4. C, 5. (A, B, C, D)

SECTION FIVE: Palliative Care and Environmental Stressors

At the completion of this section, the learner will be able to examine the role of palliative care in the high-acuity environment and identify environmental stressors, their impact on high-acuity patients, and strategies to alleviate those stressors.

Definition of Palliative Care

Palliative care is an interdisciplinary approach to relieve suffering and improve quality of life. The care is directed toward patients with life-threatening illness and toward their families. Nursing and medical treatments are combined with control of pain and symptoms. Common symptoms addressed by the team include shortness of breath, fatigue, constipation, nausea, loss of appetite, and difficulty sleeping. It is important for the high-acuity nurse to explain to patients and their families that palliative care may be provided at the same time that medical treatment is directed toward a cure. Palliative care programs incorporate the services of medical and nursing specialists, social workers, and chaplains (Meier, Spragens, & Sutton, 2004). Most insurance companies, including Medicare and Medicaid, often cover part or all of the costs for palliative care treatment. This may even include medical supplies and equipment (Center to Advance Palliative Care, 2007).

Why Palliative Care?

Unmet needs of dying patients and concerns about the cost of high-acuity care and limited bed availability have fueled the growth of palliative care in hospital settings. The number of people who live with complex illnesses is growing. To meet the needs of these patients and their families, hospitals must find a way to deliver high-quality, cost-effective care. In the past, hospitals have adapted a model that embraces treatment and quick discharge. Not all patients fit this model (Kuehn, 2007). Palliative care, as a systematic approach to patient care lowers cost, increases bed capacity, and raises quality.

High-Acuity Patients and Palliative Care

Cancer is the disease often associated with palliative care. However, many other serious illnesses cause pain and symptoms, which interfere with quality of life. These may include cardiac disease, chronic respiratory disorders, renal failure, and neurological diseases. The goal is to improve quality of life (Rice & Betcher, 2007). A nurse, physician, family member, patient, social worker, or case manager may initiate a referral to the palliative care team. Meier et al. (2004) identified several reasons that a high-acuity patient should be referred to the palliative care team (Table 2–8).

Barriers to Providing Palliative Care

The high-acuity nurse faces barriers to caring for patients who can most benefit from palliative care. Patients, families, and members of the health care team often have inflated expectations of the outcome of medical therapies. They find it difficult to move from a process of curing to a process of caring. This delays attention to palliative needs. The high-acuity environment has been a place where health care professionals work in "silos." Nurses, physicians, and other disciplines work in parallel pursuing independent goals and their paths do not intersect (Nelson, 2006). The high-acuity patient is often the recipient of fragmented care and ineffective, inconsistent communication.

To overcome these barriers, health care professionals must be educated and trained on all aspects of palliative care. Changing belief systems from denial of death and a culture of rescue in the high-acuity areas may seem like an insurmountable endeavor. Education must focus on the limitations of critical care therapies, embracing treatment goals that are attainable, and the benefits of palliative interventions. Not only does the health care team need education, the public at large must be included in the process. As availability of palliative care teams continues to increase, the evidence suggests that involvement of the team in patient care will result in positive outcomes for patients and families. The incorporation of palliative care has demonstrated improvement in symptom management, higher level of consumer satisfaction, lower rates of in-hospital death, shorter length of stay, and substantial savings in direct and indirect hospital costs (Nelson, 2006).

A Multi-Disciplinary Approach

When a patient has been referred to a palliative care team, the high-acuity nurse and other team members formulate a plan of care to meet the patient's psychological, social, cultural, and spiritual needs. Team meetings and family conferences are instrumental. During the family conference, goals are clarified, the decision-making process is supported, and communication is facilitated. The palliative care plan for the high-acuity patient is comprehensive and must address the multifaceted needs of the patient. Items to be addressed, as summarized by Meier et al. (2004), are listed in Table 2–9.

Environmental Stressors in the High-Acuity Environment

Sensory input involves all five senses: visual, auditory, olfactory, gustatory, and tactile. Individual perceptions of stimuli to the senses vary. Usually, people select stimuli that are most acceptable to them. However, during acute illness, the patient does not have control over the choice of the environment and its stimuli. Very young, very old, and postoperative or

TABLE 2–8 Reasons to Refer a High-Acuity Patient to a Palliative Care Team

- Team/patient/family needs help with decision making and determination of goals
- Uncontrolled/unacceptable level of pain (or other symptom) for more than 24 hours
- Uncontrolled psychological or spiritual issues
- Frequent emergency room visits—more than once per month for the same diagnosis
- Frequent admission to the hospital—more than once per month for the same diagnosis
- Prolonged length of stay without evidence of progress—greater than 5 days
- Prolonged ICU stay or transfer between ICU settings without evidence of progress
- ICU setting with documented poor progress

TABLE 2–9 Components of a Palliative Care Plan

- Management of symptoms and side effects
- Patient/family understanding of disease status
- Patient/family preferences regarding treatment goals
- Patient/family hopes for medical care outcomes
- Do not resuscitate status
- Advanced directives
- Religious/cultural preferences/rituals
- Wishes for care before and at time of death
- Care setting—is it meeting the needs of the patient/family?
- Goals of medical care
- Decision-making needs/priorities
- Discharge options

unresponsive patients are at greatest risk of experiencing **sensory perceptual alterations** (SPAs). Acutely ill patients who develop SPAs may be at risk for the development of additional complications.

A combination of sensory overload and deprivation can exist. The patient is deprived of normal sensory stimuli while being exposed to continuous strange stimuli. The nurse should assess what sounds are in the patient's normal environment and expose the patient to these sounds, if possible (through tape recordings). Visitors can be effective by discussing familiar topics with the patient. Unresponsive patients are particularly challenging because information about the patient's normal environment must be collected through a third person. It is difficult to assess whether unresponsive patients are experiencing sensory alterations because they cannot communicate.

Sensory overload may occur when the patient is exposed to noise for continuous periods. The background environmental noise in a high-acuity unit includes annoying and frightening alarms, ringing telephones, pagers, staff conversations, loud overhead announcement systems, ventilators, cardiac monitors, the bubbling of chest tubes, and other strange and foreign sounds. However, patients report they are most disturbed by the staff's loud voices, especially at night when they interrupt sleep (Honkus, 2003). The Environmental Protection Agency recommends hospitals maintain noise levels below 45 decibels (dBA) during the day and 35 dBA at night. Because normal human conversation is usually around 60 dBA, it is important to see why keeping staff conversations to a minimum in the direct patient care areas is essential to promoting rest.

Sensory perceptual alterations or other physical disruptions may cause **delirium** in the high-acuity patient. Although most clinicians would recognize delirium as an abnormal state, it is important for the nurse to ascertain the cause of the delirium. Features of delirium include an acute onset of fluctuating awareness, impaired ability to attend to environmental stimuli, and disorganized thinking (Kaplan, 2007). Hypoxemia, alcohol or barbiturate withdrawal, hyponatremia, drug adverse reactions, infections, and liver dysfunction can cause delirium. It is extremely important to rule out and treat any underlying causes of delirium rather than merely medicating the patient to control behavior. Many times, delirium is preceded by anxiety and restlessness that escalate to confusion and agitation and finally delirium.

Alterations in the light/dark cycle, pain, environmental noise, caregiver interruptions, and stress can contribute to the inability of hospitalized patients to get adequate sleep and rest. Sedative hypnotics are often the preferred method for sleep disturbances, but this method has been linked to an increase in falls, delirium, and functional decline in patients, particularly in the elderly (King, 2006). Interventions that contribute to the nonpharmacologic induction of sleep should be implemented. Planned rest periods that allow for two hours of uninterrupted sleep are essential to promoting rapid eye movement (REM) sleep. REM sleep facilitates protein anabolism, restores the immune system, and promotes healing. Providing the patient with a few hours of REM sleep can be beneficial. Nurses should recognize this and act as a patient advocate to control the patient's environment to ensure adequate sleep and rest periods throughout the day and night. Closing and posting a sign on the patient's door is often effective. Other nursing interventions include the following:

- Provide relaxing music of the patient's choice, or earplugs for those who prefer silence.
- Control the patient's pain (essential to promoting REM sleep).
- Care providers should place pagers on vibrate mode.
- Turn down (or turn off) the volume of the overhead announcement system in patient care areas.
- Decrease the volume of alarms on equipment.
- Adjust light levels and offer eye masks to patients.
- Encourage ancillary services, such as physical therapy or respiratory therapy, to return after the patient has rested, if appropriate.
- Limit visitation during quiet time.
- Help the patient prepare mentally for quiet time through therapeutic touch or massage, guided imagery, or aromatherapy.
- Plan a daily schedule for the patient that includes a quiet time every day so the patient can look forward to a time of relaxation and rest.

Communicating with mechanically ventilated patients is very important to prevent SPA and promote a therapeutic nurse–patient relationship. The patient's inability to talk may cause high levels of stress, insecurity, and even panic. For many patients, the family can promote a sense of security and relaxation (Happ, 2007). However, patients and families can also become frustrated because they cannot understand lip reading. An experienced nurse is often helpful because he or she has more experience using lip reading techniques with an intubated patient. Although many nurses use nonverbal communication with their patients, most of that communication is at a very concrete level—pertaining only to physical care and including short task-oriented communication which does not provide emotional support.

Patients use a variety of forms of nonverbal communication. Vital signs, such as an elevated heart rate or blood pressure, are one form of nonverbal communication. Facial expressions, such as smiling, grimacing, or even crying and laughing, can be valuable forms of communication. Hand gestures, such as grabbing the nurse's arm or holding hands, or even moving legs around, use movement as a method of communication. Some patients are able to write messages very clearly, whereas others attempt to write and simply become frustrated as they experience fine-motor difficulty or cannot see clearly. Large pen markers may be easier than thin pens or pencils for the patient to manipulate. Using computer keyboards or pointing to letters on alphabet boards requires gross-motor skills. A coded eye blink system may be used for patients who are unable to move anything else.

SECTION FIVE REVIEW

1. Palliative Care is a systematic approach to patient care that results in the following (choose all that apply)
   A. decreased bed availability
   B. increased bed availability
   C. improved quality
   D. decreased cost
2. Components of a palliative care plan should include
   A. management of symptoms and side effects
   B. patient and family preferences regarding treatment goals
   C. advanced directives
   D. all of the above
3. A frequently cited annoying noise among high-acuity patients is
   A. an ambulance siren
   B. staff's loud voices
   C. television
   D. equipment noise
4. REM sleep
   A. facilitates protein anabolism
   B. restores the immune system
   C. promotes healing
   D. all of the above
5. Which of the following nursing interventions would support the patient's REM sleep?
   A. dimming lights during normal sleep time
   B. putting up a wall clock in the patient's room
   C. decreasing environmental noise
   D. A and C

Answers: 1. (B, C, D), 2. D, 3. B, 4. D, 5. D

SECTION SIX: End-of-Life Care

At the completion of this section, the learner will be able to examine personal values as they relate to the nurse's role in working with acutely ill patients and discuss end-of-life issues to be considered in caring for high-acuity patients.

Assessment of Sources of Conflict

The American Nurses Association (ANA) *Standards of Clinical Nursing Practice* states that essential components of professional nursing practice include care, cure, and coordination (ANA, 2001b). The American Association of Critical Care Nurses (AACN) position is that nurses who work with acutely ill patients should base their practice on individual professional accountability; thorough knowledge of the interrelatedness of body systems; recognition and appreciation of a person's wholeness, uniqueness, and significant social–environmental relationships; and appreciation of the collaborative role of all health team members (AACN, 2002). While working with patients in high-acuity areas, nurses are often faced with ethical dilemmas, such as those discussed in Section Two of Module One, High-Acuity Nursing. The exposure to death and the saving of human life requires the nurse to frequently evaluate personal values. Personal values often influence decision making. It is important for the nurse to fully understand his or her personal values.

Evaluation of one's personal philosophy can improve satisfaction with working with acutely ill patients. Clarification of one's values helps to anticipate problems that may be encountered in the practice setting and supports the development of positive coping strategies. This knowledge is carried with the professional nurse throughout his or her career regardless of the practice setting or age of the patient being cared for.

It is important that the nurse be careful not to impose his or her own value system onto that of the patient. The health care team should honor any end-of-life cultural and religious preferences of the patient (Wingate & Wiegand, 2008). There may be circumstances in which conflicts occur between the nurse's worldview and that of the patient, such as in decisions regarding withholding or withdrawing life-sustaining treatment. In these circumstances, the nurse should transfer care of the patient to another qualified high-acuity nurse (ANA, 2003).

The Patient Self Determination Act, passed as part of the Omnibus Budget Reconciliation Act of 1990, requires that all patients be given information about their right to formulate advanced directives of two types: treatment directives (living wills) and appointment directives (power of attorney for health care). This has increased the role of the patient and family in making end-of-life decisions. Nurses have a primary role in ensuring that the patient makes informed decisions regarding end-of-life care (ANA, 1991). The nurse working with high-acuity patients serves as a patient advocate and intercedes for patients who cannot speak for themselves and supports the decisions of the patient or the patient's designated surrogate (American Association of Colleges of Nursing, 2002). Nurses are also directed to uphold the choices and values of the patient even when these wishes conflict with those of health care providers and families (ANA, 2003).

An acutely ill patient was once clearly distinguished from a terminally ill patient. Nurses and physicians focused their efforts on saving lives and not providing end-of-life care. Despite advances in technology, it is impossible to predict which patients will die in the acute care setting and which will live. There may not be a period of time when it is clear that care needs to shift from a cure-oriented to a comfort-oriented approach (Wingate & Wiegand, 2008). Therefore, it is incumbent on the high-acuity nurse to provide care that is comprehensive. This includes attending to comfort needs of patients and families. Patients attempting to prolong life as well as those who are at the end-of-life must have their pain controlled and receive ongoing communication regarding their prognosis. End-of-life care and high-acuity care must converge and not conflict (Wingate & Wiegand, 2008).

Emerging Evidence

- Implementation of palliative care processes alongside aggressive, life-threatening critical care led to earlier consensus around patient-appropriate use of life support technology, resuscitation, and no change in mortality rates *(Mosenthal, Murphy, Barker et al., 2008).*
- Family members feel more support and are more satisfied with decision-making processes when spirituality is addressed during a family conference *(Gries, Curtis, Wall et al., 2008).*
- Patients who receive interdisciplinary palliative care services report greater satisfaction with care, have fewer ICU readmissions, and lower total health care costs after hospital discharge *(Gade, Venohr, Conner et al., 2008).*

Barriers to End-of-Life Care in the High-Acuity Environment and Recommendations for Change

High-acuity nurses want to ensure patients at the end of life will die with dignity and peace. Beckstrand, Callister, and Kirchhoff (2008) identified barriers to providing end-of-life care in the high-acuity environment (Table 2–10).

The Institute of Medicine (IOM) recommended that end-of-life care be improved (IOM, 1997). While issues related to end-of-life have been in the media, very little has been done to change the culture in high-acuity environments. Often, the health care team does not know patients' preferences for resuscitation and advanced directives have minimal impact on treatment decisions. High-acuity nurses report that their basic nursing education did not adequately prepare them for end-of-life care (Beckstrand et al, 2008). Suggestions for improving end-of-life care, as summarized by Beckstrand and colleagues (2008), are listed in Table 2–11.

TABLE 2–10 Barriers to End-of-Life Care

- Nursing time constraints
- Staffing patterns
- Communication challenges
- Treatment decisions based upon physician and not patient needs

TABLE 2–11 Nursing Suggestions for Improving Care at the End-of-Life

- Changing the environment to accommodate families (beds, showering facilities, music, place for meditation and family gathering)
- Improved management of pain and discomfort (in accordance with advanced directives)
- Knowledge of patient wishes for end-of-life care (advanced directives that are legally binding)
- Earlier cessation of treatments or not initiating aggressive treatments (when continued medical care seems futile)

Allow Natural Death

Patient and families are often confused and frightened by terms such as *do not resuscitate* (DNR), *do not intubate* (DNI), and *comfort measures only* (CMO). Families interpret this to mean that nothing will be done for their loved one and the nurse may not be equipped to provide adequate explanations. In 2000 the term *Allow Natural Death* (AND) was introduced (Knox & Vereb, 2005). Using this term implies that the patient is dying and that everything possible is being done to keep the patient comfortable and allow the dying process to occur naturally. The goal of AND is to prevent unnecessary suffering and allow nature to take its course. While AND is not different from DNR, the language is more acceptable to patients and families (Knox and Vereb, 2005).

Educational Focus

Educational programs must be developed to address end-of-life care for all members of the health care team. The education must be directed toward those individuals already in the workforce as well as those who are completing their basic education requirements. The American Association of Colleges of Nursing (2002) has developed the End-of-Life Nursing Education Consortium Curriculum Modules (www.aacn.nche.edu/ELNEC/ELNECSeries.htm).

The high-acuity nurse can make a positive impact on patients and their families at the end of life because of the constant presence at the bedside. The nurse, the critical link to moderating discussion of difficult issues, can facilitate discussions about treatment preferences and management of signs and symptoms at the end-of-life. Nursing actions and interventions for end-of-life care, as identified by Wingate and Wiegand (2008) are summarized in Table 2–12.

TABLE 2–12 Summary of Nursing Actions/Interventions at the End-of-Life

TOPIC	INTERVENTION
Changes in treatment plan	■ Ask questions about starting/stopping treatments, withdrawal or withholding life sustaining therapies ■ Review/adjust oral meds if patient is to be discharged
End-of-life discussions	■ Keep communication open ■ Include key members of health care team ■ Build on previous discussions ■ Provide clear basic information about current condition and prognosis ■ Establish goals of care ■ Establish regular family meetings
Treatment decisions	■ Involve patient in decision making if capable ■ Use advance directives if available ■ Assist patients and families in shared decision making

(continued)

TABLE 2–12 (continued)

End of life	▪ Honor patient's preference for location of death, religious/cultural preferences, presence of family members or pets ▪ Remove non-essential monitors and equipment ▪ Turn off alarms on remaining equipment ▪ Administer analgesics and sedatives as needed to prevent discomfort ▪ Administer anxiolytics to decrease anxiety ▪ Administer oxygen, place patient in a position of comfort, and use fans to circulate air to decrease dyspnea ▪ Prepare patients family for course of dying process and physical changes to expect in the patient's body ▪ Provide families unlimited access to the patient
Bereavement	▪ Provide resources as available: pastoral care, follow-up appointments with care providers, follow-up telephone calls ▪ Consider participating in group sessions for staff members who cared for the patient

SECTION SIX REVIEW

1. Nurses should reflect on their own personal values for the following reasons (choose all that apply)
   A. to teach the patient better values
   B. to gain an understanding of the factors that may limit reasoning
   C. to understand when they might not be suitable for being a patient advocate
   D. to be careful not to impose a personal value system on that of the patient
2. Which of the following interventions improves care at end of life?
   A. providing beds for family members
   B. providing a place for family gatherings
   C. earlier cessation of treatments
   D. all of the above
3. Allow Natural Death (AND) is
   A. the same as do not resuscitate (DNR)
   B. more restrictive than DNR
   C. confusing to patients and families
   D. not acceptable for high-acuity patients
4. End-of-life care
   A. has no place in the high-acuity environment
   B. is taught extensively in undergraduate programs
   C. advocates respect of the patient's wishes
   D. is not an issue in the media
5. End-of-life nursing interventions would include
   A. ensuring monitor alarms are on
   B. removing non-essential monitors and equipment
   C. avoiding analgesics and sedatives
   D. excluding family members from decision making

Answers: 1. B, C, D, 2. D, 3. A, 4. C, 5. B

POSTTEST

1. A patient is crying about a below-knee amputation sustained as a pedestrian in a pedestrian–vehicle crash. She expresses fears about ambulating in physical therapy. This behavior is a sign of which stage of illness?
   A. denial
   B. awareness
   C. restitution
   D. resolution
2. A patient was recently admitted to the ICU after a heart attack. The family wants to meet with the nurse. It is important for the nurse to recognize at this stage of illness, most family members need (choose all that apply)
   A. frequent communication about the patient's condition
   B. to know why interventions are initiated
   C. food and shelter
   D. to know the name of the health care provider
3. Imagery is beneficial for (choose all that apply)
   A. a patient undergoing a painful dressing change
   B. a patient undergoing a minor surgical procedure
   C. a patient undergoing an endoscopy
   D. a patient being intubated
4. Which of the following CATs is a risky strategy?
   A. humor
   B. aromatherapy
   C. massage therapy
   D. guided imagery
5. High-acuity patients have a right to know and understand what procedures are being done to and for them. The nurse knows that the initial goals when teaching high-acuity patients are to (choose all that apply)
   A. decrease stress
   B. promote comfort
   C. increase knowledge
   D. facilitate recall
6. A patient is ready to be transferred from ICU to a high-acuity unit. He expresses he is anxious about leaving the ICU. The nurse's best response would be
   A. You should not worry about this. It's not good for you to worry right now.
   B. You are right. You will not get the same care you get here in ICU.

C. Your stay here in the ICU is a temporary stage in the illness continuum. You have made so much progress.
D. I can give you some medication to relieve your anxiety.

7. Which of the following interventions would support family-centered care?
A. finding the family a hotel room
B. inviting the family to join health care team rounds
C. visitation ten minutes every two hours
D. restriction of children visiting family members in high-acuity units

8. The nurse is performing an admission assessment on a patient who is an immigrant. It is important for the nurse to demonstrate cultural competence. Which of the following skills demonstrate cultural competence? (choose all that apply)
A. show respect
B. assess differences
C. show sensitivity
D. provide care with humility

9. Socioeconomic status may have a strong influence on
A. length of stay
B. health care beliefs
C. ethnicity
D. sexual orientation

10. Which of the following is the term used to describe an interdisciplinary approach to patient care to relieve suffering and improve quality of life?
A. cultural competence
B. family-centered care
C. palliative care
D. death with dignity

11. Which of the following patients may benefit from palliative care? (choose all that apply)
A. a patient with lung cancer
B. a patient with chronic obstructive lung disease
C. a patient who has just had an appendectomy
D. a patient with right lower lobe pneumonia

12. A 75-year-old female had a colon resection and colostomy two days ago for Stage IIIB adenocarcinoma of the colon. She has a patient controlled analgesia pump for pain management. She received lorazepam at 11 A.M. for anxiety. Five hours later she yells for help. She has pulled out her nasogastric tube. She is combative and resists the assistance of the nurse. The nurse should recognize that the patient is exhibiting symptoms of which condition?
A. delirium
B. sleep deprivation
C. sensory perceptual disorder
D. overdose of narcotics

13. A nurse's values conflict with that of the patient's family regarding withdrawal of life sustaining treatment. What nursing intervention is essential for patient care in this situation?
A. The nurse has a duty to care for the patient no matter what.
B. The nurse must try to help the family reverse their decision.
C. The nurse should ask for a reassignment.
D. The nurse should call the HCP to write an order for AND.

14. A patient has an order for "allow natural death." Upon entering the patient's room, the nurse notes the patient's heart rate has decreased from 80 bpm to 30 bpm. What is the best initial action by the nurse?
A. Stay with the patient and have someone get the family from the waiting room.
B. Call the code team.
C. Initiate CPR.
D. Call the HCP.

Posttest answers with rationale are found on MyNursingKit.

PEARSON
EXPLORE mynursingkit™

MyNursingKit is your one stop for online chapter review materials and resources. Prepare for success with additional NCLEX®-style practice questions, interactive assignments and activities, web links, animations and videos, and more!

Register your access code from the front of your book at **www.mynursingkit.com.**

REFERENCES

Abbott, K. H., Sago, J. G., Breen, C. M., et al. (2001). Families looking back: one year after discussion of withdrawal or withholding life support. *Critical Care Medicine, 29*, 197–201.

American Association of Colleges of Nursing. (2002). *End-of-life competency statements for a peaceful death.* Washington, D.C., American Association of Colleges of Nursing.

American Association of Critical Care Nurses. (2002). Practice resources: Critical care nursing fact sheet. Available at: http://www.aacn.org. Accessed April 24, 2008.

American Nurses Association. (1991). Nursing and the patient self-determination acts. Available at: http://nursingworld.org/MainMenuCategories/HealthcareandPolicyIssues/ANAPositionStatements/EthicsandHumanRights.aspx. Accessed April 24, 2008.

American Nurses Association (2001a). *Code for nurses.* Washington D.C.: American Nurses Publishing.

American Nurses Association. (2001b). *Standards of clinical nursing practice* (2nd ed.). Washington, D.C.: American Nurses Publishing.

American Nurses Association. (2003). Nursing care and do-not-resuscitate orders. Available at: http://nursingworld.org/MainMenuCategories/HealthcareandPolicyIssues/ANAPositionStatements/EthicsandHumanRights.aspx. Accessed April 24, 2008.

Auerbach, S., Kiesler, J., Wartella, J., et al. (2005). Optimism, satisfaction with needs met, interpersonal perceptions of the healthcare team and emotional distress in patients' family members during critical care hospitalization. *American Journal of Critical Care*, 14, 202–210.

Beckstrand, R., Callister, L., & Kirchhoff, K. (2008). Providing a "good death": critical care nurses' suggestions for improving end-of-life care. *American Journal of Critical Care*, 15, 38–45.

Broome, B. & McGuiness, T. (2007). A CRASH course in cultural competence for nurses. *Urology Nursing*, 27(4), 292–294.

Carmen, S., Teal, S., & Guzzetta, C. (2008). Development, testing and national evaluation of a pediatric patient-family-centered care benchmarking survey. *Holistic Nursing Practice.* 22(2), 61–74.

Center to Advance Palliative Care (2007). What should you know about palliative care?. Available at: www.getpalliativecare.org. Accessed April 10,2008.

Chaboyer, W., James, H., & Kendall, M. (2005). Transitional care after the intensive care unit: Current trends and future directions. *Critical Care Nurse, 25*, 16–28.

Chaboyer, W., Thalib, L., Aleorn, K., and Foster, M. (2007). The effect of an ICU liaison nurse on patients and family member's anxiety prior to transfer to the ward: an intervention study. *Intensive and Critical Care Nursing, 23*, 362–369.

Chlan, L. L. (1998). Effectiveness of a music therapy intervention on relaxation and anxiety for patients receiving ventilatory assistance. *Heart and Lung, 27*, 169–176.

Counsell, C., & Guin, P. (2002). Exploring family needs during withdrawal of life support in critically ill patients. *Critical Care Nursing Clinics of North America, 14*, 187–191.

Davidson, J. E., Powers, K., Hedayat, S. M., et al. (2007). American College of Critical Care Medicine Task Force 2004–2005. Society of Critical Care Medicine clinical practice guidelines for support of the family in the patient centered ICU. *Critical Care Medicine, 35*, 605–622.

Deng, G., Cassileth, B., Cohen, L., et al. (2007). Integrative oncology practice guidelines. *Journal of the Society for Integrative Oncology*, 5(2), 65–84.

Ernst, E., Pittler, M., Wider B. (eds.) (2006). *The desktop guide to complementary and alternative medicine: an evidence-based approach.* Second edition. Mosby/Elsevier, Edinburgh.

Farrell, M. E., Joseph, D. H., Schwartz-Barcott, D. (2005). Visiting hours in ICU: finding the balance among patient, visitor, and staff needs. *Nursing Forum, 40*, 18–28.

Flowers, D. (2004). Culturally competent nursing care. *Critical Care Nurse.* 24(4), 48–52.

Fumagalli, S., Boncinelli, L., Lo Nostro, A., et al. (2006). Reduced cardiocirculatory complications with unrestrictive visiting policy in an intensive care unit: Results from a pilot, randomized trial. *Circulation*, 113, 946–952.

Gade G, Venohr, I., Conner, D., et al. (2008). Impact of an inpatient palliative care team: a randomized controlled trial. *Journal of Palliative Medicine, 11*(2), 180–190.

Garrouste-Orgeas, M., Philippart, F., Timsit, J, et al. (2008). Perceptions of a 24-hour visiting policy in the intensive care unit. *Critical Care Medicine*, 36(1), 30–35.

Gries, C. J., Curtis, R. J., Wall, R. J., et al. (2008). Family members satisfaction with end of life decision making in the ICU. *Chest, 133*(3), 704–712.

Halm, M. (2008). Essential oils for management of symptoms in critically ill patients. *American Journal of Critical Care*, 17, 160–163.

Happ, M., Swigart, V., Arnold, R., et al. (2007). Family presence and surveillance during weaning from prolonged mechanical ventilation. *Heart and Lung*, 36(1), 47–57.

Heidrich, D. E. (2007). Delirium: an under-recognized problem. *Clinical Journal of Oncology Nursing* 11(6), 805–807.

Honkus, V. (2003). Sleep deprivation in critical care units. *Critical Care Nursing Quarterly*, 26(3), 179–189.

Ihlenfeld, J. (2006). Should we allow children to visit ill parents in intensive care units. *Dimensions in Critical Care*, 25(6), 269–271.

Institute of Medicine (1997). *Approaching Death: improving care at the end of life.* New York, NY: National Academy Press.

King, B. (2006). Functional decline in hospitalized elders. *MEDSURG Nursing*, 15(5), 265–271.

Kleinpell, R. M. (2008). Visiting hours in the intensive care unit: more evidence that open visitation is beneficial. *Critical Care Medicine, 36*, 334–335.

Knox, C., & Vereb, J. (2005). Allow natural death: a more humane approach to discussing end-of-life directives. *Journal of Emergency Nursing*, 31(6), 560–561.

Kuehn, B. (2007). Hospitals embrace palliative care. *JAMA*, 298(11), 1263–1265.

Lee, M. D., Friedenberg, A. S., Mukpo, D. H. (2007). Visiting hours in New England intensive care units: strategies for improvement. *Critical Care Medicine, 35*, 497–501.

Lipson, J., Dibble, S., & Minarikm P. (eds.). (2001). Culture & Nursing Care: A Pocket Guide UCSF Nursing Press, San Francisco.

Liu, Y., & Tonks, N. (2008). The role of massage therapy in relief of cancer pain. *Nursing Standard*, 22(21), p35–40.

Marco, L., Bermejillo, I., Garayalade, N., et al. (2006). Intensive care nurses' beliefs and attitudes towards the effect of open visiting on patients, families and nurses. *Nursing Critical Care*, 11, 33–41.

Meier, D., Spragens, L., & Sutton, S. (2004). A guide to building a hospital based palliative care program. Center to Advance Palliative Care, a national program office of the Robert Wood Johnson Foundation.

Mosenthal, A. C., Murphy, P. A., Barker, L. K., et al. (2008). Changing the culture around end of life in the trauma ICU. *Journal of Trauma 64*(6), 1587–1593.

Nelson, J. (2006). Identifying and overcoming the barriers to high-quality palliative care in the intensive care unit. *Critical Care Medicine*, 34(11) s324-s331.

Palazzo, M. O., (2001). Teaching in crisis. patient and family education in critical care. *Critical Care Clinics of North America, 13*, 83–92.

Penson, R., Partridge, R., Rudd, P., et al. (2005). Schwartz center rounds, laughter: the best medicine? *Oncologist*, 10(8), 651–660.

Quinio, P., Savry, C., Deghelt, A., et al. (2002). A multicenter survey of visiting policies in French intensive care units. *Intensive Care Medicine, 28*, 1389–1394.

Rice, E., & Betcher, D. (2007). Evidence base for developing a palliative care service. *MEDSURG Nursing*, 16(3), 143–149.

Roberts, S. L. (1976). Transfer anxiety. *Behavioral concepts and the critically ill.* Englewood Cliffs, Ca: Prentice Hall., 224–253.

Rust, G., Kondawani, K., Martinez, R., et al. (2006). A crash course in cultural competence. *Ethnicity and Disease.* 12(2, suppl.3), S3-29–36.

Steele, S., & Harmon, V. (1983). *Values clarification in nursing.* Norwalk, CT: Appleton-Century Crofts.

Suchman, E. (1965). Stages of illness and medical care. *Journal of Health and Human Behavior*, 6, 114.

Tracy, M., Lindquist, R., Savik, K., et al. (2005), Use of complementary and alternative therapies: a national survey of critical care nurses. *American Journal of Critical Care*, 14, 404–415.

Twibell, R., Siela, D., Riwitis, C., et al. (2008). Nurses' perceptions of their self-confidence and the benefits and risks of family presence during resuscitation. *American Journal of Critical Care*, 17(2), 101–111.

White, J.M. (2000). State of the science of music interventions. *Critical Care Clinics of North America, 12*, 219–225.

Wingate, S. & Wiegand, D. (2008). End-of-life care in the critical care unit for patients with heart failure. *Critical Care Nurse, 28*(2), 84–94.

Wong, H. L. C., Lopez-Nahas, V., & Molassiatis, A. (2001). Effects of music therapy on anxiety in ventilator dependent patients. *Heart and Lung, 30*, 376–387.

MODULE

3 The Older Adult High-Acuity Patient

Kristine L'Ecuyer, Helen Lach, Melanie Hardin-Pierce

OBJECTIVES Following completion of this module, the learner will be able to:

1. Describe the characteristics of the aging population.
2. Identify age-related changes in neurologic, and neurosensory function.
3. Explain the age-related changes in cardiovascular and pulmonary function.
4. Discuss the age-related changes in integumentary and musculoskeletal function.
5. Describe age-related changes in gastrointestinal and genitourinary function.
6. Explain age-related changes in endocrine and immune function.
7. Differentiate between dementia, delirium, and depression and describe their impact on high-acuity patients and their families.
8. Discuss functional decline, pain, and pharmacology as factors that impact hospitalization in the older patient.
9. Describe common geriatric assessment tools.
10. Discuss nursing management of older patients with high-risk injuries and trauma.
11. Explain special situations including the culture of care for older adults and end-of-life care.

An increasing percentage of hospital and high-acuity patients are older adults. They are a vulnerable group, needing skilled care. A number of typical changes occur as a normal result of the aging process, and while these changes do not cause illness or disability, they do put the older adult at risk for complications and negative outcomes during hospitalization. The high-acuity nurse needs to be aware of these changes and risks in order to properly assess patients and provide interventions to improve outcomes for older adults. This module reviews key aging changes and common problems nurses are likely to encounter in the older high-acuity patient, and provides strategies for improving nursing management of these challenging patients.

The module consists of eleven sections. Section One addresses the demographic characteristics of the growing aging population. Sections Two through Six focus on the normal age-related changes in the body systems and strategies for nursing management. Section Seven describes cognitive conditions of dementia, delirium, and depression that are common and can cause challenges for the patient in the high-acuity setting. Section Eight discusses physical conditions impacting the high-acuity patient including functional decline, pain, and pharmacology. In Section Nine, assessment tools are provided for evaluating the conditions described in the previous sections. In Section Ten, care of the older adult with trauma and high risk injuries is discussed. Finally, Section Eleven discusses special high-acuity situations for the older adult, including resuscitation and end of life. Each section includes a set of review questions to help the learner evaluate his or her understanding of the section's content before moving on to the next section. All Section Reviews include answers. It is suggested that the learner review those concepts answered incorrectly in the review questions before proceeding to the next section.

PRETEST

1. The population of older adults will increase by how much over the next 25 years?
   A. 10 percent
   B. 20 percent
   C. It will double.
   D. It will triple.
2. The most common chronic diseases in older adults include (choose all that apply)
   A. heart disease
   B. respiratory diseases
   C. diabetes
   D. Parkinson's disease

3. Which of the following is a normal aging change?
A. decreased cardiac output
B. memory loss
C. depression
D. arthritis

4. Skin changes in the older patient that affect nursing care include which of the following? (choose all that apply)
A. thinning of the dermis and epidermis
B. decreased sweat glands
C. decreased pigmentation
D. decreased elasticity

5. Hypoxia may occur in the older patient because of which of the following physiologic changes associated with aging?
A. hyperventilation
B. decreased alveolar surface area
C. ineffective airway clearance
D. decreased anterior-posterior chest diameter

6. Which of the following respiratory changes increases the older patient's risk of infection?
A. decreased elasticity
B. decreased mucus production
C. calcification in the lung wall
D. decreased alveolar surface

7. Which of the following laboratory tests values is **not** altered in the typical older patient?
A. serum protein
B. thyroid hormone
C. BUN
D. glucose tolerance

8. The most dependable sign of an infection in the older patient is
A. fever
B. change in mental status
C. pain
D. decreased breath sounds

9. Which of the following is the biggest risk factor for delirium in the older patient?
A. syncope
B. underlying dementia
C. blood loss
D. incontinence

10. What is the most common cause of dementia in the older adult?
A. Lewy body disease
B. vascular disease
C. Alzheimer's disease
D. Parkinson's disease

11. Loss of function during hospitalization
A. occurs slowly and insidiously
B. eventually occurs in all persons
C. is defined as organ malfunction
D. is rapid and may not be reversed

12. Which of the following drugs should be avoided in the older patient with sleep problems? (choose all that apply)
A. diphenhydramine
B. temazepam
C. acetaminophen
D. amitriptyline

13. Older adults are more susceptible to drug side effects and toxicity due to (choose all that apply)
A. changes in absorption
B. changes in renal filtration
C. changes in metabolism of drugs
D. changes in hearing

14. Pain medication should be avoided in the older patient because it can cause mental status changes.
A. True
B. False

15. Mr. Moore, age 79, was in a motor vehicle crash and had a loss of consciousness. He is confused at present. All of the following may explain his confusion except
A. delirium
B. closed head injury
C. hypovolemia
D. decreased reflexes

16. Because of his age, Mr. Moore is at risk for a(n)
A. epidural hematoma
B. subdural hematoma
C. subarachnoid bleed
D. skull fracture

17. Mr. Moore is taken to the operating room for a craniotomy. He is given a general anesthesia. He is at greater risk for
A. prolonged absorption and elimination of the anesthetic agent
B. breakthrough pain
C. hyperthermia
D. hypoglycemia

18. Care for the patient who is not expected to survive is considered
A. palliative care
B. restorative care
C. medical futility
D. ethical care

Pretest answers are found on MyNursingKit.

SECTION ONE: Characteristics of the Older Population

At the completion of this section, the learner will be able to describe the characteristics of the aging population.

Demographic Characteristics

The older population is growing in and out of the hospital setting (See Fig. 3–1). With advancements in sanitation, technology, and medicine over the past century, people are living longer. In the United States, the population aged 65 and over

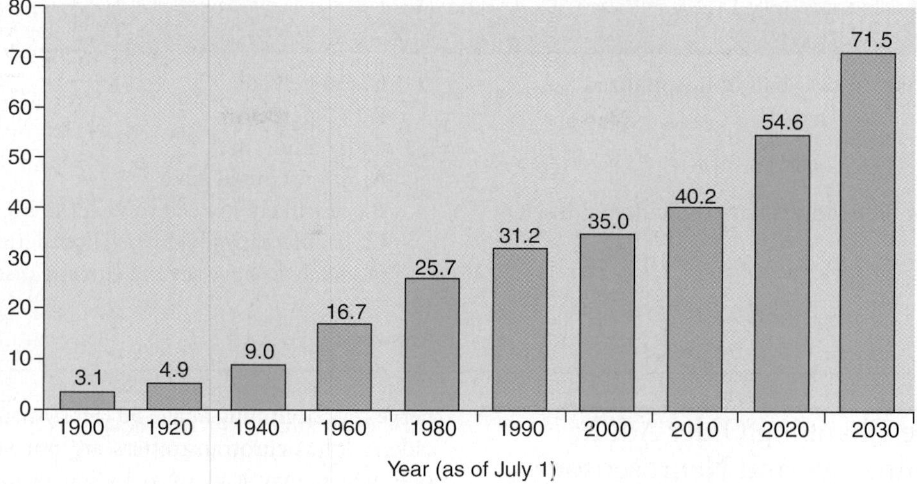

Figure 3–1 ▪ Aging population statistics. Number of persons 65+, 1900-2030 (numbers in millions). *Administration on Aging.*

is expected to double in size within the next 25 years (NIA, 2006). By 2030, almost one out of every five Americans, or over 72 million people, will be 65 years or older. There are more than 70,000 centenarians (AOA, 2007) or people over the age of 100! The fastest-growing group is people over the age of 85, who have the highest utilization of health care resources. This "age wave" will peak in 2040 when most of the baby boomers are over 65. Because older adults use a disproportionate amount of our health care resources, this has implications for all professionals in health care, including nurses in high-acuity settings.

Health

Older adults have a disproportionate amount of chronic disease; 82 percent have at least one chronic condition and many have more than one (AOA, 2007). The most common chronic diseases include hypertension, arthritis or joint problems, heart disease, cancer, diabetes, stroke, asthma, and chronic bronchitis. All of these may be the cause of hospitalization or need to be considered when treating the older patient with acute illness. The high rates of chronic disease are related to high levels of disability, with over half of older adults having some difficulty with daily activities or self-care (AOA, 2007). These rates of disease and disability increase with age.

While older adults have more health problems than younger people, it is important to remember that as an age group they are very diverse. For example, 20 percent of older adults don't have *any* chronic diseases (AOA, 2007) and 35 percent of people over 75 report their health as very good or excellent (Pleis & Lethbridge-Cejku, 2007). Only 5 percent of older adults are living in a nursing home at any given time (AOA, 2007), although more will spend some time in a nursing home during their lifetime. Younger people today may age in more healthy ways and avoid some of the problems experienced by the current generation. As a result, the nurse has to assess each older adult individually to determine his or her baseline health and functional state prior to illness, and strive to return the individual to this prior health state if possible.

Health Care

Older adults will make up a majority of nursing practice in the general hospital setting: 60 percent in the hospital (DeFrances & Hall, 2004) and about 55 percent in the intensive care unit (Angus et al., 2000). The Institute of Medicine's 2008, *Retooling for an Aging America: Building the Health Care Workforce,* describes the increased use of health care services by the older population. Emergency department visits by older people may nearly double by 2013, and these patients are more likely than younger people to be admitted to the hospital and have complications. As noted earlier, older adults make up more than half of intensive care days. Unfortunately, a high percentage of health resources are used in the last year of life, including critical care services. So the number of high-acuity patients who are at the end of life is likely to increase.

Diversity

Another change in the aging population is increasing racial and ethnic diversity. Approximately 17 percent of older adults were non-Hispanic whites in 2003, and this diverse group will increase to 28 percent by 2030 (NIA, 2006). With the growing immigrant and minority populations, nurses will need to strive to provide culturally competent care and meet the needs of a growing diverse population.

SECTION ONE REVIEW

1. Older adults make up over half of hospitalized patients.
   A. True
   B. False
2. What percent of older adults have difficulty with self-care activities?
   A. 5 percent
   B. 25 percent
   C. 50 percent
   D. 75 percent
3. Older adults are
   A. pretty much alike
   B. less likely to need to visit the ER
   C. an increasingly diverse population
   D. likely to have several chronic diseases

Answers: 1. A, 2. C, 3. C

SECTION TWO: The Changing Older Adult: Neurologic and Neurosensory Systems

At the completion of this section, the learner will be able to identify age-related changes in neurologic and neurosensory function.

The Older Adult Patient

Aging affects physical, psychological, social, spiritual, and economic aspects of a person's life experience. Lifestyle as well as genetic and environmental influences may impact the aging process. Nurses working in high-acuity areas should understand the age-related characteristics that make older patients vulnerable to complications and that may impact the outcome of their hospitalization. Physical characteristics are affected during the aging process and are marked by a gradual loss of function in all organ systems. The challenge for nurses centers on an ability to distinguish between changes associated with normal aging and those that occur due to a pathological process. Physiologic changes as well as other comorbidities impact the ability to respond to a current illness and thus are important factors which determine the outcome and recovery.

Older adults may present with common problems in uncommon ways: symptoms are less predictable, they may have multiple other comorbidities or chronic conditions and numerous medications, and they are at greater risk for permanent disability (Moore & Duffy, 2007). In addition, older adults have reduced physiologic reserve of most body systems; they have reduced homeostatic mechanisms, which affect temperature control and fluid and electrolyte balance; and they may have impaired immunologic function, which puts them at greater risk for infection (Fletcher, 2007).

Older adults may endure an increased length of hospital stay, institutionalization, and even death as a result of an acute illness and hospitalization. Early identification of high-risk patients as well as greater vigilance is needed in the care of older adults (Moore & Duffy, 2007). The application of early and appropriate interventions can improve care, promote optimal function, prevent complications, and provide for the best possible outcomes for hospitalized elderly patients.

Neurologic System

The central nervous system (CNS) regulates the cognitive, behavioral, sensory, and homeostatic functions of the body, with loss of nerve cells beginning at age 30 (Hooyman & Kiyak, 2008). In the older adult, neurotransmitters are not synthesized at the same rate, which may lead to a decline in sympathetic and a catecholamine response. This change may cause a decreased cardiac compensation in conditions such as fever, hypovolemia, or stress. Additionally, there may be declines in nervous system conduction responsible for slower reflex responses. Memory processes are slower and learning takes longer. The blood brain barrier is more permeable, so that medications may cross into the brain easily, increasing the risk of side effects or toxicity. Additionally, there is dilation of the ventricles and a decrease in brain volume (probably due to loss of water), which essentially increases the cranial dead space. Therefore, elderly persons may sustain a significant amount of hemorrhage after an injury-induced intracranial bleed, before symptoms are apparent. Table 3–1 summarizes changes in the central nervous system in the older adult.

Nursing Implications for Central Nervous System Changes

In the high-acuity area, age-related central nervous changes impact the neurologic exam. Nurses assess mental status and level of consciousness (LOC), ability to communicate and follow commands, as well as short-and long-term memory (see discussion of assessment tests in Section Five). Hypoxia, electrolyte imbalances, and medications are other factors that impact CNS

TABLE 3–1 Physiologic Changes of Aging: Central Nervous System

AGE RELATED CHANGES	PHYSIOLOGIC EFFECTS
Loss of functioning neurons	
Altered neurotransmitter synthesis	Altered sympathetic and catecholamine response
Decreased nervous system response	Decreased reflexes
Decrease brain volume and weight	Slower motor and sensory processing
Formation of neurofibrillary tangles, and senile plaque formation	Delayed onset of symptoms after intracranial bleeding Susceptibility to cognitive decline, Alzheimer's disease Shorter attention span, poorer short term memory

Data from Fletcher (2007), Hooyman & Kiyak (2008), Linton & Lach (2007).

assessment (Urden et al., 2006). Changes in fine and gross motor function, such as handgrip strength and reflexes, may be due to changes in CNS function. Nurses should be aware of the impact of CNS changes on the ability to perform self-care as well as the ability to follow instructions or interpret instructions regarding self-care. In the high-acuity setting, age-related neurologic changes along with acute medical conditions and the environmental issues associated with high-acuity settings contribute to a risk for postoperative cognitive dysfunction, falls, restraint use, over-sedation, and delirium.

Sensory System

As individuals age, there is a decline in all of the sensory receptors. Although there is a great deal of diversity among individuals in the rate and severity of sensory perception decline, the decline begins in the second decade of life, with a rapid decline after the ages of 45 to 65 (Hooyman & Kiyak, 2008). Visual acuity and depth perception decrease. Pupils are smaller, and pupillary response to light is decreased. The cornea becomes thicker, flatter, and more irregular in shape. The lens becomes more opaque and cataracts or glaucoma are common, which further complicates the accuracy of a sensory exam.

The sensitivity to smells is diminished and older adults have more difficulty discriminating between varying intensities of a flavor, which affects taste sensation (Hooyman & Kiyak, 2008). Auditory function declines, and there is decreased sensitivity to sound. An increase in cerumen impactions due to a decrease in function of the hair fibers of the ear canal cause blocking of sound, and can affect hearing ability (Cacchione, 2008). Additionally, older adults may have difficulty hearing high-pitched sounds and hearing rushed speech, especially when there is background noise, and may require more time to process and respond to auditory stimuli. Touch sensitivity in the fingertips, palms, and lower extremities also deteriorates with aging. There is a decline in proprioception, balance, and postural control. These physiologic changes combine to alter the older adult's ability to adapt to changes in the environment (Rosenthal and Kavic, 2004). In addition, these changes affect safety, and contribute to increased vulnerability for confusion and depression, falls, and traumatic injuries, and negatively impact the older adults' ability to interact in their environment (Cacchione, 2008).

SECTION TWO REVIEW

1. In the older patient, the diminished rate of neurotransmitter synthesis leads to
   A. hypertension
   B. more rapid respiratory rate
   C. increased cardiac response to stressors
   D. decreased sympathetic nervous system response
2. In the older patient, there is increased risk for development of neurologic side effects or toxicity from drug therapies related to
   A. a smaller brain volume
   B. a more permeable blood brain barrier
   C. a loss of water content in the brain
   D. atherosclerotic vascular changes
3. Older patients can have delayed manifestations of cranial bleeding due to which age-related change?
   A. more dead space in the cranium
   B. delays in reflex responses
   C. decreased compensatory mechanisms
   D. altered perceptions of pain
4. When checking the pupils in the older patient, the nurse should be aware of which pupillary changes as an age-related change?
   A. increased response to light
   B. larger pupils
   C. decreased response to light
   D. no pupil size change

Answers: 1. D, 2. B, 3. A, 4. C

SECTION THREE: The Changing Older Adult: Cardiovascular and Pulmonary Systems

At the completion of this section, the learner will be able to explain the age-related changes in cardiovascular and pulmonary function.

Cardiovascular

Coronary heart disease (CHD) is the leading cause of death in America, and 82 percent of people who die of CHD are age 65 or older (American Heart Association, 2008). Anatomic and physiologic cardiovascular changes alter the function of both the myocardium and the peripheral vasculature. Cardiovascular changes include decreased elasticity, and increased stiffness of the arterial walls. Heart muscle is replaced with fat; there is a loss of elastic tissue and an increase in collagen (Hooyman & Kiyak, 2008). The result may be ventricular hypertrophy, arteriosclerosis, increased systolic blood pressure, and/or a decline in ventricular compliance which can impair diastolic filling and myocardial relaxation. The presence of an S4 heart sound may indicate decreased ventricular compliance. Fibrosis can lead to calcification, valve incompetence, and conduction abnormalities. Nurses monitor for murmurs and electrocardiogram (ECG) changes. The arterial and peripheral vessels undergo a loss of elasticity and fat accumulation in the intima of the vessel wall, creating atherosclerosis. Atherosclerosis is exacerbated in individuals whose diets include large quantities of saturated fats (Hooykman and Kiyak, 2008).

Neurohormonal changes including decreased vasomotor tone and baroreceptor response result in altered compensatory responses, hypertension, and decreased cardiac output. Paired with age-related changes in body composition, metabolic rate, and general state of fitness, age associated physiologic changes combine to impact cardiovascular function, and result in an increased prevalence of peripheral vascular disease and coronary heart disease (CHD) in older adults.

Increases in prevalence of coronary heart disease occur in women as well as men, but begin at a later age in women. The same risk factors associated with atherosclerosis in younger adults (lipid abnormalities, smoking, hypertension, diabetes) are predictive in older individuals as well. Modification of these risk factors can be effective in reducing the risk of atherosclerosis in older patients. Other risk factors for the development of coronary heart disease are discussed in Module 16, Alterations in Myocardial Tissue Perfusion. Table 3–2 provides a summary of age-related changes in the cardiovascular system and their physiologic effects.

Nursing Implications for Cardiovascular Changes: Perfusion

Normally, when myocardial demands increase, compensation occurs by an increased blood flow to the coronary arteries. If blood flow is limited due to pre-existing cardiovascular disease, a patient is more vulnerable to myocardial ischemia and infarction. Elderly patients with cardiac ischemia and acute myocardial infarction (AMI) may present atypically. They may complain of shortness of breath or abdominal, throat, or back pain. Additionally, they may have symptoms such as syncope, acute confusion, flu-like syndromes, stroke, and/or falls, which may delay or confuse their diagnosis and treatment.

Diagnostic tests may be less reliable in the older patient. A normal electrocardiogram does not rule out cardiac ischemia since 50 percent of elderly patients do not have ST-T wave changes in ischemia (Roseborough, 2006). Creatine kinase levels are lower in the elderly, therefore, in ischemia, even though levels may elevate, the elevation may not be greater than the upper limits of normal, particularly if the patient delays seeking help.

Advances in cardiac anesthesia and myocardial protection during cardiac surgery and in surgical techniques have improved morbidity and mortality statistics for older adults (Rosborough, 2006). Therapeutic treatments such as thrombolytic therapy, percutaneous transluminal coronary angioplasty, coronary artery bypass grafts (CABG), and valve replacements are applicable to the older adult although some modifications may be considered. For example, because cardiac tissues may be more frail, careful handling would be particularly important in the older adult. Elderly patients may benefit from off-pump CABG, and other minimally invasive techniques (Rosborough, 2006). Physiologic age of an individual as well as chronological age should be assessed.

TABLE 3–2 Physiologic Changes of Aging: Cardiovascular and Pulmonary Systems

AGE RELATED CHANGES	PHYSIOLOGIC EFFECTS
Cardiovascular	
Heart valve fibrosis and thickening	Hemodynamic alterations: Reduced cardiac output, increased blood pressure, increased peripheral vascular resistance, decreased compliance of the left ventricle, increased incidence of murmurs, and extra heart sounds (S3 and S4)
Myocardial hypertrophy	Increased incidence of atherosclerotic events
Increased lipid content in artery walls	Decreased ability to increase heart rate or blood pressure in response to stressors
Progressive thickening of arterial walls	Increased prevalence of arrhythmias
Loss of vasomotor tone	Prolonged PR interval
Decreased baroreceptor sensitivity	Predisposed to orthostatic hypotension
Thickening of SA node	
Decreased number of pacemaker cells	
Increased time of AV node conduction	
Pulmonary	
Decreased elasticity of lung tissue	Decreased chest wall compliance
	Increased AP diameter
Calcification of thoracic wall	Blunted response to hypoxia/hypercapnia
Reduced sensitivity of respiratory center	Retention of secretions
Decreased cough reflex	Ineffective cough, inefficient cilia
Atrophy of cilia	Decreased PaO_2 (4mmHg decrease per decade)
Decreased alveolar surface area	Reduced ventilatory efficiency
Decreased strength of respiratory muscles	Increased susceptibility to aspiration, atelectasis, infection
	Decreased maximal breathing capacity, decreased vital capacity

Data from Fletcher (2007), Hooyman & Kiyak (2008), and Linton & Lach (2007).

The older adult cardiac patient will require vigilant clinical assessment and monitoring to prevent complications related to therapeutic interventions. Hemodynamic monitoring may be more challenging in the older adult. Older adults require higher filling pressures to maintain adequate stroke volume and cardiac output (Balas, et al., 2008). In addition, volume assessment is imperative as older adults are sensitive to hypovolemia; at the same time, hypervolemia can lead to systolic failure, poor organ perfusion, and hypoxemia leading to diastolic dysfunction.

Pulmonary

Physiological changes in the respiratory system associated with aging may result from changes in compliance of the chest wall or the lung tissue. As the costal cartilage that connects the rib cage undergoes calcification, kyphosis may develop which reduces chest wall compliance. Other structural changes may include vertebral collapse from osteoporosis, and increased anteroposterior (AP) diameter. Loss of lung elasticity leads to increased alveolar compliance and collapse of small airways, which may cause a decrease in alveolar surface area, uneven alveolar ventilation, air trapping, decreased PaO_2 levels, and an altered ability to respond to hypoxia or hypercapnia. Decreased rib mobility and decreased strength of respiratory muscles leads to a decline in maximum inspiratory and expiratory force by as much as 50 percent (Rosenthal & Kavic, 2004). Loss of epithelial cells results in a decrease in protective mucus, increasing risk for infections (Connolly, 2003). In addition, surface area of the lungs is decreased resulting in less capacity. Refer to Table 3–2 for a summary of age-related pulmonary changes and their physiologic effects.

Nursing Implications for Pulmonary Changes: Ventilation

Respiratory disorders are commonly encountered in patients in high-acuity areas. Potential nursing concerns are the risk for aspiration, atelectasis, and pneumonia, particularly in older adults recovering from surgery, suffering from rib fractures or chest injuries, or those receiving narcotics, those with artificial airways, or who are deconditioned or have altered nutritional or hydration status (Smith & Cotter, 2008). Deep breathing and coughing exercise for older adults is an important nursing focus as respiratory muscles are weaker, the cough reflex is less effective, and the ciliary function is decreased. Nurses need to be able to accurately assess respiratory status to determine adequacy of gas exchange, ventilation and perfusion, and to identify worsening respiratory function.

A number of issues relate to the increased complexity of care of the elderly patient on a mechanical ventilator. The elderly patient is at increased risk of nosocomial pneumonia directly related to mechanical ventilation. Ventilator associated pneumonia (VAP) is a bacterial pneumonia that occurs in patients on a ventilator for greater than 48 hours, and is thought to be due to migration of oral pathogens into the lungs. VAP prevention guidelines are commonly implemented to avoid complications and associated increased morbidity and mortality (CDC, 2003a). Nursing care of the mechanically ventilated patient to prevent VAP includes keeping the HOB elevated greater than 30 degrees, providing frequent oral care, maintaining adequate cuff pressure, assessing the need for ulcer prophylaxis, and turning the patient frequently (Balas et al., 2008).

Changes in respiratory structure and function occur with aging, and should be considered when older patients are placed on a mechanical ventilator. The older patient may experience greater difficulty weaning from a ventilator, due to poor respiratory muscle function, altered respiratory mechanics, as well as altered hemodynamics. Nurses monitor for signs of respiratory muscle fatigue (e.g., rapid shallow breathing, accessory muscle use, diaphoresis, and restlessness) with increased vigilance, when attempts are made to wean an older patient from a ventilator in the high-acuity area.

SECTION THREE REVIEW

1. Which description of the heart best describes the changes that occur related to aging?
   - **A.** loss of elastic tissue and replacement of cardiac muscle by fat.
   - **B.** loss of collagen with ventricular hypertrophy.
   - **C.** increased ventricular compliance with increased systolic blood pressure.
   - **D.** increased valve flexibility resulting in heart murmurs.
2. The atypical presentation of some older patients experiencing an acute myocardial ischemia/infarction may include which manifestations? (choose all that apply)
   - **A.** hypothermia
   - **B.** falls
   - **C.** flu-like syndromes
   - **D.** higher than usual elevations of creatine kinase
   - **E.** acute confusion
3. When monitoring the hemodynamic status of the older patient, the nurse needs to be aware that higher filling pressures are needed to maintain normal stroke volume and cardiac output.
   - **A.** True
   - **B.** False
4. In the older patient, there is an increased risk for development of pulmonary infections for which reason?
   - **A.** increased lung elasticity
   - **B.** increased alveolar surface area
   - **C.** decreased chest anteroposterior (AP) diameter
   - **D.** loss of pulmonary epithelial cells
5. When caring for the older patient, which intervention(s) needs to be focused on for prevention of airway clearance and gas exchange complications?
   - **A.** deep breathing and coughing exercises
   - **B.** high fluid intake
   - **C.** monitoring of respiratory rate and depth
   - **D.** assessing for adventitious breath sounds
6. In mechanically ventilated older patients, weaning is often more difficult for which major reason? (choose all that apply)
   - **A.** weak respiratory muscle function.
   - **B.** confused mental state makes weaning procedures more difficult.
   - **C.** altered respiratory mechanics
   - **D.** changes in hemodynamics

Answers: 1. A, 2. (B, C, E), 3. A, 4. D, 5. A, 6. (A, C)

SECTION FOUR: The Changing Older Adult: Integumentary and Musculoskeletal Systems

At the completion of this section, the learner will be able to discuss the age-related changes in integumentary and musculoskeletal function.

Integumentary

The continuous aging process is manifested in the changes in the appearance and function of the skin. Common cosmetic changes such as wrinkling and sagging are due to a loss of elasticity of connective tissues as well as environmental influences. There is a loss of skin turgor, and because of loss of subcutaneous tissue, fragility of capillaries, flattening of the capillary bed, and frequent aspirin or blood thinner use, older adults are prone to ecchymosis; so skin becomes more transparent and underlying veins are more visible. Because skin pigmentation declines, pallor is a less reliable sign of anemia or illness.

Lean body mass in muscle tissue is lost. The proportion of body fat increases as the proportion of body weight contributed by intracellular body water decreases (Hooyman & Kiyak, 2008). There is a loss of dermal and epidermal thickness, skin becomes thin, and is more prone to skin breakdown and injury (Fletcher, 2007). Untreated skin problems can lead to discomfort, systemic infection, or functional impairments. The number and efficiency of sweat glands decreases with aging, predisposing the patient to hypothermia, and hyperthermia, as well as fluid and electrolyte imbalances (Linton, 2007a). Table 3–3 provides a summary of the age-related changes in the integumentary system and their physiologic effects.

TABLE 3–3 Physiologic Changes of Aging: Integumentary and Musculoskeletal Systems

AGE RELATED CHANGES	PHYSIOLOGIC EFFECTS
Integumentary	
Loss of dermal and epidermal thickness	Paper-thin skin prone to breakdown and injury Decreased sweating, altered thermoregulation
Atrophy of sweat glands	Dryness
Decreased vascularity of skin	Increased wrinkling
Decreased elasticity	Reduced insulation
Loss of subcutaneous tissue and fat	Slower wound healing Increase vulnerability to hypo and hyperthermia
Musculoskeletal	
Decreased lean body mass	Decreased muscle strength and exercise tolerance
Increased fat content	
Deterioration of joint cartilage	Pain and decreased mobility of skeletal joints
Compression of spinal column	Predisposed to osteoporosis, loss of height
Bone demineralization	Susceptible to bone fractures Predisposed to osteoarthritis

Data from Fletcher (2007), Hooyman & Kiyak (2008), and Linton & Lach (2007).

Nursing Implications for Integumentary Changes

Nurses should complete a thorough skin assessment to monitor for changes in skin integrity. Skin disorders are common in the elderly. It is important to identify potentially life-threatening rashes as well as cellulitis. Rashes may be a side effect of a medication, and cellulitis may be due to a contamination of the deep layer of skin. An existing break in the skin allows bacteria to travel through the lymphatic system, where it can spread to deeper tissues or the bloodstream. Skin assessment can also provide information regarding blood supply and venous drainage.

Because the skin of an older adult is thin and fragile, the elderly are at risk for skin breakdown. Comorbidities and immobility contribute to the problem. Compression of soft tissues under bony prominences, friction, and shearing, can lead to tissue ischemia. Prevention and treatment of pressure ulcers is an important aspect of nursing care for vulnerable older adults. The development of a pressure ulcer can cause significant delays in recovery, prolong hospitalization, and greatly impact quality of life. Routine turning and repositioning is essential. Although a common position for an adult in the high-acuity setting, nurses should understand that when a patient is lying on his or her back with the head of the bed (HOB) elevated, there is increased weight placed on the coccyx. Additionally, if the patient slides down in bed, repositioning is required, which often involves friction and shearing forces on the skin. As little as a few hours on a backboard for an older trauma patient, or a few hours on an operating room table may alter skin integrity. Evidence suggests that the most important strategies to prevent pressure ulcers include using support surfaces, repositioning the patient frequently, optimizing nutritional status, and moisturizing sacral skin (Reddy, Gill & Rochon, 2006).

Because of age-related skin changes, older adults can have difficulty with thermoregulation. Nursing care incorporates methods to prevent heat loss by monitoring room temperature, keeping the patient covered while bathing, and using warmed blankets when necessary. Nursing care of IV sites includes close monitoring for infiltrations, the use of non-restrictive dressings and paper tape to promote skin integrity. When patients are at a high risk for altered skin integrity, specialty beds with pressure reducing surfaces may be warranted.

Musculoskeletal

Decreased muscle mass, bone demineralization, increased joint stiffness, and decreased joint mobility are common musculoskeletal issues in the older adult. In addition, decreased muscle strength is common with loss of selected muscle fibers, including the respiratory muscles. Numerous age-related changes in other subsystems, such as reductions in neuron-muscular innervation, insulin activity, estrogen, testosterone and growth hormone levels, as well as weight loss, protein deficiency, and physical inactivity, can contribute to loss of muscle mass and strength (Smith & Cotter, 2008).

Assessment of the musculoskeletal system must include data from patient history, such as the presence of osteoporosis, osteomalacia, or osteoarthritis. These conditions can contribute to potential complications such as fractures and falls and have implications for patient mobility, which may require adaptations in patient care. Primary osteoporosis is a common result of aging, independent of disease and medication use, while secondary osteoporosis is caused by a disease process or medication (Nyhart, 2007). Prevention of osteoporosis is accomplished through adequate intake of calcium, vitamins, smoking cessation and, most importantly, physical exercise.

Osteoarthritis is the most common arthritic condition among older adults, and affects 12.1 percent of U.S. adults (Nakasato, 2007). Interestingly, the pathophysiology of osteoarthritis is not directly related to the aging process, and predisposing factors include obesity, female sex, quadriceps weakness, major joint injury, poor proprioception, heavy physical activity, and genetics (Nakasato, 2007). Osteoarthritis is a dysfunction disorder in which cartilage between joints becomes irregular, and eventually is diminished. Pain and loss of function are complications. Many patients with osteoarthritis are prescribed non-steroidal anti-inflammatory medications (NSAIDs), which put them at risk for peptic ulcer disease and other complications, particularly if they have other comorbidities or are taking anticoagulants as well (Nakasato, 2007), and are poorly tolerated by older patients.

Many conditions, such as degenerative stenosis (narrowing of the spinal canal), thinning of the cartilage between the vertebrae, and development of bone spurs around the vertebrae, lead to compression of the spinal column or the spinal nerves, and result in a variety of symptoms, including pain and deformity. Spinal fractures are more common in older adults. Refer to Table 3–3 for a summary of the age–related musculoskeletal changes and their physiologic effects.

Nursing Implications for Musculoskelatal Changes

The presence of degenerative arthritis and other musculoskeletal alterations has important implications for the care of patient in high-acuity settings. Posture, gait, balance, symmetry of body parts, and alignment of extremities may be altered (Smith & Cotter, 2008). The threat to mobility is the most important challenge as patients suffer from weakness and joint related pain, which may be chronic and imposes limitations on comfort, recovery, and physical therapy. Fractures are more common, particularly the pelvis and femur which can be associated with significant blood loss.

SECTION FOUR REVIEW

1. The older patient is more susceptible to skin breakdown for which reasons? (choose all that apply)
   A. thinning of the skin
   B. increased subcutaneous tissue
   C. loss of elasticity
   D. flattening of capillary beds
2. When caring for the older patient, which common nursing intervention is most likely to result in skin breakdown?
   A. elevate head of bed 30 degrees.
   B. turn every two hours.
   C. use support surfaces
   D. moisturize sacral skin
3. When gathering a nursing history on an older patient, what information, if stated by the patient, would indicate an increased risk for upper GI bleeding?
   A. "I have been under intense stress lately."
   B. "I take my prescription non-steroidal anti-inflammatory drug daily."
   C. "I stopped taking my calcium supplement because it was difficult to swallow."
   D. "I drink about four cups of coffee each day."
4. Fractures of the pelvis and femur are common in older patients and associated with mild-to-moderate blood loss.
   A. True
   B. False
5. Which musculoskeletal condition is the most prevalent in the older adult?
   A. gout
   B. rheumatoid arthritis
   C. osteoarthritis
   D. fractures

Answers: 1. (A, C, D), 2. A, 3. B, 4. B, 5. C

SECTION FIVE: The Changing Older Adult: The Gastrointestinal and Genitourinary Systems

At the completion of this section, the learner will be able to describe age-related changes in gastrointestinal and genitourinary function.

Gastrointestinal (GI) System

Physiologic changes in the GI system include changes in the oral cavity, esophagus, stomach, small and large intestine, pancreas, and liver. Oral cavity changes that affect the teeth include wearing of tooth surfaces, thinning of enamel, cracking of teeth, tooth loss, and periodontal disease, all of which can affect appearance, swallowing, nutrition, and quality of life. Oral tissues become more fragile and salivary production may be altered due to drug side effects, disease states, or altered nutrition. Other possible conditions include osteoporosis or atrophy of the jaw bone. Changes in the motility of the esophagus and esophageal sphincter function have not been found to be normal age-related changes, and therefore patients having difficulty swallowing or experiencing significant problems with reflux, should be referred for further evaluation. However, a higher prevalence of neurological diseases in older people may contribute to altered esophageal motility (Linton, 2007b).

In the stomach, the secretion of digestive juices is diminished. Also, gastric acidity decreases, possibly due to chronic infection with *Helicobacter pylori*, which gradually destroys the secretory glands and parietal cells that produce gastric acids. The reduced acidity of the gastric pH increases the risk for growth of bacteria in the stomach, which increases the risk of aspiration pneumonia in the older high-acuity patient. The absorptive capacity of cells of the small intestine is altered and impacts the absorption of vitamins and minerals. Changes in the large intestine include histological changes in the colon that contribute to muscle atrophy, slower transit rate, diminished sphincter tone, and diminished compliance of the rectum. The exocrine function of the pancreas is decreased and has important implications for the patient in the high-acuity setting. Blood flow to the liver is reduced, hepatocyte number is decreased, and hepatic regeneration is reduced. Although the liver has many functions, the most important age-related change in liver function is the decrease in the capacity to metabolize drugs. Table 3–4 provides a summary of age-related gastrointestinal changes and their physiologic effects.

TABLE 3–4 Physiologic Changes of Aging: Gastrointestinal and Genitourinary Systems

AGE-RELATED CHANGES	PHYSIOLOGIC EFFECTS
Gastrointestinal	
Atrophy of salivary glands, taste buds	Dry membranes become prone to injury
Decreased ability to swallow	Decreased thirst sensation
Decreased gastric acid secretions	Change in nutritional intake
Delay in esophageal emptying, altered esophageal sphincter function	Delay in vitamin and drug absorption Predisposed to indigestion, aspiration
Decreased GI muscle tone, decreased stool transit time	Altered motility
Decreased calcium absorption	Predisposed to constipation, altered bowel habits
Decreased basal metabolic rate	Altered bone formation
Decrease size and blood flow to liver	Altered calorie utilization Decreased liver storage capacity increases vulnerability to toxins, adverse drug reactions
Renal/Genitourinary	
Loss of number and function of nephrons	Decreased ability to concentrate and conserve water
Decreased glomerular filtration rate	Decreased secretion of sodium, water, urea, ammonia, and drugs
Decreased kidney efficiency	Predisposed to dehydration, hypernatremia, fluid overload, medication reactions
Decreased intracellular body water	Increased residual urine, nocturnal urination
Reduced bladder tone, capacity	Risk for incontinence

Data from Fletcher (2007), Hooyman & Kiyak (2008), and Linton & Lach (2007).

Nursing Implications for Gastrointestinal Changes: Nutrition

Because of age-related GI alterations, digestion may be affected and has important consequences for the nutritional status of an elderly patient. Because jaw bone changes and tooth loss affects chewing, nurses should assess this important foundation to healthy dietary intake. A thorough assessment includes a history of oral hygiene, diet, altered sensory perception, as well as elimination habits. Symptoms of concern that relate to the health of the GI system and that can impact nutritional status include pain, dysphagia, dyspepsia, nausea, vomiting, anorexia, weight loss, changes in stool characteristics, and gastrointestinal bleeding. Nurses should encourage adequate hydration, advocate for early enteral/parenteral nutrition, and monitor for delayed gastric emptying, and signs of fecal impaction (Balas et al., 2008).

There is increased incidence of gastric ulcer development in older adults when compared with younger adults. Older adults are at greater risk for stomach and colon cancer (Hooyman & Kiyak, 2008). Medications that may affect the GI system include anticholinergics, laxatives, calcium channel blockers, aspirin and other NSAIDs, antacids, opioids, and antiemetics. Past problems of note include a history of surgical procedures involving the GI tract, GERD, peptic ulcer disease, cancer, hepatitis, gallstones, and diabetes mellitus (Linton, 2007b). Nurses can advocate for stress ulcer prophylaxis and monitor for signs of bleeding. Rectal tubes should be avoided (Balas et al., 2008).

Constipation is a significant concern in the older adult population. Many factors contribute to constipation, and include: sedentary life style, poor diet, dehydration, systemic illness, and medications (Rosenthal & Kavic, 2004). Nurses can assure steps are taken to promote bowel function during times of immobility.

Genitourinary (GU)

Changes that affect the kidneys, ureters, urinary bladder, urethra, and prostate, can impact the function of the genitourinary system. As an individual ages, renal blood flow decreases by 50 percent due to atrophy of the efferent and afferent arterioles, sclerotic glomeruli, and a decrease in number and size of nephrons. These changes will lead to a decline in glomerular filtration rate, and a decrease in creatinine clearance. As renal tubular function declines, the ability to conserve sodium and excrete hydrogen ions is diminished, which affects the ability to regulate fluid and acid-base balance (Rosenthal & Kavic, 2004). The ureters are vulnerable to reflux of the vesicoureteral junction, leading to reflux of urine. In the bladder, muscles weaken which may lead to incomplete emptying, while collagen content increases limiting distensibility. Bladder capacity decreases and frequency of urination increases.

Decreased circulating levels of estrogen and decreased tissue responsiveness to estrogen cause changes in the urethral sphincter in women, and prostatic hypertrophy in men, contributing to delayed bladder emptying and urinary incontinence. Problems in the urination process may be due to altered sphincter muscles, neural controls, outlet size, muscle strength, obstruction, or sensation of the need to void (Linton, 2007c). A number of variables, such as increased prevalence of atherosclerosis, hypertension, heart failure, diabetes, infection, and exposure to nephrotoxins, can contribute to altered genitourinary function in the older adult. Refer to Table 3–4 for a summary of the age-related genitourinary changes and their physiologic effects.

Nursing Implications for Genitourinary Changes

Nursing implications for GU changes are numerous and include fluid balance, renal failure, urinary tract infections (UTIs) incontinence, and sexual dysfunction. Multiple factors contribute to increased vulnerability to fluid and electrolyte imbalances in the older adult, including decreased urine concentrating ability, limitations in excretion of water, sodium, potassium, and hydrogen ions as well as the GU system's declining ability to compensate. The kidneys have a decreased ability to absorb glucose which contributes to problems of dehydration and hyponatremia (Hooyman & Kiyak, 2008).

Urinary tract infections are responsible for most community-acquired cases of **bacteremia**; and in the hospital, UTIs are attributed to the presence of indwelling catheters. Assessment for urinary tract infections is an important nursing task, as often symptoms are not apparent. The older adult patient may present with atypical manifestations of UTI, such as mental changes, confusion, nausea and vomiting, or abdominal pain rather than the classic symptoms of frequency, urgency, dysuria, and suprapubic or flank pain. This can result in delay in diagnosis of urinary tract infection in this patient population. Because of the many confounding comorbidities associated with alterations in GU function, renal disease may be overlooked. Nurses should perform routine assessments of hemoglobin, hematocrit, BUN, serum creatinine, urine albumin, glucose, pH, microscopic examination of urinary sediment, and screening for bacteruria. A history of medications as well as urinary symptoms, such as nocturia, dysuria, frequency, urgency, and incontinence should be considered (Linton, 2007b).

SECTION FIVE REVIEW

1. In the older adult high-acuity patient, altered gastric pH increases the risk for development of which complication?
   - A. gastric ulcers
   - B. hepatitis
   - C. gastric cancer
   - D. pneumonia
2. The urinary system in the older adult alters in which of the following ways?
   - A. decreased glomerular filtration rate
   - B. increased size of nephrons
   - C. decreased ureter lumen size
   - D. increased creatinine clearance
3. A physiologic alteration in the kidneys of older adults that contributes to problems of dehydration and hyponatremia is
   - A. altered neural controls
   - B. changes in the urethral sphincter
   - C. declining renal tubule function
   - D. increased concentration of urine
4. The atypical presentation of urinary tract infection often seen in the older adult patient includes (choose all that apply)
   - A. confusion
   - B. high fever
   - C. nausea and vomiting
   - D. abdominal pain

Answers: 1. D, 2. A, 3. C, 4. (A, C, D)

SECTION SIX: The Changing Adult: The Endocrine And Immune Systems

At the completion of this section, the learner will be able to explain age-related changes in endocrine and immune function.

Endocrine System

Age-related changes in the endocrine system contribute to menopause as well as altered metabolism of glucose and thyroid dysfunction. There is a decreased production of estrogen and progesterone, as well as testosterone, thyroid hormones, growth hormones, and insulin (Hooyman & Kiyak, 2008). The pancreas secretes less insulin and there is an increase in insulin resistance, which results in a decreased ability to metabolize glucose. There is an increase in the prevalence of diabetes mellitus (DM) with approximately 38 percent of the population with diabetes aged 65 years and older (CDC, 2007a). As the aging body uses less thyroid

TABLE 3–5 Physiologic Changes of Aging: Endocrine and Immune Systems

AGE-RELATED CHANGES	PHYSIOLOGIC EFFECTS
Endocrine	
Decreased production of estrogen, progesterone, testosterone, thyroid, growth hormone, and insulin	Increased insulin resistance Decreased glucose metabolism Increased blood sugar levels Hypothyroidism Decreased basal metabolic rate
Immune System	
Changes in cell-mediated immunity, decreased T-cell function	Delayed hypersensitivity reactions
Decreased production of lymphocytes	Increased susceptibility to infections
Decrease in CD3, CD4, CD8, CD28	Reactivation of latent infections
Impaired humoral immune and antibody responses, decreased production of B cells by bone marrow	Slower and less efficient antibody production
Appearance of autoantibodies	Increased prevalence of autoimmune disorders

Data from Fletcher (2007), Hooyman & Kiyak (2008), and Linton & Lach (2007).

hormone and the thyroid gland atrophies, the result is a decrease in T4 production and an increased risk for hypothyroidism. TSH values may be elevated in the older adult, although the significance is debated (Campbell, 2007). Basal metabolic rates decrease. Table 3–5 provides a summary of age-related endocrine changes and their physiologic effects.

Nursing Implications for Endocrine Changes

Nurses should monitor blood glucose carefully in the older patient with special attention to patients with diabetes. Illness, medications, and nutritional alterations influence glucose metabolism. The assessment of the older adult with diabetes includes a review of macrovascular, microvascular, and retinal complications (Margolis & Reed, 2007). Macrovascular complications of coronary, carotid, and peripheral atherosclerosis prompt symptoms such as transient neurological symptoms, syncope, chest pain, exertional dyspnea or fatigue, and claudication. Older adults with diabetes are particularly vulnerable to foot complications and foot ulcers, therefore foot assessment and care requires attention in the high-acuity area. A comprehensive approach to the care of the older adult with diabetes includes the involvement of a certified diabetic educator, pharmacist, and dietician who can instruct patients about nutrition, glucose monitoring, and recognition and prevention of hypoglycemia (Ham et al., 2007).

Thyroid dysfunction as well as lipid abnormalities may be related to depression in the older adult. Hypothyroidism is associated with a slowing of mental and physical function, intolerance to cold, weight gain, constipation, alterations in blood pressure, and anemia (Campbell, 2007). Hyperthyroidism may be associated with irregular heart rhythms (tachycardia and atrial fibrillation), congestive heart failure, weight loss, fatigue, and muscular weakness. Because these conditions often overlap with other clinical syndromes, thyroid conditions are often undiagnosed. Thyroid storm is a dangerous complication of hyperthyroidism and is related to an increased risk of death due to the associated fever, tachycardia, nausea, vomiting, mental status changes, and heart complications (Campbell, 2007).

Immune System

The immune system of an older person is more vulnerable, and careful attention to basic infection control measures should be adhered to. Cell-mediated immunity declines with aging and T-cell function decreases. Humoral-mediated immunity and antibody responses are impaired (Hooyman & Kiyak, 2008). Numerous age-related physiologic changes exist that also predispose an older adult to infection (see Table 3–6). Infection may present itself atypically in an older person. Because elderly patients have a lower basal temperature, fever (normally an early sign of infection) may be absent. The nurse must assess infection by carefully examining sputum, urine, and wounds for color and texture changes. Changes in mental status, functional decline, hypothermia, unexplained hypo- or hyperglycemia, acidosis, tachycardia, and even falls could be related to an infectious process, and should be considered.

Pneumonia and influenza remain among the top ten causes of death for older adults (CDC, 2006). Because infection is difficult to treat in the elderly, and is associated with increased morbidity and mortality, it is important to prevent infection through administration of immunizations. Table 3–7 reviews guidelines for immunizations for older adults.

TABLE 3–6 Age-Related Changes that Predispose to Infection

- Urinary retention
- Prostatic hypertrophy
- Decreased bladder tone
- Delayed gastric emptying
- Decreased cough strength
- Reduced ciliary action
- Flattened diaphragm
- Reduced muscle mass
- Stiffened thoracic cage
- Decreased skin elasticity
- Increased insulin resistance
- Decreased insulin secretion
- Decreased serum albumin (depending on nutritional state)

TABLE 3–7 Guidelines for Immunizations for Older Adults

IMMUNIZATION	OLDER ADULT INDICATIONS	FREQUENCY
Influenza	Age 50 years and older Long-term care residents Chronic medical diseases Health care workers	Annually, preferably between September and November (Can be given as late as January)
Pneumonia	Age 65 years and older Certain chronic health problems Altered immune function Alaskan Native or certain Native American populations	Once in a lifetime. Certain individuals require a booster 5 years after the initial dose: ▪ age 65 and older who received the vaccine before age 65 ▪ post transplant ▪ chronic kidney disease ▪ altered immune system
Tetanus toxoid booster	A booster dose of tetanus and diphtheria toxoid-containing vaccine should be administered to adults who have completed a primary series and if the last vaccination was received more than 10 years previously.	Every 10 years.

Data from CDC (2008).

Nursing Implications for Immunologic Changes: Infection and Sepsis

Nurses must anticipate patients at high risk for infection and assess them appropriately. Nurses consider preexisting illnesses, recent history of diagnostic tests involving invasive or indwelling lines, and implement careful monitoring of clinical signs. Because homeostasis is altered in an older adult during illness, the ability to generate a fever may be diminished. Breath sound assessment and monitoring of oxygen status is vital to identifying pneumonia early. A vaccination history is important to obtain since influenza and pneumococcal vaccines decrease the risk for pneumonia.

The presence of bacteremia (bacteria in the blood) increases the vulnerability for the development of **sepsis**, a syndrome characterized by a systemic inflammatory response (SIRS), to infection, which can further deteriorate to **severe sepsis** and **septic shock**. The incidence of SIRS in older adults is significant. Up to 60 percent of those who develop sepsis in the United States are 65 years or older (Girard, Opal & Ely, 2005). Older adults are vulnerable from bacteremia to sepsis. Important risk factors include short and long-term institutionalization, pressure sores, methicillin-resistant *S. aureus*, MRSA, bacteremia hospitalization in the last six months, antimicrobial use in the past three months, and indwelling catheters (Girard & Ely, 2007).

Because older patients do not exhibit the typical clinical manifestations of infection, the diagnosis may be delayed. Symptoms such as altered mental status (delirium, somnolence, and coma), tachypnea, anorexia, malaise, generalized weakness, falls, and urinary incontinence may be nonspecific expressions of infections in older adults (Girard & Ely, 2007). Practice guidelines have been developed that outline the recommendations for treating patients with severe sepsis, and recent evidence indicates that older adults may respond well to treatment when interventions are implemented in a timely manner (Dellinger, et al., 2008).

SECTION SIX REVIEW

1. Age-related changes in the thyroid gland increases the risk for development of which thyroid-related problem in the older patient?
   A. hyperthyroidism
   B. thyrotoxic storm
   C. hypothyroidism
   D. elevated basal metabolic rate
2. In the older patient, there is decreased ability to metabolize glucose caused by decreased insulin secretion and increased insulin resistance.
   A. True
   B. False
3. The nurse caring for an older patient would be suspicious of possible hypothyroidism if the patient developed which manifestation?
   A. intolerance to heat
   B. slowing of mental functions
   C. unexplained weight loss
   D. tachycardia and elevated blood pressure
4. Atypical signs of infection that may be present in older patients include (choose all that apply)
   A. metabolic alkalosis
   B. functional decline
   C. altered mental status
   D. unexplained hypo- or hyperglycemia
5. The older patient may not develop a fever as an early sign of infection due to
   A. lower basal temperature
   B. hyperthyroidism
   C. elevated humoral immune function
   D. increased circulating T-lymphocytes
6. Risk factors for development of sepsis in older patients include (choose all that apply)
   A. institutionalization
   B. pressure sores
   C. altered mental status
   D. indwelling urinary catheters

Answers: 1. C, 2. A, 3. B, 4. (B, C, D), 5. A, 6. (A, B, D)

SECTION SEVEN: Cognitive Conditions Impacting Hospitalization: Dementia, Delirium, and Depression

At the completion of this section, the learner will be able to differentiate between dementia, delirium and depression and describe their impact on high-acuity patients and their families.

The older adult is at high risk for three overlapping geriatric syndromes that can impact their hospital course: dementia, depression, and delirium. Often called the "3 Ds," these are common and often missed by health professionals or mistaken for one another. Table 3–8 provides key features of each. An important consideration for the nurse is to recognize that loss of memory, confusion, and low mood are *not* a normal part of aging. The normal older adult retains memory and thinking abilities throughout life! So when the older patient exhibits these symptoms, a thorough evaluation and appropriate treatments are in order. The nurse needs to be on the lookout for any changes in orientation, mood or thinking ability, and closely monitor the patient with these problems as they are very high risk for complications and safety problems in the hospital. There can be added a fourth "D" to this rubric, namely, **functional decline**. This fourth "D" is another common geriatric problem.

Dementia

Dementia is the term for the symptom of cognitive impairment seen in people with Alzheimer's disease or other conditions that cause loss of memory and thinking ability. Alzheimer's disease is responsible for the largest percentage of dementia in older adults and will be described in more detail, but Lewy body disease, vascular dementia, or small strokes are other causes. In a small percentage of people, dementia has a reversible cause such as hypothyroidism, B12 deficiency, depression, or delirium. Currently 5.2 million people have Alzheimer's disease, and since the rate increases with age (to 25 percent in people over 85), this number may more than triple by the year 2050 (Alzheimer's Association, 2008).

Alzheimer's disease causes progressive and irreversible brain damage, characterized by amyloid plaques and neurofibrillary tangles in the brain (NIA, 2007). While the mechanisms are not completely clear, damage occurs slowly, and symptoms may take years to develop. The individual gradually loses ability to make decisions, to complete self-care activities, and to communicate. In the late stages the individual may be bedridden and need complete care. Often a diagnosis is not made until problems with memory and thinking affect the older person's ability to function in daily life. This means that patients with dementia may be admitted to the hospital without a diagnosis. The nurse may be the first to recognize the problem, so it is important to communicate findings to other health professionals. Red flags the nurse might notice include poor recall of information the patient is expected to know, disorientation, failing to follow instructions, or difficulty finding the right words or completing sentences (Maslow & Mezey, 2008).

In the past, little could be done to address memory loss from Alzheimer's disease or other causes, and still no cure is available. However, current treatments can improve symptoms and slow the progression of the disease, so early diagnosis and treatment has become valuable (NIA, 2007). More important, when a dementia is determined, patients and families can begin to deal with the problem, learn how to help their loved one, and get referrals for help to organizations such as the Alzheimer's Association. For the hospitalized patient, recognizing the problem can help the nurse plan care to keep the patient safe and avoid problems such as agitation, falls and other adverse

TABLE 3–8 Differentiating Dementia, Depression, and Delirium

	DEMENTIA	DEPRESSION	DELIRIUM
Onset	Gradual, months to years	Weeks, may have past history	Sudden, hours-to-days with fluctuating course
Memory	Poor, worse for recent events	Poor, inability to concentrate	Poor, inattention
Thought	Disoriented, unable to understand complicated information	Apathy or lack of motivation, disoriented	Disoriented, unable to concentrate, may have hallucinations or illusions
Mood/speech	Repeats, often socially appropriate until later stages	Low mood, quiet or verbalizes negative thoughts	May be incoherent
Behavior	Usually appropriate until stress threshold is surpassed, then may exhibit agitation and increased confusion	Usually appropriate but slow, less often agitation	Can be hyperactive and agitated, but some are hypoactive and less obvious, disturbed sleep
Nursing care approaches	Report memory problems and Mini-Cog score Give frequent gentle reminders and reassurance Avoid overstimulation Provide opportunity for rest, sleep, and quiet time Treat discomfort which is often the cause of agitation	Report low mood and score on the GDS Provide support and encouragement Encourage family involvement in care to extent possible	Report changes in mental status on evaluation and CAM score Avoid over-medication e.g. benzodiazepines Use similar approaches to those for patients with dementia

GDS=Geriatric Depression Scale; CAM=Confusion Assessment Method.

events. Importantly, people with dementia are at high risk to develop delirium, an acute emergent condition.

Delirium

Delirium, sometimes called acute confusion, is the rapid onset of problems with cognition, characterized by fluctuating symptoms of inattention and confusion. Delirium is caused by an insult to the brain as a result of acute illness. This may occur in the healthy older adult after a major injury or illness, but in the older adult who is frail, has underlying chronic illnesses, or who has a dementia, even a minor illness can precipitate delirium. Delirium often indicates a change in status, and may be the first sign of a complication such as infection, bladder distention, or drug toxicity. Studies suggest that delirium develops in 11 to 42 percent of older people in the hospital overall, and up to half of postoperative older patients (Young & Inouye, 2007). Delirium increases the risk of long length of stay, readmission, nursing home placement, and even death. The good news is that delirium can be prevented in up to one third of patients (Young & Inouye, 2007) and many times delirium is reversible. Identifying and treating the problem can improve outcomes for older patients.

The older adult with delirium can have many symptoms, ranging from lethargy and inattentiveness to agitation, restlessness and even combativeness, making detection confusing. Nurses readily identify those patients with "hyperactive" symptoms because their behavior is noticeable. However, those with hypoactive delirium may not be noticed and/or considered either depressed or sedated. This "quiet" delirium seems to be more common in the older patients, but can be detected with routine assessment and monitoring (Peterson et al., 2006).

The key to management of delirium is to identify potential causes and try to remove or minimize them (see Table 3–9). Just some of the potential causes are infection, pain, fever, sleep disturbance, immobility, sensory disturbance (missing glasses or hearing aids), hypoxia, and dehydration (Young & Inouye, 2007). Medications are a common cause of delirium and challenging to resolve. For example, pain medication can induce delirium but so can untreated pain (see Section Four of this module for discussion of medications for pain). Other frequently used problem drugs are benzodiazepines and those with anticholinergic effects. Nurses should be diligent in trying to uncover the cause of a delirium and eliminating or preventing the causes when possible.

Depression

Depression is the third cognitive problem and another common illness in the older adult, characterized by low mood. In the older adult, depression can be a lifelong problem, the result of losses common in this age group (retirement, widowhood, social isolation), chronic stress, or related to illness. Depression is found in 8 to 20 percent of community-dwelling older adults (CDC, 2007b) and rates are higher among those in institutional settings. Depression has a significant impact on the older adult's life and can be a life-threatening condition. The highest rate of suicide of any age group is among older men.

The patient with depression may have difficulty sleeping, poor appetite, or feelings of hopelessness. Other common symptoms are apathy, difficulty concentrating, and low self-esteem. Older adults also may present with physical symptoms such as aches and pains. Diagnosis is based on the presence of persistent symptoms that are not related to a recent loss and is very common in older people with conditions causing pain or disabling conditions.

While depression may not be addressed when the patient is in the high-acuity state, the nurse should be aware of low mood or changes in mood and report concerns. For example,

TABLE 3–9 Strategies for Preventing and Managing Delirium

COMMON CAUSES	INTERVENTION
Immobility	Early mobilization and active range of motion, minimize equipment and restraints limiting mobility.
Sensory reduction	Provide glasses and hearing aids, regular communication to promote orientation, speak loudly and clearly, encourage family visits.
Metabolic disorders (hypoxia, hypercapnia, hyperglycemia, hypoglycemia, hyponatremia)	Address imbalances and monitor status.
Nutritional deficits	Monitor laboratory tests (albumin, pre-albumin) and provide enteral or parenteral nutrition as needed.
Sleep disturbance, noise	Promote a comfortable environment modifying the light, room temperature, reduce noise or provide white noise or comforting sounds.
Alcohol or drug intoxication	Identify admitting drug problems. Avoid drugs that affect CNS, particularly benzodiazepines and anticholinergic drugs, diphenhydramine, meperidine. Note: Use only low doses of antipsychotics when needed to manage severe symptoms of hallucinations or extreme agitation; use sparingly.
Dehydration, hypovolemia	Monitor fluid status and replace lost fluids.
Bowel/bladder problems	Monitor bowel and bladder function, particularly for constipation or bladder distention.

an exacerbation of depression may be triggered by withdrawal from treatment with hospitalization or acute illness. A depression can also be triggered by severe illness, such as stroke. Once the patient is stabilized, treatment of depression can be addressed.

Depression can become more important later by delaying recovery from illness, and studies have shown worse outcomes for patients with depression (CDC, 2007b). Depression is very treatable in the older adult and the newer medications produce few side effects making them safe to use in this age group. Treatment should be initiated when the patient is stabilized. Long-term treatment should include socialization, and it should be noted that counseling is very effective in this age group (Kurlowicz & Harvath, 2008).

Too often, geriatric patients admitted to hospitals experience a significant decline in function, or loss of the ability to perform activities of daily living. Factors associated with functional decline include preexisting chronic illness, delirium, immobility, malnutrition, depression, and uncontrolled pain. In the ICU, sleep deprivation may accelerate decline. In the community setting, alcoholism and substance abuse can cause severe functional decline. Health promotion activities can help to prevent functional decline in the elderly. Scientific evidence supports the fact that functional disability is not caused by aging, per se, but results from illnesses and diseases that are related to unhealthy lifestyle decisions (Criddle, 2009). This creates an opportunity for nurses to improve the quality of life for the elderly client through evidence-based health promotion activities.

SECTION SEVEN REVIEW

1. Alzheimer's disease is
   - **A.** an acute problem with memory and thinking
   - **B.** the most common cause of dementia
   - **C.** the result of brain inflammation
   - **D.** part of Lewy Body Disease
2. The following are interventions to prevent delirium (choose all that apply)
   - **A.** help the patient get adequate sleep
   - **B.** early mobilization
   - **C.** identify and treat hypoxia
   - **D.** administer pain medications
3. Depression is difficult to treat in the older patient
   - **A.** True
   - **B.** False

Answers: 1. B, 2. (A, B, C, D), 3. B

SECTION EIGHT: Factors Impacting Hospitalization: Functional Decline, Pain, and Pharmacotherapy

At the completion of this section, the learner will be able to discuss functional decline, pain, and pharmacology as factors that impact hospitalization in the older patient.

Functional Decline

Older adults are at high risk for developing problems with their functional ability during hospitalization (Graf, 2006). Many older adults already have difficulty with self-care activities due to chronic disease, pain, injury, or experience muscle weakness from being out of shape. In geriatrics, the key functional abilities to examine are activities of daily living (ADLs: bathing, dressing, eating, mobility, toileting) and instrumental activities of daily living (IADLs: cooking, housekeeping, laundry, transportation, telephone use, medication management, and finances). The patient's ability to live alone and their options for placement after hospitalization are based on what they can do for themselves and what help they can get from family or paid assistance.

Functional issues are typically not of immediate concern when the patient is severely ill. But the nurse needs to keep in mind that older adults lose strength and functional ability quickly from illness and immobility. For example, nearly 5 percent of muscle strength is lost with each day of bedrest, leading older adults to experience what has long been called the "cascade to dependence" (Creditor, 1993; Criddle, 2009). During hospitalization, many older patients have a decrease in ability to care for themselves; some *never* return to their pre-hospital level of functioning after acute illness (Graf, 2006). Nearly 15 percent of older adults over 75 are discharged to a skilled nursing facility, many to regain strength and function so they can return home (Criddle, 2009).

In the high-acuity setting, the nurse should pay attention to early mobilization of patients by getting them up and moving as quickly as possible. Range of motion is critical. When the patient is able to participate, active range of motion is best to help maintain muscle tone and maintain strength throughout acute illness. Avoiding restraints is another way to reduce loss of function, as this further decreases mobility, as does avoiding any excess equipment that decreases movement.

Functional ability is a key factor for discharge planning. Anticipatory planning for transfer and discharge should begin as soon as possible so that families can help older patients plan for next steps. Factors include the patient's pre-hospital state, type of illness, potential for recovery, rehabilitation needs, and expected duration of acute illness. Most importantly, the nurse needs to share this information when the patient is transferred to a lower level of care. This will save the nurses in the new area significant time in recollecting information and figuring out the details about the patient. Continuity in care can reduce loss of functional ability and maximize recovery time.

Pain

Pain is a common concern of older adults in acute care settings. Because of the variety of types of pain, the causes of pain, and the physical manifestations of pain, achieving adequate pain control for the older adult in the high-acuity setting can be challenging. Pain affects the older adult's ability to function as well as their quality of life. Pain can be due to either an acute condition such as a fracture, postoperative pain, or a chronic disease such as osteoarthritis, back pain, and bone and joint disorders. A particular concern for the older adult is chronic pain, which can affect all aspects of life, health, and safety. Chronic pain also increases health care costs (Baird, Keen & Swearingen, 2005).

Age-related changes such as changes in cognition and sensory perception impact the ability to perceive pain and report pain. The ability to discriminate between painful stimuli declines with age (Hooyman & Kiyak, 2008) and can impact the ability to accurately assess pain. Barriers to pain assessment and management are numerous and include the individual's beliefs about pain and potential alterations in sensory and cognitive function which interfere with communication and the reporting of pain. A thorough nursing assessment is required. Although many pain scales and pain assessment tools exist, it is equally important to assess nonverbal behavior such as facial expressions and body language.

Pain medication should be given routinely to avoid severe pain necessitating higher levels of medication, and which interferes with recovery from acute conditions. Under treatment of pain is commonly described among older adults, and leads to depression, social isolation, gait problems, and sleep disturbances (Baird, Keen & Swearingen, 2005), all of which have implications for high-acuity settings. Other problems can be agitation, immobility, delirium, and self-extubation. Nursing interventions such as promoting sleep, maintaining a calm and peaceful environment, and promoting comfort, help to create a healing environment and decrease the perception of pain.

Pain medications present a challenge in the older patient. Nonsteroidal and anti-inflammatory drugs have increased risks and meperidine should be completely avoided because it commonly causes neurotoxicity in older patients (Holzer, 2007). Frequent pain assessment and regular administration of appropriate pain medication at the lowest dose needed to treat pain may prevent or improve delirium. Nurses need to be vigilant in monitoring and treating pain and evaluating the patient for any untoward reactions to treatments.

NURSING CARE: The Older Adult Higher Acuity Patient offers a summary of nursing care considerations specific to this patient population.

NURSING CARE: The Older Adult High-Acuity Patient

Expected Patient Outcomes and Related Interventions

Outcome 1: Preserve organ function

Assess and compare to established norms, patient baselines, and trends

- Assess for co-morbidities that are present in addition to admitting diagnosis
- Monitor organ status:
  - Neurologic – Cognitive status, pupillary response, Glasgow coma scale (GCS)
  - Cardiovascular – Blood pressure, heart rate, heart rhythm (cardiac monitoring), heart sounds
  - Pulmonary – Respiratory rate and depth, lung sounds, pulse oximetry, ABG as warranted
  - Gastrointestinal – Bowel sounds, bowel palpation, nutrition status, bowel movements, signs of occult or gross GI bleeding
  - Hepatic – Liver size by palpation, liver function tests (LFT)
  - Renal – Intake and output, renal function tests (BUN, creatinine)

Interventions to support organ function

- Maintain adequate mean arterial pressure (> 60 mmHg)
  - Measures to support blood pressure – careful use of fluids or vasopressors
  - Careful monitoring of:
    - Intake and output balance (avoid over or under hydration)
    - Cardiac rhythm (monitor for cardiac dysrhythmias and treat as needed)
- Maintain adequate oxygenation:
  - Oxygen therapy, as ordered
  - Turn every 2 hours
  - Elevate head of bed 30 degrees
  - Deep breathing exercises; incentive spirometry every 2-4 hours
- Decrease energy expenditure
  - Alternate rest and active periods
  - Maintain comfortable room temperature (prevent chilling)
  - Maintain normothermia (reduce fevers, warming blankets if hypothermic)
  - Assist with physical activities as needed
- Early ambulation as tolerated (reduce stasis problems)
- Avoid drug-induced organ injury (related to polypharmacy)
  - Careful monitoring of drug dosage, interactions and toxicities
    - Adjust drug dosages as needed
    - Periodic monitoring of drug levels
    - Monitor closely for signs/symptoms of toxicities
  - Avoid drug combinations with same-organ toxicities
  - Monitor liver and kidney function

Related nursing diagnoses

- Activity intolerance
- Altered thought processes

(*continued*)

NURSING CARE (continued)

Altered tissue perfusion
Decreased cardiac output
Fluid volume excess (fluid volume deficit)
Impaired gas exchange
Nutrition: less than body requirements
Risk for impaired tissue integrity

Outcome 2: Minimize impact of delirium

Assess and compare to established norms, patient baselines, and trends

Monitor for early signs of delirium or other cognitive changes
Consider administering the CAM-ICU test

Interventions to reduce impact of delirium

Treat pain, anxiety, and agitation to promote adequate rest
Treat pain with lowest effective dose of analgesic
Avoid drugs that are associated with delirium in the elderly
Decrease environmental stimuli
Maintain nutrition and hydration
Enlist significant others to help in maintaining patient orientation
Investigate possible drug-induced causes of delirium

Related nursing diagnoses

Anxiety
Confusion
Pain

Outcome 3: Skin breakdown prevented

Assess and compare to established norms, patient baselines, and trends

Assess for co-morbidities that increase risk for problems of skin integrity (e.g., diabetes mellitus, chronic heart failure, dehydration, malnutrition)
Monitor skin color, temperature, skin integrity, evidence of stasis ulcers
Assess pressure points frequently (e.g., heels, spine, coccyx, elbows, back of head)
Monitor nutrition and hydration status

Interventions to prevent skin breakdown

Reposition frequently especially if head of bed is elevated
Handle gently, avoiding shearing forces
Use pressure reducing surfaces
Use skin cleansers that are non-drying
Use lotions to keep skin lubricated
Consult with skin specialist as needed

Related nursing diagnoses

Altered tissue perfusion
Nutrition: less than body requirements
Risk for impaired tissue integrity

Data partially from Criddle (2009).

Pharmacotherapy

The administration of medications to the older adult is complicated and related to several problems. Major concerns for nurses are drug toxicities and medication errors. The elderly are at risk for drug toxicity for a variety of physiologic reasons involving multiple body systems (Fig. 3–2). In addition, medication errors or adverse drug reactions (ADRs) can be due to potentially inappropriate medications (PIMs), normal age-related physiologic changes that affect pharmacokinetics and pharmacodynamics, polypharmacy, self medication, and patient-family non-compliance (Ferrario, 2008).

When medications are given to an older adult, conditions that could potentially affect drug absorption, distribution, metabolism, and excretion should be considered. Factors that affect absorption include decreased surface area of the small intestine, decreased splanchnic blood flow, altered gastric pH, and decreased gastric motility. Distribution is affected by a decrease in lean body mass, increase in fat content, and decrease in total body water content. Altered liver and kidney function affect metabolism and excretion. Drugs metabolized by the liver or kidneys will remain present and active for a longer period of time, with an increased opportunity to produce side effects. In addition, tolerance for medications such as penicillin, tetracycline, and digoxin, may be altered due to a decrease in renal filtration (Hooyman & Kiyak, 2008). Medications may be active in an older person's system longer and may be more potent. Therefore, drug dosage and frequency of administration may need to be altered or adjusted frequently. The therapeutic window may be narrow, with one dose not being effective, but a higher dose causing side effects. Typical signs of drug toxicity in the elderly may involve CNS changes, orthostatic hypotension, falls, and incontinence rather than the more commonly seen nausea, vomiting, diarrhea, and rash.

The older adult may have several chronic illnesses that require management with numerous medications. These medications may counteract or interact with each other, or cause side effects if withdrawn during hospitalization. Nurses should be aware of the physiologic changes of the elderly and how they may impact the metabolism of specific drug groups (see Table 3–10). It is essential to obtain a thorough medication history in elderly patients. Prescription medications, over-the-counter medications, vitamins and minerals, alcohol, caffeine, and tobacco use as well as home remedies should be considered. Nursing care includes evaluating the effects of medications, monitoring drug levels, and anticipating side effects and interactions.

Important research by experts in gerontology and pharmacology has been done to identify inappropriate medication use in older adults. The goal is to identify medications, which when administered, increase the risk for adverse drug reactions in specific clinical conditions. The Beers' Criteria for Potentially Inappropriate Medication Use in the Elderly can assist in the identification of medications that should be avoided, or if used, will require frequent monitoring of the patient. (Fick et al., 2003). Table 3–11 provides some common medications that cause side effects in the elderly and are not recommended for use in this age group.

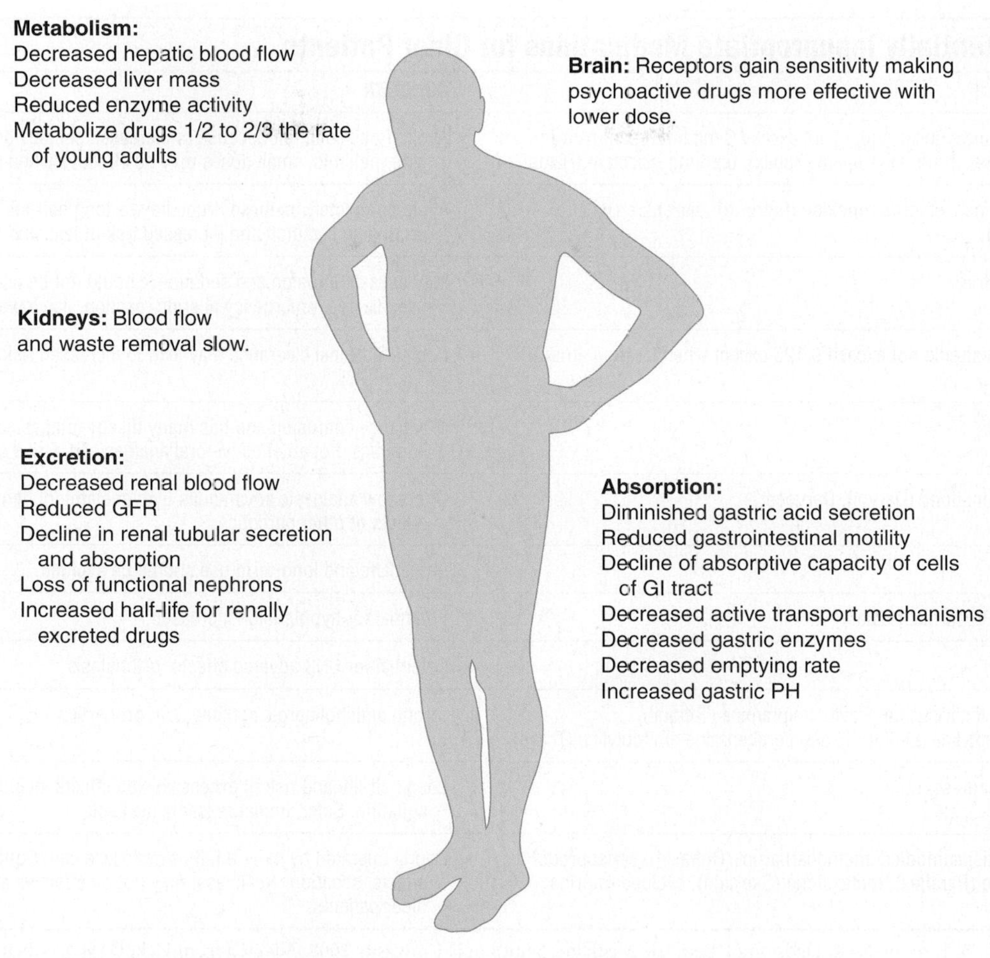

Figure 3–2 ■ Aging body and drug use.

When an older adult receives a new medication, the advice is to "start low and go slow." In other words, a low dose should be used first, and the dosage increased slowly as the patient's reaction is determined. The therapeutic window may be narrow in the older patient for all the reasons discussed above, with one dose not being effective, but a higher dose causing side effects. Nurses should monitor patient reactions to any new medication and report any untoward changes, particularly changes in mental status.

Multiple sensory issues may be present that cause problems with patient management of a medication regime. Short-term memory impairment may cause a person to take incorrect dosages, multiple doses, or skip doses. Impaired vision may affect dosage. Impaired agility in opening containers may lead to missed doses. Financial factors and transportation issues may keep the patient from filling prescriptions.

TABLE 3–10 Physiologic Changes and Associated Drug Effects

PHYSIOLOGIC CHANGES	EFFECTS
Heart is dependent upon endogenous catecholamines for effective pumping	**Beta-blocking** agents may precipitate heart failure
Dopamine-making capacity of neurons decreases	**Phenothiazines** further block dopamine uptake, precipitating Parkinson-like symptoms.
Dependence on prostacyclin-mediated renal vasodilation to maintain glomerular blood flow	**Nonsteroidal anti-inflammatory agents (NSAIDs)** that block prostacyclin may decrease renal blood flow and precipitate acute renal failure
Dependence on elevated rennin levels to maintain renal perfusion	**Angiotensin-converting enzyme (ACE) inhibitors** may decrease renal blood flow and precipitate acute renal failure
Increased body fat	Prolonged effects of fat-soluble drugs (e.g., sedatives/hypnotics) due to increased distribution volume in fat tissue
Less body water	Higher blood levels of water-soluble drugs (e.g., alcohol) due to decreased distribution volume

TABLE 3–11 Potentially Inappropriate Medications for Older Patients

DRUG	CONCERN
Short-acting benzodiazepines: doses should not exceed 3 mg lorazepam (Ativan), 60 mg oxazepam (Serax), 2 mg temazepam (Xanax), 0.25 mg triazolam (Haldol).	Avoid if possible, but because of increased sensitivity to these drugs in older patients, small doses may be effective when needed.
Long acting benzodiazepines: chlordiazepoxide (Librium), diazepam (Valium), clorazepate (Tranxene)	Avoid completely as these drugs have a long half-life in the elderly, producing sedation and increased risk of falls and fractures.
Diphenhydramine (Benadryl)	May cause confusion and sedation. Should not be used as a hypnotic. When used to treat emergency allergic reaction, use lowest dose possible.
Digoxin (Lanoxin): doses should not exceed 0.125 except when treating atrial arrhythmias	Decreased renal clearance may lead to increased risk of toxic effects.
Meperidine (Demerol)	May cause confusion and has many disadvantages compared to other narcotics; not an effective oral analgesic in doses commonly used.
Propoxyphene and combinations (Darvon, Darvocet)	Offers few analgesic advantages over acetaminophen, yet has adverse side effects of other narcotics.
Ketorolac (Toradol)	Immediate and long-term use should be avoided.
Short acting nifedipine (Procardia, Adalat)	Potential for hypotension increased.
Clonidine (Catapres)	Potential for CNS adverse effects, orthostasis.
Tricyclic antidepressants: Amitriptyline (Elavil), imipramine (Tofranil), chlordiazepoxide-amitriptyline (Limbitrol), and perphenazine-amitriptyline (Triavil)	Strong anticholinergic and sedation properties
Fluoxetine (Prozac) antidepressant	Long half-life and risk of excessive side effects including sleep disturbance, agitation. Safer antidepressants available.
Muscle relaxants and antispasmodics: methocarbamol (Robaxin), carisoprodol (Soma), chlorzoxazone (Paraflex), metaxalone (Skelaxin), cyclobenzaprine (Flexeril).	Poorly tolerated by older adults since these cause anticholinergic adverse effects, sedation, weakness; may not be effective at low doses tolerated by older patients.

Data from Flaherty, J. H., & Tumosa, N. K. Division of Geriatric Medicine, Saint Louis University 2008. Adapted from Fick, D. M. Cooper, J. W., Wade, W. E. et.al. (2003). Updating the Beers Criteria for potentially Inappropriate Medication Use in Older Adults: Results of a U.S. consensus panel of experts. *Archives of Internal Medicine*, 163(22), 2716–2724. Reprinted with permission.

SECTION EIGHT REVIEW

1. All of the following are common causes of functional decline in the older hospitalized patient: (choose all that apply)
   A. restraints
   B. medications
   C. bedrest
   D. pain
2. Medications are not absorbed as well in the older adult due to (choose all that apply)
   A. decreased gastric motility
   B. decreased splanchnic blood flow
   C. GERD
   D. decreased gastric pH
3. Age-related changes may affect which of the following factors of pharmacodynamics? (choose all that apply)
   A. absorption
   B. distribution
   C. metabolism
   D. excretion
4. The best choice for severe pain in the older patient is
   A. opioids
   B. non-steroidal anti-inflammatories
   C. meperidine
   D. acetaminophen

Answers: 1. (A, B, C, D), 2. (A, B, D), 3. (A, B, C, D), 4. A

SECTION NINE: Geriatric Assessment Tools for the High-Acuity Nurse

At the completion of this section the learner will be able to describe common geriatric assessment tools.

Geriatric assessment tools are commonly used to screen for problems in older patients. This section describes the most important tools for the high-acuity setting for the disorders described in Section Seven: dementia, delirium, and depression. Additional assessment tools for physical issues are also described. These screening tools take only a few minutes and have been widely used in clinical settings. The shortest versions of the tools are described here so they are easy to use in practice. Assessment tools are available to screen for other common geriatric problems, such as ADLs and IADLs. These are less often used in the high-acuity setting and are beyond the scope of this module.

Mental Status Assessment

The nurse can easily assess mental status using a geriatric assessment test to detect dementia. One simple test is the "Mini-Cog" (Borson et al., 2000). It takes just three minute to administer, and tests the patient's memory, ability to concentrate, and ability to follow directions (see Table 3–12). To take this test, the patient must be able to talk and write. The nurse first asks the patient to repeat and recall three items, then draw the face of a clock, with numbers and hands on a piece of paper. When the clock is finished, the patient is asked to repeat the three items. A simple scoring method makes it easy to determine if the person has normal cognition. If a patient has an abnormal score, the nurse should always try to determine if there has been a problem with memory or function before, and if the change has been gradual or sudden.

Delirium Assessment

Delirium is diagnosed through identification of symptoms that are consistent with the diagnosis. A screening instrument that walks the nurse through the patient assessment is the Confusion Assessment Method (CAM) (Inouye et al., 1990). The patient should have an acute onset of the symptoms, a fluctuating course, and inattention. In addition to these features, the patient must show either an altered level of consciousness (anything other than "0" on the Richmond Agitation and Sedation Scale (RAS)) or disorganized thinking. The Richmond Agitation and Sedation Scale (RASS) is one instrument that can be used to measure level of consciousness. An ICU version of the CAM (Ely et al., 2001) provides specific tasks the nurse can have the patient complete to help determine cognitive status; if unable to speak, for example squeezing the nurse's hand when certain letters are recited (see Table 3–13). A positive CAM score indicates a rescue situation and should be reported immediately to the physician.

TABLE 3–12 Mini-Cog Mental Status Test

1. Ask the patient to listen carefully to and remember three unrelated words, and then to repeat the words.
2. Instruct the patient to draw the face of a clock, either on a blank sheet of paper or on a sheet with a clock circle already drawn on the page.
3. Ask the patient to repeat the three previously stated words. Each word is worth one point.
4. Scoring: Give one point for each recalled word after completing the clock.
   - If none are recalled, score = 0 and the patient is classified as demented
   - If all three are recalled, score = 3 and the patient is classified normal
   - If one to two are recalled, classify based on the clock (abnormal = dementia; normal = not dementia).
   - The clock is considered normal if all numbers are present in the correct sequence and position, and the hands legibly display the requested time.

From Borson, S., Scanlan, J., Brush, M., Viatallano, P., & Dokmak, A. (2000). The Mini-Cog: A cognitive 'vital signs' measure for dementia screening in multilingual elderly. *International Journal of Geriatric Psychiatry*, 15(11), 1021–1027.
Note: Sit the patient up when possible, make sure glasses are in place and there is enough light to see during testing, and avoid excess background noise.

TABLE 3–13 Confusion Assessment Method–ICU Version (CAM-ICU)

FEATURE 1: ACUTE ONSET AND FLUCTUATING COURSE Positive if "you" answer "yes" to either 1A or 1B.	**POSITIVE**	**NEGATIVE**
1A: Is the patient different than his/her baseline mental status? **Or** **1B:** Has the patient had any fluctuation in mental status in the past 24 hours as evidenced by fluctuation on a sedation scale (e.g., RASS, GCS) or previous delirium assessment?	Yes	No
FEATURE 2: INATTENTION Positive if either score for 2A or 2B is less than 8.	**POSITIVE**	**NEGATIVE**
Attempt the ASE letters first. If patient is able to perform this test and the score is clear, record this score and move to Feature 3. If patient is unable to perform this test or the score is unclear, then perform the ASE Pictures. If you perform both tests, use the ASE Pictures' results to score the Feature.		
2A: ASE Letters: record score (enter NT for not tested) Directions: Say to the patient, *"I am going to read you a series of 10 letters. Whenever you hear the letter "A," indicate by squeezing my hand."* Read letters from the following letter list in a normal tone. **S A V E A H A A R T** Scoring: Errors are counted when patient fails to squeeze on the letter "A" and when the patient squeezes on any letter other than "A."	Number Correct < 8	Number Correct > 8
2B: ASE Pictures: record score (enter NT for not tested) Directions are included on the picture packets.		
FEATURE 3 DISORGANIZED THINKING Positive if the combined score is less than 4	**POSITIVE**	**NEGATIVE**
3A: Yes/No Questions (Use either Set A or Set B, alternate on consecutive days if necessary): **Set A Set B** 1. Will a stone float on water? 1. Will a leaf float on water? 2. Are there fish in the sea? 2. Are there elephants in the sea?		

(*continued*)

TABLE 3–13 (*continued*)

3. Does one pound weigh more than 3? Do two pounds weigh two pounds? More than one pound? 4. Can you use a hammer to pound a nail? 4. Can you use a hammer to cut wood? **Score** ___(Patient earns 1 point for each correct answer out of 4).	Number Correct < 2	Number Correct > 2
3B:Command Say to patient: "Hold up this many fingers" (Examiner holds two fingers in front of patient) "Now do the same thing with the other hand" (Not repeating the number of fingers). *If patient is unable to move both arms, for the second part of the command ask patient "Add one more finger.") **Score** ___(Patient earns 1 point if able to successfully complete the entire command)		
FEATURE 4: ALTERED LEVEL OF CONSCIOUSNESS Positive if the Actual RASS score is anything other than "0" (zero)	**POSITIVE**	**NEGATIVE**
Overall CAM-ICU Score Features 1 and 2 and either Feature 3 or 4	**POSITIVE**	**NEGATIVE**

Adapted from Ely, E. W., Inouye, S. K., Bernard, G. R. Gordon, S., Francis, J., Mey, L. et al., (2001). Delirium in mechanically ventilated patients: Validity and reliability of the confusion assessment method for the intensive care unit (CAM-ICU). *Journal of the American Medical Association*, 286, 2701–2710.

Geriatric Depression Scale

The Geriatric Depression Scale (GDS) has been widely used to screen for depressive symptoms in older adults (Yesavage et al., 1983). It has short forms that have been validated, so that administration can be as efficient and easy as possible, including a five-item version (see Table 3–14). To assess depression, the nurse asks the patient to respond "yes" or "no" to a series of questions about their mood over the past two weeks. The score is based on the number of depressed answers. When a very poor score is identified, the patient should be queried about suicidal ideation; has the patient thought about or planned suicide? A positive score and particularly suicidal comments should be reported to other health professionals for follow up.

TABLE 3–14 Geriatric Depression Scale (GDS)

"I am going to ask you about your mood and how you have been feeling. Choose the best answer for how you have felt over the past week or so:"

1.*	Are you basically satisfied with your life?	YES / NO
2.	Have you dropped many of your activities and interests?	YES / NO
3.	Do you feel that your life is empty?	YES / NO
4.	Do you often get bored?	YES / NO
5.*	Are you in good spirits most of the time?	YES / NO
6.	Are you afraid that something bad is going to happen to you?	YES / NO
7.*	Do you feel happy most of the time?	YES / NO
8.	Do you often feel helpless?	YES / NO
9.	Do you prefer to stay at home, rather than going out and doing new things?	YES / NO
10.	Do you feel you have more problems with memory than most?	YES / NO
11.*	Do you think it is wonderful to be alive now?	YES / NO
12.	Do you feel pretty worthless the way you are now?	YES / NO
13.*	Do you feel full of energy?	YES / NO
14.	Do you feel that your situation is hopeless?	YES / NO
15.	Do you think that most people are better off than you are?	YES / NO

Number of underlined answers: ___________________

Score ≥ 4 suggests depression for 15-item version

Score ≥ 2 suggests depression for 5-item version; if positive, ask all 15 items to increase accuracy.

* Notes which items are on the 5-item version of the GDS.

Adaptations from Sheikh, V. I. & Yesavage, V. A. (1986). Geriatric Depression Scale: Recent evidence and development of a shorter version. In T. L. Brink (Ed). *Clinical gerontology: a guide to assessment and intervention* (pp. 165–174). New York: Haworth.

Adaptations from Weeks, S. K., McGann, P. E. Michaels, T. K., et al. (2003). Comparing various short form geriatric depression scales leads to the GDS 5/15. *Journal of Nursing Scholarship*, 35, 133–137.

Adaptations from Hoyle, M. T., Alessi, C. A., Harker, J. O et al. (1999). Development and testing of a five-item version of the geriatric depression scale. *Journal of the American Geriatrics Society*, 47, 873–878.

Skin Assessment

Because of the changes in skin in the older adult as already described, use of a standardized skin assessment will identify those at high risk for problems. Assessment of risk for skin breakdown begins at admission, and continues with daily assessment and reevaluation of skin integrity. The Braden Scale for Predicting Pressure Sore Risk © (Prevention Plus, 2001) is used in most acute care settings. The subscales of sensory, perception, moisture, mobility, nutrition, and friction and shear are scored based on descriptive criteria. A lower score on the assessment tool indicates a higher the risk for pressure sore development (Bergstrom, Braden, Laguzza & Holman, 1987; Bergstrom & Braden, 2002). When a patient is identified at risk, nursing interventions are initiated to prevent ulcers by reducing the risk factors (Stotts and Horng-Shiuann, 2007).

Falls and Mobility Assessment

Most acute care settings also conduct routine fall risk assessment; the most common tools are the Morse Fall Scale and Hendrich II Fall Risk Model. Similar to skin assessment, the tools help identify patients at risk for falling and must be used on admission and at the very least, after any change in condition or procedure. Many facilities conduct daily screening. Key risk factors from the Hendrich II Fall Risk Model include: confusion or disorientation, depression, altered elimination, dizziness, male, antiepileptic drugs or benzodiazepines, and difficulty getting up and walking around (Hendrich, Bender & Nyhuis, 2003). The Morse Fall Scale includes the following risk factors: history of falling, multiple conditions, mental status changes, need for a walking aid or walking problems, and presence of IV therapy (Morse, Morse & Tylko, 1989).

The nurse can use the assessment tools to identify what interventions to use, such as assisting with transfers, therapy to increase muscle strength, frequent toileting, or heavy surveillance for delirious patients. Monitoring of fall events can help identify risks for specific units, as these can vary. Even in the high-acuity setting, restraints do not prevent falls and increases the risk of injuries (Mion et al., 2008).

Pain Assessment

Because of the lack of objective measures of pain, researchers have developed pain intensity scales using faces or word descriptors in visual analog scales that ask the patient to rate the severity of pain from zero (no pain) to 10 (the worst possible pain). Consistent use of any scale brings objectivity to pain assessment and bridges a gap between the patient's pain experience and the nurse's ability to monitor the pain experience and the effects of nursing interventions aimed at decreasing the level of pain. The most important consideration in the assessment of the presence and severity of pain is the patient's account of the pain. If cognitive or communication problems are suspected, the assessment of pain should be supplemented with information from family and caregivers (Baird, Keen, & Swearingen, 2005). It is important to assess pain in relationship to its impact on the older adult's ability to function. In the high-acuity setting, it is important to assess pain in relationship to its impact on the older adult's ability to recover from the present health condition which has caused admission into the current setting. Once pain has been quantified, nurses work with patients to set goals for pain management.

Assessment Laboratory Data

The slow decline in organ function seen in the older adult patient results in alterations in laboratory findings and what constitutes an "acceptable" range. It is important for the high-acuity nurse to be aware of the age-related alterations in laboratory trends. Table 3–15 lists common laboratory tests, their normal ranges, and expected age-related changes.

TABLE 3–15 Laboratory Values in the Older Adult

LAB TEST	NORMAL VALUE	CHANGES WITH AGE
Urinalysis		
Protein	0–5 mg/100mL	Rises slightly ■ Normal change due to aging ■ Urinary tract infection ■ Renal pathology
Glucose	0–15 mg/100ml	Declines slightly ■ Glycosuria noted after high serum glucose levels
Specific gravity	1.0005–1.020	Lower maximum in elderly of 1.016-1.022 ■ Declining renal function impairs ability to concentrate urine
Hematology		
Erythrocyte sedimentation rate (ESR)	MEN: 0–20 WOMEN: 0–30	Significant increase ■ Mild elevations are age related ■ Changes are influenced by changes in hematocrit, therefore, increases are not specific ■ Helpful in identifying malignancy, infection, and connective tissue disorders
Hemoglobin	MEN: 13–18g/100mL WOMEN: 12–16g/100mL	MEN: 10-17 g/mL WOMEN: change not specified ■ Anemia is very common in elderly and is multifactorial
Hematocrit	MEN: 45–52% WOMEN: 37–48%	Slight decrease ■ Decline in hematopoiesis
Leukocytes	4,300–10,800/cu mm	Decrease to 3,100-9,000/cu mm ■ Medications ■ Sepsis ■ Decreases should not be immediately attributed to age
Lymphocytes	500–2,400 T cells/cu mm 50–200 B cells/cu mm	T cells and B cells decrease ■ Increases risks of infection ■ Immunizations warranted
Platelets	150,000–350,000	No change

(continued)

TABLE 3–15 (*continued*)

Blood Chemistry		
Albumin	3.5-5.0/100mL	Decreases ■ Related to a decreased in liver size and enzymes ■ Protein energy malnutrition is common
Total serum protein	6.0-8.4g/100mL	No change ■ Decreases may be indicative of malnutrition, infection, or liver disease Decreases
Blood urea nitrogen (BUN)	MEN: 10-25 mg/100mL WOMEN: 8-20 mg/100mL	Increases significantly up to 69mg/100mL ■ May be attributed to decreased glomerular filtration rate or a decreased cardiac output
Creatinine	0.6-1.5 mg/100mL	Increases to 1.9 mg/100mL ■ Related to decrease in lean body mass
Creatinine clearance	104-124 mL/min	Decreases 10% per decade after age 40 ■ Guideline for dosages of medications excreted by kidney
Glucose tolerance	62-110 mg/dL fasting <120 mg/dL 2 hours postprandial	Slight increase of 10 mg/dL per decade after age 30 ■ Increased prevalence of diabetes Mellitus in older adults ■ Medications may be the cause of glucose intolerance
Triglycerides	40-150 mg/100mL	Normal range alters: 20-200 mg/100mL
Cholesterol	120-220 mg/100mL	Total Cholesterol increases between ages 60-90, especially in women. Decreases after age 90. ■ Risks for CHD
Thyroxine (T4)	4.5-13.5 mcg/100mL	No age-related changes ■ Changes may be due to thyroid disease, acute or chronic illnesses, or caloric deficiencies
Triiodothyronine (T3)	90-220 ng/100mL	Decrease of 25%
Thyroid-stimulating hormone (TSH)	0.5-5.0 mcg/mL	Slight increase ■ Sensitive indication of thyroid disease
Alkaline phosphate	13-39 iu/L	Increase by 8-10 iu/L ■ Increase greater than 20% usually due to disease ■ Elevations may be found with bone abnormalities, drugs (narcotics), and eating a fatty meal

Data from Fletcher, K. R. (1999). Physical and laboratory assessment in J. T. Stone, J. F. Wyman, S. A. Salisbury (eds). *Clinical gerontological nursing: a guide to advanced practice.* 2e Philadelphia: Saunders.

SECTION NINE REVIEW

1. Testing for dementia, depression or delirium requires
A. a great deal of training
B. at least twenty minutes
C. a brief geriatric assessment tool
D. none of the above

2. The best tool for assessing delirium in the high-acuity older adult is the
A. CAM ICU
B. CAM
C. GDS
D. Mini-Cog

3. Skin assessment should be conducted
A. daily
B. after changes in condition
C. at least weekly
D. once per shift

4. The most important consideration in the assessment of the presence and severity of pain is
A. the documentation of the previous shift
B. the report of the patient's family members
C. the patient's account of the pain
D. the physician's assessment of the pain

Answers: 1. C, 2. A, 3. A, 4. C

SECTION TEN: High-Risk Injuries and Complications of Trauma

At the completion of this section, the learner will be able to discuss nursing management of older patients with high-risk injuries and trauma.

Traumatic Injury

Traumatic injuries are a leading cause of death in the elderly. Factors such as altered sensory function; changes in motor strength, postural stability, balance, and coordination; exacerbations of medical conditions; and medication therapies;

combine to increase the vulnerability of an older adult to environmental hazards, and increase the risk of falls and other traumatic injuries. While falls are the most common cause of injury, motor vehicle crashes (MVCs) account for the most fatalities. Additionally, burns have a high mortality rate in the elderly.

Nursing care is aimed at stabilizing the injuries and preventing complications. The older patient has more difficulty compensating for injury or trauma and is at greater risk for complications. Priorities for the care of the elderly patient in the high-acuity area include assessment of airway, breathing, and circulation. Oxygenation status is monitored via peripheral oxygen saturation, lactic acid levels, arterial blood gases, and mixed venous oxygen saturation. Older adults do not tolerate hypoperfusion, which can quickly deteriorate to cardiogenic shock (Meiner & Lueckenotte, 2006). Early hemodynamic monitoring is important. Hemodynamic status is monitored noninvasively via urine output, level of consciousness (LOC), pedal pulses, or invasively with cardiac output measurements. Assessment of hypovolemic shock is more challenging. Tachycardia, normally an early sign of hypovolemia, is often obscured as the heart rate may not respond to blood loss. Volume overload is an additional concern, particularly in a patient with cardiac and renal disease. Thermoregulatory mechanisms may be impaired and therefore, heat loss should be prevented by simply using warm IV solutions, warm blankets, and careful environmental control (Meiner & Lueckenotte, 2006).

An in-depth history should be performed to obtain information about past medical and surgical history, immunization status, and information about chronic diseases such as renal failure, respiratory diseases, cirrhosis, diabetes, heart disease, and previous myocardial infarctions. Previous cardiovascular disease and treatment for hypertension may precipitate a syncopal episode from either decreased cardiac output or inadequate cerebral circulation. Syncopal episodes require an in-depth assessment (Table 3-16). Cardiac dysrhythmias may be a contributing factor to the injury, and could be related to numerous factors such as anemia, or hormonal or electrolyte imbalances. Other risk factors for injury to consider are diminished senses such as vision, hearing, diminished reflexes, agility, and coordination. It may be difficult to determine if confusion or agitation, if present, is due to preexisting sensory deficits, hypovolemia, or a head injury.

A thorough medication history may reveal medications that increase the risk of injury such as antihypertensives, oral hypoglycemic agents that may induce syncope, or diuretics without potassium supplements, that may precipitate dysrhythmias and hypotension. Additionally, beta-blocking agents are known to decrease the sympathetic nervous system response to hypovolemia, and therefore they alter the usual compensatory responses to injury and shock.

Injuries that are considered high-risk injuries due to an associated increase in morbidity and mortality in the older adult include falls; head and spine injuries; chest, abdominal, and pelvic injuries; and burns. Falls may result in significant fractures such as the hip, femur, humerus, or wrist or head and spine injuries. Early stabilization of all fractures is important to prevent complications of immobility (e.g. pneumonia, pulmonary emboli).

TABLE 3–16 Assessment of Syncope in the Older Adult

Focus Area: Decreased Perfusion

1. History of palpitation, shortness of breath, diaphoresis, chest pain?
2. History of previous AMI, CVA?
3. Dizziness or loss of balance upon arising or changing position?
4. History of vomiting, diarrhea, GI bleeding?
5. Lack of food and/or fluid intake?

Focus Area: Neurologic

1. Any weakness, tingling, or numbness?
2. Prior trouble with walking or balance?
3. Trouble completing ADLs?
4. Any difficulty with speech or communication?

Focus Area: Illness

1. Any history of diabetes; if so, how treated? Last meal, activity, and medication?
2. Any history of cancer; if so, how treated? Last radiation, chemotherapy treatment, CBC, platelet count?
3. Any infection: fever, respiratory symptoms, change in urination, and/or urine output?

Focus Area: Medications

1. Use of alcohol or recreational drugs?
2. Use of antihypertensives?
3. Use of antihistamines?
4. Use of sedatives?
5. Use of pain medications?
6. Use of OTC medications?
7. Use of herbal or homeopathic remedies?

AMI=acute myocardial infarction; CVA=cerebrovascular accident; GI=gastrointestinal; ADL=activities of daily living; CBC=complete blood count; OTC=over the counter.

Head and Spine Injuries

Subdural hematomas occur more frequently in the older adult following a head injury. The age-related loss of brain volume and increased intracranial space between the brain and the dura permit a large amount of bleeding before the appearance of symptoms of intracranial bleeding. Additionally, the classic signs of headache and vomiting due to increased intracranial hypertension may be absent due to cerebral atrophy. Nurses caring for older adults after an injury should assess for subtle LOC changes and cranial nerve deficits.

Chest Injuries

Chest injuries are associated with fractured ribs in the elderly because of osteoporosis. Pre-existing pulmonary disease and diminished pulmonary reserve increase the risk of pulmonary failure, and the necessity of intubation and mechanical ventilation.

Abdominal Injuries

Abdominal trauma in the elderly has a high mortality rate due to postoperative, pulmonary, and infectious complications. The elderly have diminished sensation and abdominal wall muscle tone, so the typical signs of peritoneal irritation, such as involuntary guarding and muscular rigidity, may be missing. Fragile ribs and a weakened abdominal wall increase the likelihood of abdominal injury with very little force.

Pelvic Injuries

Pelvic fractures are associated with great blood loss. Because the elderly have fewer compensatory responses to combat hypovolemic shock, early control of hemorrhage is essential. Embolization of major pelvic arteries may need to be performed as well as early stabilization with external fixation.

Burns

The mortality of a burn in an older adult is very high. Flame injuries associated with cooking, and scald injuries associated with bathing are common. The elderly tend to have greater depth and size of burn due to their thinner skin, slower reaction times, reduced mobility, and diminished sensations. Prolonged healing is also a factor particularly in the presence of malnutrition prior to injury. The elderly do not scar as much as younger patients, and therefore pressure garments are not essential.

SECTION TEN REVIEW

1. Which of the following increase the older adult's risk of traumatic injuries?
   A. increasing age
   B. sensory changes
   C. decreased glomerular filtration
   D. decreased cough reflex
2. Subdural hematoma is a common complication of head injury in the older patient because of
   A. increase in intracranial space between the brain and dura
   B. decreased reaction time
   C. decreased sympathetic nervous system response to hypovolemia
   D. decreased muscle tone
3. Older patients with trauma are more likely to need intubation and mechanical ventilation than younger patients.
   A. True
   B. False

Answers: 1. B, 2. A, 3. A

SECTION ELEVEN: Special considerations: A culture of caring and end-of-life care

At the completion of this section the learner will be able to explain special situations including the culture of care for older adults and end-of-life care.

A Culture of Care for Older Adults

Numerous specialty organizations have recently engaged in efforts to ensure that nurses in their organizations provide exemplary care to older adults (Resnick, 2007). One example is a group initiative from the American Academy of Nursing Expert Panel on Acute and Critical Care, which addressed and outlined evidenced based strategies for reducing deterioration in hospitalized elders by creating a "culture of care" (Kleinpell, 2007). Nurses working in high-acuity areas can use these strategies to form a framework for practice. Eight goals for elder care were identified and are listed in Table 3-17.

TABLE 3–17 Eight Goals for Elder Care

- Promote recovery
- Optimize reserve
- Maximize safety
- Support independence
- Uphold dignity
- Maintain vigilance
- Cultivate responsiveness
- Improve access

Data from: Kleinpell (2007).

Older adults are more vulnerable to adverse outcomes and are at greater risk for functional decline or a loss of independence as a result of a hospitalization. For this reason, special attention must be given to the needs of this patient population to improve outcomes. Table 3-18 provides a summary of key steps for the nurse to provide better care of the older high-acuity patient.

Emerging Evidence

- Advanced age alone is not a valid reason to refuse ICU care, but the benefits received from intensive care seem to decrease with aging in terms of quality of life years. 97 percent of elderly survivors of critical care lived at home and 88 percent of them considered their quality of life to be satisfactory or good after hospital discharge in a cross sectional survey to assess mortality, quality of life, and quality adjusted life years for critically ill elderly patients ($n=882 \geq 65$ years of age) in a 10-bed medical surgical ICU in a large university hospital compared to a control group of 1,827 patients who were < 65 years of age *(Kaarlola, Tallgren, & Pettila, 2006).*
- In patients older than 70 years, hospital admission with a diagnosis of heart failure was associated with a mortality rate of 4 percent to 7 percent and high risk for subsequent admissions with the same diagnosis. Mortality rate was significantly higher when comorbidities were present, particularly renal failure or cardiogenic shock *(Dar & Cowie, 2008).*
- A study measuring prevalence of device removal and self-removal of devices (e.g., self-extubation) in the ICU setting was not associated with being elderly, restraint rates, or being male *(Mion, Minnick, Leipzig, Catrambone, & Johnson, 2007).*

TABLE 3–18 Steps to Better Care of the Older High-Acuity Patient

1. Find out what the patient was like prior to the current illness, particularly the functional and cognitive states. The patient could have been living alone and completely independent or, conversely, in a nursing home. This can have a major impact on how the nurse views the patient, as during critical illness, the nurse may make incorrect assumptions about the patient's prehospitalization state.
2. Identify preadmission conditions and medications that may impact the patient's response to the current illness.
3. Expect the unexpected. Older adults often have an altered presentation of diseases so any change in vital signs or cognitive state could indicate a new problem such as infection, delirium, or complications. The nurse may need to use good nursing detective skills to figure out what is really going on.
4. Pay special attention to basic nursing care. Pressure sores, falls, and incontinence are common geriatric syndromes and are as preventable or manageable with good skin care, turning, and attention to voiding. Medicare will stop paying for preventable complications such as these, increasing hospital attention to these problems.
5. Maximize the person's ability to communicate by having the patient's glasses and hearing aids available and in place when possible. Communication is also facilitated by speaking slowly and loudly (avoiding shouting or using a higher pitched voice) while facing the patient when speaking.
6. Learn key aging changes that may impact older patients in the high-acuity area.
7. Use appropriate brief geriatric assessment tools (e.g. Mini-Cog Mental Status Test) to identify common problems, particularly dementia, delirium, and depression.
8. Work with other members of the team to address problems – the complex problems of the older adult need complex interventions. Bring in social workers, geriatric physicians, physical or occupational therapists, dieticians, and psychologists or other professionals to assist in meeting the patient's needs.

End-of-Life Care

In most acute care settings, the focus of patient care is of a curative nature and therefore the needs of the elderly person at the end of life are often neglected (Dawson, 2008). Palliative care can and should be integrated into acute care settings, including critical care units. As technology exists to postpone death, it contributes to an imbalance between curative and palliative care (Dawson, 2008). Nurses are challenged with the task of blending high-tech and high-touch care in order to enhance the quality of life of older adults at the end of life. Many hospitals or systems offer specialists who can consult on appropriate palliative care to increase comfort for patients and families and advise staff on appropriate therapies, such as pain medication.

Resuscitation

Ethical Issues. Numerous ethical issues surround resuscitation efforts in all patients, not just the elderly. Issues for debate regarding resuscitation surround the topics of benefits, likelihood of failure or adverse effects, futility, and decision making. There has been a great deal of debate surrounding the patient's wishes at the end of life and an individual's rights to determine medical treatment decisions at the end of life. For example, in the later stages of dementia, intensive treatments may not be appropriate and health care providers should help families make decisions about resuscitation and heroic measures for patients who may not benefit. In the absence of planning, families may be making decisions while dealing with high-acuity illness. Even healthier older patients may reach the point where continued intensive treatments are not likely to benefit them. Nurses provide education and information about patient status and provide supportive care to families making difficult decisions. Nurses can ensure that patients and families are well educated on the issues of cardiopulmonary resuscitation (CPR) and "do not resuscitate" (DNR) and other advanced directives.

Physiological Issues. During resuscitation efforts of an older adult, a number of physiologic factors should be considered. An increase in heart rate is a normal compensatory response to low cardiac output states; however, the heart rate of an older adult has less ability to increase in response to stressors. Vasopressors or inotropes may be required when the cardiac output is low and the heart rate does not increase. The lack of chronotropic response has implications in fluid and electrolyte imbalance as tachycardia may not occur in hypovolemia. Nurses must rely on other indicators of hypovolemia such as changes in hemodynamic values and decreased blood pressure. Additionally, older adults are unable to increase their metabolic rates in proportion to the metabolic demands of increased heat production. Decreased muscle mass and decreased peripheral vasoconstriction prevents heat conservation in the elderly, and therefore nurses must monitor for hypothermia. A warm environment and warmed IV fluids may be warranted. Consideration of age should be incorporated into standard resuscitation protocols to assure the best outcome for older patients.

SECTION ELEVEN REVIEW

1. It is appropriate to incorporate palliative care into high-acuity settings.
   A. True
   B. False
2. The following are topics of ethical concerns surrounding resuscitation (choose all that apply)
   A. futility
   B. likelihood of failure
   C. paternalism
   D. decision making
3. The chronotropic response to stress in the older adult is:
   A. unchanged
   B. decreased
   C. increased
   D. does not apply

Answers: 1. A, 2. (A, B, D), 3. B

POSTTEST

1. Older adults make up at least 40 percent of patients in the general hospital setting.
   A. True
   B. False
2. Because older patients are very diverse in their baseline health, history and ethnicity, the nurse needs to do which of the following? (choose all that apply)
   A. obtain a good history from the patient or family
   B. use standardized care plans
   C. individualize care
   D. monitor patients closely
3. The main cause of urinary tract infection in the hospitalized older patient is
   A. decreased glomerular filtration rate
   B. immobility
   C. weak bladder muscles
   D. indwelling catheter
4. The following age-related changes make evaluation of cardiac status in the older patient more difficult (choose all that apply)
   A. increased time of AV conduction
   B. prolonged PR interval
   C. lack of ST-T wave changes in ischemia
   D. thickening of arterial walls
5. Ventilator acquired pneumonia (VAP) prevention includes which of the following?
   A. check for gastric acidity
   B. decreasing cuff pressure
   C. frequent oral care
   D. rapid weaning
6. Normal age-related changes in the gastrointestinal system result in
   A. risk for poor nutrition
   B. constipation
   C. GERD
   D. dehydration
7. A slightly elevated erythrocyte sedimentation rate (ESR) is a reliable indicator of inflammation.
   A. True
   B. False
8. The following increase risk for infection in the older patient? (choose all that apply)
   A. urinary retention
   B. prostatic hypertrophy
   C. decreased bladder tone
   D. delayed gastric emptying
9. Older adults need influenza vaccination annually. Which two other immunizations are important?
   A. pneumococcal
   B. meningitis
   C. tetanus
   D. pertussis
10. The key feature differentiating delirium from dementia is
    A. confusion
    B. changes in behavior
    C. sudden onset
    D. inability to follow directions
11. You suspect your patient has Alzheimer's disease and you want to test his mental status. The best evaluation for the high-acuity older adult to determine dementia is the
    A. orientation
    B. RASS
    C. CAM-ICU
    D. Mini-Cog
12. An important nursing intervention for older patients with altered cognitive status is
    A. report changes in cognition from baseline
    B. identify preferences for bedtime
    C. keep the patient immobilized
    D. withhold medications
13. Depression is common with which of the following conditions (choose all that apply)
    A. pain
    B. widowhood
    C. urinary tract infection
    D. chronic illness
14. Which of the following is the main result of changes in pharmacokinetics and pharmacodynamics in the older patient?
    A. pain medications are not as effective
    B. medications last longer in the system increasing their effect
    C. lower blood levels of most medications
    D. increase in renal blood flow
15. The following pain medications should be avoided in the older patient (choose all that apply)
    A. opioids
    B. meperidine
    C. propoxyphene
    D. ketorolac
16. What symptom of delirium is often missed by health professionals?
    A. hyperactive
    B. quiet (hypoactive)
    C. combative
    D. restlessness
17. Which of the following can cause syncope and falls in the older adult
    A. orthostatic hypotension
    B. acetaminophen
    C. physical deconditioning
    D. poor glucose tolerance
18. Pain assessment in older patients can be complicated by which of the following? (choose all that apply)
    A. changes in cognition
    B. changes in sensory perception
    C. setting
    D. difficulty reporting symptoms

19. Monitoring the older trauma victim should include which of the following? (choose all that apply)
- **A.** oxygenation status
- **B.** hemodynamics
- **C.** level of consciousness
- **D.** tachycardia

20. Resuscitation should always be performed in the high-acuity area.
- **A.** True
- **B.** False

Posttest answers with rationale are found on MyNursingKit.

EXPLORE PEARSON **mynursingkit**™

MyNursingKit is your one stop for online chapter review materials and resources. Prepare for success with additional NCLEX®-style practice questions, interactive assignments and activities, web links, animations and videos, and more!

Register your access code from the front of your book at **www.mynursingkit.com.**

REFERENCES

Administration on Aging (AOA). (2007). *A Profile of Older Americans: 2007.* Retrieved April 15, 2008 from *http://www.aoa.gov/prof/Statistics/profile/profiles.asp.*

Alzheimer's Association. (2008). *Alzheimer's disease.* Retrieved May 10, 2008 from *http://www.alz.org/national/documents/topicsheet_alzdisease.pdf.*

American Heart Association. (2008). *Older Americans and Cardiovascular Diseases – Statistics.* Retrieved April 11, 2008 from *http://www.americanheart.org/presenter.jhtml?identifier53000936*

Angus, D.C., Kelley, M. A., Schmitz, R. J., White, A., Popovich, J., Jr., & the Committee on Manpower for Pulmonary and Critical Care. (2000). Current and projected workforce requirements for care of the critically ill and patients with pulmonary disease: can we meet the requirements of an aging population? *Journal of the American Medical Association,* 284 (21), 2726–2770.

Baird, M., Keen, J., & Swearingen, P. (2005). *Manual of critical care nursing,* 5th ed. St. Louis: Elsevier.

Balas, M. C., Casey, C. M., & Happ, M. B. (2008). Comprehensive assessment and management of the critically ill. In E. Capezuti, D. Zwicker, M. Mezey, T. Fulmer (eds.) *Evidence-based geriatric nursing protocols for best practice.* 3rd ed. New York: Springer.

Bergstrom, N., Braden, B. J., Laguzza, A., & Holman, V. (1987). The Braden Scale for predicting pressure sore risk. *Nursing Research,* 36(4), 201–210.

Bergstrom, N. & Braden B. J. (2002). Predictive validity of the Braden Scale among black and white subjects. *Nursing Research,* 51(6), 398–403.

Borson, S., Scanlan, J., Brush, M., Vitallano, P., & Dokmak, A. (2000). The Mini-Cog: A cognitive 'vital signs' measure for dementia screening in multi-lingual elderly. *International Journal of Geriatric Psychiatry,* 15(11), 1021–1027.

Cacchione, P. Z. (2008). Sensory changes. In E. Capezuti, D. Zwicker, M. Mezey, T. Fulmer (eds.) *Evidence-based geriatric nursing protocols for best practice.* 3rd ed. New York: Springer.

Campbell, J. W. (2007). Thyroid Disorders. In R. J. Ham, P. D. Sloane, G. A. Warshaw, M. A. Bernard, & E. Flaherty (eds.) *Primary care geriatrics: a case-based approach.* Philadelphia: Mosby.

CDC (Centers for Disease Control and Prevention). (2003a). *Guidelines for preventing health-care-associated pneumonia: recommendations of CDC and the Healthcare Infection Control Practices Advisory Committee (HICPAC).* Retrieved March 3, 2008 from *www.cdc.gov/ncidod/hip/pneumonia/default.htm.*

CDC (Centers for Disease Control and Prevention). (2006). *Trends in causes of death among older persons in the United States.* Retrieved June 5, 2008 from *http://www.cdc.gov/nchs/data/ahcd/agingtrends/06olderpersons.pdf.*

CDC (Centers for Disease Control and Prevention). (2007a). *Diabetes Surveillance System,* Data and Trends. Retrieved June 24, 2008 from *http://www.cdc.gov/ diabetes/Statistics/prev/national/figpersons.htm.*

CDC (Centers for Disease Control and Prevention). (2007b). *Health-related behaviors.* Retrieved May 21, 2008 from *http://www.cdc.gov/aging/info.htm.*

CDC (Centers for Disease Control and Prevention). (2008). *Recommended Adult Immunization Schedule—United States, October 2007–September 2008.* Retrieved May 21, 2008 from *www.cdc.gov/mmwr/pdf/wk/mm5641-Immunization.pdf.*

Connolly, M. J. (2003). Age-related changes in the respiratory system. In R. J. Tallis & H. M. Fillit (Eds). *Brocklehurst's Textbook of Geriatric Medicine and Gerontology.* London: Churchill Livingstone.

Creditor, M.C. (1993). Hazards of hospitalization of the elderly. *Annals of Internal Medicine,* 118(3), 219–223.

Criddle, L.M. (2009). Caring for the critically ill elderly patient. In K.K. Carlson (ed.). *AACN: Advanced Critical Care Nursing,* (pp. 1372–1400). St. Louis: Saunders/Elsevier.

Dar, O., & Cowie, M.R. (2008). Acute heart failure in the intensive care unit: epidemiology. *Critical Care Medicine, 35*(1), S3–8.

Dawson, K. S. (2008). Palliative care for critically ill older adults. *Critical Care Nursing Quarterly, 31*(1): 19–23.

DeFrances, C. J. & Hall, M. J. (2004). *National Hospital Discharge Survey: advance data from vital and health statistics* (No. 324). Hyattsville, MD: National Center for Health Statistics.

Dellinger, R. P., Levy, M. M., Carlet, J. M., Bion, J., Parker, M. M., Jaeschke, R., Reinhart, K., Angus, D. C., Crun-Buisson, C., Beale, R., Calandra, T., Dhainaut, J., Gerlach, H., Harvey, M., Marini, J. J., Marshall, J., Ranieri, M., Ramsay, G., Sevransky, J., Thompson, T., Townsend, S., Vender, J. S., Zimmerman, and J. L. Vincent, J. (2008). Surviving sepsis campaign: international guidelines for management of severe sepsis and septic shock. *Critical Care Medicine,* 36, 296–327.

Ely, E. W., Inouye, S. K., Bernard, G. R. Gordon, S., Francis, J., Mey, L. et al., (2001). Delirium in mechanically ventilated patients: validity and reliability of the confusion assessment method for the intensive care unit (CAM-ICU). *Journal of the American Medical Association,* 286, 2701–2710.

Extermann, M., and Hurria, A. (2007). Comprehensive geriatric assessment of older patients with cancer. *Journal of Clinical Oncology, 25,* 1824–1831.

Ferrario, C. G. (2008). Geropharmacology: A primer for advanced practice acute care and critical care nurses, Part I. *AACN Advanced Critical Care, 19* (1):23–27.

Fick, D. M., Cooper, J. W., Wade, W. E., Waller, J. L., Maclean, J. R., & Beers, M. H. (2003). Updating the Beers criteria for potentially inappropriate medication use in older adults: results of a U.S. consensus panel of experts. *Archives of Internal Medicine,* 163, 2716–2724.

Fletcher, K. (2007). Optimizing reserve in hospitalized elderly. *Critical Care Nursing Clinics of North America, 19,* 285–302.

Girard, T. D., and Ely, E. W. (2007). Bacteremia and sepsis in older adults. *Clinics in Geriatric Medicine,* 23, 633–647.

Girard, T. D., Opal, S. M., and Ely, E. W. (2005). Insights into severe sepsis in older patients: from epidemiology to evidence-based management. *Aging and Infectious Diseases,* 40, 719–727.

Graf, C. (2006). Functional decline in hospitalized older adults. *American Journal of Nursing,* 106(1), 58–65.

Hendrich, A. L., Bender, P.S. & Nyhuuis, A. (2003). Validation of the Hendrich II Fall Risk Model: a large concurrent case/control study of hospitalized patients. *Applied Nursing Research,* 16(1), 9–21.

Hendrich, A., Nyhuuis, A., Kippenbrock, T., & Soga, M. E. (1996). Hospital falls: development of a predictive model for clinical practice. *Applied Nursing Research,* 8, 129–139.

Holzer, C. (2007). Perioperative care. In R. J. Ham, P. D. Sloane, G. A. Warshaw, M. A. Bernard, & E. Flaherty (eds.) *Primary care geriatrics: A case-based approach.* Philadelphia: Mosby.

Hooyman, N. R. & Kiyak, H. A. (2008). *Social gerontology: a multidisciplinary perspective,*. 8th ed. Boston: Allyn & Bacon.

Inouye, S. K., van Dyck, C. H., Alessi, C. A., Balkin, S. Siegal, A. P., & Horwitz, R. I. (1990). Clarifying confusion: the confusion assessment method. a new method for detection of delirium. *Annals of Internal Medicine,* 113(12), 941–948.

Institute of Medicine. (2008). *Retooling for an aging America: building the health care workforce.* National Academy of Sciences.

Kaarlola, A., Tallgren, M., & Pettila, V. (2006). Long-term survival, quality of life, and quality adjusted life-years among critically ill elderly patients. *Critical Care Medicine, 34*(8):2120–2126.

Kleinpell, R. (2007). Preface. *Critical Care Nursing Clinics of North America,* 19:ix–x.

Kurlowicz, L. H. & Harvath, T. A. (2008). Depression. In E. Capezuti, D. Zwicker, M. Mezey, T. Fulmer, D. Gray-Miceli, & M. Klugers (Eds.), (3rd ed., pp. 57–82). *Evidence-Based Geriatric Nursing Protocols for Best Practice,* 3rd ed. New York: Springer Publishing.

Linton, A. D. (2007a). Integument system. In A. D. Linton & H. W. Lach (eds.). *Matteson and McConnells' gerontological nursing: concepts and practice.* St. Louis: Saunders/Elsevier.

Linton, A. D. (2007b). Gastrointestinal system. In A. D. Linton & H. W. Lach (eds.). *Matteson and McConnells' gerontological nursing: concepts and practice.* St. Louis: Saunders/Elsevier.

Linton, A. D. (2007c). Genitourinary system. In A. D. Linton & H. W. Lach (eds). *Matteson and McConnells' gerontological nursing: concepts and practice.* St. Louis: Saunders/Elsevier.

Margolis, S. A. & Reed, R. L. (2007). Thyroid disorders. In R. J. Ham, P. D. Sloane, G. A. Warshaw, M. A. Bernard, & E. Flaherty (eds.). *Primary care geriatrics: a case-based approach.* Philadelphia: Mosby.

Maslow, K., & Mezey, M. (2008). Recognition of dementia in hospitalized older adults. *American Journal of Nursing,* 108(1), 40–49.

Meiner, S. E. and Lueckenotte, A.G. (2006). *Gerontologic nursing,* 3rd ed. St.Louis: Mosby/Elsevier.

Merrill, C. T. & Elixhauser, A. (2005). *Hospitalization in the United States, 2002: HCUP fact book no. 6.* Rockville, MD: AHRQ.

Mion, L. C., Halliday, B. L., & Sandhu, S. K. (2008). Physical restraints and side rails in acute and critical care setting: Legal, ethical and practice issues. In E. Capezuti, D. Zwicker, M. *Evidence-Based Geriatric Nursing Protocols for Best Practice,* 3rd ed. New York: Springer.

Mion, L., Minnick, A., Leipzig, R., Catrambone, C., & Johnson, M. (2007). Patient-initiated device removal in intensive care units: a national prevalence study. *Critical Care Medicine,* 35(12), 2714–2720.

Moore, S. M. and Duffy, E. (2007). Maintaining vigilance to promote best outcomes for hospitalized elders. *Critical Care Nursing Clinics of North America,* 19:313–319.

Morse, J. M., Morse, R. M., Tylko, S. J. (1989). Development of a scale to identify the fall-prone patient. *Canadian Journal on Aging,* 8(4), 366–367

Nakasato, Y. (2007). Arthritis and related disorders. In R. J. Ham, P. D. Sloane, G. A. Warshaw, M. A. Bernard, & E. Flaherty (eds.) *Primary care geriatrics: A case-based approach.* Philadelphia: Mosby.

National Institute on Aging. (2007). *Alzheimer's disease fact sheet.* Retrieved May 20, 2008 from *http://www.nia.nih.gov/Alzheimers/Publications/adfact.htm.*

National Institute on Aging. (2006). *65+ in the United States: 2005.* Retrieved April 25, 2008 from *http://www.census.gov/prod/2006pubs/p23-209.pdf.*

Nau, K. C., & Congdon, H. B. 02007). Diabetes mellitus. In R. J. Ham, P. D. Sloane, G. A. Warshaw, M. A. Bernard, & E. Flaherty (eds.). *Primary care geriatrics: A case-based approach.* Philadelphia: Mosby.

New York University. (2008). Try This Series. Last accessed June 5, 2008.

Neyhart, B. (2007). Osteoporosis. In R. J. Ham, P. D. Sloane, G. A. Warshaw, M. A. Bernard, & E. Flaherty (eds.). *Primary care geriatrics: a case-based approach.* Philadelphia: Mosby.

Peterson, J. F., Pun, B. T., Dittus, R. S., Thomason, J. W. W., Jackson, J. C., Shintani, A. K., & Ely, E. Wesley. (2006). Delirium and its motoric subtypes: a study of 614 critical patients. *Journal of the American Geriatrics Society,* 54, 479–484.

Pleis, J. R., & Lethbridge-Cejku, M. (2007). *Summary health statistics for U. S. adults: national health interview survey,* 2006. Hyattsville, MD: NCHS.

Prevention Plus. (2001). Accessed 6/5/20008 @ www.bradenscale.com.

Reddy. M., Gill, S. S., and Rochon, P. A. (2006). Preventing pressure ulcers: a systematic review. *Journal of American Medical Association,* 296, 974–984.

Resnick, B. (2007). Nurse competence in aging: from dream to reality. *Geriatric Nursing,* 28(6S) 7–8.

Rosborough, D. (2006). Cardiac surgery in elderly patients: strategies to optimize outcomes. *Critical Care Nurse,* 26(5): 24–31.

Rosenthal, R. A. and Kavic, S. M. (2004). Assessment and management of the geriatric patient. *Critical Care Medicine,* 32(4): S92–S105.

Sheikh, V. I. & Yesavage, V. A. (1986). Geriatric Depression Scale: recent evidence and development of a shorter version. In T. L. Brink (ed.). *Clinical Gerontology: a guide to assessment and intervention* (pp. 165–174). New York: Haworth.

Smith, C. M. and Cotter, V. (2008). In E. Capezuti, D. Zwicker, M. Mezey, T. Fulmer (eds.). *Evidence-based geriatric nursing protocols for best practice.* 3rd ed. New York: Springer.

Stotts, N. A. and Horng-Shiuann, W. (2007). Hospital recovery is facilitated by prevention of pressure ulcers in older adults. *Critical Care Nursing Clinics of North America, 19*:269–275.

Urden, L. D., Stacy, K. M., and Lough, M. E. (2006). *Thelan's critical care nursing; diagnosis and management,* 5th ed. Mosby: St. Louis:Mosby/Elsevier.

Yesavage, J. A., Brink, T. L., Rose, T. L., Lum, O., Huang, V., Adey, M., & Leirer, V. O. (1983). Development and validation of a geriatric depression screening scale: a preliminary report. *Journal of Psychiatric Research,* 17, 37–49.

Young, J., & Inouye, S. K. (2007). Delirium in older people. *British Medical Journal,* 334, 842–846.

MODULE

4 Acute Pain in the High-Acuity Patient

Donna Jarzyna, Kathleen Dorman Wagner, Jill Arzouman

OBJECTIVES Following completion of this module, the learner will be able to

1. Identify the basic physiology involved in the transmission of pain.
2. Explain the multifaceted nature of pain.
3. Describe potential sources and effects of pain.
4. Discuss pain assessment.
5. Describe effective management of pain for the high-acuity patient.
6. Discuss issues related to the undertreatment of pain.
7. Identify considerations associated with pain management in special populations.
8. Discuss the nursing management of patients undergoing conscious/moderate sedation.

The focus of this module is on the concept of acute pain rather than chronic pain. The module is composed of eight sections. Section One provides a brief discussion of the physiology involved in the transmission of pain. Section Two defines acute pain and presents a multifaceted model of pain. Section Three discusses potential sources of pain and the effects of pain on the body. Section Four presents a variety of pain assessment tools, including unidimensional and multidimensional assessment tools. Sections Five, Six, and Seven focus on the management of pain. Information covered in these sections includes pharmacologic and nonpharmacologic approaches to pain management, reasons for undertreatment of acute pain, and special considerations regarding pain management in special patient populations. Finally, Section Eight presents an overview of conscious (moderate) sedation as it applies to the high-acuity patient. Each section includes a set of review questions to help the learner evaluate his or her understanding of the section's content before moving on to the next section. All Section Reviews include answers. It is suggested that the learner review those concepts answered incorrectly in the review questions before proceeding to the next section.

Author's Note: The Agency for Health Care Policy and Research (AHCPR) developed federal guidelines in 1992 and 1994 for "Acute Pain Management: Operative or Medical Procedures and Trauma". This was a remarkable initiative. The guidelines were developed by an independent multidisciplinary panel of experts whose recommendations were based primarily on the published scientific data available at the time. The wisdom and philosophy of these guidelines provide the direction for the standard of care today. Although comprehensive and generically intact, the guidelines no longer reflect the state of current medical and nursing research relevant to pain. The National Guideline Clearinghouse is now available as a public resource for more current evidence based guidelines.

PRETEST

1. The five types of sensory receptors include (choose all that apply)
   A. chemoreceptors
   B. nociceptors
   C. thermoreceptors
   D. odoreceptors
2. The A nerve fibers have which of the following characteristics?
   A. myelinated
   B. primitive
   C. transmit slowly
   D. transmit aching sensations
3. Acute persistent pain is associated with
   A. a short duration
   B. a rapid healing process
   C. chronic pain conditions
   D. a distinct organic pathology
4. A second-degree burn on the arm is an example of what type of noxious stimulus?
   A. thermal
   B. physiologic
   C. chemical
   D. mechanical

5. When the stress response becomes too high, it is associated with which physiologic changes? (choose all that apply)
   A. organ hypoperfusion
   B. enhanced hormone function
   C. increased vascular shunting
   D. elevated blood endorphin levels
6. The clinician would anticipate a masking of the sympathetic symptoms of pain by increased parasympathetic response under which of the following circumstances?
   A. fractured ribs
   B. leg amputation
   C. injury to the bowel
   D. severe pneumonia
7. If a patient is mildly confused, the nurse should initially try to assess pain using
   A. vital signs
   B. self-report
   C. facial expression
   D. body posturing
8. A major weakness of multidimensional tools is that
   A. the nurse performs the assessment
   B. they measure only pain intensity
   C. the patient must comprehend the vocabulary
   D. they are unable to measure degree of anxiety
9. Which of the following statements is correct regarding nonopioid therapy?
   A. nonopioids have more severe side effects than opioids
   B. nonopioids are harder to access than opioids
   C. nonopioids can manage pain as effectively as opioids
   D. combining opioids with nonopioids enhances analgesia effectiveness
10. The most common route used for patient-controlled analgesia (PCA) is
    A. intramuscular
    B. intravenous
    C. subcutaneous
    D. epidural
11. Which of the following statements is correct regarding opioid use and respiratory depression?
    A. respiratory depression precedes onset of sedation
    B. respiratory depression worsens as tolerance develops
    C. sedation occurs before respiratory depression
    D. respiratory depression is a common problem in hospitalized patients
12. Accumulation of morphine metabolites in the blood secondary to renal dysfunction can cause
    A. seizures
    B. tachycardia
    C. central nervous system (CNS) stimulation
    D. severe respiratory depression
13. Elderly patients have fewer endogenous receptors and neural transmitters than younger patients. The primary clinical significance of this statement is
    A. pain relief using opioids is less effective
    B. pain relief using opioids is more unpredictable
    C. smaller doses of opioids are required to achieve pain relief
    D. larger doses of opioids are required to achieve pain relief
14. When managing acute pain in a patient with a history of chronic pain and tolerance to opioids, it is most effective to
    A. Discontinue the patient's home medication and change to intravenous medication.
    B. Focus on the use of adjuvant medication since the patient is tolerant to opioids.
    C. Continue the patient's home opioid dose as a baseline dose and titrate a short acting opioid or IV opioid to treat the acute pain.
    D. Convert the patient's home dose to an IV equianalgesic dose and infuse continuously.
15. The hierarchy for assessment of pain in the cognitively impaired adult based on the ASPMN Position Statement published in 2006 includes the following categories in which order? (Correctly reorder the four categories below.)
    A. behavioral assessment of pain behaviors
    B. patient self report
    C. surrogate report
    D. assume pain is present when a pathological condition exists that would create pain
16. Conscious sedation is classified as which level of sedation on the American Society of Anesthesiologist's sedation-analgesia continuum?
    A. Level 1
    B. Level 2
    C. Level 3
    D. Level 4
17. The major purpose of conscious sedation is which of the following?
    A. to decrease anxiety in high-acuity patients
    B. to sedate the patient to decrease oxygen consumption
    C. to tolerate uncomfortable procedures without altering respiratory and cardiovascular function
    D. to reduce level of consciousness in patients who are receiving a neuromuscular blockade drug concurrently

Pretest answers are found on MyNursingKit.

SECTION ONE: Pain Physiology – A Review

At the completion of this section, the learner will be able to identify the physiology involved in the transmission of pain.

A review of pain sensory receptors and their pathways is presented to provide a basic understanding of the assessment and management of the patient in acute pain. A description of the transmission of pain impulses is presented to provide a foundation for understanding the numerous problems involved in the effective management of pain.

The three major types of pain are *somatic pain,* which arises from stimulation of receptors in the skin, muscle, joints, and tendons; *visceral pain,* which arises from stimulation of receptors in the viscera; and *neuropathic pain,* which is due to abnormal signal processing in the nervous system. Sensory stimuli, such as cold, heat, touch, and pain, are communicated to the nervous system through sensory receptors. There are five types of sensory receptors, each one with the ability to detect changes in a specific type of sensory input (Table 4–1). Sensory receptors require a certain level of excitation (called the threshold) before they will transmit input. Once the sensory threshold has been achieved, the nerve fiber is stimulated and the impulse travels the length of the associated sensory nerve (Guyton & Hall, 2006b).

Pain Nerve Fibers

The nerves that carry pain impulses are categorized in terms of their size and whether a myelin sheath is present. Nerves termed *A beta fibers* are large in diameter and have a **myelin sheath.** *A delta fibers* are small in diameter and are also myelinated. *C fibers* are small in diameter and are usually unmyelinated. Impulses are conducted more quickly over large, myelinated nerves in comparison to small or unmyelinated nerves. For example, A delta fibers conduct impulses rapidly. Sharp, pinprick-like pain is conducted along these fibers. C fibers, however, have a slow conduction rate and transmit aching, throbbing sensations.

Pain Transmission

Pain impulses initiated at receptor sites are transmitted to the brain along multiple pathways. A major dual pathway consists of the neospinothalamic tract and paleospinothalamic tract.

TABLE 4–1 Sensory Receptors

RECEPTOR	FUNCTION
Pain receptors (nociceptors)	Detection of tissue damage
Thermoreceptors	Detection of temperature changes
Electromagnetic receptors	Detection of light on eye retina
Chemoreceptors	Detection of smell, taste, concentration of arterial blood oxygen and carbon dioxide, and others
Mechanoreceptors	Detection of mechanical changes in cells adjacent to receptors (e.g., position and tactile senses)

An example of this dual pathway is as follows: A delta pain fibers primarily transmit thermal and mechanical pain through the neospinothalamic tract. The theory underlying the A delta route of transmission is that pain impulses travel along first-order neurons to the dorsal horn of the spinal cord, terminating primarily in the lamina marginalis. Upon reaching the lamina marginalis in the dorsal horn, the impulse excites second-order neurons and immediately crosses to the opposite side of the spinal cord. The impulse then ascends through the brain stem to the thalamus, where it is consciously acknowledged. From the thalamus it travels to the cerebral cortex, where analysis of pain quality takes place. The slower-transmitting C fibers travel along a cruder, more primitive pain pathway, the paleospinothalamic tract, which primarily terminates in a broad area of the brain stem, with less than a quarter of the fibers passing on through to the thalamus (Smith, 2003).

Sensitization

Pain transmission is a complex process. Both the peripheral and the central nervous system can be sensitized to persistent stimulation.

Peripheral Sensitization

Injury activates the peripheral nervous system by the release of a variety of inflammatory mediators. With continuing input, high threshold mechanoreceptors are sensitized to a lower threshold of pain and adjacent receptors are recruited for pain transmission resulting in increased input to the central nervous system.

Central Sensitization

Persistent exposure to peripheral input at the spinal nerves results in overresponsiveness to the usual stimuli and sensitization at the central nervous system as well. Persistent central pain can result in **neuroplasticity** (actual changes in the structure and function of the spinal segment of the nervous system), creating long-term changes in the cell's response to stimuli. This can lead to the development of chronic pain syndromes (de Leon-Casasola, 2006).

Endogenous Analgesia System

Although the transmission of the impulse along the spinothalamic pathways appears relatively simple and straightforward, the process is complex. Guyton and Hall (2006a) explain that the body has its own analgesia system that significantly influences how each person reacts to pain. There are three components to this system (in order of their location in the CNS): (1) the periventricular and periaqueductal gray (PAG) areas, located in the third ventricle, hypothalamus, and upper brain stem; (2) the raphe magnus nucleus, located in the brain stem; and (3) the pain inhibitory complex, located in the spinal cord's dorsal horns. Stimulation of the PAG or raphe magnus nucleus causes significant suppression of extremely strong pain signals that

TABLE 4–2 Endogenous Opiates

GROUP	PRIMARY LOCATION	COMMENTS
Enkephalins	Spinal cord and brain stem	Most widely distributed in body Effects last minutes to hours Serotonin causes enkephalin release at dorsal horn
Beta-endorphins	Hypothalamus and pituitary gland	Most like morphine
Dynorphins	Spinal cord and brain stem	Present in minute quantities Extremely powerful (perhaps 200 times more powerful than morphine)

Data from Guyton & Hall (2006).

are coming in through the dorsal spinal roots. Pain signals that primarily stimulate the periventricular and PAG areas are suppressed, but to a lesser degree. Pain signals that are blocked by the pain inhibitory complex in the spinal cord are suppressed at that level and may not be transmitted on to the brain.

The analgesia system secretes special pain-modulating neurotransmitters that influence pain impulses at various stages of transmission. These endogenously produced analgesic substances are called endogenous opioid peptides. When these substances are released, they bind to special receptor sites along the ascending pain pathway and modify the pain transmission. Three types of endogenous opioid peptides have been identified as enkephalins, beta-endorphins, and dynorphins. These substances modulate pain transmission in response to specific physiologic events, such as pain and stress (Curtis et al., 2002; Smith, 2003; Hawthorn & Redmond, 1998; Way et al., 2001). Table 4–2 provides a brief summary of the endogenous opioid peptides.

In addition, theorists Melzack and Wall (1965), in their classic work on pain mechanisms, contended that the substantia gelatinosa acts as a gate for pain impulses. Whether the gate is open (allowing impulses to continue along the pain pathway) or closed depends on whether large-fiber firing or small-fiber firing predominates. Large-fiber firing causes the gate to close, whereas small-fiber firing opens the gate.

SECTION ONE REVIEW

1. The five types of sensory receptors include (choose all that apply)
   A. odoreceptors
   B. nociceptors
   C. thermoreceptors
   D. chemoreceptors
2. Which of the following characteristics are associated with type A nerve fibers?
   A. myelinated
   B. primitive
   C. transmit slowly
   D. transmit aching sensations
3. Pain is analyzed in which part of the brain?
   A. cerebellum
   B. thalamus
   C. cerebral cortex
   D. brain stem
4. When pain is suppressed at the pain inhibitory complex, it
   A. moves on to the PAG
   B. is blocked at the spinal cord level
   C. transfers to the raphe magnus nucleus
   D. is ultimately suppressed in the hypothalamus
5. The neospinothalamic pain pathway terminates in the
   A. cerebral cortex
   B. brain stem
   C. dorsal horns
   D. substantia gelatinosa
6. The paleospinothalamic tract
   A. is the primary pain pathway
   B. terminates throughout the brain stem
   C. transmits signals to specific sensory areas
   D. transmits signals identically to the fast pathway

Answers: 1. (B, C, D), 2. A, 3. C, 4. B, 5. A, 6. B

SECTION TWO: The Multifaceted Nature of Pain

At the completion of this section, the learner will be able to explain the multiple facets of pain.

A Working Definition of Acute Pain

McCaffery has defined **pain** as "whatever the experiencing person says it is, existing whenever the experiencing person says it does" (McCaffery & Pasero, 1999, p. 17). The AHCPR Guidelines

(1992, p. 95) state that pain is "an unpleasant sensory and emotional experience associated with actual or potential tissue damage or described in terms of such damage." The complexity of pain is described in the following definition: "Pain is the resulting product of cellular, molecular, genetic, physiologic, psychologic, and social factors processing the signal to create the circumstances that a person designates as pain" (Lamberg, 1998, p. 122). The commonality of all definitions remains, that pain is a subjective experience and that there is no test to prove its presence. The patient's report of pain must be believed; although pain is subjective, it is real to that patient.

Acute pain has been defined as pain that is continually changing and transient. It is accompanied by a high level of emotional and autonomic nervous system arousal and is usually associated with tissue pathology or surgery. It can be further divided into two types—brief acute pain (short duration, minutes to days) and acute persistent pain (longer duration, weeks to months). Acute persistent pain is primarily associated with a distinct organic pathology and a slow healing process (Chapman & Syrjala, 1990). Acute pain serves a major protective function by acting as an early warning system of impending or actual tissue injury and typically diminishes as the injury heals.

A Multifaceted Model of Pain

Loeser and Cousins (1990) propose that pain is multifaceted and composed of nociception, pain, suffering, and pain behaviors. Only the outermost facet, pain behaviors, can be observed by someone other than the person experiencing the pain. The other three facets are completely personal and can only be inferred by another person. The relative contribution of each of the four facets to the pain experience is variable. Each facet is present to some degree in any pain experience. This multifaceted model of pain remains useful to describe the pain experience. Special problems that impact the psychological aspect of pain are uncertainty of diagnosis, the degree of success in management or control of pain, the impact of pain on daily activities, and the projected future course of pain (Main, Spanswick, 2000). In general, the noxious stimulus and the process of nociception predominate during acute pain.

Noxious (pain causing) stimuli may be mechanical, thermal, or chemical, and they have the potential to excite pain receptors. These stimuli must exist in sufficient quantities to trigger the release of biochemical mediators that activate the pain response (nociception). Activation of the pain response may also be triggered

- In response to what would typically be defined as nonnoxious stimuli;
- In response to sympathetic discharge (sympathetically maintained pain); or
- Spontaneously.

The First Facet: Nociception

Nociception refers to the activation of pain receptors called **nociceptors** and the pain pathway by a noxious stimulus of sufficient strength to threaten tissue integrity. Under normal circumstances, it leads to the sensation of pain. Acute pain is primarily of nociceptive origin. Nociception does not, however, always lead to pain. Certain factors or conditions can alter or eliminate the sensation of pain even when the person is subjected to extremely noxious stimuli. Such factors include severe nerve damage (spinal cord injury, peripheral neuropathy), anesthesia, and strong analgesia therapy. Pain can also occur without nociception, and may be found in patients with neuropathic pain and other chronic pain conditions (Loeser & Cousins, 1990).

The Second Facet: Pain

According to Loeser and Cousins (1990), pain "is the perception of a noxious stimulus dependent upon events in the neurons of the spinal cord and brain stem" (p. 179). A person can perceive pain only when transmission of the noxious stimulus terminates within the brain. It is unknown whether the patient's ability to perceive pain remains intact when cortical function is compromised or when cortical function has been chemically altered by sedative-hypnotics. It is clear that the negative physiologic outcomes related to the activation of the body's stress response occur regardless of whether the patient perceives pain at the cortical level.

The Third Facet: Suffering

The multifaceted model describes the term *suffering* as a negative affective response that is generated in the higher nervous centers of the brain. It further states that suffering can be caused by pain or a variety of situations such as stress, anxiety, fear, loss of a loved one, and depression. The concept of suffering seems closely connected to the personal meaning of the pain. The clinician's objective assessment of suffering is restricted to observing for the presence or absence of pain behaviors. According to Loeser and Cousins (1990), suffering is particularly associated with chronic pain. The complex concept of suffering has received increased attention over the past decade, and there is a growing body of literature in this area.

The Fourth Facet: Pain Behaviors

It is no coincidence that the outside circle of the multifaceted model of pain is pain behavior. **Pain behavior** refers to a person's physical reaction to the conscious perception of pain; it is what leads the observer to conclude that pain is being experienced. There are two types of pain behaviors: those that are intended to communicate pain (pain-expressing behaviors) and those that are intended to lessen or control the pain (pain-controlling behaviors). Common pain-expressing behaviors include groaning, rubbing the painful part, or lying motionless. It is often difficult for the observer to differentiate pain-controlling from pain-expressing behaviors. For example, rubbing or massaging the painful part may be a means of moderating the sensory input (pain-controlling behavior) rather than a means of communicating (expressing) the pain to others. Pain behaviors are discussed further in Section Four, "Pain Assessment."

SECTION TWO REVIEW

1. Acute persistent pain is associated with
   A. a short duration
   B. a rapid healing process
   C. chronic pain conditions
   D. a distinct organic pathology
2. A second-degree burn on the arm is an example of what type of noxious stimulus?
   A. thermal
   B. physiologic
   C. chemical
   D. mechanical
3. The activation of pain receptors and the pain pathway by a noxious stimulus of sufficient strength to threaten tissue integrity is known as
   A. acute pain
   B. suffering
   C. nociception
   D. neuropathy
4. Suffering is most commonly associated with which type of pain?
   A. acute
   B. persistent acute
   C. slow chronic
   D. intermittent
5. Behaviors that are intended to convey the presence of pain are called what type of pain behaviors?
   A. expressing
   B. heralding
   C. controlling
   D. communicating

Answers: 1. D, 2. A, 3. C, 4. C, 5. A

SECTION THREE: Acute Pain in the High-Acuity Patient

At the completion of this section, the learner will be able to discuss potential sources and effects of pain.

Potential Sources of Pain

High-acuity patients are at risk for brief acute, as well as, persistent acute types of pain. The initial insult requiring admission to the hospital is often linked to acute pain (e.g., traumatic injury, organ ischemia, surgical manipulation). In addition, high-acuity patients commonly have invasive lines and tubes inserted (e.g., chest tubes, intravenous lines, endotracheal and tracheostomy tubes), all of which irritate delicate tissues and cause varying degrees of pain. The patient may also be required to undergo painful procedures such as lumbar puncture or endoscopic examinations. Forced immobility because of the serious or critical nature of an illness and attachment to multiple tubes may exacerbate more chronic conditions, such as back or arthritic pain.

Acute pain is usually accompanied by some degree of anxiety, which may be further aggravated by the stress associated with the hospital or critical care environment. High-anxiety states are associated with an increase in pain perception and may decrease pain tolerance. Pain may also be a contributor to patient confusion and inadequate sleep.

The Effects of Stress and Pain on the Body

In the high-acuity patient, pain can result from a variety of sources, such as tissue injury, ischemia, metabolic or chemical mediators, inflammation, or muscle spasm. Pain is also affected by stress. The stress response is a crucial part of self-preservation. It initiates events that increase the body's chances of survival. When the body experiences a massive insult, however, the stress response can become too high, which can cause physiological changes that are associated with poor patient outcomes. A high-stress response increases vascular shunting, resulting in hypoperfusion of vital organs. It also increases serum levels of endogenous opioid peptides, which may result in counterregulation of hormonal responses. Tissue injury is a strong stress response stimulus. The acute pain created by injured tissue initially increases both hormonal and sympathetic nervous system responses. However, if the pain becomes prolonged, the sympathetic response to pain diminishes as a result of a parasympathetic rebound effect, which results in the vital signs returning more toward normal. This is an important consideration when assessing pain in the high-acuity patient. Although the sympathetic response is important to assess, reliance on it as the sole indicator of acute pain may significantly misrepresent the intensity of pain.

Patients experiencing moderate to high levels of pain are often at increased risk for developing stasis-related complications because of immobility. Pain is associated with a natural limiting of activity that encourages a person to rest and, therefore, aids in the healing process. This decrease in activity, however, is also associated with negative outcomes, such as pulmonary complications and deep-vein thrombosis (DVT). Pulmonary complications, such as atelectasis and stasis pneumonia, result from splinting that decreases spontaneous ventilatory movement and oxygenation. For example, pulmonary complications are frequently noted in patients who have had thoracic surgery, abdominal surgery, or trauma, and prolonged bedrest is a significant risk factor in the development of DVT. By decreasing the level of pain, patients may become more active earlier in their recovery period, thus significantly decreasing the risk of developing stasis complications.

SECTION THREE REVIEW

1. Which statement reflects the relationship between pain, stress, and anxiety?
   A. increased levels of stress and anxiety worsen pain
   B. increased levels of stress worsen pain but anxiety has no significant effect
   C. increased levels of anxiety worsen pain but stress has no significant effect
   D. there is no significant relationship between pain, stress, and anxiety
2. The stress response is
   A. an avoidable reaction
   B. a maladaptive response to crises
   C. a crucial part of self-preservation
   D. an unpredictable reaction to pain
3. When the stress response becomes too great, it is associated with which physiologic changes? (choose all that apply)
   A. organ hypoperfusion
   B. enhanced hormone function
   C. increased vascular shunting
   D. elevated blood endorphin levels
4. If acute pain is sustained for a prolonged period of time, the
   A. sympathetic response diminishes
   B. parasympathetic response diminishes
   C. pain threshold increases
   D. pain tolerance decreases

Answers: 1. A, 2. C, 3. (A, C, D), 4. A

SECTION FOUR: Pain Assessment

At the completion of this section, the learner will be able to discuss pain assessment in the high-acuity patient.

Pain is a complex, subjective, multidimensional response. The patient's self-report is the most reliable indicator of the existence and intensity of adult pain, and yet it has been shown that nurses' attitudes frequently alter the assessment by subjectively interpreting the patient's self-report of pain (McCaffery & Pasero, 1999; Stephenson, 1994). The use of objective pain assessment tools may improve the subjectivity of pain assessment. Young et al. (2006) found that the value nurses place on pain assessment tools is positively correlated with nursing education but not with years of nursing experience. Nursing education must emphasize the application of the nursing process if acute pain is to be managed effectively because pain is an ongoing process that requires continual reassessment and reevaluation using objective rather than subjective evaluation.

Pain levels vary in each individual primarily because of the biopsychological nature of pain. To manage pain effectively, it is essential to use self-report pain assessment tools whenever possible. These assessment tools help clinicians establish baseline criteria for evaluating pain and facilitate the development of appropriate comfort interventions. The ongoing challenge for caregivers and researchers is to find an effective alternative means of assessment for unconscious patients and other patients who for some reason cannot self-report their levels of pain (e.g., incoherent).

Pain History

The patient's pain history provides valuable information regarding preexisting pain experiences, treatment modalities, and medication history. In addition, it may also be used for obtaining information regarding the patient's usual pain behaviors and pain relief methods used at home. Knowledge of an individual's usual pain behaviors would be of particular value if the patient should lose the ability to communicate during hospitalization. Table 4–3 lists important information that can be obtained through a pain history.

TABLE 4–3 Pain History

Drug allergies
Prior acute pain experiences
Chronic pain problems—location? Description of pain? How often? For how long?
Activity level maintained during pain?
Any recent changes in usual pain/discomfort pattern?
How does the patient express pain at home (e.g., paces, lies motionless, cries, distraction, etc.)?
How does the pain make the person feel (e.g., sad, angry, frustrated, etc.)?
Usual relief measures: Drug therapy—which drug(s)? How much? How often? Level of relief? Nonpharmacologic—what type (e.g., hot water bottle, ice, heating pad, etc.)? Level of relief?

Unidimensional and Multidimensional Pain Assessment

Unidimensional pain assessment tools provide the patient with a means to rate a single pain dimension, such as pain intensity, affective distress, or the subjective meaning of the pain. When the specific cause of pain is apparent (e.g., postsurgical incisional pain), a unidimensional pain assessment tool is often considered sufficient. Unidimensional tools are especially useful in evaluating the effectiveness of interventions used to decrease the pain. These tools are simple to use and take little time to administer. Examples of unidimensional pain assessment tools include the Visual Analog Scale (VAS); the Numeric Rating Scale (NRS); and verbal descriptor scales, such as the Adjective Rating Scale (ARS). Unidimensional tools can also be used as part of a multidimensional pain assessment.

Multidimensional pain assessment tools provide the patient with a means to express the affective and evaluative aspects of the

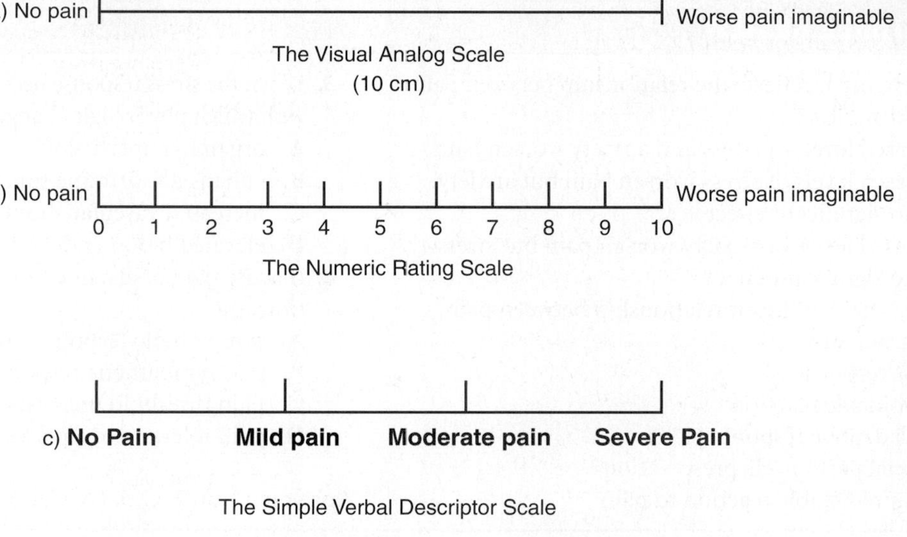

Figure 4–1 ■ Examples of undimensional pain assessment.

pain experience in addition to the sensory aspect. These tools work best for patients with more complex pain such as pain of unknown origin or chronic pain. Examples of multidimensional tools include the McGill Pain Questionnaire (MPQ) and the short-form McGill Pain Questionnaire (SF-MPQ), the Multidimensional Affect and Pain Survey (MAPS), and the Brief Pain Inventory (Mace, S., Ducharme, J., Murphy, M., 2006).

Unidimensional Pain Assessment

Visual Analog Scale (VAS). The VAS has been shown to be an effective measurement of pain intensity. There are several variations of the VAS. The most common is a horizontal or vertical line with one end labeled "no pain" and the opposite end labeled "worst pain imaginable." The patient self-reports the level of pain is along this line. The line is usually 10 cm in length. Once the patient has indicated the point on the scale that best represents the current level of pain, a centimeter ruler is placed on the scale and a numeric rating of 0 to 10 is given. On some VAS variations, a numeric scale is present on the reverse side, with a slide rule type of device for converting the VAS to a numeric score. Figure 4–1a illustrates an example of a VAS.

Numeric Rating Scale (NRS). The NRS (Fig. 4–1b) is a variation of the VAS. It uses a sequence of numbers from which the patient chooses. The most common use of the NRS is measurement of pain intensity based on a continuum of pain, with 0 being "no pain" and the extreme opposite number (5, 10, or 100) being the "worst pain imaginable." The most common and clinically proven NRS is the 0 to 10 scale. The NRS has also been used to rate numerically other dimensions of pain. An advantage of using the NRS is that the directions for using it have been translated into a variety of languages (McCaffery & Pasero, 1999; Herr et al., 2006; Dunwoody et al., 2005).

Verbal Descriptor Scales. As a unidimensional assessment tool, a verbal descriptor scale, such as the ARS, may be used to measure any of the pain dimensions. For example, as a sensory dimension measure, the scale might include a list of adjectives, such as sharp, cutting, and lacerating (from the MRQ, in Mace, Ducharme, & Murphy, 2006). Using this list of words, the patient is asked to choose the adjective that best describes his or her current pain. The words should reflect different levels of the dimension being measured. Using this type of tool has several potential disadvantages. First, careful choice of descriptor words is necessary if this type of scale is to be a useful pain assessment tool. Second, patients have a tendency to choose words from the middle of the scale rather than choosing from either end (Chapman & Syrjala, 1990). The Verbal Descriptor Scale (Fig. 4–1c) is a useful scale for use with older adults who are unable to rate their pain using the numeric rating scales (Herr et al., 2004).

Wong–Baker Faces Scale (Faces). The Faces Scale has been shown to be popular with both children and adults (Carey et al., 1997). It consists of six facial drawings ranging from smiling to crying. Each face is assigned a number from 0 to 5 or 0 to 10. The patient simply points to the face that represents his or her current level of pain. Directions for the Wong–Baker Faces Scale have also

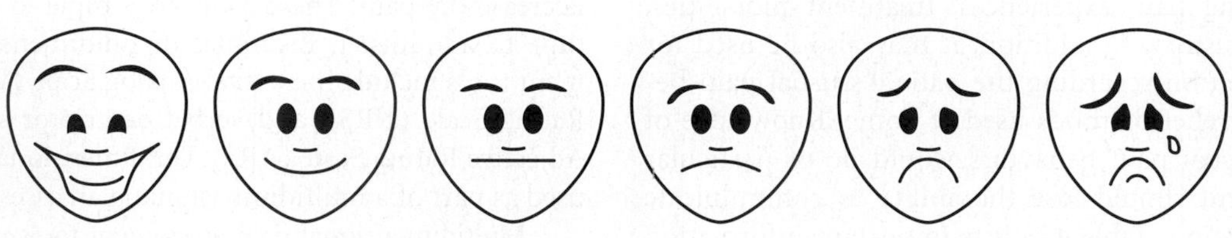

Figure 4–2 ■ Example of a faces pain scale.

been translated into a variety of languages (McCaffery & Pasero, 1999). Figure 4–2 shows an example of a faces scale. The faces scale "may trigger assessment of a broader concept of pain than pain intensity" (Herr et al., 2004, p 18), such as suffering or sadness.

Adapting the Unidimensional Pain Assessment Tool for the Severely Ill Patient

A patient who is extremely ill or weak may be able to use unidimensional tools with the nurse's assistance. For example, the nurse can run a pencil along a VAS and have the patient nod or indicate in some way where the "point" of pain is on the scale. Sometimes, the patient may be able to point to the number on an NRS or to the location on the line of a VAS that best indicates the intensity of pain. As an alternative, the patient may be able to raise the number of fingers that indicate the level of pain, with no fingers raised being "no pain" and 5 or 10 fingers raised being the "worst pain imaginable."

Nurses frequently assume that extreme illness, weakness, or mild confusion prevents the patient from being able to self-report pain. This is not necessarily true. Self-report methods should be attempted in this patient group even though it may require patience and flexibility on the part of the nurse. If the nurse is to be successful using these methods, brief but clear directions must be given and repeated as needed during the assessment procedure.

It has been shown that even when nurses use self-report tools, they rely more on their own nursing observations of behavioral cues in determining whether the patient is in pain (Ferrell et al., 1991). This may result in the nurse's applying a numeric value based on nursing observation and estimation of the patient's level of pain intensity (e.g., documenting a patient as rating a 5 out of 10 based strictly on nursing observation). This is an inappropriate use of the unidimensional self-report tools.

Both types of tools have strengths and limitations associated with their use. Table 4–4 summarizes the advantages and disadvantages of using unidimensional and multidimensional pain assessment tools. The clinician also should be aware that discrepancies may exist between the patient's self-reported level of pain and nurse-observed pain behaviors. For example, a patient may describe pain intensity as a 7 out of 10 while watching television or talking on the phone. This individual may be using coping skills that subjectively do not reflect high-pain scores. A patient's use of distraction and relaxation techniques can be misinterpreted as stoicism or exaggeration of self-reported pain levels (AHCPR, 1992).

TABLE 4–4 Advantages and Disadvantages of Pain Assessment Tools

UNIDIMENSIONAL TOOLS	
Advantages	**Disadvantages**
Provide baseline data	Measure only one dimension of the pain experience
Provide a means of comparing pre- and postintervention pain intensity	Unable to measure degree of anxiety or stress accompanying the pain
Provide a standardized method for assessment of pain intensity	Require relatively high cognitive level
Can be clearly documented and reported	Require some means of communication
Adaptable for patients who cannot verbalize	
Easy to perform	
Short assessment time	
MULTIDIMENSIONAL TOOLS	
Advantages	**Disadvantages**
Provide baseline data	Valid only if patient understands vocabulary
Provide a standardized method for assessment of pain	Long length of completion time (McGill Pain Questionnaire)
Can be clearly documented and reported	Require a high cognitive level
Assess multiple aspects of the pain experience	
Provide data for choosing nonpharmacologic interventions	
Adaptable for patients who cannot verbalize	

Multidimensional Pain Assessment

The most frequently used measurement of sensory and affective pain is the MPQ. This questionnaire measures four aspects of the pain experience: sensory, affective, evaluative, and miscellaneous. Each pain category is measured using a cluster of descriptive words. The patient's choice of words assists the clinician in determining which category the pain is originating from and aids the clinician in choosing a therapeutic pain regimen that is individualized to the patient's needs. The SF-MPQ is recommended for conscious patients in the critical care area. The SF-MPQ takes two to five minutes to administer. It is more practical for many high-acuity patients, assuming that vocabulary is not a problem and that the patient is functioning at a sufficiently high cognitive level. The words are simple and are understood by most patients. Administration of the SF-MPQ can be adjusted for patients who cannot communicate verbally (e.g., intubated patients) by having them either point to desired descriptive words or, if they are too weak, use a head nod when the nurse reads the desired descriptive word. In addition to the McGill tools, the clinician can develop a simple word list using words describing emotions and sensations that would be appropriate for a particular patient or patient population.

Assessment of Pain in the Adult with Altered Cognitive Status

High-acuity patients have many reasons for experiencing acute pain, and a significant number are at risk for undertreatment because of their inability to self-report pain. Many high-acuity patients have altered communication abilities for a variety of reasons, such as altered levels of consciousness and extreme weakness. Figure 4–3 is an example of an alternative pain assessment tool that has been developed by nurses for use with all patients.

University of Kentucky Hospital
Chandler Medical Center
Lexington, Kentucky

PAIN ASSESSMENT/MANAGEMENT FLOW SHEET

Addressograph

Date________ Use the following codes to document assessments of patients with c/o pain AND REASSESS these patients within a reasonable time frame following interventions.

Pain Rating Scales: 0/10 FACES FLACC Behavioral Other__________ Pain Management Goal: ______________________

Time	*Body Site (s)	*Description	*Pain Level before INTV	*Intervention(s)	*Pain Level after INTV	*Level of Arousal (S-4)	*Behavior Patterns	*SE from INTV	*Tx for SE	Comments: See Nsg Notes (Place check mark)	Nurse Initials
2400-0100											
0100-0200											
0200-0300											
0300-0400											
0400-0500											
0500-0600											
0600-0700											
0700-0800											
0800-0900											
0900-1000											
1000-1100											
1100-1200											
1200-1300											
1300-1400											
1400-1500											
1500-1600											
1600-1700											
1700-1800											
1800-1900											
1900-2000											
2000-2100											
2100-2200											
2200-2300											
2300-2400											

Codes

Body Sites

A=Abdomen
C=Chest
F=Face
H=Head
J=Jaw
N=Neck
A=Arm (R or L)
L=Leg (R or L)
T=Throat
UB=Upper Back
LB=Lower Back
Other: ________

Description

A=Ache
B=Burning
D=Dull
P=Pressure
S=Sharp
St=Stabbing
T=Throbbing

Pediatrics:
O="Owie" or "boo=boo"
H="Hurt"
Other: ________

Level of Arousal

S=Sleeping, Easily Aroused
1=Awake & Alert
2=Occasionally Drowsy
3=Freq. Drowsy, drifts off to sleep easily
4=Somnolent, Minimal or No Response to Stimuli

Interventions (INTV)

D=Distraction
GI=Guided Imagery
H=Heat
M=Massage
Med=Medication (see MAR of PCA sheet)
R=Reposition
Rel=Relaxation
T=Teaching (i.e., PCA use)

Pediatrics:
C=Cuddling or holding
Mu=Music
NP=Non-pharmacologic (i.e., bubbles, pinwheel, etc.)
P=Play

Behavior Patterns

A=Anxious
G=Grimacing
P=Peaceful, Calm, Restful
R=Restless, Thrashing
I=Inconsolable
U=Unnoticeable
APP=Assumed pain present
Other: ________

Side Effects (SE)

C=Confusion
I=Itching
N=Nausea
R=Resp. Depression
U=Urinary Retention
V=Vomiting

Treatment of SE

A=Med Adjustment
C=In & Out Catheter
F=Foley Catheter
Med=Medication
S=Safety Measures
Other: ________

Signature	Initials	Signature	Initials	Signature	Initials
Signature	Initials	Signature	Initials	Signature	Initials

8/02

Figure 4–3 ■ Pain assessment/management flow sheet. (Adapted from "Pain assessment/management flow sheet," developed by Pain Committee (2003). University Hospital, University of Kentucky.)

Visual Analog Scale

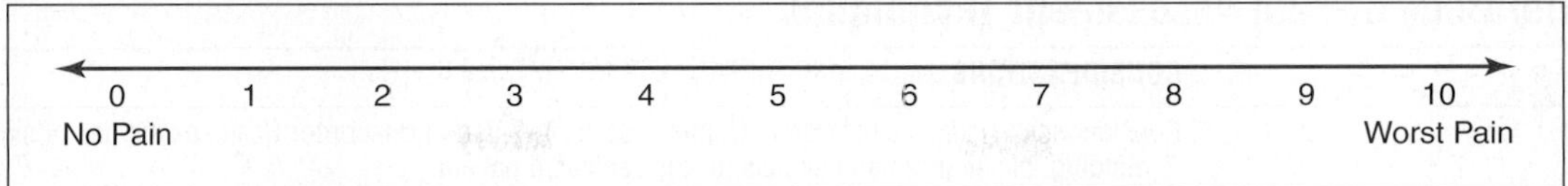

Faces Pain Rating Scale

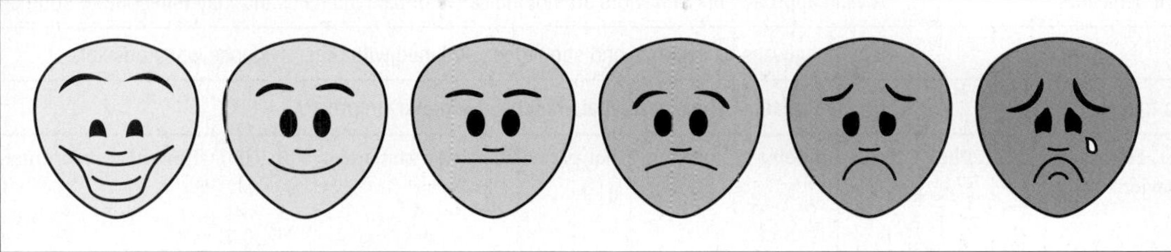

Descriptive Scale

No Pain	Mild	Moderate	Severe	Excruciating

Behavioral Observation Scale

Observed Behavior	0	1	2
Restlessness	Calm, cooperative	Slightly restless, consolable	Very restless, agitated, inconsolable
Muscle tension	Relaxed	Slight tenseness	Extreme tenseness
Facial expression	No frowning or grimacing, composed	Slight frowning or grimacing	Constant frowning or grimacing
Vocalization	Normal tone, no sound	Groans, moans, cries out in pain	Cries out, sobs
Wound guarding	No negative response to wound	Reaching/gently touching wound	Grabbing vigorously at wound

Behavioral Observation Scale Directions

- This scale can be used with very young children and patients who are unable to speak because of injury, mental status, medications, or treatment.
- Assess each of the areas identified in the Observed Behavior column, rating each behavior using the 0, 1, or 2 rating. Add the ratings together for each observed behavior.
- Assign a numerical score to the designated observations.
- Record the score on the pain assessment record or designated place on the documentation sheet.
- A low score indicates a low or acceptable level of pain and a high score (maximum score = 10) indicates the most pain.

Figure 4–4 ■ Pain assessment tools. (Adapted from "Pain assessment tools," developed by Pain Committee (2003). University Hospital, University of Kentucky.)

Figure 4–4 shows the various pain scales that accompany this tool including a 10-point behavioral pain scale, which is used for vulnerable patients, such as those in critical care settings. It is used with any adult who is unable to self-report pain level.

Patients who cannot communicate their pain rely on the nurse to advocate and intervene for them. Examples of such patients are those who are ventilated and sedated or those whose cognitive status precludes a report of pain such as the older adult with dementia. The negative patient outcomes created by the physiologic stress response to pain occur despite the inability of the patient to cognitively interpret the meaning of a painful event and possibly even to communicate the level of pain being experienced.

Review of the patient's medical history provides information on chronic pain conditions, routine home medications or non-drug interventions currently being utilized by the patient for painful conditions (e.g., application of heat or cold, wears a brace). The omission of acetaminophen, muscle relaxants, or agents being used for neuropathic pain such as anticonvulsants or tricyclic antidepressants could have a distressful outcome in terms of increased pain or even withdrawal. The American

TABLE 4–5 Hierarchy of Pain Assessment Techniques

ACTION	CONSIDERATIONS
Self-report	Consider scales such as the Verbal Numeric Scale, The Verbal Descriptor Scale, or the use of signals such as nodding, blinking or hand signals for the ventilated patient.
Search for potential causes of pain	Pathological conditions may create pain without triggering a behavioral or physiological response.
Observation of patient behaviors	A valid approach but behaviors are not indicative of pain intensity and may reflect other sources of distress.
Surrogate reporting	May not always be accurate and should be combined with other evidence when possible.
Attempt an analgesic trial	Provide a cautious analgesic trial. Pain behaviors may improve.

Reprinted from 7(2), Herr, K., et al., (2006) Pain assessmemt in the nonverbal patient: Position statement with clinical practice recommendations, p.45, with permission from Elsevier.

Society of Pain Management Nursing published a position paper regarding nursing assessment of pain in this population. The authors describe the dilemma as follows: "No single objective assessment strategy such as interpretation of behaviors, pathology or estimates of pain by others is sufficient by itself" (Herr, 2006, p. 45). Their recommendations are listed in a hierarchy based on McCaffery and Pasero's guidelines (1999, p. 94) (see Table 4–5).

Nurses frequently use physiologic indicators (e.g., change in heart rate or blood pressure) as evidence of pain. Absence of these indicators does not preclude pain. Patients with chronic pain, for example, adapt to the stress response and do not demonstrate the same physiologic changes. Additionally, pharmacologic interventions may prevent such changes.

Most behavioral pain scales use patient behaviors (cues) that may indicate the presence of pain. These behaviors can be divided into three main groups: vocal, facial, and body posturing. Sympathetic nervous system response should also be considered but may become less of an indicator over time. Some scales also include compliance with ventilation instead of verbalization as an indicator of pain for intubated patients (Payen et al., 2001). Vocal behaviors are sounds, such as crying, moaning, or grunting. The primary facial cues that suggest pain are facial grimacing and a crying expression (tears may be noted). Certain body posturing behaviors are associated with the presence of pain. Typical observations include agitation or lying completely still, guarding, splinting respirations, withdrawing or localizing to invasive modalities and procedures, stiffening, and repetitive/rhythmic activity of a body part (such as rocking or tapping). Acute pain is associated with stimulation of the sympathetic nervous system response, which causes elevation of heart rate, blood pressure, and respiratory rate, and increased pallor and diaphoresis. Although it is of value in assessing short-term acute pain, the use of the sympathetic response criteria for assessing the presence of pain loses validity over time. The sympathetic response is known to adapt rapidly, within 24 hours, even in the patient experiencing severe pain.

SECTION FOUR REVIEW

1. The Numeric Rating Scale is most commonly used to measure what part of the pain experience?
   - **A.** affective
   - **B.** evaluative
   - **C.** intensity
   - **D.** coping
2. If a patient is mildly confused, the nurse should initially try to assess pain using
   - **A.** vital signs
   - **B.** self-report
   - **C.** facial expression
   - **D.** body posturing
3. A major weakness of multidimensional tools is that
   - **A.** the patient must comprehend the vocabulary
   - **B.** they measure only pain intensity
   - **C.** the nurse performs the assessment
   - **D.** they are unable to measure degree of anxiety
4. Examples of vocal pain behaviors include (choose all that apply)
   - **A.** grunting
   - **B.** moaning
   - **C.** guarding
   - **D.** crying

Answers: 1. C, 2. B, 3. A, 4. (A, B, D)

SECTION FIVE: Management of Acute Pain

At the completion of this section, the learner will be able to describe effective pain management for the high-acuity patient.

Organized Approach to Pain Management

Effective pain management is facilitated by use of an organized, systematic approach. The World Health Organization (WHO) Analgesic Ladder provides an example of such an approach. The

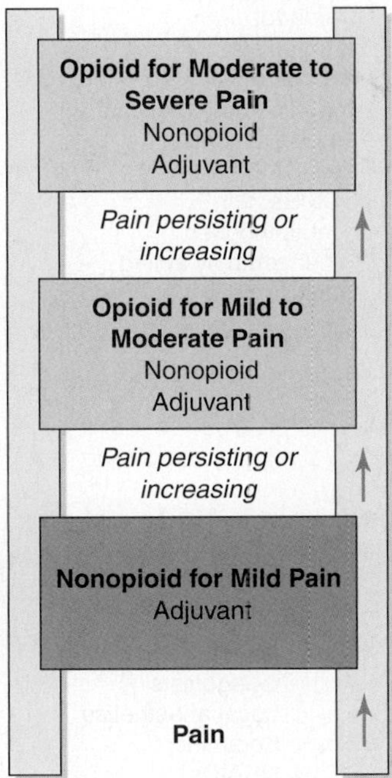

Figure 4–5 ■ The WHO ladder (Adapted from WHO. [1996]. Cancer pain relief, (2nd ed.) Geneva Switzerland: World Health Organization.)

ladder (Fig. 4–5) suggests general pain management choices based on the level of pain (i.e., mild, mild-to-moderate, or moderate-to-severe). In addition, it provides a step-by-step approach to adjusting the pharmacologic choices if the patient's pain is persistent or increases.

The high-acuity patient is particularly at risk for moderate to severe pain; thus, discussion will focus on management at this level of the ladder. Opioids are generally the drugs of choice for pain management at this level. In addition, the ladder recommends consideration of nonopioid and adjuvant therapies to further enhance the effects of opioid therapy.

Pharmacologic Pain Management

The pharmacologic management of pain involves modulation of pain transmission at different levels of the nervous system. For example, opioids bind with opioid receptors in such areas as the spinal cord, peripheral nervous system, and central nervous system. Nonsteroidal anti-inflammatory drugs (NSAIDs) may relieve pain by working peripherally at the site of injury, by inhibiting the formation of prostaglandins, proteolytic enzymes, and bradykinins. They may also have a CNS effect.

Nonopioid Therapy

Effective pain management can be enhanced by a combination of opioid and nonopioid therapy. A better level of analgesia is often achieved in combination than when either is administered alone. Nonopioids include such drugs as acetaminophen, aspirin, and in particular, NSAIDs. Nonopioids are associated with fewer side effects than opioids.

Adjuvant Therapy

Adjuvant therapy includes drugs that can assist in reducing certain types of pain. Their assistance may be indirect (by decreasing other symptoms associated with the underlying condition) or direct, as a coanalgesic. These drugs are generally used in addition to opioid and nonopioid analgesics. Several specific examples of adjuvant drugs include corticosteroids for cancer related pain, and antidepressants (e.g., amitriptyline [Elavil®]) or anticonvulsants (e.g., gabapentin [Neurontin®]) for treatment of neuropathic pain (Lussier, Huskey & Portenoy, 2004).

Opioid Therapy

Therapeutic use of opioids begins with the selection of a specific opioid drug and route of administration. After the choice of drug and route are determined, decisions are made regarding the suitable initial dose; frequency of administration; optimal doses of nonopioid analgesics, if these are to be given; and incidence and severity of side effects. The importance of careful adjustment of these medications for therapeutic effects cannot be overemphasized because dosing needs and analgesic responses vary greatly among individual patients (AHCPR, 1992).

Multimodal Therapy

Multimodal or **balanced analgesia** is described as a balanced approach to pain treatment that targets numerous pain signaling pathways and matches the treatment to the type of pain (Kehlet, Werner & Perkins, 1999). *Preemptive pain treatment* is treatment initiated prior to tissue injury (surgery) with the goal of reducing postoperative hypersensitivity (sensitization). Both nonsteroidals such as Celebrex® and the anticonvulsant Neurontin® have been found to be opioid sparing and to reduce pain related to surgical procedures (Reuben & Buvanendran, 2007). A multimodal approach to pain management takes advantage of the additive or synergistic effects of different classes of analgesics. Multimodal regimens may include a combination of local anesthetics (epidurals, regional or peripheral nerve blocks, wound infiltration), nonsteroidals, acetaminophen, anticonvulsants, and Alpha$_2$ agonists (Clonidine®) with opioids.

Postoperatively, bimodal therapy (use of an opioid with a second agent) has been demonstrated to be opioid sparing and to decrease patient reports of pain but have not yet demonstrated a decrease in the incidence of opioid related side effects. A multimodal approach is most likely required to reduce opioid related adverse effects (Elia et al., 2005). Figure 4–6 illustrates the relationship between various analgesics and adjuvants to the route of nociception.

Routes of Administration

There are many routes available for administration of analgesia. The oral, subcutaneous, intramuscular, and intravenous (IV) routes can be accessed by the nurse. Most other routes require initial access by an anesthesiologist.

The oral route is most commonly used for opioids. This route is also the most inexpensive and convenient. For the high-acuity patient, however, the oral route may not be available because of a nothing-by-mouth status. Although these

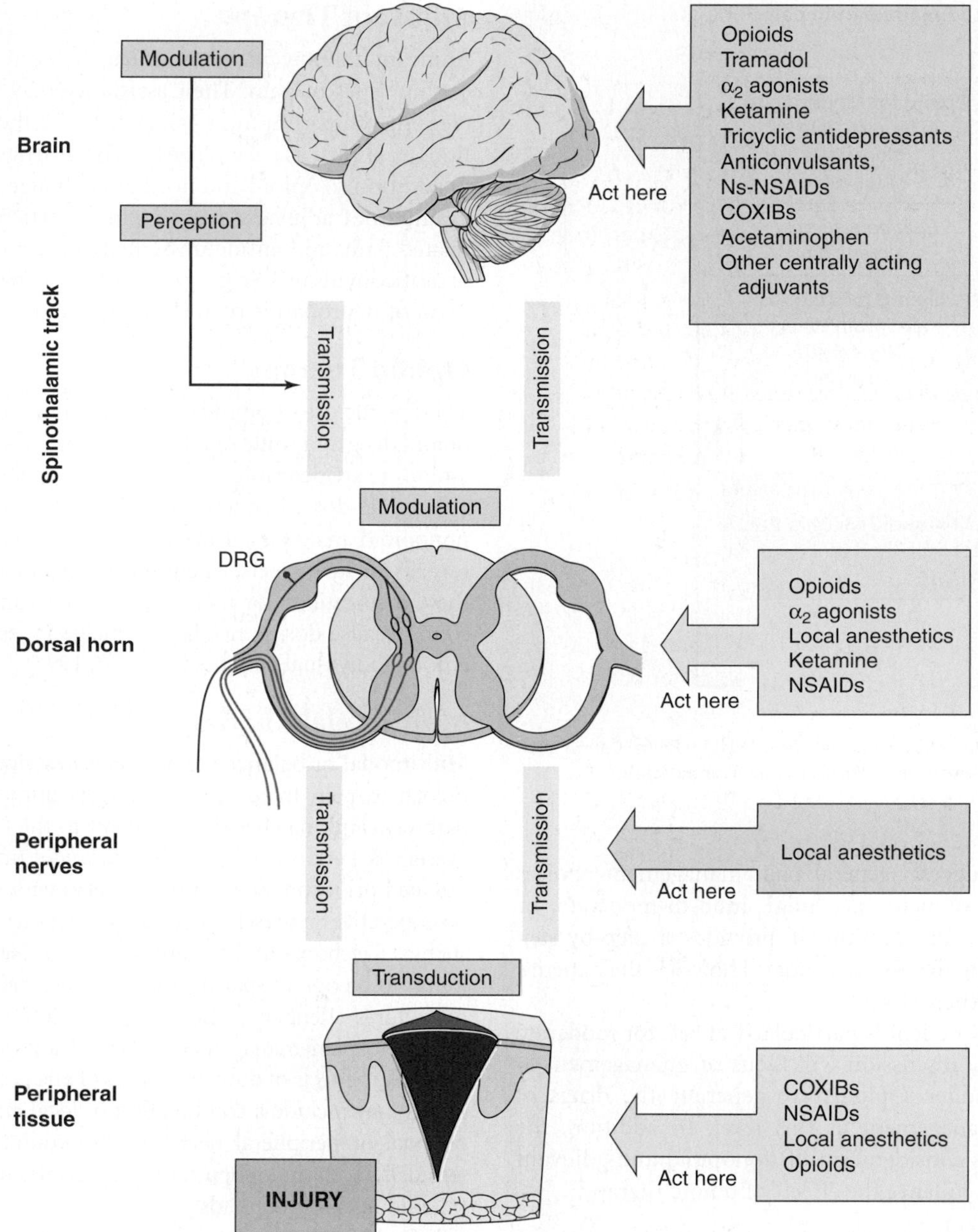

Figure 4–6 ▪ Anatomic scheme of nociception route coupled with the antinociceptive sites of various analgesics. This figure was published in *Cancer Pain: Pharmacological, Interventional and Palliative Care Approaches*, by O. DeLeon–Casasola, p. 257, Copyright Elsevier (2006).

individuals are not able to take medications orally, many have feeding tubes that act as an alternate medication route.

AHCPR guidelines state that when IV access is not possible, the rectal or sublingual routes should be considered in preference to the traditional use of subcutaneous and intramuscular routes. Repeated use of the subcutaneous and intramuscular routes is painful to the patient and may cause tissue trauma. In addition, the lag time between injection and absorption into the circulation makes these injection routes less desirable alternatives (AHCPR, 1992).

The intravenous route can be used by the nurse or self-administered by the patient using intravenous patient-controlled analgesia (PCA). The most common method of PCA allows the patient to self-dose intravenously by pushing a button that is attached via a cord to an infusion device. The infusion device can be programmed for the patient to self-administer doses of opioid without becoming overly sedated (AHCPR, 1992). Other forms of PCA are subcutaneous, intramuscular, and epidural.

Intraspinal opioids can be administered in a variety of ways:

- Single-dose epidural or intrathecal
- Intermittent scheduled dose epidural or intrathecal
- Intermittent patient-controlled epidural (PCEA) or intrathecal
- Continuous infusion of opioid alone or in combination with local anesthetic epidural or intrathecal
- Continuous infusion plus patient-controlled opioid alone or in combination with local anesthetic (American Pain Society, 2003)

Intraspinal insertion requires an anesthesiologist or a certified nurse anesthetist.

The **epidural** route requires insertion of a small catheter into the space located just before the dura mater. An opioid, or a combination of opioid and local anesthetic, is delivered using an infusion device. The opioids diffuse across the dura mater and bind at opioid receptors. The local anesthetic selectively blocks sensory nerve fibers that make up the spinal nerve roots, acting as a neural blockade. The spinal nerve roots pass through the epidural space to the spinal cord, thus making the epidural space a convenient place to infuse drugs. Combinations of opioid and local anesthetic agents are used to modulate the transmission of pain at different sites. This route requires low doses of analgesic, whether administered alone or in combination. This route also minimizes the potential for side effects. Neural blockade provides analgesia without the central nervous system effects of sedation, drowsiness, and respiratory depression that can occur when analgesics are given systemically (oral [PO], IV, or intramuscular [IM]).

The **intrathecal** route for analgesia requires the passage of a small catheter into the cerebrospinal fluid (CSF) space. Opioid flows through the CSF and rapidly binds to opioid receptors in the spinal cord. Smaller amounts of an intrathecally administered drug are required to achieve the same effects as epidural administration. This method places the spinal cord at some degree of risk, however, because of the potential for mechanical or chemical irritation or damage. There is also a higher risk of infection than with the epidural route. Many methods are available to deliver intrathecal medications, including percutaneous catheters, implanted ports, and implanted pumps. Use of the epidural or intrathecal routes requires close communication between anesthesiology and nursing staff and careful monitoring of the patient.

Peripheral nerve blocks and pleural infusion routes also require an anesthesiologist. When a **peripheral nerve block** is performed, the peripheral nerve path that is transmitting the pain is located, and local anesthetic is injected medial to the point of pain origin. The sites most frequently used for peripheral nerve blocking are the intercostal nerves medial to the insertion site of chest tubes and the femoral nerve prior to total knee arthroplasty. The duration of the analgesia depends on the half-life of the local anesthetic that has been injected.

The **pleural infusion** route primarily is used when multiple rib fractures are present. A small catheter is placed into the pleural space (between the visceral and parietal pleura) and a local anesthetic is injected. By administering a local anesthetic via this route, multiple intercostal nerves can be blocked at one time without repeated needlesticks to the skin.

Whenever local anesthetics are administered, it is important for the health care provider to monitor the patient for systemic anesthetic toxicity. Signs and symptoms of this complication include a 25 percent drop in baseline heart rate, tinnitus, slurred speech or thick tongue, and mental confusion. Table 4–6 provides a comparison of pharmacologic pain interventions.

TABLE 4–6 Pharmacologic Interventions

TYPE/ROUTE OF ANALGESIA	ADVANTAGES	LIMITATIONS
Nonsteroidal anti-inflammatory drugs (NSAIDs)		
Oral (alone)	Effective for mild-to-moderate pain.	Relatively contraindicated in patients with renal disease, risk of or actual coagulopathy and risk of or active GI bleeding. May mask fever.
Oral (as an adjunct to opioid)	Potentiating effect results in opioid sparing.	Cautions as above.
Parenteral (ketorolac)	Effective for moderate to severe pain. Expensive. Useful where opioids are contraindicated especially to avoid respiratory depression and sedation. May advance to opioid.	Cautions as above.
Opioids		
Oral (PO)	As effective as parenteral in appropriate doses. Route of choice. Noninvasive, inexpensive. Use as soon as oral medication tolerated.	Oral route may not be available for high-acuity patients. Slower onset of action.
Intramuscular	Avoid when other routes available.	Injections painful and absorption unreliable. May cause tissue trauma.
Subcutaneous	Less painful and preferable to IM especially when slow infusion technique (1–3 ml/hr) utilized. Can place a butterfly needle for continuous infusions.	Bolus injections painful and absorption unreliable.
Transdermal fentanyl patch	Useful when oral route unavailable. Noninvasive.	Difficult to titrate due to delay of effective blood fentanyl concentrations.

(continued)

TABLE 4–6 (*continued*)

TYPE/ROUTE OF ANALGESIA	ADVANTAGES	LIMITATIONS
Rectal	Does not require functional IV. May be appropriate in the patient unable to tolerate oral medications.	Absorption may be unpredictable, affected by defecation. May not be acceptable to all patients. Contraindicated in patients with painful anal conditions or who are at risk for infection (neutropenia).
Intravenous	Parenteral route of choice after major surgery or when oral route unavailable. Suitable for titrated bolus or continuous infusion.	Requires intravenous access. Requires monitoring, significant risk of respiratory depression with inappropriate dosing.
Patient-controlled analgesia (PCA)	Can be used with intravenous, subcutaneous, or epidural routes. Provides steady level of analgesia. Provides patient control. Avoids peaks and troughs.	Requires special infusion pumps and staff education. Requires monitoring, significant risk of respiratory depression with inappropriate dosing.
Epidural and intrathecal	Provides good analgesia. May be utilized for surgical or for cancer pain in specific circumstances. May be used as a one-time injection (bolus) or as a continuous infusion.	Requires special infusion pumps and staff education. Requires daily follow-up by experienced physician or pain team. Requires monitoring, risk of respiratory depression higher with bolus dose than with continuous infusion.
Local Anesthetics Epidural and intrathecal	Effective regional analgesia. Opioid sparing. Addition of opioid to local will improve analgesia. Usually used continuously.	Require daily follow up by experienced physician or pain team. Requires careful monitoring, special pumps and staff education. Risk of hypotension, weakness, and numbness.
Peripheral nerve block	Effective regional analgesia. Used postoperatively or for trauma pain. Opioid sparing. May be one time injection or continuous infusion.	Requires careful monitoring, special pumps and staff education.

Data from Ballantyne (2002).

Nonpharmacologic (Complementary) Interventions

Nonpharmacologic therapies, often referred to as complementary therapies, can be used concurrently with medications to manage pain. The role of the clinician is to assist the patient in identifying effective alternative interventions to be systematically incorporated into the care plan. All clinicians involved in the patient's care have a role in providing the necessary support for utilization of these therapies as outlined in the care plan. Guidelines for choice of nonpharmacologic interventions include pain problem identification, effectiveness for a specific patient, and the skill of the clinician. Table 4–7 lists examples of nonpharmacologic interventions for the management of pain.

McCaffery and Pasero (1999) emphasize the individual response of the patient to nonpharmacologic interventions to pain. In general, especially with acute pain, nonpharmacologic interventions are useful in combination with analgesia and do not take the place of analgesics. Nondrug therapies can be initiated when pain is under reasonable control.

Assessment of the patient's past experience with nondrug therapies is beneficial as patients may have experience with therapies that are not only compatible with their coping style but have been helpful in the past. The provision of adequate support materials (written or audio tapes) will increase the benefit of such interventions. A patient who is fatigued, frightened, or in considerable pain will not be able to concentrate well enough to follow instructions or to perform time-consuming or complicated interventions.

Emerging Evidence

- Capnography may help identify early changes in respiratory function better than pulse oximetry and respiratory rate with the administration of opioid analgesia *(Hutchison and Rodriguez, 2008)*.
- The use of naloxone to reverse opioid-induced respiratory depression is rare but more prevalent in older patients, those receiving central nervous system depressants, and in patients with the development of other conditions such as pneumonia and renal failure *(Gordon and Pellino, 2005)*.
- In acute and critical care adult patients undergoing painful procedures, pain was the greatest during the procedure regardless of age; however, rating of procedural distress was higher in younger patients. In addition, younger patients received more analgesia during procedures than did older patients even though pain was rated similarly regardless of age *(Stotts, Puntillo, Stanik-Hut, et al., 2007)*.
- Patients in acute respiratory failure are increasingly being treated using noninvasive positive pressure ventilation (NPPV). Sedation and analgesia practices vary widely in patients receiving NPPV. In the United States, a combination of sedation and analgesia was often employed, using intermittent sedation administered by the nurses without use of a sedation protocol or sedation scale *(Devlin, 2007)*.

TABLE 4–7 Nonpharmacologic Interventions

Simple Relaxation (begin preoperatively)	
Interventions:	Jaw relaxation, progressive muscle relaxation, and simple imagery.
Comments:	Effective in reducing mild to moderate pain and as an adjunct to analgesic drugs for severe pain. Use when patients express an interest in relaxation. Requires 3 to 5 minutes of staff time for instructions.
Intervention:	Music
Comments:	Effective for reduction of mild to moderate pain. Requires appropriate equipment.
Complex Relaxation (begin postoperatively)	
Intervention:	Biofeedback
Comments:	May be effective in reducing mild to moderate pain and operative site muscle tension. Requires skilled personnel and special equipment.
Intervention:	Imagery
Comments:	May be effective for reduction of mild to moderate pain. Requires skilled personnel.
Education/Instruction (begin preoperatively)	
Comments:	Effective for reduction of pain. Should include sensory and procedural information and instruction aimed at reducing activity-related pain. Requires 5 to 15 minutes of staff time.
TENS (transcutaneous electrical nerve stimulation)	
Comments:	Effective in reducing pain and improving physical function. Requires skilled personnel and special equipment. May be useful as an adjunct to drug therapy.

Data from McCaffery and Pasero (1999).

SECTION FIVE REVIEW

1. The World Health Organization (WHO) Analgesic Ladder provides the clinician with
   - **A.** general pain management choices based on level of pain
   - **B.** nonpharmacologic interventions based on level of pain
   - **C.** specific pain management choices based on severity of pain
   - **D.** pharmacologic and nonpharmacologic pain management choices
2. Which of the following statements is correct regarding nonopioid therapy?
   - **A.** nonopioids have more severe side effects than opioids
   - **B.** nonopioids are harder to access than opioids
   - **C.** nonopioids can manage pain as effectively as opioids
   - **D.** combining opioids and nonopioids enhances analgesia effectiveness
3. The most common route used for PCA is
   - **A.** intramuscular
   - **B.** intravenous
   - **C.** subcutaneous
   - **D.** epidural
4. A major advantage of using the epidural route for analgesia is that it
   - **A.** can be accessed by the nurse
   - **B.** uses only nonopioid analgesics
   - **C.** blocks a specific peripheral nerve path
   - **D.** provides analgesia without CNS side effects
5. The guidelines for choosing appropriate nonpharmacologic interventions include (choose all that apply)
   - **A.** skill of clinician
   - **B.** effectiveness for patient
   - **C.** pain problem identification
   - **D.** type of opioid being used

Answers: 1. A, 2. D, 3. B, 4. D, 5. (A, B, C)

SECTION SIX: Issues in Inadequate Treatment of Acute Pain

At the completion of this section, the learner will be able to discuss issues related to the undertreatment of pain.

Strassels, McNicol, and Suleman (2008) state that undertreatment of pain has remained a persistent challenge for the medical and nursing professions despite advances in scientific knowledge regarding pain and its treatment. They suggest that the undertreatment problem is multifactorial and involves complex social and health care system issues, as well as inadequate attention being given to pain education in many pharmacy, medicine, and nursing educational professional programs. The authors conclude that "Important clinical, human, and economic consequences of this shortcoming include altered immune system functioning, diminished ability to function, increased risk for chronic pain, needless suffering, and higher health care costs" (p. 276). This section provides a brief overview of some of the major pain-related misconceptions that often lead to undertreatment.

Definitions

It is important to differentiate among tolerance, dependence, and addiction, terms that are misused and have potentially negative connotations. The definitions of the early AHCPR guidelines remain current and are often referenced in current literature. These terms are defined as follows:

- **Tolerance.** A common physiologic result of chronic opioid use; it means that a larger dose of opioid is required to maintain the same level of analgesia (AHCPR, 1994).
- **Physical dependence.** A physical adaptation of the body to the presence of opioids, existing when rapid drug withdrawal produces signs and symptoms (Hawthorn & Redmond, 1998).
- **Psychological dependence (addiction).** A pattern of compulsive drug use characterized by a continued craving for an opioid and the need to use the opioid for effects other than pain relief (or other medical indications) (AHCPR, 1994).
- **Opioid pseudoaddiction.** A term applied to patients who develop behaviors that mimic those associated with addiction. The individual may be labeled as drug craving or drug seeking. Pseudoaddiction, however, results from inadequate pain management, not psychological dependence. A variety of responses are noted in patients who experience unrelieved pain, from acceptable drug-seeking to pathologic behaviors. Unfortunately, it is often extremely difficult for nurses and physicians to discriminate between these two types of behaviors, particularly in situations in which patient–physician/nurse contact is limited, such as in the emergency department. Behaviors that suggest undertreatment of pain but are frequently misread as drug seeking rather than pain relief seeking include demands for different or more pain medications that escalates, clock watching, preoccupation with obtaining pain medications, anger, and others (ASAM, 2001; ASPMN, 2002). Pseudoaddiction results in a patient's distrust and suspicion of staff and avoidance of the patient by staff (ASPMN, 2002). Pseudoaddiction is distinguishable from actual addiction by resolution of aberrant behaviors when pain is relieved (ASAM, 2001).

Reasons for Opioid Undertreatment of Pain

The practice of treating pain with minimal drug use is known as **oligoanalgesia** (Mace et al., 2006). Physicians underprescribe opioids by two methods: prescribing subtherapeutic doses and prescribing time intervals for drug doses that are less than the pharmacologic duration of action. Nurses undertreat pain by administering less than what the patient can receive per physician orders and administering opioids at longer intervals than prescribed. Patients often contribute to their own undertreatment of pain by not requesting as needed (PRN) pain medications, taking medication at longer-than-ordered intervals, taking less than the amount prescribed, or refusing to take the drug at all (McCaffery & Pasero, 1999).

Inadequate treatment of pain is a complex problem based on misconceptions widely held by physicians, nurses, and patients. There are four common misconceptions regarding opioid use that contribute to inadequate treatment: fear of addiction, physical dependence, tolerance, and respiratory depression.

Fear of Addiction (Psychological Dependence)

Fear of addiction is probably the major cause of undertreatment of pain. The term **opiophobia** has been used to describe the irrational fear of prescribing (or consuming) adequate amounts of opiates for therapeutic results. In fact, very few hospitalized patients who receive opioids become addicted; as the pain subsides, so does the use of the opioids. The term **addiction** should be used with extreme caution. The indiscriminate labeling of a person who uses drugs as being an addict carries a strong social stigma that may label an individual negatively (McCaffery & Pasero, 1999). The National Institute of Drug Abuse (NIDA) in its Research Report Series, has this to say regarding use of opioids in treating pain:

> Most patients who are prescribed opioids for pain, even those undergoing long-term therapy, do not become addicted to the drugs. The few patients who do develop rapid and marked tolerance for and addiction to opioids usually have a history of psychological problems or prior substance abuse. In fact, studies have shown that abuse potential of opioid medications is generally low in healthy, nondrug-abusing volunteers. One study found that only 4 out of about 12,000 patients who were given opioids for acute pain became addicted. In a study of 38 chronic pain patients, most of whom received opioids for 4 to 7 years, only 2 patients became addicted, and both had a history of drug abuse (NIDA, 2008).

Fear of Physical Dependence

Some of the fear associated with **physical dependence** is generated from the belief that opioid withdrawal is life-threatening, the symptoms associated with physical dependence are difficult to control, and the presence of symptoms of physical dependence prevent decreases in opioid doses as the pain decreases. In addition, many people believe that addiction is the natural progression of physical dependence. It is true that any patient who receives repeated doses of opioids is at risk for some degree of withdrawal symptoms if the opioid is suddenly stopped. These symptoms, however, can be effectively managed by gradual reduction in opioid dosage as the patient's pain subsides (McCaffery & Pasero, 1999).

Fear of Tolerance

Fear of tolerance is usually seen in patients with long-term pain associated with either a disease process or painful treatments (e.g., patients with burns, cancer, or life-threatening illnesses). Patients, physicians, and nurses have expressed fear that opioids lose their effectiveness over time and may not work when really needed. A part of this fear is the belief in an imaginary dose ceiling, beyond which the patient cannot be taken. In fact, this feared dose ceiling does not seem to exist. As tolerance to an opioid develops, so does the patient's tolerance to the side effects of sedation and respiratory depression. Tolerance is treated by decreasing the dose interval or increasing the dose. Nursing management should focus on patient education about the concept of tolerance, and monitoring for the therapeutic and nontherapeutic effects of the adjusted dosage (McCaffery & Pasero, 1999).

Fear of Respiratory Depression

Physicians and nurses are particularly sensitive to the fear of respiratory depression. All opioids have the capability of causing respiratory depression, yet it need not be a life-threatening problem and should not prevent therapeutic opioid use. In the majority of hospitalized patients, respiratory depression has not been shown to be a significant problem. Nursing management should focus on close observation of the patient's response. **Sedation** develops before respiratory depression; therefore, the nurse should observe and document the patient's sedation level (e.g., wide awake, drowsy, dozing intermittently, mostly sleeping, or awakens only when aroused). Respiratory depression is dose related, and low doses are generally considered safe. It is impossible, however, to know what dose of an opioid will cause respiratory depression in any given patient. It is more important to watch the individual's response, especially to the first dose (McCaffery & Pasero, 1999).

Nursing Approach in Acute Pain Management

The way in which an analgesic is used is probably more important than which drug is used (McCaffery & Pasero, 1999). In the acute care setting, the nurse maintains significant control over how analgesics are used. Nursing activities that have an impact on therapeutic pain management include the following:

- Selecting an appropriate opioid or nonopioid from the analgesics ordered
- Evaluating when to administer the analgesic
- Evaluating how much analgesic to administer
- Obtaining a change in prescription when required

Effective pain management requires objective assessment skills and specific knowledge of opioids and nonopioids. In addition, the nurse must individualize the care plan to best meet the patient's individual comfort needs.

There are two major approaches to effective pain management: the preventive and the titration approaches.

Preventive

Using the preventive approach, analgesics are administered before the patient complains of pain. For example, when pain is occurring consistently over a 24-hour period, administering analgesics on a regular around-the-clock (ATC) schedule is more effective than administering them as needed (PRN). This method helps to maintain a consistent therapeutic level of analgesic in the bloodstream and diminishes the likelihood of undertreatment of pain. Administering pain medication on a PRN basis can cause prolonged delays in treating the patient's pain. If PRN analgesia is to be used, it is important for the clinician to know the half-life and effectiveness of the medication being administered in order to predict when the patient is likely to need another dose. Maintaining awareness of pain by offering pain medication on a routine basis is more effective for pain control than requiring the patient to ask for medication (PRN). The patient may wait for the pain to become severe before requesting analgesia, or the clinician may be delayed in getting the drug to the patient. Either situation makes adequate pain relief more difficult to obtain.

There are times when PRN administration is an acceptable option, for example, changing to PRN late in the postoperative course to help decrease side effects; or when the pain is incidental, intermittent, or unpredictable (AHCPR, 1992; McCaffery & Pasero, 1999). In addition, PRN analgesics may be used as supplemental doses to regularly scheduled analgesics, primarily when a certain known activity causes pain (e.g., ambulation, sitting up in a chair, coughing, and deep breathing).

As the patient's advocate, it is recommended that the nurse be alert to the patient's comfort status and be proactive in consulting with the physician regarding changing the PRN order to ATC if a more effective analgesia schedule is required. The nurse also has an important role in educating the patient and family regarding effective analgesia scheduling.

Titration

The titration approach calls for adjusting and individualizing therapy based on the effects the drug is having on the patient rather than the milligrams being administered. The goal is to gain the desired level of pain relief with minimum side effects. When using this approach, the clinician should consider the following:

- Dose. Analgesic potency helps provide a rational basis for choosing the appropriate starting dose (AHCPR, 1992).
- Interval between doses. Assess the patient regarding the amount of time it takes for the pain to increase. For example, if the nurse is administering an analgesic every four hours and the patient notices that the pain increases quickly after three hours, the interval should be changed to three hours.
- Route of administration. Use a conversion chart for equal analgesic dosing when switching from one route to another (see Table 4–8). Dosing conversion factors based on relative potency estimates may differ between patients (AHCPR, 1992).
- Choice of drug. Opioids are classified as full (pure) opioid agonists, partial agonists, or mixed agonist–antagonists. Full agonists are more potent than partial agonists. Agonist–antagonists activate one type of opioid receptor and at the same time block another type (AHCPR, 1992). Withdrawal-like symptoms can occur when switching a patient from a pure agonist to an agonist–antagonist.

Regardless of the approach chosen to treat pain, undertreatment can still occur. Improved education for all health care professionals about pain and its treatment is a crucial first step in reversing this problem. Further, the high-acuity nurse must act as the patient's advocate through open communication with the other interdisciplinary team members when there is perceived undertreatment of pain.

TABLE 4–8 Equianalgesic Doses of Selected Opioids

DRUG	TRADE NAME	ROUTES	EQUIANALGESIC DOSE (MG)	DURATION (HOURS)
Morphine	Generic	IM/IV	10	4–6 (IM)
		PO/R	30	4–7
Hydromorphone	Generic; Dilaudid	IM/IV	1.5	4–5 (IM)
		PO/R	7.5	4–6
Codeine	Generic; 2 APAP; Tylenol 3, etc.	IM/IV	130	4–6 (IM)
		PO	200[a]	4–6
Oxycodone	Generic; w/APA; Percocet w/ASA; Percodan	PO	20	3–5
Fentanyl	Generic; Sublimaze; Duragesic	IM/IV	0.1	1–2
		Topical		
Oxymorphone	Numorphan	IM	1	4–6
		R	10	4–6
Meperidine[b]	Generic; Demerol (not recommended)	IM/IV	75	4–5 (IM)
		PO	300	4–6

[a]The dose of codeine may be lowered when administered as a combination product containing aspirin or acetaminophen, which work synergistically.
[b]Meperidine has very limited use, as the toxic metabolite, normeperidine, builds to unacceptable levels in the CNS.

SECTION SIX REVIEW

1. A common physiologic consequence of chronic opioid use that results in a person's requiring an increasing dose of opioids to maintain the same level of analgesia is the definition of
   A. pseudoaddiction
   B. tolerance
   C. psychologic dependence
   D. physical dependence
2. Which of the following statements is correct regarding opioid use and respiratory depression?
   A. respiratory depression precedes the onset of sedation
   B. respiratory depression worsens as tolerance develops
   C. sedation occurs before respiratory depression
   D. respiratory depression is a common problem in hospitalized patients
3. PRN analgesics are appropriately used in which situations? (choose all that apply)
   A. when pain is intermittent
   B. when pain is consistent
   C. when pain is unpredictable
   D. when used as a supplement to scheduled doses
4. When the titration approach to pain management is used, the emphasis is on
   A. the patient's analgesic response
   B. total milligrams per day
   C. physical dependence
   D. psychological dependence

Answers: 1. B, 2. C, 3. (A, C, D), 4. A

SECTION SEVEN: Pain Management in Special Patient Populations

At the completion of this section, the learner will be able to identify considerations associated with pain management in special populations.

Several important patient-focused factors influence acute pain management. These factors include age, concurrent medical disorders, and history of substance abuse. A basic understanding of these factors helps to facilitate effective pain management.

Pharmacology and Aging

The relationship that exists between aging and adverse drug reactions is much more ambiguous and complex than once thought (Gurwitz & Avorn, 2001). Chronologic age does not have a direct relationship with deterioration of organ function; thus aging individuals vary greatly in their capacity to absorb, metabolize, and excrete drugs. It can be stated, however, that as a group, older adults are at higher risk for drug toxicity than younger adults for a variety of reasons (Fig. 4–7). Drug reactions may be dose-related

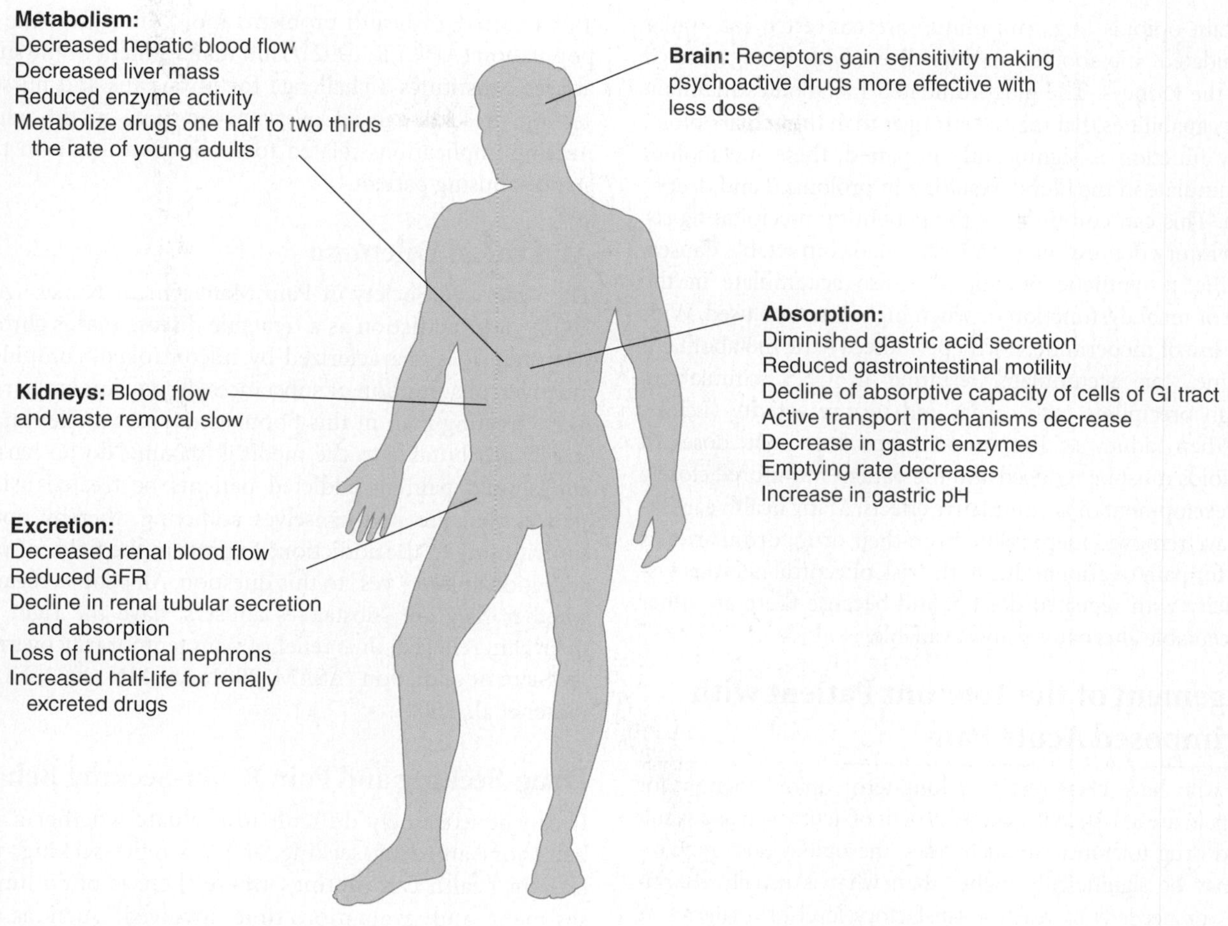

Figure 4–7 ■ Pharmacologic-related alterations in the aging body.

or the result of the drug's interaction at the cellular level. Older adults tend to take more drugs, including analgesics, on a long-term basis often related to the presence of chronic illnesses that require drug therapy. These medications may interact, producing symptoms. Older adults tend to have less body water and increased body fat. Less body water causes high blood levels of water-soluble drugs because of decreased distribution volume. Increased body fat causes prolonged effects of fat-soluble drugs because of increased distribution volume in fat tissue (Stassels, McNicol, & Suleman, 2008). Other complicating factors that increase the risk of adverse reactions or subtherapeutic dosing include the fact that short-term memory impairment may cause a person to take incorrect dosages, miss doses, or take multiple doses. Impaired vision may lead to overdosage. Impaired agility in opening containers may encourage a patient to miss a dose. Financial factors as well as limited transportation may keep the patient from filling prescriptions.

In obtaining a medication history, the nurse should ask about prescription and over-the-counter (OTC) preparations, OTC supplements, alcohol, caffeine and tobacco use, and home remedies. The nurse should be aware that certain drugs often prescribed for older adults, such as diuretics, anticholinergics, and sedatives, have a great number of undesirable side effects in this patient population. In assessing the older adult, symptoms suggesting drug toxicity frequently include delirium, depression, worsening dementia, orthostatic hypotension, falls, and incontinence, rather than the more commonly seen nausea, vomiting, diarrhea, and rash.

According to Katzung (2006), opioid use in the older adult is associated with variable alterations in pharmacokinetics. This patient population is particularly at risk for respiratory depression; thus opioids should be initiated with caution until sensitivity is determined. Studies have shown that opioids are underutilized in older patients who could significantly benefit from their use. Katzung suggests that there is no justification for this underutilization if opioids are administered according to an appropriate pain management plan.

Patients with Concurrent Medical Disorders

High-acuity patients frequently have more than one dysfunctioning organ at any single time. Impaired function of the liver and kidneys has serious implications for analgesic therapy. Analgesics are primarily metabolized in the liver, with a small percentage being excreted unchanged. The kidneys have the major responsibility for opioid excretion. When either of these organs has decreased functioning, serum drug levels increase, placing the patient at increasing risk for the development of adverse effects.

Certain opioids (e.g., morphine) are converted into polar glucuronidated metabolites in the liver and then excreted through the kidneys. The glucuronidated metabolites maintain analgesic capabilities that may be stronger than the actual opioid. If kidney function is significantly impaired, these metabolites may accumulate in the blood, resulting in prolonged and deeper analgesia. This can compromise the patient by precipitating severe respiratory depression, deep sedation, or intractable nausea. Meperidine, a synthetic opioid, may also accumulate in the presence of renal dysfunction or when high doses are used. With repeated use of meperidine, normeperidine, a toxic metabolite of meperidine, can accumulate, resulting in CNS stimulation, which can precipitate tachycardia and seizure activity (Lehne, 2007). When kidney or liver impairment is present, doses of most opioids must be reduced and the patient monitored closely for the development of accumulative effects. Many health care facilities have removed meperidine from their drug formularies as a choice for pain treatment due to the risk of central nervous system toxicity with repeated dosing, and because there are other more acceptable alternatives now available.

Management of the Tolerant Patient with Superimposed Acute Pain

Patients who have been receiving long-term opioid therapy for chronic pain are at risk for undertreatment of acute pain as a result of opioid drug tolerance. In such cases, the opioid dose requirements may be significantly higher than what is usually recommended (or needed) to reach a satisfactory level of analgesia. A thorough pain history provides valuable information regarding the potentially altered dose requirements of this patient population. Consensus recommendations are to consider a patient's home routine opioid dose as a baseline to which additional opioid is titrated to manage the incidence of acute pain (Mehta & Langford, 2006; Rozen & Grass, 2006; Mitra et al., 2004; and Carroll et al., 2005). When the patient is able to take oral medications, this can easily be accomplished by continuation of the patient's home opioid dose in a long acting oral form and titration of either short-acting oral opioid or patient-controlled analgesia for acute pain coverage. A patient restricted to intravenous therapy requires conversion from the home oral opioid dose to an hourly intravenous dose. Patient-controlled analgesia can then be delivered starting with a conservative continuous PCA dose with additional opioid delivered in the patient incremental format. The continuous dose and the incremental dose can be slowly titrated upward to control pain while monitoring for over sedation or respiratory depression. Interpatient variability requires individual dose titration. Use of a multimodal approach will improve the effectiveness of this regimen while decreasing the opioid dose required.

The Known Active or Recovering Substance Abuser as Patient

Pain management of the high-acuity patient who is either an active or recovering substance abuser has important nursing implications. Substance abusers experience traumatic injuries and a variety of health problems more often than the general population (AHCPR, 1992). Pain management of the substance abuser constitutes a challenge for physicians and nurses. This section presents a brief overview of some of the issues and nursing implications related to dealing with pain in the substance-abusing patient.

An Ethical Dilemma

The American Society of Pain Management Nurses (ASPMN, 2002) views addiction as a treatable disease that is chronic and relapsing. It is characterized by uncontrolled, compulsive use and overconsumption of substances despite known harmful effects. Treating pain in this population poses a dilemma that is largely attributable to the medical maxim, "do no harm." Can and should pain in addicted patients be treated using substances that are in themselves addicting, thereby potentially contributing to the addiction? Experts in the fields of pain and addiction answer "yes" to this question. All people, regardless of whether they are substances abusers, have the right to have their pain relieved; thus relief of pain temporarily overrides the problem of addiction (ASAM, 2001; ASPMN, 2002; NCI, 2003; Prater et al., 2002).

Drug-Seeking and Pain Relief-Seeking Behaviors

It can be extremely difficult to evaluate whether a person's behaviors are drug-seeking or pain relief-seeking, particularly in health care settings where there is often limited assessment and evaluation time involved, such as walk-in clinics and emergency departments (Mace et al., 2006; Kurtz, 2003). However, it is also true that pain relief-seeking and drug-seeking behaviors are often interchangeable when pain is not adequately relieved, regardless of whether a person is an active substance abuser.

Health care providers should be aware of behaviors and evidence that suggest active addiction. Table 4–9 lists some of the more common behaviors and evidence of active substance abuse. The problem of discriminating between pseudoaddiction and addiction-driven behaviors may become even more difficult if the person has previously experienced inadequate pain relief when seeking medical help (Prater et al., 2002). Previous negative pain relief-seeking experiences tend to foster more maladaptive behaviors that can be misconstrued by the health care team and perpetuate suspicion and distrust, and encourage the practice of oligoanalgesia. One way to differentiate between drug-seeking and pain relief-seeking behaviors is that pseudoaddiction behaviors cease when pain relief is achieved, whereas addiction behaviors continue when the primary motivation is drug seeking rather than pain relief (Kurtz, 2003; Prater et al., 2002). It is crucial then, to closely observe and document changes in behavior prior to and during pain relief interventions.

The probability of opioid abuse has been tied to certain risk factors. This has led to the development of screening tools to help determine which patients may have higher risk factors in order to determine the appropriate level of monitoring to

TABLE 4–9 Evidence Suspicious of Active Substance Abuse

Behavioral Evidence
Frequent occurrences of significant impairment in communication or physical abilities
Swings in mood and changes in personality
Drug hoarding
Withdrawal or alienation from family or friends
Heavy alcohol use in social settings
Obtaining drugs from others
Use of multiple pharmacies
Forging prescriptions
Change in appetite, unexplained weight change
Changes in speech pattern (e.g., slurred, rapid)
Fatigue or drowsiness (depressants); restlessness, irritability (stimulants)
Impaired memory
Altered appearance and hygiene
Physical Evidence
Inappropriately dilated or constricted pupils
Red or watery eyes
Hand tremors, stumbling gait
Altered sleep patterns
Persistent inflammation of nostrils, runny nose
Deteriorating health
Altered vital signs (elevated [stimulants]; decreased [depressants])
Evidence of substance abuse (e.g., needle marks)

prevent abuse during opioid treatment in chronic pain. Two such tools are the Opioid Risk Tool (ORT) and the Screener and Opioid Assessment for Patients with Pain (SOAPP). The authors of both tools emphasize that all patients deserve treatment for pain despite the level of risk or the presence of aberrant behaviors. These tools are proposed to be used solely to determine the level of monitoring required (Butler et al., 2004; and Webster, 2005).

Major Considerations in Pain Management

Kurtz (2003) emphasizes the importance of not confusing physical dependence with the addiction when considering how best to manage pain in the active or the recovering addict. Although treatment may renew physical dependence, it does not necessarily foster a relapse to active addiction (Heit, 2002). In fact, failure to relieve pain increases the likelihood of relapse (Kurtz, 2003). Stress is known to increase substance craving and inadequate pain relief often increases stress, which may result in an escalation of substance use in the acute abuser or relapse in the recovering abuser. Although managing pain in this population may be difficult, it is not impossible. Employing recommendations of experts, such as those developed by the ASPMN, can be useful in guiding medical and nursing pain interventions in this population. Table 4–10 provides a list of recommendations based on ASPMN's position paper, *Pain Management in the Patient with Addictive Disease.*

Clinical Management Considerations

NCI (2003) offers guidelines that can be applied to pain treatment of the high-acuity patient with a history of substance abuse:

- Involve a multidisciplinary team.
  - Substance abuse is complex and requires interdisciplinary care, such as pain expert physicians, nurses, social workers and, if available, an addiction medicine expert.
- Set realistic goals for therapy.
  - The risk of relapse increases with the heightened stress associated with life-threatening disease. Prevention of relapse may be impossible, requiring altered goal setting for management to include structured therapy, support, and limit setting.
- Evaluate and treat comorbid psychiatric disorders.
  - The substance abuser is at extreme risk for anxiety, personality disorders, and depression. Presence of these disorders may require treatment during acute disease states.
- Prevent or minimize withdrawal symptoms.
  - Obtain a complete drug history, keeping in mind that many patients abuse multiple drugs. Laboratory drug screening tests can provide a baseline of currently abused substances. Health care professionals should be familiar with the manifestations of commonly abused substances (see Table 4–11).
- Consider the impact of tolerance.
  - Substance abusers may require significantly higher doses (one-and-a-half times or more) of analgesia to achieve the same level of pain relief as a nonabuser (Kurtz, 2003). This varies widely among individuals.
- Apply appropriate pharmacologic principles to treat chronic pain.
  - Analgesic dose individualization is an important principle; focusing on dose size rather than pain relief achievement may result in pain undertreatment and subsequent development of pseudoaddiction behaviors.
- Use a multimodal approach to treatment when possible.
  - Recognize specific drug abuse behaviors (see Table 4–9).
- Use nondrug approaches as appropriate.
  - These may include further patient education, relaxation and coping techniques, and other complementary pain relieving interventions.

TABLE 4–10 Recommendations of the ASPMN: Patients with Addictive Disease

Recommendations for all patients with addictive disease:

- Identify and use resources available to assist in the diagnosis and treatment of both addiction and pain.
- Encourage the patient to use support systems, such as family, significant others, or a rehabilitation sponsor; offer additional resources, such as an addiction counselor.
- Involve the patient in pain management planning and, with the patient's consent, include family and significant others.
- Provide the patient with verbal and written information on the pain management plan, including what the patient can expect from caregivers and what the patient's responsibilities are.
- Ensure consistency in the implementation of the pain management plan.
- Educate the patient, family, and significant others on the differences among addiction, physical dependence, and tolerance.
- Help the patient make informed choices regarding medications by educating the patient, family, and significant others on medication options.
- Select and titrate analgesics based on pain assessment, side effects, and function, as well as sleep and mood.
- Be prepared to titrate opioid analgesics and benzodiazepines to doses higher than usual. The patient may have developed tolerance to some medications, or drug use may have caused sensitivity to pain.
- Benzodiazepines, phenothiazines, or other sedating medications that do not relieve pain should not be used as substitutes for analgesics.
- If pain is present most of the time, provide analgesics around the clock.
- Use the oral route and long-acting analgesics when possible.
- Consider the use of IV or epidural patient-controlled analgesia for acute pain management.
- Record and discuss with the patient any behavior suggestive of inappropriate medication use, especially of controlled substances.
- When opioids, benzodiazepines, or other medications with a potential for physical dependence are no longer needed, taper them very slowly to minimize withdrawal symptoms.
- Consider nonpharmacologic methods of treatment for pain, but do not use them in place of appropriate pharmacologic approaches.

Recommendations for patients who are actively using alcohol or other drugs, in addition to the recommendations for all patients with addictive disease:

- Distinguish between pseudoaddiction (an iatrogenic syndrome created by the undertreatment of pain, characterized by behaviors such as anger and escalating demands for more or different medications; distinguished from true addiction in that the behaviors resolve when pain is effectively treated) and addiction. This may be difficult in the presence of unrelieved pain.
- Assess for and treat symptoms of withdrawal from alcohol or other drugs.
- If the patient acknowledges inappropriate use of prescribed medications or nonprescribed substances, openly discuss this and encourage the patient to express any fear of how this may affect pain management and treatment by staff.
- Assess for psychiatric comorbidity, such as anxiety and depression, and obtain treatment if needed.
- If the patient is physically dependent on morphine-like opioids, do not treat pain with opioid agonist–antagonists, such as nalbuphine, butorphanol, buprenorphine, or pentazocine, because it will precipitate acute withdrawal.
- Once pain is controlled, provide information on options for treatment of addictive disease.

Recommendations for patients in recovery, in addition to the recommendations for all patients with addictive disease:

- Explain any intent to use opioids or other psychoactive medications.
- Explain the health risks associated with unrelieved pain, including increased risk of relapse.
- Encourage the patient, family, and significant others to discuss concerns about relapse, and offer assistance.
- Respect the patient's decision about whether to use opioids or other psychoactive medications. Reassure the patient that other methods of pain relief, such as nonsteroidal anti-inflammatory drugs and regional or local anesthetics, can be used if the patient prefers not to use opioid analgesics.
- Encourage a therapeutic plan in case relapse occurs.
- If relapse occurs, intensify recovery efforts; do not terminate pain care.

Recommendations for patients on methadone maintenance treatment, in addition to the recommendations for all patients with addictive disease:

- Initiate and continue regular discussions of the pain management plan with methadone treatment providers.
- Methadone doses used for methadone maintenance in the treatment of opioid addiction should be continued but not relied on for analgesia. When opioid analgesics are appropriate for pain management, two options are available:
  1. Add another opioid on an around-the-clock basis, or
  2. Give additional methadone doses. Methadone given for analgesia must be given more than once a day.

Visit the ASPMN Web site for the ASPMN Position Statement on Pain Management in Patients with Addictive Disease and references for managing the care of this patient population.

Adapted from ASPMN, Patients with Addictive Disease (ASPMN Position Paper, Sept 2002).

TABLE 4–11 Commonly Abused Substances and Withdrawal Manifestations

SUBSTANCE	COMMON EXAMPLES	COMMON STREET NAMES	WITHDRAWAL ONSET AND MANIFESTATIONS
Opiates (CNS depressant)	Codeine, hydromorphone (Dilaudid), morphine, oxycodone (Percodan), others Heroin, opium	Morphine: morph, M Dilaudid: little D, dillies, lords Percodan: percs Heroin: horse, smack, H Opium: hop, tar	**Onset:** 4–6 hours following last dose **Manifestations:** Mild initially and becoming more severe; dilated pupils, runny nose, diarrhea, abdominal pain, chills, gooseflesh, insomnia, aching joints and muscles, nausea and vomiting, muscle twitching and tremors (may become severe), mental depression

Alcohol (CNS depressant)	Beer, wine, whiskey, many others	Liquor, beer, booze, wine	**Onset:** 12–48 hours **Manifestations:** Headache, anxiety, depression, nervousness, shakiness, irritability, depression, fatigue, clouded thinking, emotionally labile; GI: nausea, vomiting, anorexia; CV: heart palpitations; EENT: enlarged, dilated pupils; skin: clammy, pale, sweaty palms; musculoskeletal: tremors, abnormal movements **Severe (complicated) withdrawal:** Rapid muscle tremors, seizures, tachycardia, cardiac dysrhythmias, profuse sweating, hallucinations, others
Barbiturates (CNS depressant)	Phenobarbital, pentobarbital	Barbs, red devils, goof balls, yellow jackets, downers	**Onset:** 12–20 hours following last dose **Manifestations:** Similar to alcohol withdrawal in the absence of alcohol; other mental changes: blank facial expression, slurred speech, flat affect; severe withdrawal can result in respiratory and heart failure, seizures, and death
Cocaine (CNS stimulant)	None	Coke, blow, snow, nose candy	**Onset:** 4–8 hours **Manifestations:** Few physical withdrawal symptoms; strong psychological symptoms, including rapid onset of depression, fatigue/sleepiness, strong craving for more cocaine, loss of pleasure; may also experience paranoia, agitation
Amphetamines (CNS stimulant)	Methylphenidate (Ritalin), pemoline (Cylert)	Speed, uppers, dexies, crank, meth, ice, crystal	**Onset:** 4–8 hours **Manifestations:** Depression, severe craving, mental confusion, insomnia, restlessness, paranoia, possible psychosis
Ecstasy (3,4-methylene-dioxymethamphetamine [MDMA])*	None	XTC, Adam, roll, E	**Onset:** Rapid **Manifestations:** depression, anxiety, panic attacks, sleeplessness, depersonalization, paranoid delusions, drug craving
Anabolic-androgenic steroids*	Depo-Testosterone, clomiphene citrate (Clomid), stanozolol	Roids, juice, Arnolds, stackers, gym candy	**Onset:** Not fully documented **Manifestations:** Mood swings, fatigue, restlessness, anorexia, insomnia, reduced sex drive, the desire for more steroids

*Additional sources for onset and manifestations information: Ecstasy: National Institute on Drug Abuse [NIDA]. (2006); Anabolic-androgenic steroids: Leshner, (2008).

Other clinical pain management suggestions include the following:

- Avoid (if possible) analgesics that have the same pharmacologic basis as the abused drug. For example, heroin is a form of opiate.
- Choose extended-release and long-acting analgesics (e.g., fentanyl and methadone) rather then short-acting ones, and restrict short-acting opiates for breakthrough pain (Kurtz, 2003).
- Avoid naloxone (Narcan) unless life-threatening toxic effects are present because use of naloxone will precipitate immediate opiate withdrawal (Kurtz, 2003).
- Administer analgesics orally rather than intravenously when possible.

SECTION SEVEN REVIEW

1. Older patients have fewer endogenous receptors and neurotransmitters than younger patients. The primary clinical significance of this statement is
   A. larger doses of opioids are required to achieve pain relief
   B. pain relief using opioids is more unpredictable
   C. smaller doses of opioids are required to achieve pain relief
   D. pain relief using opioids is less effective
2. Accumulation of morphine metabolites in the blood because of renal dysfunction can cause
   A. severe respiratory depression
   B. seizures
   C. tachycardia
   D. CNS stimulation
3. Accumulation of the metabolite of meperidine (normeperidine) in the blood can result in
   A. severe sedation
   B. bradycardia
   C. severe respiratory depression
   D. seizures
4. The known substance abuser who is hospitalized
   A. should receive no opioids
   B. may require higher-than-usual opioid dose ranges
   C. should receive only one type of opioid
   D. may require lower-than-usual opioid dose ranges
5. Substance abusers may require significantly higher doses of analgesia to achieve the same level of pain relief as a nonabuser.
   A. True
   B. False
6. Amphetamine withdrawal is associated with which manifestation?
   A. depression
   B. nausea and vomiting
   C. severe headache
   D. muscle twitching

Answers: 1. C, 2. A, 3. D, 4. B, 5. A, 6. A

SECTION EIGHT: Conscious Sedation

At the completion of this section, the learner will be able to discuss the nursing management of patients undergoing conscious/moderate sedation.

Conscious sedation, also referred to as moderate sedation, is classified as a "sedation level two" on the American Society of Anesthesiologists' (ASA) sedation-analgesia continuum. Most often it is used to induce relaxation with minimal variation in vital signs when patient cooperation is needed for a procedure (Harrington, 2006). Conscious sedation is produced by the administration of pharmacological agents, primarily through the intravenous route. A patient who is undergoing conscious sedation has an altered level of consciousness but is still able to maintain a patent airway and respond to verbal and environmental stimuli (American Association of Critical Care Nurses, 2002).

The terminology of sedation has changed considerably over the years. Both medical and dental specialties have used conflicting terms to describe the continuum of consciousness, which ranges from awake and alert to death. It is important that the high-acuity nurse have a clear understanding of the different stages of consciousness to effectively communicate with members of the health care team. Clarification of terms leads to increased patient safety. The Ramsay Sedation Scale was developed in 1974 to assess sedation in the intensive care unit. Recently this scale was modified to correlate with sedation definitions that have been outlined by TJC. A comparison of these definitions is summarized in Table 4–12.

Purpose of Conscious Sedation

A high-acuity patient who is moderately sedated can tolerate uncomfortable procedures such as diagnostic colonoscopy, endoscopic retrograde cholangiopancreatography (ERCP), upper endoscopy, or electrical cardioversion. The patient is able to breathe spontaneously and maintain his airway, cough and swallow reflexes remain intact, and cardiovascular function is not affected (Harrington, 2006). The number and types of procedures done outside of the operating room are increasing and nurses often provide the sedation. Nurses may administer conscious sedation only in the presence of a physician (American Society of Pain Management Nurses [ASPMN], 2008).

TABLE 4–12 Ramsay Sedation Scale Modified to Correlate with TJC Definitions of Minimal Sedation, Moderate Sedation, Deep Sedation, and General Anesthesia

SCORE	MODIFIED RAMSAY SEDATION SCALE SCORE DEFINITION	TJC SEDATION DEFINITION
1	Awake and alert, minimal or no cognitive impairment	**Minimal sedation (anxiolysis)** is a drug-induced state during which patients respond normally to verbal commands. Although cognitive function and coordination may be impaired, ventilatory and cardiovascular functions are unaffected.
2	Awake but tranquil, purposeful responses to verbal commands at conversational level	**Moderate sedation/analgesia**: A drug-induced depression of consciousness during which patients respond purposefully to verbal commands, either alone or accompanied by light tactile stimulation. No interventions are required to maintain a patent airway and spontaneous ventilation is adequate. Cardiovascular function is usually maintained.
3	Appears asleep, purposeful responses to verbal commands at conversational level	
4	Appears asleep, purposeful responses to commands but at a louder than usual conversational level, requiring light glabellar tap, or both	
5	Asleep, sluggish purposeful responses only to loud verbal commands, strong glabellar tap, or both	**Deep sedation/analgesia** is a drug-induced depression of consciousness during which patients cannot be easily aroused but respond purposefully following repeated or painful stimulation. The ability to independently maintain ventilatory function may be impaired. Patients may require assistance in maintaining a patent airway, and spontaneous ventilation may be inadequate. Cardiovascular function is usually maintained.
6	Asleep, sluggish purposeful responses only to painful stimuli	
7	Asleep, sluggish withdrawal to painful stimuli only (no purposeful responses)	
8	Unresponsive to external stimuli, including pain	**General anesthesia** is a drug-induced loss of consciousness during which patients are not arousable, even by painful stimulation. The ability to independently maintain ventilatory function is often impaired. Patients often require assistance in maintaining a patent airway, and positive pressure ventilation may be required because of depressed spontaneous ventilation or drug-induced depression of neuromuscular function. Cardiovascular function may be impaired.

From Mace, S. E., Ducharme, J., and Murphy, M. F. (2006). *Pain Management and Sedation: Emergency Department Management.* New York: McGraw-Hill. With permission.

Nursing Management of the Consciously Sedated Patient

Institutions that provide conscious sedation are required to abide by strict policies, clinical guidelines, and protocols. The policies must contain age-appropriate considerations and should include: necessary equipment and supplies; mandatory education requirements; process for validating competency; interface with Risk Management and Quality Improvement; and required documentation (ASPMN, 2008). Those administering the sedation must be trained to rescue patients who become unstable during the procedure or progress to deeper states of sedation (Pino, 2007). For example, if a patient is undergoing a procedure with moderate sedation and he progresses to a state of deep sedation, the nurse must be prepared to manage the compromised airway by providing oxygenation and ventilation. If that same patient progresses to a state of general anesthesia, the nurse must be competent to manage oxygenation and ventilation as well as an unstable cardiovascular system.

Before the Procedure

Prior to beginning any procedure that requires conscious sedation, the nurse must verify that the patient or family, if indicated, has given informed consent and the physician has explained the procedure to them. This includes, but is not limited to, the medications to be administered, risks, benefits, possible adverse reactions, and alternative treatments (Harrington, 2006).

It is essential that the nurse managing the care of the patient undergoing conscious sedation has no additional responsibilities during this time that might result in leaving the patient unattended or compromise continuous monitoring (AACN, 2002). Nurses must be specifically trained in the care of these patients and have a working knowledge of the legal liability of administering conscious sedation (AACN, 2002). The high-acuity nurse who administers medications for procedural sedation must have an understanding of the principles of respiratory physiology and will be required to monitor oxygenation and ventilation (American Society of Pain Management Nurses [ASPMN], 2008).

During the Procedure

Continuous monitoring of oxygen saturation using pulse oximetry (SpO_2) is the standard of care (Guliano & Higgans, 2005). Other physiologic measurements that must be monitored during the sedation and recovery period include respiratory rate, blood pressure, heart rate and rhythm, and level of consciousness (AACN, 2002). Capnometry has been recommended for conscious sedation but is not mandated (Mace et al., 2006). The equipment listed in Table 4–13 must be available prior to the start of the procedure. Back-up personnel trained in airway management, intubation, and advanced cardiac life support (ACLS) should be readily available in the event of an emergency. If available, the respiratory therapist may provide an extra set of hands if needed for airway management.

TABLE 4–13 Equipment Needed for Conscious Sedation

Intravenous access
Pulse oximeter
Blood pressure monitor
Cardiac monitor
Emergency medications
Emergency cart with defibrillator
Suction equipment
Positive pressure breathing device (Ambu bag)
Supplemental oxygen
Appropriate artificial airways (e.g., oral airways, endotracheal tubes)

Post-Procedure

The high-acuity nurse must monitor the patient's level of consciousness and vital signs until the patient is fully awakened from the sedation. Depending upon the procedure performed, the nurse will also assess for pain, wound drainage, nausea, vomiting, intake and output, and neurovascular status. Following the procedure, the patient may report a brief period of amnesia. Other side effects may include headache, hangover, or unpleasant memories of the diagnostic procedure (American Association of Nurse Anesthetists [AANA], 2008). No patient should be sent to an unsupervised area such as X-ray until he has returned to the previous state of sedation. In the event the patient does need to leave the area to have another procedure before he is fully recovered, the nurse must accompany him (Mace et al., 2006).

Drugs Used for Conscious Sedation

A wide variety of drugs are available for use to attain a state of conscious sedation. This may include but is not limited to etomidate, propofol, ketamine, fentanyl, and midazolam. Drugs used for conscious sedation are summarized in the Related Pharmacotherapy box. Medications that produce a state of sedation may not control pain. Often, a combination of analgesics and sedatives is selected. To achieve the best results, these intravenous medications should be administered through separate intravenous lines. The patient's level of pain should be assessed using a behavioral pain rating scale, and analgesics should be administered as indicated by the patient's condition (Harrington, 2006).

Because of the multiple uses for these drugs, it is important to focus on the goal of therapy rather than on the specific drug (ASPMN, 2008). The use of single large-bolus doses of any medication carries more risk for respiratory and cardiovascular depression than titrated intravenous administration to a defined end point. Titratable drugs have rapid onset and offset and allow for adjustments in dose and dose interval (Mace et al., 2006). Administration of the drugs and monitoring of the patient is typically the responsibility of the nurse while the procedure is being performed.

Possible Complications of Conscious Sedation

Deep Sedation

Sedation is a continuum and it is not always possible to predict how a patient will respond to the medication. Therefore, the nurse who is administering moderate sedation must be

RELATED PHARMACOTHERAPY: Short-Acting Intravenous Anesthetics Used for Conscious Sedation

Hypnotics/Sedative Hypnotics

Etomidate (Amidate)
Propofol (Diprivan)

Actions and Uses

Short-acting hypnotics/sedative hypnotics that induce and maintain anesthesia. If concurrent analgesia is desired it may be given with short-acting opioid, such as fentanyl.

Major Side/Adverse Effects

- Cardiovascular and respiratory depression
- Nausea and vomiting
- Etomidate: Seizure-like activity is possible during induction.
- Overdose: Severe cardiopulmonary depression (hypotension, apnea, cardiopulmonary arrest)

Nursing Implications

- Etomidate: Suppresses adrenal cortex function causing temporary reduction in steroid hormone synthesis, such as cortisol.
- Propofol: Cautious use with hypovolemic states and in elderly and patients with poor cardiac function. **Increased infection risk**: Vials carry high risk for infection due to composition of the solution which makes it an excellent bacterial growth medium. Discard open vial within six hours. Store unopened vials at 22°C.

Opioids

Fentanyl (Sublimaze)

Actions and Uses

Narcotic analgesic that causes CNS depression. Useful for short-term analgesia needed for painful procedures or treatments. Often used in conjunction with short-term anesthesia agents.

Major Side/Adverse Effects

- Cardiovascular and respiratory depression
- Overdose: apnea, cardiovascular collapse, cardiopulmonary arrest, others

Nursing Implications

- Monitor patient for opioid toxicity (severe respiratory depression, pinpoint pupils, and coma).
- Cautious use in elderly as it may result in severe respiratory depression.

Benzodiazepines

Midazolam (Versed®)

Actions and Uses

Short-acting benzodiazepines are CNS depressants that can produce an unconscious state and amnesia. They are useful for inducing anesthesia and for conscious sedation. For the purpose of conscious sedation, they are often used in combination with a short-acting opioid analgesic, such as fentanyl.

Major Side/Adverse Effects

- Cardiac and respiratory depression (hypotension, cardiac dysrhythmias, airway obstruction, apnea, respiratory arrest, and others)
- Nausea and vomiting, hiccups
- Overdose: deep sedation, unstable vital signs

Nursing Implications

- For sedation purposes: drug should be delivered slowly (over at least two minutes) to minimize adverse cardiac and respiratory complications
- Contraindicated in patient with glaucoma or if patient has vital signs that are abnormally low.

Dissociative Anesthetic

Ketamine (Ketalar®)

Actions and Uses

Ketamine places the patient in a dream-like state that is dissociated from his or her environment. Other actions include analgesia, amnesia, sedation, and immobility. It is most useful for pediatric use during minor procedures or diagnostic tests.

Major Side/Adverse Effects

- Cardiovascular and respiratory stimulation
- Sensory and neuro: nystagmus and diplopia, increased muscle tone (may develop seizure-like activity).
- Nausea and vomiting
- Adverse psychological reactions: may develop hallucinations, confusion, excited state, and delirium lasting for approximately one hour.

Nursing Implications

- Adverse psychological reactions: most common in 15-65 age range. To minimize, maintain patient in a quiet, low stimulus environment. Premedicating patient with a benzodiazepine prior to ketamine induction reduces risk of this reaction.
- Use is contraindicated in patients with severe hypertension or known hypersensitivity.

Data from Gahart & Nazareno (2008); Lehne (2007).

prepared to rescue a patient who progresses to a state of deep analgesia (sedation) (Mace et al., 2006). The Joint Commission (TJC) recommends that health care personnel administering conscious sedation be qualified to rescue a patient from unintentional deep sedation. This includes the ability to manage a compromised airway and provide ventilation if necessary. Placing a call to the Rapid Response Team in such an emergency does not meet this standard (Harrington, 2006). If the patient progresses to a deeper state of sedation than required for the procedure, all efforts must be focused on returning the patient to the original level of sedation. It is not acceptable to continue the procedure if the patient is over-sedated (Mace et al, 2006).

Other Possible Complications

Adverse events may include cardiopulmonary arrest, airway compromise, hypoxemia, aspiration, significant hypotension, significant brady/tachycardia, prolonged sedation, or death (Mace et al, 2006). If necessary, the nurse should be prepared to initiate resuscitative measures, including CPR, cardioversion, or defibrillation if indicated (American Society of Pain Management Nurses [ASPMN], 2008). Untoward events must be documented and reported according to established protocols. Reporting of adverse events through the proper channels allows for follow-up and continuous quality improvement.

SECTION EIGHT REVIEW

1. When a patient is sedated at level two (conscious sedation), the nurse would expect to assess which patient level of response?
   A. fully conscious but pain free
   B. altered level of consciousness but able to respond to verbal stimuli
   C. not responsive to verbal stimuli but able to maintain a patent airway
   D. does not respond to verbal or environmental stimuli
2. During a procedure in which conscious sedation is used, which parameters are usually monitored?
   A. arterial blood gases, 12-lead ECG, and vital signs
   B. level of consciousness, arterial blood gases, and ECG rhythm
   C. pulse oximetry, vital signs, cardiac rhythm, and level of consciousness
   D. vital signs, serum electrolytes, pulse oximetry, and level of consciousness
3. Equipment that should be available during a procedure in which conscious sedation is employed includes
   A. emergency cart with defibrillator, suction equipment, and Ambu bag
   B. central intravenous access, pulse oximeter, and blood pressure monitor
   C. supplemental oxygen, ABG-obtaining equipment, emergency equipment
   D. emergency medications, suction equipment, and mechanical ventilator on stand-by
4. When propofol (Diprivan) is used, the nurse can expect that the unused vial will require
   A. special handling with gloves
   B. protection from the sunlight
   C. disposal after six hours
   D. placement in a freezer after two hours
5. A patient receives ketamine (Ketalar) as anesthesia. The nurse is aware that to minimize the chance of adverse psychological reactions
   A. A sedative may be required.
   B. Frequent stimulation is required.
   C. A reversal drug will be administered.
   D. A quiet, low stimulation environment needs to be maintained.
6. A major complication of conscious sedation that must be monitored for is development of
   A. unintentional deep sedation
   B. anaphylactic reaction
   C. status epilepticus
   D. hypertensive crisis

Answers: 1. B, 2. C, 3. A, 4. C, 5. D, 6. A

POSTTEST

The following posttest is constructed in a case study format. A patient is presented, and questions are asked based on available data. New data are presented as the case study progresses.

Marcos M., 32-years-old, was involved in a pedestrian–car crash in which he sustained multiple injuries. It is now four days after open reduction of his left femur and left humerus; a splenectomy was also necessary. He is complaining of severe sharp pain at his abdominal incision site.

1. His sharp pain is transmitted through
   A. A fibers
   B. B fibers
   C. C fibers
   D. D fibers
2. Marco's acute pain sensation is transmitted up the spinal cord and terminates in the
   A. thalamus
   B. substantial gelatinosa
   C. cerebral cortex
   D. brain stem
3. The type of pain that Marcos is most likely experiencing at this time is
   A. brief acute
   B. acute persistent
   C. chronic
   D. chronic intermittent

4. Which of the following statements is correct regarding suffering?
   A. It is related to the personal meaning of pain.
   B. It is measurable.
   C. It is associated with acute pain.
   D. It bears no relations to stress and anxiety.

The nurse notes Marcos continues to be in a high anxiety state and continues to require analgesia at regular intervals.

5. Which statement reflects the relationship between pain and anxiety?
   A. anxiety increases pain tolerance
   B. anxiety decreases pain complaints
   C. anxiety decreases pain-related stress
   D. anxiety increases pain perception
6. If Marco's stress response becomes too high, it can result in (choose all that apply)
   A. counterregulation of hormone responses
   B. decreased vascular shunting
   C. hypoperfusion of vital organs
   D. initial elevation in levels of blood endorphins

The nurse notes that Marcos is becoming increasingly agitated and he has begun rhythmically hitting his right foot on the rail of the bed.

7. The nurse's initial intervention should consist of
   A. administering his ordered analgesic
   B. contacting the physician
   C. having him indicate his pain level on a VAS
   D. documenting his new behaviors
8. The best method of assessing Marcos for pain is by
   A. self-report
   B. facial cues
   C. vital sign changes
   D. body posturing changes

Marcos is bilingual, with Spanish as his first language. His understanding of spoken English is only fair and he states that he does not read English well.

9. Based on Marco's language status, which of the following assessment approaches would be most valid (assuming all assessments are written in English)?
   A. Short-Form McGill
   B. VAS/NRS
   C. McGill Pain Questionnaire
   D. nurse observation
10. Marcos describes his pain as being severe and sharp. He is grimacing and continues to tap his foot on the bed rail. The nurse assigns him a pain intensity score of 8/10 (8 out of a possible 10) This method of assigning a score is
    A. probably accurate in reflecting his pain
    B. an acceptable alternative pain assessment tool
    C. acceptable only under special circumstance
    D. an inappropriate use of a unidimensional tool

Marcos is complaining of pain at a level of 7 /10. The nurse notes that his vital signs are normal and he is watching television. He is requesting pain medication.

11. Based on this new information, the nurse should
    A. contact his physician
    B. wait for one hour and recheck his vital signs
    C. administer his ordered analgesic
    D. suspect that he is exaggerating

Marcos has the following pain management orders: morphine 10 mg (IM) every 3 to 4 hours PRN; ibuprofen 400 mg (PO) every 6 hours.

12. Marco's combination pain therapy is ordered for which primary purpose?
    A. to enhance the level of analgesia
    B. to increase sedation effects
    C. to decrease respiratory depressive effects
    D. to significantly reduce opioid dose

Marcos is switched to intravenous patient controlled analgesia (PCA).

13. The primary advantage for switching Marcos from injections to intravenous PCA is that PCA
    A. decreases the number of painful injections
    B. decreases the frequency of patient assessment
    C. allows Marcos to gain some control over his analgesia
    D. reduces the risk of severe respiratory depression
14. If the epidural route for analgesia had been chosen, the nurse would focus the pain assessment on the degree of
    A. sedation
    B. respiratory depression
    C. pulse decrease
    D. pain relief

Marcos is interested in trying some nonpharmacologic interventions.

15. The AHCPR guidelines support use of nonpharmacologic in patients who (choose all that apply)
    A. are comatose
    B. have prolonged pain
    C. express fear or anxiety
    D. would benefit from reducing drug therapy

Marcos has been receiving morphine on a regular basis for several weeks. He is now complaining that the usual dose he has been receiving is no longer relieving his pain as effectively.

16. Assuming nothing has changed in Marco's condition, the nurse would suspect that Marcos is
    A. exaggerating his level of pain
    B. becoming psychologically dependent
    C. developing tolerance to the morphine
    D. needs to have the morphine discontinued

17. The term pseudoaddiction refers to behaviors that mimic those associated with addiction but are motivated by:
    A. drug craving
    B. drug tolerance
    C. PRN drug administration
    D. pain undertreatment
18. Marcos is refusing to take any more morphine because he is afraid he will stop breathing. The nurse teaches Marcos about opioid therapy based on which facts? (choose all that apply)
    A. opioid use places him at high risk for respiratory depression
    B. sedation occurs before respiratory depression
    C. respiratory depression is dose-related
    D. his level of sedation and respiratory rate will be closely monitored
19. If Marcos develops renal function impairment while receiving morphine, he will need to be monitored closely for
    A. tachycardia
    B. severe tachypnea
    C. seizure activities
    D. severe respiratory depression

Posttest answers are with rationale found on MyNursingKit.

REFERENCES

AHCPR [Agency for Health Care Policy and Research]. (1992). *Acute pain management: Operative or medical procedures and trauma. Clinical Practice Guideline No. 1.* Rockville, MD: U.S. Department of Health and Human Services. [AHCPR Publication No. 92–0032.]

AHCPR [Agency for Health Care Policy and Research]. (1994). *Management of cancer pain. Clinical Practice Guideline No. 9.* Rockville, MD: U.S. Department of Health and Human Services. [AHCPR Publication No. 94–0592.]

American Association of Critical Care Nurses [AACN]. (2002). AACN Position Statement. Role of the registered nurse (RN) in the management of patients receiving conscious sedation for short-term therapeutic, diagnostic or surgical procedures. Available at: www.aacn.org/AACN/practice.nsf/Files/o2s/$file/2002%201%20Sedation.doc. Accessed February 20, 2008.

American Association of Nurse Anesthetists. (2008). Conscious Sedation: What the Patient Should Expect. Available at : http://www.aana.com/forpatients.aspx. Accessed March 20, 2008.

American Pain Society. (2003). *Principles of analgesic use in the treatment of acute pain and cancer pain* (5th ed.). Glenview, IL: Author.

ASAM. (2001). American Academy of Pain Medicine. Public Policy of ASAM: Definitions related to use of opioids in pain treatment. Available at: www.asam.org/ppol/paindef.htm. Accessed February 11, 2004.

ASPMN [American Society of Pain Management Nurses]. (2008). Procedural Sedation Consensus Statement. Available at: http://www.aspmn.org/organization/documents/PS_-2-11-08.pdf. Accessed March 2, 2008.

ASPMN [American Society of Pain Management Nurses]. (2002). ASPMN position statement: Pain management in patients with addictive disease. Available at: www.aspmn.org/html/PSaddiction.htm. Accessed February 11, 2004.

Ballantyne, J., Fishman, S., Abdi, S., (2002), *The Massachusetts General Hospital Handbook of Pain Management,* 2d ed. New York: Lippincott, Williams and Wilkins.

Carey, S. J., Turpin, C., Smith, J., et al. (1997). Improving pain management in an acute care setting. *Journal of Orthopedic Nursing, 16*(4), 29–36.

Carroll, I. R, Angst, M. S., Clark, I. K. (2005) Management of perioperative pain in patients chronically consuming opioids, *Regional Anesthesia and Pain Medicine,*

Chapman, C. R., & Syrjala, K. L. (1990). Measurement of pain. In J.J. Bonica (ed.), *The management of pain, vol. 1,* 2d ed., pp. 480–594. Philadelphia: Lea & Febiger.

Curtis, S., Kolotylo, C., & Broome, M. E. (2002). Somatosensory function and pain. In C.M. Porth (ed.), *Pathophysiology: concepts of altered health states* (5th ed., pp. 1091–1122). Philadelphia: J. B. Lippincott.

DeFriez, C., & Huether, S. (2008). Pain, temperature, sleep, and sensory function. In S.E. Huether & K. L. McCance (eds.). *Understanding pathophysiology,* 4th ed., pp. 305–330. St. Louis: Mosby/Elsevier.

DeLeon-Casasola, O. (2006). *Cancer pain: pharmacological, interventional and palliative care approaches.* New York: Saunders-Elsevier.

Dunwoody, C., Krenzischek, D., Pasero, D., Polomano, R., Rathmell, J. (2005). Assessment, Physiological Monitoring and Consequences of Inadequately Treated Pain, *Pain Management Nursing,* 9(1) pp. S11–S21.

Elia, N., Lysakowski, C., Tramer, M. R. (2005) Does Multimodal Analgesia with Acetaminophen, Nonsteroidal Antiinflammatory Drugs or Selective Cyclooxygenase-2 Inhibitors and Patient-Controlled Analgesia Morphine Offer Advantages over Morphine Alone? Meta-analyses of Randomized trials, *Anesthesiology,* 103, 1296–1304.

Ferrell, B. R., McCaffery, M., & Grant, M. (1991). Clinical decision making and pain. *Behavior Research and Therapy, 30*(1), 71–73.

Gahart, B. L. and Nazareno, A. R. (2008). *Intravenous Medications,* 24th ed. St. Louis: Mosby/Elsevier.

Giuliano, K. and Higgans, T. (2005). New Generation Pulse Oximetry in the Care of Critically Ill Patients. *American Journal of Critical Care,* 14(1), 26–39.

Gordon, D., Pellino, T. (2005). Incidence and character of naloxone use in postoperative pain management: a critical examination of Naloxone use as a potential quality measure. *Pain Management Nursing,* 6(1). 30–36.

Gurwitz, J. H., & Avorn, J. (2001). The ambiguous relation between aging and adverse drug reactions. *Annals of Internal Medicine, 114*(11), 956–966.

Guyton, A. C., & Hall, J. E. (2006a). Somatic sensations II: pain, headache, and thermal sensations. In A. C. Guyton & J.E. Hall (eds.), *Textbook of medical physiology,* 11th ed. (pp. 598–609). Philadelphia: Elsevier/Saunders.

Guyton, A. C., & Hall, J. E. (2006b). Somatic sensations: I. general organization, the tactile and position senses. In A. C. Guyton & J. E. Hall (eds.), *Textbook of medical physiology,* 11th ed. (pp. 585–597). Philadelphia: W. B. Saunders.

Harrington, L. (2006). Staying alert about NAPS. *Nursing Management,* Suppl., 2–6.

Heit, H.A. (2002, December). The best methods of managing pain in the recovering patient. *Counselor, 3*(6), 28–32.

Herr, K., Coyne, P. J., Key, T., Manworren, R., McCaffery, M., Merkel, S., Pelosi-Kelly, J., Wild, L. (2006). Pain assessment in the nonverbal patient: position statement with clinical practice recommendations, *Pain Management Nursing* 7(2)44–52.

Herr, K., Spratt, K., Mobily, P. R., Richardson, G. (2004). Pain intensity assessment in older adults: use of experimental pain to compare psychometric properties and usability of selected pain scales with younger adults, *The Clinical Journal of Pain,* 20(4)207–219.

Hutchison, R., Rodriguez, L. (2008). Capnography and respiratory depression. *American Journal of Nursing, 108*(2), 36–39.

Katzung, B. G. (2006). Special aspects of geriatric pharmacology. In B. G. Katzung (ed.), *Basic & clinical pharmacology,* 10th ed. (pp. 983–990). New York: McGraw Hill Medical.

Kehlet, H., Werner, M., Perkins, F. (1999), Balanced analgesia: what is it and what are its advantages in postoperative pain?, *Drugs,* 56(5)793–797.

Kurtz, D. R. (2003). Managing acute pain in admitted or suspected substance abusers. *Physician Assistant, 27*(7), 36–44.

Lamberg, L. (1998). Venus orbits closer to pain than Mars: Rx for one sex may not benefit the other. *The Journal of the American Medical Association, 280*(2). 120–128.

Lehne, R. A. (2007). *Pharmacology for nursing care,* 6th ed.. Philadelphia: Saunders/Elsevier.

Leshner, A. (2000 Revised). Anabolic Steroid Abuse. The NIDA Research Report Series, retrieved from www.drugabuse.gov/PDF/RRSteroi.pdf on 4/15/2008.

Loeser, J. D., & Cousins, M. J. (1990). Contemporary pain management. *The Medical Journal of Australia, 153,* 208–212, 216.

Lovering, S. (2006). Cultural attitudes and beliefs about pain. *Journal of Transcultural Nursing, 17*(4). 389–395.

Lussier, D., Huskey, A., Portenoy, R. K. (2004). Adjuvant analgesia in cancer pain management, *The Oncologist,* 9, 571–591.

Mace, S. E., Ducharme, J. and Murphy. M. F.(eds.) (2006). *Pain management and sedation: emergency department management* (pp.1–21). New York: McGraw-Hill, Medical Publishing Division.

Mace, S. E., Ducharme. J., Murphy, M. F. (2006). *Pain management and sedation: emergency department management,* New York, McGraw-Hill.

Main, C., Spanswick, C. (2000). *Pain management: an interdisciplinary approach,* London: Churchill Livingston.

McCaffery, M., & Pasero, C. (1999). *Pain: clinical manual for nursing practice,* 2d ed. St. Louis: C. V. Mosby.

McCaffery, M., Grimm, M., Pasero, C., Ferrell, B., Uman, G. C. (2005). On the meaning of "drug seeking." *Pain Management Nursing, 6*(4), 122–136.

Mehta, V., Langford, R. M. (2006) Acute pain management for opioid dependent patients, *Anaesthesia,* 61(3)269–276.

Melzack, R., & Wall, P. (1965). Pain mechanisms: a new theory. *Science, 150*(699), 971–979.

Mitra, S., Sinatra, R. (2004). Perioperative management of acute pain in the opioid-dependent patient. *Anesthesiology, 101*(1), 212–227.

National Institute on Drug Abuse [NIDA]. (2006). MDMA (Ecstasy). Retrieved from http://www.nida.nih.gov/InfoFacts/ecstasy.html accessed on 5/10/2008.

NCI [National Cancer Institute]. (2005). Substance abuse issues in cancer (PDQ®). Available at: www.cancer.gov/cancertopics/pdq/supportivecare/substanceabuse. Accessed May 13, 2008.

Payen, J. F., Bru, M. D., Bosson, J. L., et al. (2001). Assessing pain in critically ill sedated patients by using a behavioral pain scale. *Critical Care Medicine, 29*(12), 2258–2263.

Pino, R. M. (2007). The nature of anesthesia and procedural sedation outside of the operating room. *Current Opinion in Anesthesiology.* 20(4), August 2007, p. 347–351.

Prater, C. D., Zylstra, R. G., & Miller, K. E. (2002). Successful pain management for the recovering addicted patient. *Journal of Clinical Psychiatry, 4*(4), 125–131.

Reuben, S. S., Buvanendran, A. (2007). Preventing the development of chronic pain after orthopaedic surgery with preventive multimodal analgesic techniques. *The Journal of Bone and Joint Surgery, 89,* 1343–1358.

Rozen, D., and Grass, G. W. (2005). Perioperative and intraoperative pain and anesthetic care of the chronic pain and cancer pain patient receiving chronic opioid therapy. *Pain Practice, 5*(1), 18–32.

Stephenson, N. A. (1994). A comparison of nurse and patient perceptions of postsurgical pain. *Journal of Intravenous Nursing, 17,* 235–239.

Stotts, N. A., Puntillo, K., Stanik-Hutt, J., Thompson, C. L., White, C., and Rietman Wild, L. (2007). Does age make a difference in procedural pain perceptions and responses in hospitalized adults? *Acute Pain, 9*(30), 125–134.

World Health Organization. (1996). *Cancer Pain Relief with a Guide to Opioid Availability,* 2d ed. Geneva, Switzerland.

Young, J., Horton, F., Davidhizar, R. (2006). Nursing attitudes and beliefs in pain assessment and management. *Journal of Advanced Nursing, 53*(4), 412–21.

MODULE

5 Determinants and Assessment of Hematologic Function

Kathleen Dorman Wagner

OBJECTIVES

Following completion of this module, the learner will be able to

1. Explain the anatomy and physiology of the hematologic system.
2. Describe erythrocytes, the cells of oxygen transport.
3. Explain the characteristics and cells of innate (natural) immunity.
4. Discuss the characteristics and cells of adaptive (acquired) immunity.
5. Describe the characteristics of antigens and antigen-antibody response.
6. Describe the origin and function of platelets and coagulation.
7. Discuss the assessment of blood cells and coagulation.

This self-study module provides the reader with foundational information on the hematologic system that will facilitate a deeper understanding of the alterations modules (Modules 6-8). The module is divided into seven sections. The first six sections present the determinants of hematologic function. Section One provides a brief review of some of the basic anatomy and physiology of blood, blood cells, and organs and tissues of the immune system. Section Two provides a review of the erythrocyte, the cellular component of oxygen transport. Section Three presents a discussion of innate (natural) immunity, highlighting neutrophils, the mononuclear phagocyte system, natural killer lymphocytes, and the complement system. Section Four focuses on adaptive (acquired) immunity, with a discussion of humoral and cell-mediated immunity highlighting the major cells of adaptive immunity, the T and B lymphocytes. Section Five provides information on antigens and the antigen-antibody response. Section Six, shifts from the immune system to focus on hemostasis with a discussion of platelets, as the cell component of hemostasis, and coagulation. Finally, Section Seven presents an overview of major laboratory tests performed to assess the status of the blood cells and coagulation. Each section includes a set of review questions to help the learner evaluate her or his understanding of the section's content before moving on to the next section. All Section Reviews include answers. It is suggested that the learner review those concepts answered incorrectly in the review questions before proceeding to the next section.

PRETEST

1. The major single component of blood is
   A. plasma
   B. cell wastes
   C. blood cells
   D. glucose
2. A fully differentiated blood cell has which characteristics? (choose all that apply)
   A. one function
   B. clones itself
   C. cannot reproduce
   D. no granules
3. The bursa equivalent is thought to be located in the
   A. spleen
   B. Peyer's patches
   C. bone marrow
   D. thymus
4. Formation of new erythrocytes is regulated by level of
   A. alveolar oxygen tension
   B. tissue oxygenation
   C. cytokine stimulation
   D. stimulation of bone marrow
5. Adequate iron is a crucial part of hemoglobin because
   A. it cements the hemoglobin chain together
   B. it facilitates the release of oxygen to the tissues
   C. the heme molecule attaches to it to make a chain
   D. the oxygen molecule attaches to it
6. Oxygen attaches to which part of the red blood cell?
   A. folate short arm
   B. the globin molecule
   C. the iron atom
   D. the heme portion of hemoglobin

7. A major function of macrophages is
   A. presenting an antigen to B cells and T cells
   B. protecting against local mucosal invasion of viruses
   C. triggering the complement system
   D. interfering with the immune response
8. To actively participate in phagocytic activities, monocytes must mature into
   A. neutrophils
   B. lysosomes
   C. cytokines
   D. macrophages
9. Which of the following immune cells is responsible for direct antigen attack and destruction?
   A. helper T cell
   B. NK cell
   C. suppressor B cell
   D. memory B cell
10. Cytokines as a group perform which overall function?
   A. directly destroy cancer cells
   B. stimulate the bone marrow to produce lymphocytes
   C. act as chemical messengers for immune system activation
   D. regulate endothelial activities throughout the body
11. A child who first had chicken pox and then is immune from that disease in the future is said to have
   A. active acquired immunity
   B. passive acquired immunity
   C. innate (natural) immunity
   D. species-specific immunity
12. The T lymphocyte that oversees many immune cell functions is the
   A. natural killer cell (NK)
   B. cytotoxic T cell (T_C)
   C. suppressor T cell (T_S)
   D. helper T cell (T_H)
13. Humoral immunity is best characterized by
   A. development of antibodies from B cells
   B. recognition of self and nonself
   C. specific recognition and memory of antigens
   D. differentiation of cellular function known as killer, helper, and suppressor cells
14. The immunoglobulin that comprises about 80 percent of the total immunoglobulin in the healthy human body is
   A. IgA
   B. IgE
   C. IgG
   D. IgM
15. The purpose of histocompatibility antigens is
   A. distinguish self from nonself
   B. muster an attack against foreign antigens
   C. present foreign antigens to phagocytes
   D. stimulate antibody production
16. Specific sites on antigens that interact with immune cells to elicit the immune response are called
   A. antigenic determinants
   B. surface cells
   C. human leukocyte antigens
   D. histocompatibility complexes
17. HLA antigens are located where on cells?
   A. cell nucleus
   B. cell cytoplasm
   C. cell surface
   D. chromosome 3
18. Which statement is correct regarding tumor associated antigens?
   A. they are highly recognizable as foreign or pathogenic
   B. they are not well recognized as being pathogenic early in tumor growth
   C. an antigen is called tumor necrosis factor (TNF)
   D. elevations of alpha-fetoprotein (AFP) suggest lung cancer
19. Platelet production is regulated by which substance?
   A. thrombopoietin
   B. platelet factor
   C. erythropoietin
   D. prostacyclin I_2
20. Which mineral ion is required throughout the coagulation cascade?
   A. Na^+
   B. K^+
   C. Fe^{++}
   D. Ca^{++}
21. During the dissolution process, a blood clot is destroyed by
   A. t-PA
   B. Plasminogen
   C. Plasmin
   D. Fibroblasts
22. An elevated reticulocyte count in the presence of anemia indicates that the
   A. red blood cells are being destroyed prematurely
   B. bone marrow is depressed
   C. red blood cells are to be sequestered in the spleen
   D. bone marrow is functioning correctly
23. Which cell component of the WBC differential count is normally the highest in percentage?
   A. lymphocytes
   B. monocytes
   C. basophils
   D. neutrophils
24. When a shift to the left occurs in the neutrophil count, it refers to a(n)
   A. elevated band level
   B. decreased band level
   C. elevated seg level
   D. decreased seg level

25. Lymphocytes make up about ______ percent of the total WBC count.
A. 5
B. 10
C. 20
D. 25

26. The INR is an international ratio measurement of
A. partial thromboplastin time
B. fibrin split products
C. prothrombin time
D. bleeding time

Pretest answers are found on MyNursingKit.

SECTION ONE: Review of Anatomy and Physiology

At the completion of this section, the learner will be able to explain the anatomy and physiology of the hematologic system.

Composition of Blood

The adult body contains about five liters of blood. Blood is composed of plasma, plasma proteins, and blood cells. Blood transports oxygen, glucose, hormones, electrolytes, and cell

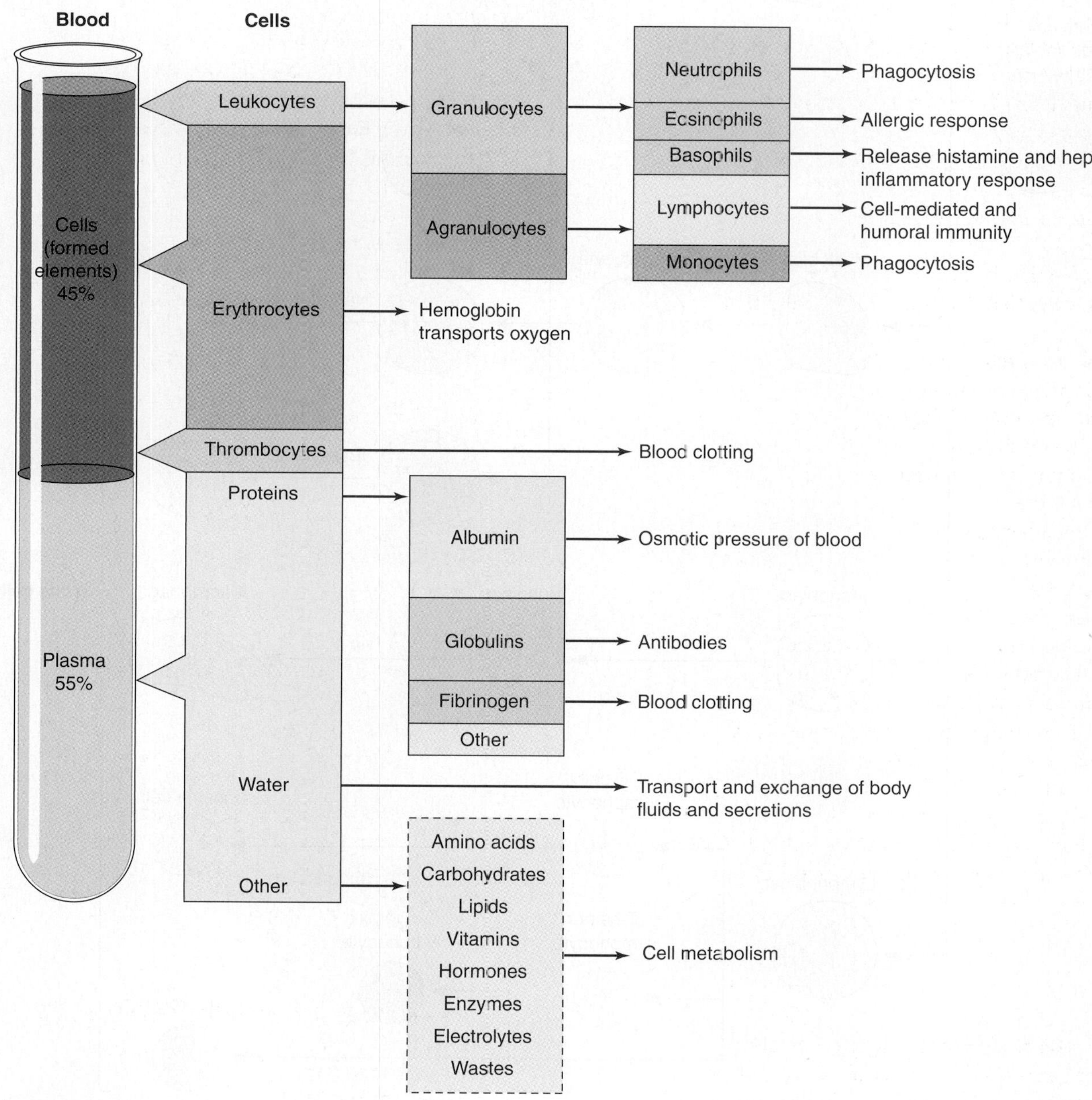

Figure 5–1 ■ Components of blood and their functions. Reprinted from Gould, B. (2002). Pathophysiology for the health professionals, (2nd ed., p.234) Copyright 2002, with permission from Elsevier.

wastes. Plasma is a clear fluid that remains after cells have been removed. Plasma makes up 55 percent of the whole blood volume. The remaining 45 percent of the whole blood volume is composed of cells (Rote & McCance, 2008). The anatomic components of blood and their physiologic functions are summarized in Figure 5–1.

By the fifth gestational month and throughout life thereafter, blood cells are formed in the bone marrow. Bone marrow

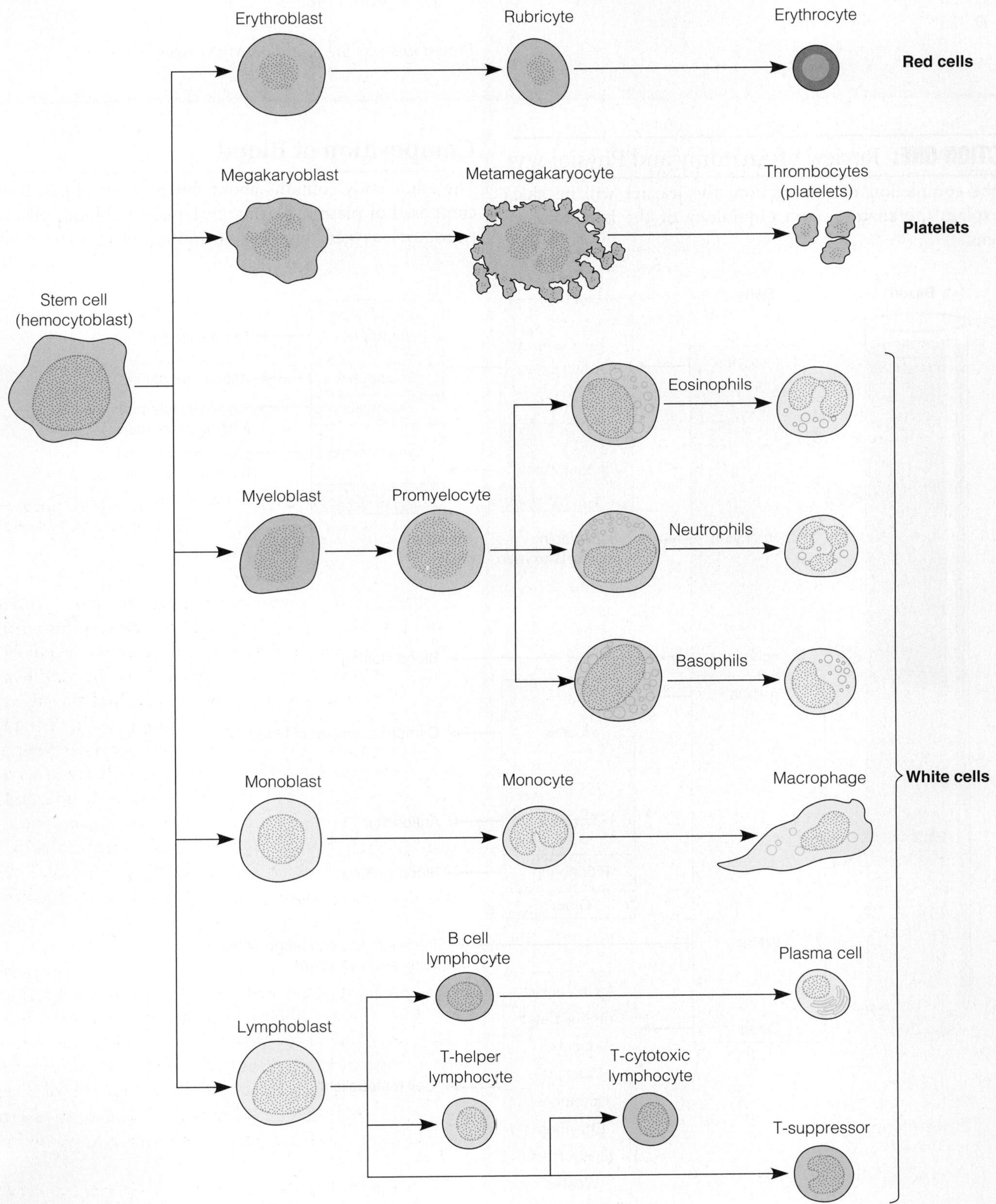

Figure 5–2 ■ Blood cell formation from stem cells. Regulatory factors control the differentiation of stem cells into blast cells. Each of the five kinds of blasts is committed to producing one type of mature blood cell. Erythroblasts, for example, can differentiate only into RBCs; megakaryoblasts can differentiate only into platelets.

exists within all bones and consists of yellow marrow (primarily composed of fat) and red marrow. It is the red marrow from which blood cells are formed. By young adulthood, red marrow (and therefore blood cell formation) is confined to specific bones, including the skull, ribs, sternum, ribs, vertebrae, and the ends (epiphyses) of the humerus and femur.

Formation of Blood Cells

Blood cells include **erythrocytes** (red blood cells), **leukocytes** (white blood cells), and **thrombocytes** (platelets). All three types of blood cells develop from the same stem cells, called **pluripotential hematopoietic stem cells (PHSC),** which reside in the bone marrow. Once appropriately induced to reproduce a particular type of blood cell, the pluripotential stem cell divides. During PHSC division, one cell may remain as a PHSC, whereas the other becomes a **committed stem cell** of either the myeloid or lymphoid cell line. This means that the newly committed cell begins to mature down a particular cell development pathway of cell growth and differentiation (Fig. 5–2). The term **cell differentiation** refers to the maturation process that a blood cell undergoes. It begins as an immature, undifferentiated (primitive) cell with no specific functions and ultimately becomes a mature, well-differentiated cell with specific cell functions. A fully differentiated (mature) blood cell has two major characteristics—it has only one function and it can no longer reproduce. The cell maturation process requires special proteins, called growth inducers and differentiation inducers. Factors external to the bone marrow trigger the formation of these special proteins. For example, chronic hypoxia induces secretion of erythropoietin, a growth factor that increases production of erythrocytes.

Organs and Tissues of the Immune System

Acting as a surveillance mechanism, the immune system monitors the internal environment of the body for foreign agents. It is a complex system of organs and cells capable of distinguishing self from nonself, remembering previous invaders, and reacting according to needs as they arise. The primary lymphoid organs are the bone marrow and the thymus, which are the major sites of lymphocyte development. The secondary lymphoid organs include the tonsils and adenoids, lymph nodes, spleen, and other lymphoid tissue. Cellular and humoral immune responses occur in the secondary lymphoid organs. The spleen responds to primary blood borne **antigens,** whereas the lymph nodes respond to antigens circulating in the lymph system. The tonsils respond to antigens, which enter through the mucosal barriers. Contributing to the immune response are lymphoid tissues in nonlymphoid organs (such as the intestinal tissue), and circulating immune cells, such as T cells, B cells, and phagocytes. Figure 5–3 shows primary organs and lymph tissue sites as well as the sites of T cell and B cell differentiation.

Lymph System

The blood is filtered continuously by the lymph system. The lymph nodes actually serve two purposes for the body. They act as a filtering system for foreign materials, and they serve as a reservoir for the specialized immunologic T cells and B cells.

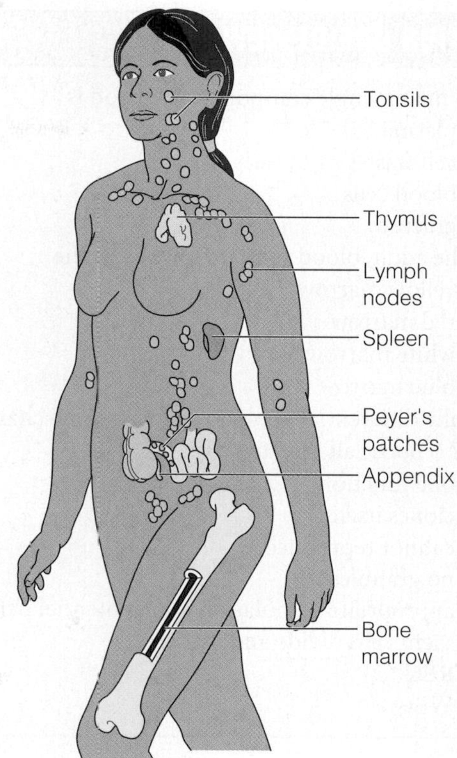

Figure 5–3 ■ The lymphoid system. The central organs of the thymus and bone marrow and the peripheral organs, including the spleen, tonsils, lymph nodes, and Peyer's patches.

Peripherally, the serous portion of the blood (excluding platelets, red blood cells, and large proteins) diffuses from the capillaries into the peripheral lymph channels, where it is progressively filtered and then returned to the cardiovascular system. Lymph ducts carry the serous fluid through lymph nodes, where it is filtered. It may be useful to think of a lymph node as a sponge, where the meshwork serves as a surface on which antigens and other foreign materials are arrested and destroyed or neutralized. Large clusters of lymph nodes are found in the axillae, groin, thorax, abdomen, and neck. With many infectious processes, these nodes become enlarged as their activity increases and defense cells proliferate. T cells are most abundant here, although B cells can be found also.

Spleen

The spleen is a small organ about the size of a fist in the left upper quadrant of the abdomen. It is protected by the ninth, tenth, and eleventh ribs and usually is nonpalpable. The spleen serves three functions, only one of which is actually immune-related. First, it is the site for the destruction of injured and worn-out red blood cells. Second, it is a reservoir for B cells, although T cells also are found there. Third, it serves as a storage site for blood, which is released from distended vessels in times of demand.

The tonsils, Peyer's patches in the intestine, and the appendix are quite similar in function and structure to the lymph nodes and the spleen. The tonsils, like the thymus, diminish in size after childhood and, unless inflamed, are difficult to distinguish from surrounding tissue in the posterior pharynx.

SECTION ONE REVIEW

1. The major single component of blood is
   - **A.** plasma
   - **B.** cell wastes
   - **C.** blood cells
   - **D.** glucose
2. In the adult, blood cells are formed in the
   - **A.** yellow marrow
   - **B.** red marrow
   - **C.** white marrow
   - **D.** blue marrow
3. A fully differentiated blood cell has which characteristics? (choose all that apply)
   - **A.** one function
   - **B.** clones itself
   - **C.** cannot reproduce
   - **D.** no granules
4. On appropriate stimulation, pluripotential hematopoietic stem cells divide and create a
   - **A.** RBC
   - **B.** WBC
   - **C.** committed stem cell
   - **D.** megakaryocyte
5. A major function of the lymph nodes is to
   - **A.** filter foreign substances
   - **B.** destroy worn-out red blood cells
   - **C.** produce lymphocytes
   - **D.** produce stem cells
6. Which function is correct regarding the spleen?
   - **A.** It destroys worn-out white blood cells.
   - **B.** It filters out foreign materials.
   - **C.** It produces the hormone thymosin.
   - **D.** It is a reservoir for B cells.

Answers: 1. A, 2. B, 3. (A, C), 4. C, 5. A, 6. D

SECTION TWO: Erythrocytes—The Cellular Component of Oxygen Transport

At the completion of this section, the learner will be able to describe erythrocytes, the cells of oxygen transport.

When compared to the total numbers of white blood cells and platelets, red blood cells (RBCs) or erythrocytes are by far the most plentiful of the blood cells. This quantity difference becomes readily apparent when looking at the laboratory blood cell counts: RBCs are measured in million per microliter (mcL), whereas white blood cells (WBCs) and platelets are measured in cells per mcL. Erythrocytes have a relatively long life span of approximately 120 days.

Erythropoiesis

The purpose of RBCs is oxygen transport via hemoglobin; and regulation is based on the level of tissue oxygenation, which is a function of tissue demand and oxygen transport. Red blood cells arise from the myeloid cell line in the red bone marrow and as reticulocytes, they mature in the blood or spleen. Erythrocyte production (**erythropoiesis**) is tightly regulated by **erythropoietin,** a circulating hormone that is primarily produced by the kidneys (about 90 percent). It is believed that erythropoietin may be produced in the renal tubular cells, which are major consumers of oxygen and are particularly sensitive to lowering oxygen levels. Erythropoietin is a critical part of an erythrocyte production feedback loop (Fig. 5–4). Erythropoietin is produced under specific conditions that decrease arterial oxygen tension and tissue hypoxia, including a reduction in RBCs or hemoglobin, decreased blood flow, or increased oxygen consumption (Rote & McCance, 2008). Once

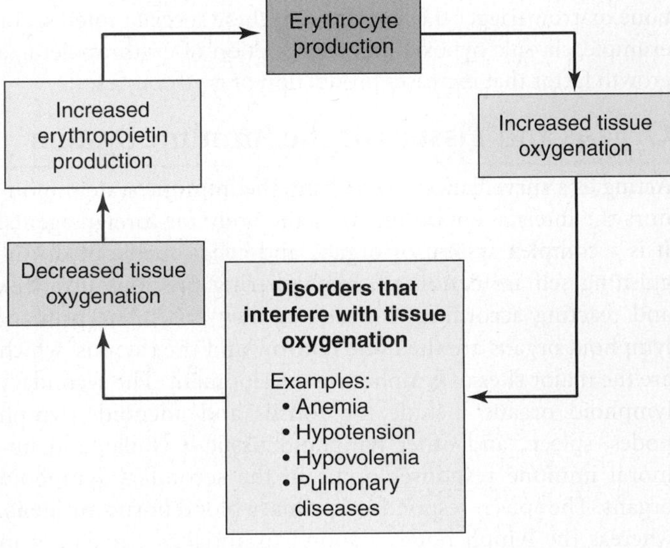

Figure 5–4 ■ Erythrocyte production feedback loop.

stimulated into production, erythrocytes take 3 to 5 days to mature. The erythrocyte maturation process is illustrated in Figure 5–5.

Production of normal RBCs requires adequate levels of certain nutrients, including protein, multiple vitamins, and minerals. Amino acids are needed to synthesize hemoglobin, which is protein-based. Vitamins B_6, B_{12}, folic acid, C, E, and others) are needed for normal RBC synthesis, development of DNA and RNA, and cell maturation. The minerals iron and copper are important for hemoglobin synthesis and strong plasma membrane.

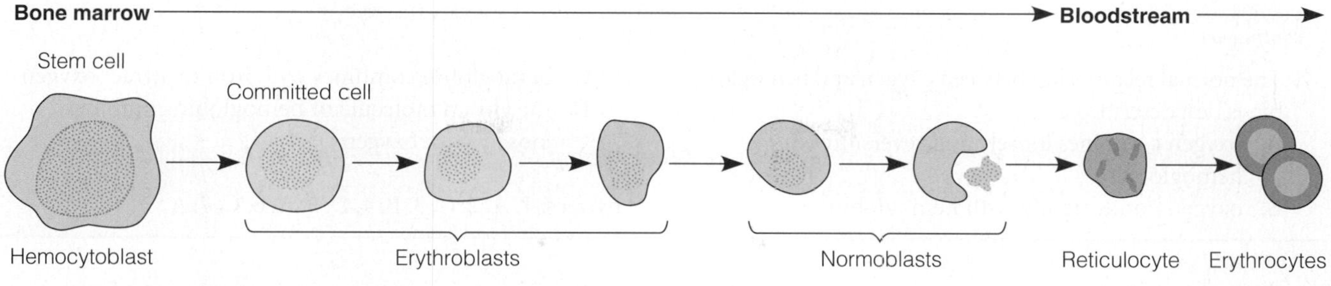

Figure 5–5 ■ Erythropoiesis. RBCs begin as erythroblasts within the bone marrow, maturing into normoblasts, which eventually eject their nucleus and organellas to become reticulocytes. Reticulocytes mature within the blood or spleen to become erythrocytes.

Hemoglobin

Hemoglobin (Hgb) is sometimes referred to as the respiratory protein because its function is to transport oxygen. The erythrocyte is uniquely structured to produce and carry hemoglobin, which constitutes about 90 percent of the total weight of an erythrocyte (Rote & McCance, 2008). Hemoglobin production begins early in the RBC maturation process and ends on maturation. As its name suggests, hemoglobin has two components—heme (nonprotein) and globin (protein) (Fig. 5–6). Each heme molecule contains one iron atom and one oxygen molecule. The oxygen molecule (O_2) located in hemoglobin is attached only to the single iron atom in the molecule; thus, when there is deficient iron in the body (e.g., iron-deficiency anemia), the oxygen-carrying capacity is significantly reduced. A heme molecule joins with a polypeptide chain to form a hemoglobin chain. It takes four hemoglobin chains, linked together, to form one hemoglobin molecule. In a normal adult male, there are about 15 grams of hemoglobin in every 100 mL of blood. Each gram of hemoglobin can bind with a maximum of about 1.34 mL of oxygen. Normally, the hemoglobin in 100 mL of blood (if fully saturated with oxygen) can bind with 20 mL of oxygen. Oxygen combines with hemoglobin loosely and reversibly. This means that oxygen can be loaded onto the hemoglobin, transported to the tissues, and then released from the hemoglobin to diffuse across the capillary membrane into the tissues.

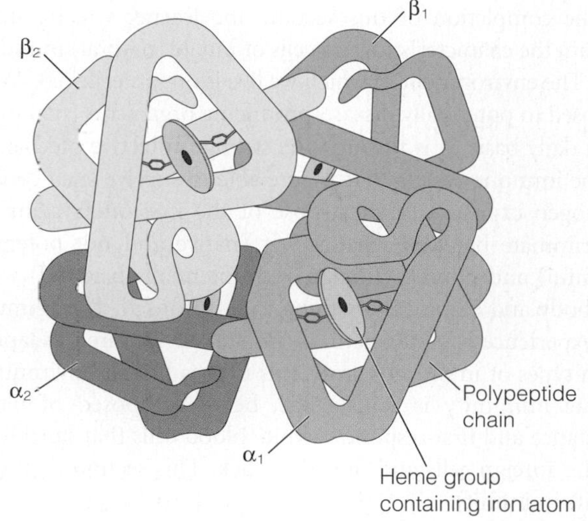

Figure 5–6 ■ The hemoglobin molecule includes globin (a protein) and heme, which contains iron. Globin is made of four subunits, two alpha and two beta polypeptide chains. A heme disk containing an iron atom (red dot) nests within the folds of each protein subunit. The iron atoms combine reversibly with oxygen, transporting it to the cells.

SECTION TWO REVIEW

1. The purpose of the erythrocyte is
   A. oxygen transport
   B. nutrient transport
   C. hemostasis
   D. protection
2. Erythropoietin is formed in which organ?
   A. lungs
   B. intestines
   C. kidneys
   D. spleen
3. Formation of new erythrocytes is regulated by the level of
   A. alveolar oxygen tension
   B. tissue oxygenation
   C. cytokine stimulation
   D. stimulation of bone marrow
4. Adequate iron is a crucial part of hemoglobin because
   A. it cements the hemoglobin chain together
   B. it facilitates the release of oxygen to the tissues
   C. the heme molecule attaches to it to make a chain
   D. the oxygen molecule attaches to it
5. Good protein nutrition is necessary for normal RBC production because it is
   A. required to synthesize hemoglobin
   B. necessary for cell maturation
   C. needed for plasma membrane development
   D. required to attract iron ions
6. Oxygen attaches to which part of the red blood cell?
   A. folate short arm
   B. the globin molecule
   C. the iron atom
   D. the heme portion of hemoglobin

(continued)

(continued)

7. The normal relationship between oxygen and hemoglobin is best described as
   A. oxygen combines loosely and reversibly with hemoglobin
   B. oxygen bonds tightly with hemoglobin
   C. hemoglobin combines with iron to attract oxygen
   D. the globin molecule of hemoglobin combines loosely with oxygen

Answers: 1. A, 2. C, 3. B, 4. D, 5. A, 6. C, 7. A

SECTION THREE: Characteristics and Cells of Innate (Natural) Immunity

At the completion of this section, the learner will be able to explain the characteristics and cells of innate (natural) immunity.

The environment in which we live is not a sterile one. We are exposed to potentially disease-producing organisms (pathogens) on a daily basis. It is through the strong protective mechanisms of the immune system that we are able to survive such constant pathogen exposure. The purpose of the immune system is to discriminate between what is self (native and not potentially harmful) and nonself (foreign and potentially harmful) within the body and eliminate anything that is nonself. The immunity we experience is either natural (innate) or acquired (adaptive). Both types of immunity protect us from a hostile environment. Innate immunity is nonspecific, being composed of natural resistance and first responder white blood cells that quickly recognize foreign cells and directly attack. This section focuses on innate immunity.

Innate (Natural) Immunity

Innate immunity is species specific; that is, human beings are immune to a variety of diseases to which certain animals are susceptible, and vice versa. For example, human beings are not vulnerable to feline leukemia and cats are not susceptible to human immunodeficiency virus (HIV). Innate immunity is natural; human beings are born with specific immunities. This innate immunity is nonspecific and provides primary protection against infection with immune cells that are incapable of developing long-term memory. Natural resistance to a particular infectious agent is not improved with repeated exposure to the agent; and includes physical barriers to disease by means of the skin and mucous membranes, and natural chemical barriers found in the gastrointestinal tract, respiratory tract, and genitourinary structures.

Phagocytosis

Phagocytosis is an important part of the innate (nonspecific) immune response whereby invading foreign materials or injured cells are ingested and destroyed by phagocytic cells (phagocytes). The major phagocytic cells include the granulocytes (neutrophils, etc.), monocyte/macrophages, and **natural killer (NK) cells.** Phagocytosis involves **chemotaxis,** the chemical attraction of phagocytic cells to antigens, as well as the engulfing of antigens for purposes of destruction or neutralization. A process known as **opsonization** modifies the antigen, making it more susceptible to phagocytosis. Two circulating factors enhance the opsonization process. The IgG immunoglobulin and C3b, a fragment of the complement system, are called **opsonins** and provide binding sites for attachment of macrophages or neutrophils to the antigen.

Cytokines

Special secreted cellular proteins, collectively called **cytokines,** are another important part of innate immunity. The cells of the immune system are regulated by cytokines, which serve as chemical messengers for activation of components of the immune system. The activities of cytokines are not restricted to the immune system; they are important in regulation of many hematopoietic functions, such as hematopoiesis and inflammation. Cytokines affect cells in several different ways. First, some cytokines activate the same cells that secrete them (autocrine actions). Others activate cells that are touching or are near the cytokine secreting cells (paracrine actions); while others are able to activate cells at distant sites (endocrine actions). Cytokine functions are redundant in that multiple cytokines perform the same function and may do so simultaneously. One major group of cytokines is produced by lymphocytes (T and B cells); and therefore can be referred to more specifically as **lymphokines.** For the purposes of this discussion, the broader term, cytokines, will be used.

There are many different cytokines that help regulate the immune system, including **interleukins (IL), interferons (INF), granulocyte monocyte colony-stimulating factors (GM-CSF),** and **tumor necrosis factor (TNF).** Many cytokines have multiple subtypes (e.g., more than 15 interleukins have been identified). Although interferons are pathogen nonspecific, they are species specific; thus, animal interferons offer little, if any, protection for human beings as vaccines. Table 5–1 summarizes the source and functions of these four cytokines.

While cytokines are crucial to normal immune function, they have also been associated with disease. For example, tumor necrosis factor (TNF) plays an active role in rheumatoid arthritis and psoriasis, and genetic modifications of TNF have been implicated in multiple diseases. Extremely high levels of TNF-alpha (in addition to several other mediators) have been found in children who died of septic shock (NCBI, 2008). The use of cytokines for therapeutic reasons continues to be of interest and a research focus, particularly in the treatment of certain diseases such as cancer and HIV/AIDS. GM-CSF is sometimes administered to patients with leukopenia to shorten WBC recovery time following chemotherapy treatment.

TABLE 5–1 Major Cytokines

CYTOKINE	SOURCE	FUNCTIONS
Interleukins (IL)	As a group, they are produced by WBCs, primarily T cells	Inflammatory mediator Lymphocyte activation, growth, and differentiation Attraction of neutrophils
Interferons (IF, IFN)	Originate from CD8 and some CD4 T cells, NK cells, and other cells.	Inhibit the synthesis of viral protein in their reproduction without inhibiting the host's protein synthesis in normal cell reproduction Macrophage activation Inflammatory mediator
Tumor necrosis factors (TNF)	Primarily produced by monocyte/macrophages and T cells	Proinflammatory Endothelial activities Involved in programmed cell death (apoptosis) Death of tumor cells (hence its name)
Granulocyte monocyte colony-stimulating factors (GM-CSF)	Primary produced by T cells	Involved in the division and differentiation of neutrophils and monocytes Acts in the bone marrow in response to inflammation and infection A proinflammatory cytokine due to its ability to stimulate secretion of TNF-alpha Different colony-stimulating factors influence the proportion of different cell types that are produced

Major Cells of Innate Immunity

The granulocytes (particularly neutrophils), NK cells (a granular lymphocyte) and the monocyte/macrophage system are the major cells responsible for innate immunity.

Neutrophils

Neutrophils, eosinophils, basophils, and monocytes have a common origin, the myelocyte; and all three are *polymorphonuclear granulocytes.* The term **polymorphonuclear** refers to the presence of multiple nuclei and explains why they are commonly referred to as *polys* or *polymorphonuclear neutrophils* **(PMNs).** Neutrophils significantly outnumber all of the other types of leukocytes, comprising 50 to 70 percent of the total leukocyte (WBC) count (Kee, 2009). The myelocyte cell lineage is illustrated in Figure 5–2 (see Myeloblast cell line).The term **granulocyte** refers to cells with granules located within the cytoplasm. The granules contain special enzymes that break down foreign and other substances. Neutrophils mature in the bone marrow and stay in reserve in the marrow for about five days before being sent into the general circulation. Once released from the bone marrow, they have a brief life span of only six to eight hours; thus, they must be reproduced at an extremely fast rate to keep up with the rapid turnover.

Neutrophils are the immune system's first line of defense in the presence of an acute infection or inflammation. They are first at the scene, within 1 to 1.5 hours of an injury event. Neutrophils are responsible for the formation of pus. As they die, neutrophil-degrading enzymes are released, causing breakdown and liquefaction of local cells as well as foreign substances. This forms **pus,** a thin liquid residue that is an important indicator of inflammation. Pus is an important consideration in the presence of neutropenia and is discussed in detail in Module 7, *Alterations in WBC Function.*

Mononuclear Phagocyte System

The mononuclear phagocyte system, sometimes referred to as the **reticuloendothelial system** or monocyte-macrophage system, refers to a group of immune cells and tissues, including monocytes, macrophages (mobile and fixed tissue), and certain endothelial cells found in the spleen, bone marrow, and lymph nodes (Guyton & Hall, 2006). This powerful system plays a major role in clearing the blood of bacteria (Rote & McCance, 2008).

Monocytes are large, single-nucleus cells that provide the second line of defense. Circulating monocytes are immature immune cells that do not actively participate in defense. They undergo maturational changes once they move into the tissues (Rote & McCance, 2008). During the maturation process, they enlarge by up to fivefold and develop a large number of lysosomes in their cytoplasm. Lysosomes provide a digestive system that can digest nutrients, bacteria, or other particles that are brought into the cell. After they have matured, the monocytes become powerful phagocytes called **macrophages.**

Monocytes act as long-term backup for neutrophils, arriving at the scene within about 5 hours of the event. Monocytes and neutrophils become the predominant cell types at the site of injury within 48 hours of the precipitating event. Monocytes live much longer than neutrophils, with a life span of four to five days. Monocytes circulate in the blood for about a day before taking up residence in a tissue, becoming tissue macrophages (histiocytes).

There are two types of macrophages, mobile and fixed. Mobile macrophages circulate in the blood supply and migrate out of the vessels into the tissues when required through the process of chemotaxis. Fixed macrophages, on leaving the circulation, affix themselves to tissues and remain there, waiting for pathogens to appear. When needed, fixed macrophages are able to break away from the tissue to initiate phagocytic activity. Tissue macrophages can remain in a fixed position within the tissue for months or years until they are required to protect the tissue through their phagocytic functions. Common examples of fixed macrophages include the Kupffer's cells in the liver and the type 1 alveolar cells in the lungs. They play important roles in protecting the organs against pathogens (e.g., bacteria or viruses, sloughing tissue or foreign particles).

Antigen-Presenting Cells. Macrophages participate in the immune response as **antigen-presenting cells (APCs)** by processing the antigen and presenting a fragment of it in such a way as to increase its recognition and reaction by the B and T lymphocytes. By means of phagocytosis, the macrophage ingests and digests the antigen; in the process, a fragment of the altered antigen is released through the macrophage cell membrane, where it attaches to receptor sites on the surface of the macrophage. It is at these receptor sites that the interaction takes place between the invading antigen and T lymphocytes. The macrophage is a critical factor in the immune response to both the T lymphocytes and the B lymphocytes and is considered the link between the inflammatory response and the specific resistance of antibody production and cell mediation by its production of interleukins. The macrophage is primarily responsible for carrying antigens to the lymph tissue, where the B lymphocytes and T lymphocytes reside. The liver, lungs, and lymph nodes contain macrophages because these areas encounter many antigens.

Migration Properties of Neutrophils and Macrophages. Circulating neutrophils and monocytes require some means of recognizing where they are needed, and then they must be able to transfer from the blood vessels to the site of injury. This process involves multiple steps, including margination, diapedesis, migration, and chemotaxis. Soon after initiation of the inflammatory response, the capillary endothelium becomes more permeable, allowing fluid to escape into the inflamed or injured area. The loss of fluid locally results in increased blood viscosity and increased concentration of cells in the local capillaries. When tissue becomes inflamed, a variety of chemicals, including chemical mediators and cytokines, are released at the site of injury. These chemical substances cause alterations of local capillary endothelial cells and stimulate leukocytes to increase their release of adhesion molecules.

Margination occurs as circulating leukocytes begin to accumulate and adhere to the capillary wall. Once the cells have adhered to the capillary wall, they develop **pseudopods** (fingerlike projections) and squeeze out of the capillary using ameboid movement, a process called **diapedesis.** After the leukocyte is outside the capillary, it requires guidance to move to the correct location. This is accomplished through chemotaxis, which refers to movement as a result of some type of chemical stimulus. When applied to leukocyte migration, chemotaxis is the movement of leukocytes along an increasing concentration of chemical stimulus (chemotactic factors) towards an area of inflammation. The leukocytes follow the signal, traveling by ameboid action to the inflammatory site. Figure 5–7 illustrates this concept.

Natural Killer Lymphocytes

Natural killer lymphocytes (NK cells) originate in the bone marrow, arising from the lymphocytic cell line. They are large in size and contain granules; thus, they are also known as large granulated lymphocytes or LGL. The NK cells comprise only about 2 percent of the total WBC count. NK cells are important in protecting the body from pathologic cells such as microbes and cancer cells through cytolytic activities and secretion of

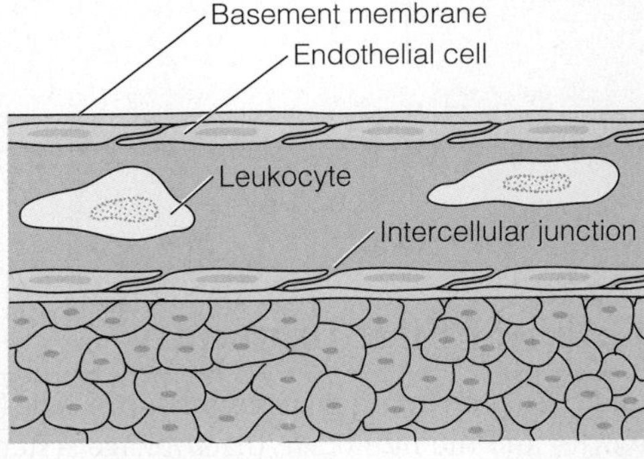

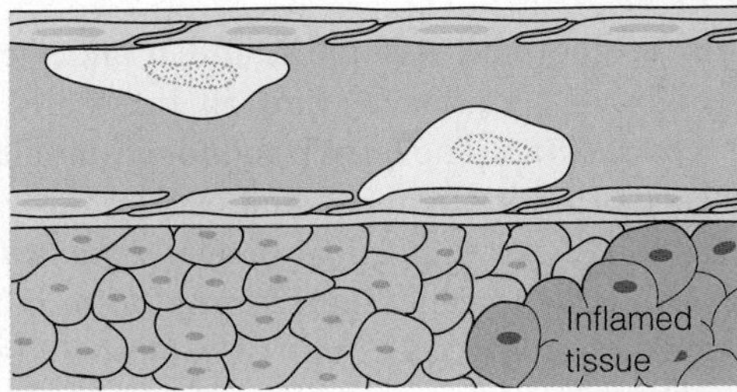

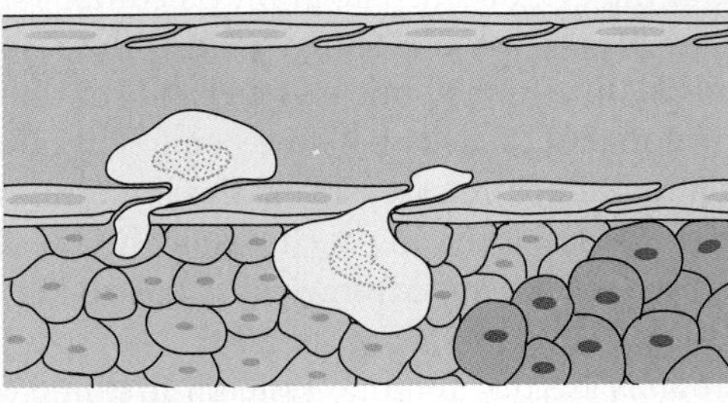

Figure 5–7 ■ The process of leukocyte emigration at the site of inflammation. A, Normal blood flow with free movement of formed elements. B, As blood flow slows, leukocytes move toward the periphery of blood stream and begin to cling to capillary endothelium, a process known as margination and pavementing. C, Leukocytes emigrate from the vessel into inflamed tissues.

cytokines (Trinchieri & Lanier, 2006). They do not require recognition of a specific antigen on target cells in order to attack and destroy them. When a NK cell comes into direct contact with a target cell, it chemically ruptures the cell membrane of the target cell, leading to cell death.

Complement System

The **complement system** is an immune mechanism that resembles the blood coagulation cascade in that, once initiated, it progresses through several sequential stages, each contributing to the immune response and resulting in cellular destruction or cytolysis. The precursors to the complement pathways are normally circulating in the bloodstream. These precursors are activated only by specific agents, such as IgG and IgM. The complement system is instrumental in facilitating phagocytosis by making antigens more susceptible to digestion, lysis of antigen cell membranes, and attraction of phagocytes to the invading antigen.

Emerging Evidence

- Higher levels of the immunoglobulin IgG were found in the cerebrospinal fluid (CSF) of African Americans (AA) with multiple sclerosis than Caucasian Americans (CA) with multiple sclerosis, suggesting a more active humoral response in the CSF in the AA group. The higher levels were not predictive of earlier disease progression *(Rinker, Trinkaus, & Naismith, 2007)*.
- Improved humoral immunity was associated with long-term use of an immune-enhancing enteral formula (IEEF). After 12 weeks of IEEF use in non-surgical patients, B-cell fraction was increased, T-cell cell fraction was decreased, and there was a significant increase in serum insulin-like growth factor-I concentration in the experimental group *(Sakurai, Oh-Oka, Kato et al., 2006)*.
- In high-risk individuals with atherosclerosis, a four-week statin regimen showed a decrease in the proinflammatory chemokine interleukin-8 (IL-8), reflecting a reduction of proinflammatory properties of neutrophils (polymorphonucleocytes) *(Guasti, Marino, Cosentino, Cimpanelli et al., 2006)*.

SECTION THREE REVIEW

1. A nonspecific immune response involves
   A. T cell differentiation
   B. recognition of nonself
   C. production of antibody
   D. recognition of a particular antigen
2. Innate (natural) immunity has which of the following characteristics?
   A. species nonspecific
   B. requires presentation by APCs
   C. has no long-term memory for antigens
   D. composed of T lymphocytes
3. A major function of macrophages is
   A. presenting an antigen to B cells and T cells
   B. protecting against local mucosal invasion of viruses
   C. triggering the complement system
   D. interfering with the immune response
4. To actively participate in phagocytic activities, monocytes must mature into
   A. neutrophils
   B. lysosomes
   C. cytokines
   D. macrophages
5. The primary purpose of granules located in the granulocyte, such as a neutrophil, is to
   A. detect the presence of infection
   B. break down foreign substances
   C. stimulate the production of monocytes
   D. initiate ameboid cell movement
6. Which immune cell is responsible for direct antigen attack and destruction?
   A. helper T cell
   B. NK cell
   C. suppressor B cell
   D. memory B cell
7. The process by which circulating neutrophils and macrophages are able to squeeze out of a capillary to go to the site of injury is called
   A. diapedesis
   B. chemotaxis
   C. margination
   D. translocation
8. Cytokines, as a group, perform which overall function?
   A. directly destroy cancer cells
   B. stimulate the bone marrow to produce lymphocytes
   C. act as chemical messengers for immune system activation
   D. regulate endothelial activities throughout the body
9. Cytokines are primarily produced by which cells?
   A. B lymphocytes
   B. T lymphocytes
   C. bone marrow
   D. lymph nodes
10. The complement system has which major innate immune function?
    A. makes antigens more susceptible to phagocytosis
    B. activates the IgG and IgM antibodies
    C. its phagocytosis system attacks and destroys antigens
    D. stimulates production of T lymphocytes
11. Interferons act by inhibiting the synthesis of _______, thus limiting abnormal cell growth.
    A. the complement system
    B. immunoglobulins
    C. lymphokines
    D. viral proteins

Answers: 1. B, 2. C, 3. A, 4. D, 5. B, 6. B, 7. A, 8. C, 9. B, 10. A, 11. D

SECTION FOUR: Characteristics and cells of Adaptive (Acquired) Immunity

Upon completion of this section, the learner will be able to discuss the characteristics and cells of adaptive (acquired) immunity.

Whereas the innate immune system is a first responder system, adaptive immunity is a second responder system. Adaptive immunity is a highly integrated adaptive process that is antigen-specific. Resistance to a particular infectious agent is significantly improved with repeated exposure to specialized cells that have been differentiated into long-term memory cells. This adaptive immunity is primarily a function of T lymphocytes (T cells), and B lymphocytes (B cells). Acquired immunity can be either passive or active.

Passive Acquired Immunity

Passive acquired immunity is a temporary immunity involving the transfer of antibodies from one individual to another or from some other source (laboratory cultures, other animals) to an individual. An infant receives passive immunity both in utero and from breast milk. A neonate does not yet have a mature immune system capable of efficient development of antibodies in response to invading agents. Passive immunity can be transferred also through vaccination either of antiserum, such as rabies; an antitoxin, such as tetanus; or as gamma globulin, which contains a variety of antibodies. One way to remember passive immunity is that a person who receives this type of immunity receives it as a gift—the recipient's own immune system is passive in the process. Passive immunity provides rapid but short-lived immunity and may be treatment of choice for an individual with increased susceptibility to infection (e.g., immunocompromised state), who is inadvertently exposed to a pathogen. For example, for an organ transplant or HIV/AIDS patient who is exposed to chicken pox, passive immunity may be the treatment of choice.

Active Acquired Immunity

Active acquired immunity develops on exposure to an antigen, such as the chicken pox virus, during which time antibodies are programmed to protect the body from illness with future exposures. These antibodies are quite specific, often providing lifetime immunity against another attack of the same antigen. Inoculation provides another means for development of active immunity through exposure to a specific antigen by introduction of a vaccine. Smallpox and polio vaccines provide a lifetime of antibody protection without an actual illness occurring. Active immunity following exposure to a specific antigen does not provide immediate protection but develops over a period of days to weeks. However, the programming of specific antibodies provides heightened protection with subsequent exposures within a matter of minutes or hours.

Both passive and active immunity create levels of antibodies circulating in the body. Many of these levels can be monitored by venipuncture blood tests to determine full immunity to a particular disease. The result of testing the level of a particular antibody is called the *antibody titer.* The titer of the specific antibody is compared with a preestablished level thought to guarantee immunity. If the individual's titer is found to be lower than the preestablished norm, he or she may require repeated immunization with the vaccine. An example of such a process is the increased scrutiny of individuals regarding their immune status to rubella.

Antigen-Specific Immunity

The immune system can be described as providing either antigen-specific or nonspecific immunity. Section Two presented antigen-nonspecific (innate) immunity. There are two types of antigen-specific immunity: humoral immunity, which is based on the activity and characteristics of the B lymphocyte, and cell-mediated immunity, which is based on the roles of the T lymphocyte.

Humoral Immunity

Humoral immunity—the recognition of antigens and the production of specific antibodies—occurs with a primary and secondary response pattern. During the **primary response,** there is a latency period before the antibody can be detected in the serum. This delay may be 48 to 72 hours after exposure. It represents the time needed for the antigen to be recognized as nonself and specifically identified, after which antibodies are formed in response to the antigen's particular molecular makeup. After this latency period, a blood test should reflect the level of antibody to a particular antigen and the degree of immune response. This level of antibody is the antibody titer. The titer normally continues to rise for about ten days to two weeks. The peak of the titer generally occurs during recovery from most infectious diseases.

The **secondary response** occurs with subsequent exposures to the same antigen. It is during this time that the memory cells of the plasma cell clones recognize the antigen almost immediately and initiate the immune response with heightened antibody formation. If a titer were to be drawn at this exposure, the antibody titer would be higher than that of the primary exposure. The follow-up booster regimen of many vaccines, such as tetanus, takes advantage of this secondary response and boosts the titer of specific antibodies to a level that will prevent the disease from occurring. This is the rationale for administering a tetanus booster within 24 hours of a new puncture wound.

Cell-Mediated Immunity

Cell-mediated immunity is based on the activity and characteristics of the T cell. During this portion of the immune response, the T cell and macrophage predominate, creating a direct attack on invading antigens. T cell immunity provides protection from intracellular organisms (such as viruses, fungi, and parasites), cancer cells, and foreign tissue. It is the T cell that is also responsible for much of the rejection phenomenon of transplanted organs and grafts. Cell-mediated immunity is one of the body's primary surveillance and attack mechanisms for protection from growth of malignant cells. Unfortunately, T cell protection is not readily transferred from one individual to another, as humoral protection is. Cell-mediated immunity depends heavily on thymus and lymph node integrity as well as a nutritionally healthy body.

Major Blood Cells of Adaptive Immunity

The lymphocytes play a pivotal role in the specific immune response to harmful cells by providing either cell-mediated (T cells) or humoral immunity (B cells).

T Lymphocytes

The **T lymphocytes** (also referred to as **T cells** or T lymphs) are formed in the bone marrow and travel to the thymus gland. The **thymus** is a flat, lobed organ located in the neck below the thyroid and extending into the upper thorax behind the sternum. During extrauterine life, the role of the thymus is to differentiate lymphocytes into various types of T cells. Reaching its peak size at puberty, the thymus steadily diminishes in size and composition until it is hardly distinguishable in adulthood. Its lymphoid tissue is gradually replaced by adipose tissue over a person's lifetime. T cells are marked by the thymus with specific surface antigens that characterize them and distinguish them from B cells. Mature, differentiated lymphocytes are released into the bloodstream, and they relocate in peripheral lymph tissue, such as lymph nodes, tonsils, intestines, and spleen, where they await a call to action in body defense.

The T lymphocytes represent approximately 70 to 80 percent of the total lymphocyte count and have a life expectancy of several years. There are several different types of T cells, each playing a unique role in the body's defense. Subsets of mature T cells are identified by a nomenclature referred to as clusters of differentiation (CD). These clusters are actually surface antigens commonly known as **CD markers.** For example, helper T cells (T_H cells) bear a CD4 marker. Approximately 70 percent of mature T cells carry the CD4 marker, and 30 percent carry the CD8 marker. The markers help to differentiate the various properties and functions of cells. Table 5–2 summarizes the types of T cells, common abbreviations, associated CD markers, and their major functions. In parentheses, it also gives common abbreviations for each T cell type.

B Lymphocytes

B lymphocytes (B cells) are larger than T cells and have a much shorter life span than T cells. They mature with exposure to an antigen. Immature B cells are stored in the bone marrow, the lymph nodes, and other lymphatic tissue. They are also found circulating in the bloodstream. Much like the thymus in T cell maturation, the bursa equivalent in the bone marrow differentiates lymphocytes into B cells (B, of bursa origin). Prior to birth, B cells develop from fetal liver tissue beginning at eight to nine weeks of gestation. Later, B cell production shifts to the bone marrow, where it continues throughout life. Once released, these immature B cells migrate to the peripheral lymph tissue (lymph nodes, spleen, and tonsils), where they mature and await the body's need for defense against foreign agents. The majority of B cells do not reach the circulation but undergo a process of programmed cell death (apoptosis).

It is the B lymphocytes that are responsible for antibody production to provide humoral immunity. Following exposure to an antigen (via presentation by APCs), mature B cells transform into plasma cells, which then secrete antibodies called **immunoglobulins (Ig).** Each plasma cell is specialized to produce only one type of antibody. This specificity is often described as a key-and-lock relationship since only a specific antigen (the key) can unlock a specific plasma cell to produce antibodies. Once activated, each plasma cell then produces identical cells capable of continuing production of antibodies in response to a particular antigen. Some of the offspring of a particular plasma cell continue to produce antibodies, while other cells of that set become memory cells for the particular antigen.

Immunoglobulins. The immunoglobulins are in the globulin fraction of the plasma protein. Each has a distinct amino acid chain that creates its specificity to react with a particular antigen. Because of this basic protein matrix of antibodies, a person's nutritional status, particularly the protein status, is a major factor in determining the adequacy of the humoral immune system. Five classes of immunoglobulins have been identified and each is active within a given course of events in the immune response. Each of the five immunoglobulins plays a particular role in the immune response (see Table 5–3).

TABLE 5–2 T Lymphocyte Types, CD Marker, and Functions

TYPE	CD MARKER	FUNCTIONS
T helper (T_H, T4 cell)	CD4	Orchestrate the activities of the other immune cells Interact with the mononuclear phagocytes and assist in the destruction of pathogens Interact with the B cells, assisting the B cells in division and production of antibodies
T suppressor (T_S cell)	CD8	Important in shutting down the immune response once a pathogen has been destroyed
T cytotoxic (T_C, killer, T8 cell)	CD8	Responsible for the destruction and lysis of the infected host cells

TABLE 5–3 Immunoglobulins in Adults

IMMUNOGLOBULIN (PERCENTAGE OF TOTAL IG)	FUNCTIONS	DESCRIPTION
IgG (80%)	Antibacterial and antiviral activities	The chief immunoglobulin Produced on secondary exposure to an antigen The only immunoglobulin that is known to cross the placental barrier and is responsible for protecting the newborn during the first few months of life.
IgA (15%)	Protection of mucous membrane from invading pathogens	Found in large quantities in secretory body fluids, such as tears; saliva; breast milk; and vaginal, bronchial, and intestinal secretions. Produced by B cells in Peyer's patches, tonsils, and other lymph tissue.
IgM (4%)	Primary immunity; produced early in the immune response to most antigens and is also important in activating the complement system	Found in secretions (respiratory, gastrointestinal, genitourinary tracts, saliva, and tears) Instrumental in forming natural antibodies (e.g., for ABO blood antigens).
IgD (0.2%)	Unknown; may influence B cell maturation	A trace antibody found primarily in the blood.
IgE (0.0002% U/mL)	Plays a role in allergy; levels elevate during hypersensitivity reactions (particularly type 1)	While it exists in the body in miniscule quantities, it is considered extremely powerful.

Data from Kee (2009).

SECTION FOUR REVIEW

1. A child who first had chicken pox and then is immune from that disease in the future is said to have
   A. active acquired immunity
   B. passive acquired immunity
   C. innate (natural) immunity
   D. species-specific immunity
2. An infant who receives temporary immunity while being breastfed has
   A. active acquired immunity
   B. natural innate immunity
   C. passive acquired immunity
   D. species-specific immunity
3. Which statement is correct regarding cell-mediated immunity?
   A. it depends on B cell and macrophage activity
   B. it is part of the surveillance mechanism for malignant cells
   C. it is readily transferred to an individual
   D. it does not protect against invading viruses
4. The T lymphocyte that oversees many immune cell functions is the
   A. natural killer cell (NK)
   B. cytotoxic T cell (T_C)
   C. suppressor T cell (T_S)
   D. helper T cell (T_H)
5. Which two lymphocytes bear the CD8 marker?
   A. helper T cell
   B. suppressor T cell
   C. cytotoxic T cell
   D. natural killer cell
6. Humoral immunity is best characterized by
   A. development of antibodies from B cells
   B. recognition of self and nonself
   C. specific recognition and memory of antigens
   D. differentiation of cellular function known as killer, helper, and suppressor cells
7. An individual whose antibody titer is greater than the preestablished level of immunity is said to
   A. require reimmunization
   B. transmit the disease as a carrier
   C. demonstrate a specific antigen–antibody complex
   D. demonstrate immunity from the disease in question
8. A major responsibility of the B lymphocytes is
   A. phagocytosis
   B. direct attack on antigens
   C. antibody production
   D. helper T cell function
9. The immunoglobulin that comprises about 80 percent of the total immunoglobulin in the healthy human body is
   A. IgA
   B. IgE
   C. IgG
   D. IgM
10. The immunoglobulin that locally protects the body at the mucosal level from invading organisms is
   A. IgA
   B. IgE
   C. IgG
   D. IgM

Answers: 1. A, 2. C, 3. B, 4. D, 5. (B, C), 6. A, 7. D, 8. C, 9. C, 10. A

SECTION FIVE: Antigens and Antigen–Antibody Response

At the completion of this section, the learner will be able to describe characteristics of antigens and antigen–antibody responses.

Antigens

Antigens are substances that are capable of triggering an immune response if they can be recognized by a B cell antibody or T cell (Male, 2001). The immune response can involve either humoral or cellular components of the immune system but commonly involves both. The degree to which an antigen stimulates an immune response is referred to as its immunogenicity or its immunogenic nature and is influenced by factors such as physical and chemical properties of the antigen, the relative foreignness of the antigen, and the person's genetic makeup. Antigens may be either foreign to the body or be important self-markers or tumor markers.

Foreign Antigens

Some foreign-body antigens are capable of causing disease and are called **pathogens** or pathogenic antigens. Many bacteria, viruses, parasites, and other microorganisms are pathogenic antigens, such as *Staphylococcus aureus, Mycobacterium tuberculosis*, herpes simplex, and HIV. Other antigens, such as vaccines, are foreign to the body but are not pathogenic microorganisms. Vaccines induce a protective immunologic response by introducing either viruses or bacteria that are killed, treated, or attenuated (selectively altered). These vaccines are incapable of inducing a disease state but effectively stimulate a mild immune response as a protective mechanism against similar live microorganisms.

A second example of a nonpathogenic antigen is a transplanted heart or kidney. The cells making up the tissues of these organs are not disease producing but are recognized by the body as being foreign (nonself); thus, the transplanted organ can precipitate an immune reaction. Although the immune system is certainly capable of distinguishing self from nonself in its natural state, it is not able to determine that a foreign material is acceptable even if that material is beneficial to the well-being of the body as a whole. This is the scenario that occurs in organ transplant rejection.

Histocompatibility Antigens

In addition to foreign materials being antigens, all nucleated cells in the body contain surface antigens, which are proteins found on the surface of a cell. These proteins distinguish an individual's tissue (self) from tissue of other persons (nonself). Surface antigens are genetically determined and are referred to as **histocompatibility antigens** or **human leukocyte antigens (HLA)**. The term *histocompatibility* comes from the Greek word *histos,* meaning tissue, and the Latin word *compati,* meaning to sympathize with. Histocompatibility, then, refers to the ability of cells and tissues to live without interference from the immune system. The HLA proteins are coded by a group of genes called the **major histocompatibility complex (MHC)** located on the sixth chromosome. They exist in pairs (called haplotypes) on the surface of cells and are genetically determined. MHC molecules that are involved in intracellular communication for self-recognition are classified into two groups: MHC I (or class I) antigens and MCH II (or class II) antigens.

- **MHC I (Class I) Antigens.** The MHC I proteins have been labeled HLA-A, HLA-B, and HLA-C. They are found on the surface of essentially all nucleated cells.
- **MHC (Class II) Antigens.** The MHC II proteins have been labeled HLA-DR, HLA-DP, and HLA-DQ. They are primarily found on the cell surfaces of macrophages and B lymphocytes.

The HLA antigens in the MHC I and II classes help the immune system distinguish self from nonself, functioning somewhat like "fingerprints" that are unique to the individual. Normally, the immune system is able to recognize its own HLA "fingerprint" as self, and the immune response is not triggered. HLA antigens are inherited; thus, each full sibling in a family will have some combination of HLA inherited from both biological parents. The closer the HLA antigen combination matches between two people, the more the "fingerprint" is recognized as self.

A multitude of combinations of pairings can occur; therefore, complete HLA matching is virtually impossible with the exception of identical twins. Because full siblings share the same biological parents, they often have some degree of HLA matching. In contrast, transplanted cadaver organs are completely unmatched when chosen randomly for an organ recipient (a person who receives an organ). For this reason, immediate family members most often make the best kidney transplant donors because they are more likely to have a better matched tissue type. Identical twins, however, have the same histocompatibility pairings and are, therefore, perfect HLA matches. In the case of identical twins, a transplanted tissue or organ is recognized as having a self-HLA fingerprint and is accepted into the recipient without an immune assault.

Tumor-Associated Antigens

Some human tumors have been found to display particular antigens (tumor-associated antigens) that distinguish normal cells from abnormally transformed cells. Identification of tumor associated antigens has progressed rapidly with technological advances in tumor immunology. Tumor-associated antigens typically do not evoke an immune response (low immunogenicity), perhaps because they are recognized as self from early development during embryonic and fetal stages. Although many of these antigens occur naturally in small quantities, an elevation of the particular antigen type can be helpful in detecting potentially abnormal cells and tracking progression of disease or regression of disease following treatment. For example, carcinoembryonic antigen (CEA) has been found to be elevated in a variety of adenocarcinomas of the colon, lung, breast, and pancreas; alpha-fetoprotein (AFP) is frequently elevated in patients with testicular and hepatic cancer; and serum elevations of prostate-specific antigen (PSA) have been found in occurrences of prostatic cancer. Serum elevations of tumor-associated antigens are also possible with several nonmalignant disease states. Success in identifying and characterizing tumor-specific antigens that are not found in other disease states or on other host cells has been less successful to date.

Antigenic Determinants

Antigens have several specific sites, called antigenic determinant sites, which interact with immune cells to elicit the immune response. These sites are quite specific in configuration, requiring a particular structure of the immunoglobulin molecule or antibody. Some molecules are so small that they cannot act as antigens until they attach to larger molecules or carriers. The immune response recognizes the antigens, and destroys and eliminates them. When the antigen is eliminated, the immune system is turned off (Male, 2001). Figure 5–8 illustrates how the immune system responds (cell-mediated and humoral immunities) to a specific antigen.

Antigen–Antibody Responsiveness

Remember, immune responsiveness may be either specific or nonspecific. A specific response requires the recognition of a particular antigen and involves the production and action of a programmed antibody for that antigen. Normally, an antibody circulates in the bloodstream until it encounters an appropriate antigen to which it can bind. Such binding results in antigen–antibody complexes, or immune complexes. The process of binding is such that the antibody binds to specifically conformed antigenic determinant sites on the antigen, which effectively prevents the antigen from binding with receptors on host cells. The overall effect is protection of the host from antigen infection or penetration.

An antigen–antibody reaction can have several consequences for the invading agent. The reaction can cause agglutination (clumping of the cells), neutralization of the antigen toxin (e.g., a bacterial toxin), cell lysis (destruction of the antigen), enhanced phagocytosis of the antigen by other cells, opsonization, or activation of the complement system.

Antigen Entry Site

The entry site of an antigen is an important consideration. Many enzymes and other secretions are important in innate immune defense. Some antigens are destroyed before they cross into the bloodstream. For example, some antigens are readily destroyed or neutralized by salivary and other digestive enzymes in the gastrointestinal tract, rendering them incapable of causing disease. Other antigens are not affected by these enzymes and can proliferate rapidly, creating pathologic states. The site of entrance also determines the strength or virulence of the antigen. For example, an antigen that is neutralized by digestive enzymes in the gastrointestinal tract might be quite virulent if entering the body through the genitourinary tract or the respiratory tract where digestive enzymes are not normally found.

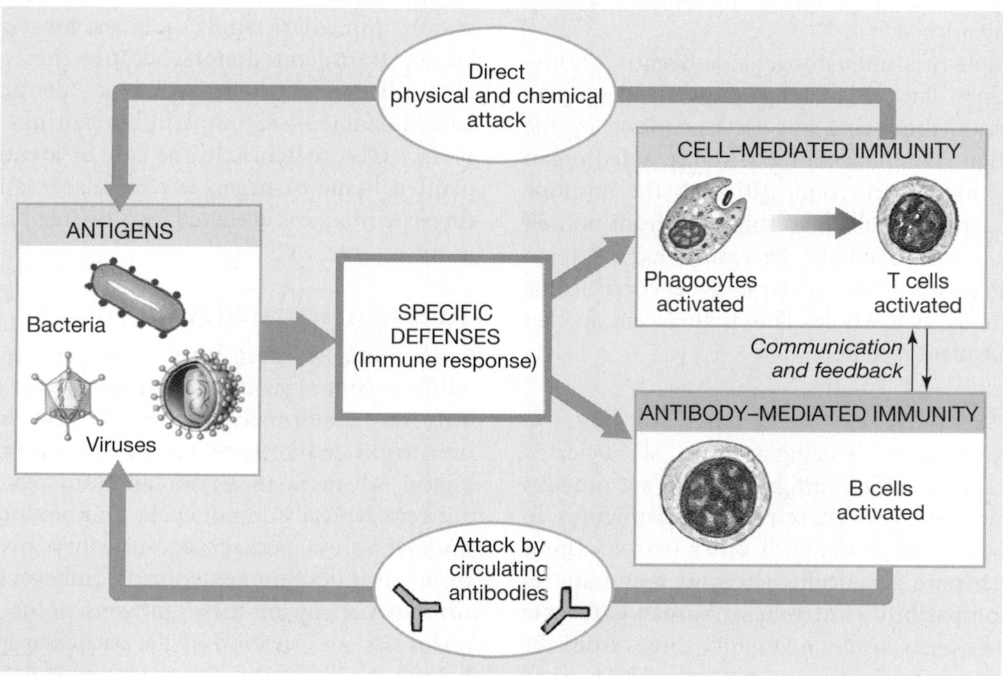

Figure 5–8 ■ An overview of the immune response. Bledsoe, Bryan E.; Martin, Frederick H.; Bartholomew, Edwin F.; Ober, William, C.; Garrison, Claire W., *Anatomy & Physiology for Emergency Care*, 2nd © N/A. Electronically reproduced by permission of Pearson Education, Inc., Upper Saddle River, New Jersey.

SECTION FIVE REVIEW

1. An antigen is defined as a substance that is capable of
   - **A.** triggering an immune response
   - **B.** causing a disease
   - **C.** creating an allergy
   - **D.** initiating an antigen-antibody reaction
2. The purpose of histocompatibility antigens is to
   - **A.** distinguish self from nonself
   - **B.** muster an attack against foreign antigens
   - **C.** present foreign antigens to phagocytes
   - **D.** stimulate antibody production
3. HLA antigens are located on
   - **A.** RNA chains
   - **B.** erythrocytes
   - **C.** chromosome 6
   - **D.** the gamma globulin protein fraction
4. Specific sites on antigens that interact with immune cells to elicit the immune response are called
   - **A.** antigenic determinants
   - **B.** surface cells
   - **C.** human leukocyte antigens
   - **D.** histocompatibility complexes
5. Antigens that precipitate disease states are called
   - **A.** immunoglobulins
   - **B.** pathogens
   - **C.** human leukocyte antigens
   - **D.** histocompatibility antigens
6. HLA antigens are located where on cells?
   - **A.** cell nucleus
   - **B.** cell cytoplasm
   - **C.** cell surface
   - **D.** chromosome 3
7. Which statement is correct regarding tumor associated antigens?
   - **A.** They are highly recognizable as foreign or pathogenic.
   - **B.** They escape immune recognition early in tumor growth.
   - **C.** An antigen is called tumor necrosis factor (TNF).
   - **D.** Elevations of alpha-fetoprotein (AFP) suggest lung cancer.
8. Which statements regarding the entry site of an antigen are correct? (choose all that apply)
   - **A.** saliva in the mouth destroys many antigens
   - **B.** digestive enzymes neutralize many antigens
   - **C.** site of entry helps determine virulence of the antigen
   - **D.** entry location does not determine strength of the antigen

Answers: 1. A, 2. A, 3. C, 4. A, 5. B, 6. C, 7. B, 8. (A, B, C)

SECTION SIX: Hemostasis

At the completion of this section, the learner will be able to describe the origin and function of platelets and the coagulation cascade.

The hematologic system is sometimes referred to as a fluid organ. Correct functioning of an organ requires that its borders remain intact. The blood vessel walls constitute the borders of the hematologic system. Vascular integrity is maintained through two closely interwoven mechanisms, hemostasis and blood coagulation.

Platelets—The Cell Component of Hemostasis

Platelets are not actually cells. They are tiny cell fragments composed of cytoplasm that are shed from megakaryocytes in the bone marrow. The mechanism by which shedding occurs is not well understood. One theory suggests that mature megakaryocytes may transform in response to some unknown signal, forming spiderlike projections called *proplatelets* (Battinelli, Willoughby et al., 2001). These tiny proplatelets break off from the megakaryocyte as a result of a shearing force when they encounter blood flow in the bone marrow sinusoids.

The normal platelet count in an adult is 150,000 to 400,000/mcL (Kee, 2009). Platelet production is regulated by thrombopoietin, which is primarily produced by the liver. Certain cytokines (e.g., GM-CSF) are also known to stimulate the production of platelets using different mechanisms (Rote & McCance, 2008). Mature platelets survive about ten days, with about two thirds being in the circulation at all times and the remaining one third being stored in the spleen. The stored platelets are continuously exchanging with circulating platelets (Rote & McCance, 2008).

Hemostasis is defined as prevention of blood loss. Platelets play a crucial role in hemostasis by creating a **platelet plug** to seal off leaking vessels. The internal structures of platelets also contain a variety of coagulation-related proteins and enzymes that interact with the coagulation process. Under normal circumstances, platelets circulate freely throughout the vascular system as inactive, smooth, disk-shaped particles. Normally, the vessel endothelium maintains platelets in an inactive state by secreting substances such as nitric oxide and prostacyclin I_2. When vessel endothelial injury occurs, special activating factors are produced, such thrombin and platelet-activating factor, that stimulate platelet hemostatic activities. On activation, the platelets undergo significant changes including adhesion and aggregation. Within one to two minutes after vascular integrity is lost, platelets begin to adhere to the collagen fibers of the damaged subendothelium (Rote & McCance,

2008). To do this, they rapidly reshape themselves, developing pseudopods along the vessel's endothelial surface. As the platelets accumulate, they begin to aggregate or clump together and eventually form a cohesive mass, called a *platelet plug.* Once the platelet plug is formed, it is stabilized and consolidated by fibrinogen, eventually forming a fibrin clot. Platelet plugs are particularly effective in rapid repair of small vascular leaks. Figure 5–9 depicts platelet plug formation and blood clotting.

Coagulation

While platelets play a crucial role in maintaining hemostasis by providing a platelet plug to seal off an injured vessel, they are only one aspect of hemostasis. The platelet plug provides rapid reduction or complete closure of an injured vessel by forming a simple plug. The injury then requires a more stable and permanent repair through formation of a thrombus, which is the function of the coagulation cascade — a complex series of chemical events. The following is a brief overview of coagulation.

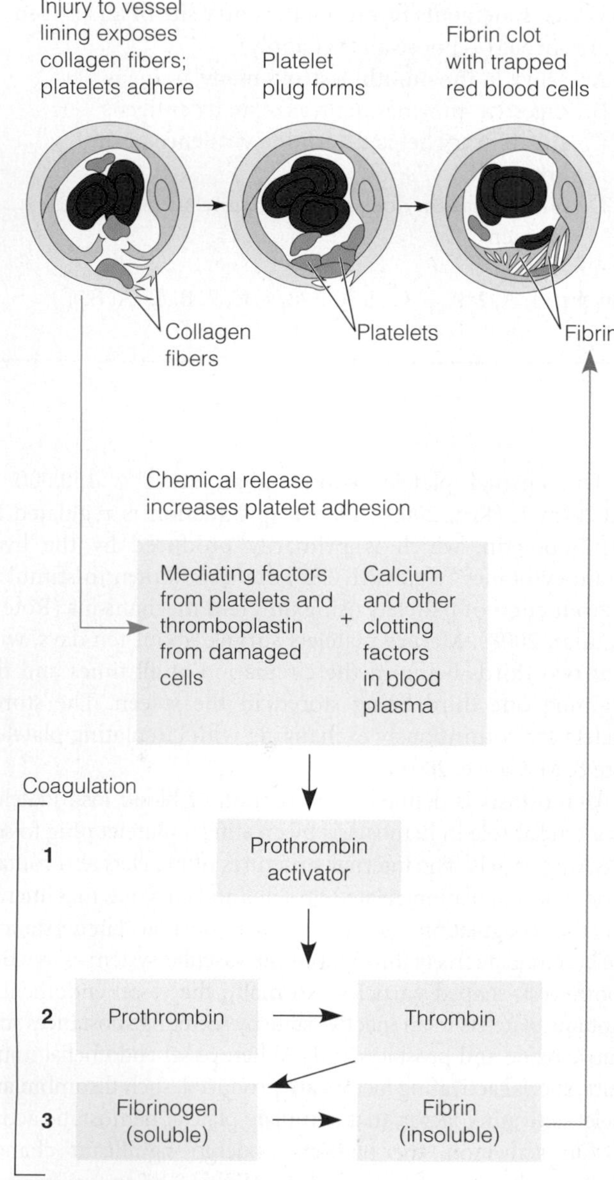

Figure 5–9 ■ Platelet plug formation and blood clotting. The flow diagram summarizes the events leading to fibrin clot formation.

The Coagulation Cascade

The coagulation process is dependent on the presence of adequate numbers of coagulation factors (plasma proteins, calcium ions, and phospholipids). Once triggered into action, a specific sequence of chemical reactions occurs that results in a clot made of fibrin strands. Table 5–4 provides a list of the coagulation

TABLE 5–4 Coagulation Factors

COAGULATION FACTOR	SOURCE	PURPOSE
I – Fibrinogen	Liver	Precursor of fibrin
II – Prothrombin	Liver; requires vitamin K	Precursor of thrombin
III –Thromboplastin (tissue factor, TF)	Found throughout tissues	Conversion of prothrombin to thrombin
IV – Ionized calcium (Ca^{++})	Blood and intracellular; consumed	Required throughout the coagulation cascade
V – Proaccelerin (labile factor)	Liver	Increases the formation of thromboplastin (factor III); triggers prothrombin-thrombin conversion
VII – Proconvertin (stable factor)	Liver; requires vitamin K	Increases prothrombin-thrombin conversion
VIII – Antihemophilic factor (A)	Reticuloendothelial cells	Required for prothrombin-thrombin conversion and production of thromboplastin (factor III)
IX – Plasma thromboplastin component (Christmas factor, antihemophilic factor B)	Liver; requires vitamin K	Required for synthesis of thromboplastin
X – Stuart-Prower factor	Liver; requires vitamin K	Important in formation of thromboplastin
XI – Plasma thromboplastin antecedent (antihemophilic factor C)	Unknown	Required in formaton of plasma-thromboplastin
XII – Hageman factor	Unknown	When activated, stimulates factor XI to continue clotting process; during fibrinolysis it converts plasminogen-plasmin
XIII – Fibrinase (fibrin stabilizing factor)	Unknown	Assists in stabilization of fibrin in forming a strong blood clot

Adapted from Kee, J. L. (2005). *Laboratory and diagnostic tests with nursing implications*, 7th ed. (pp. 177–178). Upper Saddle River, N.J.: Pearson/Prentice Hall.

factors, where they are synthesized, and their purpose. The liver is the major source of most of the factors and many require vitamin K for synthesis by the liver.

There are several different models of how the coagulation cascade works. The classic model visualizes two coagulation pathways that join into a common pathway. In this model, coagulation is triggered by either the direct exposure of blood to subendothelial vascular tissue (collagen)—the **intrinsic pathway,** a slower process; or blood is exposed to extravascular tissues—the **extrinsic pathway,** a rapid process. The pathways join into a common pathway which results in clot formation. The normal clot formation cascade maintains homeostasis by balancing stimulating and inhibiting factors. Figure 5–10 illustrates the classic model of two pathways of

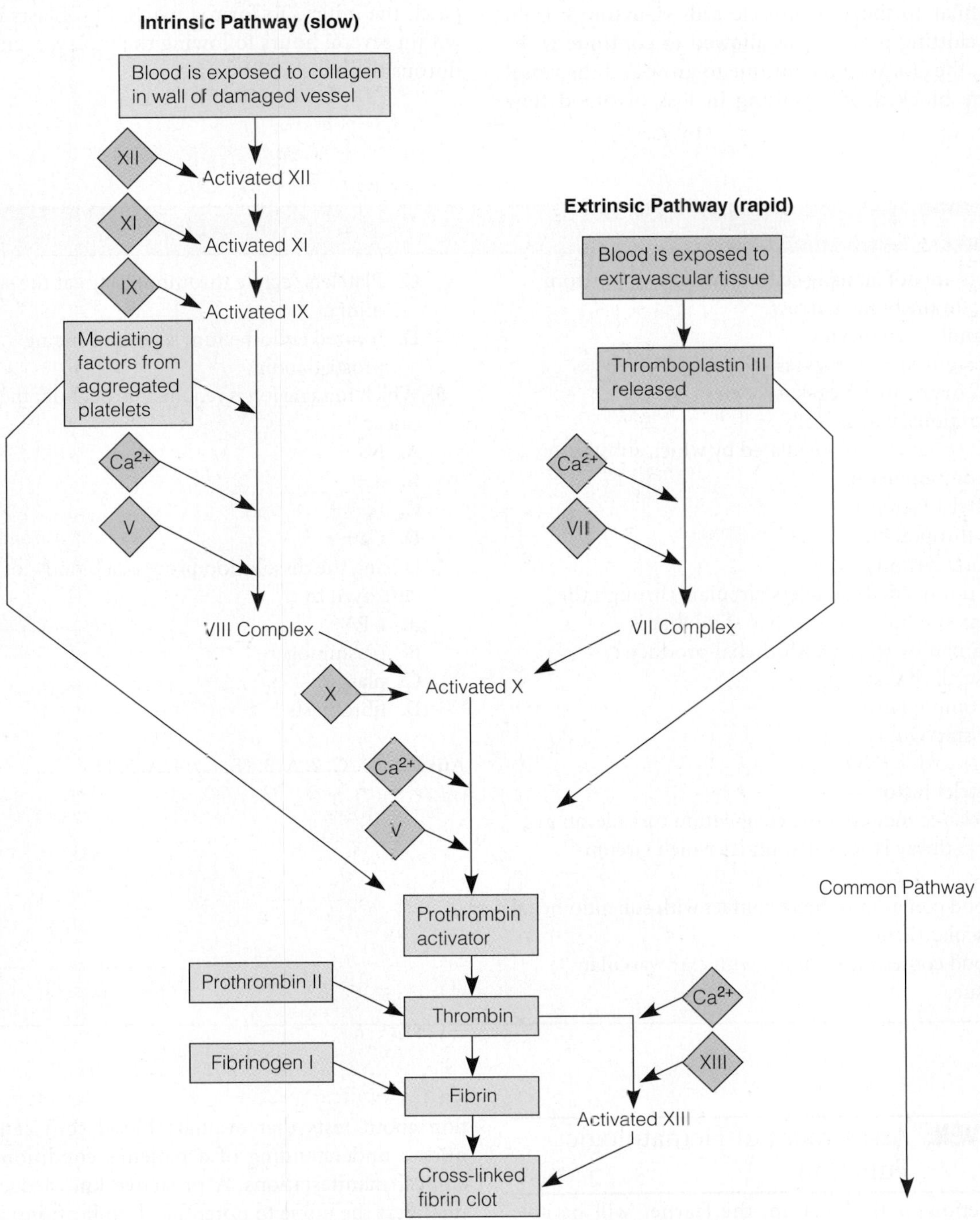

Figure 5–10 ■ Clot formation. Both the slower intrinsic pathway and the more rapid extrinsic pathway activate factor X. Factor X then combines with other factors to form prothrombin activator. Prothrombin activator transforms prothrombin into thrombin, which then transforms fibrinogen into long fibrin strands. Thrombin also activates factor XIII, which draws the fibrin strands together into a dense meshwork. The complete process of clot formation occurs within 3 to 6 minutes after blood vessel damage.

the coagulation cascade. Note the distinct activation sequence of events to produces a clot.

Clot Retraction and Dissolution

Hemostasis does not end with formation of the fibrin clot. Shortly after the clot has formed, it contracts (called retraction), drawing the torn vessel walls into closer proximity, reducing leakage. Clot retraction is largely a function of platelets, which contain contractile proteins in their cytoplasm similar to those of muscle cells (Guyton & Hall, 2006). If the clotting process was allowed to continue without restraints, the clot would continue to grow and the vessel would become blocked off resulting in loss of blood flow distal to the clot. When the clot has finished forming, it begins to alter in one of two ways. First, it can dissolve (called dissolution). A blood clot contains lytic plasma proteins (plasminogen) that when activated becomes plasmin, a powerful protein busting (proteolytic) enzyme that destroys clotting factors contained in the clot (Guyton & Hall, 2006). The plasminogen-to-plasmin conversion results from the slow release of tissue plasminogen activator (t-PA) by the injured vessel endothelium. Second, it can form connective tissue to patch the injury. To form a patch, fibroblasts invade the clot within several hours following the injury, eventually forming fibrous tissue.

SECTION SIX REVIEW

1. Platelets are not actually cells; they are ______ from ______ in the bone marrow.
   - **A.** granules; leukocytes
   - **B.** lysosomes; erythrocytes
   - **C.** cell fragments; megakaryocytes
   - **D.** secretions; plasma cells
2. Platelet production is regulated by which substance?
   - **A.** thrombopoietin
   - **B.** platelet factor
   - **C.** erythropoietin
   - **D.** prostacyclin I_2
3. When not needed, platelets circulate through the vascular system in an inactive state that is maintained by which endothelial products? (choose all that apply)
   - **A.** thromboplastin
   - **B.** prostacyclin I_2
   - **C.** nitric oxide (NO)
   - **D.** platelet factor
4. In the classic model of the coagulation cascade, an intrinsic pathway is activated under which circumstances?
   - **A.** Blood comes into direct contact with subendothelial vascular tissue.
   - **B.** Blood comes into contact with extravascular tissue.
   - **C.** Platelets secrete thromboplastin at the site of injury.
   - **D.** Injured endothelium stops producing prostaglandin.
5. Which mineral ion is required throughout the coagulation cascade?
   - **A.** Na+
   - **B.** K+
   - **C.** Fe++
   - **D.** Ca++
6. During the dissolution process, a blood clot is destroyed by
   - **A.** t-PA
   - **B.** plasminogen
   - **C.** plasmin
   - **D.** fibroblasts

Answers: 1. C, 2. A, 3. (B, C), 4. A, 5. D, 6. C

SECTION SEVEN: Assessment of Hematologic Function

At the completion of this section, the learner will be able to discuss the assessment and diagnosis of hematologic disorders.

In the high-acuity setting, it is often the nurse who first sees a patient's laboratory test results. Learning some basic information about tests that evaluate blood cells can facilitate the nurse's understanding of a patient's condition and cause of clinical manifestations. A proactive knowledge of such tests may alert the nurse to potential complications so that preventative or corrective measures can be taken in a timely manner. Table 5–5 provides a summary of normal blood cell ranges and common causes of abnormal complete blood count (CBC) results.

TABLE 5–5 Normal Complete Blood Cell (CBC) Values and Causes of Abnormal Results

TYPE	REFERENCE VALUE	DECREASED LEVEL	ELEVATED LEVEL
Red Blood Cells (RBCs)			
RBC count (mcL)	Adult: M: 4.5–6.0 Fe: 4.0–5.0 Elderly: M: 3.7–6.0 Fe: 4.0–5.0	Hemorrhage Anemias Hemodilution (overhydration)	Hemoconcentration (dehydration) Polycythemia vera
Hgb (g/dL)	Adult: M: 13.5–18.0 Fe: 12.0–16.0 Elderly: M: 11.0–17.0 Fe: 11.5–16.0	Anemias: Iron deficiency, aplastic, hemolytic, Acute blood loss Hemodilution	Hemoconcentration (dehydration) Polycythemia vera
Hct (%)	Adult: M: 40–54 Fe: 36–41 Elderly: M: 38–42 Fe: 38–41	Anemias: Aplastic, hemolytic, folic acid deficiency, pernicious, sickle cell	Hemoconcentration (dehydration) Polycythemia vera
MCV (mcm^3)	Adult: 80–98 Elderly: M: 74–110 Fe: 78–100	Microcytic anemia: Iron deficiency	Macrocytic anemias: Aplastic, hemolytic, pernicious
RDW (Coulter S)	11.5–14.5	NA (evaluated in terms of normal or high & compared with MCV levels)	Anemias: Iron deficiency, anemia, megaloblastic anemias
White Blood Cells (WBC) with Differential			
WBC count (mcL)	Adult: 5,000–10,000 Elderly: M: 4,200–16,000 Fe: 3,100–10,000	Anemias: Aplastic, pernicious	Anemias: Hemolytic, sickle cell
Neutrophils (%)	Adult: 50–70 Elderly: 45–75	Anemias: Aplastic, folic acid deficiency, iron deficiency	Anemia: Acquired hemolytic
Basophils (%)	Adult: 0.5–1.0	Steroid therapy, stress, pregnancy	Healing or inflammatory process, leukemia
Lymphocytes (%)	Adult: 25–35 Elderly: Ave: 30	Cancer, agranulocytosis, aplastic anemia, renal failure	Lymphocytic leukemia, chronic and viral infections, hepatitis
Monocytes (%)	Adult: 4–6 Elderly, Ave: 10	Anemias: Aplastic, iron deficiency, folic acid deficiency	Anemias: Sickle cell, hemolytic
Platelets			
Platelet count (mcL)	Adult: 150,000–400,000	Idiopathic thrombocytopenia purpura, leukemias, anemias, disseminated intravascular coagulation (DIC)	Polycythemia vera, Acute blood loss

Adapted from Kee, J. L. (2005). *Laboratory and diagnostic tests with nursing implications*, 7th ed. Upper Saddle River, NJ: Pearson/Prentice Hall.

Evaluation of Erythrocytes

Basic information about the size, shape, and concentration of erythrocytes is easily obtained by performing peripheral blood smears. Tests that are commonly used to evaluate erythrocytes include reticulocyte count, mean corpuscular volume (MCV), total RBC count, hemoglobin and hematocrit, and evaluation of erythrocyte color. Table 5–6 provides a summary of the red blood cell indices.

Reticulocyte Count

Reticulocytes are immature erythrocytes that are easily detected and measured. Under normal circumstances, only about 1 percent of circulating erythrocytes are reticulocytes that have entered the circulation to replace dying mature erythrocytes. There are two general reasons why the reticulocyte count rises: (1) an increase in circulating reticulocytes or (2) a reduction in circulating red cells. A common type of

TABLE 5–6 Description of Red Blood Cell Indices

RED BLOOD CELL COUNT	BASIS	DESCRIPTION
Mean corpuscular volume (MCV)	Red blood cell size	Microcytic = small size—Iron deficiency anemia and thalassemia Normocytic = normal size—Anemia of chronic disease Macrocytic = large size—Pernicious and folic acid anemia
Mean corpuscular hemoglobin (MCH)	Weight	Indicates the weight of hemoglobin
Mean corpuscular hemoglobin concentration (MCHC)	Hemoglobin concentration	Indicates the hemoglobin concentration per unit volume of RBCs
RBC distribution width (RDW)	Size difference	RDW is the measurement of the width of the distribution curve on a histogram. An elevated RDW indicates iron deficiency, folic acid deficiency, and vitamin B_{12} deficiency anemias.

Data from Kee (2009).

reticulocyte count is the "corrected" count that corrects for the presence of anemia. The corrected reticulocyte count is calculated as follows:

$$\%\text{ reticulocytes} \times \frac{\text{Hct (patient)}}{\text{Hct (normal)}}$$

Obtaining a corrected reticulocyte count helps differentiate between types of anemia. An elevation (greater than 1.5 percent) occurs when the bone marrow is stimulated by erythropoietin to produce more reticulocytes. As a result of erythropoietin stimulation, reticulocytes are produced and released from the bone marrow at a faster rate. An elevated reticulocyte count is present in types of anemia where the bone marrow is functioning normally (e.g., blood loss and extrinsic hemolytic anemias). A reduced reticulocyte count suggests that the bone marrow is unable to respond to the increased demand (e.g., aplastic anemia, bone marrow depression, or failure).

Mean Corpuscular Volume

Measurement of **mean corpuscular volume (MCV)** evaluates the size (volume) of the RBCs. Using MCV criteria, anemias can be divided into three categories: microcytic, normocytic, and macrocytic. A low MCV value indicates the presence of **microcytic** RBCs, which are smaller than normal in size and are present in such conditions as iron deficiency anemia and thalassemia. **Normocytic** RBCs are normal in size and are present in blood loss anemia, renal insufficiency, and early iron-deficiency anemia. **Macrocytic** RBCs are larger than normal in size and are found in conditions such as vitamin B_{12} or folate deficiency and drug-induced anemias. Anemias associated with chronic illness are generally either microcytic or normocytic.

Total RBC Count

The healthy adult has between 4 million and 6 million/mcL $\times 10^{12}$ red blood cells (Kee, 2009). Men normally have higher RBC counts than women or children. Abnormally low levels (erythrocytopenia) are associated with specific anemias (e.g., blood loss, chronic renal failure), alcoholic cirrhosis, and other conditions. Abnormally high levels (erythrocytosis) may be seen in posthemorrhage states, leukemias, sickle cell and hemolytic anemias, and other conditions.

Hemoglobin and Hematocrit

Hemoglobin (Hgb). Higher-than-normal Hgb levels may result from hemoconcentration (e.g., dehydration), polycythemia (primary or secondary, discussed in Module 6), and severe burns. Lower-than-normal levels may result from certain anemias (e.g., aplastic, iron deficiency), hemorrhage, hepatic cirrhosis, leukemias, and many other conditions. Refer to Section Two for a deeper discussion of hemoglobin.

Hematocrit (Hct). The hematocrit is a concentration measurement. It is the volume (in milliliters) of packed red blood cells in 100 mL of blood and is stated as a percentage. An elevated hematocrit suggests dehydration situations (e.g., severe diarrhea or hypovolemia), polycythemia vera, secondary polycythemia (as seen with late chronic obstructive pulmonary disease [COPD]), and other problems. A lower-than-normal hematocrit is most commonly associated with leukemias and anemias.

Evaluation of Erythrocyte Color

Laboratory descriptions of erythrocytes as well as descriptions of erythrocytes in anemias usually include the descriptive terms *hypochromic* or *normochromic.* Normally, the color of the biconcave disk-shaped RBC is pinkish-red in color in the outer two thirds of the disk and very pale in the center third (called the *central pallor*). This 2:1 (dark-to-light) ratio gives the RBC its "healthy" appearance, reflecting the presence of adequate levels of hemoglobin. The normal color appearance is called **normochromic.** In certain anemia types, the 2:1 ratio is lost, and the central pallor extends beyond its one-third border. This extended pallor gives the RBC a pale or **hypochromic** appearance. Hypochromic RBCs are most commonly seen in iron-deficiency anemia. Color alterations can also reflect cell immaturity, if the immature RBC has not yet taken in all of its hemoglobin.

Red Cell Mass

Red cell mass, also called red cell volume, is used to make a differential diagnosis of polycythemia. To perform this serum test, the patient has about 25 mL of blood drawn. The blood sample is radiolabeled with chromium (Cr-51) and a known quantity of the labeled blood is then reinjected into the patient's bloodstream. After one hour, a second blood specimen is obtained. The second sample is then appropriately prepared and the circulating blood volume is calculated. Patients with polycythemia have an abnormally high circulating red cell mass.

Red Cell Distribution Width

The red cell distribution width (RDW) is a recent addition to erythrocyte laboratory tests. According to Kee (2009), it is an index of RBC size variation and is calculated using a histogram. The normal RDW range is 11.5 to 14.5 percent. An elevated level (greater than 14.5 percent) has been associated with anemias caused by deficiencies in folic acid, B_{12}, or iron; and hemolysis. Although it maintains an independent relationship with MCV, the RDW is often used in comparison with MCV values. The RDW value is an earlier indicator of nutritional deficiencies than the MCV value. Comparisons of the two tests can also help distinguish among types of anemia. For example, iron-deficiency anemia results in a high RDW and a normal to low MCV, and anemia associated with chronic disease results in a normal RDW and a normal to low MCV.

Erythrocyte Sedimentation Rate (ESR)

Although the erythrocyte sedimentation rate (ESR) is not part of the CBC count, it is of interest to the high-acuity patient. The ESR is commonly referred to as "sed rate" or "sedimentation rate." It is a measure of how rapidly RBCs settle in unclotted blood. ESR is a nonspecific screening measure of inflammation or infection; however, elevated levels also result from a variety of other problems. When ESR is abnormal, more specific diagnostic testing is indicated for making a differential diagnosis. ESR is measured in millimeters per hour (mm/hr) and increases with aging. Abnormally high ESR is associated with acute myocardial infarction, cancer, hepatitis, and rheumatic-type problems, such as rheumatic fever or rheumatoid arthritis. Abnormally low levels may be seen in patients with congestive heart failure, angina pectoris, or polycythemia vera (Kee, 2009).

Evaluation of Leukocytes

Although a simple WBC count is often adequate for general screening purposes, it is not sufficient for gaining an in-depth understanding of the patient's infectious or inflammatory status. This information is obtained through the WBC differential count. The differential cell count breaks out the constituent cells of the WBCs: neutrophils (immature and mature), monocytes, eosinophils, basophils, and lymphocytes.

Neutrophils

Neutrophils are measured in the serum as a percentage of maturity versus immaturity. The mature neutrophils are called **segmented cells** or **segs** (referring to a segmented nucleus). Immature neutrophils, called **bands** or **stabs** (referring to the band- or horseshoe-shaped nucleus), normally make up 5 percent or less of the total WBC count (Kee, 2009). When called into action, neutrophils are produced at a faster rate by the bone marrow to meet the new demand. During periods of extremely high neutrophil production (e.g., severe infection), the bone marrow releases immature neutrophils. The elevated band level (**bandemia**) is referred to as a "shift to the left." The neutrophil count increases (neutrophilia) in response to inflammatory disorders (including cancer), acute bacterial infections, and tissue necrosis. An abnormally low neutrophil count (neutropenia) can occur under circumstances involving increased destruction or decreased production. Neutrophil counts are monitored closely in critically ill patients, as severe neutropenia significantly increases mortality.

Monocytes

Monocytes comprise about 4 to 6 percent of the total WBC count (Kee, 2009). Elevated levels of monocytes are associated with chronic infections (e.g., bacterial endocarditis and tuberculosis), rickettsial diseases (e.g., malaria), and inflammatory bowel disease. Monocytosis is also seen in acute and chronic monocytic leukemia. Two examples of disorders with low levels of monocytes are aplastic anemia and lymphocytic leukemia (Kee, 2009).

Eosinophils

Eosinophils comprise 1 to 3 percent of the total WBC count (Kee, 2009). The eosinophil count increases during many types of allergic responses (e.g., asthma and drug reactions) and parasitic infections. It also increases with certain types of neoplastic disorders, such as Hodgkin's disease. The eosinophil count decreases with elevated steroid levels of endogenous or exogenous origin.

Basophils

Basophils comprise only 0.4 to 1 percent of the total WBC count (Kee, 2009). An elevated basophil count may be caused by a myeloproliferative disease such as leukemia, an allergy or inflammation, or an infection. A lower than normal basophil count may be caused by stress, hyperthyroidism, and hypersensitivities (Kee, 2009), glucocorticoids and ovulation (Galli et al., 2006).

Lymphocytes

Lymphocytes make up about 25 percent of the total WBC count. Increased levels occur with viral infections (e.g., infectious mononucleosis and hepatitis), chronic infections, and lymphocytic leukemia. Abnormally low levels are associated with many diseases, such as cancers, leukemia, aplastic anemia, and multiple sclerosis (Kee, 2009).

Evaluation of Hemostasis

In the high-acuity setting, the most common tests measuring some aspect of hemostasis are tests of clotting times, such as prothrombin time, INR, partial thromboplastin time, and platelet count. Furthermore, certain disorders of hematologic function require other coagulation testing. For example, disseminated intravascular coagulation (DIC), a coagulopathy that arises as a complication of critical illness requires evaluation of clotting times and factor I (fibrinogen), fibrin split products, plasminogen and others. Table 5–7 provides a summary of major measurements of hemostasis in the adult.

Platelets

The number of platelets (thrombocytes) is measured using the platelet count, which is usually obtained as part of the complete blood cell (CBC) count. Another useful test of platelet function is the bleeding time, a test that is performed when a platelet abnormality is suspected. A prolonged bleeding time is associated with such disorders as thrombocytopenia (from any cause) and DIC.

Tests of Clotting Time

Prothrombin Time (PT) and INR. Prothrombin time (Pro-Time or PT) is a measure of factor II: prothrombin, which is synthesized by the liver. Recall that factor II is activated in the common pathway of the coagulation cascade and is one of the final steps in forming a fibrin clot and is frequently used to evaluate the anticoagulant status of patients on warfarin therapy. It is now recommended that prothrombin time be documented as an International Normalized Ratio (INR) value because the ratio is an internationally standardized measure of long-term warfarin anticoagulant therapy; however, it should only be used until the patient has been stabilized on warfarin (Kee, 2009). Many diseases and drugs can alter prothrombin time; therefore the patient's medical and medication history are important to consider when interpreting PT.

TABLE 5–7 Measures of Hemostasis in the Adult

TEST	ADULT NORMAL RANGE
Platelet Count	150,000 to 400,000 mcL
Bleeding Time	3 to 7 minutes
Prothrombin Time (PT)	10–13 seconds Desired levels in warfarin therapy: 1.5–2.0 times the control
INR (measure of PT)	Target in warfarin therapy: 2 to 3 Target in mitral valve replacement: 2.5 to 3.5
Partial Thromboplastin Time (PTT) and Activated PTT	PTT: 60 to 70 seconds APTT: 20 to 35 seconds
Fibrin Split Products	2 to 10 mcg/mL
D-dimer (Fibrin degradation fragment)	Negative

Data from Kee (2009).

Partial Thromboplastin Time (PTT) and Activated Partial Thromboplastin Time (APTT). The PTT and APTT tests can be used as a screening test for factors VII, XIII, and platelets (Kee, 2009). Both tests are more sensitive to minor coagulation deficiencies than is the prothrombin time (PT) test; and the APTT test is even more sensitive than the PTT. Both are useful in monitoring heparin anticoagulant therapy and in evaluation of clotting factor deficiencies.

D-dimer. D-dimer, or fibrin degradation fragment, is a measure of fibrin degradation, confirming that fibrin split products (FSP) are present (Kee, 2009). It is a nonspecific test that one or more clots are being broken down somewhere in the body. D-dimer is a useful tool in diagnosing disseminated intravascular coagulation (DIC) and may be of use in ruling out pulmonary embolism or other thrombosis. D-dimer values also increase as a result of fibrinolytic therapy such as tissue plasminogen activator (t-PA) treatment for acute myocardial infarction.

Fibrin Split (Degradation) Products. Fibrin split products (FSP), also referred to as fibrin degradation products, is a measurement of anticoagulation caused by the breakdown of clots via the clot dissolution portion of the coagulation process. The split products of fibrin act as anticoagulants. When FSP is elevated, prolonged bleeding results; thus the FSP is frequently used in emergency hemorrhage situations such as in severe trauma or shock (Kee, 2009). It is also useful in diagnosis of DIC.

Evaluation of Bone Marrow

The bone marrow aspiration (biopsy) is used to rule out, confirm, or make a differential diagnosis of a disorder involving the bone marrow. It is often performed after suspicious cells are found in the peripheral blood. The biopsy is usually performed by needle aspiration and is usually taken from the iliac crest in an adult. The bone marrow is examined for the presence, number, and type of abnormal cells, or the absence of normal cells. When assisting with a bone marrow aspiration, prior to the procedure the nurse should assure that the patient has received an explanation of the procedure and that the appropriate consent form has been signed. Following the procedure, vital signs should be monitored as ordered and the patient's aspiration site should be observed for bleeding. An analgesic may be needed to relieve postprocedure discomfort.

SECTION SEVEN REVIEW

1. An elevated reticulocyte count in the presence of anemia indicates that the
   - A. red blood cells are being destroyed prematurely
   - B. bone marrow is depressed
   - C. red blood cells are being sequestered in the spleen
   - D. bone marrow is functioning correctly
2. An example of a condition that is associated with microcytic red blood cells (a low MCV) is
   - A. aplastic anemia
   - B. vitamin B_{12} deficiency anemia
   - C. iron-deficiency anemia
   - D. blood loss anemia
3. A higher-than-normal hemoglobin level can result from
   - A. dehydration
   - B. aplastic anemia
   - C. hepatic cirrhosis
   - D. leukemia
4. Segmented neutrophils normally make up ______ percent of the total WBC count.
   - A. 20 to 35
   - B. 35 to 50
   - C. 50 to 70
   - D. 65 to 80
5. When a shift to the left occurs in the neutrophil count, it refers to a(n)
   - A. elevated band level
   - B. decreased band level
   - C. elevated seg level
   - D. decreased seg level
6. An elevated monocyte (monocytosis) level is associated with
   - A. early bacterial infection
   - B. aplastic anemia
   - C. hemolytic anemia
   - D. chronic infections
7. Elevated levels of lymphocytes develop in the presence of which disorders?
   - A. hypersensitivity reactions
   - B. viral and chronic infections
   - C. aplastic anemia
   - D. renal failure
8. Which cell component of the WBC differential count is normally the highest in percentage?
   - A. lymphocytes
   - B. monocytes
   - C. basophils
   - D. neutrophils
9. Abnormally low monocyte levels are found when which disease is present?
   - A. aplastic anemia
   - B. chronic infections
   - C. inflammatory bowel disease
   - D. acute monocytic leukemia
10. Lymphocytes make up about ______ percent of the total WBC count.
    - A. 5
    - B. 10
    - C. 20
    - D. 25
11. A blood sample for bleeding time is most likely to be drawn when which type of disease is suspected?
    - A. pulmonary embolism
    - B. thrombocytopenia
    - C. deep vein thrombosis
    - D. stroke
12. The INR is an international ratio measurement of
    - A. partial thromboplastin time
    - B. fibrin split products
    - C. prothrombin time
    - D. bleeding time
13. The D-dimer is a measure of which of the following?
    - A. presence of fibrin split products
    - B. platelet function
    - C. plasminogen activation
    - D. factor II

Answers: 1. D, 2. C, 3. A, 4. C, 5. A, 6. D, 7. B, 8. D, 9. A, 10. D, 11. B, 12. C, 13. A

POSTTEST

Melinda T., 42-year-old, is brought into the emergency room by her husband with complaints of severe weakness and hematemesis. She has just completed a second round of chemotherapy for treatment of ovarian cancer. Blood work is drawn.

1. The nurse is aware that Melinda's blood cells all come from the same cell, which is called a
   - A. pluripotential hematopoietic stem cell
   - B. committed stem cell
   - C. myeloid precursor stem cell
   - D. lymphoblast cell
2. Melinda's RBC count is significantly lower than normal. This will result in problems of
   - A. nutrient transport
   - B. bone marrow stimulation
   - C. iron transport
   - D. tissue oxygenation

3. The nurse asks Melinda about any history of kidney problems and Melinda states that her kidney function has always been normal. This is important for which reason?
A. RBCs can be destroyed by abnormally functioning nephrons.
B. Erythropoietin is produced by the kidneys.
C. Amino acids produced by the kidneys are needed for hemoglobin development.
D. Vitamin B_{12} is synthesized by the renal nephrons.

Melinda's WBC differential count shows a WBC of 2,000/mcL, neutrophil count of 600/mcL (30%), and a monocyte count of 400 (2%).

4. These WBC results suggest what about her innate immune system?
A. insufficient data
B. it is adequate
C. it is deficient
D. nothing, need to look at T cell values

5. Melinda's abnormal WBC values increase her risk for
A. infection
B. bleeding
C. tissue hypoxia
D. seizure activity

Melinda informs the nurse that she was exposed to chicken pox virus and that she has never had chicken pox. It is decided to administer gamma globulin.

6. The primary reason Melinda was given an injection of gamma globulin against chicken pox virus is
A. her age
B. her cancer
C. her gender
D. her immunodeficient state

7. Administering gamma globulin to Melinda is an example of which type of immunity?
A. active acquired
B. natural innate
C. passive acquired
D. non-specific

8. An antibody titer is drawn on Melinda. The best definition of antibody titer is the
A. presentation of processed T lymphocytes
B. amount of a specific antibody in a serum
C. synthesis of circulating immunoglobulins
D. molecular weight of an antigenic determinant

It is decided to give Melinda cytokine therapy using GM-CSF.

9. Cytokines, such as GM-CSF are sometimes given therapeutically, because they
A. activate components of the immune system
B. reduce inflammation
C. increase all bone marrow activity
D. increase immunoglobulin production

10. In its role as an antigen-presenting cell (APC), the macrophage presents a fragment of an antigen where?
A. within its cytoplasm
B. fragment breaks away
C. on its cell membrane
D. inside of its granules

11. Neutrophils and macrophages arrive at a site of inflammation through chemotaxis, which is
A. accumulation of leukocytes along a capillary wall near an inflammatory site
B. movement along an increasing concentration of chemotactic factors towards the area of inflammation
C. leukocytes squeezing through a capillary using an ameboid movement
D. adherence of leukocytes to the capillary wall near the site of inflammation

12. Cell-mediated immunity is best characterized by
A. specific recognition and memory of antigen
B. primary and secondary response patterns
C. subsets of IgG, IgA, IgE, IgM, and IgD
D. direct attack on invading antigens

13. Which immunoglobulin is found in large quantities in secretory body fluids?
A. IgA
B. IgE
C. IgG
D. IgM

14. The best definition of the complement system is
A. a nonspecific immune response of engulfing and ingesting foreign antigens by neutrophils
B. the body's first line of defense against viruses
C. the body's surveillance system for malignant cells
D. a progressive, sequential immune response activated by IgG and IgM

15. Some tumor-associated antigens can be used for what purpose?
A. as therapy against tumor growth
B. as serum markers of possible cancer
C. to monitor transplanted organs
D. to "turn off" cancer cells

16. The antigen–antibody response can result in which set of consequences against an invading pathogen? (choose all that apply)
A. agglutination
B. neutralization
C. cytokine attack
D. enhanced phagocytosis
E. complement activation

17. The primary storage area for platelets is which organ?
A. liver
B. pancreas
C. spleen
D. general circulation

18. The reason that platelets, under normal conditions, do not adhere and clump to the endothelial lining of vessels is
    A. The endothelium secretes certain substances that maintain the platelets in an inactive state.
    B. The endothelium secretes thrombin and platelet-activating factor to maintain the platelets in an inactive state.
    C. Inactive platelets secrete plasminogen to discourage adherence and clumping.
    D. Circulating platelets secrete minute quantities of t-PA to prevent adherence and clumping.
19. Coagulation factors are primarily synthesized by the liver, and many require which substance for synthesis?
    A. folic acid
    B. vitamin B_{12}
    C. ascorbic acid
    D. vitamin K
20. A patient's reticulocyte count is 30,000/mcL, which is abnormally low. This value makes you suspicious that the patient may be experiencing
    A. overproduction of RBCs in bone marrow
    B. microcytic, hypochromic RBCs
    C. bone marrow depression or failure
    D. rapid hemolyzation of RBCs
21. A laboratory report on a patient returns describing a patient's red blood cells as being hypochromic. This means that the RBC is
    A. pale in color
    B. smaller than normal
    C. abnormally shaped
    D. missing a nucleus
22. A patient who had a recent coronary artery bypass surgery has an erythrocyte sedimentation rate (ESR) drawn. The level comes back elevated. The significance of this is
    A. It suggests that the patient is dehydrated.
    B. It suggests that there is premature death of RBCs occurring.
    C. It suggests that the patient is experiencing an active inflammatory process.
    D. It suggests that the patient may have developed a viral infection.
23. A patient's neutrophil count shows a left shift (an abnormally high percentage of bands). This suggests
    A. bone marrow depression
    B. presence of a severe infection
    C. presence of a viral infection
    D. decreased thymus activity

Posttest answers with rationale are found on MyNursingKit.

PEARSON

EXPLORE mynursingkit™

MyNursingKit is your one stop for online chapter review materials and resources. Prepare for success with additional NCLEX®-style practice questions, interactive assignments and activities, web links, animations and videos, and more!

Register your access code from the front of your book at **www.mynursingkit.com.**

REFERENCES

Battinelli, E., Willoughby, S. R., Foxall, T. Valeri, R., & Loscalzo, J. (2001). Induction of platelet formation from megakarycytotoid cells by nitric oxide. *PNAS (Proceeding of the National Academy of Sciences of the United States of America), 98*(2): 14458–14463.

Galli, S. J., Metcalfe, D. D., Arber, D. A. and Dvorak, A. M. (2006). Basophils and mast cells and their disorders. In M. A. Lichtman, E.Beutler, T. J. Kipps, et al., *Williams hematology* (7th ed., pp. 879–897). New York: McGraw-Hill Medical.

Guasti, L., Marino, F., Cosentino, M., Cimpanelli, M., Maio, R., et al. (2006). Simvastatin treatment modifies polymorphonuclear leukocyte function in high-risk individuals: a longitudinal study. *Journal of Hypertension, 24*(12), 2423–2430.

Gould, B. (2002). *Pathophysiology for the health professions,* 2d ed. Philadelphia: W. B. Saunders.

Guyton, A. C., and Hall, J. E. (2006). Hemostasis and blood coagulation. In A. C. Guyton and J. E. Hall, *Textbook of Medical Physiology* (11th ed., pp. 457–468). Philadelphia: Elsevier/Saunders.

Kee, J. L. (2005). *Laboratory and diagnostic tests with nursing implications* (7th ed.). Upper Saddle River, N.J.: Prentice Hall.

Kee, J. L. (2009). *Prentice Hall handbook of laboratory and diagnostic tests with nursing implications*, 6th ed.. Upper Saddle River, N.J.: Prentice Hall.

NCBI (National Center for Biotechnology Information). (2008). Accessed 6/27/2008 at http://www.ncbi.nlm.nih.gov/entrez/dispomim.cgi?id=191160.

Rinker, J. R., Trinkaus, K., & Naismith, R. T. (2007). Higher IgG index found in African Americans versus Caucasians with multiple sclerosis. *Neurology, 69*(1), 68–72.

Rote, N. S. & McCance, K. L. (2008). Structure and function of the hematologic system. In S. E. Huether and K. L. McCance, *Understanding pathophysiology* (4th ed., pp. 481–507). St. Louis: Mosby/Elsevier.

Sakurai, Y, Oh-Oka, Y., Kato, S., Suzuki, S., Hayakawa, M., Masui, T., et al. (2006). Effects of long-term continuous use of immune-enhancing enteral formula on nutritional and immunologic status in non-surgical patients. *Nutrition, 22*(7/8), 713–21.

Trinchieri, G. and Lanier, L. (2006). Functions of natural killer cells. In M. A. Lichtman, E. Beutler, T. J. Kipps, U. Seligsohn, K. Kaushansky, and J. T. Prachal, *Williams Hematology* (7th ed., pp. 1077–1082). Philadelphia:McGraw-Hill Medical.

MODULE

6 Alterations in Red Blood Cell Function and Hemostasis

Kathleen Dorman Wagner

OBJECTIVES Following completion of this module, the learner will be able to

1. Describe anemia, including types, etiology, pathophysiology, clinical manifestations, and management.
2. Explain sickle cell disease, including etiology, pathophysiology, clinical manifestations, complications, diagnosis, and management.
3. Discuss polycythemia, including types, etiology, pathophysiology, clinical manifestations, complications, diagnosis, and management.
4. Describe thrombocytopenia, including types, etiology, pathophysiology, clinical manifestations, complications, diagnosis, and management.
5. Explain disseminated intravascular coagulation, including the etiology, pathophysiology, clinical manifestations, diagnosis, and management.
6. Discuss blood and blood component products as replacement therapy in the treatment of hematologic problems.
7. Describe the nursing assessment the patient with actual or potential problems of erythrocytes or hemostasis.

This self-study module presents the pathophysiologic processes involved in hematologic disorders of the red blood cells, platelets, and hemostasis. The module is composed of seven sections. Sections One and Two focus on disorders of too few erythrocytes. Section One presents various types of anemia and their clinical manifestations. Section Two profiles the inherited erythrocyte disorder, sickle cell disease, with an emphasis on the crises that can place this patient population in a high-acuity setting. The reader's attention is then turned to disorders of too many erythrocytes with a discussion of polycythemia in Section Three. Sections Four and Five shift the focus away from erythrocyte disorders to problems of hemostasis including disseminated intravascular coagulation. Section Six presents an overview of blood component therapy in the adult. Finally, in Section Seven, the focused assessment for problems of erythrocytes or hemostasis is provided. Each section includes a set of review questions to help the learner evaluate her or his understanding of the section's content before moving on to the next section. All Section Reviews include answers. It is suggested that the learner review those concepts answered incorrectly in the review questions before proceeding to the next section.

PRETEST

1. The clinical manifestations of the anemias are primarily attributable to
   A. decreased cardiac output
   B. impaired oxygen transport
   C. decreased blood volume
   D. impaired bone marrow function
2. Loss of intrinsic factor (IF) causes development of which form of anemia?
   A. megaloblastic
   B. hemolytic
   C. aplastic
   D. iron-deficiency
3. The premature destruction of RBCs causing hemolytic anemia is usually caused by
   A. infectious agents
   B. an immune disorder
   C. physical agents
   D. a microangiopathy
4. Anemia of inflammation (AI) is characterized as a low serum iron level in the presence of
   A. chronic bleeding
   B. increased iron-binding capacity
   C. adequate bone marrow iron stores
   D. premature death of RBCs

5. In a healthy infant, hemoglobin F (Hb F) is replaced by which type of hemoglobin at about 6 months of age?
   A. hemoglobin A (Hb A)
   B. hemoglobin B (Hb B)
   C. hemoglobin C (Hb C)
   D. hemoglobin S (Hb S)
6. When sickle hemoglobin experiences a deoxygenated state, it results in
   A. release of iron from hemoglobin
   B. stiff fibrous polymers
   C. inability of oxygen to attach to iron
   D. destruction of normal RBCs by the spleen
7. Appropriate nursing care of the patient in sickle cell crisis includes
   A. administer aspirin 300 mg P.O.
   B. restrict fluids to one liter or less per 24 hours
   C. transfuse blood to achieve hematocrit greater than 40 percent
   D. administer oxygen at 2-4 L/minute by nasal cannula
8. The two major features of polycythemia are
   A. elevated red cell mass and hematocrit
   B. larger than normal erythrocytes
   C. polymerization of red blood cells
   D. premature destruction of red blood cells
9. Which statement is correct regarding polycythemia vera?
   A. It is a rapidly progressive neoplastic disease.
   B. It affects all of the blood cells in the myeloid cell line.
   C. It tends to become milder over time.
   D. It only affects the RBCs in the myeloid cell line.
10. A major complication of severe primary and secondary of polycythemia is
    A. thrombosis and tissue ischemia or infarction
    B. bleeding peptic ulcer
    C. eventual onset of leukemia
    D. chronic obstructive pulmonary disease
11. The typical bleeding pattern of thrombocytopenia involves bleeding into the
    A. joints
    B. peritoneum
    C. internal organs
    D. skin and mucous membranes
12. Idiopathic thrombocytopenia purpura is believed to be
    A. of autoimmune origin
    B. caused by a drug reaction
    C. closely associated with splenomegaly
    D. of antibody–antigen immune complex origin
13. The paradoxical thromboembolism associated with immune-mediated heparin-induced thrombocytopenia (HIT type II) is caused by
    A. activated platelet prothrombotic activities
    B. heparin–platelet complexes
    C. accumulation of leukocytes
    D. red blood cell aggregation
14. Which statement is correct regarding disseminated intravascular coagulation (DIC)?
    A. Vessels become occluded because of vasospasm.
    B. Clot formation uses up all available platelets.
    C. DIC is a disease that causes acute myocardial infarction.
    D. DIC is caused only by activation of the intrinsic pathway.
15. DIC is called a coagulation paradox because
    A. platelets are being destroyed while fibrinolysis is occurring
    B. coagulation factors are being produced at the same rate as platelets
    C. blood is coagulating at the same time that clots are being dissolved
    D. thrombin is excessively produced while platelet production is decreased
16. The most important first step in treating DIC is
    A. initiate heparin therapy
    B. aggressive cryoprecipitate therapy
    C. initiate large doses of fresh-frozen plasma
    D. vigorous treatment of the underlying disease
17. The primary recommended use for whole blood is
    A. hypotension secondary to massive trauma
    B. when massive arterial vasodilatation is present
    C. hypovolemic shock from massive loss of blood
    D. when a patient has developed sensitivity to packed red cells
18. Once thawed, fresh frozen plasma (FFP) needs to be completely infused within which time frame?
    A. 4 hours
    B. 10 hours
    C. 24 hours
    D. 36 hours
19. Cryoprecipitate is an important therapy for treatment of
    A. hemophilia A
    B. hypofibrinogenemia
    C. Von Willebrand disease
    D. DIC
20. Transfusion-related acute lung injury (TRALI), associated with critical illness, usually presents with
    A. rapid onset of bacterial pneumonia
    B. acute onset of fever, chills & progressive respiratory distress
    C. cardiogenic pulmonary edema and left heart failure
    D. slow, insidious onset of fever, cough and unilateral pulmonary infiltrates
21. Which of the following causes the neurologic manifestations associated with anemia?
    A. leukostasis
    B. bleeding
    C. tissue hypoxia
    D. increased intracranial pressure
22. The activity intolerance created by some of the hematologic disorders is specifically related to
    A. intravascular fluid volume loss
    B. O_2 supply and demand imbalance
    C. decreased systemic blood flow
    D. inadequate secondary defenses

Pretest answers are found on MyNursingKit.

SECTION ONE: Acute Anemias: Disorders of Inadequate Erythrocytes

At the completion of this section, the learner will be able to describe anemia, including types, etiology, pathophysiology, clinical manifestations, and management.

The term **anemia** literally means "without blood"; however, its definition more specifically refers to a reduction of or dysfunction in **erythrocytes** (RBCs). It can be clinically expressed in terms of reduced levels of RBCs, hematocrit, or hemoglobin. Anemia is not a disease; rather, it is an important sign of some underlying disorder. This section focuses on the acute forms of anemia seen in high-acuity patients.

Clinical Manifestations

When caring for the patient with anemia, the ongoing nursing assessment focuses on the patient's oxygenation status. This is because regardless of the cause, the clinical manifestations of anemia are primarily attributable to one problem—*impaired oxygen transport*, which affects all body systems. Figures 6–1 and 6–2 illustrate the multisystem affects of anemia. Additional manifestations may be present, related to the rate of onset of the anemia, the hematocrit level, and the underlying cause. Table 6–1 summarizes the pathophysiologic basis of major manifestations.

Tissue Hypoxia Manifestations

Impaired oxygen transport causes tissue hypoxia. During an anemia episode, some degree of hypoxia is necessary to continue to stimulate the various compensatory mechanisms. Two factors determine the severity of clinical manifestations, rate of onset, and the underlying cause. It is important to include questions that investigate these two factors while taking the nursing history.

Rate of Onset. The speed with which the anemia occurs is an important factor in determining the severity of symptoms. When a mild-to-moderate anemia develops slowly, the person often remains asymptomatic as long as the body is not stressed (increasing oxygen demand). Given a slow enough onset, a person may remain relatively asymptomatic (if sedentary) with a hemoglobin as low as 7 or 8 g/dL (Adamson & Longo, 2005). When the onset of anemia is rapid (e.g., hemorrhage), there is insufficient time for adequate compensatory mechanisms to activate, which can potentially result in severe hypoxemia and tissue ischemia.

Underlying Cause. The patient's clinical manifestations usually reflect both the underlying disorder and the anemia. For example, a person with end-stage renal failure will have manifestations related to anemia plus any additional manifestations resulting from severe renal dysfunction. Some of the anemias also have their own unique manifestations. For example, sickle cell anemia (sickle cell disease) has many unique symptoms related to microvascular occlusion. In aplastic anemia, the decreased RBC level is just one part of a pancytopenia problem (involving two or more blood cell types). If pancytopenia is present, the patient will also develop the clinical manifestations of deficiencies in the other cell types.

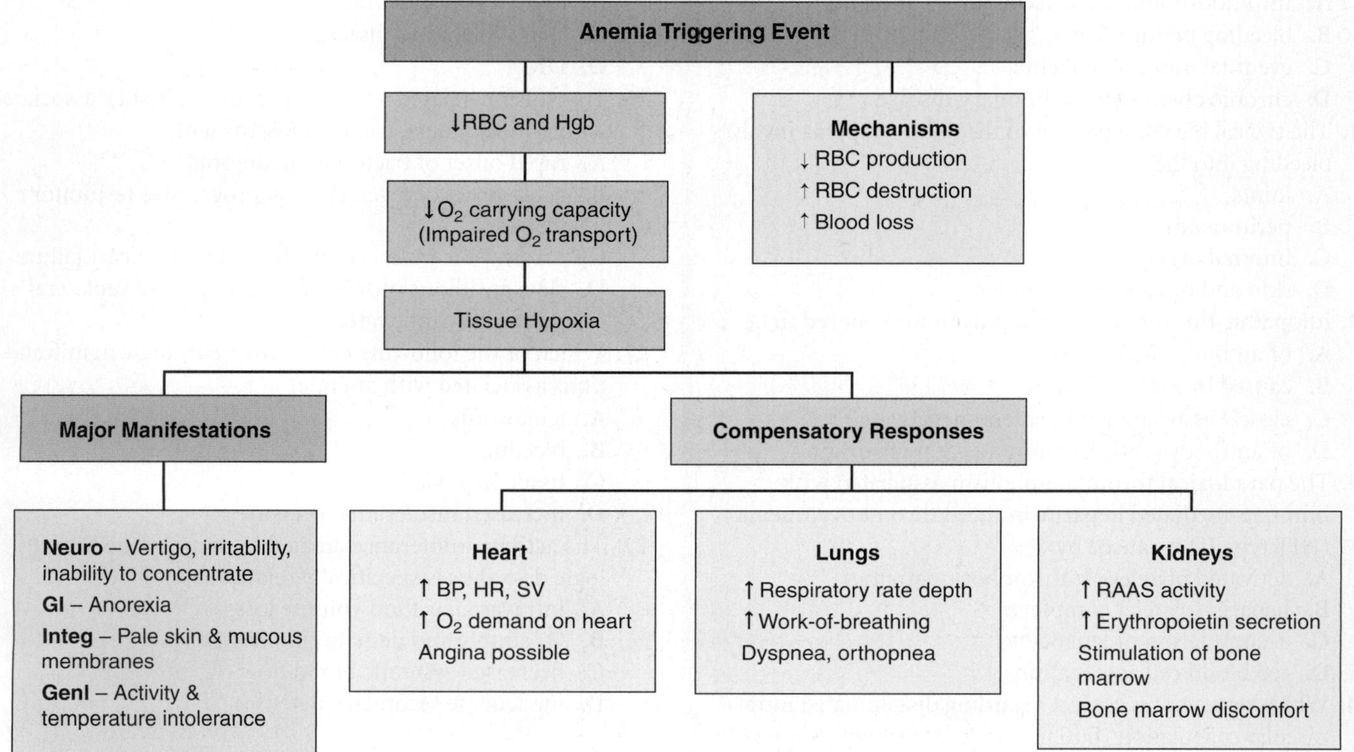

Figure 6–1 ■ The physiologic basis for the manifestations of anemia. ***KEY:*** *SV, stroke volume; RAAS, renin angiotensin aldosterone system*

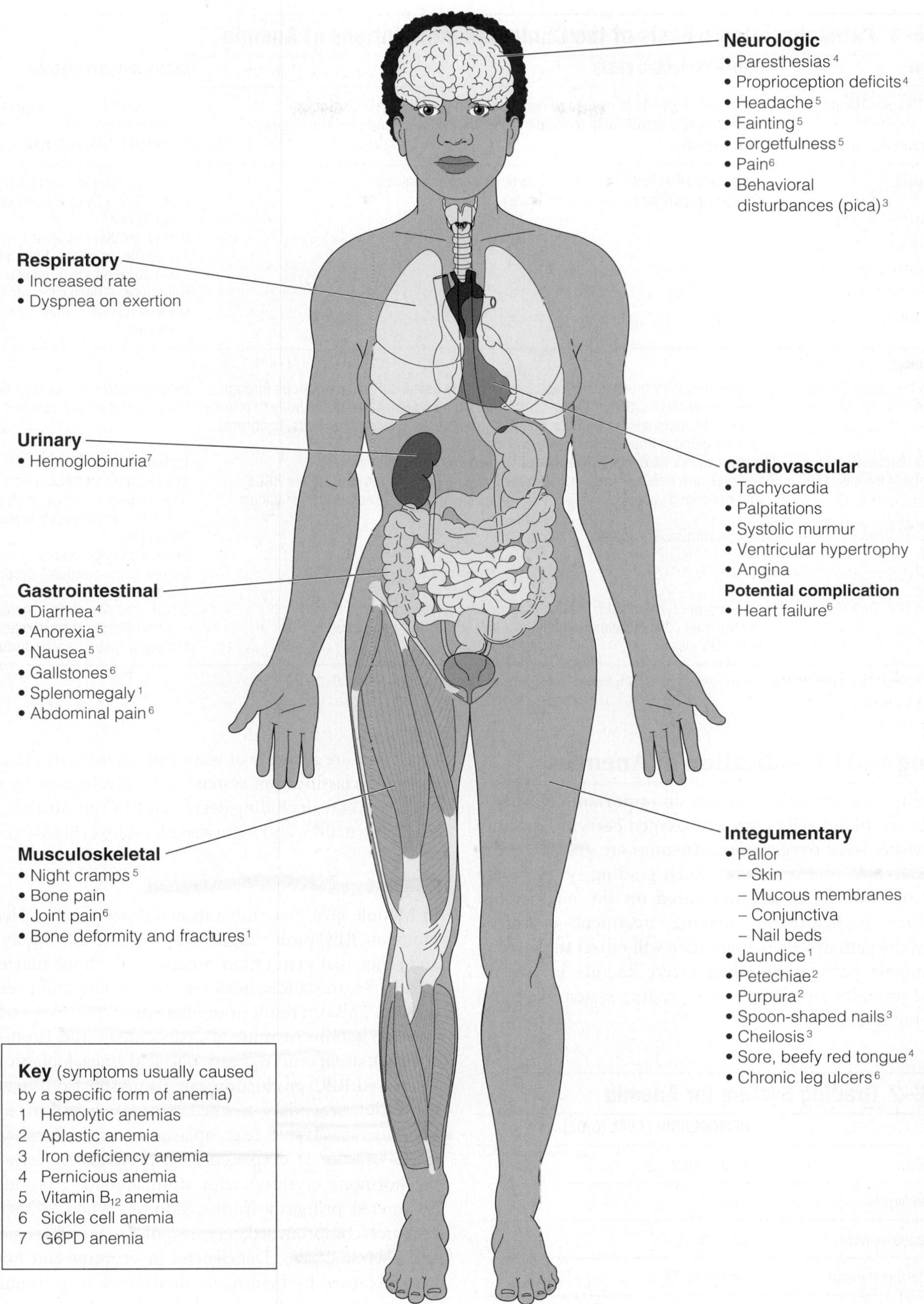

Figure 6–2 ■ The multisystem effects of anemia. Reprinted from LeMone, P. & Burke, K. *Medical–Surgical Nursing* (4th ed., p. 1104). © 2008, with permission from Pearson Education, Inc., Upper Saddle River, New Jersey.

TABLE 6–1 Pathophysiologic Basis of the Clinical Manifestations of Anemia

ALTERATION	PATHOPHYSIOLOGIC BASIS	SIGNS AND SYMPTOMS
Decreased Oxygen Affinity	The decreased affinity of oxygen to hemoglobin improves oxygen extraction from available hemoglobin to maintain adequate delivery and maintain tissue oxygenation.	A right shift on oxyhemoglobin-dissociation curve. Decreased P_VO_2 and S_VO_2
Tissue Hypoxia	Hypoxia-related symptoms develop if hypoxia becomes severe (oxygen supply and demand imbalance).	General – Fatigue (common) Pulmonary – Dyspnea on exertion (or at rest) Cardiovascular – Angina Peripheral vascular – Intermittent claudication; night muscle cramps Neurologic – Headache, lightheadedness Gastrointestinal – abdominal cramping, nausea
Compensatory:		
▪ Selective Increased Tissue Perfusion	As a compensatory mechanism, selective increased tissue perfusion develops through selective vasoconstriction that shunts blood from nonvital areas of the body to priority organs. In acute anemia blood is shunted from mesenteric and iliac beds. In chronic anemia blood is shunted from skin and kidneys.	Pale skin and mucous membranes Urine output usually remains normal
▪ Increased Cardiac Output (in absence of increased BP)	The heart works harder to deliver oxygen; a hyperdynamic cardiac output. Blood pressure does not increase because blood viscosity is reduced (fewer RBCs) and peripheral vascular resistance becomes lower due to selective vasodilatation.	Tachycardia Systolic flow murmur Severe anemia: angina, high output heart failure, cardiomegaly is possible
▪ Increased Pulmonary Function	Develops with severe anemia	Tachypnea Decreased a-A gradient Severe state: exertional dyspnea and orthopnea
▪ Increased RBC Production	Production of erythropoietin maintains an inverse relationship with the hemoglobin concentration to maintain a balance of RBC production with RBC loss	Stress reticulocytosis – increased number and proportion of reticulocytes Increased bone marrow discomfort

Key: P_VO_2=partial pressure of venous oxygen; S_VO_2=saturation of venous oxygen. Data from Prchal (2006).

Grading and Classification of Anemias

The severity of a patient's anemia is an important consideration since red blood cells represent oxygen carrying capacity and therefore tissue oxygenation. Anemias are graded by degree of severity (mild to severe). Such grading systems help quantify the severity of anemia based on the hemoglobin level, which is helpful in making treatment decisions. Clinically, the patient's assessment data will reflect the severity of the anemia particularly when severe anemia is present. Table 6–2 provides an example of a grading system based on hemoglobin levels.

TABLE 6–2 Grading System for Anemia

SEVERITY	HEMOGLOBIN LEVEL (G/DL)
Grade 1 (Mild)	10.0 to 10.9
Grade 2 (Moderate)	8.0–9.9
Grade 3 (Serious/severe)	6.5–7.9
Grade 4 (Life-threatening)	Less than 6.5

Adapted from: The National Cancer Institute and Cooperative Oncology Groups Grading System for Anemia. AHRQ (2001). *Uses of Epoetin for Anemia in Oncology.* Summary, Evidence Report/Technology Assessment: Number 30. AHRQ Publication Number 01-E008, March 2001. Agency for Healthcare Research and Quality, Rockville, MD. http://www.ahrq.gov/clinic/epcsums/epoetsum.htm.

There are a variety of ways that anemias are classified. One common classification system is the mechanism by which the anemia occurs, including decreased RBC production, increased RBC destruction, and increased blood loss (Fig. 6–3).

Decreased RBC Production

In Module Five, Determinants and Assessment of Hematologic Function, RBC proliferation was presented as a tightly regulated and sequential maturation process in the bone marrow. Under certain circumstances, however, RBC proliferation becomes depressed. This can result from inadequate intake or absorption of certain vitamins or minerals, particularly iron (iron-deficiency anemia); or vitamin B_{12} and folic acid (megaloblastic anemias). Decreased RBC production can also result from bone marrow depression secondary to chemotherapy, infection, or primary bone marrow failure (e.g., aplastic anemia). Renal failure also causes anemia of decreased RBC production. Remember that the hormone erythropoietin stimulates RBC production and is secreted primarily by the kidneys. When kidney function becomes compromised, erythropoietin is no longer secreted and anemia ensues. Deficiencies in vitamins and minerals are usually caused by inadequate intake and are chronic forms of anemia; therefore, they are only briefly profiled here.

Iron-Deficiency Anemia. Iron-deficiency anemia is the most common form of anemia found worldwide. Iron deficiency is caused by inadequate dietary intake (e.g., iron-poor diet),

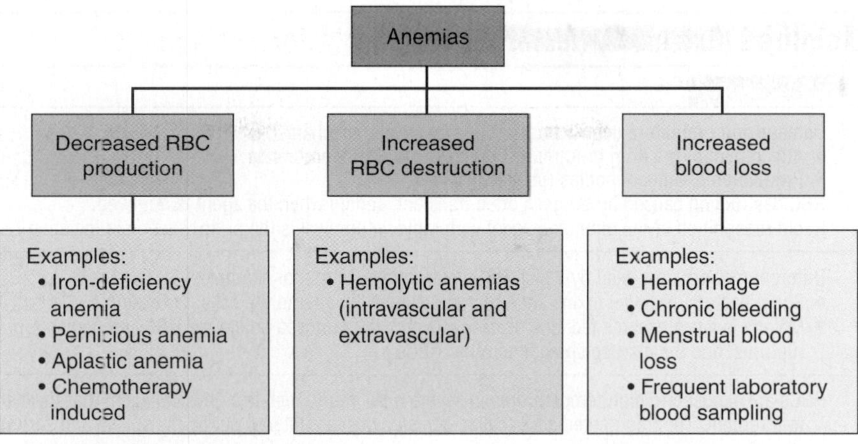

Figure 6–3 ■ Classification of anemias.

increased demand for iron (e.g., pregnancy or lactation), increased loss of iron (e.g., acute or chronic bleeding or menstrual blood loss), or a problem of iron uptake. Iron is the atom that oxygen attaches to on the hemoglobin molecule; therefore, a reduction in available iron atoms means a reduction in oxygen molecules attached to hemoglobin.

Megaloblastic Anemias. The term *megaloblastic* refers to the large size of the RBCs. These abnormal cells typically have large immature nuclei and have fragile membranes that are prone to rupture (Guyton & Hall, 2006). Vitamins B_{12} (cobalamin) and folic acid are essential components of RBC development. While inadequate intake is the major cause of these anemias, vitamin B_{12} deficiency can also result from malabsorption. Vitamin B_{12} requires a gastric secretion, intrinsic factor (IF), to protect it from being destroyed in the GI tract before it arrives at its absorption site in the terminal ileum. Loss of intrinsic factor from any cause (e.g., autoantibodies) leads to vitamin B_{12}-deficiency anemia (pernicious anemia).

Acquired Aplastic Anemia. Aplastic anemia is characterized by decreased production of blood cells from bone marrow failure (bone marrow aplasia). It has two peak incidence periods: a major peak in young adults (ages 15 to 25) and a lesser peak in the elderly (ages 65 to 69) (Segel & Lichtman, 2006). Because the entire bone marrow is usually affected, it results in a pancytopenia (all blood cell lines are diminished). Fatty tissue replaces the normal hematopoietic tissue in the bone marrow.

Etiology. In the high-acuity patient, it may be seen as part of bone marrow depression or failure secondary to some acquired (extrinsic) mechanism, such as a viral infection, drug, radiation, or autoimmunity mechanism. While the etiology is often unknown, aplastic anemia has been associated with several different causes

- Benzene
- Drugs (e.g., chloramphenicol, phenylbutazone, gold salts, phenytoin, and cytotoxic chemotherapeutic agents)
- Infections (rare; e.g., Epstein-Barr virus, hepatitis B and C)
- Ionizing radiation

When the etiology remains unknown, the condition is referred to as *idiopathic* aplastic anemia. When acquired aplastic anemia is suspected, it is important to investigate possible etiologies while taking the patient's history. A good starting point is asking questions that target the known etiologies.

Pathophysiology. Aplastic anemia develops when damaged or impaired stem cells inhibit red blood cell production. The severity of aplastic anemia varies widely from mild to severe and the prognosis is based on the severity of the disease. At its most severe, aplastic anemia is a relentless disease with rare spontaneous remissions. If left untreated, the prognosis is poor, with most patients dying within 6 months of onset. Even with effective treatment, life expectancy is often only a few years.

Treatment. The treatment for aplastic anemia focuses on three general areas: supportive, immunosuppressive, and hematopoietic stem-cell replacement. Supportive therapy includes blood transfusions to replace RBCs and platelets, and antibiotic therapy to protect from infection. Immunosuppressive therapy frequently consists of antithymocyte globulin (ATG) or a combination of ATG, steroids, and/or cyclosporine. These drugs are used when hematopoietic stem-cell transplantation is not planned. Hematopoietic stem-cell transplantation (HSCT) is the definitive treatment for aplastic anemia in younger patients. If the patient is a candidate for HSCT, blood transfusions will be limited and with no transfusions coming from potential stem-cell donors. This helps reduce both the risk of hypersensitivity reactions and potential stem-cell rejection.

Increased Destruction of RBCs

The term **hemolytic anemia** refers to all anemias that are caused by premature destruction of red blood cells, either intravascularly or within the **reticuloendothelial system.** Hemolytic anemia can result from intrinsic (e.g., congenital) problems or, more commonly, from extrinsic (acquired) problems. The majority of high-acuity patients are much more at risk for acquired problems. An exception to this is sickle cell crisis, a potentially life-threatening complication of sickle cell anemia. The acquired hemolytic anemias are often categorized by the

TABLE 6–3 Types of Acquired (Extrinsic) Hemolytic Anemia

TYPE	DESCRIPTION
Drug-induced (Examples: alpha-methyldopa, sulfonamides)	Damage and premature destruction of RBCs by several mechanisms: ■ Attachment of the drug or immune complexes to RBC membranes ■ Production of autoantibodies (usually IgM) RBC destruction caused by drugs is often transient, ending when the agent is removed. Rapid recognition of the offending agent with rapid withdrawal is the priority action in initiating treatment.
Infectious agent-induced	Different mechanisms exist by which RBC destruction occurs, for example: ■ Some bacteria produce toxins and other substances that hemolyze cells, for example, *Clostridium perfringens* infections. ■ Malaria is a protozoan infectious disease in which the protozoa enters the RBC and begins reproducing. Eventually, the RBC ruptures, and the disease spreads to other RBCs.
Physical agent-induced	RBCs are exposed to high temperatures in severe burn injury. Heat is a physical agent that makes RBCs fragile and causes them to fragment. The fragmented cells (called *schistocytes*) are filtered out by the spleen and serum RBC levels drop significantly.
Microangiopathy-Induced	Involves the fragmentation of RBCs as they move through damaged small blood vessels. Microangiopathy occurs in such problems as ■ Disseminated intravascular coagulation (DIC) ■ Thrombotic thrombocytopenic purpura (TTP) ■ Malignant hypertension ■ Pregnancy complications (e.g., HELLP syndrome and eclampsia) ■ Damage caused by administration of certain drugs (e.g., cyclosporine and mitomycin-c) ■ RBC fragmentation caused by artificial heart valve trauma is sometimes classified under this category The schistocytes are easily found on peripheral blood smears.

condition or agent that causes the RBC destruction, including immune disorders, drugs, infectious agents, physical agents, and conditions associated with microangiopathy.

Hemolytic Anemia. Premature destruction of RBCs by the immune system is a major cause of hemolytic anemia. Antibodies or complement (or sometimes both) coat the red blood cell membrane, causing premature death of the cell. The antibodies can be autoimmune-induced, isoimmune-induced, or drug-induced (e.g., sulfonamides). Autoimmune-induced hemolytic anemia (AIHA) results from production of autoantibodies against the person's own red blood cells. The cause is unknown, but it is believed that the autoimmune reaction may at times result from an infectious agent, such as infectious mononucleosis. Isoimmune-induced hemolytic anemia is primarily seen in two situations. It most commonly results from ABO blood type incompatibility between mother and baby. It can also result from **Rh incompatibility** in newborn infants. Table 6–3 summarizes types of extrinsic hemolytic anemia; sickle cell disease is presented in detail in the next section of this module.

Increased Blood Loss

Anemia caused by blood loss is a common problem of high-acuity patients. Blood loss can be acute (rapid onset) or chronic (slow, insidious onset), and can involve gross or occult bleeding. These two sets of factors largely determine the patient's clinical presentation. Problems of acute blood loss seen in high-acuity patients are presented here.

Trauma is a major cause of acute blood loss. It is also associated with surgery and acute gastrointestinal (GI) bleeding. The clinical manifestations of acute blood loss are usually more severe than those associated with chronic blood loss because of the body's inability to muster sufficient compensatory mechanisms in an acute situation. The effects of acute blood loss can be classified into stages of hemorrhage, as noted in Table 6–4.

During acute bleeding, early laboratory studies can be deceptive. Hemoglobin and hematocrit do not initially reflect anemia because plasma as well as cells are equally lost. As bleeding continues, fluid begins to shift from the extravascular spaces into the intravascular space. This fluid shift causes dilution of the remaining blood cells. In addition, as fluid resuscitation is initiated, the intravascular space is loaded with fluids, which further increases the dilutional effect. The end result is a significant reduction in serum hemoglobin and hematocrit. The full extent of the bleed cannot be evaluated using Hgb and Hct values until 48 to 72 hours after the acute bleed. The reticulocyte count becomes elevated within several days of the bleeding event as the bone marrow begins to produce and release the immature RBCs at a rapid rate.

TABLE 6–4 Patient Signs Associated with Stages of Hemorrhage

STAGE	BLOOD LOSS	VASOCONSTRICTION	VITAL SIGNS HR	BP	RR
+1	< 15%	↑	↑	→	→
2	15–25%	↑↑	↑↑	→	↑
3	25–35%	↑↑↑	↑↑↑	↓	↑↑
4	>35%	↓↓	Variable	↓↓↓	↓

HR=heart rate; BP=blood pressure; RR=respiratory rate. Adapted from Bledsoe, B., Porter, R. & Cherry, R. (2004). *Intermediate Emergency Care: Principles & Practice*, (p. 651). Upper Saddle River, N.J.: Pearson/Prentice Hall.

Treatment of blood loss anemia is largely based on the hemoglobin level. As with other forms of anemia, the underlying cause should be corrected if possible, or at least controlled. The hemodynamic status of the patient is supported as needed through fluid resuscitation and vasopressors. In severe cases of blood loss anemia, blood transfusions may be considered. Exactly what constitutes the appropriate use of blood transfusion has become controversial. Evidence suggests that using a restricted transfusion strategy (goal Hgb of 7 g/dL) may lead to improved outcomes for the patients (Shorr & Jackson, 2005; Hebert et al., 1998). Blood transfusions are presented in more detail in Section Six of this module.

Timouth, McIntyre & Fowler (2008) explain that recombinant erythropoietin therapy (e.g., Procrit or Epogen) has been used for some time for treatment of chronic anemias of renal failure and cancer and is now gaining popularity in the critical care environment. Investigations in use of erythropoietin therapy in the critical environment to date have failed to show a decrease in mortality or a decrease in use of blood transfusions.

Anemia of Inflammation and Critical Illness

Anemia has been associated with many chronic diseases and, until recently, was called "anemia of chronic disease." New research has shed light on the pathogenesis associated with this mild-to-moderate form of anemia; and to more accurately reflect the cause of the anemia, it has been renamed *anemia of inflammation (AI)*. The primary characteristic of anemia of inflammation is deficient RBC production in the presence of low serum iron and reduced iron-binding capacity despite adequate bone marrow iron stores (Ganz, 2005). In other words, the body does not sufficiently increase its production of RBCs to sufficiently cover increased RBC losses.

Anemia of inflammation is believed to exist worldwide in individuals with chronic inflammation and infections. Some of the major inflammatory and infective disorders that are now considered to be AI disorders include:

- Inflammatory – Inflammatory bowel diseases, rheumatoid disorders, and systemic inflammatory response syndrome (SIRS)
- Infective – Sepsis, chronic abscesses, and HIV/AIDS (Ganz, 2005)

The anemia of inflammation process is not fully understood but is believed to involve multiple factors, including increased RBC destruction, blunted erythropoiesis and resistance to erythropoietin, as well as **hypoferremia** (low iron blood levels; a defining feature).

Anemia of Critical Illness

Anemia of critical illness is a subtype of anemia of inflammation that develops rapidly, within days of illness onset. It is estimated that over 90 percent of critically ill patients develop anemia by the third day post admission to ICU (Tinmouth, McIntyre & Fowler, 2008). The anemia of inflammation pathologic processes are involved but accompanied by additional factors that are more unique to critical illness, such as iatrogenic blood loss through blood sampling, acute blood loss, occult blood loss through stress-related mucosal injury, and chemotherapy-related factors. Iatrogenic blood loss through diagnostic blood sampling has been studied since the 1980s. Critically ill patients may have blood withdrawn up to 24 times/day with mean blood loss estimates that range from 41.5 to 377 mL/day (Tinmouth, McIntyre & Fowler, 2008). Acute blood loss can result from a variety of problems, such as initial postsurgical bleeding, gastrointestinal bleeding (e.g., stress ulcers), or trauma-related hemorrhage. Disease-related factors often involving use of chemotherapeutic agents can suppress the bone marrow (e.g., steroid or other immunosuppressant therapy).

Emerging Evidence

- A quality-of-life measure for adults with sickle cell disease was tested and validated. The instrument is called Sickle Cell Impact Measurement Scale (SIMS). The investigators concluded that SIMS was a valid, reliable, and responsive instrument for measuring the health-related quality of life in this patient population *(Adams-Graves, Johnson, & Corley, 2008)*.
- In a study of 2,420 patients who received heparin for four or more successive days, a significant number (36.4 percent) developed thrombocytopenia. There was a higher incidence of death, acute MI, and heart failure in those who developed thrombocytopenia. The greatest predictor of death was a relative reduction in the platelet count of greater than 70 percent from the admission level *(Oliveria, Crespo, Becker, Honeycutt et al., 2008)*.
- In a study of the efficacy and safety of epoetin alpha in patients with critical illnesses, patients received a placebo or epoetin alpha to evaluate whether use of epoetin alpha reduced the number of red cell transfusions administered. Investigators concluded that use of epoetin increased the incidence of thrombotic events and did not decrease the use of red cell transfusion therapy. They also concluded that use of epoetin may reduce mortality associated with trauma *(Corwin, Gettinger, Fabian, May et al., 2007)*.
- In an investigation of elderly surgical mostly male patients (veterans), those with preoperative anemia Hct of <39.0 percent or polycythemia with Hct greater than 51 percent) were at increased risk of death or a cardiac event within 30 days postoperatively *(Wu, Schifftner, Henderson, Eaton et al., 2007)*.

Nursing Considerations

The high-acuity nurse needs to be mindful of any risk factors that a patient may have for development of anemia in the high-acuity setting, particularly in the critical care environment. Care of the patient with anemia centers on treating the cause and improving oxygenation. Regardless of the underlying cause of the anemia, the nurse will largely focus on monitoring the patient's oxygenation status and supporting tissue oxygenation. Major assessments and interventions that apply to the anemic patient are provided in the box, *NURSING CARE: The patient with anemia.*

NURSING CARE: The Patient with Anemia

Expected Patient Outcomes and Related Interventions

Outcome: Maintain adequate oxygenation

Assess and compare to established norms, patient baselines, and trends

- Monitor for signs and symptoms of anemia/reduced oxygenation
  - Cardiopulmonary
    - Tachycardia, systolic flow murmur, angina
    - Tachypnea, orthopnea, dyspnea, low pulse oximetry
  - Peripheral vascular
    - Intermittent claudication, night muscle cramps
  - Neurologic
    - Impaired thought processes, headache, dizziness
  - Integumentary/Skeletal
    - Pale mucous membranes, skin pallor, cyanosis, cold sensitivity, bone marrow discomfort
  - Gastrointestinal
    - Anorexia, abdominal cramping, nausea
  - Laboratory tests
    - Low RBC, high reticulocyte count, low hemoglobin and hematocrit
    - Low PaO_2, SaO_2

Investigate potential etiologies of anemia

- Obtain thorough nursing history including dietary, recent and chronic illnesses, medications, environmental exposure

Administer related drug therapy and monitor for therapeutic and nontherapeutic effects

- Oxygen therapy, synthetic erythropoietin therapy
- Nutritional supplements to support RBC development as ordered (e.g., iron, vitamin B_{12}, folic acid)

Interventions to support adequate oxygenation

- Decrease energy expenditure
  - Alternate rest and active periods
  - Maintain comfortable room temperature for patient (prevent chilling)
  - Maintain normothermia (reduce fevers, warming blankets if hypothermic)
  - Assist with physical activities as needed
- Administer oxygen at 2–4 L/min per nasal cannula, as ordered

Related Nursing Diagnoses

- Activity intolerance
- Altered tissue perfusion
- Nutrition: less than body requirements

Data taken from: Hamilton & Janz (2006); and Benz (2005).

SECTION ONE REVIEW

1. The clinical manifestations of the anemias are primarily attributable to
   A. decreased cardiac output
   B. impaired oxygen transport
   C. decreased blood volume
   D. impaired bone marrow function
2. The severity of symptoms associated with anemia largely depends on the
   A. type of anemia
   B. total blood volume
   C. speed with which it develops
   D. degree of bone marrow involvement
3. An adult patient with a hemoglobin of 7.8 g/dL would be classified as which grade?
   A. 1 (mild)
   B. 2 (moderate)
   C. 3 (serious/severe)
   D. 4 (life-threatening)
4. The most common form of anemia found worldwide is
   A. megaloblastic anemias
   B. iron-deficiency anemia
   C. aplastic anemia
   D. blood loss anemia
5. Loss of intrinsic factor (IF) causes development of which form of anemia?
   A. megaloblastic
   B. hemolytic
   C. aplastic
   D. iron-deficiency
6. The form of anemia that usually involves pancytopenia is
   A. aplastic
   B. hemolytic
   C. megaloblastic
   D. iron-deficiency
7. The definitive treatment for aplastic anemia in younger patients is
   A. blood transfusions
   B. antibiotic therapy
   C. immunosuppressant therapy
   D. hematopoietic stem-cell transplant
8. The premature destruction of RBCs causing hemolytic anemia is usually caused by
   A. infectious agents
   B. an immune disorder
   C. physical agents
   D. a microangiopathy

9. The most common cause of acute blood loss anemia is
   A. alcohol abuse
   B. menorrhagia
   C. trauma
   D. GI bleeding
10. When a patient is hemorrhaging, the vital signs begin to fail (decreased BP, increased heart rate and respirations) at which stage of hemorrhage?
    A. Stage 1 (less than 15 percent blood loss)
    B. Stage 2 (15-25 percent blood loss)
    C. Stage 3 (25-35 percent blood loss)
    D. Stage 4 (greater than 35 percent blood loss)
11. Anemia of inflammation (AI) is characterized as a low serum iron level in the presence of
    A. adequate bone marrow iron stores
    B. increased iron-binding capacity
    C. chronic bleeding
    D. premature death of RBCs
12. Iatrogenic blood loss as a factor in anemia of critical illness refers to blood lost resulting from
    A. stress ulcer erosions
    B. laboratory sampling
    C. trauma-related surgery
    D. mild disseminated intravascular coagulation

Answers: 1. B, 2. C, 3. C, 4. B, 5. A, 6. A, 7. D, 8. B, 9. C, 10. C, 11. A, 12. B

SECTION TWO: Sickle Cell Disease – A Disorder of Abnormal RBCs

At the completion of this section, the learner will be able to explain sickle cell disease, including etiology, pathophysiology, clinical manifestations, complications, diagnosis and management.

To better understand sickle cell disease, it is important to have a basic understanding of types of hemoglobin. Babies are born with RBCs that contain fetal hemoglobin (Hb F). As the Hb F-containing RBCs naturally age and die off, they are normally replaced by RBCs that contain Hb A (adult hemoglobin). After the first six months of age, 95 to 98 percent of hemoglobin should be Hb A, with Hb F levels dropping down to no more than 1 to 2 percent (Kee, 2005). Sickle cell disease refers to a group of inherited disorders characterized by abnormal hemoglobin, called "sickle hemoglobin" or hemoglobin S (Hb S), that develops rather than Hb A to replace fetal hemoglobin. Sickle cell disease results from an autosomal recessive mutation in the β-globin gene whereby the sixth amino acid (glutamic acid) is replaced by another (valine) (Benz, 2005). There are variations of the disease based on inheritance patterns. This section focuses on the most severe form, sickle cell anemia, which has the homozygous inheritance pattern. Table 6–5 provides a brief summary of two major forms of the disease, sickle cell anemia (the most serious form) and sickle cell trait (the carrier form), and Figure 6–4 shows the inheritance pattern for sickle cell anemia.

TABLE 6–5 Two Major Forms of Sickle Cell Disease

TYPE	DESCRIPTION
Sickle Cell Anemia	Hemoglobin is predominantly Hb S (75–95%) Inheritance pattern: Homozygous (Inherit Hb S from both parents, HbS/S)) Most severe form of disease
Sickle Cell Trait	Hemoglobin is Hb A/S (a mixture of Hb A and Hb S) Inheritance pattern: Heterozygous (Hb S inherited from one parent and Hb A [normal] inherited from other parent) Carrier state Rarely develop clinical manifestations

Epidemiology

Sickle cell disease is most prevalent in equatorial Africa, where the prevalence for the heterozygous form is estimated to be about 20 to 40 percent (Beutler, 2006a). It also has a higher frequency in tropical parts of India and the Mediterranean (Kline, 2008). In the United States, the disease is primarily found in the African American population with a frequency of about 8 percent (Beutler, 2006a). The fact that the disease is most prevalent in countries

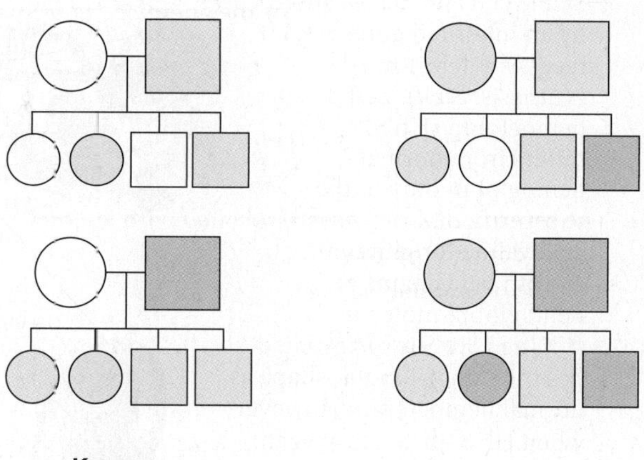

Figure 6–4 ■ The inheritance for sickle cell anemia. Reprinted from LeMone, P. & Burke, K. *Medical–Surgical Nursing* (4th ed., p. 1107). © 2008, with permission from Pearson Education, Inc., Upper Saddle River, New Jersey.

where malaria is endemic, suggests that the sickle cell mutation may have resulted as a genetic adaptation against malaria (*Plasmodium falciparum* infection). The sickle cell trait form (heterozygous) is the most advantageous because there are usually no clinical manifestations of the disease; yet it reduces the severity and duration of malaria (Beutler, 2006a).

Pathophysiology of Hb S

In a normal, well-oxygenated state, sickle hemoglobin (Hb S) functions normally. The problem arises when the PaO_2 and SaO_2 drop, producing a deoxygenated state. The relative hypoxic state causes the mutated hemoglobin to polymerize, forming fibrous polymers (Benz, 2005). The realignment of polymers is what gives the RBC its sickled shape. While sickled, RBCs take on two important characteristics. First, the polymer realignment makes the RBC membrane stiffer, which can slow down or obstruct flow in the small capillaries. Second, while sickled, the RBC membrane is sticky, allowing cells to adhere to the endothelium of vessel walls. Together, these two characteristics can cause microvascular occlusion, the major characteristic of sickle cell anemia. Figure 6–5 illustrates the polymerization process of Hb S.

Hemoglobin S has a significantly shortened life span of only 10 to 20 days (rather than the usual 120 days), with elevated erythropoiesis (5 to 8 times normal) that compensates for the premature RBC hemolysis (Kline, 2008). The abnormal RBCs sequester in and are destroyed by the spleen. Over time, the pooling of abnormal cells in the spleen can cause tissue ischemia and infarction that eventually destroys the spleen (autosplenectomy). When the underlying cause of the hypoxic event is relieved, most of the sickled cells return to their normal shape; however, with sickle cell anemia, a significant number (up to 30 percent of Hb S) cannot revert back to normal and are destroyed by the spleen (Kline, 2008).

Clinical Manifestations of Sickle Cell Anemia

The clinical manifestations of sickle cell anemia develop between the ages of 6 months to one year old, when Hb S becomes the predominant RBC type. Chronic hemolytic anemia and intermittent episodes of microvascular occlusion (vaso-occlusive crisis) become the sources of many of the manifestations of sickle cell anemia.

Manifestations of Microvascular Occlusion

Occlusion in the microvasculature causes ischemic pain (called painful crises) and possible dysfunction of the tissue or organs in which the occlusion is occurring. Table 6–6 provides a summary of the effects of micro-obstruction and infarction of some of the organs targeted by vascular occlusion in sickle cell anemia.

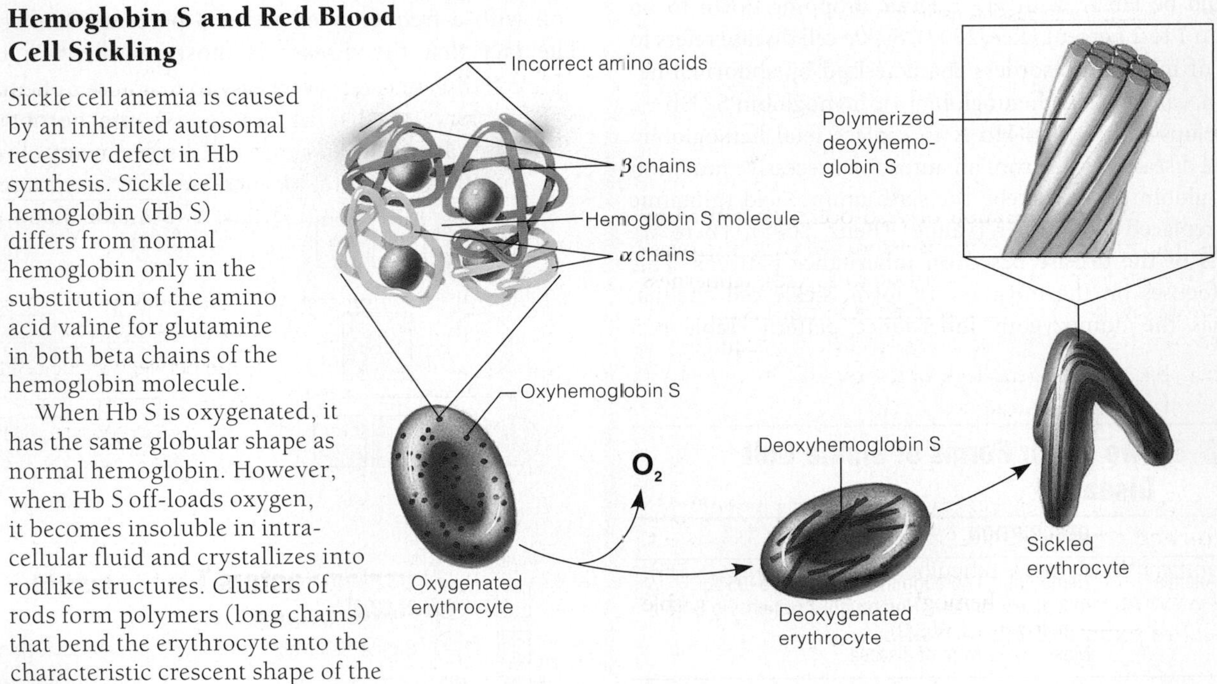

Figure 6–5 ▪ The polymerization process of Hb S. Reprinted from LeMone, P. & Burke, K. *Medical–Surgical Nursing* (4th ed., p. 1108). © 2008, with permission from Pearson Education, Inc., Upper Saddle River, New Jersey.

TABLE 6–6 Effects of Micro-Obstruction and Infarction on Organs

ISCHEMIC ORGAN/TISSUE	RESULTS
Brain	Stroke (most common in children; often hemorrhagic)
Retina	Hemorrhage, retinopathy Retinal detachment
Lungs	Acute chest syndrome ▪ A type of acute lung injury ▪ Presentation: chest pain, tachypnea, fever, cough, oxygen desaturation, chest infiltrates ▪ Cause of about 25% of deaths [Hamilton & Janz, 2006] Pulmonary hypertension and cor pulmonale (common cause of death in adults) Pulmonary embolism
Liver	Infarction Hepatitis (secondary to transfusions)
Spleen	Infarction and destruction (usually within 18–36 months of age) Loss of the spleen increases susceptibility to infections (esp. pneumococci)
Kidneys	Papillary necrosis with isosthenuria Global renal necrosis Renal failure in adults (a common adult cause of death)
Bone and joints	Aseptic necrosis (especially humeral and femoral heads) Bone infarctions Chronic arthropathy Osteomyelitis Hand-foot syndrome (painful inflammation and infarction of digits)
Male genitalia	Priapism with possible tissue infarction Permanent impotence
Integument	Lower leg stasis ulcers

Data from Benz (2005) and Hamilton & Janz (2006).

Figure 6–6 provides an illustration of vaso-occlusion caused by sickled cells. The major manifestations associated with microvascular occlusion are pain (can be moderate to severe), tenderness of the affected area, tachycardia, and fever. Pain can develop anywhere, based on the location of the vaso-occlusion (frequently in the abdomen, back, chest, arms, legs, or knees). Painful crisis lasts anywhere from a few hours to several weeks.

Manifestations of Hemolytic Anemia

A person with sickle cell anemia usually maintains a hemoglobin of 7-10 g/dL and a hematocrit ranging from 15 to 30 percent, with a significantly elevated reticulocyte count (Benz, 2005). Given this abnormal range of hemoglobin, it is understandable that hypoxia is a common trigger for sickle cell crises.

Sickle Cell Crises

The adult with sickle cell anemia is at risk for two disease-related crises:

- **Vaso-occlusive (painful) crisis** – By far the more common. It involves ischemic tissue pain from sickled cells occluding microcirculation. The duration of a painful crisis is usually less than a week but some episodes last several weeks. Repeated crises cause tissue damage that accumulates over time, resulting in end-organ damage.
- **Aplastic crisis** – A severe degree of anemia resulting from the inability of erythropoiesis to meet the high demand for new RBCs due to the short life span of abnormal RBCs. Global tissue hypoxia results from the compromised oxygen delivery to the tissues.

Table 6–7 lists common factors that can trigger a sickling crisis.

Morbidity and Mortality

Sickle cell anemia is a life-shortening disease; however, the survival time is unpredictable (ranging from childhood to the mid-twenties). The major cause of death is infection. About 10 percent of young children develop sepsis and meningitis by age 5 with a mortality rate of about 25 percent (Benz, 2005). Certain factors are known to increase morbidity and decrease survival, including:

- Three or more hospital admissions in a year for treatment of crises
- A history of splenic sequestration or hand-foot syndrome
- More than one episode of acute chest syndrome
- History of stroke (increases the risk for repeated strokes)
- Chronic neutropenia (Benz, 2005)

Diagnosis and Treatment

Diagnosis

Sickle cell disease is relatively easy to diagnose. A hematologic family history (mother and father) should be obtained. A positive family history of sickle cell disease in any of its forms is an important indicator of increased sickle cell disease risk for any child born to that family. Two major blood tests for Hb S include:

- Sickle cell screening test (e.g., Sickledex test) – A screening blood test that is read as positive or negative for Hb S. A positive result cannot differentiate between sickle cell trait and sickle cell anemia. A false negative reading can occur if the hemoglobin is less than 10 g/dL or hematocrit is less than 30 percent (Kee, 2005).

TABLE 6–7 Common Factors That Promote Painful Crises

Abrupt temperature changes
Anxiety
Excessive exercise
Fever
Hypoxia (including sleep apnea)
Infection
Smoking
Stress

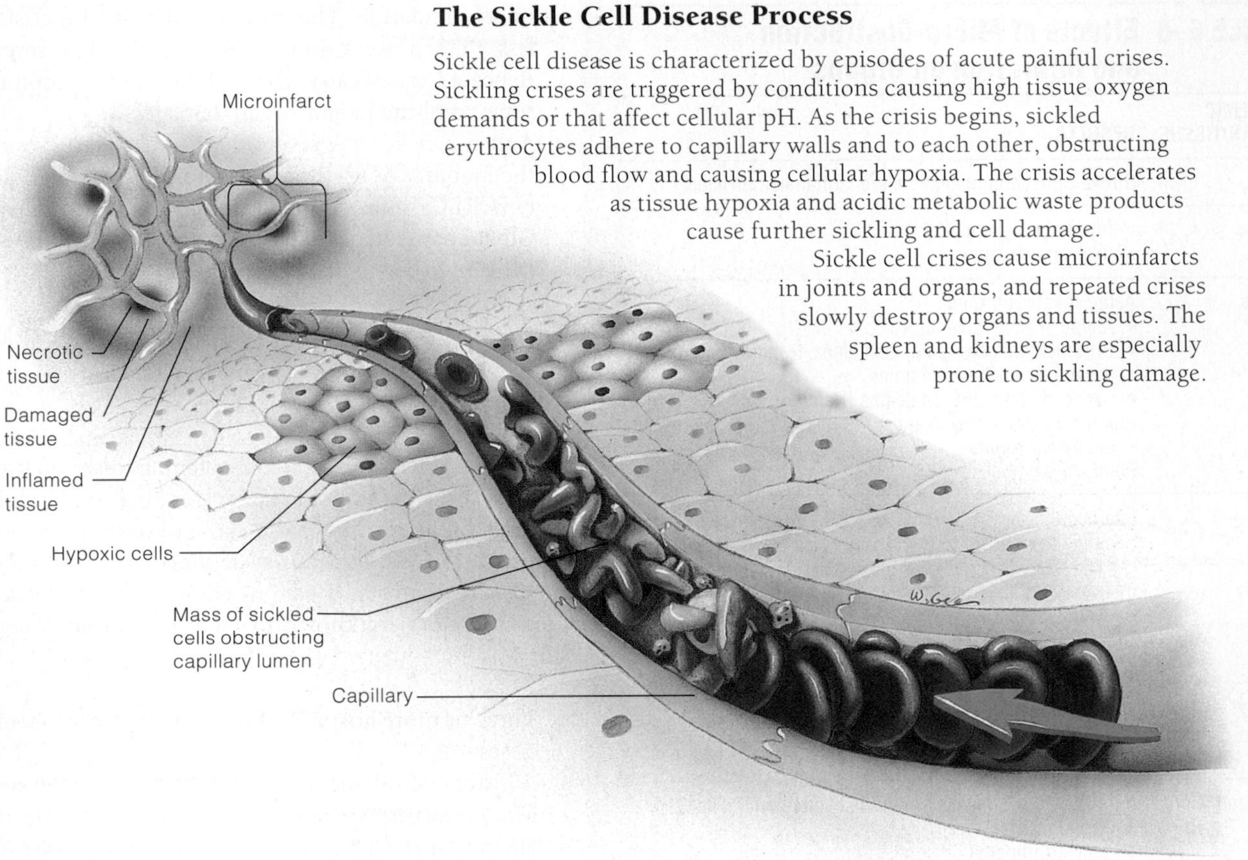

The Sickle Cell Disease Process

Sickle cell disease is characterized by episodes of acute painful crises. Sickling crises are triggered by conditions causing high tissue oxygen demands or that affect cellular pH. As the crisis begins, sickled erythrocytes adhere to capillary walls and to each other, obstructing blood flow and causing cellular hypoxia. The crisis accelerates as tissue hypoxia and acidic metabolic waste products cause further sickling and cell damage.

Sickle cell crises cause microinfarcts in joints and organs, and repeated crises slowly destroy organs and tissues. The spleen and kidneys are especially prone to sickling damage.

Microinfarct
Necrotic tissue
Damaged tissue
Inflamed tissue
Hypoxic cells
Mass of sickled cells obstructing capillary lumen
Capillary

Figure 6–6 ■ Vaso-occlusion caused by sickled cells.
Reprinted from LeMone, P. & Burke, K. *Medical–Surgical Nursing* (4th ed., p. 1108). © 2008, with permission from Pearson Education, Inc., Upper Saddle River, New Jersey.

- Hemoglobin electrophoresis – Ordered when the sickle cell screening test is positive. It is a blood test that differentiates between the various subtypes of hemoglobin. Confirmation of a diagnosis of sickle cell trait or anemia focuses on the percentages of Hb S, Hb A, and possibly Hb F (Kee, 2005). When sickle cell anemia is present, the Hb S ranges between 75 to 95 percent of the total hemoglobin.

Treatment

General supportive goals for managing sickle cell anemia include providing disease-related education to the patient and family; avoiding sickle cell crises; preventing anemia complications; providing psychological support; and encouraging genetic counseling. If the spleen has been removed, prophylactic antibiotics may be ordered prior to any invasive procedures (e.g., dental procedures, etc.). Vaccinations against *H. influenza* and pneumococcal pneumonia may be recommended. Educating the patient and family on preventing sickling crises is a major emphasis, since the tissue damaging effects of the crises are cumulative and result end-organ damage or destruction. The box *NURSING CARE: The patient with sickle cell (sickling) crisis* for a summary of the nursing management of a patient who develops sickle cell crisis.

A major breakthrough in pharmacologic therapy for treatment of sickle cell anemia is the antisickling agent hydroxyurea (see *Related Pharmacotherapy: Antisickling Agent*). Allogenic hematologic stem-cell transplantation (HSCT) may be considered as a possible curative treatment for sickle cell anemia in children; however, the death rate is around 10 percent and there is increased risk of eventual malignancy secondary to long-term immunosuppression chemotherapy (Ferri, 2008).

NURSING CARE: The Patient with Sickle Cell (sickling) Crisis

Expected Patient Outcomes and Related Interventions

Outcome 1: Optimize hydration

Assess and compare to established norms, patient baselines, and trends

Intake and output balance

Monitor for S & S of fluid volume excess

Administer related drug therapy and monitor for therapeutic and nontherapeutic effects

Intravenous hydration – dextrose 5% / 0.5% normal saline – initial rate 150–200 mL/hr

Encourage good oral hydration

Drink at least 8 glasses of water/day

Related nursing diagnoses

Alteration in fluid volume: deficit

Risk for alteration in fluid volume: excess

Outcome 2: Optimize oxygenation

Assess and compare to established norms, patient baselines, and trends

PaO_2, SaO_2, SpO_2

Administer oxygen at 2–4L/min per nasal cannula

Related nursing diagnoses

Altered tissue perfusion

Outcome 3: Control pain (in painful crises)

Assess and compare to established norms, patient baselines, and trends

Location and level of pain

Administer related drug therapy and monitor for therapeutic and nontherapeutic effects

Example emergency department painful crisis analgesic protocol:

- Morphine sulfate (IV) –
  - Bolus (0.15 mg/kg per dose) with 10 mg per dose limit
  - 1–2 hours prior to stopping morphine infusion: 60-mg dose of oral morphine sulfate or equivalent
- At 6 hours, patient decides - inpatient vs. outpatient therapy
  - Outpatient therapy: 4 to 6 days of oral analgesic (Hamilton & Janz, 2006).

Bone pain – ketorolac 30 – 60 mg initially, 15–30 mg q 6–8 hours (Benz, 2005)

Other analgesics:

- NSAIDs, acetaminophen, aspirin

Investigate and reverse underlying cause of crisis

Related nursing diagnoses

Altered comfort: pain

Outcome 4: Rapid diagnosis and treatment of infections

Assess and compare to established norms, patient baselines, and trends

Monitor for infection and fever

Administer related drug therapy and monitor for therapeutic and nontherapeutic effects

Antibiotic therapy: e.g., cephalosporin and erythromycin

Treat suspected infections (high risk for salmonella, osteomyelitis, and pneumococcal infections)

Related nursing diagnoses:

Potential for infection

Altered body temperature: Hyperthermia

Outcome 5: Reverse sickling crisis

Assess and compare to established norms, patient baselines, and trends

Monitor reticulocyte count and serial hemoglobins closely

Administer blood and monitor for therapeutic and nontherapeutic effects

Transfusions to increase hematocrit to greater than 30 percent

Emergency exchange transfusions if SaO_2 is less than 90 percent

Longer term transfusion program (3 to 4 weeks)

- Goal: Reduce Hb S to less than 25 percent (Hamilton & Janz, 2006)

Related nursing diagnosis

Altered tissue perfusion

Outcome 6: Avoid repeated sickling crises

Assess knowledge level of patient and family

Teach importance of avoiding sickling conditions, including:

Infections

Dehydration

Hypoxia

Acidosis

Administer related drug therapy and monitor for therapeutic and nontherapeutic effects

Antisickling agent: hydroxyurea (goal: Reduce sickling episodes)

Related nursing diagnosis:

Knowledge deficit

Data from Hamilton & Janz (2006) and Benz (2005).

RELATED PHARMACOTHERAPY: Antisickling Agent

Antisickling/Antimetabolite
Hydroxyurea (Hydrea, Droxia)

Action and Uses
Hydroxyurea inhibits DNA synthesis through RNA reductase inhibition but it does not interfere with RNA synthesis. Its primary use is for cancer therapy and it is also useful in treatment of polycythemia vera. In relatively low doses it reduces the number of vaso-occlusive crises, by increasing the level of fetal hemoglobin (Hb F), reducing the reticulocyte count; decreasing vascular adhesion, and improving hydration of RBCs (Benz, 2005). It is considered to be a major advancement in the treatment of sickle cell anemia.

Major Adverse Effects
Generally well tolerated
Most common: Neutropenia – mild and reversible
Potentially life-threatening: Suppression of bone marrow

Nursing Implications
Monitor CBC and platelet count closely
Monitor kidney and liver function periodically
Teach patient/family:
- Cannot take during pregnancy due to teratogenic nature of drug
- Signs and symptoms of bone marrow suppression (neutropenia and thrombocytopenia)
- Signs and symptoms of infection

SECTION TWO REVIEW

1. In a healthy baby, hemoglobin F (Hb F) is replaced by which type of hemoglobin at about 6 months of age?
   A. hemoglobin A (Hb A)
   B. hemoglobin B (Hb B)
   C. hemoglobin C (Hb C)
   D. hemoglobin S (Hb S)
2. Sickle cell anemia has which characteristic?
   A. hemoglobin is a mixture of Hb S and Hb A
   B. carrier state
   C. rarely develop clinical manifestations
   D. homozygous inheritance pattern
3. When sickle hemoglobin experiences a deoxygenated state, it results in
   A. release of iron from hemoglobin
   B. stiff fibrous polymers
   C. inability of oxygen to attach to iron
   D. destruction of normal RBCs by the spleen
4. The term *painful crises* in patients with sickle cell anemia refers to
   A. loss of a digit from tissue necrosis
   B. sequestration of blood in the liver and spleen
   C. ischemic pain from microvascular occlusion
   D. failure of the bone marrow to meet the high demands for new RBCs
5. Which of the following tests is used for initial screening for sickle cell disease?
   A. red cell mass
   B. sickle cell test
   C. hemoglobin electrophoresis
   D. complete blood cell count
6. Appropriate nursing care of the patient in sickle cell crisis includes
   A. administer aspirin 300 mg P.O.
   B. restrict fluids to one liter or less per 24 hours
   C. transfuse blood to achieve hematocrit greater than 40 percent
   D. administer oxygen at 2-4 L/minute by nasal cannula
7. The antimetabolite, hydroxyurea (Hydrea) is useful in treating sickle cell disease for which reason?
   A. It reduces Hb S.
   B. It increases Hb F.
   C. It increases the reticulocyte count.
   D. It increases vascular adhesion.

Answers: 1. A, 2. D, 3. B, 4. C, 5. B, 6. D, 7. B

SECTION THREE: Polycythemia: A Disorder of Excessive RBCs

At the completion of this section, the learner will be able to discuss polycythemia, including types, etiology, pathophysiology, clinical manifestations, complications, diagnosis, and management.

Polycythemia refers to the production and presence of an abnormally high number of red blood cells (erythrocytosis). Its distinct hematologic features include an elevated red cell mass and abnormally elevated hematocrit (men, Hct greater than 51 percent; women, Hct greater than 48 percent) (Prchal, 2005). There are two major forms of polycythemia: primary and secondary. This section provides a brief overview of primary polycythemia and focuses on secondary polycythemia, a more common disorder.

Primary Polycythemia (Polycythemia Vera)

Primary polycythemia, called *polycythemia vera (PV),* is a rare clonal myeloproliferative disease involving the pluripotential hematopoietic stem cells (PHSC). It involves excessive production of all three cell types but the degree of RBC proliferation is particularly striking. Polycythemia vera is a chronic disease that exists on a continuum from mild to severe but tends to worsen over many years. It is a disorder of older age and affects more men than women. The cause is unknown, but certain risk factors have been identified, such as chemical exposure and unclear genetic influences. The disease is characterized by

- Significant increase in the RBC mass
- Elevated hematocrit
- Hypervolemia
- Increased viscosity of the blood
- Splenomegaly from pooling of RBCs

The major clinical manifestations primarily revolve around the extreme RBC proliferation. The life span of patients with polycythemia vera is variable, and is largely dependent on prevention of thrombotic complications which, in turn, is greatly dependent on controlling the red blood cell mass. The two major causes of polycythemia vera-related death are **thrombosis** and acute leukemia (especially acute myelocytic leukemia), which develops in about 19 percent of patients (Prchal & Beutler, 2006).

Secondary Polycythemia

Secondary polycythemia, or *erythrocytosis,* is not a disease; rather, it is a symptom of some underlying pathology or environmental factor. In the high-acuity patient, secondary "appropriate" polycythemia frequently occurs as an appropriate compensatory response to chronic tissue hypoxia. Compensatory secondary polycythemia can result from

- Environmental factors (e.g., living at a high altitude)
- Chronic cardiac or pulmonary diseases (e.g., congenital heart disease or COPD)
- Smoking

In the presence of chronic tissue hypoxia, the kidneys produce more erythropoietin (EPO), which then stimulates the bone marrow to produce more RBCs (erythrocytosis). The elevated RBC count results in increased oxygen-carrying capacity of the blood and, ultimately, increased oxygen to the tissues. Some diseases can cause an "inappropriate" secondary polycythemia, whereby EPO is secreted without the proper tissue hypoxia stimuli. Such is the case with some renal tumors.

Clinical Manifestations

The clinical manifestations of secondary polycythemia are often milder than those of polycythemia vera; and frequently the patient's symptoms reflect the underlying disease rather than the polycythemia. When symptoms are present, they reflect the elevated red cell mass, hyperviscosity, and thrombosis (see Table 6–8). Smoking-related polycythemia is generally asymptomatic; however, there is increased risk for thrombotic episodes that may be more related to smoking than the polycythemia. Not all secondary polycythemias are mild. For example, some renal diseases are associated a significant increase in EPO secretion causing severe polycythemia accompanied by increased thrombotic episodes, hypertension, and heart failure (Prchal & Beutler, 2006). Table 6–9 lists possible complications of severe polycythemia.

TABLE 6–8 Common Manifestations of Polycythemia

- Headache, vision disturbances, dizziness, weakness
- Hypertension
- Plethora (ruddy [red] colored: face, ears, mucous membranes, hands and feet)
- Night sweats
- Manifestations of chronic tissue hypoxia
- Elevated erythropoietin (EPO) levels

Data partially from Adamson & Longo (2005) and Rote, McCance, & Mansen (2008).

Diagnosis

Obtaining a good history is crucial to diagnosing secondary polycythemia, as the patient's history usually is positive for chronic conditions that result in chronic hypoxia—for example, a history of smoking, chronic heart disease, sleep apnea syndrome, or chronic lung disease (Adamson & Longo, 2005). History of renal disease should also be pursued. Diagnostic laboratory tests will minimally include CBC, red cell mass, and erythropoietin. A CBC usually shows an elevation of RBCs, hemoglobin, and hematocrit without elevations in leukocytes or platelets, which helps differentiate it from primary polycythemia. An arterial blood gas confirms chronic hypoxemia. A carboxyhemoglobin level may be drawn if smoking-related polycythemia is suspected.

Treatment

Treatment of secondary polycythemia focuses on eliminating or reducing the underlying problem. Phlebotomy is recommended only in severe situations. If the polycythemia is due to an EPO-secreting tumor, removal of the tumor should relieve the problem.

TABLE 6–9 Complications of Polycythemia

Thrombotic Episodes Transient ischemia attacks (TIA) and ischemic strokes (major arterial complications) Acute myocardial infarction Deep vein thrombosis (DVT) Pulmonary embolus Hepatic vein thrombosis Ischemia of the digits
Bleeding (gingival bleeding, easy bruising, GI bleeding, hemorrhage)
Angina, heart failure
Pulmonary hypertension

SECTION THREE REVIEW

1. The two major features of polycythemia are
   A. elevated red cell mass and hematocrit
   B. larger than normal erythrocytes
   C. polymerization of red blood cells
   D. premature destruction of red blood cells
2. Polycythemia vera is a myeloproliferative hematopoietic disorder that affects which patient population the most?
   A. younger women
   B. older women
   C. younger men
   D. older men
3. Which statement is correct regarding polycythemia vera?
   A. It is a rapidly progressive neoplastic disease.
   B. It affects all of the blood cells in the myeloid cell line.
   C. It tends to become milder over time.
   D. It only affects the RBCs in the myeloid cell line.
4. The underlying cause of secondary polycythemia is
   A. depletion of erythropoiesis
   B. myeloproliferative disease
   C. chronic tissue hypoxia
   D. chronic obstructive pulmonary disease
5. A major complication of severe secondary polycythemia is
   A. thrombosis and tissue ischemia or infarction
   B. bleeding peptic ulcer
   C. eventual onset of leukemia
   D. chronic obstructive pulmonary disease
6. The major therapy used to control the high RBC counts associated with polycythemia is
   A. immunosuppressant therapy
   B. splenectomy
   C. cancer chemotherapy
   D. periodic phlebotomy

Answers: 1. A, 2. D, 3. B, 4. C, 5. A, 6. D

SECTION FOUR: Thrombocytopenia: A Problem of Hemostasis

At the completion of this section, the learner will be able to describe thrombocytopenia, including types, etiology, pathophysiology, clinical manifestations, complications, and diagnosis and management.

This section focuses on platelets, the cellular component of hemostasis. Discussion is focused on disorders associated with abnormally low levels of platelets—thrombocytopenia.

Thrombocytopenia is clinically defined as a platelet count of less than 150,000 cells/mcL. The major complication of thrombocytopenia is bleeding. The bleeding associated with thrombocytopenia is different from bleeding caused by other coagulopathies. Thrombocytopenia typically manifests itself as petechiae and purpura on the skin and mucous membranes. Epistaxis is a common finding of patients that have severe thrombocytopenia. Two important assessments of epistaxis are the length of time required to stop the epistaxis and the involvement of one or both nostrils. Epistaxis in one nostril is probably caused by a local vascular abnormality rather than thrombocytopenia. Coagulopathies caused by missing or abnormal coagulation factors tend to cause internal bleeding. Thrombocytopenia is usually not a life-threatening condition unless it is severe (less than 10,000 to 20,000 cells/mcL); however, the underlying disorder that is causing it may be serious or life-threatening (Howell & Rothman, 2001). Thrombocytopenia can be intrinsic (e.g., a hereditary disorder) or acquired. This section focuses on acquired types of thrombocytopenia.

Causes of Thrombocytopenia

Four general conditions cause thrombocytopenia, including decreased platelet production, increased destruction, increased utilization, and problems with distribution. In addition, the commonly used anticoagulant heparin can cause a potentially life-threatening condition called immune-mediated heparin-induced thrombocytopenia (HIT type II).

Problems of Decreased Production

Any problem that injures the bone marrow can result in a temporary or permanent reduction in megakaryocytes; for example, chemicals, drugs, and irradiation. A thorough drug history is important because many drugs may affect platelet number and function. Nonprescription drugs, such as aspirin; nonsteroidal anti-inflammatory drugs; and some herbal supplements may affect platelet function and bleeding time. Production can also be decreased by problems with thrombopoiesis, as is seen with megaloblastic anemia.

Problems of Increased Destruction

In adults premature destruction of platelets usually results from several types of immune reactions:

- Antibody–platelet antigen response or complement activation – Seen with certain drugs or toxins, such as quinidine, heroin, morphine; or snake venom
- Antigen–antibody immune complex formation - Seen with certain types of bacterial sepsis

Problems of Increased Utilization

Increased platelet consumption most commonly results from **idiopathic (immunologic) thrombocytopenia purpura (ITP).** ITP is more common in children than in adults. In adults, it usually develops in young women as a chronic disorder of autoimmune origin, with formation of platelet autoantibodies (usually Immunoglobulin G [IgG]), and it sometimes develops in conjunction with the autoimmune disorder systemic lupus erythematosus (SLE). Treatment may be warranted if the thrombocyte

TABLE 6–10 Idiopathic (Immunologic) Thrombocytopenia Purpura (ITP)

Pathophysiology

Immune-mediated (IgG) destruction of platelets; involves formation of platelet autoantibodies that attack and destroy platelets

Characteristics

Normal bone marrow
Abnormally low platelet count
No splenomegaly
No identifiable cause of thrombocytopenia

Clinical Manifestations

Platelet count less than 20,000: petechiae (usual presenting sign)
Platelet count less than 10,000: petechiae, cutaneous bleeding, epistaxis, gingival bleeding, hematuria, menorrhagia
Rare: spontaneous or post-traumatic intracranial hemorrhage or internal bleeding

Treatment

Platelet count less than 20,000–30,000:
Glucocorticoids (prednisone)
Immune anti-D antibody or dexamethasone (intravenous)
Intravenous immune globulin (IVIG) if not responding to steroid therapy; for active bleeding; or preparation for splenectomy
Splenectomy (laparoscopic) if unresponsive to other therapy
Platelets: not usually recommended; considered if needed to reverse hemorrhage
Factor VIIa: may be considered to treat intracranial hemorrhage

Data from Soliman & Broadman (2006).

count drops below 20,000-30,000 (Soliman & Broadman, 2006). The spleen is a major destroyer of the antibody-coated platelets and splenectomy is usually recommended for patients who either do not respond to corticosteroid therapy or who cannot be maintained on low doses. As an alternative to splenectomy, splenic radiation may be performed if the patient is a poor surgical risk. The characteristics, clinical manifestations, and treatment of ITP are summarized in Table 6–10.

Problems of Platelet Distribution

In the presence of splenomegaly, the spleen can hold vast numbers of platelets, which significantly reduces the numbers in the circulating blood. The total number of platelets may increase by two to three times normal to compensate for those pooled in the spleen. Disorders associated with this problem include cirrhosis (posthepatic or alcoholic), leukemias, lymphomas, and others.

Immune-Mediated Heparin-Induced Thrombocytopenia (HIT type II)

Immune-mediated heparin-induced thrombocytopenia (HIT type II) is a potentially life-threatening complication of heparin anticoagulant therapy. It is estimated that about 0.5 to 5 percent of patients treated with heparin therapy develop HIT, with the frequency being greatly dependent on the type of heparin used and type of patient population rather than the dose or route of administration (see Table 6–11 for risk factors) (Levy & Hursting, 2007).

Pathogenesis of HIT

There are two types of HIT. Type I HIT is a benign, transient decrease in the platelet count of patients receiving heparin therapy and is not an immune-mediated problem. Type II HIT, however, is a potentially devastating immune-mediated complication that involves not only decreased platelet counts but also formation of thrombi. HIT can present as thrombocytopenia with or without a thrombotic episode that typically occurs one to two weeks after heparin therapy was initiated. The thrombocytopenia is usually moderate (median platelet count of 50,000 to 80,000) (Levy & Hursting, 2007). When only the thrombocytopenia component is present, it is referred to as "isolated HIT".

The prothrombotic pathogenesis of type II HIT is complex. Heparin has a high affinity for **platelet factor 4 (PF4)**, a platelet protein. Heparin and PF4 bind, forming a "heparin-PF4 complex" that the immune system recognizes as a foreign antigen and stimulates antibody production. The antibody (IgG) then binds with the heparin-PF4 complex creating a new "antibody-heparin-PF4 complex." It is the antibody-heparin-PF4 complex that activates the platelets, causing them to initiate their prothrombotic activities that lead to formation of potentially life-threatening thrombi (Levy & Hursting, 2007). Thrombocytopenia develops as aggregated platelets are removed from the circulation.

The thrombotic threat associated with HIT does not end when heparin therapy is withdrawn. The risk remains days to weeks after the platelet count returns to normal (Levy & Hursting, 2007). Reported thrombotic episodes

TABLE 6–11 Risk Factors for Development of HIT

Type of Heparin Used

Unfractionated heparin

Type of Patient Population

Cardiac transplant
Hemodialysis
Surgeries: Orthopedic, cardiac, neurologic

Data from Levy & Hursting (2007).

resulting from HIT include stroke, acute myocardial infarction, pulmonary embolus, arterial occlusion of a limb, and disseminated intravascular coagulation (DIC) (Levy & Hursting, 2007).

Treatment. Treatment usually consists of discontinuing the heparin and immediately initiating alternative anticoagulation therapy until the platelet count normalizes. Alternative anticoagulant therapy is necessary to reduce the prothrombotic component of the HIT phenomenon. Warfarin is not recommended as an initial alternative anticoagulant, as it may worsen the thrombosis problem. If warfarin is being used at the time of making the HIT diagnosis, vitamin K should be initiated. Cautious initiation of warfarin may be considered once the HIT episode has resolved if long-term anticoagulation is needed.

For alternative anticoagulation therapy during the HIT episode, direct thrombin inhibitor agents such as argatroban (Argatroban) or lepirudin (Refludan) are recommended. Both of these drugs have been shown to improve outcomes when used as treatment for HIT and have been approved as therapy for HIT (Levy & Hursting, 2007). The direct thrombin inhibitor agents do not trigger heparin-PF4 antibody production or interact with existing heparin-PF4 antibodies. Following an episode of HIT, heparin is generally avoided when possible but may be tolerated for short periods, such as during cardiac surgery. Heparin should not be reintroduced until the heparin-PF4 antibodies are no longer detectable in the blood. Argatroban and another direct thrombin inhibitor agent, bivalirudin (Angiomax), have been approved in the United States for prophylactic use during percutaneous coronary intervention (PCI) (Levy & Hursting, 2007).

SECTION FOUR REVIEW

1. Thrombocytopenia is clinically defined as a platelet count of less than _______ cells/mcL.
   - A. 50,000
   - B. 100,000
   - C. 150,000
   - D. 200,000
2. The typical bleeding pattern of thrombocytopenia involves bleeding into the
   - A. joints
   - B. peritoneum
   - C. internal organs
   - D. skin and mucous membranes
3. An example of decreased platelet production caused by a reduction in thrombopoiesis is
   - A. megaloblastic anemia
   - B. hemolytic anemia
   - C. sequestration of platelets in spleen
   - D. idiopathic thrombocytopenia purpura
4. The most common mechanism of platelet destruction by drugs is
   - A. autoimmune reaction
   - B. drug antibody–platelet antigen reaction
   - C. antigen–antibody immune complex reaction
   - D. direct toxic effect
5. Idiopathic thrombocytopenia purpura is believed to be
   - A. of autoimmune origin
   - B. caused by a drug reaction
   - C. closely associated with splenomegaly
   - D. of antibody–antigen immune complex origin
6. The major treatment of idiopathic thrombocytopenia purpura is
   - A. alkylating chemotherapy
   - B. platelet transfusions
   - C. corticosteroid therapy
   - D. bone marrow transplant
7. The paradoxical thromboembolism associated with immune-mediated heparin-induced thrombocytopenia (HIT type II) is caused by
   - A. activated platelet prothrombotic activities
   - B. heparin–platelet complexes
   - C. accumulation of leukocytes
   - D. red blood cell aggregation
8. In the presence of HIT type II, if anticoagulation must be continued, which type of drug therapy is now recommended?
   - A. warfarin
   - B. vitamin K
   - C. low-dose heparin
   - D. direct thrombin inhibitors
9. Certain types of surgeries have been associated with increased risk for development of HIT type II, including
   - A. orthopedic
   - B. intestinal
   - C. hepatic
   - D. splenic

Answers: 1. C, 2. D, 3. A, 4. B, 5. A, 6. C, 7. A, 8. D, 9. A

SECTION FIVE: Disseminated Intravascular Coagulation: A Problem of Hemostasis

At the completion of this section, the learner will be able to explain disseminated intravascular coagulation, including the etiology, pathophysiology, clinical manifestations, and diagnosis and management

Acute disseminated intravascular coagulation (DIC), also called consumptive coagulopathy, is a systemic activation of the coagulation cascade (Levi, 2007). It is a complication of some underlying acute condition rather than a disease in itself. Sepsis (usually gram negative or gram positive) is the most common (about 35 percent) underlying cause of DIC (Levi, 2007). Table 6–12 lists common disorders associated with DIC. The development of severe acute

TABLE 6–12 Major Risk Factors for Development of Acute DIC

Most Common
Sepsis (particularly gram-negative)
Severe trauma or burns
Shock (any type)
Abruptio placenta
Other
ABO incompatibility blood transfusion reaction
Severe liver disease
Disseminated cancer or leukemia

Data from Seligsohn & Hoots (2006).

DIC is a critical setback for the patient because it significantly increases mortality. The widespread deleterious effects of DIC can result in multiple organ dysfunction syndrome (MODS).

The Coagulation Cascade and DIC

The normal coagulation cascade maintains homeostasis by balancing clot stimulating and inhibiting factors and clot formation is activated and controlled locally rather than systemically. In DIC this balance is lost, causing a coagulation paradox of excessive systemic clotting (with depletion of clotting factors) followed by excessive bleeding. An underlying pathology (e.g., sepsis) stimulates cytokines, such as interleukins and tumor necrosis factor, to activate the clotting cascade. Platelet activation, clot formation, and fibrinolysis are three important homeostatic activities of the normal coagulation process; but in the presence of DIC they are an integral part of the pathology of DIC.

Platelet Activation

When a vessel is injured, the coagulation cascade is activated and platelets become sticky, making them capable of attaching to the injured endothelial cells or lining. The adherence of the platelets to the vessel wall stimulates platelet degranulation. The platelet granules contain mediators (e.g., serotonin, histamine, adenosine diphosphate, and thromboxane A2) that are released (Geiter, 2003). As a group, activation of these mediators results in rapid formation of a platelet plug through local vasoconstriction, increased adherence of nearby platelets, and activation of more chemical mediators. The injured vascular endothelium releases prostacyclin (a prostaglandin), which counteracts the effect of platelet mediators. This action limits (and localizes) vasoconstriction, platelet aggregation, and degranulation to the area of injury.

When disseminated intravascular coagulation (DIC) develops, platelet activation inappropriately becomes systemic and massive numbers of circulating platelets are activated, resulting in development of microvascular occlusions that can cause tissue ischemia or necrosis. Eventually, the available platelet supply is exhausted (used up) causing thrombocytopenia and bleeding.

Clot Formation

The coagulation cascade converts prothrombin to thrombin, which then converts fibrinogen to fibrin and stimulates platelet aggregation. Fibrin binds the platelets, white blood cells, and red blood cells when a clot is formed and functions to stabilize the clot (Geiter, 2003). In DIC, the amount of thrombin becomes excessive and increases clot formation in the microcirculation. Widespread thromboses develop in the microvasculature that can compromise organ blood supply and result in organ injury or organ failure (Levi, 2007).

Fibrinolysis

When the coagulation cascade is stimulated, tissue plasminogen activator (tPA) dissolves the clot by activating plasminogen to convert to plasmin (Geiter, 2003). The plasmin digests fibrinogen and fibrin in clots and in the circulation. DIC is a coagulation paradox—the blood is coagulating at the same time that clots are being dissolved, which results in bleeding from the consumption of platelets and coagulation factors and tissue ischemia and possible necrosis from occlusive microthrombi. Figure 6–7 provides an illustration of the sequence of events involved in DIC.

Clinical Findings of DIC

Not all cases of disseminated intravascular coagulation are severe. Some are mild, discovered only on laboratory data. Mild cases are often self-limiting and require no interventions. In severe cases, the clinical manifestations reflect the volume of blood being lost and organ-related manifestations. Bleeding is often the first and most obvious sign of DIC with oozing seen from partially healed puncture wounds, old intravenous insertion sites, or incision sites. Extensive ischemic organ dysfunction results from microthrombi formation, for example, renal ischemia may result from microthrombosis of the afferent glomerular arterioles or from hypotension related to acute tubular necrosis. The lungs may develop a range of problems from mild (transient hypoxemia) to severe (ARDS or hemorrhage). The cerebral vasculature is at risk for ischemic problems or hemorrhage; thus, changes in mental status are monitored closely. Infectious disease and prolonged hypotension contribute to hepatocellular dysfunction which results in jaundice as bilirubin levels increase. Finally, shock is a possible complication resulting from either DIC or from the underlying pathology (Seligsohn & Hoots, 2006). Table 6–13 summarizes some of the more common clinical findings associated with DIC.

Laboratory Studies

Diagnosis of DIC requires close examination of the clinical condition and laboratory results of the patient. The underlying disease may also affect the lab values so the tests should be repeated every 6 to 8 hours. In severe DIC the patients are critically ill. The exact group of laboratory tests needed to diagnose and monitor DIC is not universally agreed upon; however, it usually includes a platelet count, tests of clotting time,

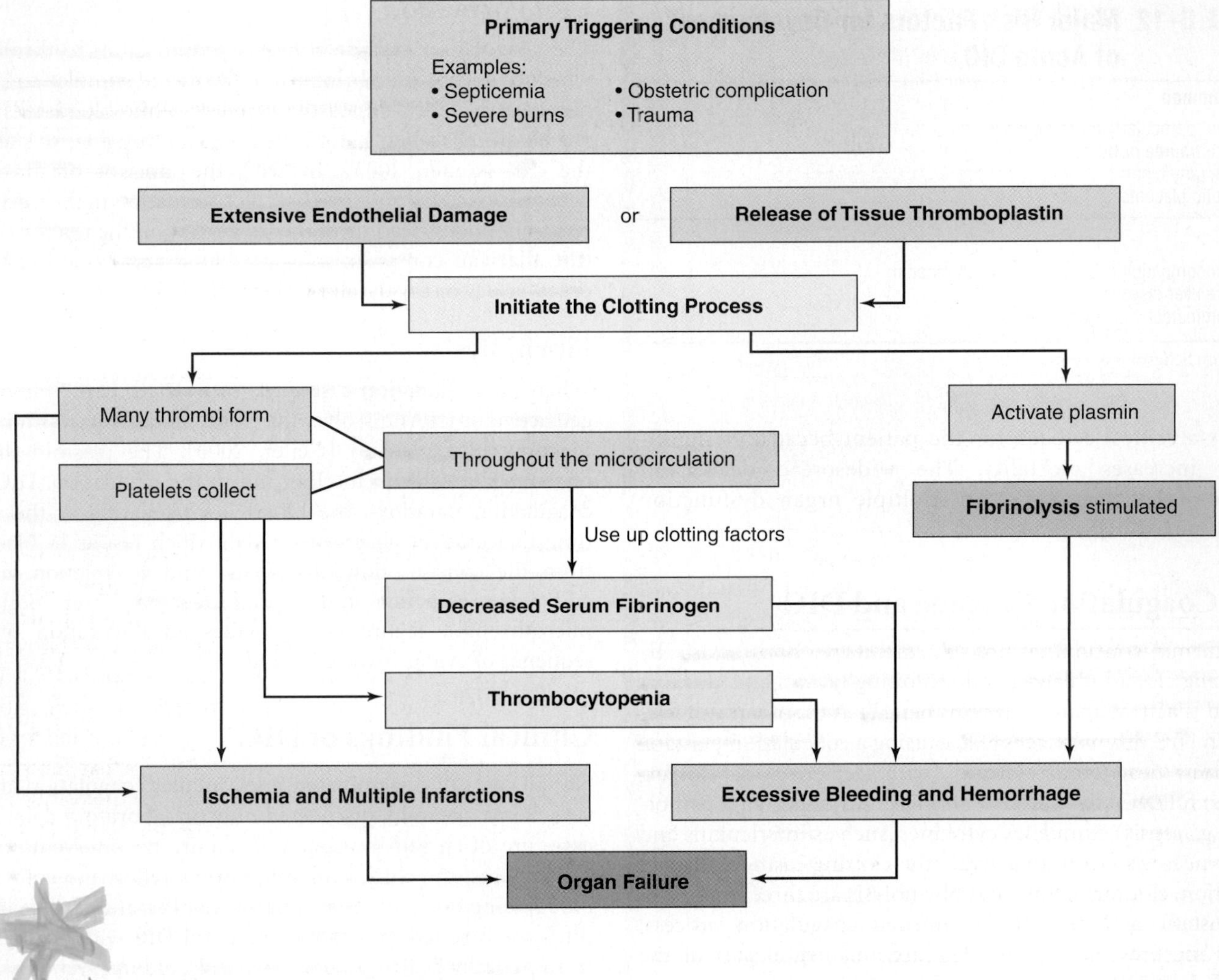

Figure 6–7 ■ Disseminated intravascular coagulation (DIC). Adapted from Gould, B. (2002). Pathophysiology for the health professions, (2nd ed., p. 252). Copyright 2002, with permission from Elsevier.

TABLE 6–13 Clinical Manifestations of DIC

BASIS OF FINDINGS	CLINICAL MANIFESTATIONS
Bleeding-Related	**Superficial bleeding** Petechiae, ecchymoses Bleeding/continuous oozing from arterial lines, catheters, and injured tissues **Internal bleeding** GI tract, lungs, and CNS (potentially life threatening)
Microthrombosis-Related	**Superficial** Cyanosis/ischemia, or gangrene of fingers, nose, and ears **Signs of organ ischemia/dysfunction** Renal: Oliguria/anuria, azotemia, hematuria Pulmonary: Transient hypoxemia, pulmonary hemorrhage, acute respiratory distress syndrome (ARDS) CNS: Delirium, coma, cerebral hemorrhage Hepatic: Jaundice

Data from Seligsohn & Hoots (2006).

thrombin time (TT), tests of fibrinogen, and a blood film to check for fragmented red cells. Table 6–14 summarizes some of the common adult DIC coagulation laboratory screening tests. In most cases, there may be changes of three or more parameters plus a decreased platelet count (Seligsohn & Hoots, 2006).

Treatment

Vigorously treating the underlying disease is imperative to correct DIC and restore the patient's vital functions. Volume replacement and correction of hypotension improve blood flow. Instituting supportive measures for the pulmonary, cardiac, and renal systems improve oxygenation, cardiac output, and fluid and electrolyte balance. Blood components, such as platelets, cryoprecipitate, and fresh-frozen plasma, may be administered if the patient is depleted of hemostatic factors, bleeding, or preparing for surgery.

Thrombocytopenia may be treated with the administration of concentrated platelets if the patient is actively bleeding or has a platelet count of less than 50,000 (Levi, 2007). Hypofibrinogenemia can be treated by administering

TABLE 6–14 Adult DIC Diagnostic Tests

TEST	NORMAL VALUE	SUGGESTIVE OF DIC	OTHER
	1–6 min	Greater than 6 min	Useful in determining abnormal function of platelets
Platelet Count	150,000–400,000	Less than 150,000	Reflects increased destruction of platelets
PT	11–15 sec	Greater than 15 sec	Tests anticoagulant therapy
aPTT	60–70 sec	Greater than 60 sec	Detects clotting factors and platelet disorders
Factor 1: Fibrinogen	200–400 mg/dL	Less than 100 mg/dL	A deficiency of fibrinogen results in bleeding
Fibrin Degradation Product (FDP)	2–10 mcg/dL	Greater than 10 mg/dL	Increased FDP usually indicative of DIC caused by severe injury or trauma
D-dimer	Negative for D-dimer fragments	Greater than 250 mg/dL	Confirms presence of FDP

Adapted from Kee, J. L. (2005). *Laboratory and diagnostic tests with nursing implications,* (7th ed., p. 735). Upper Saddle River, N.J.: Prentice Hall.

cryoprecipitate and fresh-frozen plasma (FFP) may be ordered if the patient is depleted of coagulation factors. Replacement therapy should be evaluated every 8 hours after reviewing the platelet count, PT, aPTT, and fibrinogen level (Seligsohn & Hoots, 2006). In most cases of severe DIC, heparin administration has not shown a reduction in mortality but may aggravate bleeding.

Administration of heparin is beneficial in some categories of DIC, for example, when DIC is secondary to metastatic carcinoma, dead fetus syndrome, and aortic aneurysm. Patients with acute DIC may respond to heparin therapy if they have not responded to blood component therapy or when thrombosis threatens to cause irreversible tissue injury. Antithrombin-III concentrate, an inhibitor of coagulation, has been used to treat patients with DIC. Levi (2007) explains that clinical trials using antithrombin-III for treatment of DIC have shown some beneficial effects (e.g., improved laboratory parameters, decreased duration of DIC, and improved organ function) but not a reduction in mortality. Use of activated protein C in treatment of cases of severe sepsis with severe DIC has demonstrated some benefit and clinical trials continue.

Nursing Implications

Early recognition and aggressive management of the underlying problem may improve outcomes; therefore, patients who are at risk for development of DIC should be monitored closely for bleeding and microthrombosis-related clinical manifestations. Care of the patient with DIC is primarily supportive. The nurse will closely monitor for early signs of complications, with particular focus on kidney, lung, and neurologic function; and for internal bleeding. There are many nursing diagnoses that may apply to the patient with DIC since bleeding and microthrombosis can develop in multiple body systems. A partial listing of priority nursing diagnoses includes:

- Anxiety
- Decreased cardiac output
- Fear
- Fluid volume excess
- Impaired gas exchange
- Impaired skin integrity
- Ineffective tissue perfusion
- Pain

SECTION FIVE REVIEW

1. Which statement is correct regarding disseminated intravascular coagulation (DIC)?
   A. Vessels become occluded because of vasospasm.
   B. Clot formation uses up all available platelets.
   C. DIC is a disease that causes acute myocardial infarction.
   D. DIC is caused only by activation of the intrinsic pathway.
2. In the presence of DIC, what happens to platelets?
   A. They lose their adherence qualities.
   B. They massively collect in the spleen, destroying it.
   C. They do not take part in the coagulation cascade.
   D. They activate throughout the microcirculation, exhausting the supply.
3. DIC is called a coagulation paradox because
   A. platelets are being destroyed while fibrinolysis is occurring
   B. coagulation factors are being produced at the same rate as platelets
   C. blood is coagulating at the same time that clots are being dissolved
   D. thrombin is excessively produced while platelet production is decreased
4. When working with a patient who is at risk for development of DIC, the nurse would be suspicious if which of the following was noted?
   A. harsh, nonproductive cough
   B. oozing from around an old IV insertion site
   C. complaints of severe generalized itching
   D. development of hives and urticaria

(*continued*)

(continued)

5. Laboratory tests that may be ordered when DIC is suspected includes
   - **A.** fibrinogen
   - **B.** lymphocyte count
   - **C.** troponin
   - **D.** myoglobin
6. The most important first step in treating DIC is
   - **A.** initiate heparin therapy
   - **B.** aggressive cryoprecipitate therapy
   - **C.** initiate large doses of fresh-frozen plasma
   - **D.** vigorous treatment of the underlying disease

Answers: 1. B, 2. D, 3. C, 4. B, 5. A, 6. D

SECTION SIX: Blood Component Therapy in the Adult

At the completion of this section, the learner will be able to discuss whole blood and blood component products as replacement therapy in the treatment of hematologic problems

Blood component therapy refers to transfusing specific blood components rather than whole blood. Use of component therapy is built on the belief that it is to the patient's advantage to be given only the specific constituent that is lacking in the blood. Blood component therapy became available as new blood retrieval, separation, and storage techniques were developed; and it is now an integral part of the management of many disorders (Fasano & Luban, 2008). A major advantage of using blood components rather than whole blood is that, when broken down into its component parts, a single unit of whole blood can be used to treat multiple problems in multiple patients. Furthermore, using only specific missing blood components, there is decreased risk for development of many of the adverse effects associated with use of whole blood. Figure 6–8 provides a simple example of how one unit of whole blood can be broken down into its component parts. National guidelines are available on storage and use of blood and blood products and hospitals also have their own institutional level blood and blood products policies, of which the nurse should be knowledgeable prior to administering any of these products.

Whole Blood

Whole blood consists of plasma; all of the cellular components of blood, including white blood cells, red blood cells, and platelets; and plasma proteins and clotting factors. One unit of whole blood is about 500 mL in volume. Whole blood is no longer routinely used for transfusions; in fact, some hospitals no longer keep whole blood in their blood banks. It is recommended that whole blood transfusions be reserved for the purpose of treatment for hypovolemic shock in which there is active bleeding with blood loss of more than 25 percent of the patient's total blood volume (Miller, 2005).

Red Blood Cell Products

Packed red blood cells (PRBCs) are obtained by separating the blood cell components from the plasma by centrifuging the whole blood. One unit of PRBCs provides the equivalent amount of hemoglobin as whole blood but in about one half the volume (250-300 mL) (Miller, 2005). Packed red cells are

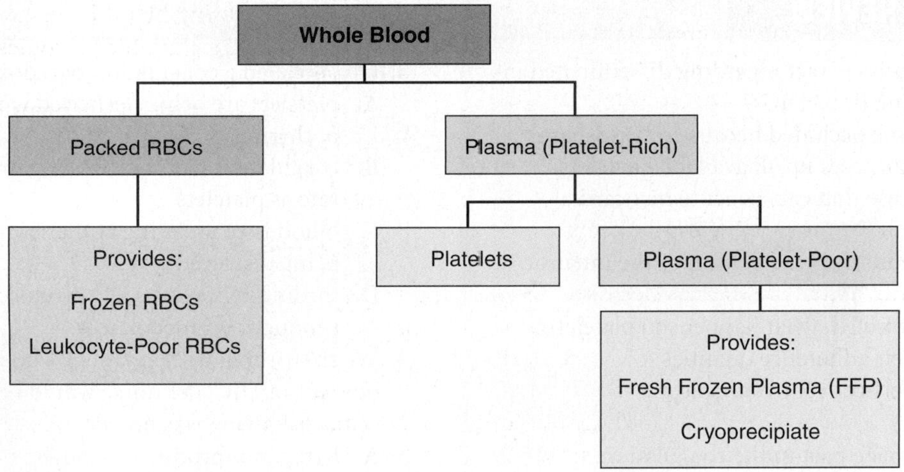

Figure 6–8 ■ Simple example of breakdown of whole blood into component parts. Various techniques such as centrifuging, freezing, and thawing are required to obtain the various blood components.

commonly used for treating significant bleeding associated with trauma and surgery. Freezing red blood cells significantly increases their shelf life, which is an advantage for blood bank stores. Using a filtration process, leukocyte-poor RBCs are available for patients who have developed sensitivity reactions to leukocytes. Red blood cells can also be washed to remove the plasma, if a patient has become hypersensitive to plasma.

Platelet Concentrates

Platelets are obtained through one of two methods, either centrifuging whole blood (random donor platelet concentrates) or through the apheresis process (apheresis platelet concentrates). When using the centrifuging method, up to 8 units of platelets, each from different units of whole blood (and different donors), may be joined together to make one unit of concentrated platelets (usually 200-400 mL). The platelet-rich plasma is allowed to settle out from the red blood cells and transferred to another sterile bag. The platelets are then separated from the plasma through centrifuge. Ideally, the same ABO blood type is used for all of the pooled units; however, in an emergent situation, ABO incompatible platelets are sometimes used, at low risk for reaction.

Using apheresis, all of the platelets come from a single donor who may be a member of the recipient's family or a volunteer compatible donor. The number of platelets obtained using apheresis varies based on donor factors and length of time used for apheresis. The U.S. Food and Drug Administration currently requires that a unit of platelets must contain more than 3.0×10^{11} platelets (Vassallo & Murphy, 2006). Platelets are primarily used for patients with severe thrombocytopenia, from any cause, to either treat acute bleeding or to prevent bleeding. Like red blood cells, leukocyte-poor platelets and washed platelets are available for patients who are hypersensitive to leukocytes or plasma, respectively.

Plasma Products

Plasma, blood's fluid component (without RBC, WBC, and platelets), is composed primarily of water (over 90 percent) and plasma proteins. These plasma proteins are important in maintaining oncotic pressure within the intravascular space. Other proteins, the plasma-derived coagulation (clotting) factors, maintain hemostasis.

Fresh Frozen Plasma

Fresh frozen plasma (FFP) is obtained by centrifuging whole blood, ending with one unit of plasma per unit of blood, with a volume of about 250 mL. After plasma has been separated from the rest of the blood, it is frozen; as fresh frozen plasma it can be stored for a year. Fresh frozen plasma is to be completely infused within 24 hours of thawing (O'Shaughnessy, Atterbury et al., 2004). It is primarily used for treatment of clotting factor deficiencies; it cannot, however, be used for platelet replacement. It is not recommended as a volume expander unless there is significant coagulopathy present concurrently.

Cryoprecipitate

Cryoprecipitate ("cryo") is derived from fresh frozen plasma through a slow-thawing process. It contains multiple coagulation factors, including fibrinogen, factor VIII, factor XIII, and von Willebrand factor (vWF). Other constituents include fibronectin, albumin, and two immunoglobulins (IgG and IgM). Each unit of cryoprecipitate is contained in about 15 mL of plasma with a typical adult dose being six bags, which provides about 1500 mg of fibrinogen. Once thawed, cryoprecipitate is to be used within four hours and if transfusion must be delayed, it should be stored at room temperature (O'Shaughnessy, Atterbury et al., 2004). Cryoprecipitate is no longer recommended for treatment of hemophilia A (factor VIII deficiency) or von Willebrand disease, except in situations where the recommended treatment is not available. It is primarily recommended for treatment of hypofibrinogenemia.

Factor Concentrates

Factor concentrates can be used for treatment of hemophilia A (missing factor VIII) and B (missing factor IX). Factor concentrates are obtained from whole blood of many donors and has a high concentration of the specific missing factor, either VIII or IX. Factor concentrate therapy may be scheduled on a regular prophylactic basis (prophylactic therapy), or it may be used during an acute bleeding episode (demand therapy). Nonemergency infusions can be performed at home or in an institutional setting; however, home therapy is generally recommended, as it is cheaper and more convenient. Laboratory developed recombinant clotting factors are also available but are much more expensive than natural sources.

Nursing Implications of Administering Blood

The nurse is usually responsible for administering blood or blood components. Blood can be administered safely and effectively by closely adhering to institution policies (see Table 6–15). Transfusing blood or its components, however, is not without risk when the blood comes from a source other than the patient. High-acuity patients may require massive replacement of one or more components during a crisis, which increases the risk for transfusion-related complications.

The Risks of Blood Transfusion

While allogeneic red blood cell transfusions can be a lifesaving therapy, they are associated with a variety of potentially severe adverse effects and complications (Sheppard & Hillyer, 2008). In general, these effects can be divided into two major categories:

- Transfusion reactions such as allergic, febrile, and acute hemolytic
- Transfusion-related complications such as infectious diseases (e.g., viral hepatitis, HIV, and bacteria); acute lung injury; and circulatory overload.

TABLE 6–15 Nursing Considerations for Transfusing Blood and Blood Components

Preparation

- Verify physician order for blood product type and number of units
- Explain procedure to patient
- Obtain signed informed consent (if required by institution)
- Verify that blood type and cross matching has been performed
- Assure that patient's name band is in place and contains blood type and crossmatch information
- Gather necessary equipment – Y intravenous tubing with filter, 0.9% normal saline (250 or 500 mL) solution bag
- Verify that blood product is ready for use (Administer within 20 minutes of leaving blood bank)
- Check and document patient vital signs

Administration

- With another RN, crosscheck the blood unit information with the information on the crossmatch slip (patient's name and ID number, blood type, Rh factor, donor number on blood unit, and expiration date). Reverify information with patient's armband.
- Apply gloves and prime tubing
- Initiate intravenous access if not already present with 18-gauge catheter
- Run in approximately 50 mL of normal saline to assure line patency
- Close normal saline clamp and open blood tubing clamp to run at keep open rate for first 15 minutes
- Take frequent vital signs (blood pressure, pulse, respirations and temperature) and observe closely for signs of transfusion reaction
  - Common signs include: Hypotension, tachycardia, respiratory distress (e.g., wheezing or tachypnea, cyanosis), fever, hives, or rashes
  - If signs of reaction are present:
    - Stop transfusion immediately
    - Remove bag and tubing
    - Flush IV line with normal saline and maintain line patency
    - Contact the ordering physician and blood bank
    - Send blood and administration tubing to lab with fresh blood and urine sample
- If no signs of reaction after 15 minutes

  Continue administering blood over a 2 to 4 hour period (or as ordered)

Documentation

- Date and time transfusion initiated
- Exact type of blood component and identification number
- Time transfusion was ended
- Patient's response

The rigorous blood-screening processes used in many countries have significantly reduced the risk of transfusion-related infectious diseases; however, when contamination does occur, it can have devastating consequences. Table 6–16 summarizes the mechanisms, clinical manifestations, and related laboratory findings of transfusion reactions and the transfusion-related complications, transfusion-related ALI (or TRALI), circulatory overload, and bacterial contamination.

TABLE 6–16 Allogeneic Red Blood Cell Transfusion Adverse Effects in Adults

TYPE OF ADVERSE EFFECT	POTENTIAL MECHANISMS	CLINICAL MANIFESTATIONS	RELATED LABORATORY FINDINGS
Transfusion Reactions			
▪ Allergic	Not well understood 1. Possible plasma protein sensitivity 2. Possible sensitivity to other agent in donor blood	Mild: (most common) Itching, hives, skin flushing (generalized), urticaria Moderate: Angioedema, cough, wheezing Severe (anaphylaxis): Pulmonary : Bronchospasm, dyspnea, cough CV: Hypotension, shock GI: Nausea and vomiting Other: Angioedema	No abnormal
▪ Febrile Nonhemolytic Transfusion Reaction (FNHTR)	1. Platelet or leukocyte sensitivity (common) 2. Hemolytic reaction 3. Pyrogens (bacterial) (rare) 4. Unknown origin	Fever – rises up to 6 hours after stopping transfusion; may persist to 12 hours Chills or rigors Headache If severe (rare): Hypotension, nausea and vomiting, chest and back pain	Presence of antibodies to WBC antigens or platelet antigens

■ Acute Hemolytic Transfusion Reaction (AHTR)	1. Intravascular breakdown – ABO incompatibility 2. Extravascular breakdown – Macrophage destruction in spleen, bone marrow, or liver	Fever, chills or rigors Pain (infusion site, flank, back, abdomen, or chest pressure) CV: Circulatory collapse, vasoconstriction and organ ischemia, shock Skin: Pruritus, urticaria, diaphoresis Hematologic: Coagulopathy – microvascular occlusions Renal: Hemoglobinuria, anuria GI: Nausea and vomiting	Hemoglobinuria or hemoglobinemia Schistocytes (peripheral smear) Increased serum bilirubin (indirect) Elevated reticulocyte count
Transfusion-Related Complications			
■ Transfusion-Related Lung Injury (TRALI)	1. Leukocyte antigen incompatibility (most common) 2. Donor antigen-recipient antibody reaction Also known to occur with other blood component therapies	Acute onset fever, chills, with progressive respiratory distress Pulmonary: Progressive hypoxemia, bronchospasm, wheezing; chest x-ray: Bilateral patchy, diffuse infiltrates (pulmonary edema) CV: Hyper- or hypotension tachycardia; no cardiac enlargement	Presence of antibodies or antigens to leukocytes
■ Circulatory Overload	Transfusing blood at rate of greater than 1 liter per 10 minutes	Manifestations of heart failure: Pulmonary edema (dyspnea, hypoxemia, cough; chest x-ray-bilateral infiltrates), hypertension, increased JVD	Elevated BNP
■ Bacterial Contamination	Citrate in transfused blood can support growth of certain organisms	Fever, and chills or rigors after 30 minutes of initiation of transfusion CV: Severe septic shock with marked hypotension GI: Abdominal cramping, nausea, vomiting Renal: Renal failure	Blood cultures positive for pathogen (e.g., *Pseudomonas*) Urine: Positive for hemoglobin

Data from Kyles (2009), Sheppard & Hillyer (2008), and Beutler (2006b).

SECTION SIX REVIEW

1. The use of blood component therapy is built on the belief that
- **A.** the body does not develop sensitivities to blood components
- **B.** blood component therapy is less expensive than using whole blood
- **C.** allogeneic whole blood transfusions carry a high risk for bacterial contamination
- **D.** the patient benefits most from only receiving the specific missing blood component

2. The primary recommended use for whole blood is
- **A.** hypotension secondary to massive trauma
- **B.** when massive arterial vasodilatation is present
- **C.** hypovolemic shock resulting from massive blood loss
- **D.** when a patient has developed sensitivity to packed red cells

3. Leukocyte-poor RBCs are sometimes ordered for which reason?
- **A.** The patient does not need any leukocyte replacement.
- **B.** The patient has developed hypersensitivity to leukocytes.
- **C.** When available, this form of pack red blood cells is now preferred.
- **D.** When clotting factors are not required by the patient.

4. When administering platelets, it is not necessary to consider ABO blood type.
- **A.** True
- **B.** False

5. The primary recommended use for platelet therapy is
- **A.** severe thrombocytopenia
- **B.** moderate to severe bleeding
- **C.** acute bleeding in DIC
- **D.** bleeding in severe trauma

6. Once thawed, fresh frozen plasma (FFP) needs to be completely infused within which time frame?
- **A.** 4 hours
- **B.** 10 hours
- **C.** 24 hours
- **D.** 36 hours

7. Cryoprecipitate is an important therapy for treatment of:
- **A.** hemophilia A
- **B.** Von Willebrand disease
- **C.** hypofibrinogenemia
- **D.** DIC

8. Which of the following statements correctly describes factor concentrates?
- **A.** a unit provides only one missing clotting factor
- **B.** a unit provides factors VII and IX, and fibrinogen
- **C.** it is a newer term for cryoprecipitate
- **D.** they are only used in emergency situations

(*continued*)

(continued)

9. The most common cause of febrile nonhemolytic transfusion reaction (FNHTR) is
   A. unknown origin
   B. presence of bacterial pyrogens
   C. macrophage destruction of RBCs
   D. hypersensitivity to platelets or leukocytes
10. Transfusion-related acute lung injury (TRALI), associated with critical illness, usually presents with
   A. rapid onset of bacterial pneumonia
   B. acute onset of fever, chills, & progressive respiratory distress
   C. cardiogenic pulmonary edema and left heart failure
   D. slow, insidious onset of fever, cough and unilateral pulmonary infiltrates

Answers: 1. D, 2. C, 3. B, 4. B, 5. A, 6. C, 7. C, 8. A, 9. D, 10. B

SECTION SEVEN: Nursing Assessment of the Patient with Problems of Erythrocytes or Hemostasis

At the completion of this section, the learner will be able to describe the nursing assessment of the patient with actual or potential problems of erythrocytes or hemostasis.

The Focused Nursing Assessment

Focused Neurologic Assessment

The neurologic status of the patient can change related to tissue hypoxia or bleeding. The nurse's neurologic assessment may include level of consciousness (LOC), pupillary checks, cranial nerve assessment, and monitoring for increased intracranial pressure. The patient's state of consciousness is a sensitive indicator of tissue oxygenation; thus, in the presence of severe anemia (oxygen transport problem), LOC should be closely monitored. Cranial bleeding may manifest itself as headache, weakness, altered LOC, pupillary changes, altered cranial nerve functions, or symptoms of increased intracranial pressure.

Focused Cardiopulmonary Assessment

Hematologic problems can cause significant alterations in the hemodynamic and oxygenation status of the high-acuity patient. In the presence of anemia, infection, or bleeding, the nurse can anticipate development of compensatory vital signs, such as tachycardia, tachypnea, and changes in blood pressure. Blood pressure may rise with oxygenation problems or may fall with hypovolemia from bleeding. The patient may develop dyspnea or orthopnea associated with tissue hypoxia. Sputum should be checked for occult blood in patients with bleeding problems. If the hematologic problem (e.g., DIC or severe thrombocytopenia) causes increased risk for hemorrhage, vital signs and hemodynamic parameters should be monitored closely for hypovolemic shock.

Focused Gastrointestinal Assessment

Hepatomegaly and splenomegaly are associated with several hematologic disorders; thus, the nurse may want to palpate for their presence. Patients with bleeding disorders should have all gastrointestinal secretions closely monitored for occult or gross bleeding. Intestinal bleeding is also associated with cramping, diarrhea, and melena.

Focused Renal Assessment

Patients with bleeding problems should have their urine routinely tested for occult blood. If hemoglobin is free in the urine, hemoglobinuria develops, with its characteristically port wine colored-urine.

Focused Integumentary Assessment

In the patient with anemia, monitoring the skin, nail beds, and mucous membranes for the presence and degree of cyanosis is important. If the patient develops thrombocytopenia, the skin and mucous membranes should be examined for petechiae, purpura, and ecchymoses. Patients experiencing hemolytic anemia should be monitored for jaundice because of excessive bilirubin from RBC destruction. The jaundice may also be accompanied by pruritus.

The Nursing Plan of Care

There are no North American Nursing Diagnosis Association (NANDA)–approved nursing diagnoses that directly address anemia, polycythemia, or thrombocytopenia. A plan of care is developed around the manifestations and complications associated with each disorder. These can be divided into four major underlying problems:

1. Tissue hypoxia
2. Hypertension
3. Stasis of blood flow
4. Bleeding

Tissue Hypoxia. Impaired oxygen transport associated with the anemias causes varying degrees of tissue hypoxia, depending on the severity of the anemia. Many of the clinical manifestations associated with tissue hypoxia are addressed as nursing diagnoses, such as

- Fatigue related to decreased energy production
- Activity intolerance related to oxygen supply-and-demand imbalance
- Altered tissue perfusion related to decreased oxygen-carrying capacity of the blood
- Ineffective breathing pattern related to decreased energy, fatigue

- Risk for injury related to tissue hypoxia
- Pain related to tissue hypoxia

Potential complications associated with tissue hypoxia include organ ischemia and infarction.

Hypertension. Hypertension is a common finding in polycythemia related to increased intravascular volume and increased RBC mass. Two nursing diagnoses that apply to hypertension include:

- Altered tissue perfusion
- Pain manifesting as headache

Potential complications associated with hypertension include stroke, heart failure or myocardial infarction, renal dysfunction, and others.

Stasis of Blood Flow. Stagnant blood flow is particularly associated with polycythemia (extreme erythrocytosis). The major nursing diagnosis that addresses this problem is altered tissue perfusion related to decreased systemic blood flow (venous stasis). Stasis of blood flow places the patient at risk for thrombus and thromboembolism complications.

Bleeding. The bleeding related to decreased platelet count (thrombocytopenia) is primarily caused by aplastic anemia, leukemia, and chemotherapy. Nursing diagnoses that apply to excessive bleeding include fluid volume deficit related to intravascular fluid volume loss and decreased cardiac output related to decreased intravascular volume.

SECTION SEVEN REVIEW

1. Which of the following causes the neurologic manifestations associated with anemia?
   A. leukostasis
   B. bleeding
   C. tissue hypoxia
   D. increased intracranial pressure
2. The compensatory vital sign changes associated with anemia, infection, and bleeding result in
   A. elevated temperature
   B. increased heart rate
   C. decreased respiratory rate
   D. decreased blood pressure
3. A nursing diagnosis that commonly addresses tissue hypoxia associated with hematologic disorders includes
   A. fatigue
   B. pain
   C. risk for infection
   D. decreased cardiac output
4. Altered tissue perfusion related to decreased systemic blood flow is a nursing diagnosis that addresses which of the following underlying problems in polycythemia vera?
   A. tissue hypoxia
   B. infection
   C. bleeding
   D. hypertension
5. The activity intolerance created by some of the hematologic disorders is specifically related to
   A. intravascular fluid volume loss
   B. O_2 supply and demand imbalance
   C. decreased systemic blood flow
   D. inadequate secondary defenses

Answers: 1. C, 2. B, 3. A, 4. D, 5. B

POSTTEST

Robin T, a 24-year-old woman, is brought to a local walk-in clinic by her husband with complaints of severe fatigue, recurrent respiratory infections accompanied by high fevers, and intermittent episodes of epistaxis. Petechiae and purpura are noted on her trunk and arms. Her history is negative for exposure to toxins, and she takes no medications other than occasional nonsteroidal anti-inflammatory drugs (NSAIDs) for headache. Blood work is drawn and shows pancytopenia, with a reticulocyte count of 30,000/mcL, neutrophil count of 1,000/mcL, and platelet count of 60,000/mcL. She is diagnosed as having idiopathic aplastic anemia.

1. Her low reticulocyte count suggests
   A. overproduction of RBCs in bone marrow
   B. small, pale RBCs
   C. bone marrow depression or failure
   D. RBCs are being rapidly hemolyzed
2. Her current hemoglobin is 5 g/dL. Which of the following descriptions is most consistent with this level of anemia?
   A. asymptomatic at rest
   B. dyspnea and palpitations
   C. spontaneous epistaxis
   D. intermittent high fevers
3. Robin's neutrophil count is most likely the cause of
   A. recurrent infections
   B. severe fatigue
   C. intermittent epistaxis
   D. petechiae and purpura

Robin complains of activity intolerance, an inability to concentrate, and orthopnea. Her heart rate is 106/min and respirations are 24 to 26/min.

4. Which of the following underlying problems best explains these manifestations?
   A. slow internal bleeding
   B. chronic infection
   C. tissue hypoxia
   D. increased bone marrow activity
5. An aspiration bone marrow biopsy is taken. In the presence of aplastic anemia, the bone marrow should primarily consist of
   A. immature cells
   B. plasma cells
   C. normal tissue
   D. fatty tissue
6. The definitive treatment for aplastic anemia in younger patients is
   A. transfusions of RBCs and platelets
   B. hematopoietic stem-cell transplant
   C. immunosuppressive therapy
   D. supportive therapy
7. If Robin is not a candidate for hematopoietic stem-cell transplantation, her supportive treatment regimen will include
   A. alpha-interferon
   B. radiation therapy
   C. immunosuppressive therapy
   D. vitamin B_{12} injections

Antwan M., a 16-year-old African-American male, is brought into the emergency department (ED) by his mother, with a chief complaint of severe chest pain. Antwan's medical history is positive for sickle cell anemia (SCA). He has been in the ED several times in the past year with other painful crises. His mother informs you that Antwan tended to be overactive sometimes, and had been playing basketball with his friends prior to the onset of his chest pain.

8. Antwan's diagnosis of sickle cell anemia means that, if you were to measure his of Hb A, it would usually range between
   A. zero and 5 percent
   B. 5 and 25 percent
   C. 25 and 50 percent
   D. 50 and 75 percent
9. What, if any, is the probable relationship between Antwan's playing basketball and the onset of his pain?
   A. A high level of activity could have precipitated a deoxygenation episode.
   B. Air pollution where he was playing may have triggered an allergic response.
   C. He drank two caffeinated drinks while playing; the caffeine could have triggered a crisis onset.
   D. His playing basketball and the onset of his chest pain probably had no relationship.
10. The severe pain associated with Antwan's sickle cell crisis is caused by
    A. elevations in bilirubin when sickled cells are destroyed by the spleen
    B. release of bradykinin from damaged RBCs
    C. microvascular occlusion with resulting tissue ischemia
    D. mechanism is not well understood

It is determined that Antwan is experiencing "Acute chest syndrome."

11. In addition to acute onset of chest pain, other common manifestations of acute chest syndrome include (choose all that apply)
    A. tachypnea
    B. cough
    C. ischemic ECG changes
    D. clear chest X-ray
    E. decreased SaO_2
12. As a patient known for painful crises of SCA, on entering the ED with a complaint of acute pain, Antwan, should immediately receive which intervention?
    A. Administer hydroxyurea.
    B. Have patient drink several glasses of water.
    C. Administer one baby aspirin per protocol.
    D. Apply oxygen therapy at 2–4 liters per minute.

Kathleen W., a 55-year-old female, is a patient in a medical intensive care unit (MICU). Her original diagnosis was cholecystitis; however, she developed complications postoperatively and is now in the MICU on the mechanical ventilator. She has required hemodialysis for about two weeks. Today, Kathleen developed an arterial occlusion in her right leg. It is suspected that she might be experiencing immune-mediated, heparin-induced thrombocytopenia (HIT type II).

13. The pathogenesis of HIT type II is best described as
    A. activation of cytokines (such as interleukins) by heparin resulting in inappropriate activation of the coagulation cascade
    B. formation of platelet-heparin-PF4 complexes that trigger increased levels of fibrinogen in the blood
    C. activation of platelets by heparin-Fc receptor complexes resulting in prothrombotic activity
    D. formation of antibody-heparin-PF4 complexes with subsequent activation of platelets by the antibody portion of the complexes
14. Assuming that Kathleen has HIT type II, which type of heparin did she most likely receive?
    A. fractionated
    B. unfractionated
    C. both fractionated and unfractionated
15. The thrombotic threat will end rapidly after Kathleen has her heparin therapy withdrawn.
    A. True
    B. False

16. Kathleen has her heparin therapy stopped. The substitute anticoagulant therapy is likely to be
    A. Argatroban
    B. warfarin (Coumadin)
    C. acetylsalicylic acid (aspirin)
    D. hydroxyurea (Hydrea)
17. In the presence of idiopathic thrombocytopenia purpura (ITP), laboratory testing would show which of the following?
    A. elevated bilirubin
    B. reduced numbers of RBCs
    C. presence of antiplatelet antibodies
    D. bone marrow depression
18. In patients with idiopathic thrombocytopenia in which the platelet count is around 20,000, the most common presenting sign is
    A. epistaxis
    B. petechiae
    C. hematuria
    D. intracranial bleeding
19. The nurse is anticipating care for a patient who has been newly diagnosed with idiopathic thrombocytopenia (ITP). The patient's platelet count is 19,250. Initial treatment is likely to include:
    A. splenectomy
    B. factor VIIa therapy
    C. platelet transfusion
    D. glucocorticoid therapy
20. Disseminated intravascular coagulation is said to be a coagulation paradox because
    A. coagulation and bleeding are occurring simultaneously
    B. the intrinsic and extrinsic coagulation pathways are both stimulated
    C. coagulation occurs throughout the vascular system
    D. a coagulation problem can result in multiple-organ failure

Posttest answers with rationale are found on MyNursingKit.

REFERENCES

Adams-Graves, P., Johnson, C., & Corley, P. (2008). Development and validation of SIMS: an instrument for measuring quality of life of adults with sickle cell disease. *American Journal of Hematology, 83*(7), 553–562.

Adamson, J. & Longo, D. (2005). Anemia and polycythemia. In D. L. Kasper, E. Braunwald, A. Fauci, S. Hauser, D. Longo, & J. Jameson, *Harrison's principles of internal medicine* (16th ed., pp. 329–336). New York: McGraw-Hill Medical.

Benz, E. (2005). Hemoglobinopathies. In D. L. Kasper, E. Braunwald, A. Fauci, S. Hauser, D. Longo, & J. Jameson, *Harrison's principles of internal medicine.* (16th ed., pp. 593–601). New York: McGraw-Hill Medical.

Beutler, E. (2006a). Disorders of hemoglobin structure: sickle cell anemia and related abnormalities. In M. A. Lichtman, E. Beutler, T. Kipps, U. Seligsohn, K. Kauschansky, & J. Prchal, *Williams hematology* (7th ed., pp. 667–700). New York: McGraw-Hill Medical.

Beutler, E. (2006b). Preservation and clinical use of erythrocytes and whole blood. In M.A. Lichtman, E. Beutler, T. Kipps, U. Seligsohn, K. Kauschansky, & J. Prchal, *Williams hematology* (7th ed. pp. 667–700). New York: McGraw-Hill Medical.

Corwin, H., Gettinger, A., Fabian, T., May, A., Pearl, R., Heard, S., An, R., Bowers, P., Burton, P., Klausner, M., & Corwin, M. (2007). Efficacy and safety of epoetin alpha in critically ill patients. *N Engl J Med, 357*(10), 965–976.

Ferri, F. (2008). Sickle cell disease. In F. Ferri, *Ferri's clinical advisor online 2008.* St. Louis: Elsevier. Retrieved from MD Consult database.

Geiter, H. (2003). Disseminated intravascular coagulopathy. *Dimensions of critical care nursing, 22*(3), 108–114.

Hamilton, G. & Janz, T. (2006). Anemia, polycythemia, and white blood cell disorders. In J. Marx, *Rosen's emergency medicine: concepts and clinical practice* (6th ed.). St. Louis: Mosby.

Harkreader, H., Hogan, M. A., and Thobaben, M. (2007). *Fundamentals of nursing: caring and clinical judgment,* 3rd ed. St. Louis: Elsevier.

Hebert, P., Wells, G., Martin C., et al. (1998). A Canadian survey of transfusion practices in critically ill patients: transfusion requirements in critical care investigators and the Canadian critical care trials group. *Crit Care Med, 26*:482–487.

Howell, C. J., & Rothman, J. (2001). The etiology of thrombocytopenia. *Dimensions of critical care nursing, 20*(4), 10–16.

Kee, J. L. (2005). *Laboratory and diagnostic tests with nursing implications,* 7th ed. Upper Saddle River, N.J.: Prentice Hall.

Kline, N. (2008). Alterations in hematologic function in children. In S. Huether and K. McCance, *Understanding pathophysiology* (3rd ed., pp. 550–566). St. Louis: Mosby

LeMone, P. and Burke, K. (2008). Nursing care of clients with hematologic disorders. In P. LeMone, and K. Burke, *Medical-surgical nursing: critical thinking in client care* (4th ed., pp. 1101–1149). Upper Saddle River, N. J.: Pearson/Prentice Hall.

Levi, M. (2007). Disseminated intravascular coagulation. *Crit Care Med, 35*(9), 2191–2195.

Levy, J. & Hursting, M. (2007). Heparin-induced thrombocytopenia, a prothrombotic disease. *Hematol Oncol Clin N Am, 21,* 65–88.

Miller, R. (2005). Blood component therapy. In R. D. Miller, *Miller's anesthesia* (6th ed.). St. Louis: Churchill Livingstone/Elsevier. Retrieved from MD Consult database.

Oliveria, G., Crespo, E., Becker, R., Honeycutt, E., Abrams, C., Anstrom, K, Berger, P., Davidson-Ray, L., Eisenstein, E., Kleiman, N., Moliterno, D., Moll, S., Rice, L., Rodgers, J., Steinhubl, S., Tapson, V., Ohman, E., & Granger, C. (2008). Incidence and prognostic significance of thrombocytopenia in patients treated with prolonged heparin therapy. *Archives of Internal Medicine, 168*(1), 94–102.

O'Shaughnessy, D. F., Atterbury, C., Bolton-Maggs, P., Murphy, M, Thomas, D., Yates, S. Williamson, L. (2004). Guidelines for the use of fresh-frozen plasma, cryoprecipitate and cryosupernatant. *Br J Haematol,* 126(1):11–28. Retrieved from National Guideline Clearinghouse database. http://www.guideline.gov/summary/summary.aspx?ss=15&doc_id=12007&nbr=6191. Accessed 8/5/08.

Perkins, J., Cap, A., Weiss, B., Reid, T., & Bolan, C. (2008). Massive transfusion and nonsurgical hemostatic agents. *Crit Care Med, 36*(7) (Suppl.), S325–S339.

Prchal, J. (2006). Clinical manifestations and classification of erythrocyte disorders. In M. A. Lichtman, E. Beutler, T. Kipps, U. Seligsohn, K. Kauschansky, & J. Prchal, *Williams hematology* (7th ed., pp. 411–418). New York: McGraw-Hill Medical.

Prchal, J. & Beutler, E. (2006). Primary and secondary polycythemias. In M.A. Lichtman, E. Beutler, T. Kipps, U. Seligsohn, K. Kauschansky, & J. Prchal, *Williams hematology* (7th ed., pp. 779–802). New York: McGraw-Hill Medical.

Rote, N. S., McCance, K. L., & Mansen, T. J. (2008). Alterations of hematologic function. In S. E. Huether and K. L. McCance, *Understanding pathophysiology* (4th ed, pp. 508–549). St. Louis: Mosby/Elsevier.

Segel G. B., and Lichtman M. A., (2006). Aplastic anemia. In M. A. Lichtman, E. Beutler, T. Kipps, U. Seligsohn, K. Kauschansky, & J. Prchal, *Williams hematology* (7th ed., pp. 419–436). New York: McGraw-Hill Medical.

Seligsohn, U. & Hoots, W. (2006). Disseminated intravascular coagulation. In M. A. Lichtman, E. Beutler, T. Kipps, U. Seligsohn, K. Kauschansky, & J. Prchal, *Williams hematology* (7th ed., pp. 1959–1979). New York: McGraw-Hill Medical.

Shorr, A., and Jackson, W. (2005). Transfusion practice in the ICU: when will we apply the evidence? *Chest, 127*(3), 702–704.

Spivak, J. (2005). Polycythemia vera and other myeloproliferative diseases. In D. L. Kasper, E. Braunwald, A. Fauci, S. Hauser, D. Longo, & J. Jameson, *Harrison's principles of internal medicine* (16th ed., pp. 626–631). New York: McGraw-Hill Medical.

Tinmouth, A., McIntyre, L., & Fowler, R. (2008). Blood conservation strategies to reduce the need for red blood cell transfusion in critically ill patients. *CMAJ, 178*(1):49–57.

Vassallo, R. & Murphy, S. (2006). Preservation and clinical use of platelets. In M. A. Lichtman, E. Beutler, T. Kipps, U. Seligsohn, K. Kauschansky, & J. Prchal, *Williams hematology* (7th ed., pp. 2175–2189). New York: McGraw-Hill Medical.

Wu, W., Schifftner, T., Henderson, W., Eaton, C., Poses, R., Uttley, G., Sharma, S., Vezeridis, M., Khuri, S., Friedmann, P. (2007). Preoperative hematocrit levels and postoperative outcomes in older patients undergoing noncardiac surgery. *JAMA, 297*(22), 2481–2488.

MODULE

7 Alterations in White Blood Cell Function

Susan Bohnenkamp, Virginia LeBaron, Kathleen Dorman Wagner

OBJECTIVES Following completion of this module, the learner will be able to:

1. Discuss the etiology, pathophysiology, clinical manifestations, and management of neutropenia.
2. Explain the theoretical concepts of the hypersensitivity and autoimmune disorders.
3. Discuss the etiology, pathophysiology, clinical manifestations, and management of leukemia.
4. Discuss human immunodeficiency virus (HIV) and acquired immunodeficiency syndrome (AIDS).
5. Describe the effects of aging, malnutrition, stress, and trauma related to the functions of the adult immune system.
6. Discuss nursing considerations pertinent to the assessment and care of the immunocompromised patient.

This self-study module presents disorders of white blood cell function that nurses caring for high-acuity patients are likely to find. Many of these disorders, such as leukemia, HIV/AIDS, and hypersensitivity responses are usually managed outside of a high-acuity setting—often on an outpatient basis. However, when complications arise, these disorders can precipitate physiologic crises, requiring intensive treatment in a high-acuity environment. Before beginning this module, it is recommended that the learner review several sections in Module Five, Determinants and Assessment of Hematologic Function: white blood cells and the immune system in sections Three, Four, and Five and assessment of leukocytes in Section Seven.

This module is composed of six sections. Section One discusses neutropenia and its management. Section Two presents disorders of hyperfunction of the immune system, including hypersensitivity responses and autoimmune disorders. Section Three provides an overview of leukemia and its management. Section Four describes HIV and AIDS including management. Section Five describes the effects of aging, malnutrition, stress, and trauma on multiple functions of the immune system. Finally, Section Six provides a discussion of the assessment and care of patients experiencing immunodeficiency. Each section includes a set of review questions to help the learner evaluate her or his understanding of the section's content before moving on to the next section. All Section Reviews include answers. It is suggested that the learner review those concepts answered incorrectly in the review questions before proceeding to the next section.

PRETEST

1. When severe neutropenia is present, the primary symptom of infection may be
   A. pus formation
   B. fever
   C. local edema
   D. local erythema
2. Decreased levels of neutrophils are associated with
   A. stress
   B. tissue necrosis
   C. infectious conditions
   D. bone marrow depression
3. About 70 percent of acute lymphocytic leukemia (ALL) cases involve proliferation of immature
   A. B cells
   B. T cells
   C. plasma cells
   D. megakaryocytes
4. The major characteristic of chronic lymphocytic leukemia (CLL) is the presence of ______ mature lymphocytes.
   A. larger than normal
   B. fewer than normal
   C. irregularly shaped
   D. abnormally small
5. The MOST common cause of death in adults with acute leukemia is
   A. hemorrhage
   B. infection
   C. tissue hypoxia
   D. brain infiltration

6. A "complete remission" is obtained when there are no leukemic cells in the
   A. lymph nodes and bone marrow
   B. lymph nodes and peripheral blood
   C. bone marrow and brain
   D. bone marrow and peripheral blood
7. The initial treatment of the acute leukemias is
   A. surgery
   B. chemotherapy
   C. radiation therapy
   D. bone marrow transplant
8. Treatment of CLL is usually initiated
   A. when the WBC count is greater than 100,000
   B. when the hemoglobin is less than 6
   C. at stage III or IV of disease
   D. at the time of diagnosis
9. Which statement BEST characterizes HIV disease?
   A. symptoms result from opportunistic pathology
   B. clinical manifestations are of a characteristic and predictable sequence
   C. the HIV virus invades cells primarily through the bloodstream
   D. individuals who test positive for the HIV virus are carriers and considered contagious
10. Which fluid is known to be a mode of transmission for the acquired immune deficiency syndrome (AIDS) virus?
   A. tears
   B. perspiration
   C. plasma
   D. saliva
11. The results of a true type I hypersensitivity response are caused by
   A. a histamine precursor causing anaphylaxis
   B. antigen–IgE–mast cell interaction
   C. antigen–antibody complexes deposited in vessel walls
   D. massive numbers of destroyed red blood cells (RBCs)
12. What characterizes the concept of autoimmune disease?
   A. recognition of self as foreign
   B. exacerbation and death
   C. accelerated production of killer T cells
   D. immunosuppression and altered cortisol levels
13. What effect does the normal aging process have on the immune system?
   A. B cell function in general is particularly depressed
   B. the immune system becomes hypervigilant to invading organisms with increasing age
   C. autoantibodies begin to diminish with increasing age
   D. T cells begin to deteriorate in functioning
14. In the acutely ill adult, which nutritional loss to the body is a critical factor in immune system integrity?
   A. protein
   B. vitamin C
   C. complex carbohydrate chains
   D. iron
15. The most important clinical manifestation associated with infection in an immunocompromised patient is
   A. elevated WBC
   B. local inflammation
   C. fever
   D. pain

Pretest answers are found on MyNursingKit.

SECTION ONE: Neutropenia

At the completion of this section, the learner will be able to discuss the etiology, pathophysiology, clinical manifestations, and management of neutropenia.

Neutrophils are first-line responders to **pathogens** and account for about 60 percent of circulating white blood cells. Bone marrow takes 10–14 days to mature a neutrophil; once released into the circulation the neutrophil lives only four to eight hours. **Neutropenia** is a reduction of these first responders, placing the patient at risk for infections and sepsis. Immediate treatment is necessary if the patient becomes febrile (Niremberg et al., 2006).

Neutropenia (granulocytopenia) refers to an abnormally low level of neutrophils. Neutropenia is not a disease; rather, it is an important symptom of some other underlying problem. Neutropenia exists when the neutrophil count drops below 50 percent of the total WBC count. It is commonly defined as a neutrophil count of less than 2,000 cells/mcL. A neutrophil count below 1,000/mcL places the neutropenic person at a high risk for developing an infection, and a count below 500/mcL is considered life-threatening (Schwartzberg, 2006)—the lower the neutrophil count, the higher the risk. The absolute neutrophil count (ANC) equals the number of white blood cells multiplied by the sum of the percentage of segmented (mature) neutrophils plus the percentage of **band** (immature) neutrophils (ANC = WBC × [segs + bands]). An ANC of less than 100 cells/mcL is referred to as **agranulocytosis.** The cause of neutropenia can be intrinsic (primary, usually caused by a genetic mutation), or acquired (secondary, from some underlying disease). The focus of this section is on acquired neutropenia, which is a relatively common problem in high-acuity illnesses. Table 7–1 is the National Cancer Institute's grading system of neutropenia.

Causes of Neutropenia

Neutropenia is usually acquired rather than intrinsic. Acquired neutropenia is associated with either premature destruction or decreased production of neutrophils.

Premature Destruction

Premature death of neutrophils is most commonly associated with a drug-induced hypersensitivity response. Certain drugs

TABLE 7–1 National Cancer Institute Neutropenia Grading Scale

GRADE	ABSOLUTE NEUTROPHIL COUNT (ANC/MM^3)	INFECTION RISK
1	Less than 2,000	Slight
2	Less than 1,500	Minimal
3	Less than 1,000	Moderate
4	Less than 500	Severe

Data from National Cancer Institute. (1999). National Institutes of Health.

(e.g., certain antibiotics) can cause development of drug–antibody immune complexes, which then attach to and destroy neutrophils. Neutropenia can also result from an isolated autoimmune process, as a complication of another autoimmune disorder, such as systemic lupus erythematosus (SLE). Furthermore, the spleen is capable of entrapping neutrophils and destroying them; this sometimes occurs with disorders that cause splenomegaly.

Decreased Production

Decreased production of neutrophils can occur by direct injury to the bone marrow (e.g., aplastic anemia), by overcrowding of normal bone marrow components from infiltration of malignant cells (e.g., leukemia), or bone marrow suppression by cancer chemotherapy or irradiation. It can also result from severe nutritional deficits (e.g., starvation), and vitamin B_{12} or folate deficiency, chemical exposure, or infectious agents such as a viral infection. Drugs that have a high occurrence of causing agranulocytosis (severe neutropenia) include propylthiouracil (PTU, antithyroid class), chloramphenicol (Chloromycetin, antibiotic class), phenothiazine (Thorazine, antipsychotic class), phenylbutazone (Butazolidin, NSAID class), and sulfonamides (antibiotic class) (Distenfeld, 2006).

Clinical Manifestations

Neutropenia causes altered responses to inflammation and infection because neutrophils are the first line of internal defense against infection and play a crucial part in the inflammatory process. The patient who develops neutropenia is at risk for infection. The source of the infection is usually from the person's own normal skin or gastrointestinal flora because the body is host to a variety of pathogens, both externally and internally. Under normal circumstances, these pathogens remain harmless, but in conditions such as neutropenia, they can invade the body and cause serious, sometimes life-threatening infections.

The clinical manifestations associated with infection are altered to the degree that the neutrophil count is compromised. In mild-to-moderate cases of neutropenia, a normal inflammatory response to infection occurs (redness, swelling, heat, pus formation, and fever). These signs and symptoms become significantly blunted or disappear when the ANC drops below 500 cells. Fever is an exception, as it is produced by proinflammatory cytokines that come from most of the leukocytes, rather than relying on sufficient numbers of neutrophils. Thus, with severe neutropenia, fever may be the only remaining sign of inflammation and infection early in an infection. A moderate fever that lasts for more than one hour may become the primary sign—often no higher than 100.4°F (38.0°C) if leukopenia is present. The absence of overt inflammation makes diagnosis of acute infections difficult. For example, a patient could have severe bacterial pneumonia for three to four days before the lungs develop sufficient pus that it is evidenced in the sputum and is visible on a chest X-ray (Antoniadou & Giamarellou, 2007). Febrile neutropenia is a potentially life-threatening event and must be treated rapidly (Schwartzberg, 2006). The clinical presentation of patients with agranulocytosis is fairly predictable and is a medical emergency. Without appropriate therapy, the patient usually develops sepsis that may be life-threatening (Distenfed, 2006). Table 7–2 summarizes the history and clinical presentation typical of the patient with agranulocytosis.

Treatment

Early discovery and aggressive treatment of the underlying cause of the neutropenia is imperative. Investigation of the cause may include antibody or bone marrow testing, or discontinuing a drug. Empiric antibiotic therapy is often initiated, with close attention being placed on monitoring for secondary infections. A G-CSF (granulocyte-colony stimulating factor) drug, either filgrastim (Neupogen) or its long-acting form, pegfilgrastim (Neulasta®) may be administered to try to stimulate the bone marrow to increase production of neutrophils. G-CSF therapy has significantly improved patient recovery from an episode of agranulocytosis (Distenfed, 2006). The box, RELATED PHARMACOTHERAPY: Severe neutropenia/agranulocytosis provides a summary of G-CSF therapy. Nursing management of the immunosuppressed patient is discussed in Section Six of this module.

TABLE 7–2 Clinical Presentation of Agranulocytosis in Adults

TYPE OF DATA	PRESENTATION
History	Rapid onset of malaise, fever, chills Stomatitis, pharyngitis with painful swallowing Patient report of: recent new drug use; exposure to chemicals or physical agents; recent viral or bacterial infection; preexisting autoimmune diseases
Physical	High-grade fever (may be 40° C or higher) Vital signs: Tachycardia and tachypnea; BP may be hypotensive if septic shock is present Oral: Swollen, painful gums; mouth ulcers Integument: Skin infections with swelling (usually without redness or pus formation)
Lab Studies	Absolute neutrophil count (ANC): Less than 100 cells/mcL

Data from Distenfeld (2006).

RELATED PHARMACOTHERAPY: Severe neutropenia/agranulocytosis

Colony-stimulating factors (GSF)
Filgrastim (Neupogen); long-acting form, Pegfilgrastim (Neulasta)

Action and Uses:
A growth factor cytokine (granulocyte colony-stimulating factor [G-CSF]). Primarily stimulates increased proliferation and differentiation of neutrophils in the bone marrow, and enhances phagocytic activities. Useful for reduction of severity and shortening recovery time from severe neutropenic episodes, including agranulocytosis. It is also used for speeding post cancer chemotherapy neutrophil recovery.

Major Adverse Effects
Most common: Bone pain, fever

Nursing Implications
Drug is initiated after a minimum of 24 hours following cytotoxic chemotherapy
Obtain baseline CBC with differential count; follow-up 2 times/week to monitor recovery; monitor platelet count
Assess for presence and level of bone pain
Monitor: Temperature; leukocytosis (an ANC of > 10,000 cells/mcL indicates need for discontinuing drug)
Filgrastim is administered IV or SC daily; Pegfilgrastim is administered once
Drug vial precautions: Store in refrigerator. Enter a single vial only once; each vial is one dose only; discard vial after 6 hours if left at room temperature. Can allow drug to warm to room temperature prior to administration – but no longer than 6 hours [Measures to minimize contamination and bacterial growth.]

SECTION ONE REVIEW

1. A neutrophil count of less than ______ cells/mcL places the patient at highest risk for development of an acute infection.
   - A. 500
   - B. 1,500
   - C. 2,000
   - D. 2,500
2. The most common cause of premature destruction of neutrophils is
   - A. environmental toxins
   - B. autoimmune disorder
   - C. drug–antibody reaction
   - D. bacterial infection
3. Decreased production of neutrophils results from which type of insult?
   - A. splenomegaly
   - B. hypersensitivity response
   - C. circulating immune complexes
   - D. bone marrow depression
4. When severe neutropenia is present, the primary symptom of infection is usually
   - A. pus formation
   - B. fever
   - C. local edema
   - D. local erythema
5. The purpose of using filgrastim (Neupogen) in the treatment of neutropenia is to
   - A. treat the underlying infection
   - B. stop the inflammatory process
   - C. speed up neutrophil count recovery time
   - D. actively heal the bone marrow

Answers: 1. A, 2. C, 3. D, 4. B, 5. C

SECTION TWO: Disorders of Hyperactive Immune Response: Hypersensitivity and Autoimmunity

At the completion of this section, the learner will be able to explain the theoretical concepts of the hypersensitivity and autoimmune disorders.

Hypersensitivity Responses

Although several types of hypersensitivity reactions are recognized as immune responses, only those particularly associated with the acutely ill adult are discussed here. Some immune responses can cause an excessive or inappropriate reaction referred to as **hypersensitivity** (Platts-Mills, 2006). Historically, hypersensitivity disorders have been described as immediate or delayed reactions based on time from exposure to symptom appearance. Since 1962, hypersensitivity disorders have been commonly described as types I, II, III, and IV (Fig. 7–1). Of these four recognized categories, types I, II, and III involve humoral (antigen-antibody) immunity and specific **immunoglobulins.** Type IV, however, is a cell-mediated response. Many hypersensitivity responses manifest themselves with mild to moderately distressful symptoms, such as watery eyes, sneezing, and nasal congestion. Strong hypersensitivity responses, however, are capable of triggering a severe response, for example, anaphylactic shock response, severe transfusion reaction, or allergic asthma response.

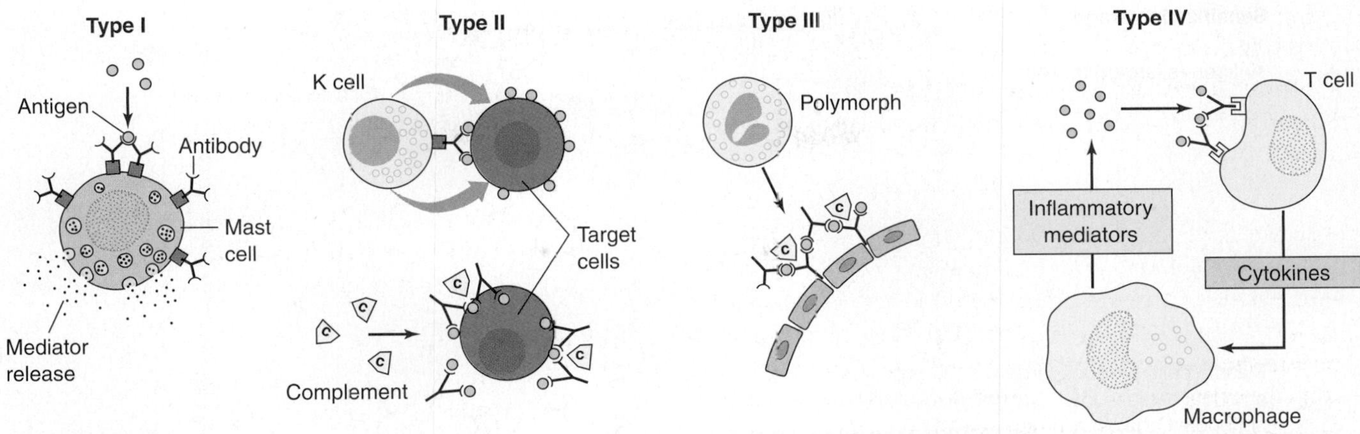

Figure 7–1 ■ Four Types of Hypersensitivity Reaction In type I, mast cells bind IgE via their Fc receptors. On encountering allergen the IgE induces degranulation and release of mediators that produce allergic reactions. In type II, antibody is directed against the antigen on an individual's own cells (target cell) or foreign antigen, such as transfused red blood cells. This may lead to cytotoxic action by natural killer (K or NK) cells, or complement-mediated lysis. In type III, immune complexes are deposited in the tissue. Complement is activated and phagocytes (polymorphs) are attracted to the site of deposition, causing local tissue damage and inflammation. In type IV, antigen-sensitized T cells release lymphokines following a secondary contact with the same antigen. Cytokines induce inflammatory reactions and activate and attract macrophages, which release inflammatory mediators. This figure was published in *Immunology*, 7th ed., p. 424, by D. Male, J. Brostoff, D. Roth & I. Roitt (Eds.), Copyright Elsevier, 2006.

Type I (IgE-Mediated) Hypersensitivity Response

The **type I hypersensitivity response** is also referred to as **allergic response** or anaphylactic response and involves an interaction between the immunoglobulin IgE and mast cells. **Mast cells** are large granule-containing tissue cells that are located in connective tissue throughout the body. The heaviest concentration of mast cells is in the skin and mucous membranes (e.g., gastrointestinal, genitourinary, and respiratory tracts), which places them in close proximity to where antigens are most likely to appear (where the internal body interfaces with the external environment) (Platts-Mills, 2006). Mast cells contain potent mediators, such as histamine, heparin, and leukotriene. When stimulated, these mediators trigger strong vascular, smooth muscle, hematologic, and other activities. Table 7–3 provides a listing of the major mediators and some of their activities.

The type I response requires repeated exposures—a sensitization (priming or *primary response)* phase and subsequent exposure. When a person initially encounters an allergen–antigen (e.g., pollen), IgE attaches itself to mast cells (e.g., pollen would involve mast cells in the respiratory tract). The mast cells are now primed for an allergic response. With subsequent exposure to the same allergen–antigen, the allergic response (antigen–IgE–mast cell) interaction is triggered (called the secondary response) causing rapid degradation of the primed mast cells and release of mediators and chemotactic factors—and the person becomes symptomatic. Figure 7–2 illustrates the type I IgE-mediated hypersensitivity response. The type I response can affect tissues at the local or systemic level.

Local Type I. Allergic asthma and allergic rhinitis (hay fever) are especially noteworthy examples of a type I response. Type I allergies tend to be atopic; that is, a particular type of allergy tends to run in families (a genetic predisposition). While common allergic rhinitis is a fairly benign process (local symptoms of stuffy and runny nose, sneezing, and watering eyes), other local type I disorders, such as allergic asthma, can cause severe, even life-threatening symptoms. In allergic asthma, the chemical mediators cause smooth muscle constriction in the bronchioles and histamine release results in edema of the bronchial tissues. The combination of bronchiolar constriction and bronchial edema, when severe, may require emergency treatment to prevent death by asphyxiation. Antihistamines may be used to block the effect of histamine release, but corticosteroids often are administered to suppress the entire immune response. Another example of local type I response that is of particular interest to health care professionals is latex glove allergy, which can cause mild to severe allergic reactions.

Systemic Type I. **Anaphylaxis** is a severe type I hypersensitivity response caused by the massive systemic release of the same mediators that are triggered in a local type I reaction. Common

TABLE 7–3 Major Mediators of Type I Hypersensitivity Response

MEDIATOR	MAJOR ACTIVITIES
Histamine	Capillary dilation, increased vascular permeability, smooth muscle constriction, bronchoconstriction, secretion of mucus
Leukotrienes[a]	Smooth muscle contraction, increased vascular permeability, leukocyte adherence to endothelium, platelet activation
Platelet-Activating Factor (PAF)	Same as leukotrienes
Prostaglandins	Increased vascular permeability, neutrophil chemotaxis, pain
Chemotactic Factors[b]	Recruit neutrophils and eosinophils

[a] Also called slow-reacting substances of anaphylaxis (SRS-A).
[b] Chemotactic factors include neutrophil chemotactic factor and eosinophil chemotactic factor of anaphylaxis (ECF-A).
Data from Rote (2008).

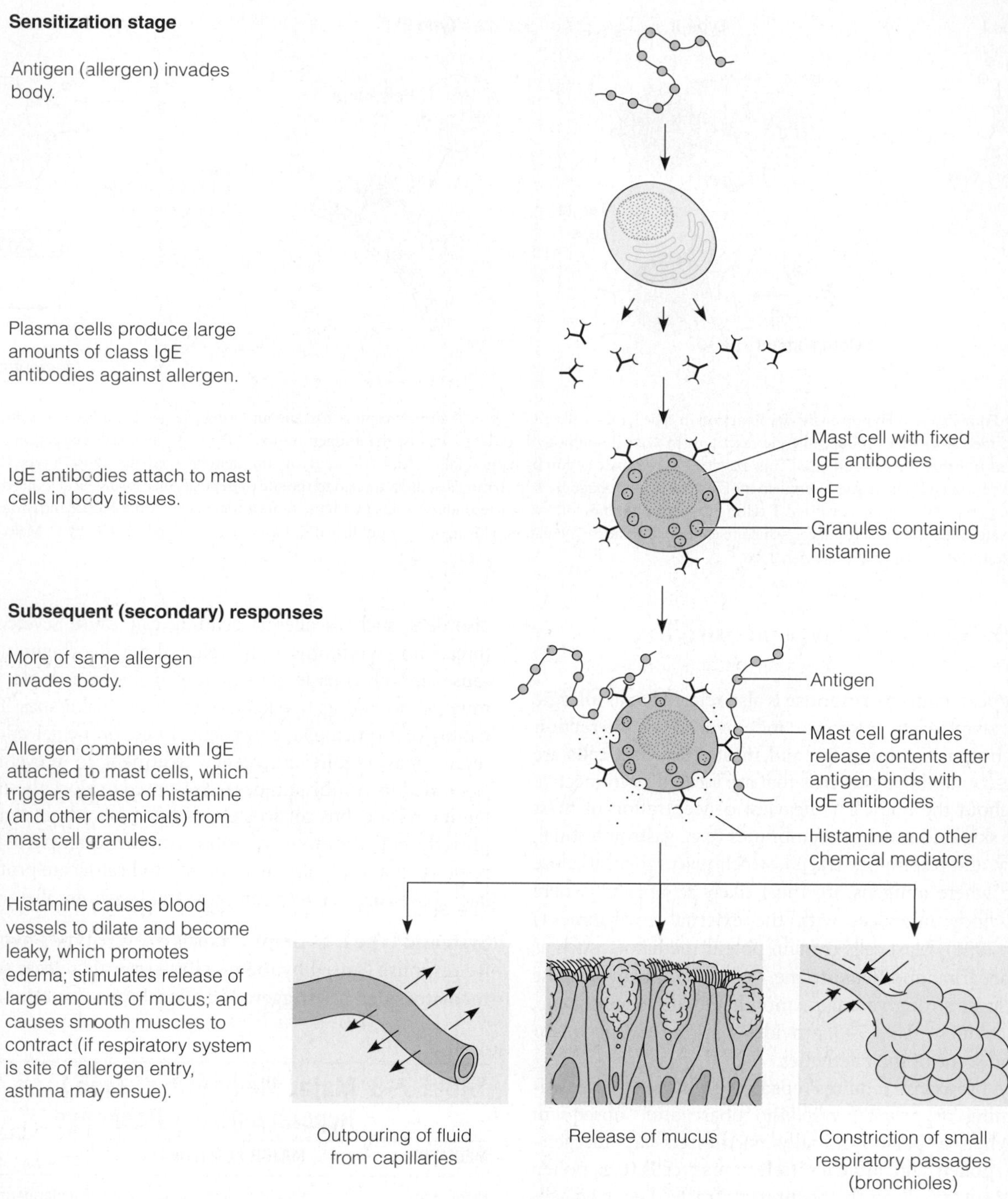

Figure 7–2 ■ Type I IgE-mediated hypersensitivity response. Reprinted from LeMone, P. & Burke, K. *Medical–Surgical Nursing* (4th ed., p. 332). © 2008, with permission from Pearson Education, Inc., Upper Saddle River, New Jersey.

type I causative anaphylaxis-triggering allergens are drugs and insect venom. Less common allergens are food proteins (e.g., peanuts, shellfish). Of significance is that the reaction lacks a genetic predisposition and may be fatal in response to prior sensitization to a minute amount of allergen.

The symptoms of anaphylaxis develop rapidly following exposure—within minutes—and simultaneously in multiple organs in response to an allergen capable of stimulating the immune system. In anaphylaxis, mast cells trigger widespread release of histamine and other mediators, which then cause widespread edema and vascular congestion. Complement is also activated, further stimulating histamine release and triggering a widespread inflammatory response. Anaphylaxis typically involves the cardiovascular, respiratory, cutaneous, and gastrointestinal systems. Urticaria or hives (Fig. 7–3) are the result of histamine release from the IgE–mast cell interaction in which receptors in cutaneous blood vessels cause the characteristic redness and swelling. Urticaria alone is not life-threatening but heralds the presence of an anaphylactic response. Assessment should include examining the patient for the potential risk of upper airway edema with asphyxiation and the risk of irreversible shock. Gastrointestinal involvement is related to smooth muscle contraction and edema of

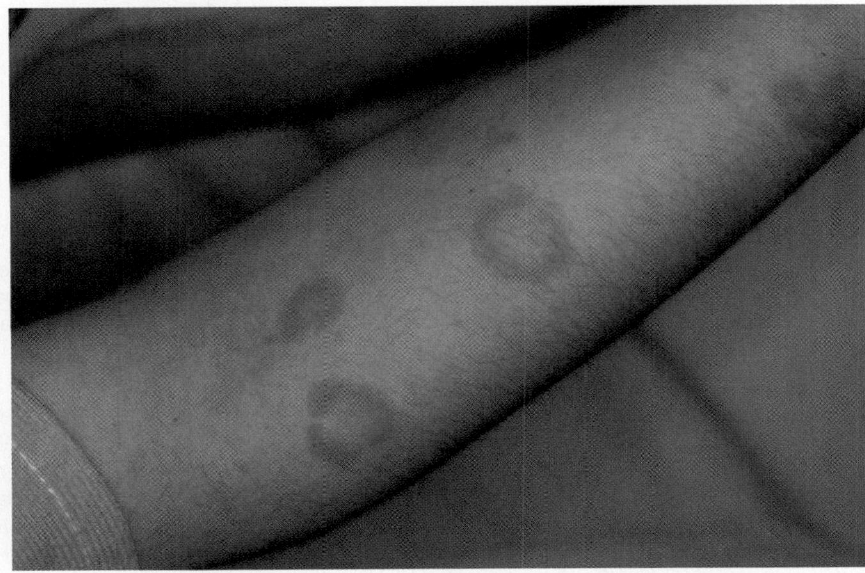

Figure 7–3 ■ Hives. Reprinted from Bledsoe, B. Porter, R., & Cherry, R. (2004). Intermediate emergency care, (3rd ed., p. 964). Charles Stewart MD FACEP, FAAEM. Copyright 2004, with permission from Prentice Hall.

the mucosa resulting in cramplike pain, nausea, and diarrhea. Similar responses can occur within the uterus, causing cramplike pelvic pain and a risk of spontaneous abortion. Figure 7–4 illustrates the effects of anaphylaxis, including clinical manifestations.

Anaphylactic shock is the extreme result of mediator-induced generalized vasodilatation and increased vascular permeability causing rapid loss of plasma into interstitial spaces. This shift of fluid causes hypovolemic shock with profound hypotension, decreased cardiac output, myocardial ischemia, and widespread organ death. Furthermore, edema and bronchoconstriction of the airway can compromise airway patency causing asphyxia. Anaphylactic shock is presented in more detail in Module 18, Alterations in Oxygen Delivery and Consumption: Shock States.

Treatment of systemic anaphylaxis must be instituted immediately and includes epinephrine (intravenous, intramuscular, or subcutaneous depending on the intensity). Laryngeal edema may require tracheostomy when edema precludes endotracheal airway placement. Oxygen and injectable antihistamines should be administered. The patient should be kept warm if shock is suspected. Glucocorticoids may be used for severe or prolonged reactions because they reduce the immune response and stabilize the vascular system. Other symptoms, such as gastrointestinal cramping and urticaria, respond well to antihistamines. After the patient has fully recovered, diagnostic skin testing may be ordered to identify the offending allergen. See the RELATED PHARMACOTHERAPY box for a summary of the drug interventions associated with anaphylaxis.

Type II (Cytotoxic) Hypersensitivity Response

A **type II hypersensitivity response** (Fig. 7–5) is referred to as a cytotoxic (or hemolytic) reaction, meaning that it destroys cells. The immunoglobulins IgM and IgG react directly with cell surface antigens, activating the complement system and producing direct injury to the cell surface. Cellular membranes are disrupted, and target cells such as erythrocytes (red blood cells [RBCs]), thrombocytes (platelets), and leukocytes (white blood cells [WBCs]), are destroyed. Transfusion reaction is a major example of this type of hypersensitivity. Other examples include Rh incompatibility in the neonate, drug reaction-induced hemolytic anemia, and hyperthyroidism caused by Graves' disease.

Hemolytic Transfusion Reaction. Transfusion reactions can be classified as febrile (fever and chills) where recipient antibodies act against the donor white blood cells; as a hypersensitivity reaction whereby recipient antibodies attack donor blood proteins; or as a hemolytic reaction, a type of type II cytotoxic response.

In a hemolytic transfusion reaction, preexisting antibodies in the recipient's serum target and attach to the ABO antigens on erythrocytes (RBC) of the transfusing donor blood, which activates the complement cascade. As the immune system is activated, phagocytes destroy the donor RBCs, causing release of hemoglobin into the circulation. The released hemoglobin follows the general circulation and eventually flows into the renal glomeruli. Hemoglobin fragments can obstruct renal tubular blood flow, increasing the risk of risk of oliguria and renal shutdown.

Symptoms of a hemolytic transfusion reaction are likely to occur within the first 2 to 5 minutes of initiation of the transfusion. Clinical manifestations that suggest this type of reaction include the sensation of heat and redness at the infusion site, nausea, headache, back pain, chills, fever, and a sense of chest heaviness with difficulty breathing. Tachycardia, hypotension, and death can follow if the transfusion is not interrupted and treatment begun to reestablish cardiovascular stability.

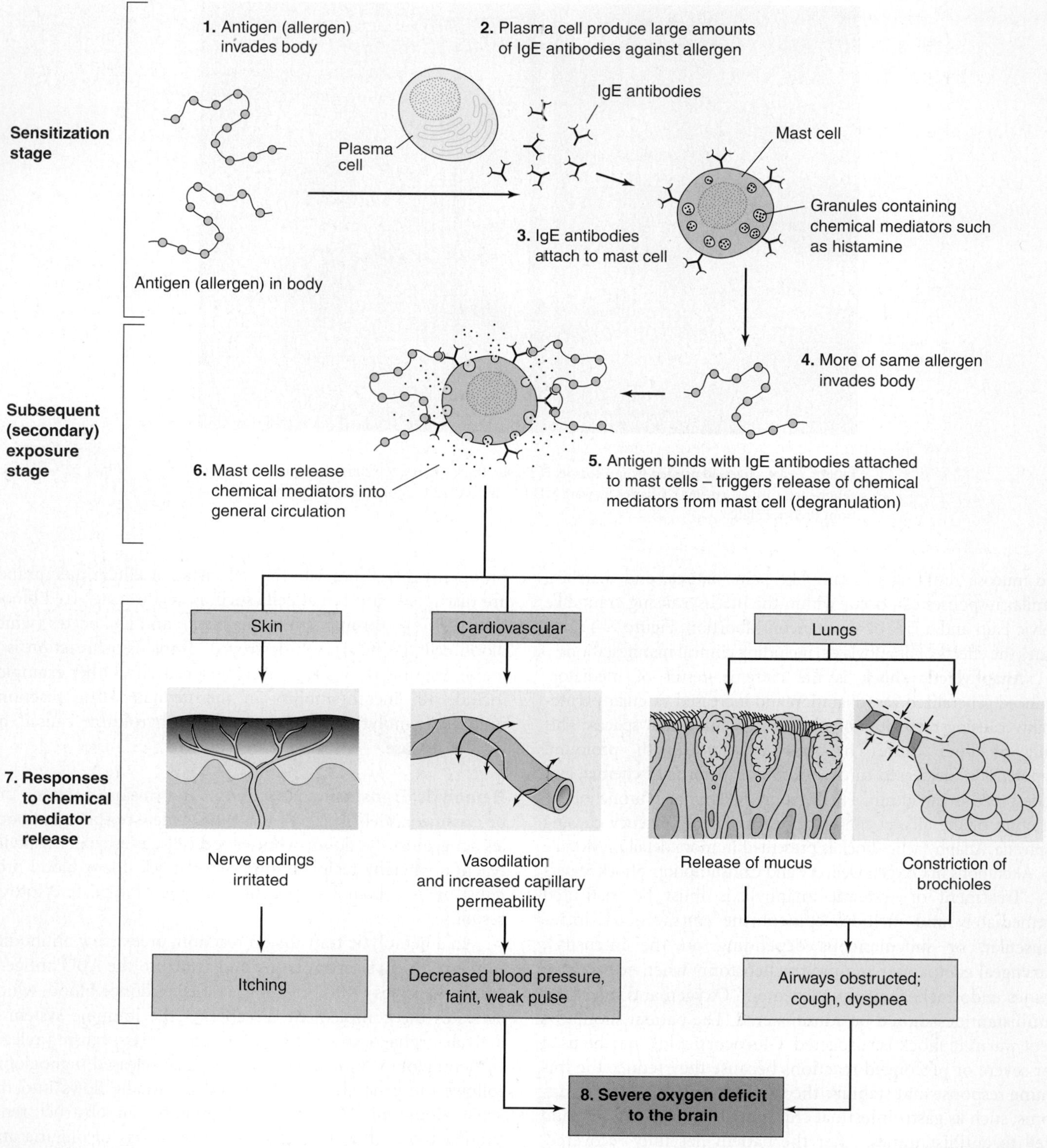

Figure 7–4 ■ The effects of anaphylaxis. This figure was published in Pathophysiology for the health professions, 32nd ed., by Gould, B. E., p. 586, Copyright Elsevier, 2006.

LeMone and Burke (2008, p. 262) recommend the following immediate response protocols to suspected transfusion reaction:

1. Stop the infusion of blood immediately, and notify the physician. Continue to infuse the saline.
2. Take vital signs and assess manifestations.
3. Compare the blood slip with the unit of blood to ensure that an identification error was not made.
4. Save the blood bag and any remaining blood for return to the laboratory for further tests to determine the cause of the reaction.
5. Follow institutional policy for collecting urine and venous blood samples.

RELATED PATHOPHARMACOLOGY: Anaphylaxis

Epinephrine

Actions and Uses:

Epinephrine is a natural catecholamine that stimulates the alpha and beta receptors with stronger alpha activity. Its actions are those of sympathetic nervous system stimulation (e.g., elevations in BP, HR, CO; bronchodilation; and inhibition of release of histamine). It is first-line treatment for anaphylaxis.

Major Adverse Effects:

Most common: Palpitations, nervousness, tremors

Potentially life-threatening: Acute myocardial infarction, pulmonary edema, ventricular fibrillation

Nursing Implications:

Be aware of correct dosage, dilution, and rate of administration. It is recommended that lowest dose be used initially and repeat until desired effect is attained. If higher dose is required, increase the dose gradually.

Can be delivered SC, IM, IV or via endotracheal tube. In an emergency situation, SC may not be advisable, as subcutaneous circulation may be impaired. IV is often used emergently.

Monitor VS and cardiac rhythm every 5 minutes.

In elderly, doses of 0.1 mg are advised.

Antihistamines

diphenhydramine HCL (Benadryl)

Actions and Uses:

Antihistamines block histamine release by competing for the histamine receptor sites. They are useful for temporary relief of allergic symptoms and are used in anaphylaxis as adjunct therapy with epinephrine. Epinephrine should be administered first.

Common Adverse Effects:

Most common: Drowsiness, tachycardia, dry mouth

Potentially life-threatening (rare): Hypersensitivity (cardiovascular collapse, anaphylactic shock)

Nursing Implications:

Check for known hypersensitivity to antihistamines.

May be delivered PO, IM, or IV. For IV administration, be aware of correct dosage, dilution, and rate of administration.

Cautious use in children and elderly – dose may require adjustment to decrease adverse effects.

Adrenocorticoid/Glucocorticoids

dexamethasone (Decadron),
hydrocortisone (Solu-Cortef)
methylprednisolone (Solu-Medrol)

Actions and Uses:

The adrenocorticoid/glucocorticoids have powerful anti-inflammatory and immunosuppressive actions. They are useful as adjunct therapy with epinephrine in treatment of acute hypersensitivity reactions, including anaphylaxis. In anaphylaxis, epinephrine should be given first.

Common Adverse Effects (acute therapy only):

Generally well tolerated in the short term; hyperglycemia, euphoria

Potentially life-threatening (rare): Hypersensitivity reaction is possible

Nursing Implications:

Check for known hypersensitivity.

Can be given IM or IV with anaphlaxis. Be aware of dosage, dilution, and rate of administration if given IV.

Monitor for desired effects.

Beta$_2$-Antagonists

albuterol (Proventil, Ventolin)

Actions and Uses:

Beta$_2$-antagonists act on the beta$_2$-receptors of smooth muscles of the airway resulting in bronchodilation. They also have an inhibitory action on histamine release from the mast cells. Inhaling albuterol is useful as adjunct therapy to open the airways during an anaphylaxis reaction.

Major Adverse Effects:

Most common: tremor, palpitations

Potentially life-threatening: hypersensitivity is possible

Nursing Implications:

Monitor for desired effects of improved ventilation.

Important interaction: Can potentiate effects of epinephrine.

---

6. Continue to monitor the client and provide prescribed interventions to treat hypersensitivity or hemolytic manifestations.

Drug Reaction-Induced Hemolytic Hypersensitivity Reaction. Drugs—especially penicillin, quinine, and sulfonamides—can also trigger a type II cytotoxic reaction. There are three mechanisms by which this can occur. First, a drug can bind to the blood cells causing antibodies to be produced against the drug; second, drug-antibody immune complexes can be absorbed onto the erythrocytes causing the RBCs to begin to breakdown; and third, the drug can induce an allergic reaction (Platts-Mills et al., 2006). Any of these mechanisms can lead to a drug-induced form of hemolytic anemia.

Type III (Immune Complex-Mediated) Hypersensitivity Response

The type III reaction involves formation of antigen–antibody complexes. These complexes form in the circulation, follow the blood flow, and eventually deposit themselves either in the tissues or on vessel walls. The actual tissue damage is caused by altered blood flow, increased vascular permeability, and destruction by

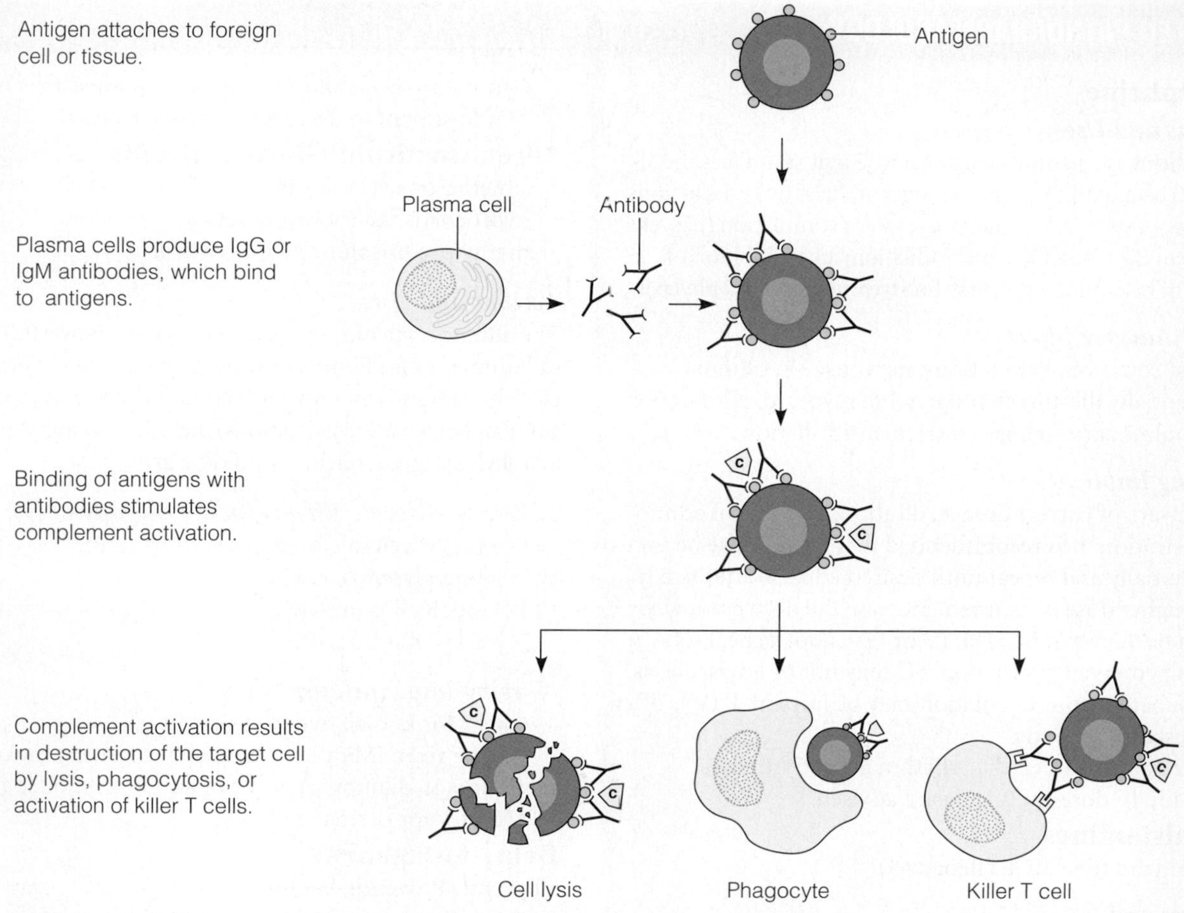

Figure 7–5 ■ Type II Cytotoxic hypersensitivity response. Reprinted from LeMone, P. & Burke, K. *Medical–Surgical Nursing* (4th ed., p. 333). © 2008, with permission from Pearson Education, Inc., Upper Saddle River, New Jersey.

inflammatory cells secondary to activation of the inflammatory response by complement, not the antigen–antibody complexes. The IgG and IgM antibodies are the major immunoglobulins involved in the type III response.

Once formed, the antigen–antibody complexes Type III reactions are characterized by deposits of antigen–antibody complexes in the epithelial lining of blood vessels, the kidneys, joints, skin, and other organs. A **type III hypersensitivity response** can develop as a type of organ transplant rejection. Although a type III response may be considered transient and treatable in many circumstances, in the case of a graft tissue rejection, the graft may become necrotic from the vasculitis and fail to recover. Type III responses can also be responsible for lung, joint, and skin damage in autoimmune disorders, such as systemic lupus erythematosus (SLE) and kidney damage in glomerulonephritis. The type III response can manifest as a local response (Arthus reaction) or as a systemic response (serum sickness).

Arthus Reaction. The Arthus reaction, or Arthus vasculitis, is localized to the skin reaction in which antigen–antibody complexes form in vessels walls, triggering an inflammatory response in the vessels (vasculitis). The reaction onset is relatively rapid, usually within one hour of exposure, and peaks within 6 to 12 hours (Rote, 2008). The clinical manifestations are those caused by the inflammatory response. The vessels become more permeable, allowing fluid to leak out, causing edema. Neutrophils are attracted to the area of inflammation and attempt to destroy the complexes, causing tissue damage. Other local vessel activities include localized hemorrhage and clotting. If severe, localized tissue necrosis can result. An Arthus (or Arthus-like) reaction can follow an injection of a drug or other substance (e.g., skin test antigens), or from an inhaled substance (e.g., farmer's lung) or the gastrointestinal tract (e.g., gluten-sensitive enteropathy found in celiac disease) (Rote, 2008).

Serum Sickness. Serum sickness is the systemic form of a type III hypersensitivity response. The onset of symptoms is slow, increasing over a week or more. The antigen–antibody complexes flow in the circulation and deposit in target tissues, usually the kidneys (glomeruli), joints, or blood vessels. The tissue destruction is the same as described in the Arthus response.

Figure 7–6 illustrates the type III immune complex-mediated hypersensitivity response.

Type IV (Delayed) Hypersensitivity Response

Cell-mediated **type IV hypersensitivity** is a delayed response involving primarily the T lymphocytes, with no antibody

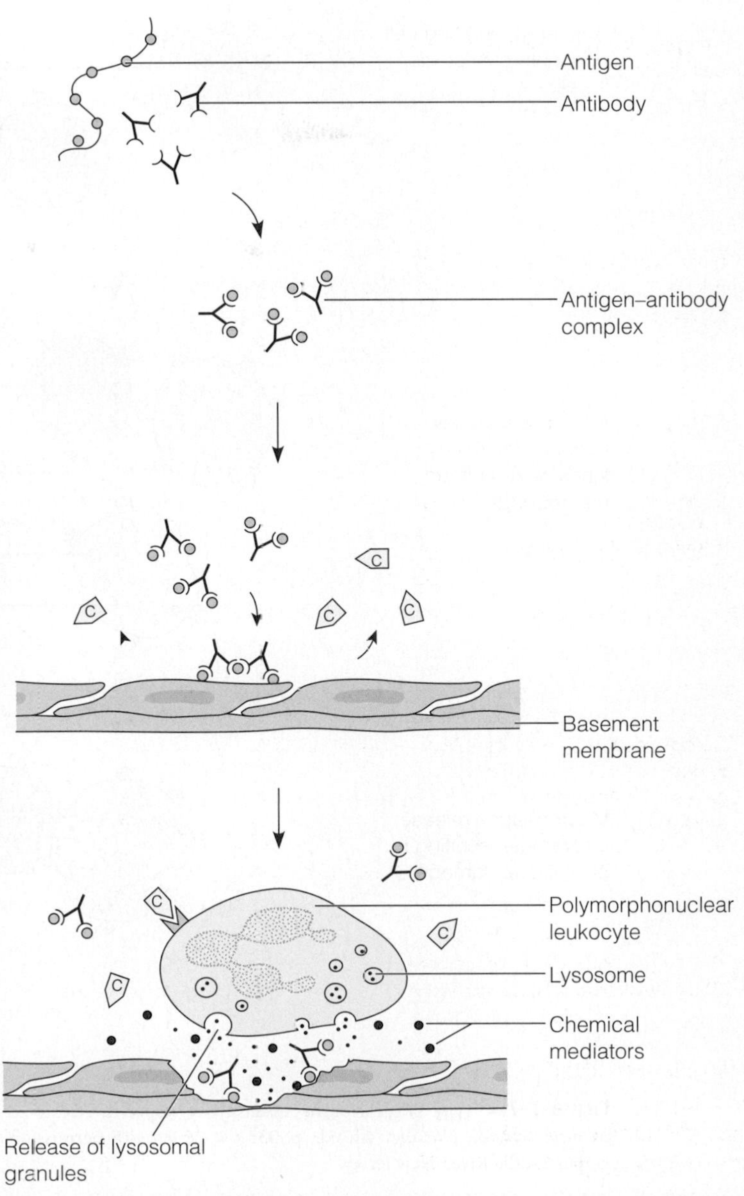

Figure 7–6 ■ Type III immune complex-mediated hypersensitivity response. Reprinted from LeMone, P. & Burke, K. *Medical–Surgical Nursing* (4th ed., p. 334). © 2008, with permission from Pearson Education, Inc., Upper Saddle River, New Jersey.

activity. In this response, sensitized T cells attack the antigen, releasing lymphokines, which attract and activate macrophages. The macrophages cause localized inflammation and edema. Tissue destruction is its hallmark, most notably through direct cellular destruction by T cell toxins, lysosomal enzymes, or phagocytosis following activation by the release of cytokines and lymphokines. If the response is excessive it can damage the host. Figure 7–7 illustrates the type IV response.

Local reaction to a type IV response can be demonstrated in the induration of a positive tuberculin test or contact dermatitis, such as poison ivy. Clinical examples include graft or organ transplant rejection in which the HLA antigen is the principal target (graft-versus-host and host-versus-graft diseases). Furthermore, some autoimmune disorders have a type IV response component, for example Hashimoto thyroiditis, rheumatoid arthritis, and type 1 diabetes mellitus (Rote, 2008).

Treatment of Hypersensitivity Responses

The severity of symptoms varies widely in hypersensitivity reactions. Often, no therapy is required when symptoms are mild to moderate and of short duration (e.g., mild poison ivy or hay fever). When treatment is desired or required to reduce or eliminate a particular hypersensitivity response, the drug therapy typically ordered includes antihistamines, glucocorticoids, or both. The delivery method of these agents may vary, as well. For example, an oral (or injection) preparation of a glucocorticoid likely would be ordered for a systemic or severe hypersensitivity drug-induced reaction, while a topical preparation likely would be ordered for a mild contact dermatitis.

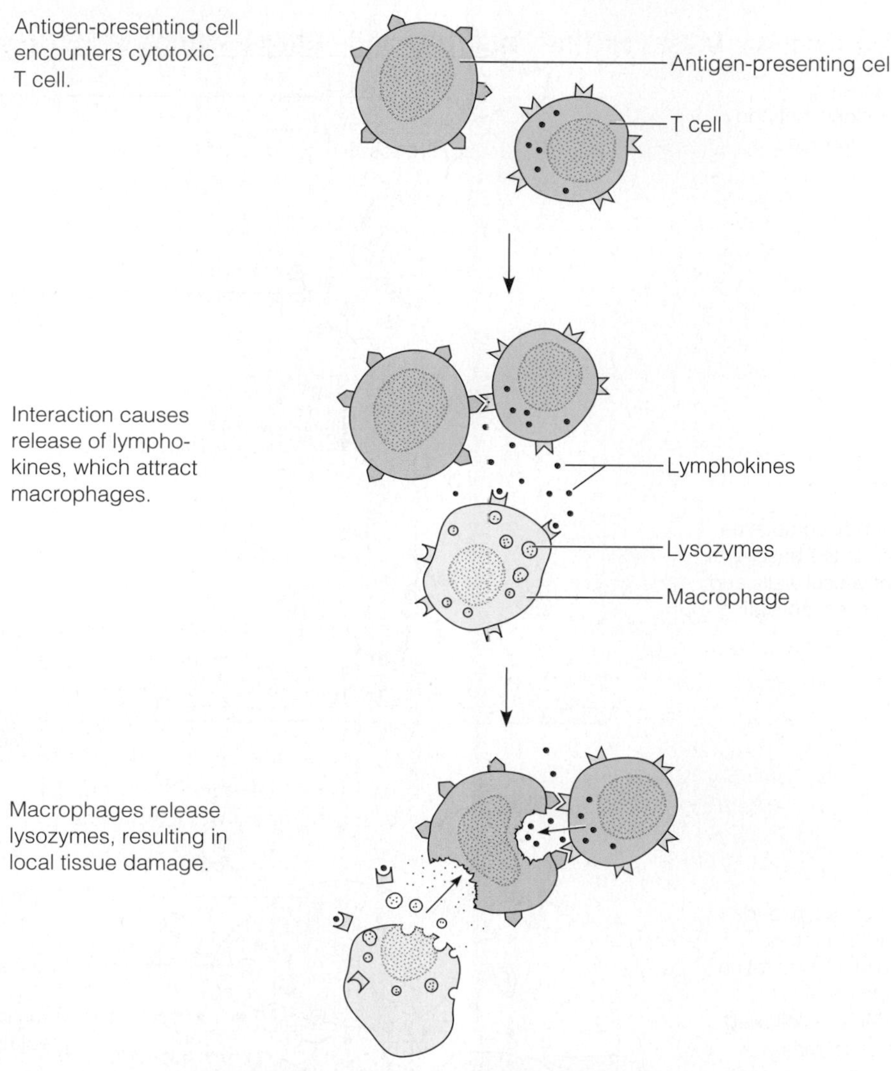

Figure 7–7 ■ Type IV delayed hypersensitivity response. Reprinted from LeMone, P. & Burke, K. *Medical–Surgical Nursing* (4th ed., p. 335). © 2008, with permission from Pearson Education, Inc., Upper Saddle River, New Jersey.

Autoimmune Disorders

Autoimmunity is an immune intolerance to one's own body tissue (self-antigens) that can involve abnormal activities of B cells, T cells, or the complement system. For reasons not fully understood, the immune system incorrectly recognizes self as foreign and initiates a destructive response against targeted tissues. Characteristic of most autoimmune disorders is B cell hyperactivity. Any of the four types of hypersensitivity response may be involved; however, types II and III are the most common. Many diseases are now attributed to an autoimmune response and many others are suspected. Table 7–4 provides a list of common autoimmune diseases that target specific body systems or tissues Other autoimmune diseases, such as systemic lupus erythematosus (SLE) target multiple body systems.

Etiology

Many autoimmune disorders seem to have a genetic predisposition (i.e., they tend to run in families); however, not all family members develop an autoimmune disease. It is theorized that many autoimmune diseases may require some type of trigger to be activated, such as a virus or chemical substance. An example of such a trigger is exposure to the sun which can trigger systemic lupus erythematosus (SLE). In addition to a positive family history, aging and gender are two other risk factors. The occurrence of autoimmune diseases increases as we age, possibly related to the decreased effectiveness of the immune system relevant to the aging body. Women develop autoimmune disorders more frequently than men; however, the reason for this is unknown but may be hormone related.

Mechanisms of Autoimmunity

Multiple theories attempt to explain how autoimmunity can develop. One such theory is molecular mimicry. The theory of molecular mimicry helps explain the development of rheumatoid heart disease, which damages the heart valves. The cell wall proteins of certain microbes (e.g., group A beta hemolytic streptococcus) structurally resemble those of specific normal cells in the body, such as the heart valves. In

TABLE 7–4 Common Autoimmune Diseases That Target Specific Body Systems or Tissues

Pulmonary System
- Goodpasture disease

Gastrointestinal System
- Ulcerative colitis
- Crohn's disease
- Pernicious anemia

Endocrine System
- Graves' disease (thyroid gland)
- Type I diabetes mellitus (pancreas)
- Addison's disease (adrenal gland)
- Partial pituitary deficiency (pituitary gland)

Renal System
- Immune-complex glomerulonephritis

Neuromuscular System
- Multiple sclerosis
- Cardiomyopathy
- Myasthenia gravis
- Rheumatic fever

Connective Tissue
- Systemic lupus erythematosus
- Scleroderma (progressive systemic sclerosis)
- Rheumatoid arthritis
- Ankylosing spondylitis

Hematologic System
- Autoimmune hemolytic anemia
- Autoimmune thrombocytopenic purpura

response to development of strep throat/rheumatic fever, the immune system musters its attack, forming antibodies against the bacteria. The antibodies destroy the initial strep infection but then misidentify the similar (twin) proteins on the normal cells of the heart valves and shift their attack to those cells, causing valve damage. It is believed that there are likely multiple mechanisms involved in autoimmunity and currently most autoimmune diseases are of idiopathic (unknown) origin.

Management

Immunodeficiency or immunosuppression may be a therapeutic goal in treating autoimmune disorders. Immune-mediated tissue damage may be suppressed through drug-induced, radiation-induced, or surgically induced immunodeficiency. Treatment of organ-specific autoimmune disorders involves metabolic control, while treatment of systemic disorders includes anti-inflammatory or immunosuppressive medications.

SECTION TWO REVIEW

1. The results of a true type I hypersensitivity response are the result of
   - **A.** a histamine precursor causing anaphylaxis
   - **B.** antigen–IgE–mast cell interaction
   - **C.** antigen–antibody complexes deposited in vessel walls
   - **D.** massive numbers of destroyed red blood cells
2. Type III hypersensitivity reactions are often characterized by
   - **A.** specific target cells
   - **B.** widespread multiorgan involvement
   - **C.** rapidly progressing symptoms
   - **D.** relatively low-risk patterns
3. Which statement is correct regarding type IV cell-mediated hypersensitivity responses?
   - **A.** It involves primarily antibody activity.
   - **B.** It does not harm body tissues.
   - **C.** T cell activity is responsible.
   - **D.** It directly interacts with cell surface antigens.
4. Disorders thought to be autoimmune in etiology include (choose all that apply)
   - **A.** chronic bronchitis
   - **B.** ulcerative colitis
   - **C.** pernicious anemia
   - **D.** diabetes mellitus (type 1)

Answers: 1. B, 2. B, 3. C, 4. (B, C, D)

SECTION THREE: Leukemia

At the completion of this section, the learner will be able to discuss the etiology, pathophysiology, clinical manifestations, and management of leukemia.

Leukemia is a malignant process in which there is a transformation of hematopoietic cells, causing unregulated clonal growth. This dysfunctional cell proliferation results in the accumulation of abnormal (leukemic) cells in the bone marrow and a decreased production of normal blood cells. Leukemias are categorized broadly as either "acute" or "chronic" with different illness trajectories, prognoses, and approaches to treatment. Acute leukemias are characterized by aggressive proliferation of immature lymphoid or myeloid **blast cells.** Examine Figure 7–8 to review the early stage of blast cells in cell development. Chronic leukemias are characterized by production of mature, differentiated cells of either lymphoid or myeloid lineage. Chronic leukemias have a more insidious long-term clinical course than the acute leukemias.

The uncontrolled production of malignant cells in the bone marrow suppresses and essentially "crowds out" the normal cells, which leads to progressive **pancytopenia.** In untreated

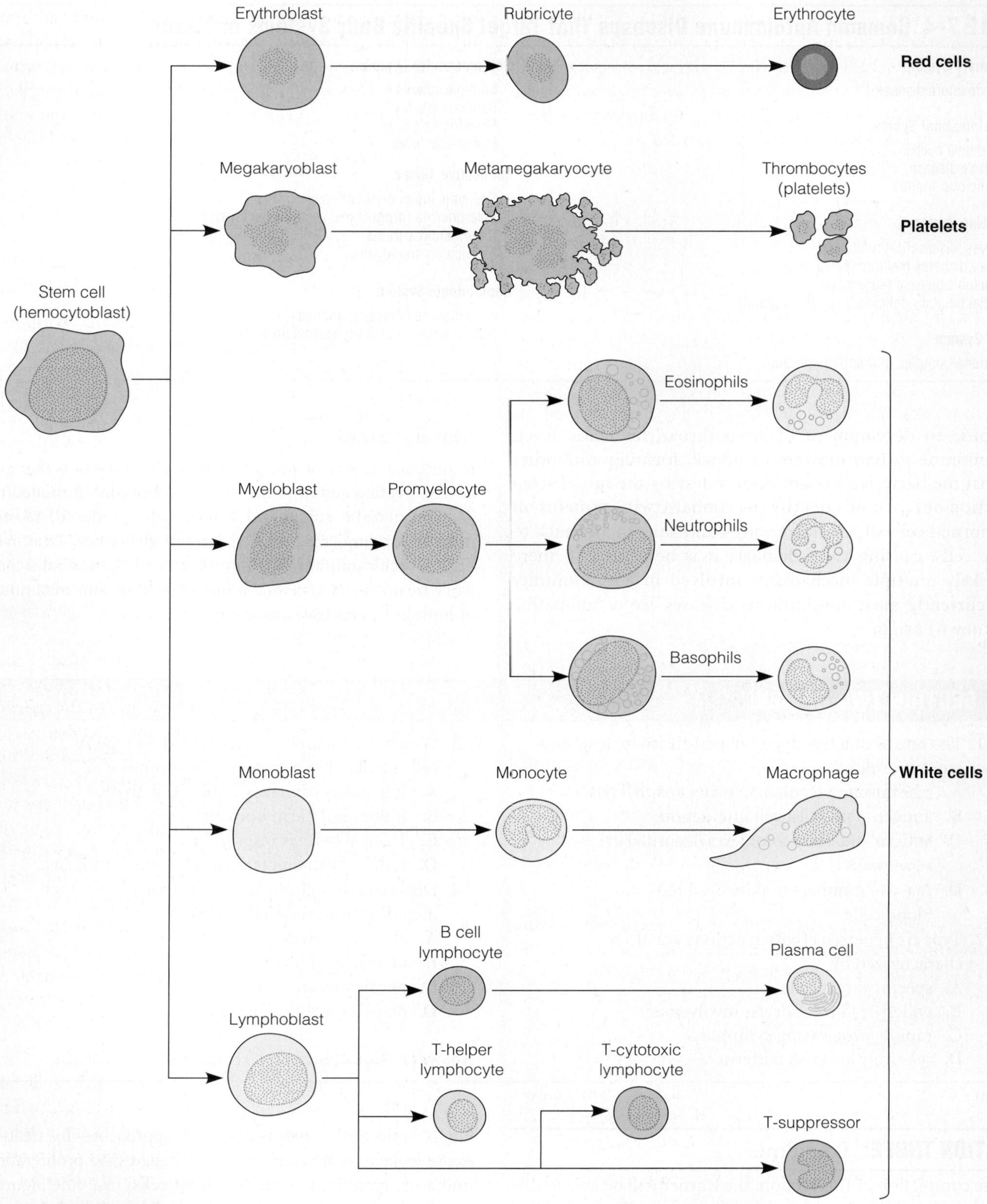

Figure 7–8 ■ Blood cell formation from stem cells. Regulatory factors control the differentiation fo stem cells into blasts. Each kind of blast cell is committed to producing one type of mature blood cell. Erythroblasts, for example, can differentiate only into RBCs; megakaryocytes can differentiate only into platelets. Reprinted from LeMone, P. & Burke, K. *Medical–Surgical Nursing* (4th ed., p. 1077). © 2008, with permission from Pearson Education, Inc., Upper Saddle River, New Jersey.

acute leukemia, the patient rapidly succumbs to complications of pancytopenia, particularly infection or hemorrhage (Gould, 2006; Linker, 2008). The acute leukemias are also associated with infiltration into other tissues, such as the gums, spleen, central nervous system, and lymph nodes, thereby creating clinical manifestations specific to each affected tissue.

Etiology

The exact causes of leukemia are unknown. It is believed that there may be multiple factors involved in the development of each of the different leukemias, including environmental and genetic factors. There is an increased incidence of leukemia with certain chromosomal abnormalities, for example, in children with Down syndrome. Furthermore, in chronic myelogenous leukemia (CML), a specific chromosomal abnormality has been isolated called the Philadelphia chromosome (Ph^1), which involves the translocation between the long arms of chromosomes 22 and 9. Certain chemical and drug exposures are associated with development of leukemia (e.g., benzene, chloramphenicol, and some antineoplastic agents), as is radiation exposure that may occur following nuclear disasters or radiation treatment for previous malignancies.

Types of Leukemia

Acute Leukemias

There are two subclassifications of acute leukemia: acute lymphocytic (lymphoblastic) leukemia (ALL) and acute myelogenous leukemia (AML). Acute leukemias are characterized by the acute onset of symptoms (e.g., fatigue, fever, and bleeding), pancytopenia (anemia, thrombocytopenia, neutropenia), more than 20 percent blast cells in the bone marrow, and the presence of blast cells in peripheral blood in the vast majority (90 percent) of patients (Linker, 2008). In essence, while the number of white blood cells is markedly elevated (leukocytosis), the functional ability of these cells is severely impaired by their lack of maturation.

Acute Lymphocytic (Lymphoblastic) Leukemia. Acute **lymphocytic leukemia** (ALL) is primarily a disease of childhood with a peak incidence between the ages 3 and 7 (Linker, 2008). It accounts for 80 percent of the acute leukemias seen in children (Linker, 2008). Acute lymphocytic leukemia is associated with proliferation of immature lymphoblasts from the B cell lineage (about 70 percent of ALL cases) or, less commonly, the T cell lineage (Linker, 2008). The leukemic cells fail to mature or differentiate any further than the stage at which they are produced; therefore, they cannot carry on normal immune functions.

Acute Myelogenous (Myelocytic) Leukemia. Acute **myelogenous leukemia** (AML) is largely a disease of adulthood. The incidence of AML is increasing in the elderly population, with a median age at presentation of 60 years and it is characterized by a proliferation of malignant blast cells from the myeloid stem cell lineage (Linker, 2008). The proliferation can involve any or all of the cells in the myeloid lineage (erythroblasts, megakaryoblasts, monoblasts, or myeloblasts). Blast cells are not programmed to die; thus, malignant blast clones can produce malignant cells indefinitely. Cells rapidly accumulate in the bone marrow and then infiltrate into other tissues. An examination of peripheral blood and the bone marrow in AML will show a predominance of myeloblastic cells, and possibly Auer rods. **Auer rods** are abnormally large granule-containing needle-like rods in the cytoplasm and are most commonly found in blast cells taken from the bone marrow and blood from patients with AML.

Chronic Leukemias

There are two subclassifications of chronic leukemia: chronic lymphocytic leukemia and chronic myelogenous leukemia.

Chronic Lymphocytic Leukemia. Chronic **lymphocytic leukemia** (CLL) is primarily a disease of middle-age to older adults, and is the second most commonly diagnosed leukemia in Western countries (Moran et al., 2007). Ninety percent of CLL cases occur after age 50, with the average age of presentation being 65 (Linker, 2008). Patients most commonly present with fatigue, lymphadenopathy, **lymphocytosis,** and enlargement of the liver or spleen (Linker, 2008; Moran et al., 2007). CLL has a variable life expectancy, ranging from two to ten years, with some patients surviving for 30 years or more. Death most commonly results from infection. About one third of persons with CLL eventually develop hemolytic anemia of autoimmune etiology. Chronic lymphocytic leukemia is almost always B lymphocyte cell type.

The major characteristic of CLL is the presence of smaller than normal mature lymphocytes in the peripheral blood and bone marrow. These cells can often be found in the spleen and lymph nodes, causing splenomegaly and lymphadenopathy. The small CLL lymphocytes often are not fully functional as immune cells, causing **hypogammaglobulinemia,** or low levels of gamma globulin in the blood; consequently the patient with CLL becomes increasingly immunodeficient and at increased risk for developing potentially fatal infections. Laboratory findings consistent with CLL include anemia and thrombocytopenia, which can be worsened if autoantibodies develop, causing premature blood cell destruction. The diagnostic hallmark of CLL is lymphocytosis (Linker, 2008). The total white blood cell count is usually greater than 20,000 cells/mcL and may be as high as several hundred thousand, with 75–98 percent of circulating lymphocytes in the peripheral blood (Linker, 2008).

Chronic Myelogenous (Myelocytic) Leukemia. Chronic **myelogenous leukemia** (CML) is also primarily a disease of adults, with the median age at presentation 55 years (Linker, 2008). A key distinguishing feature of CML is the presence of the Ph^1 (Philadelphia) chromosome abnormality. This translocation of chromosomes 9 and 22 results in the transfer of the Abelson (ABL) oncogene to an area on chromosome 22 called the *breakpoint cluster region* (BCR). This abnormal hybrid gene, BCR-ABL, produces a protein that causes accelerated cell growth and decreased cell death, and subsequently results in the malignant proliferation of the blood cells (D'Antonio, 2005). Chronic myelogenous leukemia, like AML, involves hyperproliferation of all cells in the myelocytic stem cell line. It is characterized by the predominance of excessive numbers of mature and immature myelocytic cells, and is a slow-onset, slowly progressive disease.

The course of CML is unique and typically runs in three phases: chronic, accelerated, and acute (blast).

Chronic phase. The patient typically initially presents with marked leukocytosis, thrombocytosis and splenomegaly (D'Antonio, 2005). The chronic phase is usually treatable and the patient remains asymptomatic. Without treatment, the chronic phase generally lasts from two to four years. With treatment, this phase may last five or more years.

Accelerated phase. Eventually, most persons with CML develop resistance to therapy, which moves the person from the chronic phase into the accelerated phase. This phase begins with the onset of increased signs and symptoms. It usually develops with or without treatment; however, treatment during the chronic phase can significantly delay onset of the accelerated phase.

Acute (blast transformation) phase. The accelerated phase generally ends with the patient's disease transforming from a chronic form of leukemia to an acute form, usually a form of acute myelocytic leukemia (AML). The acute phase is characterized by the onset of a "blast crisis" in which the leukocytes are no longer able to differentiate into their more mature forms, resulting in blast cell predominance in the bone marrow and peripheral blood. This final phase is typically resistant to treatment and usually results in death within a few months.

Laboratory findings consistent with CML depend on the phase of the disease. Overall, however, CML is characterized by extreme leukocytosis and the existence of any combination of mature and immature myelogenous cells in the bone marrow and blood. The total leukocyte count may exceed 300,000, placing the patient at high risk for complications of leukostasis (Linker, 2008). At the time of initial presentation, the patient is normally not anemic and the platelet count is often normal, or sometimes markedly elevated. As the disease progresses, however, progressive anemia and thrombocytopenia can occur (Linker, 2008).

Clinical Manifestations of Leukemia

The initial clinical presentation of a person at the onset of acute leukemia is often dramatic, and can include complaints of fever, easy fatigability, bruising, bleeding, bone pain, and persistent/frequent infections (Linker, 2008; Rizzieri et al, 2005). The major clinical manifestations of the leukemias can be categorized into two groups: those that are caused by pancytopenia and those that are caused by expansion and infiltration of malignant cells into other tissues. Table 7–5 provides a summary of manifestations.

TABLE 7–5 Clinical Manifestations of Leukemia

CATEGORY	COMMON CLINICAL MANIFESTATIONS
Pancytopenia	Leukopenia (immunodeficiency) ▪ Frequent infections ▪ Fever Thrombocytopenia (bleeding tendencies) ▪ Epistaxis, bleeding gums ▪ Petechiae and ecchymosis Erythrocytopenia (anemia) ▪ Pale mucous membranes ▪ Fatigue, activity intolerance, malaise ▪ Intolerance to cold ▪ Tachycardia, tachypnea
Malignant Cell Expansion	Bone ▪ Bone tenderness or pain Vascular system ▪ Leukocytosis and leukostasis ▪ Impaired circulation (particularly brain and/or lungs)

Infiltration	CNS
	▪ Headache, nausea, and vomiting
	▪ Seizures, coma
	▪ Papilledema, cranial nerve palsies
	Liver and spleen
	▪ Hepatomegaly and splenomegaly
	  ▪ Abdominal discomfort
	  ▪ Worsening thrombocytopenia/pancytopenia

Pancytopenia Manifestations

Recall that leukemia causes overcrowding in the bone marrow resulting in decreased production of all normal blood cell types. As the red blood cell count decreases, the person with leukemia becomes increasingly anemic, demonstrating all of the manifestations of that problem. As the normal leukocyte count decreases, the patient becomes increasingly immunodeficient and at high risk for development of infections. However, if significant neutropenia is present, the typical clinical picture associated with infection may be diminished or absent. Infection is the most common cause of death in adults with acute leukemia (Gould, 2006; Moran et al, 2007). Fever is commonly related to infection and increased metabolism of the malignant cells (Gould, 2006). Finally, as platelet numbers decrease, the patient develops bleeding problems, particularly petechiae and ecchymosis on the skin, as well as epistaxis and bleeding gums.

Malignant Cell Expansion and Infiltration Manifestations

As the malignant cells proliferate in the bone marrow, their expanding volume increases the pressure inside the bone. The increased pressure causes bone tenderness or pain. Malignant cells can infiltrate into the central nervous system (CNS), leading to multiple CNS-related manifestations, such as nausea and vomiting, headache, seizures, coma, papilledema, and possible cranial nerve palsies (Gould, 2006). Infiltration of malignant cells into the spleen and liver gives rise to splenomegaly and hepatomegaly, which can cause general abdominal discomfort and worsening pancytopenia, particularly thrombocytopenia.

Leukostasis. Gucalp and Dutcher (2005) explain that **leukostasis** (or leukostasis syndrome) is a potentially fatal complication of extreme elevations (greater than 100,000 cells/mcL) of circulating leukocytes (usually blast cells). It is primarily associated with AML but can occur with ALL. It is not associated with the chronic forms of leukemia. The massive load of blast cells in the circulation increases the blood viscosity and aggregation (clumping) of leukemic cells, which leads to sluggish blood flow through the capillaries. The end result is impaired capillary circulation. Some of the leukemic cells escape the endothelium and may cause hemorrhage. The brain and lungs are most commonly affected. Neurologic symptoms include headache, dizziness, and altered level of consciousness that can range from mild confusion to deep coma. Pulmonary manifestations include hypoxemia, respiratory distress, and possible respiratory failure. The multiple body system effects of leukemia are shown in Figure 7–9.

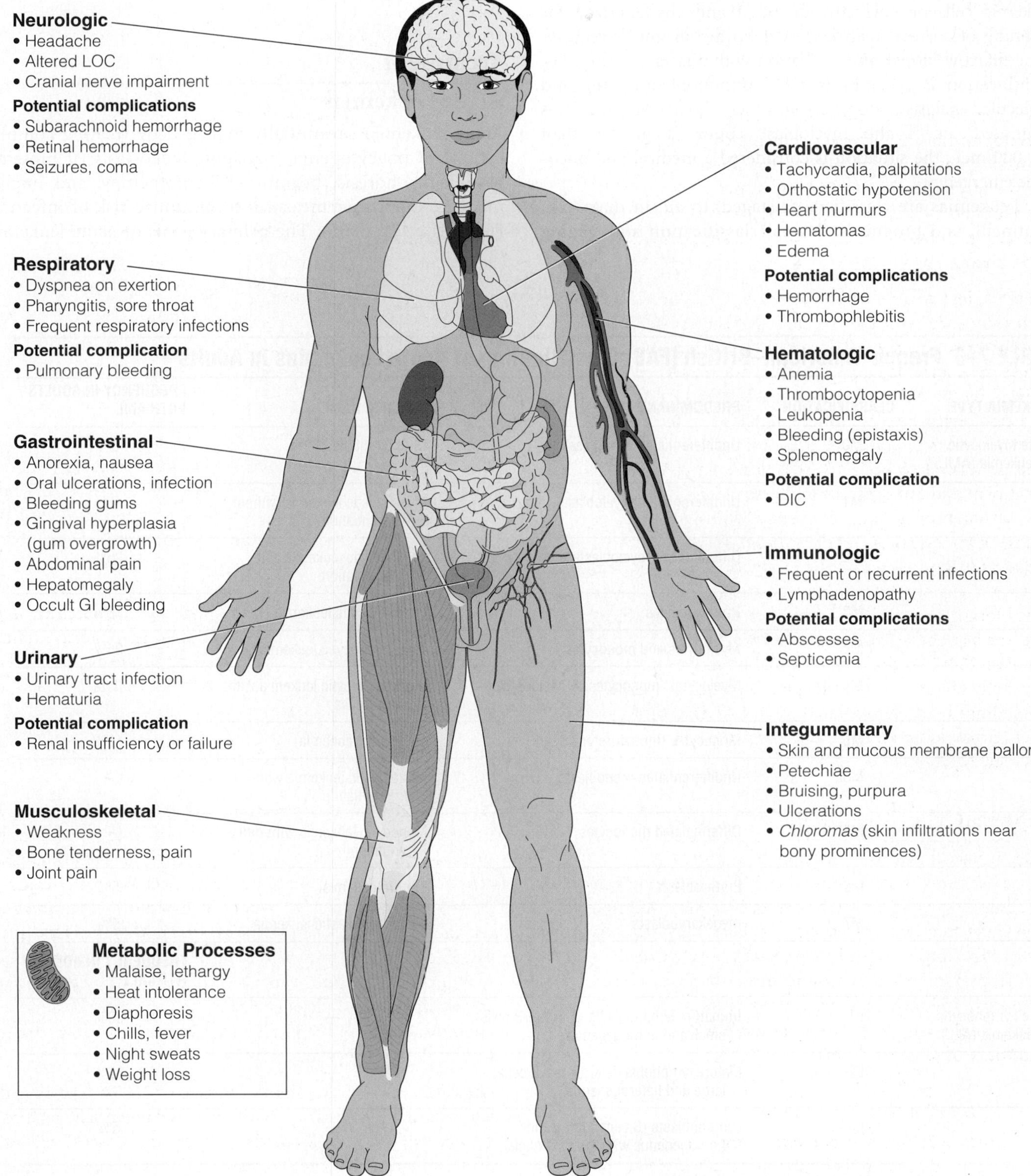

Figure 7–9 ■ The multiple body system effects of leukemia. Reprinted from LeMone, P. & Burke, K. *Medical–Surgical Nursing* (4th ed., p. 1210). © 2008, with permission from Pearson Education, Inc., Upper Saddle River, New Jersey.

Diagnosis

Diagnosis of the exact subtype of leukemia requires prompt and thorough clinical evaluation, and may be complicated by the fact that the blast cells are so primitive as to make it difficult to determine whether the malignant cell clones are of myelocytic or lymphocytic origin (Gould, 2006). It is critical that the leukemic cells be correctly identified and characterized for planning of correct treatment. A definitive diagnosis requires bone marrow biopsy and aspiration with analysis of the cells. Identification is accomplished by immunophenotyping and molecular analysis (cytogenetics). When either AML or ALL is diagnosed, or if the myeloblast count is greater than 100,000/mcL, the situation is considered a medical and oncologic emergency.

Leukemias are classified, or staged, to aid in diagnosis, treatment, and prognosis. Several classification and staging systems have been developed over the years to aid in diagnosis and treatment. The French–American–British (FAB) classification system was developed to differentiate acute leukemias by morphology and remains the most commonly used classification system in the clinical setting (Table 7–6) and provides invaluable morphologic guidance in diagnosing acute leukemia.

Treatment

Acute Leukemias

Acute leukemias are initially managed by treating complications of pancytopenia, managing leukostasis (if present) with leukophoresis, beginning chemotherapy, and implementing supportive measures to minimize risk of infection (Rizzieri et al., 2005). The primary goals of acute leukemia

TABLE 7–6 French–American–British (FAB) Classification of Acute Leukemias in Adults

LEUKEMIA TYPE	CLASSIFICATION	PREDOMINANT CELLS	SPECIFIC NAME	FREQUENCY IN ADULTS WITH AML
Acute Myelocytic Leukemia (AML)	M0	Undifferentiated myeloblasts	Undifferentiated AML	5%
	M1	Undifferentiated myeloblasts	Myeloblastic leukemia without differentiation	15%
	M2	Differentiated myeloblasts	Myeloblastic leukemia with differentiation	25%
	M3	Promyelocytes	Promyelocytic leukemia (APL)	10%
	M4	Myelocytes and monocytes	Myelomonocytic leukemia	25%
	M4 eos	Myelocytes, monocytes, & eosinophils	Myelomonocytic leukemia with eosinophilia	Rare
	M5	Monocytes (immature or mature)	Monocytic leukemia	10%
	M5a	Undifferentiated monoblasts	Monoblastic leukemia without differentiation	—
	M5b	Differentiated monocytes	Monocytic leukemia with differentiation	—
	M6	Erythroblasts	Erythroleukemia	5%
	M7	megakaryoblasts	Megakaryoblastic leukemia	5%
				FREQUENCY IN ADULTS WITH ALL
Acute Lymphocytic Leukemia (ALL)	L1	Immature lymphoblasts (T or pre-B cells); small and homogeneous	—	30%
	L2	Mature lymphoblasts (T or pre-B cells); large and heterogeneous	—	65%
	L3	Lymphoblasts (B cells); large and homogeneous with multiple nuclei	—	5%

Data from American Cancer Society (2008), Seiter, K. (2006a), and Seiter, K. (2006b).

therapy are to eliminate the malignant cells, restore normal hematopoiesis, and produce complete remission (Rizzieri et al., 2005). This is typically achieved through aggressive chemotherapy, which may require multiple courses of treatment that may last for two years. The optimal treatment approach depends on the patient's age, overall clinical status and presence of comorbidities, and the cytogenetic and molecular profile of the patient's leukemia type (Linker, 2008).

Induction Chemotherapy. The initial phase of chemotherapy is referred to as *induction,* which lasts for approximately one week. Patients may stay in the hospital for about a month until the blood counts recover and it is safe for the patient to be discharged. While in the hospital, many patients are given intravenous antibiotics, and blood products may be ordered to support the patient through the therapy. Most patients with AML are treated with combination chemotherapy of an anthracycline plus cytarabine, resulting in an initial complete remission in 80 percent of patients under age 60 and in 50-60 percent of older patients (Linker, 2008). Chemotherapy induction in the ALL patient usually requires a combination drug approach and may include prednisone, L-asparaginase, vincristine, and other therapeutic agents. Induction therapy aims at creating a state of complete remission—the absence of leukemic cells in the bone marrow or peripheral blood. In children with ALL, induction is associated with complete remission for more than five years in about 90 percent of cases.

Consolidation Chemotherapy. Induction therapy may be followed by *consolidation* chemotherapy, which aims to solidify the remission response and eradicate any remaining leukemic cells. It frequently includes the same chemotherapeutic agents used during induction but at lower doses and for shorter durations.

Maintenance Chemotherapy. The final phase of chemotherapy is called *maintenance* chemotherapy, which is primarily required for treatment of ALL. During this phase, the patient with ALL may have intrathecal (drugs injected into the cerebrospinal space, typically done through a lumbar puncture) prophylactic treatment of the CNS and possibly brain radiation. Hematopoietic stem-cell transplantation may be the curative treatment of choice, particularly in patients with AML or relapsed ALL, and is addressed later in this section.

Chronic Leukemias

The development of targeted molecular therapies has revolutionized the control and treatment of chronic leukemias. Chronic myelogenous leukemia (CML) was traditionally treated with interferon and chemotherapy drugs such as hydroxyurea with variable response (D'Antonio, 2005). However, the treatment of CML has been transformed with the advent of tyrosine kinase inhibitor agents, specifically imatinib mesylate (Gleevec). This novel oral agent specifically inhibits the tyrosine kinase activity of the bcr/abl oncogene and was approved in 2002 as first-line therapy for newly diagnosed CML (D'Antonio, 2005). Imatinib mesylate is generally well tolerated with infrequent and mild side effects and results in nearly universal (98 percent) hematologic control of the disease (Linker, 2008). Additional promising targeted molecular therapies are currently in development for treating resistant or relapsed CML (D'Antonio, 2005). Allogeneic stem-cell transplant remains the only definitive curative option for CML, but now is reserved for patients who fail therapy with imatinib mesylate. The best results with stem-cell transplants occur in patients who are younger than 40 years of age, are transplanted within a year of diagnosis, and use a HLA-matched sibling as the donor (Linker, 2008; D'Antonio, 2005).

Treatment of CLL may be reserved until the patient moves into the advanced stages (III and IV) of the disease, develops pancytopenia, and/or becomes symptomatic (Linker, 2008). Chemotherapy is the usual initial form of therapy, often using a combination of chemotherapeutic agents such as fludarabine (Fludara), cyclophosphamide (Cytoxan), and the antibody rituximab (Rituxan) (Linker, 2008). Chlorambucil, an oral alkylating agent, given with or without prednisone, was the standard of care prior to the development of fludarabine and remains a viable treatment option for patients who are not candidates for intravenous chemotherapy (Linker, 2008; Moran et al., 2007). The monoclonal antibody, alemtuzumab, has been approved for treating refractory CLL, but can produce significant immunosuppression and its role in managing CLL remains to be determined (Linker, 2008).

Radiation therapy may be used to reduce the size of bulky masses in the lymph nodes or spleen, and splenectomy may be performed, in conjunction with administration of prednisone and rituximab if autoimmunity develops. Preventing, identifying, and treating infections in CLL is paramount in managing the disease (Moran et al., 2007). Antimicrobial therapy is ordered as necessary to treat infections, and patients may benefit from prophylactic infusions of gamma globulin (Linker, 2008).

Hematopoietic Stem-Cell Transplantation

Hematopoietic stem-cell transplantation (HSCT), formerly referred to as *bone marrow transplantation,* is an intensive therapy used to eradicate hematological malignancy from the bone marrow and promote the return of a normal functioning immune system. HSCT can be used for a variety of disorders, including leukemia, multiple myeloma, autoimmune disorders such as systemic lupus erythematosus (SLE), and aplastic anemia (Copelan, 2006). In some disorders, such as relapsed AML, it is the only potentially curative therapeutic option. HSCT is discussed in detail in Module 8, Alteration in Immune Response: Solid Organ and Hematopoietic Stem Cell Transplantation.

SECTION THREE REVIEW

1. The myelocytic leukemias differ from lymphocytic leukemias in that both forms of myelocytic leukemias involve
   A. more than one type of blood cell
   B. a predominance of mature blood cells
   C. red blood cells
   D. plasma cell proliferation
2. In general, the cause of death in the patient who has untreated acute leukemia is
   A. infection
   B. tissue hypoxia
   C. thrombocytopenia
   D. hemorrhage
3. About 70 percent of ALL cases involve proliferation of immature
   A. B cells
   B. T cells
   C. plasma cells
   D. megakaryocytes
4. The presence of Auer rods in the cytoplasm is primarily found in which type of leukemia?
   A. ALL
   B. AML
   C. CLL
   D. CML
5. CML is associated with a final-stage *blast crisis,* which is best described as occurring when
   A. the disease transforms from a chronic to an acute form
   B. blast cells obstruct the circulation
   C. bone marrow completely fails
   D. blast cells infiltrate the brain
6. The term *leukostasis* refers to
   A. infiltration of brain and lungs by blast cells
   B. inability of leukocytes to move out of bone marrow
   C. loss of vision or stroke caused by stagnant blood flow
   D. impaired circulation as a result of capillary congestion by blast cells
7. A "complete remission" is obtained when there are no leukemic cells in the
   A. lymph nodes and bone marrow
   B. lymph nodes and peripheral blood
   C. bone marrow and lymph nodes
   D. bone marrow and peripheral blood
8. The initial treatment of acute leukemias is
   A. surgery
   B. chemotherapy
   C. radiation therapy
   D. bone marrow transplant
9. Treatment of ALL may include "maintenance" therapy, which commonly includes
   A. intrathecal chemotherapy
   B. total body irradiation
   C. bone marrow transplantation
   D. corticosteroid therapy

Answers: 1. A, 2. A, 3. A, 4. B, 5. A, 6. D, 7. D, 8. B, 9. A

SECTION FOUR: HIV Disease: A Disorder of Immunodeficiency

At the completion of this section, the learner will be able to discuss human immunodeficiency virus (HIV) and acquired immunodeficiency syndrome (AIDS).

The immune system can be subject to inadequate development, disease, and injury from illness or treatments that can result in impaired immune activity. Such a situation is called an **immunodeficiency state.** Immunodeficiency results from a loss of function of one or more components of the immune system, and the problem may be acute or chronic. Human immunodeficiency virus/acquired immunodeficiency disease syndrome (HIV/AIDS) is the most common disease associated with secondary (acquired) immunodeficiency. This section provides a broad overview of HIV/AIDS, including cellular manifestations characterizing HIV disease, epidemiology and transmission, viral invasion, phases of infection, screening, clinical manifestations, and treatment approaches.

Types of Immunodeficiency

There are two types of immunodeficiency: primary and secondary. **Primary immunodeficiency** involves a failure of immune system without evidence of some other underlying disorder to explain its presence. Primary immunodeficiency is rare, and results from an embryonic anomaly, genetic predisposition, or congenital failure of the immune system to develop. **Secondary, or acquired, immunodeficiency** refers to loss of the immune response secondary to another disease or therapy from an external cause and may occur at any age. The causes include infection, splenectomy, malnutrition, liver disease, use of immunosuppressive drugs in patients with organ transplants, and chemotherapy and radiation for cancer treatment. HIV/AIDS differs from primary immunodeficiency in that it is not genetically transmitted, nor is it embryonic in the sense of lymphoid tissue failing to develop adequately.

Epidemiology

HIV/AIDS was first recognized in the United States in 1981 and initially thought to be a disease solely affecting homosexual males. Studies now show that the disease has become widely disseminated to include heterosexual groups and all races and ethnic groups represented in the United States. Currently, an estimated 950,000 Americans are infected with HIV, and the global pandemic continues, especially in sub-Saharan Africa and Southeast Asia, with nearly 40 million people infected worldwide. There is also increasing concern with the rapidly growing number of women infected with HIV (Zolopa & Katz, 2008).

Transmission

The mode of transmission is predominantly through infected blood and body secretions, generally excluding saliva and tears. The HIV virus is fragile and cannot survive outside of the body;

thus it requires direct contact for transmission to occur, such as secretion-secretion, secretion-blood, or blood-blood. The most common modes of transmission include sexual contact (greater than 70 percent), administration of contaminated blood and blood products, contaminated needles, and mother-to-fetus (vertical transmission). Transmission of HIV by infected blood products is now unlikely with the sophisticated cross-matching and antibody screening precautions used in the United States, but this remains a significant concern in countries where this technology is not available. Individuals who require specific blood components (such as factor VIII and frequent plasma replacement) may be at increased risk because of the large numbers of donors needed to produce adequate quantities of these components. Successful transmission also requires a sufficient viral load; that is, the amount of virus that enters the blood. The higher the initial viral load, the higher the risk of developing the actual HIV infection.

HIV Screening

The antibody to HIV has been identified and can be used for screening purposes. The point at which serum antibodies are measurable in the blood is called **seroconversion,** which generally occurs within 6 to 14 months of infection onset (Rote, 2008). A prolonged latency period associated with HIV infection effectively reduces the accuracy and immediacy of host identification. Screening for the antibody is helpful to the extent that individuals can be identified who have been exposed to HIV; however, not all of these individuals actually carry the virus, nor will all of them show signs of illness. Several types of human–HIV relationships are possible.

- **Exposure.** An individual may be exposed to the virus but may neither carry it nor contract the disease
- **Carrier.** The individual may carry the virus with the capability of infecting others but without accompanying signs and symptoms
- **Terminal disease.** The individual may be infectious, symptomatic, and terminal

Pathophysiology

Cellular Characteristics of HIV Disease

The immunodeficiency state that eventually develops with HIV infection involves elements of both cell-mediated and humoral-mediated immunodeficiency (Zolopa & Katz, 2008). The cellular immune deficiency characterizing HIV disease is manifested by markedly depressed T lymphocyte functioning, with a reduction of helper T cells (T_H, $CD4^+$), impaired cytotoxic T cell (T_C, $CD8^+$) activity, and increased suppressor T cells (T_S, $CD8^+$). By selectively invading and infecting T cells (particularly T_H cells), the HIV virus damages the very cells whose function it is to orchestrate the identification and destruction of the virus as antigen. Eventually, the individual's supply of functional T cells becomes depleted. In a person with a competent immune system, the number of T_H cells ranges from 600 to 1,200 cells/mcL, whereas the patient with HIV might have a T_H cell count of zero to 500 cells/mcL. The humoral response in producing antibodies is less directly affected by the HIV virus. B cell production does not seem to be decreased, but the induction and regulation of the humoral response may be affected by the lack of T cell regulators (e.g., T_H and T_S cells), subsequently depressing B cell responses to new antigen challenges (Zolopa & Katz, 2008).

Viral Invasion

HIV is a type of retrovirus, carrying genetic information in ribonucleic acid (RNA) rather than in deoxyribonucleic acid (DNA). The virus infects the T lymphocyte by binding to it at the $CD4^+$ T cell receptor site and penetrating the T cell membrane. Through an enzyme called reverse transcriptase, the viral RNA is copied as a double-stranded DNA and inserted into the host cell chromosome. When the T cell is activated to reproduce, such as with other viral infections or stresses, the viral genetic information is programmed to produce more of the infectious HIV virus, and the number of functional T cells diminishes rapidly. Viral load and $CD4^+$ T cell counts are reflective of viral activity and disease progression.

Reverse transcriptase is highly error-prone and may produce multiple mutations during each replication of the HIV virus, which can make targeted therapy difficult. Most antiviral drugs currently being tested or used in treatment regimens work by inhibiting the action of reverse transcriptase or by inhibiting an enzyme (protease) needed at a later stage of the HIV's course. To date, there are two forms of HIV: HIV-1 and HIV-2. HIV-1 is the major cause of AIDS globally. HIV-2 has been isolated in West African patients and is currently rarely found in the United States (Zolopa & Katz, 2008). The HIV-2 virus has been found to cause AIDS, but seems less virulent, less transmissible, and creates lower proportions of infected cells (Gould, 2006). The course of HIV/AIDS is illustrated in Figure 7–10.

Progression of HIV Infection

The progression of HIV disease in adults is monitored and categorized by the grouping of clinical manifestations or on $CD4^+$ T cell levels, both of which reflect disease progression. For ease of discussion, it can be grouped into three general stages: early, progressive, and overt AIDS.

Early-Stage HIV Disease

Early-stage HIV disease can be further broken down into two periods: an acute viral syndrome and the latent (window) period.

Acute Viral Syndrome. Within several weeks of exposure to the virus, transient flu-like or mononucleosis-like symptoms develop. The infected person then becomes asymptomatic. During this period, the virus is not lying dormant; rather, it is actively replicating, thereby increasing the serum viral load. If the blood is tested for HIV during this time, the results would be negative for antibodies (seronegative). Usually within 2 to 10 weeks of exposure, sufficient antibodies have developed against the virus to be measureable in the blood (seroconversion). This event ushers in the next stage of the disease.

Latent (Window) Period. The latent (or window) period of the disease is usually long, often ten years or more, with a mean time frame of approximately 10 years between exposure and development of AIDS (Zolopa & Katz, 2008). The infected person is often asymptomatic during latency; however, if symptoms are present, they are usually mild. The virus is primarily sequestered in the lymph nodes and continues to actively replicate in the

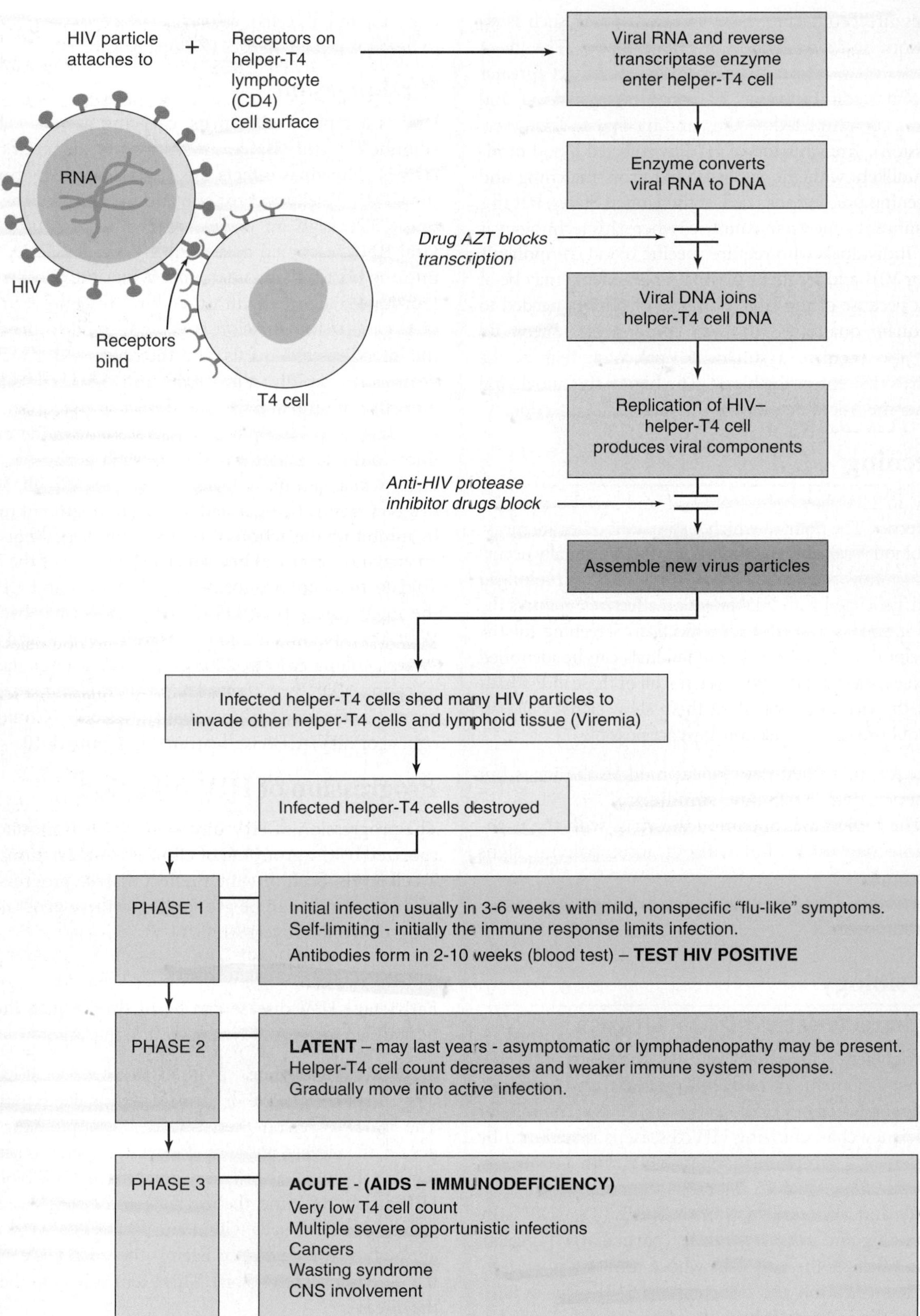

Figure 7–10 ■ The course of HIV-AIDS. This figure was published in Pathophysiology for the health professions, 3rd ed., by Gould, B. E., p. 257, Copyright, Elsevier, 2006.

nodes during this phase. $CD4^+$ cell levels remain adequate and viral load may become insignificant.

Progressive HIV Disease and AIDS

Eventually, the latency period ends, heralded by an increasing HIV viral load with a subsequent decline in $CD4^+$ (T_H) cell levels. The clinical manifestations associated with HIV/AIDS worsen as the active disease progresses and the potential for infection increases as the immune protection afforded by the $CD4^+$ cells becomes increasingly compromised. Eventually, the infected individual meets the AIDS defining criteria.

Defining characteristics of AIDS were established in 1981 by the Centers for Disease Control and Prevention (CDC). The most up-to-date 1993 revision defines AIDS as:

- Seropositive HIV infection with
- A $CD4^+$ T cell count of less than 200 cells/mL, OR
- The presence of at least one "AIDS-defining" illness.

The most common AIDS-defining illnesses in the United States are *Pneumocystis jiroveci* pneumonia (PJP) (previously called *Pneumocystis carinii* [PCP]), Cytomegalovirus (CMV), and *Mycobacterium avium-intracellulare* complex (MAC). Without appropriate antiviral drug therapy, a person with AIDS usually dies within two to three years. Figure 7–11 illustrates the progression of HIV infection.

Clinical Manifestations

The clinical presentation of HIV/AIDS patients varies depending largely on which opportunistic infections are present. Some of the more common general clinical manifestations of progressive disease and AIDS are summarized in Table 7–7. Eventually, the patient dies of complications of end-stage AIDS, usually uncontrollable infection (Gould, 2006). Figure 7–12 shows a person with wasting disease.

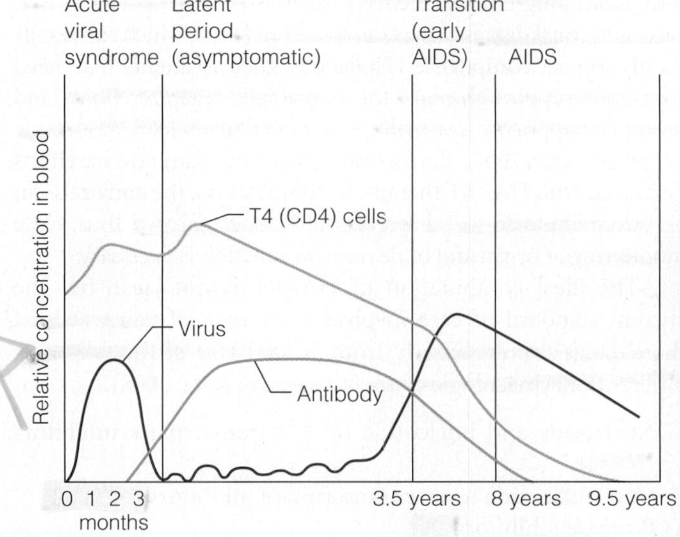

Figure 7–11 ■ The progression of HIV infection. Acute illness develops shortly after the virus is contracted, corresponding with a rapid rise in viral levels. Antibodies are formed and remain present throughout the course of the infection. Late in the disease, viral activation results in a marked increase in virus while CD4 (T4) cells diminish as they are destroyed with viral replication. Antibody levels gradually decrease as immune function is impaired. Reprinted from LeMone, P. & Burke, K. *Medical–Surgical Nursing* (4th ed., p. 351). © 2008, with permission from Pearson Education, Inc., Upper Saddle River, New Jersey.

TABLE 7–7 General Clinical Manifestations of Progressive HIV Disease and AIDS

DISEASE PHASE	COMMON CLINICAL MANIFESTATIONS
Progressive HIV Disease ($CD4^+$ is less than normal but greater than 200 cells/mcL; absence of any AIDS-defining illness)	No AIDS-defining illness present Manifestations are variable, may include: Lymphadenopathy Mouth lesions Anemia or thrombocytopenia Neurological symptoms
Overt AIDS ($CD4^+$ is less than 200 cells/mcL and presence of at least one AIDS-defining illness)	Wasting syndrome (10% or greater weight loss; may also include fevers, general weakness, diarrhea) (see Fig. 7–12) Neurological symptoms: Dementia, tremors, encephalitis Malignancies and opportunistic infections/conditions Increasing debilitation and severe fatigue Lymphadenopathy Pharyngitis

Data partially from Gould (2006).

Diagnosis of HIV

Laboratory testing to diagnose HIV infection relies predominantly on the presence of the antibody to antigen p24, a major protein found in HIV. The p24 protein is an antigen that is capable of triggering a detectable immune system response to HIV. Antibodies to the p24 antigen can be detected in the blood using several testing methods, such as polymerase chain reaction (PCR). However, these tests are prohibitively expensive as primary screening tools for adults. They can, however, be useful in detecting the virus during the latency period, or in cases in which antibody tests are not conclusive. PCR is generally used only as a first-line diagnostic tool in infants.

When HIV exposure is suspected, a screening test using the enzyme-linked immunosorbent assay (ELISA) is usually repeated at three- and six-month intervals. If the screening test becomes positive or questionable, a Western blot test is performed. This can be accomplished with a blood sample or through a sample of

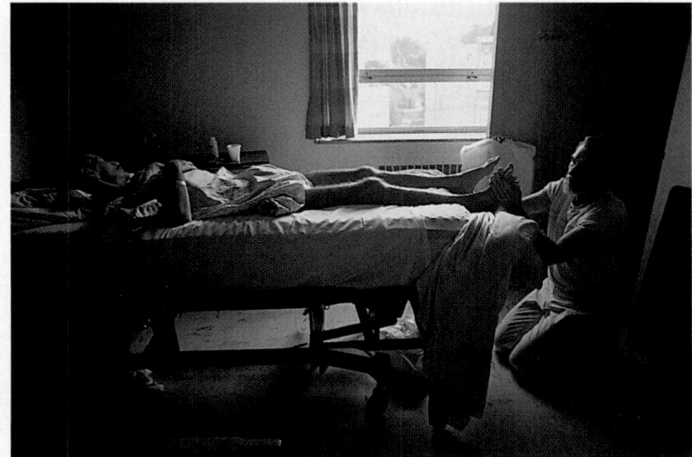

Figure 7–12 ■ HIV-AIDS patient with wasting disease. Reprinted from LeMone, P. & Burke, K. *Medical–Surgical Nursing* (4th ed., p. 353). © 2008, with permission from Pearson Education, Inc., Upper Saddle River, New Jersey.

oral mucosa transudate. The noninvasive oral saliva test is thought to be as reliable as blood tests using the regular Western blot. The enzyme-linked immunosorbent assay (ELISA) is 95 to 99 percent accurate in identifying the presence of an antibody. A false-positive ELISA result can occur as a result of cross-reactive antibodies to HLA antigens, hepatic disease, gamma globulin injections, and some malignancies. A positive ELISA must be confirmed with another antibody-reliant test known as the Western blot test. A confirmed diagnosis of HIV requires:

- Two positive ELISA tests AND
- One positive Western blot test

Specialized Tests

Serum Lymphocytes. Periodic testing of serum lymphocytes is a valuable tool for monitoring the progress or effectiveness of therapy in HIV/AIDS and autoimmune diseases. This test (also called lymphocyte marker studies) allows measurement of the subsets of lymphocytes, the T and B cells. Normally, T cells comprise about 60 to 80 percent of the total lymphocyte count and B cells comprise about 4-16 percent (Kee, 2005).

CD4+ (T4, helper T cells, T_H). Periodic testing of the CD4+ (every three to six months) helps monitor the immune system status in regard to the body's fight against an immune system damaging disease such as HIV. Normally, CD4+ cells comprise about 40 percent of T cells.

Viral Load Count. Like the CD4+ count, regular testing of the viral load monitors the progress of the disease. The viral load is a measurement of plasma HIV RNA. Once seroconversion occurs, the viral load diminishes significantly until the patient moves into the progressive (symptomatic) phase of HIV/AIDS at which time, viral load increases and CD4+ counts decrease.

Viral Hepatitis Testing. The risk factors for development of HIV/AIDS are essentially the same as those of HBV and HCV. Many patients who are positive for HIV also are positive for viral hepatitis (particularly HCV); thus, viral hepatitis testing is common.

CD8 (T8, cytotoxic T cells, T_C) Counts. The HIV virus also has an affinity for CD8+ cells but to a lesser extent than its attraction to CD4+ cells. As HIV disease progresses, the phenotype of CD8+ cells changes, causing impaired cytotoxic cell function. A CD4+-to-CD8+ (CD4:CD8) ratio is sometimes measured. Normally, the ratio is greater than one but as HIV/AIDS progresses toward AIDS, the ratio lowers significantly.

Treatment

To date, there is no predictable course of curative treatment, and the AIDS mortality rate continues to be approximately 95 percent for symptomatic individuals. Two variables that predict outcomes (i.e., time to AIDS or time to death) include viral load and CD4+ count.

Treatments for HIV/AIDS can be divided into four broad categories: antiretroviral therapy, treatment for opportunistic infections and malignancies, prophylaxis of opportunistic infections, and hematopoietic stimulating factors (Zolopa & Katz, 2008).

Various approaches to treatment have been theorized and tested. Restoration of immune function has been attempted by bone marrow transplant, transfusions of white blood cells, and interferon treatments. Unfortunately, the newest healthy cells are quickly infected by the virus. The structure of HIV is so variable (much like the variations of flu virus) that a medication formulated against one genetic mutation of the virus may not provide protection against other strains.

Antiviral Therapy

Pharmacological approaches using combination antiretroviral therapy rather than monotherapy (one drug) have been successful in maintaining viral load suppression and in treating AIDS as a long-term chronic disease in adults. Antiviral therapy, known as highly active antiretroviral therapy (HAART), can reduce the viral replication but cannot kill the virus (Gould, 2006). With HAART, combinations of three to five drugs in a "cocktail" are used to prolong the asymptomatic phase as well as to reduce the viral load in the overt AIDS phase (Gould, 2006). Viral suppression is considered effective when it is less than 400 to 500 copies/mL. Rising viral load indicates disease progression (5,000 to 10,000 copies/mL) as do falling $CD4^+$ levels (less than 500 cells/mcL) (Kee, 2005).

HAART has become a mainstay of treatment management for patients with HIV/AIDS. The optimal time to begin HAART has not been clearly established, and there are multiple factors to consider before initiating therapy. However, general treatment guidelines suggest beginning HAART for asymptomatic HIV disease when the $CD4^+$ cell count drops below 350 cells/mcL, or for symptomatic HIV disease (Zopola & Katz, 2008). A critical aspect of HAART is the importance of continuing the drug therapy without interruption to reduce the chance of developing drug resistance. Antiretroviral drug resistance is one of the most difficult challenges in HIV management.

Incomplete HIV suppression can result in HIV resistance to treatment; therefore, long-term, uninterrupted antiviral therapy is required for HIV inhibition. HAART drugs have a host of troubling short- and long-term side effects, such as peripheral neuropathy, gastrointestinal distress, rash, and hyperlipidemia, which can significantly impact compliance (Hollander, 2005). Patients may need adherence support through the use of pill organizer boxes and prompts, supportive counseling, or daily supervision of therapy (Zopola & Katz, 2008). Furthermore, there are many adverse effects associated with HAART therapy. In combination, the antivirals can be extremely toxic to the organs and bone marrow; thus, close monitoring of organ and bone marrow function is necessary.

The ideal combination of HAART is not clear, but the current standard of care involves a regimen of using at least three drugs simultaneously from at least two of the following different pharmacologic classes (Zolopa & Katz, 2008):

- Nucleoside and nucleotide reverse transcriptase inhibitors (NRTI)
- Non-nucleoside reverse transcriptase inhibitors (NNRTI)
- Protease inhibitors (PI)
- Entry inhibitors

New classes of drugs, such as the integrase inhibitors, are in development and the tech-pharmacologic management of HIV/AIDS will continue to evolve. Table 7–8 provides an example of a four drug HAART approach to therapy.

Drug prophylaxis protocols for opportunistic infections of HIV/AIDS have shown promise in delaying or avoiding

TABLE 7–8 Example of HAART Therapy

ANTIVIRAL DRUG	CLASSIFICATION
Lopinavir	Protease inhibitor (PI)
Ritonavir	Protease inhibitor (PI)
Zidovudine	Nucleoside reverse transcriptase inhibitor (NRTI)
Lamivudine	Nucleoside reverse transcriptase inhibitor (NRTI)

symptomatic infections. The goal of primary prophylaxis is to avoid or delay the onset of disease symptoms, and secondary prophylaxis seeks to prevent or delay recurrent symptomatic infection. Other treatment approaches are symptomatic, and still others continue to be under experimental investigation.

The most common infectious manifestation of the immunosuppressed HIV patient is *Pneumocystis jiroveci* pneumonia (PJP) and its recurrence. This type of pneumonia was originally called *Pneumocystis carinii* pneumonia (PCP); however, the name was changed to denote the specific form found in humans. This disease was one of the first opportunistic infections to be identified as an AIDS-defining illness. Since its prevalence in the AIDS population has been followed, it continues to be the most life-threatening opportunistic infection to both adult and pediatric AIDS patients. Although the PJP organism is not considered particularly pathogenic in the immunocompetent individual, its virulence increases as the T_H cell ($CD4^+$) count falls below 200 cells/mcL in the adult and 1,500 cells/mcL in the child. The infected patient presents with fever, fatigue, and weight loss months before actual respiratory symptoms develop. Coughing, shortness of breath, hypoxemia, and abnormal pulmonary function studies contribute to the clinical picture of progressive illness. Prophylaxis therapy for PJP is indicated when the $CD4^+$ cell count falls below 200 to 300 cells/mcL in the adult HIV-1 patient. Typical preventive and treatment therapy for PJP includes trimethoprim-sulfamethoxazole (TMP-SMX, Bactrim, and Septra) or an aerosol of pentamidine.

Prevention of other opportunistic infections such as toxoplasmosis, tuberculosis, *Mycobacterium avium* complex (MAC), cytomegalovirus (CMV), and fungi is crucial, and with the advent of HAART the need for prophylaxis therapy is largely guided by the patient's CD4 count (Zolopa & Katz, 2008). High-priority vaccine recommendations include pneumonia and influenza. Other vaccines, such as measles, mumps, and rubella (MMR) and chicken pox (varicella zoster), may be contraindicated because of their imposed risk as live viruses. Granulocyte stimulants, such as filgrastim (Neupogen), may be given to counteract the neutropenia related to antiretroviral therapy or to the HIV itself.

Holistic Care

It is critical to holistically support the patient and caregivers coping with HIV/AIDS along the illness trajectory. Counseling should be offered at time of screening, and continue as needed. Despite advances in the management of HIV/AIDS, it remains an illness with a significant symptom burden, both physically and emotionally, and, unfortunately, lingering societal stigma. Not all patients with HIV/AIDS have access to care or the expensive drugs needed to manage their illness, and this reality, along with the growing numbers of infected individuals, will present challenges for our global health care community.

HIV Exposure in the Health Care Professional. Although relatively few health care professionals are at risk for HIV, treatment approaches and protocols for occupational exposure to needle sticks, blood and body fluids, or contaminated instruments have been developed. Post-exposure prophylaxis protocols include determining the source and severity of the exposure, determining HIV status of the source, and recommendations for treatment. The risk of acquiring HIV infection from a needle stick with infected blood is approximately 1:300 (Zolopa & Katz, 2008). It is important to remember that the HIV virus is fragile, is easily destroyed by chemical disinfectants, and cannot survive outside of the human body. A basic post-exposure prophylactic (PEP) regimen begins within hours (not days) after exposure and includes either a two- or three-drug HAART combination for four weeks (CDC, 2005). The most up-to-date PEP recommendations and protocols can be found on the Centers for Disease Control (CDC) website, www.cdc.gov.

SECTION FOUR REVIEW

1. Immunodeficiency originating from embryonic anomaly, genetic predisposition, or congenital failure is categorized as
   - **A.** primary
   - **B.** secondary
   - **C.** acute
   - **D.** chronic
2. Which statement best characterizes HIV disease?
   - **A.** Symptoms result from opportunistic pathology.
   - **B.** HIV invades cells only through the bloodstream
   - **C.** Clinical manifestations are in a characteristic and predictable sequence.
   - **D.** People testing positive for HIV are carriers and contagious.
3. Fluids known to be modes of transmission for HIV include
   - **A.** tears
   - **B.** perspiration
   - **C.** plasma
   - **D.** saliva
4. AIDS-defining illnesses include (choose all that apply)
   - **A.** PJP
   - **B.** CMV
   - **C.** MAC
   - **D.** Rubella (measles)
5. Hepatitis B (HBV) testing may be conducted at the time of HIV testing for which reason?
   - **A.** Low CD4+ cell levels increase the risk for HBV.
   - **B.** Risk factors of HIV are the same as for HBV and HCV.
   - **C.** The HIV virus can bind with HBV virus.
   - **D.** Active HBV makes CD4+ cells more vulnerable.

Answers: 1. A, 2. A, 3. C, 4. (A, B, C), 5. B

SECTION FIVE: Aging, Malnutrition, Stress, Trauma, and the Immune System

At the completion of this section, the learner will be able to describe the effects of aging, malnutrition, stress, and trauma related to the functions of the adult immune system.

The immune system has an amazing ability to protect against many insults; however, it is also a vulnerable system that is significantly altered by certain factors such as aging, malnutrition, stress, and trauma. This section provides a brief overview of how these four factors alter immune system function.

Aging

The functionality of the immune system declines with age. The thymus gland, where T lymphocytes mature and differentiate, begins to atrophy early in life and continues to shrink until a person reaches middle age. Although T lymphocytes continue to be produced, their maturation and differentiation into the various functional T cells (e.g., T helper [T_H] cells) decreases. This places the older patient at higher risk for increased frequency and severity of infections accompanied by a decreased ability to resolve the infection. Macrophages continue to function throughout life; however, the length of time it takes them to clear the pathogens significantly increases with age. The ability of the immune system to discriminate between antigens that are "self" from those that are "nonself" also declines with aging, which increases the incidence of autoimmune diseases by middle age and older. In addition, the immune system also becomes significantly less efficient at recognizing and destroying mutated (tumor) cells, which at least partially accounts for the increased incidence of cancer in the older adult. B lymphocyte response to antigens also declines in cell numbers and efficacy with aging. Production of the immunoglobulin IgM decreases; however, production of IgA and IgG increases, possibly related to autoantibody responses to self-antigens.

Malnutrition

Although nutritional deficiencies can occur at any age, the older adult, particularly the frail elderly, are at particular risk. Many factors can contribute to the development of malnutrition in this patient population, including decreased appetite, loss of social supports, decreased accessibility to grocery stores, and impaired functional status. The possibility of malnutrition should be considered by the nurse whenever an acutely ill older adult is admitted because it can have a profound impact on the immune system, and subsequently on the patient's overall prognosis. Basic components of calorie and protein intake play key roles in the formation and integrity of T cells and immunoglobulins (antibodies). Malnutrition contributes to immunocompromise by causing impaired response of lymphocytes to pathogens, to vaccines, and to components of defense, such as the complement and macrophage functions (Gould, 2006). Zinc plays a major role in the structure and function of both B cells and T cells and in collagen synthesis for wound healing. As a cofactor, zinc is required for the normal function of lymphocytes in their production of enzymes. Although zinc deficiencies are rare in those with regular diets, there can be significant loss through the gastrointestinal tract with malabsorption syndromes or inflammatory bowel disease. It also can be lost through the skin in burn victims. Vitamins, such as A, E, pyridoxine, folic acid, and pantothenic acid, serve as cofactors in enzyme production and, in malnourished states, can affect the function of both T cells and B cells.

Malnutrition is also believed to contribute to sepsis as the malnourished gut becomes atrophied and more permeable to bacteria following trauma. When bacteria seep out of the gut, immune system mediators are released and trigger systemic lymphocyte activity. Tumor necrosis factor (TNF), a major immune mediator, is primarily responsible for precipitating multiple organ dysfunction syndrome (MODS). Early enteral feedings, which prevent gut atrophy in the acutely ill patient, can prevent sepsis by reducing circulating immune mediators and subsequent multiple organ dysfunction in the critically ill patient (Gould, 2006).

Stress

Stress affects the immune system primarily through the effects of cortisol. During periods of stress, either physical or psychological, the adrenal glands produce more cortisol in response to perceived need. However, cortisol has a direct suppressing effect on the immune system. Normally, when an antigen enters the body, a series of reactions takes place: the antigen is recognized as non-self; it is presented to T cells by macrophages; the macrophages secrete interleukin-1 (IL-1), which activates helper T cells; these helper T cells produce interleukin-2 (IL-2), which stimulates more T cell production; and finally, B cells may be stimulated to program antibodies to the antigen. Cortisol inhibits the production of IL-1 and IL-2, thus decreasing the T cell response and the subsequent B cell response.

Trauma

Trauma, both intentional (such as surgery/anesthesia) and unintentional (such as burns, motor vehicle crashes, and falls), suppresses T cell and B cell activity and compromises immune function (Gould, 2006). Trauma can cause cellular dysfunction, characterized by decreased chemotactic and phagocytic activities and decreased antibody and lymphocyte levels (Gould, 2006). Impaired T cell activity and depressed lymphokines have been linked to multiple organ dysfunction and poor clinical outcomes in the trauma patient (Gould, 2006). Although the degree of immunosuppression directly correlates with the severity of the injury, the cause for such changes is not fully understood. Hypovolemic shock has also been found to decrease antigen-specific antibody production, cellular immunity, and macrophage function for approximately two weeks following hemorrhage (Gould, 2006). The high-acuity trauma patient enters the intensive care unit immunosuppressed from the outset because of a stress response to the injury, hemorrhage, and shock. Subsequent malnutrition, organ dysfunction, hypoxia, and multiple invasive procedures all create a potential scenario of vulnerability to pathogens.

SECTION FIVE REVIEW

1. What is the function of zinc in the competent immune system?
   - **A.** It is required for normal lymphocyte function.
   - **B.** It protects B cells from being destroyed by macrophages.
   - **C.** T cells require zinc for production of gamma globulin.
   - **D.** Macrophages are composed primarily of zinc.
2. What effect does the normal aging process have on the immune system?
   - **A.** B cell function in general is particularly depressed.
   - **B.** T cells begin to deteriorate in functioning.
   - **C.** Autoantibodies begin to diminish with increasing age.
   - **D.** The immune system becomes hypervigilant to invading organisms.
3. In the acutely ill adult, which of the following nutritional losses is a critical factor in immune system integrity?
   - **A.** iron
   - **B.** vitamin C
   - **C.** complex carbohydrate chains
   - **D.** protein
4. Stress primarily affects the immune system through the effects of
   - **A.** lymphokines
   - **B.** interleukin
   - **C.** cortisol
   - **D.** epinephrine

Answers: 1. A, 2. B, 3. D, 4. C

SECTION SIX: Care of the Immunocompromised Patient

At the completion of this section, the learner will be able to discuss nursing considerations pertinent to the assessment and care of the immunocompromised patient.

Focused Assessment

The physical examination for level of immunocompetence primarily reflects the patient's nutritional status because the proper functioning of the immune system depends on nutritional status. Consequently, if the patient is malnourished, the immune status will be negatively affected. Physical assessment techniques and critical thinking must be focused on seeking evidence of infection, either acute or chronic. This includes assessing for skin lesions, open wounds, the presence of adventitious breath sounds and abnormal sputum, enlarged liver or spleen, or palpable lymph nodes or masses.

Nursing History

The patient history gives important clues to possible altered immunocompetence. Carpenito-Moyet (2008) suggests obtaining the following historical data:

- Complaints of fever, fatigue, weakness, swollen glands, lightheadedness, visual disturbances
- Loss of appetite and weight loss
- Slow wound healing history
- Unexplained rashes, mouth sores, or oral patches
- Presence of increased levels of stress, infection, malignancy, or autoimmune disease
- History of exposure to infectious diseases
- Changes in menstrual patterns, unusual bleeding or bruising (reflective of platelet dysfunction)
- Recent use of immunosuppressant drugs
- Allergy history
- Burn injury
- Exposure to work environment chemicals
- At-risk factors for development of HIV/AIDS
  - Homosexual orientation or sexual partner of homosexual orientation
  - Transfusion of blood or blood products
  - IV illegal drug users or sexual partner of drug user
  - Child born of mother with AIDS
- Family history of autoimmune disorders or cancer

Immunocompetence in the High-Acuity Patient

The high-acuity patient is at high risk for development of immunocompetence problems secondary to prolonged stress, severe infections, malnutrition, diabetes, and other problems. The nurse must monitor the patient for critical cues that suggest altered immune function. Some of these major critical cues include the presence of:

- Fever
- Poor wound healing
- Joint pain
- White oral patches
- Level of consciousness and mental status changes
- Abnormal complete blood count (CBC) with differential
- Abnormal coagulation studies
- Recurrent, prolonged, or severe infections
- Secondary infections
    - Other at-risk factors, such as splenectomy, diabetes mellitus, chronic alcohol abuse, malnutrition, or renal failure
- Immunosuppressive drug therapy, such as corticosteroids or cytotoxic drugs

Laboratory Findings

Laboratory testing is the major diagnostic tool for establishing immune status. Tests may include common ones, such as the WBC with differential and total lymphocyte count (TLC) as well as tests establishing nutritional status, such as serum albumin or prealbumin. These tests are relatively inexpensive and easy to perform and are used as screening tests for general immune status. The nurse should be able to monitor these levels for abnormal trends.

A variety of cell-specific and disorder-specific laboratory tests are available if further evaluation of immunocompetence is necessary. Many of these tests, however, are both time consuming and expensive. Immunoglobulins, T cells, and B cells can be measured both quantitatively and functionally. Skin testing may be ordered to evaluate cellular immunocompetence. Protein and immunoglobulin levels through electrophoresis can help detect diseases associated with excess or deficient immune function. The ELISA can show exposure to HIV, to rheumatoid factor, and to lupus cells (Kee, 2005).

Emerging Evidence

- In a retrospective study of 90 patients with acute leukemia who were admitted to an intensive care unit (none were status post stem-cell transplant), the major reason for admission was pulmonary distress. Most of those admitted (68 percent) required mechanical ventilation and half required vasopressor therapy. During the course of their ICU stay, 32 percent improved and resumed leukemic management; 27 percent survived through discharge from the hospital. The 12-month overall survival was 16 percent. Predictors of poor outcomes were: higher APACHE II scores, pressor use, ongoing stem-cell transplantation preparation; and cytogenetics issues (*Thakkar, Sweetenham, Mciver, et al, 2008*).
- In a review of retrospective studies of HIV patients, the incidence of thromboembolism (VTE) was 1 percent to 2 percent, which is 10 times what is expected in people who do not have HIV disease. Recent hospitalization was the primary risk factor found for development of VTE in this patient population (*Ahonkhai, Gebo, Streiff et al., 2008*).
- In a case report of six patients who developed anaphylactic shock, vasopressin was required to stabilize hemodynamic status after more traditional therapy (epinephrine, IV fluids, discontinuing of trigger) failed to reduce the process. The authors concluded that vasopressin may play a pivotal role when anaphylactic shock is refractory to other therapy (*Schummer, Wirsing et al., 2008*).
- In a review of medical records of 39 patients who presented to the hospital with food-induced anaphylaxis, 16 percent required a second dose of epinephrine to relieve symptoms. Patients requiring two doses had developed anaphylaxis from peanut or tree nut exposure, and had experienced hypotension. The authors concluded that additional studies are needed to determine whether two doses of epinephrine rather than one dose should be carried by individuals with severe food-induced allergies (*Oren, Banerji, & Camargo, 2007*).
- A prospective study investigated adverse reactions to N-acetylcysteine (NAC) during treatment of acetaminophen overdose. The study examined the relationship between serum acetaminophen concentration and the occurrence of NAC reaction. Patients with higher serum acetaminophen levels had a lower incidence of NAC anaphylactoid reaction, suggesting that acetaminophen may have some protective quality (*Waring, Stephen et al., 2008*).

Nursing Management

General Goals

The goals for care of the immunocompromised patient include the goals appropriate to the malnourished patient. Additional goals include reestablishing immunocompetence and preventing and treating complications.

Collaborative Interventions

1. **Laboratory testing.** Various tests may be ordered to evaluate immune status. Initially, a CBC with differential count is usually obtained. Because many of the cell-specific blood tests are not commonly performed and are both expensive and time consuming to obtain or measure, the nurse should clarify nursing responsibilities and expectations regarding the tests before drawing samples or having them drawn to prevent nursing error.
2. **Drug therapy.** Two types of drugs have a direct impact on the immune system: immunosuppressive therapy agents and agents that enhance immunity. Immunosuppressants decrease immune function. Uses include control of chronic inflammatory problems, prevention of organ transplant rejection, and others. Examples of immunosuppressant drugs are steroids and cyclosporin A. Drugs that enhance immune function in some way include immunotherapy agents, primarily used in cancer therapy; monoclonal antibodies, antibodies that act against specific antigens; and interleukin, a lymphokine used to enhance immune responses.
3. **Environmental protection.** Severe leukopenia places the patient at high risk for infection. The severely immunocompromised patient is placed in a controlled environment. Hospitals have protocols establishing the exact nature of the environmental protection. A private room is ordered. Some hospitals have special positive airflow rooms that diminish airflow of possibly contaminated air into the protected patient's room.

Independent Nursing Interventions

When caring for the immunocompromised patient, the nurse's role centers around monitoring for and preventing infection, regaining or maintaining adequate nutrition, and meeting the psychosocial needs of the patient and family. Remember that the severely neutropenic (agranulocytosis) patient will not be able to muster a normal immune response, which significantly alters the clinical findings. For example, the inability to form pus (a by-product of normal neutrophil activity) significantly reduces common infection findings, such as

- Cloudy urine
- Purulent sputum and adventitious breath sounds
- Purulent wound drainage

Patient and family teaching to prevent and recognize infection is essential. Monitoring for infection should focus on the mucous membranes, skin, and lungs, which are the most common sites of infection in this patient population.

Oral complications associated with severe neutropenia negatively impact the patient's ability to take in nutrition. Common oral complications include infection-related fungal infection, mouth ulcers, and **stomatitis** (inflammation of any or all of the oral mucous membranes [i.e., tongue, gums, pharynx, lips, and cheeks]). Oral complications are common nursing management problems when working with severely immunocompromised patients that can compromise the patient's ability to take in oral nutrition.

The two nursing diagnoses that apply to problems of infection and nutrition are:

- *High risk for infection:* related to deficient immune protection
- *Alteration nutrition:* in less than body requirements

The box, NURSING CARE: The immunodeficient patient provides a summary of the nursing care related to infection and oral complications for a patient with immunodeficiency, including neutropenia. Be aware that many other nursing diagnoses are potentially applicable to the immunosuppressed patient based on individual physiologic and psychosocial needs. Some of the more common ones include the following:

- High risk for injury
- Anxiety
- Coping, ineffective individual
- Pain
- Knowledge deficit
- Powerlessness
- Activity intolerance
- Social isolation
- Self-care deficit

NURSING CARE: The Immunodeficient Patient

Expected Patient Outcomes and Related Interventions

Outcome 1: No evidence of infection[a]

Assess and compare to established norms, patient baselines, and trends.

Monitor patient every 2 to 4 hours for any signs and symptoms of infection.

Fever in the immunosuppressed patient – a persistent fever of 100.5°F (38 °C) or higher for more than 1 hour may be the only sign of infection (severe neutropenia).

Signs and symptoms of inflammation, such as pain, redness, heat, or swelling (some or all of these may be absent if neutrophils are too low).

Skin or mucous membrane lesions - Check all skin folds, mouth, and perianal area; check wounds, mucous membranes and skin fold areas for yeast invasion (white patches).

Gastrointestinal lesions - Check all stools for occult blood; monitor for diarrhea or constipation.

Genitourinary problems - Check urine for color, odor; monitor patient for pain or fever.

Respiratory - Monitor for adventitious breath sounds, cough, dyspnea, pain; early in the course of a pulmonary infection, the patient may only develop dyspnea, tachypnea, and fever.

Invasive line/tube sites - Observe all sites closely for signs or symptoms of actual or potential infection.

Institute measures to protect the patient environmentally

Place in private room; keep door closed

Screen all persons coming into contact with patient for signs and symptoms of infection; apply mask if respiratory infection is suspected or confirmed

Excellent hand washing before contact (gloves recommended)

Maintain strict aseptic technique for all sterile procedures

Minimize foods and objects brought into the room from outside environment: fresh fruits and vegetables may need to be washed or peeled before being taken into the room; flowers and vases with standing water may be restricted.

Special daily room cleaning with disinfectants is recommended.

[a] *Finding evidence of infection may be extremely difficult in severely immunosuppressed patients, as any signs and symptoms of infection may be delayed, subdued, or completely absent, making this goal a particular challenge for the caregiver.*

(continued)

NURSING CARE: (continued)

Provide ongoing protection against development of infection

- Monitor hydration status every shift.
- Turn every 1 to 2 hours.
- Skin care
  - Thorough bathing every day.
  - Keep skin clean and lubricated at all times.
- Keep linens clean and wrinkle free.
- Pulmonary exercises every 4 hours
  - Incentive spirometry, deep breathing
  - As ordered: percussion, postural drainage, vibration (percussion is contraindicated if coagulopathy exists)
- Minimize invasive procedures: no rectal temperatures or enemas and no injections.
- Protect against injury by instructing patient as follows:
  - No straining
  - No sharp objects: use electric razor
  - Report any infection signs and symptoms
  - Brush teeth with very soft bristle brush or toothette at least every 4 hours.
- Meticulous central line care (if present)
- Cook all foods thoroughly; no raw fruits or vegetables

Institute measures that foster drug regimen compliance

- Clarify critical importance of regimen to prevent development of drug resistance.
- Tailor medication regimen to patient lifestyle.
- Direct observation, as needed.
- Help patient and family plan ahead for changes in routine.

Administer related drug therapy and monitor for therapeutic and nontherapeutic effects

- G-CSF (Filgrastim) therapy (cytokine therapy to decrease severity of symptoms and increase rate of neutrophil recovery from moderate-to-severe neutropenia) (Distenfeld, 2006)
- Antibiotic therapy, as ordered (For rapid control of infections; third-generation cephalosporin or equivalent) (Distenfeld, 2006)

Related Nursing Diagnoses:

High risk for infection related to deficient immune protection

Outcome 2: Maintain nutritional status

Assess and compare to established norms, patient baselines, and trends.

- Examine oral mucous membranes, tongue, and pharynx for fungal growths, ulcers, redness, and swelling at least every shift (more often if pain, ulcers, or fungal growths are present).
- Assess for presence and level of oral pain at least every shift and before meals (more often if pain is present).

Administer related drug therapy and monitor for therapeutic and nontherapeutic effects.

- Saline, hydrogen peroxide, or chlorhexidine mouth rinses every 3 to 4 hours
- Nystatin oral rinse every 6 hours (Q.I.D.) (If oral fungal infection is present.) If esophagitis is also present, nystatin can be swished and swallowed.
- Anesthetic throat lozenges, gels, or gargles

Perform actions to minimize oral pain at mealtime.

- Mouth care before mealtime
- Provide a liquid or soft food diet with frequent small meals.

Related Nursing Diagnoses:

Alteration in nutrition: Less than body requirements r/t oral pain

SECTION SIX REVIEW

1. Common patient complaints associated with altered immunocompetence include (choose all that apply)
   A. abnormal bleeding
   B. pain
   C. swollen glands
   D. fatigue

2. A severely immunocompromised hospitalized patient should receive environmental protection, including
   A. screening visitors for infection
   B. using bedding brought from home
   C. wearing clean gloves for dressing changes
   D. placement in semiprivate room with door closed

3. Nursing actions that provide ongoing protection against development of infection in a patient with neutropenia include
   A. restricting patient's fluid intake
   B. turning patient every one to two hours
   C. bathing patient every third day
   D. encouraging patient's use of incentive spirometer once per shift

Answers: 1. (A, C, D), 2. B, 3. B

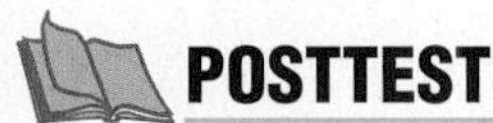

POSTTEST

Marian M., 32-years-old, presents at her primary care physician's office with complaints of recurrent fevers, chills, and malaise. Blood work is ordered, including a CBC with differential count. Lab results include: WBC, 2,600; segs, 15 percent; and bands, 20 percent.

1. Based on a calculation of her absolute neutrophil count (ANC) her grade of neutropenia (according to National Cancer Institute) would be
   A. 1
   B. 2
   C. 3
   D. 4

Marian reports that she just completed radiation therapy for treatment of ovarian cancer. Prior to that, she had received several rounds of cancer chemotherapy.

2. Based on her history, the most likely underlying cause of Marian's neutropenia is
   A. decreased production of neutrophils
   B. drug-induced hypersensitivity response destroying neutrophils
   C. premature destruction of neutrophils
   D. destruction of neutrophils by the spleen
3. If Marian's ANC continues to fall and drops below 500 cells, she would be at high risk for development of what complication of neutropenia?
   A. bone marrow failure
   B. sepsis
   C. splenomegaly
   D. liver dysfunction

Joseph P., 16-year-old, is brought into the clinic by his mother. He has a high fever associated with a persistent respiratory infection that has been treated multiple times with antibiotic therapy. His mother states that he is no longer able to play with his friends but lies on the couch or in a chair for most of the day. The nurse notes petechiae on Joseph's trunk and arms. He has had several episodes of epistaxis and bleeding gums that are difficult to control. A complete blood count (CBC) shows a pancytopenia present. Following further blood work, a diagnosis of acute lymphoblastic leukemia (ALL) is made.

4. The pancytopenia associated with Joseph's leukemia is caused by which problem of the bone marrow?
   A. crowding out of normal cells
   B. bone marrow failure
   C. proliferation of fatty tissue
   D. hemolysis by antigen–antibody complexes
5. Which of the following statements best reflects leukemic cell maturation?
   A. they mature at an accelerated rate
   B. they differentiate slower than normal cells
   C. they differentiate in an unpredictable manner
   D. they do not mature beyond the stage at which they are produced
6. Joseph's leukocyte count climbs to 105,000/mcL. He develops dyspnea, confusion, and severe headache. These manifestations are most consistent with which complication of leukemia?
   A. leukostasis
   B. severe neutropenia
   C. CNS infiltration
   D. bone marrow failure
7. Joseph is now receiving "consolidation" chemotherapy. The goal of this drug regimen is best described as
   A. production of a complete remission
   B. halting all bone marrow cell production
   C. elimination of leukemic cells from the CNS
   D. solidification of remission/elimination of remaining leukemic cells
8. An example of a type IV hypersensitivity reaction is
   A. blood transfusion reaction
   B. host transplant rejection
   C. allergic asthma
   D. Arthus reaction
9. Which of the following is commonly thought of as being an autoimmune phenomenon?
   A. transplant rejection
   B. polio
   C. *Pneumocystis jiroveci*
   D. ulcerative colitis
10. How do increased levels of cortisol released during stress affect the immune system?
    A. It increases the production of glycogen.
    B. Stimulation of T cell production is enhanced by cortisol.
    C. Cortisol inhibits the production of interleukin-1 and -2.
    D. Higher levels of cortisol cause accelerated production of immunoglobulins by B cells.
11. Zinc plays a major role in B cell and T cell production. For what reasons might an acutely ill adult have a zinc deficiency?
    A. third-space fluid deficit
    B. hyperosmolar dehydration
    C. prolonged periods of IV potassium replacement
    D. malabsorption syndromes with severe diarrhea
12. In what ways is the immune system compromised in the patient with extensive burns?
    A. Zinc levels may become dangerously high, with extensive epidermal loss.
    B. The patient's serum contains substances that suppress all immune functions.
    C. T cells are suppressed, but B cell activity and antibody production generally are unaffected.
    D. Dehydration creates an imbalance between humoral and cell-mediated immunity.
13. For which reason has HIV treatment been largely disappointing?
    A. Treatment against one genetic strain may not provide protection against other evolving strains.
    B. The virus does not attach to immunoglobulin antigenic sites as other antigens do.
    C. The HIV blocks the complement system.
    D. HIV invades B cells and sequesters itself from view of the body's immune system.

14. Why are individuals who receive specific blood components more at risk for acquiring HIV than the average person who receives whole blood or packed cell transfusion?

A. The screening procedures lack the sophistication of whole blood testing.

B. The risk increases with the large numbers of donors required to produce therapeutic amounts.

C. HIV is more difficult to detect in blood components than in whole blood or packed cells.

D. The virus attaches to large amounts of factor VIII and platelets.

15. The nurse should suspect an infection in an immunodeficient patient if the patient's temperature is above ______ for more than an hour.

A. 100°F (37.8°C)

B. 100.4°F (38°C)

C. 101°F (38.3°C)

D. 101.5°F (38.6°C)

16. A patient experiencing significant immunosuppression may develop which symptoms EARLY in the course of a pulmonary infection? (choose all that apply)

A. dyspnea

B. tachypnea

C. adventitious breath sounds

D. fever

Posttest answers with rationale are found on MyNursingKit.

REFERENCES

Ahonkhai, A., Gebo, K., Streiff, M., Moore, R., & Segal, J. (2008). Venous thromboembolism in patients with HIV/AIDS: a case-control study. *J Acquir Immune Defic Syndr, 48*(3), 310–314.

American Cancer Society. (2008). Accessed 10/30/08 at http://www.cancer.org.

Antoniadou, A. & Giamarellou, H. (2007). Fever of unknown origin in febrile leucopenia. *Infect Dis Clin N Am, 21,* 1055–1090.

Carpenito-Moyet, L. J. (2008). *Nursing diagnosis: application to clinical practice.* Philadelphia: Lippincott Williams & Wilkins.

Centers for Disease Control and Prevention (CDC). (1992). Revised classification system for HIV infection and expanded surveillance case definitions for AIDS among adolescents and adults. *MMWR, 41* RR 17–19. Available at http://www.cdc.gov/mmwr/preview/mmwrhtml/00018871.htm. Accessed on 3/29/08.

Centers for Disease Control and Prevention (CDC). (2005). Updated U.S. Public Health Service guidelines for the management of occupational exposures to HIV and recommendations for postexposure prophylaxis. *MMWR,* 2005; 54(No. RR09). Available at http://www.cdc.gov/mmwr/preview/mmwrhtml/rr5409a1.htm. Accessed on March 29, 2008.

Centers for Disease Control and Prevention (CDC). (2002). Guidelines for preventing opportunistic infections among HIV-infected persons. *MMWR, 52,* RR 08 1–46.

Copelan, E. (2006). Hematopoietic stem-cell transplantation. *New England Journal of Medicine,* 354(17), 1813–1826.

D'Antonio (2005). Chronic myelogenous leukemia. *Clinical Journal of Oncology Nursing,* 9(5), 535–538.

Distenfeld, A. (2006). Agranulocytosis. Available at http://www.emedicine.com/med/TOPIC82.HTM. Accessed on 7/18/08.

Gould, B. E. (2006). Immunity and abnormal responses. In B. E. Gould, *Pathophysiology for the health professions* (3rd ed., pp. 44–75). Philadelphia: W. B. Saunders.

Hollander, H. (2005). Signs, symptoms, and laboratory abnormalities in HIV disease. In R. Wachter, L. Goldman, & H. Hollander (eds.). *Hospital medicine* (2d ed., pp 719–727). Philadelphia: Lippincott, Williams & Wilkins.

Kee, J. L. (2005). *Laboratory and diagnostic tests with nursing implications* (7th ed.). Upper Saddle River, N.J.: Prentice Hall.

LeMone, P., & Burke, K. (2008). Nursing care of clients with altered immunity. In P. LeMone & K. Burke (eds.), *Medical-surgical nursing: critical thinking in client care* (4th ed., pp 328–367). Upper Saddle River, N.J.: Pearson/Prentice Hall.

Linker, C. (2008). Blood disorders. In S. McPhee, M. Papadakis, & L. Tierney (eds.), *Current medical diagnosis and treatment* (47th ed., pp. 439–450). New York: McGraw Hill Medical.

Moran, M., Browning, M. & Buckby, E. (2007). Nursing guidelines for managing infections in patients with chronic lymphocytic leukemia. *Clinical Journal of Oncology Nursing, 11*(6), 914–923.

NCI. (1999). Grading scale on neutropenia. National Cancer Institute. Available at: www.nci.nih.gov. Accessed on February 22, 2008.

NCCN and ACS. (2006). Fever and neutropenia: treatment guidelines for patients with cancer. Available at www.cancer.org/downloads/CRI/Fever. Accessed on May 9, 2008.

Nirenberg, A., Bush, A. P., Davis, A., Friese, C., Gillespie, T. W., Rice, R. D. (2005). Neutropenia: state of the knowledge Part I, *Oncology Nursing Forum, 33*(6), 1193–1208.

Oen, E. Banerji, A, Clark, S, & Camargo, C. (2007). Food-induced and repeated epinephrine treatments. *Annals of Allergy, Asthma & Immunology, 99*(5), 429–32.

Platts-Mills, T. (2006). Hypersensitivity type 1. In D. Male, J. Brostoff, D. Roth & I. Roitt (eds.), *Immunology* (7th ed., pp. 423–447). Edinburgh: Mosby.

Rizzieri, D., Long, G., & Chao, N. (2005). Leukemia. In Wachter, R., Goldman, L. & Hollander, H. (Eds.). *Hospital medicine* (2d ed., pp. 929–936). Philadelphia: Lippincott, Williams and Wilkins.

Seiter, K. (2006a). Acute lymphoblastic leukemia. Available at http://www.emedicine.com/med/TOPIC3146.HTM. Accessed on 10/30/08.

Seiter, K. (2006b). Acute myelogenous leukemia. Available at http://www.emedicine.com/med/topic34.htm. Accessed on 10/30/08.

Shummer, C., Wirsing, M., & Schummer, W. (2008). The pivotal role of vasopressin in refractory anaphylactic shock. *Anesthesia and Analgesia, 107*(2), 620–624.

Schwartzberg, L. S. (2006). Neutropenia: etiology and pathogenesis. *Clinical Cornerstone, 8,* (5): S5–S11.

Thakkar, S., Fu, A., Sweetenham, J., Mciver, A., Mohan, S., Ramsingh, G., Advani, A., Sobecks, R., Rybicki, L., Kalaycio, M., & Sekeres, M. (2008). Survival and predictors of outcome in patients with acute leukemia admitted to the intensive care unit. *Cancer, 112*(10), 2233–2240.

Waring, W., Stephen, A., Robinson, O., Dow, M., & Pettie, J. (2008). Lower incidence of anaphylactoid reactions to N-acetylcysteine in patients with high acetaminophen concentrations after overdose. *Clinical Toxicology, 46*(6), 496–500.

Zolopa, A. & Katz, M. (2008). HIV infection and AIDS. In S. McPhee, M. Papadakis & L. Tierney (eds.), *Current medical diagnosis and treatment* (47th ed., pp. 1150–1177). New York: McGraw Hill Medical.

MODULE

8 Alteration in Immune Response: Solid Organ and Hematopoietic Stem Cell Transplantation

Kathleen Dorman Wagner, Diana Thacker

OBJECTIVES Following completion of this module, the learner will be able to

1. Discuss the history of organ transplantation.
2. Describe types of grafts and donors.
3. Explain the general organ procurement process and organ procurement.
4. Discuss donor and organ management and organ preservation.
5. Explain the immunologic considerations of organ transplantation.
6. Describe the determination of transplant need.
7. Discuss the major complications associated with organ transplantation.
8. Discuss hematopoietic stem cell transplantation.
9. Describe immunosuppressant therapy for prevention of graft rejection.
10. Discuss the general concepts related to transplantation of selected organs, including postprocedure management implications.

This self-study module provides the learner with a broad picture of solid-organ transplantation and hematopoietic stem cell transplantation. The module is organized into two parts. As an introduction, Section One presents a brief history of solid organ transplantation.

The first part of this module, which is composed of Sections Two through Four, focuses on the organ donor. Section Two differentiates between the various types of grafts and donors and includes a brief summary of some of the major laws intended to protect the donor and establish procurement protocols. Section Three explains organ procurement and includes discussions of establishing brain death, suitability for organ donation, obtaining consent, and working with the family to obtain consent. It concludes with the typical sequence of events involved in the procurement process. Section Four discusses management of the donor prior to organ removal and organ preservation.

The second part of the module focuses on the organ recipient. Sections Five through Eight present specific recipient topics. Section Five explains immunologic considerations, such as histocompatibility and donor–recipient compatibility testing. Section Six describes how the need for an organ transplant is determined. Key concepts include determination of need and transplant recipient evaluation. Section Seven discusses posttransplantation complications, dividing them into three categories: technical, organ rejection, and immunosuppressant related. Section Eight presents an overview of hematopoietic stem cell transplantation, including types of grafts, the sources of hematopoietic stem cells, and the transplant procedure from preparation through posttransplantation management. Section Nine describes some of the major immunosuppressants currently in use for prevention of graft rejection. Finally, Section Ten paints a broad picture of selected organ transplants, including kidney, heart, heart–lung, liver, pancreas, pancreas–kidney, and small bowel. The discussion of each type of organ transplant includes major indications for transplantation, preparation of the recipient, postoperative management, and evaluation of organ function. Each section includes a set of review questions to help the learner evaluate his or her understanding of the section's content before moving on to the next section. All Section Reviews include answers. It is suggested that the learner review those concepts answered incorrectly in the review questions before proceeding to the next section.

PRETEST

1. The early focal point of interest for organ transplantation was the
   A. lung
   B. kidney
   C. heart
   D. liver
2. Skin grafts were first experimented with as a treatment for
   A. leg ulcers
   B. traumatic injury
   C. skin cancer
   D. burn injury

3. The specific term referring to transplantation between identical twins is
   A. isograft
   B. autograft
   C. heterograft
   D. allograft
4. Segmental (partial) live-organ donations are usually between
   A. identical twins
   B. husband and wife
   C. parent and child
   D. human and ape
5. Under what circumstance should the nurse refer a patient to the organ procurement coordinator when death is imminent?
   A. after the patient's heart stops
   B. after the patient is pronounced brain dead
   C. when the patient is admitted to the hospital
   D. when the Glasgow Coma Score is 6 or less
6. The major advantage of early notification of the organ procurement coordinator when a potential donor has been identified is that ______ can be initiated.
   A. family counseling
   B. life-support measures
   C. signing of the consent form
   D. preliminary evaluation for suitability
7. Major management goals for caring for the donor patient include which of the following? (choose all that apply)
   A. maintaining stable hemodynamic status
   B. maintaining infections at minimum level
   C. maintaining fluid and electrolyte balance
   D. maintaining optimal oxygenation status
8. The most common underlying cause of hypotension in the donor is
   A. dehydration
   B. cardiac failure
   C. fluid overload
   D. increased systemic vascular resistance
9. Histocompatibility antigens are also known as
   A. monocytes
   B. macrophages
   C. human leukocyte antigens
   D. polymorphonuclear lymphocytes
10. Human leukocyte antigens (HLAs) are important because they
    A. are the source of donor organ rejection
    B. indicate the degree of organ failure
    C. are identical only within the same species
    D. reflect the need for transplantation
11. General guidelines for determination of organ transplant need include which of the following? (choose all that apply)
    A. severe functional disability
    B. end-stage organ failure
    C. psychological readiness
    D. additional serious health problems
12. The decision as to whether a person is placed on the organ transplant waiting list as a potential recipient is usually made by
    A. the patient/family
    B. a multidisciplinary committee
    C. the organ procurement team
    D. the potential recipient's physician
13. Which of the following are examples of technical complications of organ transplantation? (choose all that apply)
    A. bleeding
    B. infection
    C. anastomosis leakage
    D. vascular thrombosis
14. Organ rejection that takes place within minutes to hours following transplantation and results from the presence of preformed graft-specific cytotoxic antibodies is called ______ rejection.
    A. subacute
    B. acute
    C. hyperacute
    D. chronic
15. Stem cell delivery into the recipient involves which process?
    A. injection of cells directly into the bone marrow
    B. intravenous transfusion of the stem cells
    C. multiple injections into various body parts
    D. surgical procedure whereby stem cells are directly implanted
16. The immunosuppressant that selectively acts against the helper T cells without affecting other types of immune cells is
    A. corticosteroids
    B. azathioprine
    C. cyclosporine
    D. OKT3
17. Long-term posttransplantation steroid therapy is particularly associated with potentially severe ______ disorders.
    A. bone
    B. heart
    C. liver
    D. blood
18. The major indication for kidney transplantation is end-stage renal disease, which most commonly results from which of the following? (choose all that apply)
    A. diabetes mellitus
    B. hypertension
    C. glomerular nephritis
    D. nephrotoxicity
19. Dysfunction of a renal graft is most commonly associated with the
    A. preoperative condition of the donor
    B. preoperative condition of the recipient
    C. length of time the organ was preserved
    D. length of time required to perform the transplant
20. Major conditions that are associated with the need for heart transplantation include (choose all that apply)
    A. myocardial infarction
    B. congenital malformations
    C. ventricular aneurysm
    D. cardiomyopathy
21. Major indications for liver transplantation include (choose all that apply)
    A. fulminant hepatic failure
    B. acute hepatotoxicity

C. malignant hepatic tumors
D. irreversible chronic liver disease

22. Liver transplant patients are at particularly high risk for development of which early complication?
A. hemorrhage
B. rejection
C. infection
D. obstruction

23. The most common complications in the immediate post-operative period of the pancreas transplant include (choose all that apply)
A. dehydration
B. metabolic acidosis
C. hyperinsulinemia
D. infection

23. The gold standard for diagnosing acute rejection in the intestinal transplant is a(n)
A. significant increase in stomal output
B. ileus
C. endoscopic mucosal biopsy
D. change in stomal color

Pretest answers are found on MyNursingKit.

SECTION ONE: Brief History of Organ Transplantation

At the completion of this section, the learner will be able to discuss the history of organ transplantation.

For centuries there have been attempts to **graft** body tissue—that is, to transfer it from one part of the body to a different part, or from another donor source. However, it was not until the dawn of the twentieth century that surgical skills and knowledge of immunology and immunosuppression became advanced enough to facilitate tissue survival following transplantation. This section highlights strategic events in the development of modern organ transplantation as described by Dr. Joseph Murray, a pioneer in transplantation (Murray, 1991).

1910 to 1930: The Beginnings

The kidney was the early focal point of interest for organ transplantation. Surgeons had struggled with young patients who, while otherwise healthy, were dying of end-stage renal failure. Prior to 1912, although there was interest in performing such transplants, surgeons had not yet developed a successful method of reconnecting the organ vasculature to make transplantation a feasible option. It was in 1912 that the Nobel Prize winner Dr. A. Carrel developed a landmark method of successfully suturing and transplanting blood vessels and organs. It was also during this period that animal research began exploring tissue survival following autografts and allografts.

1930 to 1950: In Search of Long-Term Success

In the early 1930s, experimentation in skin grafting as a treatment for burns contributed greatly to the advancement of transplantation knowledge. It was noted that, although no skin grafts survived for long, skin grafts from family member **donors** survived longer than those provided by nonfamily members. In 1937, it was discovered that skin grafting between identical twins could provide permanent graft survival. This discovery rekindled interest in organ and tissue replacement, although the reasons for tissue acceptance or **rejection**—the activation of the immune response against the transplanted tissue—were still unknown.

In the late 1940s renal transplantation programs began to develop in earnest. Following World War II, research began to focus on allograft rejection. A common antigen was discovered between kidney and skin allografts that would cause sensitization of a **recipient** for subsequent graftings. Scientists knew that for renal transplantation to be a feasible option they must find a way to get around the immunologic problems experienced thus far. By the end of the 1940s, transplanted kidneys were surviving for up to six months. Long-term organ transplant survival remained just out of reach.

1950 to 1960: The Isograft and Immunosuppressant Discovery Years

In 1954, the first **isograft**—a transplant occurring between identical human twins—took place. Tissue matching was performed by cross skin grafting between two twin brothers. The success of this isograft, a renal transplant, demonstrated that identical twins provided a method of bypassing the tissue incompatibility problem.

Research continued toward solving the problem of tissue incompatibility. Total body X-ray was performed experimentally as a means to depress the immune system. After the X-ray treatments were completed, bone marrow infusions were performed and the renal allograft transplant was completed. This method, however, had only marginal success in the short term and little success in the long term.

During this decade, research also focused on developing **immunosuppressants**—drugs that curb the body's immune response. In 1959, animal experimentation began using 6-mercaptopurine, an antimetabolite, with encouraging success. It was during the next year that azathioprine (Imuran) was introduced. Early use of azathioprine was associated with patient death from high-dose–related complications, although after the correct dose was established azathioprine was very successful during human clinical trials and continues to be a major form of immunosuppression therapy today. Not long after initiating the use of azathioprine, corticosteroids were introduced as adjunctive therapy.

In 1957, Dr. E. Donnall Thomas documented the first allogeneic hematopoietic marrow transplantations, which he performed on several patients with cancer (Applebaum, 2007). His initial attempts were not successful, primarily due to the lack of scientific knowledge at that time about **histocompatibility.** However, after years of research, by 1969 Dr. Thomas finally realized success by using well-matched sibling marrow in patients with leukemia.

1961 to 1979: The Expansion Years

The 1960s saw a rapid increase in transplant knowledge. Renal transplant survival rates increased dramatically. New forms of immunosuppressive therapy were discovered. Organ procurement programs were initiated, both regionally and nationally. There was great enthusiasm to take what was learned from the renal transplantation programs and expand it to transplantation of other organs.

The mid-to-late 1960s saw important expansion in organ transplantation, as it is during this period that pancreas/kidney, isolated pancreas, liver, and heart transplantation were first successful. Early attempts at heart transplantation did not have a high success rate. Cardiac transplantation is highly successful today, in part because of tissue typing and improved immunosuppressant therapy.

1980 to the Present

Following on the heels of successes in the area of cardiac transplantation, surgeons turned to perfecting the heart–lung, single-lung, and double-lung transplants in the early1980s. In 1989, a transplantation milestone was achieved with the first successful living-donor liver transplantation; and in 1990 the first successful living-donor lung transplant was performed.

SECTION ONE REVIEW

1. The early focal point of interest for organ transplantation was the
   A. kidney
   B. lungs
   C. heart
   D. liver
2. Skin grafts were first experimented with as a treatment for
   A. leg ulcers
   B. traumatic injury
   C. burn injury
   D. skin cancer
3. One of the earliest immunosuppressants to be successfully used on transplant patients was
   A. cyclosporine
   B. azathioprine
   C. corticosteroids
   D. 6-mercaptopurine
4. Early attempts at organ and hematopoietic cell transplantation failed for which underlying reason?
   A. use of nonhuman donors
   B. postoperative infections
   C. primitive surgical techniques
   D. lack of knowledge about histocompatibility

Answers: 1. A, 2. C, 3. B, 4. D

The Organ Donor

SECTION TWO: The Graft and Donor

At the completion of this section, the learner will be able to describe types of grafts and donors.

The term **graft** refers to the transfer of tissue from one part of the body to a different part, or from another donor source. There are three major types of grafts: the autograft, the heterograft, and the allograft.

The Autograft

The **autograft** is the transplantation of tissue from one part of a person's body to another part of the body. It is the ideal situation for tissue compatibility and graft survival. A common example of autografting is the skin autograft. For example, when a person receives severe burns, healthy tissue can be removed from an undamaged body area and transplanted over the burned area to promote healing and recovery. Autografting is not used for organ transplantation and thus will not be discussed further in this section.

The Heterograft

The **heterograft,** also called a **xenograft,** refers to transplantation of tissue between two different species. Examples of heterografts are porcine skin grafts and experimental baboon heart transplants. At this time, heterografts are primarily used as temporary transplantations until a permanent allograft becomes available. Tissue rejection occurs rapidly because of the dissimilarities of tissues between species.

The Allograft

The **allograft** (also known as *homograft)* refers to tissue that is transplanted between members of the same species. One form of allograft, the **isograft** or **syngraft,** refers to transplantation between identical twins. The allograft is the most common type of organ transplantation. With the exception of isografts, allografts trigger an immune reaction that will cause rejection of the graft. Allografts are obtained either from live or cadaver donors.

The Living Donor

The **living donor** is a person who volunteers to have an organ, part of an organ, or hematopoietic stem cells removed for transplantation into another person while still alive. Ideally, the living donor is related to the recipient as part of the immediate family (e.g., parents, siblings). Related donors are preferred because of increased histocompatibility and, therefore, longer graft life. When a related donor is not available, a nonrelated living donor is used. If an isograft (between identical twins) is used, no rejection is expected because the two tissues are completely histocompatible.

The kidney is the primary solid organ that is recovered in its entirety from a living donor. Segmental (partial) organ donation, such as one lobe of a liver or lung or part of the pancreas, is also performed using a living donor. Initially, segmental organ donation was primarily used for pediatric patients, often parent-donor to child-recipient. There is an increasing trend towards adult-to-adult living donors due to scarcity of whole organ resources, since the size of the organ waiting list continues to increase while the number of available donors has remained fairly constant. For example, the waiting list for liver transplantation (as of August, 8, 2008) was 16,712 while available donor livers over the same period of time was 2,974: 2,866 from cadavers and 108 from living donors (OPTN, 2008).

Murphy & Byrne (2007) explain that becoming a living donor is not without risk. For example, a living kidney donor may develop postoperative complications, such as infection and thromboembolism, and in some cases the donor has died. Furthermore, there have been cases where a live kidney donor has eventually developed disease of the remaining kidney, requiring a kidney transplant. Another concern relative to the live donor initiative in general is the potential for coercion or fear of rejection by family members if the donor refuses. It is important that the potential live donor and the recipient are both well informed of the risks and benefits associated with live organ transplantation.

The Cadaver Donor

The **cadaver donor** is one whose organs or tissues are recovered after death. Cadaver donors are most commonly healthy individuals who die as the result of a traumatic event or a sudden death. Cadaver donors comprise the majority of solid organ donors. Potential cadaver donors are initially evaluated for suitability. There are two types of potential cadaver donors: those who die of cardiac death and those who die of brain death.

Donors Who Die of Cardiac Death. Cardiac death refers to death by termination of cardiac and respiratory function. Transplantable tissues may be limited to heart valves, corneas, eyes, saphenous veins, skin, and bones. These tissues are to be recovered within 12 to 24 hours postdeclaration of death. On occasion, organs may be recovered following cardiac death. This must be initiated within minutes of cardiac arrest with the appropriate personnel available to complete the organ recovery.

Donors Who Die of Brain Death. Brain death refers to the cessation of the entire brain and brainstem function. Loss of brainstem function destroys the vital centers for blood pressure, temperature, and respiratory control, making cardiopulmonary death imminent. Organ donations resulting from brain death comprise the majority of cadaver organs. Transplantable tissues from this group of donors include tissues as well as solid organs, such as the kidneys, lungs, heart, liver, pancreas, and small bowel. Strict laws and formal procurement protocols have been established to protect the potential donor's rights.

Legal Aspects of Donation and Transplantation

Many laws are in place at both the national and state levels to protect the potential organ donor and to organize and facilitate organ procurement and distribution. The following are examples of some of this legislation in the United States.

Uniform Anatomical Gift Act

The Uniform Anatomical Gift Act (UAGA) authorizes the donation of all or part of the human body following death for a variety of uses (research, transplantation, and education). The act also includes guidelines regarding who can donate, how donation is to be carried out, and who can receive the organ donation. The act provides for the donor card as a means for individuals to convey their desire to be donors. The act also includes liability protection for health care providers. All states have passed the UAGA.

Required-Request Legislation

A section of the UAGA, called "Routine Inquiry and Required Request; Search and Notification," stipulates hospitals responsibilities toward identifying potential donors and providing donor information to families to make them aware of their opportunities to donate. Hospitals that do not comply with the required-request stipulations may be open to penalties or administrative actions.

National Organ Transplant Act

The National Organ Transplant Act set up the National Organ Procurement and Transplantation Network (OPTN). The OPTN establishes national registries to track potential recipients and posttransplantation organ recipients. It also provides for a national system to match organs and potential recipients. In addition, the act prohibits selling of human organs and tissues. This act has been adopted in all 50 states.

Uniform Determination of Death Act

The Uniform Determination of Death Act has been enacted as a guideline for states to establish a legal definition of death. Most states have adopted some form of this act. For example, in Kentucky, KRS 446.400: Determination of death; minimal conditions to be met, states:

> For all legal purposes, the occurrence of human death shall be determined in accordance with the usual and customary standards of medical practice, provided

that death shall not be determined to have occurred unless the following minimal conditions have been met: (1) When respiration and circulation are not artificially maintained, and there is a total and irreversible cessation of spontaneous respiration and circulation; or (2) When respiration and circulation are artificially maintained, and there is a total and irreversible cessation of all brain function, including the brain stem and that such determination is made by two licensed physicians.

Medicare Conditions of Participation

Enacted in 1998, two bills (A-0369 and JCAHO 42 CFR 482.110) established guidelines that specifically address the responsibilities of hospitals toward notifying and working with their organ procurement organization (OPO). Specifically, hospitals must report all deaths and imminent deaths to the OPO in a timely manner. If the OPO finds a patient meets criteria for organ donation, the hospital is to ensure that the family is offered the donation option. Those who communicate with the family about donation must be employed by the OPO or have received training from the OPO on best practices for donation communication. Care must be provided to the donor to allow for donation to occur while testing and placement of organs and tissues take place. Death record reviews are completed collaboratively by the OPO and hospital, and the OPO provides education to the hospital as needed. In addition, if the hospital performs organ transplants, data must be submitted to the Secretary of Health and Human Services when requested. Providing patient information to OPOs is not in violation of patient confidentiality, since OPOs are HIPAA-exempt. The OPOs, however, are still held to a standard of confidentiality in regard to patient information.

SECTION TWO REVIEW

1. Tissue that is transplanted between members of the same species is the definition of
   A. autograft
   B. heterograft
   C. xenograft
   D. allograft
2. The specific term referring to transplantation between identical twins is
   A. isograft
   B. autograft
   C. heterograft
   D. allograft
3. Segmental (partial) live-organ donations are usually between
   A. identical twins
   B. husband and wife
   C. parent and child
   D. human and ape
4. The major legislation that authorizes the donation of all or part of the human body following death is called the
   A. National Organ Transplant Act
   B. Uniform Anatomical Gift Act
   C. Uniform Determination of Death Act
   D. Omnibus Reconciliation Act

Answers: 1. D, 2. A, 3. C, 4. B

SECTION THREE: Organ Procurement

At the completion of this section, the learner will be able to explain the general organ procurement process.

The specific procedures used to procure and distribute organs differ among transplant programs and organizations. This section will provide information regarding the procurement process in general.

Establishing Death

The Uniform Determination of Death Act defines how death is determined. Death can either be pronounced by cardiac standstill criteria or brain death criteria. Each state legislates specific criteria to be met for a death pronouncement. An example is Kentucky's legislation (KRS 446.440):

> When artificial respiration and circulation are not maintained and there is irreversible cessation of spontaneous respiration and circulation (Cardiac Standstill Death).
>
> When respiration and circulation are artificially maintained and there is total and irreversible cessation of all brain and brain stem function (Brain Death). Two licensed physicians must determine brain death.

When cardiac standstill occurs, tissue donation is possible. Tissues that can be recovered include corneas; eyes; skin from anterior and posterior torso, buttocks, and thighs; bone from the upper and lower extremities; leg veins; heart for valves; and mandible. Tissues must be recovered within 12 to 24 hours of cardiac standstill.

When brain death occurs, both organs and tissues can be donated. Organ recovery can include heart, lungs, liver, pancreas, small bowel, and kidneys. Organ perfusion and oxygenation must be maintained to allow for organ donation. The brain-dead patient continues to have a beating heart and is maintained on a ventilator, sometimes requiring medications to promote adequate blood pressure and hemodynamic stability. This artificial supportive care must continue through the organ recovery to prevent ischemia and cellular death within the organs. Brain death most often occurs within a few diagnostic categories, including traumatic brain injury, bleeding in the brain, anoxia, and cerebral tumors and infections.

In 1968, the Ad Hoc Committee on Brain Death of Harvard Medical School published the report *A Definition of Irreversible Coma.* In this report, the criteria for brain death included apneic coma and an absence of elicited responses for a period of 24 hours using electroencephalogram (EEG) recordings. Its exclusions for brain death included hypothermia and drug intoxication. In 1981, the President's Commission for the Study of Ethical Problems submitted a report to the President and Congress defining death. The Commission's final report was published as the *Guidelines for the Determination of Death,* which has become the guidelines for legislation in all states with regard to brain death. This document includes exclusion for hypotension.

There are several conditions that can make a patient appear brain-dead when he or she is not; therefore, when brain death is suspected, three factors must be known before brain death testing is initiated. These three factors are as follows:

- Cause of unresponsiveness must be known
- Absence of metabolic central nervous system (CNS) depression
- Absence of toxic CNS depression

Determining the cause of unresponsiveness is necessary to rule out a condition that might be reversible. Metabolic CNS depression can occur if the patient is hypotensive or hypothermic or has severe acid–base imbalances. The President's Commission has recommended that the patient must have an adequate blood pressure related to the patient's age and size (adults should have a systolic blood pressure of at least 90 mm Hg), a PaO_2 greater than 60 mm Hg, and a temperature greater than 32.2°C (90.0°F). If these parameters are not met, they must be corrected before brain-death testing begins. Toxic CNS depression can occur from sedatives, alcohol, or neuromuscular blockades, which depress cranial nerve responses as well as cerebral electrical activity. In cases where any of these substances are present, there are two options available. First, the health care team can wait until the substances are eliminated from the body and then proceed with clinical or electroencephalograph (EEG) testing. Second, cerebral blood flow studies can be used to determine brain death immediately.

Brain-death testing determination can be done by a clinical exam, cerebral blood perfusion study, or EEG. The type of testing used is determined by the physician with consideration of the patient's injuries and hemodynamic stability and whether toxic or metabolic CNS depression is present.

Clinical Examination

Clinical examination is probably the most cost-effective testing that can be used to determine brain death and can be completed at the bedside. It cannot be used if the patient has toxic or metabolic CNS depression. Clinical exams should not be used if the patient has an inability to initiate respiration as a result of other injuries or pathology. Examples of this include the patient with C1–C2 quadriplegia or amyotrophic lateral sclerosis (commonly known as Lou Gehrig disease, or ALS) requiring ventilator assistance. Each hospital should have policies in place outlining how many clinical tests are required, and how often to test for brain death (e.g., two clinical exams 12 hours apart, with continued observation between the two exams).

The following criteria must be observed with all of the reflexes being absent.

- No response to any painful or verbal stimuli. The patient's Glasgow Coma Score is 3.
- No pupillary response to light.
- No eye movement (doll's eyes reflex) with head rotation.
- No eye movement to iced water calorics.
- No blink response to cornea irritation.
- No cough response to deep suctioning.
- No gag response to oral-pharyngeal stimulation.
- Apnea

Apnea Testing. Apnea testing is typically performed once, at the time of the final clinical exam. The purpose of apnea testing is to allow the $PaCO_2$ to rise sufficiently to stimulate the respiratory drive center. If the $PaCO_2$ is above 60 mm Hg and no respiratory movement is noted, the patient is considered apneic. This testing is approached with caution and close monitoring, as the patient can become hypoxic or cardiac dysrhythmias may develop during the test. To optimize oxygenation during the test, several procedures are followed. First, prior to initiating the test, the patient is preoxygenated with 100 percent oxygen concentration. Second, during the test, passive oxygenation is maintained through an endotracheal or tracheostomy tube.

The procedure is as follows. The patient is removed from the ventilator and observed for any respiratory movement while allowing a rise in the $PaCO_2$. If any respiratory effort is seen, the patient is reconnected to the ventilator and care is continued, as this indicates continued brain function in the medulla. If no respiratory effort is seen, after ten minutes an arterial blood gas (ABG) is drawn and the patient is reconnected to the mechanical ventilator. During the test, if the patient develops cardiac dysrhythmias, hypotension, or the oxygen saturation falls below 70 percent, an arterial blood gas is immediately drawn and the patient is reconnected to the ventilator. In situations where the patient requires reconnection to the ventilator before apnea testing is complete and the patient's $PaCO_2$ is less than 60 mm Hg at the time of ventilator reconnection, another type of testing may be considered or the apnea test is repeated after the patient is stabilized.

Cerebral Blood Flow

Brain death can be determined if cerebral blood flow is absent. A cerebral angiogram, cerebral nuclear flow study, or transcranial doppler can be used. The patient must have an adequate blood pressure to allow cerebral blood flow. If cerebral blood flow is absent, no further testing or observation is required. Use of this test can be expensive, but it provides immediate results.

Electroencephalogram

The EEG measures electrical activity of the cerebrum. Publicly, it is the most recognized test used to determine brain death. Electrodes are placed on the patient's head to monitor for electrical activity while the patient receives different levels of stimulation. Hospital policies vary regarding how EEGs can be used in determining brain death. Many policies require that multiple EEGs be performed over a specific period of time (e.g., two EEGs over a 48-hour interval). Electrocerebral silence or a "flat" EEG and a clinical exam with no brainstem activity are adequate for brain death determination.

Referral to the OPO

The Medicare conditions of participation state all imminent deaths should be referred to the OPO. Imminent death refers to the potential brain-dead patient, although the Department of Health and Human Services (DHHS) defines imminent death as that of a severely brain-injured patient with a Glasgow Coma Score of 5 or less. After the referral, the OPO will then make a determination of suitability for organ donation and develop a plan of care with the medical staff regarding patient and family care. Should the patient become brain-dead, the early notification and evaluation facilitates a timely communication with the family and OPO.

It is often the emergency room or critical care nurse who first identifies the patient as a potential organ donor. To facilitate the referral process, there are certain data the nurse can have available to help the OPO begin the evaluation process (see Table 8–1).

Determination of Patient's Suitability for Organ Donation

Several factors must be considered in determining if a patient is a candidate for donation. Some of these factors include the patient's medical and social history, compliance with medical treatments, and current hemodynamic stability or instability. Past medical and social history considers the patient's illnesses, and behaviors that affect the body's function and influence the transmission of diseases. This information is important for the transplant surgeon to consider in determining the risks posed to a potential organ recipient. Factors that can prevent donation from occurring include human immunodeficiency virus (HIV), acquired immune deficiency syndrome (AIDS), or active hepatitis B (HbSaG). Certain other factors, although not necessarily precluding donation, are important to take into consideration, including sepsis and any high-risk behaviors for disease transmission (e.g., IV drug abuse; male-to-male sex; extended time in jail; hemophilia; blood contact with a person who has HIV, AIDS, or HbSaG). Having cancer does not necessarily eliminate a person as a potential donor, particularly if the cancer is in remission, localized, and not blood borne. If the extent of the potential donor's history is unknown, he or she should still be considered a potential organ donor.

Hemodynamic status is also assessed on each potential donor patient. Some degree of hemodynamic instability usually develops related to a sequelae of physiologic events that occur with brain death. These include diabetes insipidus, initial hypertension followed by hypotension, inability to regulate body temperature, and neurogenic pulmonary edema. Although most patients go through periods of hemodynamic instability as brain death occurs, it is often sufficiently correctable to maintain adequate perfusion of the organs. The goals of management are to maintain the potential donor within the normal hemodynamic parameters (Table 8–2). However, failing to meet those criteria does not mean donation cannot occur. The OPO reviews the hemodynamics and makes a determination if the instability is significant.

Obtaining Consent

The Uniform Anatomical Gift Act defines the order of priority of those who give consent for donation. Individuals can indicate their wish for donation by registering on their state's donor registry or having it designated in a legal document. If the patient has not indicated a wish for donation in a legal document, the responsibility of consent lies with the legal next-of-kin. Most states have legislation that states if a patient has indicated a wish for donation on a

TABLE 8–1 Donor Referral Initial Nursing Database

Patient's name
Age, sex, race
Cause of brain injury
Height and weight
Current Glasgow Coma Score (GCS)
Past medical and social history
Laboratory data (if available)
Serum electrolytes, BUN, creatinine, AST, ALT, alk phos, WBC, Hgb, Hct
Hemodynamic status (blood pressure, heart rate, O_2 saturation)
Urine output (mL/hr)
Current inotropic support (drug name and dose)
Plan of care (brain death testing scheduled, DNR status)

TABLE 8–2 Hemodynamic Parameters of the Adult Potential Organ Donor

Blood pressure	Greater than 100 mm Hg (systolic) or MAP greater than 75 mm Hg
Heart rate	80–110/min
SaO_2	Greater than 95%
CVP	8–12 mm Hg
PCWP	10–12 mm Hg
SVR	800–1,200 dynes/sec/cm^5
Cardiac index	Greater than 2.0 L/m/m^2

MAP=mean arterial pressure; SaO_2=arterial oxygen saturation; CVP=central venous pressure; PCWP=pulmonary capillary wedge pressure; SVR=systemic vascular resistance registry or legal document, the decedent's wish is to be honored and cannot be declined by other family or friends. When the legal next of kin is to be approached, the order is, the spouse, followed by adult children, either parent, adult sibling(s), or a guardian.

The Medicare Conditions of Participation states that only persons employed by the OPO or those who have received training from the OPO in best practices in the consent process should discuss donation. OPO staff will provide support to the family after receiving the patient referral. The OPO staff's initial interactions focus heavily on facilitating the family's understanding of the patient's brain injury, poor prognosis, and imminent death. A significant amount of time is devoted to helping the family understand the concept of brain death and understanding that death has occurred although the patient will sustain a heartbeat for a period of time. Only after the family develops the understanding that brain death is true death should conversations about donation begin. This process is called *decoupling*. Decoupling is the separation of conversations about brain death and its understanding by the next of kin before donation is requested. In a study conducted by Kentucky Organ Donor Affiliates (KODA, 1994), it was determined that if a family's acceptance of brain death did not occur before donation was requested, consent rates for donation were 18 percent. However, if the family understood and accepted brain death as actual death and subsequently donation was mentioned, the consent rate rose to 65 percent.

Donor Testing

After consent is obtained, care of the donor is transferred to the OPO and an OPO coordinator will initiate orders. A thorough organ evaluation is initiated as each organ is evaluated to ensure suitability for transplant. Serologic testing is performed to determine the absence or presence of transmittable diseases. Blood type and human leukocyte antigen (HLA) typing are determined. After these tests are completed, the information is entered into the United Network for Organ Sharing (UNOS) system to identify matching recipients.

The heart evaluation includes assessment for any positive cardiac history and injury. An electrocardiogram (ECG), chest X-ray, and echocardiogram may be done to determine the current cardiac function and measurements. If the patient is more than 45 years of age or has a medical history consistent with the development of coronary artery disease, a cardiac catheterization may be done. If no cardiac dysfunction is present, matching a heart recipient is initiated.

The lung evaluation includes assessment for any positive pulmonary history including smoking or injury. An arterial blood gas, chest X-ray, and sputum gram stain are obtained. If the results of these tests are adequate, a bronchoscopy is completed; after which, if no pulmonary dysfunction is noted, matching a lung recipient(s) search is initiated.

Liver function is evaluated through investigation of any positive hepatic history, including alcohol and drug use to evaluate whether any hepatic injury has occurred. Electrolyte and liver function tests will be initiated. If hepatic function is adequate, matching a liver recipient search is initiated.

The pancreas is evaluated by history, including diabetes and any pancreatic injury. The serum glucose, amylase, and lipase are monitored. If the patient is 10 to 60 years of age and pancreatic function is adequate, pancreas matching is initiated.

Evaluation of the kidneys includes medical history, injuries, and laboratory findings, such as blood urea nitrogen (BUN) and serum creatinine. A recipient match is identified after HLA typing is completed and the evaluation confirms adequate kidney function.

A specific algorithm matches each organ to a recipient. In addition to matching the donor and recipient blood and tissue types, the final choice of recipient is dependent on additional factors, such as a recipient's status of illness and distance of the donor from the recipient. In general, priority is given to recipients within the donor's local area. A significant factor for initial function and long-term survival of a transplanted organ is a decreased cold ischemic time, the time when circulation to the organ is stopped in the donor and restored in the recipient. If a matching recipient is not found within the local area, the search continues in the region followed by a national search.

It is routine for the OPO coordinator to find recipients for the organs prior to the donor organ recovery. If the donor patient becomes hemodynamically unstable and stability cannot be established, organ placement will occur during and after the recovery completion. During the recovery, the surgeon observes the organ for its functioning in the donor and assures that anatomically, all is well. Should the recovery process begin and a terminal disease process be found (such as cancer), the donation will be halted.

The Organ Recovery Process

Once the recipients are located, the donor organ recovery is scheduled. Each transplant team receiving an organ from the donor may be present for the organ recovery or ask a transplant recovery team from the donor's location to recover the organ. Each recovery team must be present in the operating room to complete the recovery together. The donor is taken to the operating room, prepped, and draped as in any procedure completed in surgery. The patient is continued on mechanical ventilation with anesthesia working to maintain hemodynamic stability. Usually an abdominal surgical team begins the recovery process with an incision from the supra-sternal notch to the symphysis pubis. The organs are prepared for removal by each recovery team. Once all organs are ready to be removed, cannulas are placed and fluid for organ preservation is prepared to flush blood from each organ. Once the blood has been removed, the organ is recovered, packaged for transport to the recipient, and transported.

Donation after Cardiac Death

Donation after cardiac death (DCD), previously known as "non-heart beating donation," is how organ donations began in the 1950s. The first kidney, liver, and heart transplants occurred after DCD donations. In the 1980s, it was recognized that organ donation after brain death offered superior organ recovery outcomes. Organs recovered from brain-dead donors were better perfused and had better long-term outcomes for recipients. For this reason, most of the United States stopped pursuing organs from DCD donors. Over the past 20 years, however, surgeons have learned improved organ preservation techniques and recovery processes, making use of DCD organs more viable; thus there has been a resurgence of interest in the DCD organ recovery option. Furthermore, as the waiting list for organs has continued to increase at a much faster rate than organ donation, there is an ever-increasing gap between the supply and demand for organs, making DCD donation a much-needed additional organ resource.

The DCD candidate is a patient with whom the decision has been made to terminate mechanical ventilation support with an expectation that death is likely to occur within a short period of time. Therefore, when decisions are being made to terminate ventilatory support, a referral should be made to the OPO and an evaluation for organ donation will be completed by the OPO. An important factor that will be considered is the likelihood of cardiac standstill once life supportive care is terminated. If it appears that cardiac standstill may occur within the hour of termination, the OPO will counsel the family regarding an organ donation opportunity. If consent is given, the same organ evaluation and search for a recipient occurs as it does in the brain-dead organ donor.

After the various preparatory procedures are completed, the patient is taken to the operating room and mechanical ventilation is terminated. The patient is observed by the primary care physician. If death occurs and the patient is pronounced dead within 60 to 90 minutes, then organ recovery can occur. Transplant physicians for the organ recovery are placed on standby to complete the recovery, should it occur. It is important to note that the transplant surgeon cannot be in the donor's operating room during the time of termination of care. Only after death is pronounced can the transplant surgeon enter the operating room. From consent until death, the primary care physician coordinates the patient's care, which may include comfort care measures utilized in palliative care treatments, as these measures do not interfere with organ donation. If cardiac standstill death does not occur within the required 60- to 90-minute period following termination of ventilatory care, organ donation cannot occur and any palliative care measures are continued; however, tissue donation can still occur after death.

SECTION THREE REVIEW

1. A major advantage of early notification of the organ procurement coordinator when a potential donor has been identified is that ______ can be initiated.
   - **A.** family counseling
   - **B.** life-support measures
   - **C.** signing of the consent form
   - **D.** preliminary evaluation for suitability
2. The topic of organ donation should not be initiated with the family until the
   - **A.** patient has died
   - **B.** family signs the consent form
   - **C.** family acknowledges the patient's death
   - **D.** family asks about possible donation
3. When apnea testing is performed on the patient, he or she is considered apneic if the $PaCO_2$ is ______ mm Hg after ______ minutes and no respiratory effort is noted.
   - **A.** 50; 5
   - **B.** 50; 10
   - **C.** 60; 5
   - **D.** 60; 10
4. Donation after cardiac death (DCD) has made a resurgence primarily because of
   - **A.** improved evaluation criteria
   - **B.** scarcity of resources
   - **C.** better transplantation results
   - **D.** family's wishes

Answers: 1. D, 2. C, 3. D, 4. B

SECTION FOUR: Donor Management and Organ Preservation

At the completion of this section, the learner will be able to discuss donor management and organ preservation.

Donor Management

Donor management focuses on maintaining organ function when brain death occurs. Close monitoring and evaluation of the patient's body system functions is crucial for maintaining organ viability for eventual transplantation. This section is organized by major body and organ functions that must be stabilized to adequately oxygenate and perfuse the organs to retain organ viability. Table 8–3 provides a summary of organ donor management.

Hemodynamic Instability

As brain death ensues, organ functions begin to deteriorate and this results in hemodynamic instability. Hemodynamic dysfunction, when recognized and treated early, can usually be controlled and hemodynamic stability restored and maintained. Many patients with brain injury arrive at the hospital in a normal hemodynamic state. Initially, the body attempts to repair the injured area of brain by increasing cerebral blood flow (CBF) and oxygen to the area of injury. The increased CBF increases cerebral edema. As cerebral edema increases, CBF eventually becomes compromised. The body responds by releasing catecholamines that increase heart rate and blood pressure in an attempt to increase cerebral blood supply. Catecholamine-induced tachycardia and hypertension continue until the body depletes its supply of catecholamines, resulting in the onset of

TABLE 8–3 Summary of Organ Donor Management

FUNCTIONAL INSTABILITY	PROBLEM	GOALS	MANAGEMENT
Hemodynamic	Hypotension	Systolic blood pressure (SBP) greater than 100 mm Hg is desired (SBP greater than 90 mm Hg may be acceptable)	IV catecholamine therapy—Intropin (Dopamine) most common choice; norepinephrine or epinephrine drip may be considered if Intropin therapy is ineffective for maintenance of blood pressure
Thermoregulatory	Hypothermia (occasionally hyperthermia)	Maintain body temperature at 96°F to 100°F (35.6°C to 37.8°C)	Warming blanket (hypothermia); cooling blanket (hyperthermia)
Renal/Fluid and Electrolyte	Dehydration and electrolyte imbalances from diabetes insipidus (DI); decreased renal perfusion resulting in organ deterioration	Maintain urine output between 100 to 300 mL/hr and serum creatinine less than 1.5 - 2 mg/dL (Powner, 2005); maintain adequate electrolyte balance	Supportive measures to maintain cardiac output and tissue perfusion (e.g., fluid resuscitation); replace ADH if necessary (DDAVP or vasopressin); IV fluids: salt-poor IV fluids and avoid hypo-osmotic fluids; placement of central line or pulmonary artery catheter; close monitoring urine output and replacement of fluid and electrolytes
Pulmonary	Neurogenic pulmonary edema	Maintain PaO_2 above 100 mm Hg	Mechanical ventilation; positive end-expiratory pressure (PEEP); bronchodilator (if bronchospasm is present)
Hematopoietic	Coagulopathy	Maintain adequate hematopoietic status	Monitor Hgb/Hct; PT, PTT and INR; replace blood as necessary
Endocrine	Loss of thyroid hormone and cortisol production; decreased insulin production	Maintain adequate hormone levels	Replace hormones as necessary—thyroid protocol: IV bolus of levothyroxine (T4), Solu-Medrol, insulin, and 50% dextrose followed by continuous T4 intravenous infusion

hypotension. The hypotensive state persists unless catecholamine stores are replaced intravenously. Intropin (dopamine) is the most common catecholamine used for this purpose, generally correcting the patient's hypotension. However, if dopamine therapy is not successful in achieving an acceptable arterial blood pressure, initiation of norepinephrine, neosynephrine, or epinephrine may be necessary. In an adult, a systolic blood pressure of 100 mm Hg is desired, although 90 mm Hg is acceptable. If the hypotension is not successfully treated, cardiac standstill is imminent, which compromises organ donation. The development of hypotension after a period of hypertension is a late sign in the brain death sequence of events and is referred to as the *herniation picture,* usually indicating brain death.

Loss of Thermoregulation

As brain death progresses, the hypothalamus is destroyed and the patient can no longer regulate body temperature. Hypothermia is seen most often and warming must be initiated. If left untreated, hypothermia can cause cardiac dysrhythmias and cardiac standstill. Occasionally, hyperthermia develops and cooling blankets must be employed. Hyperthermia results in vasodilatation and worsening hypotension if untreated. The temperature should be maintained at 96°F to 100°F (35.6°C to 37.8°C).

Fluid and Electrolyte Instability

As the pituitary gland ceases functioning, antidiuretic hormone (ADH) is no longer secreted. The absence of ADH results in diabetes insipidus (DI). Symptoms of DI include urine outputs greater than 4 mL/kg/hr, urine specific gravity of less than 1.005, and urine osmolality of less than 300 mOsm/kg. Placing a central line or pulmonary artery catheter can be helpful in the measurement and treatment of adequate fluid replacement. Replacement of ADH may be necessary to manage an appropriate fluid balance. Desmopressin acetate (DDAVP) or vasopressin is the usual drug of choice in treating DI. Urine output should be maintained at 1 to 2 mL/kg/hr.

When diabetes insipidus is present, choosing the correct IV fluid can be challenging. IV fluids need to be salt poor. If large amounts of dextrose-containing IV fluids are used, a hyperosmolar diuresis can develop; therefore, serum glucose levels must be closely monitored and treated appropriately. Care should be taken to avoid hypo-osmotic fluids, such as sterile water, because administration of large volumes of this type of fluid can result in rhabdomyolysis (renal damage caused by myoglobin). The rapid loss of urine from diabetes insipidus can result in significant electrolyte and acid–base imbalances. Potassium, calcium, phosphorus, and magnesium are lost, whereas sodium is retained. Unresolved hypernatremia eventually causes liver dysfunction, which may result in primary liver nonfunction if transplanted. Serum electrolytes need to be closely monitored and replaced as necessary to maintain optimal cell and organ function.

Pulmonary Dysfunction

Occasionally, brain death may precipitate *neurogenic* pulmonary edema. This is characterized by rhonchi, pink frothy secretions, a decreasing PaO_2, and a normal to low central venous pressure (CVP). The chest X-ray shows "whited out" lungs. Judicious treatment with ventilator support is required, maximizing the F_IO_2 and positive end-expiratory pressure (PEEP) to maintain the PaO_2 above 100 mm Hg. In addition, low tidal volumes are used to minimize alveolar damage. Bronchospasms are likely to occur in the acute burn patient who developed smoke-inhalation–related anoxia. In such cases, a bronchodilator may be indicated.

If symptoms of pulmonary edema are present but the CVP is high, the pulmonary edema is likely from fluid overload. To treat this problem, restricting fluids, administering diuretics, and discontinuing vasopressin may be necessary, which can cause pulmonary vasoconstriction.

Hematopoietic Dysfunction

Coagulopathies are common in the patient with a traumatic brain death. As brain death occurs, large amounts of tissue plasminogen activator (tPA), a thrombolytic enzyme, are released. Long-term hypothermia increases the likelihood of coagulopathy. Hemograms, prothrombin time (PT), partial thromboplastin time (PTT), and international normalized ratio (INR) should be monitored. Blood replacement should occur if needed.

Loss of Endocrine Function

Progressing brain death results in a loss of thyroid hormone production. In addition, cortisol production ceases and insulin production decreases. A combination of these processes causes a shift from aerobic to anaerobic metabolism. The myocardial cells become oxygen depleted and cellular death begins. OPOs now use a thyroid protocol to reverse this process. Levothyroxine (T4), Solu-Medrol, insulin, and 50 percent dextrose are given in a bolus. A T4 drip is started and continued throughout the organ recovery process.

Preservation of Organs

A single donor may provide one or multiple organs and tissues. At a prearranged time agreed on by all the transplant teams involved, the donor is taken to the operating room and prepared for surgery. When the donor is brought to the OR, the chart must have the correct documentation present: date and time of the death declaration and the signed or recorded consent form. In addition, the hospital may require a signed death certificate or other documentation. The procedures followed in the OR are similar to those in any other surgery. The anesthesiologist monitors and maintains the donor's cardiopulmonary and renal status and the fluid and electrolyte balance throughout the organ recovery period. There may be more than one organ recovery team in the OR, with each team being responsible for recovering a particular organ or organ set. The donor's attending physician cannot be part of the recovery teams.

During the organ recovery surgery, the transplant surgeon(s) makes one incision from the suprasternal notch to the symphysis pubis. The surgeon inspects the donor for the presence of any unexpected disease, such as an undiagnosed cancer, and then begins the process of dissecting each organ from its surrounding anatomical structures. When all of the organs are ready to be removed, cannulas are placed in the thoracic aorta, pulmonary artery, portal vein, and abdominal aorta. A clamp is placed on the aorta and perfusion of the organs begins with a cold preservation solution. The solution runs through each organ, removing the blood from the organ. This procedure slows the organ's metabolic rate and preserves it until the organ is transplanted. Once removed from the donor, the organ is packaged in the preservative solution and sterile triple bagged. It is then placed on ice and transported to the recipient's hospital. Table 8–4 lists the allowed cold ischemic times for each organ.

TABLE 8–4 Organ Preservation and Transplantation Time Frames

ORGAN	TRANSPLANTATION TIME FRAME (HRS)
Heart	4–6
Lungs	4–6
Liver	12–24
Pancreas	12–24
Kidneys	24–48
Small bowel	12–24

SECTION FOUR REVIEW

1. Major management goals in caring for the donor patient include maintaining (choose all that apply)
   A. a stable hemodynamic status
   B. infections at a minimum level
   C. fluid and electrolyte balance
   D. optimal oxygenation status

2. The most common underlying cause of hypotension in the donor is
   A. dehydration
   B. cardiac failure
   C. fluid overload
   D. increased systemic vascular resistance

3. Which of the following statements best reflects procedures related to organ recovery in the operating room?
   A. An anesthesiologist is not necessary.
   B. The recipient's physician must be part of the recovery team.
   C. Only one organ recovery team can be present in the operating room.
   D. The donor's physician is not part of the recovery team.

4. The organ preservation method that is common to all organs is
   A. hypothermia
   B. concentration of electrolytes
   C. type of diuretic
   D. preservation formula

Answers: 1. (A, C, D), 2. A, 3. D, 4. A

The Organ Recipient

SECTION FIVE: Immunologic Considerations

At the completion of this section, the learner will be able to explain the immunologic considerations of organ transplantation.

Histocompatibility

Recall from Section Five of Module 5, Determinants and Assessment of Hematologic Function that histocompatibility refers to immunologic similarities between cells that allow the body to distinguish self from nonself. In humans, this is accomplished through special cell surface antigens called human leukocyte antigens (HLA). Before the scientific discovery of HLA, organ transplants were for the most part unsuccessful in the long term since a mismatch of HLA between the organ donor and recipient resulted in organ rejection. Tests of histocompatibility performed on the donor and recipient are crucial for optimizing success in organ transplantation. A perfect HLA match is only possible between identical twins; however, the HLA matching between first-degree relations (parents and siblings) generally is a much better match than non-relations.

Donor–Recipient Compatibility Testing

Three common tests used to evaluate the compatibility of the donor's tissues to the recipient's are tissue typing, crossmatching, and ABO typing.

Tissue Typing

Tissue typing refers to the identification of the HLA (histocompatibility) antigens of both the donor and the recipient. It evaluates the degree to which the two sets of tissues are HLA matched. The closer the HLA match is between the donor and the recipient, the better chance for long-term transplant success. The opposite is true, as well.

Crossmatching

Crossmatching tests the potential recipient for antidonor (preformed) antibodies. When such preformed antibodies are present, the patient is referred to as presensitized. Histocompatibility can be tested by evaluating the degree of reactivity of the immune response to crossmatch testing of donor and recipient cells and serum. When a serum crossmatching is performed, a sample of the recipient's serum is subjected to the serum of a sample of the prospective donor's blood. The serum is analyzed for the formation of preformed antibodies (PRA). The normal value is 0 percent. A prospective crossmatch is performed immediately prior to the transplant on those patients with a PRA of 10 percent or higher. In order to suppress the preformed antibodies, the patient awaiting a transplant may undergo one or more treatment modalities, such as plasmapheresis, intravenous immunoglobulin (IVIg), or immunosuppressant therapy. A recipient can become sensitized to foreign HLA antigens for a variety of reasons, such as prior organ transplantation, blood transfusions, and pregnancy. In such cases, the reintroduction of a new organ containing the sensitized HLA antigens can cause rapid organ rejection and possibly death.

ABO Typing

ABO typing identifies the blood group of the donor and the recipient. ABO compatibility is an initial criterion for transplantation. The rules for blood type matching are the same as for transfusions: Unmatched protein types will cause a rapid immune reaction. The type O allograft is considered the universal transplant donor type because it can be transplanted safely into a recipient with any blood type. Type AB is considered to be the universal organ recipient because it can receive an allograft from all blood types. Types A and B can only receive an allograft from their own blood type or type O donors. Table 8–5 summarizes ABO compatibility.

TABLE 8–5 Organ Donor and Recipient ABO Compatibility

	COMPATIBLE POTENTIAL
RECIPIENT'S BLOOD TYPE	DONOR'S BLOOD TYPE
A	A or O
B	B or O
AB (universal recipient)	A, B, or O
O	O only

SECTION FIVE REVIEW

1. Histocompatibility antigens are also known as
   - A. monocytes
   - B. macrophages
   - C. human leukocyte antigens
   - D. polymorphonuclear lymphocytes
2. HLA antigens are located on (in) the cell
   - A. surfaces
   - B. nucleus
   - C. cytoplasm
   - D. mitochondria
3. The best histocompatibility matching is found between
   - A. siblings
   - B. identical twins
   - C. parent and child
   - D. fraternal twins
4. The identification of the histocompatibility antigens of both the donor and the recipient is called
   - A. crossmatching
   - B. ABO typing
   - C. antigen classifying
   - D. tissue typing
5. A recipient can become sensitized to foreign HLA antigens through which of the following ways? (choose all that apply)
   - A. pregnancy
   - B. donating blood
   - C. prior organ transplantation
   - D. receiving blood transfusions

Answers: 1. C, 2. A, 3. B, 4. D, 5. (A, C, D)

SECTION SIX: Determination of Transplant Need

At the completion of this section, the learner will be able to describe the determination of transplant need.

The scarcity of organ resources along with the physical and financial costs involved make determination of transplant need a major issue. In August of 2008, there were 99,160 patients on the waiting list for transplants (UNOS, 2008). Solid-organ transplantation is expensive—the first-year posttransplant expenses can range from $210,000 to more than $800,000 and the cost of antirejection drugs can range between $9,000 to $13,000 per year (Cavanaugh & Martin, 2007).

Determining who will receive an organ is not a simple decision. Hundreds or possibly thousands of patients are on the national waiting list for the same organ at any one time. Many of those on the waiting list will succumb to their disease before a donor organ becomes available. Organs are allocated to recipients based on a point system established by UNOS.

Determination of Need

The criteria used for determination of need are multifaceted. Specific guidelines vary among transplant programs, but the general guidelines are fairly consistent and include end-stage organ failure, short life expectancy, severe functional disability, no additional serious health problems, and psychological readiness.

End-stage organ disease is the primary indicator for transplantation need and is established by evaluation of organ function. The short life expectancy criterion is generally considered 6 to 12 months. Measurement of functional disability evaluates the potential recipient's ability to lead a reasonable lifestyle (e.g., ability to work or perform activities of daily living). This can be evaluated by interviewing the patient and family, observation, and cardiopulmonary exercise testing. Psychological readiness is established through interviewing, assessing known history, and possible psychological testing. Because of the highly stressful nature of transplantation, the presence of additional serious medical problems increases the risk of postoperative complications and is associated with a higher mortality rate.

Transplant Recipient Evaluation

The patient is considered as a potential transplant candidate only after maximum medical therapy has become ineffective, leaving transplantation as the final option. Evaluation of the potential recipient is an extensive process. Many factors must be thoroughly evaluated prior to placing the patient on the UNOS national patient waiting list for organ transplantation. These factors usually include the potential recipient's clinical, nutritional, psychological, and financial status.

Clinical Status

Organ-specific diagnostic studies and laboratory testing are conducted; preexisting or concurrent medical problems (risk factors for transplantation) are closely scrutinized and discussed with the patient and family. Table 8–6 summarizes common major studies and tests for organ transplantation preparation.

Nutritional Status

Malnourished patients awaiting an organ transplant are at high risk for perioperative complications such as wound infection, graft failure, cytomegalovirus (CMV) infection, and bacterial infection. Nutritional intervention is crucial in the pretransplant stage and may even require enteral or parenteral feedings. Assessments should include regular physical assessments, weights, anthropometric measurements, and laboratory tests.

TABLE 8–6 Common Organ Evaluation Studies and Tests

ORGAN	STUDIES/TESTS
General tests common to all transplant candidates	**Immune specific** ABO, HLA tissue typing, presensitization, crossmatching, HIV profile
	General Complete blood count (CBC) with differential, blood chemistries, coagulation studies, urinalysis; serum creatinine; diabetic patients (HbA1c, estimated GFR, urine protein)
	Cardiovascular ECG, echocardiogram, cardiac catheterization (if risk for heart disease)
	Radiographic Chest x-ray
	Other Blood typing and crossmatching, examination and testing for infection (e.g., culturing of blood, urine, etc.), viral titers, tuberculin skin tests, colonoscopy, gender specific tests (PSA, mammogram, PAP smear)
Kidneys	**Radiographic** Gastrointestinal X-rays, abdominal ultrasound, voiding cystourethrogram
Heart, heart–lung, and lung	**Cardiovascular** Endomyocardial biopsy (to rule out myocarditis and sarcoidosis), echocardiogram, cardiac catheterization
	Pulmonary Arterial blood gas, chest x-ray, pulmonary function testing, ventilation/perfusion scan, computed tomographic (CT) scan of chest, exercise testing
	Other Doppler study, legs duplex scan
Liver	**Laboratory Tests** Liver function tests, drug and alcohol screening tests
	Other Portal vein sonogram and Doppler, abdominal CT scan, liver biopsy, endoscopic retrograde cholangiopancreatography (ERCP)
Pancreas	**Laboratory Tests** Pancreatic enzymes, hemoglobin A1c
	Other Nerve conduction studies, gastric emptying scan, ophthalmology exam
Intestines	**Laboratory Tests** Iron studies, lipid profile
	Radiographic Gastrointestinal contrast studies, abdominal ultrasound
	Other Nutritional and metabolic assessments

Psychological Status

Chronic illness and its treatment are known to have profound long-term psychological effects on the patient and family. These psychological effects may have an impact on the long-term success of the transplant. In addition, the stresses associated with organ transplantation can further strain the coping abilities of this population. For these reasons, the potential organ recipient, and possibly the family, will undergo a psychological evaluation. If problems are assessed, appropriate counseling is initiated.

Financial Status

The total cost of organ transplantation varies with the organ being grafted. Costs that are factored in include pretransplantation evaluation, interim transplantation, and posttransplantation care. Medicare, state medical programs, and private health insurance coverage vary widely. Coverage is often differentiated by the type of organ being transplanted. If financial resources are questionable, financial options are explored. In addition, the patient may be required to relocate close to the transplant center for a designated time period both pre- and posttransplant, adding an additional financial strain.

Once the decision is made to accept a patient as a suitable transplant candidate, the patient's name and vital information are entered into the computer bank at the United Network for Organ Sharing (UNOS). This organization is charged with distributing organs in an equitable and nondiscriminatory manner. The potential recipient remains on the UNOS organ waiting list until an organ becomes available, the patient is removed from the list, or dies. Periodic reevaluation of the transplant candidate's health status is recommended. For example, the International Society for Heart and Lung Transplantation (ISHLT) recommends reevaluation using specific criteria every six months and yearly as a part of organ waitlist management (Ohler, 2007). It is also recommended that transplant candidates have a yearly malignancy and serology screening (Ohler, 2007).

SECTION SIX REVIEW

1. General guidelines for determination of organ transplant need include (choose all that apply)
   A. severe functional disability
   B. end-stage organ failure
   C. psychological readiness
   D. additional serious health problems
2. The decision as to whether a person is placed on the organ transplant waiting list as a potential recipient is usually made by
   A. the patient/family
   B. a multidisciplinary committee
   C. the organ procurement team
   D. the potential recipient's physician
3. The determination of end-stage organ failure is primarily based on which of the following criteria?
   A. tissue biopsy
   B. patient history
   C. functional disability
   D. age/gender
4. A potential transplant recipient has his or her psychological status thoroughly assessed because
   A. there is a risk of posttransplant psychosis
   B. a depressed state is a major contraindication for transplantation
   C. there is a higher mortality associated with psychological distress
   D. stress associated with transplantation strains coping abilities

Answers: 1. (A, B, D), 2. B, 3. A, 4. D

SECTION SEVEN: Posttransplantation Complications

At the completion of this section, the learner will be able to discuss the major complications associated with organ transplantation.

Although each type of organ transplant has many unique features, they also have commonalities; this is true also of organ transplant complications. Three major types of complications are associated with transplantation:

- Technical complications
- Graft rejection
- Immunosuppressant-related problems

Technical Complications

The technical procedures involved in performing the transplantation are not without risks. Three major groups of technical complications are associated with the surgical procedure: vascular thrombosis, bleeding, and anastomosis leakage.

Vascular Thrombosis

Vascular thrombosis is a fairly rare complication that usually develops during the early postoperative period. It refers to the development of a blood clot in the vascular system. As a complication of organ transplantation, it refers to a blood clot in the vasculature of the graft, often the major artery. The presence of a thrombosis may not be detected initially because the patient is frequently asymptomatic. Diagnostic tests may be performed soon after surgery (e.g., duplex ultrasonography) to assure arterial patency. Early detection and immediate thrombectomy are essential if the graft is to survive. Even then, the graft is at high risk for failure. Any delay in detection of thrombosis frequently leads to loss of the graft.

Bleeding

Postoperative transplantation bleeding is managed in a fashion similar to other postsurgery patients, with the exception of liver transplants. In the liver transplant patient, it is often difficult to differentiate bleeding that is secondary to coagulopathy associated with a dysfunctional liver from bleeding that has resulted from a surgical (technical) problem. Postoperatively, a transplanted liver may have some degree of coagulopathy present, which makes control of otherwise normal postoperative bleeding extremely difficult. The decision must be made as to whether to allow bleeding to continue until the coagulopathy resolves as liver function returns or whether to take the patient for exploratory surgery immediately under the assumption that the cause is surgical.

Anastomosis Leakage

The term **anastomosis** refers to the site at which the graft is sutured into the recipient. Problems at the anastomosis site usually occur one to three weeks following transplantation. The problem may be failure of the anastomosis to seal completely, usually at the epithelial layer, which results in leakage of fluids (e.g., urine following a postrenal graft, or air as in bronchial dehiscence). An anastomosis leak usually results from inadequate healing, possibly as a result of a deficient blood supply or steroid therapy. Anastomosis leaks usually require surgical exploration and repair.

Graft Rejection

Graft rejection refers to the activation of the immune response against a transplanted tissue or organ. It is the result of the body recognizing the new tissue as nonself, which then triggers an autoimmune system attack to eliminate the invader. Graft rejection is primarily the result of T lymphocyte and B lymphocyte activities. The three types of graft rejection are based on the time and speed of onset and are called hyperacute, acute, and chronic.

Hyperacute Rejection

Hyperacute rejection is a type III (Arthus) hypersensitivity response; that is, it is a humoral response in which the B lymphocytes are activated to produce antibodies. It occurs within minutes to hours following transplantation and results from the presence of preformed graft-specific cytotoxic antibodies. Because the antibodies are already formed, as soon as the graft is placed, the immune system recognizes the foreign tissue and increases graft-specific antibody production. In turn, the antibodies accumulate rapidly and trigger agglutination of platelets, activation of the complement system, and phagocytic activities. Fortunately, hyperacute rejection is now rare in countries such as the United States, where improved donor–recipient screening and matching procedures are performed.

Acute Rejection

Acute rejection is characterized by its sudden onset and usually occurs within days or months following the transplant. Acute rejection begins as a type IV hypersensitivity response; that is, it is a cell-mediated immune response in which the T lymphocytes and macrophages of the host (recipient) attack and destroy the graft (donor) tissue. The graft's HLA antigens are recognized as foreign (nonself), thereby triggering T lymphocyte proliferation and attack. As the acute rejection continues, graft-specific cytotoxic antibodies are produced, which further aggravates the acute rejection process.

Chronic Rejection

Chronic rejection is a humoral immune response in which antibodies slowly attack the graft. Chronic rejection may begin at any time following transplantation and may take years to render the graft nonfunctional. The antibodies trigger the same immune response as seen with hyperacute rejection but at a very low level. In time, the organ becomes ischemic and dies.

Immunosuppressant-Related Problems

Immunosuppressants are the cornerstone to successful long-term transplantation; however, this group of drugs is associated with side effects that can cause serious problems, such as infection, organ dysfunction, malignancy, and steroid-induced problems such as hyperglycemia.

Infection

Infection is a leading cause of morbidity and mortality in posttransplantation patients. In the past, specific types of infection developed at fairly predictable times following surgery; thus the patient could be monitored for anticipated infections. Today, the predictability of posttransplant infections has been altered, with improved antibiotic and immunosuppressant therapies available (Fischer, 2006). This reduced predictability, when accompanied by a stunted immune response to infection, makes infection more difficult to recognize. During the initial weeks following surgery, nosocomial infections, such as pneumonia, urinary tract infections, and wound infections, are the most common source of infections.

Common sources of infection within the first few weeks following the transplantation surgery include nosocomial infection (most common), infected donor organ transmitted to recipient, contaminated donor organ, and infection contracted prior to hospitalization (Fischer, 2006). Common sources of postsurgical nosocomial infections include IV catheter infections, pneumonia, urinary tract infections, and surgical wound infection (Fischer, 2006).

Treatment of the infections with repeated runs of antibiotics may precipitate a superinfection (e.g., *Clostridium difficile* or *Candida*) or development of a resistant strain of bacteria such as ganciclovir-resistant cytomegalovirus (CMV), methicillin-resistant *S. aureus* (MRSA), or vancomycin-resistant *enterococcus* (VRE) (Stitt, 2003). There is a particular risk for development of a CMV infection. The CMV may have already been present in the recipient or it may have been introduced in conjunction with the transplant. CMV-seropositive patients may develop reactivation of the virus as a result of their immunosuppressed state. CMV infections may be mild or severe. A severe CMV infection can potentially cause dysfunction of multiple organs. This is especially a problem in seronegative recipients who received a seropositive organ or CMV-positive blood products. These patients may receive CMV prophylaxis therapy for three or more months following surgery to prevent activation of CMV until the immune system as had time to stabilize (Fischer, 2006).

The mold *Aspergillus*, while not as common in occurrence as *Candida*, is an important infection in the posttransplant patient, and is seen more in heart, lung, and liver transplant patients than in renal transplant patients. *Aspergillus* can become invasive, resulting in abscesses, pneumonia, skin infections, or it can become widely disseminated in the body (Fischer, 2006). It usually develops within the first six months following organ transplantation.

Infection is a major posttransplantation problem because immunosuppressant therapy compromises the immune system in some way. The immunosuppressed patient is unable to muster the same response to acute infection as a person who is immunocompetent; therefore, infection presents itself in more subtle ways. The primary symptom of infection in this population is the presence of a fever that is often low grade (about 100.5°F [38°C]). Other assessments may include tachypnea, fatigue, tachycardia, and pain. Development of a fever requires a rapid but thorough search for the source of the infection and aggressive treatment. The lungs and urinary tract are the most common sources of nosocomial infection.

Organ Dysfunction

Almost all solid organ transplant patients receive a similar regimen of immunosuppressant therapy. Immunosuppressants are associated with multiple side effects, many of which target specific organs. Some degree of graft dysfunction is common immediately following organ transplantation. Development of nephrotoxicity and hepatotoxicity can occur with any organ transplant but are considered especially serious in kidney and liver transplants, respectively. The combination of the adverse effects of the drug and postgraft dysfunction may precipitate a severe graft crisis. Immunosuppressant therapy is discussed in Section Nine.

Malignancy

Patients on long-term immunosuppressant therapy are at increased risk for development of some form of malignancy. The most common malignancies that have been associated with organ transplantation include nonmelanoma skin cancers (most commonly squamous cell cancer), posttransplant lymphoproliferative disorders (PTLD), and Kaposi's sarcoma (Ojha et al., 2008; Azfar et al., 2008). The incidence of cancer at 20 years post-renal transplantation may be as high as 40 percent; and cancer is the reported cause of death 26 percent of patients who die within 10 years of renal transplant (Zafar et al., 2008). Posttransplant lymphoproliferative disorders (PTLD) result from reactivation of the Epstein-Barr virus (EBV). Categories of PTLDs range from hyperplasia and mild-infectious mononucleosis-like disorders to a variety of lymphomas such as B-cell, T-cell, and Hodgkin's lymphomas. Kaposi's sarcoma (KS), an opportunistic disease often associated with the AIDS epidemic, may affect up to 6 percent of solid organ transplant recipients, which is about 500 times higher than seen in the general population (Zafar et al., 2008).

Posttransplant Diabetes Mellitus

In a review of research literature, Driscoll (2007) reported that the post solid organ transplant patient is at significant risk for development of new-onset diabetes mellitus and impaired glucose tolerance. For example, studies of post-renal transplant patients estimate that up to 24 percent develop diabetes within three years and about 30 percent within 15 years of their kidney transplant.

Diabetes develops in approximately 40 percent of liver transplant patients within three years of surgery. The pathogenesis of this phenomenon is not well understood but may be related to decreased insulin secretion and increased insulin resistance. Risk factors for development include age (older than 40 years), ethnicity (higher in nonwhite people), weight (weight gain following transplantation), positive family history for diabetes, hepatitis C infection, immunosuppression, organ rejection, underlying disease, and possibly CMV infection.

Steroid-Induced Problems

Long-term steroid therapy carries with it multiple potentially serious side effects. Steroid-induced hyperglycemia, significant weight gain, and metabolic bone disease are common problems especially in the first year. Steroid therapy is discussed further in Section Nine.

SECTION SEVEN REVIEW

1. Which of the following are examples of technical complications of organ transplantation? (choose all that apply)
   A. bleeding
   B. infection
   C. anastomosis leakage
   D. vascular thrombosis
2. Organ rejection that takes place within minutes to hours following transplantation and results from the presence of preformed graft-specific cytotoxic antibodies is called ______ rejection.
   A. subacute
   B. acute
   C. hyperacute
   D. chronic
3. Posttransplant patients are at particular risk for developing a ______ infection either from being seropositive prior to the transplant or by receiving a seropositive organ or blood transfusion.
   A. cytomegalovirus
   B. pneumonia
   C. hepatitis A
   D. wound
4. Posttransplant patients are at increased risk for development of malignancies secondary to ______.
   A. organ toxicity
   B. preexisting conditions
   C. underlying tissue incompatibility
   D. prolonged immunosuppressant therapy

5. Risk factors for development of posttransplant new onset diabetes mellitus include (choose all that apply)
   A. organ rejection
   B. age: older than 60
   C. ethnicity: non-white population
   D. gender: female
   E. history of Hepatitis C infection

Answers: 1. (A, C, D), 2. C, 3. A, 4. D, 5. (A, C, E)

SECTION EIGHT: Hematopoietic Stem Cell Transplantation

On completion of this section, the learner will be able to discuss hematopoietic stem cell transplantation.

Hematopoietic stem cell transplantation (HSCT), formerly referred to as "bone marrow transplantation," is a technique that can restore normal bone marrow function in patients who have a hematologic malignancy or bone marrow failure. HSCT can be used to treat a variety of disorders, including leukemia, multiple myeloma, lymphomas, autoimmune disorders (e.g., systemic lupus erythematosus [SLE]), and aplastic anemia (Copelan, 2006). In some disorders, such as relapsed acute myelogenous leukemia (AML), it is the only potentially curative therapeutic option. With the advent of HSCT, the physician is able to use high-dose therapies to eradicate a disease, such as cancer; after which healthy stem cells are reintroduced to restore bone marrow function and speed up hematologic recovery time (LLS, 2008).

Types of HSCT

There are two types of HSCT: autologous and allogeneic. Each is useful under certain circumstances.

Autologous Transplantation

Autologous stem cells come from the recipient's own blood or bone marrow, which provides the perfect HLA match; thus, no graft-rejection complications and a significantly reduced morbidity and mortality. To qualify for autologous stem cell transplantation, the patient's blood and bone marrow need to be free of malignant cells. The stem cells are not harvested until all tests are negative for malignant cells during a full disease remission period. The primary drawback of autologous transplantation is the high incidence of malignancy relapse due to reintroduction of small (undetectable) numbers of the patient's own malignant cells when the autologous cells are reintroduced. Research is continuing in search of better ways to process the harvested stem cells to reduce the occurrence of malignancy relapse.

Allogeneic Transplantation

Allogeneic stem cells come from a carefully selected donor other than the patient. Close HLA matching is essential, and when possible, the patient's siblings are tested first, as they are likely to provide the best HLA match. If a related donor cannot be found, the donor can be unrelated. In allogeneic transplants, the goal is to first eradicate the cancer and then perform the transplant to stimulate a graft-vs-tumor (GVT) effect. This effect, primarily due to donor-provided lymphocytes, helps destroy any remaining cancer cells (LLS, 2008). Unfortunately, grafting allogeneic stem cells can precipitate the complication, graft-versus-host disease (GVHD).

Sources of Hematopoietic Stem Cells

The two major sources of hematopoietic stem cells are the bone marrow and the peripheral blood. Umbilical cord blood is a recent addition to potential sources; however, it is not a common source at this time.

Bone Marrow

The bone marrow was the original source for obtaining hematopoietic stem cells. The procedure is performed under general anesthesia and requires about two hours. The volume removed varies with the recipient's size; however, up to a liter of bone marrow may be aspirated. The National Marrow Donor Program Guidelines recommend that the volume of bone marrow aspiration be limited to 15 mL/kg of donor weight (Samavedi et al., 2007). A large bore needle is inserted multiple times into easily accessible bone marrow locations, usually the iliac crests (see Fig. 8–1). Complications to this procedure are rare and include bleeding and infection. The patient may complain of localized discomfort at the site of the harvesting.

Peripheral Blood

Harvesting hematopoietic stem cells from the peripheral blood is now the major source of stem cells for transplantation. Stem cells can be identified and measured through their CD marker, the CD34 antigen; thus they are referred to as CD34+ cells. These CD34+ cells normally exist in the peripheral circulation but only in small numbers; however, these numbers can be increased significantly using growth factors, such as granulocyte colony-stimulating factor (G-CSF) (e.g., Filgrastim®). There is a wait period for the stem cells to be mobilized after the growth factors have been administered. During the wait period (usually four to nine days), daily blood samples are taken to measure the number of CD34+ cells. Hematopoietic stem cell engraftment requires a CD34+ count of 1 to 2 $\times 10^6$ cells/kg (Samavedi et al., 2007). When a sufficient number of cells are present, cell harvesting is accomplished by **apheresis,** which can be performed in an ambulatory setting, such as a blood bank facility. It takes about three to four hours and requires no anesthesia. The cells can then be frozen for extended periods of time.

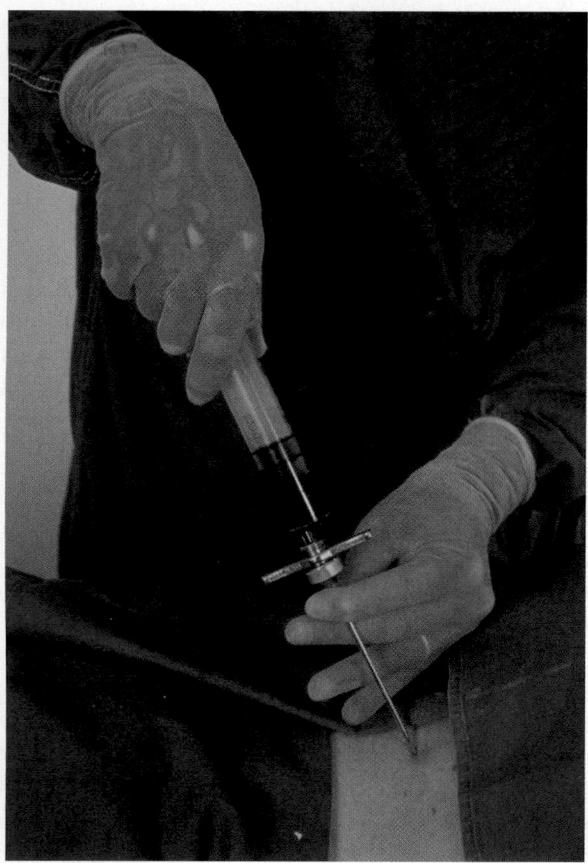

Figure 8–1 ▪ Allogeneic bone marrow transplant. Bone marrow from the donor is aspirated, then filtered and infused into the recipient. From Fraser, Simon/Photo Researchers, Inc.

Transplanting Procedure

Preparing for HSCT

Preparation for stem cell engraftment (called "conditioning") involves eradication of the disease for which the person is to receive the HSCT, and immunosuppression to prevent rejection of the graft (Samavedi et al., 2007). In general, disease eradication procedures include a regimen of high-dose chemotherapy and radiation therapy, which often includes total body irradiation (TBI). Total body irradiation is accomplished by using multiple small daily doses to minimize side effects (LLS, 2008). There are many different protocols for the preparative regimen, but the overriding goal is to essentially clear the patient's dysfunctional bone marrow of as much disease as possible—and optimize the engraftment potential of the donor's hematopoietic stem cells (Copelan, 2006).

Stem Cell Delivery and Engraftment

The donor stem cells are delivered to the patient through a simple transfusion process, much like a blood transfusion. By mechanisms that are poorly understood, the donor's stem cells migrate to the patient's bone marrow. After transplantation, there is a period of waiting for engraftment—for the donor's stem cells to take hold in the patient's marrow and start producing normal hematopoietic cells. Engraftment can take as long as five weeks, during which time the allogeneic transplant patient is maintained in a protective environment, described later in this section.

Post-HSCT Outcomes and Prognosis

The primary desired outcome of allogeneic HSCT as curative cancer therapy is graft-vs-tumor (the donor marrow effectively attacks and destroys any remaining cancer cells). The major negative outcomes and complications include graft failure (the donor marrow does not successfully "take hold" or engraft); graft-vs-host disease (the donor marrow sees the patient as "foreign" and attacks the patient's own tissues). Graft failure occurs in about 1 to 5 percent of matched-sibling donor grafts and about 15 percent of matched-unrelated donor grafts (Samavedi et al., 2007). Results of allogeneic HSCT depend on multiple factors, such as the patient's overall clinical status, age, disease process, and compatibility of the donor.

Graft-vs-Host Disease

Graft-vs-host disease (GVHD) is a complication that develops in allogeneic HSCT patients. It occurs when donor T-cells, along with the hematopoietic stem cells, are infused into the host (the recipient). The donor T-cells recognize the recipient's tissues as being nonself (foreign) and muster an attack. The incidence of GVHD is highest when a matched unrelated donor is used. Graft-vs-host disease can be acute or chronic, and is difficult to treat successfully; thus, prophylactic drug therapy is generally initiated soon after grafting to prevent development of GVHD.

Despite the significant progress that has been made in the area of HSCT, approximately 40 percent of patients with advanced cancer who undergo allogeneic transplantation will die from complications (Copelan, 2006). Table 8–7 summarizes the common complications of HSCT, including clinical manifestations, and treatments.

Management of the Immediate Post-Allogeneic HSCT Patient

Until engraftment occurs and bone marrow function adequately recovers, the allogeneic HSCT patient is at extreme risk of contracting fatal infections, particularly lethal fungal or viral infections. For this reason, many transplant centers have specific units that house only transplant patients; alternatively, the patient may be placed in an intensive care unit. Both of these settings are able to provide the specialized protective and supportive care required for these patients. Within two to three days after the transplant, the patient's

TABLE 8–7 Clinical Manifestations and Management of Major Complications of HSCT

COMPLICATION	CLINICAL MANIFESTATIONS	MANAGEMENT
Mucositis (oral or intestinal)	Oropharyngeal pain Nausea, abdominal cramping, diarrhea	Pain control: ■ Topical analgesics ■ Systemic opioids Prophylactic: ■ Growth factors (e.g., palifermin, amifostine)
Severe Pancytopenia	Leukopenia ■ < 500 cells/mcL (often < 100) ■ Prolonged neutropenia (2-4 weeks) Thrombocytopenia ■ $< 50,000$ (often $<10,000$) Erythrocytopenia (anemia)	Prophylaxis ■ Recombinant hematopoietic growth factors (e.g., filgrastim) ■ Recombinant erythropoietin ■ Antibiotic, antifungal, and/or antiviral therapy Infection ■ Empiric broad-spectrum antibiotics, antifungals, antivirals Thrombocytopenia ■ Platelet transfusions Anemia ■ RBC transfusions Other infection prophylaxis: ■ Positive-air-pressure sealed rooms with HEPA-filter ■ Strict hand hygiene
Graft-versus-Host Disease (GVHD) (Mild, moderate, or severe)	Acute ■ Skin rash & blisters (similar to burns) ■ Abdominal pain (severe) ■ Severe diarrhea ■ Hyperbilirubinemia, jaundice (liver injury) Chronic ■ Onset: after 3rd month posttransplant ■ Skin rash and itching; possible loss of patches of skin ■ Skin texture and color changes ■ Skin scarring ■ Dry oral mucous membranes and eyes ■ Hyperbilirubinemia (liver injury)	Prophylaxis to reduce occurrence: ■ T-cell depletion of graft Immunosuppressant therapy (e.g., cyclosporine, tacrolimus, methotrexate) Treatment: ■ Corticosteroids ■ Cyclosporine (Successful treatment is often disappointing, making prophylaxis a better option)
Graft Failure (Poor function or complete failure)	Severe pancytopenia Clinical manifestations of ■ Infection ■ Anemia ■ Thrombocytopenia	Prevention ■ Well HLA matched donor Improving marrow function ■ Growth factors (e.g., G-CSF) ■ Erythropoietin Second stem cell infusion

Data from LLS (2008) and Samavedi et al. (2007).

bone marrow function drops to its lowest level (from the conditioning treatment regimen), placing the patient at significant risk for infection; thus a protective environment must be provided (LLS, 2008). The protective environment includes a positive-air-pressure sealed room with special HEPA filters, and protective protocols to guard against potential contamination from people and the hospital environment.

SECTION EIGHT REVIEW

1. The ability to do allogeneic hematopoietic stem cell transplantation in treatment of cancer has had which major advantage?
   A. It can cure all types of leukemia.
   B. It has fewer complications than other treatments for cancer.
   C. Remaining cancer cells can be filtered out during apheresis.
   D. A high-dose chemotherapy regimen can now be used to eradicate the cancer.

2. The major drawback of using autologous stem cells for transplantation is
   A. a higher risk for graft rejection than allogeneic grafts
   B. increased risk of reintroducing malignant cells into the blood
   C. requires high doses of immunosuppressant drug therapy
   D. not as effective as allogeneic stem cell transplant in restoring marrow function

(continued)

(continued)

3. When an allogenic stem cell transplant is desired, the first choice of donor is
   A. a sibling
   B. a parent
   C. a grandparent
   D. a well-matched unrelated donor
4. When a donor's peripheral blood is to be used as the source of hematopoietic stem cells for grafting purposes, what step must be taken before cells are harvested?
   A. The final round of cancer chemotherapy has been completed.
   B. Growth factors are administered to mobilize stem cells.
   C. Total body irradiation therapy must be completed.
   D. Immunosuppressants are administered to decrease the numbers of immune cells.
5. When bone marrow is the source of hematopoietic stem cells, the usual site for cell harvesting is
   A. the sternum
   B. the greater trochanter
   C. the humerus
   D. the iliac crest
6. Hematopoietic stem cells carry which CD marker?
   A. CD4
   B. CD24
   C. CD34
   D. CD44
7. The conditioning treatment necessary to prepare a patient for the hematopoietic stem cell transplant, usually includes (choose all that apply)
   A. high-dose chemotherapy
   B. administration of growth factor
   C. total body irradiation
   D. administration of erythropoietin
8. Stem cell delivery into the recipient involves which process?
   A. injection of cells directly into the bone marrow
   B. intravenous transfusion of the stem cells
   C. multiple injections into various body parts
   D. surgical procedure whereby stem cells are directly implanted
9. Graft failure is a potential negative outcome of HSCT therapy. The risk of this problem can be reduced by
   A. using a matched-sibling donor graft
   B. administering immunosuppressant therapy prior to grafting
   C. holding the conditioning treatments until after the grafting
   D. using a matched-unrelated donor graft
10. Which statement regarding graft-vs-host disease (GVHD) is correct?
   A. It usually targets the heart and lungs.
   B. It is treated using apheresis.
   C. It requires aggressive antibiotic therapy.
   D. It is difficult to successfully treat.

Answers: 1. D, 2. B, 3. A, 4. B, 5. D, 6. C, 7. (A, C), 8. B, 9. A, 10. D

SECTION NINE: Immunosuppressant Therapy

At the completion of this section, the learner will be able to describe immunosuppressant therapy.

The long-term success of organ transplantation has been made possible by use of immunosuppressant therapy. Prior to the discovery and refinement of immunosuppressant therapy, tissue transplantation was considered only a short-term therapy with the exception of identical twin grafts. This section presents an overview of some of the major drug groups and drugs administered for their ability to alter immune function. A summary of the actions and uses, major adverse effects, and nursing implications of the major immunosuppressants is provided in the RELATED PHARMACOTHERAPY: Immunosuppressant agents box. Figure 8–2 shows sites of action of the immunosuppressive agents.

Cyclosporine

Cyclosporine (Sandimmune®, Neoral®), a unique drug of fungal origin, was the major immunosuppressant agent for prevention of allograft rejection for many years. Cyclosporine comes in two forms, Neoral (a microemulsion) and Sandimmune. These two forms are not interchangeable as they are not bioequivalent. Cyclosporine is notable for being highly incompatible with other drugs and great care should be taken to avoid incompatibilities, which can be life-threatening.

Corticosteroids

Corticosteroids are steroid hormones. Prednisone is a synthetic corticosteroid that is commonly used as adjunct immunosuppressant therapy following organ transplantation. Corticosteroids have both anti-inflammatory and immunosuppressant capabilities. In

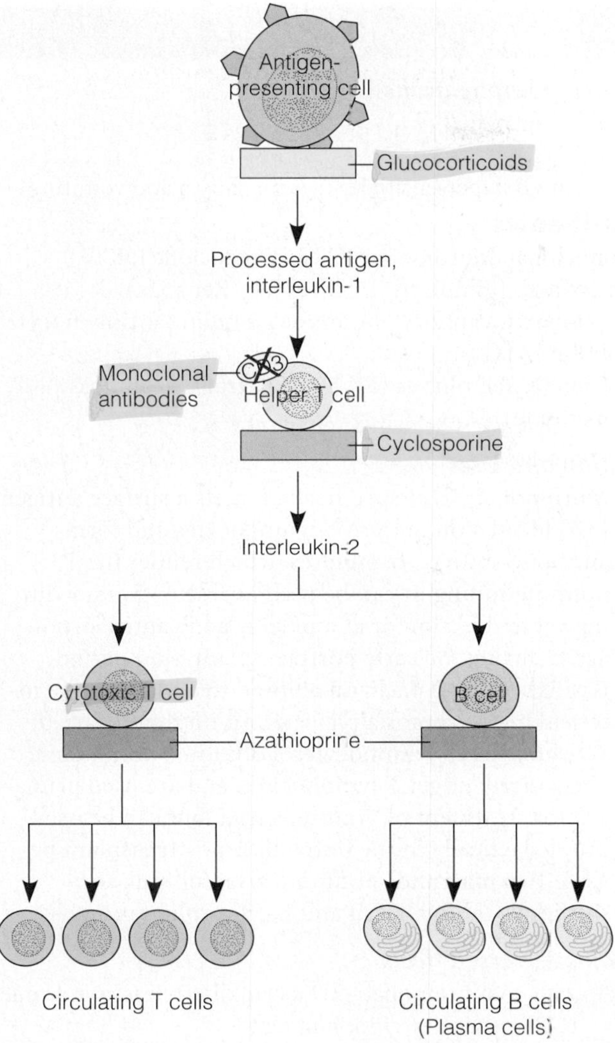

Figure 8–2 ■ Sites of action of immunosuppressive agents. Reprinted from LeMone, P. & Burke, K. *Medical–Surgical Nursing* (4th ed., p. 344), © 2008, with permission from Pearson Education, Inc., Upper Saddle River, New Jersey.

the posttransplant patient, corticosteroids are administered primarily for their immunosuppressant activities; however, long-term use is associated with severe bone disorders, diabetes mellitus, and cataracts.

Antimetabolites

Antimetabolites are **cytotoxic agents** that have the capability of destroying target cells. Certain drugs target immunocompetent cells and thus are of use as immunosuppressants. Two commonly used cell cycle-specific cytotoxic agents are azathioprine and mycophenolate. Before the introduction of cyclosporine, azathioprine was the drug of choice for prevention of graft rejection. Now it mainly has been replaced by mycophenolate or sirolimus as part of combination immunosuppressant therapy. Its action is not specific to lymphocytes and can also inhibit proliferation of all blood cell lines; therefore, the patient can develop anemia and thrombocytopenia, as well as leukopenia. A common product name for azathioprine is Imuran. Mycophenolate, a newer drug than azathioprine, is a less toxic alternative to azathioprine therapy.

Antibodies

Several preparations have been produced specifically as antilymphocyte antibodies. There are two major antibody preparations: monoclonal and polyclonal antibodies. Both types of antibodies are formed from foreign proteins that may cause recipient antibodies to form against them, resulting in sensitization of the patient and possible development of serum sickness or anaphylactic reactions.

Monoclonal and Polyclonal Antibodies

Monoclonal antibodies (mAb) were developed, in part, to increase the specificity of attack by targeting the lymphocyte subsets responsible for the immune rejection reaction. Ideally, this would allow the majority of the immune system to remain intact. Muromonab-CD3 (OKT3), a murine antihuman-CD3

RELATED PHARMACOTHERAPY: Immunosuppressant Agents

Calcineurin Inhibitors

Cyclosporine (Sandimmune, Neoral); tacrolimus (FK-506, Prograf)

Action and Uses

Cyclosporine's powerful immunosuppressant activities are directed against the helper T cells without affecting other types of immune cells, such as macrophages, B cells, granulocytes, and suppressor T cells. The high degree of specificity of cyclosporine allows the immune system to maintain some degree of protection from infection, especially bacterial infections. It may be used as sole or combination therapy in prevention of rejection. It is also an effective agent in treating graft-versus-host disease (GVHD).

Major Adverse Effects

Renal injury with reduced GFR (most common)
Hepatotoxicity, neurotoxicity
Hyperglycemia, hirsutism, gingival hyperplasia

Nursing Implications

Monitor:
- For hypersensitivity reaction
- Kidney and liver function
- Cyclosporine blood levels

Should not be administered concurrently with other immunosuppressants except adrenocortical steroids

Glucocorticoids

Deltasone, Solu-Medrol

(continued)

RELATED PHARMACOTHERAPY *(continued)*

Action and Uses

Corticosteroids significantly decrease the number of lymphocytes, particularly T lymphocytes, by interfering with the production and secretion of interleukin-2. In addition, large doses of corticosteroids suppress immune globulin production, particularly IgG and IgA, and significantly impair monocyte–macrophage function. Steroid therapy is useful for prevention of rejection and is used in rescue therapy for organ rejection; however, long-term use is associated with severe bone disorders, diabetes mellitus, and cataracts.

Major Adverse Effects

- When used postoperatively to prevent rejection
  - Can cause decreased wound healing, increased risk of dehiscence, or tearing of the anastomosis
- Long term
  - Cushing's syndrome (hyperglycemia, bruising, redistribution of fat, bone weakening, and multi-system problems)
  - Gastric ulcers

Nursing Implications

- Patient teaching:
  - Take with milk or food.
  - Do not stop taking drug abruptly.
  - Take same time every day.
- Monitor
  - Serum glucose
  - Blood pressure, weight
  - Serum electrolytes

Antimetabolites

Azathioprine (Imuran, AZA), Mycophenolate mofetil (CellCept, MMF)

Action and Uses

Azathioprine is a prodrug derivative of 6-mercaptopurine that exerts its immunosuppressive activity through its metabolite, 6-thioguanine. It inhibits DNA and RNA synthesis, which ultimately causes suppression of cell-mediated immunity. Azathioprine primarily targets T lymphocytes but has some effect on B cells and, therefore, exerts a degree of inhibition on the humoral immune response. It may be used as adjunct immunosuppressive therapy following transplantation. Mycophenolate mofetil interferes with cell proliferation by inhibiting deoxyribonucleic acid (DNA) and ribonucleic acid (RNA) synthesis. B and T cell lymphocytes are targeted. MMF has been shown to be more effective than azathioprine in preventing acute rejection and is effective in rejection rescue therapy.

Major Adverse Effects

- Bone marrow suppression, hepatotoxicity
- Gastrointestinal - abdominal pain, nausea, diarrhea
- Gastrointestinal hypersensitivity reaction possible

Nursing Implications

- Monitor:
  - CBC, liver enzymes
  - For GI hypersensitivity (severe nausea and vomiting)

Antibodies

Monoclonal: Muromonab-CD3 (Orthoclone OKT3), Basiliximab (Simulect), Daclizumab (Zenapax)
Polyclonal: Lymphocyte immune globulin (antithymocyte globulin [ATG])
Macrolide: Tacrolimus (FK 506, Prograf), sirolimus (Rapamune)

Action and Uses

Muromonab-CD3 specifically targets a surface antigen (T3) located on mature T lymphocytes and forms antibody–antigen complexes, which render the T3 nonfunctioning. It can be used as rescue therapy during acute rejection or as a prophylactic antirejection agent during the early posttransplantation period. Basiliximab and daclizumab bind to and block the interleukin-2 receptor alpha subunit on the surface of activated T cell lymphocytes. Polyclonal antibodies particularly target T lymphocytes and are used primarily for treatment of graft rejection, but can be used prophylactically in the immediate posttransplant period. Two macrolide antibiotics, tacrolimus and sirolimus, inhibit T cell and B cell proliferation.

Major Adverse Effects

- Specific to muromonab-CD3: cytokine-release syndrome (CRS) – see description in text
- Anaphylaxis
- Renal injury, pulmonary injury
- Gastrointestinal (abdominal discomfort, nausea, diarrhea)
- Hypo- or hypertension, tachycardia, fever
- Neurotoxicity
- Specific to tacrolimus: Diabetes mellitus (potentially reversible)
- Specific to sirolimus: Hyperlipidemia, hepatotoxicity, nephrotoxicity, hyperglycemia

Nursing Implications

- Muromonab-CD3: Administer prophylactic drugs to minimize CRS symptoms; monitor closely for development of CRS; have cardiopulmonary resuscitation equipment available
- Sirolimus: Should not be administered within four hours of cyclosporine
- Monitor for:
  - Hypersensitivity reactions
  - Hyperglycemia, hyperlipidemia
  - Gastrointestinal disturbances
  - CNS disturbances
  - Renal and hepatic injury

monoclonal antibody, is the primary agent currently in use, although two new induction agents have recently been added to the immunosuppressant drug arsenal.

Basiliximab (Simulect®) and Daclizumab (Zenapax®) are two newer generation monoclonal antibodies available and are used for induction therapy. These IL-2 receptor antagonists are modified monoclonal antibodies with most of the murine portion replaced with human antibody component (Gelone & Lake, 2002; Smith, 2002). Unlike OKT3, the IL-2 receptor antagonists do not trigger the cytokine-release syndrome (CRS), have relatively mild side effects, and exhibit few drug interactions.

Cytokine-release syndrome (CRS) is a reaction that is associated with initiation of monoclonal antibody therapy, particularly OKT3. When first described, it was called "first-dose response" because it typically develops within the first hour following the initial dose of OKT3. CRS is caused by the release of cytokines following an initial activation of T lymphocytes. Cytokines are cell mediators that are responsible for cell function and growth regulation. CRS can be mild or life-threatening. Severe flulike symptoms are the most common, such as chills, fever, and headache. Additional symptoms may include nausea, vomiting, and diarrhea. CRS symptoms usually diminish with each day of treatment. Severe symptoms are rare and may include pulmonary edema, hypotension, neurotoxicity, nephrotoxicity, and thrombosis. Premedication with diphenhydramine, methylprednisolone, and acetaminophen is usually given 30 minutes prior to OKT3 administration. Symptoms typically disappear after 2 to 3 days of therapy. Cardiopulmonary resuscitation equipment should be kept available when initiating OKT3.

Whereas monoclonal antibodies are derived from one cell line, **polyclonal antibodies** come from multiple cell lines. Polyclonal antibodies, such as lymphocyte immune globulin (antithymocyte globulin), are typically obtained from animal sources.

Macrolide Antibiotics

Macrolides are a class of drugs (usually antibiotics) like erythromycin and clarithromycin that bind to cell membranes and cause changes in protein function leading to bacteria cell death. There are two major immunosuppressant drugs in this class, tacrolimus and sirolimus. Tacrolimus (Prograf®, FK-506) was originally derived from a soil fungus. Although unrelated to cyclosporine, it acts in a similar fashion in its attack on helper T lymphocytes and has largely replaced cyclosporine therapy in many transplant programs. Sirolimus (Rapamune®), approved in 1999, was originally developed as a potential antifungal drug. Hyperlipidemia is the most notable side effect, especially when paired with cyclosporine and prednisone. Concomitant use with cyclosporine potentiates the nephrotoxicity effect of cyclosporine leading the manufacturer to recommend that sirolimus be given four hours after cyclosporine.

SECTION NINE REVIEW

1. The immunosuppressant that selectively acts against the helper T cells without affecting other types of immune cells is
   A. corticosteroids
   B. azathioprine
   C. cyclosporine
   D. OKT3
2. Long-term posttransplantation steroid therapy is particularly associated with potentially severe ______ disorders.
   A. heart
   B. bone
   C. liver
   D. blood
3. The major gastrointestinal side effect common to almost all immunosuppressant drugs is
   A. nausea and vomiting
   B. heartburn
   C. abdominal cramping
   D. constipation
4. Monoclonal antibodies are unique in that they target
   A. B cells
   B. helper T lymphocytes
   C. suppressor T lymphocytes
   D. specific lymphocyte subsets
5. The MOST common symptoms associated with CRS include which of the following?
   A. chills
   B. vomiting
   C. diarrhea
   D. hypotension
6. When a patient has orders to receive sirolimus and cyclosporine, which administration rule applies?
   A. They should be administered simultaneously.
   B. They cannot be given within four hours of each other.
   C. They should be administered in separate veins.
   D. They cannot be administered within six hours of each other.

Answers: 1. C, 2. B, 3. A, 4. D, 5. A, 6. B

SECTION TEN: Overview of Selected Organ Transplantation

At the completion of this section, the learner will be able to discuss the general concepts related to transplantation of selected organs, including postprocedure management implications.

This section presents a brief overview of selected solid organ transplants, including kidney, heart, heart–lung, lung, liver, pancreas, pancreas–kidney, and small intestine. Postprocedure management and evaluation of organ function are also discussed.

Emerging Evidence

- A study of survival of intestinal transplantation candidates showed that use of home parenteral nutrition was a satisfactory option for treatment of intestinal failure and timely intestinal transplantation was a potentially life-saving option for those candidates who develop parenteral nutrition failure (*Piroi, Forbes, Joly et al., 2008*).
- In a study of level of education as a potential determinant of access to kidney transplantation and outcomes following kidney transplant, the findings suggested that mortality following kidney transplantation was not associated with level of education; however, death rates following allograft kidney failure were associated with less education (*Schaeffner, Mehta, & Winkelmayer, 2008*).
- In a study of liver transplant candidates, investigators concluded that candidates could benefit from earlier referral to a liver transplant center for the purposes of improved management of advanced renal disease and addressing psychosocial issues (*Aranda-Michel, et al, 2008*).
- A study of renal function following solitary pancreas transplantation investigated deterioration of kidney function following transplantation. The findings suggested that transplant patients with a baseline GFR below 60 prior to transplantation were at increased risk for post transplant renal complications. Researchers suggested that better selection of transplant candidates based on GFR might reduce the incidence of kidney complications (*Odorico, et al., 2008*).

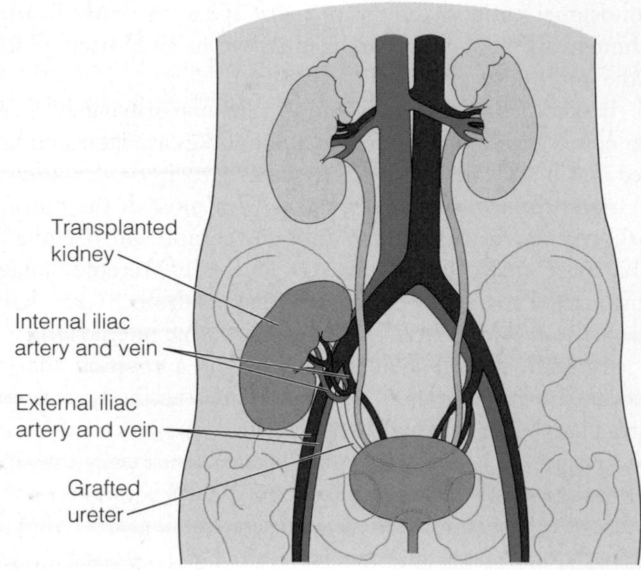

Figure 8–3 ■ Placement of a transplanted kidney in the iliac fossa with anastomosis to the hypogastric artery, iliac vein, and bladder. Reprinted from LeMone, P. & Burke, K. *Medical–Surgical Nursing* (4th ed., p. 921), © 2008, with permission from Pearson Education, Inc., Upper Saddle River, New Jersey.

Kidney Transplantation

Kidney transplants have been in the literature since the early 1930s, when a kidney was transplanted into the thigh of a young woman in Russia. Today, kidney transplants are a highly successful mode of therapy. A diagnosis of end-stage renal disease (ESRD) does not necessitate renal transplantation because dialysis can be used as an alternative therapy for ESRD. A patient who is being considered for transplantation is carefully screened to determine whether the probability of a successful transplant is sufficient to warrant transplantation rather than continuing use of dialysis. When a renal transplant is successful, it is significantly less costly than long-term dialysis therapy.

Major Indications for Transplantation

ESRD is the primary indicator for a renal transplant. ESRD can result from many problems, the three most common causes being hypertension, diabetes mellitus, and glomerulonephritis. These three conditions comprise more than half of all causes of ESRD. As of August 2008, there were more than 76,500 patients on the national waiting list for renal transplants (UNOS, 2008).

Preparation of the Recipient

When a kidney becomes available, the recipient is admitted to the hospital and pretransplant orders are initiated. Admission may be the day before a scheduled surgery if there is a living donor. If a cadaver donor is made available, preparatory time is much shorter. On notification, the patient is admitted to the transplant center, with surgery rapidly following admission. Preoperative hemodialysis is often performed to normalize fluid and electrolyte balance. Before the patient goes to surgery, crossmatching is performed. If the results are negative, an initial dose of an immunosuppressant and prophylactic antibiotics are administered either before or after the patient is transferred to the operating room. Figure 8–3 provides an illustration of a renal transplant.

Postoperative Management

Following transplantation, the patient is monitored closely for the first 24 hours, often in an intensive care setting. Medical and nursing priorities depend on the level of graft function and development of any complications. Typical postoperative orders for the first 24 hours include the following:

- IV fluids at a rate sufficient to keep urine output greater than 100 mL/hr; rate may also be titrated based on hourly urine outputs
- Diuretic therapy
- Daily weights
- Vital signs and central venous pressure readings
- Prophylactic antibiotic therapy
- Close monitoring of:
  - laboratory values: serum creatinine trends, electrolytes (particularly potassium, sodium, bicarbonate, calcium, and phosphorous), hemoglobin and hematocrit, serum glucose, blood urea nitrogen (BUN), arterial blood gases (ABGs), and white blood cell (WBC) count
  - intake and output balance with hourly urine output
  - blood clots, which can obstruct the urinary catheter
  - signs and symptoms of fluid volume excess
  - signs and symptoms of acute infection
- Blood levels of immunosuppressant drugs (e.g., C_sA, tacrolimus, and sirolimus)

Graft dysfunction is more commonly noted in cadaver grafts than in live ones. In the cadaver transplant, organ ischemia is more likely a result of the increased length of time the organ was preserved. Renal ischemia may lead to acute tubular necrosis, which causes oliguria or anuria. If the dysfunction lasts more than 48 hours, hemodialysis may be necessary until the graft begins functioning sufficiently. Recovery of the graft takes approximately two weeks.

Hypertension is a common problem in the kidney transplant patient. This condition can be exacerbated during the postoperative recovery period because of fluid volume imbalances precipitated by the high volume of IV fluids used to maintain a high urine flow. Antihypertensive agents may be ordered preoperatively and postoperatively to maintain the blood pressure within an acceptable range for the patient.

Evaluation of Renal Function

In addition to laboratory tests, several other procedures can be performed to evaluate function of the renal graft. A needle biopsy using ultrasound is performed to examine renal tissue. This is considered the most valuable indicator of renal function. Ultrasound of the kidney may be ordered to look for hydronephrosis, obstruction, or collections of fluid. A renal scan using radioactive isotopes also evaluates renal function.

Postrenal Transplant Complications

General complications associated with organ transplantation are presented in Section Seven. The one-year graft survival rate for cadaver renal transplants is about 88 percent, and for living-donor transplants the graft survival rate is about 95 percent (UNOS, 2005). The most common long-term complication of renal transplantation is graft rejection.

Heart, Heart–Lung, and Lung Transplantation

Dr. Christiaan Barnard performed the first heart transplant in 1967 in South Africa (Augustine & Masiello-Miller, 1995). The first single-lung transplant was performed by Hardy in 1963, and the first successful heart–lung transplant was performed at Stanford University in 1981 (Owens & Wallop, 1995). The early history of heart, lung, and heart–lung transplants was one of poor graft success rates. Organ rejection, inadequate healing, and infection were major obstacles to success. It was not until the late 1970s (heart) and early 1980s (lung and heart–lung) that technical and immunosuppressant therapy improvements made these transplants a successful surgical option. The introduction of the immunosuppressant cyclosporine played a major role in the eventual success of these transplants.

Major Indications for Transplantation

General criteria for determination of transplant need were presented in Section Six. Specific major conditions that are associated with heart, lung, or heart–lung transplantation are listed in Table 8–8. As of August 2008, there were about 2,650 patients on the heart transplant waiting list, about 2,100 patients on the lung transplant waiting list, and about 100 on the heart–lung waiting list (UNOS, 2008).

TABLE 8–8 Major Heart and Lung Conditions Associated with Organ Transplantation

ORGAN	MAJOR CONDITIONS
Heart	Cardiomyopathy, valvular heart disease, ventricular aneurysm, viral myocarditis, congenital malformations, arteriosclerotic coronary artery disease
Lung	*Single lung:* End-stage pulmonary fibrosis, chronic obstructive pulmonary disease, pulmonary hypertension secondary to Eisenmenger's syndrome, primary pulmonary hypertension
	Double lung: Cystic fibrosis, bronchiectasis, primary pulmonary hypertension
Heart–lung	Primary pulmonary hypertension (no known cause), congenital heart disease, Eisenmenger's syndrome

Preparation of the Recipient

After the patient has been found suitable for organ transplantation and he or she has been placed on the transplant waiting list, the major management focus becomes maintaining the patient's cardiac and/or lung status. If the patient lives any distance from the transplant center, he or she may be asked to find lodging close to the transplant center to be readily available. In some cases, the patient may carry a pager, cell phone or other communication device to facilitate quick communication and availability.

During the waiting period, the patient may require multiple admissions into the hospital to control cardiac or respiratory failure problems. Health maintenance is promoted through rest; control of cardiac arrhythmias, heart failure, and sodium and fluid intake; and monitoring of drug therapy for therapeutic effects. Lung transplant candidates will have pulmonary function closely monitored and controlled through bronchodilators; IV diuretics; oxygen supplementation; steroid therapy; and pulmonary vasodilator therapy, such as prostacyclin to control pulmonary hypertension. Some heart patients may require more aggressive therapy, such as IV inotropic drugs; a pacemaker-cardioverter-defibrillator; or mechanical circulatory assistance, such as the intra-aortic balloon pump (IABP) or a left ventricular assist device (LVAD) as a bridge to transplantation. Unfortunately, some patients die before they can receive a transplant because of rapid worsening of heart or lung failure, or scarcity of organ resources.

When a donor organ is available, the recipient is immediately brought to the hospital and initially prepared with appropriate laboratory tests and a chest X-ray. Preoperative teaching (transplant teaching) begins and the patient may receive an initial dose of immunosuppressant therapy and prophylactic antibiotics. Blood is drawn for a retrospective HLA crossmatch with the donor.

As part of the transplant teaching, the patient and family are informed that the surgery will not be performed until the donor organs have been examined and have been determined to be suitable for transplantation. More specifically, the patient is taken to the operating room and intubated but the incision is not made until the procurement team has visualized the organs to be transplanted and they have given the "go-ahead." If the

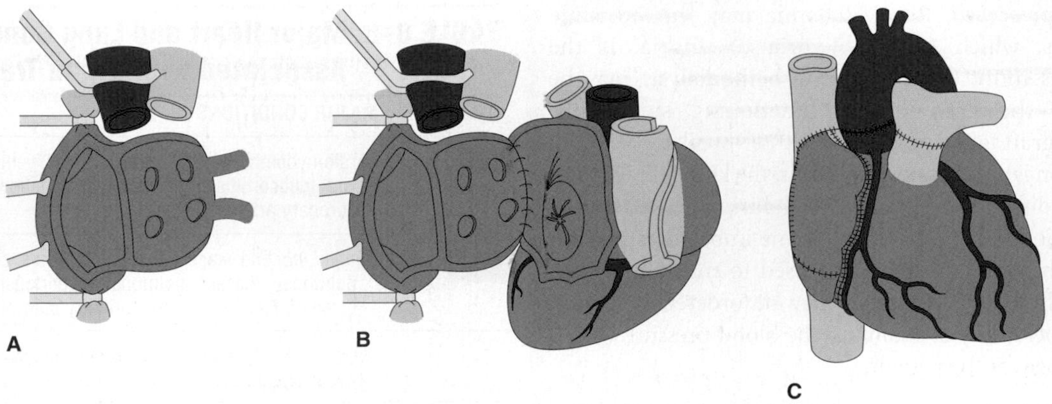

Figure 8–4 ■ Cardiac transplantation. A, The heart is removed, leaving the posterior walls of the atria intact. The donor heart is anastomosed to the atria, B; and the great vessels, C. Reprinted from LeMone, P. & Burke, K. *Medical–Surgical Nursing* (4th ed., p. 1035), © 2008 with permission from Pearson Education, Inc., Upper Saddle River, New Jersey.

donor organs are determined to be not suitable, the recipient surgery is canceled. Figure 8–4 provides an illustration of a cardiac transplant.

Postoperative Management

Postoperative management of the heart and heart–lung transplant patient is similar to that of all open-heart surgery patients with the exception of denervation of the transplanted heart. Loss of cardiac autonomic innervation alters the heart's ability to respond to hypovolemia, hypotension, exercise, and certain drugs (e.g., atropine). In addition, a resting tachycardia is usually present because of the lack of vagal innervation. These patients generally do not experience chest pain with cardiac ischemia and infarction. Typical postoperative management includes the following:

1. Maintaining or correcting problems associated with cardiac function and denervation, including
   - Hemodynamic and cardiac monitoring for cardiac failure, cardiac dysrhythmias, perioperative myocardial infarction, cardiac tamponade, and hemorrhage
   - Pharmacologic therapy based on cardiac status, possibly including diuretics, vasodilators, inotropic agents, and cardiac dysrhythmic agents
2. Maintaining or correcting problems with fluid and electrolyte balance, including
   - Monitoring intake and output balance and electrolyte trends
   - Intravenous fluid therapy titrated to fluid balance status and cardiac function status
   - Electrolyte replacement as indicated
3. Maintaining and correcting problems with renal function, including
   - Monitoring patient's urine output and renal laboratory value trends

The heart–lung and lung transplant patient is at risk for development of problems associated with pulmonary dysfunction. Denervation of the transplanted lung leads to impaired cough and mucociliary clearance resulting in infections, retained secretions, and mucous plugs (Schulman, 2001). Bronchoscopic exams, called "surveillance bronchoscopies," are often performed in the immediate postoperative period to remove retained secretions and mucous plugs, and visually assess the anastomotic site for possible dehiscence, necrosis, or stenosis. The following are management considerations related to the lungs:

1. Maintaining pulmonary function
   - Administer diuretic therapy
   - Fluid restriction
   - Early weaning from mechanical ventilator with reintubation, if required
   - Monitor fluid balance: intake and output, daily weights
   - Monitor ABGs, pulse oximetry, and S_vO_2
   - Bronchodilator therapy, as required
   - Early ambulation
   - Incentive spirometry
2. Preventing infection
   - Strict aseptic suctioning technique
   - Aggressive postextubation pulmonary toilet
   - Cough and deep-breathing exercises
   - Incentive spirometry
   - Percussion and postural drainage
   - Early removal of invasive lines and tubes
   - Close monitoring of trends in temperature, chest x-ray, and peak expiratory flow. Although the white blood cell count will be monitored, it is anticipated that it will increase significantly for several days postop secondary to drug therapy

Evaluation of Organ Function

Postoperative organ function will be evaluated in a variety of ways, including laboratory tests, electrocardiograms, pulmonary function testing, and tissue biopsies. Organ rejection in the heart transplant patient may present as malaise, shortness of breath, new onset of peripheral edema, weight gain, or new onset of atrial fibrillation/flutter. Rejection in the lung and heart–lung transplant may be exhibited by shortness of breath, hypoxia, decrease in spirometry, elevated WBC, or a chest X-ray infiltrate (Nathan & Ohler, 2002).

The Biopsy

Heart Biopsy. A biopsy of the right ventricular wall is obtained approximately one week posttransplantation. A special device called an endomyocardial bioptome is inserted into the right ventricle by way of the right jugular vein. The procedure is generally performed in the cardiac catheterization laboratory. The biopsy results can definitively indicate whether rejection is present and to what degree. Immunosuppressant therapy can then be adjusted to halt the rejection process. Biopsies are performed periodically to continue monitoring the graft status.

Lung Biopsy. Pulmonary tissue can be obtained by biopsy during a bronchoscopy procedure. In patients who have had a heart–lung transplant, the lung is usually biopsied first because rejection occurs more frequently in the lungs.

Liver Transplantation

Liver transplantation was first attempted in a human being in 1963 by Dr. Thomas Starzl. It was not until the early 1980s that the procedure became a long-term option. This change was largely because of the introduction of cyclosporine, which rapidly increased graft survival rates to approximately 79 percent at three years posttransplantation by 2005 (UNOS, 2005). Improvements in immunosuppressant therapy and better surgical and donor organ preservation techniques played important roles in increasing survival rates.

Major Indications for Transplantation

Three major liver problems that are referred for possible liver transplantation include chronic irreversible liver disease, liver and biliary tree primary malignant tumors, and fulminant hepatic failure. Cirrhosis is the most common indicator for liver transplantation in adults. In children, indications include such disorders as biliary atresia, Alagille syndrome, and inborn errors of metabolism.

Preparation of the Recipient

As with other patients on the waiting list for organs, the waiting period is an extremely stressful period. Patients may experience anger, fear, depression, and hopelessness as their condition worsens. The patient and the family members need psychological support and possibly counseling during this period. When available, patients and their families may be encouraged to join a transplant support group at the transplant medical center.

The patient's hepatic function and nutritional status are monitored intermittently, usually including laboratory tests. The patient may require admission into the hospital for interim treatment if hepatic function decreases significantly. Preoperative teaching is often initiated during the waiting period because time is short once an organ becomes available for transplantation.

Alternative Transplant Approaches

Not all recipients receive an entire donor liver. Two alternative types of liver grafts may be used: split-liver transplants and living-related donor transplants. The split-liver transplant divides a single donor liver into two pieces to provide a graft for two recipients. Scarcity of resources and the fact that a small child recipient cannot take an entire adult donor liver triggered the original interest in split-liver transplants. The operation is extremely complex and a high morbidity and mortality rate has made this option a limited one at this time. The living-related donor transplant usually involves a donation from a parent to a small child.

Postoperative Management

Immediate postoperative management in the critical care unit focuses on prevention of complications, particularly those associated with liver dysfunction, abnormalities of fluid and electrolytes, infection, and rejection. Early management also centers on support of the other systems, such as cardiopulmonary, renal, gastrointestinal, and neurologic. The complexity of the liver transplant procedure places the recipient at risk for development of many complications. Nursing care in the intensive care unit setting requires intense multiple system monitoring and rapid analysis of abnormal assessment data.

In addition to the typical postoperative management associated with all transplant patients, the major management goal that is unique to liver transplantation is maintaining normal liver function, which includes the following assessments:

- Monitor bile drainage appearance and quantity
- Monitor laboratory tests that reflect liver function:
  - Prothrombin time (PT) and partial thromboplastin time (PTT)
  - Alanine aminotransferase (ALT) and aspartate aminotransferase (AST), alkaline phosphatase
  - Bilirubin (total and direct), ammonia levels
  - Glucose
- Monitor neurologic status

Evaluation of Organ Function

The general function of the graft is routinely monitored through laboratory testing. **Rejection** typically presents itself as elevations in liver function indicators, such as serum transaminases, bilirubin, alkaline phosphatase; and an elevated WBC count. In addition, the patient may experience general malaise, a mild fever, disorientation, hepatomegaly, and right upper quadrant pain/tenderness. An ultrasound of the abdomen may be ordered to investigate the general condition of the liver. Liver biopsy, however, is the only means of making the definitive diagnosis of rejection.

Pancreas and Pancreas-Kidney Transplantation

William Kelly and Richard Lillehei pioneered human pancreas transplantation in 1966 at the University of Minnesota. Even though this allograft was unsuccessful, the nine combination kidney–pancreas transplants performed over the subsequent two years were successful. Because of the success of the dual-organ transplantation, pancreas transplantation was abandoned in favor of the kidney–pancreas transplant. The pancreas transplantation success rate has improved dramatically over the past decade because of improved donor selection and immunosuppressive therapy, advanced organ retrieval and preservation techniques, and modifications in pancreatic exocrine secretion management.

Major Indications and Types of Transplants

Type 1 diabetes mellitus is the leading cause of end-stage renal disease, blindness, and amputation. To date, pancreas transplantation is the single most effective physiologic method of controlling glucose metabolism, slowing the progression of end-stage organ disease and improving the quality of life in type 1 diabetes patients (Dimercurio et al., 2002; Cowan et al., 2002). The degree of nephropathy determines the type of pancreas transplant. Available options include simultaneous pancreas–kidney transplant (SPK), pancreas transplant alone (PTA), or pancreas transplant after a kidney transplant (PAK). Figure 8–5 provides an illustration of a simultaneous pancreas–kidney transplant surgery. In August 2008, there were over 1,500 patients on the pancreas wait list, and more than 2,250 on the pancreas-kidney organ wait list. (UNOS, 2008).

Preparation of the Recipient

Pretransplant care for the pancreas–kidney transplant candidate is similar to that for the patient awaiting a kidney transplant. Monitoring of common diabetic complications, such as nephropathy, retinopathy, and hyperglycemia, is followed closely by the transplant team. Depending on the degree of nephropathy present, the pretransplant patient may require renal dialysis prior to transplantation. Education is initiated during this period, focusing on the surgical procedure and method of exocrine drainage, immunosuppressant drugs, and organ rejection.

Postoperative Management

In the critical care unit, postoperative care focuses on prevention and treatment of infection, thrombosis, dehydration, metabolic acidosis, hyperinsulinemia, acute rejection, and graft dysfunction. In addition, management of pancreatic exocrine secretions (digestive enzymes) is essential to prevent and control enzyme-related complications. Use of the "systemic bladder" surgical technique predisposes the transplant patient to bladder infections, pyelonephritis, graft pancreatitis, and dehydration with intractable metabolic acidosis. The "portal-enteric" technique is more physiologic with normal carbohydrate and lipid metabolism. Fasting hyperinsulinemia and metabolic acidosis are avoided as are urinary tract infections, hematuria, and reflux pancreatitis. Postoperative monitoring includes:

- Serum glucose, amylase, HbA1c, C-peptide levels, CBC, and electrolytes
- Urinary amylase levels if bladder drainage of exocrine secretions is employed
- Hourly urine, nasogastric, and wound drainage measurements
- Aggressive fluid volume and electrolyte replacement
- Daily weights
- Vital signs with central venous pressure readings
- Observation for signs and symptoms of infection, especially urinary tract infections and pancreatitis
- Hematuria
- Serum drug levels to maintain therapeutic levels of immunosuppressant therapy (e.g., C_sA, tacrolimus, sirolimus)

Graft dysfunction or loss may be attributed to thrombosis, pancreatitis, organ preservation, or surgical techniques. Typical signs and symptoms include pain/tenderness over the graft site, fever, elevated serum glucose and amylase levels, and decreased urinary amylase levels.

Evaluation of Organ Function

Early detection of pancreas rejection in the PAK and PTA transplant recipient remains difficult because of a lack of specific clinical markers. Signs and symptoms often mimic pancreatitis. Elevated laboratory values may be a result of

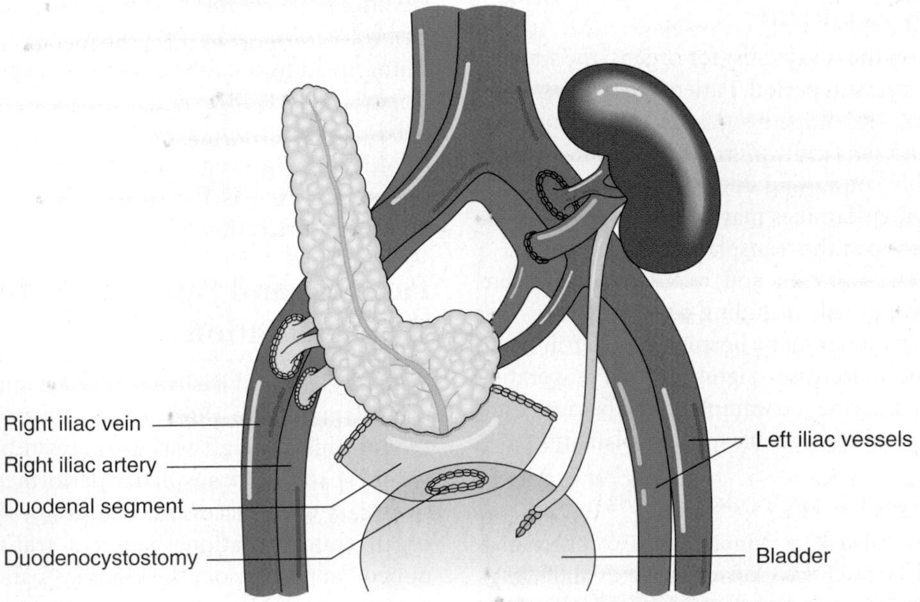

Figure 8–5 ■ Surgical technique of combined pancreas kidney transplantation.

drug toxicity, high dose steroids, and diuretic therapy. An elevated serum glucose occurs late in the rejection episode and is not considered a reliable indicator of rejection. The definitive diagnosis can only be made by ultrasound or CT-guided needle biopsy through a cystoscopy for bladder drained grafts or a percutaneous biopsy. In the SPK transplant a rise in the serum creatinine is an early indicator for kidney rejection and a surrogate marker for pancreas rejection because both organs reject at approximately the same time. In this case a kidney biopsy is performed to determine the grade of rejection.

Intestine Transplantation

Not until the introduction of tacrolimus in 1989 did small bowel transplantation emerge as a successful option for patients with permanent intestinal failure dependent on total parenteral nutrition (TPN). Prior to this time technical complications, sepsis from the intestinal bacterial load, and lack of effective immunosuppressive therapy against the massive lymphoid tissue prevented any long-term success. The small intestine is unique in that it is the largest immune organ in the body, is prone to infection because its contents are not sterile, and has no clinical tests to assess function of the transplanted organ. As of August 2008 approximately 230 patients were waiting for an intestinal transplant (UNOS, 2008). Significant progress has been made in transplant success since 1989, with an approximate 80 percent survival rate of graft and recipient at one year post transplantation (O'Keefe, 2006).

Major Indications and Types of Transplants

The major indication for intestinal transplantation is permanent and irreversible intestinal failure as a result of short gut syndrome, which is further divided into structural and functional failure. *Intestinal failure* is the inability of the gut to maintain sufficient nutrition, fluid, and electrolyte balance. *Functional failure* is associated with severe dysmotility of the gut leading to malabsorption and TPN dependency, such as chronic intestinal pseudo-obstruction syndrome (CIPS), congenital enteritis, and radiation enteritis. *Structural failure* results from trauma, bowel resection, or other abnormalities that shorten the length of the small intestine. Crohn's disease and necrotizing enterocolitis are examples of diseases that can eventually cause structural failure.

Currently, there are three types of surgical procedures performed, depending on the needs of the patient. The isolated intestinal transplant is indicated in irreversible intestinal failure accompanied by poor quality of life, failure to thrive, permanent dependence on TPN for survival, and limited central venous access for TPN therapy. Combined intestinal and liver transplantation is necessary for patients with both irreversible intestinal failure and TPN-induced liver dysfunction/failure (Park, 2002; Williams et al., 2002). Global dysmotility of the GI tract results in the need for a multivisceral transplant (small bowel with liver, stomach, and/or pancreas).

Preparation of the Recipient

After the patient is placed on the waiting list, the focus shifts to maintaining optimum nutrition and preventing infection, especially at the vascular access site. TPN provides the needed caloric intake in addition to enteral and oral feedings, if tolerated. Blood chemistries, coagulation studies, liver function tests, and vitamin levels are assessed on a regular basis. Vascular line access for TPN therapy must remain patent and free of infection because these lines may be needed for several months posttransplant for ongoing nutritional therapy. Teaching begins with the patient and family to prepare them for prolonged daily management and care, and the change in body image associated with the ileostomy.

Postoperative Management

Postoperative management of the intestinal transplant patient presents a unique challenge to the ICU nursing staff in maintaining a balance between the appropriate level of immunosuppressive therapy and the predisposition to infections in the gut. In addition, denervation of the transplanted intestine has a significant effect on water and electrolyte absorption and motility function leading to diarrhea and malabsorption. Based on these issues, priorities in the immediate postoperative period include

- Strict intake and output including enteric output from the ileostomy, nasogastric tube, jejunostomy tube, and rectum
- Daily weights
- Vital signs and hemodynamic monitoring
- Assessment of postoperative ileus, which should resolve after 5 days
- Monitoring for rejection and infection
- Frequent monitoring of labs: electrolytes, vitamins, mineral and trace elements, protein, albumin, magnesium, bicarbonate, CBC, liver function tests
- Strict management of IV fluids to meet demands of stomal output
- Caloric support to meet the metabolic demands
- Maintenance of skin integrity around stomal site
- Daily monitoring of serum levels of immunosuppressive drugs (cyclosporine, tacrolimus, and sirolimus)

With improved nutritional therapies now available, many intestinal transplant patients can eventually attain nutritional autonomy; and initiation of early, progressive enteral feedings should be considered, using complex polymeric formula (Matarese, Costa, Bond et al., 2007).

Evaluation of Organ Function

Unlike the kidney and liver transplants, the intestinal transplant lacks a serum marker to suggest rejection. Clinically, patients may exhibit significant increase or decrease in stomal output, fever, decreased or absent bowel sounds, abdominal pain/distention, irritability, and/or change in stomal color. Surveillance endoscopy with tissue biopsy is performed as often as twice weekly through the ileostomy to diagnose rejection.

SECTION TEN REVIEW

1. The major indication for kidney transplantation is end-stage renal disease, which most commonly results from which problems? (choose all that apply)
   A. diabetes mellitus
   B. hypertension
   C. glomerulonephritis
   D. nephrotoxicity
2. Dysfunction of a renal graft is most commonly associated with the
   A. preoperative condition of the donor
   B. preoperative condition of the recipient
   C. length of time the organ was preserved
   D. length of time required to perform the transplant
3. The most common cause of renal graft failure is
   A. rejection
   B. hypoperfusion
   C. hypertension
   D. nephrotoxicity
4. Major conditions that are associated with the need for heart transplantation include (choose all that apply)
   A. myocardial infarction
   B. congenital malformations
   C. ventricular aneurysm
   D. cardiomyopathy
5. While the patient is waiting for a lung transplant, health maintenance particularly focuses on the ______system.
   A. cardiopulmonary
   B. renal
   C. hepatobiliary
   D. neurologic
6. Postoperative management of the patient with a heart transplant includes the goal of preventing infection. Which of the following interventions most directly addresses this goal?
   A. early ambulation
   B. monitor urine output and laboratory trends
   C. monitor ABGs, pulse oximetry, SVO_2
   D. aggressive postextubation pulmonary toilet
7. Approximately 1 week following a heart transplant, a heart biopsy is performed to evaluate the recipient for
   A. anastomosis leak
   B. rejection
   C. infection
   D. ischemic tissue
8. Major indications for liver transplantation include (choose all that apply)
   A. fulminant hepatic failure
   B. acute hepatotoxicity
   C. malignant hepatic tumors
   D. irreversible chronic liver disease
9. Liver transplant patients are at particularly high risk for development of which early complication?
   A. hemorrhage
   B. rejection
   C. infection
   D. obstruction
10. A split-liver type of transplant refers to
    A. a parent-to-small-child liver donation
    B. splitting normal from abnormal parts of liver
    C. dividing a cadaver donor liver between two recipients
    D. splitting lobes of a live donor liver between several recipients
11. Postoperative monitoring of liver function typically includes which of the following? (choose all that apply)
    A. bilirubin
    B. ammonia
    C. prothrombin time
    D. blood urea nitrogen
12. The major indication for a pancreas transplant is
    A. type 1 diabetes mellitus
    B. end-stage renal disease
    C. diabetic retinopathy
    D. peripheral neuropathy
13. Use of the systemic bladder technique to manage the pancreatic exocrine secretions predisposes the recipient to which complications? (choose all that apply)
    A. graft pancreatitis
    B. thrombosis
    C. hematuria
    D. pyelonephritis
14. The most common complications in the immediate postoperative period of the pancreas transplant include (choose all that apply)
    A. hemorrhage
    B. metabolic acidosis
    C. hyperinsulinemia
    D. dehydration
15. Clinical signs and symptoms of pancreatic graft dysfunction exhibited by the patient include which of the following? (choose all that apply)
    A. fever
    B. tenderness over graft site
    C. decreased serum amylase
    D. elevated blood sugar
16. Irreversible intestinal failure is the primary indication for intestine transplantation. Which of the following conditions can result in intestinal failure? (choose all that apply)
    A. Crohn's disease
    B. gastroesophageal reflux disease
    C. radiation enteritis
    D. trauma to the intestine
17. Denervation of the transplanted small intestine results in
    A. malabsorption
    B. decreased caloric requirements
    C. constipation
    D. elevated serum sodium

18. The gold standard for diagnosing acute rejection in the intestinal transplant is
   A. a significant increase in the stomal output
   B. an ileus
   C. an endoscopic mucosal biopsy
   D. a change in stomal color

Answers: 1. (A, B, C), 2. C, 3. A, 4. (B, C, D), 5. A, 6. D, 7. B, 8. (A, C, D), 9. A, 10. C, 11. (A, B, C), 12. A, 13. (A, C, D), 14. (B, C, D), 15. (A, B, D), 16. (A, C, D) 17. A, 18. C.

POSTTEST

The following Posttest is constructed in a case study format. A patient is presented. Questions asked are based on available data. New data are presented as the case study progresses.

Kathy S. is a critically ill 23-year-old college student who recently sustained multiple trauma in a motor vehicle crash. The health care team is currently initiating evaluation of Kathy for establishing brain death.

1. If it is decided that Kathy may be a potential organ donor, she will be evaluated for suitability as a donor. Before contacting the organ procurement organization (OPO) for a referral, you should gather what information? (choose all that apply)
   A. age, sex, and race
   B. past medical history
   C. cause of brain injury
   D. details of the crash
2. Potential donors such as Kathy are protected by law. The legislation that gives specific guidelines regarding how donation is to be carried out is the
   A. National Organ Transplant Act
   B. Uniform Anatomical Gift Act
   C. Uniform Determination of Death Act
   D. required-request legislation
3. Brain-death testing at the bedside is performed on Kathy. Required brain-death criteria include which of the following? (choose all that apply)
   A. Glasgow Coma Scale of 5
   B. negative ice calorics
   C. no doll's eye reflex
   D. no CNS depressants
4. The manner in which Kathy's family is approached about organ donation is important. It is strongly suggested that her family not be approached until
   A. Kathy has been declared legally dead
   B. they have asked the physician about possible donation
   C. they have acknowledged that Kathy is brain dead
   D. it is determined whether Kathy has signed a uniform donor card
5. Prior to discussing donation with Kathy's family, she may have a preliminary evaluation performed by the donor procurement coordinator/team. Initial evaluation is performed primarily to
   A. save time
   B. evaluate for unsuitability
   C. guarantee suitability
   D. meet legal requirements

Kathy has been found suitable as a potential organ donor. Although her family has been in close contact with the physician and nurses, they are unable to be at Kathy's bedside for the next several days. They have expressed an interest in organ donation, but consent has not been given.

6. Kathy meets all of the criteria for brain death and she has not signed an organ donor card. The health care team is anxious to obtain consent to initiate donor supportive measures. Which of the following statements is correct regarding obtaining consent?
   A. any member of Kathy's family can come in to sign a consent form
   B. consent is not mandatory if the family is not available
   C. consent could be obtained over the telephone
   D. her sister who is at the hospital can give the approval.

Kathy is now legally established as a donor.

7. As a donor, maintaining Kathy's fluid and electrolyte balance is a priority. Nursing interventions to accomplish this goal may include (choose all that apply)
   A. maintaining urine output at 20 to 25 mL/hr
   B. mL/mL replacement of urine output with IV fluid
   C. monitoring for therapeutic effects of Pitressin
   D. maintaining blood pressure above 90 mm Hg systolic

Kathy is taken to the operating room for organ recovery to be performed.

8. Operating room procedures for donor organ recovery may include (choose all that apply)
   A. several recovery teams in the operating room
   B. Kathy's physician not in the operating room
   C. aseptic procedures not required
   D. the anesthesiologist performing functions

Juan C., 46-year-old, has a long history of chronic renal problems. He has been receiving hemodialysis for the past 5 years. Mr. C., his family, and his physician have been discussing the possibility of renal transplantation.

9. Mr. C. has no siblings. Assuming that he eventually does undergo a renal transplant, he will most likely receive a(n) ______.
   A. autograft
   B. allograft
   C. isograft
   D. heterograft

10. Mr. C. and his son (a possible kidney donor) have tissue typing done. Their HLA matching is likely to be
A. partially matched
B. identical
C. totally unmatched
D. unpredictable

11. Kathy's kidney is being considered for transplantation into Mr. C. He will have a sample of his blood subjected to a sample of Kathy's blood to check for preformed antibodies. This test is called
A. antigen testing
B. ABO typing
C. tissue typing
D. crossmatching

12. Mr. C. has type A blood and Kathy's blood type is O. This combination of donor and recipient blood types is a(n)
A. unacceptable match
B. questionable match
C. acceptable match
D. ideal match

13. If Mr. C. develops a technical type of complication associated with his kidney transplantation, it could include which of the following problems? (choose all that apply)
A. urine leakage at the anastomosis site
B. vascular thrombosis of the renal artery
C. perioperative or postoperative bleeding
D. type III hypersensitivity response

14. If Mr. C. develops a cytomegalovirus infection following the surgery, he would most likely develop it through
A. incorrect suctioning procedures
B. reactivation of preexisting CMV
C. infiltration in wound infections
D. contamination via invasive tubes

15. Mr. C. develops symptoms of acute rejection. This complication of organ transplantation initially involves which type of hypersensitivity response?
A. a humoral response in which B cells form antibodies that attack and destroy the donor organ
B. a cell mediated response in which the T cells and macrophages attack and destroy the donor organ
C. preformed antibodies rapidly recognize and attack the donor organ
D. a humoral response in which antibodies slowly attack and injure the graft

16. Mr. C. is currently receiving cyclosporine. The major advantage of using this drug is that it
A. affects only helper T cells
B. directs its action against B cells
C. is a cell-cycle specific cytotoxic agent
D. has anti-inflammatory and immunosuppressant capabilities

17. If Mr. C. is started on muromonab-CD3 (OKT3) therapy, the nurse will need to monitor him closely for the first 48 hours for ______, in addition to the usual assessments.
A. infection
B. renal failure
C. nausea and vomiting
D. cytokine-release syndrome

Additional history on Mr. C.: History of type 1 diabetes mellitus since age 5. Several episodes of staphylococcal pneumonia as a child. He is 5 foot 10 and weighs 150 pounds (68.2 kg). Several months ago, he was treated for a severe infection with gentamicin. He has a history of hypertension that has been well controlled with antihypertensive therapy.

18. Mr. C.'s end-stage renal disease most likely resulted from
A. hypertension
B. type 1 diabetes mellitus
C. complications of staphylococcal pneumonia
D. recent antibiotic therapy

19. If Mr. C. develops failure of his transplanted kidney, it is most likely going to be because of
A. nephrotoxicity
B. hypertension
C. hypoperfusion
D. rejection

20. Following his transplant, Mr. C. will need periodic reevaluation of kidney function. Which test would specifically evaluate the condition of the kidney?
A. needle biopsy of the grafted kidney
B. complete blood cell count
C. a 24-hour urine output
D. kidney ultrasound

Posttest answers with rationale are found on MyNursingKit.

REFERENCES

Appelbaum, F. R. (2007). Hematopoietic-cell transplantation at 50. *N Engl J Med, 357*(15), 1472-1475.

Aranda-Michel, J., Dickson, R., Bonatti, H., Crossfield, J., Keaveny, A., & Vasquez, A. (2008). Patient selection for liver transplant: 1-year experience with 555 patients at a single center. *Mayo Clinic Proceedings, 83*(2), 165-168.

Augustine, S. M., & Masiello-Miller, M. (1995). Heart transplantation. In M. T. Nolan & S. M. Augustine (eds.), *Transplantation nursing: acute and long-term management* (pp. 109–140). Norwalk, CT: Appleton & Lange.

Cavanaugh, T., & Martin, J. (2007). Update on pharmacoeconomics in transplantation. *Progress in Transplantation,15*(2), np.

Cowan, P. A., Wicks, M. N., Rutland, T. C., Ammons, J., & Hathaway, D. K. (2002). Pancreas transplantation. In S. L. Smith, Organ transplantation: concepts, issues, practice, and outcomes. *Medscape Transplantation, 2002.*

Dimercurio, B., Henry, L., & Kirk, A. D. (2002). Simultaneous kidney-pancreas transplantation. In S. A. Cupples & L. Ohler (eds.), *Solid organ transplantation: a handbook for primary health care providers* (pp. 223–239). New York: Springer-Verlag.

Driscoll, C. J. (2007). Risk factors for posttransplant diabetes mellitus: a review of the literature. *Progress in Transplantation, 17*(4), 295–301.

Fischer, S. A. (2006). Infections complicating solid organ transplantation. *Surg Clin N Am, 86,* 1127–1145.

Gelone, D. K., & Lake, K. D. (2002). Transplantation pharmacotherapy. In S. A. Cupples & L. Ohler (eds.), *Solid organ transplantation: A handbook for primary health care providers* (pp. 88–130). New York: Springer-Verlag.

KODA. (1994). Materials provided by Kentucky Organ Donor Affiliates (KODA). Lexington, KY: Author.

Matarese, L., Costa, G., Bond, G., Stamos, J., Koritsky, D., O'Keefe, S., and Abu-Elmagd, K. (2007). Therapeutic efficacy of intestinal and multivisceral transplantation: survival and nutrition outcome. *Nutrition in Clinical Practice, 22*(5), 474–481.

Murphy, F., and Byrne, G. (2007). Ethical issues regarding live kidney transplantation. *British Journal of Nursing, 16*(19). 1224–1229.

Murray, J. E. (1991). Nobel Prize lecture: The first successful organ transplants in man. In P. I. Terasaki (ed.), *History of transplantation: thirty-five recollections* (pp. 123–138). Los Angeles: UCLA Tissue Typing Laboratory.

Nathan, S., & Ohler, L. (2002). Lung and heart-lung transplantation. In S. A. Cupples & L. Ohler (eds.), *Solid organ transplantation: a handbook for primary health care providers* (pp. 240–260). New York: Springer-Verlag.

Odorico, J., Voss, B., Munoz Del Rio, A., Leverson, G., Becker, Y., Pirsch, J., Hoffman, R., and Sollinger, H. (2008). Kidney function after solitary pancreas transplantation. *Transplantation Proceedings, 40*(2), 513–515.

Ohler, L. (2007). Waitlist management (editorial). *Progress in Transplantation, 17*(4), 254–256.

Ohler, L. (2002). Appendix: Review of transplant immunology for community health care providers. In S. A. Cupples & L. Ohler (eds.), *Solid organ transplantation: a handbook for primary health care providers* (pp. 394–400). New York: Springer-Varlag.

O'Keefe, S. J. (2006). Candidacy for intestinal transplantation. *American Journal of Gastroenterology, 101*(7), 1644–1646.

Owens, S. G., & Wallop, J. M. (1995). Heart–lung and lung transplantation. In M. T. Nolan & S. M. Augustine (eds.), *Transplantation nursing: Acute and long-term management* (pp. 141–163). Norwalk, CT: Appleton & Lange.

Park, B. K. (2002). Intestine transplantation. In S. L. Smith, Organ transplantation: concepts, issues, practice, and outcomes. *Medscape Transplantation, 2002.* Available at: http://www.medscape.com/viewarticle/436543. Accessed October 1, 2003.

Pironi, L., Forbes, A., Joly, F., Colomb, V., Lyszkowska, M., Van Gossum, A., Baxter, J., Thul, P., Hebuterne, X., Gambarara, M., Gottrand, F., Moreno Villares, J., Messing, B., Goulet, O., & Staun, M. (2008). Survival of patients identified as candidates for intestinal transplantation: a 3-year prospective follow-up. *Gastroenterology, 135*(1), 61–71.

Powner, D. J. (2005). Variables during care of adult donors that can influence outcomes of kidney transplantation. *Progress in Transplantation, 15*(3), 219–225

Schaeffner, E., Mehta, J., & Winkelmayer, W. (2008). Educational level as a determinant of access to and outcomes after kidney transplantation in the United States. *American Journal of Kidney Diseases, 51*(5), 811–818.

Schulman, L. L. (2001). Physiology of the transplanted lung. In D. J. Norman & L. A. Turka (eds.), *Primer on transplantation* (2d ed., pp. 674–680). Mt. Laurel, NJ: American Society of Transplantation.

Smith, S. L. (2002). Immunosuppressive therapies in organ transplantation. In S. L. Smith, *Organ transplantation: concepts, issues, practice, and outcomes.* Medscape Transplantation, 2002.

Stitt, N. L. (2003). Infection in the transplant recipient. In S. L. Smith, Organ transplantation: concepts, issues, practice, and outcomes. *Medscape Transplantation, 2003.*

UNOS [United Network for Organ Sharing]. (2008). Critical data. United Network for Organ Sharing. Available at: http://www.unos.org/. Accessed August 8, 2008.

Williams, L., Horslen, S. P., & Langnas, A. N. (2002). Intestinal transplantation. In S. A. Cupples & L. Ohler (eds.), *Solid organ transplantation: a handbook for primary health care providers* (pp. 292–333). New York: Springer-Verlag.

Zafar, S., Howell, D., & Gockerman, J. (2008). Malignancy after solid organ transplantation: an overview. *The Oncologist, 13*(7), 769–778.

MODULE

9 Determinants and Assessment of Pulmonary Gas Exchange

Kathleen Dorman Wagner, Beth Augustyn

OBJECTIVES Following completion of this module, the learner will be able to

1. Explain the conducting airway and the concept of ventilation.
2. Discuss external respiration and pulmonary gas diffusion.
3. Describe pulmonary perfusion.
4. Identify mechanisms that the body uses to compensate for acid–base imbalances, and differentiate between respiratory acidosis and alkalosis, and metabolic acidosis and alkalosis.
5. Identify normal values for and interpret arterial blood gases.
6. Recognize mixed acid–base disorders.
7. Describe a focused respiratory nursing history and assessment.
8. Describe tests used to evaluate pulmonary function.
9. Discuss noninvasive and invasive methods of monitoring gas exchange and applications.

This self-study module provides foundational knowledge of pulmonary physiology and assessment of pulmonary function to provide the learner with a deeper understanding of pulmonary disease. It is divided into nine sections. Sections One through Three discuss the underlying principles involved in the respiratory process, including the mechanics of breathing—ventilation, external respiration and pulmonary diffusion, and pulmonary perfusion. Section Four describes acid–base physiology and disturbances, including respiratory and metabolic alkalosis and acidosis. Section Five provides a systematic approach to interpretation of arterial blood gases and Section Six introduces the advanced concept of mixed acid–base disorders and provides basic instruction on the interpretation of more complex arterial blood gases. Section Seven focuses on collection of nursing history and physical assessment data as they apply to the high-acuity patient. Section Eight describes a variety of common pulmonary function tests used to evaluate ventilatory status. Finally, Section Nine provides an overview of two common noninvasive monitoring methods, including pulse oximetry and end-tidal carbon dioxide monitoring and an invasive method using arterial catheterization. All Section Reviews include answers. It is suggested that the learner review those concepts answered incorrectly in the review questions before proceeding to the next section. The module also includes a set of arterial blood gas interpretation exercises.

PRETEST

1. Ventilation is best defined as
   A. movement of gases across the alveolar–capillary membrane
   B. mechanical movement of gases in and out of the lungs
   C. transport of gases through the blood to and from the tissues
   D. movement of gases down a pressure gradient
2. During inspiration, air is drawn into the lungs because intrapulmonary pressure is
   A. below atmospheric pressure
   B. equal to intra-abdominal pressure
   C. above alveolar–capillary pressure
   D. above intrathoracic pressure
3. Which of the following factors affect pulmonary diffusion? (choose all that apply)
   A. gradient
   B. thickness
   C. surface area
   D. barometric pressure
4. If the ventilation–perfusion $\dot{V}/\dot{Q}$ ratio is low, it will affect arterial blood gases in which way?
   A. decreased $Pa{O_2}$
   B. decreased $Pa{CO_2}$
   C. increased $Pa{O_2}$
   D. increased pH
5. Pulmonary shunt refers to
   A. blood that bypasses the heart
   B. blood that bypasses the lungs

C. blood that does not take part in gas exchange
D. blood that does not release carbon dioxide

6. Normal tidal volume in an average-sized adult male would be how many mL/kg?
A. 3 to 4
B. 4 to 5
C. 5 to 7
D. 7 to 9

7. Common factors affecting gas exchange include (choose all that apply)
A. partial pressure
B. oxyhemoglobin dissociation
C. mixed venous saturation
D. diffusion

8. Which partial statement reflects the natural movement of gas diffusion?
A. from low to high pressure
B. from high to low pressure
C. from equal to unequal pressure
D. from negative to positive pressure

9. The body compensates for acid–base imbalances by which mechanisms? (choose all that apply)
A. buffering
B. hepatic compensation
C. respiratory compensation
D. excretion of bicarbonate

10. Respiratory compensation involves excretion or retention of
A. CO_2
B. HCO_3
C. H_2O
D. K^+

11. Normal values for arterial blood gases (ABGs) include
A. pH 7.5
B. $Pa{CO_2}$ 20 mm Hg
C. HCO_3 26 mm Hg
D. $Sa{O_2}$ 75 mm Hg

12. According to the oxyhemoglobin dissociation curve, at a $Pa{O_2}$ of less than 60 mm Hg, a large decrease in $Pa{O_2}$ should produce what response in the $Sa{O_2}$?
A. a small increase
B. a large increase
C. a small decrease
D. a large decrease

13. Respiratory acidosis is caused by
A. alveolar hypoventilation
B. alveolar hyperventilation
C. excessive perfusion
D. inadequate perfusion

14. Patient situations associated with respiratory alkalosis include
A. sedation
B. anxiety
C. pulmonary edema
D. neuromuscular blockade

15. Metabolic disturbances are reflected by changes in
A. HCO_3, $Sa{O_2}$
B. $Pa{O_2}$, base excess
C. base excess, HCO_3
D. HCO_3, $Pa{O_2}$

16. Metabolic acidosis results in
A. increased $Pa{CO_2}$
B. decreased pH
C. increased base excess
D. increased HCO_3

17. A patient has the following ABG results: pH 7.48, $Pa{CO_2}$ 38 mm Hg, HCO_3 30 mEq/L. The correct acid–base interpretation of this ABG is
A. uncompensated respiratory alkalosis
B. partially compensated respiratory acidosis
C. uncompensated metabolic alkalosis
D. partially compensated metabolic acidosis

18. A patient has the following ABG results: pH 7.48, $Pa{CO_2}$ 33 mm Hg, HCO_3 26 mEq/L, $Pa{O_2}$ 68 mm Hg. The correct interpretation of this ABG is
A. acute respiratory alkalosis with hypoxemia
B. uncompensated respiratory acidosis with normal oxygenation status
C. acute metabolic alkalosis with normal oxygenation status
D. partially compensated metabolic acidosis with hypoxemia

19. Which statement most accurately describes a mixed acid–base disorder?
A. it can have a nullifying effect on the pH
B. it has no predictable effect on the pH
C. it is primarily associated with respiratory disorders
D. it has a respiratory as well as a metabolic acid–base component

20. The key to recognizing mixed acid–base disorders on an arterial blood gas is
A. looking for pH extremes
B. recognizing abnormal base excess levels
C. knowing the predicted compensation relationships
D. the presence of abnormal HCO_3 with a normal pH

21. Pulse oximetry measures
A. mixed venous saturation
B. transcutaneous oxygen saturation
C. venous oxygen capillary hemoglobin saturation
D. arterial oxygen capillary hemoglobin saturation

22. The end-tidal CO_2 is an indicator of alveolar
A. ventilation
B. acid–base state
C. oxygenation
D. compensation

Pretest answers are found on MyNursingKit.

SECTION ONE: Mechanics of Breathing—Ventilation

At the completion of this section, the learner will be able to explain the conducting airway and the concept of ventilation.

The respiratory process has three vital components: ventilation, diffusion, and perfusion. The next three sections of this module discuss each of these concepts and their importance to the entire respiratory process. This section provides an overview of ventilation.

The Conducting Airway

The respiratory tract can be divided into the conducting and respiratory airways. The conducting airways consist of the nasal passages, mouth, pharynx, larynx, trachea, bronchi, and bronchioles. These airways serve as an air conduit to move air to and from the atmosphere and alveoli. They also provide important protective functions by humidifying, filtering, and warming air passing through them. In addition, much of the conducting airway contains a mucociliary system that removes pathogens and foreign materials by capturing them on the mucus layer and removing them through ciliary movement that transports foreign particles toward the pharynx where they can be swallowed and destroyed in the stomach. In high-acuity patients who require an artificial airway (e.g., tracheostomy or endotracheal tube), the initial conducting airway is bypassed, which significantly reduces the protective functions, placing patients at increased risk of aspiration and ventilator associated pneumonia (VAP). In such cases, the protective functions are artificially replaced using special equipment that provides humidity, warmth, and in some cases, filtering services.

The tracheobronchial tree consists of the trachea, which branches into the right and left bronchi. It may be helpful to think of the trachea as being the base of the tree and the alveoli as being the tiny terminal fruit clusters of the tree. At the junction of the "Y" formed by the two primary bronchial branches is the **carina.** This structure is heavily enervated and extremely sensitive to stimulation. The carina becomes clinically significant when touched by a suction catheter (or other device), which can trigger bronchospasm or severe coughing. The right bronchus is shorter and larger in diameter than the left bronchus, and is at almost a straight angle with the trachea. The left bronchus is longer, smaller in diameter, and at a more acute angle than the right bronchus. The bronchial anatomic structure has clinical significance because the size and positioning of the right bronchus makes it more vulnerable to the introduction of pathogens and foreign particles as well as for the misplacement of an endotracheal tube. The trachea and bronchial walls contain a C-shaped cartilage structure, which is present down to the bronchiole level. The cartilage gives structure and protection to the larger airways.

Toward the terminal end of the bronchial tree are the bronchioles, which are surrounded by smooth muscle but lack cartilage. "Bronchioles are to the respiratory system what arterioles are to the circulatory system" (Martini & Bartholomew, 2003, p. 463). This statement refers to the fact that bronchioles (like arterioles) have the ability to regulate resistance to flow by causing constriction or dilation, thus controlling airflow distribution. However, arterioles control blood flow via vasoconstriction and vasodilation, whereas the bronchioles control airflow through bronchoconstriction and bronchodilation. Figure 9–1 provides an illustration of the anatomy of the respiratory system.

Ventilation

Ventilation is the first of the three components of the respiratory process and is defined as the mechanical movement of airflow to and from the atmosphere and the alveoli. Ventilation involves the actual work of breathing and requires nervous system control and adequate functioning of the lungs and conducting airways, thorax, and ventilatory muscles. Decreased functioning of any one of these factors will affect the body's ability to ventilate properly.

Ventilation is accomplished through a bellows-like action. Air is able to move in and out of the lungs as a result of the changing size of the thorax caused by ventilatory muscle activity. When the thorax enlarges, the intrapulmonary pressure drops to below atmospheric pressure. Air then moves from the area of higher pressure to the area of lower pressure, resulting in air flowing into the lungs (inspiration) until the pressure in the lungs becomes slightly higher than atmospheric pressure. At this point, air flows back out of the lungs (expiration) until once again pressures are equalized.

Lung tissue has a constant tendency to collapse because of several important properties. First, the fluid lining of the alveoli has a naturally high surface tension, creating a tendency for the alveolar walls to collapse. To prevent this, special cells (type II cells) in the alveoli secrete a lipoprotein called **surfactant.** Surfactant has a detergent-like action that reduces the surface tension of the fluid lining the alveolar sacs (Fig. 9–2), thereby decreasing the tendency toward collapse. Second, the lungs are composed of elastic fibers. The elastic force of these fibers constantly seeks to return to a resting state (i.e., collapsed lungs). To maintain the lungs in an inflated state, the elastic forces must constantly be overcome by opposing forces.

The thorax is the primary opposing force that maintains the lungs in an expanded state. The thoracic bony structure provides a cage-like framework that maintains the lungs in a baseline inflated state even at rest because of the attraction that exists between the visceral and parietal pleura. The pleura are slick-surfaced, moist membranes. The **parietal pleura** adheres to the thoracic walls, diaphragm, and mediastinum; and the **visceral pleura** adheres to the lung parenchyma. To understand the pleural attraction, it may help to think of placing two moistened sheets of smooth glass together. Although it would be relatively easy to glide one sheet over the other in a parallel fashion, it would be very difficult to pull them directly apart at a 180° angle. The glass sheets represent the two pleurae. Under normal circumstances (a negative intrapleural state), the parietal and visceral pleura act as one membrane. Therefore, as the thorax increases and decreases in size, so will the lungs increase and decrease in volume.

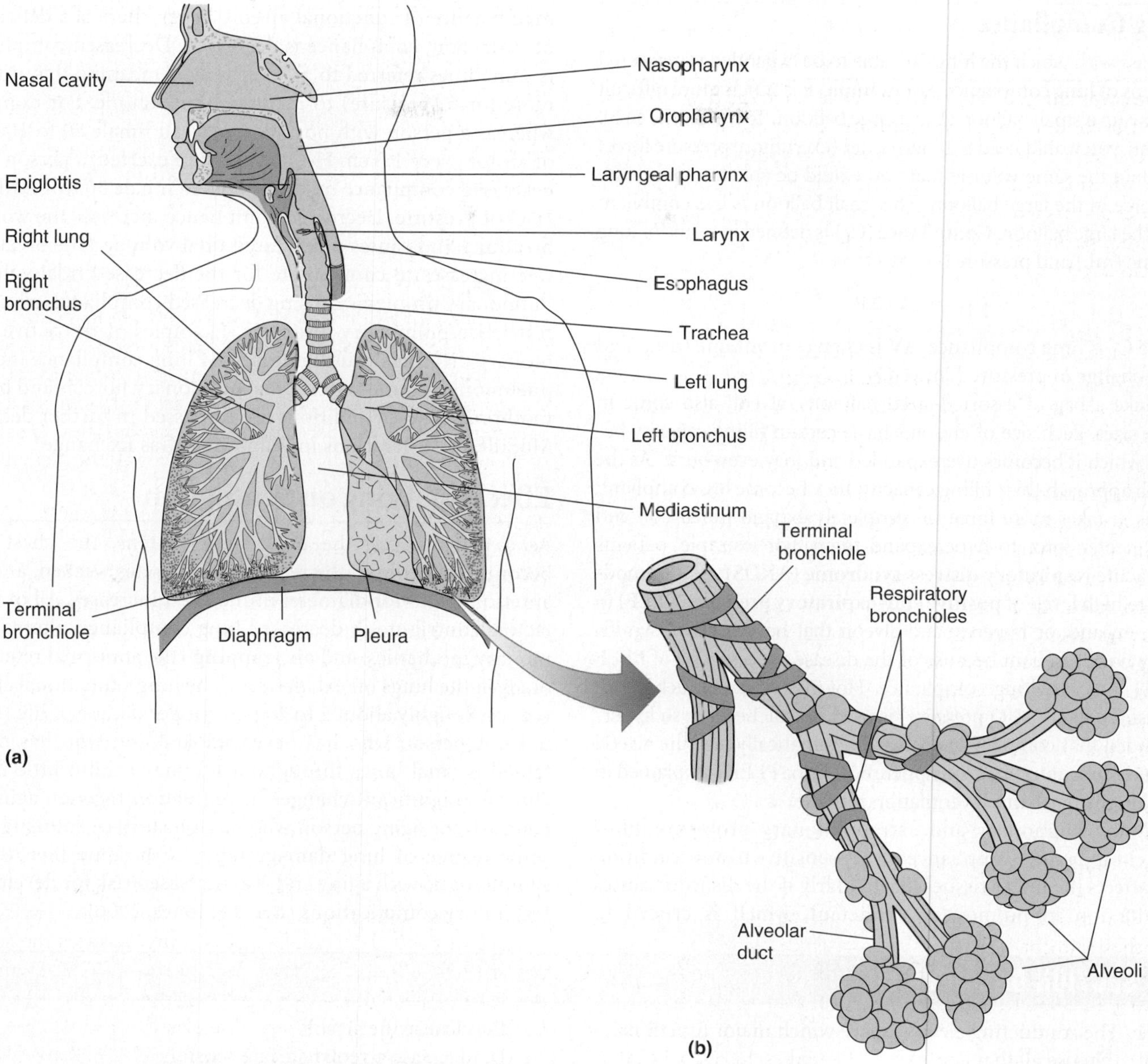

Figure 9–1 ■ Anatomy of the respiratory system. (a) Major anatomic features; (b) Terminal airways.

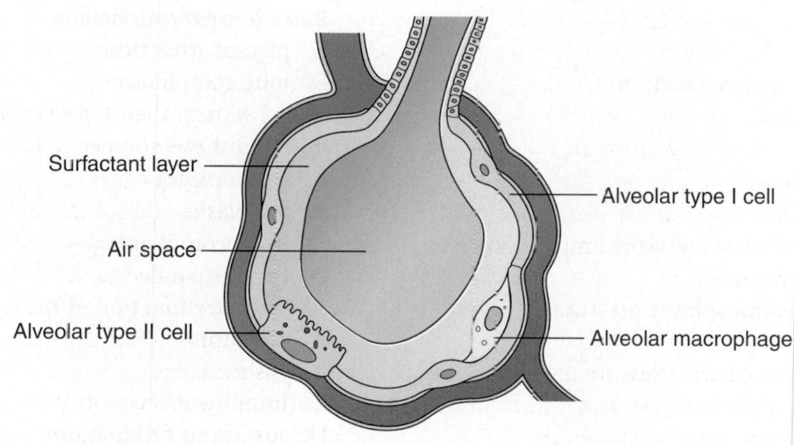

Figure 9–2 ■ The surfactant layer. Type II cells secrete surfactant, a lipoprotein that lines the inner wall of the alveoli, reducing surface tension to prevent alveolar collapse.

Lung Compliance

The ease with which the lungs are able to be expanded is measured in terms of lung compliance. For example, it is much more difficult to blow up a small balloon than a large balloon. To inflate the small balloon, you would need to blow harder (exert more pressure force) to obtain the same volume that you would be able to obtain with less force in the large balloon. The small balloon is less compliant than the large balloon. **Compliance (C_L)** is defined in terms of lung volume (mL) and pressure (cm H_2O) as

$$C_L = \Delta V/\Delta P$$

where C_L is lung compliance, ΔV is change in volume (mL), and ΔP is change in pressure (cm H_2O).

Like a bag of assorted-sized balloons, alveoli also come in many sizes. Each size of alveolus has a certain filling capacity beyond which it becomes overexpanded and may even burst. As the alveoli approach their filling capacity, they become less compliant; that is, it takes more force to completely expand the alveoli and even greater force to hyperexpand them. For example, patients with **acute respiratory distress syndrome (ARDS)** require moderate to high levels of **positive end–expiratory pressure (PEEP)** to open, expand, or hyperexpand alveoli that have become significantly noncompliant because of the disease process. Use of PEEP ideally increases lung compliance. However, if too much PEEP (measured in cm H_2O pressure) is used, alveoli become so hyperexpanded that compliance decreases dramatically and the alveoli are at risk of rupture, causing pneumothorax. PEEP is explained in detail in the mechanical ventilation module.

Many pulmonary and extrapulmonary problems influence compliance. Compliance is very sensitive to any condition that affects the lung's tissues, particularly if the disorder causes a reduction in pulmonary surfactant, which is crucial to maintenance of functional alveoli. When there is a deficiency of surfactant, compliance is decreased. Decreased compliance is sometimes referred to as "stiff lungs," meaning that it takes more force (pressure) to increase lung volume. For example, whereas a person with normal lungs can inhale 50 to 100 mL of air for every 1.0 cm H_2O of pressure exerted, a person with decreased compliance might be able to inhale 30 to 40 mL/cm H_2O of pressure. Decreased compliance increases the work of breathing and causes a decreased tidal volume. The breathing rate increases to compensate for the decreased tidal volume. Pulmonary problems causing decreased compliance are called restrictive pulmonary disorders. Examples of restrictive pulmonary disorders causing decreased lung compliance include pneumonia, pulmonary edema, pulmonary fibrosis and pneumothorax. These conditions are discussed in further detail in Module 10, "Alterations in Pulmonary Gas Exchange".

Effects of Aging on Ventilation

As a person ages, the diaphragm flattens, the chest wall becomes more rigid, the respiratory muscles weaken, and the anterior–posterior diameter of the chest increases. All of these factors contribute to decreased lung compliance, altered pulmonary mechanics, and **air trapping** (the abnormal retention of air in the lungs on exhalation). The lung's functional ability reduces roughly about 5 to 20 percent per decade of life (Ross, n.d.). A person who has never smoked and who has maintained normal lungs throughout life may exhibit little if any clinically significant changes in ventilation through aging. In contrast, the aging person who has a history of smoking with some degree of lung damage tends to become increasingly symptomatic with aging and is at increased risk for developing respiratory complications (Beers & Jones, 2006).

SECTION ONE REVIEW

1. The conducting airways serve which major functions? (choose all that apply)
   A. gas exchange
   B. filtering
   C. immune
   D. humidifying
   E. warming
2. The elastic force of lung tissue seeks to
   A. keep lungs expanded
   B. collapse the lungs
   C. flatten the diaphragm
   D. decrease thorax size
3. During expiration, air flows out of the lungs because the intrapulmonary pressure
   A. increases to above atmospheric pressure
   B. is equal to perfusion pressure
   C. drops to below atmospheric pressure
   D. is equal to alveolar pressure
4. The purpose of surfactant is to
   A. decrease lung compliance
   B. increase alveolar surface tension
   C. cleanse the alveoli
   D. decrease alveolar surface tension
5. The lungs adhere to the thoracic walls because of
   A. elastic forces
   B. pulmonary surfactant
   C. pleural attraction
   D. lung compliance
6. As alveoli near their filling capacity, they become
   A. less compliant
   B. less elastic
   C. more compliant
   D. hyperexpanded
7. The primary function of the type II alveolar cells is
   A. filtration
   B. gas exchange
   C. immune protection
   D. surfactant production

Answers: 1. (B, D, E), 2. B, 3. A, 4. D, 5. C, 6. A, 7. D

SECTION TWO: Pulmonary Gas Exchange—Respiration and Diffusion

At the completion of this section, the learner will be able to discuss external respiration and pulmonary gas diffusion.

The Cardiopulmonary Circuit and Respiration

Respiration is the process by which the body's cells are supplied with oxygen and carbon dioxide (cellular waste product) is eliminated from the body. Respiration can be further divided into internal and external respiration. **Internal respiration** refers to the movement of gases across systemic capillary–cell membranes in the tissues. Internal respiration is presented in detail in Module 17, Determinants and Assessment of Oxygen Delivery and Oxygen Consumption. **External respiration** refers to the movement of gases across the alveolar–capillary membrane (i.e., pulmonary gas exchange) and is the focus of this module. Both external and internal respiration use diffusion as their means of exchanging gases. To understand diffusion, it is helpful to first understand the concept of partial pressure and the oxyhemoglobin dissociation curve. Figure 9–3 illustrates the cardiopulmonary circuit and respiration.

Diffusion

Diffusion is the second of the three components of the respiratory process. Oxygenation of tissues is dependent on the process of diffusion as the vital mechanism for both external and internal respiration. **Diffusion** is the movement of gases down a pressure gradient from an area of high pressure to an area of low pressure. The alveolar–capillary membrane is very thin (0.5 mcm), offering little resistance to diffusion in normal circumstances. The membrane can thicken when pulmonary pathologic processes exist, reducing diffusion (e.g., pulmonary edema, acute respiratory distress syndrome). When diffusion is reduced, the carbon dioxide tension may remain at normal levels initially because carbon dioxide diffuses 20 times faster than oxygen; however, the oxygen tension decreases rapidly. Four factors affect diffusion through the alveolar–capillary membrane: partial pressures and gradient, surface area, thickness, and length of exposure. In addition, the oxyhemoglobin dissociation curve plays an important role in determining the affinity of oxygen to hemoglobin, which directly affects diffusion.

Partial Pressures and Gradient

Atmospheric air is composed of molecules of nitrogen, oxygen, carbon dioxide, and water vapor. The combination of all of these gases exerts about 760 mm Hg of pressure at sea level.

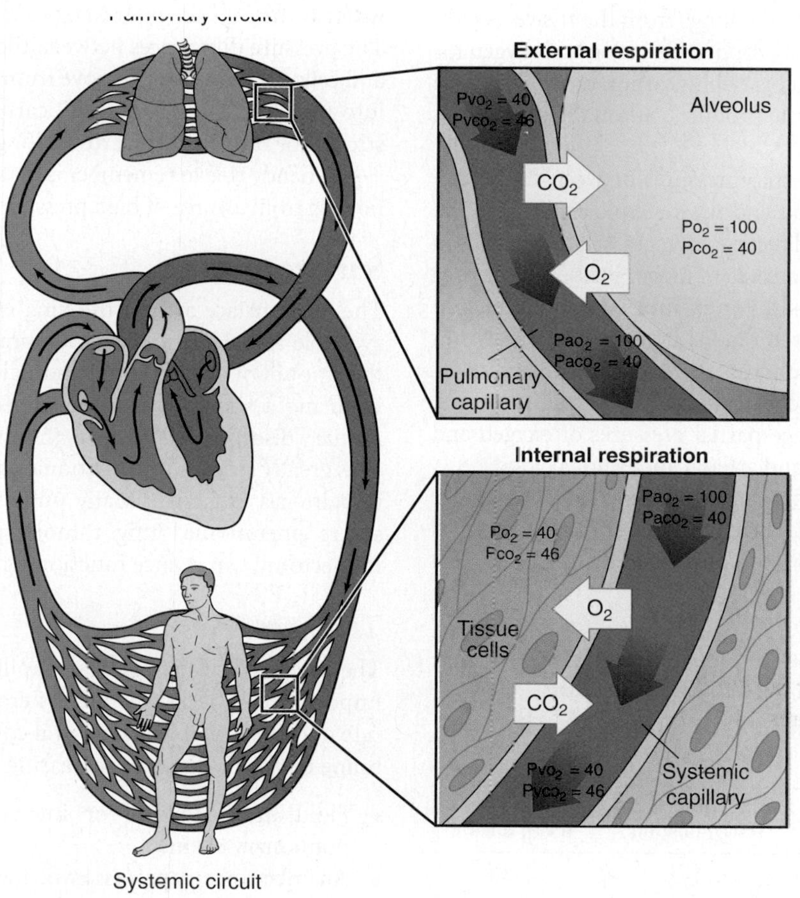

Figure 9–3 ■ Cardiopulmonary circuit and external and internal respiration.

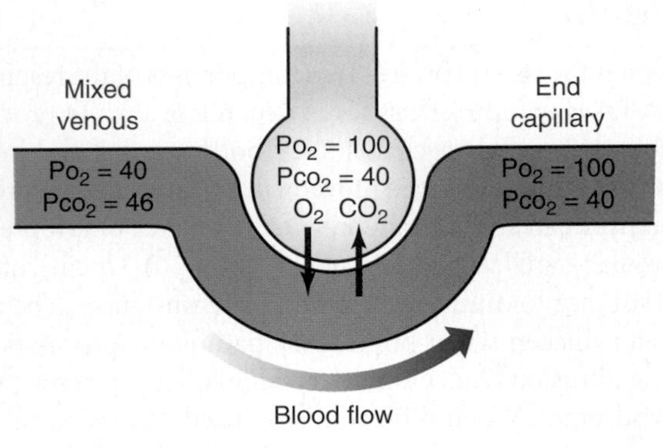

Figure 9–4 ■ Gas distribution.

The respiratory process, however, does not actively involve the use of the water vapor or nitrogen. It is concerned with exchange of oxygen and carbon dioxide.

Oxygen and carbon dioxide both exert a certain percentage of the total air pressure. Oxygen in the alveoli exerts an average of 100 mm Hg pressure, and this **partial pressure** of oxygen is called Po_2, or oxygen tension. When the Po_2 refers to oxygen in the alveoli, it is more precisely referred to as PAo_2. When it refers to arterial blood, it is abbreviated as Pao_2, and when it refers to venous blood, it is specified as Pvo_2. Carbon dioxide in the alveoli exerts an average of 40 mm Hg of pressure. This partial pressure is called Pco_2. The abbreviation alterations of A, a, and v used for describing Po_2 also apply to Pco_2.

Venous blood returning to the lungs from the tissues is oxygen poor because the blood has dropped off its load of oxygen for use by the tissues. Venous blood is rich in carbon dioxide because of transport of the cellular waste product, carbon dioxide (CO_2), for removal from the lungs.

The differences in gas partial pressures between the alveoli and pulmonary capillary blood and the systemic capillary blood and the tissues dictate which direction each gas will flow based on the law of diffusion (i.e., from an area of higher pressure to an area of lower pressure) (see Fig. 9–4). For example, if alveolar oxygen (PAo_2) is 100 mm Hg and mixed venous oxygen (Pvo_2) is 40 mm Hg, alveolar oxygen will diffuse across the alveolar-capillary membrane into the capillary blood to equalize the partial pressures. Table 9–1 compares the average partial pressures of oxygen and carbon dioxide in the alveoli, and arterial and venous blood.

Henry's law states that when a gas is exposed to liquid, some of it will dissolve in the liquid. The partial pressure of the gas and its solubility determine the amount of gas that dissolves. Oxygen is not very soluble in plasma and only 3 percent of the total oxygen content dissolves in blood. It is the partial pressure of gases (oxygen and carbon dioxide) flowing in the arterial system that is measured in an arterial blood gas sample (see Fig. 9–5).

The difference between the partial pressures is called the **pressure gradient.** In external respiration, a pressure gradient (difference) exists between the atmosphere and the alveoli and between the alveoli and the pulmonary capillaries. The greater the pressure difference, the more rapid the flow of gases. Multiple factors can increase the gradient; for example, exercise, positive pressure mechanical ventilation, and intermittent positive pressure breathing (IPPB). Air enters the alveoli from the atmosphere because the atmospheric air pressure is slightly higher than alveolar pressure, which creates a pressure gradient.

In external respiration, a pressure gradient exists between the alveoli and the pulmonary capillaries, causing flow of gases across the alveolar–capillary membrane. For example, Patient X has a Pvo_2 (oxygen–poor blood returning to the heart) of 45 mm Hg and a $Pvco_2$ of 55 mm Hg, whereas his alveolar Po_2 (P_Ao_2) is 100 mm Hg and $Paco_2$ is 25. Because the oxygen tension in the alveolus is much higher than in the capillary, oxygen will diffuse down the gradient from the alveolus into the blood passing by. The carbon dioxide tension, however, is lower in the alveolus than it is in the blood, causing a pressure gradient that will diffuse CO_2 out of the blood and into the alveolus.

In internal respiration, the process is reversed. The arterial blood is rich (high) in oxygen and poor (low) in carbon dioxide, whereas the cells are poor in oxygen and rich in carbon dioxide. The pressure differences between the Po_2 and Pco_2 in the blood and cells cause oxygen to move from the circulating hemoglobin into the cells. The cells release carbon dioxide into the bloodstream for transport back to the lungs for excretion.

A handy rule to remember is that gradients seek to equalize by flowing from an area of high pressure to an area of low pressure.

TABLE 9–1 Comparison of Average Partial Pressures in the Alveoli, and Arterial and Venous Blood

	ALVEOLI (Pao_2) (mmHg)	ARTERIAL BLOOD (Pao_2) (mmHg)	VENOUS BLOOD (Pvo_2) (mmHg)
Oxygen	100	100	40
Carbon Dioxide	40	40	46

Surface Area

The total surface area of the lung is very large. The greater the available alveolar–capillary membrane surface area, the greater the amount of oxygen and carbon dioxide that can diffuse across it during a specific time period. Emphysema is a major pulmonary disorder that destroys the alveolar–capillary membrane. This greatly reduces the functional surface area and consequently impairs gas exchange. Many pulmonary conditions, including severe pneumonia, lung tumors, pneumothorax, and pneumonectomy, can reduce functioning surface area significantly.

Thickness

The thickness of the alveolar–capillary membrane is of major importance—the thinner the membrane, the more rapid the rate of diffusion of gases. Several conditions can increase membrane thickness, thereby decreasing the rate of diffusion:

- Fluid in the alveoli or interstitial spaces or both (e.g., pulmonary edema)
- An inflammatory process involving the alveoli (e.g., pneumonia)
- Lung conditions that cause fibrosis (e.g., ARDS or pneumoconiosis)

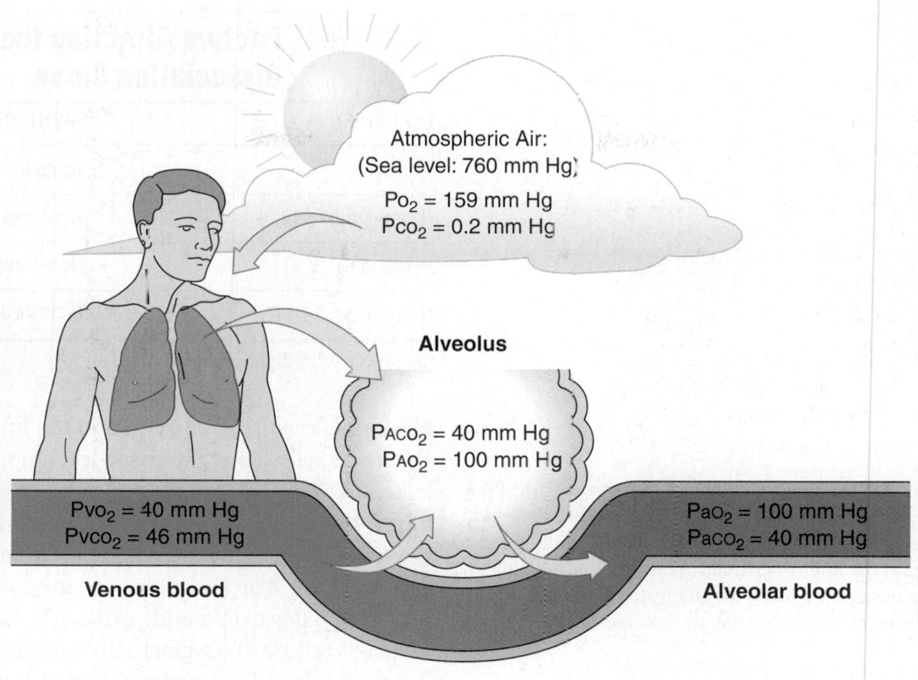

Figure 9–5 ■ Partial pressure-atmosphere, alveoli, and blood.

Length of Exposure

During periods of rest, blood flows through the alveolar–capillary system in approximately 0.75 second. Diffusion of oxygen and carbon dioxide requires about 0.25 second to reach equilibrium (the balance between alveolar and capillary gas levels). During periods of high cardiac output, such as occurs with heavy exercise or stress, blood flow is faster through the alveolar–capillary system. Under these circumstances, diffusion takes place during a shortened exposure time. In healthy lungs, oxygen exchange is usually not impaired with high cardiac output states; however, hypoxemia may result if diffusion abnormalities are present, such as pulmonary edema, alveolar consolidation (e.g., pneumonia), or alveolar fibrosis.

Oxyhemoglobin Dissociation Curve

Hemoglobin is the primary carrier of oxygen in the blood. It has an affinity or attraction for oxygen molecules. In the pulmonary capillaries, oxygen binds loosely and reversibly to hemoglobin, forming oxyhemoglobin for transport to the tissues where it can be released. The amount of oxygen that loads onto hemoglobin is expressed as a percentage of hemoglobin saturation by oxygen (percent Sao_2). The affinity of hemoglobin for oxygen varies, depending on certain physiologic factors. The **oxyhemoglobin dissociation curve** represents the relationship of the partial pressure of arterial oxygen (Pao_2) and hemoglobin saturation (Sao_2). The curve (Fig. 9–6) is depicted as an S-curve rather than a straight line, showing that the percentage saturation of hemoglobin does not maintain a direct relationship with the Pao_2.

The top portion of the curve (Pao_2 greater than 60 mm Hg) is flattened into a horizontal position. In this portion of the curve, a large alteration in Pao_2 produces only small alterations in the percentage of hemoglobin saturation. For example, note that a 10 mm Hg decrease of a patient's Pao_2 from 80 mm Hg to 70 mm Hg would produce very little change in Sao_2 (see Fig. 9–6). Clinically, this means that although administering supplemental oxygen may significantly increase the patient's Pao_2, the resulting Sao_2 increase will be small in proportion. The patient's oxygenation status is better protected at the top of the curve.

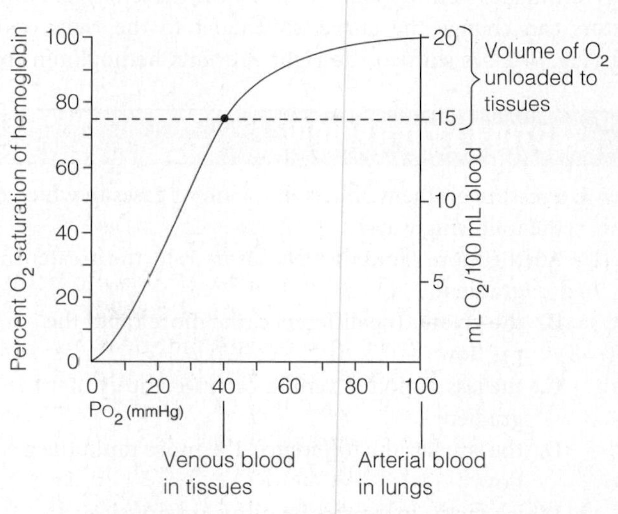

Figure 9–6 ■ Oxyhemoglobin dissociation curve. The percent O_2 saturation of hemoglobin and total blood oxygen volume are shown for different oxygen partial pressures (Po_2). Arterial blood in the lungs is almost completely saturated. During one pass through the body, about 25% of hemoglobin-bound oxygen is unloaded to the tissues. Thus, venous blood is still about 75% saturated with oxygen. The steep portion of the curve shows that hemoglobin readily off-loads and on-loads oxygen at Po_2 levels below the 50mmHg.

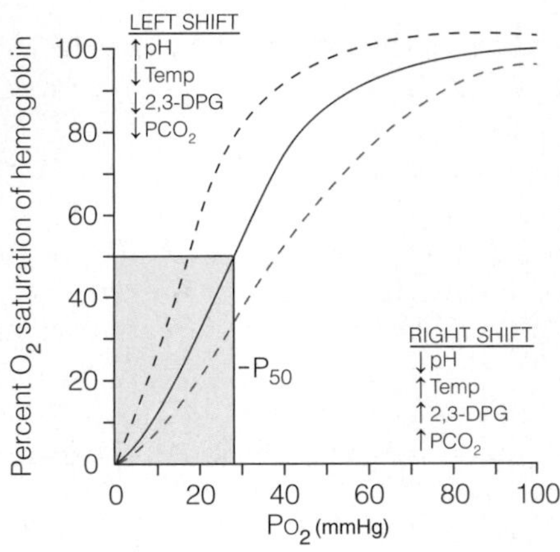

Figure 9–7 ▪ Oxyhemoglobin dissociation curve right and left shifts. Normally, when hemoglobin is 50 percent saturated with oxygen (P_{50}) the Pa_{O_2} will be 27 mm Hg. The P_{50} changes when physiologic factors are altered, shifting the curve. A shift to the left increases the affinity of oxygen to hemoglobin, inhibiting its release to tissues. A shift to the right decreases the affinity of oxygen to hemoglobin, making it release to tissues more readily. LeMone & Burke. *(2008)*.

The bottom portion of the curve (Pa_{O_2} less than 60 mm Hg) is steep. In this portion, any alteration in Pa_{O_2} yields a large change in percentage of hemoglobin saturation (Sa_{O_2}). For example, a 10 mm Hg decrease in Pa_{O_2} from 60 mm Hg to 50 mm Hg decreases the Sa_{O_2} from about 85 percent to about 75 percent (a decrease of approximately 10). Clinically, this means that administration of supplemental oxygen sufficient to increase the Pa_{O_2} should yield large increases in Sa_{O_2}. However, abnormalities in the ventilation–perfusion relationship may exist, interfering with reoxygenation.

Low Pa_{O_2} at the tissue level stimulates oxygen release from hemoglobin to the tissues. High Pa_{O_2} at the pulmonary capillary level stimulates hemoglobin to bind with more oxygen. Other factors can change the curve, shifting it to the right or the left (Fig. 9–7). A shift to the right prevents hemoglobin from binding as readily with oxygen in the lungs, although oxygen is able to be released at the tissue level more readily. A shift to the left causes hemoglobin to bind more readily with oxygen in the lungs, but inhibits release at the tissue level. Factors that shift the curve to the right and left are listed in Table 9–2. Slight shifts are adaptive. For example, an increased body temperature increases oxygen demand, causing a slight right shift, which increases release of oxygen to the tissues to meet increasing tissue oxygen demand. Severe or rapid shifts, however, can produce life-threatening tissue hypoxia.

TABLE 9–2 Factors Affecting the Oxyhemoglobin Dissociation Curve

LEFT SHIFT	RIGHT SHIFT
Alkalosis	Acidosis
Hypothermia	Hyperthermia
Hypocapnia	Hypercapnia
Decreased 2,3-DPG[a]	Increased 2,3-DPG

[a]2,3-DPG = 2,3-diphosphoglycerate.

The Effects of Aging on Diffusion

As a person ages, total lung surface area decreases, the alveolar–capillary membrane thickness increases, and alveoli are destroyed because of aging processes. These changes result in decreased diffusion across the alveolar–capillary membrane, altering the ventilation–perfusion relationship. Overall, gas exchange becomes less efficient, placing the high-acuity older patient at risk for hypoxemia and/or hypercapnia problems. Additionally, over time, the airways become larger, increasing dead space ventilation and terminal airways lose supportive structures, which can result in air trapping. Both of these physiologic changes can lead to carbon dioxide retention.

SECTION TWO REVIEW

1. Pressure gradient affects diffusion of gases in which of the following ways?
   A. the more rapid the ventilatory rate, the greater the gradient
   B. the greater the difference, the more rapid the gas flow
   C. the less rapid the ventilatory rate, the greater the gradient
   D. the smaller the difference, the more rapid the gas flow
2. Which factor increases the diffusion pressure gradient?
   A. increased exercise
   B. decreased activity
   C. negative pressure ventilation
   D. amount of lung surface area
3. The normal partial pressure of alveolar oxygen is approximately
   A. 60 mm Hg
   B. 80 mm Hg
   C. 100 mm Hg
   D. 110 mm Hg
4. Surface area as a factor affecting diffusion refers to the
   A. size of the alveoli
   B. conducting airways
   C. functional capillary perfusion
   D. functional alveoli and surrounding capillaries
5. An example of a disease process that would increase the thickness of the alveolar–capillary membrane is
   A. pneumothorax
   B. pneumonia
   C. lung tumor
   D. pneumonectomy

6. Which statement regarding diffusion is correct?
   A. diffusion refers to capillary pressure
   B. diffusion refers to alveolar pressure
   C. gas flows up a pressure gradient
   D. gas flows down a pressure gradient
7. Which statement is correct regarding the normal relationship between oxygen and hemoglobin?
   A. oxygen binds loosely and reversibly to hemoglobin
   B. hemoglobin is attracted to oxygen molecules
   C. the affinity of hemoglobin to oxygen is constant
   D. the relationship is expressed in mm Hg (pressure)
8. On the oxyhemoglobin dissociation curve, at a Pao_2 less than 60 mm Hg, any change in Pao_2 yields a large change in Sao_2.
   A. True
   B. False
9. External respiration refers to
   A. movement of air from the atmosphere to the alveoli
   B. diffusion of gases across the alveolar–capillary membrane
   C. movement of air from the alveoli to the atmosphere
   D. diffusion of gases across the tissue–capillary membranes

Answers: 1. B, 2. A, 3. C, 4. D, 5. B, 6. D, 7. A, 8. A, 9. B

SECTION THREE: Pulmonary Gas Exchange—Perfusion

At the completion of this section, the learner will be able to describe pulmonary perfusion.

Perfusion is the third and final component of the respiratory process. For our purposes, **perfusion** refers to the pumping or flow of blood into tissues and organs. Perfusion can be divided into two circulatory systems: the systemic system and the pulmonary system. The *systemic system* is vast, running from the aorta through the right atrium of the heart. The *pulmonary system* is much smaller, beginning with the pulmonary artery in the right ventricle, running through the lungs and back into the left ventricle. The pulmonary system is dependent on adequate perfusion in the systemic system and adequate perfusion in both systems is required for oxygenation of the tissues in the entire body. Both of these perfusion systems are composed of a complex network of blood vessels of varying sizes and functions (Fig. 9–8).

Pulmonary perfusion depends on three factors: cardiac output (CO), gravity, and pulmonary vascular resistance (PVR).

Cardiac Output

Cardiac output (CO) is a function of stroke volume (SV) and heart rate (HR) – $CO = SV \times HR$. Normal cardiac output is between 4 and 8 liters per minute. Stroke volume is a function of ventricular preload, afterload, and contractility. A common measurement that is used clinically to reflect adequacy of perfusion is the mean arterial pressure (MAP). This can be approximated using the equation: $MAP = [2(P_{dias}) + P_{sys}]/3$, where P_{dias} is diastolic blood pressure and P_{sys} is systolic blood pressure. Ideally, the MAP is maintained between 65 and 110 mmHg. It is known that a MAP of less than 60 mmHg is inadequate for perfusing major organs, such as the brain, heart, and kidneys. Typically, the clinical goal is to maintain the MAP at 70 or above to prevent organ hypoperfusion, which can result in organ ischemia and **multiple organ dysfunction syndrome (MODS).** Systemic perfusion, including cardiac output and mean arterial pressure, are presented in detail in Module 12, Determinants and Assessment of Cardiac Output.

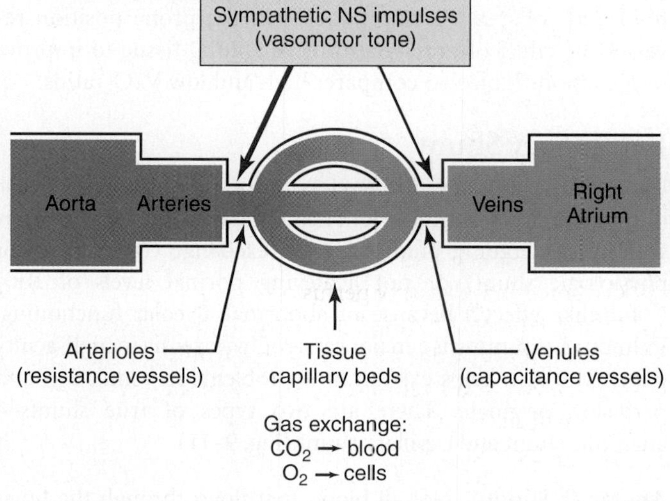

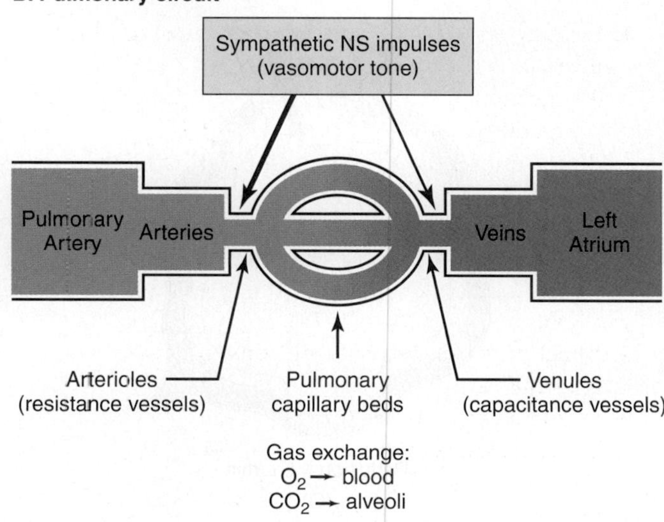

Figure 9–8 ■ Two perfusion system. A, systemic and B, pulmonary.

Gravity

The effects of gravity on blood are an important consideration in pulmonary gas exchange. Because blood has weight, it is gravity dependent; thus it naturally flows toward (and is greatest) in dependent areas of the body. Gravity has a major influence on the relationship between ventilation and pulmonary perfusion.

Ventilation–Perfusion Relationship

Normal diffusion of gases requires a certain balance of alveolar ventilation (movement of gas into the alveoli) and pulmonary perfusion (blood flow through the pulmonary capillaries). Should a significant imbalance in this relationship develop, normal gas exchange cannot take place in the affected areas. For this reason, it is important to gain a basic understanding of the relationship of ventilation (V) to perfusion (Q). This relationship is expressed as a ratio of alveolar ventilation to pulmonary capillary perfusion (**$\dot{V}/\dot{Q}$ ratio**). For ideal gas exchange to occur, we might expect that for every liter of fresh air coming into the alveoli, 1 liter of blood would flow past it, creating a 1:1 ratio of ventilation to perfusion. In reality, for approximately every 4 liters of air flowing into the alveoli, about 5 liters of blood flows past (an average ratio of 4:5, or 0.8) (Fig. 9–9).

The balance of ventilation to perfusion is greatly affected by the $Pa{O_2}$ and $Pa{CO_2}$. This balance depends on adequate diffusion of oxygen and carbon dioxide across the alveolar–capillary membrane, and movement of oxygen into and carbon dioxide out of the alveoli.

Although normal values are given for $Pa{O_2}$ (100 mm Hg) and $Pa{CO_2}$ (40 mm Hg), these numbers only express an average. The actual partial pressures of oxygen and carbon dioxide vary throughout the lungs because ventilation is not distributed evenly because of gravity-dependent factors. In an upright person, alveolar ventilation is moderate in the apices of the lungs because of increased negative pleural pressures in the apices in relation to the lung bases. This makes the alveoli in the lung apices more resistant to airflow during inspiration. When breathing spontaneously, airflow naturally moves toward the diaphragm, which results in more air movement into the bases and peripheral lung during inspiration (airflow follows the path of least resistance). Pulmonary capillary perfusion is gravity dependent, making perfusion greatest in the dependent areas of the lungs (the bases in an upright person). Consequently, because ventilation and perfusion are both greatest in the bases of the lungs, the greatest amount of gas exchange occurs in this portion of the lung fields.

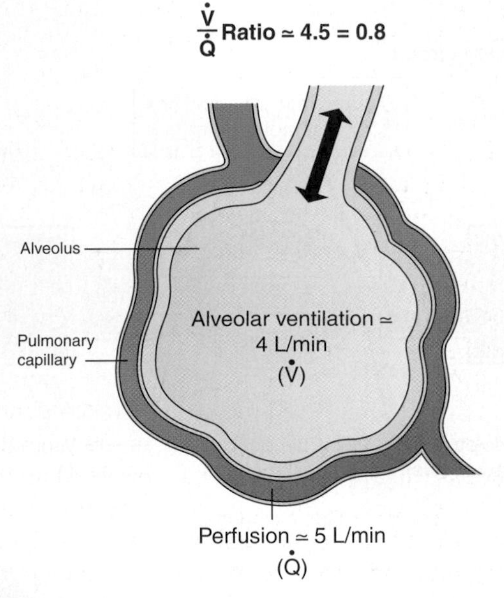

Figure 9–9 ■ The relationship of ventilation to perfusion.

In the upper lungs, there is moderate alveolar ventilation and significantly reduced perfusion, making an excess of ventilation to available perfusion. This results in a "high" $\dot{V}/\dot{Q}$ ratio; that is, a $\dot{V}/\dot{Q}$ ratio that is higher than the average of 0.8. In the lower lungs, there is a moderate increase in ventilation with a significant increase in perfusion. This results in a "low" $\dot{V}/\dot{Q}$ ratio (lower than the average of 0.8).

The clinical significance of ventilation–perfusion balance becomes apparent when considering its implications in high-acuity patients. This patient population generally requires prolonged bedrest, usually in a relatively horizontal position. Because blood is gravity dependent, it will shift from the lung bases to whichever lung area is now in the dependent position; however, air continues to be drawn toward the diaphragm (Fig. 9–10).

Keeping the principles of $\dot{V}/\dot{Q}$ ratio in mind, what could happen if a patient is positioned on the right side when there is significant pneumonia in the right lung fields? Because the patient is lying on the right side, maximum pulmonary capillary perfusion will be on the right. Pneumonia is associated with secretions and other factors that cause obstruction to airflow into the affected right lung alveoli. Therefore, because airflow follows the path of least resistance, it will avoid the diseased right lung area. This combination of a significant decrease in ventilation in the presence of normal-to-increased perfusion causes a mismatching of ventilation to perfusion, creating a low $\dot{V}/\dot{Q}$ ratio. If sufficient mismatching occurs, $Pa{O_2}$ and oxygen saturation levels can decrease significantly. Positioning this patient on the left side may be tolerated better because $\dot{V}/\dot{Q}$ matching would be improved. This, then, is one reason why some high-acuity patients tolerate being turned on one side more than another. For patients in acute respiratory distress syndrome (ARDS), prone positioning may improve oxygenation. When supine, blood gravitates to the posterior lung fields causing alveoli to fill with fluid and collapse. Placing patients in the prone position reverses the effect of gravity and recruits lung tissue to improve oxygenation. Table 9–3 compares high and low $\dot{V}/\dot{Q}$ ratios.

Pulmonary Shunt

The term **pulmonary shunt** refers to the percentage of cardiac output that flows from the right heart and back into the left heart without undergoing pulmonary gas exchange (**true shunt,** or physiologic shunt) or not achieving normal levels of $Pa{O_2}$ ("shuntlike effect") because of abnormal alveolar functioning. Pulmonary shunting is a major cause of hypoxemia in high-acuity patients. It also helps explain how problems in ventilation and perfusion originate. There are two types of true shunts—anatomic shunt and capillary shunt (Fig. 9–11).

Anatomic Shunt. Not all blood that flows through the lungs participates in gas exchange. **Anatomic shunt** refers to blood that

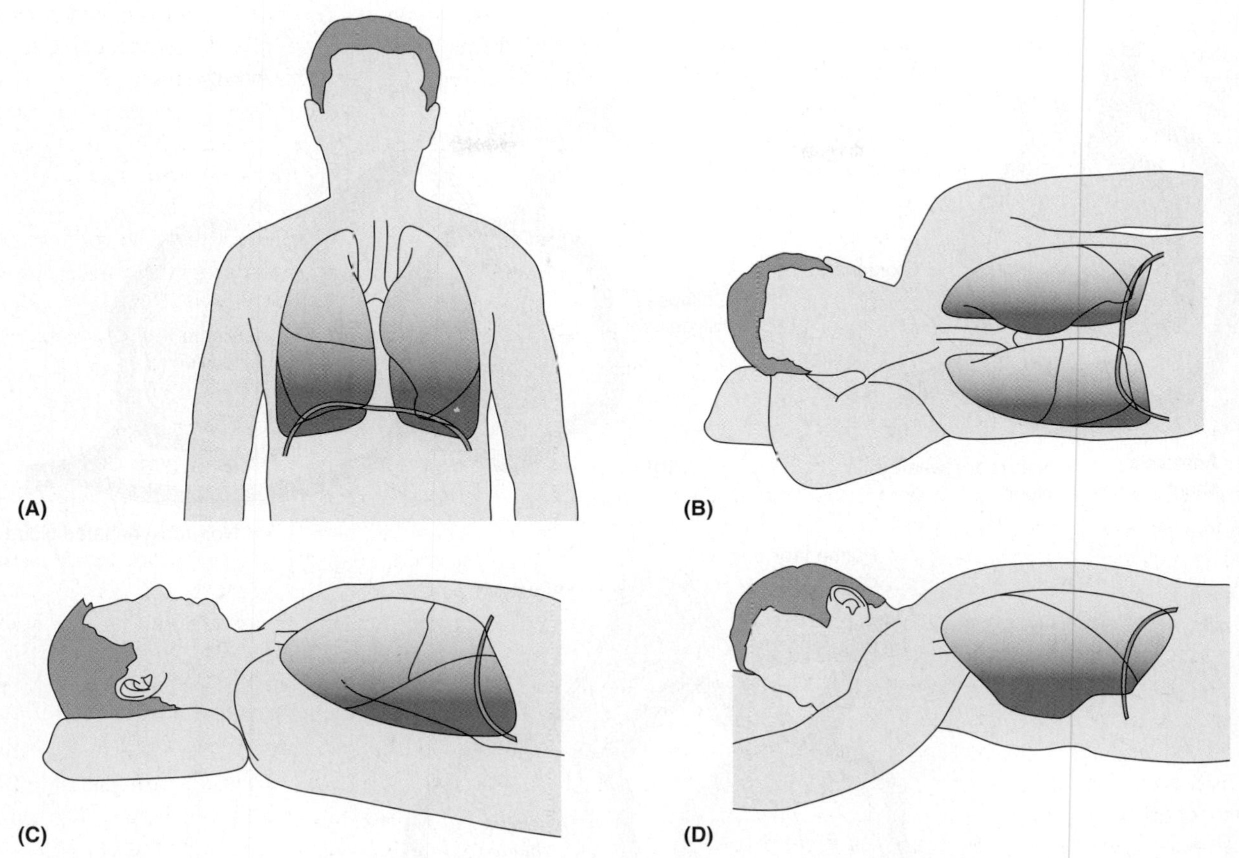

Figure 9–10 ■ Positioning and ventilation-to-perfusion relationship. (**A**) Upright position—Air moves towards diaphragm and blood gravitates to bases. Best $\dot{V}/\dot{Q}$ match (**B**) Side lying position—Air moves towards diaphragm while blood gravitates to lateral dependent lung fields. (**C**) Supine position—Air moves towards diaphragm while blood gravitates to posterior dependent lung fields. (**D**) Prone position—Air moves towards diaphragm while blood gravitates to the anterior dependent lung fields.

moves from the right heart and back into the left heart without coming into contact with alveoli. Normally, this is approximately 2 to 5 percent of blood flow. Normal anatomic shunting occurs as a result of emptying of the bronchial and several other veins into the lung's own venous system. Abnormal anatomic shunting can occur because of heart or lung problems; for example, a ventricular septal defect (a hole in the heart wall dividing the right and left ventricles), in the presence of pulmonary hypertension, shunts venous blood from the right heart directly into the arterial blood in the left heart. Traumatic injury to pulmonary blood vessels and tissues and certain types of lung tumors can also cause abnormal anatomic shunting.

TABLE 9–3 Comparison of High and Low $\dot{V}/\dot{Q}$ Ratios

HIGH $\dot{V}/\dot{Q}$ RATIO	LOW $\dot{V}/\dot{Q}$ RATIO
Normal to increased alveolar ventilation associated with decreased perfusion	Decreased alveolar ventilation associated with normal to increased perfusion
Alveolar gas effect	**Alveolar gas effect**
Increased cardiac output Decreased alveolar CO_2 Normally exists in upper lung fields	Decreased oxygen in alveoli Increased carbon dioxide in alveoli Normally exists in lower lung fields
Abnormally present with	**Abnormally present with**
Decreased cardiac output Pulmonary emboli Pneumothorax Destruction of pulmonary capillaries	Hypoventilation Obstructive lung diseases Restrictive lung diseases
Arterial blood gas effects	**Arterial blood gas effects**
Increased Pao_2 Decreased $Paco_2$ Increased pH	Decreased Pao_2 Increased $Paco_2$ Decreased pH

Capillary Shunt. **Capillary shunt** is the normal flow of blood past completely unventilated alveoli. This means that the blood flowing by the affected units will not take part in diffusion. Capillary shunt results from such conditions as consolidation or collapse of alveoli, atelectasis, or fluid in the alveoli.

The combined amount of anatomic shunt and capillary shunt is called **absolute shunt.** The total percentage of cardiac output involved in absolute shunt has important clinical implications. Lung tissue that is affected by absolute shunt is unaffected by oxygen therapy because it involves nonfunctioning alveoli. No matter how much oxygen is administered, diffusion cannot take place if alveoli are completely bypassed or nonfunctioning. Shunting of more than 15 percent of cardiac output can result in severe respiratory failure. In fact, patients with acute respiratory distress syndrome (ARDS) generally have an absolute shunt of more than 20 percent of their cardiac output. The hallmark of ARDS is refractory hypoxemia (hypoxemia that is not

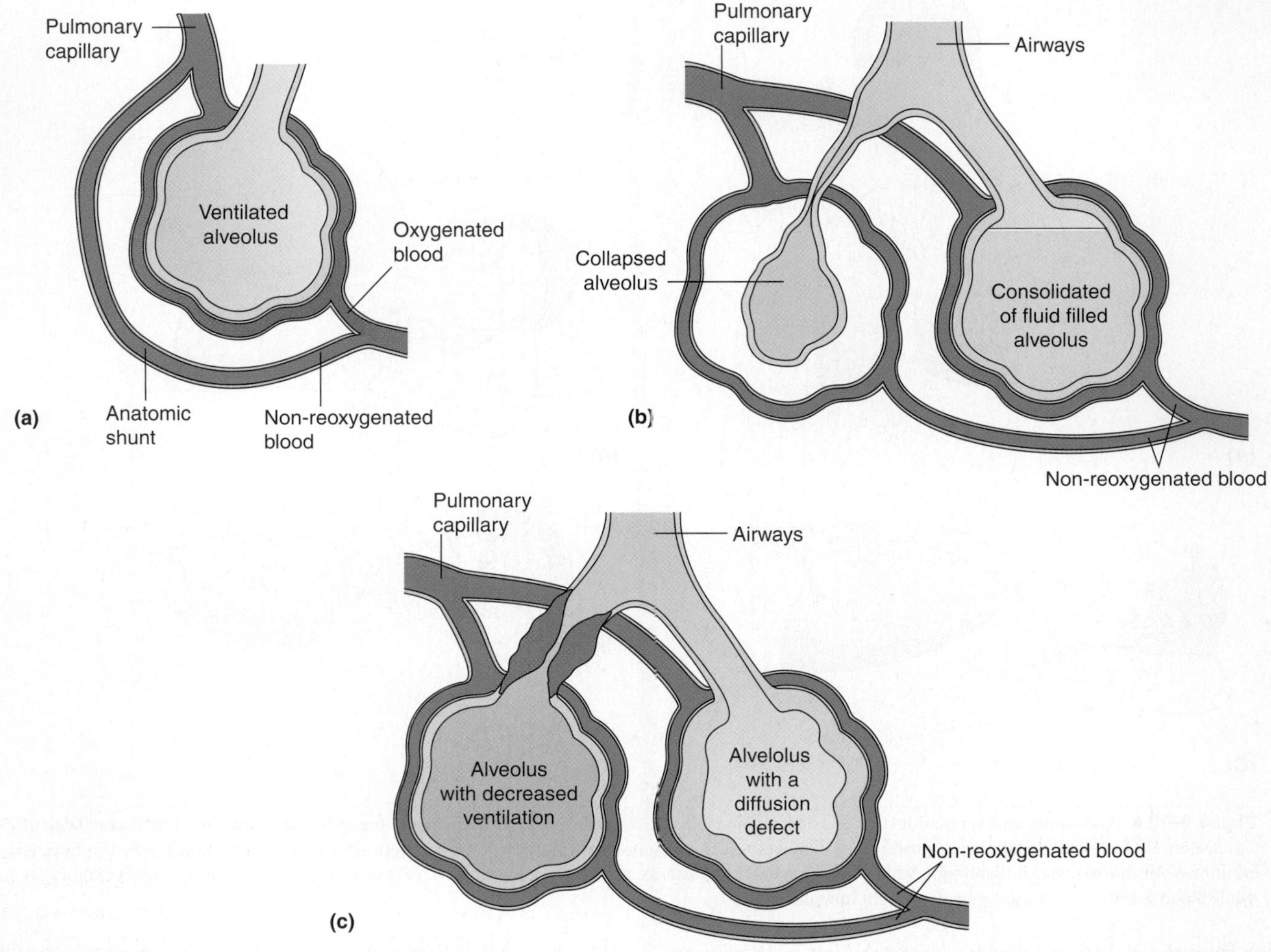

Figure 9–11 ▪ Types of physiologic shunt. (a) Anatomic shunt; (b) Capillary shunt; (c) Shuntlike effects—Alveoli with decreased ventilation may respond well to oxygen therapy.

significantly affected by administration of increasing levels of oxygen), which is consistent with the clinical picture of absolute shunt. Estimates of the amount of shunt can be made using relatively easy calculations.

Shuntlike Effect. **Shuntlike effect** is not a true shunt because the shunting is not complete. Shuntlike effect exists when there is an excess of perfusion in relation to alveolar ventilation–in other words, when alveolar ventilation is reduced but not totally absent. Common causes include bronchospasm, hypoventilation, or pooling of secretions. Fortunately, because the alveoli are still functioning to some extent, hypoxemia secondary to shuntlike effect is very responsive to oxygen therapy.

Venous Admixture. **Venous admixture** refers to the effect that pulmonary shunt has on the contents of the blood as it drains into the left heart and out into the system as arterial blood. Beyond the shunted areas, the fully reoxygenated blood (from normal alveolar units) mixes with the completely or relatively unoxygenated blood (from true or shuntlike effect alveolar units). The oxygen molecules remix in the combined blood to establish a new balance, resulting in a PaO_2 that is higher than that which existed in blood affected by shunt but lower than what it would be if the alveoli were normal (Fig. 9–12).

Estimating Intrapulmonary Shunt

A variety of calculations are available that provide significant information regarding the oxygenation status of the high-acuity patient. Increasingly, nurses who take care of this patient population are expected to have a basic understanding of these calculations and their significance. Calculating the P/F (PaO_2/FiO_2) ratio is the simplest way to estimate intrapulmonary shunt. It is best used when the patient's $PaCO_2$ is stable because it is not sensitive to changes in that value. Table 9–4 shows how to calculate a P/F ratio.

Pulmonary Vascular Resistance

Pulmonary vascular resistance (PVR) measures the resistance to blood flow in the pulmonary vascular system, which is a low-resistance system. In effect, it represents right ventricular afterload in much the same way that systemic vascular resistance (SVR) represents left ventricular afterload (a high-resistance system). The right ventricle pumps oxygen-poor blood into the pulmonary capillaries by way of the pulmonary artery. The amount of right ventricular force required to pump the blood into the lungs depends on the resistance to flow present in the pulmonary vascular system. This resistance to flow is called pulmonary vascular resistance.

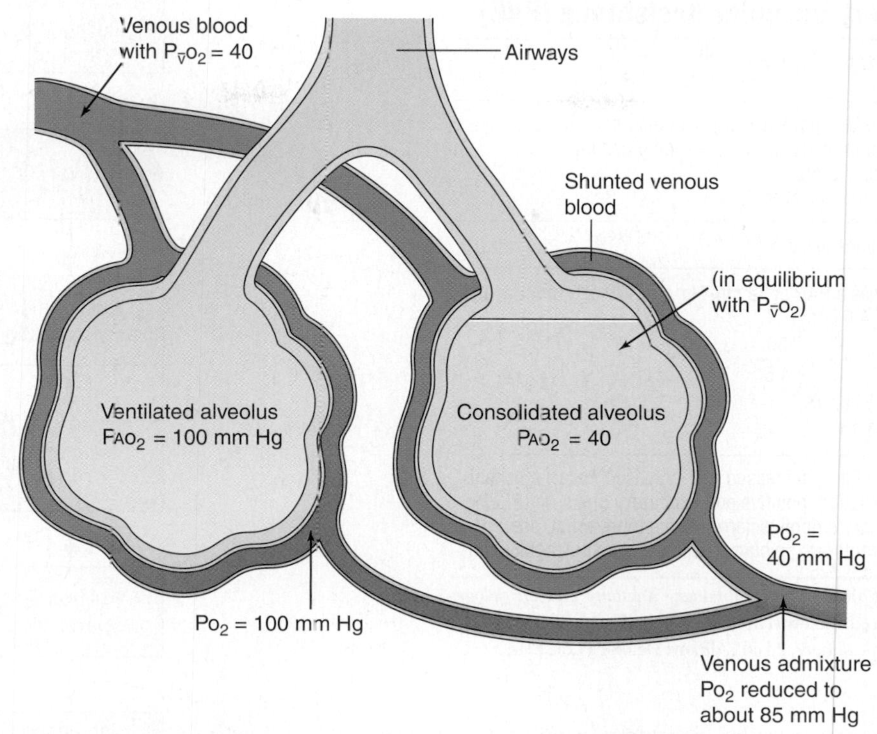

Figure 9–12 ■ Venous admixture. Venous admixture occurs when reoxygenated blood mixes with nonreoxygenated blood distal to the alveoli.

Three main factors determine the amount of pulmonary resistance: the length and radius of the vessels and the viscosity (thickness) of the blood. Of these factors, the major determinant of pulmonary vascular resistance is vessel radius (caliber).

Vessel Radius Determinants

Vessel radius refers to the diameter (caliber) of the vessels. Vessel radius is altered by

- The volume of blood in the pulmonary vascular system
- The amount of vasoconstriction
- The degree of lung inflation

Factors related to the volume of blood in the pulmonary vascular system include capillary recruitment and distention. Of these factors, recruitment is the most influential. The small pulmonary capillaries open up (are recruited) in response to an increase in blood flow. Under circumstances in which pulmonary blood flow is low (e.g., shock), the smaller capillaries may receive so little blood that they collapse. The concept of pulmonary capillary recruitment is similar to the recruitment and collapse of alveoli based on volume of airflow. The second factor, distention, occurs in response to increased cardiac output or increased intravascular fluid volume. By distending, the capillaries are able to accommodate the increased flow. Distention of the capillaries decreases PVR.

Pulmonary vasoconstriction occurs in response to hypoxia, hypercapnia, and acidosis. Vasoconstriction is a major cause of increased PVR in the high-acuity patient, and hypoxia is the strongest stimulant for pulmonary vasoconstriction. When an area of the lung becomes hypoxic, such as is seen in shunt, vasoconstriction is triggered. This response effectively diverts blood flow to more functional areas of the lungs and results in a reduction in the impact of shunt. Unfortunately, in cases involving a generalized pulmonary disease process (e.g., late-stage emphysema), pulmonary vasoconstriction becomes global and PVR increases significantly. The elevated PVR requires the right heart to work against elevated pressures. In response to this increased workload, the right heart hypertrophies and cor pulmonale develops.

The degree of lung inflation also has an impact on the diameter of the pulmonary capillaries. As the lung inflates, capillaries become stretched. In states of high lung inflation, capillaries become compressed, which decreases their diameter and increases PVR. The opposite is also true, lower lung volumes are associated with decreased PVR.

TABLE 9–4 P/F (Pa_{O_2}/Fi_{O_2}) Ratio

EQUATION[a]	$\frac{Pa_{O_2}}{Fi_{O_2}}$
Components	Pa_{O_2} = partial pressure of arterial oxygen (mm Hg) Fi_{O_2} = fraction of inspired oxygen (O_2 concentration) (decimal)
Normal values	350–450 Minimum clinically acceptable level = 286 Inverse relationship: The lower the ratio value drops below normal, the more intrapulmonary shunt worsens
Example	A patient has a Pa_{O_2} of 92 mm Hg on a Fi_{O_2} of 0.60 $\frac{92}{0.60} = 153$ This is below the minimum acceptable level.

[a]This formula is best used when Pa_{CO_2} is stable.
Normal value from Pilbeam (2006).

TABLE 9–5 Pulmonary Vascular Resistance (PVR)

EQUATION	$PVR = (\overline{PAP} - PCWP) \times \frac{80}{CO}$
Components	$\overline{PAP}$ = mean pulmonary artery pressure PCWP = pulmonary capillary wedge pressure CO = cardiac output 80 = conversion factor
Normal values	50–150 dynes·sec·cm^{-5}
Example	A patient has a $\overline{PAP}$ of 22 mm Hg, a PCWP of 9 mm Hg, and a CO of 4.5 L/min $PVR = 22 - 9 \times \frac{80}{4.5}$ PVR = 13 × 17.78 PVR = 231.14
Factors associated with increased PVR	Decreased Pao_2, decreased pH, increased $Paco_2$; mechanical ventilation, positive end expiratory pressure (PEEP); pulmonary emboli, scleroderma, emphysema, pneumo- and hemothorax; histamine, prostaglandin, angiotensin

Data from Des Jardins, T.R. (2008). *Cardiopulmonary anatomy and physiology: essentials for respiratory care,* 5th ed. Albany: Thomson Delmar Learning; and Chang, D.W. (1998). *Respiratory care calculations,* 2d ed.. Albany: Delmar Publishers.

Calculating pulmonary vascular resistance requires the presence of a flow-directed pulmonary artery catheter. The calculation measures resistance, which is a function of pressure and flow. Pressure is determined by the mean pulmonary artery pressure and the pulmonary capillary wedge pressure. Flow is measured as the cardiac output. Table 9–5 summarizes the calculation of pulmonary vascular resistance.

Cor Pulmonale

Cor pulmonale refers to right ventricular hypertrophy and dilation secondary to pulmonary disease. It is a complication of both restrictive and obstructive pulmonary diseases. Cor pulmonale can cause right heart failure and is a major cause of death in the chronic obstructive pulmonary disease (COPD) patient. It is the result of a sequence of events precipitated by pulmonary hypertension. Pulmonary vessels normally function in a low-pressure system. Many pulmonary conditions cause pressures to increase in the vascular bed, creating a state of pulmonary hypertension. When this occurs, PVR increases. Pressure in the pulmonary artery is increased, making it more difficult to push blood out of the right heart during systole. The right heart becomes congested because less blood is moved out with each contraction. Over time, this congestion causes the right heart chambers to dilate. The right heart muscle hypertrophies to compensate for the required increased work of contraction. Figure 9–13 shows how the heart is affected by pulmonary hypertension.

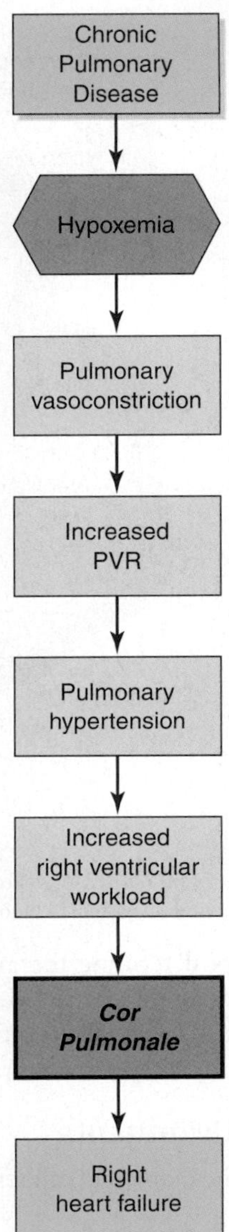

Figure 9–13 ▪ Cor pulmonale. Severe chronic pulmonary diseases are associated with a pattern of increasing hypoxemia that causes the lungs to vasoconstrict. The pulmonary vascular vasoconstriction increases PVR, which results in pulmonary hypertension. The right heart is required to work harder to pump blood into the pulmonary vascular system, and, over time, the right ventricle dilates and hypertrophies in response to the increased PVR. The adaptation of the right ventricle is called *cor pulmonale.*

SECTION THREE REVIEW

1. Which statement is true regarding the relationship of ventilation to perfusion in an upright person?
   A. It varies throughout the lung.
   B. Ventilation is best in the apices.
   C. Perfusion is best in peripheral lung areas.
   D. It maintains a 1:1 relationship.

2. During spontaneous breathing, air flows toward
   A. the apices
   B. the diaphragm
   C. the higher-pressure gradient
   D. higher-resistance areas

3. Mr. M. has left lower lobe pneumonia. His remaining lung fields are clear. It is time to reposition Mr. M. in bed. Of the following positions, which is most likely to optimize the ventilation–perfusion relationship?
   A. Place him on his right side.
   B. Place him supine.
   C. Place him on his left side.
   D. Place him horizontal in the bed.
4. When ventilation–perfusion mismatching occurs, it can be detected by which parameter?
   A. hemoglobin (Hgb) level
   B. oxygen saturation level (Sa_{O_2})
   C. partial pressure of arterial carbon dioxide (Pa_{CO_2})
   D. arterial sodium bicarbonate level (HCO_3)
5. A decrease of airflow to the apices of the lungs is caused by increased
   A. natural airflow toward lung periphery
   B. negative pleural pressure in bases
   C. negative pleural pressure in apices
   D. positive pleural pressure in apices
6. Which statement best describes the term *true shunt*?
   A. alveoli that have no airflow
   B. alveoli that have air trapped in them
   C. blood that does not take part in pulmonary gas exchange
   D. blood entering the right heart without being oxygenated
7. The normal percentage of cardiac output as a result of anatomic shunt is
   A. 0 to 5 percent
   B. 2 to 5 percent
   C. 10 to 30 percent
   D. 20 to 40 percent
8. Anatomic shunt would be most increased with which disorder?
   A. pneumonia
   B. pulmonary edema
   C. tuberculosis
   D. ventricular septal defect
9. Normal blood flow past completely unventilated alveoli is the definition of
   A. physiologic shunt
   B. anatomic shunt
   C. capillary shunt
   D. venous admixture
10. Oxygen therapy is most effective in treating
   A. shuntlike effect
   B. anatomic shunt
   C. capillary shunt
   D. absolute shunt
11. A patient who is receiving oxygen at 40 percent (Fi_{O_2} of 0.4) has an ABG drawn that shows a Pa_{O_2} of 76 mmHg. What is this patient's P/F ratio and what is its significance? (fill in the blanks)
   P/F Ratio: ______
   Significance: ______
12. The nurse is calculating a patient's pulmonary vascular resistance (PVR). The latest hemodynamic values are PAP, 30 mm Hg; PAWP, 15 mm Hg; CO 5.2 L/min. What is the PVR and what is its significance? (fill in the blanks)
   PVR: ______
   Significance: ______

Answers: 1. A, 2. B, 3. A, 4. B, 5. C, 6. C, 7. B, 8. D, 9. C, 10.A, 11. P/F Ratio=190; Significance: Abnormally low-suggests a significant shunt, 12. PVR = 230.7; Significance = abnormally high PVR

SECTION FOUR: Acid–Base Physiology and Disturbances

At the completion of this section, the learner will be able to identify mechanisms that the body uses to compensate for acid–base imbalances, and differentiate between respiratory acidosis and alkalosis, and metabolic acidosis and alkalosis.

The acid–base status is another type of determinant of gas exchange because the lungs are heavily invested in maintaining acid–base homeostasis and they are also the source of severe acid–base imbalances in the presence of certain pulmonary disease states. This section provides an overview of acid–base physiology and disturbances.

Acid–Base Physiology

Acid–base balance is crucial to the effective functioning of the body systems. Severe imbalances can be lethal to the patient. The body contains many acid and base substances. **Acids** are substances that dissociate or lose ions. **Bases** are substances capable of accepting ions. A **buffer** is a substance that reacts with acids and bases to maintain a neutral environment of stable pH. The **pH** represents the free hydrogen ion (H^+) concentration. An increase in H^+ concentration lowers pH and increases acidity. A decrease in H^+ concentration increases pH and increases alkalinity.

The body's acids include volatile acids and nonvolatile acids. **Volatile acids** can convert to a gas form for excretion (carbonic acid). Carbonic acid rapidly converts to carbon dioxide for excretion from the lungs. The lungs excrete a very large amount of acid each day in this manner. **Nonvolatile (metabolic) acids** cannot be converted to gas so they must be excreted through the kidneys. Examples of nonvolatile acids include lactic acid and ketones. Unlike the lungs, the kidneys are capable of excreting only a small amount of acid each day and respond slowly to changes. Hydrogen ions are excreted in the proximal and distal tubules of the kidneys in exchange for sodium.

Maintaining Acid–Base Balance: Buffer Systems and Compensation

Buffer Systems

The body is intolerant of wide changes in pH and works constantly to maintain the pH range between 7.35 and 7.45 (Fig. 9–14).

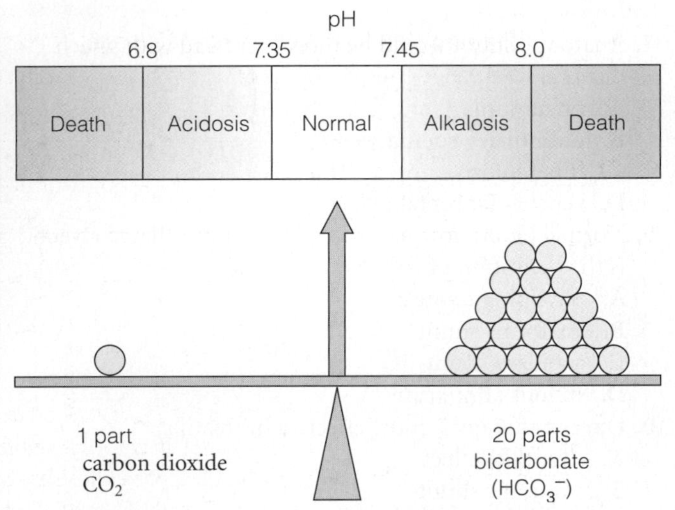

Figure 9–14 ■ The normal ratio of bicarbonate to carbon dioxide is 20:1. As long as this ratio is maintained, the pH remains within the normal range of 7.35 to 7.45. LeMone & Burke. *(2008)*.

A normal pH is maintained if the ratio of bicarbonate (HCO_3) to carbon dioxide (CO_2) remains at approximately a 20:1 (HCO_3/CO_2) ratio. The body has three mechanisms to maintain acid–base balance: the buffering mechanism, the respiratory compensation mechanism, and the metabolic or renal compensation mechanism.

Compensation

Compensation is the process whereby an abnormal pH is returned to within normal limits through counterbalancing acid-base activities. Compensation occurs over time; thus, it is referred to in terms of the degree (or level) to which the body has achieved compensation. There are four levels of compensation: uncompensated (acute), partially compensated, compensated (chronic), or corrected. An **uncompensated** (acute) acid-base state is one in which the pH is abnormal because other buffer and regulatory mechanisms have not begun to correct the balance. A **partially compensated** acid-base state is one in which the pH is abnormal; however, the body buffers and regulatory mechanisms have begun to respond to the imbalance. A **compensated** acid-base state is one in which the pH has returned to within normal limits, with the acid-base imbalance being neutralized but not corrected. Finally, a **corrected** acid-base state is one in which all acid-base parameters have returned to normal ranges after a state of acid-base imbalance. Table 9–6 summarizes the characteristics and provides examples of the levels of compensation.

Buffering mechanisms represent chemical reactions between acids and bases to maintain a neutral environment. Bases react with excess hydrogen ions (H^+) and acids react with excess HCO_3 to prevent shifts in pH. The buffering mechanisms are triggered quickly in response to any change in pH.

Metabolic (Renal) Compensation Mechanism. The bicarbonate buffer system is the major buffering system in the body. Its components are regulated by the lungs (CO_2) and kidneys (HCO_3). The following reversible reaction (carbonic acid equation) represents the shifts that occur as carbonic acid (H_2CO_3) is shifted depending on body needs (left shift makes pH more acid and right shift makes pH more alkaline):

$$H^+ + HCO_3 \leftrightarrow H_2CO_3 \leftrightarrow CO_2 + H_2O$$
$$\text{More Acid} \quad \leftrightarrow \quad \text{More Alkaline}$$

Additional nonbicarbonate buffers include hemoglobin, serum proteins, and the phosphate system, the latter of which is mainly

TABLE 9–6 Levels of Compensation

LEVEL OF COMPENSATION	CHARACTERISTICS	EXAMPLE
Uncompensated (acute)	Abnormal pH with one abnormal value and one normal value.	pH 7.20, $Paco_2$ 60 mm Hg, HCO_3 24 mEq/L. *Interpretation:* The pH and $Paco_2$ match (acid). HCO_3 is normal. No compensation is occurring. An uncompensated (acute) acidosis state exists.
Partially compensated	Abnormal pH with two abnormal values ($Paco_2$ and HCO_3 are moving in opposite directions).	pH 7.30, $Paco_2$ 60 mm Hg, HCO_3 30 mEq/L. *Interpretation*: The pH and $Paco_2$ match (acid). HCO_3 is alkaline or moving in the opposite direction from the $Paco_2$. The pH is still abnormal. A partially compensated acidosis state exists.
Compensated (chronic)	Normal pH plus two abnormal values ($Paco_2$ and HCO_3 are moving in opposite directions).	pH 7.38, $Paco_2$ 50 mm Hg, HCO_3 30 mEq/L. *Interpretation*: The pH and $Paco_2$ match (acid). HCO_3 is alkaline (opposite of $Paco_2$). pH is normal. A (chronic) compensated acidosis state exists.
Corrected	Normal pH and two normal values. No acid–base disturbance currently exists.	pH 7.36, $Paco_2$ 43 mm Hg, HCO_3, 26 mEq/L. *Interpretation*: A normal acid-base state in a person who, until recently, had an acid-base disturbance.

a function of the kidneys. The bicarbonate system is a relatively slow responding system, taking hours-to-days to respond to acid–base disturbances.

The metabolic compensation mechanism controls the rate of elimination or reabsorption of hydrogen and bicarbonate ions in the kidney. In situations of increased acid loads (acidosis), H^+ elimination and bicarbonate reabsorption are increased. In alkalosis, H^+ is reabsorbed and HCO_3^- is excreted. Metabolic compensation is slow. It begins in hours but takes days to reach maximum compensation. This delayed compensatory mechanism helps explain why so many respiratory problems initially cause acute (uncompensated) acid-base disturbances.

Respiratory (Pulmonary) Compensation Mechanism. The respiratory buffer system is the rapid-response compensatory mechanism for metabolic acid–base disturbances. It responds within minutes of development of a metabolic acid-base disturbance. The lungs have two ways in which they compensate: (1) alveolar hypoventilation in response to metabolic alkalosis and (2) alveolar hyperventilation in response to metabolic acidosis. Hypoventilation (slow and/or shallow breathing) retains CO_2, which is then available to shift the carbonic acid equation toward the left (see the preceding discussion), resulting in shifting the pH toward acid. Hyperventilation (rapid and/or deep breathing) blows off CO_2, which then shifts the carbonic acid equation back toward the right, resulting in driving the pH up, toward alkaline.

Respiratory Acid–Base Disturbances

Primary respiratory disturbances are reflected by changes in the $PaCO_2$, being either above normal as in respiratory acidosis, or below normal as in respiratory alkalosis.

Respiratory Acidosis

Respiratory acidosis occurs when the $Paco_2$ rises above 45 mm Hg and the pH drops below 7.35. **Hypercapnia,** elevated carbon dioxide (CO_2), indicates alveolar hypoventilation. The lungs are not blowing off enough carbon dioxide, causing a carbonic acid excess. Carbon dioxide is considered an acid because it combines with water to form carbonic acid. It is essential to determine the cause of hypoventilation and then to correct it when possible. Table 9–7 lists some of the major causes of acute respiratory acidosis.

A "chronic" abnormal acid–base state means that a state of compensation exists. Chronic respiratory acidosis usually is associated with a chronic obstructive pulmonary disease, such as chronic bronchitis or emphysema. The elevation of carbon dioxide occurs gradually over many years; therefore, the body is able to compensate to maintain a normal pH by elevating the bicarbonate. Because these individuals have little respiratory reserve, additional stressors can cause decompensation, which produces respiratory failure. Table 9–8 compares the effects of acute and chronic acidosis on ABG levels.

TABLE 9–7 Common Causes of Acute Respiratory Acidosis

Alveolar hypoventilation, caused by

Respiratory depression
- Oversedation
- Overdose
- Head injury

Decreased ventilation
- Respiratory muscle fatigue
- Neuromuscular diseases
- Mechanical ventilation (underventilation)

Altered diffusion/ventilation–perfusion mismatch
- Pulmonary edema
- Severe atelectasis
- Pneumonia
- Severe bronchospasm

TABLE 9–8 Comparison of Acute and Chronic Respiratory Acidosis

	UNCOMPENSATED	COMPENSATED	
PARAMETER	ACUTE	PARTIAL	CHRONIC
pH	↓	↓	Normal
$Paco_2$	↑	↑	↑
HCO_3	Normal	↑	↑

Respiratory Alkalosis

Respiratory alkalosis occurs when the $Paco_2$ falls below 35 mm Hg with a corresponding rise in pH to greater than 7.45. The decreased carbon dioxide indicates alveolar hyperventilation. The lungs are eliminating too much carbon dioxide, creating a carbonic acid deficit. In the presence of respiratory alkalosis, there is insufficient carbon dioxide available to combine with water to form carbonic acid (H_2CO_3). The key to effective treatment of respiratory alkalosis is to determine the cause of the hyperventilation and provide the intervention necessary to correct the problem. Common causes of acute respiratory alkalosis are listed in Table 9–9.

Chronic respiratory alkalosis is uncommon. The same factors causing acute respiratory alkalosis could cause a chronic state if the problem remained uncorrected. Table 9–10 compares the effects of acute and chronic respiratory alkalosis on ABG levels.

TABLE 9–9 Common Causes of Acute Respiratory Alkalosis

Alveolar hyperventilation, caused by

Anxiety, fear
Pain
Hypoxia
Head injury
Fever
Mechanical ventilation (overventilation)

TABLE 9–10 Comparison of Acute and Chronic Respiratory Alkalosis

	UNCOMPENSATED	COMPENSATED	
PARAMETER	ACUTE	PARTIAL	CHRONIC
pH	↑	↑	Normal
$Paco_2$	↓	↓	↓
HCO_3	Normal	↓	↓

TABLE 9–11 Comparison of Acute and Chronic Metabolic Acidosis

	UNCOMPENSATED	COMPENSATED	
PARAMETER	ACUTE	PARTIAL	CHRONIC
pH	↓	↓	Normal
$Paco_2$	Normal	↓	↓
HCO_3	↓	↓	↓

Metabolic Acid–Base Disturbances

While the focus of this module is on the pulmonary system, a discussion of acid-base imbalances would not be complete without also presenting metabolic imbalances. Primary metabolic disturbances are reflected by abnormal base excess (BE) levels and changes in bicarbonate (HCO_3) levels.

Base Excess

Base excess (BE) is a measure of the amount of buffer required to return the blood to a normal pH state. The normal range is ± 2 mEq/L. Base excess is considered a purely nonrespiratory measurement because it is not affected by carbonic acid concentrations. A base excess is present if the BE is greater than +2mEq/L, reflecting either an excess of base or a deficit of fixed acids. It signals the presence of a metabolic alkalosis state. A base deficit is present if BE is less than −2 mEq/L, reflecting an excess of fixed acids or a deficit in base in the blood. It signals the presence of a metabolic acidosis state.

Metabolic Acidosis

Metabolic acidosis can be defined clinically as HCO_3 less than 22 mEq/L, pH less than 7.35, with a base deficit (less than −2). Metabolic acidosis can be caused by an increase in metabolic acids or excessive loss of base.

Examples of conditions that can cause an increase in hydrogen ion (H^+) concentration include

- Diabetic acidosis as a result of elevated ketones
- Uremia associated with increased levels of phosphates and sulfates
- Ingestion of acidic drugs, such as aspirin (salicylate) overdose
- Lactic acidosis caused by increased lactic acid production

Examples of conditions that precipitate a decrease in bicarbonate (HCO_3) levels include

- Diarrhea, which causes loss of alkaline substances
- Gastrointestinal fistulas leading to loss of alkaline substances
- Loss of body fluids from drains below the umbilicus (except urinary catheter) causing loss of alkaline fluids
- Drugs causing loss of alkali, such as laxative overuse
- Hyperaldosteronism, which causes increased renal loss

Lactic Acidosis. Currently, there is increased clinical interest in evaluating metabolic acidosis that is precipitated by elevated lactate levels. Acid metabolites, such as lactic acid (lactate), result from cellular breakdown and anaerobic metabolism. The normal range for serum lactate is 0.5 to 2.0 mEq/L. High-acuity patients are at particular risk for developing elevated levels of lactate because lactic acidosis is closely associated with shock and other severe physiologic insults. During a shock episode, cellular hypoxia drives serum lactate levels up rapidly, usually greater than 5 mEq/L. This rise often precedes decompensatory signs, such as decreased urine output and decreased blood pressure, and thus may be an indicator of impending shock. Other conditions that can cause lactic acidosis include severe dehydration, severe infection, severe trauma, diabetic ketoacidosis, and hepatic failure (Kee, 2005).

Table 9–11 compares the effects of acute and chronic metabolic acidosis on arterial blood gases.

Metabolic Alkalosis

Metabolic alkalosis can be defined clinically as a bicarbonate (HCO_3) level greater than 26 mEq/L, pH greater than 7.45, and a base excess (greater than +2). Metabolic alkalosis occurs when the amount of alkali (base) increases or excessive loss of acid occurs.

A common cause of increased alkali is ingestion of alkaline drugs associated with the overuse of antacids or over-administration of sodium bicarbonate during a cardiac arrest emergency. Examples of conditions that result in a decrease in acid include:

- Loss of gastric fluids from vomiting or nasogastric suction
- Treatment with steroids, especially those with mineralocorticoid effects
- Diuretic therapy with certain drugs, such as furosemide (Lasix), causing loss of potassium
- Binge–purge syndrome

Table 9–12 compares the effects of acute and chronic metabolic alkalosis on arterial blood gases.

TABLE 9–12 Comparison of Acute and Chronic Metabolic Alkalosis

	UNCOMPENSATED	COMPENSATED	
PARAMETER	ACUTE	PARTIAL	CHRONIC
pH	↑	↑	Normal
$Paco_2$	Normal	↑	↑
HCO_3	↑	↑	↑

SECTION FOUR REVIEW

1. The body compensates for acid–base imbalance with which mechanisms? (choose all that apply)
   A. buffering
   B. hepatic compensation
   C. respiratory compensation
   D. excretion of bicarbonate
2. Respiratory compensation involves excretion or retention of
   A. CO_2
   B. HCO_3
   C. H_2O
   D. K^+
3. Metabolic compensation involves changes in renal excretion or reabsorption of
   A. H^+, CO_2
   B. HCO_3, H^+
   C. glucose, HCO_3
   D. CO_2, HCO_3
4. The body's buffering system continually works toward maintenance of a bicarbonate/carbon dioxide ratio of
   A. 1:5
   B. 1:20
   C. 5:1
   D. 20:1
5. Respiratory acidosis is caused by
   A. alveolar hyperventilation
   B. alveolar hypoventilation
   C. mechanical ventilation
   D. inadequate perfusion
6. Which parameter change occurs as a result of acute respiratory acidosis?
   A. Po_2 increases
   B. pH decreases
   C. CO_2 decreases
   D. HCO_3 decreases
7. Respiratory alkalosis results from which problem?
   A. alveolar hyperventilation
   B. alveolar hypoventilation
   C. metabolic alkalosis
   D. inadequate perfusion
8. Patient situations associated with respiratory alkalosis include
   A. sedation
   B. neuromuscular blockade
   C. pulmonary edema
   D. anxiety
9. Metabolic disturbances are reflected by changes in
   A. HCO_3, Fio_2
   B. Pao_2, Sao_2
   C. HCO_3, BE
   D. BE, Pao_2
10. Metabolic acidosis results in
    A. increased $Paco_2$
    B. decreased BE
    C. increased pH
    D. increased HCO_3
11. A condition that may cause metabolic acidosis because of decrease in bicarbonate levels is
    A. diarrhea
    B. uremia
    C. aspirin ingestion
    D. diabetic ketoacidosis
12. Metabolic alkalosis is caused by a (an) ______ in acid or a (an) ______ in base.
    A. increase, increase
    B. decrease, decrease
    C. decrease, increase
    D. increase, decrease

Answers: 1. (A, C, D), 2. A, 3. B, 4. D, 5. B, 6. B, 7. A, 8. D, 9. C, 10. B, 11. A, 12. C

SECTION FIVE: Arterial Blood Gases

At the completion of this section, the learner will be able to identify normal values for and interpret arterial blood gases.

Interpretation of arterial blood gases provides valuable information on the patient's acid-base and oxygenation status.

Determinants of Acid–Base Status

Remember from Section Four that acid-base status is determined by the pH, $PaCO_2$ and bicarbonate (HCO_3) levels. Base excess can give important clues regarding the presence of a metabolic derangement. All of these parameters are included in the arterial blood gas results.

Determinants of Oxygenation Status

Pao_2

Pao_2 represents the partial pressure of the oxygen dissolved in arterial blood (3 percent of total oxygen) (normal value 80 to 100 mm Hg), not the total amount of oxygen available. Though it accounts for only a small percentage of total oxygen in the blood, it is an important indicator of oxygenation because Pao_2 and oxygen saturation (Sao_2) maintain a relationship. This relationship is reflected in the oxyhemoglobin dissociation curve, which was discussed in Section Two.

Sao_2

Oxygen saturation (Sao_2) is the measure of the *percentage* of oxygen combined with hemoglobin compared with the total amount it could carry (normal value greater than 95 percent). The degree of saturation is important in determining the amount of oxygen available for delivery to the tissues.

Hemoglobin

Hemoglobin (Hgb or Hb) is the major component of red blood cells (normal values 12 to 15 g/dL in women, 13.5 to 17 g/dL in men). It is composed of protein and heme, which contains iron. Oxygen binds to the iron atoms located on the four heme groups of each hemoglobin molecule. Hemoglobin is the major carrier of oxygen in the blood and is, therefore, an important factor in tissue oxygenation.

TABLE 9–13 Normal Arterial Blood Gas Values

COMPONENT	RANGE
Acid–base	
pH	7.35–7.45
$Paco_2$	35–45 mm Hg
HCO_3	22–26 mEq/L
BE	±2 mEq/L
Oxygenation Status	
Pao_2	80–100 mm Hg
Sao_2	95–100%
Hgb*	13.5–17 g/dL (males) 12–15 g/dL (females)

*Values from Kee (2009).

Arterial Blood Gas

Arterial blood gas (ABG) normal values typically are reported as normal at sea level (760 mm Hg) partial pressures, room air (21 percent oxygen), and a blood temperature of 37°C (98.6°F). Significant alterations in any of these factors need to be considered during interpretation. Age also affects normal ABG values. For example, newborns have a lower Pao_2 (40 to 70 mm Hg), as do elderly people, whose Pao_2 decreases approximately 10 mm Hg per decade (in the 60- to 90-year age range). Normal ABG values are ranges for normal, healthy adults. It is important to establish a baseline for the individual because abnormal values become "normal" (acceptable) for some individuals. For example, a patient with chronic lung disease may have a Pao_2 of 60 mm Hg with a $Paco_2$ of 50 mm Hg as a normal baseline. Attempts to return this individual's ABG values to those of a normal, healthy person would have serious consequences.

Table 9–13 provides a summary of normal ABG values.

TABLE 9–14 Steps in Determining Acid–Base and Oxygenation Status

STEP	NORMAL VALUES	QUESTIONS
Acid-Base Interpretation		
Step 1: Evaluate pH	pH = 7.35 to 7.45; midpoint = 7.40. If less than 7.40 = acid. If greater than 7.40 = alkaline.	Ask: ■ Is the pH within normal range? ■ Is pH on acid or alkaline side of 7.40?
Step 2: Evaluate $Paco_2$	$Paco_2$ = 35 to 45 mm Hg. If less than 35 mm Hg = alkaline. If greater than 45 mm Hg = acid.	Ask: ■ Is $Paco_2$ within normal range? ■ If not, does it deviate to acid or alkaline side?
Step 3: Evaluate HCO_3	HCO_3 = 22 to 26 mEq/L. If less than 22 mEq/L = acid. If greater than 26 mEq/L = alkaline.	Ask: ■ Is HCO_3 within normal range? ■ If not, does it deviate to alkaline or acid side?
Step 4: Determine Acid–Base Status	The acid–base status has now been determined for the individual components of $Paco_2$ and HCO_3.	Ask: ■ Which individual component matches the pH acid–base state? ■ The match determines the *primary* acid–base disturbance.
Oxygenation Status Interpretation		
Step 5: Evaluate Pao_2	Pao_2 = 80 to 100 mm Hg.	Ask: ■ Is it within normal range? ■ What is this person's baseline? ■ Is it within acceptable range for this person? ■ If not, is it too low or too high?
Step 6: Evaluate Sao_2	Sao_2 = greater than 95%.	Ask ■ Is it within acceptable range?
Step 7: Evaluate Hgb	Hgb = 12 to 15 g/dL (females) and 13.5 to 17 g/dL (males).	Ask: ■ Are there enough oxygen carriers?
Step 8: Evaluate patient	Although ABG interpretation is an important adjunct to assessing a patient's status, it cannot take the place of direct evaluation of the patient.	Ask: ■ Does patient's clinical picture match the acid–base and oxygen interpretation? ■ Does the patient have a chronic disorder that is associated with long-term alterations in ABGs? ■ Are there any acute processes occurring that need to be taken into consideration? ■ Does the patient have a fever?

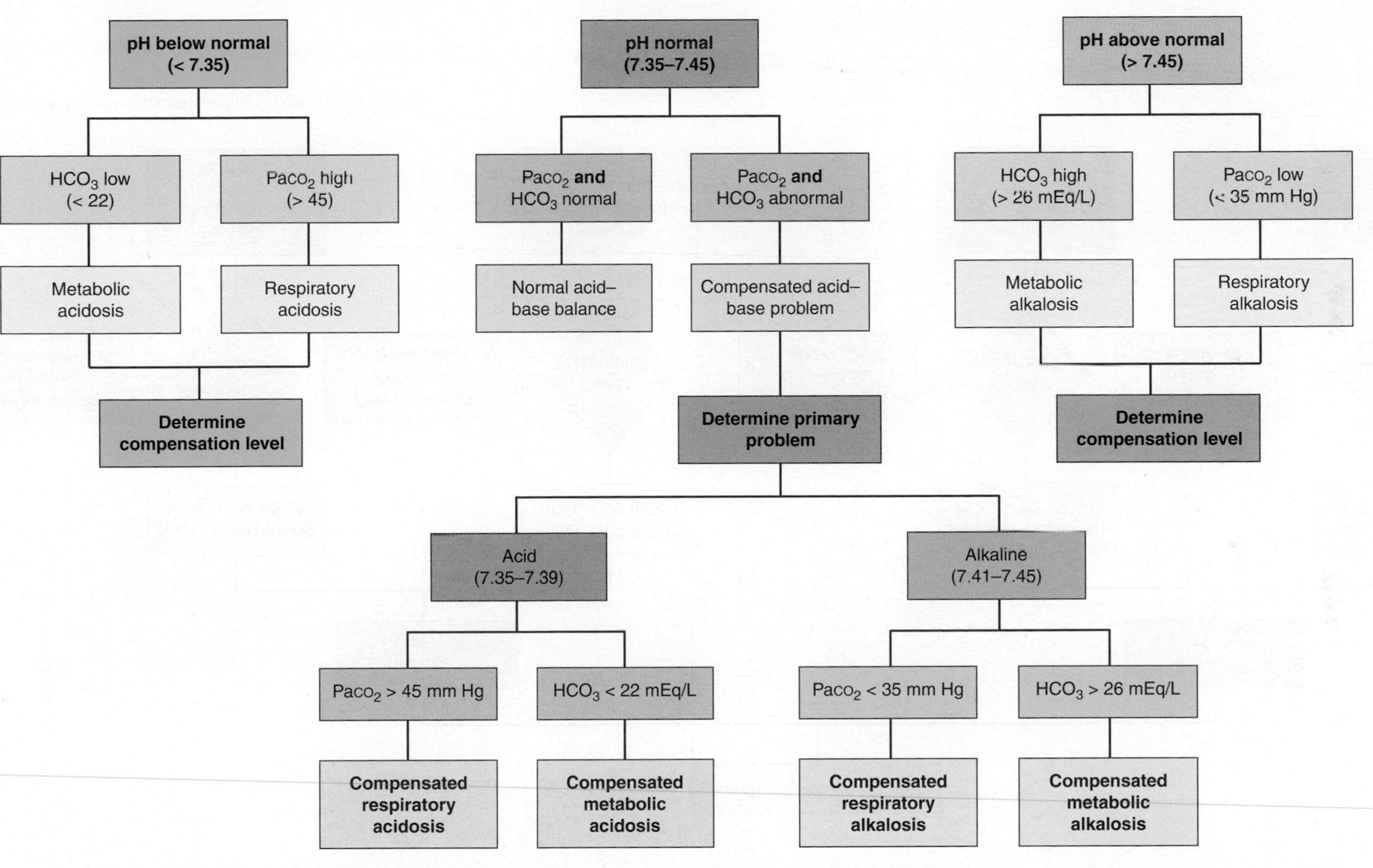

Figure 9–15 ■ Algorithm for interpreting primary acid-base disturbances.

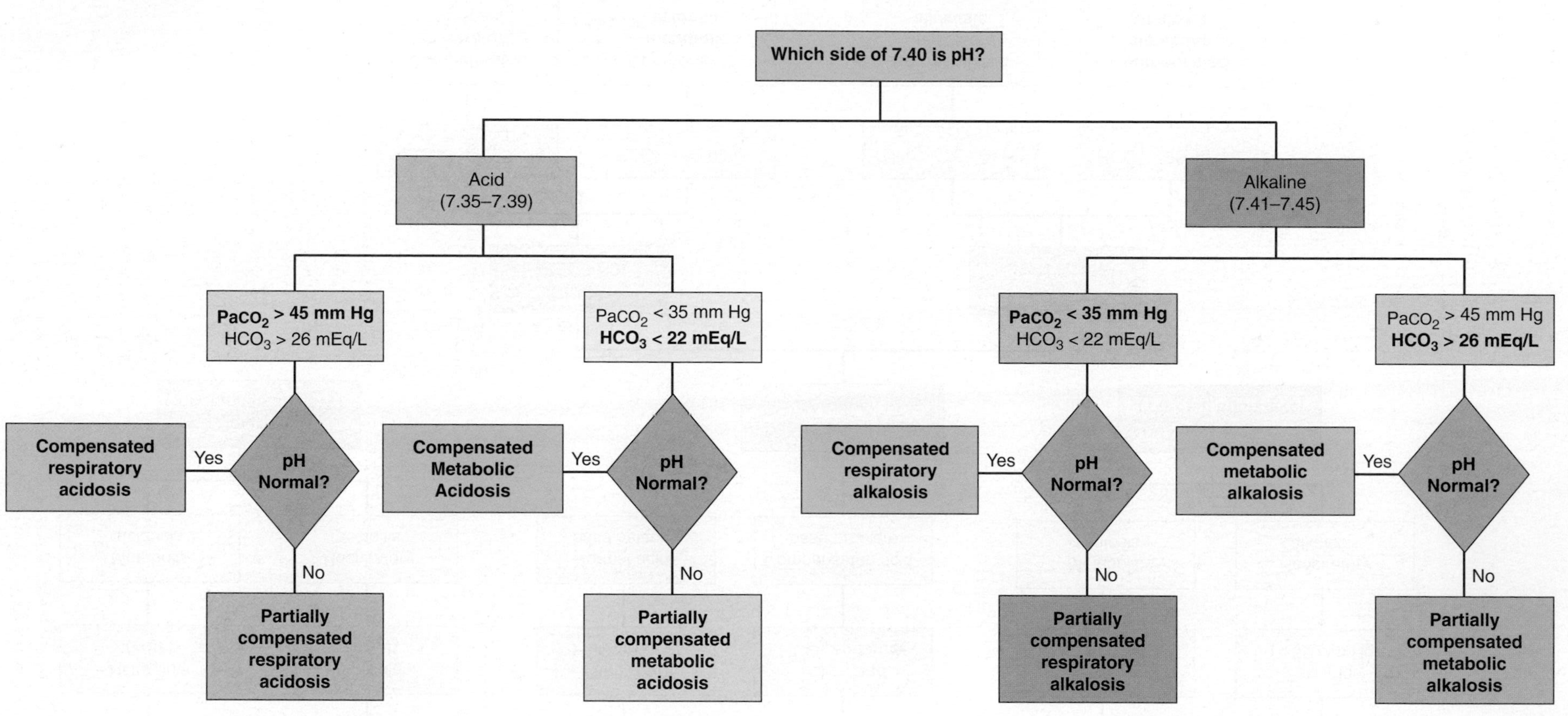

Figure 9–16 ■ Algorithm for interpreting degree of compensation.

Arterial Blood Gas Interpretation

A single ABG measurement represents only a single point in time. Arterial blood gases are most valuable when trends are evaluated over time, correlated with other values, and incorporated into the overall clinical picture. Interpretation of ABGs includes determination of acid–base state, level of compensation, and oxygenation status. Determination of the acid-base state was presented in Section Four. The oxygenation status reflects alveolar ventilation, the amount of oxygen available in arterial blood for possible tissue use, oxygen-carrying capacity, and oxygen transport. The severity of hypoxemia is frequently referred to in terms of being mild, moderate, or severe; however, the exact associated PaO_2 levels are somewhat arbitrary and vary between experts. For the purposes of this chapter, the levels of hypoxemia are defined as:

- Mild hypoxemia: PaO_2 60 to 75 mm Hg
- Moderate hypoxemia: PaO_2 45 to 59 mm Hg
- Severe hypoxemia: PaO_2 of less than 45 mm Hg

A step-by-step process for ABG interpretation evaluates each component to determine acid–base balance and oxygenation status, presented in Table 9–14). Although acid–base balance determination is presented first, oxygenation status often is analyzed first, based on the needs of the patient and the preference of the person performing the analysis. Figures 9–15 and 9–16 provide algorithms for interpreting primary acid–base disturbances and level of compensation.

Supplemental ABG exercises are available at the end of this module. Take the time to practice determining acid-base states and oxygenation status using the steps and algorithms provided in this section.

SECTION FIVE REVIEW

1. Normal values for arterial blood gases include
   A. pH 7.5
   B. $PaCO_2$ 20 mm Hg
   C. HCO_3 26 mm Hg
   D. SaO_2 75 mm Hg
2. An increase in bicarbonate would cause the pH to become more
   A. acidic
   B. alkaline
   C. neutral
   D. no change
3. $PaCO_2$ is the ______ component, and HCO_3 is the ______ component.
   A. oxygenation, metabolic
   B. respiratory, metabolic
   C. metabolic, respiratory
   D. hepatic, oxygenation
4. In people over the age of 60, PaO_2 decreases about ______ mm Hg per decade.
   A. 4
   B. 6
   C. 8
   D. 10
5. What factor must you always evaluate to place ABGs in the proper context?
   A. laboratory values
   B. oxygen supplemental therapy
   C. mode of ventilation
   D. patient

Answers: 1. C, 2. B, 3. B, 4. D, 5. D

SECTION SIX: Advanced Interpretation: Mixed Acid–Base Disorders

At the completion of this section, the learner will be able to recognize and discuss mixed acid–base disorders.

It is not always clear whether the patient is experiencing a simple acid–base disorder with compensation or a mixed acid–base disorder. Recognition and analysis of mixed acid–base disorders is a more complex skill than basic blood gas analysis. This section focuses on the basic concepts involved in recognition of mixed acid–base disorders and provides four rules that help differentiate mixed acid–base disorders from simple (single) disorders with compensation.

The majority of acid–base disturbances have one primary origin with a single secondary acid–base compensatory response. The high-acuity patient, however, is at increased risk for more complex acid–base disorders and may have several different primary acid–base disturbances at the same time. For example, a patient with diabetic ketoacidosis (DKA), a primary metabolic acidosis, might also develop respiratory failure, a primary respiratory acidosis. This situation represents a mixed acid–base disorder. Mixed disorders can have an additive effect, such as is seen with the preceding example (two forms of acidosis), which results in a major derangement in pH. Mixed disorders can also have a nullifying effect (e.g., a primary metabolic alkalosis in the presence of a primary respiratory acidosis), which may rebalance the pH. Table 9–15 lists some complex health problems frequently involved in mixed acid–base disorders.

Identifying a Mixed Acid–Base Disorder

Initial Recognition

Before the nurse can attempt to analyze an ABG for the presence of a mixed acid–base disorder, she or he must first recognize the characteristics of a mixed disorder. When either the $PaCO_2$ or the HCO_3 value appears to be out of the ordinary boundaries, a mixed disorder should be suspected. The following rule summarizes the initial recognition:

RULE: A mixed acid–base disorder is present when either the $PaCO_2$ or the HCO_3 value is

TABLE 9–15 Examples of Clinical Problems Associated with Mixed Acid–Base Disorders

CLINICAL PROBLEM	ASSOCIATED MIXED DISORDERS
Cardiac arrest	Metabolic acidosis and respiratory acidosis
Salicylate toxicity	Metabolic acidosis and respiratory alkalosis
Renal failure with vomiting	Metabolic acidosis and metabolic alkalosis
Vomiting with chronic obstructive pulmonary disease	Metabolic alkalosis and respiratory acidosis
COPD with mechanical ventilation	Metabolic alkalosis and chronic respiratory acidosis
Gram negative sepsis	Metabolic acidosis and respiratory alkalosis
COPD with acute pneumonia	Chronic respiratory acidosis AND acute respiratory acidosis

1. In a direction opposite to its predicted direction, or
2. Not close to the predicted value, during normal compensatory activity (see Table 9–16).

For example, a patient with diabetic ketoacidosis (DKA) has an ABG drawn, which shows a pH of 7.05 and an HCO_3 of 16. In this instance, both the pH and the HCO_3 are acidotic. Depending on the level of compensation, one would predict that the $Paco_2$ level should be either normal or predictably alkaline, as a secondary acid–base response to this situation. If, however, the same DKA patient develops ventilatory failure (hypercapnia), the $Paco_2$ will also be acidotic (indicating respiratory acidosis), which is not a predicted alteration. The presence of both an acid HCO_3 and $Paco_2$ is an example of an additive type of mixed acid–base problem, which would drop the pH significantly.

A second example is one that presents a situation in which a nullifying mixed acid–base problem might develop. Assume that the same acute DKA patient develops severe vomiting or diarrhea, causing metabolic alkalosis. This patient, then, will have metabolic acidosis (caused by DKA) plus metabolic alkalosis (caused by vomiting or diarrhea). The opposing metabolic disturbances represent a nullifying mixed acid–base problem. In this situation, the pH will lean toward the predominant problem, but it will not be as severely deranged as one would predict based on the patient's DKA status. As a result of these opposing metabolic derangements, the patient's $Paco_2$ compensatory changes will reflect the predominant acid–base disorder. The degree of $Paco_2$ compensation, however, will not be as would be predicted for either metabolic disturbance existing alone. In this complex clinical situation, evaluation of the patient's condition must be an integral part of the acid–base assessment. In addition, the base excess and anion gap can be obtained to assist in the analysis of the situation. This type of complex interpretation is generally beyond the nurse's responsibility. It is more important that the nurse (1) recognizes that the patient's clinical picture does not coincide with the ABG results and (2) contacts the physician to report the concern.

> The key is learning how to predict the "normal" compensation relationships between $Paco_2$, HCO_3, and pH so that you can recognize when the relationships are abnormal.

Systematic Evaluation

Once a mixed acid–base problem is suspected, a systematic approach should be used to interpret the disorder. The first two steps are common to all blood gas analyses. It is at Step 3 that mixed acid–base analysis begins. Table 9–17 summarizes a four-step interpretation approach.

Expected Compensatory Responses

Three pairs of relationships require analysis when seeking to differentiate the nature of a mixed acid–base disorder: (1) pH to HCO_3, (2) pH to $Paco_2$, and (3) $Paco_2$ to HCO_3.

Each pair is accompanied by a rule that defines the relationship. If the calculated (predicted) values are similar to the actual values, a simple acid–base disturbance with compensation is present. If, however, the calculated (predicted) values are not similar to the actual values, a mixed disorder is present.

The pH to HCO_3 Relationship. If a metabolic disturbance is present, the pH and HCO_3 should maintain a stable relationship.

RULE: If the acid–base problem is purely metabolic, a pH change of 0.15 will result in a corresponding change in HCO_3 of approximately 10 mEq/L (Pilbeam, 2006).

TABLE 9–16 A Comparison of Mixed Acid–Base Disorders[a]

PARAMETER	MIXED DISORDERS: MATCHING DERANGEMENTS		MIXED DISORDERS: OPPOSITE DERANGEMENTS		
	Metabolic acidosis + Respiratory acidosis	Metabolic alkalosis + Respiratory alkalosis	Metabolic acidosis + Respiratory alkalosis	Metabolic alkalosis + Respiratory acidosis	Metabolic acidosis + Metabolic alkalosis
pH	↓↓	↑↑	NL, ↓, or ↑	NL, ↓, or ↑	NL, ↓, or ↑
$Paco_2$	↑	↓	↓	↑	↓, or ↑
HCO_3	↓	↑	↓	↑	NL, ↓, or ↑

[a]The Matching Derangements columns on the left illustrate the direction of the value trends when both primary disorders are the same (acidotic or alkalotic). This situation results in a severely deranged pH (as shown by two arrows). The Opposite Derangements columns on the right illustrate the direction of value trends when the primary disorders are the opposite of each other (one is acidotic and the other is alkalotic). When opposite primary derangements coexist, they may fully or partially nullify the impact of the pH. If one disorder is predominant, the pH will lean toward the pH associated with that disorder, but to a lesser degree (as shown by single arrows). NL = normal.

TABLE 9–17 Interpretation of Mixed Blood Gases

The First Two Steps Are Common to all Blood Gas Analyses. Step 3 Begins Mixed Acid–Base Analysis.

STEP	QUESTIONS	EXAMPLES/DISCUSSION
Step 1: Identification of primary disorder	Ask: ■ Does pH indicate acidosis or alkalosis? ■ To which side of 7.40 does pH lean?	pH less than 7.40? ■ Acid side of normal pH greater than 7.40? ■ Alkaline side of normal
Step 2: Identification of primary disorder (continued)	Ask: ■ Which value ($Paco_2$ or HCO_3) matches the acid–base state of pH? ■ Discussion: If both values match the pH, a mixed acid–base disturbance is present. Several primary disorders are at work.	pH less than 7.30, $Paco_2$ greater than 50 mm Hg, HCO_3 less than 20 mEq/L. All three indicators are acidotic; thus, the problem is a mixed acid–base disorder.
Step 3: Estimate expected compensatory responses using appropriate rule[a]	Ask: ■ Is the relationship between pH and $Paco_2$ (respiratory component) as predicted? ■ Is the relationship between pH and HCO_3 (metabolic component) as predicted? ■ Is the relationship between $Paco_2$ and HCO_3 as predicted? ■ If the relationships are not as predicted, has there been sufficient time for compensation to have taken place?	Use the appropriate rule related to one of the three blood gas relationships: ■ pH to HCO_3 relationship ■ pH to $Paco_2$ relationship ■ $Paco_2$ to HCO_3 relationship See examples in text.
Step 4: Compare ABG with patient's clinical status	Ask: Is the patient at risk for ■ Alveolar hyper- or hypoventilation? ■ Lactic acidosis? ■ Ketoacidosis? ■ Loss of bicarbonate?	Knowledge of patient's clinical status and risk factors for possible metabolic and respiratory disorders is essential when attempting to interpret mixed acid–base problems.

[a]See "Expected Compensatory Responses" in Section Six.

Example 1: Max W had an ABG drawn revealing a pH of 7.55 and an HCO_3 of 34 mEq/L. The pH difference between the initial standard of 7.40 and Max's ABG pH of 7.55 is 0.15. The HCO_3 difference between the initial standard of 24 mEq/L and Max's HCO_3 is 10 mEq/L. Therefore, because Max's pH and HCO_3 altered within the parameters of the rule, the relationship has been maintained, indicating that a pure metabolic acidosis is present.

The pH and $Paco_2$ Relationship. If the acid–base problem may have a primary respiratory origin, the relationship of pH to $Paco_2$ can be estimated.

RULE: For every 20 mm Hg increase in $Paco_2$ above 40, the pH will decrease by 0.10 unit. For every 10 mm Hg decrease in $Paco_2$ below 40, the pH will increase by 0.10 unit. pH decreases as $Paco_2$ increases; pH increases as $Paco_2$ decreases (Pilbeam, 2006).

Example 2: Jill B's $Paco_2$ is 60 mm Hg, which is 20 mm Hg above the standard of 40 mm Hg. In response, her pH should predictably decrease by 0.10 unit, dropping from 7.40 to 7.30.

Example 3: Lee C's $Paco_2$ is 30 mm Hg, which is 10 mm Hg below the standard of 40 mm Hg. In response, his pH should increase to 7.50 (an increase of 0.10 unit).

Example 4: Eva T has a $Paco_2$ of 60 mm Hg, which is 20 mm Hg above the standard of 40 mm Hg, and a pH of 7.20. Her pH is NOT close to the predicted pH value of 7.30. Assuming that there has been sufficient time for compensatory mechanisms to take effect, a mixed disorder is present.

The $Paco_2$ to HCO_3 Relationship. Under normal conditions the $Paco_2$ and HCO_3 maintain a stable relationship.

RULE: For every increase of 10 mm Hg in $Paco_2$, there is a corresponding increase of 1.0 mEq/L of HCO_3. For every decrease of 10 mm Hg in $Paco_2$, there is corresponding decrease of 2.0 mEq/L of HCO_3 (Pilbeam, 2006).

Example 5. Richard C has an ABG drawn. The $Paco_2$ was 60 mm Hg and the HCO_3 was 31.2 mEq/L. The difference between his $Paco_2$ (60 mm Hg) and the standard of 40 mm Hg is 20 mm Hg. The predicted HCO_3 is 26 mEq/L. Richard's actual HCO_3 compensatory response level is 31.2 mEq/L, which is significantly different from the predicted answer. Assuming that his compensatory mechanisms have had sufficient time to take effect, a mixed disorder is present.

Example 6: Joseph B has an ABG drawn. The $Paco_2$ was 35 mm Hg and the HCO_3 was 26 mEq/L. The difference between Joseph's $Paco_2$ (35 mm Hg) and the standard is 5 mm Hg. This means that for a $Paco_2$ of 35 mm Hg, the predicted HCO_3 compensatory response level would be approximately 25 mEq/L. Joseph's HCO_3 is close to the predicted level. The appropriate level of compensation suggests a simple acid–base disorder.

SECTION SIX REVIEW

1. A mixed acid-base disorder should be suspected when either the $Paco_2$ or the HCO_3 value is
   A. in a direction opposite of its predicted direction.
   B. close to the predicted value during normal compensatory activity.
   C. either significantly alkalotic or acidotic.
   D. impossible to interpret.
2. Mixed acid-base disorders may have what two effects on the pH? (short answer)
   1.
   2.
3. When evaluating a possible mixed acid-base problem, it is crucial to
   A. Obtain a second arterial blood gas.
   B. Contact the physician immediately.
   C. Assess patient's current clinical picture.
   D. Initiate oxygen therapy.
4. The relationship between pH and HCO_3 is best reflected in which statement?
   A. A pH change of 0.15 will result in an opposite change in HCO_3 of about 10 mEq.
   B. A 10 mEq increase in HCO_3 will result in approximately 0.15 increase in pH.
   C. A pH decrease of 0.30 will result from a HCO_3 decrease of about 10 mEq.
   D. The relationship is unpredictable.
5. Which statement is correct regarding the relationship between pH and $Paco_2$?
   A. There is no predictable relationship.
   B. If a patient's $Paco_2$ increases from 41 to 61, the pH will increase 0.10 units (e.g., from 7.39 to 7.49).
   C. If a patient's $Paco_2$ decreases from 39 to 29, the pH will decrease 0.10 units (e.g., from 7.40 to 7.30).
   D. If a patient's $Paco_2$ increases from 41 to 61, the pH will decrease 0.10 units (e.g., from 7.39 to 7.29).
6. The normal relationship $Paco_2$ to HCO_3 is best reflected in which statement?
   A. For every increase of 10 mm Hg in $Paco_2$, there is a corresponding decrease of 1.0 mEq/L in HCO_3.
   B. For every decrease of 10 mm Hg in $Paco_2$, there is a corresponding decrease of 1.0 mEq/L in HCO_3.
   C. For every increase of 10 mm Hg in $Paco_2$, there is a corresponding increase of 1.0 mEq/L in HCO_3.
   D. There is no stable relationship.

Answers: 1. A, 2. additive and nullifying, 3. C, 4. B, 5. D, 6. A

SECTION SEVEN: Focused Respiratory Nursing History and Assessment

At the completion of this section, the learner will be able to describe a focused respiratory nursing history and assessment.

Nursing History

When a patient is admitted to the hospital in acute distress, the nurse initially assesses airway, breathing, and circulation (ABCs), and immediately takes appropriate action based on those assessments. As soon as is feasible, information regarding the immediate events leading to admission should be obtained. A recent history gives important clues as to the etiology and chain of events related to the current problem.

The presence of severe respiratory distress limits the amount of health history information a patient is able to relate. Minimize questions directed to the patient to reduce the stress on breathing, stating all inquiries in such a way that they require very brief answers.

Historical data of particular importance to assess in the patient with acute pulmonary problems include the following.

Social History

Assess tobacco and alcohol use. Tobacco use is associated with many pulmonary diseases, and current use may further aggravate acute pulmonary problems. The number of cigarettes smoked per day and the number of years a patient has smoked should be assessed. Alcohol use in association with prescribed drug therapy may adversely affect the patient's respiratory condition. Problems with alcohol withdrawal can complicate the cardiopulmonary status should delirium tremens develop.

Nutritional History

The nutritional state of a pulmonary patient is crucial to assess because malnutrition is contributory to the development of respiratory failure. Furthermore, many patients with chronic pulmonary disorders are admitted to the hospital in a malnourished state, which negatively impacts patient outcomes. There are several ways in which this can happen. First, a protein–calorie deficit weakens muscles, including the respiratory muscles. Second, malnutrition is associated with a weakened immune system, which increases susceptibility to infection and makes it harder to fight against existing infections. The increased stress associated with an acute infection can precipitate acute respiratory failure. Third, a high-carbohydrate diet increases the overall carbon dioxide load in the body. This may lead to ventilatory complications in certain patients. If there is concern that malnutrition is present, a nutritional assessment, laboratory testing of proteins and a nutrition consult may be considered.

Cardiopulmonary History

Because the lungs, heart, and blood vessels comprise a common circuit, factors that alter any part of the circuit can cause a subsequent alteration in other parts. It is often difficult to differentiate between problems of pulmonary and cardiovascular etiology. Because of this, obtaining sufficient data regarding the cardiovascular system will be invaluable in planning the management of the patient. Of particular importance is data concerning preexisting cardiovascular conditions such as a history of hypertension, coronary artery disease, or previous myocardial infarction. Preexisting pulmonary problems such as asthma or emphysema as well as prehospital activity tolerance can also help to differentiate pulmonary and cardiac problems.

Sleep–Rest History

Pulmonary problems frequently interfere with sleep and rest for a variety of reasons. If the respiratory problem is severe enough to cause hypoxia, the patient often exhibits restlessness associated with inadequate oxygenation of the brain. Pulmonary disorders often increase the work of breathing, which can interfere with rest and sleep. Patients in respiratory distress may sleep poorly because they fear that they will cease to breathe when they are unaware. Others cannot sleep because of their level of general discomfort. Dyspnea and air hunger are anxiety-producing and threatening experiences for pulmonary patients.

Common Complaints Associated with Pulmonary Disorders

If a respiratory problem is suspected, the nurse should focus on obtaining information concerning the most common respiratory complaints: dyspnea, chest pain, cough, sputum, and hemoptysis. This can be accomplished by interviewing the patient and/or family (subjective data) and by performing a nursing assessment (objective data). Regular assessment of the common respiratory symptoms is also important in monitoring the patient for acute changes in respiratory status.

Dyspnea

Subjective Data. **Dyspnea** is a subjective (patient-based) symptom. It refers to the feeling of difficulty breathing or shortness of breath. Physiologically, dyspnea is associated with increased work of breathing—a supply-and-demand imbalance. Increased work of breathing occurs when ventilatory demands go beyond the body's ability to respond. Progressive dyspnea is noted commonly in both restrictive and obstructive pulmonary disorders. **Orthopnea** is a type of dyspnea closely associated with cardiac problems or severe pulmonary disease. It refers to a state in which the patient assumes a head-up position to relieve dyspnea. Orthopnea may be mild (the patient may need several pillows to sleep comfortably in bed), or it may be severe (the patient may need to sit upright in a chair or in bed). When taking the patient's history, it is important to ask how many pillows are required for breathing comfortably while at rest. Additional pillows required for breathing comfortably while lying down is sometimes referred to as "pillow orthopnea." For example, a patient who states that three pillows are required for sleep would have three-pillow orthopnea.

One type of dyspnea is of particular interest in differentiating cardiac from pulmonary disorders. **Paroxysmal nocturnal dyspnea (PND)** is associated with left heart failure. The typical patient report is that of waking during the night, after being asleep for several hours, with a sudden onset of severe orthopnea. On sitting up or getting out of bed, the dyspnea is relieved, and the patient is able to resume sleep. Paroxysmal nocturnal dyspnea is a form of transient mild pulmonary edema. It is believed that fluids that have been congested in the lower extremities during the day because of gravity drainage shift to the heart and lungs, causing a fluid volume overload when the person becomes horizontal (as in sleep) for several hours.

Objective Data. Objectively, the nurse may note tachypnea, nasal flaring, use of **accessory muscles** in the neck, chest, or abdomen, or abnormal arterial blood gases. The patient may voluntarily assume a high-Fowler sitting position secondary to orthopnea. Severe tachypnea, a respiratory rate of more than 30 breaths per minute, significantly increases the work of breathing. If allowed to continue for a prolonged period of time, respiratory muscle fatigue can occur, which may ultimately cause acute respiratory failure.

Chest Pain

Subjective Data. When assessing chest pain it is important to note how long the pain has been present, if it radiates, and what are the triggering and alleviating factors. The type of chest pain the patient describes can be helpful in differentiating cardiogenic (originating from the heart) from pleuritic (originating from the pleura) pain. Cardiogenic pain generally is described as dull, pressure like discomfort often radiating to the jaw, back, or left arm. If asked to point to the painful area, the patient often uses the palm of the hand, indicating a somewhat general area. Cardiogenic pain is unaffected by breathing. Pleuritic pain frequently is described as sharp and knifelike, and the patient is able to point to the pain focal area with one finger. When the patient is between breaths or the breath is held, pain decreases or ceases. The pain increases with deep breathing but does not radiate. A pleural friction rub may sometimes be auscultated at the focal pain point.

Most pulmonary disorders affecting only the lung parenchyma (lung tissue) are not associated with chest pain as an early symptom because the parenchyma is insensitive to pain. For example, lung cancer frequently goes undetected until a routine chest x-ray is taken or the tumor impinges on innervated thoracic structures, causing deep pain. Like lung tissue, the attached visceral pleura is insensitive. The parietal pleura, however, is well innervated, and when inflammation (called **pleurisy** or **pleuritis**) occurs, it can trigger the sharp pain as previously described.

Objective Data. Objective data the nurse may note include splinting, shallow respirations, tachypnea, facial changes associated with pain, and increased blood pressure and pulse.

Cough

Subjective Data. Coughing is an important reflex activity that assists the mucociliary escalator in removing secretions and foreign particles from the lower airway. It is triggered by irritation, the presence of foreign particles, or obstruction of the airway. The patient should be asked to provide the following information about cough: frequency, character (dry, productive, congested), duration, triggers, and pattern of occurrence and alleviating factors.

Objective Data. The nurse can observe the strength, character, and frequency of the cough.

Sputum

Subjective Data. It is important to obtain a description of sputum production in a pulmonary patient. If the patient has a disease that is associated with chronic production of sputum, he or she should be asked to describe the usual quantity, characteristics, and color. It is important to get the patient to describe any changes in sputum associated with the current pulmonary problem.

Objective Data. Sputum may consist of a variety of substances, such as mucus, pus, bacteria, or blood. Sputum should be monitored on a regular basis for quantity, characteristics (thin, thick, tenacious), color, and odor. Careful attention to sputum changes should be noted and documented because they may reflect a change in the patient's pulmonary status. Normal secretions are thin and clear. Sputum color varies depending on the underlying problem (Table 9–18).

Hemoptysis

Subjective Data. **Hemoptysis** refers to expectoration of bloody secretions. It is important to determine the source of the bleeding, which may be from the upper airway (e.g., the oral cavity or nose) or the lower airway (e.g., the lungs). In patients who are experiencing respiratory problems, the presence of hemoptysis can be a significant finding and may be of cardiovascular or pulmonary origin.

Common causes of cardiovascular-related hemoptysis include pulmonary embolism and cardiogenic pulmonary edema secondary to left heart failure. The most common source of hemoptysis, however, is lung disease, particularly as a result of infection and neoplasms. Lung diseases associated with hemoptysis include bronchitis, bronchiectasis, pneumonia, tuberculosis, fungal and parasitic infections, and lung tumors. Information to obtain concerning hemoptysis includes color, consistency and quantity, and frequency and duration.

Objective Data. When hemoptysis is noted, it should be assessed for color, consistency, and quantity. The frequency and duration also should be noted and documented.

Focused Respiratory Physical Assessment

The initial general nursing assessment focuses on all body systems in detail. Once the initial assessment is completed and baseline data are documented, the nurse conducts more specific shift assessments. These frequent bedside assessments often are focused on organ systems (or functional patterns) that have the potential for changing rapidly, indicating a status change in actual or potential patient problems.

Skin coloring should be inspected closely for cyanosis. Observe the lips, earlobes, and beneath the tongue for central cyanosis, which may indicate prolonged hypoxia. In patients with dark skin tones, cyanosis can be observed on the lips and tongue, which will appear ashen-gray. Cyanosis is not a reliable indicator of hypoxia because it is dependent on the amount of reduced hemoglobin present. Its value, therefore, is as supportive rather than diagnostic data. When present, cyanosis is a late sign of respiratory distress. Inspect the shape of the chest and observe chest movement for symmetry of expansion and the rate, depth, and pattern of breathing. Note use of accessory muscles to assist in breathing. If the patient has sustained chest trauma or has chest tubes in place, the chest should be observed for changes in appearance and palpated for subcutaneous emphysema and areas of tenderness. The chest also may be palpated for tactile fremitus and chest expansion. Chest percussion is useful for detecting the presence of air, fluid, or consolidation under the area being percussed.

TABLE 9–18 Sputum Color and Consistency and Underlying Problems

COLOR AND CONSISTENCY	UNDERLYING PROBLEM
Yellow-green	Bacterial infection (e.g., pneumonia, bronchitis, sinusitis)
White, tenacious, mucoid	Acute asthma
Rust colored/blood-tinged	Trauma of coughing, pneumonia, pulmonary infarction
Frothy, pink-tinged	Pulmonary edema, pulmonary embolism, tuberculosis
White-clear	Common cold, bronchitis, other viral infection

Auscultation

Auscultation is one of the most important pulmonary assessments. The diaphragm of the stethoscope is best for hearing most breath sounds, auscultating in a pattern that allows comparison of one lung to the other.

Normal Breath Sounds. There are three types of normal breath sounds: vesicular, bronchial (tubular), and bronchovesicular. Table 9–19 differentiates the various normal sounds.

Abnormal Breath Sounds. The chest should be auscultated routinely for diminished or absent sounds in any field. The presence of abnormal breath sounds is associated with a change in lung status, such as partial or complete obstruction of a part of the airway by secretions or fluid, or loss of elasticity in the lung fields. Adventitious breath sounds are heard on top of other breath sounds. They are never considered normal. Adventitious sounds may be caused by fluid or secretions in the airways or alveoli, by alveoli opening or collapsing, or by bronchoconstriction. When abnormal breath sounds are present, the nurse should assess and document the location and when in the respiratory cycle they are heard. Adventitious sounds are classified as crackles, rhonchi, wheeze, pleural rub, and diminished or absent lung sounds.

Crackles (previously called *rales*) are heard as relatively discrete, delicate popping sounds of short duration. They are associated with either fluid or secretions in the small airways or alveoli, or opening of alveoli from a collapsed state. Crackles are heard most commonly during inspiration. Crackles may be described as fine or coarse. Fine crackles are delicate and high pitched and are of short duration. The classic description of crackles is that they sound similar to the noise that can be made by rubbing hair between the fingers next to the ear. Conditions such as atelectasis and pneumonia are associated with fine crackles. Coarse or loud crackles are louder, lower-pitched sounds of longer duration than fine crackles, making a sound similar to Velcro separating. They are heard in conditions such as bronchitis and pulmonary edema.

TABLE 9–19 Normal Breath Sounds

BREATH SOUND	INSPIRATORY/ EXPIRATORY PATTERN	NORMAL LOCATION	DESCRIPTION
Vesicular	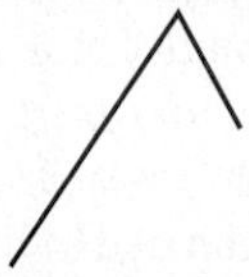	Peripheral lung fields	Whispering, rustling quality; quiet and low pitched; inspiratory phase is longer than expiratory phase; no distinct pause between inspiration and expiration
Bronchial (tubular)	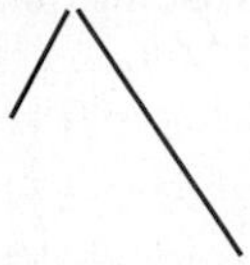	Over the trachea and larynx	High-pitched, loud sound; pause heard between inspiratory and expiratory phases; expiration phase is longer than inspiration (abnormal if heard in peripheral lung; may indicate a consolidation, such as pneumonia)
Bronchovesicular	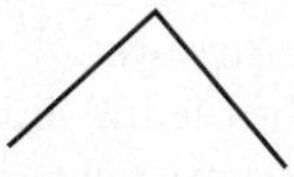	In all lobes near major airways	Sound is between vesicular and bronchial

Rhonchi are heard as coarse, "bubbly" sounds. They are most commonly present during expiration and are auscultated over the larger airways. Rhonchi are associated with an accumulation of fluid or secretions in the larger airways, such as in pneumonia.

Wheeze is caused by air passing through constricted airways. The constriction may be caused by bronchospasm, fluid, secretions, edema obstructing the airway, or the presence of an obstructing tumor or foreign body. Wheeze has a musical quality that may be high pitched or low pitched. It may be heard on inspiration or expiration and is of long duration. **Stridor** is a type of wheeze caused by upper airway obstruction from inflamed tissue or a foreign body. It is described as a high pitched inspiratory wheeze heard louder over the neck than the chest wall. In high-acuity adult patients, it may develop from airway edema resulting from such problems as thermal burn inhalation injury or airway trauma during extubation.

Pleural rub is caused by an inflammation of the pleural linings (membranes). When inflammation occurs, the linings become resistant to free movement. The characteristic sound is heard during breathing and ceases between breaths or with breath holding. Also referred to as a pleural friction rub, it has been described as sounding like leather rubbing together or creaking.

Decreased or absent breath sounds are caused by diminished or absent air flow to an area of the lungs. Loss or diminished sounds in discreet lung areas often results from problems such as lung consolidation as seen with pneumonia, tumors, or pneumothorax. When assessed, the nurse should document the location. In patients with lung hyperinflation disorders such as chronic obstructive pulmonary disease (COPD) and acute asthma, generalized loss of breath sounds may indicate a potentially life-threatening hypoventilation situation.

Vital Signs and Hemodynamic Values

Vital signs and hemodynamic values give crucial baseline data and are important indicators of changing patient status when trended over time. Vital signs include arterial blood pressure, pulse rate and rhythm, respiratory rate and rhythm, and temperature. In addition to vital signs, a pulse oximeter reading should be obtained. If a pulmonary artery catheter is in place, important hemodynamic monitoring assessments include central venous pressure (CVP), pulmonary artery pressure, pulmonary artery wedge pressure, mean arterial pressure, and cardiac output. Hemodynamic monitoring generally is initiated when cardiac involvement is suspected or fluid status is questioned. If the patient's condition is purely pulmonary in nature, data collected from hemodynamic monitoring may be of insufficient use to warrant such an invasive procedure. The presence of pulmonary hypertension can alter hemodynamic measurements.

Focused Respiratory Assessment

The onset of acute respiratory distress can be rapid and severe. The nurse should be alert to changes from previously assessed baseline data and data trends. A rapid respiratory assessment should be immediately conducted, focusing on key data that strongly suggest an acute alteration in respiratory function. Table 9–20 provides a list of key abnormal data.

TABLE 9–20 Key Abnormal Data Suggesting Altered Respiratory Function

Suspicious Assessment Data

- Suddenly increased restlessness and agitation (hypoxia)
- Suddenly decreased level of responsiveness, increased lethargy (hypercapnia)
- Significant change in pattern of breathing:
  - Respiratory rate less than 10/min or greater than 30/min
  - Shallow or erratic breathing
- Increased cyanosis or duskiness
- Increased use of accessory muscles
- Increased dyspnea or orthopnea
- Increase in adventitious breath sounds or development of abnormal breath sounds
- Changing trends in vital signs (blood pressure, pulse, respirations):
  - Increasing trends indicate that compensation is occurring
  - Decreasing trends indicate that decompensation activities may be occurring
- Presence of pain

SECTION SEVEN REVIEW

1. When a patient is admitted in acute respiratory distress, the initial history should focus on which priority?
   A. smoking history
   B. events leading to current admission
   C. nutritional history
   D. events leading to previous admissions
2. The most common complaints associated with pulmonary disease include (choose all that apply)
   A. cough
   B. sputum
   C. dyspnea
   D. a chest pain
3. Chest pain that is typical of pleuritic pain can be best characterized as
   A. sharp
   B. pressure-like
   C. radiating
   D. dull
4. Normal sputum should appear
   A. white and tenacious
   B. yellow-green
   C. clear and thin
   D. frothy and pink-tinged
5. Breath sounds that are auscultated in the peripheral lung fields and have a whispery, rustling quality are
   A. vesicular
   B. bronchovesicular
   C. bronchial
   D. wheezes
6. Crackles are caused by
   A. secretions in the large airways
   B. an inflammation of the pleural linings
   C. air passing through constricted airways
   D. fluid or secretions in the small airways or alveoli

Answers: 1. B, 2. (A, B, C, D), 3. A, 4. C, 5. A, 6. D

SECTION EIGHT: Pulmonary Function Evaluation

At the completion of this section, the learner will be able to briefly describe tests used to evaluate pulmonary function.

The medical team generally initiates orders for pulmonary function testing to assist in diagnosing a pulmonary problem or updating or evaluating a patient's pulmonary status. Actual implementation and interpretation of the tests often becomes an interdisciplinary undertaking.

Pulmonary Function Tests

Ventilation is measured in a variety of ways using pulmonary function tests (PFTs). These tests provide baseline data and also provide a means to monitor the progress of functional impairments associated with pulmonary diseases. They help differentiate a restrictive pulmonary problem from an obstructive problem. In addition, PFTs are useful for monitoring the effectiveness of therapeutic interventions (see Figure 9–17). Diagnostic pulmonary function testing is usually conducted in a pulmonary laboratory using special computerized equipment that accurately measures pulmonary volumes, capacities, and air flow. Simpler measures of pulmonary function, however, can be easily measured at the bedside using a spirometer.

Bedside Pulmonary Function Measurements

High-acuity patients with or without direct pulmonary involvement are at risk of developing pulmonary complications associated with immobility and respiratory muscle fatigue.

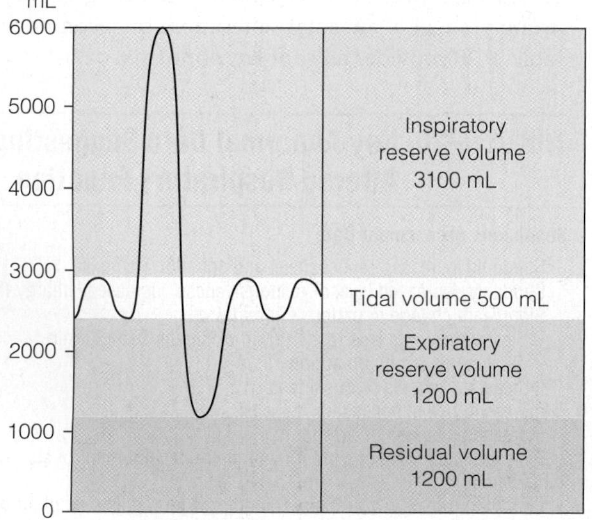

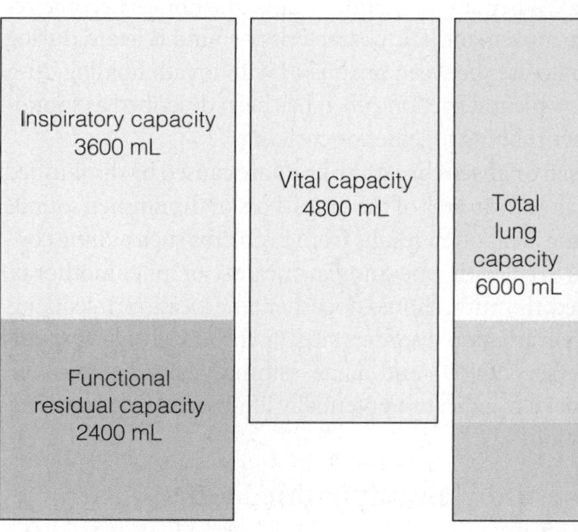

Figure 9–17 ■ Pulmonary function tests. The relationship of lung volumes and capacities. Volumes (mL) shown are for an average adult male.

TABLE 9–21 Pulmonary Function Measurements

MEASUREMENT	NORMAL ADULT RANGE/VALUE
Tidal volume (V_T, Tv)	7–9 mL/kg (IBW)
Vital capacity (VC)	4,800 mL (average young adult man) 3,200 mL (average young adult woman)
Minute ventilation $\dot{V}_E$	5–10 mL/min

Pulmonary function may be monitored in patients who are at particular risk for ventilatory decompensation. Of particular interest are tidal volume, vital capacity, and minute ventilation. Both tidal volume and vital capacity help monitor respiratory muscle strength. As the patient experiences respiratory muscle fatigue, these values will decrease. Both of these PFTs can be easily measured using a respiratory spirometer and frequently are used as part of weaning criteria during mechanical ventilation. Table 9–21 lists the normal values for common bedside pulmonary function tests (PFTs).

Tidal volume (V_T or TV) is the amount of air that moves in and out of the lungs with each normal breath. When V_T drops below 4 mL/kg, a state of alveolar hypoventilation develops because the patient rebreathes deadspace air in the conducting airways rather than exchanging gases with the atmosphere. Acute respiratory failure results when hypoventilation becomes severe and results in hypercapnia.

Vital capacity (VC) is the maximum amount of air expired after a maximal inspiration. Normal vital capacity differs with a person's gender, height, weight, and age. It decreases with age and in the presence of acute or chronic restrictive pulmonary diseases.

Minute ventilation ($\dot{V}_E$) is the total volume of expired air in 1 minute. It is used as a rapid method of measuring total lung ventilation changes, but it is not considered to be an accurate measure of alveolar ventilation. Minute ventilation is not a direct measurement but a simple calculation,

$$\dot{V}_E = VT \times f$$

where f = frequency, breaths per minute. Normal minute ventilation is 5 to 10 L/min. When it increases to greater than 10 L/min, the work of breathing is significantly increased. Minute ventilation less than 5 L/min indicates that the patient is at risk for problems associated with hypoventilation.

Forced Expiratory Volumes

Forced expiratory volumes (FEVs) are important diagnostic measurements that help differentiate restrictive pulmonary problems from obstructive problems and measure airway resistance. They are also important in determining the severity of obstructive diseases. FEVs measure how rapidly a person can forcefully exhale air after a maximal inhalation, measuring volume (in liters) over time (in seconds). Patients who have a restrictive airway problem are able to push air forcefully out of their lungs at a normal rate, whereas persons who have an obstructive disorder have a delayed emptying rate (a reduced rate of expiratory air flow). FEV testing generally is not conducted routinely at the bedside as a bedside trending parameter.

SECTION EIGHT REVIEW

1. In the acutely ill patient, pulmonary function testing helps monitor for
   A. impending ventilatory failure
   B. acute hypoxemia
   C. acute metabolic acidosis
   D. impending oxygenation failure
2. Minute ventilation ($\dot{V}_E$) is calculated using which formula?
   A. $\dot{V}_E = VC \times f$
   B. $\dot{V}_E = VT/f$
   C. $\dot{V}_E = VC \times VT$
   D. $\dot{V}_E = VT \times f$
3. Patients who have obstructive pulmonary disease will have which pattern of FEVs?
   A. increased FEVs
   B. delayed FEVs
   C. normal FEVs
   D. variable FEVs
4. Normal tidal volume in an average-sized adult male would be ______ mL/kg.
   A. 3 to 4
   B. 4 to 5
   C. 5 to 7
   D. 7 to 9

Answers: 1. A, 2. D, 3. B, 4. D

SECTION NINE: Noninvasive and Invasive Monitoring of Gas Exchange

At the completion of this section, the learner will be able to discuss noninvasive and invasive methods of monitoring gas exchange and applications.

Pulse Oximetry

Pulse oximetry is a noninvasive technique for monitoring arterial capillary hemoglobin saturation (SpO_2) and pulse rate. It uses light wavelengths to determine oxyhemoglobin saturation. It also detects pulsatile flow to differentiate between venous and arterial blood. A sensor is placed on a finger, nose, or ear, and an oximeter provides a constant assessment of arterial oxygen saturation (see Fig 9–18). A forehead sensor is now available that may be of particular use in patients with low cardiac index (Fernandez, Burns, Calhoun et al., 2007). Fingers are most commonly used for sensor placement; however, adequacy of peripheral circulation must be taken into consideration when choosing the best sensor location. Pulse oximetry is best used as an adjunct to a variety of assessment modalities in providing continuous information for evaluation of oxygenation status. Ideally, the continuous arterial oxygen saturation readings reflect the patient's oxygenation status and alert the clinician to subtle or sudden changes. In some patients, use of oximetry may decrease the frequency of invasive ABG measurements if acid–base and ventilation are not problems.

Causes of Inaccurate Readings

Many factors can alter the accuracy of pulse oximetry in high-acuity patients. In general, these factors can be divided into problems of technical (mechanical) origin and those of physiologic origin. Technical problems include motion artifact, external light sources, and improper sensor placement. Motion artifact refers to patient movement that the sensor misinterprets as being a pulse. It is a major cause of false alarms and inaccurate readings (Booker, 2008; Walters, 2007). New technologies are being developed to be more tolerant of motion. Bright light sources within the patient's immediate environment can compete with the pulse oximetry sensor light source. When this is a problem, the sensor must be covered up to protect it from the external lighting. An improperly placed sensor may not be able to register arterial pulsations because of lack of sufficient arterial flow. Nail polish or artificial nails may also interfere with the pulse oximeter's light source.

Physiologic factors that alter the accuracy of Spo_2 to predict blood oxygen content (and ultimately delivery of oxygen to the tissues) include hemoglobin level, acid–base imbalance, and vasoconstrictive situations (e.g., peripheral vascular disease, hypothermia, shock, hypovolemia, and vasopressors in high doses). Cardiac dysrhythmias such as slow atrial fibrillation can also cause inaccurate measurements (Giuliano, 2006). The level of hemoglobin greatly affects the oxygen content of the blood. When a patient is severely anemic, the Spo_2 may remain high, indicating sufficient oxygen saturation of available hemoglobin. The actual oxygen content of the blood, however, may be inadequate to meet tissue oxygenation needs, thus increasing the risk of tissue hypoxia. Hemoglobin levels should be monitored and taken into consideration when analyzing Spo_2 measurements.

When an acid–base imbalance exists, acidosis may cause a lower saturation reading and alkalosis may cause a higher reading because of shifts in the oxyhemoglobin dissociation curve. Severe peripheral vasoconstriction creates a low-flow arterial state in which the pulsatile force is too weak to be accurately read by pulse oximetry. When severe vasoconstriction is present, the sensor may read more accurately if it is removed from distal sites (fingers, toes) and attached to a more central location, such as the bridge of the nose or the ear lobe. The hypothermic patient generally requires warming to normothermic levels before pulse oximetry can be used. In addition, patients who have abnormal levels of carboxyhemoglobin (carbon dioxide and carbon monoxide) may have a high Spo_2 even though the oxyhemoglobin level is very low. This false reading occurs because pulse oximetry cannot differentiate carboxyhemoglobin from oxyhemoglobin.

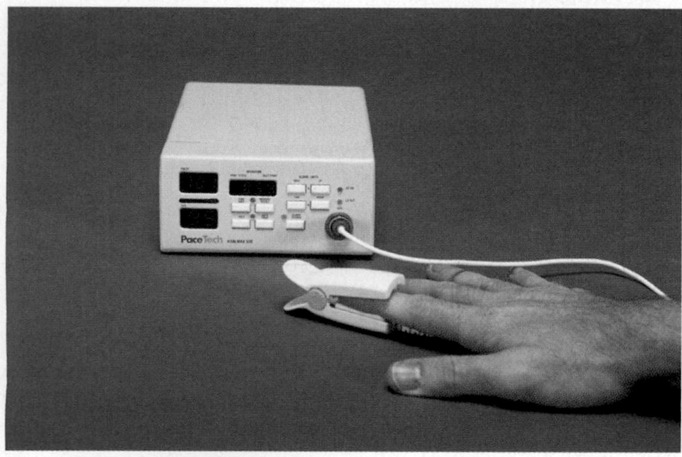

Figure 9–18 ■ Pulse oximetry.

Emerging Evidence

- A study investigated the prevalence of sleep-disordered breathing in patients with right ventricular dysfunction secondary to pulmonary hypertension. Investigators concluded that sleep-disordered breathing (i.e., Cheyne-Stokes respiration, central sleep apnea, and obstructive sleep apnea) were common. They further concluded that in this patient population, use of pulse oximetry to detect sleep apnea was not reliable for detecting these episodes *(Ulrich, Fischler, Speich, & Bloch, 2008).*
- A prospective trial, investigators compared pulse oximetry or capnography and assessment of respiratory rate to detect respiratory depression in opioid-naïve postoperative patients taking opioids. They concluded that capnography was more sensitive in detecting respiratory depression in postsurgical high-risk patients but additional research was needed to confirm this finding *(Hutchison & Rodriguez, 2008).*
- A study investigated use of sublingual capnometry ($SLCO_2$) for diagnosing hemorrhagic shock and monitoring resuscitation adequacy in hypotensive trauma patients. Investigators concluded that $SLCO_2$ was equivalent to measurements of serum lactate levels and base deficit in predicting survival in this patient population *(Baron, Dutton, Zehtabchi et al., 2007).*
- A survey of critical care nurses' knowledge regarding pulse oximetry technology and monitoring, found that nurses' knowledge had improved when compared to a previous studies. The investigators caution that the study did not address nurses' clinical application of this knowledge *(Giuliano & Liu, 2006).*

End-Tidal Carbon Dioxide Monitoring

Capnometry is the noninvasive measurement of carbon dioxide (CO_2) concentration in expired gas. It results in a single value measurement called the **P_{ETCO_2}** (partial pressure of end-tidal CO_2). Continuous bedside monitoring of CO_2 is accomplished using infrared light absorption or mass spectrometry. Infrared analyzers measure carbon dioxide based on its strong absorption band at a distinctive wavelength. A **capnogram** displays the capnometry measurements as a continuous waveform that can be read, breath by breath, throughout the breathing cycle. CO_2 can be sampled using either sidestream or mainstream techniques. Figure 9–19 shows an example of a capnograph monitor.

Sidestream Technique

When a sidestream analyzer is used, a small volume of exhaled gas is diverted from the main airway circuit through a small tube and is analyzed in a special chamber apart from the airway circuit. This causes a time delay between the carbon dioxide sampling and the display of data. There are two disadvantages associated with using sidestream technique. First, the capnogram is averaged and the P_{ETCO_2} can be underestimated, particularly if breathing rates are rapid or the sampling catheter is long. Second, the small tubing may become obstructed with secretions or water. The major advantage of using this technique is that sidestream analysis devices can be applied to nonintubated patients as well as those who are intubated.

Mainstream Technique

Mainstream infrared analyzers use a technology that is similar to sidestream analyzers. Mainstream analyzers, however, are placed inline as part of the airway circuit, and continuous P_{ETCO_2} analysis occurs in-line. Their major advantage is that they provide rapid response readings. There are several disadvantages to the mainstream technique. The mainstream devices are relatively heavy and cumbersome additions to the artificial airway circuit that increases dead space. Airway secretions can interfere with the sensor resulting in false high readings or failure to detect the waveform. Furthermore, there is a slight risk of burning because of heating of the analyzer. This type of analyzer is primarily used on intubated patients.

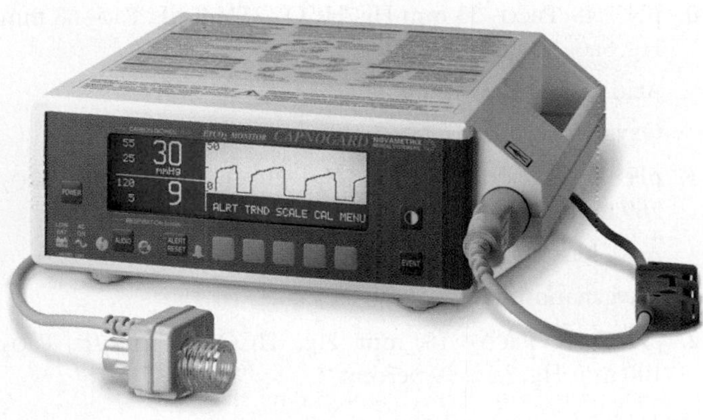

Figure 9–19 ■ Example of a capnograph monitor. Measures and displays end tidal carbondioxide (P_{ETCO_2}), SpO_2, and respiratory and pulse rates. (Image courtesy of Respironics, Inc., Murrysville, PA)

The Capnogram. The normal capnogram shows a P_{ETCO_2} within several mm Hg of arterial $PaCO_2$ at the end of the plateau phase (the end-tidal CO_2). In a normal capnogram, the carbon dioxide concentration is zero at the beginning of expiration, gradually rising until it reaches a plateau (Fig. 9–20). The end-tidal carbon dioxide is the highest concentration at the end of exhalation. End-tidal carbon dioxide (P_{ETCO_2}) monitoring is used in the clinical setting as a noninvasive indirect method of measuring $PaCO_2$. In a normal person, P_{ETCO_2} is 30–43 mmHg, typically 4 to 6 mm Hg below $PaCO_2$.

End-tidal carbon dioxide monitoring may be used to assess ventilatory status to provide an early warning of changes in ventilation. An abnormally low P_{ETCO_2} (less than 30 mm Hg) most commonly is associated with hyperventilation. Increased P_{ETCO_2} (greater than 44 mm Hg) is associated with increased production of carbon dioxide or problems causing hypoventilation (e.g., respiratory center depression, neuromuscular diseases, COPD). Use of the capnogram may help detect improper intubation, ventilation patterns, mechanical problems, or failure in ventilators. Certain capnographic patterns are associated with hyperventilation, incomplete exhalation, and a variety of disease states. Anesthesiologists frequently use capnography in the operating room, and new applications continue to be explored in critical care, emergency care, and outpatient care. Monitoring P_{ETCO_2} has also proven helpful in protection of the brain in acute cerebral injury. Cerebral hypocapnia ($PaCO_2$ less than 35) can constrict cerebral vessels sufficiently to cause cerebral ischemia; while an abnormally high $PaCO_2$ can increase intracranial pressure through cerebral artery vasodilatation. In acute head injury, the $PaCO_2$ is ideally maintained between 35–40 mmHg through manipulation of the mechanical ventilator. Continuous P_{ETCO_2} monitoring is recommended as an early warning tool to detect swings in $PaCO_2$ levels that might prove harmful to the brain injured patient (Albano, Comandante & Nolan, 2005).

In patients with ventilation–perfusion abnormalities, the P_{ETCO_2} may not accurately reflect $PaCO_2$. However, it still may be helpful if a correlation between $PaCO_2$ and P_{ETCO_2} can be established and used for trending. Unfortunately, many high-acuity

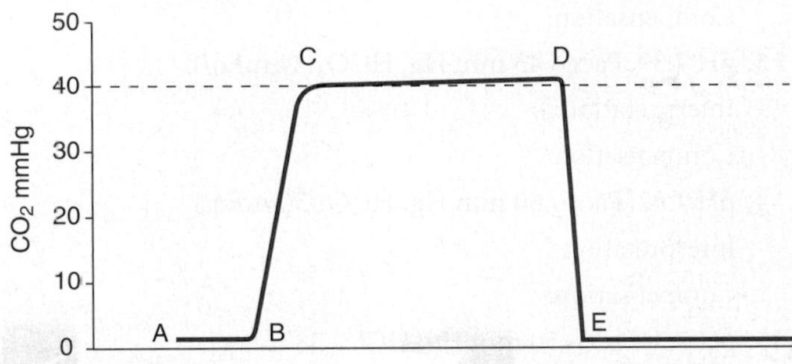

A to B – Beginning of expiration, anatomical deadspace with no measurable CO_2
B to C – Mixed CO2, rapid rise in CO_2 concentration
C to D – Alveolar Plateau, all exhaled gas that took part in gas exchange
D to E – Inspiration, CO_2 drops off rapidly

Figure 9–20 ■ Normal Capnogram Pattern. (Courtesy of Respironics, Inc., Murrysville, PA)

patients develop ventilation–perfusion abnormalities, which may limit the usefulness of P_{ETCO_2} monitoring.

Invasive Blood Gas Monitoring

The arterial catheter (commonly called an "arterial line" or "art line") is an invasive means to monitor a patient's hemodynamic status (e.g., blood pressure, mean arterial pressure, heart rate) as well as pulmonary gas exchange status. Arterial catheters are most commonly inserted into a radial artery but can also be inserted into a femoral or other artery. A major advantage of drawing blood, including arterial blood gases from the arterial line is that frequent samples can be obtained without causing additional trauma and pain to the patient from repeated needle sticks. Insertion and nursing care of arterial catheters is discussed in detail in Module 17, Determinants and Assessment of Oxygen Delivery and Oxygen Consumption.

SECTION NINE REVIEW

1. Pulse oximetry measures
   A. mixed venous saturation
   B. transcutaneous oxygen saturation
   C. venous oxygen capillary hemoglobin saturation
   D. arterial oxygen capillary hemoglobin saturation
2. Conditions that impair the accuracy of pulse oximetry include (choose all that apply)
   A. excessive movement
   B. vasodilation
   C. hypothermia
   D. improper sensor placement
3. P_{ETCO_2} is used as a reflection of
   A. arterial carbon dioxide
   B. $\dot{V}/\dot{Q}$ ratio
   C. oxygenation status
   D. venous carbon dioxide
4. P_{ETCO_2} is an indicator of alveolar
   A. acid–base state
   B. compensation
   C. oxygenation
   D. ventilation

Answers: 1. D, 2. (A, C, D), 3. A, 4. D

SUPPLEMENTAL ABG EXERCISES

Interpret the acid–base status as normal, metabolic or respiratory, alkalosis or acidosis. Indicate the state of compensation as being uncompensated (acute state), partially compensated, or compensated (chronic state). Indicate the oxygenation status as adequate or inadequate, when indicated. Answers are found on MyNursingKit.

1. pH 7.58, $Paco_2$ 38 mm Hg, HCO_3 30 mEq/L
   Interpretation:
   Compensation:
2. pH 7.20, $Paco_2$ 60 mm Hg, HCO_3 26 mEq/L
   Interpretation:
   Compensation:
3. pH 7.39, $Paco_2$ 43 mm Hg, HCO_3 24 mEq/L
   Interpretation:
   Compensation:
4. pH 7.32, $Paco_2$ 60 mm Hg, HCO_3 30 mEq/L
   Interpretation:
   Compensation:
5. pH 7.5, $Paco_2$ 50 mm Hg, HCO_3 38 mEq/L
   Interpretation:
   Compensation:
6. pH 7.45, $Paco_2$ 30 mm Hg, HCO_3 20 mEq/L
   Interpretation:
   Compensation:
7. pH 7.40, $Paco_2$ 40 mm Hg, HCO_3 24 mEq/L
   Interpretation:
   Compensation:
8. pH 7.37, $Paco_2$ 48 mm Hg, HCO_3 29 mEq/L, Pao_2 80 mm Hg, Sao_2 95 percent
   Acid–base state:
   Oxygenation status:
9. pH 7.48, $Paco_2$ 30 mm Hg, HCO_3 24 mEq/L, Pao_2 90 mm Hg, Sao_2 98 percent
   Acid–base state:
   Oxygenation status:
10. pH 7.48, $Paco_2$ 33 mm Hg, HCO_3 25 mEq/L, Pao_2 68 mm Hg, Sao_2 98 percent
    Acid–base state:
    Oxygenation status:
11. pH 7.38, $Paco_2$ 38 mm Hg, HCO_3 24 mEq/L, Pao_2 269 mm Hg, Sao_2 100 percent
    Acid–base state:
    Oxygenation status:
12. pH 7.17, $Paco_2$ 18 mm Hg, HCO_3 7 mEq/L, Pao_2 100 mm Hg, Sao_2 99 percent
    Acid–base state:
    Oxygenation status:

Answers are found in the Appendix.

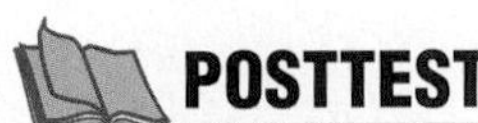

POSTTEST

The following Posttest is constructed in a case study format. A patient is presented, and questions are asked based on available data. New data are presented as the case study progresses.

Margaret Jameson is a 60-year-old high-school teacher. She is active and considers herself fairly healthy.

1. When Ms. Jameson inhales, air moves into her lungs because
   A. intrapulmonary pressure has dropped below atmospheric pressure
   B. intrapleural pressure has dropped below atmospheric pressure
   C. intrapulmonary pressure has risen above atmospheric pressure
   D. intrapleural pressure has risen above atmospheric pressure
2. If her surfactant production would cease, how would it affect the lungs and alveoli?
   A. decrease work of breathing
   B. increase lung compliance
   C. alveoli would collapse
   D. alveoli would have decreased surface tension
3. Should Ms. Jameson develop a pulmonary problem that decreases her lung compliance, it would
   A. increase her tidal volume
   B. increase her work of breathing
   C. decrease her oxygen consumption
   D. decrease her carbon dioxide level

Ms. Jameson becomes ill. She develops a productive cough and fever. She is diagnosed as having right middle lobe pneumonia.

4. Her pneumonia can affect pulmonary diffusion by increasing membrane thickness as a result of
   A. atelectasis
   B. inflammation
   C. bronchial secretions
   D. surfactant deficiency
5. Ms. Jameson has crackles present on auscultation. The nurse knows that these are discrete, noncontinuous sounds that are
   A. caused by fluid or secretions in the small airways or alveoli
   B. caused by fluid or secretions in the large airways
   C. caused by air passing through constriction in the airways
   D. caused by inflammation of the pleural lining
6. Ventilation will decrease in her affected lung area because
   A. pressure gradient is increased
   B. gas moves from low-pressure to high-pressure areas
   C. decreased perfusion causes decreased ventilation
   D. gas follows the path of least resistance
7. Ms. Jameson has developed a pulmonary shunt. What clinical manifestation would you expect?
   A. hypercapnia
   B. infection
   C. hypoxia
   D. pleuritis
8. Her shunt is an absolute shunt. Oxygen therapy has been initiated per venti-mask. Considering this type of shunt, her hypoxemia will ______ with oxygen therapy?
   A. remain the same
   B. worsen
   C. be relieved
   D. initially improve and then worsen
9. Which position would optimize $\dot{V}/\dot{Q}$ matching for Ms. Jameson?
   A. laying on right side
   B. laying on left side
   C. laying supine
   D. positioning will not affect $\dot{V}/\dot{Q}$ matching
10. Ms. Jameson has pulmonary function tests performed. Both her tidal volume and vital capacity are below normal. Inadequate tidal volume and vital capacity most likely indicate
    A. respiratory muscle fatigue
    B. increased atelectasis
    C. loss of pulmonary surfactant
    D. hyperventilation
11. In the presence of cor pulmonale, the nurse can anticipate that pulmonary vascular resistance (PVR) will be
    A. low
    B. unchanged
    C. high
    D. vacillating
12. Pulmonary vascular resistance (PVR) increases in response to
    A. hypocapnia
    B. alkalosis
    C. hypoxemia
    D. low lung volumes

Una W, a 21-year-old college student, is admitted to the hospital with complaints of severe chest pain and dyspnea. She has an oral temperature of 38.3° C (101°F).

13. When a pulmonary disorder is suspected, obtaining a nutritional history is important for which reason?
    A. hypoglycemia weakens respiratory muscles
    B. high-carbohydrate diets decrease carbon dioxide levels
    C. high-carbohydrate intake weakens respiratory muscles
    D. poor nutritional status increases susceptibility to infection
14. Una continues to complain of feeling dyspneic. Which clinical manifestation is most compatible with a worsening clinical state?
    A. increased respiratory rate
    B. tachycardia
    C. agitation
    D. cyanosis

Juanita M., a 32-year-old female with a medical history of asthma, was admitted to the hospital last night with fever and a diagnosis of left lower lobe pneumonia was made. She was started on oxygen via an aerosol face tent.

15. Juanita's febrile state would cause the oxyhemoglobin dissociation curve to shift away from the normal curve. Based on the direction of the shift associated with fever, which statement is correct?
A. Oxygen binds rapidly to hemoglobin.
B. Carbon dioxide binds rapidly to hemoglobin.
C. Hemoglobin readily releases its oxygen to tissues.
D. Hemoglobin is prevented from releasing its oxygen to tissues.

Juanita has a complete blood count (CBC) and ABG drawn. Her Hgb is currently 10 g/dL. Her latest temperature was 102.4 F. The ABG was: pH 7.47, $Paco_2$ 32 mm Hg, HCO_3 25 mEq/L, BE 1.5, Pao_2 74 mm Hg, Sao_2 89 percent. She is started on 40 percent oxygen.

16. If Juanita has normal gas exchange, her predicted response to initiation of 40 percent oxygen therapy would be an increased Pao_2 to about
A. 100 mm Hg
B. 150 mm Hg
C. 200 mm Hg
D. 250 mm Hg

17. The underlying problem associated with Juanita's acid-base status is
A. alveolar hyperventilation
B. alveolar hypoventilation
C. hypercapnia
D. metabolic acidosis

18. Upon auscultation, Juanita has bilateral expiratory wheezes. The nurse knows wheezes occur when
A. air moves through fluid or secretions in the large airways
B. air moves through the inflamed pleural lining
C. air moves through fluid or secretions in the small airways or alveoli
D. air moves through a narrowed airway

19. Juanita becomes lethargic and tachypneic. A repeat ABG is done. Which finding is most indicative of impending respiratory failure?
A. Pao_2 90 mm Hg
B. pH 7.40
C. $Paco_2$ 65 mm Hg
D. Sao_2 96 percent

Thomas J., a 46-year-old type 1 diabetic, is admitted to the hospital with a serum glucose of 650 mg/dL and positive serum ketones. He is diagnosed with DKA. He has blood gases drawn with the following results: pH 7.25, $Paco_2$ 36 mm Hg, HCO_3 14 mEq/L.

20. Thomas' current pH is most likely due to
A. metabolic acidosis
B. respiratory acidosis
C. respiratory alkalosis
D. metabolic alkalosis

21. What changes in Thomas' ABG would you see with compensation?
A. low pH, low $Paco_2$
B. elevated pH, low HCO_3
C. low pH, high $Paco_2$
D. normal range of pH, low $Paco_2$

22. A compensatory mechanism seen in patients experiencing metabolic acidosis is
A. deep, gasping respirations
B. prolonged expiratory effort
C. several short breaths followed by apnea
D. shallow respirations

23. Joshua has the following ABG results: pH 7.50, $Paco_2$ 30 mm Hg, HCO_3 20 mEq/L, Pao_2 88 mm Hg, Sao_2 98 percent. The nurse would correctly interpret this ABG as
A. compensated metabolic acidosis
B. partially compensated metabolic acidosis
C. partially compensated respiratory alkalosis
D. compensated respiratory acidosis

24. Carrie has the following ABG results: pH 6.83, $Paco_2$ 50 mm Hg, HCO_3 20 mEq/L. The nurse would correctly interpret this ABG as
A. suspicious of a mixed acid-base disorder
B. acute metabolic acidosis
C. acute respiratory acidosis
D. compensated respiratory acidosis

25. Adam is in hypovolemic shock secondary to a massive gastrointestinal bleed. The best location for a pulse oximetry sensor in this patient is
A. toe
B. earlobe
C. fingertip
D. forearm

26. Beverly has been in the ICU intubated for one week. She has P_{ETCO_2} monitoring attached to her mechanical ventilator circuit. This type of monitor is used to assess
A. early tissue metabolic changes
B. oxygenation failure
C. early changes in ventilation
D. ventilatory dependency

27. Mr. Jones comes to the emergency room complaining of shortness of breath and chest pain. The ABG results are as follows: pH 7.45, $Paco_2$ 35 mm Hg, Pao_2 60 mm Hg, HCO_3 24 mEq/L. The nurse's first intervention should be
A. set up for intubation
B. no intervention required
C. place the patient on oxygen
D. administer sodium bicarbonate

28. The adequacy of oxygenation is most accurately measured by
A. hemoglobin
B. pulmonary function tests

C. pulse oximetry
D. arterial blood gas

29. If Mr. Jones begins to hypoventilate, the nurse would monitor the patients ABG for the development of
A. respiratory alkalosis
B. respiratory acidosis
C. metabolic alkalosis
D. metabolic acidosis

Posttest answers with rationale are found on MyNursingKit.

PEARSON

EXPLORE mynursingkit™

MyNursingKit is your one stop for online chapter review materials and resources. Prepare for success with additional NCLEX®-style practice questions, interactive assignments and activities, web links, animations and videos, and more!

Register your access code from the front of your book at **www.mynursingkit.com.**

REFERENCES

Albano, C., Comandante, L., and Nolan, S. (2005). Innovations in management of cerebral injury. *Crit Care Nurs Q, 28*(2), 135–149.

Baron, B. J., Dutton, R. P., Zehtabchi, S., Spanfelner, J., Stavile, K. L., Khodorkovsky B. et al. (2007). Sublingual capnometry for rapid determination of the severity of hemorrhagic shock. *Journal of Trauma, 61*(1), 120–124.

Beers, M. H., & Jones, T. V. (eds.). (2006). Aging and the lungs. *The Merck manual of geriatrics.* Available at: http://www.merck.com/mkgr/CVMHighLight?file=/mkgr/mmg/sec10/ch75/ch75a.jsp%3Fregion%3Dmerckcom&word=lungs&domain=www.merck.com#hl_anchor. Accessed May 19, 2008.

Booker, R. (2008). Pulse oximetry. *Nursing Standard, 22*(30), 39–41.

Chang, D. W. (1998). *Respiratory care calculations* (2d ed.). Albany, NY: Delmar Publishers.

Des Jardins, T. R. (2008). *Cardiopulmonary anatomy and physiology: essentials for respiratory care* (5th ed.). Albany, N. Y.: Thomson Delmar Learning.

Fernandez, M., Burns, K., Calhoun, B., Gorge, S., Martin, B., & Weaver, C. (2007). Evaluation of a new pulse oximeter sensor. *American Journal of Critical Care, 16*(2), 146–152.

Giuliano, K. K., and Liu, L. M. (2006). Knowledge of pulse oximetry among critical care nurses. *Dimensions of Critical Care Nursing, 24*(1), 44–49.

Hutchison, R., and Rodriguez, L. (2008). Capnography and respiratory depression: is capnography a good way to monitor at-risk postsurgical patients? a prospective trial examines the question. *American Journal of Nursing, 108*(2), 35–39.

Kee, J. L. (2005). *Laboratory and diagnostic tests with nursing implications* (7th ed.). Upper Saddle River, N. J.: Pearson/Prentice Hall.

Kee, J. L. (2009). *Prentice Hall handbook of laboratory and diagnostic tests with nursing implications* (6th ed.). Upper Saddle River, N. J.: Pearson/Prentice Hall.

Martini, F. H., & Bartholomew, E. F. (2003). *Essentials of anatomy & physiology* (3rd ed.). Upper Saddle River, N.J.: Prentice Hall Pearson Education.

Pilbeam, S. P. (2006). *Mechanical ventilation: Physiological and clinical applications* (4th ed.). St. Louis: Mosby/Elsevier.

Ross, B. K. (n.d.). Aging and the respiratory system. American Society of Anesthesiologists. Available at: www.asahq.org/clinical/geriatrics/aging.htm. Accessed May 19, 2008.

Ulrich, S., Fischler, M., Speich, R., & Bloch, K. E. (2008). Sleep-related breathing disorders in patients with pulmonary hypertension. *CHEST, 133*(6), 1375–1380.

Walters, T. P. (2007). Pulse oximetry knowledge and its effects on clinical practice. *British Journal of Nursing, 16*(21). 1332–1340.

MODULE

10 Alterations in Pulmonary Gas Exchange

Gail Priestley, Kathleen Dorman Wagner

OBJECTIVES Following completion of this module, the learner will be able to

1. Explain the basic difference between restrictive and obstructive pulmonary diseases.
2. Discuss the pathophysiologic basis of respiratory failure.
3. Describe acute lung injury (ALI)/acute respiratory distress syndrome (ARDS).
4. Explain the types, pathophysiology, and management of acute pulmonary embolism.
5. Discuss the types, pathophysiology, and management of acute bacterial and viral pneumonias.
6. Describe the principles and management of patients undergoing thoracic surgery and chest drainage.
7. Develop a general plan of care for a patient with an acute alteration in respiratory function.

The module is composed of seven sections. Section One differentiates pulmonary diseases on the basis of restrictive versus obstructive processes with a discussion of status asthmaticus. Section Two describes the pathophysiologic basis of acute respiratory failure. Section Three provides an in-depth discussion of acute lung injury (ALI)/acute respiratory distress syndrome (ARDS). Section Four discusses acute pulmonary embolism, with an emphasis on thromboembolism. Section Five presents an overview of acute bacterial and viral pneumonias. Section Six provides an overview of the management of the patient who has had thoracic surgery and chest tubes. Finally, Section Seven describes respiratory-focused nursing diagnoses and how they apply to patients with restrictive and obstructive pulmonary disorders. Each section includes a set of review questions to help the learner evaluate his or her understanding of the section's content before moving on to the next section. All Section Reviews include answers. It is suggested that the learner review those concepts answered incorrectly in the review questions before proceeding to the next section.

PRETEST

1. The primary ventilatory problem associated with obstructive pulmonary disease is
   A. delay of airflow out of the lungs
   B. obstruction to perfusion
   C. decreased diffusion of gases
   D. inability to achieve normal tidal volumes
2. Restrictive pulmonary diseases are associated with
   A. increased lung expansion
   B. increased lung compliance
   C. decreased lung expansion
   D. decreased airflow into lungs
3. Lung compliance is increased with which disorder?
   A. chest burns
   B. pneumonia
   C. pneumothorax
   D. emphysema
4. The nurse would expect a person who has respiratory insufficiency to have which arterial blood gas conditions?
   A. pH below normal
   B. $Paco_2$ below normal
   C. pH normal
   D. $Paco_2$ normal
5. Classic symptoms associated with hypercapnia would include
   A. weak, thready pulse
   B. flushed, wet skin
   C. hypotension
   D. slow, shallow breathing
6. The most common indirect predisposing disorder of ALI/ARDS is
   A. sepsis
   B. severe trauma

C. gastric aspiration
D. pneumonia

7. The pulmonary edema associated with ALI/ARDS is caused by
A. capillary microembolism
B. left ventricular failure
C. loss of surfactant
D. injured alveolar–capillary membrane

8. Which clinical finding is typically present with ALI/ARDS?
A. decreased P/F (PaO_2/FiO_2) ratio
B. increased lung compliance
C. decreased airway resistance
D. increased functional residual capacity

9. Which type of embolism manifests itself as dyspnea, tachypnea, neurological symptoms, AND petechiae?
A. venous air
B. fat
C. thrombus
D. amniotic

10. Venous (endothelial) injury is one of three major factors that cause formation of deep vein thrombosis. This type of injury can result from
A. immobility
B. sepsis
C. surgery
D. varicose veins

11. One definitive test to diagnose a pulmonary embolism is
A. angiography
B. $\dot{V}/\dot{Q}$ scan
C. D-dimer
D. compression ultrasound

12. The most common pneumonia pathogen in the United States is
A. *H. influenzae*
B. *S. pneumoniae*
C. *S. aureus*
D. *Mycoplasma pneumoniae*

13. Which statement is correct regarding MRSA pneumonia in high-acuity patients?
A. It causes a chronic, low-level pulmonary infection.
B. It increases the risk for bacteremia and septic shock.
C. It has a low mortality risk.
D. About 50 percent of cases require hospitalization.

14. Aspiration of low pH gastric contents into the lungs results in
A. destruction of pulmonary capillaries
B. growth of gastric pathogens
C. consolidation from flooding the lungs
D. damage via the inflammatory response

15. The pathogen that causes SARS is a unique form of which virus?
A. hantavirus
B. coronavirus
C. rhinovirus
D. influenza-A virus

16. The SARS virus is known to be transmitted by
A. contaminated feces
B. blood contact
C. tears
D. airborne droplet

17. Pneumothorax caused by positive end expiratory pressure (PEEP) represents which type of injury?
A. procedural rupture
B. chest contusion
C. spontaneous bleb rupture
D. barotrauma induced

18. Common clinical findings associated with pneumothorax include (choose all that apply)
A. tachypnea
B. bradycardia
C. respiratory acidosis
D. shortness of air
E. decreased PaO_2

19. The purpose of the water-seal chamber in a three-chamber chest drainage system is to
A. facilitate drainage from the chest tube
B. prevent airflow back into the patient
C. facilitate control of level of negative suction
D. prevent fluid from draining into the suction chamber

20. Nursing interventions that would assist in maintaining effective airway clearance would include
A. restrict fluids to 1 liter per day
B. cough and deep breathe every 1 to 2 hours
C. minimize use of opioid analgesics
D. restrict activities

Pretest answers are found on MyNursingKit.

SECTION ONE: Review of Restrictive and Obstructive Pulmonary Disorders

At the completion of this section, the learner will be able to explain the basic differences between restrictive and obstructive pulmonary diseases.

Pulmonary diseases may be divided into acute and chronic problems. Acute problems have a rapid onset, are episodic, and frequently are confined to the lungs. In contrast, chronic problems usually have a slow, often insidious onset, and the pulmonary impairment either does not change or slowly worsens over an extended period. Chronic pulmonary problems generally involve other organs as part of the disease process. Patients with chronic pulmonary problems, such as emphysema, may develop an acute problem (e.g., pneumonia) that may further stress their pulmonary status.

Pulmonary diseases may be divided further into problems of inflow of air (restrictive) and problems of outflow of air (obstructive). By being able to differentiate between obstructive and restrictive pulmonary diseases, the nurse can apply appropriate nursing diagnoses regardless of the medical diagnosis of the specific pulmonary disease process.

Restrictive Pulmonary Disorders

Restrictive disorders are associated with decreased lung compliance (C_L) and decreased lung expansion. They may be caused by internal problems, such as a decrease in the number of functioning alveoli (e.g., atelectasis or pneumonia) or lung tissue loss (e.g., pneumonectomy or lung tumors), or by external problems (e.g., chest burns or morbid obesity). Table 10–1 provides a more complete listing of restrictive disorders.

Restrictive disorders are problems of volume (the amount of air measured in mL or L that flows in and out of the lungs) rather than airflow (the rate or speed at which air moves into or out of the lungs). In other words, the volume of air that is inhaled can be exhaled at a normal rate of flow. The patient with a restrictive disorder will have a reduced **tidal volume (VT)** and **total lung capacity (TLC)**. Air cannot move into the alveoli as readily as it should because of limited expansion (decreased lung compliance), which can lead to alveolar hypoventilation. Hypoxemia will result if alveolar oxygen diffuses into the blood at a faster rate than it is replaced by ventilation. When this occurs, the Pa_{O_2} falls at approximately the same rate as the Pa_{CO_2} rises, assuming that diffusion is normal.

Restrictive pulmonary problems often disturb the relationship of ventilation to perfusion ($\dot{V}/\dot{Q}$ ratio). In mild-to-moderate restrictive disease, the $\dot{V}/\dot{Q}$ ratio may stay normal because both ventilation and perfusion may be fairly equally disturbed. In many acute restrictive diseases, perfusion becomes diminished because of edema that results from an inflammatory process. Perfusion can also become reduced by compression or blockage of the pulmonary vasculature. In severe disease, a low $\dot{V}/\dot{Q}$ ratio may develop because ventilation is greatly diminished, whereas perfusion may be fairly normal or moderately disturbed. A low $\dot{V}/\dot{Q}$ ratio is associated with hypoxemia with a decreasing pH and increasing Pa_{CO_2}. Table 10–2 lists the typical signs and symptoms associated with restrictive pulmonary disorders.

TABLE 10–1 Common Restrictive Pulmonary Disorders

EXTERNAL PROBLEMS	INTERNAL (PARENCHYMAL) PROBLEMS
Obesity	Pneumonia
Neuromuscular diseases	Atelectasis
Myasthenia gravis	Congestive heart failure
Muscular dystrophy	Pulmonary edema
Guillain–Barré syndrome	Pulmonary fibrosis
Spinal cord trauma	Pulmonary tumors
Chest wall disorders	Pneumothorax
Extensive chest burns	Asbestosis
Scoliosis	
Flail chest	

TABLE 10–2 Signs and Symptoms of Restrictive Pulmonary Disorders

Increased respiratory rate
Decreased tidal volume (VT)
Normal to decreased Pa_{O_2}
Shortness of air
Cough
Chest pain or discomfort
Fatigue
History of weight loss

Obstructive Pulmonary Disorders

Chronic obstructive pulmonary disease (COPD) is the term commonly applied in the clinical setting to pulmonary disorders that hinder expiratory airflow. The more accurate and preferred term for these disorders, however, is *chronic airflow limitation.* Currently, these two terms are often used interchangeably. Some of the major obstructive disorders include

- Emphysema
- Chronic bronchitis
- Asthma
- Cystic fibrosis

In **obstructive pulmonary disorders,** air is able to flow into the lungs but then becomes trapped, making it difficult to rid the lungs of the inhaled air. The inability to exhale rapidly causes a prolongation of expiratory time. If expiratory time becomes significantly prolonged, the alveoli are unable to empty before the person inhales again, trapping CO_2 within them. Expiratory times are measured using **forced expiratory volume (FEV)** testing, which is a measure for dynamic lung function. FEV testing determines how rapidly a person can forcefully exhale air after a maximal inhalation.

Obstructive problems may be caused by airway narrowing, such as bronchospasm, bronchoconstriction, and edema; or by airway obstruction, such as is seen with pooling of secretions or destruction of bronchioles and alveoli. Obstructive disorders are associated with increased lung **compliance** (hyperinflated lungs) accompanied by a loss of elastic recoil. The $\dot{V}/\dot{Q}$ ratio may be disturbed with this group of disorders. In disease processes that do not destroy alveoli, such as chronic bronchitis, a low $\dot{V}/\dot{Q}$ ratio may exist (i.e., ventilation is reduced, whereas perfusion remains normal). If lung tissue is actually destroyed, such as occurs with emphysema, the $\dot{V}/\dot{Q}$ ratio may remain normal because both

TABLE 10–3 Clinical Manifestations of Obstructive Pulmonary Disorders

Mucus hypersecretion (except with pure emphysema)
Wheezes, rhonchi
Dyspnea (episodic or progressive)
Diminished breath and heart sounds
Barrel chest (increased AP diameter)
Progressive hypercapnia and respiratory acidosis
Progressive or episodic hypoxemia (particularly in later stages)
Cor pulmonale
Accessory muscle use
Increased expiratory time (expiration time longer than inspiration time)
Pulmonary function tests (PFTs): Normal to increased TLC, increased FRC, decreased FEV, decreased VC

TLC=total lung capacity; FRC=functional residual capacity; FEV=forced expiratory volume; VC=vital capacity

ventilation and perfusion are equally impaired. A normal $\dot{V}/\dot{Q}$ ratio does not necessarily indicate healthy lungs. It indicates only that a balance exists between ventilation and blood flow. Table 10–3 lists the typical clinical manifestations associated with obstructive pulmonary disorders.

Restrictive and obstructive diseases differ in the effect on lung volumes, air flow, pathophysiology, blood gas disturbances and physical assessment. Table 10–4 compares these two disease processes.

Status Asthmaticus

Asthma differs from the other obstructive pulmonary diseases in that the airflow obstruction is episodic rather than continuous. For many years, asthma was considered to be a reversible disease in that lung function and gas exchange were thought to return to normal with treatment. Today, however, experts know that the process is not always completely reversible with some patients (particularly those with frequent exacerbations) eventually developing permanent remodeling of the airways (National Heart Lung and Blood Institute, 2007). Physiologic changes that characterize acute asthma exacerbations include inflammation that causes airway edema with narrowing of airway passages and hyperresponsiveness of airways to irritants that result in bronchospasm and mucous plugging. While it was once thought to be a reversible process between exacerbations, it is now known that the process is not always completely reversible and may result in eventual permanent remodeling of the airways. The classic triad of asthma symptoms includes paroxysmal episodes dyspnea, wheeze, and cough triggered by a stimulus (McFadden, 2005). Some of the more common triggering stimuli include allergens, exercise, stress, and infections. Commonly, asthma is managed with combinations of inhaled corticosteroids and bronchodilators.

Status asthmaticus refers to a severe exacerbation of asthma signs and symptoms that does not respond to the usual drug therapy. If it persists, status asthmaticus can become a life-threatening emergency from airway obstruction. Death from status asthmaticus is rare but is usually due to suffocation-related hypoxia. The ability to rapidly recognize a life-threatening episode of status asthmaticus is crucial for health care professionals who work in emergency settings (McFadden, 2005). Table 10–5 lists some of the major features of life-threatening status asthmaticus. A particularly ominous clinical finding is sudden decrease in wheezing or loss of breath sounds, which may indicate complete airway obstruction from mucus plugs and impending cardiopulmonary arrest.

TABLE 10–4 Comparison of Pulmonary System Alterations in Restrictive and Obstructive Pulmonary Diseases

RESTRICTIVE DISORDERS	OBSTRUCTIVE DISORDERS
Characteristics	
Decreased lung expansion Decreased lung compliance Normal airflow	Increased lung expansion Increased lung compliance Decreased expiratory airflow; prolonged expiratory time
Pulmonary Function Testing	
Decreased total lung capacity (TLC) Decreased tidal volume	Decreased forced expiratory volumes (FEVs)
Pathologic Disturbances	
Internal Problems Decreased functioning alveoli Loss of pulmonary tissue Loss of respiratory muscle strength	Bronchoconstriction Bronchospasm Airway edema Airway obstruction Airway collapse Pooling of copious secretions
External Problems Disorders that decrease lung compliance external to the lungs	
Associated Blood Gas Disturbances	
Decreased Pa_{O_2} Normal to low $\dot{V}/\dot{Q}$ ratio Increased intrapulmonary shunt Increased Pa_{CO_2} and decreased pH if ventilatory pump failure is present	Increased Pa_{CO_2} Decreased pH (if not compensated) Normal to decreased Pa_{O_2} (may stay stable until severe disease state)
Associated Lung Sounds	
Crackles (most common) Rhonchi, if secretions build up in large airways	Wheezes (most common) Rhonchi, if secretions build up in large airways Diminished breath sounds (severe bronchospasm)

TABLE 10–5 Major Features of Life-Threatening Status Asthmaticus

Pulsus paradoxus of 25 mmHg or greater
Use of accessory muscles
Significant lung hyperinflation
ABG showing hypoxemia with or without hypercapnia
Reduced peak expiratory flow rate or FEV_1 (20% or less of predicted value)
Sudden onset of decreased wheezing or reduced (or no) breath sounds

Recommendations for treatment of status asthmaticus include oxygen, intravenous corticosteroids, and possibly inhalation of heliox (a combination of helium and oxygen) to improve air flow (National Asthma Education and Prevention Program Expert Panel Report 3, 2007) and repeated doses of a short-acting sympathomimetic inhalation agent such as albuterol (McFadden, 2005). Development of ventilatory failure (hypercapnia) is unusual but can result from fatigue due to the increased work of breathing. Fatigue and decreasing level of consciousness may signal the need for mechanical ventilation (Oddo et al., 2006). Mechanical ventilation in acute asthma is avoided if at all possible due to the risks of intubation and challenges of ventilator management. The RELATED PHARMACOTHERAPY: Agents Used for Treatment of Pulmonary Diseases box provides a summary of some of the major drugs used in treatment of disorders such as asthma.

RELATED PHARMACOTHERAPY: Agents Used for Treatment of Pulmonary Diseases

Beta Agonists

Short-acting: Albuterol (Proventil, Ventolin, ProAir), Pirbuterol (Maxair), Levalbuterol (Xopenex), Racemic epinephrine (Vaponefrin)
Long-acting: Salmeterol (Serevent), Formoterol (Foradil)

Action and Uses

- Stimulate Beta 2 adrenergic (epinephrine) receptors in the lung
- Relaxes bronchial smooth muscle and causes bronchodilation
- Used for obstructive diseases (asthma, exercise-induced asthma, COPD)
- Short-acting drugs used as "Rescue" medications for asthma
  - May be used hourly or as continuous nebulizer for acute exacerbations
- Long-acting drugs used routinely for control and night-time symptoms

Major Adverse Effects

- Tachycardia, hypertension, tremors
- Potential paradoxical response of increased bronchospasm
- Hypokalemia (primarily in higher doses)

Nursing Implications

- Document heart rate and blood pressure, therapeutic response (improved airflow, wheezing), side effects
- Patient education: correct use of inhalers, spacers, nebulizers
- Patient education: long-acting inhalers not to be used as rescue medications, risk of toxicity
- Drugs available as metered-dosed inhaler, dry powder inhaler and small volume nebulizer

Anti-Cholinergic Bronchodilators

Short-acting: Ipratropium bromide (Atrovent)
Long-acting: Tiotropium (Spiriva)
Combination Ipratropium bromide and albuterol (Combivent)

Action and Uses

- Bronchodilation; blockade of cholinergic-induced bronchoconstriction.
- Maintenance therapy primarily for COPD

Major Adverse Effects

- Poor absorption via inhalation limits systemic side effects (anxiety, dizziness, headache, nervousness)
- Cough, dry mouth (more common)

Nursing Implications

- Avoid eye exposure during nebulizer treatments (pupil dilation)
- Caution: older meter-dose inhalers contained soy base (soy and peanut allergy)
- Caution in patients with narrow-angle glaucoma, prostatic hypertrophy
- Document heart rate and blood pressure, therapeutic response, side effects
- Patient education: correct use of inhalers, nebulizers
- Assess history for soy/peanut allergy: assure formulation does not contain soy
- Drugs available as metered-dosed inhaler, dry powder inhaler and small volume nebulizer

Corticosteroids

IV: Methylprednisolone (Solu-Medrol), Hydrocortisone (Solu-Cortef)
Oral: Prednisone
Inhaled: Beclomethasone dipropionate (QVAR)
- Flunisolide (AeroBid)
- Fluticasone (Flovent)
- Budesonide (Pulmicort)
- Combinations of steroid and beta agonists (Advair)

Action and Uses

- Anti-inflammatory agents, reduce airway edema (reduces airway obstruction) associated with asthma, COPD
- Used as a "controller" for asthma and COPD to reduce airway inflammation
- Additional higher doses IV given for acute exacerbations

Major Adverse Effects

- Fewer side effects with inhaled steroids
- Systemic (IV and oral formulations): insomnia, mood changes (euphoria or delirium possible), hypertension, hyperglycemia, hypokalemia, fluid retention, adrenal suppression, poor wound healing, GI bleeding, immune suppression / infection especially fungal, acute adrenal insufficiency with sudden withdrawal after long-term use
- Local: oral/pharyngeal fungal infections, cough, hoarse voice, bronchospasm

Nursing Implications

- High-acuity formulation is primarily intravenous; oral and inhaled used for stable patients
- Onset of effect is hours; used as a "controller" for asthma and COPD, not rapid response for bronchospasm

Use with spacer/reservoir device for inhaled steroids to prevent oral thrush; brush teeth, rinse mouth after dosing.
Patient education: oral hygiene, use of spacer, inhaler technique to reduce oral infections and hoarseness
Drugs available primarily as metered-dosed inhaler and dry powder inhaler
Avoid stopping systemic corticosteroids abruptly and monitor for acute adrenal insufficiency (e.g., hypotension, shock)

Methylxanthines

Theophylline (Slo-bid, Theo-Dur)

Action and Uses

Bronchodilation by blocking phosphodiesterase
Stimulates ventilation
Used as a third-line bronchodilator for chronic obstructive disease, occasionally used in acute care settings

Major Adverse Effects

Multiple: tachycardia, dysrhythmias, anxiety, insomnia, seizures, tremors, nausea, vomiting, anorexia
Severe adverse effects have limited use in recent years

Nursing Implications

Monitor serum theophylline levels (goal = 5–15 mcg/ml), toxicity common if level greater than 20 mcg/ml
Monitor I & O (diuretic effect), heart rate, blood pressure, cardiac rhythm
Assess for therapeutic effect, side effects
Administer IV loading dose by infusion, slowly over 20–30 minutes. Maximum 20–25 mg/minute or continuous infusion

Mucolytics

Acetylcysteine (Mucomyst)
Dornase alfa (Pulmozyme) also called "DNase"

Action and Uses

Decreases viscosity of respiratory secretions
Acetylcysteine: Used acutely to improve airway clearance in diseases with thick mucus production (bronchitis, bronchiectasis) and during bronchoscopy to clear mucous plugs
Dornase: synthetic pancreatic enzyme, breaks down DNA material from neutrophils (DNase)
Used chronically in some diseases (cystic fibrosis)

Major Adverse Effects

Acetylcysteine: bronchospasm (do not use for asthma), bad odor and taste, nausea
Dornase Alfa: pharyngitis, chest pain,

Nursing Implications

Assess for effectiveness on cough, clearance of secretions, possible bronchospasm, and side effects
Administer bronchodilator prior to acetylcysteine

Pulmonary Vasodilators

Inhaled: Nitric oxide (iNO) off-label use in ARDS for adults, Iloprost (pulmonary hypertension)
Intravenous: epoprostenol (Flolan), treprostinil (Remodulin)
Subcutaneous: treprostinil (Remodulin)
Oral: Bosentan, sildenafil

Action and Uses

Specialized treatment (rescue therapy for life-threatening hypoxemia) and pulmonary hypertension
Selectively vasodilate pulmonary vasculature
Reduce pulmonary hypertension
Improve oxygenation; $\dot{V}/\dot{Q}$ matching improves due to improved perfusion to ventilated alveoli

Major Adverse Effects

Multiple, depending on agent
Nitric oxide: hypotension, methemoglobinemia
Treprostinil: hypotension, headache, flushing, jaw pain

Nursing Implications

Monitor heart rate, blood pressure, therapeutic effects and side effects
iNO: observe for rebound pulmonary hypertension and hypoxemia as dose is tapered
Treprostinil (prostaglandin) therapy for pulmonary hypertension is specialized and complex: refer to specialized literature

SECTION ONE REVIEW

1. Restrictive pulmonary diseases are associated with
A. increased lung expansion
B. increased lung compliance
C. decreased lung expansion
D. decreased airflow into lungs

2. Which pulmonary disorder is considered a restrictive disease?
A. pneumonia
B. asthma
C. emphysema
D. chronic bronchitis

3. Obstructive pulmonary diseases are associated with decreased
A. lung expansion
B. lung compliance
C. airflow into lungs
D. expiratory airflow

4. An example of an obstructive pulmonary disorder is
A. multiple sclerosis
B. asthma
C. tuberculosis
D. pneumonia

(*continued*)

(continued)

5. Lung compliance is increased with which disorder?
   A. emphysema
   B. pneumonia
   C. pneumothorax
   D. chest burns
6. A patient who has cor pulmonale will have
   A. left heart dilation
   B. right heart hypertrophy
   C. pulmonary fibrosis
   D. left ventricular hyperplasia
7. The nurse monitoring a patient experiencing a degree of status asthmaticus would become particularly concerned if which clinical finding developed?
   A. Pao_2 of 78 mmHg
   B. respiratory rate of 30 breaths/minute
   C. $Paco_2$ of 30 mmHg
   D. no breath sounds

Answers: 1. C, 2. A, 3. D, 4. B, 5. A, 6. B, 7. D

SECTION TWO: Acute Respiratory Failure

At the completion of this section, the learner will be able to discuss the basis of respiratory failure.

Cardiopulmonary System

In Module 9, perfusion was described in terms of two circuits—pulmonary and systemic. For the purposes of this module, it is helpful to reconsider these circuits in a slightly different manner. That is, to view the heart and lungs as a complex integrated cardiopulmonary system that shares volume and pressure with the rest of the systemic circulation—whatever affects one part of the system potentially affects the whole. The cardiopulmonary system is very sensitive to pressure changes within it, requiring compensatory adjustments to maintain homeostasis. Primary problems of cardiac origin can create secondary pulmonary problems. For example, left heart failure can cause cardiogenic pulmonary edema. The opposite is also true as pulmonary problems can affect cardiac status, for example, cor pulmonale (right heart failure of pulmonary origin). If a pulmonary disorder decreases the ability of the lungs to maintain adequate acid–base balance and oxygenation, the heart must work harder to make more blood available for diffusion, causing a compensatory increase in vital signs (increased blood pressure and pulse). The patient's lungs work harder by the respiratory rate (tachypnea) and depth (hyperventilation).

Respiratory Insufficiency and Failure

Respiratory disorders vary greatly in the way they affect lung function. The amount of diffusion surface area that becomes impaired is a major factor in altering gas exchange. The extent of impairment coupled with the rate of disease onset contributes greatly to the ability of the body to cope adequately through compensatory mechanisms. The terms *chronic (compensated) respiratory insufficiency* and *acute respiratory failure* are used to differentiate the level of compensation.

Chronic Respiratory Insufficiency

Respiratory insufficiency is a state in which an acceptable level of gas exchange is maintained only through cardiopulmonary compensatory mechanisms. Chronic pulmonary problems have a slow onset and often are progressive in nature. The body has time to compensate for growing pulmonary deficits, thereby maintaining an adequate level of oxygenation and acid–base balance until late stage disease. A person can lead a relatively normal life in a state of chronic respiratory insufficiency. Arterial blood gases typically noted when chronic respiratory insufficiency exists include a normal pH, an elevated $Paco_2$, accompanied by an elevated HCO_3 (a compensated respiratory acidosis), and a normal to low Pao_2. Respiratory insufficiency, with its compensated arterial blood gas status, is not a normal state and should be considered impending respiratory failure, particularly in unstable patients.

High-acuity patients often walk a fine line between respiratory insufficiency and respiratory failure and their ability to compensate is not infinite. Decompensation results from any stressor (such as acute infection) that is severe enough to push patients beyond their ability to meet the added demands; that is, they develop a supply and demand imbalance and develop respiratory muscle fatigue and impending respiratory failure. Without rapid recognition and timely interventions to relieve the underlying problem, the patient's condition often deteriorates rapidly into acute respiratory failure. The nurse plays a crucial role in early recognition of impending respiratory failure. Clinical signs suspicious of impending failure include tachypnea, tachycardia, increased use of accessory respiratory muscles (e.g., trapezius, sternocleidomastoid, or abdominals), nasal flaring, abnormal chest wall movements, labored breathing, and a decreasing Spo_2. The patient may also be diaphoretic, orthopneic, complain of air hunger, and appear anxious. When a patient's clinical signs suggest increased respiratory muscle fatigue or impending respiratory failure, an ABG is usually ordered. Early recognition of impending respiratory failure coupled with aggressive interventions to treat the underlying cause, decrease oxygen demands, and increase oxygen supply will often improve patient outcomes.

Acute Respiratory Failure

Respiratory failure is a life-threatening state in which the cardiopulmonary system is unable to maintain adequate gas exchange. Acute respiratory failure is caused by an imbalance in supply and demand. Normally, the cardiopulmonary system is able to meet the demands of the body by increasing its work to supply adequate oxygen and ridding the body of carbon dioxide. If the body's demands become higher than the cardiopulmonary system can supply, the system will fail, precipitating acute respiratory failure.

Components of Acute Respiratory Failure

The term *acute respiratory failure* is a general one that pertains to both gas exchange gases: oxygen and carbon dioxide. To better understand the complexity of respiratory failure, it is helpful to break it down into its two component parts: failure of oxygenation and failure of ventilation. Sometimes, both failure components are present initially; however, more commonly, a failure of one or the other system occurs initially, causing respiratory failure. For this reason, it is important to be able to differentiate the two failure components.

Failure of Oxygenation. When a state of **oxygenation failure** exists, the primary problem is one of hypoxemia. Carbon dioxide (CO_2) is able to diffuse across the alveolar–capillary membrane approximately 20 times more rapidly than is oxygen. For this reason, CO_2 levels may remain normal when diffusion is interfered with, even though the patient is showing signs of moderate to severe hypoxemia. Conditions that can cause oxygenation failure are frequently restrictive pulmonary disorders, such as acute respiratory distress syndrome (ARDS) and pneumonia. Should these conditions worsen or should the patient develop respiratory muscle fatigue, CO_2 levels will rise due to hypoventilation, which may result in development of ventilatory failure. Hypoxemia is accompanied by multiple compensatory mechanisms that work to regain an adequate oxygenation state. Clinically, it is important to maintain the PaO_2 at 60 mm Hg or above because of oxygen's decreased affinity to hemoglobin at a PaO_2 less than 60 mm Hg. At this crucial point, any further decrease in PaO_2 will result in a large decrease in hemoglobin saturation (SaO_2). The clinical manifestations and clinical definition of oxygenation failure are presented in Table 10–6.

Failure of Ventilation. **Ventilatory failure** (acute respiratory acidosis) is caused by alveolar hypoventilation; that is, the inability to move air adequately out of the alveoli, allowing a buildup of carbon dioxide. Ventilatory failure can be caused by any problem that interferes with adequate movement of airflow (e.g., neuromuscular disorders, respiratory muscle fatigue, and COPD).

Clinical manifestations of ventilatory failure reflect hypercapnia (elevated carbon dioxide). Most of the symptoms associated with hypercapnia are the result of the strong vasodilator effect of carbon dioxide. The term **CO_2 narcosis** is sometimes used to describe ventilatory failure based on its anesthetic effects. The clinical manifestations and clinical definition of ventilatory failure are presented in Table 10–6.

TABLE 10–6 Acute Respiratory Failure and Its Components

TYPE OF FAILURE	CLINICAL DEFINITION	CLINICAL MANIFESTATIONS
Acute respiratory failure	$PaCO_2$ greater than 50 mm Hg with a pH less than 7.30 and/or PaO_2 less than 60 mm Hg	See below
Oxygenation failure	PaO_2 less than 60 mm Hg	Pulmonary: dyspnea, tachypnea, increased pulmonary vascular resistance Cardiovascular: increased blood pressure, heart rate, cardiac dysrhythmias, cyanosis; weak, thready pulse Central nervous system: altered level of responsiveness; restlessness, confusion
Ventilation failure	$PaCO_2$ greater than 50 mm Hg with a pH less than 7.30 (acute respiratory acidosis)	Pulmonary: tachypnea Vascular: headache; flushed, wet skin Cardiovascular: bounding pulse, increased blood pressure and heart rate Central nervous system: anesthetic effects of carbon dioxide: lethargy, drowsiness, coma (CO_2 narcosis)

Complications of Respiratory Failure

Acute respiratory failure can affect virtually all body systems by causing organ hypoxia. If the respiratory failure is coupled with decreased cardiac output, the patient is at particular risk for development of hypoperfusion/hypoxic organ shock complications, such as those seen with multiple organ dysfunction syndrome (MODS), including acute lung injury/ acute respiratory distress syndrome (ALI/ARDS). The presence of hypercapnia, with its accompanying respiratory acidosis and vasodilation states, adds an additional pathophysiologic burden on the body because cellular function rapidly becomes impaired in acidotic states. In addition, the generalized vasodilatory effects can increase intracranial pressure and decrease cardiac output and systemic vascular resistance. As a general rule, ventilation failure is considered a more serious problem than oxygenation failure. Acute respiratory acidosis can quickly deteriorate to systemic acidosis, which is poorly tolerated by the body. Oxygenation failure, however, is associated with better compensatory mechanisms and, therefore, is better tolerated.

Pathogenesis of Respiratory Failure

The sequence of events that leads to the development of respiratory failure is a complicated one. It is initiated by the presence of a disease process that either directly (e.g., pneumonia) or indirectly (e.g., Guillain-Barré syndrome) interferes with normal lung function. As pulmonary function deteriorates, the patient develops $\dot{V}/\dot{Q}$ ratio abnormalities and decreasing PaO_2. The body recognizes increased oxygen demand and responds by increasing the rate and depth of respirations to move more air into and out of the alveoli (compensation). This compensatory mechanism increases the PaO_2 and decreases the $PaCO_2$ to regain an adequate level of oxygenation and acid–base balance. Compensatory mechanisms (including increased work of breathing) require more energy; thus, the body's metabolic rate increases. As the metabolic rate increases, more oxygen is consumed by the tissues and more carbon dioxide is produced as an end product of metabolism. The overall effect of the sequence is a progressive increase in arterial carbon dioxide and a decrease in arterial oxygen. A state of acute respiratory failure exists when the patient meets the clinical criteria (i.e., $Paco_2$ greater than 50 mm Hg with a pH of less than 7.30 and/or a Pao_2 of less than 60 mm Hg).

Should the sequence of events that precipitated the acute respiratory failure not be corrected adequately, the level of respiratory failure worsens, causing a further increase in the work of breathing. As the work of breathing increases, the patient develops respiratory muscle fatigue, which can eventually lead to respiratory muscle failure and decompensation with worsening of both ventilation and oxygenation. If this sequence of events is allowed to continue, arterial blood gas concentrations steadily deteriorate, leading to death of the patient.

Management of the Patient with Acute Respiratory Failure

Management goals for the patient in acute respiratory failure include:

- Treat the underlying cause
- Support the patient
- Prevent or treat complications

Detailed information on the management of patients with specific pulmonary disorders are found in the remaining sections of this module. Section Seven presents nursing considerations for caring for patients with pulmonary disorders organized around the three respiratory specific nursing diagnoses: *ineffective breathing patterns, impaired gas exchange*, and *ineffective airway clearance.*

SECTION TWO REVIEW

1. Which arterial blood gas pH results would the nurse most commonly note with respiratory insufficiency?
   A. pH within normal limits
   B. pH above normal range
   C. pH below normal range
   D. variable pH
2. Which arterial blood gas pH results, when noted by the nurse, would be most suspicious of acute respiratory failure?
   A. normal pH
   B. pH higher than normal
   C. pH lower than normal
   D. variable pH
3. Failure to oxygenate refers to which of the following primary problems?
   A. ventilation
   B. hypoxemia
   C. arterial pH
   D. carbon dioxide
4. Which symptom, if noted by the nurse, would suggest that the patient is experiencing failure to oxygenate?
   A. bounding pulse
   B. headache
   C. flushed skin
   D. restlessness
5. The primary problem associated with failure to ventilate is
   A. alveolar hypoventilation
   B. capillary hypoperfusion
   C. alveolar hyperventilation
   D. capillary hyperperfusion
6. Many of the common clinical manifestations that are typically noted in patients with ventilatory failure are primarily the result of
   A. vasoconstriction
   B. hypoxemia
   C. vasodilation
   D. acidosis
7. The result of increased metabolic demand is
   A. decreased oxygen consumption
   B. decreased carbon dioxide production
   C. increased oxygen consumption
   D. increased carbon dioxide consumption

Answers: 1. A, 2. C, 3. B, 4. D, 5. A, 6. C, 7. C

SECTION THREE: Acute Lung Injury/Acute Respiratory Distress Syndrome

At the completion of this section, the learner will be able to discuss acute lung injury and acute respiratory distress syndrome.

Adult respiratory distress syndrome (ARDS) was first described in 1967 as a respiratory failure syndrome characterized by bilateral pulmonary filtrates (Ashbaugh et al., 1967). Until recently it was referred to as "adult" RDS to differentiate it from infant hyaline membrane disease. As the disorder became better understood, the word *adult* was replaced by *acute* to acknowledge the similarities between the adult and child versions of the disorder. Currently, **acute respiratory distress syndrome** is conceptualized as the most severe expression of **acute lung injury** (ALI); thus, it is frequently referred to as ALI/ARDS. Acute lung injury can be viewed as a continuum of severity from mild, subclinical injury at one end of the continuum to severe injury (ARDS) at the opposite end. ALI and ARDS are "syndromes with a spectrum of increasing severity of lung injury defined by physiologic and radiographic criteria in which widespread damage to cells and structures of the alveolar capillary membrane occurs within hours to days of a predisposing insult" (Matthay et al., 2003, p. 1027). The ARDS Network (n.d.) further defines ARDS as, "a devastating, often fatal, inflammatory disease of the lung characterized by the sudden onset of pulmonary edema and respiratory failure, usually in the setting of other acute medical conditions resulting from local (e.g., pneumonia) or distant (e.g., multiple trauma) injury.

Etiologic Factors

ARDS is predominantly a complication of systemic disease processes. As the ARDS Network definition implies, ARDS can be precipitated by a variety of direct or indirect pulmonary injuries. Table 10–7 provides a list of some of the more common predisposing factors (Atabai & Matthay, 2002). Predisposing factors have one thing in common—all of them are known to trigger a systemic inflammatory response that, if sufficiently strong, may involve the lungs, leading to diffuse lung injury (Crouser & Fahy, 2009). Currently, there is no explanation as to why, in similar pathologic conditions, a few people develop ARDS when most do not. It is suggested that the determination of who actually develops ARDS depends to some extent on the characteristics and severity of the primary injury, and the presence of coexisting risk factors (Crouser & Fahy, 2009).

Gastric aspiration and septic shock (sepsis with refractory hypotension) are associated with a greater than 25 percent risk of ARDS, whereas the administration of multiple blood transfusions carries a risk of ARDS of less than 5 percent. The risk of ARDS appears to be additive when multiple risk factors are present (Crouser & Fahy, 2009, p. 573). Furthermore, it is suspected that there are other, yet unknown, factors that influence who develops ARDS—some of which may be genetic (Matthay et al., 2003).

Diagnosis

Defining ARDS and differentiating it from other acute pulmonary disorders has been a difficult task since it was first described. In 1992, the American–European Consensus Conference on ARDS defined ALI/ARDS on the basis of clinical criteria (often referred to as "ARDS consensus criteria"). Using the consensus criteria, ALI is differentiated from ARDS based on the ratio of Pao_2 to Fio_2 (P/F ratio) (see Table 10–8).

TABLE 10–7 Common Predisposing Disorders of ALI/ARDS

DIRECT	INDIRECT
Pneumonia[a]	Sepsis[a]
Gastric aspiration[b]	Severe traumatic injury with shock requiring massive blood transfusions[b] (Each factor alone [traumatic injury, shock, massive blood transfusions] can lead to ALI/ARDS; the combination increases the risk significantly)
Near drowning	Severe head injury
Direct severe chest contusion	Acute pancreatitis
Inhalation injury	Drug overdose

[a]Most common predisposing disorders.
[b]Common predisposing disorders.

TABLE 10–8 ARDS Consensus Criteria: Definition of ALI/ARDS (1992 American–European Consensus Conference on ARDS)

Acute onset
Bilateral infiltrates on chest X-ray (frontal view)
Pulmonary artery wedge pressure (PAWP) 18 mm Hg or less and/or no left atrial hypertension (CHF)
Oxygenation status measured as P/F ratio (regardless of PEEP level): ALI = 300 mm Hg or less ARDS = 200 mm Hg or less

These criteria are still commonly used in clinically defining and diagnosing ALI/ARDS. Differentiating the pulmonary edema of ARDS from that of congestive heart failure (CHF) can be difficult because both cause pulmonary edema. It is important, however, to make this differentiation because therapy differs between the two distinct disease states. There are several criteria that assist in making a differential diagnosis:

1. **Pulmonary artery wedge pressure (PAWP).** A PAWP of 18 or greater is suggestive of heart failure (HF), whereas a PAWP of less than 18 is suggestive of ARDS.
2. **Bronchoalveolar lavage (BAL) fluid.** Bronchoalveolar fluid is obtained during a bronchoscopic examination into a lung lobe. BAL fluid present in heart failure (hydrostatic pulmonary edema) is protein poor and lacks inflammatory cells, whereas BAL fluid present in ARDS pulmonary edema is protein rich and contains inflammatory cells (Crouser & Fahy, 2009).
3. **Chest radiography.** Heart enlargement is typically noted in heart failure, whereas it is not typically noted in ARDS. Pulmonary infiltrates noted in heart failure are usually greatest in the dependent lung fields; whereas pulmonary infiltrates noted in ARDS are more diffuse (throughout the lung fields). Pulmonary effusions may be noted in HF, whereas they are not common in ARDS.

There is also investigational interest in finding serum molecular markers that measure acute lung injury similar to measuring serum troponin for myocardial cell injury (Moss, 2006). Ware and colleagues (2007) studied markers of coagulation and fibrinolysis in ARDS patients. Abnormalities in protein C and plasminogen activator inhibitor-1 correlated with mortality. Their results are encouraging but more extensive research is required before its usefulness can be determined.

ALI/ARDS has also been diagnosed using the Modified Lung Injury Score. The Modified Lung Injury Score clinically defines ARDS as the presence of bilateral infiltrates by chest X-ray with a decreased P/F ratio of less than 175 mm Hg. The Modified Lung Injury Score and the American–European Consensus Conference on ARDS clinical criteria are both considered predictive of ARDS (Atabai & Matthay, 2002).

Pathogenesis

ALI/ARDS is not a disease but a pattern of pathophysiological lung changes resulting in a corresponding pattern of clinical manifestations (i.e., a syndrome). It is a distinct type of acute lung injury resulting in severe respiratory failure. ALI/ARDS is caused by diffuse inflammatory injury to the alveolar–capillary membrane, resulting in disruption of both the pulmonary capillary endothelium and the alveolar epithelium. Invasion of lung tissue by neutrophils (PMNs), which activate a variety of inflammatory by-products, is believed to be central to the inflammatory injury. Disruption of the pulmonary capillary endothelium allows plasma proteins and fluid to escape into the pulmonary interstitial spaces. Injured alveolar epithelial linings permit fluid and plasma proteins to flood into the alveoli, resulting in nonhydrostatic pulmonary edema (Crouser & Fahy, 2009; Matthay & Zimmerman, 2005). Figure 10–1 provides a graphic map of one possible explanation of the pathogenesis of this form of pulmonary edema.

The hydrostatic pulmonary edema of heart failure (HF) has a different pathogenesis. Crouser and Fahy (2009) explain that, normally, hydrostatic pressure in the alveoli is greater than the pressure in the pulmonary interstitium, which protects the alveoli from abnormal inflow of interstitial fluid. In situations where left heart pressures create an elevated backup pressure into the pulmonary veins (as seen in CHF), the resulting elevated hydrostatic capillary pressure causes increased flow out of the capillaries into the interstitium because fluid passes through a semipermeable membrane (alveolar-capillary membrane) from greater pressure to lower pressure. Eventually, if interstitial pressures become sufficiently elevated, the alveoli can begin to take in fluid as well (the mechanism for this form of alveolar flooding is not fully understood). Although the pathophysiology of lung edema in ARDS is due to increased permeability, the edema of ARDS can be worsened by increased hydrostatic pressures resulting from fluid overload (Matthay & Zimmerman, 2005).

ARDS can be triggered either from a local (pulmonary) inflammatory problem or from a distant systemic problem (particularly sepsis or systemic inflammatory response syndrome [SIRS]). ARDS is the lung's expression of this widespread inflammatory event. No matter what initial direct or indirect insult triggers the onset of ALI/ARDS, the subsequent sequence of events remains relatively predictable. Figure 10–2 provides a theoretical pathogenesis pathway of ARDS.

Crouser and Fahy (2009) describe two phases of ARDS, the exudative phase and the fibroproliferative phase. These phases reflect the early phase of acute injury followed by a phase of lung repair, and are summarized in Table 10–9.

Clinical Presentation

There are two patterns of clinical presentation based on the preexisting health state of the individual and time of ARDS diagnosis. These patterns impact prognosis and should be taken into consideration. In otherwise healthy individuals, onset of ALI/ARDS

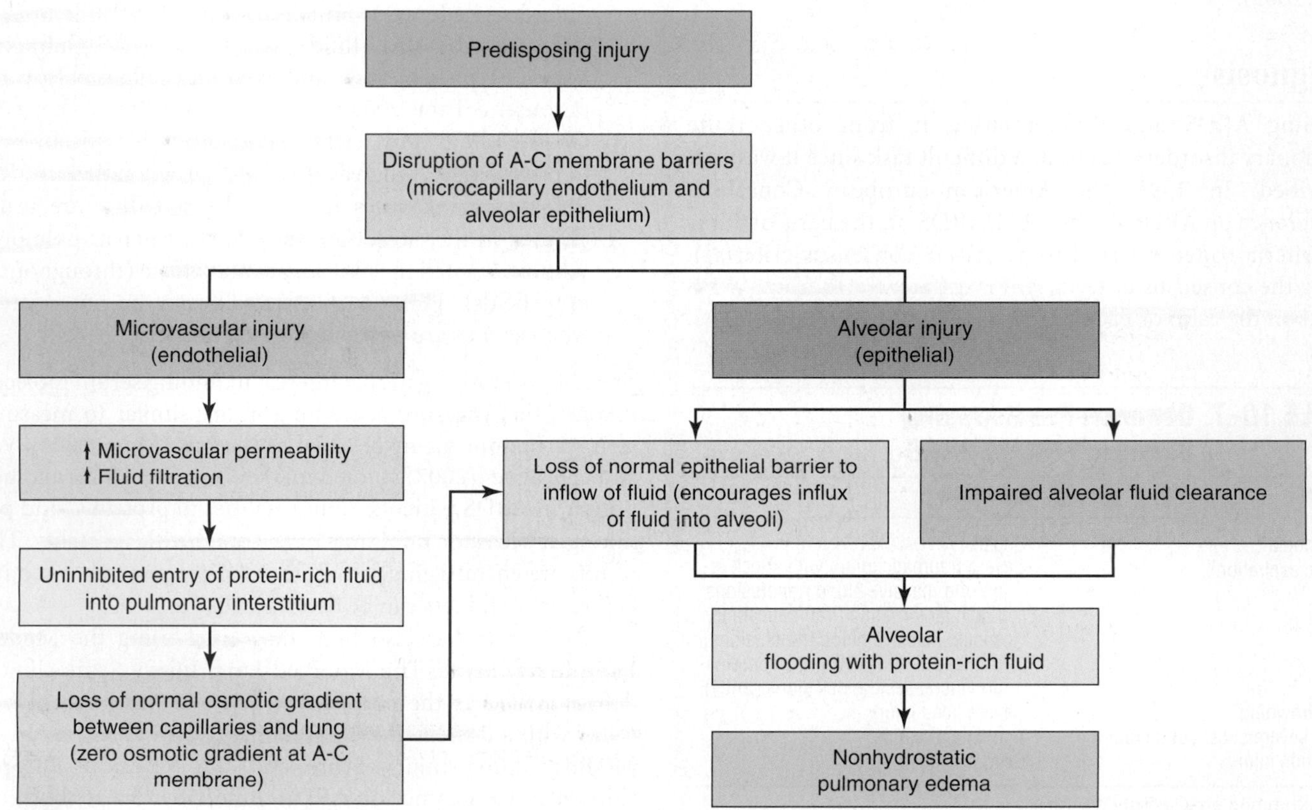

Figure 10–1 ■ Pathogenesis of nonhydrostatic pulmonary edema. Data from Crouser & Fahy (2009).

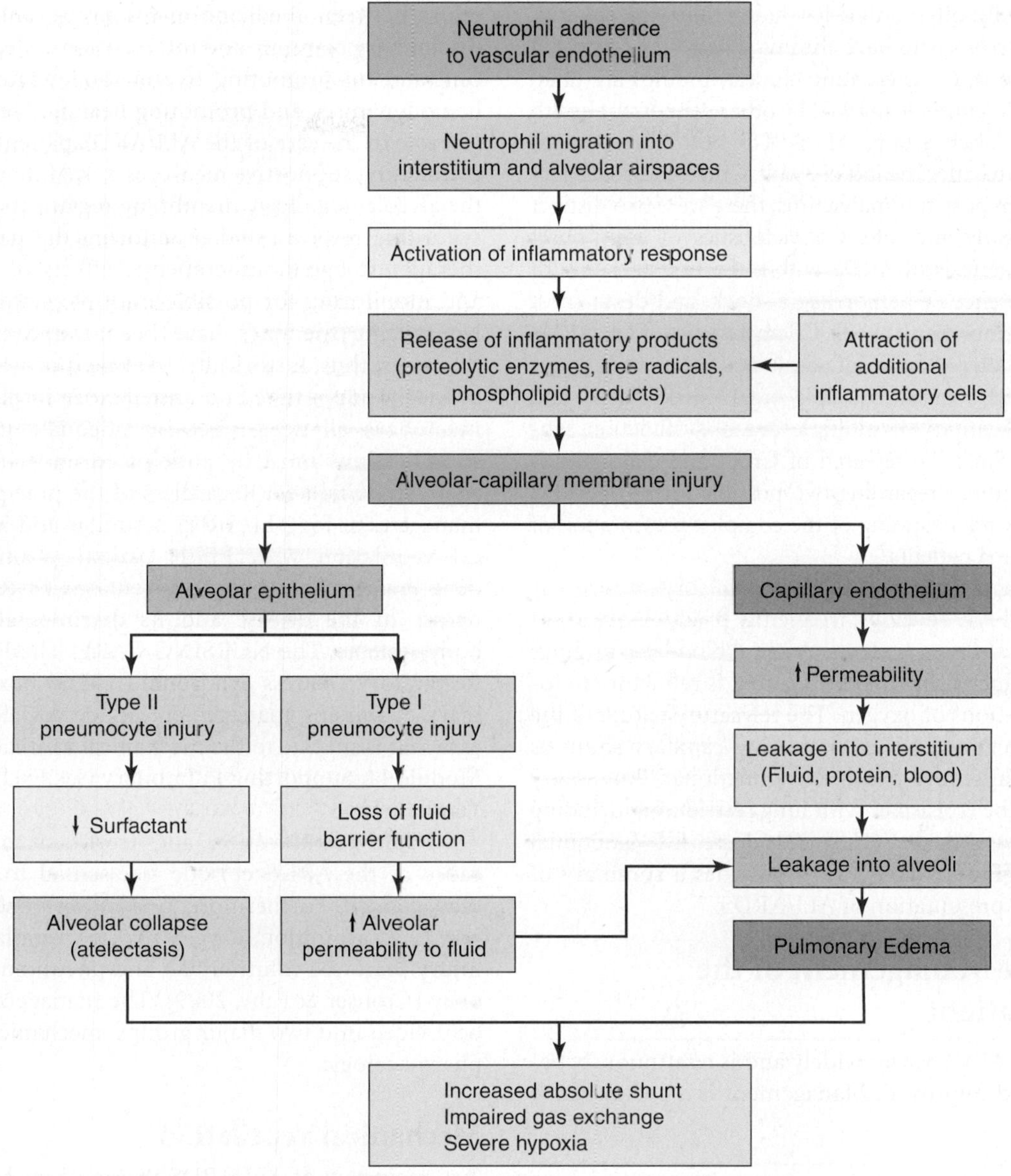

Figure 10–2 ■ Theory of pathogenesis of ARDS. Data from Suratt & Parsons (2006).

TABLE 10–9 Phases of ARDS

PHASE	CHARACTERISTICS	PATHOLOGY
Exudative phase (1 to 3 days)	Diffuse microvascular injury and alveolar damage Invasion of inflammatory cells into interstitium Development of hyaline membranes[a] in alveolar spaces	Destruction of type I pneumocytes
Fibroproliferative phase (3 to 7 days)	Lung repair period Degree of recovery is dependent on: 1. Severity of primary lung injury 2. Influence of secondary forms of injury (e.g., barotrauma, nosocomial infection, oxygen toxicity)	Hyperplasia of type II pneumocytes Proliferation of fibroblasts in basement membrane of alveoli Development of intra-alveolar and interstitial fibrosis[b] Lung remodeling Degree of lung repair is variable Full repair of lung architecture - Return to normal compliance and gas exchange over 6- to 12-month period Permanent damage to lung architecture - Occurs if basement membrane becomes disrupted—cannot repair correctly

[a]Hyaline membranes consist of plasma proteins and cellular debris.
[b]Severity of pulmonary disability in survivors of ARDS depends on extent of fibrosis.
Data from Crouser & Fahy (2009).

usually occurs rapidly, often only a few hours following the triggering insult. In persons who have chronic illnesses or comorbid pathologic conditions, the presenting clinical findings are often more insidious, being initially masked by other concurrent health problems. In the latter group, ALI/ARDS becomes apparent within 24 to 48 hours after the initial insult. Croce and colleagues (1999) noted that in post-trauma victims, there were two distinct forms of ARDS, early and late. Characteristics of early onset ARDS included diagnosis of ARDS within the first 48 hours of admission, the presence of hemorrhagic shock, and death most commonly from hemorrhagic shock. Characteristics of late ARDS included diagnosis after 48 hours of admission, presence of pneumonia prior to ARDS onset, multiple organ involvement, and death from complications of multiple organ dysfunction syndrome (MODS). While the research of Croce and colleagues is rather old, their findings regarding two possible forms of ARDS have added to the understanding of the complex presentation of ARDS in post-trauma patients.

As ARDS progresses, cyanosis and accessory muscle use may be noted. A cough develops, frequently producing sputum that is typical of pulmonary edema. Arterial blood gas findings show a pattern of increasing hypoxemia that is refractory to increasing concentrations of oxygen. The refractory nature of the hypoxemia is largely a result of increasing capillary shunt as alveolar units collapse and become dysfunctional. Pulmonary function tests will be consistent with lung restriction, including decreased lung compliance (CL) and decreased functional residual capacity (FRC). Table 10–10 provides a summary of the typical clinical presentation of ALI/ARDS.

Collaborative Management of the ALI/ARDS Patient

Treatment of ALI/ARDS varies widely and is continuously being researched and improved. Management is a collaborative effort between medicine and nursing and requires multidisciplinary planning and interventions. Medical therapy concentrates on promoting oxygenation, maintaining adequate hemodynamics, and promoting healing. Nursing plays a crucial role in the care of the ALI/ARDS patient, focusing on implementing supportive measures to maintain the patient until the alveolar–capillary membrane regains its integrity and the syndrome resolves; and monitoring the patient's status, the therapeutic and nontherapeutic effects of medical therapy; and monitoring for possible multiple system complications. No specific therapies have been found that directly heal the lungs; thus, historically, treatment of ALI/ARDS has been primarily supportive and anticipatory in nature. The patient must have all needs met for adequate lung healing, and complications must be anticipated and either prevented or aggressively treated. Regardless of the precipitating event, the management for ALI/ARDS is similar and includes mechanical ventilation with PEEP, patient positioning strategies, drug therapy, and other interventions based on the complex nature of the disease and its detrimental effect on other body systems. The NURSING CARE: The Patient with Acute Respiratory Distress Syndrome (ARDS) box provides a summary of nursing management of the ARDS patient. Nursing care that is specific to the mechanical ventilator is presented in Module 11, Supporting Pulmonary Gas Exchange: Mechanical Ventilation.

Rapid identification and treatment of the underlying cause of the ARDS episode is essential to successful ARDS management. Furthermore, prevention of secondary lung injury (e.g., aspiration, oxygen toxicity, ventilator-induced lung injury [baro- or volutrauma], and pneumonia) is a major priority (Crouser & Fahy, 2009). The management of ARDS can be divided into two major groups: mechanical ventilation and pharmacologic.

TABLE 10–10 Common Clinical Presentation of ARDS

Early Onset

Onset: Within first 24 to 48 hours postadmission
Chest radiograph: Initially normal
Increasing respiratory distress, tachypnea, and dyspnea
Initial ABGs: Respiratory alkalosis (secondary to hyperventilation); PaO_2 normal or mild hypoxemia

Late Onset

Onset: After 24 to 48 hours postadmission
Chest radiograph: May show evidence of pneumonia
Labs: Reflect multiple body system dysfunction
Rate of onset: May be insidious (related to overall poor condition)

Progressive Manifestations

Cyanosis
Cough (productive)
Increasing use of accessory muscles
ABGs: Pattern of increasing hypoxemia (refractory to oxygen therapy)
Pulmonary function tests: Increasing pulmonary restriction (e.g., decreasing lung compliance, decreasing FRC)

Mechanical Ventilation

Two mainstays of ALI/ARDS therapy have been positive pressure mechanical ventilation and positive end expiratory pressure (PEEP) to adequately overcome low lung compliance and refractory hypoxemia.

Protective Ventilation. Until recently, a high tidal volume (10 to 15 mL/kg body weight) was recommended for treatment of ALI/ARDS. Unfortunately, high tidal volumes are known to cause ventilator-induced lung injury (VILI) (ARDS Network, 2000; Malhotra, 2007). Current research suggests that using a low tidal volume (6 mL/kg body weight) with a plateau pressure of 30 cm H_2O or less significantly reduces mortality as well as ventilator days in ALI/ARDS patients regardless of the precipitating cause (ARDS Network, 2000; Wheeler & Bernard, 2007).

Positive End Expiratory Pressure (PEEP). A major complicating factor in ALI/ARDS is the massive collapse of alveoli, which causes a significant shunt, decreased lung compliance, and severe hypoxemia. This explains the refractory nature of

NURSING CARE: The Patient with Acute Respiratory Distress Syndrome (ARDS)

Expected Patient Outcomes and Related Interventions

Outcome 1: Support of Pulmonary Gas Exchange

Assess and compare to established norms, patient baseline, and trends

- Vital signs, lung sounds, chest X-ray, P/F ratio, peak airway pressure, Spo_2, ABG, CBC, intake and output, daily weights, hemodynamic parameters (particularly left atrial pressure), ET tube position, secretions (amount and consistency)

Interventions to decrease lung fluid

- Conservative fluid therapy, as ordered (Goal: prevent fluid overload while maintaining adequate CO)
- Diuretic therapy, as ordered

Interventions to increase pulmonary gas exchange

- Mechanical ventilation
- Least PEEP therapy, as ordered (Goal: maintain Pao_2 of 60 mmHg at Fio_2 of 0.6 or less) -
  - Monitor for desired and adverse effects
- Protective ventilation (VT of 6 mL/kg or less IBW) (Goal: prevent ventilator-induced lung injury [VILI])
- Frequent body position changes (Goal: improve $\dot{V}/\dot{Q}$ relationship)
  - Reposition every 2 hours (if other alternative position therapy not being used)
  - Alternative positioning
    - Prone positioning or CLRT therapy, as ordered
      - Prevent accidental dislodgement of ET tube
      - Monitor for development of pressure ulcers
      - Monitor closely for adverse effects

Interventions to maintain airway patency and protect airway

- Secure ET tube with tape or other stabilizing device
- Suction ET tube and mouth as needed
- Maintain ET tube cuff pressure

Administer related drug therapy and monitor for therapeutic and nontherapeutic effects

- Diuretic agents (e.g., furosemide [Lasix])
- Corticosteroids (e.g., methylprednisolone)
- Nitric oxide (iNO) therapy
- Surfactant replacement therapy
- Beta-adrenergic agonist therapy (e.g., IV albuterol) (IV use is not yet available in U.S.)
- *N*-Acetylcysteine therapy

Related nursing diagnoses

- Alteration in respiratory function
  - Impaired gas exchange
  - Ineffective airway clearance
- Decreased cardiac output
- Activity intolerance
- Alterations in fluid volume (excess or deficit)

Outcome 2: Optimize Oxygen Delivery to Body Systems

Assess and compare to established norms, patient baseline, and trends

- Arterial blood pressure, heart rate, temperature, mean arterial pressures (MAP), CBC, hemodynamic parameters, pain and anxiety

Interventions to maintain adequate oxygen delivery (Do_2) to body systems (Crouser & Fahy, 2009)

- Maintain MAP greater than 70 mmHg; BP greater than 90 mm Hg systolic
- Maintain adequate urine output
- Correct lactic acidosis
- Maintain adequate levels of hemoglobin

Interventions to reduce metabolic demands

- Maintain afebrile state
- Control pain and anxiety
- Reduce extraneous body movements

Administer related drug therapy and monitor for therapeutic and nontherapeutic effects

- Vasopressor agents (e.g., dopamine, dobutamine)
- Sedation agents (e.g., midazolam, lorazepam, propofol)
- Analgesic agents (e.g., morphine, fentanyl)
- Neuromuscular blockade (e.g., cisatracurium, pancuronium)

Related nursing diagnoses

- Altered comfort: Pain
- Altered tissue perfusion
- Anxiety
- Decreased cardiac output

Outcome 3: Maintain Nutritional Balance

Assess and compare to established norms, patient baseline, and trends

- Daily weights, temperature, serum electrolytes, CBC, serum albumin, prealbumin, renal function tests (BUN, creatinine), nitrogen balance (e.g., metabolic cart study), edema, bowel sounds, bowel movements

Interventions to maintain nutritional balance

- Provide nutritional support: Enteral nutrition (Goal: initiate within 24 hours of intubation)
  - Monitor tube tip placement
  - Elevate head of bed 30 degrees or greater
  - Frequent oral care: Oral airway cleaning and suctioning

Administer related drug therapy and monitor for therapeutic and nontherapeutic effects

- Agents to reduce metabolic demand (see Outcome 2)
- Intravenous fluids, as ordered
- Bowel regimen agents: Stool softeners, bulking agents, laxatives
- Oral hygiene agents (e.g., chlorhexidine)

(*continued*)

NURSING CARE *(continued)*

Related nursing diagnoses
- Altered nutrition: less than body requirements
- Potential for aspiration
- Altered bowel elimination
- PC: electrolyte imbalance

Outcome 4: Minimize pain and anxiety, promote sleep

Assess and compare to established norms, patient baselines and trends
- Patient self-assessment of pain, anxiety, lack of sufficient rest; when patient cannot communicate – evaluate for signs of pain or anxiety (e.g., facial grimacing, restlessness); assess for presence of pain producing invasive tubes or lines or altered skin integrity

Interventions to reduce anxiety and promote rest
- Cluster activities to provide periods of undisturbed rest
- Maintain a restful environment (e.g., turn down lights between procedures; reduce environmental noise levels)
- Explain all procedures and treatments
- Keep call light within patient reach, as appropriate

Administer related drug therapy and monitor for therapeutic and nontherapeutic effects
- Sedation agents (e.g., midazolam, lorazepam, or propofol)
- Analgesic agents (e.g., morphine, fentanyl)

Related nursing diagnoses
- Altered comfort: pain
- Anxiety
- Fatigue
- Self-care deficits: total
- Sleep pattern disturbance

Outcome 5: Promote communication and provide family support

Assess and compare to established norms, patient baselines, and trends
- Glasgow Coma Scale, mental status, ability to communicate through alternative means

Interventions to promote communication and provide family support
- Frequent reminders that patient is unable to talk at present time
- Frequent reorientation of family members to ventilator equipment
- Ask yes/no questions
- Use alternative communication boards (e.g., alphabet or picture boards, writing boards)
- Provide patient and family with updates on patient status

Related nursing diagnoses
- Altered family processes
- Altered role performance
- Alteration in family or individual coping
- Impaired social interaction
- Impaired verbal communication

ALI/ARDS to conventional oxygen therapy. Recall that atelectasis is a type of capillary shunt, which is absolute in nature. Regardless of the oxygen concentration delivered, the gas never enters into the affected alveoli for gas exchange. Until positive end expiratory pressure (PEEP) became available there was no way to force alveoli open once they had collapsed.

PEEP applies positive pressure into the patient's airway at the end of expiration such that the alveoli are prevented from closing. PEEP maintains the alveoli in an open state throughout the breathing cycle, which increases gas diffusion time, thereby increasing gas exchange. PEEP also reduces shunt by recruiting collapsed alveoli (popping them open). Once open, PEEP may prevent another type of damage to alveoli from the stress of opening and closing with each ventilator cycle termed "atelectrauma" (Malhotra, 2007). The goal in using PEEP is to achieve an adequate PaO_2 (usually at least 60 mm Hg) while reducing the inspired oxygen concentration (FiO_2) to less than 0.6 (60 percent) because high concentrations of oxygen eventually cause oxygen toxicity. The level of desired PEEP is individually evaluated. Current recommendations are to use the least amount of PEEP to achieve oxygenation goals and avoid toxic oxygen levels (Crouser & Fahy, 2009). Although PEEP has been invaluable for treatment of ALI/ARDS, it is not without hazards, including decreased cardiac output, overdistention of alveoli, and pneumothorax, among others. PEEP is further described in Module 11, Supporting Pulmonary Gas Exchange: Mechanical Ventilation.

Alternative mechanical ventilation options may be initiated when conventional therapy has not been effective in attaining adequate gas exchange. Some of the more common alternatives include pressure control ventilation, reverse I:E ratio ventilation, airway pressure release ventilation, high-frequency ventilation, and BiLevel ventilation. It is important to note, however, that while some of these alternative mechanical ventilation options have the advantage of decreasing problems of barotrauma and volutrauma, none of them stand out as being superior for use in ARDS in the adult population.

Table 10–11 summarizes mechanical ventilation settings that strive to support oxygen exchange while protecting the lungs.

Patient Positioning Strategies

There has been increasing interest in the effects of various types of patient positioning in improving patient outcomes. Two

TABLE 10–11 Protective Mechanical Ventilation Settings to Reduce Ventilator-Induced Lung Injury (VILI)

PARAMETER	SETTING
Tidal Volume (VT)	6 to 10 mL/kg (IBW)
PEEP (least PEEP)	Minimum level that achieves Sa_{O_2} 90% or greater at Fi_{O_2} of 0.6 (60%) or less
Permissive Hypercapnia[a]	No specific settings. Goal: Maintain peak airway pressure (PAP) less than 40 to 45 cm H_2O
Mean airway pressure	35 cm H_2O or less

[a]Permissive hypercapnia—VT, f, VE, and other settings can be manipulated to allow Pa_{CO_2} to elevate, keeping the pH within specified acidotic parameters (such as 7.25–7.30) to reduce PAP to within desired range; contraindicated in patients with unstable intracranial pressure or hemodynamic status.
Data from Crouser & Fahy (2009).

major types of therapy, continuous lateral rotation therapy and prone positioning, are briefly described here.

Continuous Lateral Rotation Therapy (CLRT). Beds that provide CLRT (also called Kinetic Therapy™ or oscillation therapy) continuously rotate the patient's body from side to side (with brief pauses), thus shifting pressure and fluid. Powers and Daniels (2004) explain that, for many years, patients on prolonged bedrest were manually turned from side to side primarily to prevent the formation of decubitus ulcers. Beginning in the 1980s, research began linking prolonged immobility with a variety of serious complications, such as pneumonia, pulmonary embolus, and deep vein thrombosis. CLRT is commonly employed in critical care units as an alternative to manual turning for the purpose of reducing stasis of fluid and gas-related complications.

Research evaluating CLRT concluded that this therapy decreases atelectasis and the incidence of ventilator associated pneumonia (VAP), but does not affect ICU length of stay or mortality (Rauen, Chulay et al., 2008; Goldhill et al., 2007). CLRT appears to be most effective when initiated early in the course of critical illness and when used for more than 18 hours per day (Rauen, Chulay et al., 2008). Figure 10–3 shows an example of a CLRT bed.

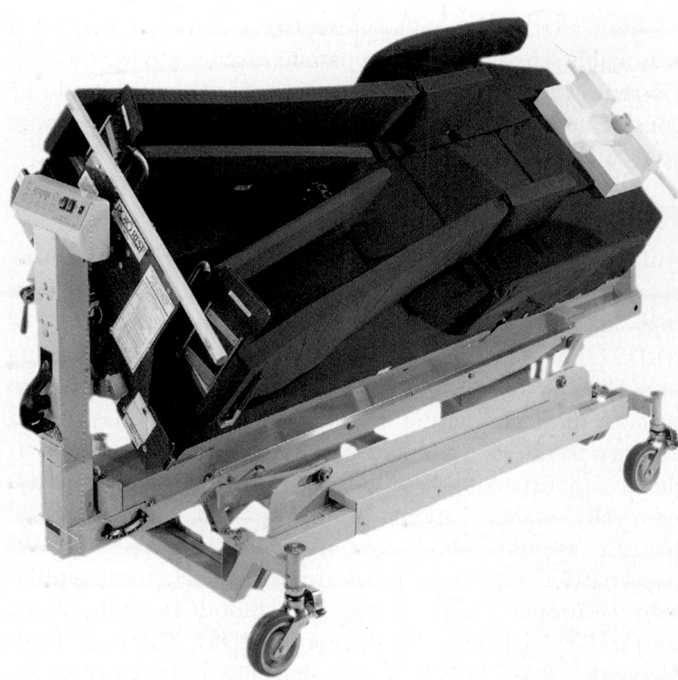

Figure 10–3 ■ RotoRest bed. A form of CLRT therapy. RotoRest Delta TM Advanced Kinetic Therapy TM (System); Courtesy of KCI Licensing, Inc. 2008.

Prone Position Therapy. Prone positioning ("proning") is the periodic placement of a patient in a face-down (prone) position for the purpose of increasing oxygenation while potentially reducing oxygen therapy concentration (Mancebo et al., 2006). While the exact mechanism for improved oxygenation is unknown, understanding the effects of supine position on the injured lung helps explain why prone position might be therapeutic. Supine position results in atelectasis in the lower, posterior (dependent) areas of the lung. Factors that may contribute to this loss of lung volume include edema, secretions and compression from the heart and abdominal organs (Galiatsou et al., 2006). At the same time, gravitational forces maintain blood flow to the now atelectatic dependent lung regions resulting in severe shunt.

Prone position may improve oxygenation by shifting edema, and recruiting alveoli (Alsaghir & Martin, 2008, Galiatsou et al., 2006) and changing pleural pressure gradients to improve ventilation (Mancebo et al, 2006). A major advantage of prone positioning is that improved oxygenation can be achieved using a noninvasive, relatively simple procedure. Evidence suggests that there is a window of opportunity in which prone positioning is therapeutic in ALI/ARDS patients, effectiveness being limited to the early phase of the disease, with up to 70 percent of patients benefiting (Gattinoni et al., 2001). Although oxygenation may improve rather dramatically, there is as yet no clear evidence that use of prone position improves survival overall, but there may be improved survival in the most severely ill patients (Alsaghir & Martin, 2008) especially when instituted early and for longer periods of the day (Mancebo et al., 2006).

Not all patients can tolerate being placed in prone position and may develop worsening oxygenation or hemodynamic instability. Proning is contraindicated in some patients, for example, those with uncontrolled intracranial pressure, or spinal injury (Vollman, 2004). Careful preparation prior to the turn is essential to minimize positioning related complications, such as accidental ET tube dislodgement, pressure ulcers, loss of venous access, or eye injury (Vollman, 2004; Bream-Rouwenhorst, Beltz et al., 2008). The optimal duration for prone positioning has not been determined. Vollman (2004) suggests that 6 to 12 hours of prone position alternating with supine/lateral rotation may be a reasonable schedule based on patient response to the therapy. Current evidence suggests that prone positioning should be considered as a position therapy option when other, more conventional therapies, have not been effective.

Fluid Management

Although the lung edema of ARDS is primarily due to increased permeability, increased hydrostatic pressure from high intravascular volume can aggravate the edema of ARDS. However, fluid resuscitation is vital to maintaining organ perfusion in this complex patient population. How to balance these competing issues of fluid balance has been a concern in the management of ARDS patients. Current evidence supports conservative fluid management in hemodynamically stable patients following initial resuscitation because avoiding fluid gain in stable patients improves oxygenation and results in less time on mechanical ventilation (National Heart, Lung, and Blood Institute Acute Respiratory Distress Syndrome (ARDS) Clinical Trials Network, 2006). Other fluid management strategies under investigation include the combination therapy of albumin and furosemide, and continuous hemofiltration (Calfee & Matthay, 2007).

Pharmacologic Therapy

Pharmacologic-based treatment of ARDS has failed to significantly improve ALI/ARDS patient outcomes (Cepkova & Matthay, 2006). Currently, there are several therapies that warrant description.

Corticosteroids. The use of corticosteroids as a treatment for ALI/ARDS remains controversial and is based on the inflammatory nature of the disease pathology. Inflammation and lung injury from the by-products of inflammation are a major source of lung destruction in the ALI/ARDS pathogenesis. Some patients recover within the first week of ARDS, but in others, the inflammation does not resolve and progresses to a fibrotic phase of the disease (Cepkova & Matthay, 2006). High-dose steroids have not been shown to be effective in the treatment of ARDS and may be harmful (Annane, 2007). Clinical trials investigating patient outcomes following medium-dose corticosteroid therapy have had conflicting results. A large randomized, controlled trial conducted by the ARDS Clinical Trials Network found improvement in oxygenation but no improvement in mortality. Of note, late steroid use (after 14 days) was associated with increased mortality and greater neuromuscular weakness and is not recommended (Steinberg, et al., 2006). More recently, Meduri et al. (2007) found early, prolonged steroids improved survival. These investigators also found frequent infections without fever in the patients receiving steroids and stressed the importance of obtaining active surveillance cultures. These studies, while conflicting, add to the body of information regarding the place of anti-inflammatory agents in the treatment of ARDS, as well as highlighting serious complications of infection and muscle weakness.

Inhaled Nitric Oxide (iNO). Nitric oxide should not be confused with nitrous oxide (N_2O, "laughing gas"), which is used for mild anesthesia. Nitric oxide, a potent vasodilator, is normally produced by the body and plays an important role in pulmonary blood flow regulation. The pathology of ALI/ARDS includes acute pulmonary hypertension as a result of pulmonary vasoconstriction in early ALI/ARDS as well as impairment of hypoxic vasoconstriction (Cepkova & Matthay, 2006). Inhalation of low doses of nitric oxide increases PaO_2 by selectively redistributing pulmonary blood flow to working alveoli (Cepkova & Matthay, 2006). iNO has been shown to improve oxygenation in the first days of use, but not to improve survival from ARDS (Adhikari et al., 2007). Lack of overall benefit plus an increased risk of acute renal failure prompted the authors of a recent meta-analysis to conclude that there is no evidence to support routine use (Adhikari et al., 2007). However, these authors, and others (Dellinger, 2006) suggest that iNO may have a role for those patients with the most severe, life threatening hypoxemia when other strategies have failed. Refer to the box, RELATED PHARMACOTHERAPY: Agents Used for Treatment of Pulmonary Diseases for additional information on iNO as a pulmonary vasodilating agent.

Surfactant Replacement Therapy. Use of surfactant therapy in treating infant distress syndrome is a well-known, highly successful therapy. Use of exogenous surfactant in adults with ALI/ARDS has not met with the same success because of the complexity of the pathology of ARDS in adults with loss of surfactant being only one part of the disease process (Cepkova & Matthay, 2006). Several features of current surfactant therapy have been identified that pose challenges, particularly the composition of the formula and the method of delivery (aerosol versus direct instillation) (Cepkova & Matthay, 2006). In a meta-analysis of the studies of surfactant in adults, Davidson et al. (2006) concluded that surfactant therapy may improve oxygenation, but not mortality. They suggest that further study is needed to explore alternative drug doses, composition, and delivery systems.

Partial Liquid Ventilation. Partial liquid ventilation is the introduction of perfluorocarbon liquid into the lungs. Perfluorocarbons are carbon-based molecules that readily dissolve oxygen and carbon dioxide. Perfluorocarbons are able to flow into the terminal airways where they enhance gas exchange, thus improving oxygenation. Partial liquid ventilation seems to be better tolerated than full liquid ventilation. Early studies were promising, suggesting that this therapy may result in reduction of the inflammatory response and lung injury and may enhance oxygenation and improve lung mechanics. However, a more recent study of liquid ventilation showed no benefit to partial or total liquid ventilation and higher complications such as barotrauma (Kacmarek et al., 2006).

Other Emerging Drug Therapy. There remains high interest in finding a drug or drugs that can effectively reduce mortality in patients with ARDS. Several drugs currently under investigation include prostaglandins, *N*-acetylcysteine, and albuterol.

Prognosis

The mortality rate associated with ARDS varies widely depending on its etiology and comorbidity factors, and ranges from estimates of about 30 percent to more than 85 percent. Until recently, the general estimate of mortality was about 50 percent regardless of advances in therapy. In general, patients who show improvement within the first week of treatment have outcomes that are more successful. Two relatively new interventions, however, have reduced the mortality rates, including low (protective) tidal volumes using mechanical ventilation, and use of activated protein C for treatment of **sepsis** (the major cause of ARDS) (Matthay et al., 2003).

There is research interest in finding methods to more accurately predict prognosis in patient with ALI and ARDS. More accurate prediction could assist teams in counseling families (Avecillas et al., 2006), in designing research studies and to identify patients likely to need more aggressive therapies (Ware, 2005). A number of patient factors such as age and underlying diseases (e.g., liver disease) have been identified. There is work underway to validate biological markers such as protein C and coagulation factors (Ware, 2005) as well as genetics (Gong et al., 2006).

Quality of life for ARDS survivors is an issue receiving a great deal of attention. For those who survive, lung repair occurs slowly and terminates by about 6 months following the onset of ARDS. Long-term, most survivors of ARDS do not have severe pulmonary dysfunction. They do report serious impairment in physical, psychological and emotional function related to persistent muscle weakness, pain, depression, anxiety and cognitive changes such as memory loss (Rubenfeld & Herridge, 2007). These post-ICU impairments have profound implications for patients' quality of life, needs for rehabilitation, family support and health care costs. Interventions that may impact long-term outcomes are not known, but research is ongoing (Hopkins & Herridge, 2006).

The elderly have become a prevalent population in the ICU setting. Historically, it was assumed that the elderly had poorer outcomes with ARDS than their younger patients but the effects of older age with ARDS outcomes has not been investigated. Eachempati, Hydo, Shou, and Barie (2007) studied patient outcomes in the elderly with ARDS. They found that while the elderly ICU population is often sicker than younger ICU patients, close hemodynamic monitoring and resuscitation interventions accompanied by stabilization and correction of organ problems, improved elderly patient outcomes.

SECTION THREE REVIEW

1. The most common indirect predisposing disorder of ALI/ARDS is
   A. gastric aspiration
   B. severe trauma
   C. sepsis
   D. pneumonia
2. The pulmonary edema associated with ALI/ARDS is caused by
   A. capillary microembolism
   B. left ventricular failure
   C. loss of surfactant
   D. injured alveolar–capillary membrane
3. Which clinical finding is typically present with ALI/ARDS?
   A. decreased P/F ratio
   B. increased lung compliance
   C. decreased airway resistance
   D. increased functional residual capacity
4. The refractory (resistant) nature of ARDS to oxygen therapy is based on the amount of
   A. anatomic shunt
   B. venous admixture
   C. capillary shunt
   D. shuntlike effect
5. The pulmonary edema of ALI/ARDS differs from pulmonary edema of CHF in which way?
   A. In CHF, PAWP is less than 18.
   B. In CHF, bronchoalveolar lavage (BAL) fluid is protein rich.
   C. In ARDS, heart enlargement is typically noted.
   D. In ARDS, BAL fluid contains inflammatory cells.
6. According to the ARDS consensus criteria, a diagnosis of ARDS requires a P/F ratio of less than ______ mm Hg.
   A. 175
   B. 200
   C. 225
   D. 300
7. Which type of inflammatory cell is believed to be the major cause of lung injury?
   A. neutrophils
   B. lymphocytes
   C. eosinophils
   D. basophils
8. The nurse would expect to see which ABG trend in an ALI/ARDS patient?
   A. low pH
   B. low PaO_2
   C. high $PaCO_2$
   D. high HCO_3

(continued)

(continued)

9. Protective ventilation uses tidal volumes of ______ mL/kg.
   A. 4
   B. 6
   C. 8
   D. 10
10. The term *permissive hypercapnia* refers to
    A. reducing peak airway pressures by allowing some increase in $PaCO_2$
    B. controlling $PaCO_2$ level at 45 to 50 mm Hg
    C. enhancing gas exchange by allowing some increase in $PaCO_2$
    D. controlling PaO_2 level by allowing hypercapnia
11. Optimal PEEP level is usually between
    A. 5 and 10 cm H_2O
    B. 6 and 12 cm H_2O
    C. 8 and 15 cm H_2O
    D. 10 and 18 cm H_2O
12. Which statement is correct regarding the primary purpose of CLRT?
    A. It prevents pneumonia.
    B. It saves manual turning time.
    C. It prevents decubitus ulcers.
    D. It prevents reduced stasis of fluid and gas.
13. When initiating prone positioning, the nurse would monitor the patient for a significant improvement in
    A. PaO_2
    B. $PaCO_2$
    C. breathing pattern
    D. level of consciousness
14. Inhaled nitric oxide is sometimes ordered because of which physiologic effect?
    A. vasoconstriction
    B. vasodilation
    C. anesthetic
    D. analgesic
15. Corticosteroid therapy may be used for the ALI/ARDS patient because of which ALI/ARDS characteristic?
    A. atelectasis
    B. pulmonary edema
    C. loss of surfactant
    D. diffuse inflammation

Answers: 1. C, 2. D, 3. A, 4. C, 5. D, 6. B, 7. A, 8. B, 9. B, 10. A, 11. C, 12. D, 13. A, 14. B, 15. D

SECTION FOUR: Pulmonary Embolism

At the completion of this section, the learner will be able to explain pulmonary embolism and its treatment.

Pulmonary embolism accounts for about 250,000 hospitalizations in the United States per year and 50,000 deaths annually (Horlander et al., 2003) and has a high mortality rate if untreated (Tapson, 2008). Although many pulmonary emboli are asymptomatic, others lead to rapid death. This section provides an overview of the types, causes, signs and symptoms, and treatment of pulmonary emboli but focuses on thromboembolism.

Pulmonary embolism is blockage of a pulmonary blood vessel caused by lodging of a thromboembolism or other blood-borne material that has passed through the venous system, into the right side of the heart and into the pulmonary artery. Emboli become lodged in the lungs because of the natural blood flow of the venous system into the lungs for gas exchange through a decreasing-size pulmonary vascular system that begins at the pulmonary artery trunk and ends in the microvasculature of the pulmonary capillary system. This system makes the lungs act as a filtering organ, stopping any material that is too large to squeeze through the tiny microvasculature (Awtry & Loscalzo, 2001). Therefore, a variety of blood-borne material can flow through the system until it can no longer move forward, lodging and obstructing flow distal to the obstruction.

Types and Causes of Emboli

There are four types of pulmonary emboli: thrombus, fat, amniotic, and venous air.

Thromboembolism

A thrombus or blood clot comprises almost all pulmonary emboli. The major source of thromboembolism is deep vein thrombosis (DVT) in the lower extremities, usually in the thigh or pelvis areas. Thromboembolism is discussed in detail later in this section.

Fat Embolism

Fat embolism occurs when fat gains access into the venous circulation. Fat embolism may be quite common, however life-threatening illness is quite rare and usually results from long bone trauma or orthopedic surgery. Fat emboli are often small and may go undetected. When symptoms are present, they usually appear within 12 to 48 hours after the predisposing event. Major criteria for fat embolism syndrome include petechiae (e.g., over the anterior neck and axilla, oral mucosa and conjunctivae), dyspnea and tachypnea, hypoxemia, neurologic symptoms (e.g., confusion, drowsiness, or coma), and diffuse bilateral shadowing on chest radiography (Husebye et al., 2006). A person experiencing this form of embolus may also exhibit a fever, tachycardia, and a variety of other signs and symptoms.

Amniotic Embolism

Normally, the fetal membranes prevent amniotic fluid from gaining access to the maternal circulation (O'Shea & Eappen, 2007). Amniotic emboli can develop during the birthing process when amniotic fluid mixes with maternal blood. Amniotic fluid embolism is not well understood, but three pathophysiological mechanisms have been suggested: mechanical obstruction caused by amniotic material; cytokine release causing vasoconstriction, coagulopathy, and ARDS; and an anaphylactic-type syndrome resulting in shock. The patient presents with sudden onset shock, severe hypoxemia and disseminated intravascular coagulation (DIC), a potentially severe coagulopathy. Neurological changes including seizures are also common. Care is supportive focusing on oxygenation, cardiovascular support with vasopressors and inotropes, and blood products to correct the coagulopathy (Stafford & Sheffield, 2007).

Venous Air Embolism

Venous air embolus (VAE) results from a bolus of air being introduced into the venous circulation. VAE is a rare but potentially lethal complication usually of iatrogenic procedures or trauma. The potentially catastrophic effects of air embolus can be better understood by visualizing venous flow into the heart. On introduction of an air embolus (air bubble) into the venous circulation, the bubble follows venous flow into the right atrium, flows into the right ventricle and then into the pulmonary artery. If the embolus is sufficiently large, it can become trapped (remember, it is a physical bubble) at the pulmonary valve in the right ventricle, blocking venous blood from entering into the lungs. Common predisposing factors for development of air embolism include venous or arterial intravenous catheters, procedures that involve insufflation of air such as laparoscopy, or penetrating chest trauma. Wittenberg, et al. (2006), explain that surgical procedures and central venous cannulization (e.g., subclavian) pose the greatest risk. The exact volume required for a lethal air bolus is unknown but volumes of 3 to 8 mL/kg can cause right heart outflow obstruction, subsequent cardiovascular collapse, and death. For example, a lethal dose in a 150-pound (68-kg) adult male would be a bolus of 204 to 544 mL of air. Smaller volumes of air can move from the right heart into the pulmonary artery system, causing pulmonary vascular injury (e.g., vasoconstriction, pulmonary hypertension, injury to the capillary endothelium, and pulmonary edema). Development of an air bolus following a central venous cannulization procedure has a mortality of about 30 percent; thus, prevention is key! The clinical manifestations of VAE are similar to thromboembolism. Recommendations for treatment include steps to prevent further air entry, administration of 100 percent oxygen and positioning on the left side in Trendelenburg position. This position encourages the embolus to float away from pulmonary valve; thus allowing blood to move into the pulmonary artery. Air embolism associated with central venous catheters can be prevented with careful technique during insertion and removal.

Predisposing Factors of Thromboembolism

More than 80 percent of pulmonary emboli (PE) originate as deep-vein thromboses (DVT) in lower extremity deep veins. Many high-acuity patients are at increased risk for development of DVT and, therefore, for development of PE. There are three major factors (called Virchow's triad) that place a person at risk for development of DVT:

- **Venous stasis.** Venous stasis refers to slowing of blood flow. It most commonly results from significantly reduced mobility, such as is seen with prolonged bedrest, severe illness, or major surgery; or immobility states, such as limb casts or paralysis. It can also develop when vein valves in the extremities are incompetent, for example, in severe varicose veins. People with polycythemia vera can also develop venous stasis because of a thickening of the blood (hyperviscosity) from a significantly elevated red blood cell count.
- **Hypercoagulability.** Hypercoagulability refers to an abnormal tendency to form thrombi that can be inherited or acquired. Acquired causes include such conditions as cancer, oral contraceptives, sepsis, and others.
- **Venous (endothelial) injury.** Endothelial injury can occur either directly or indirectly. It can result from such predisposing events as surgery or trauma, infection, and central venous catheters.

Table 10–12 lists the most common predisposing factors for development of thromboembolism.

TABLE 10–12 Common Predisposing Factors for Thromboembolism

- Immobilization (three or more consecutive days in the past month)
- Recent surgery (within past three months)
- Malignancy
- Prolonged travel (longer than four hours in past month)
- Previous history of thrombophlebitis

Data from Stein, Beemath et al. (2007).

Emerging Evidence

- In a study of high-acuity patients with heart failure, the combination of acuity level, presence of venous thrombosis risk factors (immobility, acute infection, and COPD), and lack of thromboembolism prophylaxis presented patients with a "triple threat" for increased risk of venous thromboembolism and subsequent right ventricular failure and pulmonary embolism *(Piazza, Seddighzadeh, & Goldhaber, 2008)*.
- The role of corticosteroid use in the treatment of acute respiratory distress syndrome (ARDS) remains controversial. A meta-analysis found that initiation of steroids at the onset of ARDS may reduce number of days on the ventilator and reduce mortality; however, use of corticosteroids as preventive therapy may actually increase ARDS risk in adults with critical illness *(Peter, John et al., 2008)*.
- Current research does not support the need for routine milking or stripping of mediastinal chest tubes after cardiac surgery. The practice of stripping chest tubes generates high negative pressures that may injure tissue and increase bleeding. Chest tube drainage is enhanced by coiling the tubing on the bed and avoiding dependent loops *(Halm, 2007)*.

Pathophysiology of Pulmonary Embolism

The severity of pulmonary embolism depends on the degree of obstruction and location of the embolus (Fig. 10–4). More than half of pulmonary emboli lodge in the main or lobar pulmonary arteries and about 36 percent lodge in the segmental branches (Quinlan et al., 2004). Figure 10–5 illustrates some of the major pathophysiologic events associated with pulmonary embolism. Pulmonary embolism creates a decreased pulmonary vascular bed area and is a major etiology of secondary pulmonary hypertension (Sharma, 2006).

Signs and Symptoms of Pulmonary Embolism

Pulmonary embolism is often a hidden killer because only about 30 percent of patients who die (directly or indirectly from PE) are diagnosed prior to their death (Clemens & Leeper, 2007) and approximately 25 percent of patients with pulmonary embolism die of sudden death (Heit, 2006). Pulmonary embolism often is not easy to recognize or diagnose, particularly when the patient's health status is deteriorating rapidly. Although the presenting manifestations of PE are frequently described in general terms (see Table 10–13), not all episodes of pulmonary embolism present in the same way. Stein and Henry (1997) identified three presenting syndromes that suggest the degree of severity of PE. The syndromes are seen in patients who survive long enough to be evaluated and diagnosed. Stein and Henry, however, also found that patients who have a history of cardiopulmonary diseases may either hide or mimic any of the syndromes. Table 10–14 summarizes three syndromes of pulmonary embolus identified by Stein and Henry (1997).

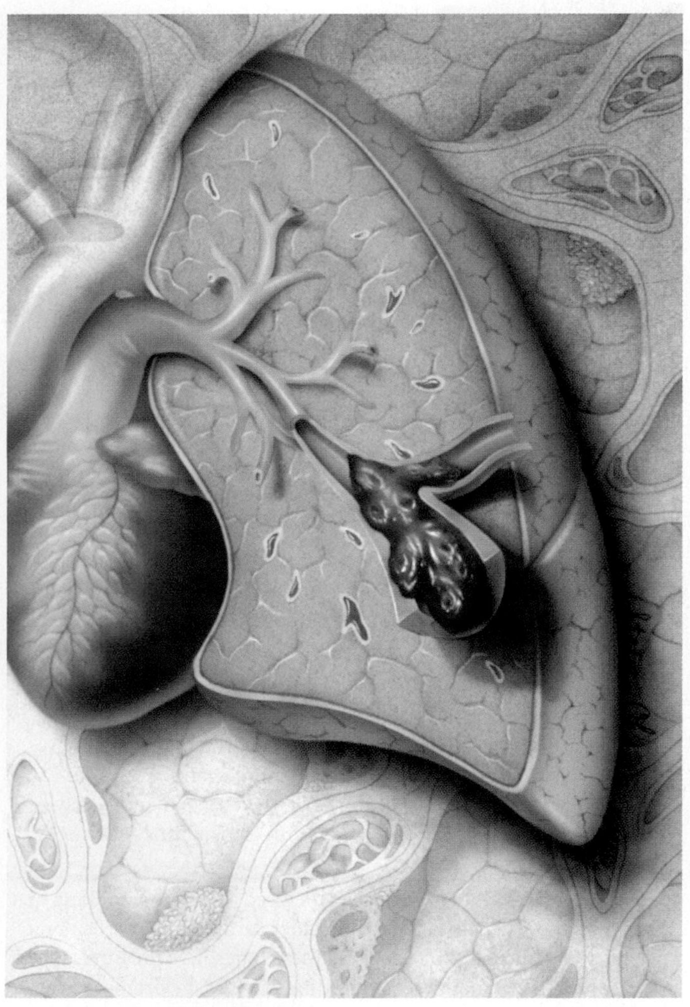

Figure 10–4 ■ A thromboembolism lodged in a pulmonary vessel. (From Phototake NYC)

TABLE 10–13 Common Signs and Symptoms of Pulmonary Embolism in Order of Frequency

Dyspnea
Tachypnea
Pleuritic pain
Cough
Unilateral leg pain and swelling (DVT findings; about 1/3 of PE cases)
Wheezing
Crackles (rales)

Data from Stein, Beemath, Matta et al. (2007).

Diagnosis

Diagnosis of pulmonary embolism frequently is not made until autopsy. The presenting manifestations may not be recognized or may be misinterpreted and there are few tests available for making a definitive diagnosis. Diagnostic testing generally is initiated based on clinical suspicion, such as a positive history and presenting signs and symptoms. A variety of tests are recommended to aid in diagnosis.

Clinical Probability Assessment

Given the difficulty of diagnosing pulmonary embolus, screening tools have been developed to estimate the probability of PE in presenting patients. Two such tools, the Wells Score and Geneva Score, have been studied (Tapson, 2008). These pretests categorize patient risk as low, intermediate, or high probability. The scores are based on presence or past medical history of DVT or PE, immobility or surgery, cancer, vital signs, and other parameters (Tapson, 2008). On calculating the score based on predicting factors, the higher the score the higher the probability of pulmonary embolus. Based on the risk stratification, further diagnostic testing may be warranted or excluded.

D-dimer

D-dimer is a specific type of fibrin degradation product (i.e., a product of fibrin clot breakdown) that increases in the blood following any thrombotic event in the body (e.g., pulmonary

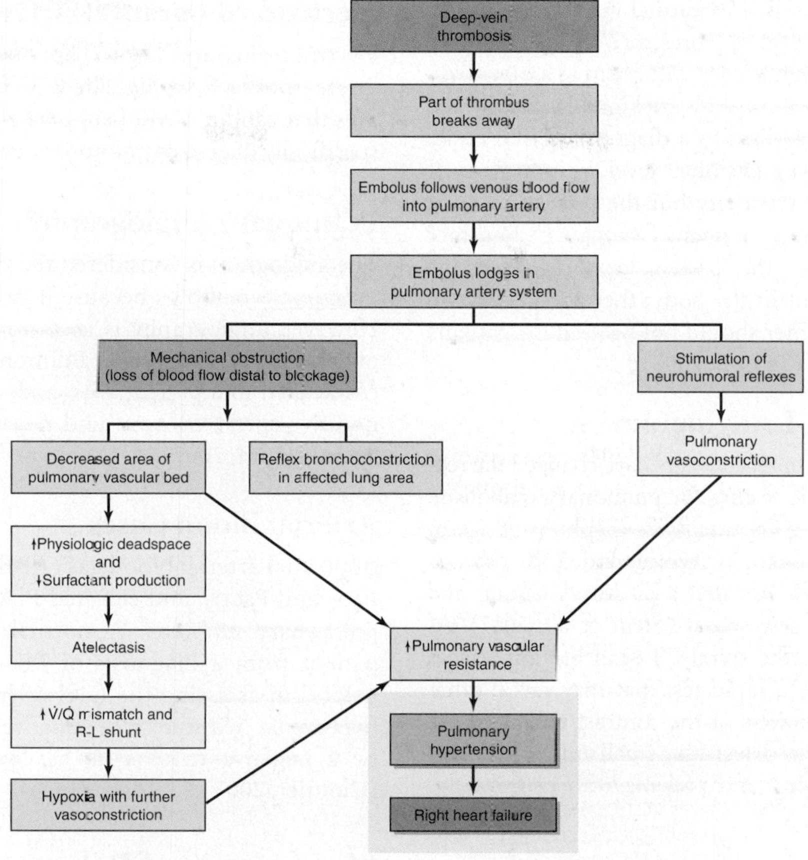

Figure 10–5 ■ Pathophysiology of pulmonary embolus.

TABLE 10–14 Three Syndromes of Pulmonary Embolus Presentation

NAME	FREQUENCY/ SEVERITY[a]	PRESENTING DEFINING CHARACTERISTICS	OTHER SUPPORTIVE DATA
Pulmonary infarction syndrome	Frequency: 65%	Pleuritic pain	Tachypnea, dyspnea, hemoptysis may be present.
	Severity: Mild	Crackles (rales)	Absence of tachycardia ECG: Normal reading is more likely seen than in isolated dyspnea syndrome Chest radiograph: May show atelectasis or lung tissue abnormality and pleural effusion (more commonly noted than in isolated dyspnea syndrome) $\dot{V}/\dot{Q}$ scan probability[b]: Usually intermediate but may be low
Isolated dyspnea syndrome	Frequency: 22% Severity: Moderate	Dyspnea Absence of pleuritic pain and hemoptysis	Tachycardia (greater than 120/min) ECG: T= wave or ST= segment changes may be present or may be normal Chest radiograph: May show atelectasis or lung tissue abnormality and pleural effusion may be present $\dot{V}/\dot{Q}$ scan probability: Usually high but may be intermediate
Circulatory collapse syndrome	Frequency: 8%	Tachycardia	ECG: Likely to show T-wave or ST-segment changes
	Severity: Severe	Hypotension or loss of consciousness	Chest radiograph: May be normal
		Complete right bundle branch block Cardiomegaly Absence of pleural effusion	$\dot{V}/\dot{Q}$ scan probability: High

The defining characteristics of each syndrome were made based on percentage of presence or absence of characteristic.
[a]Frequency is the percentage of occurrence in the study.
[b]$\dot{V}/\dot{Q}$ scan probability: The probability of a positive PE reading on $\dot{V}/\dot{Q}$ scan.
Data from Stein & Henry (1997).

embolus, venous thrombosis, or myocardial infarction). In patients with low or moderate pretest scores, a D-dimer assay may be performed to eliminate pulmonary embolism as a diagnosis. D-dimer levels of less than 1.0 mcg/mL are highly predictive for exclusion of pulmonary embolism as a diagnosis (Hirai et al., 2007). An elevated (positive) D-dimer level is indicative of the presence of thrombolytic activity but the test is too nonspecific to indicate a location. A normal (negative) D-dimer level strongly suggests that the patient has no detectable thrombolytic activity present in the body; therefore, no active pulmonary embolism. D-dimer should not be used for patients with a high-risk Wells score (Tapson, 2008).

Contrast-enhanced CT Angiogram

Technological developments in recent years have changed the recommendations for diagnostic testing for pulmonary embolism. A contrast-enhanced, spiral computed tomographic angiogram (also known as a **spiral CT scan**) is recommended for patients with low- to moderate risk scores and a positive D-dimer and for patients with high risk assessment (Stein et al., 2007). As described by Tapson (2008), the spiral CT scan has advantages over traditional $\dot{V}/\dot{Q}$ scan as a rapid test that may reveal other pulmonary pathology. Limitations of the contrast enhanced CT angiogram include inability to detect very small emboli (subsegmental) in the lung periphery; and patients with contrast dye allergy or renal insufficiency.

Ventilation–Perfusion ($\dot{V}/\dot{Q}$) Scan

A $\dot{V}/\dot{Q}$ scan may be ordered if the D-dimer assay is positive for thrombolytic activity. The $\dot{V}/\dot{Q}$ scan provides information on ventilation and perfusion relationships in areas of the lung. An intermediate- or high-probability abnormal $\dot{V}/\dot{Q}$ scan result supports a diagnosis of PE but is not specific to this diagnosis. $\dot{V}/\dot{Q}$ scan is a diagnostic option for patients with allergy to IV contrast and renal insufficiency when spiral CT scan is contraindicated (Stein et al., 2006).

Compression Ultrasound

Evaluating the patient for DVT is important because of the high percentage of PE being attributed to DVT; thus, ultrasound of both lower extremities may be ordered to rule it out. This test is often performed if the spiral CT scan or $\dot{V}/\dot{Q}$ scan is nondiagnostic. A positive result suspicious of DVT occurs when the vein cannot be fully compressed. This test, in conjunction with unilateral lower extremity swelling, tenderness, redness, and a positive Homan's sign, are strongly suggestive of DVT.

Chest Radiography

Chest X-rays are frequently normal early in the course of a pulmonary embolus and, depending on the severity of the PE, they may remain normal. Atelectasis, pleural effusions, or pulmonary tissue abnormalities may be noted but are nonspecific for PE. For these reasons, chest radiographs are not considered a good diagnostic tool but may be helpful when accompanied by other tests.

Electrocardiograms (ECGs)

Electrocardiograms (ECGs) are often normal and may only indicate sinus tachycardia. The ECG may show certain abnormalities that can be used to support a diagnosis of PE but cannot specifically diagnosis pulmonary embolism.

Pulmonary Angiography

The angiogram is considered the definitive diagnostic test for pulmonary embolus because it can pinpoint the blockage(s). However, angiography is invasive, carries serious risks of its own, and is expensive. Pulmonary angiography may be considered in a patient with high-risk pretest assessment but negative spiral CT scan and negative lower extremity ultrasound (Hunt, 2007).

Arterial Blood Gases

Abnormal arterial blood gas (ABG) results typical of PE (low PaO_2 and $PaCO_2$, and elevated $P[A\text{–}a]O_2$) are nonspecific for pulmonary embolus. A normal PaO_2 cannot exclude the patient from a diagnosis of PE. However, ABG results are helpful in assessing the level of hypoxia present, and severe hypoxemia without wheezing (e.g., asthma) accompanied by a negative chest x-ray is considered suspicious of PE (Cloutier, 2007).

Management of Pulmonary Embolism

Proper management of pulmonary embolism is contingent on diagnosing it, which is often difficult. On diagnosis of pulmonary embolism, a variety of therapy options become available; the issue is in making the diagnosis. Table 10–15 summarizes the major medical treatment options of pulmonary embolism.

Nursing Considerations

Prevention of pulmonary embolism is a priority of nursing care in all high-risk patients. Since the major cause of pulmonary embolism is deep vein thrombosis (DVT), management should center on interventions to prevent DVT. Preventive measures include: early ambulation, anticoagulant therapy, antiembolism stockings, compression boots, elevation of injured leg above heart level, and frequent assessment of injured leg for signs of DVT for early recognition and treatment. Deep vein thrombosis may not have any signs or symptoms; however, when present they may include unilateral leg swelling, pain or tenderness, or cramping.

Pulmonary embolism is a potential complication (PC) rather than a nursing diagnosis; therefore, it requires a collaborative practice model. This means that, in addition to addressing any appropriate nursing diagnoses, the nurse also focuses on administering treatments as ordered by the physician or the advanced practice nurse, monitoring for status changes, and monitoring for the therapeutic and nontherapeutic effects of prescribed treatments.

TABLE 10–15 Summary of Medical Treatment Options for Pulmonary Embolism

MEDICAL THERAPY	TREATMENT/COMMENTS
General	Hospitalization recommended for anyone suspected of pulmonary embolism Oxygen therapy and airway management (as required) Management of shock (as required)
Anticoagulant therapy	Time of initiation: Immediately when diagnosis of pulmonary embolism is established Type ■ Heparin (either UH or LMWH) ■ Usually administered for five to six days. Discontinued when INR has been therapeutic for two days consecutively ■ Loading dose followed by continuous IV drip. ■ May be ordered for home management (subcutaneously) ■ Unfractionated heparin (UH) ■ First 24 hours—use sliding scale dose based on APTT ■ Draw APTT every six hours for first 24 hours then once daily ■ Low-molecular-weight heparin (LMWH) ■ Routine lab monitoring may not be required ■ Warfarin ■ May also be initiated at same time as heparin therapy ■ Goal: Maintain prothrombin time at INR 2.0–3.0 ■ May be ordered for three to six months or indefinitely
Vena Cava Filter	Indications: Situations in which patients cannot be anticoagulated (e.g., GI bleeding); major bleeding while on anticoagulation; recurrent PE on therapy. Recent advancement: temporary removable filters
Thrombolytic therapy	Indication: Circulatory collapse; emergency situation Risks: Bleeding, especially intracranial hemorrhage
Embolectomy	Catheter embolectomy Indication: Massive PE with shock, thrombolytic therapy contraindicated. Surgical Embolectomy: Indication: If emergency thrombolytic therapy is not successful, requires cardiopulmonary bypass; often used as a last resort to save patient; associated with high mortality

UH=Unfractionated Heparin; LMWH=Low-molecular-weight Heparin; INR=International Normalized Ratio; APTT=Activated Partial thromboplastin time.
Data from Piazza & Goldhaber (2006).

Carpenito-Moyet (2008) suggests the following interventions for pulmonary embolism (not including potential interventions unique to air or fat embolism):

- Monitor for signs and symptoms of pulmonary embolism
- Initiate shock protocols if manifestations of PE develop
- Initiate O_2 therapy and monitor SpO_2 or SaO_2
- Monitor labs: ABG, CBC, Electrolytes, BUN
- Initiate thrombolytic therapy as ordered
- Initiate and monitor heparin therapy as ordered following thrombolytic therapy
- Monitor clotting times
- Monitor closely for abnormal bleeding when patient is receiving thrombolytics or anticoagulant therapy

The major nursing diagnoses that are typically appropriate in care of the patient with pulmonary embolism include:

- Immobility
- Impaired gas exchange
- Risk for ineffective peripheral tissue perfusion
- Risk for ineffective respiratory function
- Ineffective breathing pattern
- Chest pain
- Fear/anxiety
- Knowledge deficit

SECTION FOUR REVIEW

1. The most common type of pulmonary embolism is
A. venous air
B. amniotic
C. thrombus
D. fat

2. Which type of embolism manifests itself as dyspnea, tachypnea, neurological symptoms, AND petechiae?
A. venous air
B. amniotic
C. thrombus
D. fat

(continued)

(continued)

3. Venous (endothelial) injury is one of three major factors that causes formation of deep-vein thrombosis. This type of injury can result from
   A. immobility
   B. sepsis
   C. surgery
   D. varicose veins
4. Which factor determines the severity of a pulmonary embolus?
   A. type of embolus
   B. degree of obstruction
   C. speed of onset
   D. general health of patient
5. The most common predisposing factor for development of thromboembolism is
   A. immobility
   B. postsurgery status
   C. malignancy
   D. coronary artery disease
6. Mechanical obstruction of a pulmonary vessel results in
   A. vasodilation
   B. atelectasis
   C. decreased vascular resistance
   D. left heart failure
7. Common signs and symptoms of pulmonary embolism include
   A. rhonchi
   B. pneumothorax
   C. dyspnea
   D. bradycardia
8. The most common clinical presentation of someone with a pulmonary embolism is seen with pulmonary infarction syndrome. The defining characteristics of the syndrome include
   A. absence of pleuritic pain
   B. pleuritic pain
   C. hypotension
   D. hemoptysis
9. Under what circumstances is surgical embolectomy usually done?
   A. if heparin therapy is unsuccessful
   B. if symptoms are severe
   C. if patient is unconscious
   D. if thrombolytic therapy is unsuccessful
10. The definitive test to diagnose a pulmonary embolism is
    A. angiography
    B. $\dot{V}/\dot{Q}$ scan
    C. D-dimer
    D. compression ultrasound
11. The major initial treatment for pulmonary embolism is
    A. thrombolytic therapy
    B. surgical embolectomy
    C. oxygen therapy
    D. anticoagulant therapy

Answers: 1. C, 2. D, 3. C, 4. B, 5. A, 6. B, 7. C, 8. B, 9. D, 10. A, 11. D

SECTION FIVE: Acute Respiratory Infections

At the completion of this section, the learner will be able to discuss the pathogenesis and management of acute respiratory infections including pneumonia and severe acute respiratory syndrome (SARS).

The lower respiratory tract is normally sterile. When the lung is exposed to pathogens, immune defenses are typically sufficient to resist infection. Microorganisms that gain access to the lung may cause infection, such as bronchitis or pneumonia when host defenses are overwhelmed. Pneumonia is the far more serious infection and poses a serious problem in the U.S. It is the leading cause of death from infection and is the sixth most common cause of death (Niederman, 2008).

Pneumonia

Classification

Traditionally, pneumonia has been classified according to the patient's location when the infection was contracted; for example, at home in the community ("community-acquired") or in the hospital ("nosocomial"). The typical microorganisms in these two categories were sufficiently different that antibiotic recommendations could be made based on the most likely pathogens. The categories were useful in guiding early and appropriate antibiotic therapy.

In recent years, there is recognition that patient location and exposures have become more complex. Patients may not be hospitalized, yet may be exposed to health-care environments such as long-term care facilities or outpatient treatment centers. Potential organisms in these settings are different than "community-acquired" in that they more closely resemble hospital bacteria and are often multi-drug resistant. Within the hospital, the distinction is also made between patients on mechanical ventilation (ventilator-associated pneumonia) and non-ventilated patients. New terminology has been developed to describe the categories (Table 10–16).

Microbiology and pathogenesis

The type of pathogen responsible for pneumonia varies somewhat by the location of the exposure. For example, in the United States, typical CAP is most likely to be *Streptococcus pneumoniae (pneumococcus)* [National Heart Lung and Blood Institute (2008)]. Other common community-acquired pathogens include *S. aureus* and *H. influenzae*. Atypical CAP pathogens include *Legionella, Mycoplasma pneumoniae*, and others. *S. pneumoniae* infections can be particularly severe, with about 50 percent of

TABLE 10–16 Classifications of Pneumonia

PNEUMONIA CATEGORIES	DESCRIPTION
Hospital-acquired (Nosocomial) Pneumonia (HAP)	Develops 48 hours or more after admiss on to the hospital and was not incubating prior to admission Highest increase in morbidity/mortality of all nosocomial infections Increases length of hospital stay Highest incidence is ICU setting while on mechanical ventilation (see VAP)
Ventilator-associated Pneumonia (VAP)	A subtype of HAP Develops at least 24 hours after intubation for mechanical ventilation and was not incubating prior to intubation Usually develops within four days of intubation Risk for developing pneumonia is six to twenty times greater in ventilated patients compared to other hospitalized patients
Healthcare-associated Pneumonia (HCAP)	Pneumonia that occurs within two days of admission when the patient has the following risk factors: ■ Resident of long-term care facility ■ Hospitalized within 30 days ■ Long-term hemodialysis
Community-acquired Pneumonia (CAP)	Pneumonia present on admission in a patient not previously hospitalized or in outpatient treatment

Data from Kollef, Shorr, Tabak, Gupta, Liu & Johannes (2005); and Marrie, Campbell, Walker, and Low (2005).

cases requiring hospital admission (Marrie, Campbell et al., 2005). The common pathogens associated with VAP include *P. aeruginosa*, *Acinetobacter*, *Enterobacter*, and others (Schmitt & Longworth, 2009). The spread of antibiotic-resistant strains of bacteria is an increasing concern for treatment of both community and hospital acquired pneumonia. The occurrence of methicillin-resistant *S. aureus* (MRSA) pneumonia is on the increase. In the critical care hospital environment, MRSA pneumonia increases the risk of bacteremia, septic shock, and death (Marrie, Campbell et al., 2005). MRSA and MSSA (methicillin-susceptible *S. aureus*) are both associated with increased mortality. Furthermore, *Enterobacteriaceae*, which accounts for about 30 percent of pneumonias in ICU is becoming resistant to cephalosporin therapy. Ventilator-associated pneumonia is presented in more detail in Module 11, *Supporting Pulmonary Gas Exchange: Mechanical Ventilation.*

To cause infection, organisms must gain access to the lung and overwhelm the defense mechanisms. Patients can become exposed to pathogens by a variety of routes, including aspiration of oral flora or gastric contents (microaspiration or large volume), airborne spread, direct inoculation (e.g., via endotracheal tube), through the bloodstream, or spread from adjacent infections (e.g., abscess). Additional factors influence the incidence and severity of pneumonia. The elderly are particularly vulnerable to viral infection, as are immunocompromised patients. Underlying chronic conditions (comorbidities) such as COPD, heart disease, and diabetes; as well as smoking and alcohol abuse are also identified risk factors (Niederman, 2008).

Clinical Presentation

The classic signs and symptoms associated with pneumonia include acute onset of cough, fever, chills, purulent sputum, pleuritic chest pain and shortness of breath (Schmitt & Longworth, 2009). There is considerable variation in presentation, however, depending on the infecting pathogen. A category of infections called "atypical pneumonias" (e.g., Legionella) may have a gradual onset over days with fever, headache, gastrointestinal symptoms, and dry cough. Pneumonia in the elderly may appear as dyspnea, confusion and heart failure without fever or cough (Schmitt & Longworth, 2009). These authors suggest that, especially in the elderly, an increased respiratory rate warrants additional assessment because it may indicate development of pneumonia.

The severity of pneumonia varies greatly as does the clinical presentation. Where to treat the patient (outpatient, general ward, ICU) is another decision that must be made. Patients with mild disease are frequently treated as outpatients with antibiotic regimens geared toward likely community-acquired pathogens. More serious symptoms or risk factors require hospital admission. Patients with severe CAP should be admitted to an ICU or high-acuity monitoring unit (Mandell et al., 2007). Evidence-based criteria are available that assist in determining the seriousness of pneumonia. Table 10–17 provides an example of criteria that can be used to quickly evaluate the need for hospitalization and possible ICU (Tazkarji, 2008; Marrie, Campbell et al., 2005). The CURB-65 is one example of a simple guide for evaluation of the severity of CAP. There are other, more complex sets of criteria available, as well (Mandell, Wunderink et al., 2007). The CURB-65 criteria include five risk factors: confusion, urea nitrogen, respiratory rate, blood pressure, and age. Each criterion has a value of one point and the patient is assigned one point for each criterion present. The higher the score, the more severe is the pneumonia. A score of 3 or greater is associated with increased mortality and hospitalization and possible ICU admission should be considered. A low serum albumin (less than 3.0 g/dL) is an additional criterion that significantly influences the seriousness of pneumonia. In the high-acuity population, hypoalbuminemia is an important risk factor for increased mortality (Tazkarji, 2008). A P/F ratio of less than 250 and the need for vasopressor therapy are also sometimes included in severe pneumonia criteria.

TABLE 10–17 CURB-65 Severe Pneumonia Criteria

CRITERIA	POINTS
C – Confusion; altered level of consciousness	1
U – BUN (greater than 19.6 mg/dL)	1
R- Respiratory rate (30 or greater breaths/minute)	1
B – Blood pressure (SBP less than 90; DBP less than 60)	1
65- Patient age is 65 or older	1

(Additional criteria to consider: serum albumin less than 3.0 g/dL; P/F ratio less than 250; vasopressor therapy for greater than four hours.)

Treatment of Pneumonia

Extensive guidelines have been written on the treatment of pneumonia (Mandell et al., 2007). For example, the Institutes for Healthcare Improvement (n.d.) recommends an adult pneumonia admission order bundle that includes blood cultures, assessment of oxygenation, screening for pneumococcal infection and influenza, smoking history and cessation information, and recommendations for admission and antibiotic regimens.

Early and appropriate antibiotic therapies are important elements to improve patient outcomes in pneumonia (Mandell et al., 2007). *Early* has been described as within four hours of diagnosis (Niederman, 2008) or while the patient is in the setting where the diagnosis is made (e.g., emergency department) (Mandell et al., 2007). Initial antibiotics are selected to cover likely organisms and high-risk infections. When microbiologic data from cultures is available, the antibiotics are changed/narrowed to cover the identified pathogens if needed.

Twenty to 40 percent of patients with pneumonia develop pleural effusions (parapneumonic effusions). Such pleural effusions may become infected and pose two problems: continued sepsis and the risk of pleural thickening from the fibrotic, inflammatory process. Large pleural effusions associated with pneumonia require sampling of the pleural fluid and drainage, usually with a chest tube, if the fluid is considered high risk for infection (Light, 2006).

Prevention of Pneumonia

Prevention strategies aimed at decreasing the incidence of community-acquired pneumonia include influenza and pneumococcal vaccines and smoking cessation. Centers for Disease Control (CDC) guidelines now require assessment of vaccination status and administration of vaccine to appropriate patients while in the hospital. Smoking is a risk factor for pneumonia; patients should be encouraged to stop smoking and offered educational materials (Mandell et al., 2007). Strategies to prevent ventilator-associated pneumonia (VAP) are presented in Module 11.

Diagnosis of Pneumonia

Diagnostic testing is done to determine whether a patient has pneumonia and to identify the causative organism (Niederman, 2008). Diagnosis of pneumonia presents several challenges depending on the organism involved. In many cases, the pathogen is never identified. Chest X-rays are important for establishing a baseline to monitor changes, and for helping differentiate pneumonia from other pulmonary disorders. The following diagnostic and laboratory tests are used in this setting to help identify the pathogen involved and the severity of disease (Table 10–18).

TABLE 10–18 Diagnostic and Laboratory Tests for the Diagnosis of Pneumonia

ROUTINE TESTS	SPECIAL DIAGNOSTIC TESTS
Chest radiograph	Bronchoscopy
Sputum culture and gram stain	Thoracentesis
Blood cultures	Lung biopsy
Complete blood count	Serology for antigens and antibodies
Blood chemistries	
Pulse oximetry, arterial blood gas	

Data from Schmitt & Longworth (2009).

Aspiration Pneumonia

Aspiration plays a particularly important role as a complication of high-acuity illnesses; thus it is presented here in greater detail. Aspiration, the entry of oral secretions or gastric contents into the lower respiratory tract, is the cause of CAP in 10 percent of all patients and up to 30 percent of patients admitted from long-term care (Shigemitsu & Afshar, 2007). There are two different aspiration syndromes: aspiration pneumonitis and aspiration pneumonia.

Aspiration Pneumonitis

Aspiration of acidic gastric contents results in aspiration pneumonitis, resulting in acute lung injury due to a chemical injury (Marik, 2005). Inflammation, not infection, results from aspiration as the acidic gastric juices trigger an inflammatory response that results in damage to exposed airway tissues.

Aspiration Pneumonia

Aspiration pneumonia may result when oral secretions or colonized gastric secretions reach the lung. Gastric contents can become colonized with bacteria when the gastric pH is alkalinized (e.g., use of acid-reducing medications or enteral feedings) (Marik, 2005). It is estimated that 50 percent of healthy people aspirate small volumes of secretions while sleeping; however, pneumonia does not normally occur because of effective lung protective mechanisms. Pneumonia results when the volume of aspirate is larger, contains pathogens, or the natural defenses are impaired.

Major risk factors for aspiration include: decreased level of consciousness, an incompetent lower esophageal sphincter (e.g., GERD); elevated pressure or volume in the stomach; and neuromuscular diseases that alter glottic closure (Marrie, Campbell et al., 2005). Two additional risk factors are poor oral hygiene, which increases the bacterial load in oral secretions, and **dysphagia** (impaired swallowing) (Palmer & Metheny, 2008). The presence of tubes through the lower esophageal sphincter (LES), such as nasogastric tubes or feeding tubes, prevents the LES from closing fully, and may contribute to aspiration risk due to reflux of gastric contents.

Clinical Manifestations of Aspiration

The exact clinical presentation depends on the type and volume of aspirant. The position of the patient at the time of aspiration will dictate where the pneumonia or pneumonitis develops (i.e., what part of the lung the aspirant locates). Table 10–19 lists some of the major clinical features of aspiration.

Prevention of Aspiration Syndromes

Reducing the incidence of aspiration requires a multidisciplinary approach (Shigemitsu & Afashar, 2007). In addition to identifying patients at risk, nurses must recognize signs of aspiration such as coughing, drooling, development of a hoarse

TABLE 10–19 Clinical Features of Aspiration Syndromes

Aspiration Pneumonitis
Acute onset of:
Tachypnea
Dyspnea
Bronchospasm
Cyanosis
Chest X-ray: Diffuse opacities
Aspiration Pneumonia
Presentation is that of bacterial pneumonias

Data from Marrie, Campbell et al. (2005).

voice or gurgling sounds associated with eating. Assessment by a speech pathologist can identify measures such as positioning and food consistency to improve swallowing (Palmer & Metheny, 2008). Oral care in all at-risk patients reduces the incidence of aspiration pneumonia (Marik, 2005) as does elevation of the head of the bed at least 30 degrees.

Viral Pneumonias

When we think of pneumonia, we tend to focus on its bacterial forms; however, pneumonia caused by viruses, particularly the influenza virus, constitutes a significant percentage of pneumonia cases that occur each year. Furthermore, there are emerging viral infections that have the potential to become the world's next viral pandemics.

Influenza Viral Pneumonia

Viral pneumonia is a serious-to-severe complication of influenza, more commonly referred to as "the flu." In 2007, over 34,000 confirmed cases of influenza were documented, with 74 percent being classified as influenza A viruses and 26 percent being influenza B viruses (CDC, 2008). There are three types of influenza-related pneumonias, including

- Primary viral pneumonia – Caused by the influenza virus
- Secondary bacterial pneumonia – Develops directly following influenza
- Mixed viral and bacterial pneumonia – Concurrent infections

Primary viral pneumonia is a complication of influenza, usually type A. While it is the least common influenza-related pneumonia, it is the most severe and deadly of the three types.

Clinical Presentation and Diagnosis. Primary viral pneumonia presents as flu that, rather than resolving after a few days, continues to become progressively worse. The patient develops progressive dyspnea that begins several days after the onset of flu symptoms; a persistent fever; and eventual onset of cyanosis (Dolin, 2005; Japanese Respiratory Society, 2006). As with most pure viral infections, sputum is scanty but blood may be present due to sloughing of necrosed airway tissue. As the pneumonia progresses, the chest x-ray usually shows diffuse infiltrates that will have a similar pattern to acute respiratory distress syndrome (ARDS). People at particular risk for primary viral pneumonia are those with cardiac disease (Dolin, 2005). Diagnosis is difficult and is usually made on the basis of a confirmed influenza virus, the presence of antigens, and elevated serum antibody titre in the absence of leukocytosis or purulent sputum (both suggest bacterial origin) (Japanese Respiratory Society, 2006).

Mixed viral and bacterial pneumonia is the most common complication of influenza. People with chronic respiratory or cardiac disease are at highest risk for developing the mixed type. The clinical presentation is more typical of bacterial pneumonia. Diagnostically, a sputum specimen will typically show influenza A and a bacterial pathogen. The chest X-ray appears patchier (more focal) than seen on primary viral pneumonia – a pattern more typical of bacterial pneumonia. In April, 2009 a novel form of the seasonal influenza type A (H1N1) was first detected. The virus is of swine origin and is believed to have originated in Mexico, rapidly spreading into the United States and internationally. As with many other seasonal influenza viruses, transmission is airborne via large-particle droplet through coughing and sneezing. The incubation is short at 1 to 7 days or less. As with all forms of influenza, certain populations are at increased risk for development of complications, particularly children less than 5 years of age and older adults over the age of 65. Complications, such as viral pneumonia are a particular risks in these vulnerable populations.

Treatment. Influenza pneumonia has a poor prognosis; however, it has shown improvement with the advancement of antiviral drug therapy. Treatment may include antiviral agents, and possible use of antimicrobials or immunoglobulin therapy (Japanese Respiratory Society, 2006).

Avian Influenza Pneumonia

Worldwide, health organizations are closely monitoring the avian (H5N1) virus, as a potential pandemic virus. Currently few humans have contracted the virus and the flu has only developed in humans with close direct contact with infected birds. The concern is that while the H5N1virus has not yet bridged the species (human-bird) barrier, it will eventually mutate sufficiently to allow human-to-human transmission; thereby triggering rapid spread as occurred with the SARS-CoV virus. Avian influenza can result in a viral pneumonia and has a poor prognosis, with a high mortality rate. As seen with SARS CoV, there is no vaccine or definitive treatment for avian influenza.

Severe Acute Respiratory Syndrome (SARS)

Severe acute respiratory syndrome (SARS) was first described in 2003 as an atypical pneumonia when it suddenly appeared. The virus that causes SARS (SARS-CoV) is actually a novel form of coronavirus (CoV), which is a major cause of the common cold worldwide, and usually affects the upper respiratory tract. The unique SARS-CoV is suspected to have originated as a nonhuman virus, possibly in bats, that jumped to humans (Gu & Korteweg, 2007). Fortunately, the SARS epidemic was short lived, lasting from November 2002 through May 2003, with 28 countries reporting a total of 8096 cases of SARS (WHO, 2004). Incidence is now low and cases are isolated. The world was caught unprepared for the sudden emergence of SARS; this is a good example of the potential seriousness of viral mutations that can spread not only quickly but lethally in pandemic proportions.

Transmission. Transmission of SARS-CoV is by airborne droplet (e.g., cough, secretions) or aerosol (e.g., humidifier) in close person-to-person contact. It may also spread by droplet without close contact and on environmental surfaces (Hirsch, 2007). Transmission of the virus to health care workers was an important feature in the outbreaks in Hong Kong and Toronto (Booth et al., 2005).

Clinical Presentation and Course. SARS presents in two stages. The most common presenting symptoms are flu-like and include fever (greater than 100.5°F, or 38°C), chills, severe myalgias, weakness, headache and, occasionally, diarrhea. These early symptoms are followed by respiratory symptoms of dry cough and dyspnea within three to seven days. Respiratory symptoms may progress to hypoxic failure requiring mechanical ventilation (Hirsch, 2007). Most patients are discharged without complications by day 14 postadmission. However, Lew and colleagues (2003) reported that about 25 percent of SARS patients in their study progressed to ALI/ARDS.

Diagnosing SARS. Diagnosing SARS is difficult because it initially presents as an atypical pneumonia. Initial diagnosis is based on history of possible exposure (major criterion), clinical presentation, and laboratory testing. Tests can identify the virus via culturing respiratory secretions and sampling secretions or blood for reverse transcriptase; further, patients are positive for antibodies within 28 days of onset (Dolin, 2005). Actual tests and diagnostic procedures primarily are those recommended for other types of pneumonia.

The worldwide outbreak of SARS was contained through the cooperation of multiple agencies. Lessons learned from SARS have application for other infectious diseases. These include the importance of public health preparation and response systems, strict implementation of infection control measures and training of personnel (Rothman et al., 2006).

SECTION FIVE REVIEW

1. Community-acquired pneumonias (CAPs) are best described as pneumonia that
   A. incubated prior to hospital admission
   B. incubated within 24 hours of hospital admission
   C. developed 48 hours or more after hospital admission
   D. does not require hospitalization
2. The most common pneumonia pathogen in the United States is
   A. *H. influenzae*
   B. *S. pneumoniae*
   C. *S. aureus*
   D. *Mycoplasma pneumoniae*
3. Which statement is correct regarding MRSA pneumonia in high-acuity patients?
   A. It causes a chronic, low level infection.
   B. It increases the risk for bacteremia and septic shock.
   C. It has a low mortality risk.
   D. About 50 percent of cases require hospitalization.
4. The effect of aspiration of low pH gastric contents has on lung tissue is
   A. destruction of the pulmonary capillaries
   B. growth of resistant gastric pathogens
   C. consolidation from flooding the lungs
   D. damage via the inflammatory response
5. Risk factors for aspiration include: (choose all that apply)
   A. incompetent lower esophageal sphincter
   B. age greater than 65 years
   C. decreased level of consciousness
   D. elevated gastric pressure
   E. gender is male
6. According to the CURB-65 severity of CAP criteria, which value is considered a risk factor?
   A. BUN of 15 mg/dL
   B. hemoglobin less than 10
   C. respiratory rate of 28 breaths/min.
   D. systolic BP less than 90 mmHg
7. Viral influenza pneumonia typically presents in which way?
   A. productive cough with purulent thick sputum
   B. progressive dyspnea and persistent fever
   C. pleuritis and copious sputum
   D. night sweats and harsh dry cough
8. People who are at greatest risk for development of viral pneumonia are those with a history of
   A. cardiac or pulmonary disease
   B. diabetes mellitus
   C. chronic renal failure
   D. previous viral pneumonia
9. The pathogen that causes SARS is a unique form of which virus?
   A. hantavirus
   B. coronavirus
   C. rhinovirus
   D. influenza–A virus
10. Which statement is correct regarding the clinical features of the SARS virus?
   A. a persistent dry cough is present
   B. the chest radiograph is usually normal
   C. the patient has been experiencing hemoptysis
   D. the incubation period is 10 days to 2 weeks
11. The SARS virus is known to be transmitted by
   A. contaminated feces
   B. blood contact
   C. tears
   D. airborne droplets

Answers: 1. A, 2. C, A 3. B, 4. D, 5. (A, C, D), 6. D, 7. B, 8. A, 9. B, 10. A, 11. D

SECTION SIX: Thoracic Surgery and Chest Tubes

At the completion of this section, the learner will be able to describe the principles and management of patients undergoing thoracic surgery and chest drainage.

Thoracic Surgery

The term "thoracic surgery" applies to procedures on the structures within the chest: heart, lungs, esophagus and great vessels. This section will focus on surgery involving the lungs. Disorders commonly treated with thoracic surgery include lung cancer, emphysema, localized infection of the lung and pleura (e.g., abscess, empyema), injuries, lung transplantation, and chest wall deformities.

Thoracic Surgery Terminology

The surgical entry into the thorax is called a thoracotomy. Thoracic surgery for lung resection is categorized by the amount of lung tissue removed, as follows:

- **Pneumonectomy**–Removal of one entire lung and creation of a "stump" (the sutured end of a main bronchus)
- Removal of smaller portions of the lung are described by the lung anatomy:
    - **Lobectomy**–Removal of one or more lobes of the lung
    - **Segmentectomy**–Removal of one or more portions (segments) of a lobe
    - **Wedge resection**–Removal of a small wedge-shaped section of the peripheral portion of the lung

Pneumonectomy

Pneumonectomy is an old procedure dating back to 1895 as a treatment for tuberculosis (TB) (Cerfolio, 2007). Today, pneumonectomy is used primarily in the treatment of lung cancer. Despite surgical improvements, pneumonectomy remains a high-risk procedure with mortality estimates of 3 percent to 12 percent for cancer surgery and higher for inflammatory diseases such as TB (Cerfolio, 2007).

In the pneumonectomy procedure, the lung and vessels are removed. When thoracotomy is performed, opening the chest wall breaks the integrity of the negative pleural space; thus, the lung on the thoracotomy side collapses. Postoperatively, the cavity fills with serosanguineous fluid and, eventually, fibrotic tissue. Because there is no remaining lung to expand, a chest tube is not required; however, one may be placed to detect postoperative bleeding. Potential complications associated with pneumonectomy include vocal cord dysfunction (nerve injury during the procedure), atrial arrhythmias, pulmonary edema, bronchopleural fistula and empyema resulting from breakdown of the stump suture line, and postpneumonectomy syndrome. Pulmonary edema may result from the dramatic change in hemodynamics with the entire blood volume now directed through the pulmonary vessels of the remaining lung. Postpneumonectomy syndrome is a tracheal obstruction caused by abnormal shifting of the intrathoracic structures.

Thoracic Incisions

Thoracotomy incisions used in thoracic procedures vary depending on the size and area to be resected. Posterolateral incisions extend from the scapula/spine to the anterior axillary line. This is the traditional incision that allows extensive view of the chest cavity. A smaller incision, axillary thoracotomy, also called "muscle sparing," is used for smaller procedures. Other approaches include anterior, median sternotomy (used for cardiac surgery) and the "clamshell" incision, used primarily for bilateral lung transplantation (Marshall, 2007).

Video-Assisted Thoracoscopic Surgery (VATS). VATS is the thoracic equivalent to minimally invasive laparoscopic abdominal surgery. Using a scope and small incisions, VATS is used for both diagnostic and therapeutic procedures. Common diagnostic procedures in which VATS is used include sampling of pleural effusions, biopsy of lung tissue, nodules, and mediastinal nodes. VATS is also used to treat persistent pleural effusions, repair pneumothorax and for lung resections. Advantages cited for the VATS procedure versus open thoracotomy include decreased pain, fewer complications and shorter length of stay in the hospital (Khraim, 2007).

Postthoracic Surgery Management

Important considerations for post surgery management are the common issues of postoperative positioning, pain management, postoperative pulmonary hygiene, and early mobilization to prevent complications.

Postoperative Positioning. Postoperative positioning for the pneumonectomy differs from other types of lung resection. These patients may be positioned on their back or lying on the operative side, but should not be turned onto the unaffected lung. Positioning the patient on the operative side results in some degree of mediastinal shift into the empty space as it fills with fluid. Placing the patient on the unaffected side could cause mediastinal and fluid shifts toward the remaining lung, potentially compromising the patient's respiratory status.Patients undergoing the other types of lung resection may be turned from side to side and will have chest tubes.

Pain Management. Postthoracic surgical pain is significant due to retraction of the ribs and in some cases rib dissection, muscle dissection, possible nerve injury, and chest tubes. Postoperative pain is controlled with PCA or epidural catheters (see Module 4, Acute Pain Management, for details on these methods). Pain control is especially important to prevent postoperative hypoventilation and impaired cough that may result in atelectasis and respiratory failure.

Pulmonary Hygiene. Optimizing pulmonary hygiene, always a concern after surgery, becomes an even greater priority following thoracic surgery. In addition to the incision and pain, these patients commonly have underlying lung disease. Assessment of pre-operative function and sputum production are important to guide treatment and evaluate the effectiveness of therapy. Effective cough is essential for adequate airway clearance, but will cause pain. Pharmacologic control of pain must be balanced to avoid over-sedation and respiratory depression.

Post-thoracic surgery patients must be able to take a deep breath and generate an exhalation sufficiently strong to clear secretions. Two modifications of the standard cough may be helpful to use for patients with chest wall pain from the surgery. The first, the

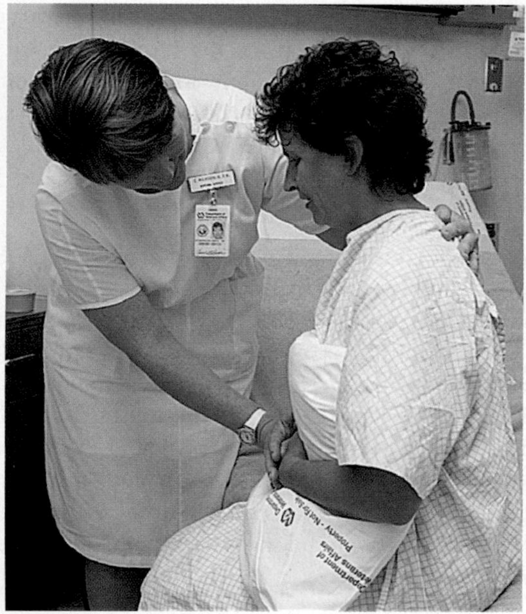

Figure 10–6 ■ Splinting abdomen while coughing.

"cascade" cough, is a series of three to four coughs on one exhalation. Repeated several time, this technique moves peripheral secretions. The "huff" cough is another modification in which the patient coughs with the glottis open. This cough is a gentler maneuver and is effective for patients with emphysema and for postoperative patients. Splinting the incisional area will also decrease pain with cough. One effective method is to use a folded towel wrapped around the chest (e.g., lateral incision). To splint, the patient crosses the hands and holds the end of the towel, pulling tighter during the cough (Fig 10–6). A modification for a posterolateral incision is to use a folded sheet wrapped over the shoulder, across the incision in back and under the arm. Again, the ends of the sheet are pulled tighter with the cough to splint the incision.

Chest Drainage Management

The remainder of Section Six provides an overview of chest drainage principles and management through presentation of two cases that will be used to describe chest drainage management.

CASE 1

Nineteen-year-old T.J. was thrown from his motorcycle onto the hood of a vehicle approaching from the opposite direction. He was stabilized at the scene by the rescue squad and rapidly transferred to a nearby hospital emergency department (ED). On arrival at the ED, a rapid assessment revealed the following: T.J. was oriented and complaining of severe left chest pain. Chest contusions were noted on the left upper chest. He was tachypneic with circumoral cyanosis noted. Chest auscultation revealed positive breath sounds on the right but negative breath sounds in the left upper lung field. A portable chest X-ray showed multiple left rib fractures and left hemopneumothorax—preparations were made for immediate chest tube placement.

CASE 2

M.T., a 55-year-old woman, was admitted to the hospital with a diagnosis of "exacerbation of COPD." She has been receiving intermittent positive pressure breathing (IPPB) therapy, oxygen at 2 L per nasal cannula, and a bronchodilator drug. This afternoon, M.T. suddenly developed sharp right side chest pain and increased shortness of breath. Her nurse was unable to auscultate breath sounds in the right upper anterior lung field during a rapid focused respiratory assessment. A portable chest X-ray was taken, showing a right upper lobe pneumothorax. Chest drainage was initiated with one chest tube being inserted on the right side of M.T.'s chest.

Chest Drainage

Chest drainage is the active or passive removal of air or fluid from the intrapleural space of the lungs or from the mediastinal compartment. Chest drainage may be a short term or intermittent therapy (e.g., aspiration of intrapleural air or fluid using a needle and syringe); or it may be relatively long-term therapy (e.g., treatment of pneumothorax or hemothorax resulting from chest trauma).

Who Requires Chest Drainage?

Both T.J. and M.T. required chest drainage, but for different reasons. Chest drainage is used to treat thoracic problems that may be external or internal in origin. External origins include blunt chest trauma, and traumatic or surgical entry into the intrapleural or mediastinal spaces, resulting in pneumothorax or hemothorax (see Fig. 10–7). **Pneumothorax** (sometimes referred to as "pneumo") refers to the abnormal presence of air in the intrapleural space, whereas **hemothorax** refers to the abnormal presence of blood in the intrapleural space. Frequently both pneumothorax and hemothorax exist simultaneously (**hemopneumothorax**). T.J.'s case is an example of an external origin problem. Internal origins of pneumothorax include spontaneous rupture of a pulmonary **bleb**, procedural rupture of the visceral pleura, or barotrauma. Bleb rupture is most commonly found in patients with chronic lung diseases. Barotrauma-induced pneumothorax results from therapies that increase airway pressure and hyperinflate the alveoli. M.T.'s

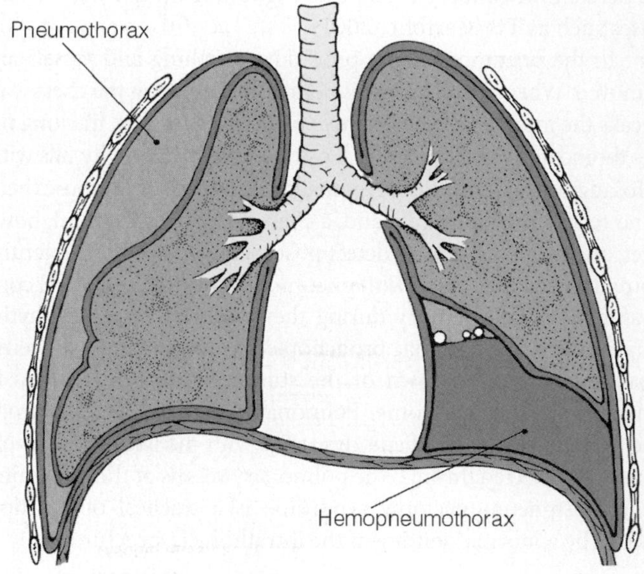

Figure 10–7 ■ Pneumothorax and hemothorax. Pneumothorax refers to air in the intrapleural space and hemothorax refers to blood in the intrapleural space around the lung. A hemopneumothorax, such as depicted here, is a combined problem of having both air and blood in the intrapleural space.

case is an example of an internal origin. Common external and internal origins of pneumothorax are listed in Table 10–20. In addition to treating pneumo- or hemothorax, chest tubes may be inserted to drain severe **pleural effusion** or **empyema** if either condition is causing significant compression of lung tissue.

Pathogenesis of a Collapsed Lung

The thorax and lungs exist as opposing forces (i.e., the thorax's natural state is expansion, whereas the lungs' natural state is collapsed). Normal lung inflation depends on the intactness of the two pleural linings, which act as a single unit because of a state of negative intrapleural pressure; thus, as the thorax expands during inhalation, the lungs expand with it. Loss of negative intrapleural pressure, either of external or internal origin, results in rapid collapse (atelectasis) of the affected lung tissue because the two pleura separate, allowing the opposing forces to come into play. The size of lung collapse depends on how much of the intrapleural space loses negative pressure. Table 10–21 summarizes the three major types of pneumothorax, including pathophysiology and manifestations.

Size of the pneumothorax and the patient's symptoms are important considerations in making the decision whether chest drainage is required. A small pneumothorax with mild symptoms does not require insertion of a chest tube, whereas a medium-to-large pneumothorax does require chest tube insertion and drainage (Currie et al., 2007).

Common Clinical Findings

Although T.J.'s case greatly differs from M.T.'s in etiology, their clinical presentation related to pneumothorax may be similar, dependent on the size of the pneumothorax. Many of the typical clinical findings are those noted with an acute hypoxia episode and reflect normal compensatory mechanisms, including tachypnea, tachycardia, agitation, and confusion. If chest pain is present, shallow respirations with splinting may be noted. In addition, the presence of tachypnea is frequently associated with initial respiratory alkalosis. Table 10–22 provides a summary of common clinical findings.

Chest Tube Insertion

The nurse frequently assists with insertion of chest tubes; hence, a brief description of necessary equipment and procedure are provided here. The following equipment is needed for chest tube insertion:

- Chest tube thoracotomy tray and drainage system
- Antiseptic solution
- Protective eyewear
- Local anesthetic (1 percent lidocaine)
- Sterile gowns, gloves, masks, caps, and drapes (Wiegand & Carlson, 2005)

Depending on the size of the pneumothorax and other circumstances, preparation for insertion may need to be rapid. It is important to prepare the patient for the procedure as thoroughly as possible based on the patient's condition and the need for speed. The nurse's role in assisting with the procedure varies but often centers on obtaining (and possibly preparing) the necessary equipment, supporting the patient, and maintaining the patient in the appropriate position during the procedure. Table 10–23 summarizes common nursing activities in preparation for and during chest tube insertion.

The Procedure

If a pneumothorax is present, the chest tube typically is inserted anteriorly at the level of the second intercostal space, which approximates the lung apex; and if a hemothorax (or fluid) is present, the chest tube typically is inserted midaxillary at the fifth or sixth intercostal space to drain the base of the lung field (Wiegand & Carlson, 2005). After the chest tube has been inserted, it is quickly connected to special extension tubing that joins with the collection chamber of the chest drainage system. The chest tube is then sutured to the patient to prevent unintentional removal. An occlusive dressing (Fig. 10–8) is applied. All connections are properly taped or banded (plastic strips tightly wrapped around connections) to prevent unintentional disconnection (Fig. 10–9). The chest drainage system is placed and maintained below heart level at all times to assure proper drainage. A chest X-ray is ordered immediately following the procedure to assure correct tube placement.

Chest Drainage System

Although there are a variety of chest drainage systems available, the most common is the disposable self-contained system such as is seen in Figure 10–10. This type of drainage system is sometimes referred to as a "three-chamber system," which includes the collection, water-seal, and suction chambers. The disposable self-contained units essentially mimic the older three-bottle chest drainage systems; however there are also one- and two-bottle systems (Fig. 10–11).

Collection Chamber. The collection chamber accepts air or fluid coming into the system through extension tubing directly attached to the patient's chest tube. The collection chamber is composed of several interconnected vertical towers that are marked in mL for ease of fluid volume measurement.

Water-Seal Chamber. The water-seal (or air-leak) chamber is located in the center of a three-chamber system. Its purpose is to act as a one-way valve to prevent airflow back into the patient. Prior to initial use, the water-seal chamber is filled with sterile water to the 2 cm mark.

TABLE 10–20 Origins of Pneumothorax

EXTERNAL ORIGINS	INTERNAL ORIGINS
Thoracic surgery (e.g., open heart surgery)	Spontaneous bleb rupture
Penetrating chest trauma (e.g., knife or bullets)	Procedural rupture of visceral pleura (e.g., lung tissue biopsy)
Unintentional catheter entry into intrapleural space during central line placement	Barotrauma (e.g., mechanical ventilation, positive end expiratory pressure)
Chest contusion	

TABLE 10–21 Types of Pneumothorax

TYPE	PATHOPHYSIOLOGY	MANIFESTATIONS
A. Spontaneous 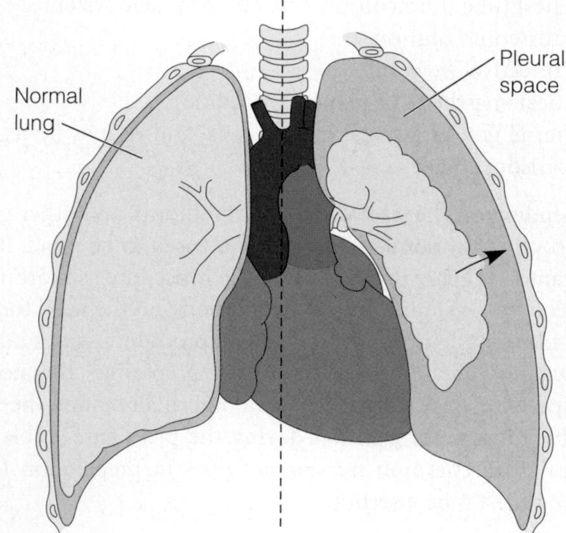	Rupture of a bleb on the lung surface allows air to enter pleural space from airways. ■ *Primary pneumothorax* affects previously healthy people. ■ *Secondary pneumothorax* affects people with preexisting lung disease (e.g., COPD).	■ Abrupt onset ■ Pleuritic chest pain ■ Dyspnea, shortness of breath ■ Tachypnea, tachycardia ■ Unequal lung excursion ■ Decreased breath sounds and hyperresonant percussion tone on affected side
B. Traumatic 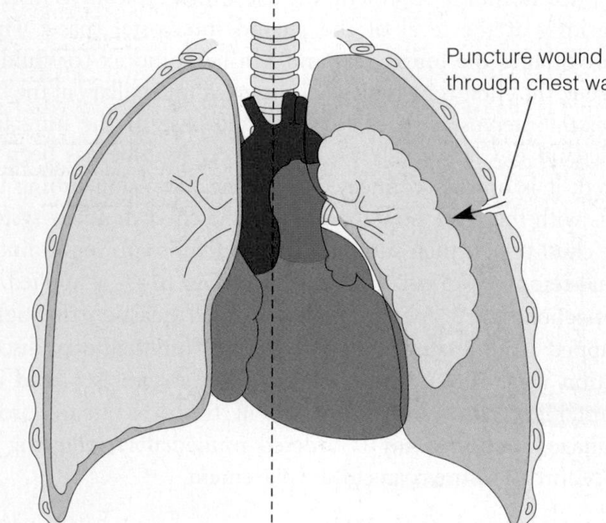	Trauma to the chest wall or pleura disrupts the pleural membrane. ■ *Open* occurs with penetrating chest trauma that allows air from the environment to enter the pleural space. ■ *Closed* occurs with blunt trauma that allows air from the lung to enter the pleural space. ■ *Iatrogenic* involves laceration of visceral pleura during a procedure such as thoracentesis or central-line insertion.	■ Pain ■ Dyspnea ■ Tachypnea, tachycardia ■ Decreased respiratory excursion ■ Absent breath sounds in affected area ■ Air movement through an open wound
C. Tension 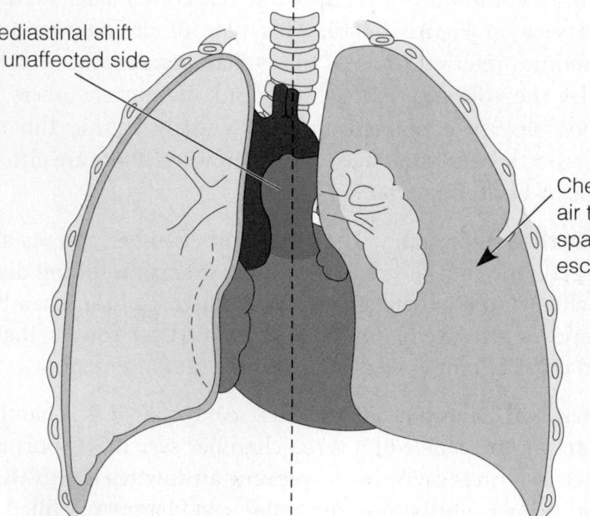	Air enters pleural space through chest wall or from airways but is unable to escape, resulting in rapid accumulation. Lung on affected side collapses. As intrapleural pressure increases, heart, great vessels, trachea, and esophagus shift toward the unaffected side.	■ Hypotension, shock ■ Distended neck veins ■ Severe dyspnea ■ Tachypnea, tachycardia ■ Decreased respiratory excursion ■ Absent breath sounds on affected side ■ Tracheal deviation toward unaffected side

TABLE 10–22 Summary of Common Clinical Findings of Pneumothorax

Signs of chest trauma (external origin)
Tachypnea, tachycardia (with possible onset of cardiac dysrhythmias)
Shortness of air
Diminished or absent breath sounds on one side (or one area of lung)
ABG: Decreased Pa_{O_2} and Sa_{O_2}, respiratory alkalosis
May complain of sharp chest pain on one side of chest (may not be present initially)
Positive chest X-ray for pneumothorax

The design of the water-seal chamber is simple but effective, being based on the one-bottle chest tube drainage system. To understand how the water-seal works, it may help to visualize a bottle filled with 2 cm (about 0.8 in.) of water (refer to Fig. 10–11). The bottle is sealed with a tight lid with two holes punched into it. A long tube is inserted into the bottle through one of the holes such that the distal tip is under water (a water-seal). The bottle is placed on the floor and the proximal end of the tube is kept at bed height. Air is drawn into the bottle through the tube because of negative gravity pull. As the air is pulled through the distal end of the tube, it bubbles through the water and escapes through the second hole in the lid. Air left in the bottle, however, cannot move back into the tube because of the presence of the water-seal and negative gravity pull. Although it is not used commonly anymore in the United States, the one-bottle system is an effective method of managing simple pneumothorax.

TABLE 10–23 Nursing Considerations for Chest Tube Insertion

Patient Preparation

Assure that the patient understands the reason for the procedure and what to expect during and following the procedure
Confirm that written consent has been obtained
Acquire and administer ordered sedation or analgesic prior to the procedure, timing the administration for the peak effect during the procedure
Assist the patient into the appropriate position (pneumothorax—lateral or supine; hemothorax—semi-Fowler)
Remind the patient not to move during the procedure (nurse may have to hold the patient in correct position)

Nurse's Role during Procedure

Pouring the antiseptic
Swabbing off lidocaine vial top with alcohol and holding vial for solution withdrawal
Supporting patient and maintaining correct patient position during procedure

Data from Wiegand & Carlson (2005).

Bubbling in the water-seal chamber indicates one of two things: (1) intermittent bubbling noted with pneumothorax suggests that air continues to be present in the intrapleural space, or (2) constant or vigorous bubbling may indicate an air leak in the system. If the patient's chest tube drainage system is not attached to external suction, the water level in the water-seal chamber should move up and down with breathing. This is a normal phenomenon called "tidling." Tidling ceases when the lung has reinflated.

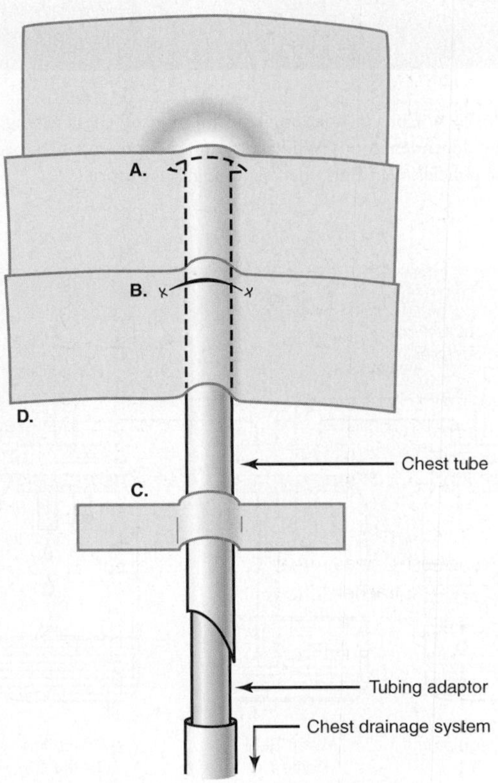

Figure 10–8 ■ Securing the chest tube. A) Incision site. B) Tube sutured to patient. C) Tube stabilized with tape. D) Occlusive dressing.

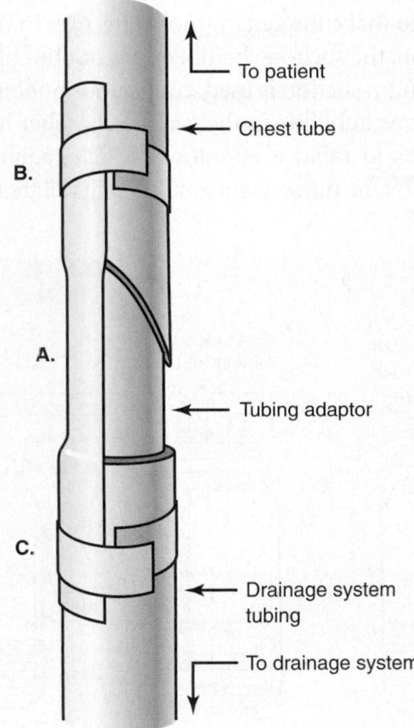

Figure 10–9 ■ Securing chest tube connections. A) Strip of cloth tape overlaps connection points along vertical axis. B and C) Strip of tape placed horizontally, overlapping vertical axis tape on both sides of connection.

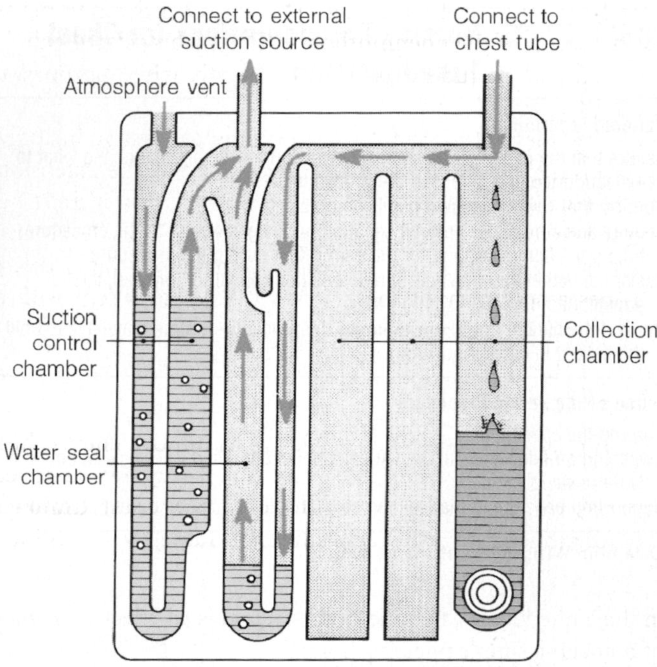

Figure 10–10 ▪ Disposable self-contained chest drainage system with wet suction control.

Suction Chamber. The suction chamber regulates the amount of negative suction pressure being exerted on the intrapleural space. The amount of negative pressure is determined by the volume of water in the suction chamber. Typically, it is set at 20 cm H_2O in the adult. The suction chamber does not require attachment to external suction (e.g., wall suction) to work, but it is commonly added to make the system more effective. In the absence of external suction, the suction chamber does not bubble; however, if additional vacuum suction is used, continuous bubbling should be present. Vigorous bubbling in the suction chamber has no advantage and results in rapid evaporation, which requires more frequent refilling by the nurse. Gentle bubbling is all that is required.

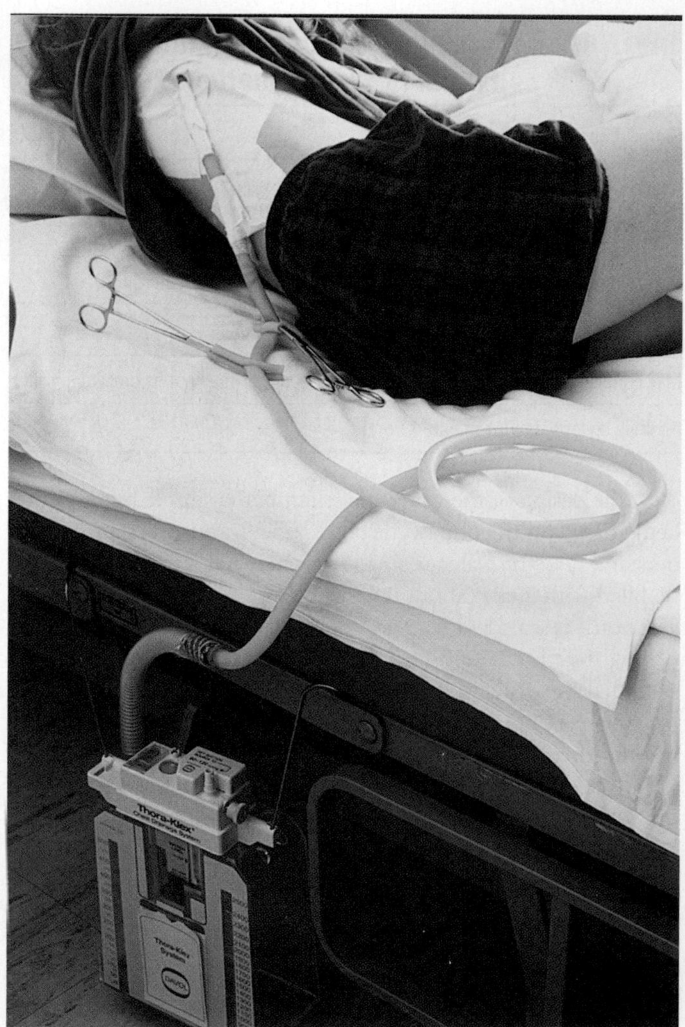

Figure 10–12 ▪ Correct horizontal positioning of chest tubing. Note that there are no dependent loops. While hemostats are present at the bedside, there are specific policies regarding when clamping is appropriate.

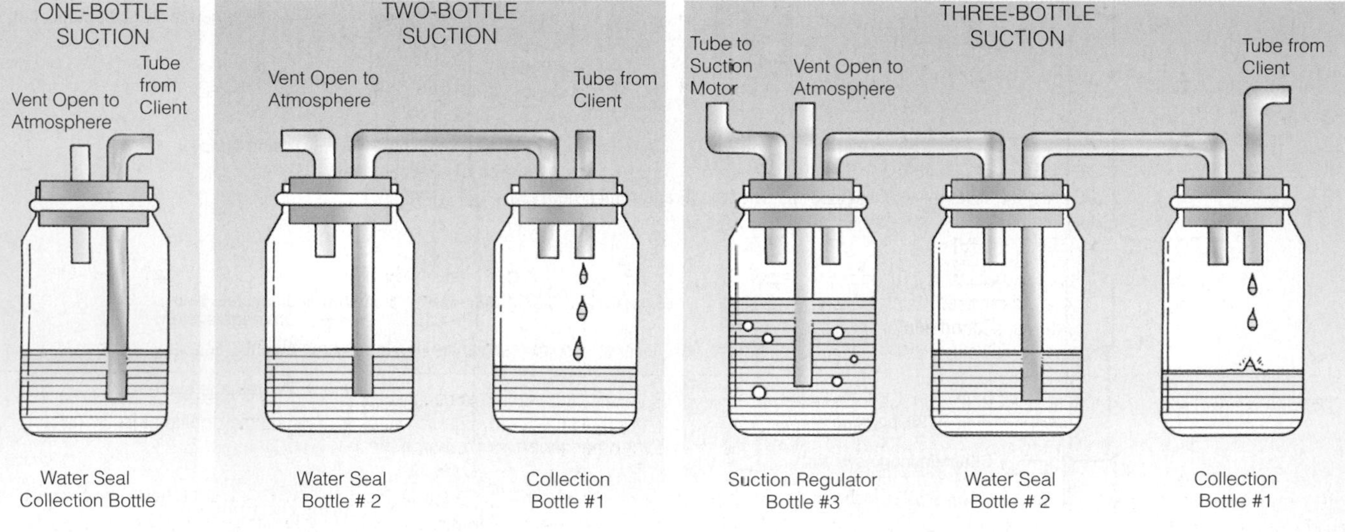

Figure 10–11 ▪ One-, two-, and three-bottle chest drainage/suction bottle systems.

Dry Chest Drainage Systems. Some chest drainage systems are "dry" in that they may not require water in the suction chamber. The amount of suction is regulated by a dial on the system and the wall suction. Depending on the design, this type of system may still require water in the water-seal chamber. Dry systems offer the advantages of easily adjusted levels of suction and are quiet (Wiegand & Carlson, 2005).

Assessment of the Patient with a Chest Tube in Place

Assessing the patient with a chest tube includes assessment of the patient as well as assessment of the chest tube and drainage system. In assessing the patient's status, vital signs and respiratory status are closely monitored, including chest auscultation and oxygenation status (e.g., level of consciousness, ABG, pulse oximetry [Spo_2], skin/mucous membrane coloring, and respiratory effort). Chest radiographs may be ordered to monitor the status of the pneumothorax. Chest tube–related pain is common and should be assessed frequently with appropriate administration of analgesia.

Assessment of the chest tube and drainage system includes the dressing and site, position and patency of the extension tubing (see Fig. 10–12), type and amount of output draining into the collection chamber, and assessment of fluid levels and activities in the water-seal and suction chambers. Table 10–24 provides a summary of the assessment of the patient with a chest tube and drainage system.

Chest Tube Removal

Nurses may assist with the procedure to remove chest tubes. Determining when a chest tube can be safely removed depends on the patient's requirement for chest drainage (e.g., pneumothorax, thoracic surgery). Table 10–25 outlines

TABLE 10–24 Nursing Assessment of the Patient with a Chest Tube Drainage System

Patient assessment	Vital signs Respiratory and oxygenation status (chest auscultation, level of consciousness, ABG, Spo_2, skin/mucous membrane coloring, and respiratory effort) Level of pain
Chest tube insertion site	Dressing should be occlusive, dry, and intact—reinforce as necessary (dressings may or may not be initially changed by the nurse based on hospital policy or physician or advanced practitioner orders) If dressing is changed, note appearance of tube insertion and suture sites Monitor for excessive bleeding through the dressing Palpate around dressing site for subcutaneous emphysema If affected area is enlarging, mark edge of area with pen to further evaluate rate and size of spread
Chest drainage system tube	**Extension tubing** Check all tubing connections to assure that they are secured to avoid unintentional disconnection Loop extension tubing horizontally on the bed to avoid excessive dependent looping, which may decrease drainage flow (see Figure 10–12) **Collection chamber** Routinely check blood or fluid output in the collection chamber Assess volume and appearance (sanguineous, serosanguineous, serous, purulent, etc.) Be aware of expected volume of bleeding for the first 24 hours following surgery and be alert for drainage above acceptable volume; a reverse appearance of drainage (serous → serosanguineous → sanguineous) as potential hemorrhage complication If clots are present, gently milk[a] the tubing to facilitate movement of clots into collection chamber Do not "strip" tubing[b] Routinely mark the volume on the outside of the collection chamber, indicating the time and date of the marking **Water-seal chamber** Assess for the presence of abnormal (constant) bubbling as an indication of a system leak Check water level to assure that it is at 2-cm level and refill if necessary **Suction chamber** Check level of water in chamber to assure that it is at 20 cm H_2O or other prescribed level and refill to prescribed level as required (to stop bubbling, temporarily pinch off the tubing that connects the drainage system to the external suction equipment) Check degree of bubbling in chamber and decrease level of external suction as needed to create gentle bubbling action
Documentation	If charting by exception, document abnormal vital signs and respiratory/oxygenation parameter; site appearance, excessive bleeding; presence of subcutaneous emphysema; abnormal chest output, such as excessive volume or change in drainage appearance (e.g., reversal of drainage appearance, or other abnormal characteristics)

[a]*Milking* refers to repeatedly squeezing the extension tubing without using a pulling motion. This is usually done starting at the proximal end (chest tube connection) and working down toward the collection chamber to encourage movement of clots. Excessive or vigorous milking can result in damage to the pleura.
[b]*Stripping* is a vigorous squeezing/pulling motion on extension tubing to move an obstructing clot. Stripping can create excessive negative intrapleural pressure that damages the pleura.

TABLE 10–25 Indications for Chest Tube Removal

Patient status improved and stable
Decreased chest tube drainage, usually less than 100 mL in 24 hours
Air leak resolved
Lung is reinflated on chest X-ray and remains inflated without recurrent pneumothorax when system is on waterseal

Data from Wiegand & Carlson (2005).

general guidelines used to make the decision to remove the tube.

Chest tube removal is a painful procedure. Pre-medication for anticipated pain is important and may be accomplished with systemic narcotic or non-steroidal medication (Puntillo & Ley, 2004). An occlusive dressing with Vaseline gauze is applied as the chest tube is removed to prevent air entry into the pleural space (Wiegand & Carlson, 2005).

Related Nursing Diagnoses

There are multiple nursing diagnoses and potential complications (PC) that frequently are applicable to the patient who requires a chest tube, including

- Anxiety
- Impaired gas exchange
- Ineffective breathing pattern
- Knowledge deficit
- Chest pain
- Risk for infection
- PC: hemorrhage
- PC: pneumothorax

SECTION SIX REVIEW

1. Currently, the primary indication for pneumonectomy is as a surgical treatment for which disease?
   A. lung cancer
   B. tuberculosis
   C. pulmonary fibrosis
   D. bronchiectasis
2. When a chest tube is placed following pneumonectomy, its primary purpose is to
   A. remove air from the surgical site
   B. reestablish negative pressure
   C. monitor the operative side for bleeding
   D. administer intrathoracic drugs
3. A patient has recently had a right pneumonectomy. The nurse should NOT position the patient in which way?
   A. to the back
   B. to the operative side
   C. to high Fowler's position
   D. to the unaffected lung side
4. The nurse decides to use the cascade cough technique to encourage an effective postthoracic surgery cough. Using this technique, the patient will cough in which pattern?
   A. while splinting the chest with a pillow
   B. three to four times during a single exhalation
   C. every hour on an escalating schedule
   D. once during each of 4 rapid breaths
5. Examples of internal origin problems that may require chest tube insertion include (choose all that apply)
   A. barotrauma
   B. penetrating chest trauma
   C. procedural rupture of visceral pleura
   D. chest contusion
   E. bleb rupture
6. Pneumothorax caused by positive end expiratory pressure (PEEP) represents which type of injury?
   A. procedural rupture
   B. chest contusion
   C. spontaneous bleb rupture
   D. barotrauma induced
7. Lung tissue collapses under which set of circumstances?
   A. increased pulmonary interstitial fluid pressure
   B. loss of negative intrapleural pressure
   C. increased pulmonary vascular resistance
   D. loss of capillary endothelium integrity
8. Common clinical findings associated with pneumothorax include (choose all that apply)
   A. tachypnea
   B. bradycardia
   C. respiratory acidosis
   D. shortness of breath
   E. decreased $Pa{O_2}$
9. The patient with a pneumothorax would most likely have a chest tube inserted at which location?
   A. midaxillary line, second intercostal space
   B. anterior chest, fourth intercostal space
   C. midaxillary line, fourth or fifth intercostal space
   D. anterior chest, second intercostal space

10. Immediately following the chest tube insertion procedure, correct placement is confirmed by
    A. arterial blood gas
    B. auscultation
    C. chest X-ray
    D. ultrasonography
11. The purpose of the water-seal chamber in a three-chamber chest drainage system is to
    A. facilitate drainage from the chest tube
    B. prevent airflow back into the patient
    C. facilitate control of level of negative suction
    D. prevent fluid from draining into the suction chamber
12. Vigorous bubbling in the water-seal chamber suggests that
    A. an air leak is present
    B. pneumothorax is still present
    C. wall suction pressure is too high
    D. the system is working correctly
13. The collection chamber is routinely assessed for (choose all that apply)
    A. fluid volume
    B. rate of volume increase
    C. drainage characteristics
    D. degree of bubbling

Answers: 1. A, 2. C, 3. D, 4. B, 5. (A, C, E), 6. D, 7. B, 8. (A, D, E), 9. D, 10. C, 11. B, 12. A, 13. (A, B, C)

SECTION SEVEN: Developing a Pulmonary Plan of Care

At the completion of this section, the learner will be able to develop a plan of care for a patient with altered respiratory function.

This section presents a standard respiratory plan of care based on the three approved nursing diagnoses from the North American Nursing Diagnosis Association (NANDA), that focus on respiratory function. Each nursing diagnosis is defined, major patient outcomes are listed, and some of the major independent nursing interventions are provided. Patient outcomes reflect the relative nature of "normal" parameters, as they apply to the high-acuity patient population, who often has chronic respiratory disorders in addition to the current acute health problem.

The Standard Respiratory Plan of Care

The three NANDA-approved respiratory nursing diagnoses are

- Breathing pattern, ineffective
- Gas exchange, impaired
- Airway clearance, ineffective

All three of the pulmonary-related nursing diagnoses may apply to high-acuity patients during a single illness. For this reason, the nurse may consider using an alternative that joins all three NANDA diagnoses, *impaired respiratory function* (Ulrich & Canale, 2001).

Breathing Pattern, Ineffective

Ineffective breathing pattern is defined as "[i]nspiration and/or expiration that does not provide adequate ventilation" (Ulrich & Canale, 2001, p. 19).

Desired Patient Outcomes. Maintenance of an effective breathing pattern is evidenced by

1. Normal respiratory rate, depth, and rhythm
2. ABGs and/or SpO_2 within normal limits for patient
3. Bilateral chest excursion
4. No dyspnea

Independent Nursing Interventions

1. Assess for ineffective breathing patterns (report abnormals)
    A. Respirations less than 8/min or greater than 30/min
    B. Increasingly shallow, labored breathing
    C. Increasing dyspnea
    D. Increasingly abnormal ABGs or pulse oximetry results
    E. Increasingly irregular breathing pattern
    F. Increasing use of accessory muscles
2. Monitor for abdominal or chest pain
3. Reduce level of abdominal or chest pain
    A. Regular administration of pain medication, as ordered (observe for respiratory depression)
    B. Splint chest or abdomen with pillow or arms for coughing and deep-breathing exercises
4. Implement respiratory muscle strengthening exercises
5. Encourage incentive spirometer use every 1 to 2 hours, as ordered
6. Encourage slow, deep breaths (as appropriate)
7. Elevate head of bed to 45 degrees or level of comfort
8. Turn (self or assisted) every two hours

Gas Exchange, Impaired

Impaired gas exchange is defined as "[e]xcess or deficit in oxygenation and/or carbon dioxide elimination at the alveolar–capillary membrane" (Ulrich & Canale, 2001, p. 35).

Desired Patient Outcomes. Maintenance of normal gas exchange is evidenced by

1. ABGs within normal (acceptable) limits for patient
2. Usual mental status
3. Breathing unlabored (or baseline for patient)
4. Respiratory rate 12 to 20/min (or usual rate for patient)
5. No use (or decreased use) of accessory respiratory muscles

Independent Nursing Interventions

1. Assess for impaired gas exchange (report abnormals)
   A. Change in mental status
      1. Increased lethargy
      2. Increased restlessness
      3. Confusion
   B. Accessory muscle use
   C. Abnormal ABGs
      1. Elevated $Paco_2$ (above acceptable limits)
      2. Decreased Pao_2 (below acceptable limits)
   D. Decreasing pulse oximetry readings
2. Turn every two hours
   A. In patients with pneumonia or other unilateral pulmonary disorder, turning to unaffected lung side may enhance oxygenation (improve $\dot{V}/\dot{Q}$ relationship) while turning to affected side may cause oxygen desaturation.
3. Encourage incentive spirometer use every one to two hours
4. Maintain position of comfort, with head of bed elevated greater than 30 degrees (assist to tripod position, if desired)
5. Monitor effects of drug therapy (including oxygen therapy) (refer to RELATED PHARMACOTHERAPY box)
6. Encourage early ambulation
7. Assist patient to sit up in chair

Airway Clearance, Ineffective

Ineffective airway clearance is defined as "[i]nability to clear secretions or obstructions from the respiratory tract to maintain a clear airway" (Ulrich & Canale, 2001, p. 13).

Desired Patient Outcomes. Maintenance of effective airway clearance is evidenced by

1. Normal or improved lung sounds
2. No cyanosis
3. Normal respiratory rate and depth
4. No dyspnea

Independent Nursing Interventions

1. Assess for ineffective airway clearance
   A. Adventitious breath sounds
   B. Ineffective cough
   C. Respirations greater than 24/min
   D. Respiratory depth shallow
   E. Presence of cyanosis
   F. Complaint of dyspnea
2. Assist patient to cough and deep breathe every one to two hours
3. Encourage fluids to 2 to 2.5 L per 24 hours or 600 to 800 mL per eight-hour shift (if not contraindicated)
4. Perform tracheal suction as necessary
5. Monitor for effects of drug therapy (expectorants, mucolytics) (refer to RELATED PHARMACOTHERAPY table)
6. Monitor for and treat acute pain
7. Administer pain medications, as needed
8. Encourage self-care as tolerated
9. Encourage activity and early ambulation

SECTION SEVEN REVIEW

1. Evaluation of the effectiveness of interventions to resolve the nursing diagnosis *ineffective breathing patterns* is best measured by which of the following desired patient outcomes?
   A. usual mental status
   B. normal or improved lung sounds
   C. absent accessory muscle use
   D. normal respiratory rate, depth, and rhythm
2. The state in which a person experiences decreased passage of oxygen and/or carbon dioxide between the alveoli and the vascular system is the definition of
   A. impaired gas exchange
   B. ineffective breathing pattern
   C. ineffective airway clearance
   D. altered respiratory function
3. Assessments for impaired gas exchange in the early stage would include (choose all that apply)
   A. confusion
   B. increased lethargy
   C. decreased restlessness
   D. change in mental status
4. Nursing interventions that would assist in maintaining effective airway clearance would include
   A. restrict fluids to 1 L/day
   B. cough and deep breathe every 1 to 2 hours
   C. minimize use of opioid analgesics
   D. restrict activities

Answers: 1. D, 2. A, 3. (A, B, D), 4. B

POSTTEST

The following Posttest is constructed in a case study format. A patient is presented, and questions are asked based on available data. New data are presented as the case study progresses.

John Huang is a 68-year-old grocery store owner. He has a 45-year history of smoking one to two packs of cigarettes per day. Approximately ten years ago he was diagnosed with COPD. Mr. Huang is admitted to the hospital with severe dyspnea and a productive cough. He is diagnosed with right lower lobe pneumonia. He is currently receiving oxygen therapy per nasal prongs at 2 L/min.

1. Based only on available data, Mr. Huang's pneumonia condition would be considered an acute
   A. restrictive disease
   B. obstructive disease
   C. respiratory failure
   D. ventilatory failure
2. Mr. Huang's pneumonia affects expiratory airflow in which way?
   A. increases
   B. decreases
   C. no effect
   D. increases or decreases
3. His obstructive pulmonary disorder is associated with
   A. decreased tidal volumes
   B. increased inspiratory times
   C. decreased inspiratory airflow
   D. increased expiratory times
4. Assuming Mr. Huang is in a state of chronic respiratory insufficiency, he would most likely exhibit which clinical finding related to his chronic condition?
   A. increased blood pressure
   B. decreased respiratory rate
   C. increased temperature
   D. decreased pulse rate
5. If Mr. Huang develops acute ventilatory failure, you would anticipate which arterial blood gas finding?
   A. PaO_2 less than 60 mm Hg
   B. $PaCO_2$ greater than 50 mm Hg
   C. PaO_2 greater than 100 mm Hg
   D. $PaCO_2$ less than 35 mm Hg
6. According to the module, respiratory failure is clinically defined as
   A. $PaCO_2$ 50 mm Hg or greater with pH 7.30 or less and/or PaO_2 60 mm Hg or less
   B. $PaCO_2$ 60 mm Hg with a pH 7.30 or less and PaO_2 less than 60 mm Hg
   C. $PaCO_2$ 45 mm Hg with a pH 7.35 and/or PaO_2 80 mm Hg
   D. $PaCO_2$ 60 mm Hg with a pH 7.35 and PaO_2 80 mm Hg
7. ARDS is a pulmonary disorder that initially causes
   A. lung destruction
   B. ventilatory failure
   C. alveolar hypoventilation
   D. oxygenation failure
8. The nurse is developing a plan of care for the nursing diagnosis *impaired gas exchange.* Of the following, which desired patient outcome most accurately measures this diagnosis?
   A. ABG within acceptable limits for patient
   B. SaO_2 greater than 95 percent
   C. usual mental status
   D. no cyanosis
9. The nurse writes the nursing diagnosis *ineffective airway clearance* on Mr. Huang's care plan. All of the following are appropriate interventions to address this diagnosis EXCEPT
   A. administer pain medications as needed
   B. cough and deep breathe every 1 to 2 hours
   C. limit fluid intake to less than 1 L/24 hours
   D. tracheal suction as necessary

A 22-year-old female, Shelida W., was admitted to Trauma ICU after sustaining severe multiple trauma injuries in an automobile–tree collision. She has multiple abrasions on her head, arms, and legs; an open right femur fracture; right humeral fracture and pelvic fractures; and a ruptured spleen. She required multiple blood transfusions as a result of the development of hypovolemic shock. Since her admission, she has been on a mechanical ventilator. On day 5 postadmission, she developed sepsis.

10. Examine Shelida's presenting history. List three factors that place her at increased risk for development of ALI/ARDS.
    1. ______
    2. ______
    3. ______

It is now day 7 postadmission. Shelida has a pulmonary artery catheter and arterial line in place. The nurse is concerned with the deterioration in Shelida's SpO_2 regardless of supportive interventions. The nurse performs assessments and then contacts the physician who orders an immediate arterial blood gas and portable chest X-ray.

11. If Shelida is developing ALI/ARDS, the nurse would anticipate which values in her hemodynamic readings?
    A. deteriorating pulmonary artery pressures
    B. normal pulmonary artery wedge pressures
    C. elevated pulmonary artery pressures
    D. elevated pulmonary artery wedge pressures

The nurse calculates Shelida's PaO_2/FiO_2 (P/F) ratio. It is 180 mm Hg.

12. Assuming that the medical team uses the ARDS consensus criteria, Shelida's PaO_2/FiO_2 (P/F) ratio meets the criterion for ARDS.
    A. True
    B. False

13. Shelida's ABG result is pH 7.48; $Paco_2$ 32, Pao_2 64, and HCO_3 25. Which statement best explains the acid–base state reflected in her ABG result?
   A. She is triggering the ventilator at 28 to 32 breaths per minute.
   B. Her heart rate and blood pressure have been steadily increasing.
   C. The oxygen concentration on her ventilator was increased 30 minutes ago.
   D. She received pain medication 30 minutes ago.
14. A bronchoalveolar lavage (BAL) fluid sample is taken from her lungs. If Shelida has ALI/ARDS, the fluid should contain
   A. no inflammatory cells
   B. low protein content
   C. high RBC content
   D. high protein content

Shelida is diagnosed with ARDS.

15. The nurse is explaining the concept of nonhydrostatic pulmonary edema to Shelida's family. Which statement, if made by the family, suggests that they understand the concept sufficiently?
   A. "Her disease has injured the membranes in her lung so that fluid is leaking into her lungs from the tiny blood vessels."
   B. "The high blood pressure in the left side of her heart is forcing fluid from her blood vessels into her lung tissue."
   C. "Infection in her lungs has harmed the small blood vessels there, causing blood to spill into the lung tissue."
   D. "The small air sacs have been destroyed, which has allowed air to enter into the blood vessels."
16. The nurse notes that Shelida's peak airway pressures are now above 50 cm H_2O. The reason for this development in the ALI/ARDS patient is
   A. onset of pneumonia
   B. development of microemboli
   C. development of $\dot{V}/\dot{Q}$ mismatch
   D. extensive atelectasis
17. Shelida is now receiving positive end expiratory pressure (PEEP). The medical team adheres to a "least PEEP" protocol. According to the module, least PEEP uses the minimum PEEP required to achieve a Sao_2 of at least ______ percent with an Fio_2 (oxygen concentration) of ______ or less.
   A. 75, 0.45 (45 percent)
   B. 80, 0.50 (50 percent)
   C. 85, 0.55 (55 percent)
   D. 90, 0.60 (60 percent)

Brian J., 32-years-old, is recovering from major surgery, in which he had left femur reconstruction performed. He has been immobilized for seven days.

18. Based on Brian's available history, which factors of Virchow's triad are in place that make him at risk for development of deep-vein thrombosis? (choose all that apply)
   A. venous stasis
   B. hypercoagulability
   C. venous (endothelial) injury

Today, the nurse becomes concerned with an acute change in Brian's pulmonary status.

19. To assess Brian for a possible pulmonary embolus, for what common signs and symptoms would the nurse monitor him? (list all that apply)
   1. ______
   2. ______
   3. ______
   4. ______
   5. ______
   6. ______
20. The physician orders a D-dimer assay. The purpose of using this test initially is to
   A. confirm the presence of a pulmonary embolism
   B. rule out pulmonary embolism
   C. check for presence of hypercoagulability
   D. rule out pulmonary edema
21. Brian has an ABG drawn. Assuming that he has a pulmonary embolism, what ABG results would the nurse anticipate seeing?
   A. acute respiratory alkalosis with hypoxemia
   B. acute respiratory acidosis with hypoxemia
   C. acute metabolic alkalosis with hypoxemia
   D. acute metabolic acidosis with hypoxemia
22. The definitive diagnostic test for the presence of pulmonary embolism is
   A. $\dot{V}/\dot{Q}$ scan
   B. angiogram
   C. compression ultrasound
   D. D-dimer assay
23. True or False: Most diagnoses of pulmonary embolism are not made until postmortem.
24. True or False: Most pulmonary emboli are small and breakdown on their own.
25. What treatment options may be considered? (short answer)

Wen Wu, 43-years-old, flew to Hong Kong to visit his family. Near the end of his visit, his sister (a nurse at a local hospital) became ill with what appeared to be a severe chest cold. Mr. Wu returned to his home in San Francisco the next day. Several days later, he became ill at work, complaining of sore muscles and feeling feverish. He was unable to work the next day and felt even worse than the day before. By day 7 of his illness, he developed a dry cough and was complaining of having difficulty breathing. His wife became alarmed and drove him to a local hospital emergency department.

26. In the emergency department, a portable chest X-ray was taken. If Mr. Wu has developed SARS, what will the chest X-ray show?
   A. presence of pneumonia
   B. enlarged right heart
   C. normal lungs
   D. pleural effusions

27. The MOST COMMON presenting manifestations of SARS include (check all that apply)
    ______ fever greater than 100°F (37.8°C)
    ______ sore throat
    ______ severe myalgias
    ______ hemoptysis
    ______ mild headache
    ______ chest pain
    ______ extreme weakness
    ______ persistent dry cough
    ______ petechiae on trunk
28. Mr. Wu has a battery of laboratory tests drawn, such as CBC with differential, blood cultures, and Gram stain and culture. For what primary reason are these tests performed in a patient who may have SARS? (short answer)

Clinical Update: Mr. Wu suddenly becomes more tachycardiac, his SpO_2 drops, and his peak inspiratory pressure increases. The nurse immediately auscultates his lungs and finds that he has no lung sounds in his right upper lung field. A chest X-ray confirms a right upper lobe pneumothorax. A chest tube is ordered.

29. The nurse is positioning Mr. Wu for the chest tube procedure. Which position would be most appropriate for insertion of a chest tube for a right pneumothorax?
    A. high-Fowler's position
    B. supine in bed or lying on left side
    C. mild Trendelenburg position on left side
    D. right side with head of bed elevated 30 degrees
30. Mr. Wu has had his chest tube in place for two days. While assessing the chest drainage system, the nurse notes continuous vigorous bubbling in the water-seal chamber. The appropriate action to take would be
    A. decrease the amount of wall suction attached to the system
    B. check all connections for a leak
    C. check for subcutaneous emphysema
    D. place Mr. Wu on his left side
31. Mr. Wu is to have his chest tube removed today. Based on recent research regarding pain control during chest tube removal, which action is most effective (assuming that orders are present)?
    A. Place warm, dry heat over the dressing site directly following tube removal.
    B. Give PO diazepam (Valium) one hour before the planned tube removal.
    C. Provide Mr. Wu with a thorough explanation of the tube removal procedure.
    D. Administer IV analgesia so that the drug's peak effect coincides with tube removal.

Posttest answers with rationale are found on MyNursingKit.

REFERENCES

Adhikari, N. K., Burns, K. E., Friedrich, J. O., Granton, J. T., Cook, D. J., & Meade, N. O. (2007). Effect of nitric oxide on oxygenation and mortality in acute lung injury: systematic review and meta-analysis. *British Medical Journal, 334*(7597), 779–782.

Alsaghir A. H., & Martin, C. M. (2008). Effect of prone positioning in patients with acute respiratory distress syndrome: a meta-analysis. *Critical Care Medicine, 36*(2), 603–609.

Annane, D. (2007). Glucocorticoids for ARDS: just do it! *Chest, 131*(4):945–946.

ARDS Network (The Acute Respiratory Distress Syndrome Network). (n.d.). Available at: http://www.ardsnet.org/index.php. Accessed June 1, 2004.

ARDS Network (The Acute Respiratory Distress Syndrome Network). (2000). Ventilation with lower tidal volumes as compared with traditional tidal volumes for acute lung injury and the acute respiratory distress syndrome. *New England Journal of Medicine, 342*(18), 1301–1308.

Ashbaugh, D. G., Bigelow, D. B., Petty, T. L., & Levine, B. E. (1967). Acute respiratory distress in adults. *Lancet, 2*(7511), 319–323.

Atabai, J. & Matthay, M. A. (2002). The pulmonary physician in critical care: acute lung injury and the acute respiratory distress syndrome: definitions and epidemiology. *Thorax, 57*(5), 452–458.

Avecillas, J. F., Freire, A. X., & Arroliga, A. C. (2006). Clinical epidemiology of acute lung injury and acute respiratory distress syndrome: Incidence, diagnosis, and outcomes. *Clinics in Chest Medicine, 27*(4), 549–557.

Awtry, E. H., & Loscalzo, J. (2001). Vascular diseases and hypertension. In C. C. J. Carpenter, R. C. Griggs, & J. Loscalzo (eds.), *Cecil essentials of medicine* (5th ed., pp. 145–163). Philadelphia: W.B. Saunders.

Booth, T. F., Kournikakis, B, Bastien, N., Ho, J., Kobasa, D., Stadnyk L., Li, Y. et al. (2005). Detection of airborne severe acute respiratory syndrome (SARS) coronavirus and environmental contamination in SARS outbreak units. *The Journal of Infectious Diseases, 191*(9), 1472–1477.

Breiburg, A. N., Aitken, L., Reaby, L., Clancy, R. L., & Pierce, J. D. (2000). Efficacy and safety of prone positioning for patients with acute respiratory distress syndrome. *Journal of Advanced Nursing, 32*(4), 922–929.

Calfee, C. S. & Matthay, M. A. (2007). Nonventilatory treatments for acute lung injury and ARDS. *Chest, 131*(3), 913–920.

Carpenito-Moyet, L. J. (2004). *Nursing diagnosis: Application to clinical practice* (10th ed.). Philadelphia: Lippincott/Williams & Wilkins.

Carpenito-Moyet, L. J. (2008). *Nursing diagnosis: Application to clinical practice* (12th ed.). Philadelphia: Lippincott/Williams & Wilkins.

CDC [Centers for Disease Control]. (2004a). Severe acute respiratory syndrome: in the absence of SARS-CoV transmission worldwide: guidance for surveillance, clinical and laboratory evaluation, and reporting version 2. Available at: www.cdc.gov/ncidod/sars/absenceofsars.htm. Accessed May 2, 2008.

CDC [Centers for Disease Control]. (2004b). Severe acute respiratory syndrome. Supplement 1: Infection control in healthcare, home, and community settings. III. Infection control in healthcare facilities. Available at: www.cdc.gov/ncidod/sars/guidance/I/pdf/healthcare.pdf. Accessed May, 2008.

Cepkova, M., & Matthay, M. A. (2006). Pharmacotherapy of acute lung injury and the acute respiratory distress syndrome. *Journal of Intensive Care Medicine, 21*(3), 119–143.

Cerfolio R. (2007). Pneumonectomy. In L. R. Kaiser, I. L. Kron, & T .L. Spray (eds.) *Mastery of cardiothoracic surgery.* (2d ed. pp. 53–63). Philadelphia: Lippincott/Williams & Wilkins.

Clemens, S., & Leeper, K. V. (2007). Newer modalities for detection of pulmonary emboli. *American Journal of Medicine, 120*(10 Suppl. 2), S2–S12.

Cloutier, L. M. (2007). Diagnosis of pulmonary embolism. *Clinical Journal of Oncology Nursing, 11*(3), 343–348.

Conrad, S. A. (2002). Venous air embolism? *E-medicine.* Available at: www.emedicine.com/emerg/topic787.htm. Accessed June 12, 2004.

Croce, M. A., Fabian, T. C., Davis, K. A., & Gavin, T. (1999). Early and late acute respiratory distress syndrome: two distinct clinical entities. *Journal of Trauma-Injury Infection & Critical Care, 46*(3), 361–367.

Crouser, E. D., & Fahy, R. J. (2009). Acute lung injury, pulmonary edema, and multiple system organ failure. In R. L. Wilkins, J. K. Stoller, & R. M. Kacmarek, *Egan's fundamentals of respiratory care* (9th ed., pp. 571–592). St. Louis: C.V. Mosby.

Currie, G. P., Alluri, R., Christie, G. L., & Legge, J. S. (2007); Pneumothorax: an update. *Postgraduate Medical Journal, 83*(981), 461–465.

Davidson, W. J., Dorscheid, D., Spragg, R., Schulzer, M., Mak, E., & Ayas, N. T. (2006). Exogenous pulmonary surfactant for the treatment of adult patients with acute respiratory distress syndrome: results of a meta-analysis. *Critical Care, 10*(2), R41.

Davies, S. (2001). Amniotic fluid embolus: A review of the literature. *Canadian Journal of Anesthesia, 48,* 88–98.

Davis, K., Johannigman, J., Campbell, R., et al. (2001). The acute effects of body position strategies and respiratory therapy in paralyzed patients with acute lung injury. *Critical Care, 5,* 81–87.

Dellinger, R. P. (2006). Inhaled nitric oxide: Should it be used in acute respiratory distress syndrome? *Critical Care Medicine, 34*(12),3035–3036.

Eachempati, S. R., Hydo, L. J., Shou, J., and Barie, P. S. (2007). Outcomes of acute respiratory distress syndrome (ARDS) in elderly patients. *J Trauma 63*(2): 344–50.

Eisner, M. D., Thompson, T., Hudson, L. D., et al., & the Acute Respiratory Distress Syndrome Network. (2001). Efficacy of low tidal volume ventilation in patients with different clinical risk factors for acute lung injury and the acute respiratory distress syndrome. *American Journal of Respiratory and Critical Care Medicine, 164,* 231–236.

Galiatsou, E., Kostanti, E., Svarna E., Kitsakos, A., Koulouras, V., Efremidis, S., et al. (2006). Prone position augments recruitment and prevents alveolar overinflation in acute lung injury. *American Journal of Respiratory and Critical Care Medicine, 174*(2), 187–197.

Gattinoni, L., Tognoni, G., Pesenti, A., et al. (2001). Effect of prone positioning on the survival of patients with acute respiratory failure. *New England Journal of Medicine, 345*(8), 568–573.

Goldhill, D. R., Imhoff M., McLean B., & Waldmann C. (2007). Rotational bed therapy to prevent and treat respiratory complications: a review and meta-analysis. *American Journal of Critical Care, 16* (1), 50–62.

Gong, M. N., Thompson, B. T., Williams, P .L., Zhou, W., Wang, M. Z., Pothier, L., et al. (2006). Interleukin-10 polymorphism in position and acute respiratory distress syndrome. *European Respiratory Journal, 27*(4), 674–681.

Gu, J., & Korteweg, C. (2007). Pathology and pathogenesis of severe acute respiratory syndrome. *American Journal of Pathology, 170*(4), 1136–1147.

Halm M. A. (2007). To strip or not to strip? physiological effects of chest tube manipulation. *American Journal of Critical Care, 16*(6), 609–612.

Heit, J. A. (2006). The epidemiology of venous thromboembolism in the community: Implications for prevention and management. *Journal of Thrombosis and Thrombolysis, 21*(1), 23–29.

Hirai, L. K., Takahashi, J. M., Yoon, H. C. (2007). A prospective evaluation of a quantitative D-dimer assay in the evaluation of acute pulmonary embolism. *Journal of Vascular and Interventional Radiology, 18*(8), 970–974.

Hirsch, M. S. (2007). Severe acute respiratory syndrome (SARS). *UpToDate.* Available at: www.utdol.com/online/content/topic.do?topicKey=viral_in/23539.

Hopkins R. O., & Herridge, M. S. (2006). Quality of life, emotional abnormalities, and cognitive dysfunction in survivors of acute lung injury/acute respiratory distress syndrome. *Clinics in Chest Medicine, 27*(4),679–689.

Horlander, K. T., Mannino, D. M., & Leeper, K. V. (2003). Pulmonary embolism mortality in the United States, 1979–1998. *Archives of Internal Medicine, 163*(14), 1711–1717.

Houston, S., Hougland, P., Anderson, J., et al. (2002). Effectiveness of 0.12% chlorhexidine gluconate oral rinse in reducing prevalence of nosocomial pneumonia in patients undergoing heart surgery. *American Journal of Critical Care 11,* (6), 567–570.

Hunt, D. (2007). Determining the clinical probability of deep venous thrombosis and pulmonary embolism. *Southern Medical Journal, 100*(10), 1015–1021.

Husebye, E. E., Lyberg, T., & Roise, O. (2006). Bone marrow fat in the circulation: Clinical entities and pathophysiological mechanisms. *Injury 37*(Suppl 4), S8–S18.

Institutes for Healthcare Improvement. (n.d.). Adult community-acquired pneumonia (CAP) order bundle. Retrieved on 11/28/08 from http://www.ihi.org/IHI/Topics/Reliability/ReliabilityGeneral/EmergingContent/AdultCommunityAcquiredPneumonia%28CAP%29OrderBundle.htm.

Jassal, D., Sharma, S., & Maycher, B. (2004). Pulmonary hypertension. *E-medicine.* Available at: www.emedicine.com/radio/topic583.htm. Accessed June 12, 2004.

Kacmarek, R. M., Wiedemann, H. P., Lavin, P. T., Wedel, M. K., Tutuncu, A. S., and Slutsky, A. S. (2006). Partial liquid ventilation in adult patients with acute respiratory distress syndrome. *American Journal of Respiratory and Critical Care Medicine, 173*(8), 882–889.

Khraim, F. M. (2007). The wider scope of video-assisted thoracoscopic surgery. *Association of Perioperative Registered Nurses, 85*(6), 1199–1208.

Kollef, M. H., Shorr, A., Tabak, Y. P., Gupta, V., Liu, L. A., & Johannes, R. S. (2005). Epidemiology and outcomes of health-care-associated pneumonia. Results from a large US database of culture-positive pneumonia. *Chest, 128*(6), 3854–3862.

Lapinsky, S. E., & Hawryluck, L. (2003). ICU management of severe acute respiratory syndrome. *Intensive Care Medicine, 29*(6), 870–875.

Lew, T., Kwek, T-K., Tai, D., et al. (2003). Acute respiratory distress syndrome in critically ill patients with severe acute respiratory syndrome. *Journal of the American Medical Association, 290*(3), 374–380.

Light, R. W. (2006). Parapneumonic effusions and empyema. *Proceedings of the American Thoracic Society, 3*(1), 75–80.

Malhotra, A. (2007). Low-tidal-volume ventilation in the acute respiratory distress syndrome. *New England Journal of Medicine, 357*(11), 1113–1120.

Mancebo J., Fernandez R., Blanch L., Rialp G., Gordo F., Ferrer M., et al. (2006). A Multicenter trial of prolonged prone ventilation in severe acute respiratory distress syndrome. *American Journal of Respiratory and Critical Care Medicine, 17*(11),1233–1239.

Mandell, L. A., Wunderink, R. G., Anzueto, A., Bartlett, J. G., Campbell, G. D., Dean, N.C., et al. (2007). Infectious Diseases Society of America/American Thoracic Society consensus guidelines on the management of community-acquired pneumonia in adults. *Clinical Infectious Diseases, 44*(Suppl. 2), S27–S72.

Marik, P. E. (2005). Aspiration pneumonitis and pneumonia. In M. P. Fink, E. Abraham, J. Vincent & P. M. Kochanek (eds.), *Textbook of Critical Care Medicine.* (5th ed, pp. 581–585). Philadelphia: Elsevier/Saunders.

Marshall, M. B. (2007). Thoracic incisions. In L. R. Kaiser, I. L. Kron, & T. L. Spray (eds.). *Mastery of Cardiothoracic Surgery.* (2d ed., pp 26–32). Philadelphia: Lippincott /Williams & Wilkins.

Matthay, M. A., & Zimmerman, G. A. (2005). Acute lung injury and the acute respiratory distress syndrome. Four decades of inquiry into pathogenesis and rational management. *American Journal of Respiratory Cell and Molecular Biology, 33*(4), 319–327.

Matthay, M. A., Zimmerman, G. A., Esmon, C., Bhattacharya, J., Coller, B., Doerschuk, C. M., et al. (2003). Future research directions in acute lung injury. summary of a national heart, lung, and blood institute working group. *American Journal of Respiratory and Critical Care Medicine, 167*(7), 1027–1035.

Matthay, M., Zimmerman, G., Esmon, C., et al. (2003). Future research directions in acute lung injury: Summary of a national heart, lung, and blood institute working group. *American Journal of Respiratory and Critical Care Medicine, 167,* 1027–1035.

Matthay, M., Zimmerman, G., Esmon, C., et al. (2003). Future research directions in acute lung injury. Summary of a national heart, lung, and blood institute working group. *American Journal of Respiratory and Critical Care Medicine, 167,* 1027–1035.

Meduri, G. U., Golden, E., Freire, A. X., Taylor, E., Zaman, M., Carson, S. J., et al. (2007). Methylprednisolone infusion in early severe ARDS. Results of a randomized controlled trial. *Chest, 131*(4), 954–963.

Mellor, A., & Soni, N. (2001). Fat embolism. *Anaesthesia, 56,* 145–154.

Moss, M. (2006). Searching for the Holy Grail of the acute respiratory distress syndrome. *Intensive Care Medicine, 32*(8), 1112–1114.

National Asthma Education and Prevention Program Expert Panel Report (2007). Guidelines for the diagnosis and management of asthma. National Heart Lung and Blood Institute, National Institutes of Health. Available at: www.nhlbi.nih.gov/guidelines/asthma/index.htm. Accessed April 24, 2008.

National Heart, Lung, and Blood Institute Acute Respiratory Distress Syndrome (ARDS) Clinical Trials Network. (2006). Comparison of two fluid-management strategies in acute lung injury. *New England Journal of Medicine, 354*(24), 2564–2575.

National Heart Lung and Blood Institute. (2007). Expert Panel Report 3: Guidelines for the diagnosis and management of asthma. Retrieved July 19, 2008 from: http://www.nhlbi.nih.gov/guidelines/asthma/asthsumm.htm.

National Heart Lung and Blood Institute. (2008). Diseases and Conditions: Pneumonia. Retrieved on 11/28/08 from: http://www.nhlbi.nih.gov/health/dci/Diseases/pnu/pnu_causes.html.

Niederman, M. S. (2008). Pneumonia: considerations for the critically ill patient. In J. E. Parrillo & R. P. Dellinger (eds.), *Critical Care Medicine. Principles of diagnosis and management in the adult.* (3rd ed., pp. 867–883) Philadelphia: Mosby.

O'Shea, A., & Eappen, S. (2007). Amniotic fluid embolism. *International Anesthesiology Clinics, 45*(1), 17–28.

Oddo, M., Feihl, F., Schaller, M. D. & Perret, C. (2006). Management of mechanical ventilation in acute severe asthma: practical aspects. *Intensive Care Medicine 32*(4), 501–510.

Palmer, J. L., & Metheny, N. A. (2008). Preventing aspiration in older adults with dysphagia. *American Journal of Nursing, 108*(2), 40–48.

Peter, J. V., John, P, Graham, P. L., Moran, J. L., George, I. A., and Bersten, A. (2008). Corticosteroids in the prevention and treatment of acute respiratory distress syndrome (ARDS) in adults: meta-analysis. *BMJ, 336*(7651):969–70.

Piazza, G., & Goldhaber, S. Z. (2006). Acute pulmonary embolism part II: treatment and prophylaxis. *Circulation, 114*(3), e42–e47.

Piazza, G., Seddighzadeh, A., and Goldhaber, S. Z. (2008). Heart failure in patients with deep vein thrombosis. *Am J Cardiol, 101*(7):1056–9.

Powers, J., & Daniels, D. (2004). Turning points: implementing kinetic therapy in the ICU. *Nursing Management, 35*(Suppl. 5), 1–7.

Puntillo, K., & Ley, S. J. (2004). Appropriately timed analgesics control chest pain due to chest tube removal. *American Journal of Critical Care, 13*(4), 292–303.

Quereshi, M., Shah, N., Hemmen, C., et al. (2003). Exposure of intensive care unit nurses to nitric oxide and nitrogen dioxide during therapeutic use of inhaled nitric oxide in adults with acute respiratory distress syndrome. *American Journal of Critical Care, 12*(2), 147–153.

Quinlan, D. J., McQuillan, A., & Eikelboom, J. W. (2004). Low-molecular-weight heparin compared with intravenous unfractionated heparin for treatment of pulmonary embolism. *Annals of Internal Medicine, 140*,(3), 175–183.

Rothman, R. E., Hsieh, Y. H., & Yang, S. (2006). Communicable respiratory threats in the ED: Tuberculosis, influenza, SARS, and other aerosolized infections. *Emergency Medicine Clinics of North America, 24*(4), 989–1017.

Rubenfeld, G. D., & Herridge, M. S. (2007). Epidemiology and outcomes of acute lung injury. *Chest, 131*(2),554–562.

Schmitt, S. K. & Longworth, D. L. (2009). Pulmonary Infections. In R. L. Wilkins, J. K. Stoller, R. M. Kacmarek,, *Egans fundamentals of respiratory care* (9th ed., pp. 483–501). St. Louis: C.V. Mosby.

Sharma, S. (2006). Pulmonary hypertension, secondary. *E-medicine.* Available at: www.emedicine.com/med/topic2946.htm. Accessed April 19, 2008.

Shigemitsu, H., & Afshar, K. (2007). Aspiration pneumonias: under-diagnosed and under-treated. *Current Opinion in Pulmonary Medicine, 13*(3), 192–198.

Stafford, I., & Sheffield, J. (2007). Amniotic fluid embolism. *Obstetrics and Gynecology Clinics of North America, 34*(3):545–553.

Stein, P. D., & Henry, J. W. (1997). Clinical characteristics of patients with acute pulmonary embolism stratified according to their presenting syndromes. *Chest, 112*(4), 974–979.

Stein, P. D., Beemath, A., Matta, F., Weg, J. G., Yusen, R. D., Hales, C. A., et al. (2007). Clinical characteristics of patients with acute pulmonary embolism: Data from PIOPED II. *The American Journal of Medicine, 120*(10), 871–879.

Stein, P. D., Woodard, P. K., Weg, J. G., Wakefield, T. W. Tapson, V. F., Sostman, H. D., et al. (2006). Diagnostic pathways in acute pulmonary embolism: Recommendations of the PIOPED II investigators. *The American Journal of Medicine, 119*(12), 1048–1055.

Steinberg K. P., Hudson, L. D., Goodman, R. B., Hough, C. L., Lanken, P. N., Hyzy, R., et al. (2006). Efficacy and safety of corticosteroids for persistent acute respiratory distress syndrome. *New England Journal of Medicine 354*(16),1671–1684.

Suratt, B. T., & Parsons, P. E. (2006). Mechanisms of acute lung injury/acute respiratory distress syndrome. *Clinics in Chest Medicine, 27*(4), 579–589.

Tapson, V. F. (2008). Acute pulmonary embolism. *New England Journal of Medicine, 358*(10), 1037–1052.

Traver, G. A. (1985). Ineffective airway clearance: Physiology and clinical application. *Dimensions of Critical Care Nursing, 4*(4),198–208.

Uchiyama, K., Takano, H., Yanagisawa, R., Inoue, K., et al. (2004). A novel water-soluble vitamin E derivative prevents acute lung injury by bacterial endotoxin. *Clinical and Experimental Pharmacology and Physiology, 31*, 226–230.

Ulrich, S. P., & Canale, S. W. (2001). *Nursing care planning guides* (5th ed.). Philadelphia: W. B. Saunders.

Vollman, K. M. (2004). Prone positioning in the patient who has acute respiratory distress syndrome: The art and science. *Critical Care Nursing Clinics of North America. 16*(3), 319–336.

Vollman, K. M., & Aulbach, R. K. (1998). Acute respiratory distress syndrome. In M. R. Kinney, S. B. Dunbar, J. A. Brooks Brunn, N. Molter, & J. M. Vitello Cicciu (eds.), *AACN clinical reference for critical care nursing* 4th ed, pp. 529–564). St. Louis: C.V. Mosby.

Ware, L. B. (2005). Prognostic determinants of acute respiratory distress syndrome in adults: impact on clinical trial design. *Critical Care Medicine, 33*(Suppl.3), S217–S222.

Ware, L. B., Matthay, M. A., Parsons, P. E., Thompson B. T., Januzzi J. L., Eisner, M. D., The National Heart, Lung, and Blood Institute Acute Respiratory Distress Syndrome Clinical Trials Network. (2007). Pathogenetic and prognostic significance of altered coagulation and fibrinolysis in acute lung injury/acute respiratory distress syndrome. *Critical Care Medicine, 35*(8),1821–1828.

Wheeler, A. P. & Bernard, G. R. (2007). Acute lung injury and the acute respiratory distress syndrome: a clinical review. *Lancet, 369*(9572), 1553–1565.

WHO. (2003). Update 95 – SARS: Chronology of a serial killer. Available at: www.who.int/csr/don/2003_07_04/en/print.html. Accessed May 2, 2008.

WHO. (2004). Summary of probable SARS cases with onset of illness from 1 November 2002 to 31 July 2003. Retrieved 5/2/2008 from www.who.int/csr/sars/country/table2004_04_21/en/index.html.

Wiegand Lynn-McHale, D.J., & Carlson, K. (eds.) (2005). *AACN procedure manual for critical care* (5th ed.). Philadelphia: Elsevier/W. B. Saunders.

Wittenberg, A. G., Richard, A. J., & Conrad, S. A. (2006). Venous air embolism. *E-medicine.* Retrieved 4/19/2008 from www.emedicine.com/emerg/topic787.htm.

MODULE

11 Supporting Pulmonary Gas Exchange: Mechanical Ventilation

Beth Augustyn, Kathleen Dorman Wagner, Gail Priestley

OBJECTIVES Following completion of this module, the learner will be able to

1. Identify criteria used to determine the need for mechanical ventilator support.
2. Discuss the equipment necessary to initiate mechanical ventilation.
3. Describe the types of mechanical ventilators, based on mechanism of force and cycling mechanism.
4. Explain the commonly monitored ventilator settings.
5. Briefly explain two methods of providing noninvasive ventilatory support.
6. Discuss the major complications of mechanical ventilation.
7. Explain the cause and prevention of artificial airway complications.
8. Describe the care of the patient requiring mechanical ventilation.
9. Describe the process of weaning a patient from mechanical ventilation and the nurse's role in this process.

This self-study module focuses on a variety of concepts related to initiation of mechanical ventilation and management of the patient on a mechanical ventilator. This module uses information covered in two other modules: Module 9, Determinants and Assessment of Pulmonary Gas Exchange, and Module 10, Alterations in Pulmonary Gas Exchange. It is suggested that the reader become familiar with the material in those two modules before completing this one.

The module is divided into nine sections. Sections One through Five include the criteria used for determination of the need for mechanical ventilation, the required equipment to initiate mechanical ventilation, an introduction to the various types of mechanical ventilators, a brief discussion of the more commonly monitored ventilator settings, and noninvasive ventilatory support. In sections Six and Seven, the focus shifts to a discussion of how mechanical ventilation and artificial airways affect various parts of the body, including information about potential complications and methods to avoid them. Section Eight describes the nursing management of the mechanically ventilated patient, focusing on respiratory-related nursing diagnoses. The final section provides an overview of the weaning process. Each section includes a set of review questions to help the learner evaluate his or her understanding of the section's content before moving on to the next section. All Section Reviews include answers. It is suggested that the learner review those concepts answered incorrectly in the review questions before proceeding to the next section.

PRETEST

1. Mechanical ventilators are responsible for
   A. diffusion
   B. ventilation
   C. perfusion
   D. respiration
2. The most common indication for use of a mechanical ventilator is
   A. pneumonia
   B. chronic obstructive pulmonary disease (COPD)
   C. acute asthmatic attack
   D. acute ventilatory failure
3. Acute ventilatory failure is associated with
   A. alveolar hypoventilation
   B. severe hypoxemia
   C. alveolar hyperventilation
   D. severe hypocarbia
4. Acute respiratory acidosis can be defined clinically as
   A. pH greater than 7.50, $Pa{O_2}$ less than 60 mm Hg
   B. pH less than 7.30, $Pa{CO_2}$ greater than 50 mm Hg
   C. pH greater than 7.50, $Pa{O_2}$ less than 35 mm Hg
   D. pH less than 7.30, $Pa{CO_2}$ less than 30 mm Hg

5. The primary purpose of the endotracheal tube cuff is to seal off the
A. lower airway from the upper airway
B. lower airway from the esophagus
C. oropharynx from the nasopharynx
D. oropharynx from the esophagus

6. The most common type of airway access used during an emergency is
A. tracheostomy
B. nasal intubation
C. pharyngeal airway
D. oral intubation

7. A major advantage of volume-cycled ventilation is that it
A. applies negative pressure to the thorax
B. overcomes changes in lung compliance
C. does not require an artificial airway
D. automatically adjusts volume of gas delivered

8. A low tidal volume is associated most closely with
A. hypoventilation
B. hypocapnia
C. hypoxia
D. hypotension

9. The fraction of inspired oxygen (FiO_2) is correctly measured in
A. decimals
B. percentages
C. centimeters of water pressure (cm H_2O)
D. millimeters of mercury (mm Hg)

10. Synchronized intermittent mandatory ventilation (SIMV) is sensitive to
A. rate of airflow
B. respiratory rate
C. concentration of oxygen
D. the patient's ventilatory cycle

11. A common side effect of positive end-expiratory pressure (PEEP) is
A. increased blood pressure
B. decreased cardiac output
C. decreased lung compliance
D. increased venous return to the heart

12. During positive pressure ventilation, airflow will be greatest
A. in areas that are diseased
B. in areas that are nondependent
C. in the peripheral lung areas
D. in the lung apices

13. In what way does positive pressure ventilation affect intracranial pressure (ICP)?
A. it has no effect
B. it decreases ICP
C. it increases ICP
D. its effects are unknown

14. What effect does positive pressure ventilation have on renal function?
A. urine output is unaffected
B. urine output is decreased
C. urine output is increased
D. its effects are unknown

15. The term *barotrauma* refers to injury caused by
A. oxygen
B. friction
C. temperature
D. pressure

16. Oxygen toxicity has what effect on lung tissue?
A. It increases surfactant production.
B. It decreases mucous production.
C. It increases macrophage activity.
D. It increases lung compliance.

17. Endotracheal cuff trauma can be avoided by maintaining cuff pressures in the range of
A. 5 to 10 mm Hg
B. 10 to 20 mm Hg
C. 20 to 25 mm Hg
D. 25 to 30 mm Hg

18. Noninvasive intermittent positive pressure ventilation (NIPPV) is most useful for patients who
A. requires only support of tidal volume
B. cannot fully support their own expiratory effort
C. requires only support for nocturnal hypercapnia and hypoxemia
D. cannot fully support their own ventilatory effort over long periods of time

19. Common complications of noninvasive methods of ventilatory support include (choose all that apply)
A. conjunctivitis
B. nasal congestion
C. hypoventilation
D. otitis media

20. The majority of difficult-to-wean patients have which problem?
A. pneumonia
B. congestive heart failure
C. acute respiratory distress syndrome
D. chronic pulmonary disease

21. The term ______ weaning is used to refer to weaning by intermittently removing the patient from the ventilator for increasing periods of time.
A. manual
B. ventilator
C. SIMV
D. pressure support

Pretest answers are found on MyNursingKit.

SECTION ONE: Determining the Need for Ventilatory Support

At the completion of this section, the learner will be able to identify criteria used for determining the need for mechanical ventilatory support.

Mechanical ventilators are life-support machines that augment and support the **ventilation** portion of the respiratory process. The decision to place a patient on a mechanical ventilator is a very serious one. The invasiveness of the artificial airway as well as the physiologic alterations associated with mechanical ventilation place the patient at substantial risk for development of major complications; therefore, the relative benefits and costs must be weighed. Mechanical ventilation is a supportive intervention only. It is meant to support the patient's oxygenation and ventilation status while interventions are initiated to correct the underlying problem. Ventilatory support is best initiated as a "semi-elective" procedure before the patient's condition becomes severely compromised (i.e., cardiopulmonary arrest). Early support is thought to improve the patient's outcome.

How then is the decision made to place a patient on a mechanical ventilator? A variety of criteria have been established by pulmonary experts to aid the health care team in rapidly determining which patients may require ventilatory support. These criteria generally are not based on specific medical diagnoses but rather on respiratory function status (see Table 11–1).

Acute Ventilatory Failure

Acute ventilatory failure (AVF) is the most common indication for ventilator support. Acute ventilatory failure is the inability of the lungs to maintain adequate **alveolar ventilation**. It is diagnosed on the basis of the acid–base imbalance it creates—acute respiratory acidosis, which is expressed as **$Paco_2$** greater than 50 mm Hg and pH less than 7.30. A variety of problems can cause AVF, such as head trauma, apnea of any etiology, neuromuscular dysfunction, and drug-induced central nervous system (CNS) depression. Essentially, any problem that decreases movement of air to and from the alveoli can precipitate AVF.

Generally speaking, AVF is a direct indication for rapid intubation and mechanical ventilatory support. A possible exception is the patient with chronic obstructive pulmonary disease (COPD, chronic airflow limitation). Patients with COPD live in a state of chronic (long-term) ventilatory insufficiency. They are at particularly high risk for development of complications if placed on a ventilator and may be difficult if not impossible to wean from mechanical ventilatory support. For this reason, physicians often are reluctant to intubate and mechanically ventilate these patients unless it is absolutely necessary. Other criteria may be used, such as level of consciousness or a particular degree of respiratory acidosis, in making the decision to initiate mechanical support for this patient population. Patients with severe COPD or other nonreversible conditions may have firm opinions as to whether or not they want life support devices such as mechanical ventilation and should have the opportunity for informed consent that includes an explanation of risks and benefits by the physician.

TABLE 11–1 Criteria for Ventilatory Support

CRITERIA	CRITICAL VALUES
Acute ventilatory failure (AVF)	$Paco_2$ greater than 50 mm Hg, pH less than 7.30
Acute hypoxemia	Pao_2 less than 60 mm Hg
Pulmonary mechanics	
Respiratory rate (f)	f greater than 35 breaths/min
Vital capacity (VC)	VC less than 15 mL/kg (normal: 65 to 75)
Maximum Inspiratory Pressure (MIP)	MIP less than –20 cm H_2O (normal: –50 to –100 cm H_2O)
Minute ventilation $\dot{V}_E$	$\dot{V}_E$ greater than 10 L/min (normal: 5 to 10 L/min)

Pulmonary mechanics data from Pilbeam (2006).

Hypoxemia

The second major indication for mechanical ventilatory support is hypoxemia, which is frequently quantified as a **Pao_2** of less than 60 mm Hg. A low ventilation–perfusion ($\dot{V}/\dot{Q}$) ratio is the most common cause of hypoxemia. A low $\dot{V}/\dot{Q}$ refers to a state in which there is an excess of perfusion in relation to ventilation. The cause of a low $\dot{V}/\dot{Q}$ often is an obstructing mucous plug in the distal airway, causing a reduction in alveolar ventilation. Examples of conditions that are associated with a low $\dot{V}/\dot{Q}$ include asthma, pneumonia, COPD, and atelectasis.

Low $\dot{V}/\dot{Q}$ is associated with a phenomenon called shunting. **Shunting** refers to the state in which pulmonary capillary perfusion is normal but alveolar ventilation is lacking. Pulmonary capillary blood that runs by a nonfunctioning alveolar unit cannot pick up oxygen from that alveolus. Although some shunting is normal, if many alveolar units become nonfunctioning, a significant decrease in oxygen saturation (Sao_2) will occur, causing hypoxemia. Severe shunting is associated with such conditions as respiratory distress syndromes of both the infant and adult and severe pneumonia.

Pulmonary Mechanics

Pulmonary function (pulmonary mechanics) testing may be used to decide if mechanical ventilatory support is needed. Such testing provides the clinician with crucial information about respiratory muscle strength and airflow. When evaluating the need for mechanical ventilation, pulmonary function tests can provide data regarding evidence of hypoventilation. Several of the more common tests used as criteria are vital capacity, maximum inspiratory pressure, and respiratory rate (f). **Vital capacity** (VC) is the maximum amount of air that is expired after a maximal inspiration; and measures a person's greatest breathing capacity. Vital capacity decreases in the presence of restrictive pulmonary diseases such as atelectasis, pneumonia, and other disorders that reduce lung **compliance. Maximum inspiratory pressure (MIP, PImax)** measures the amount of negative pressure that a person is able to generate resulting from a maximal inspiratory effort. It reflects the strength of the respiratory muscles. Abnormally low MIP levels develop with respiratory muscle fatigue or neuromuscular diseases. A sustained respiratory rate of over 35 breaths per minute significantly increases the work of breathing, leading to respiratory muscle fatigue. Pulmonary mechanics also play a crucial role in determining readiness for removal from mechanical ventilation and will be discussed further in Section Nine.

Special Considerations

Age-related changes in pulmonary physiology place the elderly at risk for respiratory failure. These changes include decreased chest wall compliance, which increases the work of breathing; decreased oxygenation because of structural lung changes; and decreased lung volume and strength, which reduce cough effectiveness and increase the risk for infection. A reduced sensitivity to hypoxia and carbon dioxide plus changes in drug metabolism may increase the respiratory depressive effects of narcotics and sedatives. Many pulmonary diseases, such as COPD, become more evident with age. Age-related changes in other organs as well as comorbid conditions such as heart and renal disease alter respiratory function. Poor nutrition and decreased muscle strength can be additional risk factors. Thus, the elderly are at risk for respiratory failure due to pulmonary and nonpulmonary reasons.

The risks and benefits of critical care for the elderly and any patient with chronic disease, especially end-stage COPD and irreversible neuromuscular diseases has generated considerable controversy. Outcomes for elderly patients are related to disease severity and comorbid conditions; age alone is not predictive of survival or recovery (Sevransky & Haponik, 2003). Patient self-determination, futility, and other ethical concepts are especially pertinent to mechanical ventilation which is the most invasive commonly used form of life support. The decision whether to institute mechanical ventilation should include a compassionate and realistic evaluation of the patient's status and wishes for care.

SECTION ONE REVIEW

1. The term *ventilatory failure* refers to the inability of the lungs to
   A. expand
   B. diffuse gases
   C. use oxygen and carbon dioxide
   D. maintain adequate alveolar ventilation
2. Acute respiratory acidosis is defined clinically as
   A. $PaCO_2$ greater than 50 mm Hg and pH less than 7.30
   B. PaO_2 less than 60 mm Hg
   C. $PaCO_2$ greater than 45 mm Hg and pH less than 7.35
   D. PaO_2 less than 80 mm Hg
3. Common causes of acute ventilatory failure include (choose all that apply)
   A. apnea
   B. head trauma
   C. myocardial infarction
   D. neuromuscular dysfunction
4. A low $\dot{V}/\dot{Q}$ exists when
   A. ventilation is in excess of perfusion
   B. perfusion is in excess of ventilation
   C. blood is shunted away from the alveoli
   D. there is an obstruction in the pulmonary capillaries
5. The term *pulmonary shunt* refers to
   A. movement of air directly from one alveolus to another
   B. normal pulmonary capillary perfusion, lacking alveolar ventilation
   C. an opening between the pulmonary artery and the heart
   D. normal alveolar ventilation, lacking pulmonary capillary perfusion

Answers: 1. D, 2. A, 3. (A, B, D), 4. B, 5. B

SECTION TWO: Required Equipment for Mechanical Ventilation

At the completion of this section, the learner will be able to describe the equipment necessary for proper mechanical ventilation.

Mechanical ventilation is a complex intervention that requires a protocol of procedures and equipment. Adequate preparation will facilitate smooth implementation.

Initial Equipment Necessary for Establishment of a Patent Airway

Mechanical ventilation requires the use of special artificial airways. Artificial airways can be divided into two groups: endotracheal tubes and tracheostomy tubes.

Endotracheal Tubes

The endotracheal (ET) tube is a specially designed semirigid radiopaque tube (Fig. 11–1). Its slightly curved shaft is designed for ease of passage through the curved upper airway. In adults, the tubes require a cuff if positive pressure ventilation is to be initiated. The cuff is a balloon that is attached to the outside wall on the distal end of the ET tube. When it is inflated, the tube seals the space between the tube and the trachea so air is directed through the tube into the lower airway ensuring a predictable tidal volume or pressure (Fig. 11–2). Neonatal and small pediatrics ET tubes do not have cuffs because in children younger than 5 years of age, the cricoid cartilage offers a sufficient seal once the tube is inserted. New models of ET tubes are available with an

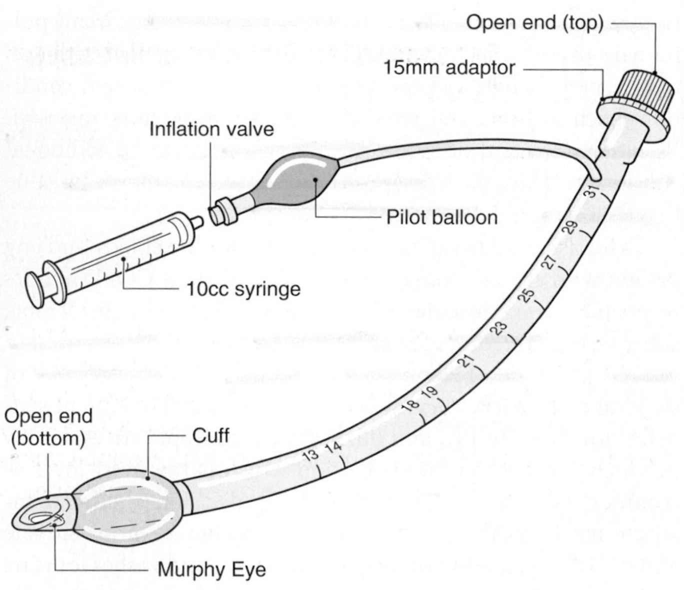

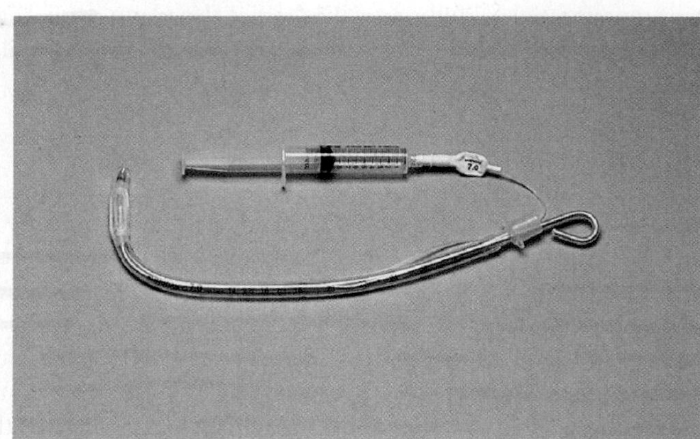

Figure 11–1 ■ Endotracheal tube. The photoimage on the right shows an endotracheal tube with a stylet (metal guide wire) in place.

evacuation lumen that opens above the cuff to suction out secretions that accumulate at the back of the throat on top of the inflated cuff (Fig. 11–3).

Choice of Endotracheal Tube Size and Route. The size of the ET tube to be inserted will depend primarily on the age of the person to be intubated. ET tube sizes range from 2 mm to 11 mm, which reflects the diameter of the inside lumen. Table 11–2 lists recommended adult ET tube sizes by gender.

In the adult, the route of entry also determines ET tube size. A smaller-sized tube is required if it is to be inserted nasally because the nasal airway passage is significantly smaller than the oral airway passage. Many brands of ET tubes designate, on the tube, which route is appropriate for each size tube (i.e., nasal, nasal/oral, or oral).

Current guidelines recommend the use of the orotracheal as opposed to the nasotracheal route. Although the nasotracheal tube may be more comfortable for the patient,

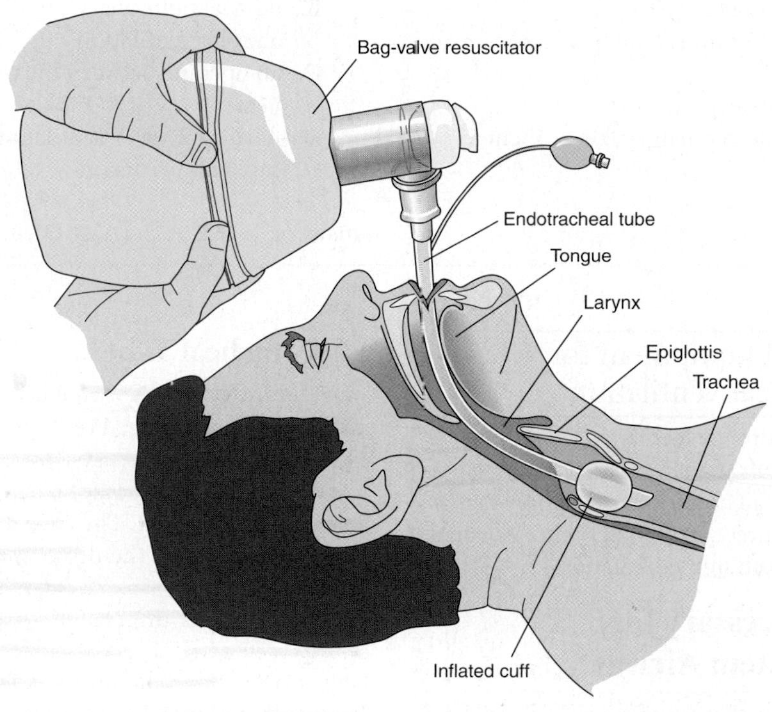

Figure 11–2 ■ Endotracheal tube with cuff inflated.

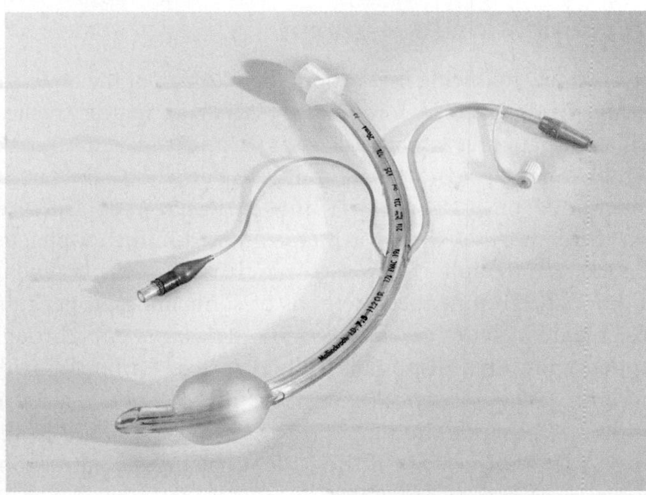

Figure 11–3 ▪ Hi-Low Evac Endotracheal Tube with Evacuation Lumen. PB 840 image used by permission from Nellcor Puritan Bennett LLC, Boulder, Colorado, part of Covidien.

it carries greater risk of sinusitis and other infections. Other problems associated with the smaller tube needed to intubate nasally includes increased **airway resistance**, increased chance of tube kinking, and more difficulty suctioning effectively. Nasotracheal intubation should be reserved for situations where facial trauma or other considerations make oral intubation impossible (NGC, n.d.).

Intubation Equipment. The endotracheal tube is inserted by a specially trained member of the health care team. The following items must be gathered before intubation:

- Soft-cuffed ET tubes (in a variety of sizes)
- Stylet
- Topical anesthetic
- Laryngoscope handle with blade attached
- Magill forceps
- Suction machine
- Suction catheters, Yankauer suction tip
- Syringe for cuff inflation
- Water-soluble lubricant
- Endotracheal tube holding device (or adhesive tape if device not available)
- Personal protective equipment
- Sedative medication

Tracheostomy Tubes

Generally, when mechanical ventilation is initiated, a tracheostomy is not the entry of choice because it is more invasive and takes longer to perform. However, tracheostomy might be performed initially if the patient has received head or neck surgery or has an upper airway obstruction resulting from severe edema (such as inhalation burns) or a tumor obstruction. Tracheostomy is more commonly performed on the patient who requires prolonged intubation because of failure to wean from the ventilator. Hospitals establish guidelines for limiting the length of time a person is allowed to have an ET

TABLE 11–2 Recommended Sizes for Endotracheal Tubes in Adults

GENDER	INTERNAL DIAMETER (MM)	LENGTH (CM)
Female	7.5–8.0	19–24
Male	8.0–9.0	20–28

tube in place before receiving a tracheostomy, usually a maximum of 2-3 weeks of intubation. Recent practice guidelines recommend early tracheostomy in trauma patients with an anticipated need for mechanical ventilator support longer than 7 days (NGC, n.d.[a]). Prolonged use of an ET tube is associated with many complications. Some of these complications can be avoided if a tracheostomy is performed in a timely manner.

Securing the Artificial Airway

Any type of artificial airway must be secured in place properly to prevent tube displacement and to minimize trauma to mucous membranes. Initially, in an emergency situation, the tube can be secured with adhesive tape; however, commercially available ET tube stabilizers are the preferred method of securing the ET tube. Figure 11–4 provides an example of a tube holder. Tracheostomy tubes commonly are secured with twill tape or a commercially available tracheostomy band. The tracheostomy tube also may be sutured in place to prevent accidental dislodgment. Once the airway is secured, a chest X-ray should be performed to confirm correct placement (2-3 cm above the carina).

Supportive Equipment

In addition to the artificial airway and mechanical ventilator, other supplies and equipment must be readily available, including:

- Two oxygen sources
  - One for the ventilator
  - One for the manual resuscitation bag, to provide 100 percent oxygen
- Suction equipment and at least one suction source

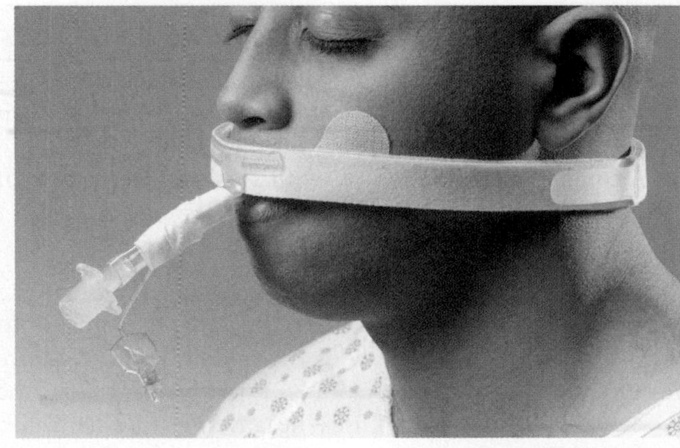

Figure 11–4 ▪ Securing the endotracheal tube. (Courtesy of Dale Medical Products.)

- Disposable sterile suction kits or sterile suction catheters, gloves, containers, sterile water
- Oral pharyngeal airway or a bite block if the oral route is used (to prevent closure of the airway if the patient should bite down on the tube)—also facilitates access to the oropharynx for suctioning
- Cuff manometer to check the ET tube cuff pressure on a regular basis
- A manual resuscitation bag to provide adequate backup in case of ventilator failure and for suctioning
- If positive end-expiratory pressure (PEEP) is to be used on the ventilator, a manual resuscitation bag with a PEEP attachment is recommended if a closed suctioning system is not to be used
- Secure intravenous access for medication administration
- Appropriate sedation and muscle relaxant agents should be readily available

Postintubation Assessment

Immediately following intubation, the position of the endotracheal tube is assessed for proper placement in the trachea. While the patient is receiving breaths via a manual resuscitation bag, both lung fields are auscultated for equal breath sounds. Air sounds or gurgling over the epigastric area indicates that the endotracheal tube is malpositioned in the esophagus. A chest radiograph is taken to confirm proper placement. Additional recommended methods of confirming proper tube placement include carbon dioxide measurement through capnography or a disposable CO_2 detector. Carbon dioxide monitors may produce false negatives if the cardiac output is too low to generate the return of CO_2 from the blood to the lungs; and false positives if the patient has ingested a carbonated beverage prior to intubation.

SECTION TWO REVIEW

1. In the adult, an inflated ET tube cuff is necessary for mechanical ventilation primarily because it
   A. prevents stomach contents from getting into the lungs
   B. seals off the nasopharynx from the oropharynx
   C. prevents air from getting into the stomach
   D. seals off the lower airway from the upper airway
2. The endotracheal tube size indicated on the tube reflects what measurement?
   A. the length of the tube
   B. the internal diameter of the tube
   C. the circumference size of the tube
   D. the length of the person's airway
3. In an emergency situation, the most common entry route for airway access is
   A. oral intubation
   B. nasal intubation
   C. tracheostomy
   D. oropharyngeal airway
4. Which of the following statements is true about securing the artificial airway?
   A. The inflated cuff provides sufficient securing.
   B. The airway is generally sutured in place.
   C. A nasotracheal tube does not require securing.
   D. Artificial airways must be secured directly to the patient.
5. When setting up a room for mechanical ventilator use, there must be
   A. one oxygen source
   B. two oxygen sources
   C. clean gloves for suctioning
   D. a backup ventilator in the room

Answers: 1. D, 2. B, 3. A, 4. D, 5. B

SECTION THREE: Types of Mechanical Ventilators

At the completion of this section, the learner will be able to describe the types of mechanical ventilators, based on mechanism of force and cycling mechanism.

A common classification of ventilators uses mechanism of force, which is either negative or positive pressure.

Negative Pressure Ventilators

Negative pressure ventilators were the first type of ventilator to be experimented with, as early as the middle 1800s. Negative pressure ventilation uses negatively applied pressure to the thorax by external means. To use a negative pressure ventilator, the patient's entire body (e.g., an iron lung) or thoracic region (e.g., a cuirass) is encased in an airtight unit. At regular intervals, the air pressure in the sealed unit is reduced to below atmospheric pressure. The resulting negative pressure is transmitted through the thorax, which results in a pressure gradient that causes air to move into the lungs. The amount of negative pressure used is based on the desired tidal volume (V_T) —the higher the desired V_T, the higher the negative pressure required. Today, negative pressure ventilators are primarily used in the home, for long-term use in patients with relatively normal lung function. Examples of patients who might benefit from negative pressure ventilation include those with chronic hypoventilation and/or respiratory failure associated with neuromuscular diseases; those who require intermittent ventilatory support, such as during sleep; and, in certain cases, those with COPD.

Positive Pressure Ventilators

Positive pressure ventilation is the mainstay of ventilatory support in acute care settings. Positive pressure ventilators most commonly require an artificial airway to deliver ventilatory support. Gases are driven into the lungs through the ventilator's circuitry, which

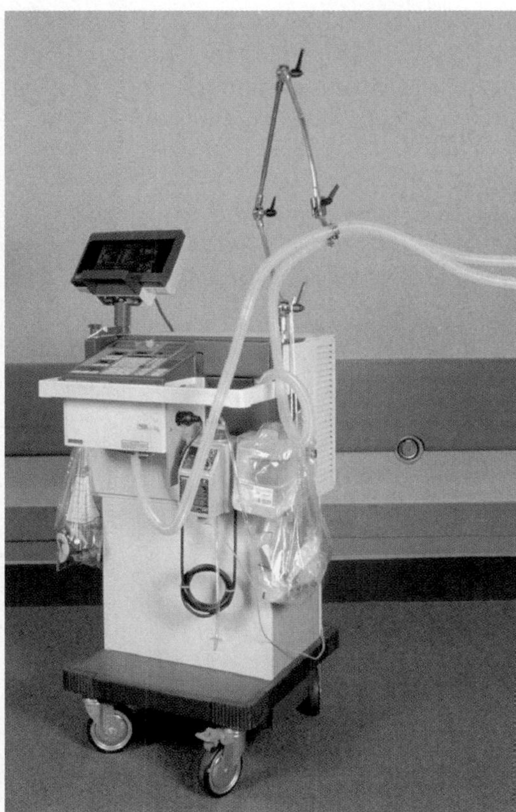

Figure 11–5 ■ Example of a mechanical ventilator.

is attached to an artificial airway (ET or tracheostomy tube). Figure 11–5 shows an example of a positive pressure ventilator.

Positive pressure ventilators are commonly described on the basis of their cycling mechanism. The term **cycle** refers to the mechanism by which the inspiratory phase is stopped and the expiratory phase is started. There are four major cycling mechanisms: pressure-cycled, volume-cycled, time-cycled, and flow-cycled.

Because the cycling mechanisms actually limit the length of inspiration, the term *cycle* is often replaced by the term *limit* (i.e., pressure-limited). The newer ventilators provide more than one cycling device; however, only one cycling mechanism can be used at a time. With this increased flexibility, the health care team can alter the type of cycling based on the changing needs of the patient without switching ventilators. Some newer ventilators switch their cycling mechanisms to meet the patient's needs. The remainder of this section briefly describes ventilators based on the cycling mechanism used.

Pressure-Cycled Ventilation

Pressure-cycled ventilation delivers a preset pressure of gas to the lungs. The pressure delivered (expressed in cm H_2O) is constant while the volume of air it delivers varies with the lung's compliance and airway resistance. This presents potentially serious support problems because stiffening lungs, a leak in the system or a partially obstructed airway can significantly alter the volume of gas delivered with each breath. Maintaining an adequate V_T is crucial for normal lung functioning. Pressure-cycled ventilation is increasingly used as a method to protect the injured lung from further damage from high pressures and is an option on most ventilators.

Volume-Cycled Ventilation

Volume-cycled ventilation delivers a preset volume of gas (measured in mL or L) to the lungs, making volume the constant and pressure the variable. Within a certain preset safety range (pressure limits), the ventilator will deliver the established volume of gas regardless of the amount of pressure it requires. This has the advantage of being able to overcome changes in lung compliance and airway resistance. For example, as lung compliance decreases or airway resistance increases, the pressure at which the gas is delivered to the lungs will increase sufficiently to deliver the desired volume of gas to the lungs. Volume ventilation has the potential to generate high pressures, especially in less compliant lungs in order to deliver the set volume. Therefore, the risk of barotrauma is greater.

Time-Cycled Ventilation

When time-cycled ventilation is used, the length of time allowed for inspiration is controlled. These ventilators hold time constant but volume and pressure may vary. Time-cycled ventilators frequently are referred to as time-cycled–pressure-limited ventilators because they also limit the maximum amount of pressure that can be delivered. The microprocessor ventilators can use time cycling and also have the advantage of being able to limit volume and pressure.

Flow-Cycled Ventilation

Pressure support ventilation (PSV) is an example of flow-cycled ventilation. A preset pressure augments the patient's inspiratory effort and continues as long as the patient continues to inhale at a certain flow rate. As the patient reaches the end of inspiration, flow decreases. At a predetermined level of flow (e.g., 25 percent of peak inspiratory flow) inspiration ends. Tidal volume, rate, and time are variable.

SECTION THREE REVIEW

1. Negative pressure ventilators adjust the tidal volume by
   A. adjusting the amount of negative airflow
   B. adjusting the amount of positive airflow
   C. altering the amount of negative pressure applied
   D. altering the amount of positive pressure applied

2. The term *cycle* as it applies to mechanical ventilation refers to the mechanism by which
   A. the ventilator turns on and off
   B. inspiration ceases and expiration starts
   C. the concentration of oxygen is controlled
   D. the rate of airflow is maintained

(continued)

(continued)

3. Volume-cycled ventilation has an advantage over pressure-cycled ventilation because it
   - A. adjusts volume as pulmonary pressure changes
   - B. increases airflow as compliance increases
   - C. decreases airflow as airway resistance decreases
   - D. can adjust pressure to changes in lung compliance
4. Pressure-cycled ventilation uses which of the following as a constant?
   - A. pressure
   - B. time
   - C. volume
   - D. flow rate
5. Time-cycled ventilation is also referred to as time-cycled ______ limited ventilation.
   - A. volume
   - B. flow
   - C. pressure
   - D. time
6. When flow-cycled ventilation is used, ______ is preset.
   - A. time
   - B. pressure
   - C. volume
   - D. rate

Answers: 1. C, 2. B, 3. D, 4. A, 5. C, 6. B

SECTION FOUR: Commonly Monitored Ventilator Settings

At the completion of this section, the learner will be able to explain the commonly monitored ventilator settings.

Positive pressure ventilators offer many variables that can be manipulated to meet precisely the individual pulmonary needs of the patient. Certain settings and values related to each variable must be monitored by anyone taking care of a mechanically ventilated patient whether in a critical care unit, on a general floor, or in the home. The most commonly monitored settings include tidal volume (VT), fraction of inspired oxygen (FiO_2), ventilation mode, respiratory rate (f), positive end-expiratory pressure (PEEP), continuous positive airway pressure (CPAP), pressure support (PS), peak inspiratory pressure (PIP), and alarms. Figure 11–6 shows the ventilator screen on a Puritan Bennett® 840™ dual-microprocessor ventilator system control panel that includes patient settings. These settings are summarized in Table 11–3.

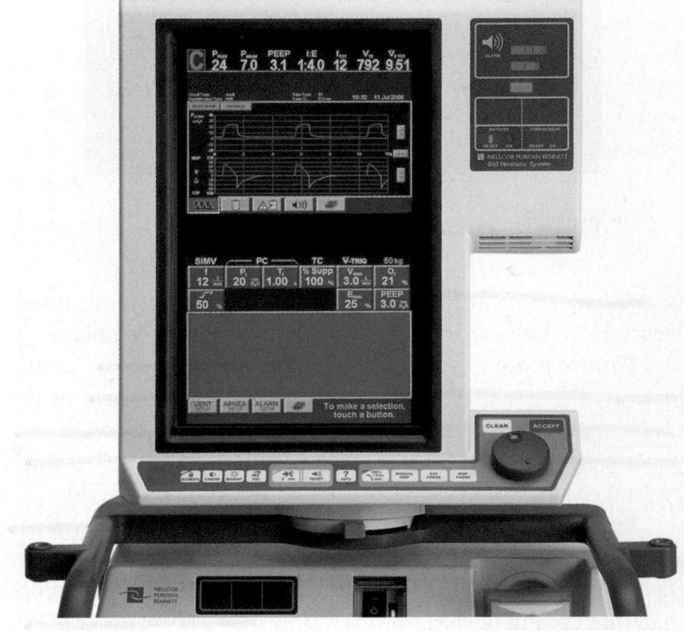

Figure 11–6 ■ Example of a mechanical ventilator control board. The Puritan Bennett® 840™ dual-microprocessor ventilator system. (PB 840 image used by permission from Nellcor Puritan Bennett LLC, Boulder, Colorado, part of Covidien.)

Tidal Volume

Tidal volume (VT or TV) is the amount of air that moves in and out of the lungs in one normal breath. Normal VT ranges from 7 to 9 mL/kg (or 500 to 800 mL in an adult). If VT is set too low, hypoventilation will occur. If VT is set too high, the patient is at risk for pneumothorax and possible depression of the cardiovascular system.

If volume-cycled ventilation is to be used, the desired VT is set when mechanical ventilation is initiated. Opinions vary regarding how high to set the VT. Current trends in ventilator management are to use smaller tidal volumes and prevent high peak airway pressures. The goal tidal volume is the maximum volume allowed to keep the peak airway pressure less than 30 mm Hg while maintaining adequate ventilation.

Adverse Effects of High Tidal Volumes

The risk of lung injury increases as peak alveolar pressure increases. Although alveolar pressure is not measured directly, it can be approximated through measurement of the plateau pressure. Plateau pressure reflects to the pressure being exerted on the alveoli during positive pressure ventilation and is easily measured at the end of inspiration by momentarily occluding the ventilatory circuit.

Barotrauma. Excessive pressure can cause **barotrauma,** an injury to pulmonary tissue. A tidal volume of more than 12 mL/kg is no longer recommended because it overdistends the alveoli, causing lung damage (Sullivan & Gropper, 2007). This damage may result in rupture of the alveolar membrane allowing air to enter the pleural space (pneumothorax) or tissue (subcutaneous emphysema).

TABLE 11–3 Commonly Monitored Ventilator Settings

SETTING	NORMAL RANGE
Minute Ventilation ($\dot{V}_E$)	5-7 L/minute
Respiratory Rate (f)	6-20 breaths/minute
Tidal volume (V_T)	5-12 mL/kg
Fraction of Inspired Oxygen (FiO_2)	0.21-1.0
Positive end expiratory pressure (PEEP)	5-20 cm H_2O
Pressure Support (PS)	5-15cm H_2O
Peak Pressure (P_{Peak}) or Peak Inspiratory Pressure (PIP)	Less than 40 cmH_2O

Volutrauma. Excessive volume can result in **volutrauma,** an injury to pulmonary tissue. The overdistension of the alveoli can cause more subtle alveolar injury through overstretching the alveolar cells, triggering release of inflammatory mediators and stimulation of the inflammatory response. Volutrauma increases the permeability of the lungs' microvasculature, which may result in pulmonary edema (Pilbeam, 2006).

Normal-Volume Settings

The selection of tidal volume may range from 4 to 12 mL/kg of ideal body weight (adult) based on the patient's lung status (Marino, 2006). Patients with normal lungs can be ventilated in the higher ranges, whereas those with restrictive or obstructive disease should be managed with lower tidal volumes. The goal is to adequately ventilate the lungs while maintaining a plateau pressure of less than 30 cm H_2O. Some patients with pulmonary diseases cannot be adequately ventilated (i.e., normal $PaCO_2$) at these lower pressures and volumes. A technique called permissive hypercapnia may be considered for use in this patient population. This technique deliberately allows hypoventilation by using low tidal volumes. The health care team must determine how high the $PaCO_2$ and how low the pH will be permitted to drift.

Sigh

The term **sigh** refers to intermittent hyperinflation of the lungs. During normal spontaneous breathing, a person naturally takes an occasional deep breath (about one sigh every 6 minutes), which improves ventilation of the lungs. Use of manual and automatic sighs during mechanical ventilation was used widely in the 1960s to prevent development of atelectasis and to decrease shunt. When the practice of high tidal volume ventilation became common, use of the sigh controls was no longer considered necessary or desirable. Use of sighing remains controversial. When used, it is commonly set at a volume of 1.5 to 2 times the patient's V_T and at a rate of 6 to 10 per hour.

Fraction of Inspired Oxygen (FiO_2)

FiO_2 means the **fraction of inspired oxygen.** It is expressed as a decimal, although clinicians often discuss it in percentages, in terms of oxygen concentrations. At sea level, the room air that is inhaled into the alveoli is composed of oxygen that is 0.21 of the total concentration of gases in the alveoli. A mechanical ventilator is able to deliver a wide range of FiO_2, from 0.21 to 1.0 (an oxygen concentration of 21 percent to 100 percent).

Initially, in an emergency situation, FiO_2 is commonly set at 0.5 to 1.0 to deliver 50 percent to 100 percent oxygen to the patient. The setting is then increased or decreased based on the patient's PaO_2 and clinical picture. The goal is to maintain the PaO_2 within an acceptable range for the individual, using the lowest level of FiO_2. Prolonged use of FiO_2 greater than 0.60 may cause complications associated with oxygen toxicity (discussed in Section Seven).

In a semielective situation, the initial FiO_2 may be set at lower levels, based on more individualized oxygenation needs. The patient who retains carbon dioxide, (e.g., advanced stage COPD) requires special consideration. When maintenance of some degree of patient-initiated breathing is desirable, care must be taken to set the FiO_2 at the lowest level that will deliver an acceptable PaO_2. The use of high concentrations of oxygen on such an individual may increase the PaO_2 excessively and obliterate the hypoxic drive to breathe.

Ventilation Modes

The ventilation mode refers to that which initiates the cycling of the ventilator to terminate expiration. The most common modes are assist-control (AC or ACMV) mode and synchronized intermittent mandatory ventilation (SIMV). Table 11–4 summarizes the positive pressure ventilator modes.

Assist-Control Mode

Most ventilators have an assist mode, a control mode, and an **assist-control mode (AC).** In assist mode, the ventilator is sensitive to the inspiratory effort of the patient. When the patient begins to inhale, the assist mode triggers the ventilator to deliver a breath at the prescribed settings (called a *ventilator* or *mechanical breath*). In the control mode, the ventilator delivers the breaths at a preset rate based on time. It is not sensitive to the patient's own ventilatory effort. Control mode generally is not used alone unless the patient is continuously apneic. A combination of assist and control modes generally is used. AC mode protects the patient in the following manner. The assist part of the mode is sensitive to spontaneous inspiratory effort of the patient, allowing the patient to maintain some control over the rate of breathing. At the same time, the control part of the mode acts as a backup should the patient decrease the breathing effort below the preset rate. When AC mode is used, every breath is a ventilator breath at the preset tidal volume. AC mode commonly is used initially, as a resting mode, particularly in patients with acute respiratory failure or respiratory muscle fatigue because it takes over the work of breathing, thereby resting the respiratory muscles and reducing oxygen consumption. The major disadvantage of AC

TABLE 11–4 Modes of Positive Pressure Mechanical Ventilation

MODE	DESCRIPTION	PATTERN
Spontaneous breathing	Client has full control of rate, tidal volume, pressures.	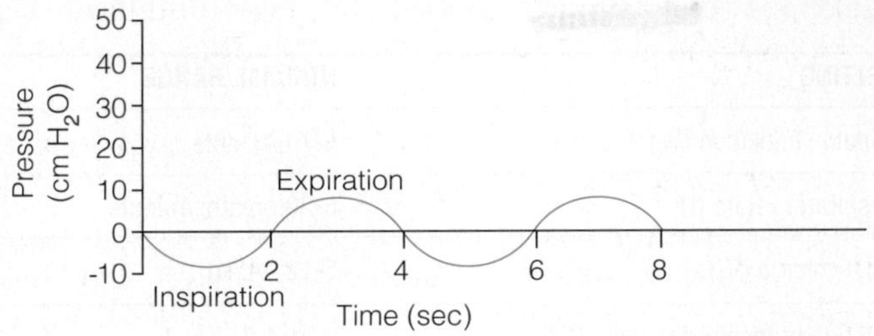
Assist-control mode ventilation (ACMV)	Client can trigger ventilator to deliver breaths at preset volume or pressure and inspiratory flow rate; breaths will be delivered at preset rate if client does not initiate.	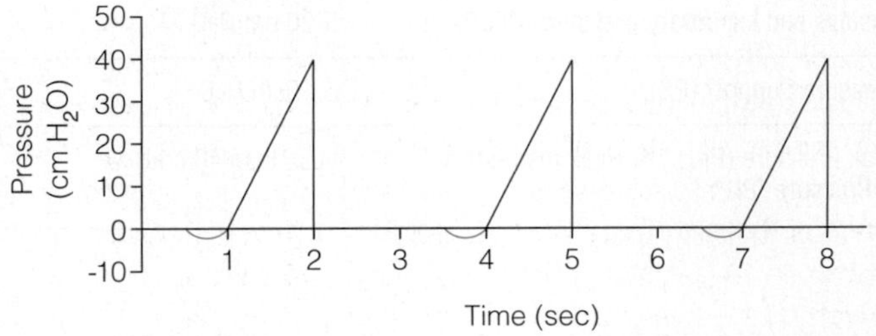
Synchronized intermittent mandatory ventilation (SIMV)	Mandatory breaths delivered by ventilator are synchronized with client's inspiratory effort.	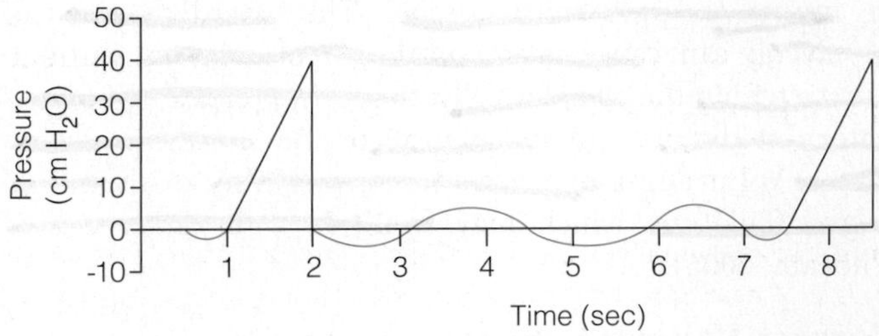
Continuous positive airway pressure (CPAP)	Positive pressure is maintained in airways; all breaths are spontaneous.	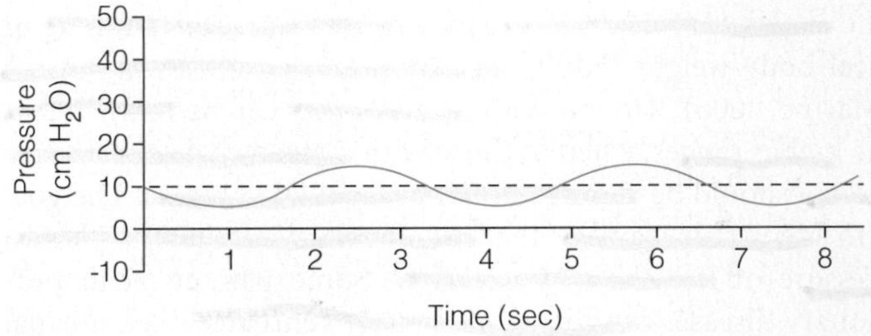
Positive end-expiratory pressure (PEEP)	Used in conjunction with other ventilator modes; positive airway pressure is maintained throughout respiratory cycle.	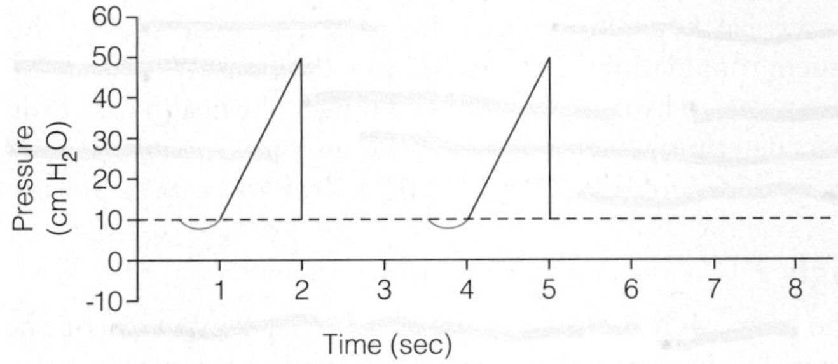
Pressure support ventilation (PSV)	Pressurized inspiratory flow supports the client's inspiratory effort, decreasing the work of breathing.	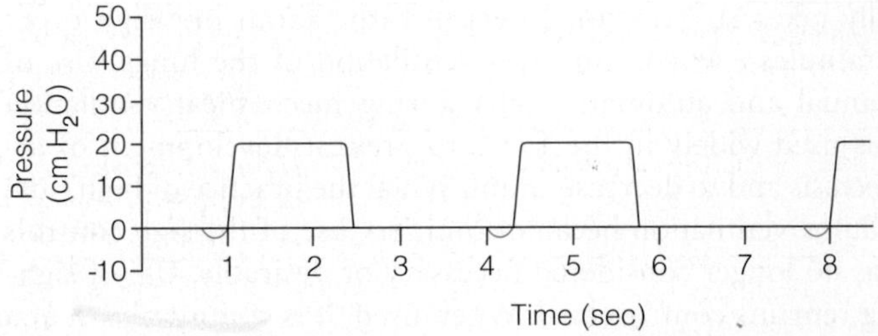

mode is development of respiratory muscle atrophy, which occurs since the ventilator is performing the work of breathing. Prolonged use of this mode can make weaning more difficult due to respiratory muscle weakness.

Synchronous Intermittent Mandatory Ventilation Mode

Using the **synchronous intermittent mandatory ventilation (SIMV)** mode, the patient spontaneously breathes through the ventilator circuit, maintaining much of the work of breathing. Interspersed at regular intervals, the ventilator provides a preset ventilator breath. The intervals are based on the SIMV rate set by the operator. For example, if the SIMV is set at 12, the ventilator will deliver a breath approximately every 5 seconds to make 12 breaths per minute. Between mandatory breaths, the patient's breathing will vary in V_T and rate because it is composed of **spontaneous breaths**, not ventilator breaths. SIMV synchronizes a mandatory breath to follow the patient's exhalation to prevent stacking of breaths (adding a ventilator breath on top of the patient's own inhalation). SIMV has certain advantages over the other modes. It decreases the risk of hyperventilation and provides a better ventilation–perfusion distribution. SIMV also facilitates the process of ventilator weaning and is often referred to as a weaning mode.

Pressure Support Ventilation Mode

Pressure support ventilation (PSV) was introduced into the United States during the mid-1980s. Pressure support ventilation is defined as an adjunct weaning mode that enhances spontaneous inspiratory effort by application of positive pressure. It is triggered by the patient's spontaneous breathing effort and decreases the effort (work) required to achieve a tidal volume. PSV applies and maintains the preset pressure throughout the entire inspiration phase.

One use for PSV is to decrease the work of breathing by overcoming increased airway resistance (R_{aw}) imposed by an artificial airway and ventilator circuitry. In this application, pressure support ventilation may be used as an aid to ventilator weaning. Patients on SIMV weaning mode are at increased risk for respiratory muscle fatigue and ventilatory failure. This is because they must breathe harder than normal to maintain adequate tidal volumes due to increased airway resistance associated with the endotracheal tube and ventilator circuitry. In these patients, PSV decreases the work of breathing by supporting the tidal volume during spontaneous breaths. It can also be used as a primary ventilatory mode to assist patients who are breathing spontaneously, including patients receiving continuous positive airway pressure (CPAP). This application requires a stable lung condition as well as reliable respiratory control. Should the patient have an apneic spell while on PSV using only an assist mode, there is no timed backup present to take over ventilation.

Three major factors determine the patient's tidal volume: the preset pressure support level, the degree of patient effort, and the level of airway resistance and lung compliance. When using desired tidal volume as the basis for manipulating the level of PSV, the PSV level is increased until the desired tidal volume is reached. When the level of PSV is used to offset the resistance imposed by the artificial airway, the PSV level commonly is adjusted to provide just enough support to overcome estimated resistance, increasing patient comfort. Pressure support ventilation frequently is adjusted in increments of 5 cm H_2O, with levels commonly ranging from 5 to 15 cm H_2O.

Pressure-Regulated Volume-Controlled Mode (PRVC)

Pressure-regulated volume-controlled (PRVC) ventilation is a dual control mode of ventilation. This mode resembles AC mode in that rate and tidal volume are preset and breaths can be initiated by the patient (assisted breath) or the ventilator (controlled breath). Like pressure support ventilation, pressure is constant throughout inspiration; however, the pressure readjusts on a breath-to-breath basis to achieve the set tidal volume. As the patient's pulmonary condition improves, the pressure required to deliver the tidal volume reduces automatically. Oxygenation is improved through a decelerating inspiratory flow pattern.

Table 11–5 provides a summary of the advantages and disadvantages of the ventilator modes.

TABLE 11–5 Advantages and Disadvantages of the Common Ventilation Modes

MODE	ADVANTAGES	DISADVANTAGES
Assist-Control (AC)	Every breath is guaranteed set tidal volume Takes over work of breathing, respiratory muscle rest	Risk of hyperventilation Respiratory muscle atrophy
Synchronized Intermittent Mandatory Ventilation (SIMV)	Prevents respiratory muscle atrophy Decreased risk of hyperventilation Better ventilation-perfusion distribution	Tachypnea and fatigue if set rate too low
Pressure Support Ventilation (PSV)	Improved patient-ventilator synchrony Prevents respiratory muscle atrophy Facilitates weaning	Requires spontaneous respiratory effort Tachypnea and fatigue if pressure support is too low
Pressure-Regulated Volume-Controlled Ventilation (PRVC)	Guaranteed $\dot{V}_E$ Improved patient-ventilator synchrony Decreased risk of barotrauma	Respiratory muscle atrophy May result in unequal ventilation-perfusion distribution

Respiratory Rate

Properly setting the respiratory (breathing) rate (f) on the ventilator is important in establishing adequate minute ventilation ($\dot{V}E$). *Minute ventilation* is the amount of air that moves in and out of the lungs in one minute. Normal $\dot{V}E$ is 5 to 7 L/min. VT (tidal volume) and f (rate) are the two variables that make up $\dot{V}E$. It can be calculated using the following equation:

$$\dot{V}_E = V_T \times f$$

These variables are significant because if either one is manipulated, it will affect $\dot{V}E$. If $\dot{V}E$ becomes too low, hypoventilation will occur, possibly precipitating acute respiratory acidosis. In the carbon dioxide–retaining COPD patient, hyperventilation that results in decreased carbon dioxide levels can complicate weaning from the mechanical ventilator. Additionally, the respiratory alkalosis produced by hyperventilation will shift the oxyhemoglobin dissociation curve to the left, impairing the release of oxygen at the tissue level.

The most therapeutic ventilator rate depends on the characteristics of the patient's lungs (Hall, Schmidt, and Wood, 2005). Three examples are provided here to show how three different lung states can alter the therapeutic tidal volume (VT) and respiratory rate (f):

- A patient with normal lungs
  VT: 8-12 mL/kg; f: 8 to 12/min
- A patient with lung disease with increased lung compliance (C_L) and airway resistance (R_{aw}) (e.g., COPD)
  VT: 8 to 12 mL/kg; f: 6 to 10/min
- A patient with restrictive lung disease (e.g., a neuromuscular disease)
  VT: 5 to 7 mL/kg or less; f: 12 to 20/min

PEEP and CPAP

For many years there has been an interest in perfecting a method to keep the alveoli open throughout the breathing cycle. Although this method (called **positive end-expiratory pressure, PEEP**) was first developed in the 1940s by the military, it was not used in medicine until the late 1960s. In the early 1970s, it was introduced as a treatment for respiratory distress syndrome in newborns. Since that time, it has become the foundation for oxygenating the lungs in newborns and adults with respiratory distress syndrome (Pilbeam, 2006).

Positive end-expiratory pressure is applied to the lungs in one of two ways, either as continuous positive airway pressure (CPAP) or positive end-expiratory pressure (PEEP). PEEP is used when a patient is being mechanically ventilated and it can be used in a variety of ventilator modes, including assist-control and SIMV. CPAP is used when a patient is spontaneously breathing. It does not require an artificial airway or a mechanical ventilator, although many ventilators have a CPAP setting. PEEP and CPAP provide the alveoli with a constant (preset) amount of positive pressure at the end of the expiratory phase of breathing, which prevents airway pressure from returning to zero. Normally, at the end of expiration, alveoli have a natural tendency to collapse. When positive pressure is provided during the expiration phase of the breathing cycle, it forces the alveoli to remain open, which (1) recruits previously collapsed alveoli, (2) prevents atelectasis, and (3) improves oxygenation.

The primary indication for use of PEEP/CPAP is the presence of refractory hypoxemia (i.e., hypoxemia that is unresponsive to increasing concentrations of oxygen). PEEP is useful in treating acute diffuse lung disease processes (e.g., acute respiratory distress syndrome and cardiogenic pulmonary edema) and in treating postoperative atelectasis. Low levels of PEEP (e.g., 5 cm H_2O) are commonly used for intubated patients to prevent atelectasis and achieve adequate oxygenation at lower FIO_2 levels.

The level of PEEP can be monitored on most ventilators by observing the airway pressure manometer. When no PEEP is being applied, the manometer needle should fall back to zero at the end of each breath. When PEEP is present, the needle should fall back to the level of PEEP. For example, if PEEP is set at 10 cm H_2O, the needle should fall to 10 ± 2 cm H_2O rather than to zero. The level of PEEP is adjusted to meet the patient's oxygenation needs. Traditionally, this has been done by increasing the PEEP level in increments of 3 to 5 cm H_2O until adequate oxygenation is achieved at a safe FIO_2. Newer methods are now available for selecting the optimal PEEP level using ventilator graphics that reflect levels of airway closure.

The level of positive pressure required depends primarily on the severity of lung injury. Mild forms of lung injury usually require between 5 and 10 cm H_2O. In cases of more severe lung injury, the patient may require 10 to 20 cm H_2O. Levels of PEEP as high as 30 cm H_2O or more have been used; however, there is a trend away from using such high PEEP (sometimes referred to as "super PEEP") levels in favor of newer ventilator strategies that limit peak inspiratory pressures and use smaller tidal volumes.

PEEP can also be used to offset **auto-PEEP**, which refers to an unintentional buildup of positive end-expiratory pressure caused by alveolar airtrapping. It is particularly associated with COPD. Airtrapping prevents the COPD patient from exhaling fully, which leaves a volume of air in the alveoli at the end of expiration. When the lungs of COPD patients become hyperinflated, the patient may not be able to inhale sufficiently to trigger the mechanical ventilator in an assist mode. Applying a small amount of PEEP externally, to match the level of auto-PEEP, can offset the effects of the auto-PEEP such that the patient can trigger the ventilator to cycle properly.

Although PEEP and CPAP are important in the treatment of severe hypoxemia, their use is associated with significant complications that can be as detrimental to patient outcomes as severe hypoxemia. The risk of complications increases as the amount of PEEP or CPAP is increased. High levels of PEEP require close cardiovascular monitoring. The complications associated with PEEP can be categorized into two groups: barotrauma to the lungs and decreased cardiac output, and are discussed in Section Six.

Peak Airway Pressure or Peak Inspiratory Pressure

When using volume-cycled ventilation, the tidal volume is preset to deliver a certain number of milliliters or liters of air.

The pressure it takes to deliver that amount of volume varies depending primarily on airway resistance and lung compliance. The amount of pressure required to deliver the volume is called the **peak airway pressure (P_{Peak})** or *peak inspiratory pressure (PIP)*. PIP is measured in centimeters of water pressure (cm H_2O) and may be visualized on an airway pressure manometer or on a data screen. In the adult, PIP volumes of less than 40 cm H_2O are considered desirable. It is known that high PIPs greatly increase the risk of barotrauma and have negative effects on other body systems (see Section Six). PIP should be recorded at regular intervals for trending—taking multiple measurements over an extended period of time to evaluate the parameter for a pattern of change.

An increasing peak inspiratory pressure (PIP) trend signifies that increasing amounts of pressure are necessary to deliver the preset tidal volume. It is most commonly indicative of increasing airway resistance or decreasing lung compliance, suggesting a worsening of the patient's pulmonary status. A decreasing peak inspiratory pressure signifies that less pressure is needed to deliver the tidal volume. It may indicate an improvement in airway resistance or lung compliance, suggesting improvement of the patient's pulmonary status.

Alarms

The patient's life depends on correct functioning of the ventilator and maintenance of a patent airway. To protect the patient, ventilators are equipped with a system of alarms to alert the caregiver to problems. Two frequently triggered alarms are the low exhaled volume and high-pressure alarms. In any alarm, the nurse should always check the patient before the ventilator. Additionally, the nurse should collaborate with the respiratory therapist to troubleshoot ventilator operation. A manual resuscitation bag should be kept at the bedside to be used for manually ventilating the patient in the event of ventilator or power failure.

Low Exhaled Volume Alarm

The low exhaled volume alarm indicates that there is a loss of tidal volume or a leak in the system. When this alarm goes off, the nurse should focus rapidly on checking to see whether the ventilator tubing has become disconnected or whether the artificial airway cuff is inadequately filled with air or has a leak. The cuff can be checked by feeling for air leaking out of the nose and mouth. The nurse may also hear gurgling sounds from the mouth. It may be noted that the patient can suddenly vocalize, which also indicates a leak or insufficiently inflated cuff. A leaking cuff may be checked by deflating and then reinflating the cuff to observe for its ability to attain and then maintain a tracheal seal. If the cuff is ruptured, the nurse must notify the medical team immediately and prepare for reintubation. If a cuff must be deflated for any reason, deep oral suctioning should precede deflation to prevent flooding the lower airway with contaminated secretions from the upper airway. The low exhaled volume alarm is commonly triggered when the patient is switched from assist-control mode to SIMV mode and the exhaled volume alarm is not reset. In this instance, the alarm sounds because the patient's spontaneous tidal volume is general lower than mechanically set tidal volume.

Box 11–1 The Golden Rules of Ventilator Alarms

- Check the patient first. If the patient looks satisfactory, then check the machine.
- If the cause of an alarm is not immediately found or cannot be corrected immediately, the patient should be removed from the ventilator and manually ventilated using a resuscitation bag until the problem is corrected.

High-Pressure Alarm

The high-pressure alarm is the most common one that is triggered. Any patient problem that increases airway resistance can trigger it. Examples of clinical conditions that cause a high-pressure alarm include coughing, biting on the tube, secretions in the airway, or water in the tubing. Clearing the airway or tubing frequently will correct the problem.

Alarms should never be ignored or turned off. Some alarms can be muted temporarily, for example, during suctioning. The The Golden Rule of Ventilator Alarms box presents the rule regarding the proper response to an alarm.

Initial Ventilator Settings

When a patient is first placed on the mechanical ventilator, certain standard settings may be used as a guideline. Initial settings will differ based on the patient's pulmonary status. Table 11–6 provides a summary of common standard initial ventilator settings. In emergent situations, the FiO_2 is often initially set at 1.0 and can be titrated by pulse oximetry to maintain adequate oxygen saturation. Arterial blood gases are checked after the initiation of mechanical ventilation and adjustments in ventilator settings are made based on the ABG results. FiO_2 is adjusted to attain and maintain a SaO_2 greater than 90 percent and PaO_2 greater than 60 mmHg (Amitai & Sinert, 2006). Tidal volume and rate may be altered to correct pH and $PaCO_2$ abnormalities.

TABLE 11–6 Standard Initial Ventilator Settings

PARAMETER	INITIAL SETTING
Minute ventilation ($\dot{V}_E$)*	Adults: Men = 4 × BSA; Women=3.5 × BSA
Tidal volume (V_T)	6 to 12 mL/kg (IBW)
Rate (f)	8 to 12/minute
Mode	AC or SIMV
FiO_2	0.5 to 1.0
Peak flow	40 to 60 L/min
Inspiratory sensitivity	−1 to −2 cm H_2O

*Determining desired $\dot{V}_E$ first will help establish f and V_T settings ($\dot{V}_E = f \times V_T$). BSA=Body Surface Area; IBW=Ideal Body Weight; Peak flow—The maximum delivery rate of gas allowed during inspiration; Inspiratory sensitivity—The amount of negative pressure required to trigger a ventilator assisted breath.

SECTION FOUR REVIEW

1. The normal tidal volume (VT) in a spontaneously breathing adult is ______ mL/kg.
   A. 2 to 5
   B. 5 to 7
   C. 7 to 9
   D. 10 to 15
2. The common VT setting range on a mechanical ventilator is ______ mL/kg.
   A. 2 to 5
   B. 6 to 12
   C. 7 to 9
   D. 10 to 15
3. If VT is set too low on the ventilator, it will cause
   A. hypoventilation
   B. pneumothorax
   C. hypoxemia
   D. hypocapnia
4. A high PaO_2 is avoided in patients with COPD when possible because it could
   A. cause hyperventilation
   B. lead to hypocapnia
   C. obliterate the hypoxic drive
   D. precipitate metabolic acidosis
5. A major advantage of initial use of AC mode is that it allows
   A. the diaphragm to exercise
   B. the patient to rest
   C. increased work of breathing
   D. maintenance of some spontaneous breathing
6. SIMV is used primarily for
   A. weaning
   B. full support
   C. acute head injury
   D. acute pulmonary diseases
7. A low minute ventilation ($\dot{V}E$) can cause
   A. acute metabolic alkalosis
   B. acute respiratory alkalosis
   C. acute metabolic acidosis
   D. acute respiratory acidosis
8. PEEP affects the alveoli by
   A. increasing alveolar fluid
   B. decreasing their relative size
   C. sealing off nonfunctioning units
   D. maintaining them open at end expiration
9. PSV is used primarily for what purpose?
   A. to increase PIP
   B. to decrease oxygen need
   C. to decrease work of breathing
   D. to prevent atelectasis
10. An increasing PIP most commonly indicates
    A. increasing airway resistance and/or decreasing lung compliance
    B. decreasing airway resistance and/or decreasing lung compliance
    C. increasing airway resistance and increasing lung compliance
    D. decreasing airway resistance and decreasing lung compliance
11. The ventilator low exhaled volume alarm will trigger when
    A. the patient is coughing
    B. there is water in the tubing
    C. the patient is biting the ET tube
    D. there is a leak in the system

Answers: 1. C, 2. B, 3. A, 4. C, 5. B, 6. A, 7. D, 8. D, 9. C, 10. A, 11. D

SECTION FIVE: Noninvasive Alternatives to Mechanical Ventilation

At the completion of this section, the learner will be able to briefly explain methods of providing noninvasive ventilatory support.

The combination of positive pressure ventilation and artificial airways places the patient at risk for multiple complications and significantly increases patient morbidity and mortality. In an effort to reduce some of the risks, several alternative noninvasive methods have been developed for delivery of positive airway pressure without requiring artificial airways. Noninvasive ventilatory methods have been shown to be effective alternatives to traditional invasive techniques in certain patient populations (Liesching et al., 2003). This section presents an overview of two major noninvasive alternatives to conventional mechanical ventilatory support: noninvasive intermittent positive pressure ventilation (NIPPV or NPPV) and continuous positive airway pressure (CPAP).

Noninvasive Intermittent Positive Pressure Ventilation

Noninvasive Intermittent Positive Pressure Ventilation (NIPPV or NPPV) is a means of providing ventilatory support without requiring intubation. It is more comfortable for the patient, is easier for the caregiver to apply and remove, and has a lower incidence of nosocomial pneumonia than conventional mechanical ventilation. It requires use of a positive pressure mechanical ventilator and an "interface," usually a mask.

Masks/Interfaces

NIPPV is applied using a variety of *interfaces*, often a mask, in place of the invasive endotracheal or tracheostomy tube. In

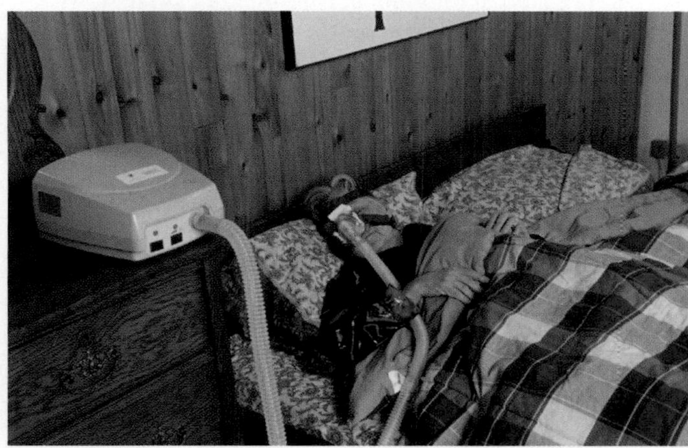

Figure 11–7 ■ A client using a nasal mask and CPAP to treat sleep apnea. (From Custom Medical Stock Photo, Inc.)

the acute care setting, the two most commonly used interfaces are oronasal and nasal masks. The oronasal mask covers both the mouth and the nose, and the nasal mask covers only the nose (see Fig. 11–7). Choice of mask primarily depends on patient comfort and effectiveness of ventilation. For example, a patient may find the oronasal mask to be claustrophobic and prefer the nasal mask. A distressed patient breathing through the mouth may get more benefit from the oronasal mask. Other interface options include nasal pillows (which fit into the nares), full-face masks, helmets, and a large, cannula-type device.

Unlike artificial airways, noninvasive interfaces commonly have air leaks. Leakage may occur at the edge of mask or through the patient's nose or mouth. Some air leakage is necessary when using a bilevel device (discussed later) because CO_2 accumulates in the single limb/hose. Air leakage is assured by the special mask design which includes an exhalation port or by a special valve on the tubing/hose.

NIPPV Mechanical Ventilator

Any positive pressure mechanical ventilator can be used for NIPPV, including standard ICU ventilators, smaller portable home ventilators, and bilevel devices.

Standard ICU Ventilators. Standard ICU ventilators offer the advantages of increased monitoring and alarms and accurate titration of oxygen. Rebreathing CO_2 is not a problem using standard ventilators because the ventilator circuit consists of two tubes. Gas from the ventilator is delivered to the patient via the inspiratory limb or tubing. Exhaled air, including CO_2, is removed by a separate expiratory limb/tubing so the patient does not rebreathe exhaled gas. ICU ventilators, however, may not be able to compensate for air leaks. Standard ventilators being used for NIPPV can be used in either volume or pressure modes (Mehta & Hill, 2001).

Portable Ventilators. Smaller portable ventilators are primarily used in the home setting for patients with chronic respiratory failure. They can be used in either volume or pressure modes, depending on the ventilator model. The smaller size makes these ventilators a convenient option for long-term use. They have fewer alarms and monitoring capabilities than standard ventilators.

Bilevel Devices. Clinicians sometimes interchange the term *bilevel* with "*bipap*," which actually refers to the trade name, *BiPAP*™, one of the first bilevel machines produced by Respironics. Bilevel devices were specifically developed for noninvasive ventilation and were designed to compensate for the required NIPPV air leak. These devices maintain a minimal PEEP level (usually about 4 cm H_2O) to continually flush CO_2 from the system. Smaller and less complex than standard ventilators, bilevel devices provide positive pressure support to the patient throughout the breathing cycle. They have a single limb/hose that carries both inspired and exhaled gas (Fig. 11–8). Gas from the bilevel device is delivered through the single limb/hose and the patient's exhaled air goes out through the same tube, making hypercapnia from rebreathing CO_2 a potential problem. To prevent hypercapnia, bilevel devices have continuous positive air flow to help expel exhaled CO_2 from the mask. In addition, either a special exhalation valve is used on the tubing, or the masks have an exhalation port. Bilevel devices are also designed to compensate for leaks. A backup breathing rate can be set for safety, but setting FIO_2 is usually less precise and the devices have fewer alarms and monitoring capabilities than a standard mechanical ventilator. Newer devices have more sophisticated monitoring and oxygen titration features.

Settings for bilevel devices use a different terminology than standard ventilators. The inspiratory positive airway pressure (IPAP) equates with the peak inspiratory pressure (PIP) and the expiratory positive airway pressure (EPAP) equates with positive end expiratory pressure (PEEP). The patient's level of support is the difference between the IPAP and EPAP.

Indications and Contraindications for Use

At home, NIPPV is used primarily for patients who cannot fully support their own ventilatory efforts for prolonged

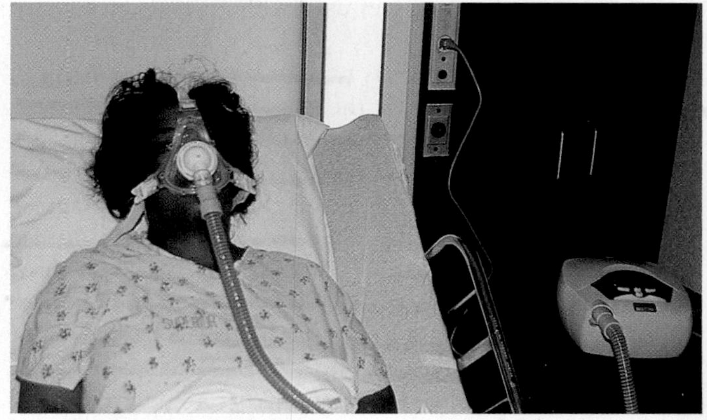

Figure 11–8 ■ Bilevel device. Patient receiving BIPAP.

periods (e.g., patients with neuromuscular disease). In the ICU setting, NIPPV is used for patients in acute respiratory distress as a treatment option to avoid intubation. Noninvasive positive pressure ventilation has been used successfully for patients with hypercapnic failure, such as those with COPD or congestive heart failure, and with postoperative patients. It has also been used for immunocompromised patients who are at increased risk of bleeding and infection with intubation and for patients who do not wish to be intubated. Furthermore, NIPPV has been used for patients with hypoxemic respiratory failure (such as ARDS and pneumonia), but the results have been mixed. Use of NIPPV in the critically ill patient requires intense monitoring so that intubation is not delayed if the patient's condition deteriorates further (Hill, Brennan et al., 2007). Use of NIPPV may be useful in supporting patients whose respiratory status has deteriorated after having been withdrawn from conventional mechanical ventilation to avoid reintubation. NIPPV is also a less invasive option for patients with irreversible disease who desire less aggressive therapy and carries less risk of certain complications such as ventilator-associated pneumonia (VAP).

There are a variety of contraindications for using NIPPV, including an unstable hemodynamic status, cardiac dysrhythmias or myocardial ischemia, apnea, the inability to clear one's own secretions or maintain airway patency, and the inability to attain a proper mask fit.

Continuous Positive Airway Pressure (CPAP)

Continuous positive airway pressure (CPAP) is a mode of mechanical assistance that is closely related to NIPPV. CPAP provides a continuous level of positive airway pressure for a spontaneously breathing person. The level of pressure remains the same throughout the breathing cycle; hence, CPAP does not provide assisted ventilation on inspiration as does NIPPV. Like PEEP, CPAP improves oxygenation by opening alveoli and is used in pressures ranging from 5 to 12.5 cm H_2O (Hill, Brennan et al., 2007). CPAP does not require a mechanical ventilator; instead, it is delivered by a special flow generator (i.e., a blower) via a nasal or facial mask (Fig. 11–9). The same type of masks/interfaces used with NIPPV can be used with CPAP.

CPAP most commonly is used to treat obstructive sleep apnea, a disorder in which the tissues of the oropharynx collapse, periodically obstructing the airway. The constant pressure of CPAP acts like a splint to hold the airway open. When employed as a treatment for obstructive sleep apnea, the desirable level of CPAP is determined through a sleep study in a laboratory setting. In establishing the correct level of CPAP, the goal is to set the CPAP level at the point at which the patient stops having the apnea episodes or when the frequency and duration of episodes is at an acceptable level. The CPAP level can also be determined at home rather than in a sleep laboratory setting. In the home setting, special equipment adjusts the level of positive pressure, and monitors apneic events, pressures, and oxygen saturation. Some of the newer CPAP units adjust airway pressure automatically, responding to snoring, apnea/hypopnea, or airflow limitation. CPAP is also used in the acute care setting to treat pulmonary edema.

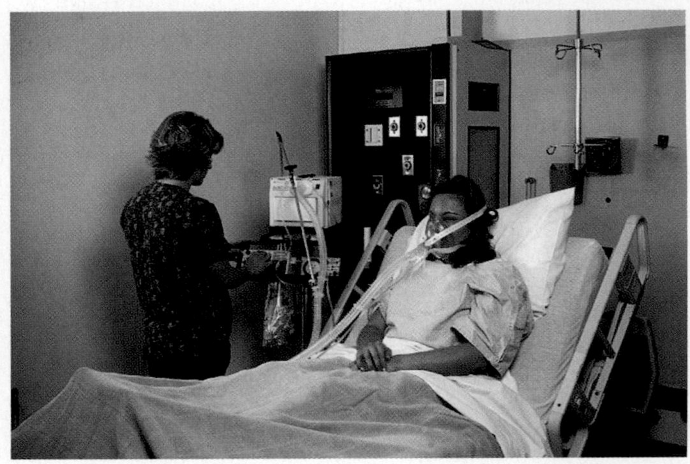

Figure 11–9 ■ Patient receiving CPAP via face mask. Machine is capable of CPAP and BIPAP.

Complications of NIPPV

Many of the potential complications of NIPPV are the same as regular positive pressure mechanical ventilation although the severity and frequency of the complications are significantly reduced with NIPPV and will be discussed in Section Six. Complications specific to delivery of positive pressure through a mask, include conjunctivitis, gastric distention, nasal problems, skin irritation, and aspiration. In addition, hypoventilation is a common complication associated with mechanical problems.

Conjunctivitis is caused by air leaking out from the mask around the bridge of the nose and blowing on the eyes. This problem may be easily corrected by adjusting the mask to eliminate the leak or fitting of a new mask. Gastric distention is caused by air swallowing. Inspiratory pressures used for NIPPV are usually less than 20 cm H_2O, which reduces air entry into the esophagus. Simethicone may be helpful in reducing gastric distention (Hill, Brennan, et al., 2007). Fortunately, with long-term use, gastric distention often becomes less of a problem. Nasal-related complaints include dryness, bleeding, and congestion. These problems may be relieved by use of heated humidification or nasal sprays. Skin irritation and pressure sores may develop under the straps and mask. To minimize or prevent this problem, masks must be fitted carefully and not strapped tightly to the face. A protective skin covering can be used over the bridge of the nose. Alternating interfaces, for example, using nasal pillows, may also reduce skin irritation. Aspiration is a rare, but serious, problem. It can be avoided by limiting NIPPV therapy to patients who can clear their own airways and who are not fed anything by mouth until stable (Hill, Brennan, et al., 2007). Hypoventilation is the major mechanical problem associated with NIPPV therapy. Hypoventilation can occur through two mechanisms: (1) when there is an inadequate seal to attain the preset pressure; or (2) when there is inadequate airflow. Improving the seal or adjusting the flow (when possible) may relieve this problem. If patients continue to hypoventilate despite NIPPV, intubation may be necessary.

Nursing Considerations

In the acute care setting, NIPPV should be instituted before the patient is severely distressed and unable to cooperate (Hill, 2001). To best assure a patient's success in using NIPPV a combination of explanations, patience, and coaching is required. The therapy should be explained and demonstrated at each step, giving the patient an opportunity to ask questions and adapt to the sensations of the masks and air pressures. The following list provides a suggested set of steps that should be included in the initiation of NIPPV (Sharma, 2006):

- Select the proper mask size
- Position head of bed at 45° angle
- Allow the patient to feel the airflow
- Hold the mask to the patient's face without straps, hose, and so forth
- Apply dressings to the nasal bridge and other pressure points
- Let the patient breathe through the mask briefly
- Connect the tubing to the mask (set IPAP low at 8 or less) to help the patient adjust to the feeling of positive airflow
- Continue to hold the mask in place
- As the patient becomes more comfortable, attach the head straps securely, avoiding too tight of a fit
- As the patient becomes more comfortable, gradually increase the pressure to the level desired

Patients are monitored for ventilator synchrony, air leaks, and patient status (e.g., comfort, relief of dyspnea). Positive patient outcomes include a decreasing respiratory rate, improved oxygenation, and decreased use of accessory muscles (Hill, Brennan et al., 2007).

Home ventilatory support therapy requires careful, thorough instructions to the patient or the primary caregiver. Teaching needs include

- Signs and symptoms of complications
- Circumstances under which to call the physician
- Proper use and maintenance of equipment
- Troubleshooting problems

Follow-up visits by a home health nurse or a respiratory therapist are usually ordered as a means of monitoring both the equipment and the patient.

SECTION FIVE REVIEW

1. Which of the following statements describes NIPPV?
   A. It requires a flow generator (blower).
   B. It combines negative and positive pressure principles.
   C. It uses a positive pressure mechanical ventilator.
   D. It independently manipulates inspiratory and expiratory pressures.
2. NIPPV is most useful for the patient who
   A. requires only support of tidal volume
   B. cannot fully support his or her own expiratory effort
   C. requires only support for nocturnal hypercapnia and hypoxemia
   D. cannot fully support his or her own ventilatory effort over long periods of time
3. Which statement best reflects nasal CPAP?
   A. It is used as a treatment of obstructive sleep apnea.
   B. It requires a positive pressure mechanical ventilator.
   C. The pressure level cannot be adjusted once it has been set.
   D. It allows manipulation of inspiratory and expiratory pressures.
4. Bilevel differs from CPAP because it
   A. requires an artificial airway
   B. can provide inspiratory positive pressure
   C. uses a standard positive pressure ventilator
   D. provides only nocturnal support
5. Common complications of noninvasive methods of ventilatory support include (choose all that apply)
   A. conjunctivitis
   B. nasal congestion
   C. hypoventilation
   D. otitis media

Answers: 1. C, 2. D, 3. A, 4. B, 5. (A, B, C)

SECTION SIX: Major Complications of Mechanical Ventilation

At the completion of this section, the learner will be able to discuss the major complications of mechanical ventilation.

Positive pressure ventilation (PPV) affects virtually all body systems. These effects can lead to multiple system complications. Table 11–7 summarizes the multisystem effects of positive pressure ventilation.

Cardiovascular Complications

During normal spontaneous inhalation, air is drawn into the lungs because of a drop in intrathoracic pressure. At the same time, the decreased intrathoracic pressure increases venous return to the heart by drawing blood into the heart and the major thoracic vessels. As blood is moved into the right heart, the right heart chamber enlarges and stretches, enhancing right ventricular preload and stroke volume. During normal

TABLE 11–7 Multisystem Effects of Positive Pressure Ventilation

SYSTEM	EFFECTS OF PPV	ASSOCIATED CLINICAL MANIFESTATIONS
Cardiovascular	Decreased cardiac output Decreased preload Decreased stroke volume	Decreased blood pressure (particularly in presence of hypovolemia); if compensation is present, normal blood pressure, increased heart rate, increased systemic vascular resistance
Pulmonary	Increased gas flow to nondependent lung and to central lung tissue Increased blood flow to peripheral lung tissues Alveolar distension with risk for barotrauma and volutrauma Lower airway contamination causing ventilator-associated pneumonia (VAP) Risk for oxygen toxicity	Decreased Pa_{O_2} Barotrauma/volutrauma manifestations: Increased agitation and coughing with frequent high pressure alarm, diminished or absent breath sounds, subcutaneous emphysema on palpation, deteriorating BP and ABG VAP manifestations: Increased adventitious breath sounds, changes in sputum color and quantity; fevers, leukocytosis; positive chest X-ray Oxygen toxicity manifestations: ARDS-like presentation
Neurovascular	Decreased venous return from the head Decreased blood flow to head if cardiac output is decreased	Possible increased intracranial pressure; possible altered level of consciousness
Renal	Redistribution of blood flow through kidneys Decreased blood flow to the kidneys associated with decreased cardiac output	Decreased urine output; increased serum sodium and creatinine levels; water retention
Gastrointestinal	Decreased blood flow into the intestinal viscera Increased risk of gastric stress ulcer formation, gastrointestinal bleed, hepatic dysfunction (increased bilirubin)	Epigastric pain or burning; occult or gross blood in stool; decreasing hemoglobin and hematocrit; increasing bilirubin

exhalation, there is an increase in the flow of blood from the pulmonary circulation to the left heart, increasing left ventricular preload and stroke volume. At the end of spontaneous exhalation, the output of blood decreases in both the right and left heart.

When PPV is used, the positive pressure exerted on the lungs causes a relative increase in intrathoracic pressure, which is then transmitted to all structures in the thorax, including the heart, lungs, and major thoracic vessels. The major vessels become compressed, which creates an increase in central venous pressure (CVP). Blood return to the right heart is reduced because of a decreased pressure gradient. The resulting reduction in venous return to the heart causes right preload and stroke volume to decrease. Left ventricular output falls as a direct result of decreased right ventricular output.

Positive pressure ventilation reduces cardiac output by decreasing venous return to the heart in three major ways. First, the presence of positive intrathoracic pressure prevents blood from being pulled into the major thoracic vessels and into the heart. Second, cardiac output is reduced through a squeezing of the heart by the lungs during the inspiratory phase of PPV. Third, the amount of pressure being exerted on the alveoli is the single most important factor influencing cardiac output when considering pulmonary influences. As the level of pressure is increased, venous return to the heart decreases. The more the heart and pulmonary capillaries are squeezed by the presence of positive pressure, the lower the cardiac output. This helps explain why high levels of PEEP can dramatically reduce cardiac output. Other factors that influence the effects of PPV on the cardiovascular system include lung and thoracic compliance, airway resistance, and the patient's volemic state.

Decreased cardiac output may be manifested as a reduction in arterial blood pressure, particularly if the patient is hypovolemic. However, a normal blood pressure frequently is maintained in PPV patients through the compensatory mechanisms of increased heart rate and increased systemic vascular resistance (SVR). Hemodynamic monitoring usually shows a decreased cardiac output, increased pulmonary artery wedge pressure, and increased right atrial pressure.

Pulmonary Complications

Normally, during spontaneous breathing, the relationship between ventilation and perfusion ($\dot{V}/\dot{Q}$) is relatively balanced, with most inhaled gases flowing toward the diaphragm. The distribution of gases to the alveoli normally favors the peripheral and dependent lung areas. Likewise, pulmonary perfusion normally is the greatest in dependent areas, thus matching the lung zones with the most ventilation with the lung zones with the most perfusion.

Altered Ventilation and Perfusion

PPV alters the relationship of ventilation to perfusion in the lungs. Gases flow through the path of least resistance, which during PPV increases ventilation to the nondependent lung areas and large airways. This is largely due to the decreased functioning and stiffening of the diaphragm associated with passive PPV. PPV gas flow increases ventilation to the healthy lung areas, whereas flow decreases to the diseased areas because it meets increased resistance in diseased lung tissue.

When PPV is used, the positive pressure is transmitted to the pulmonary vessels, pushing the blood to the peripheral lung and to dependent areas. Because perfusion is now the greatest in the periphery and in the dependent lung areas and ventilation is greatest in the nondependent and larger airways, the relationship of ventilation to perfusion is altered to some degree. In areas with the most perfusion, there is decreased ventilation, and in areas with adequate ventilation, perfusion is reduced. This can create problems with oxygenation because of increased shunting, which can be reflected in deteriorating Pa_{O_2} levels. Under certain circumstances, shunt and $\dot{V}/\dot{Q}$ matching can significantly improve during PPV. This is typically seen when PEEP is applied to treat refractory hypoxemia associated with increased shunt and decreased functional residual capacity (e.g., ARDS). In such a situation, shunt is often reduced, $\dot{V}/\dot{Q}$ matching is improved, and Pa_{O_2} levels may significantly improve.

Barotrauma/Volutrauma

There is increasing evidence that the pulmonary injury associated with PPV results from alveolar distention created by a combination of excessive alveolar pressure (barotrauma) and volume (volutrauma). The higher the positive pressure or volume applied, the greater the risk of trauma. Patients who are at the highest risk for development of barotrauma/volutrauma are those requiring high levels of PEEP and high peak airway pressures (PAP, PIP) or high tidal volumes. Barotrauma/volutrauma can manifest itself as pneumothorax, subcutaneous emphysema, or pneumomediastinum. Clinically, it should be suspected if (1) the patient has a sudden onset of agitation and cough associated with a frequent high-pressure alarm, (2) the blood pressure and ABG rapidly deteriorate, (3) breath sounds suddenly are diminished or absent, or (4) subcutaneous emphysema can be palpated on the anterior neck or chest. If a pneumothorax or pneumomediastinum is diagnosed by chest X-ray, insertion of a chest tube should be anticipated.

Oxygen Toxicity

Oxygen toxicity is associated with the use of an oxygen concentration of 60 percent or greater (Fi_{O_2} of 0.6 or greater) for more than 48 hours. The use of 100 percent oxygen concentration (Fi_{O_2} of 1.0) can cause pulmonary changes within 6 hours. Oxygen toxicity damages the endothelial lining of the lungs and decreases alveolar macrophage activity. It also decreases mucous and surfactant production. If it is allowed to continue for more than 72 hours, the patient may develop a pattern of symptoms similar to ARDS. The early signs and symptoms of oxygen toxicity are nonspecific (malaise, fatigue, and substernal discomfort). Because early symptoms are difficult to assess, the nurse should be aware of who is at risk for developing oxygen toxicity on the basis of the length of time that the patient has received an O_2 concentration of 60 percent or higher. Unfortunately, the signs and symptoms of oxygen toxicity are similar to changes that may be due to the underlying disease process or ventilator-induced lung injury (VALI). Although every effort should be made to decrease oxygen concentrations to nontoxic levels, the need to maintain adequate oxygenation and safe ventilatory pressures is paramount (Hall, Schmidt, & Wood, 2005).

Nosocomial Pulmonary Infection: Ventilator-Associated Pneumonia (VAP)

Nosocomial pulmonary infection is a common major complication of mechanical ventilation that develops in patients intubated for more than 48 hours. The passing of an ET tube from the upper airway into the lower airway introduces upper-airway contaminants into the lower airway. The presence of an artificial airway bypasses the normal upper airway defense mechanisms, reduces cough effectiveness, stimulates mucous production, and decreases the mucociliary motion that helps to remove bacteria from the lower airway. Dental plaque and oropharyngeal secretions are emerging as important factors in ventilator-associated pneumonia (VAP) (Berry et al., 2007). Upper airway secretions pool above the ET tube cuff forming a biofilm that provides an environment in which bacteria can multiply. The biofilm can become dislodged and disseminated into the lungs by ventilator induced breaths.

Because of the increased mortality and morbidity caused by ventilator-associated pneumonia (VAP), many studies have examined the factors that contribute to these infections (Augustyn, 2007). Risk factors can be divided into three categories: device-related, host-related, and personnel-related. Device-related risk factors include nasogastric and orogastric tubes, either of which can interrupt the gastroesophageal sphincter leading to increased gastroesophageal reflux and provide a route for bacteria to translocate from the stomach to the upper airway. Enteral feedings increase gastric pH and gastric volume, increasing the risk of aspiration. Medications that prevent stress ulcer formation create an alkaline pH in which bacteria multiply. The endotracheal tube itself is a risk factor for VAP. Secretions pool above the ET tube cuff and can be aspirated into the lungs. Host-related risk factors include underlying medical conditions such as COPD and immunosuppression. The patient's mental status and ability to cough and clear secretions is important in the prevention of VAP. Positioning the patient upright decreases the risk of lower airway contamination by endotracheal secretions. Personnel-related risk factors include improper hand washing and not wearing appropriate personal protective equipment while working with mechanically ventilated patients.

Signs and symptoms of a pulmonary infection include development of adventitious breath sounds and changes in sputum color or quantity. Systemically, infection may be evidenced by fever and increased white blood cell (WBC) count. Positive chest X-ray and sputum culture findings are important diagnostic tools. Reduction of oral bacteria and secretions is crucial to prevention of VAP; thus, effective oral hygiene should include brushing, rinsing, and frequent removal of oral secretions (Berry et al., 2007). Many institutions have developed VAP bundled orders that include elevating head of the bed, oral hygiene, and other interventions.

Neurovascular Complications

PPV can cause a change in neurovascular status through two major mechanisms: increased intracranial pressure (ICP); and decreased cerebral perfusion pressure (CPP). Patients who have existing intracranial or neurovascular problems are at particular risk when moderate-to-high ventilation pressures are required. The increased intrathoracic pressure associated with PPV decreases venous return from the head. The higher the pressure required to ventilate the patient, the greater the effects on the ICP.

Blood flow to the head (cerebral perfusion pressure) may be reduced. If cardiac output drops sufficiently to reduce systolic blood pressure, cerebral perfusion may become compromised. CPP is influenced by two factors: ICP and mean arterial pressure (MAP). This relationship is expressed as follows:

$$CPP = MAP - ICP$$

MAP is determined by the systolic and diastolic blood pressures. Therefore, as systolic blood pressure decreases, so will MAP, causing a reduction in CPP. If CPP drops too low, cerebral hypoxia can result.

Renal Complications

PPV is associated with decreased urinary output. The mechanisms for this decrease are multiple, and some are unclear; however, three major mechanisms that may contribute to decreased renal function include decreased cardiac output, redistribution of renal blood flow, and hormonal alterations (Kuiper, Groeneveld et al., 2005).

Decreased Cardiac Output

When cardiac output significantly drops, perfusion to organs, including the kidneys is reduced, which in turn lowers the glomerular filtration rate, causing lower urine output. Fortunately, in most mechanically ventilated patients, arterial blood pressure is maintained adequately through compensatory mechanisms.

Redistribution of Renal Blood Flow

Positive pressure ventilation increases internal pressures not only in the thorax, but also in the abdomen, creating a redistribution of intrarenal blood flow. Renal perfusion may be altered by decreased blood flow to the outer renal cortex and increased flow to the inner cortex and outer medullary tissue, where the juxtamedullary nephrons are located. The blood flow redistribution can result in a significant decrease in urinary output, and less sodium and creatinine are excreted. When sodium is reabsorbed, water also is reabsorbed to maintain homeostasis, thus reducing urine output.

Hormonal Alterations

Finally, the cardiovascular changes induced by positive pressure may stimulate the release of antidiuretic hormone (ADH), renin, aldosterone, atrial natriuretic factor, and catecholamines. These hormones may affect renal blood flow and renal function but observed effects vary with a patient's clinical status, hydration, and underlying disease (Groeneveld et al., 2005).

Gastrointestinal Complications

Gastrointestinal bleeding occurs in approximately 25 percent of patients on mechanical ventilators through development of stress ulcers. Stress ulcers develop as a result of either gastric hyperacidity or, more commonly, from a transient visceral hypoxic episode. In the mechanically ventilated patient, the tissue hypoxia may be related to acute respiratory failure or may be the result of increased resistance to blood flow in the viscera. Stress ulcers, which usually are shallow erosions in the mucosal lining, often cause slow, insidious bleeds and may, therefore, not be diagnosed early in their development. For this reason, it is important to check stools for guaiac. In addition, some patients with no history of liver disease develop hepatic dysfunction.

Clinically, the patient who develops a stress ulcer exhibits a decreasing hematocrit and guaiac positive stools. If bleeding becomes significant, the stools may be black or dark red. If the ulcer is in the stomach, nasogastric aspirate will be guaiac positive, and the aspirate appears bright red to dark red. Because mechanical ventilation for greater than 48 hours has been identified as a risk factor for stress ulcers, preventive interventions are recommended. These include the use of antacids, histamine (H_2) antagonists, or proton pump inhibitors to maintain a gastric pH of greater than 3.5. Alternatively, sucralfate provides mucosal protection without pH alteration and may have advantages in reducing bacterial overgrowth in the stomach.

SECTION SIX REVIEW

1. PPV affects the cardiovascular system by
   - **A.** increasing cardiac output
   - **B.** decreasing venous return to the heart
   - **C.** increasing arterial blood pressure
   - **D.** increasing venous return to the heart
2. Changes in cardiac output resulting from positive pressure ventilation are associated with which manifestation?
   - **A.** increased arterial blood pressure
   - **B.** increased urinary output
   - **C.** decreased arterial blood pressuredec
   - **D.** decreased pulse rate
3. Positive pressure ventilation (PPV) alters the relationship of ventilation to perfusion in what way?
   - **A.** Ventilation increases in nondependent lung areas.
   - **B.** Ventilation increases in the small airways.
   - **C.** Perfusion increases in the nondependent lung areas.
   - **D.** Perfusion increases near the large airways.

4. Which manifestation of pulmonary barotrauma/volutrauma is secondary to mechanical ventilation?
   A. onset of increased lethargy
   B. increase in arterial blood pressure
   C. increase in breath sounds over a lung field
   D. increased cough with high-pressure alarm triggering
5. In which way does oxygen toxicity affect the pulmonary tissue?
   A. by decreasing macrophage activity
   B. by increasing mucous production
   C. by increasing surfactant production
   D. by decreasing peak inspiratory pressure (PIP)
6. Patients receiving mechanical ventilation are at increased risk of developing a nosocomial pulmonary infection because
   A. the lower airway is defenseless
   B. macrophage activity has been bypassed
   C. normal upper airway defenses are bypassed
   D. normal pulmonary mechanics have been altered
7. Positive pressure ventilation (PPV) influences intracranial pressure by
   A. decreasing intrathoracic pressure
   B. increasing cerebral perfusion pressure
   C. decreasing venous drainage from the head
   D. increasing mean arterial blood pressure
8. The kidneys are affected by positive pressure ventilation in what way?
   A. decreased sodium retention
   B. redistribution of renal blood flow
   C. renal effects of increased cardiac output
   D. redistribution of urine flow through the kidneys
9. The gastrointestinal system may be adversely affected by positive pressure ventilation as a result of
   A. increased visceral vascular resistance
   B. increased blood supply to the viscera
   C. increased venous pooling in the viscera
   D. decreased visceral vascular resistance
10. Gastrointestinal bleeding secondary to mechanical ventilation most frequently manifests itself as
   A. grossly bloody stools
   B. guaiac-positive stools
   C. grossly bloody nasogastric drainage
   D. guaiac-negative nasogastric drainage

Answers: 1. B, 2. C, 3. A, 4. D, 5. A, 6. C, 7. C, 8. B, 9. A, 10. B

SECTION SEVEN: Artificial Airway Complications

At the completion of this section, the learner will be able to explain the cause and prevention of artificial airway complications.

Artificial airways have their own set of complications that are primarily related to pressure damage.

Nasal/Oral Damage

While nasotracheal intubation provides a more stable and comfortable lower airway access, it is not without drawbacks. Placing an artificial airway through the nasal passage can traumatize nasal mucous membranes during the passing of the tube. After the nasotracheal tube is in place, ischemia and possibly necrosis of the nares may develop as a result of the pressure the tube exerts on the internal nasal wall. For this reason, choosing the proper size tube is crucial in minimizing the risk of damage. Anchoring the tube to the cheeks rather than to the top of the nose also helps prevent pressure damage. Furthermore, a nasotracheal tube can occlude the eustachian tubes, which increases the risk of development of ear pressure problems or inner ear infection. The oral intubation approach can also cause damage. Pressure from the oral ET tube may cause ulcerations and possible necrosis of the inner cheek or lip. Oral endotracheal tubes should be repositioned on a regular basis to prevent pressure damage to the lips and mouth (Scott & Vollman, 2005).

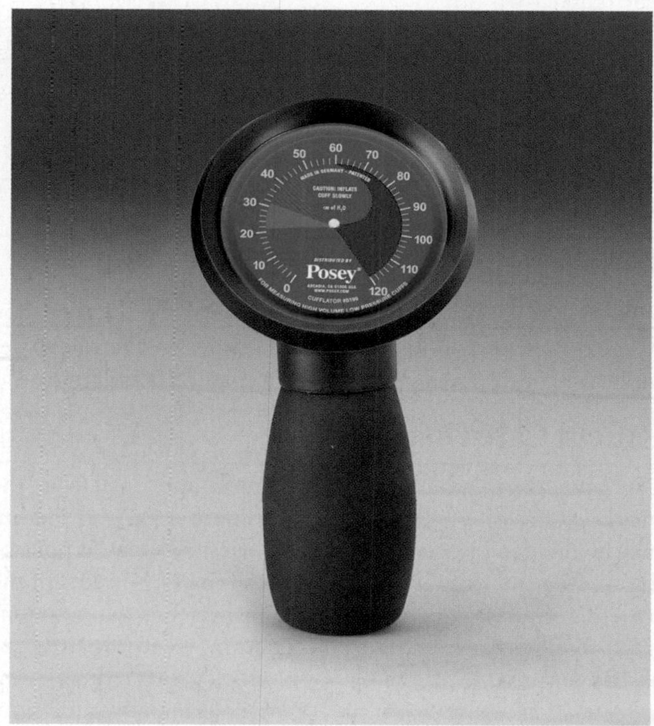

Figure 11–10 ■ Example of a cuff manometer. (Courtesy of Posey Company).

Cuff Trauma

Although the use of tracheal cuffs is necessary to mechanically ventilate the patient properly, cuffs can cause potentially severe tracheal and laryngeal injuries. The use of excessive cuff pressures is the major contributing factor in these injuries. Arterial capillary blood flow pressure through the trachea is low (less than 30 mm Hg). A high-pressure force, such as is delivered by an overinflated cuff, exerts a pressure that is higher than tracheal capillary pressure, causing circulation in the cuffed area to be compromised. Decreased or obliterated blood flow to an area of tissue causes ischemia, which, if allowed to continue for an extended period, can produce necrosis. Necrosis of the trachea, larynx, or both can result in development of fistulas, fibrosis, and ulceration.

Proper monitoring and control of cuff pressures decreases the risk of complications significantly. Cuff pressures must be monitored at least once every shift via a cuff manometer (Fig. 11–10). Safe cuff pressure ranges from 20 to 25 mm Hg (27 to 34 cm H_2O). A minimum occluding pressure technique may also be used to reduce the risk of pressure-related cuff damage. Using this technique, the cuff is inflated only to the point at which it seals the airway during the mechanical ventilation. Cuff pressure should be regularly checked using the minimum occluding pressure technique and should not exceed 20 to 25 mm Hg.

Artificial airways can damage one or both vocal cords as a result of the traumatic introduction of the tube or damage can be caused by the pressure of the tube against the cords. Fistula formation is also a major concern. Should tracheal injury from a cuff cause a fistula to form between the trachea and esophagus, gastric secretions can be aspirated into the lungs. Tracheoesophageal (TE) fistulas should be suspected if tube feeding or food is aspirated during tracheal suctioning. This infrequent, but serious, complication is diagnosed with computed tomography (CT) scan and contrast studies. Proper cuff inflation technique and use of correct tube size can minimize cuff-related complications.

SECTION SEVEN REVIEW

1. The presence of a nasotracheal tube can affect the ears because it can
   - **A.** occlude the eustachian tubes
   - **B.** exert direct pressure on the inner ears
   - **C.** cause inner ear ischemia
   - **D.** directly damage the eustachian tubes
2. High endotracheal tube cuff pressures can damage the trachea when cuff pressure is
   - **A.** increased during coughing
   - **B.** reduced due to a leak
   - **C.** lower than surrounding capillary pressure
   - **D.** higher than surrounding capillary pressure
3. Normal tracheal capillary pressure is less than
   - **A.** 10 mm Hg
   - **B.** 20 mm Hg
   - **C.** 30 mm Hg
   - **D.** 40 mm Hg
4. Safe tracheal cuff pressure ranges are ______ mm Hg.
   - **A.** 10 to 15
   - **B.** 15 to 20
   - **C.** 20 to 25
   - **D.** 25 to 30
5. TE fistula formation secondary to tracheal cuff complications can cause
   - **A.** sepsis
   - **B.** aspiration pneumonia
   - **C.** gastric ulcerations
   - **D.** esophageal varices

Answers: 1. A, 2. D, 3. C, 4. C, 5. B

SECTION EIGHT: Care of the Patient Requiring Mechanical Ventilation

At the completion of this section, the learner will be able to describe care of the patient requiring mechanical ventilation.

Patient Care Goals

The general goals and outcome criteria appropriate to the management of a patient receiving mechanical ventilation may be divided into two major categories: support of physiologic needs and support of psychosocial needs. Support of the patient's physiologic needs is accomplished through interventions that promote optimal oxygenation, treat impaired gas exchange, provide adequate ventilation, protect the airway, support tissue perfusion, and provide adequate nutrition. Support of the patient's psychosocial needs centers around interventions to reduce anxiety and pain, provide a balance of sleep and activity, promote communication, and support the family.

Nursing Management of Physiologic Needs

The patient's nursing management is planned around interventions to attain the patient care goals. The first three goals—promote optimal oxygenation, provide adequate ventilation, and protect the patient's airway—are all addressed through implementation of the three pulmonary-related nursing diagnoses. An additional goal in which the nurse takes a pivotal role is to prevent complications associated with mechanical ventilation (and critical illness), particularly ventilator-associated pneumonia (VAP), stress-induced mucosal injury (SIMI), and deep vein thrombosis (DVT). The NURSING CARE box Prevention of Common Complications in the Patient on Mechanical

NURSING CARE: Prevention of Common Complications in the Patient on Mechanical Ventilation

Expected Patient Outcomes and Related interventions

Outcome: The patient experiences no complications of mechanical ventilation

Assess and compare to established norms, patient baseline, and trends

Monitor for signs of pneumonia
- Fever, increased WBC, increased adventitious sounds
- Change in color and consistency of secretions
- Positive chest X-ray
- Worsening ABG trends

Monitor for signs of stress-induced mucosal injury (SIMI)
- Occult or gross blood in GI secretions or stool
- Decreasing hemoglobin, hematocrit, and RBC counts

Monitor for signs of deep vein thrombosis (DVT)
- Assess for risk factors on admission (e.g., recent immobilization for 3 or more consecutive days within past month, recent surgery, malignancy, prolonged travel, or previous history of thrombophlebitis, or vascular injury)
- Monitor for signs and symptoms of DVT
  - Unilateral lower extremity swelling, tenderness, redness

Interventions to prevent common complications of mechanical ventilation

Institute ventilator bundle orders
- Head-of-bed elevated 30 degrees or higher unless contraindicated[1]
- Use ET tube with continuous suction above cuff if patient is to be intubated more than 48 hours; no routine changing of ventilator circuits[1]
- Oral hygiene two or more times per day[2]
  - Brush teeth, gums and tongue with soft toothbrush; oral moisturizing to oral mucosa and lips q 2-4 hours
  - During perioperative period in adults undergoing cardiac surgery: Use chlorhexidine gluconate (0.12 percent) oral rinse twice per day
- Deep vein thrombosis prophylaxis[3]
  - Mechanical prophylaxis: Graduated compression stockings; intermittent pneumatic compression devices. Assure proper fit.
- Other interventions to prevent DVT:
  - Early ambulation, anticoagulant therapy, antiembolism stockings, compression boots, elevation of injured leg above heart level

Administer related drug therapy and monitor for therapeutic and nontherapeutic effects

- Antisecretory therapy – either histamine 2 receptor agonist (H2RA) or proton pump inhibitor (PPI)
- Mucosal protectant therapy - sucralfate
- Anticoagulant therapy[3] – Heparin (unfractionated or low dose unfractionated heparin or low-molecular-weight heparin [type depends on degree of risk])
- Monitor for signs of heparin-induced thrombocytopenia (HIT)

Related nursing diagnoses

- Immobility
- Impaired gas exchange
- Ineffective airway clearance
- Risk for ineffective peripheral tissue perfusion
- Risk for injury
- Altered tissue perfusion
- Anxiety
- Altered comfort: Pain

[1]*AACN (2008). AACN Practice Alert: Ventilator Associated Pneumonia*
[2]*AACN (2007). AACN Practice Alert: Oral Care in the Critically Ill*
[3]*AACN (2005). AACN Practice Alert: Deep Vein Thrombosis Prevention*

Ventilation, provides a summary of some of the major assessments, interventions, and nursing diagnoses specifically focusing on these potential complications.

Ineffective Airway Clearance

The patient who requires conventional positive pressure ventilation will have an endotracheal or tracheostomy tube inserted to access and seal off the lower airway. The length and relatively small internal diameter of ET tubes make it difficult, if not impossible, for the patient to clear his or her own airway. The problem of airway clearance is often compounded by general weakness and fatigue or diminished level of responsiveness, any of which also hinders airway clearance.

Airway clearance is a top-priority nursing goal in management of the patient with an artificial airway. If airway patency is not maintained, the patient's breathing and cardiovascular status eventually will fail as a result of hypoxia or hypercapnia.

> Remember to apply the ABCs—Airway, Breathing, Circulation—in that order.

The primary reason that airway patency becomes compromised is airway obstruction caused by excessive, thick, or pooled secretions. Each of these situations must be managed properly by the nurse.

Excessive Secretions. Excessive secretions are removed by suctioning the artificial airway on an as-necessary basis, which may be every few minutes during initial intubation or several times a shift in chronic intubation. The patient's breath sounds should be assessed every one to two hours for the presence of secretions. If adventitious breath sounds are auscultated in the large airways, suctioning should be performed. Coughing, regardless of whether it sets off the ventilator's high-pressure alarm, may indicate a need for suctioning. The nurse often can hear the secretions without the use of a stethoscope, particularly during coughing. Coughing, however, can occur as a result of tracheal irritation or bronchospasm or because the tip of the airway is touching the carina. The last two situations can precipitate severe coughing spasms. Because coughing may occur without the presence of secretions in the large airways, the nurse should assess the situation first. Unnecessary suctioning causes needless trauma to the delicate mucous membranes in the trachea and also depletes oxygen levels. Good rules to apply are as follows:

- Assess before suctioning.
- Do not suction unnecessarily.
- Follow approved protocols for suctioning.
- Monitor the patient closely for adverse effects of suctioning, such as arrhythmias and hypoxia.

In most circumstances, the nurse will maintain Pao_2 levels during suctioning if the following common protocol is maintained.

Step 1: **Hyperoxygenate/hyperventilate.** Deliver 100 percent oxygen accompanied by one of two methods:

1) Manual method: manually ventilate the patient with a manual resuscitation (Ambu) bag for four to five breaths (two-handed ventilating will deliver significantly larger breaths than one-handed ventilating).

2) Machine method: most mechanical ventilators have a 100 percent button that will deliver oxygen at 100 percent for two minutes (particularly important if closed suction systems are being used).

Step 2: **Suction.** Use moderate, not high, suction pressure. Apply suction only on withdrawal, rotating the catheter while using intermittent suction and withdrawing the catheter within 10 seconds. Repeat steps 1 and 2 until the airway is cleared.

Step 3: **Return the patient to the ventilator.** If an in-line closed system suction unit is used, relock access valve.

There are many variations to suctioning protocols. Some hospitals only hyperoxygenate by temporarily increasing the ventilator's oxygen concentration (Fio_2) to 100 percent (for 1 to 5 minutes). Hyperventilation may be part of such a policy. Hyperventilation can be accomplished through a sigh or other intermittent large inhaled volume mechanism on the ventilator that, when manually triggered, will deliver a breath that is 1.5 to 2 times the patient's set tidal volume. In patients with acute neurologic injury, protocol may call for initial hyperoxygenation/hyperventilation for 1 or more minutes before initiation of the suctioning protocol. Newest guidelines for suctioning recommend that saline not be instilled into the airway prior to

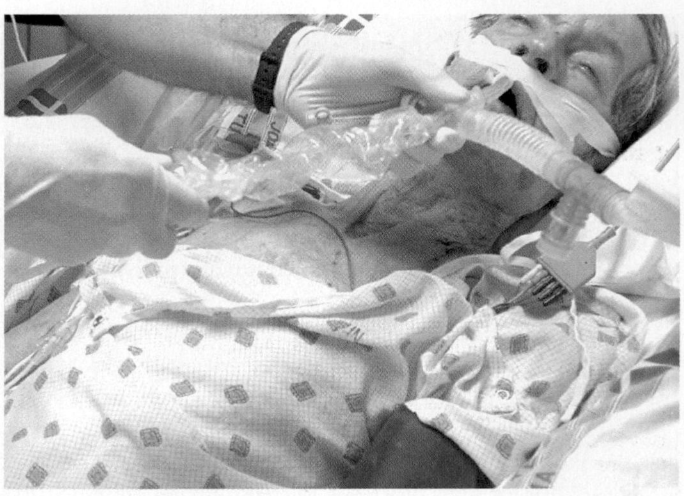

Figure 11–11 ▪ Intubated client with in-line closed suction catheter being advanced.

suctioning. This common practice does not facilitate secretion removal, increases the risk of bacterial contamination of the lower airways, and may precipitate hypoxemia (Halm & Krisko-Hagel, 2008).

Suction catheters can be divided into two major groups: open and closed systems. Both systems are used for suctioning artificial airways, but only open systems are used without an artificial airway in place. Each type of system has its own suctioning protocol. Closed system catheters are self-contained within a sheath attached directly to the artificial airway (see Fig. 11–11). A closed-catheter system remains in the artificial airway system between suctioning, allowing it to be used multiple times. Open systems generally are single-use catheters and require introduction of the catheter into the artificial airway from outside the artificial airway system.

If the patient is receiving PEEP, a different suctioning protocol may be required. Patients on PEEP often do not tolerate being detached from the ventilator for any reason. Loss of PEEP can precipitate oxygen desaturation and may make the patient hemodynamically unstable. Several airway suctioning approaches may be used: (1) the usual suctioning protocol; (2) the usual suctioning protocol using a manual resuscitation bag that has a special PEEP attachment that is set at the prescribed PEEP level; or (3) suctioning without removing the patient from the ventilator by either an in-line closed-suction system or introducing a suction catheter into the closed system through a special port on top of the ventilator adaptor nozzle. Research is continuing on which type of suctioning system and protocol is best in specific situations. All types of suctioning have associated problems, including infection, hypoxia, cardiac arrhythmias, trauma to mucous membranes, and others.

Thick Secretions. Thick secretions are a common challenge to maintaining effective airway clearance. Properly hydrating the patient is the most important means of thinning secretions because secretions are composed primarily of water. Mechanically ventilated patients receive warmed, humidified gases that facilitate liquefying secretions.

Pooled Secretions. Pooled secretions can cause obstruction of major airways or can plug the tip of the artificial airway. Methods to improve cough effectiveness such as the assisted cough technique are used for specific populations (e.g., spinal cord injury patients).

Oral secretions also pool above the cuff of the endotracheal tube, presenting a risk of ventilator-associated pneumonia (VAP). Frequent oral care and oropharyngeal suctioning are important to reduce the volume of these secretions. Special endotracheal tubes are available that permit continuous removal of subglottic secretions via an additional suction port located just above the cuff. These tubes have been shown to decrease the incidence of VAP by 50 percent (Craven, 2006).

Impaired Gas Exchange

Treatment of impaired gas exchange is the major reason for placing patients on a mechanical ventilator (i.e., impending ventilatory failure or acute respiratory failure). Ventilators can manipulate carbon dioxide levels directly by causing alveolar hyperventilation or hypoventilation.

Alveolar Hyperventilation. Hyperventilation is associated with decreasing carbon dioxide levels and respiratory alkalosis. It can be patient induced if the patient is on the AC mode and is hyperventilating for any reason (e.g., anxiety, pain, head injury) because the patient can blow off too much carbon dioxide. It also can be induced mechanically by setting the rate or tidal volume too high on the ventilator. Sometimes, as in patients with increased intracranial pressure, mild respiratory alkalosis is induced intentionally to facilitate cerebral vasoconstriction through reduced carbon dioxide levels.

Alveolar Hypoventilation. Hypoventilation is associated with increasing carbon dioxide levels and respiratory acidosis. Hypoventilation may be patient induced, for example, in the patient on SIMV mode (or other spontaneous breathing mode) whose breathing is too shallow. It also can be induced mechanically by setting the rate or tidal volume too low on the ventilator.

A changing ABG trend may indicate destabilization of the patient's respiratory or metabolic status; and the underlying cause should be investigated. It is the nurse's responsibility to monitor the ABG trends, observe the patient's condition, notify the physician of increasing abnormalities, follow up on orders received, and monitor the ventilator settings at established intervals. The nurse also can facilitate gas exchange by taking actions to maintain airway clearance and effective breathing patterns.

Ineffective Breathing Patterns

Patients may be placed on the mechanical ventilator because of ineffective breathing patterns, which consist of any significant changes in the breathing rate, rhythm, or depth from the patient's baseline normal values (e.g., tachypnea, bradypnea, apnea, hypoventilation, and hyperventilation). Changes in breathing patterns can affect oxygenation and acid–base status, as previously described.

Breathing patterns that remain too rapid must be controlled after the patient is placed on the ventilator to prevent hyperventilation problems. The nurse should assess for possible causes of the rapid pattern and take steps to relieve the problem when possible. Rapid breathing patterns may stem from fear, anxiety, pain, or such physiologic problems as acid–base imbalance or head injury.

Protection of the Airway

Protecting the airway is a major goal in caring for the mechanically ventilated patient. Any artificial airway can be fairly easily dislodged, either partially or completely. Because of this, steps must be taken to minimize the possibility of dislodgment, which could precipitate respiratory compromise. During bedside care, dislodgment is at the highest risk while moving the patient from side to side in bed or when transferring the patient into or out of bed.

If the patient is not fully oriented or is uncooperative, he or she may pull the airway out. Interventions to reorient and remind the patient are indicated as well as measures to relieve pain and anxiety. When less restrictive measures are not sufficient, soft wrist restraints may be necessary. When restraints are in use, neurovascular checks are performed routinely distal to the restraints. The purpose of the restraints must be explained and intermittently reinforced to both the patient and family, emphasizing that the restraints are in place for protection of the airway. Patients and families frequently view restraints as a punishment or unnecessary restriction of freedom.

Alteration in Cardiac Output

The general goal, supporting tissue perfusion, can be addressed using the nursing diagnosis of *decreased cardiac output.* Positive pressure ventilation profoundly affects the normal hemodynamics of the body by increasing intrathoracic pressures and decreasing venous return to the heart, which decreases cardiac output. The use of PEEP further compromises cardiac output by further decreasing venous return. These effects are described in detail in Section Six.

Hemodynamic Effects of Mechanical Ventilation. While on the mechanical ventilator, the patient may have a pulmonary artery flow-directed catheter inserted to closely monitor hemodynamic status, particularly if there is a history of cardiovascular problems. Table 11–8 shows the hemodynamic trends associated with mechanical ventilation.

If the patient does not have a pulmonary artery catheter inserted, the nurse can assess for the clinical manifestations of decreased cardiac output, such as confusion, restlessness, decreased urine output, flattened neck veins, and clammy, cool skin. Management of abnormal hemodynamics depends on the underlying cause of the instability; however, attaining and maintaining optimal hydration is a major factor in achieving

TABLE 11–8 Hemodynamic Effects of Mechanical Ventilation

MEASURED PARAMETER	TREND
Right atrial pressure (RAP)	Increased
Pulmonary artery pressure (PAP)	Increased
Pulmonary artery wedge pressure (PAWP)	Usually increased
Left atrial pressure (LAP)	Usually increased
Peripheral arterial pressure (BP)	Unchanged or decreased
Cardiac output (CO)	Decreased

hemodynamic stability. Management of the patient with decreased cardiac output is described in detail in the perfusion modules of the textbook.

Alteration in Nutrition

Many patients who require mechanical ventilation have preexisting malnutrition associated with their chronic illness or inadequate nutritional support during hospitalization or a combination of both. This patient population is at high risk for altered nutrition (less than body requirements). During the acute phase of illness, the patient will receive nothing orally. The presence of an ET tube, even with a properly inflated cuff, places the patient at high risk for aspiration of microparticles that can leak around the endotracheal cuff and contaminate the lower airway. This leakage can precipitate complications associated with aspiration.

A malnourished state with its negative nitrogen balance significantly decreases the patient's chances of successful weaning from the mechanical ventilator because of respiratory muscle atrophy and weakness. Regaining nutritional integrity is a crucial aspect of care management because it has a direct impact on the patient's ability to improve his or her condition.

Pulmonary patients may require special consideration of carbohydrate loading because of the high carbon dioxide byproduct produced, which can further complicate acid–base balance. In such cases, special low carbohydrate tube feedings may be ordered. Constipation with abdominal distention can develop during mechanical ventilation due to immobility, illness, and narcotics used for comfort.

Nursing Management of Psychosocial Needs

The psychosocial needs of the high-acuity patient are presented in depth in Module 2, Holistic Care of the High-Acuity Patient and Family. The following is a brief discussion of psychosocial needs specific to the patient requiring mechanical ventilation.

Anxiety and Pain

The patient who is being mechanically ventilated is usually experiencing a high level of anxiety associated with the insertion of the ET tube, the mechanical ventilator, and the critical care environment. Anxiety is a common complaint of patients who have chronic respiratory problems. Many chronic pulmonary diseases are progressive in nature; thus, a pattern of increasing disability is experienced. As many chronic pulmonary diseases progress, patients experience an increasing pattern of hospital admissions for complications of their diseases. Ultimately, at end-stage disease, these patients most commonly die of complications of their diseases, such as severe respiratory failure or cor pulmonale.

When patients are experiencing acute respiratory distress, they often are anxious. Severe dyspnea frequently is associated with fear of suffocation or dying. All energy is focused toward breathing when acute distress exists. Being placed on a mechanical ventilator may be received by the patient either with relief or with an increased state of anxiety. Anxiety in the high-acuity setting may be associated with the unfamiliar environment, invasive breathing assist device, loss of control, painful procedures, lack of understanding or procedures, and fear of dying.

Critically ill patients may also experience pain related to their underlying illness, procedures, immobility, and routine care, including the endotracheal tube and suctioning. Patients should be assessed for pain using self-report methods when possible and by nonverbal indicators when they cannot communicate (Lindgren and Ames, 2005).

Management of the patient's anxiety and pain while on the mechanical ventilator combines collaborative and independent nursing interventions. Sedation commonly is ordered to decrease anxiety levels, which, in turn, helps the patient breathe with the ventilator. When oxygen consumption is significantly elevated, it may be decided to use a neuromuscular blocking agent to paralyze the respiratory muscles, producing rapid apnea and total skeletal muscle paralysis. Neuromuscular blocking agents do not alter the responsiveness level of the patient. Therefore, while in the paralyzed state, this group of patients should receive intermittent IV sedation and analgesia at regular intervals to reduce anxiety, relieve pain, and enhance mental rest.

Sleep Pattern Disturbance

While on the ventilator, the patient experiences interruptions throughout the 24-hour day. Airway clearance and other maintenance nursing interventions frequently require disturbing a resting or sleeping high-acuity patient. Cabello et al. (2007) investigated sleep deprivation in patients in critical care units and concluded that critically ill patients have alterations in sleep architecture and fragmented sleep.

Communication and Sensation

The presence of an artificial airway prevents the patient from communicating verbally. The patient who is fully responsive may become very frustrated when he or she cannot be understood. Alternative communication methods are available. To evaluate appropriate types of communication alternatives, the nurse must evaluate the patient's visual status. If eyesight is poor or glasses are not available, communication alternatives are reduced significantly.

Patience on the part of the nurse is a major component of successful communication with a mechanically ventilated patient. Simple needs often can be expressed through lip reading or hand signals. It is easier to lip read with a patient who has a nasotracheal tube rather than one with an orally placed tube.

Family Support

The psychosocial needs of the patient's family cannot be forgotten while the patient is being managed on the ventilator. Families vary on how they perceive the ventilator. The family may express relief that the patient's breathing status is now protected. This is particularly true of families of patients who have had several past intubations. The patient's family initially may find the presence of the artificial airway and mechanical ventilator a frightening experience. The frequent alarms and the patient's inability to communicate verbally are the basis of many of the questions asked of the nurse.

SECTION EIGHT REVIEW

1. The primary reason that airway patency becomes compromised in the mechanically ventilated patient is
   A. ineffective cough
   B. oversedation
   C. airway obstruction
   D. dehydration
2. Unless contraindicated, the patient should receive a fluid intake of ______ to ______ L/day to combat thick secretions.
   A. 1, 1.5
   B. 2, 2.5
   C. 3, 3.5
   D. 4, 4.5
3. The mechanically ventilated patient can develop respiratory alkalosis if the ______ and ______ settings on the mechanical ventilator are set too high.
   A. rate, tidal volume
   B. peak airway pressure, rate
   C. O_2 concentration, peak airway pressure
   D. tidal volume, O_2 concentration
4. A mechanically ventilated patient who is malnourished is at high risk for failure to wean because of
   A. impaired gas exchange
   B. decreased cardiac output
   C. increased airway resistance
   D. respiratory muscle weakness
5. To treat the nursing diagnosis, *sleep pattern disturbance*, while managing the care of a mechanically ventilated patient, the best nursing action would be to
   A. cluster activities
   B. administer sedatives
   C. administer neuromuscular blocking agents
   D. space activities evenly throughout the 24-hour day

Answers: 1. C, 2. B, 3. A, 4. D, 5. A

SECTION NINE: Weaning the Patient from the Mechanical Ventilator

At the completion of this section, the learner will be able to describe the process of weaning a patient from mechanical ventilation and the nurse's role in this process.

The term mechanical ventilator weaning includes all the activities involved in withdrawing a patient from mechanical ventilator support and attaining total independence from the ventilator. Withdrawing this support is a multidisciplinary effort that requires coordination among the physician, respiratory therapist, nurse, and patient. Ventilator weaning may be a relatively simple and rapid withdrawal process or it may be complex and extremely slow. The majority of patients requiring mechanical ventilator support are weaned rapidly with little difficulty. The remaining few are those who require prolonged weaning or are unable to wean. This small but significant group primarily consists of patients who have a history of chronic pulmonary disease or who have required prolonged mechanical ventilation. This section presents a brief overview of the weaning process to familiarize the learner with major assessments and interventions that are an integral part of the process.

Patients who are being evaluated for ventilator weaning fall into one of three categories (MacIntyre, 2007):

1. Patients whose removal is rapid when the reason for mechanical ventilation is resolved
2. Patients whose removal is slow and gradual and require more deliberate planning than the usual routine weaning activities
3. Patients who are considered unweanable (ventilator dependent) and may require long-term ventilatory support

The Weaning Process

Just as criteria are used in making the decision to place a patient on a mechanical ventilator, criteria are used when determining readiness for withdrawal from ventilator support. Successful weaning involves using a systematic approach, including determination of readiness to wean, weaning, and **postextubation** (removal of the artificial airway) follow-up.

Emerging Evidence

- Ventilator associated pneumonia (VAP) when of MRSA origin requires longer ventilator support before resolution than VAP infections by other pathogens such as MSSA, *H. influenzae*, or *P. aeruginosa (Vidaur, Plana, et al., 2008).*
- In a study of patient outcomes, the majority of critically ill patients who required prolonged mechanical ventilation were able to be weaned and on discharge demonstrated improved health over time; however, a significant percentage of the critically ill patient cohort did not wean and died within the first year of critical illness onset, primarily from consensual life support withdrawal after a lengthy hospital stay *(Bigatello, Stelfox et al., 2007).*
- Use of three assessment parameters, (mental status [EMV 10 or less], preextubation Pa_{CO_2} [44 mm Hg or greater], and endotracheal secretions [moderate-to-copious volume]), was predictive of extubation failure regardless of successful spontaneous breathing trials *(Mokhlesi, Tulaimat et al., 2007).*
- In a study investigated prediction of extubation success using a new method of measuring minute ventilation recovery time following a spontaneous breathing trial. The minute ventilation recovery time was significantly longer in medical and surgical ICU patients who experienced extubation failure (15 minutes) when compared to those who experienced extubation success (2 minutes) *(Seymour, Halpern, Christie et al., 2008).*

Determination of Readiness to Wean

Successful weaning depends largely on the physiologic and psychologic readiness of the patient. A variety of criteria are used to determine readiness; these criteria can be divided into initial and comprehensive patient screenings.

Initial Patient Screening. Consideration for readiness for weaning begins when the cause of respiratory failure is resolved or a significantly improved. Other necessary criteria include adequate oxygenation (while receiving Fi_{O_2} less than 0.50 and PEEP less than 8), hemodynamic stability, and spontaneous ventilatory effort.

Comprehensive Patient Screening. The decision of when it is appropriate to begin the weaning process is not necessarily a clear one. Generally, prior to making a final decision, a multisystem assessment review is conducted, focusing on those physiologic systems that are particularly associated with ventilator dependence (respiratory, cardiovascular, CNS, renal, and metabolic).

A comprehensive, multidisciplinary approach to weaning is crucial for successful weaning (MacInytre, 2007). Table 11–9 presents an example of a combined simple and comprehensive assessment form that might be used in helping to determine readiness for weaning. Note the number of criteria that focus on nutrition and metabolic function.

TABLE 11–9 Mechanical Ventilator Weaning Criteria

CRITERIA	RESPONSES
I. Initial Criteria	
A. Is the patient clinically stable?	Yes/No
B. Is the patient's clinical condition improving?	Yes/No
C. Is the precipitating problem resolved?	Yes/No
D. Is $\dot{V}_E$ less than 10 L/min on AC or SIMV of 14 or less?	Yes/No
E. Is Sp_{O_2} greater than 90% or greater at 0.40 Fi_{O_2} or less?	Yes/No
F. Is A-a gradient less than 100 mm Hg?	Yes/No
If any "No" answers, quit here. Patient does not qualify for initiation of weaning. Reevaluate in 48 hours.	
II. Comprehensive Criteria	
Is the patient:	
A. Hemodynamically stable?	
1. SBP 100–150, DBP 60–90 mm Hg at rest?	Yes/No
2. Heart rate 60–100 beats/min at rest?	Yes/No
3. Usual ECG pattern?	Yes/No
B. Systemically hydrated?	
1. Intake = Output	Yes/No
2. Urinary output greater than 620 mL/24 hr	Yes/No
3. BUN and creatinine: within normal limits	Yes/No
C. Without fever or new/unresolved pulmonary infection? (Chest X-ray within past 48 hr; temp. less than 100°F (37.8°C) orally)	Yes/No
D. Receiving support for nutritional status?	Yes/No
E. Have drugs been discontinued that	
1. Decrease respiratory drive?	Yes/No
2. Increase muscle weakness?	Yes/No
3. Increase anxiety?	Yes/No

III. Laboratory Values

Are the following parameters in at least minimal acceptable ranges and current within the past 24 hours? Specify "Yes" if replacement therapy is occurring if value is below normal range.

A. K (normal, 3.5–5.0 mEq/L)	Yes/No
B. Na (normal, 135–145 mEq/L)	Yes/No
C. PO_4 (normal, 3.0–4.5 mg/dL, acceptable greater than 2.0)	Yes/No
D. Ca (normal, 8.5–10.5 mg/dL)	Yes/No
E. Mg (normal, 1.5–4.5 mg/dL)	Yes/No
F. Prealbumin (normal, 24–30 mg/dL, acceptable 10 or higher)	Yes/No
G. CBC with differential, specifically:	
WBC (normal, 5,000–10,000/L)	Yes/No
Hgb (normal, greater than 10 g/dL)	Yes/No
Hct (normal, greater than 30 g/dL)	Yes/No
Calculated total lymphocyte count (normal, 1,500 or 2,000/mcL or greater)	Yes/No
H. Theophylline level (normal, less than 20 mcg/dL)	Yes/No
I. ABG while on ventilator within the past 12 hours:	
pH = 7.35–7.45	Yes/No
PO_2 = 60 mm Hg or greater on Fio_2 of 0.4 or less	Yes/No
PCO_2 = less than 50 mm Hg or within 10 mm Hg of baseline	Yes/No
Sao_2 = 90% or greater at 0.40 Fio_2 or less	Yes/No

If any answers to the criteria in Sections II and III are "No", the decision to initiate weaning will be closely evaluated. If the problem is easily correctable, appropriate interventions will be taken to correct the problem and the patient will be reevaluated after 24 hours.

SBP=systolic blood pressure, DBP=diastolic blood pressure.

Assessment data provided by simple and comprehensive patient screenings identify potential barriers to successful weaning and actions that must be taken to resolve each problem. It is at this point in the weaning process that actions vary widely. Barriers to successful weaning are not necessarily considered equal and experts disagree regarding which criteria are absolute and which are relative contraindications. For this reason, weaning may be initiated on patients who do not meet all the simple or comprehensive criteria (e.g., presence of active but improving pneumonia; improving but not corrected malnutrition).

Alternative Indications of Readiness to Wean

The traditional criteria for readiness to wean are similar to the criteria used in deciding to place the patient on the mechanical ventilator. In addition to the comprehensive criteria presented in Table 11–9, there are a group of bedside tests commonly used to assess a patient's readiness to be weaned from mechanical ventilation. This group of tests is referred to as "weaning parameters." Table 11–10 provides a summary of the bedside weaning parameters.

TABLE 11–10 Bedside Weaning Parameters

PARAMETER	TARGET RANGE	COMMENTS
Rapid Shallow Breathing Index (RSBI, f/V_T)	Less than 60 to 105 breaths/min/L (spontaneous breathing)	Obtain 1 minute after disconnection
Vital Capacity (VC)	Greater than 15 mL/kg (IBW*)	Requires patient cooperation; is not a consistent predictor of readiness to wean
Breathing Rate (f)	Less than 35 spontaneous breaths/min	Breathing greater than 35/min. is a negative indicator for weaning success
Spontaneous Tidal Volume (V_T)	Greater than 4 to 6 mL/kg (IBW)	
Maximum Inspiratory Pressure (MIP, P_{Imax}) (or Negative Inspiratory Force [NIF])	Less than -20 to -30 cm H_2O	Measured after 20 sec. of airway occlusion Cease if desaturation or cardiac dysrhythmias develop
Minute Ventilation ($\dot{V}_E$)	Less than 10 to 15 L/min.	
Airway Occlusion Pressure ($P_{0.1}$ or P_{100})	Less than -6 cm H_2O	Upper airway pressure is measured after airway occluded for 100 msec during inspiratory phase. Requires special valve systems

*IBW=Ideal Body Weight

Data from Pilbeam (2006) and Shelledy (2003).

Weaning

Rapid Weaning (Short Term)

Frequently, a patient with no significant lung disease requires short-term mechanical ventilation (e.g., surgery, drug overdose). Once the underlying problem is corrected (e.g., reversal of anesthesia effects), the patient is evaluated for weaning. If weaning criteria are met, the patient is placed on CPAP or removed from the ventilator and placed on a T-piece (or blow-by) for 30 to 120 minutes. During the trial period, the patient is monitored for comfort, cardiac rhythm status, and ABG status. If these criteria remain within acceptable limits (stable PaO_2, and pH above 7.30), the patient is extubated. Rapid weaning may also be accomplished using low levels of PSV or CPAP. The patient is given a brief trial period and then extubated. Figure 11–12 illustrates a typical T-piece (blow-by) configuration.

Slow Weaning (Long Term)

Patients who have underlying chronic lung disease (e.g., emphysema or pulmonary fibrosis) that is complicated by some acute problem (e.g., pneumonia) and patients who have had a prolonged illness frequently cannot be weaned as rapidly as patients with normal lungs. Slow weaning is performed on patients who are unable to wean for a variety of reasons. Problems associated with difficult weaning include excessive respiratory muscle work of breathing, respiratory muscle fatigue, anemia, malnutrition, excessive secretions, infection, unstable hemodynamic state, fear, and anxiety. Difficult-to-wean patients often are in a poorer state of general health than the fast-weaning group. Their ability to make the transition back to spontaneous negative pressure breathing from long-term positive pressure breathing is slow and requires retraining and strengthening of the respiratory muscles.

Slow weaning is a complex and difficult process for all involved. Over time, multiple weaning alternatives (SIMV, mandatory minute ventilation [MMV], PSV, manual weaning/ spontaneous breathing trials) may need to be employed in response to changes in the patient's clinical status. Long-term weaning requires close monitoring of the patient's multisystem functions, as well as psychosocial status. Rapid, aggressive management of problems as they arise significantly improves the chances for successful weaning.

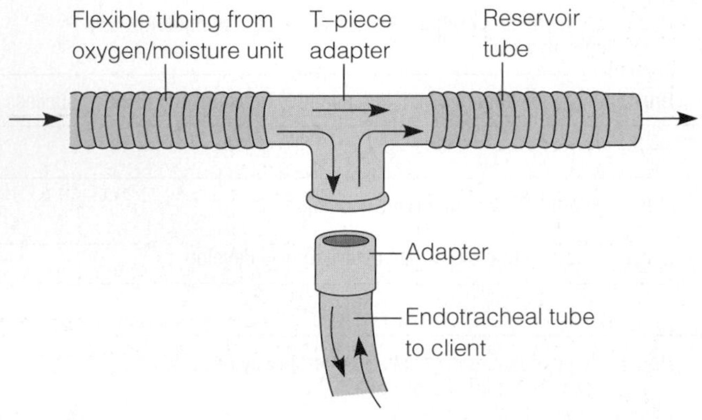

Figure 11–12 ■ T-piece (blow-by) configuration.

Methods of Weaning

Manual Weaning/Spontaneous Breathing Trials

The original method of withdrawing a patient from a ventilator is manual weaning, and it is still used today. Manual weaning is accomplished by following a schedule of removal from the mechanical ventilator for increasingly longer periods of time. When this method is used, the patient is taken off the ventilator and the artificial airway is attached to a humidified oxygen source using a T-piece. The nurse is responsible for closely monitoring the patient for signs of weaning intolerance; for example, respiratory rate greater than 30/min, a significant increase in blood pressure and pulse (often more than 10 mm Hg and 10/min, respectively), a minute ventilation of more than 10 L/min, cyanosis, or a decrease in oxygen saturation on pulse oximetry to below the patient's acceptable level. Other indicators of fatigue include diaphoresis, use of accessory muscles, and abdominal paradox.

Manual weaning requires close patient contact throughout the weaning period because the nurse plays a crucial part in patient monitoring and coaching correct breathing rate and depth for the trial period. The nurse's calm reassurance is instrumental in assisting the patient past the period of anxiety often associated with removal from the mechanical ventilator. Manual weaning is performed on an increasing schedule either throughout the 24-hour period or throughout the day and evening hours and maintaining the patient on mechanical ventilation throughout the night for rest. The amount of time the patient is kept off the ventilator may start at 5 minutes and increase to the entire day, except at night, before full independence. Manual weaning must be individually designed, based on the patient's changing status from day to day.

Manual weaning is a strengthening exercise for the respiratory muscles. Complete removal from the ventilator forces the respiratory muscles to take over complete work of breathing, without any assistance from the ventilator for increasing blocks of time. Muscle strength is increased through use of the weaning procedure and good nutrition and hydration. There are several disadvantages to manual weaning. First, it may be a frightening experience for the patient, who is more accustomed to positive pressure breathing. Abrupt removal from the ventilator may precipitate high anxiety, which can hinder the weaning process. Second, manual weaning is time consuming for the nurse. During the period that the patient is off the ventilator, particularly in the early stages of weaning, the nurse is needed directly at the bedside to coach and monitor, and to give encouragement.

Ventilator Weaning

Spontaneous breathing trials can also be done using the ventilator. Rather than placing the patient on a T-piece, the patient is placed on CPAP with or without low levels of pressure support. The length of time of spontaneous breathing is increased as tolerated, similar to T-piece weaning (MacIntyre, 2007). Using the ventilator for spontaneous trials offers the advantages of maintaining CPAP, which may be important for some patients, and ventilator monitoring for safety.

Today, ventilator weaning (use of a ventilator mode) is more common than manual weaning. It is generally thought to be less traumatic for the patient because it does not involve intermittent removal from the ventilator. A variety of alternative modes are used for ventilator weaning, the most common ones being SIMV, PSV, and MMV (mandatory minute ventilation). The choice of weaning mode is based on the clinician's preferences, the type of mode available based on equipment constraints, and the patient's needs and clinical status.

SIMV Weaning. The following is a brief description of one ventilator weaning protocol using SIMV. Using this ventilator mode, the patient is given mandatory mechanical (ventilator) breaths at preset intervals every minute. Between the mechanical breaths, the patient is able to exercise the respiratory muscles spontaneously. Initially, the SIMV rate may be set fairly high, near the patient's own respiratory rate. The rate of mandatory breaths is then decreased by two-breath increments one to two times per day (as tolerated) until the SIMV rate is down to four breaths per minute. Once the mandatory rate is at four breaths per minute, a spontaneous mode (such as PSV) or a T-piece trial is attempted for a minimum of 30 minutes. If the patient tolerates the weaning procedure and all parameters remain within acceptable boundaries, he or she can be extubated.

Table 11–11 provides a summary of the common manual and ventilator weaning modes.

SIMV weaning is an endurance exercise for the respiratory muscles. The muscles work continuously over the entire day except when the SIMV breath triggers a positive pressure breath, which allows a single breath rest. Some patients do not tolerate decreasing SIMV rates. This tolerance may change on a day-to-day basis. Weaning often is not a smooth undertaking. In patients with underlying disease, changing status can require temporary cessation of weaning. This is particularly true if the patient should develop pneumonia. Such a status change may first manifest itself in a sudden intolerance to weaning.

Whatever the method used, evidence supports a comprehensive approach to weaning. Success using structured, multidisciplinary protocols helps guide the weaning process and ongoing patient assessments (Lindgren & Ames, 2005). Continuing efforts are made to optimize all aspects of care. During weaning, the respiratory therapist is generally in charge of making setting changes to the mechanical ventilator while the nurse closely monitors the patient for signs of failure-to-wean (see Table 11–12). If failure-to-wean signs develop, the patient should be returned to the preweaning ventilator settings.

TABLE 11–11 Common Weaning Modes

WEANING MODE	DESCRIPTION	ADVANTAGES	DISADVANTAGES
T-Piece (manual)	Patient is provided supplementary oxygen and humidity. Time off of the ventilator is gradually increased.	Strengthening exercise for respiratory muscles	All breaths are spontaneous Potential for apnea Requires close monitoring, one-on-one nursing care Can cause patient anxiety
SIMV	Frequency of mandatory ventilator breaths is slowly decreased, which requires the patient to gradually take over own work of breathing.	Maintains respiratory muscle strength and reduces atrophy Maintains more normal gas distribution Reduces cardiovascular side effects Maintains some of the work of breathing	May increase the work of breathing as a result of demand valve system Rate must be manually manipulated
PSV	Provides positive pressure during the inspiration phase to support tidal volumes and decrease work of breathing.	Decreased work of breathing Increased patient comfort Minimal cardiovascular side effects	All breaths are spontaneous Flow pattern may not be adequate Inspiratory flow rate may be too high or too low
MMV	Guarantees an ongoing stable level of minute ventilation $\dot{V}_E$: As the patient increases or decreases ventilatory effort, the ventilator adjusts itself automatically to continue to provide the same level of $\dot{V}_E$.	Good control of Pa_{CO_2} Protection from hypoventilation during weaning Facilitates transition from ventilator to spontaneous breathing	May not respond quickly enough to an apneic episode Potential for development of hypercapnia in presence of a rapid shallow breathing pattern

Data from Pilbeam (2006).

TABLE 11–12 Common Failure-to-Wean Criteria

PARAMETER	CRITICAL VALUE
Tidal Volume (V_T)	Less than 100 mL/breath
ABG:	
pH	Less than 7.30
$Paco_2$	Greater than 50 mmHg
Pao_2	Less than 55 mmHg
Spo_2	Less than 90%
Clinical signs	Increased dyspnea, signs of respiratory muscle fatigue, unstable vital signs, development of cardiac dysrhythmias

Special Considerations for the Elderly

The elderly can have similar outcomes from mechanical ventilation as younger patients (El Solh & Ramadan, 2006). However, in the elderly, common complications of critical illness, such as delirium, side effects of sedative agents, and deconditioning, adversely prolong ventilation and length of stay. Higher mortality rates and poorer functional outcomes occur in patients with multiple organ failure or prolonged intubation. The best mode for weaning elderly patients has not been identified.

The elderly, without significant comorbid illness, become frail in the high-acuity setting and vulnerable to complications. El Solh and Ramadan (2006) identified two major approaches to care of the older patient: avoiding fatigue and preventing complications. To avoid fatigue, nursing care and procedures should be spaced at intervals allowing time for rest. Sleep can be enhanced by obtaining information on and trying to maintain the patient's usual schedule, promoting a day–night schedule, reducing noise, and following nonpharmacologic approaches.

Priorities for care include cautious use of sedative/hypnotic agents that can cause confusion because the elderly are at increased risk for developing delirium. All medications should be evaluated for potential adverse drug interactions. Efforts can be made to enhance quality stimulation and communication. Hearing aids and eyeglasses should be used if needed by the patient. Malnutrition may be present on admission or develop while the patient is in the hospital and can contribute to muscle weakness. Early aggressive reconditioning and physical therapy are needed to limit muscle atrophy from prolonged bedrest. Therapy may even include ambulation using a manual resuscitation bag (Pruitt, 2006). These approaches are not limited to the care of the elderly, but represent important care for any high-acuity patient. In the elderly, however, the approaches assume a greater imperative given the vulnerability of the aged and their reduced capacity to recover from severe insults.

Postextubation Follow-up

Extubation is usually carried out as soon as it is determined that the patient can sustain spontaneous breathing. Removal of the artificial airway, however, requires that patient be able to maintain their own airways and cough adequately to mobilize secretions. An "air leak" test is helpful to evaluate the potential for airway obstruction postextubation (Walz, Zayaruzny, & Heard, 2007). To conduct an air leak test, the oropharynx is suctioned, the ET cuff is deflated, and the patient is evaluated for the ability to breathe around the tube. When these criteria are met, rapid tube removal is recommended. Quick tube removal is important because the ET tube increases the work of breathing.

Following extubation, particular attention must be given to excellent pulmonary hygiene, including a routine of coughing, deep breathing, and incentive spirometry. Various aerosol therapies, percussion, and postural drainage may be ordered to prevent or treat complications, if necessary. Noninvasive ventilation may be helpful for patients at high risk for fatigue and reintubation (Caples & Gay, 2005).

Stridor is a potential postextubation complication resulting from glottic edema and can be mild or severe. When severe, it can cause total obstruction of the airway requiring reintubation. Patients are also at risk postextubation for aspiration as a result of swallowing dysfunction. There is a high incidence of aspiration (up to 50 percent) in patients who had been intubated for more than 48 hours (Postma, McGuirt et al., 2007). Many of these patients develop silent aspiration, in that they do not cough normally. Aspiration may contribute to postextubation respiratory failure. Patients must be monitored carefully when oral intake is resumed and a formal swallow evaluation may be appropriate for high-risk patients.

SECTION NINE REVIEW

1. The vast majority of patients requiring mechanical ventilation are weaned
   - A. rapidly, with difficulty
   - B. rapidly, without difficulty
   - C. slowly, with difficulty
   - D. slowly, without difficulty
2. The majority of difficult-to-wean patients have which condition?
   - A. pneumonia
   - B. congestive heart failure
   - C. acute respiratory distress syndrome
   - D. chronic pulmonary disease
3. Initial patient screening criteria for weaning eligibility include
   - A. Is the urinary output greater than 620 mL/24 hr?
   - B. Is the prealbumin 10 mg/dL or greater?
   - C. Is the patient's clinical condition improving?
   - D. Have drugs been discontinued that decrease the respiratory drive?

4. Traditional weaning criteria most effectively predict readiness in patients who
   A. are elderly
   B. are relatively healthy
   C. have chronic pulmonary disease
   D. require prolonged mechanical ventilation
5. The term ______ weaning is used to refer to weaning by intermittently removing the patient from the ventilator for increasing periods of time.
   A. manual
   B. ventilator
   C. SIMV
   D. pressure support ventilation
6. SIMV weaning primarily is a(n) ______ exercise for the respiratory muscles.
   A. supportive
   B. resistance
   C. strengthening
   D. endurance

Answers: 1. B, 2. D, 3. C, 4. B, 5. A, 6. D

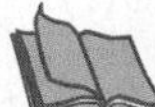

POSTTEST

The following Posttest is constructed in a case study format. A patient is presented, and questions are asked based on available data. New data are presented as the case study progresses.

Mary R., 55 years of age, has a 20-year history of smoking. She has been treated medically for emphysema for several years. Mary weighs 115 pounds. She is admitted to the hospital with a diagnosis of acute respiratory failure.

1. To be clinically called acute ventilatory failure, which of the following arterial blood gas (ABG) results must be present?
   A. PH less than 7.35
   B. $PaCO_2$ greater than 50mm Hg
   C. PaO_2 less than 60 mm Hg
   D. HCO_3 less than mm Hg
2. Mary has a low ventilation-perfusion ratio as a result of pulmonary shunting. What is the ABG result that would indicate a shunt is present?
   A. PaO_2 55mm Hg
   B. pH 7.30
   C. $PaCO_2$ 30 mm Hg
   D. PaO_2 100 mm Hg

Mary is showing evidence of ventilatory fatigue. It is decided that she will require intubation and mechanical ventilation.

3. Mary is tachypneic and hypoxic. She requires emergent intubation. The nurse can expect which of the following artificial airways to be inserted?
   A. oral endotracheal tube
   B. nasotracheal tube
   C. tracheostomy tube
   D. oral pharyngeal airway
4. The nurse can expect which procedure to be performed to confirm the endotracheal tube is correctly placed?
   A. end tidal CO_2 monitoring
   B. chest X-ray
   C. auscultation of breath sounds
   D. pulse oximetry reading of 95 percent
5. Mary is placed on volume-cycled ventilation. The nurse recognizes that volume-cycled ventilation is used to
   A. overcome changes in airway resistance
   B. avoid placement of an artificial airway
   C. automatically alter volume as pressure changes
   D. deliver higher levels of oxygen
6. Mary is placed on 10 cm H_2O of PEEP. What would the nurse see on the ventilator to indicate the patient is receiving this amount of PEEP?
   A. The airway pressure manometer needle should fall to 10 cm H_2O during inspiration.
   B. The airway pressure manometer needle should fall to 5 cm H_2O during expiration.
   C. The airway pressure manometer needle should fall to 10 cm H_2O during expiration.
   D. The airway pressure manometer needle should remain at 10 cm H_2O during the entire ventilatory cycle.
7. Mary is placed on the following ventilator settings: tidal volume 700 mL, rate 8 breaths per minute, FiO_2 50 percent. Her $PaCO_2$ has increased from 45 mm Hg to 55 mm Hg. What ventilator setting can the nurse expect to be altered to decrease the $PaCO_2$?
   A. decrease rate to 6 breaths per minute
   B. increase FiO_2 to 60 percent
   C. decrease tidal volume to 600 mL
   D. increase rate to 12 breaths per minute
8. Mary has improved and is to begin weaning from the ventilator. She is placed on synchronous intermittent mandatory ventilation (SIMV) with a pressure support of 10 cm H_2O. The nurse explains that pressure support is used to
   A. make inspiration easier
   B. make expiration easier
   C. keep alveoli open during the breathing cycle
   D. improve oxygenation

9. While on SIMV, Mary has the following changes: respiratory rate 32/min, oxygen saturation 88 percent, and use of accessory muscles. The nurse would expect
   A. weaning to continue
   B. Mary to be extubated
   C. Mary to be placed back on ventilatory support
   D. FIO_2 to be increased
10. Mary develops a fever of 101.0° F, her sputum is green, and chest auscultation reveals right lower lobe crackles. The nurse should suspect she has developed
    A. stress ulcer
    B. pulmonary embolism
    C. ventilator associated pneumonia
    D. pneumothorax
11. The low exhaled tidal volume alarm on Mary's ventilator keeps triggering. If the problem is not found immediately, the nurse should
    A. call the physician
    B. manually ventilate the patient
    C. check ventilator connections
    D. put air into the endotracheal tube cuff
12. Mary is successfully weaned using a slow T-piece mode. The nurse can explain to her family that the T-piece supports weaning by
    A. requiring Mary to gradually take over her own work of breathing
    B. supporting Mary's tidal volume during inspiration
    C. assuring that Mary maintains a stable minute ventilation
    D. supporting Mary by maintaining open alveoli at end expiration
13. Mary's endotracheal tube cuff pressure should be maintained at 20-25 mm Hg to
    A. allow secretions from the upper airway to enter the lower airway
    B. prevent necrosis of the trachea
    C. allow for air movement around the cuff
    D. increase circulation
14. The nurse can expect the following changes in heart rate and blood pressure secondary to changes in cardiac output with the use of positive pressure ventilation
    A. decreased blood pressure, increased pulse
    B. increased blood pressure, increased pulse
    C. decreased blood pressure, decreased pulse
    D. increased blood pressure, decreased pulse
15. A patient on mechanical ventilation has a decreasing hemoglobin and hematocrit, with dark and tarry stools. The nurse can expect to
    A. administer an enema
    B. give iron supplements
    C. stop proton pump inhibitor
    D. test the stool for blood
16. Noninvasive positive pressure ventilation should be considered as an alternative to intubation in which patient?
    A. an unresponsive patient with a stroke
    B. a patient in acute congestive heart failure
    C. a patient with pneumonia and hypoxia with a weak cough
    D. a patient who has frequent periods of apnea
17. The nurse is having difficulty clearing secretions from the endotracheal tube. To facilitate clearing of secretions the nurse can take which action?
    A. increase the frequency of suctioning
    B. increase fluid intake
    C. instill saline into the endotracheal tube prior to suctioning
    D. stop nebulizer treatments
18. A patient's ventilator settings were changed as follows: Tidal volume increased from 500 mL to 700 mL; rate (f) increased from 14 breaths to 16 breaths per minute. What ABG changes would the nurse expect?
    A. increasing pH
    B. increasing $PaCO_2$
    C. decreasing pH
    D. decreasing SaO_2
19. A 70 kg patient is intubated and placed on mechanical ventilation. The nurse can expect the initial tidal volume to be:
    A. 350 mL
    B. 560 mL
    C. 840 mL
    D. 250 mL
20. After an hour of being on noninvasive positive pressure ventilation (NIPPV) a patient with COPD has the following ABG changes:

Pre NIPPV	Post NIPPV
PH 7.25	pH 7.32
$PaCO_2$ 66 mm Hg	$PaCO_2$ 46 mm Hg
PaO_2 90 mm Hg	PaO_2 92 mm Hg
HCO_3 23 mm Hg	HCO_3 24 mm Hg.

    The nurses' initial action should be
    A. increase the oxygen
    B. plan for immediate intubation
    C. increase the expiratory pressure
    D. check the mask for an air leak
21. A patient with a pulmonary embolus is intubated and placed on mechanical ventilation. When suctioning the endotracheal tube, the nurse should
    A. apply suction while inserting the catheter
    B. hyperoxygenate with 100 percent oxygen before and after suctioning
    C. suction the patient every hour
    D. suction two or three times in quick successions

Posttest answers with rationale are found on MyNursingKit.

REFERENCES

AACN. (2008). AACN practice alert: ventilator associated pneumonia. Retrieved 12/08/2008 from http://www.aacn.org/WD/Practice/Docs/Ventilator_Associated_Pneumonia_1-2008.pdf.

AACN. (2007). AACN practice alert: oral care in the critically ill. Retrieved 12/08/2008 from http://www.aacn.org/WD/Practice/Docs/Oral_Care_in_the_Critically_Ill.pdf.

AACN. (2005) AACN practice alert: deep vein thrombosis prevention. Retrieved 12/08/2008 from http://www.aacn.org/WD/Practice/Docs/DVT_Prevention_12-2005.pdf.

Ackerman, M. H. (1993). The effect of saline lavage prior to suctioning. *American Journal of Critical Care, 2*(4): 326–30.

Amitai, A. and Sinert, R. (2006). Ventilator management. Accessed online on 5/27/08 at http://www.emedicine.com/emerg/TOPIC788.htm.

Augustyn, B. (2007). Ventilator-associated pneumonia: risk factors and prevention. *Critical Care Nurse, 27* (4): 32–39.

Berry, A. M., Davidson, P. M., Masters, J. & Rolls, K. (2007). Systematic literature review of oral hygiene practices for intensive care patients receiving mechanical ventilation. *American Journal of Critical Care*, 16(6): 552–562.

Bigatello, L. M., Stelfox, H. T., Berra, L., Schmidt, U, and Gettings, E. M. (2007). Outcome of patients undergoing prolonged mechanical ventilation after critical illness. *Critical Care Medicine, 35*(11): 2491–2497.

Cabello, B., Parthasarathy, S. & Mancebo, J. (2007). Mechanical ventilation: let us minimize sleep disturbances. *Current Opinions in Critical Care, 13*: 20–26.

Caples, S. M. & Gay, P. C. (2005). Noninvasive positive pressure ventilation in the intensive care unit: a concise review. *Critical Care Medicine, 33*(11): 2651–2658.

El Solh, A. A. & Ramadan, F. H. (2006). Overview of respiratory failure in older adults. *Journal of Intensive Care Medicine, 21*(6): 345–351.

Hagler, D. A., Traver, G. A. (1994). Endotracheal saline and suction catheters: sources of lower airway contamination. Am J Crit Care, *3*: 444–447.

Hall, J. B., Schmidt, G. A. & Wood, L. D. H (2005). *Principles of Critical Care* (3rd edition). New York: McGraw-Hill.

Halm, M. A., & Krisko-Hagel, K. (2008). Instilling normal saline with suctioning: beneficial technique or potentially harmful sacred cow? *American Journal of Critical Care, 17*(5), 469–472

Hill, N. S., Brennan, J., Garpestad, E., & Nava, S. (2007). Noninvasive ventilation in acute respiratory failure. *Critical Care Medicine, 35*(10): 2402–2407.

Kinloch, D. (1999). Instillation of normal saline during endotracheal suctioning: effects on mixed venous oxygen saturation. Amer J Crit Care, *8*: 231–240.

Kuiper, J. W., Groeneveld, J., Slutsky, A. S., & Plotz, F. B. (2005). Mechanical ventilation and acute renal failure. *Critical Care Medicine, 33*(6): 1408–1415.

Liesching, T., Kwok, H., & Hill, N. (2003). Acute applications of noninvasive positive pressure ventilation. *Chest, 124*: 699–713.

Lindgren, V. & Ames, N. (2005). Caring for patients on mechanical ventilation: what research indicates is best practice. *American Journal of Nursing, 105* (5): 50–60.

MacIntyre, N. (2007). Discontinuing mechanical ventilatory support. *Chest, 132* (3): 1049–1056.

Marino, P. (2006). *The ICU book* (3rd edition). Philadelphia: Lippincott Williams & Wilkins.

Martin, L. (1987). *Pulmonary physiology in clinical practice: the essentials for patient care and evaluation.* St. Louis: C. V. Mosby.

Mehta, S., & Hill, N. (2001). Noninvasive ventilation. *American Journal of Respiratory and Critical Care Medicine, 163*: 540–577.

Mokhlesi, B., Tulaimat, A., Gluckman, T. J., Wang, Y., Evans, A. T., & Corbridge, T. C. (2007). Predicting extubation failure after successful completion of a spontaneous breathing trial. *Respiratory Care, 52*(12): 1710–1717.

NGC (National Guideline Clearinghouse). (n.d.). Guidelines for preventing health-care-associated pneumonia, 2003: recommendations of CDC and the Healthcare infection Control Practices Advisory Committee. Retrieved July 22, 2008 from: National Guidelines Clearinghouse, http://www.guideline.gov/summary/summary.aspx?doc_id=4872&nbr=003506&string=nasotracheal+AND+intubation.

NGC (National Guidelines Clearinghouse). (n.d.[a]). Practice management guidelines for the timing of tracheostomy. Retrieved 12/02/08 from http://www.guideline.gov/summary/summary.aspx?doc_id=10171&nbr=005355&string=tracheostomy.

Pilbeam, S. P. (2006). *Mechanical ventilation: physiological and clinical applications* (4th ed.). St. Louis: Mosby/Elsevier.

Postma, G. N., McGuirt, W. F., Butler, S. G., Rees, C. J., Crandall, H. L., & Tansavatdi, K. (2007). Laryngopharyngeal abnormalities in hospitalized patients with dysphagia. *The Laryngoscope, 117*(10): 1720–1722.

Pruitt, B. (2006). Weaning patients from mechanical ventilation. *Nursing, 36*(9): 36–41.

Scott, J. M. & Vollman, K. M. (2005). Endotracheal tube and oral care. In D. J. Lynn-McHale Wiegand & K. K. Carlson (eds.), *AACN Procedure Manual for Critical Care* (5th edition, pp 28–33). St. Louis: Elsevier Saunders.

Sevransky, J., & Haponik, E. (2003). Respiratory failure in elderly patients. *Clinical Geriatric Medicine, 19*: 205–224.

Seymour, C. W., Halpern, S., Christie, J. D., Gallop, R., and Fuchs, B.C. (2008). Minute ventilation recovery time measured using a new, simplified methodology predicts extubation outcome. J Intensive Care Med, *23*(1): 52–60.

Sharma, S. (2006). Ventilation, noninvasive. Accessed online on April 16, 2008 at http://www.emedicine.com/med/topic3371.htm.

Shelledy, D. C. (2003). Discontinuing ventilatory support. In R. L. Wilkins, J. K. Stoller, and C. L. Scanlan, *Egan's Fundamentals of Respiratory Care* (8th ed., pp. 1121–1154). St. Louis: Mosby.

Sullivan, K. & Gropper, M.A. (2007). Mechanical ventilatory support in 2006: getting the most from the ventilator. *ASA Refresher Courses in Anesthesiology,* 35(1):185–193.

Tullmann, D., & Dracup, K. (2000). Creating a healing environment for elders. *AACN Clinical Issues, 11*: 34–50.

Vidaus, L. Planas, K., Sierra, R, Dimopoulos, G., Ramirez, A., Lisboa, T., and Rello, J. (2008). Ventilator-associated pneumonia: impact of organisms on clinical resolution and medical resources. *Chest, 133*(3): 625–632.

Walz, J. M., Zayaruzny, M. & Heard, S.O. (2007). Airway management in critical illness. *Chest, 131*(2): 608–620.

MODULE

12 Determinants and Assessment of Cardiac Output

Karen L. Johnson

OBJECTIVES Following completion of this module, the learner will be able to

1. Define and state adult normal values for cardiac output, cardiac index, heart rate, and stroke volume.
2. Discuss how preload, contractility, and afterload impact stroke volume.
3. Describe the relationship of stroke volume and preload in terms of the Frank–Starling law.
4. Describe the relationship among pressure, flow, and resistance and how these impact cardiac output.
5. Discuss factors that influence myocardial contractility.
6. State some of the conditions that affect heart rate, preload, contractility, and afterload.
7. Identify the common clinical assessments that evaluate heart rate, preload, contractility, and afterload.
8. Describe various cardiovascular diagnostic procedures used to evaluate the components of cardiac output.
9. Discuss nursing responsibilities in caring for a patient receiving cardiovascular diagnostic procedures.

This self-study module is intended for the novice nurse caring for the high-acuity patient. This module focuses on the physiologic concepts that influence the function of the cardiovascular system, with particular focus on the heart. An understanding of these concepts will allow the nurse to apply them to a variety of clinical situations in order to understand assessment findings related to cardiovascular health and disease.

The module is composed of eight sections that define terms and normal values, describe key relationships among variables, identify common clinical conditions that influence these variables, and present the clinical assessments that can be made using these variables. Each section includes a set of review questions to help the learner evaluate his or her understanding of the section's content before moving on to the next section. All Section Reviews include answers. It is suggested that the learner review those concepts answered incorrectly in the review questions before proceeding to the next section.

PRETEST

1. Stroke volume multiplied by heart rate equals the
   A. cardiac output
   B. cardiac index
   C. pulse pressure product
   D. left ventricular stroke work index
2. The normal cardiac output for an adult at rest is approximately
   A. 1.2 L/min
   B. 3.4 L/min
   C. 5.0 L/min
   D. 10.0 L/min
3. The resistance against which the heart must pump blood is known as
   A. preload
   B. afterload
   C. upload
   D. download
4. The most effective mechanism to increase cardiac output is to
   A. increase heart rate
   B. decrease contractility
   C. increase afterload
   D. decrease preload
5. The Frank–Starling law states that within physiologic limits, the heart will
   A. beat no faster than the body's demand for oxygen dictates
   B. pump the volume it receives
   C. completely empty of blood with each beat
   D. extract only the amount of oxygen needed from its blood supply
6. Too much preload results in a(n)
   A. decrease in heart rate
   B. increase in heart rate
   C. decrease in cardiac output
   D. increase in afterload

7. Blood pressure is the product of
   A. flow and volume
   B. cardiac output and afterload
   C. viscosity and resistance
   D. viscosity and volume
8. When afterload increases
   A. blood pressure decreases
   B. cardiac output decreases
   C. blood pressure increases
   D. both B and C are correct
9. Which of the following depresses myocardial contractility?
   A. epinephrine
   B. digitalis
   C. sympathetic nervous system activity
   D. hypoxemia
10. Which of the following increase(s) myocardial contractility?
   A. dopamine
   B. dobutamine
   C. digoxin
   D. all of the above
11. Profound hemorrhage initially results in
   A. decreased afterload
   B. decreased preload
   C. increased preload
   D. decreased heart rate
12. Which of the following conditions dilate arterioles?
   A. septic shock
   B. spinal cord injury
   C. anaphylactic shock
   D. all of the above
13. The number of heartbeats too weak to be transmitted to the periphery is measured by
   A. pulse pressure
   B. brachiopopliteal gradient
   C. electrocardiogram
   D. apical–radial pulse deficit
14. Which of the following is consistent with diminished preload to the right ventricle?
   A. ascites
   B. jugular venous distention
   C. hepatic engorgement
   D. poor skin turgor
15. Conscious sedation is required for which of the following cardiovascular diagnostic procedures?
   A. stress test
   B. transesophageal echocardiogram
   C. transthoracic echocardiogram
   D. electrocardiogram

Pretest answers are found on MyNursingKit.

SECTION ONE: Cardiac Output

At the completion of this section, the learner will be able to define and state adult normal values for cardiac output, cardiac index, heart rate, and stroke volume. These definitions and values will be applied to the content of later sections.

Cardiac output (CO) is the amount of blood pumped by the heart each minute. It is a critical aspect of cardiovascular function in both health and illness. Knowledge of how CO changes in response to various conditions permits an understanding of pertinent physical assessment findings when there is an alteration in cardiac output.

The normal CO is approximately 4.0 to 8.0 liters/minute (L/min). Normal CO for individuals can vary significantly depending on body size. Therefore, when CO is measured it is corrected to account for body size. The correction is calculated by dividing CO by **body surface area (BSA)** and is called the **cardiac index (CI).** Normal CI is 2.4 to 4.0 L/min/m^2. The BSA is calculated using the patient's height and weight. Extreme values of BSA in morbidly obese patients demonstrate the need for using CI rather than CO. For example, patient A is 70 inches tall and weighs 320 pounds and has a BSA of 2.5. Patient B is 70 inches tall and weighs 170 pounds and has a BSA of 2.0. Both patients have a "normal" CO of 5 L/min. However, when a CO of 5 L/min is indexed to BSA, patient A has a CI of 2.0 L/min/m^2 and patient B has a CI of 2.5 L/min/m^2. Both patients have a CI below normal.

The volume of blood pumped with each heartbeat is called the **stroke volume (SV).** CO is the product of SV and heart rate (HR). Given a normal heart rate of approximately 72 beats per minute (bpm) (range, 60 to 100) and CO of approximately 5 L/min, it is possible to determine that the usual stroke volume for an adult is 5,000 mL/min divided by 72 bpm = 69 mL/beat or approximately 70 mL per beat.

Changes in either the HR or SV will alter CO. Fortunately, the body uses the interrelationship between these two factors to maintain a normal CO. For example, if SV falls, HR increases to compensate and maintain CO. Conversely, if HR drops, SV increases to compensate and maintain CO. Of course, there is a limit to the capacity of the body to use these compensatory efforts to maintain CO.

SECTION ONE REVIEW

1. The volume of blood pumped by the heart each minute is the
   A. stroke volume
   B. cardiac output
   C. cardiac index
   D. ejection fraction
2. A normal cardiac output for an adult at rest is approximately
   A. 1.0 to 2.5 L/min
   B. 2.5 to 4.0 L/min
   C. 4.0 to 8.0 L/min
   D. 7.0 to 9.0 L/min

(continued)

(continued)

3. Mr. Z has a CO of 5 L/min and a BSA of 2.5. What is his CI?
   A. 2.0 L/min/m^2
   B. 3.0 L/min/m^2
   C. 4.0 L/min/m^2
   D. 5.0 L/min/m^2
4. Which value is a normal adult stroke volume?
   A. 7 mL
   B. 17 mL
   C. 70 mL
   D. 700 mL
5. A patient has a stroke volume of 60 mL and a heart rate of 70 bpm. What is his cardiac output?
   A. 420 mL/min
   B. 1.1 L/min
   C. 4.2 L/min
   D. 150 mL/min

Answers: 1. B, 2. C, 3. A, 4. C, 5. C

SECTION TWO: Components of Stroke Volume

At the completion of this section, the learner will be able to define *preload, contractility,* and *afterload* and discuss how each of these components impact stroke volume.

There are four determinants of CO. Any condition or disease that affects one determinant causes a change in another determinant in an effort to maintain CO. The four determinants of CO are as follows:

- Heart rate (HR)
- Preload
- Contractility
- Afterload

Where is stroke volume? SV is determined by the interplay of preload, contractility, and afterload:

$$CO = SV \times HR$$

Preload Afterload Contractility

Heart Rate

If SV is held constant, any change in HR results in an immediate change in CO. For example, if the SV is 70 mL and the HR drops from 70 to 50 bpm, the CO drops from 4.9 L/min to 3.5 L/min. If HR increases from 70 bpm to 100 bpm and SV remains at 70 mL, CO increases from 4.9 L/min to 7.0 L/min.

The most effective mechanism to increase CO is to increase HR; however, this mechanism has limitations. A severe increase in HR causes SV to decrease. A heart beating this fast spends too little time in diastole and the ventricles do not have time to fill with blood. Recall that the ventricles fill during diastole. Therefore, the faster the HR, the shorter the time spent in diastole, the less time available for ventricular filling, and less ventricular filling results in decreased preload and decreased SV.

Preload

Preload is the amount of stretch in the myocardial fibers at the end of diastole. Because blood volume affects the stretch of myocardial fibers, preload represents the volume of blood in the ventricle at end diastole. The greater the volume of blood in the ventricle, the greater the amount of stretch that the fibers experience. Preload is greatly affected by the volume of blood delivered to the heart from the venous system. If a large volume of blood returns from the venous system to the ventricle, the myocardial fibers will be stretched so that they are far apart. This represents a high preload. If a small volume of blood returns from the venous system to the ventricle, there will be less stretch and, therefore, less preload. High preload corresponds to high volume; low preload corresponds to low volume. Preload is discussed in greater detail later in Section Three.

Contractility

Contractility is defined as the force of myocardial contraction. Contractility reflects the ability of the heart muscle to work independently of preload and afterload; the ability to function as a pump. If the heart contracts forcefully, it pumps out most of the blood in the ventricle. If the heart pumps poorly, it pumps out less blood. Many variables affect the force with which the heart muscle contracts; however, anything that enhances or diminishes the ability of myocardial fibers to contract vigorously affects contractility. Contractility is discussed in further detail in Section Five.

Even when working perfectly, the ventricle does not eject all the blood it contains. Usually, the ventricle ejects only 60 percent of the blood that it contains at the end of diastole. **Ejection fraction** is a measure of the percent of blood ejected with each stroke volume and is used as an index of myocardial function. The ejection fraction is the stroke volume divided by end diastolic volume. A normal ejection fraction is 60 percent.

Afterload

Afterload is the resistance against which the ventricle pumps blood. An optimal amount of resistance is necessary for the system to work properly. If afterload increases, stroke volume decreases because the ventricle is meeting increased resistance and cannot effectively pump out its volume. The major influence on afterload is the mechanical resistance to flow offered by the arterial system. If the arterial vessels are constricted, afterload to the left ventricle increases and stroke volume decreases. Other variables include the pulmonic and aortic valves, which may become stenotic and unable to fully open during systole. Afterload is discussed in greater detail in Section Four of this module.

SECTION TWO REVIEW

1. The degree of stretch of myocardial fibers at the end of diastole is known as
   A. preload
   B. contractility
   C. compliance
   D. distensibility
2. A HR of 150 bpm would have what effect on CO?
   A. increase
   B. decrease
   C. no effect
   D. none of the above
3. The vigor of myocardial fibers' activities is known as
   A. automaticity
   B. conduction
   C. contractility
   D. afterload
4. The resistance against which the ventricle pumps blood is known as
   A. preload
   B. blood pressure
   C. compliance
   D. afterload
5. An increase in afterload has what effect on stroke volume?
   A. increase
   B. decrease
   C. no effect
   D. none of the above

Answers: 1. A, 2. B, 3. C, 4. D, 5. B

SECTION THREE: Preload

At the completion of this section, the learner will be able to describe the relationship of SV and preload in terms of the Frank–Starling law.

Within limits, the heart pumps the amount of blood it receives with each beat. This is known as the Frank–Starling law of the heart. In other words, as preload increases, so does SV, and as preload decreases, SV falls (Fig. 12–1a). Unfortunately, this law only applies within a certain range.

Note that until a critical point is reached, as preload increases, so does SV. An optimal preload results in optimal SV. Once past this point, an increase in preload results in a decrease in SV (Fig. 12–1b). If the heart receives too much preload, it cannot effectively pump out that volume and SV decreases. SV decreases because too much volume causes excessive stretching of the myocardial fibers and the ventricles cannot effectively contract.

A key assessment in high-acuity patients is to determine how much preload provides an optimal SV. The nurse must be able to recognize assessment findings that indicate the patient has gone past that optimal point of preload and now has decreased SV. This will be discussed in greater detail in Section Seven.

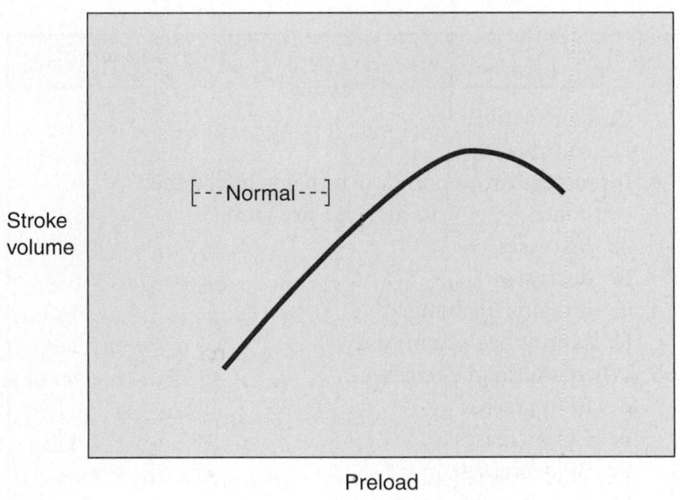

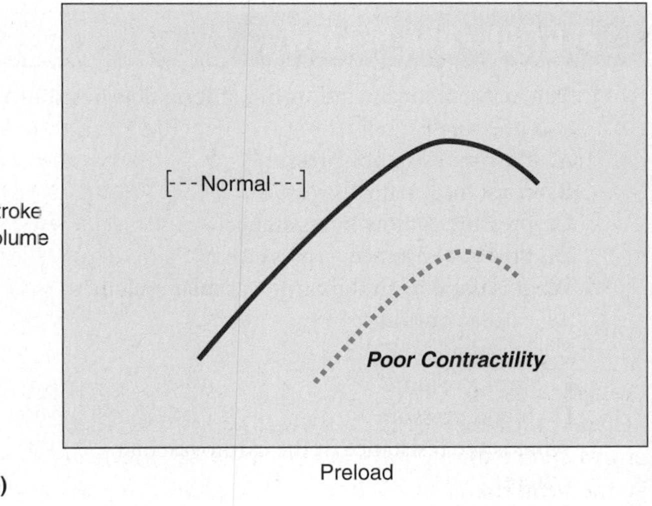

Figure 12–1 ■ Graphs demonstrating the Frank–Starling law of the heart.

SECTION THREE REVIEW

1. The Frank–Starling law states that within physiologic limits the heart
   A. pumps as fast as it receives more blood
   B. pumps as much blood as it receives
   C. pumps less blood as it receives more blood
   D. pumps an unchanging amount of blood regardless of how much it receives
2. Disease may decrease the contractility of the myocardium. This means that if the preload decreases, SV
   A. increases
   B. decreases
   C. stays the same
   D. cannot be determined from this information
3. An increase in preload results in a(n)
   A. increase in SV
   B. decrease in contractility
   C. increase in HR
   D. decrease in afterload

Answers: 1. B, 2. B, 3. A

SECTION FOUR: Afterload

At the completion of this section, the learner will be able to describe the relationship among pressure, flow, and resistance. This will help explain the relationship between cardiac output, vascular resistance, and blood pressure. These relationships are often manipulated in acutely ill patients.

Recall from Section Two that afterload is the resistance the heart meets when it pumps out its SV. Most of the resistance the heart meets is related to the "size" of the arterial blood vessels—whether they are vasoconstricted or vasodilated. If they are vasoconstricted, afterload to the ventricle increases and SV decreases. If the vessels are vasodilated, afterload to the ventricle decreases and SV increases.

Imagine a system with a pump, a rigid tube, and a valve some distance from the pump, as shown in Figure 12–2. If the valve is half closed, the pressure in the tube increases as the rate of the liquid pumped increases. If the pump runs very fast and the valve is partially closed, the pressure in the pipe is high. If, however, the pump output remains constant and the valve is opened completely, there is little pressure in the tube. This relationship among flow, resistance, and pressure is expressed in Ohm's law:

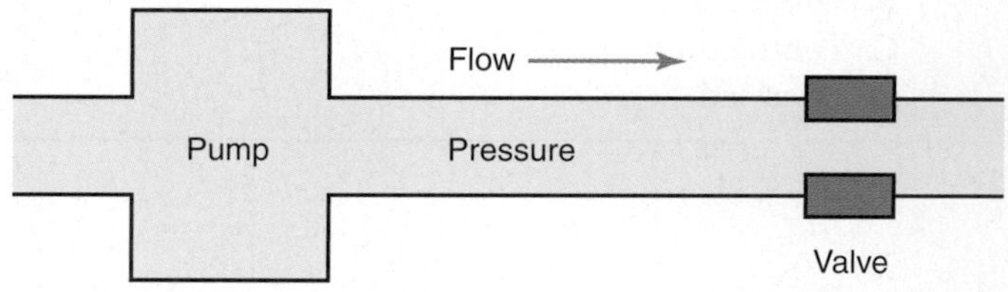

Figure 12–2 ■ Diagram demonstrating the hemodynamic concept of the relationship between flow, pressure, and resistance.

$$\text{Pressure} = \text{Flow} \times \text{Resistance}$$

Just as SV and HR compensate to maintain CO, flow and resistance compensate to maintain blood pressure (BP). Flow in the cardiovascular system is CO, resistance is afterload, and pressure is BP. Therefore, BP is the product of CO and afterload. When afterload increases (e.g., vasoconstriction), CO decreases and BP increases. This is what happens to patients with hypertension. When afterload decreases (e.g., vasodilation), CO increases and BP decreases. This is what happens to patients in septic shock. The relationship between BP, CO, and afterload have important clinical implications which are discussed in further detail in Modules 13 through 19.

SECTION FOUR REVIEW

1. The mathematical relationship among flow, resistance, and pressure is
   A. flow = resistance/pressure
   B. resistance = flow/pressure
   C. pressure × flow = resistance
   D. flow × resistance = pressure
2. What is the flow in the cardiovascular system?
   A. cardiac output
   B. heart rate
   C. stroke volume
   D. blood pressure
3. What is the resistance in the cardiovascular system?
   A. preload
   B. afterload
   C. contractility
   D. compliance
4. If pressure drops and flow remains unchanged, resistance ______ to increase pressure.
   A. increases
   B. decreases
   C. remains unchanged
   D. cannot be determined
5. When afterload decreases
   A. BP increases
   B. CO increases
   C. BP decreases
   D. both B and C are correct

Answers: 1. D, 2. A, 3. B, 4. A, 5. D

SECTION FIVE: Contractility

At the completion of this section, the learner will be able to discuss factors that influence myocardial contractility.

Contractility refers to the ability of the heart to function as a pump. The contractile state is determined by biochemical and biophysical properties that govern the actin–myosin crossbridge formations and largely depends on the influx of calcium ions (Porth, 2005). Increased calcium release allows for greater interaction between actin and myosin filaments, resulting in greater contraction. Cardiac muscle does not store calcium like skeletal muscle; cardiac muscle contraction depends on this influx of calcium. Therefore, it is important for the nurse to recognize that when a patient's serum calcium is low, contractility of the heart may be decreased. Many drugs are given to increase calcium influx to produce greater myocardial contractility.

Factors that influence contractility are known as **inotropes.** Factors that increase myocardial contractility have a positive inotropic effect. Factors that decrease contractility have a negative inotropic effect. Positive inotropes include sympathetic nervous system stimulation, increased calcium release, and the administration of inotropic drugs, such as digoxin and dobutamine. Contractility decreases with hypoxemia; therefore, hypoxemia is considered to be a negative inotrope.

In high-acuity settings, inotropic drugs are often used to augment cardiac output. Digoxin, dopamine, and dobutamine are the most common medications used to increase CO by improving myocardial contractility.

SECTION FIVE REVIEW

1. What electrolyte is important to cardiac contraction?
   A. calcium
   B. chloride
   C. sodium
   D. zinc
2. Sympathetic nervous system activation has what effect on myocardial contractility?
   A. increases myocardial contraction
   B. decreases myocardial contraction
   C. has no effect on contractility
   D. decreases heart rate, therefore, decreases cardiac output
3. Dobutamine is an example of a
   A. positive inotropic agent
   B. negative inotropic agent
   C. sympathomimetic
   D. B adrenergic blocking agent
4. Which of the following statements is true?
   A. Cardiac muscle stores calcium.
   B. Skeletal muscle does not store calcium.
   C. Cardiac muscle does not store calcium.
   D. Both A and B are true.
5. Which of the following is a negative inotrope?
   A. dopamine
   B. dobutamine
   C. digoxin
   D. hypoxemia

Answers: 1. A, 2. A, 3. A, 4. C, 5. D

SECTION SIX: Conditions That Affect Cardiac Output

At the end of this section, the learner will be able to state some of the conditions that affect heart rate, preload, contractility, and afterload.

Heart Rate

Heart rate is controlled by the heart's pacemaker sites, which are influenced by the interplay of the sympathetic and parasympathetic nervous systems. The sympathetic nervous system causes the fight-or-flight reaction, in which the body's resources are mobilized to counteract a real or perceived threat. The cardiovascular effects of sympathetic nervous system stimulation include increased HR, increased contractility, and vasoconstriction. The parasympathetic nervous system causes the opposite effects of decreased HR and decreased contractility.

Any stressors that activate the sympathetic nervous system cause an increase in HR. Such stressors may include events or conditions perceived as threats, for example, speaking in front of large groups or fleeing a burning house. In the hospital environment, stimuli that activate the sympathetic nervous system include pain, anxiety, and sensory overstimulation, in addition to the physiologic causes. On a physiologic level, anything that causes a decrease in SV is likely to cause an increase in HR in an effort to compensate and hold CO constant. In addition, there are numerous other causes of increased HR, including cardiac conduction system dysfunction, drug effects, and hormone imbalances.

Heart rate is decreased by increased activity of the parasympathetic nervous system. There are numerous causes of low HR, ranging from drug effects and poisoning to straining hard to have a bowel movement. Other sources of a low HR include impaired impulse generation or conduction in the heart. Heart rate may also be slowed by administration of drugs that either block sympathetic activity (beta blockers) or that inhibit calcium influx into myocardial fibers (calcium channel blockers). Conditions that affect HR are further discussed in Module 14, Assessment of Cardiac Rhythm: Basic Electrocardiographic/Rhythm Interpretation.

Preload

Recall that preload is the amount of stretch of myocardial fibers at the end of diastole, and preload can be thought of as being the amount of blood in the ventricle at end diastole. Preload is altered by a change in the amount of blood delivered to the heart from the venous system.

A decrease in blood volume in the ventricle results in a decrease in preload. Loss of blood volume from hemorrhage, dehydration, diuretic use, or movement of fluid out of the vascular space into the extravascular compartment results in a decrease in preload. Diminished preload also can be caused by failure of an atrioventricular (AV) valve (either tricuspid or mitral) to allow free flow of blood into the ventricle. Vasodilation of the venous system causes the venous vessels to hold more blood, which results in less blood entering the ventricle and a decrease in preload. In addition, very fast HR shortens diastolic filling time. Therefore, there is insufficient time for the ventricle to fill adequately and the result is a decrease in preload.

An increase in blood volume results in an increase in preload. Conditions that cause an increase in blood volume include renal failure, fluid overload from IV therapy, increased aldosterone secretion (with retention of sodium and water), and excess sodium in the diet. Increased preload also occurs when the ventricle is unable to pump out its volume of blood. When this happens, there is still excess blood volume in the ventricle after ejection. When the ventricle fills during diastole, it already has a residual volume and now also has the blood volume recently pumped from the atria. At some point, the ventricle can no longer pump out all this volume and blood volume begins to "back up." This is precisely what happens in congestive heart failure: The heart pumps less blood than is delivered to it, and there is congestion in the venous system that drains into the affected ventricle. If the left ventricle fails, congestion occurs in the pulmonary vascular bed. If the right ventricle fails, the congestion occurs in the systemic venous system. These concepts are further discussed in Module 15, Alterations in Cardiac Output.

Contractility

Contractility is much like HR in that it is strongly influenced by the autonomic nervous system. Sympathetic stimulation of the heart results in increased contractility, and, conversely, parasympathetic stimulation causes decreased contractility. Other major determinants of contractility include oxygenation (hypoxia or ischemia decrease contractility), myocardial disease (myocarditis, cardiomyopathy), and drug effects (many narcotics and anesthetic agents are direct myocardial depressants). Drugs that increase myocardial contractility include digitalis, epinephrine, and dobutamine.

Afterload

The major determinant of afterload is the resistance to flow caused by the arterial system. Most of the arterial resistance is caused by constriction of arterioles. Anything that changes arteriolar vascular tone changes afterload. For example, stimulation of the sympathetic nervous system causes constriction of the arterioles and an increase in afterload. Drugs that dilate or constrict the arterioles cause a prompt change in afterload. The arterioles are dilated during septic shock, spinal cord injury, or anaphylactic shock. These concepts are further discussed in Module 18, Alterations in Oxygen Delivery and Oxygen Consumption: Shock States. Further resistance to flow can be caused by failure of the pulmonic or aortic valve to allow free flow of blood from the ventricle to the artery. In this case, the stenosed valve causes an increase in afterload.

SECTION SIX REVIEW

1. Decreased HR can be caused by
   A. decreased SV
   B. anxiety
   C. parasympathetic stimulation
   D. pain
2. Increased preload may occur with
   A. mitral stenosis
   B. vasodilation of venous vessels
   C. very fast HRs
   D. renal failure
3. Increased contractility can be caused by
   A. ischemia
   B. hypoxia
   C. cardiomyopathy
   D. sympathetic stimulation
4. Increased afterload can be caused by
   A. sympathetic stimulation
   B. septic shock
   C. anaphylaxis
   D. spinal cord injury
5. Decreased preload can be caused by
   A. too much IV fluid
   B. hemorrhage
   C. diuretics
   D. both B and C

Answers: 1. C, 2. D, 3. D, 4. A, 5. D

SECTION SEVEN: Assessment of Cardiac Output

At the completion of this section, the learner will be able to identify common clinical assessments that evaluate heart rate, preload, contractility, and afterload.

Hemodynamic monitoring provides a means for invasive monitoring of CO which is discussed in Module 13, Assessment of Hemodynamic Status: Hemodynamic Monitoring. The first part of this section concentrates on the focused assessment of CO. The second part of this section focuses on diagnostic procedures that may be used to evaluate CO in acutely ill patients, and the nursing responsibilities associated with patients undergoing these diagnostic tests.

Focused Nursing Assessment

The key to accurately determining cardiac output lies in the assessment skills of the nurse. Assessment begins on admission. The nurse must obtain subjective data on admission, conduct a complete physical assessment, interpret lab results, use bedside monitoring equipment effectively, and apply knowledge gained via various diagnostic procedures. The nursing process, particularly in high-acuity care, depends on a thorough assessment.

Nursing History

On admission, airway, breathing, and circulation are assessed prior to obtaining a nursing history to assure that the patient is sufficiently stable to be interviewed. This initial assessment is generally a rapid, limited one that may take no more than a minute. Appropriate priority interventions are then performed based on the assessed priority needs. Once the patient's safety and comfort has been attended to, the nurse obtains a nursing history including the patient's present illness and medical history. It is important to assess perfusion regardless of whether the patient has a previous history of perfusion abnormalities.

Present Illness and Medical History

At the time of admission, the nurse may be interviewing the patient, a family member, or other person or persons. Eliciting a recent history of the present illness (i.e., the events leading up to this admission) provides the clinician with important data regarding the problem and possible etiologies, and the patient's ability to compensate for a cardiovascular stressor. Recent history information also helps identify areas where the patient may need external support in order to increase myocardial oxygen supply and decrease myocardial demand in order to regain or maintain a state of compensation.

A detailed patient history at the time of admission helps determine the plan of care. By using a variety of interviewing techniques and therapeutic communications, the nurse obtains demographic data, family history, diet, functional status, and prior medical history. Demographic data includes the patient's age, sex, race, and weight. Cardiovascular risk factors such as smoking history, exercise pattern, stress level, and obesity are assessed. Obesity (defined as body mass index greater than 30 g/m^2 in adults) is an independent risk factor for cardiovascular disease (Poirier et al., 2006). Obesity affects the heart through its influence on risk factors such as hypertension, glucose control, inflammatory mediators, dyslipidemia, obstructive sleep apnea and a prothrombotic state. Both obesity and being overweight (body mass index 25-29.9 g/m^2) predisposes one to, or are associated with, coronary artery disease, heart failure, and sudden death (Braun, 2006). In addition, family history of cardiovascular disease and diet history are important data to elicit from the patient during the nursing history.

Emerging Evidence

- American Indians with uncontrolled hypertension have 2.77 times greater risk of developing cardiovascular disease when compared with normotensive individuals *(Wang, Lee, Fabsitz et al., 2006).*
- In patients with coronary artery disease, regular physical activity has been shown to improve exercise capacity and quality of life while reducing symptoms and the risk of new coronary events *(Scrutinio, Bellotto, Lagioia et al., 2005).*
- The 2006 Surgeon General's Report concludes that second hand smoke has immediate adverse effects on the cardiovascular system and causes coronary heart disease *(U.S. Department of Health and Human Services, 2006).*
- Despite the increased awareness of smoking, more than 20 percent of adults in the United States continue to smoke *(CDC, 2005).*

Knowledge about functional status prior to onset of illness allows for setting realistic goals of therapy and patient/family education. The patient's prior medical history provides information about comorbidities, medication and herbal use, and other interventions that have been used to maintain health. Certain medications impact physical assessment findings including changes in heart rate, blood pressure, and urine output.

Complaints of chest pain must be assessed as pain of cardiac origin or pain of pulmonary origin. The mnemonic PQRST is helpful in organizing assessment data related to pain. Eliciting information about precipitating factors (P), quality (Q), radiation and region (R), associated symptoms (S), and timing and treatment strategies (T) help the nurse determine the origin of the pain. Pain may not always be present in all patients with perfusion disorders. Diabetic patients and the elderly may not feel pain. Women may have "atypical" pain such as abdominal pain and fatigue. Chest pain is described in greater detail in Module 16, Alterations in Myocardial Tissue Perfusion.

A patient with a perfusion disorder may complain of **palpitations,** often described as a "skipping" or "thumping" of the heart. This symptom is related to the occurrence of premature cardiac beats. Palpation of the pulse will reveal premature beats. There will be irregular pulse amplitude because of the decreased blood volume associated with premature beats and the larger-than-normal volume of the beat immediately after the premature beat related to prolonged diastolic filling. The best way of detecting premature beats is by obtaining an electrocardiogram (ECG) and monitoring the patient's cardiac rhythm. These assessments are described in greater detail in Module 14, Assessment of Cardiac Rhythm: Basic Electrocardiographic Rhythm Interpretation.

A patient with a perfusion disorder may experience a change in level of consciousness related to a decreased CO or blockage of cerebral circulation. A diminished level of consciousness, confusion, or agitation may be signs of decreased perfusion to cerebral tissue. The patient may experience **syncope** (a temporary loss of consciousness, followed by complete, spontaneous recovery).

Nursing Physical Assessment

Techniques of physical assessment of cardiac output include inspection, palpation, and auscultation. Because of the rapid changes that can occur in the acute care setting, cardiac output is assessed frequently. By developing a systematic method of physical assessment, the nurse rapidly ascertains changes in hemodynamic status. Data obtained from technological means must be corroborated with physical assessments. Overreliance on the monitoring equipment alarms may lead to complacency, and subtle physical changes may be missed.

Inspection of the precordium may demonstrate rhythmic movement. Abnormal movement may be visualized in the aortic, pulmonic, or tricuspid areas. Normal movement is found in the area of the mitral valve. This is the apical impulse. It is usually seen in the area of the left 5th intercostal space along the midclavicular line.

Inspection and palpation of the periphery can also indicate variations in the patient's cardiac output. Changes in skin color are a late sign of hemodynamic compromise, as is clubbing of the fingers. A cooling of the skin is brought about by the vasoconstriction of the arterioles as blood is shunted to the internal organs. A decrease in cardiac output may be the cause. Cool distal extremities may be a useful marker of decreased CO. Delayed capillary refill is often associated with decreased CO. However, capillary refill as an indicator of the adequacy of CO is controversial. It may be useful as a marker of hypovolemia and poor myocardial function in children, but in elderly patients it may not be as useful.

The kidney is sensitive to changes in intravascular volume; therefore, the amount of urine output is frequently used to assess the adequacy of CO. Theoretically, a decrease in CO results in a decrease in urine output. However, there are conditions in which urine output does not reflect the adequacy of CO. These conditions may affect patients in compensatory shock states (see Module 18, Alterations in Oxygen Delivery and Consumption: Shock States) and the elderly. The elderly may have chronic disease states and use medications that affect urine output.

The presence of peripheral edema may indicate too much preload to the right side of the heart. Edema is a palpable swelling produced by an accumulation of interstitial fluid volume. Pathophysiologic mechanisms that cause edema are listed below. Edema can be generalized or localized. Localized edema in the calf may indicate an obstruction of venous blood flow from a clot in a leg vein. Generalized edema is a physical assessment finding associated with congestive heart failure. See Module 25, Determinants and Assessment of Fluid and Electrolyte Balance, for a more detailed discussion of edema.

Pathophysiologic mechanisms that cause edema include:

- Increase in capillary hydrostatic pressure
- Decrease in capillary colloid pressure
- Increase in capillary permeability that creates an increase in interstitial colloid pressure
- Obstruction of lymphatic flow

The effects of edema are determined by its location: brain, larynx, lungs, hands, feet, face, or abdomen. Life-threatening situations occur with edema of the brain, larynx, or lungs. Edema of the extremities can interfere with mobility and can impair perfusion by compression on arterial vessels. Pitting edema occurs with an increase in capillary hydrostatic pressure, which pushes fluid from the vascular to the interstitial spaces. Nonpitting edema occurs with an increase in interstitial colloid pressure.

There are several methods to assess for edema including visual assessment by inspection, palpation, measurement of the affected part, and daily weight. Finger pressure can be used to assess the degree of pitting edema. Edema is measured on a 1-to-4 scale, with 4 being the most severe. Daily weights are helpful in monitoring trends in water gain or losses. One liter of water weighs 1 kilogram or 2.2 pounds. If a patient's weight increases in 24 hours by 1 kilogram, the interpretation is that the patient has gained 1 liter of fluid. If diuretics are given and the patient is weighed 24 hours later and has lost 1 kilogram, then the patient has diuresed 1 kilogram of water. Weights are particularly important for patients receiving renal dialysis because they provide an index of water balance before and after dialysis.

The presence of jugular venous distention may indicate too much preload to the right side of the heart. Jugular venous distention (JVD) may indicate a fluid distribution problem. The venous system is a low-pressure system, and it is sensitive to right atrial pressure. Retention of blood in the right side of the heart (as in the case of heart failure or cor pulmonale) will increase right atrial pressure and subsequently produce jugular venous distention as a result of backflow through the vena cava. In assessing for venous distention, elevate the head of the bed to approximately 45 degrees. The patient's head is turned slightly away from the examiner. A penlight is used to shine a light tangentially across the neck (Fig. 12–3).

Palpation gives the nurse a tactile indication of cardiac output. Rolling the patient onto the left side moves the heart closer to the surface of the body. Precordial palpation may produce a vibration, also known as a thrill. This may correspond to a murmur, valvular stenosis, or increased afterload. The point of maximal impulse (PMI) corresponds to the location of the apical impulse. Heaves and lifts also indicate ventricular hypertrophy on either side. On the periphery, palpation of pulses is indicative of CO. Pulses should be of regular rate, strength, and rhythm. A hyperkinetic (bounding) pulse may indicate increased cardiac output because of thyrotoxicosis, fever, pain, or anxiety. A hypokinetic pulse may be the result of decreased cardiac output, with causes such as dysrhythmias, damaged myocardium, or cardiomyopathy. Severely depressed cardiac function may cause **pulsus alterans,** which is evidenced by alternating weak and strong pulses in a regular rhythm.

Auscultation is another technique to assess cardiac output. Knowledge of the auditory indicators of valvular dysfunction is essential. Recall, the function of heart valves is to provide unidirectional flow of blood through the heart. With valve dysfunction there is turbulent or decreased blood flow through the heart, resulting in a decrease in CO. Heart valve disorders are discussed in greater detail in Module 15, Alterations in Cardiac Output.

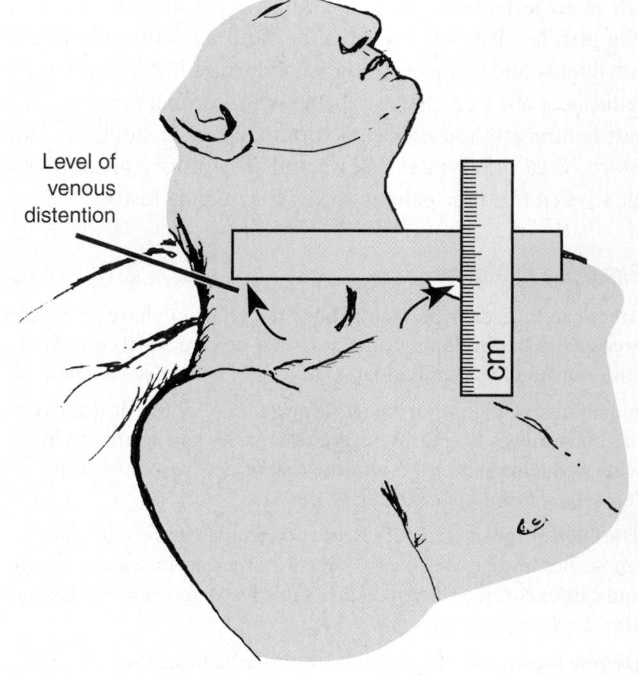

Figure 12–3 ■ Measurement of jugular venous distention.

TABLE 12–1 Grading System Used to Classify Murmurs

I/VI	Very faint
II/VI	Faint
III/VI	Loud; moderate in intensity
IV/VI	Loud; palpable thrill
V/VI	Loud enough to be heard with head of stethoscope partially off chest wall; palpable thrill
VI/VI	Loud enough to be heard with head of stethoscope completely off chest wall; palpable thrill

Auscultation of the precordium must be systematic and performed using both the bell and the diaphragm of the stethoscope. The pattern of auscultation begins at the base of the heart using the diaphragm in the area of the aortic valve, and proceeds to the pulmonic, tricuspid, and mitral valves in order. Once completed, the bell is used in reverse sequence. Various extra heart sounds may be heard, such as high- and low-frequency murmurs, or extrasystolic sounds, such as clicks and rubs. Heart murmurs are evidence of turbulent blood flow, and can be due to stenotic or incompetent valves. They can be heard during systole or diastole. Table 12–1 outlines the grading system used to classify murmurs.

Diastolic filling sounds may help determine why cardiac output is reduced. The S3 sound, heard early in diastole, is a ventricular filling sound caused by decreased ventricular compliance and is a sign of early heart failure. It is also known as **ventricular gallop.** S4 is also a ventricular filling sound but occurs late in diastole. It is heard during atrial contraction, and it, therefore, is known as **atrial gallop.** It is a result of myocardial infarction, ventricular hypertrophy, and increased afterload. A **summation gallop,** when both S3 and S4 sounds are heard, is often indicative of severe heart failure.

Shortness of breath results from fluid movement out of the pulmonary capillaries and into the lung interstitial space, thereby decreasing oxygen diffusion from the alveoli into the pulmonary capillaries. The presence of wet-sounding crackles (rales) on auscultation of the lungs indicates pulmonary edema. Severe pulmonary edema is associated with frothy, pink sputum production.

Ausculatory techniques can also be used on the peripheral vasculature system. Bruits along the carotid arteries may indicate areas of occlusion. These partial blockages represent potential compromise to the cerebral vasculature and account for some signs and symptoms also attributable to decreased cardiac output. Renal artery bruits may indicate renal artery stenosis, which leads to systemic hypertension. The resulting increase in afterload may compromise cardiac output. A dialysis graft should be auscultated. The bruit heard indicates patency of the graft and corresponds to the thrill described earlier.

Diagnostic Laboratory Tests

There are numerous diagnostic lab parameters used to assess CO, which is adversely affected by myocardial damage. When the myocardium is damaged as a result of ischemia, myocardial cells die and release their intracellular contents, including enzymes, into the general circulation. Since the enzymes are not normally present in the blood, elevated serum levels are indicative of myocardial cell death. These enzymes will be briefly described in this module and are described in greater detail in Module 16, Alterations in Myocardial Tissue Perfusion.

Creatine kinase-myocardial band (CK-MB) is a myocardial enzyme that is released 4 to 12 hours after the onset of myocardial necrosis and is very specific for myocardial damage. Because of these varying times of release, CK-MB and other cardiac enzymes are often obtained on a serial basis, meaning they are assessed every couple of hours over the course of 24 hours after the patient complains of chest pain. Serial CK-MB measurement resulting in an elevation or upward trend is a cardiac marker for acute myocardial infarction or "heart attack." The major limitation of CK-MB is that levels do not start to rise until four hours after the onset of myocardial damage. This can delay diagnosis and treatment of myocardial infarction.

Troponin is a protein found in cardiac muscle. It is part of a protein complex for the binding of myosin and actin, the myofilaments that regulate contraction. The troponin complex varies among three distinct proteins, designated as troponin-T, troponin-C and troponin-I. Troponin can appear in the blood as early as three to four hours after myocardial damage. Troponin has a higher sensitivity and specificity for identifying even minor myocyte necrosis than CK-MB. The higher the troponin level and/or the longer the troponin levels remain elevated, the greater the size of myocardial damage and the severity of injury (Howie & White, 2008). Caution must be used when interpreting abnormal troponin levels because they are released in a number of other situations in which myocardial injury has not occurred, such as pulmonary embolism, sepsis, myocarditis and acute stroke (Fromm, 2007).

C-reactive protein (CRP) is a peptide released by the liver in response to systemic inflammation, infection, and tissue damage. Atherosclerosis is considered to be a chronic inflammatory process and studies have shown CRP levels increase with the atherosclerotic disease process. Several large studies have shown CRP to be predictive of coronary disease in postmenopausal women (Ridker et al., 2000), the elderly (Kop et al., 2002), and in individuals with average levels of cholesterol (Ridker et al., 2001). The American Heart Association suggests that in patients with stable coronary disease, CRP measurement may be useful as a marker of prognosis for myocardial injury and death (Pearson et al., 2003). Normal CRP levels are 0.02 – 8 mg/L (Dakin, 2008).

B-type natriuretic peptide (BNP) is a hormone released from the ventricles. This peptide, which is released in response to increased preload, causes urinary excretion of sodium and diuresis, and counteracts the effects of the renin–angiotensin–aldosterone system. This results in a reduction of preload. When BNP is present in the blood, it is indicative of heart failure (Module 15, Alterations in Cardiac Output). Several factors can affect plasma BNP levels. Females have higher BNP levels than men, obese patients have lower BNP levels, and patients with renal disease have higher BNP levels (Kreiger, 2007). Therefore, results in these patients should be interpreted cautiously.

Hyperlipidemia, high levels of lipids in the blood, is associated with high risk for coronary heart disease. High-risk lipids include elevated total cholesterol, increased low-density lipoprotein (LDL) cholesterol, decreased high-density lipoprotein (HDL), and elevated triglycerides. HDLs are the "good" cholesterol (remember H stands for "high"). LDLs are the "bad" cholesterols (remember L stands for "low"). Higher levels of HDLs than LDLs are desirable. The ratio should be at least 1:5 with 1:3 being ideal. These lab values are discussed in greater detail in Module 16, Alterations in Myocardial Tissue Perfusion.

There are several electrolytes that affect cardiac output and are important to monitor. These include potassium, calcium, magnesium, and sodium. Imbalances of potassium, calcium, and magnesium often produce changes in heart rate and rhythm and are often detected by an ECG (see Module 14, Assessment of Cardiac Rhythm: Basic Electrocardiographic Rhythm Interpretation).

Assessment of Specific Components of Cardiac Output

Preload, like contractility and afterload, are difficult to assess at the bedside because the cardiovascular structures where these exist are embedded deeply in the chest and are unavailable for examination. Direct measures of these determinants of CO require invasive monitoring devices (such as a pulmonary artery catheter) and are discussed in Module 13, Assessment of Hemodynamic Status: Hemodynamic Monitoring. Without invasive monitoring devices, the nurse must use indirect measures that permit an estimation of preload, contractility, or afterload.

Heart Rate

Evaluating HR is relatively easy. A simple count of the radial pulse is useful for determining the number of heartbeats that are strong enough to reach the periphery. A count of the apical HR is useful to determine the total HR. Usually, these two rates are equal, but there may be a deficit between the apical rate and the radial rate caused by irregular heart rhythms that result in SV varying from beat to beat, which results in some beats being too weak to be felt at the radial artery (this is called the **apical–radial pulse deficit**). For example, a radial pulse would give a better indication of the adequacy of peripheral perfusion in a person complaining of dizziness than an apical pulse. It is recommended that the clinician use a 60-second counting interval when assessing a patient for the first time, if the patient is unstable, if the cardiac rhythm is irregular, or treatment decisions are based on HR.

Preload

Preload for the right ventricle is assessed by evaluating the systemic venous system. The assessment findings of increased and decreased right ventricular preload are summarized in Table 12–2. Increased preload to right heart typically manifests as signs of too much fluid in the peripheral tissues and organs as fluid backs up from the right side of the heart. Preload for the left heart is assessed by evaluating the pulmonary venous system. Assessment findings are summarized in Table 12–3. Increased preload to the left heart typically manifests as signs of too much fluid in the pulmonary circulation as fluid backs up from the left side of the heart.

TABLE 12–2 Assessment of Right Heart Preload

INCREASED RIGHT HEART PRELOAD	DECREASED RIGHT HEART PRELOAD
Jugular venous distention (JVD)	Poor skin turgor (immediate sign)
Ascites	Dry mucous membranes
Hepatic engorgement	Orthostatic hypotension
Peripheral edema	Flat jugular veins

Unfortunately, there are no noninvasive assessments currently available that specifically indicate diminished left ventricular preload. Usually, if the left heart has insufficient preload, the right heart has the same situation, and signs of diminished right ventricular preload are present. In some situations S1 and S2 may be muffled.

Contractility

Assessing the force of myocardial contraction is done by assessing the quality of the heartbeat when isolated from HR. The character of the pulse is noted at the radial artery. Increased contractility will demonstrate a bounding, vigorous pulse, whereas diminished contractility will demonstrate a weak, thready pulse. A splitting of S2 indicates that one ventricle is emptying earlier or later than the other, usually because of a structural (e.g., valve defect), mechanical (e.g., heart failure), or electrical (e.g., alternate pacemaker) problem. Contractility may be diminished. It is important to note that contractility is difficult to measure indirectly by physical signs because so many other factors may alter the character of the pulse. Decreased contractility usually is determined by exclusion of other causes of poor cardiac output.

The **pulse pressure** is the difference between diastolic and systolic blood pressures. It reflects how much the heart is able to raise the pressure in the arterial system with each beat. Pulse pressure increases when SV increases or in arteriole vasoconstriction. Pulse pressure drops with decreased SV or vasodilation (e.g., some shock states). The normal pulse pressure is approximately 30 to 40 mm Hg. Within the restrictions noted, the pulse pressure can be a useful, objective, and noninvasive indicator of myocardial contractility.

Afterload

Recall that indirect assessment of right ventricle afterload is difficult because of the location of the pulmonary arterial system deep in the chest. However, it is possible to assess the systemic arterial

TABLE 12–3 Assessment of Increased Left Heart Preload

INCREASED LEFT HEART PRELOAD
Dyspnea
Cough
Third heart sound (S3)
Fourth heart sound (S4)

system for signs of increased or decreased afterload. Even though signs of altered afterload may be present in some patients, they are not present in all patients with altered afterload. It is necessary to remember once again that all of these determinants of CO are interrelated, and it can be difficult to isolate individual factors at the bedside without invasive diagnostic tests.

Signs of increased systemic afterload include cool, clammy extremities. These signs may indicate that peripheral arterioles are constricted. Nonhealing wounds and thick brittle nails are indicators of chronic poor perfusion of the extremities. Signs of decreased systemic afterload include warm, flushed extremities, which may indicate peripheral vasodilation.

SECTION SEVEN REVIEW

1. Pitting edema is associated with
   - A. an increase in capillary hydrostatic pressure
   - B. an increase in interstitial colloid pressure
   - C. obstruction of lymph flow
   - D. B and C are correct
2. Mr. Z gains 2 kg over the past 24 hours. Estimate the amount of fluid he has retained.
   - A. one-half liter
   - B. 1 liter
   - C. 2 liters
   - D. unable to determine with data provided
3. JVD may be a sign of
   - A. elevated left ventricular preload
   - B. decreased left ventricular preload
   - C. hypertension
   - D. elevated right ventricular preload
4. Which of the following cardiac enzymes appear in the blood within three hours of myocardial cell death?
   - A. ANP
   - B. BNP
   - C. CK-MB
   - D. troponin
5. Signs of decreased contractility include
   - A. bounding pulse
   - B. diminished pulse pressure
   - C. ascites
   - D. poor skin turgor
6. Signs of increased afterload for the left ventricle include
   - A. cool, clammy extremities
   - B. thin, flexible toenails
   - C. liver engorgement
   - D. peripheral edema

Answers: 1. A, 2. C, 3. D, 4. D, 5. B, 6. A

SECTION EIGHT: Cardiovascular Diagnostic Procedures

At the end of this section, the learner will be able to describe various cardiovascular diagnostic procedures used to evaluate the components of cardiac output and discuss nursing responsibilities in caring for a patient receiving these diagnostic procedures.

Imaging Techniques

A chest X-ray is used to view the size and position of the heart. Pulmonary edema caused by decompensated heart failure may be visualized. An enlarged cardiac silhouette may be evidence of cardiac tamponade or dilated cardiomyopathy. Chest X-rays may be taken daily for patients with acute cardiovascular problems. Patients who require continuous ECG monitoring but are stable do not typically require a daily chest X-ray unless there is a change in status. It is important for the nurse to help the patient with proper positioning when the X-ray is obtained to ensure a high-quality film.

Magnetic resonance imaging (MRI) technology has improved to where coronary mapping, blood flow, and cardiac structures can be visualized. The patient cannot wear any metal, and patients with cardiac pacemakers are prohibited from having the procedure performed.

Radionuclide testing can be used to evaluate myocardial perfusion and left ventricular function. A small amount of a radioisotope is injected intravenously and the heart is scanned with a radiation detector. Ischemic or infarcted cells in the myocardium do not absorb the radioisotope.

Exercise Electrocardiogram

Exercise ECG, commonly known as a "stress test," evaluates heart muscle and its blood supply during physical stress (exercise). This can identify myocardial ischemia that may not be present at rest. If for some reason the patient cannot tolerate exercise, a simulated stress is given to the heart muscle by the administration of dobutamine, a positive inotropic drug.

Prior to the procedure, the patient may be anxious and may fear having a heart attack during the test. The patient should be assured of close monitoring during the procedure.

The stress test consists of the patient exercising on either a stationary bicycle or a treadmill. The patient's blood pressure and ECG are closely monitored as the exercise workload is increased. The patient is reminded to let the health care team know if chest pain, palpitations, or dyspnea occur. The test is discontinued when a predetermined heart rate is reached and maintained, signs of insufficient cardiac output appear, or ECG changes occur. The nurse conducting the exam must be familiar with cardiac dysrhythmias and emergency procedures. Emergency medications and a defibrillator should be present. Once the patient has returned to baseline hemodynamic status, the patient either returns to the hospital room or is allowed to go home. Some outpatients are admitted to the hospital for further diagnostic testing if they have unfavorable results from the exercise ECG. ECG and telemetry monitoring are discussed in detail in Module 14, Assessment of Cardiac Rhythm: Basic Electrocardiographic Rhythm Interpretation.

Echocardiogram

Another common cardiovascular diagnostic test is the echocardiogram. There are two forms of this test: transthoracic echocardiogram and transesophageal echocardiogram (TEE). Echocardiograms are particularly useful for visualizing blood, cardiac valves, the myocardium, and the pericardium. Ultrasound technology can be used to assess and diagnose cardiomyopathies, valvular function, cardiac tumors, and left ventricular function. An estimate of ejection fraction is also obtained.

Transthoracic echocardiograms are noninvasive tests that can be performed at the bedside or in the outpatient setting by a technologist. The patient is usually placed in a semifowler, left lateral, or supine position. The position is determined by the patient's overall condition, the patient's ability to tolerate the position, and the position that will give the best view of the structures to be visualized. Lubricant is placed on the skin and a transducer is placed on the skin. The transducer emits ultrasound waves and receives a signal back from the reflected waves. Nursing responsibilities may include dimming of the lights in the room and ensuring patient privacy and warmth.

The TEE is much more invasive. An ultrasound probe is inserted orally into the patient's esophagus and advanced until it is close to the heart. The TEE provides a more definitive representation of the heart. TEE produces images of intracardiac structures and the entire thoracic aorta. It produces high-quality images of both atrial chambers and is the procedure of choice to detect clots in the left atrium, atrial septal defects, infections on valve leaflets, and valve dysfunction.

Conscious sedation is used with the TEE, so nursing care is much more involved. Prior to the procedure, the nurse reviews the patient's chart, obtains a detailed history, and inserts a peripheral intravenous catheter. Suction equipment should be available in case the patient vomits. During the procedure, the nurse administers sedation, monitors vital signs and pulse oximetry saturations every three to five minutes, adjusts fluid and oxygen, and documents patient condition. During and immediately after the procedure, the nurse monitors for complications, which include respiratory depression and aspiration. Movement of the probe in the esophagus may stimulate the vagus nerve resulting in bradycardia or hypotension. Vital signs are monitored as the patient awakens from the procedure. The patient recovers in one to two hours. If the transesophageal echocardiogram was performed in an outpatient setting, the patient must be released to a responsible adult, in case there are residual effects of the sedation.

Cardiac Catheterization

Cardiac catheterization is performed to determine the presence and extent of coronary artery disease, evaluate left ventricular function, and to evaluate valvular or myocardial disorders (Harper, 2007). The catheterization can be performed on either the left or right side of the heart. Catheterization of the left side of the heart is primarily performed to determine the patency of the coronary vessels, but it can also be used to observe blood flow through the chambers and valves of the heart or to deliver a thrombolytic agent directly into the coronary vessels. Chamber pressures may also be measured.

The nurse in the prep area is responsible for initial assessment and history, vital signs, initiating intravenous access, and placing electrocardiogram leads. A thorough review of the patient's medications and allergies is required. The dye used during this fluoroscopic procedure is iodine based, so inquiries as to a patient's allergies to iodine or seafood are imperative. Because this is an invasive procedure, informed consent must be obtained.

An interventional cardiologist, who is assisted by a nurse and a cardiovascular technician, performs the procedure. The nurse prepares the insertion site, monitors vital signs, and gives medications for conscious sedation. Patients may experience slight discomfort during the procedure given that the purpose of the sedation is to ensure that patients are awake enough to report the onset of chest pain caused by the coronary artery reocclusion (Beddoes, Botti, Duke, 2007).

The procedure is conducted via the arterial system. The most common insertion route is the femoral artery. After local anesthesia is given, a femoral arterial sheath is inserted. Anticoagulation is required to prevent acute thrombotic closure of coronary vessels which can occur during insertion of the interventional devices (Sabo, Chlan, & Savik, 2007).

If a lesion is discovered, then an intervention is performed. This intervention is called an *angioplasty* or percutaneous transluminal angioplasty (PCTA). For this intervention, a balloon is inserted and inflated, then a stent (wire basket) is placed to hold the vessel lumen open (Fig. 12–4). If this type of intervention is performed, the patient stays overnight for

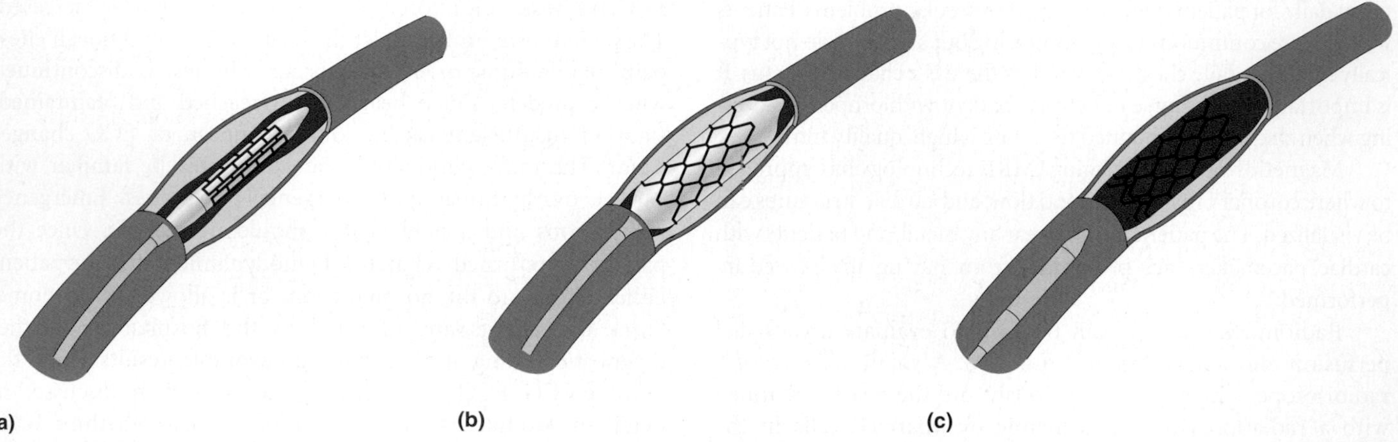

Figure 12–4 ▪ Placement of balloon expandable intracoronary stent. (a) and (b) The balloon catheter with the stent is threaded into the affected coronary artery. The stent is positioned across the blockage and expanded. (c) The balloon is deflated and removed, leaving the stent in place.

observation of potential complications, such as bleeding, dysrhythmias, or signs of vessel reocclusion.

After the cardiac catheterization procedure the patient remains in the cardiovascular lab for frequent nursing assessments until the patient is discharged to home or to the telemetry unit. The patient is monitored postprocedure for complications. Vascular complications include peripheral artery thrombosis or embolus, dye allergy, acute myocardial infarction, acute renal failure, ischemic stroke and death (Harper, 2007). The nurse monitoring the patient postprocedure assesses the access site for bleeding or hematoma formation. Pedal pulses are assessed bilaterally. One important assessment is to check the patient's flanks for signs of retroperitoneal bleeding. This complication is difficult to diagnose and can be life threatening. The patient is required to remain supine for the first hour postprocedure. The patient must be reminded to keep the procedural leg straight to reduce stress on the procedure site. For example, the patient should be instructed to compress the insertion with her or his hand when coughing.

Bedrest is maintained for four to six hours after the procedure to promote healing of the puncture site. The femoral sheath is removed when the whole blood thrombin is less than 120 seconds, generally after four to six hours after the last dose of heparin (Sabo et al., 2007). The nurse compresses the femoral artery after removal of the sheath. Methods for compression include manual pressure, C-clamp, or FemoStop (Radi Medical Systems, Uppsala, Sweden). Compression of the femoral artery can lead to the development of vascular complications including ecchymosis, hematoma, and oozing. Patients who are older in age and smaller in size may be at an increased risk of developing these complications (Sabo et al., 2007).

Electrophysiology Study

The electrophysiology study (EPS) is another invasive procedure that evaluates the cardiac conduction system and helps classify cardiac arrhythmias. The findings from this study help to determine if the patient would benefit from further interventions such as a pacemaker, implantable cardiodefibrillator, radiofrequency ablation or medication therapy (Crean, 2007) (these will be discussed further in Module 14, Assessment of Cardiac Rhythm: Basic Electrocardiographic Rhythm Interpretation).

The patient is usually given moderate sedation and analgesia. The electrophysiologist inserts a needle to access the vein or artery. Under fluoroscopy, electrode catheters are inserted into the heart. These catheters conduct electrical impulses to and from the heart. Electrical impulses are used to trigger abnormal heart rhythms (this is discussed in greater detail in Module 14, Assessment of Cardiac Rhythm: Basic Electrocardiographic Rhythm Interpretation). These rhythms usually disappear after removal of the electrical stimuli. After completion of the procedure, the catheters are removed. Firm pressure is applied for 10-20 minutes to the insertion site to achieve hemostasis. The entire procedure can last 1-5 hours. After the procedure, the patient will remain flat for four to six hours or as ordered to prevent bleeding from the insertion site (Crean, 2007).

Other Cardiology Diagnostic Tests

Other diagnostic tests used to diagnose cardiac dysfunction include the multigated angiographic (MUGA) scan, myocardial nuclear perfusion imaging (Persantine-thallium test), positron emission tomography (PET) scans, and impedance cardiography (ICG). Nursing care is focused on the patient and is dependent on the invasiveness of the procedure. The more risk of complications, the greater the involvement of the nurse in monitoring the patient. The nursing roles have been detailed previously.

SECTION EIGHT REVIEW

1. Which of the following patients is prohibited from having an MRI scan performed?
   A. the 77-year-old patient four days postcardiac catheterization
   B. the 24-year-old woman with dilated cardiomyopathy
   C. the 17-year-old patient with a titanium plate in his skull
   D. the 55-year-old man with type II diabetes currently on Metformin (Glucophage)
2. The nurse preparing a patient for cardiac catheterization must notify the cardiologist when
   A. the diabetic patient's fasting blood glucose is 244 mg/dL
   B. the patient states he has an allergy to shellfish
   C. the patient's Warfarin has been held for five days
   D. the patient complains of nervousness
3. The primary complication the nurse must monitor for after a cardiac catheterization is
   A. bleeding
   B. paresthesia
   C. increased urine output
   D. pain at the site of vascular access
4. The transthoracic echocardiogram is
   A. an invasive procedure requiring an overnight stay in the hospital postprocedure
   B. used to directly measure ejection fraction
   C. used to evaluate structures within the heart, such as the septum and valves
   D. the primary means of evaluating pulmonary artery pressures
5. The EPS is used to
   A. determine cardiac output
   B. determine cause of arrhythmias
   C. measure intracardiac pressures
   D. evaluate blockages with the coronary artery system

Answers: 1. C, 2. B, 3. A, 4. C, 5. B

POSTTEST

1. A patient has morbid obesity. He is receiving inotropic medications to improve cardiac output. Which outcome measure is the best to use in this patient to evaluate the efficacy of these medications in this patient?
   A. CO
   B. CI
   C. SV
   D. HR
2. The nurse cares for a patient with excess preload. The nurse identifies which nursing diagnosis is the priority?
   A. altered tissue perfusion
   B. ineffective breathing patterns
   C. alterations in fluid volume (deficit)
   D. alterations in fluid volume (excess)
3. The nurse is caring for a patient with increased afterload. Which finding is the patient most likely to exhibit? (choose all that apply)
   A. normal HR
   B. decreased SV
   C. hypertension
   D. hypotension
4. An 85-year-old male with a medical history of coronary artery disease presents to the ED with dehydration. He is given 5 liters of IV fluid. The nurse understands that the patient is at greatest risk for which of the following problems? (choose all that apply)
   A. excess preload
   B. decreased SV
   C. increased SV
   D. decreased preload
5. The nurse cares for a patient with hypertension. The nurse identifies that the patient is at risk to develop:
   A. decreased HR
   B. decreased resistance
   C. increased CO
   D. decreased CO
6. A patient has decreased CO from decreased myocardial contractility. Which treatment should the nurse anticipate implementing? (choose all that apply)
   A. digoxin
   B. oxygen
   C. calcium
   D. dobutamine
7. A patient is admitted to the high-acuity unit with dehydration. The nurse understands that this patient has decreased preload and is at greatest risk for developing which of the following?
   A. decreased CO
   B. decreased afterload
   C. decreased heart rate
   D. heart failure
8. A patient is placed on dobutamine, a positive inotropic agent. The nurse determines that the care is appropriate if which of the following is observed?
   A. increased preload
   B. increased cardiac output
   C. decreased afterload
   D. decreased heart rate
9. A patient with a history of palpitations states he feels his heart is skipping beats. Which assessment data warrants immediate intervention by the nurse?
   A. heart rate 60 bpm, pulse is regular
   B. S1 and S2 heart sounds present
   C. patient complains of feeling light-headed and dizzy
   D. S3 heart sound present
10. What intervention is most important to include in the nursing care plan of a patient who is started on a diuretic?
    A. daily weights
    B. offer foods high in calcium
    C. ambulate three times per day
    D. turn, cough, and deep breath every two hours
11. A patient is admitted with unstable angina. What information about the patient requires the most immediate action by the nurse?
    A. elevation of BNP levels
    B. S3 heart sounds
    C. auscultation of a carotid bruit
    D. elevation of serum troponin levels
12. A patient returns to the high-acuity unit after a cardiac catheterization. It is important for the nurse to question which of the following orders by the HCP?
    A. assess left groin insertion site for bleeding or hematomas
    B. assess bilateral pedal pulses
    C. ambulate ad lib
    D. keep left leg straight for one hour
13. The nurse can anticipate that conscious sedation will be used during which of the following cardiovascular diagnostic procedures? (choose all that apply)
    A. transesophageal echocardiogram
    B. cardiac catheterization
    C. exercise electrocardiogram
    D. magnetic resonance imaging

Posttest answers with rationale are found on MyNursingKit.

REFERENCES

Braun, L. T. (2006). Cardiovascular disease: strategies for risk assessment and modification. *Journal of Cardiovascular Nursing, 21* (6 suppl 1), S20-S42.

Centers for Disease Control and Prevention (CDC). (2005). State specific prevalence of cigarette smoking and quitting among adults in the United States. *MMWR Morb Mortal Wekly Report, 54*, 1124–1127.

Crean, C. A. (2007). How can electrophysiology help your patient? *Nursing, 37*(7), 60–61.

Dakin, C. L. (2008). New approaches to heart failure in the emergency department. *American Journal of Nursing, 108*(3), 68–71.

Fromm, R. E. (2007). Cardiac troponins in the intensive care unit: common causes of increased levels and interpretation. *Critical Care Medicine, 35*(2), 584–588.

Harper, J. P. (2007). Post diagnostic cardiac catheterization: development and evaluation of evidence-based standard of care. *Journal for Nurses in Staff Development, 23*(6), 271–276.

Howie-Esquivel, J. & White, M. (2008). Biomarkers in acute cardiovascular disease. *Journal of Cardiovascular Nursing, 23*(4), 124–131.

Kop, W. J., Gottdiener, J. S., Tangen, C., et aL (2002). Inflammation and coagulation factors in persons over 65 years of age with symptoms of depression but without evidence of myocardial ischemia. *American Journal of Cardiology, 89*, 419–424.

Kreiger, G. (2007). A basic guide to understanding plasma B-type natriuretic peptide in the diagnosis of congestive heart failure. *MedSurg Nursing, 16*(2), 75.

Pearson, T. A., Mensah, G. A., Alexander, R. W., et al. (2003). Markers of inflammation and cardiovascular disease. Application to clinical and public health practice: a statement for health care professionals from the Centers for Disease Control and the American Heart Association. *Circulation, 107*, 499–511.

Poirier, P., Giles, T. D., Bray, G. A., et al. (2006). Obesity and cardiovascular disease: pathophysiology, evaluation and effect of weight loss. *Circulation, 113*, 898–918.

Porth, C. (2005). Control of cardiovascular function. In C. Porth, (ed.), *Pathophysiology: concepts of altered health states* (7th ed.). Philadelphia: Lippincott Williams & Wilkins.

Prahash, A., & Lunch, T. (2004). B-type natriuretic peptide: a diagnostic, prognostic, and therapeutic tool in heart failure. *American Journal of Critical Care, 13*, 47–55.

Ridker, P. M., Hennekens, C. H., Buring, J. E., & Rifai, N. (2000). C-reactive protein and other markers of inflammation in the prediction of cardiovascular disease in women. *New England Journal of Medicine, 342*, 836–843.

Ridker, P. M., Rifai, N., Clearfield, M., et al. (2001). Air Force/Texas coronary atherosclerosis prevention study investigators: measurement of c-reactive protein for the targeting of statin therapy in the primary prevention of acute coronary events. *New England Journal of Medicine, 344*, 1959–1965.

Scrutinio D., Bellotto F., & Lagioia, R. (2005). Physical activity for coronary artery disease: cardioprotective mechanisms and effects on prognosis. *Monaldi Arch Chest Dis*, 64, 77–87.

United States Department of Health and Human Services. (2006). The health consequences of involuntary exposure to tobacco smoke: a report of the Surgeon General – Executive summary.

Wang, W., Lee, E. T., Fabsitz, R. R., et al. (2006). A longitudinal study of hypertension risk factors and their relation to cardiovascular disease. *Hypertension, 47*, 403–409.

MODULE

13 Assessment of Hemodynamic Status: Hemodynamic Monitoring

Kara Adams Snyder

OBJECTIVES Following completion of this module, the learner will be able to

1. Describe the purpose and functional components of a basic pulmonary artery (PA) catheter.
2. Explain how cardiac output is measured in the clinical setting.
3. Relate right ventricular preload to right atrial pressure, recognize a normal right atrial waveform, and identify common physical findings and nursing interventions related to abnormal right atrial pressures.
4. Recognize the normal right ventricular (RV) waveform, and identify appropriate nursing interventions related to RV waveforms.
5. Recognize a normal PA waveform and identify common physical findings and nursing interventions related to abnormal PA pressures.
6. Recognize a normal pulmonary artery wedge pressure waveform (PAWP), relate left ventricular preload to PAWP, and identify common physical findings and appropriate nursing interventions related to abnormal PAWP pressures.
7. Discuss the physiology underlying the systemic arterial waveform and identify the components of a normal systemic arterial waveform.
8. Discuss the implications of selected derived hemodynamic parameters and calculate the following derived hemodynamic parameters: cardiac index, stroke volume index, mean arterial pressure, systemic vascular resistance, and pulmonary vascular resistance, left ventricular stroke work index, and right ventricular stroke work index.
9. Describe newer hemodynamic monitoring technologies.

The high-acuity patient has complex nursing needs. This self-study module focuses on the integration of hemodynamic concepts and physical findings in the nursing assessment of the high-acuity patient. The nurse requires a working knowledge of the determinants of cardiac output: preload, afterload, and contractility (Module 12, Determinants and Assessment of Cardiac Output). These determinants of cardiac output are linked to the data available through hemodynamic monitoring systems, such as a pulmonary artery catheter. This knowledge, coupled with astute observation and sharp assessment skills, guides critical thinking at the bedside and provides a high level of nursing care for the high-acuity patient. Each section includes a set of review questions to help the learner evaluate his or her understanding of the section's content before moving on to the next section. All Section Reviews include answers. It is suggested that the learner review those concepts answered incorrectly in the review questions before proceeding to the next section.

PRETEST

1. Filling pressure of the right ventricle (right ventricular preload) is measured through the pulmonary artery catheter port opening into the
   A. superior vena cava
   B. right atrium
   C. right ventricle
   D. pulmonary artery
2. Potential risks associated with insertion of a PA catheter include
   A. acute respiratory failure
   B. pneumothorax
   C. arrhythmias
   D. B and C
3. Bolus thermodilution cardiac output measurements should be taken
   A. during inspiration
   B. at end expiration
   C. randomly throughout the respiratory cycle
   D. every two minutes
4. Continuous cardiac output measurements would be MOST beneficial for a patient with
   A. fluid volume excess
   B. fluid volume deficit
   C. fever
   D. septic shock

5. Which of the following conditions lead to an elevated right atrial pressure? (choose all that apply)
   A. sepsis
   B. pulmonic valve stenosis
   C. pulmonary hypertension
   D. cardiac tamponade
6. The right ventricular end-diastolic pressure is marked in the RAP tracing by the
   A. *a* wave
   B. *v* wave
   C. *x* deflection
   D. *y* deflection
7. The greatest potential for dysrhythmias occurs when the pulmonary artery catheter passes through the
   A. superior vena cava
   B. right atrium
   C. right ventricle
   D. pulmonary artery
8. RV diastolic pressure remains essentially the same as
   A. RV systolic pressure
   B. RAP
   C. PAWP
   D. B and C
9. Which of the following pressures fall within the normal range?
   A. PAP = 40/22, PAWP = 18
   B. PAP = 26/12, PAWP = 10
   C. PAP = 18/7, PAWP = 3
   D. PAP = 34/26, PAWP = 23
10. The dicrotic notch on the pulmonary artery waveform represents
    A. atrial contraction
    B. closure of the pulmonic valve
    C. closure of the aortic valve
    D. the beginning of ventricular systole
11. The right atrial waveform and the ______ waveform are similar in appearance.
    A. pulmonary artery wedge
    B. right ventricular
    C. pulmonary artery
    D. systemic arterial
12. Preload of the left ventricle is measured indirectly by
    A. cardiac output
    B. pulmonary artery systolic pressure
    C. pulmonary artery diastolic pressure
    D. pulmonary artery wedge pressure (PAWP)
13. Normal MAP is
    A. 60 to 70 mm Hg
    B. 140/80 mm Hg
    C. 70 to 90 mm Hg
    D. 100 to 120 mm Hg
14. The dicrotic notch on the systemic arterial pressure waveform represents
    A. closure of the aortic valve
    B. closure of the pulmonic valve
    C. opening of the aortic valve
    D. mean arterial pressure
15. The left ventricular stroke work index is compared with which of the following when assessing left ventricle function?
    A. right atrial pressure
    B. cardiac output
    C. cardiac index
    D. pulmonary artery wedge pressure
16. Afterload to the left ventricle is estimated by determining the
    A. PAWP
    B. right atrial pressure
    C. cardiac index
    D. systemic vascular resistance

Pretest answers are found on MyNursingKit.

Hemodynamic Parameters and Normal Values

HEMODYNAMIC PARAMETERS	NORMAL VALUES
CI = CO/BSA	2.4 to 4.0 L/min/m^2
CO = HR × SV	4 to 8 L/min
LVSWI = [(MAP – PAWP) × (SVI) × (0.0136)]	50 to 62 g/m^2/beat
MAP = [(SBP) + 2 (DBP)]/3	70 to 90 mm Hg
Mean PAP = [(systolic) + 2 (diastolic)]/3	12 to 20 mm Hg
PAS	20 to 30 mm Hg
PAD	8 to 15 mm Hg (2 to 5 mm Hg higher than PAWP)
PAWP	4 to 12 mm Hg
PVR = [(Mean PAP) – (PAWP) × 80]/CO	50 to 250 dynes · sec · cm^{-5}

HEMODYNAMIC PARAMETERS	NORMAL VALUES
PVRI = [(Mean PAP) – (PAWP) × 80]/CI	255 to 315 dynes · sec · cm^{-5}/m^2
RAP	2 to 6 mm Hg
RV pressures (RV systolic/RV diastolic)	20 to 30 mm Hg/2 to 8 mm Hg
RVSWI = [(Mean PAP – RAP) × (SVI) × (0.0136)]	7.9 to 9.7 g/m^2/beat
SVI = CI/HR	25 to 45 mL/beat/m^2
SV = CO/HR	50 to 100 mL/beat
SVR = [(MAP) – (RAP) × 80]/CO	800 to 1,200 dynes · sec · cm^{-5}
SVRI = [(MAP) – (RAP) × 80]/CI	1,970 to 2,390 dynes · sec · cm^{-5}/m^2

SECTION ONE: The Pulmonary Artery Catheter

At the completion of this section, the learner will be able to describe the purpose and functional components of a basic pulmonary artery catheter.

Various terms are used by health care professionals to refer to a pulmonary artery catheter, including right heart catheter, Swan or Swan–Ganz catheter, flow-directed thermodilution catheter, and pulmonary artery catheter. This module uses the term *pulmonary artery catheter.*

Purpose

The pulmonary artery (PA) catheter is an invasive diagnostic tool that can be used at the bedside for the following purposes:

1. To determine the pressures within the right heart and PA, and for indirect measurement of left heart pressures
2. To determine cardiac output (CO)
3. To sample mixed venous blood (Svo_2) from the PA
4. To infuse fluids

Hemodynamic data are used to make clinical management decisions in high-acuity patients. There are three steps of hemodynamic assessment with the PA catheter that the nurse must follow (Adams, 2004).

1. Obtain accurate data. It is a nursing responsibility to ensure the proper calibration of the equipment used for hemodynamic monitoring.
2. Correctly perform waveform analysis.
3. Integrate the data with other assessment parameters.

These three steps will be discussed in further detail throughout this module.

Basic Construction

The PA catheter is constructed of a radiopaque polyvinylchloride. Several sizes and various options are available. Most have a heparin coating to reduce the risk of thrombus formation. All PA catheters have color-coded extrusions or "ports" on the proximal end that provide access to the various catheter lumens. The catheter is marked at 10-cm intervals to facilitate correct placement. A typical PA catheter has five lumens, as shown in Figure 13–1.

Special Pulmonary Artery Catheters

Special PA catheters are also available and are almost identical to the one pictured in Figure 13–1. However, additional options are present. One special catheter has an integrated port for pacing wires that allows for synchronized atrial and ventricular pacing. Another catheter uses special technology to provide continuous monitoring of the cardiac output, as opposed to the individual "spot check" measurements traditionally obtained by the clinician. This technology is discussed in Section Two. Another special PA catheter allows for continuous measurement of the mixed venous oxygen saturation. Keep in mind that these special catheters provide all the functions of the basic catheter described in this section but include special features that permit additional functions.

Components and Pertinent Points

Following are discussions of each section of the basic PA catheter. When indicated, special nursing considerations are included with the descriptive information.

Proximal Injectate Lumen/Hub

- This lumen terminates in the most proximal chamber of the heart, the right atrium.
- Most catheter manufacturers imprint the word *proximal* on either the hub or the tubing close to the hub. Be sure to look for it.
- On most catheters, the tubing of this port is blue for rapid visual identification. One way to remember this is to link the blue tubing of this port to the "blue" desaturated blood found in the right atrium.
- This port allows for monitoring or sampling of the right atrial pressure (RAP) when it is connected to a transducer.

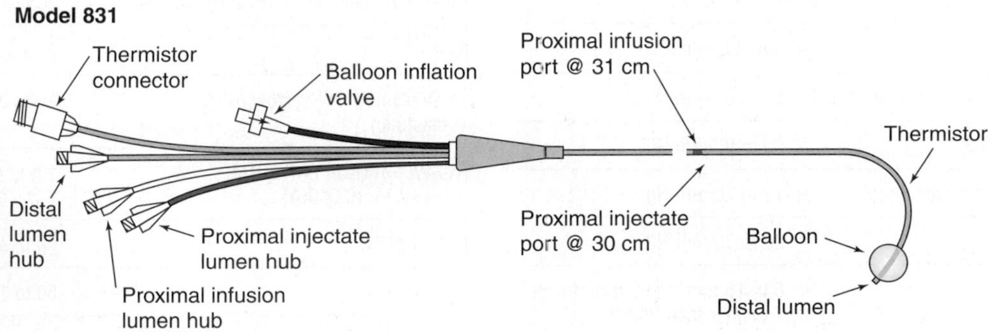

Figure 13–1 ■ A five-lumen pulmonary artery catheter. (Reprinted with permission. Copyringt © 2000 Edwards Lifesciences. Swan-Ganz® is a trademark of Edwards Lifesciences Corporation, registered in the U.S. Patent and Trademark Office)

- The injectate used to determine cardiac output is pushed through this lumen.
- IV fluids can also be infused through this port. To avoid inadvertent bolus of potent medications, do not infuse vasoactive medications through this lumen when it is used for thermodilution cardiac output measurements.

Proximal Infusion Lumen/Hub (Optional)

- When present, this extra lumen terminates in the right atrium and is labeled *infusion* on the hub or the tubing near the hub.
- On most catheters, the tubing of this port is white or clear for rapid visual identification.
- This port is primarily used as the "central line" for IV fluid infusions such as total parenteral nutrition. This is especially helpful in patients with poor peripheral venous access.
- This port can be used for obtaining cardiac output determinations if the proximal injectate lumen occludes. However, the individual values obtained from this port may not be as reproducible as those obtained from the proximal injectate port. To avoid inadvertent bolus of potent medications, do not infuse vasoactive medications through the lumen selected for bolus thermodilution cardiac output determinations.

Distal Lumen/Hub

- This lumen terminates in the PA.
- Most catheter manufacturers imprint the word *distal* on either the hub or the tubing close to the hub. Look for it.
- On most catheters, the tubing of this port is yellow for rapid visual identification.
- This port is always connected to a transducer for continuous monitoring of the PA pressure (PAP) and waveform.
- Pulmonary artery wedge pressure (PAWP) is obtained through this port by careful balloon inflation. This will be discussed later in the module.
- Mixed venous blood oxygen saturation (SvO_2) is obtained or "sampled" from this port. Remember that this port terminates in the PA. The venous blood returning from all parts of the body has been "well mixed" in the right atrium and ventricle before it is pumped into the PA.
- Medications and IV solutions are not infused through this port, except under certain conditions when indicated by a physician.

Thermistor

- The thermistor wire terminates near the tip of the catheter and is exposed to the blood flowing through the PA.
- This wire detects changes in the temperature of the blood, which is an essential part of cardiac output determination.
- It allows for continuous monitoring of core body temperature.
- The proximal end attaches (connects) to a cable linking it with the device used for measuring cardiac output. This will either be a cardiac output module compatible with the bedside monitoring system or a freestanding cardiac output computer.

Balloon Inflation Lumen/Valve

- This lumen is contiguous with the small balloon at the distal end of the catheter.
- A "gate valve" mechanism on the hub locks this port in an open or closed position.
- The balloon is slowly inflated using a syringe provided with the catheter while the PA waveform is continuously monitored. Inflation is stopped as soon as the waveform changes to a PA wedge waveform.
- The maximum recommended inflation volume provided with catheter instructions should not be exceeded.
- Deflation is always passive. Manual deflation may damage balloon integrity.
- Never leave the balloon in the inflated position.

Hemodynamic Monitoring Equipment

A typical hemodynamic monitoring set is shown in Figure 13–2. Except for the catheter, the system components are the same as for pulmonary arterial pressure monitoring or systemic arterial pressure monitoring (see Section Seven).

Transducer

Measurement of pressures within the heart and PA is accomplished using a transducer. A transducer is a "translator." It translates mechanical energy sensed by the catheter and converts it to electrical energy, displayed on the monitor screen as a waveform. It is the nurse's responsibility to ensure the transducer is translating correctly. To that end, the nurse must level and zero the catheter according to unit or hospital policies and procedures. Leveling the transducer corrects for hydrostatic pressure changes in vessels above and below the heart. Zeroing the transducer corrects for any drift or deviation from baseline that may occur in the transducer. Current transducers have minimal zero drift and therefore routine rezeroing is unnecessary.

The **phlebostatic axis** approximates the level of the right atrium and is considered to represent the level of the catheter tip. The transducer is referenced (or leveled) and zeroed at the phlebostatic axis. In the supine position, the external landmark for the right atrium is the 4th intercostal space, one half the anterior and posterior diameter of the chest (AACN, 2004). Improper positioning of the transducer leads to very different readings. Every time the patient's position changes, the transducer should be re-referenced to assure that the readings are taken in the same place each time.

Pressure Bag

To overcome the arterial pressure and prevent blood from backing up into the pressure tubing, a pressure bag is placed around the flush solution bag and inflated to 300 mm Hg. Depending on hospital policy, the flush solution may or may not contain heparin.

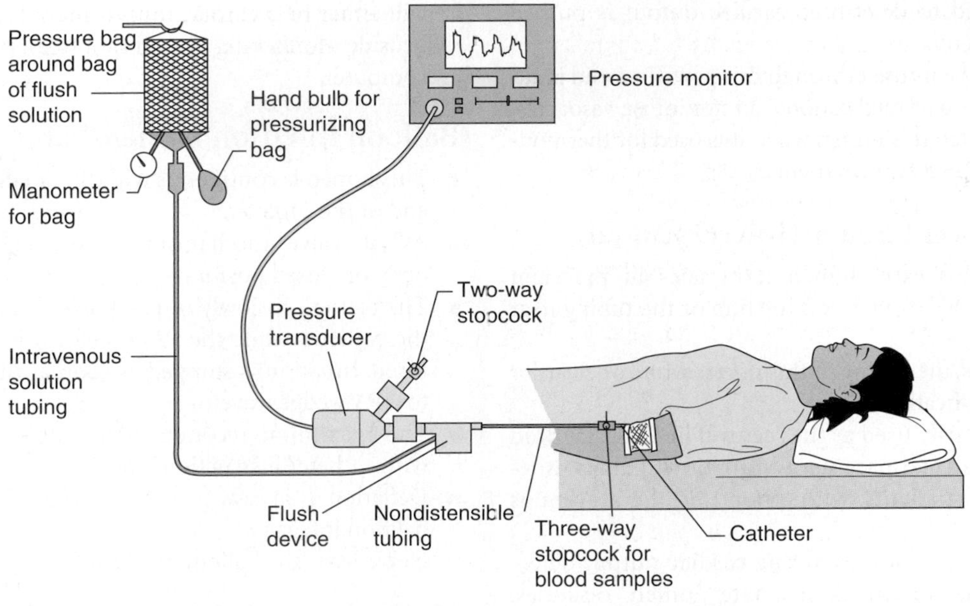

Figure 13–2 ▪ Hemodynamic monitoring equipment.

Insertion

Insertion of a PA catheter is performed in critical care units, cardiac catheterization laboratories, and operating rooms. The complication rate related to this procedure is low; however, the insertion of a PA catheter is not without risks. Potential risks include pneumothorax, damage to the blood vessels or heart, arrhythmias, infection or bleeding, bleeding at the insertion site, and death. Except in emergency situations, informed consent should be obtained prior to catheter insertion.

Prior to insertion, several steps are taken that help to assure that insertion is completed with ease and that good data are produced. Here are some key steps (Bridges, 2006):

- Gather all supplies (isotonic sodium chloride solution, pressure monitoring kit, 10mL syringe, pressure bag, PA Catheter with percutaneous introducer).
- Prime the pressure monitoring system to remove all air.
  - Be sure to prime through all stopcocks and to remove all air from the IV bag of fluid before priming the system.
  - Perform an additional flush with 10mL of IV fluid by attaching the syringe to the stopcock at the transducer and quickly flushing the tubing with the syringe. This will help flush out any remaining air bubbles.
- Inspect the tubing to be sure that all air bubbles have been removed. Repeat fast flush with syringe if needed.
- Place the IV bag in the pressure bag and inflate to 300 mm Hg.
- Connect to the bedside monitor.

The insertion of a PA catheter is always a sterile procedure. All persons in the room should perform hand hygiene prior to the procedure and should each wear a hat and mask. The nurse also ensures that the person inserting the line is wearing a sterile gown and gloves and that the patient has a full-body drape. The patient's skin is prepared with a 2 percent chlorhexidine gluconate solution. Along with the health care provider, the nurse is responsible for careful observation and monitoring of the patient during the insertion process.

Patients may be awake when the catheter is inserted, and it can be a frightening experience if the patient does not know what to expect. The patient should know that the purpose of the catheter is to assess heart function and fluid status, allowing more precise management of his or her condition. Explain to the patient that the site will be scrubbed with an antiseptic solution, and that a pinch, sting, or burning sensation may be felt when the local anesthetic is injected. A temporary sensation of pressure should be expected when a large IV catheter (the sheath) is inserted into the subclavian, jugular, or femoral vein. Once positioned, the sheath is typically secured in place. The patient should know that the long, thin, balloon-tipped catheter will not be felt as it is threaded through the sheath, floated through the right heart, and positioned in the PA. Most patients find it helpful during the procedure to receive general information on how things are going and an estimated time to completion. After the procedure, the patient should expect to be attached to multiple IV lines that will restrict some freedom of movement. In addition, postprocedure, the family should be prepared to see additional equipment during their next visit with the patient.

After the catheter has been inserted, the nurse assumes responsibility for patient safety, comfort, and system maintenance. The nurse is responsible for catheter site maintenance, documentation of pressures in the heart and PA, and obtaining valid cardiac output measurements. Postprocedure, a chest X-ray is obtained to confirm catheter position and to assess for pneumothorax. Until proper placement of the catheter has been confirmed by chest X-ray, the catheter is not used for infusion of medications or fluids. It is the nurse's responsibility to recognize abnormal waveforms and trends, and intervene appropriately, including notification of the physician when indicated. The nurse must know and follow unit-specific policies and procedures related to hemodynamic monitoring.

Several complications, including infection, may occur as a result of invasive hemodynamic monitoring. Air emboli or thromboembolism can occur from loose connections or improper flushing, respectively. Fluid overload may result from fluid infusion through multiple lumens or lack of surveillance of IV pumps. Exsanguination may occur if a stopcock remains open or tubing becomes disconnected.

Provider Competency

Hemodynamic monitoring in the high-acuity patient population requires competency in both technical and physiological aspects. As is true for all diagnostic tests, the information obtained is only as good as the data collected. Assessment of the hemodynamic profile is taken in three steps:

1. **Obtain accurate data.** This includes appropriate leveling and zeroing, use of minimal transducer tubing, maintenance of system patency free from air bubbles, square wave testing, and patient position.
2. **Assess the waveform.** Studies suggest that assessment of waveforms is best performed when printed graphically and correlated with the electrocardiogram (ECG) and respiratory cycles (AACN, 2004). Certain modes of mechanical ventilation and rapid and spontaneous respirations make locating end-expiration difficult. There is some evidence to support the use of capnography to identify physiological end expiration (Ahrens & Sona, 2003).
3. **Integrate data with the patient assessment.** Integration is accomplished by looking at all the data in the hemodynamic profile collectively. Data in the hemodynamic profile will be discussed in detail in this module; however, recognize that this data must be correlated with findings in the physical assessment of CO. Refer to Module 12, Determinants and Assessment of Cardiac Output.

It is important to recognize that ongoing education is needed to ensure patient safety and positive clinical outcomes. Resources for ongoing education are outlined in the NURSING CARE box: Hemodynamic Monitoring: Educational Resources.

Interpretation of Data

Data collection is not the end point of hemodynamic monitoring. Abnormal pressures and changes in trends must be recognized, correlated with the patient's condition, and acted on. Careful clinical assessment, integrated with the data collected from a PA catheter, provides a basis for nursing interventions and manipulation of potent vasoactive medications or fluids.

The following guidelines are used when interpreting readings.

1. Always look at patient trends and not an isolated reading.
2. Question abnormal readings. Recheck the reading after zeroing and calibrating the equipment. Assess the patient for additional data to support the reading.
3. Compare the patient's readings with his or her normal values and *not* with the normal values listed in a textbook.
4. Do not be fooled by normal readings. The patient may have normal readings temporarily because of compensatory mechanisms. Continue to assess the patient.
5. Assess the interrelationships among the readings. The goal is to obtain a picture of the patient's hemodynamic status and not simply a number.

Patient Positioning

Studies in a variety of patient populations have found that PAP and RAP measurements are accurate when the head of the bed is elevated to any angle between 0 and 60 degrees, as long as the patient is in the supine position and the transducer has been referenced to the level of the right atrium at the phlebostatic axis (AACN, 2004).

Reading at End Expiration

Changes in intrathoracic pressure during respiration significantly alter hemodynamic pressures. Obtaining accurate measurements requires reading pressure waveforms at end expiration. Digital readouts on the bedside monitor reflect pressures obtained throughout the respiratory cycle (AACN, 2004). These pressures are significantly different from end-expiratory pressures. Therefore, pressures should be read at end expiration (AACN, 2004).

NURSING CARE: Hemodynamic Monitoring

Educational Resources

Pulmonary artery catheter education project: http://www.pacep.org

American Association of Critical Care Nurses: Pulmonary Artery Measurement Practice Alert: http://www.aacn.org/WD/Practice/Docs/PAP_measurement

American Association of Critical Care Nurses: Measurement of Pulmonary Artery Pressures Education Session: http://www.aacn.org/WD/Practice/Content/practicealerts/PAPmeasurement education ppt.

American Association of Critical Care Nurses: Essentials of critical care education (ECCO)

American Association of Critical Care Nurses: Protocols for practice: hemodynamic monitoring series

SECTION ONE REVIEW

1. Which port of the PA catheter is used to obtain RAP?
   A. proximal port
   B. distal port
   C. thermistor wire port
   D. balloon inflation port
2. Which lumen is used for obtaining CO determinations?
   A. proximal port lumen
   B. distal port lumen
   C. thermistor wire lumen
   D. balloon inflation port lumen
3. The pressure reading from which lumen is always continuously monitored?
   A. proximal
   B. distal
   C. thermistor wire
   D. balloon port
4. Why should vasoactive drugs never be infused through the port used for thermodilution CO determinations?
   A. The size of the lumen is too small.
   B. A bolus injection of a potent drug will occur every time CO is obtained.
   C. CO readings will be less accurate.
   D. Some vasoactive drugs are not compatible with the catheter material.
5. What is the best way to deflate the balloon on the PA catheter?
   A. Slowly pull back on the syringe plunger.
   B. Quickly pull back on the plunger to limit inflation time.
   C. Allow the balloon to deflate passively.
   D. Remove the syringe from the hub directly after inflation.

Answers: 1. A, 2. A, 3. B, 4. B, 5. C

SECTION TWO: Hemodynamic Monitoring and Determination of Cardiac Output

At the completion of this section, the learner will be able to explain how cardiac output is measured in the clinical setting.

Recall from Module 12, Determinants and Assessment of Cardiac Output that *cardiac output (CO)* is the amount of blood ejected from the heart into the circulation each minute. It is expressed in liters per minute.

The formula used to derive the CO is simple. CO is the product of the heart rate (HR) multiplied by the *stroke volume* (SV) (i.e., the amount of blood ejected by each heartbeat). The formula for CO is CO = HR × SV. Changes in heart rate will affect CO; in fact, acceleration of heart rate is one of the first compensatory mechanisms when CO decreases. Stroke volume is also variable and is altered by the effects of preload, afterload, and contractility. These terms were introduced in Module 12 and will be briefly reviewed here, given that an understanding of these concepts is key to understanding hemodynamic monitoring.

Preload

Preload is the pressure or stretch exerted on the walls of the ventricle by the volume of blood filling the ventricle at the end of diastole. Preload is typically used as an indication of the volume status of the patient. Too little preload (volume) will not adequately stretch the ventricular muscle to get the best contraction (i.e., the best stroke volume). Too much preload acts to overstretch the ventricular muscle, resulting in poor contractility, a reduced stroke volume, and a drop in CO. Preload, then, has to be "just right" to maximize Frank-Starling's law to get the best ventricular contraction and the most optimal CO. Although emphasis is often placed on left ventricular preload, keep in mind that both ventricles have the property of preload.

An estimate of preload is obtained from a PA catheter. For the left heart, the **pulmonary artery wedge pressure** (PAWP) is used as an indirect measure of pressure in the left ventricle at the end of diastole (or left ventricular end-diastolic pressure, LVEDP). LVEDP provides an estimate of the "volume status" of the patient. It is obtained from the distal port after the catheter balloon has been inflated and allowed to float into "wedge" position. The normal range of the PAWP is 4 to 12 mm Hg; however, every patient must be considered in the context of his or her health history. Patients with impaired myocardial function (myocardial infarction) may need more volume to stretch an impaired ventricle to get the best contraction. Consequently, a higher PAWP of 15 mm Hg may be necessary to get the best possible contraction of the ventricle. Right heart preload is obtained by using a transducer to measure the RAP from the proximal port of the PA catheter. When the tricuspid valve is open, the RAP is used as a proxy for right ventricular end-diastolic pressure (RVEDP). Like the LVEDP (measured by the PAWP), the RVEDP (measured by the RAP) is an estimate of volume status of the patient. The normal range of the RAP is 2 to 6 mm Hg. RAP and PAWP are the topics of Sections Three and Six, respectively.

Afterload

Afterload is the resistance to ventricular contraction. Simply stated, afterload is the pressure the ventricle has to overcome to open the aortic or pulmonic valve and eject blood out of the ventricle into the systemic or pulmonary circulation. An estimate of afterload to the left heart is obtained by using a formula to calculate the **systemic vascular resistance** (SVR). An estimate of afterload to the right heart is obtained by using a formula to calculate the **pulmonary vascular resistance** (PVR). These measures are discussed further in Section Eight.

Afterload can be viewed as the pressure in the aorta pushing against the valve to hold it in the closed position. However, fixed lesions, such as aortic stenosis, and anomalies, such as coarctation of the aorta, also represent afterload the ventricle must overcome before it can eject the stroke volume. When looking at the formula for SVR or PVR, it is notable that these anatomical changes are not part of the formula, yet can greatly affect afterload. As afterload increases, the heart works harder, which requires more oxygen. When afterload is high, the ventricle does not fully empty, which translates into a reduced stroke volume and low CO.

Afterload can also be too low. When the pressure or resistance in the aorta is low, the left ventricle needs to generate very little pressure to open the aortic valve and eject blood into the circulation. It will not contract vigorously. The net effect is a weak contraction, resulting in a reduced CO and a low systolic blood pressure. Similar to preload, afterload needs to be "just right" for the best CO.

Contractility

Contractility is the property of the heart that allows it to shorten muscle fibers and contract. A vigorous contraction will improve CO by increasing the SV. When contractility is compromised, as in heart failure or hypovolemia, the amount of blood volume that is ejected with each beat is reduced and reflected in the SV. A normal stroke volume is 50 to 100 mL/beat. This value may be indexed to body size, known as the **stroke volume index** (SVI) (25 to 45 mL/beat/m^2). Stroke volume or stroke volume index must be assessed in the context of both the cardiac output and the preload values.

Contractility is optimized when preload and afterload are optimized. If the CO remains low after both preload and afterload have been optimized, inotropic agents to improve CO may be considered. Increasing the contractile force of a weak ventricle improves SV and CO. Contractility is assessed by calculating a parameter called the **ventricular stroke work index**. The ventricular stroke work index is the work involved in ejecting blood from the ventricle with each heartbeat against afterload. This will be further discussed in Section Eight.

Preload, afterload, and contractility interact to determine the CO by their effects on stroke volume (Fig. 13–3). Traditionally, primary emphasis has been placed on the left ventricle because it is the capacity of the left ventricle to function as a pump that determines oxygen delivery. It is important to keep in mind that these properties are important to the function of both ventricles.

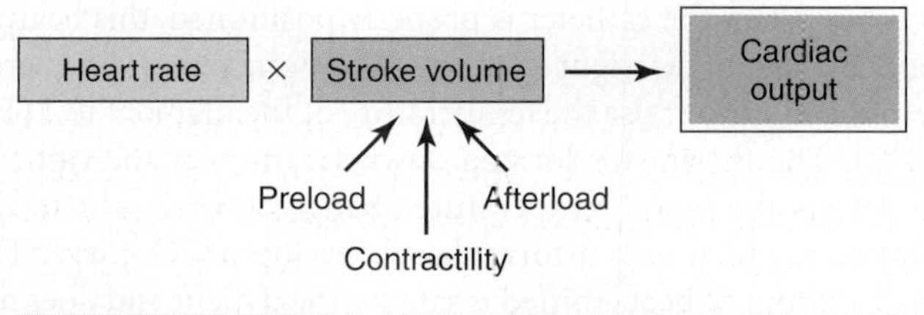

Figure 13–3 ■ The determinants of cardiac output.

Cardiac Output

The normal range for CO is 4 to 8 L/min. Recall from Module 12 that this important parameter does not address the effect of body size on CO requirements. Consider the CO required by a large and muscular professional football player versus the CO needed by a petite female bank president. If each has a CO of 4 L/min, technically, both COs fall within the normal range of 4 to 8 L/min. A quick bedside physical assessment would tell us that more information is needed. Although 4 L/min may well serve the needs of the petite female, it would likely be inadequate for the needs of a large, muscular professional football player.

The *cardiac index* (CI) references the CO to body size. This information is more useful because the CO is now individualized to a specific patient. The CI is obtained by dividing the CO by the patient's body surface area (BSA) to individualize the CO to the patient. A normal CI is 2.4 to 4.0 L/min/m^2. Most monitors calculate the CI if the patient's height and weight are entered. The CI is far more meaningful than the CO for bedside clinical decision making. As a derived parameter, the CI will be discussed further in Section Eight.

How Is Hemodynamic Monitoring Used to Guide Clinical Decisions?

According to Pinsky (2007), there are three functional questions that must be asked when patients are hemodynamically unstable. First will cardiac output increase with fluid administration and if so by how much? Meaning how much preload is needed? Second, if the patient is hypotensive, is it because arterial vasomotor tone is increased, decreased, or normal? Third, is the heart capable of sustaining an effective cardiac output, once arterial pressure is restored without going into failure? There are additional patient specific questions that should be asked and addressed, but these three fundamental questions should be the first addressed when a patient becomes hemodynamically unstable.

How Is Cardiac Output Obtained?

While various methods are used to determine CO this section will focus on the traditional "bolus" **thermodilution** method of CO measurement. With this method, intermittent "spot" checks of CO are obtained at the discretion of the clinician or by a schedule dictated by policy or procedure. Other methods of obtaining CO will be briefly discussed at the end of this section.

The thermodilution method uses temperature change over time to calculate CO. The distal end of the thermistor wire terminates in an exposed bead 1.6 in. (4 cm) below the tip of the catheter (refer to Fig. 13–1). This thermistor bead is exposed to the blood flowing past it in the PA. It senses the temperature of the blood and allows for constant monitoring of core body temperature. It also monitors changes in the temperature of the blood and the duration of the temperature change. This information is relayed to the computer through a special cable attached to the thermistor connector at the proximal end of the PA catheter.

In the traditional method of thermodilution CO, a 10-mL bolus of fluid is injected through the proximal injectate port of the PA catheter into the right atrium. The temperature of this fluid is cooler than blood temperature. The injectate fluid temperature is sensed by an in-line temperature probe and then relayed to the CO computer. The CO computer has two temperatures stored in it: the temperature of the blood and the temperature of the fluid bolus. The injection of the fluid bolus must be smooth, rapid, and completed within a 4-second interval. This fluid "bolus" mixes with blood as it is pumped through the right ventricle and into the PA. The mixture of the cooler fluid bolus with the blood results in a transient drop in the temperature of the blood flowing through the PA. As blood continues to be pumped into the PA, the blood temperature will warm to the prebolus level. The blood temperature change and the duration of the blood temperature change are sensed by the exposed thermistor bead positioned in the PA. This information is relayed to the CO computer where it is analyzed and a time–temperature CO "curve" is formed (Fig. 13–4). The area under the curve represents the CO.

This area is calculated by the computer and displayed digitally in liters per minute (L/min). There is an inverse relationship between the size of the curve and the CO. A small curve indicates a rapid return of the blood to its baseline temperature and, therefore, a high CO. A large curve indicates a slow return to baseline temperature and, therefore, a low CO. A notched or uneven curve indicates poor injection technique, and the value obtained should not be accepted.

Equipment Preparation

Obtaining valid CO determinations is an important nursing responsibility. To calculate CO accurately, the computer must know the catheter model, fluid bolus volume, and fluid temperature selected for use. A number or "constant" that represents this information is entered into the computer before starting. This constant is obtained from a chart on a package insert provided with the catheter. It is important that the correct constant is entered prior to obtaining COs. If the volume or temperature of the injectate is changed during the course of hemodynamic monitoring, a new constant is entered or the CO determinations will be inaccurate.

Fluid Bolus

Normal saline is used as the injectate fluid. The volume of the bolus injectate used varies according to hospital policy and patient condition. The most common volume is 10 mL; however, if volume overload is a problem, 5 mL can be used. The literature reports that a 10-mL bolus provides the most reproducibility (Albert, 2005). An important nursing consideration is to be consistent and not vary the volume of the bolus. It is common practice to obtain three sequential CO measurements, using 10 mL of saline for each determination. If one of the CO results varies more than 10 percent from the others, it is rejected. An average of at least two "similar" values (within 10 percent of each other) is accepted for the CO.

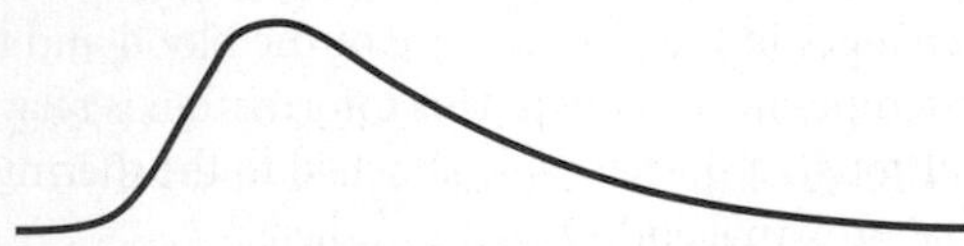

Figure 13–4 ▪ A normal cardiac output curve. (Reprinted with permission. Copyright © 2000 Edwards Lifesciences. Swan-Ganz® is a trademark of Edwards Lifesciences Corporation, registered in the U.S. Patent and Trademark Office)

Bolus Temperature

Selection of either room temperature or iced injectate is generally considered acceptable (according to unit policy) as long as the proper constant is entered into the CO computer. Although there is some controversy, research suggests that there is no significant difference between iced injectate and room temperature injectate. In hypothermia, the temperature difference between the injectate and the patient's temperature may not be wide enough to ensure accuracy. Once the choice is made to use either iced or room temperature injectate, the decision should be followed through the course of that patient's hemodynamic monitoring. If the injectate temperature is changed, a new constant must be entered into the CO computer.

Timing of Bolus Injection

The timing of the bolus injection must coincide with the end-expiratory phase of the patient's breathing cycle. This is thought to provide more consistency in the results.

Conditions Affecting Pulmonary Artery Temperature

Many conditions produce a change in venous return that can alter the PA temperature. These include coughing, restlessness, shivering, and the administration of peripheral IV fluids of a different temperature through the venous infusion port of the PA catheter.

Method of Bolus Injection

The bolus injection should be rapid and smooth. The entire bolus should be injected within a 4-second interval at end expiration. Improper injection technique affects accuracy of the data.

Continuous Cardiac Output Measurement

There are several limitations with traditional bolus thermodilution CO measurements. They are, in essence, "snapshots" of CO. They take time to obtain, are subject to operator error, and require administration of additional fluid, which may be contraindicated in some patients. Because of these limitations, a PA catheter for the determination of CO on a continuous basis was developed. This type of catheter uses a modified thermodilution method. Similar to a traditional catheter, there is a balloon tip, a proximal injectate port, an infusion port, a thermistor wire, and a distal port. The primary difference is a thermal filament on the exterior of the catheter between the infusion port and the balloon tip. When the catheter is properly positioned, this heating filament lies in the right ventricle. Random pulses of energy from the monitor raise the temperature of the filament to 111°F (44°C). The thermistor located downstream near the catheter tip detects the blood temperature change and relays it to the computer, which uses a formula to develop a CO curve. The small amount of heat emitted is safe for the patient and does not have an adverse effect on blood cells.

The CO is continuously displayed on the bedside monitor and values are updated every three minutes. The displayed values represent an average of the CO of the previous three minutes. By entering the patient's height and weight, a continuous CI is displayed. The accuracy of this modified technique, using heat "pulses" to replace the traditional fluid bolus, is not dependent on user technique. The patient is spared multiple fluid boluses. Several research studies compared this method to the traditional intermittent bolus thermodilution method. Data support the fact that these two methods to obtain CO agree (Ott, 2001).

SECTION TWO REVIEW

1. The thermodilution method of CO determination is based on
   A. a change in blood temperature over time
   B. the length of time it takes for dye to be circulated
   C. the temperature of the injectate
   D. the volume of the injectate
2. To increase the accuracy of CO determinations, which of the following techniques is used?
   A. Inject slowly and smoothly over 1 minute.
   B. Inject smoothly within a 4-second interval.
   C. Inject rapidly over 8 seconds.
   D. Intermittently inject the volume over 30 seconds.
3. Which of the following are disadvantages associated with bolus thermodilution CO measurements?
   A. They are time consuming.
   B. Multiple measurements may subject patients to fluid overload.
   C. Accuracy is affected by user technique.
   D. All of the above.
4. Continuous CO measurements
   A. are less accurate than bolus thermodilution CO measurements
   B. provide two updates on CO readings every hour
   C. depend on user technique for accuracy
   D. agree with bolus thermodilution measurements
5. Mr. S. has fluid volume overload and pulmonary edema. A PA catheter is inserted to monitor his CO. Which method would you recommend to obtain CO measurement in this patient?
   A. bolus thermodilution with 10 mL of normal saline
   B. continuous cardiac output monitoring
   C. bolus thermodilution with 10 mL of dextrose
   D. A and C

Answers: 1. A, 2. B, 3. D, 4. D, 5. B

SECTION THREE: Right Atrial Pressure

At the completion of this section, the learner will be able to relate right ventricular preload to right atrial pressure, recognize a normal right atrial waveform, and identify common physical findings and nursing interventions related to abnormal right atrial pressures.

Right atrial pressure (RAP) is obtained from the proximal port of the PA catheter, which opens into the right atrium. The RAP is always read as a mean pressure, and the normal range is 2 to 6 mm Hg (Fig. 13–5).

RAP is an estimate of right ventricular preload (i.e., the volume status of the right heart). Recall from Section Two that preload is the stretch exerted on the walls of the ventricle by the volume of blood filling the ventricle at the end of diastole. RAP is an estimate of right ventricular end-diastolic pressure (RVEDP). Measurement of RVEDP is possible because the tricuspid valve remains open until the end of right ventricular diastole, allowing right ventricular pressure to be transmitted to the right atrium. For this reason, RAP can be used as a measure of RVEDP.

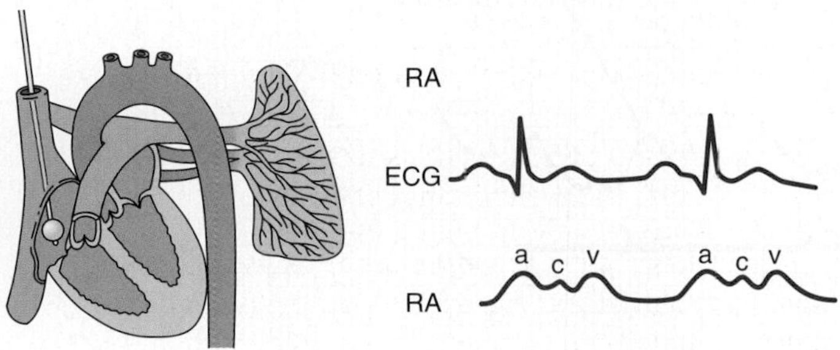

Figure 13–5 ▪ A right atrial waveform with the *a* and *v* wave components identified. (Reprinted with permission. Copyright © 2000 Edwards Lifesciences. Swan-Ganz® is a trademark of Edwards Lifesciences Corporation, registered in the U.S. Patent and Trademark Office)

Obtaining RAP Measurements

The RAP waveform is monitored by attaching a transducer to the proximal (blue) port of the PA catheter. The right atrial waveform has a characteristic undulating pattern, consisting of three positive and two negative excursions. These undulations are a result of mechanical events in the cardiac cycle. The positive excursions consist of *a*, *c*, and *v* waves. The rise in atrial pressure during atrial systole forms the *a* wave. Closure of the tricuspid valve early in systole produces the *c* wave (not always well visualized). The *v* wave is produced by an increase in pressure from passive atrial filling that occurs against a slightly bulging atrioventricular valve during ventricular systole. The negative excursions consist of the *x* and *y* deflections. The *x* descent follows both the *a* and *c* waves and results from the drop in atrial pressure after atrial systole. The y descent is a result of passive right atrial emptying into the right ventricle when the tricuspid valve opens just prior to atrial systole. Figure 13–6 illustrates a labeled atrial waveform.

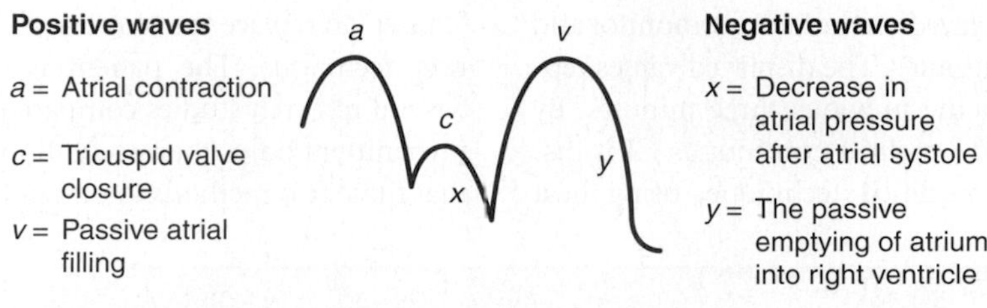

Figure 13–6 ■ A labeled right atrial waveform.

Assessment of the waveform begins with obtaining a graphic readout from either the bedside or central monitoring system. This printout should include both the ECG and RAP tracings in order to correlate the mechanical events of the heart (RAP tracing) with the electrical events (ECG tracing). The *a* wave is a ventricular diastolic event whereas the *v* wave is a systolic event. The *c* wave marks the end of diastole. The RVEDP is marked in the RAP tracing by the *c* wave when visible. The *c* wave marks end-diastole and may be located on the monitor strip (simultaneous printout of the ECG and RAP tracings) by drawing a line straight down from the *QRS* complex. If the *c* wave is not visible, the *a* wave may be used. The *a* wave represents atrial systole and, therefore, follows the *P* wave on the ECG tracing. Find the correlation between the *a* wave and the *P* wave in Figure 13–5.

Any pressure in the thoracic cavity is transmitted to the great vessels and the cardiac chambers. Thus, measurement of the right atrial pressure is obtained at end-expiration to eliminate intrathoracic pressures. Spontaneously breathing patients generate a negative pressure breath on inspiration. This is reflected in the RAP waveform as a downward deflection. Patients on a ventilator with mandatory positive pressure breaths show a rise in their RAP waveform on inspiration. Addition of positive end-expiratory pressure greater than 10 cm H_2O may result in elevation of the entire waveform above the baseline pressure. Interpretation of the RAP is based on trends in data and not the absolute number. Find the end-expiration phase of the RAP waveform in the mechanically ventilated patient in Figure 13–7.

Conditions Leading to an Elevated RAP

Pressure and volume are proportional: An increase in volume can generate an increase in pressure. This is the basis for using pressures as proxies for volume status. There are circumstances, however, where an increase in pressure may occur without an increase in volume. Consider a balloon that is inflated with a given volume of water. Imagine squeezing the balloon: The pressure inside the balloon increases, but the volume does not change. Clinically, this is seen in circumstances such as cardiac tamponade or tension pneumothorax.

Pulmonic Valve Stenosis

The right ventricle has to overcome the fixed resistance (fixed afterload) of a stenotic or "tight" pulmonary valve to eject the stroke volume into the PA. As a result, there is reduced emptying of the right ventricle and an increase in the resistance to further ventricular filling. This is reflected by an elevated RAP.

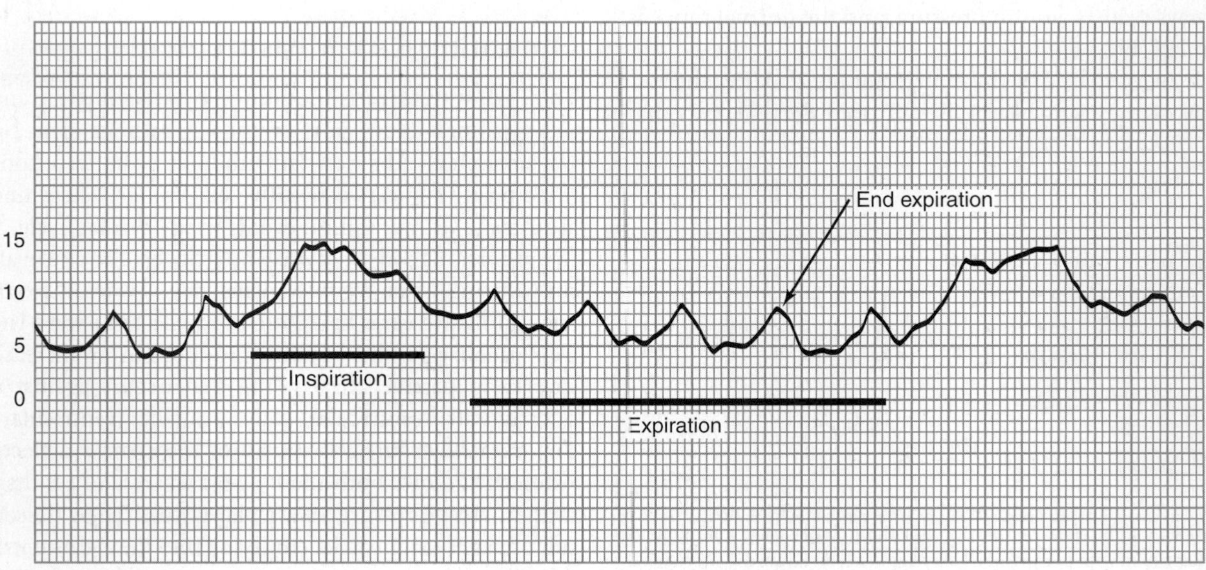

Figure 13–7 ■ End expiration phase on RAP waveform in a patient receiving mechanical ventilation.

Pulmonary Hypertension

Pulmonary hypertension increases the afterload to the right ventricle. As a result of higher afterload in the pulmonary circuit, there is reduced emptying of the right ventricle, and this is reflected by an elevated RAP.

Chronic or Severe Left Heart Failure

Inadequate cardiac output from the left ventricle results in "backward failure." The increased volume in the pulmonary circulation results in inadequate emptying of the right ventricle and increased resistance to ventricular filling. An elevated RAP will be seen.

Cardiac Tamponade

The right heart is a low-pressure system. As a result of this, any rapid fluid buildup in the pericardial space results in resistance to right ventricular filling. The RAP will be elevated.

Clinical Findings Associated with Elevated RAP

Clinical findings associated with an increased RAP vary according to the cause and duration. Signs and symptoms may include all or some of the following: distended neck veins, tachycardia, a right ventricular gallop (S3, S4, or both), right upper quadrant tenderness from liver engorgement, dependent or generalized edema, and ascites.

When elevated RAP is a result of left heart failure, signs and symptoms of left ventricular failure also will be found. These are discussed later in this module.

Collaborative and Independent Interventions for Elevated RAP

Interventions for elevated RAP are determined by the cause. In general, care is directed toward optimizing preload by reducing volume, for example by adding diuretic therapy. Overall goals are to decrease venous return to the right heart, increase contractility, and decrease the workload of the heart. Preload is reduced by fluid and sodium restrictions, and administration of diuretics or vasodilating medications.

Nursing care includes careful and frequent assessment of the patient's response to interventions. This includes keeping meticulous intake and output records, and obtaining daily weights. A care plan designed to decrease patient energy requirements is implemented. A dietary consult is obtained to provide patient and family education on sodium and fluid restrictions. Patient education includes information on the purpose and importance of all medications.

Conditions Leading to a Low RAP

A low right atrial pressure indicates low preload of the right heart. This is the result of either an actual or relative hypovolemia. Poor venous return to the heart for any reason is demonstrated in a low RAP.

Fluid Deficit

There are two types of fluid deficit. First, an actual hypovolemia results from loss of volume from the vascular system. Causes include hemorrhage, diuresis, dehydration from vomiting or diarrhea, and loss of body fluids from extensive burns.

Second, a relative hypovolemia results from vasodilation. Certain medications cause vasodilation, including IV and oral nitrates, some calcium channel blockers, angiotensin converting enzyme (ACE) inhibitors, hydralazine, and analgesics (morphine). Although intravenous nitroprusside is primarily used for its action on the arterioles, it is included here because it also dilates the venous bed. Use of these medications may cause a relative hypovolemia; fluid volume is not lost but only temporarily displaced in the venous system. This reduces venous return to the right heart and produces a low RAP, reflecting low preload.

Some conditions have also been associated with a relative hypovolemia. Liver failure results in loss of protein which causes an egress of fluid into the interstitium. Neurogenic shock, as in the case of a spinal cord injury, causes venous pooling in the extremities (below the level of the lesion). Anaphylaxis causes mediator release which results in vasodilation. A systemic inflammatory response syndrome, caused by burns, trauma, pancreatitis, or infections, can cause a relative hypovolemia due to inflammatory mediator release. In these conditions, mediators are released from bacterial cell walls which cause dilation of the vascular smooth muscle that lines the arterioles and increase intravascular permeability that allows third spacing. Fevers, often associated with these infections, may also be present. These conditions produce a relative hypovolemia as more fluid stays in the peripheral vascular system and less returns to the right atrium (See Module 18, Alterations in Oxygen Delivery and Oxygen Consumption: Shock States).

Clinical Findings Associated with Decreased RAP

Clinical findings accompanying decreased RAP depend on the severity of the condition. Typical findings include tachycardia, hypotension, diminished pulse amplitude, flat neck veins in a supine position, reduced CO, thirst, poor skin turgor, dry mucous membranes, and decreased urine output. If right heart preload (volume) is severely reduced, the signs and symptoms of shock also will be present (See Module 18, Alterations in Oxygen Delivery and Consumption: Shock States).

Interventions for Decreased RAP

Interventions for a low RAP are determined by the cause. Interventions are directed toward optimizing preload by restoring volume. Dehydration from overly vigorous diuresis, burns, vomiting, or diarrhea is corrected by oral replacement when possible or by careful intravenous hydration. Hemorrhage may need surgical correction. Crystalloid IV fluids and blood products replace volume lost by hemorrhage. The hypovolemia or low-preload state related to sepsis is treated with replacement fluids; the administration of appropriate antibiotics to treat the sepsis; and careful adjustment of vasoconstricting medications, such as dopamine and norepinephrine. Vasodilating medications are also a potential cause of low preload because pooling of blood in a dilated vascular system reduces venous return to the heart. Intravenous nitrates and nitroprusside are typically titrated by the nurse, based on physician orders. Oral medications with vasodilating properties should be identified and administration of these agents should be discussed with the physician prior to administration. As previously mentioned, the nurse provides careful and frequent assessment of the patient's response to the interventions described here. Intake and output are monitored and evaluated, and changes in the patient's weight provide important information.

SECTION THREE REVIEW

1. RAP is measured through which port of the catheter?
   - **A.** proximal port
   - **B.** distal port
   - **C.** thermistor wire port
   - **D.** balloon inflation port
2. RAP is a reflection of
   - **A.** PAWP
   - **B.** preload of the right heart
   - **C.** afterload of the right heart
   - **D.** left heart function
3. Normal mean RAP is
   - **A.** less than 4 mm Hg
   - **B.** 2 to 6 mm Hg
   - **C.** 6 to 12 mm Hg
   - **D.** 14 to 20 mm Hg
4. Right heart failure results in a RAP that is
   - **A.** lower than normal
   - **B.** above normal
   - **C.** within normal range
   - **D.** unchanged
5. Hypovolemia results in a RAP that is
   - **A.** lower than normal
   - **B.** above normal
   - **C.** within normal range
   - **D.** unchanged

Answers: 1. A, 2. B, 3. B, 4. B, 5. A

SECTION FOUR: Right Ventricular Pressure

At the completion of this section, the learner will be able to recognize the normal right ventricular (RV) waveform, and identify appropriate nursing interventions related to RV waveforms.

RV pressure is not continuously monitored with a traditional PA catheter but is observed and documented during insertion of the catheter. It is the responsibility of the nurse to recognize a RV waveform.

The normal RV systolic pressure is 20 to 30 mm Hg. This represents the pressure necessary to exceed the pressure in the PA (RV afterload), open the pulmonary valve, and eject blood into the pulmonary circulation. RV diastolic pressure range is low (2 to 8 mm Hg). This right end-diastolic pressure directly reflects the preload status of the right ventricle and should approximate the RAP.

The RV waveform has a characteristic pattern. It consists of a steep upstroke and a sharp downstroke (Fig. 13–8). Compare this waveform to the right atrial waveform in Figure 13–5.

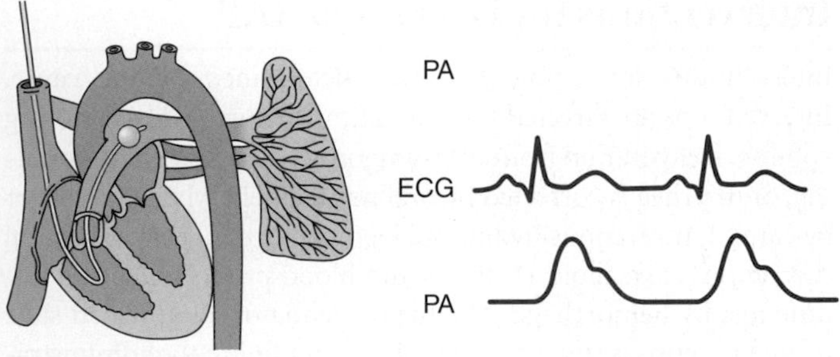

Figure 13–8 ■ Right ventricular (RV) Waveform. (Reprinted with permission. Copyright © 2000 Edwards Lifesciences. Swan-Ganz® is a trademark of Edwards Lifesciences Corporation, registered in the U.S. Patent and Trademark Office)

Although there is a marked increase in systolic pressure, the RV diastolic pressure remains essentially the same as the RAP. That is important information in identifying the waveform of a catheter that has slipped back into the right ventricle.

The RV waveform is typically seen on only two occasions:

1. During insertion, as the catheter is floated through the RV
2. If the catheter tip retreats from its proper position in the PA into the RV

Observation of this waveform at any time other than insertion indicates that the catheter tip has retreated from its proper position in the PA. This has important implications from both a technical perspective and from a patient safety consideration. All parameters obtained from the catheter, including the CO, are incorrect. Most importantly, the patient is at risk for cardiac arrhythmias. Irritation of the right ventricular endothelium by the catheter tip causes abnormal cardiac rhythms (premature ventricular contractions, ventricular tachycardia; refer to Module 14, Assessment of Cardiac Rhythm: Basic Electrocardiographic Rhythm Interpretation). In addition, the right bundle branch portion of the cardiac conduction system lies close to the surface of the right ventricular septum. Therefore, irritation can cause cardiac conduction disturbances such as heart block and bundle branch blocks (for a discussion, see Module 14). For these reasons, it is important to recognize the RV waveform and its corresponding pressures.

The cardiac rhythm and waveforms are monitored by the nurse as the catheter is floated into the PA. Once the catheter has been properly positioned in the PA, a change to an RV waveform should be reported immediately to the physician to expedite repositioning of the catheter. Some hospitals or units have specific nursing protocols to follow when a PA catheter retreats into the RV. It is the responsibility of the nurse to be aware of unit policy and state licensure guidelines related to manipulating the catheter to a different location. In addition to observing for arrhythmias and notifying the physician for repositioning, some facilities have specific protocols that instruct the nurse to pull the catheter back into the right atrium or inflate the balloon to foster flotation of the catheter tip back into the PA.

Once the catheter has been inserted, the exposed portion of the catheter is considered contaminated and should not be advanced unless a sterile sleeve was placed over the catheter before insertion. Use of these optional sleeves allows repositioning of the catheter without increasing the risk of infection.

SECTION FOUR REVIEW

1. The normal range for RV systolic pressure is
   A. 10 to 20 mm Hg
   B. 20 to 30 mm Hg
   C. 30 to 40 mm Hg
   D. 40 to 50 mm Hg
2. The normal range for RV diastolic pressure is
   A. 2 to 8 mm Hg
   B. 4 to 10 mm Hg
   C. 6 to 12 mm Hg
   D. 8 to 14 mm Hg
3. The BEST description of an RV waveform is
   A. a soft undulating pattern
   B. a steep upstroke followed by a sharp downstroke
   C. sharply notched with a slow downstroke
   D. almost flat
4. The greatest potential for abnormal cardiac rhythms occurs when the PA catheter is in the
   A. superior vena cava
   B. right atrium
   C. right ventricle
   D. PA
5. The RV waveform is typically seen by the nurse
   A. during insertion of the PA catheter
   B. if the catheter retreats from its original position in the PA
   C. on a continuous basis
   D. A and B

Answers: 1. B, 2. A, 3. B, 4. C, 5. D

SECTION FIVE: Pulmonary Artery Pressure

At the completion of this section, the learner will be able to recognize a normal PA waveform and identify common physical findings and nursing interventions related to abnormal PA pressures.

Pulmonary artery pressure (PAP) is read as a systolic and diastolic pressure. It is obtained from the distal port of the PA catheter. Under normal conditions, the PAP is considered to reflect both right and left heart pressures.

The **pulmonary artery systolic** (PAS) **pressure** reflects the highest pressure generated by the RV during systole. The normal range is 20 to 30 mm Hg. The **pulmonary artery diastolic** (PAD) **pressure** is normally 2 to 5 mm Hg higher than the pulmonary artery wedge pressure (PAWP). In the absence of chronic obstructive pulmonary disease, pulmonary embolism, mitral stenosis, and heart rates greater than 125 beats per minute (BPM), the PAD pressure is used to estimate the left ventricular preload status. This is possible because there are no valves to impede the transmission of left atrial pressure to the PA. The normal range for PAD pressure is 8 to 15 mm Hg. After the PAD pressure has been demonstrated to correlate with the PAWP, it is used to monitor left ventricular preload status.

Taking Measurements

The PA waveform is monitored continuously by a transducer attached to the distal port of the catheter. The PA waveform has a characteristic pattern (Fig. 13–9). It consists of a steep upstroke and a downstroke that is distinguished by a dicrotic notch formed by the closure of the pulmonic valve.

On entering the PA from the right ventricle, the top of the waveform stays essentially the same height, but the bottom or diastolic portion of the waveform elevates. Another identifying feature of the PA waveform is the dicrotic notch on the downstroke. The dicrotic notch is formed by the closure of the pulmonic valve. If the catheter tip retreats into the right ventricle, the diastolic pressure drops, and the dicrotic notch is lost. Knowledge of these waveform properties allows the nurse to identify catheter position correctly. This is important because catheter retreat into the right ventricle could result in dysrhythmias (see Section Four of this module).

The PA pressure waveform represents arterial pressure on the right side of the heart. The systolic upstroke of the PA pressure tracing represents right ventricular ejection and is preceded by ventricular electrical depolarization. The PA pressure may be obtained clinically by printing out both the ECG and PA pressure tracings. The PA systolic pressure will follow the *QRS* wave of the ECG. Correlate the ECG with the PA pressure tracing in Figure 13–9.

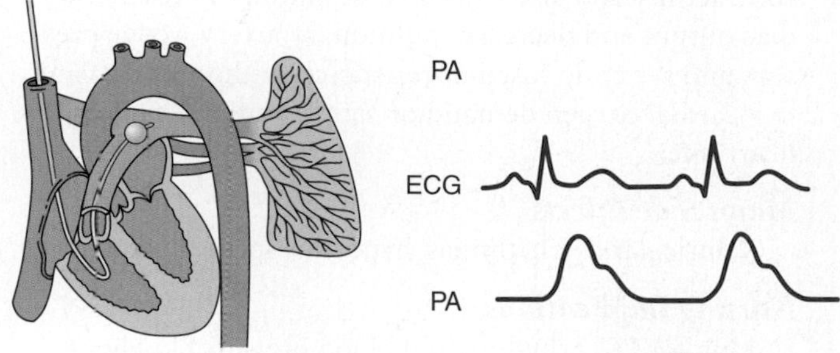

Figure 13–9 ■ PA Waveform. (Reprinted with permission. Copyright © 2000 Edwards Lifesciences. Swan-Ganz® is a trademark of Edwards Lifesciences Corporation, registered in the U.S. Patent and Trademark Office)

Elevated Pulmonary Artery Systolic Pressure

The PA pressure is generated by the right ventricle. Anything that increases the afterload of the right ventricle (i.e., increases the pulmonary vascular resistance) results in an elevated PAS pressure. Examples include pulmonary hypertension from any cause, including chronic lung disease, pulmonary embolism, and hypoxemia.

Clinical Findings

Symptoms vary according to the cause, severity, and duration of the elevated pressure. Assessment of the patient with pulmonary hypertension may reveal signs of right heart failure, including distended neck veins, peripheral edema, a tender liver, and ascites. Palpation may reveal a right ventricular lift. Auscultation may reveal S3 and S4 heart sounds. Patients with chronic lung disease have a chronically elevated PAS pressure. A pulmonary embolus increases PAS pressure. The patient with a pulmonary embolus may present as a medical emergency with dyspnea, chest pain, hemoptysis, and hemodynamic instability.

Elevated Pulmonary Artery Diastolic Pressure

Conditions that affect the left heart, such as angina or myocardial infarction, fluid overload, mitral stenosis, and left-to-right intracardiac shunts, are associated with a high PAD pressure.

Clinical Findings

Clinical findings associated with left heart failure may result in some or all of the following signs and symptoms: dyspnea, tachycardia, S3 or S4, and bilateral crackles in the lungs. CO is reduced and PAWP is elevated.

Interventions

Interventions for an elevated PAS or PAD pressure are determined by the cause. In general, care is directed toward reducing preload by administering diuretics and restricting fluid and sodium intake. Additionally, there are some novel therapies aimed at pulmonary vascular vasodilation that have been discovered to treat pulmonary hypertension. Cardiac contractility is improved by the use of inotropic medications, such as digoxin, dobutamine, dopamine, and amrinone. (See RELATED PHARMACOTHERAPY box) When indicated, the use of an intra-aortic balloon pump reduces the afterload of a failing heart as well as increases the blood supply to the heart by augmenting the patient's diastolic pressure. Nursing care includes careful administration of potent medications, intake and output measurements, and daily weights. Care is focused on reducing the workload of the heart by planning physical activities that are followed by rest periods.

Low Pulmonary Artery Diastolic Pressure

Low PAD pressure typically indicates a low preload state related to inadequate venous return to the left heart.

Clinical Findings

Clinical findings associated with low preload states include tachycardia, flat neck veins, clear lungs, dry oral mucosa, poor skin turgor, hypotension, and decreased urine output. If severe, the signs and symptoms of advanced shock, such as cool and clammy skin, also may be seen.

Interventions

Interventions are directed toward improving left ventricle (LV) preload through volume replacement. Nursing care includes managing fluid replacement through an ongoing assessment of the patient's hydration status and hemodynamic parameters. Changes in patient weight and intake and output data are important to assess.

RELATED PHARMACOTHERAPY: Inotropic Agents

Phosphodiesterase Inhibitors
Milrinone (Primacor)

Action and Uses
Inhibitory action against cyclic-AMP phosphodiesterase in cardiac and smooth vascular muscle. Increases cardiac contractility and also causes vasodilation. Increases cardiac output and decreases pulmonary artery wedge pressure and systemic vascular resistance, without increasing myocardial oxygen demand or significantly increasing heart rate.

Major Side Effects
Ventricular dysrhythmias, hypotension, headache.

Nursing Implications
Monitor ECG rhythms and blood pressure closely.

Beta-Adrenergic Agonists
Dobutamine (Dobutrex)

Action and Uses
Acts on myocardial beta receptors and alpha-adrenergic receptors. Increases cardiac output and decreases pulmonary wedge pressure and total systemic vascular resistance with little or no effect on BP. Can increase conduction through AV node.

Major Side Effects
Increased heart rate and blood pressure, anginal pain, headache.

Nursing Implications
Monitor therapeutic effectiveness. At any given dosage level, drug takes 10-20 minutes to produce peak effects.
Monitor ECG and BP continuously during administration.
Marked increases in blood pressure and heart rate, or the appearance of dysrhythmias or other adverse cardiac effects are usually reversed promptly by reduction in dosage.

SECTION FIVE REVIEW

1. The normal range for PAS pressure is
   A. 10 to 20 mm Hg
   B. 20 to 30 mm Hg
   C. 30 to 40 mm Hg
   D. 40 to 50 mm Hg
2. The normal range for PAD pressure is
   A. 2 to 8 mm Hg
   B. 4 to 10 mm Hg
   C. 6 to 12 mm Hg
   D. 8 to 15 mm Hg
3. The BEST description of a PA waveform is a
   A. soft undulating pattern
   B. steep upstroke followed by a sharp downstroke
   C. sharply notched upstroke with a steep downstroke
   D. steep upstroke and a downstroke distinguished by a dicrotic notch
4. Under normal conditions, a high PAD pressure suggests
   A. hypovolemia (low preload)
   B. hypervolemia (high preload)
   C. good left heart function
   D. right heart failure
5. A PAD is 2 mm Hg. The nurse should anticipate which of the following interventions?
   A. administer diuretics and implement fluid restrictions
   B. volume replacement
   C. administer a positive inotropic agent
   D. no intervention because 2 mm Hg is acceptable

Answers: 1. B, 2. D, 3. D, 4. B, 5. B

SECTION SIX: Pulmonary Artery Wedge Pressure

At the completion of this section, the learner will be able to recognize a normal pulmonary artery wedge pressure waveform (PAWP), relate left ventricular preload to PAWP, and identify common physical findings and appropriate nursing interventions related to abnormal PAWP pressures.

Preload is defined as the pressure or stretch exerted on the wall of the ventricle by the volume of blood filling it at end diastole. The Frank-Starling law of the heart states that the greater the myocardial fibers are stretched during diastole, the more they will shorten (contract) during systole, and the greater the force of contraction will be until a physiologic limit has been reached (refer to Module 12, Determinants and Assessment of Cardiac Output). The way myocardial fibers are stretched is through preload or volume.

This concept of preload applies to both the right and left ventricles, but emphasis is placed on the left ventricle because it is the capacity of the left ventricle to function as a pump that determines patient outcome. Left ventricular preload is measured directly only during a cardiac catheterization or following open heart surgery when a left atrial line is placed. Left ventricular preload is indirectly measured with a PA catheter through measurement of PAWP. It is obtained through the distal port of the PA catheter. The normal range is 4 to 12 mm Hg. Similar to the RAP, when the *c* wave is not visible (as is the usual case with the PAWP tracing) the PAWP is read as the mean of the *a* wave. The PAWP waveform (Fig. 13–10) is similar in appearance to the right atrial waveform shown in Figure 13–5.

To obtain a PAWP, the catheter balloon is inflated slowly, allowing the catheter to float and "wedge" in a small branch of the PA. Inflation of the balloon is stopped as soon as the characteristic PAWP pattern is observed (Fig. 13–11). The inflated balloon stops the forward flow of blood through that vessel.

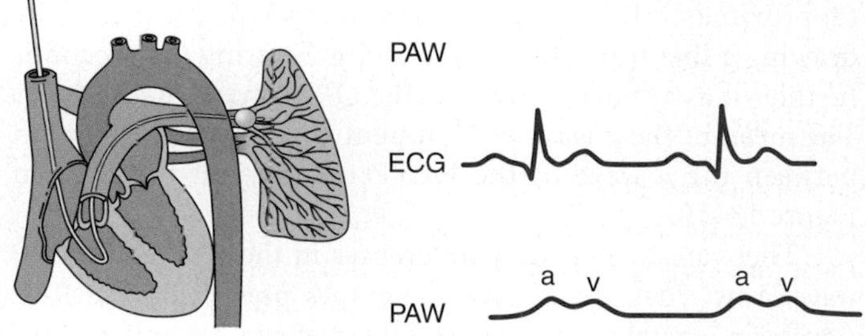

Figure 13–10 ■ Pulmonary artery wedge waveform. (Reprinted with permission. Copyright © 2000 Edwards Lifesciences. Swan-Ganz® is a trademark of Edwards Lifesciences Corporation, registered in the U.S. Patent and Trademark Office)

Because there are no valves in the pulmonary circulation, the catheter sitting in the PA "sees" through the pulmonary capillaries, pulmonary vein, left atrium, and into the left ventricle. Because the mitral valve remains open until the end of ventricular diastole, the left atrium and ventricle essentially function as one open chamber until the mitral valve closes. This is why the PAWP reflects the pressure in the left ventricle at end diastole. In the absence of mitral valve disease, the PAWP is considered an accurate estimate of left ventricular preload. It provides information about the volume status of the left ventricle and aids in the evaluation of left ventricular compliance. An elevated PAWP suggests a stiff, noncompliant

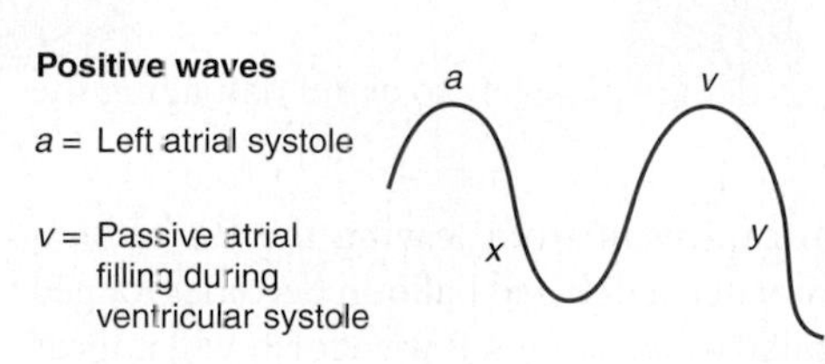

Figure 13–11 ■ A labeled PAW waveform.

left ventricle that contracts poorly. A low PAWP indicates that preload is low.

PAWP Waveform Analysis

The first positive wave is the *a* wave, produced by the rise in atrial pressure caused by left atrial contraction. The second positive wave is the *v* wave, formed as the left atrium fills during ventricular systole. The *c* wave, not typically seen on the PAWP waveform, is produced by closure of the mitral valve at the initiation of ventricular systole.

The two negative PAWP waveforms are the *x* and *y* descents. The first negative descent is the *x* wave, which reflects decreased volume in the left atrium after atrial systole. The *y* descent results from the pressure drop in the left atrium when the mitral valve opens just prior to atrial contraction, permitting passive emptying of the left atrium (as seen in Fig. 13–11).

Obtaining the PAWP is done in the same manner as that for the RAP. The tracing is printed out simultaneously with the ECG. Similar to the RAP, the *a* wave is found following the *P* wave of the ECG. Because the left side of the heart is more muscular, depolarization takes slightly more time (approximately 0.20 seconds) so the *a* wave may be located by drawing a line from the *P* wave and measuring 0.20 seconds further or as a "buried" wave in the *QRS* wave (Quaal, 2001). The mean of the *a* wave is documented. Find the correlation between the *a* wave of the PAWP tracing and the ECG in Figure 13–10.

There are two primary differences in the RAP and PAWP waveforms. First, the *c* wave sometimes present on the RAP waveform is rarely seen on a PAWP waveform. Second, normal PAWPs are higher than normal RAPs.

Key Points to Follow When Obtaining Pulmonary Artery Wedge Pressure

There are several technical points the nurse must consider when obtaining a PAWP measurement.

- Observe the waveform constantly during inflation, and stop inflation as soon as the PAWP is identified.
- Use the smallest inflation volume possible, and do not exceed the maximum recommended volume (typically less than 1.25 mL). This reduces the risk of balloon rupture.
- Maintain inflation only long enough to obtain a stable reading.
- Obtain the PAWP at end expiration, when intrathoracic pressure is most stable and less affected by respiratory variation.
- If resistance is felt during balloon inflation, stop! **Do not continue!** Allow the balloon to passively deflate. Call the health care provider.
- Allow the balloon to deflate passively to avoid damaging the balloon.

Pulmonary infarction can result from leaving the PA balloon inflated for too long or when a deflated balloon becomes lodged in the pulmonary capillary bed. A PAWP waveform will appear on the monitor. The patient should be turned or made to cough to relieve a lodged balloon. Open the stopcock on the port and remove the syringe to allow passive deflation of the balloon. The balloon may rupture from repeated overfilling. If you are unable to obtain a PAWP waveform after instilling the proper amount of air through the PA catheter balloon port, turn the balloon lumen off to the patient. Label the lumen "**Do not use.**" Notify the physician.

Elevated Pulmonary Artery Wedge Pressure

Any condition that increases the left ventricular end-diastolic blood volume results in an elevated PAWP. The following conditions are associated with elevated PAWP:

- **Fluid overload.** Occurs with overly aggressive fluid replacement, although normal kidneys usually compensate. Patients with acute and chronic renal failure often have fluid overload.
- **Left ventricular failure.** Poor contractility results in inadequate emptying of the ventricle.
- **Ischemia.** An ischemic myocardium becomes "stiff" and resistant to ventricular filling.
- **Mitral stenosis.** Mitral stenosis creates a high left atrial pressure, which is transmitted back into the pulmonary vasculature (for a discussion of mitral stenosis, see Module 15).
- **Cardiac tamponade.** Accumulation of fluid between the pericardium and the heart results in resistance to ventricular filling. The RAP, PAD, and PAWP elevate, and all three values are similar. This is known as diastolic equalization and is a hallmark of cardiac tamponade.

Clinical Findings

Clinical findings related to an elevated PAWP vary according to the degree of elevation but typically include tachycardia, exertional dyspnea, orthopnea, paroxysmal nocturnal dyspnea, crackles in the lung fields, and an S3 or S4 gallop at the apex. Neck veins are distended.

Interventions

Interventions are directed toward optimizing preload by administration of diuretics and vasodilators along with sodium and fluid restrictions. Intravenous and oral nitrates dilate the venous bed and displace fluid, which lower preload by reducing the venous return to the heart. Control of dysrhythmias helps the heart to pump more effectively. Afterload is reduced by administration of arteriole vasodilators, such as nitroprusside (Nipride), and ACE inhibitors, such as captopril (Capoten). By dilating the peripheral arterioles, these drugs reduce afterload, promote emptying of the ventricle, and effectively reduce cardiac work and myocardial oxygen requirements. Contractility is enhanced by careful titration of inotropic medications, such as digoxin, dobutamine (Dobutrex), and amrinone (Inocor). If these interventions fail to improve PAWP and CO, an intra-aortic balloon pump may be required (See Module 18, Alterations in Oxygen Delivery and Oxygen Consumption: Shock States).

The nurse is responsible for careful titration of potent vasoactive medications to improve hemodynamics. Manipulation of medications and treatments is based on astute physical assessments correlated with current hemodynamic parameters obtained from the PA catheter. Critical thinking at the bedside is crucial to improved patient outcomes. Frequent nursing assessments, meticulous intake and output records, and daily weights are crucial to follow the response to treatment.

Low Pulmonary Artery Wedge Pressure

A low PAWP typically is related to inadequate circulating blood volume.

Clinical Findings

Clinical findings include flat neck veins, clear lungs, low pulse pressure, decreased urine output, hypotension, tachycardia, and likely complaints of thirst.

Interventions

Interventions include careful replacement of fluid or blood products by correlating the PAWP with an ongoing assessment of the patient's response to treatment. Hourly urine output, careful intake and output records, and daily weights are indicated.

SECTION SIX REVIEW

1. What is the normal range of the PAWP?
   A. 2 to 10 mm Hg
   B. 4 to 12 mm Hg
   C. 8 to 16 mm Hg
   D. 10 to 18 mm Hg
2. The BEST description of a PAWP waveform is a
   A. soft undulating pattern
   B. steep upstroke followed by a sharp downstroke
   C. sharply notched with a slow downstroke
   D. sawtooth pattern
3. In a hypovolemic patient, the PAWP is
   A. well within the normal range
   B. low-normal or below normal range
   C. high-normal or above normal range
   D. high or low
4. In congestive heart failure, the expected PAWP is
   A. well within the normal range
   B. low-normal or below normal range
   C. high-normal or above normal range
   D. high or low
5. Which waveform most closely resembles the PAWP waveform?
   A. right atrial waveform
   B. right ventricular waveform
   C. PA waveform
   D. systemic arterial waveform

Answers: 1. B, 2. A, 3. B, 4. C, 5. A

SECTION SEVEN: Systemic Arterial Pressure

At the completion of this section, the learner will be able to discuss the physiology underlying the systemic arterial waveform and identify the components of a normal systemic arterial waveform.

Blood pressure is a function of blood flow (CO) and the elasticity of the blood vessels. Systolic blood pressure normally ranges between 100 and 140 mm Hg. Systolic pressure reflects the highest pressure exerted by the left ventricle as it ejects the stroke volume into the aorta. Diastolic blood pressure normally ranges between 60 and 80 mm Hg. The **mean arterial pressure** (MAP) is the average arterial pressure throughout the cardiac cycle. It normally ranges between 70 and 90 mm Hg (see Section Eight). Advantages of direct (invasive) blood pressure monitoring in the high-acuity patient include the following:

- Knowledge of minute-to-minute changes in blood pressure
- Increased accuracy of measurement in the hypotensive patient
- More precise titration of medications and fluids
- The capacity to obtain arterial blood gases (ABGs) and blood samples without pain and discomfort to the patient

The equipment needed to monitor systemic arterial blood pressures is the same as the equipment used to monitor PA pressures, except a small catheter is used and inserted into a peripheral artery or femoral artery.

The arterial waveform has a characteristic morphology that is related to the cardiac cycle (Fig. 13–12). When the aortic valve opens, blood is ejected into the aorta. This forms a steep upstroke on the arterial waveform, called the anacrotic limb. The top of this limb represents the peak, or highest systolic pressure, which appears digitally on the monitor as the systolic pressure. After this peak pressure, the waveform descends. This descent forms the dicrotic limb and represents systolic ejection of blood that is continuing at a reduced force. The descending, or dicrotic, limb is disrupted by the dicrotic notch, which is an important point on the waveform. The dicrotic notch represents closure of the aortic valve and the beginning of ventricular diastole. The lowest portion of the waveform (baseline) represents the diastolic pressure and is reflected digitally on the monitor.

Arterial pressure monitoring is common in high-acuity settings. The nurse typically is responsible for setting up the equipment for catheter insertion, calibrating the equipment to ensure

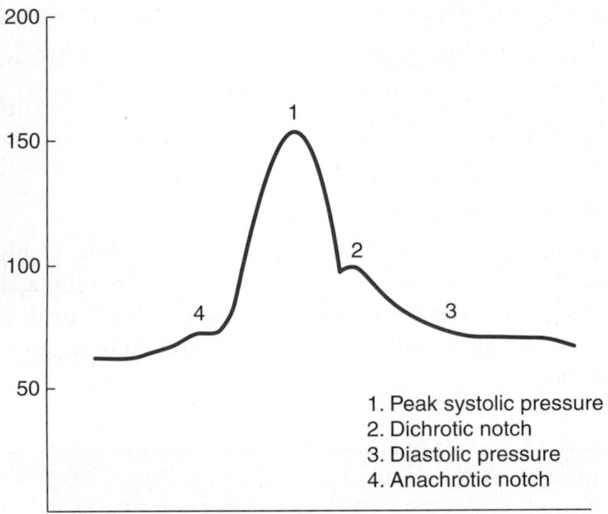

Figure 13–12 ■ Components of the systemic arterial pressure waveform. (Reprinted with permission. Copyright © 2000 Edwards Lifesciences. Swan-Ganz® is a trademark of Edwards Lifesciences Corporation, registered in the U.S. Patent and Trademark Office)

accurate readings, and assisting the physician with the procedure. The two most common insertion sites for arterial monitoring include the radial and femoral arteries.

Once the arterial catheter is in place, the nurse is responsible for patient safety and comfort, and maintenance of the system as discussed in Section One. Securing the pressure tubing to prevent dislodgement and possible exsanguination is an important nursing responsibility. Safety measures for monitoring to prevent exsanguination include covering all caps along the monitoring system, securing all connections, and ensuring that all monitor alarms are on.

Monitoring circulation distal to the insertion site is another important nursing function. The skin color and temperature and all pulses distal to the insertion site are regularly assessed and documented. Any alteration in circulation is promptly brought to the attention of the physician. The site is observed frequently for signs of infection: redness, warmth, edema, and drainage. Unit-specific protocols and responsibilities related to arterial monitoring are typically described in hospital policy and procedure manuals.

Arterial monitoring provides the capacity to monitor the patient's blood pressure on a continuous basis. Depending on specific monitor characteristics, digital blood pressure readings are usually updated at 4- to 6-second intervals. This allows the nurse to monitor the patient's response to interventions without having to disturb the patient to take a manual blood pressure reading.

The common practice of comparing systemic arterial pressure measured with the arterial line against a noninvasive blood pressure is not supported by the literature (Bridges & Middleton, 1997). Each patient should be assessed to determine which system is appropriate for monitoring blood pressure and then the system is optimized. The two pressures do not always agree. The arterial catheter measures blood pressure and the noninvasive blood pressure cuff measures blood flow. Blood pressure does not always equal blood flow, especially when the patient has vasoconstriction (see Ohm's law, discussed in Module 12, Determinants and Assessment of Cardiac Output).

SECTION SEVEN REVIEW

1. The dicrotic notch on the descending limb of the arterial waveform represents
   - **A.** opening of the aortic valve
   - **B.** closure of the aortic valve
   - **C.** the beginning of ventricular systole
   - **D.** the diastolic pressure
2. The highest point on the arterial waveform denotes the
   - **A.** anacrotic limb
   - **B.** peak systolic pressure
   - **C.** mean arterial pressure
   - **D.** diastolic pressure
3. The lowest point on the arterial waveform represents the
   - **A.** anacrotic limb
   - **B.** peak systolic pressure
   - **C.** mean arterial pressure
   - **D.** diastolic pressure
4. The indentation on the descending limb of the arterial waveform is called the
   - **A.** anacrotic limb
   - **B.** dicrotic notch
   - **C.** peak systolic pressure
   - **D.** dicrotic limb
5. Which of the following is a common insertion site for monitoring arterial blood pressure?
   - **A.** carotid artery
   - **B.** radial artery
   - **C.** femoral artery
   - **D.** B and C

Answers: 1. B, 2. B, 3. D, 4. B, 5. D

SECTION EIGHT: Derived Parameters

At the completion of this section, the learner will be able to discuss the implications of selected derived hemodynamic parameters and calculate the following derived hemodynamic parameters: cardiac index, stroke volume index, mean arterial pressure, systemic vascular resistance, and pulmonary vascular resistance, left ventricular stroke work index, and right ventricular stroke work index.

Cardiac Index

As discussed in Section Two, CO is the amount of blood ejected from the heart in one minute. The normal range is 4 to 8 L/min. As a generic or raw value, the CO does not take the size of the patient into account. The cardiac index (CI) individualizes the CO to the patient by taking body size into consideration. Knowledge of the CO and body surface area (BSA) are all that is necessary to determine the CI. The formula is

$$CI = CO/BSA$$

The normal CI is 2.4 to 4.0 L/min/m^2. The BSA is simply a function of height and weight. Most monitors will calculate the BSA when the patient's height and weight are entered. The following example demonstrates the importance of calculating the CI.

	Patient A	Patient B
Height	6 feet	5 feet
Weight	216 lb	118 lb
BSA	2.22 m^2	1.50 m^2
CO	4.0 L/min	4.0 L/min
CI	1.89 L/min/m2	2.4 L/min/m^2

Both patients have a CO of 4.0 L/min, which falls within the normal range, but the CI of patient A is well below normal and suggests a shock state. Using the CO alone does not indicate the gravity of the patient's hemodynamic status. The CI provides meaning to the CO and is the more important parameter to consider when making clinical decisions.

Stroke Volume and Stroke Volume Index

As discussed in Section Two, the stroke volume (SV) and stroke volume index (SVI) are used to assess cardiac function and cardiac contractility. With the traditional PA catheter, the SV is not directly measured. Stroke volume is a helpful parameter in interpreting the hemodynamic profile. A decreased stroke volume is seen in hypovolemia, cardiac failure, increased afterload, or in patients with cardiac valve problems. An increase in the stroke volume is seen with a reduction in afterload values. The cardiac output and cardiac index are assessed in the context of the preload values as well as the SV and SVI.

SV = Cardiac output/HR (normal SV = 50 to 100 mL/beat)
SVI = Cardiac index/HR (normal SVI = 25 to 45 mL/beat/m^2)

Mean Arterial Pressure

The MAP is an approximation of the average pressure in the systemic circulation throughout the cardiac cycle. The normal range is 70 to 90 mm Hg. The MAP is provided as a digital readout when an arterial line or automatic blood pressure equipment is in use. The MAP obtained from an arterial line is the most accurate because the mean actually is measured rather than calculated.

When direct arterial monitoring is not available, the MAP must be calculated. Keep in mind that MAPs calculated from cuff pressures (automatic or manual) have a potential for error because of extraneous factors, such as incorrect cuff size, differences in hearing, sensitivity of the instrument, and patient movement.

The formula for MAP reflects the components of the cardiac cycle. In normal heart rates, systole accounts for one third of the cycle and diastole for two thirds of the cycle.

$$MAP = SBP + 2(DBP)/3$$

Use the MAP formula to calculate the MAP for a patient with a blood pressure of 90/40 mm Hg. The correct answer is 57 mm Hg.

Systemic Vascular Resistance and Systemic Vascular Resistance Index

Systemic vascular resistance (SVR) is an estimate of left ventricular afterload. It represents an average of the resistance of all the vascular beds. Recall from Section Two that afterload is the resistance the left ventricle must overcome to open the aortic valve and eject the stroke volume into the systemic circulation. Afterload is one of the primary determinants of myocardial oxygen demand. The harder the heart works to pump blood out of the ventricle, the higher the myocardial oxygen requirements. A high SVR can reduce SV and CO. This is an important aspect to consider during regulation of potent vasoactive medications. These medications may improve MAP and afterload, but may also decrease SV.

Most monitors will calculate the SVR; however, it is helpful to understand the components that make up the formula. Recall from Module 12 that Ohm's law describes afterload. Left ventricular afterload is the product of a change in pressure (MAP – RAP) divided by flow (CO): (80 is a conversion factor).

$$SVR = \frac{(MAP - RAP) \times 80}{CO}$$

The SVR is expressed in dynes · sec · cm^{-5}, and the normal range is 800 to 1,200 dynes · sec · cm^{-5}. To individualize SVR to the patient, the CI is substituted for the CO in the formula. The formula for the SVR index (SVRI) is

$$SVRI = \frac{(MAP - RAP) \times 80}{CI}$$

The normal range for the SVRI is 1,970 to 2,390 dynes · sec · cm^{-5}/m^2. The indices of CI and SVRI are far better indicators of the patient's hemodynamic status than the CO and SVR alone because the indices are referenced to body size.

Elevated Systemic Vascular Resistance

A high SVR may be the result of multiple causes. In hypothermia, peripheral vasoconstriction occurs as a compensatory mechanism to keep core body temperature warm. In this circumstance, warming the patient may be the only intervention necessary to dilate the constricted peripheral vasculature, normalize SVR, and improve CO.

Hypovolemia can produce an elevated SVR due to the compensatory mechanisms that are activated. Inadequate circulating blood volume induces vasoconstriction. This mechanism results in the shunting of as much peripheral blood volume as possible back to the vital organs (heart, lungs, and brain). Careful fluid replacement normalizes the SVR.

In cardiac failure, hypotension initiates similar compensatory mechanisms. The peripheral vascular beds constrict in an attempt to increase the blood return to the heart, thereby increasing the blood pressure. However, in this situation, returning more blood (more preload) to an already failing heart does not help. The vasoconstriction itself results in an increased afterload, which means the already-struggling heart must now overcome more pressure to open the aortic valve and eject the stroke volume. This patient needs help on both preload and afterload reduction. Diuretics and nitrates reduce preload. Afterload reduction is done cautiously in a patient with low blood pressure. A vasodilator such as nitroprusside, or an ACE inhibitor, such as captopril, may be administered (see the RELATED PHARMACOTHERAPY box: Vasodilating Agents). Milrinone is an inotrope that improves myocardial contractility and causes vasodilation to reduce both afterload and preload. Reducing afterload makes it easier for the heart to eject SV, lessens cardiac work and myocardial oxygen demand, and improves CO.

Low Systemic Vascular Resistance

Physiologic responses to shock states, such as sepsis, neurogenic shock, and anaphylactic shock, initiate vasodilation. This results in low SVR. Low SVR results in low blood pressure. (Treatment of specific shock states is discussed in Module 18, Alterations in Oxygen Delivery and Consumption: Shock States.) SVR is improved with careful titration of vasoconstricting medications, such as dopamine, phenylephrine, or norepinephrine (Levophed).

Pulmonary Vascular Resistance

Pulmonary vascular resistance (PVR) is an estimate of right ventricular afterload. It represents an average of the resistance of pulmonary vascular beds. A high PVR reduces right ventricular SV and CO. Most monitors calculate PVR. However, it is helpful to understand the components that make up the formula. Recall from Module 12, Ohm's law describes afterload. Right ventricular afterload is the product of change in pressure (mean PAP – PAWP) divided by flow (CO): (80 is a conversion factor)

$$\text{PVR} = \frac{(\text{Mean PAP} - \text{PAWP}) \times 80}{\text{CO}}$$

The normal range is 50 to 250 dynes · sec · cm^{-5} (much less than SVR). To individualize PVR to the patient, CI is substituted for CO in the formula. The formula for the PVR index (PVRI) is

$$\text{PVRI} = \frac{(\text{Mean PAP} - \text{PAWP}) \times 80}{\text{CI}}$$

The normal range for the PVRI is 255 to 315 dynes · sec · cm^{-5}/m^2.

PVR or PVRI is elevated with acute lung injury, acute respiratory distress syndrome, pulmonary hypertension, and pulmonary congestion. Like SVR, vasodilators decrease PVR.

Left Ventricular Stroke Work Index

Left ventricular stroke work index (LVSWI) is the amount of work involved in moving blood in the left ventricle with each heartbeat. A lot of information goes into calculating the LVSWI because it represents work performed that is influenced by both pressure the heart beats against and the volume the heart must pump. Variables in the calculation of LVSWI are first collected. These include SVI, MAP, and PAWP. Once all the information is obtained, it is placed in the following equation:

$$\text{LVSWI} = [(\text{MAP} - \text{PAWP}) \times (\text{SVI}) \times (0.0136)]$$

MAP – PAWP = a measure of the pressure the left ventricle is ejecting against
SVI = the volume the left ventricle must eject
0.0136 = a constant that converts work to pressure

Normal values for LVSWI range from 50 to 62 g/m^2/beat. There are situations in which it helps to compare the LVSWI with the PAWP. PAWP reflects volume. LVSWI

RELATED PHARMACOTHERAPY: Vasodilating Agents

Non-Nitrate Vasodilator
Nitroprusside (Nitropress)

Action and Uses
Acts directly on vascular smooth muscle to produce peripheral vasodilation, with consequent lowering of arterial BP, associated with slight increase in heart rate, mild decrease in cardiac output, and moderate lowering of systemic vascular resistance.

Major Side Effects
Thiocyanate toxicity (profound hypotension, tinnitus, blurred vision, fatigue, metabolic acidosis, pink skin color, absence of reflexes, faint heart sounds, loss of consciousness).

Nursing Implications
Monitor constantly to titrate IV infusion rate to BP response.
Relieve adverse effects by slowing IV rate or by stopping drug; minimize them by keeping patient supine.
Monitor blood thiocyanate levels in patients receiving prolonged treatment or in patients with severe kidney dysfunction.

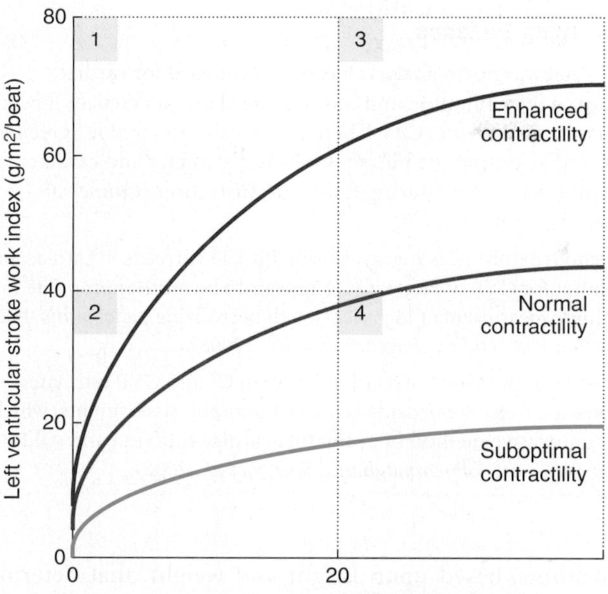

Figure 13–13 ■ Ventricular function curve.

represents pressure. When the left ventricle becomes stiffer (decreased compliance), the PAWP does not accurately reflect the workload of the left ventricle because the relationship between volume and pressure is not direct. It is best to calculate LVSWI.

Once the LVSWI is obtained, it is plotted on the *y* axis of a ventricular function curve (Fig. 13–13). PAWP is plotted on the *x* axis. This provides a picture of how the left ventricle is performing in light of the pressure and volume conditions. As noted in the diagram, an LVSWI between 40 and 60 g/m^2/beat, and a PAWP between 8 and 20 mm Hg, is best for left ventricular ejection.

Low LVSWI may be an indication that the patient is hypovolemic or has cardiac failure. In situations in which both the LVSWI and the PAWP are low, more volume may be needed to improve contractility. High LVSWI may be an indication of hypervolemia. In situations in which both the LVSWI and the PAWP are high, diuretics and vasodilators may be needed.

Right Ventricular Stroke Work Index

Right ventricular stroke work index (RVSWI) is the amount of work involved in moving blood in the right ventricle with each beat. The formula represents the pressure generated (mean PAP) multiplied by the volume pumped (SVI). Similar to LVSWI, the RVSWI increases or decreases because of changes in either pressure (mean PAP) or volume pumped (SVI). Normal values are 7.9 to 9.7 g/m2/beat. Increased and decreased values are treated much the same as for LVSWI.

$$RVSWI = [(meanPAP) - (RAP) \times (SVI) \times (0.00136)]$$

SV COMPONENT	RIGHT HEART	LEFT HEART
Preload	RAP	PAWP
Afterload	PVR, PVRI	SVR, SVRI
Contractility	RVSWI	LVSWI

SECTION EIGHT REVIEW

1. Normal range for MAP is
   A. 60 to 80 mm Hg
   B. 70 to 90 mm Hg
   C. 80 to 100 mm Hg
   D. 90 to 110 mm Hg
2. Using the following hemodynamic parameters: MAP = 90 mm Hg, RAP = 6 mm Hg, CO = 6.2 L/min, BSA = 1.8 m^2, calculate the CI.
   A. 2.00
   B. 3.44
   C. 4.50
   D. 2.96
3. Using the hemodynamic parameters in question 2, calculate the SVR.
   A. 1,832 dynes · sec/cm^{-5}
   B. 622 dynes · sec/cm^{-5}
   C. 1,083 dynes · sec/cm^{-5}
   D. 1,274 dynes · sec/cm^{-5}
4. Calculate the SVRI.
   A. 3,200 dynes · $sec/cm^{-5}/m^2$
   B. 1,020 dynes · $sec/cm^{-5}/m^2$
   C. 2,195 dynes · $sec/cm^{-5}/m^2$
   D. 1,953 dynes · $sec/cm^{-5}/m^2$
5. What is the normal range for the SVRI?
   A. 800 to 1,200 dynes · $sec/cm^{-5}/m^2$
   B. 250 to 680 dynes · $sec/cm^{-5}/m^2$
   C. 1,970 to 2,390 dynes · $sec/cm^{-5}/m^2$
   D. 1,200 to 1,500 dynes · $sec/cm^{-5}/m^2$
6. The LVSWI should be used instead of the PAWP in assessing left ventricular function in cases of
   A. hypovolemia
   B. congestive heart failure
   C. decreased compliance
   D. hypervolemia

Answers: 1. B, 2. B, 3. C, 4. D, 5. C, 6. C

SECTION NINE: Advances in Hemodynamic Monitoring Technologies

At the completion of this section, the learner will be able to describe newer hemodynamic monitoring technologies.

Several studies have questioned the efficacy of the pulmonary artery catheter (Connors et al., 1985; Peters et al., 2003). While the PA catheter continues to be in use, the industry has developed several newer technologies in an effort to avoid the complications associated with the pulmonary artery catheter. The ideal cardiac output monitor should be noninvasive, valid, and reliable under various hemodynamic situations, easy to use, continuous, and cost-effective. To date, there is not a single technology that meets all of these criteria. A brief description of the following technologies is presented: doppler, pulse contour analysis, and impedance cardiography.

Emerging Evidence

- Arterial waveform analysis has been proposed for cardiac output determination and monitoring (FloTrac/Vigileo; Edwards Lifesciences, Irvine, CA). There is clinically acceptable agreement in cardiac output via pulmonary artery catheter and cardiac output via FloTrac during fluid administration *(Cannesson, Attof, Rosamel et al., 2007).*
- Hemodynamic measurements using PiCCO correlate to cardiac index but not for CVP or Hct. PiCCO appears to be more appropriate for volume measurement in patients with necrotizing pancreatitis than CVP or Hct *(Huber, Umgelter, & Reindl, 2008).*
- There is significant correlation between CI and CVP estimates obtained from the bedside echocardiographic assessments, which is a noninvasive method of evaluating cardiac function and volume status *(Gunst, Ghaemmaghami, Sperry et al., 2008).*

Doppler

Doppler ultrasound is a technology first used in the 1840s and continues to be widely used in clinical practice today. Doppler ultrasound measures blood flow velocity in the vessel. When applied to hemodynamic monitoring, the doppler ultrasound can help to determine cardiac output, preload, afterload, and contractility status. Hemodynamic monitoring technologies using Doppler ultrasound have specific algorithms, based upon height and weight, that determine the cross sectional area of the vessel or valve. When the doppler probe is placed over the specific area, the blood flow velocity and heart rate are measured. With the blood flow velocity and the predetermined cross sectional area of the vessel or valve known, the stroke volume may be calculated. Calculating the cardiac output becomes simple based upon the CO formula, where CO = HR × SV. Table 13–1 reviews the different doppler ultrasound technologies.

TABLE 13–1 Newer technologies for hemodynamic monitoring

TECHNOLOGY	DESCRIPTION OF DEVICE	EXAMPLES OF PRODUCTS AND COMPANIES

Doppler	■ Technology is based upon Doppler echocardiography.
	■ Measures blood flow velocity in the vessel using a Doppler signal.
	■ Stroke volume is determined as a product of the velocity time integral and the cross-sectional area of the vessel or valve. The velocity time integral represents the distance a column of blood travels with every stroke.
	■ Calculates aortic flow time and peak velocity of blood flow.
	  ■ The flow time is corrected for heart rate and is a preload value.
	  ■ Peak velocity of blood flow is a contractility measurement.
	■ Esophageal probe	

	■ The esophagus lies in close proximity to the ascending aorta ■ An esophageal probe (the size of an 18 gauge NGT) is inserted into the esophagus orally. ■ Calculates aortic flow and peak velocity of blood flow.	*CardioQ*, Deltex Medical
	■ The noninvasive Doppler probe is placed on the suprasternal or left parasternal position to obtain waveforms. ■ Uses aorta and pulmonary artery outflow tracts to determine flow time and peak velocity.	*USCOM* Doppler
	■ Continuous cardiac output is monitored via an artery ■ Each technology uses a proprietary algorithm (mathematical) to determine the hemodynamic indicators.	
Pulse contour analysis	■ Requires that a central artery and central vein be used. ■ A special arterial thermodilution catheter in the femoral, axillary, or brachial artery is placed ■ Measures continuous CO by analysis of the arterial pulse contour. ■ An initial calibration and recalibration using transpulmonary thermodilution is required	*PiCCO* Pulsion Medical Systems
	■ Measures arterial pulse contour analysis using a special blood flow sensor ■ No special arterial catheter is needed: any arterial line may be used. ■ No thermodilution CO is needed for calibration	*FloTrac* Edwards Lifesciences, LLC
Impedance Cardiography	■ Noninvasive technology using 4 to 6 external skin electrodes ■ Uses high-frequency, low-amplitude current to measure the resistance to electrical current flow ■ Used to measure directly volume of electrically participating tissue and indirectly stroke volume, cardiac output, contractility indicators.	*IQ* Noninvasive medical technologies *BioZ* Cardiodynamics *RS-205* RS Medical Monitoring

Pulse Contour Analysis

Pulse waveforms are generated by many monitors, including pulse oximeters, arterial lines, or pulmonary artery catheters. The use of the pulse contour analysis is based upon the principle that the stroke volume may be measured by assessing the beat to beat changes in the amplitude of the pulse pressure as displayed on the waveform. Stroke volume affects systolic blood pressure. Consider the patient who is mechanically ventilated. With the positive pressure breath, volume returning to the heart is reduced due to the increased intrathoracic pressure encountered with the positive pressure breath. With a reduction in stroke volume, a change is seen in the beat to beat pulse amplitude (or variation in stroke volume). This change in pressure has been shown to be more sensitive to volume-related changes in cardiac index than the pulmonary artery wedge pressure (Bennett-Gurrero, et al., 2002).

Impedance Cardiography

Also known as bioimpedance cardiography, impedance cardiography is used to assess cardiac function through the use of a high-frequency, low-amplitude current to measure the resistance to flow of the electrical current. This is based upon the principle that electricity travels better through fluid than it does through bone, tissue, and air. Less impedance is then experienced in patients who are hypervolemic than those that are euvolemic or hypovolemic. Many settings use this technology in both the office and hospital setting. It has been also used to aid in diuretic therapy titration (Folan & Funk, 2008).

SECTION NINE REVIEW

1. Doppler ultrasound hemodynamic monitors measure the
   - a. pulmonary artery wedge pressure
   - b. blood flow velocity
   - c. pulse pressure variation
   - d. systolic blood pressure
2. Using the pulse contour analysis hemodynamic monitors, stroke volume is measured by assessing
   - a. the cardiac output
   - b. beat to beat changes in pulse amplitude
   - c. heart rate
   - d. central venous pressure
3. Impedance cardiography is based upon the principle that electrical current
   - a. travels best through air
   - b. travels best through bone
   - c. travels best through water
   - d. travels best through tissue

Answers: 1. B, 2. B, 3. C

POSTTEST

1. IV fluids can be infused through which port on the PA catheter?
   - A. proximal port
   - B. distal port
   - C. yellow port
   - D. balloon port
2. A PA catheter is an invasive diagnostic tool used to
   - A. determine right and left heart pressures
   - B. determine CO
   - C. sample $S\bar{v}O_2$
   - D. all of the above
3. In viewing a CO curve, a large curve indicates
   - A. a normal CO
   - B. a high CO
   - C. a low CO
   - D. an error in technique
4. CI is more specific than CO because
   - A. CI is a direct measurement instead of an estimate.
   - B. CI takes the size of the patient into consideration.
   - C. CO can be affected by afterload.
   - D. CO depends on patient position.
5. The hemodynamic measurement for right heart preload is
   - A. PAWP
   - B. PAS pressure
   - C. RAP
   - D. CO
6. Which of the following conditions cause a decreased RAP?
   - A. sepsis
   - B. cardiac tamponade
   - C. pulmonary hypertension
   - D. pulmonic valve stenosis
7. It is important to recognize a right ventricular waveform because
   - A. a catheter in the right ventricle can induce dysrhythmias
   - B. this pattern is the one that should be monitored constantly
   - C. this is the best indicator of hemodynamic status
   - D. this is the patient's pulmonary end diastolic pressure

8. The nurse notes an RV waveform on the bedside monitor during routine hemodynamic monitoring. Which of the following actions should the nurse institute?
A. nothing; this is normal
B. assess for altered CO
C. auscultate lungs for crackles
D. notify the physician immediately

9. A normal PA pressure waveform demonstrates which of the following characteristics?
A. a soft undulating pattern
B. a steep upstroke followed by a sharp downstroke
C. a sharply notched upstroke with a steep downstroke
D. a steep upstroke and a downstroke distinguished by a dicrotic notch

10. Which of the following clinical findings are associated with elevated PAD pressures? (choose all that apply)
A. dyspnea
B. S3 or S4
C. crackles
D. flat neck veins

11. PAWP is the hemodynamic measurement for
A. right ventricular preload
B. right ventricular contractility
C. left ventricular preload
D. left ventricular afterload

12. The nurse would expect the primary intervention for a symptomatic patient with a PAWP of 3 mm Hg to be
A. fluid restriction
B. decreasing preload
C. volume replacement
D. decreasing afterload

13. The dicrotic notch on the systemic arterial pressure waveform represents
A. left ventricular end-diastolic volume
B. right ventricular end-diastolic volume
C. beginning of ventricular diastole
D. beginning of ventricular systole

14. Important nursing interventions for the patient with arterial pressure monitoring include
A. calibrating the equipment
B. promoting patient safety and comfort
C. securing the tubing to prevent dislodgement
D. monitoring circulation distal to the insertion site

15. To assess the afterload status of the left ventricle, one should
A. calculate the pulmonary vascular resistance
B. calculate the systemic vascular resistance
C. determine the mean arterial pressure
D. determine the CI

16. Which is the most important parameter to follow when titrating inotropic drugs on a patient with poor left ventricular function?
A. CO
B. CI
C. MAP
D. RAP

Posttest answers with rationale are found on MyNursingKit.

REFERENCES

AACN (2004). Pulmonary Artery Pressure Measurement Practice Alert. Available at http://www.aacn.org/WD/Practice/Docs/PAP_Measurement_05-2004.pdf

Adams, K. L. (2004). Hemodynamic assessment: The physiologic basis for turning data into clinical information. *AACN Clinical Issues, 15*, 534–546.

Ahrens, T., & Sona, C. (2003). Capnography application in *acute* and critical care. *AACN Clinical Issues, 14*, 123–132.

Alpert, N. M. (2005). Cardiac output measurement techniques: Invasive. In D. Lynn-McHale Weigand & K. Carlson (eds.), *AACN procedure manual for critical care* (5th ed., pp. 482–497). St. Louis: Elsevier Saunders.

Bartz. B., Maroun, C., & Underhill. S. (1988). Differences in midanterior posterior level and midaxillary level of patients with a range of chest configurations. *Heart Lung*, 17(3), 309.

Bennett-Guerrero E., Kahn, R. A., Moskowitz, D.M., et al. (2002). Comparison of arterial systolic pressure variation with other clinical parameters to predict the response to fluid challenges during cardiac surgery. *Mt Sinai J Med,* 69(1–2), 96–100.

Bridges, E. J., & Middleton, R. (1997). Direct arterial versus oscillometric monitoring of blood pressure: Stop comparing and pick one. *Critical Care Nurse, 17*(3), 58–72.

Bridges, E. J. (2008). Arterial pressure-based stroke volume and functional hemodynamic monitoring. *J Cardiovasc Nurs 23*(2); 105–112.

Cannesson., M., Attof, Y., Rasamel, P., et al. (2007). Comparison of FloTrac cardiac output monitoring system in patients undergoing coronary artery bypass graft with pulmonary artery cardiac output measurements. *Eur J Anaesthesiol 24*(10), 832–839.

Connors, A. F., Castele, R. J., Farhat, N. Z,. et al. (1995). Complications of right heart catheterization: A prospective autopsy study. *Chest,* 88:567–572

Folan, L. & Funk, M. (2008). Measurement of thoracic fluid content in heart failure: The role of impedance cardiography. *AACN Advanced Critical Care, 19*(1), 47–55.

Gunst, M., Ghaemaghami, V., Sperry J., et al. (2008). Accuracy of cardiac function and volume status estimates using the bedside echocardiography assessment in trauma and critical care. *J Trauma 65*(3), 509–516.

Huber, W., Umgelter, A., Reindel, W., (2008). Volume assessment in patients with necrotizing pancreatitis: a comparison of intrathoracic blood volume index, central venous pressure, hematocrit and their correlation to cardiac index and extravascular lung water index. *Crit Care Med 36*(8), 2348–2354.

Keckeisen, M., Chulay, M., & Gawlinski, A. (1998). Pulmonary artery pressure monitoring. In *AACN's protocols for practice: Hemodynamic monitoring series.* Aliso Viejo, CA: AACN.

Ott, K., Johnson, K. L., & Ahrens, T. S. (2001). New technologies in the assessment of hemodynamic parameters. *Journal of Cardiovascular Nursing, 15*(2), 41–55.

Peters S. G., Afessa B., Decker P. A., et al. (2003). Increased risk associated with pulmonary artery catheterization in the medical intensive care unit. *J Crit Care, 18*,166–171)

Pinsky, M. R. (2007). Hemodynamic evaluation and monitoring in the ICU. *Chest 132*;2020–2029.

MODULE

14 Assessment of Cardiac Rhythm: Basic Electrocardiographic Rhythm Interpretation

Angela C. Muzzy

OBJECTIVES

Following completion of this module, the learner will be able to

1. Explain membrane permeability changes in cardiac cells and discuss the relationship between membrane permeability and serum electrolyte levels.
2. Describe the cardiac conduction system, the normal electrocardiogram (ECG) complex, and identify nursing responsibilities for the patient who requires cardiac monitoring.
3. Identify a system for interpreting ECG patterns.
4. Identify factors that place a person at risk for developing dysrhythmias.
5. Identify common dysrhythmias arising from the SA node and describe the treatment of these dysrhythmias.
6. Identify basic atrial dysrhythmias and describe appropriate treatment.
7. Identify common junctional dysrhythmias and describe the treatment of these dysrhythmias.
8. Compare and contrast atrial and ventricular premature beats, identify their origin, and describe the treatment of these premature beats.
9. Identify common ventricular dysrhythmias and describe treatment of these dysrhythmias.
10. Distinguish the four conduction abnormalities and describe the treatment of these abnormalities.
11. Discuss pharmacologic and countershock interventions and their nursing implications.
12. Identify indications for pacemaker and implantable cardioversion/defibrillation therapy, types of devices, and nursing implications for the patient receiving these therapies.

This self-study module is written at an introductory knowledge level for individuals who provide nursing care for high-acuity patients. It translates the cardiac cycle in order to promote understanding of the implications of cardiac dysrhythmias, including guidelines for electrocardiogram (ECG) interpretation. The module also provides a systematic approach to understanding automaticity and conduction that can then be applied to practical situations. While the module profiles basic cardiac dysrhythmias of atrial, junctional, and ventricular origin it is not intended as a comprehensive lesson in every potential dysrhythmia a nurse may encounter in the clinical setting.

The module is divided into 12 sections. Section One discusses cellular membrane permeability. Section Two covers cardiac conduction, the normal ECG, and the nursing care of patients who require ECG monitoring. Section Three provides the reader with guidelines that can be used to interpret ECG patterns and normal sinus rhythm. Section Four addresses factors that place a person at risk for developing dysrhythmias. Sections Five through Ten introduce the reader to basic dysrhythmia interpretation. Section Eleven discusses pharmacologic interventions and implications. Section Twelve provides an overview of long term electrical therapy. All Section Reviews include answers. It is suggested that the learner review those concepts answered incorrectly in the review questions before proceeding to the next section.

PRETEST

1. The cell is ready to be depolarized during what phase of an action potential?
   - **A.** phase 1
   - **B.** phase 2
   - **C.** phase 3
   - **D.** phase 4
2. Closure of fast sodium channels occurs during
   - **A.** depolarization
   - **B.** early repolarization
   - **C.** plateau phase
   - **D.** repolarization
3. Which of the following statements are accurate about the *QRS* complex? (choose all that apply)
   - **A.** *QRS* complex reflects ventricular depolarization.
   - **B.** *QRS* complex reflects atrial repolarization.
   - **C.** The shape of the *QRS* complex can vary between individuals.
   - **D.** Normal *QRS* complex is less than 0.10 seconds.

4. You measure the *PR* interval. It is 0.24 seconds. This represents
   A. a normal *PR* interval
   B. atrial fibrillation
   C. a conduction delay
   D. delayed conduction in the ventricles
5. The horizontal axis of ECG graph paper reflects
   A. strength of the contraction
   B. electrical activity
   C. voltage
   D. time
6. The *PR* interval is determined to be 0.30 seconds. What does this mean?
   A. This is a normal finding.
   B. The SA node is not serving as the primary pacemaker.
   C. There is a delay in conduction between the atria and ventricles.
   D. There is a heart block.
7. Hyperkalemia produces
   A. tall, peaked *T* waves
   B. absent *T* waves
   C. flat *T* waves
   D. inverted *T* waves
8. Hypothermia is associated with what ECG changes? (choose all that apply)
   A. tachycardia
   B. prolongation of *PR* interval
   C. prolongation of *QT* interval
   D. thin *QRS* complex
9. Pharmacologic treatment of sinus tachycardia includes (choose all that apply)
   A. atropine
   B. cardioversion
   C. defibrillation
   D. analgesics
10. Sinus bradycardia is identified on ECG by (choose all that apply)
    A. regular *P* waves before each *QRS*
    B. heart rate less than 60 bpm
    C. prolonged *PR* interval
    D. widened *QRS* complex
11. Junctional rhythms commonly occur
    A. as a protective mechanism in sinoatrial (SA) node abnormalities
    B. in response to ventricular escape beats
    C. as an indication of reperfusion in thrombolytic therapy
    D. when a pacing device fails to capture
12. Which of the following is/are true about *P* waves in a junctional dysrhythmia? (choose all that apply)
    A. *P* wave may be inverted.
    B. *P* wave may precede *QRS*.
    C. *P* wave may follow *QRS*.
    D. *P* wave is indistinguishable.
13. A junctional rhythm is characterized by (choose all that apply)
    A. rate 40-60 bpm
    B. rate greater than 100 bpm
    C. inverted *P* waves
    D. absent *P* waves
14. When the SA node fails to fire, the AV nodes acts as a backup. This results in
    A. normal sinus rhythm
    B. junctional dysrhythmia
    C. heart block
    D. asystole
15. A PAC is associated with (choose all that apply)
    A. irregular *QRS* complexes
    B. absent *T* waves
    C. a noncompensatory pause
    D. a compensatory pause
16. A PVC is associated with (choose all that apply)
    A. a premature *P* wave
    B. a regular rhythm
    C. a noncompensatory pause
    D. a compensatory pause
17. In ventricular tachycardia, the
    A. *P* waves are inverted
    B. *QRS* complexes are less than 0.12 seconds
    C. R–R interval is irregular
    D. *P* waves are not discernable
18. Which of the following dysrhythmias is the most common cause of sudden death?
    A. ventricular defibrillation
    B. ventricular tachycardia
    C. atrial fibrillation
    D. atrial flutter
19. The nurse notes the following on an ECG rhythm strip: HR 80 bpm, rhythm regular. There are a group of beats, then a pause. The *PR* interval gradually prolongs until a *QRS* is dropped. The *QRS* interval is 0.08 seconds. What is this rhythm?
    A. first-degree heart block
    B. second-degree heart block
    C. third-degree heart block
    D. left bundle branch block
20. A patient with second degree AV block who becomes hypotensive may be treated with
    A. dopamine
    B. cardioversion
    C. atropine
    D. isoproterenol
21. Which of the following antiarrhythmic categories are contraindicated in patients with asthma?
    A. class I
    B. class II
    C. class III
    D. class IV
22. Which of the following is used to treat ventricular tachycardia in an unresponsive patient?
    A. cardioversion
    B. defibrillation
    C. permanent pacemaker
    D. transcutaneous pacemaker

23. A DDD pacemaker would have pacing leads in the (choose all that apply)
A. atria
B. ventricles
C. epicardium
D. endocardium

24. The ICU can prevent
A. heart block
B. cardiac arrest
C. atrial fibrillation
D. complete heart block

Pretest answers are found on MyNursingKit.

SECTION ONE: Cellular Membrane Permeability

At the completion of this section, the learner will be able to explain membrane permeability changes in cardiac cells and discuss the relationship between membrane permeability and serum electrolyte levels.

Electrolytes, particularly sodium and potassium, affect cardiac function. Under resting conditions intracellular potassium concentration is greater inside the cell than outside. Sodium concentration outside the cell is greater than inside the cell. There is a higher concentration of calcium outside the cell. As a result, during the resting state, the inside of the cell is more electrically negative relative to the outside of the cell.

The resting cardiac cell is negatively charged, or **polarized.** A change in polarity is produced by an **action potential.** The action potential is a five-phase cycle that produces changes in the cell membrane's electrical charge. It is caused by stimulation of cardiac cells that extend across the myocardium to produce contraction or relaxation.

When the cell receives an electrical stimulus, sodium rushes into the cell and potassium leaks out, causing the cell to become positively charged, or depolarized. **Depolarization** should result in cardiac muscle contraction. As the cell recovers, ions move back to their original places and the cell returns to a negative charge, or **repolarization.** Repolarization should result in cardiac muscle relaxation. Figure 14–1 illustrates the action potential of a cardiac cell.

There are five phases of an action potential as shown in Figure 14–2: depolarization (phase 0), early repolarization (phase 1), **plateau phase** (phase 2), repolarization (phase 3), and **resting membrane potential** (phase 4). During depolarization, the cell is almost impermeable to sodium unless a stimulus occurs. This stimulus may be electrical in origin, such as the firing of the sinoatrial (SA) node, (an internal stimulus), or **defibrillation** (an external stimulus). Chemical changes also may precipitate depolarization.

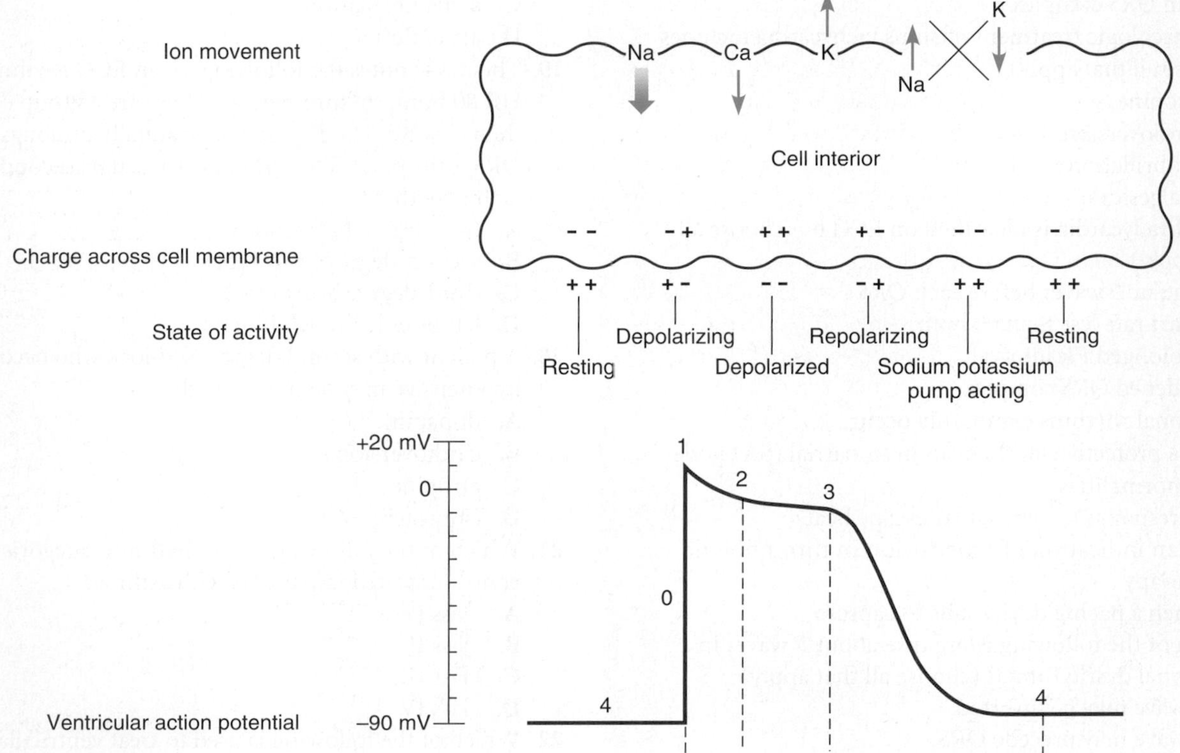

Figure 14–1 ■ Action potential of a cardiac cell. In the resting state (phase 4), the cell membrane is polarized: the cell's interior has a negative charge compared to that of extracellular fluid. On depolarization (phase 0), sodium ions diffuse rapidly across the cell membrane into the cell, and calcium channels open. In the fully depolarized state (phase 1), the cell's interior has a net positive charge compared to its exterior. During the plateau period (phase 2), calcium moves into the cell and potassium diffusion slows, prolonging the action potential. In phase 3, calcium channels close, the sodium-potassium pump removes sodium from the cell, and the cell membrane again becomes polarized with a net negative charge.

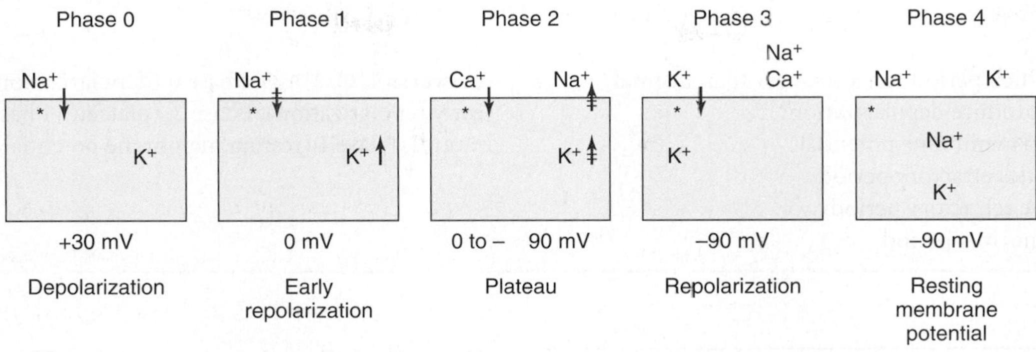

Figure 14–2 ■ Membrane permeability changes in nonpacemaker myocardial cells.

Hypoxemia respiratory acidosis and pharmaceutical agents (e.g., sodium bicarbonate) may serve as chemical stimuli. In depolarization, more sodium moves into the cell through the fast sodium channels and creates a fast response action potential. The inside of the cell becomes positively charged.

The process of repolarization takes place over phases 1, 2, and 3 (Fig. 14–2). In early repolarization, sodium channels close. During the plateau phase, calcium channels open. These channels are slow in relation to the preceding sodium channels. The influx of calcium maintains the positive charge (depolarization) a little longer. Chemical blockage of the channels is used to treat cardiac abnormalities. In phase 3, repolarization, potassium moves back into the cell to create the original electrochemical gradient.

During the resting membrane potential phase (phase 4), repolarization is completed, and the original electrochemical gradient is in place. The cell is ready to be depolarized again. The absolute refractory period begins in phase 0 and lasts until the midpoint of phase 3. During this period, the cell cannot respond to another stimulus regardless of the strength of the stimulus. The cell cannot deal with a new impulse, it is "resistant" to stimuli because it is still dealing with the last one. The **relative refractory period** begins at the midpoint of phase 3 and lasts until the beginning of phase 4. A stronger than normal stimulus can produce depolarization. During the **supranormal period** (phase 4), a weaker than normal stimulus can produce depolarization. It does not take much to cause depolarization. A common example of a stimulus producing depolarization during the supranormal or relative refractory period is premature atrial or ventricular beats. These are discussed later in the module. Table 14–1 summarizes the phases of the action potential. The **pacemaker** cells in the sinoatrial node have a constant sodium influx; thus, they slowly depolarize at a steady rate until threshold is reached and an action potential created. This is referred to as **automaticity.** Through the characteristic of **conductivity,** this impulse is then transmitted to the surrounding myocardium (Ellis, 2007).

TABLE 14–1 Phases of an Action Potential

Phase 0	Depolarization	Movement of sodium into cell (fast channels open)
Phase 1	Early repolarization	Closure of fast sodium channels
Phase 2	Plateau	Calcium moves into cell (slow channels open)
Phase 3	Repolarization	Potassium moves into cell
Phase 4	Resting membrane potential	Electrochemical gradient returned to normal potential Sarcolemma almost impermeable to sodium

SECTION ONE REVIEW

1. Depolarization may occur in direct response to (choose all that apply)
   A. hypoxemia
   B. firing of the SA node
   C. defibrillation
   D. hyperglycemia
2. Under resting conditions, which of the following electrolytes has a higher concentration inside the cell, relative to outside the cell?
   A. potassium
   B. sodium
   C. calcium
   D. chloride
3. Match the phase of the action potential with the electrical event.
   __Phase 0 a. repolarization
   __Phase 1 b. plateau
   __Phase 2 c. depolarization
   __Phase 3 d. resting membrane potential
   __Phase 4 e. early repolarization
4. During the plateau phase, which of the following channels are open?
   A. potassium
   B. sodium
   C. calcium
   D. chloride

(continued)

(continued)

5. During which period can a stronger than normal stimulus produce depolarization?
   A. resting membrane potential
   B. absolute refractory period
   C. relative refractory period
   D. supranormal period

Answers: 1. C, 2. A, 3. Phase 0 (depolarization), Phase 1 (early repolarization), Phase 2, (plateau), Phase 3 (repolarization), Phase 4 (resting membrane potential); 4. C, 5. C

SECTION TWO: Cardiac Conduction and the Electrocardiogram

At the completion of this section, the learner will be able to describe the cardiac conduction system, the normal electrocardiogram (ECG) complex, and identify nursing responsibilities for the patient who requires cardiac monitoring.

Electrical Conduction of the Heart

The cardiac cycle is perpetuated by an intrinsic electrical circuit in the heart. Specialized areas of myocardial cells influence this electrical pathway. A thorough understanding of the electrical conduction system is an essential component of learning and understanding ECG interpretation (Fig. 14–3).

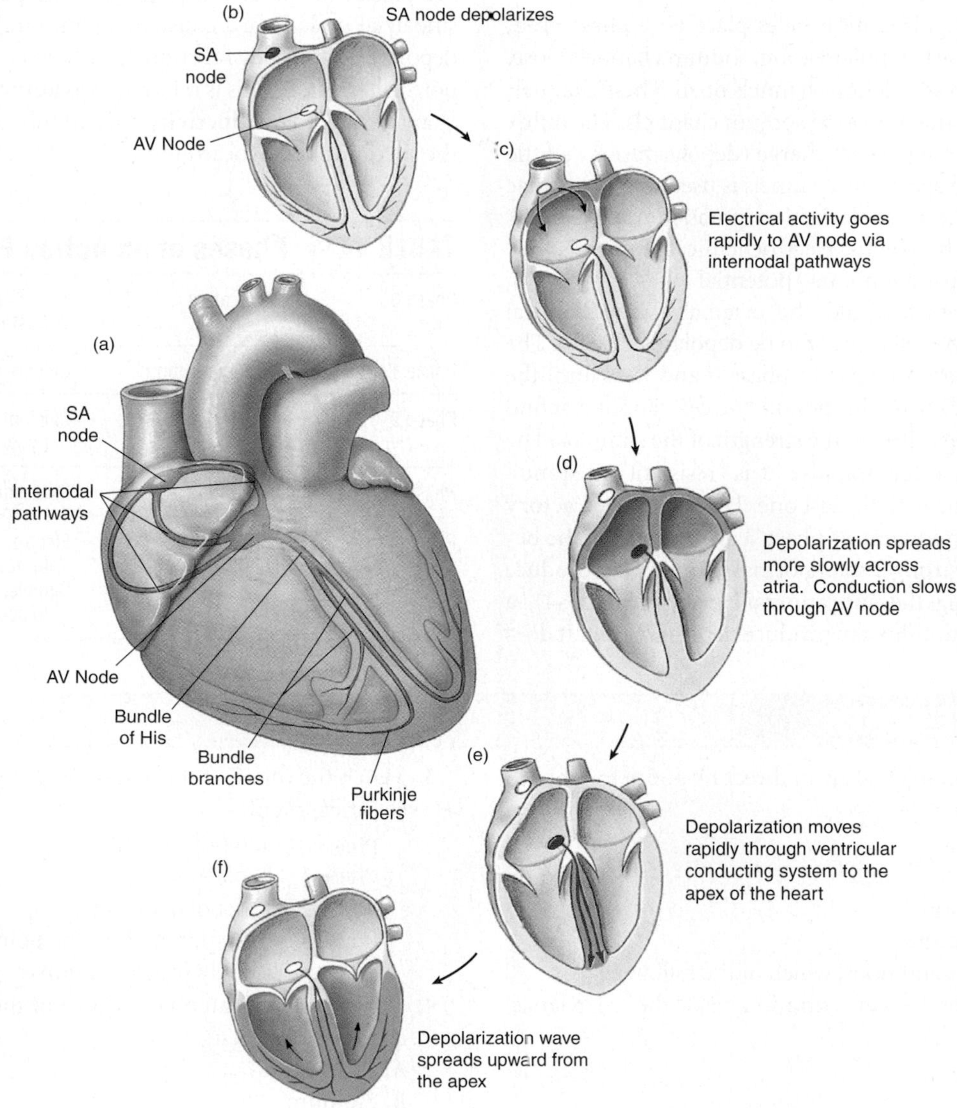

Figure 14–3 ■ Electrical conduction system in the heart. (From Beasley, B. M. [2003]. EKG's: A Practical Approach [2nd ed.]).

The SA node is the primary pacemaker of the heart because it controls the heart rate normally between 60 and 100 beats per minute (bpm). Should the firing of the SA node fail, the AV node will generally take over as the pacemaker of the heart, firing between 40-60 bpm. The impulse from the SA node is transmitted from the atria to the ventricles along a cardiac conduction pathway. The conduction pathway that leads out of the AV node is the bundle of His. This specialized group of cells has the ability to self-initiate electrical activity at a rate of 40-60 bpm. From the bundle of His, a network of fibers called Purkinje's fibers, carry electrical impulses directly to ventricular muscle cells. The firing rate of the Purkinje fibers is normally within the range of 20-40 bpm.

The Electrocardiogram

The ECG is a graphic representation of the electrical activity of the heart (Fig. 14–4). It is important to remember the ECG is a graphic tracing of the electrical, not mechanical, activity of the heart. The normal ECG complex consists of several components The *P* wave indicates atrial depolarization, stimulated by the firing of the SA node. The *P* wave is a smooth rounded upward deflection. The *PR* interval depicts conduction of the impulse from the SA node and downward to the ventricles. The normal length of the *PR* interval is 0.12 to 0.20 seconds. A longer *PR* interval suggests a conduction delay, usually in the area of the AV node.

The *QRS* complex reflects ventricular depolarization and atrial repolarization. Atrial repolarization is overpowered by ventricular depolarization because the ventricular muscle mass is larger than that of the atria. Therefore, atrial repolarization is not seen on the ECG. The normal QRS is spiked in appearance. The shape of the *QRS* complex can vary between individuals and not all three waves are necessarily present. The *QRS* segment is 0.10 second or less in length. A prolonged *QRS* complex indicates abnormal impulse conduction through the ventricles (i.e. bundle branch block).

The *ST* segment represents the completion of ventricular depolarization and the beginning of ventricular repolarization. The segment should be **isoelectric,** or consistent with the baseline. There should be no deflections present because positive and negative charges are balanced. Deflections in the *ST* segment usually indicate ventricular muscle injury. The *T* wave depicts ventricular repolarization. The *T* wave is normally seen as a slightly asymmetrical, slightly rounded, positive deflection. The *T* wave is often referred to as the resting phase of the cardiac cycle. It represents the absolute and refractory periods. *T* waves also are affected by ventricular muscle injury because of interference with repolarization. An example of a clinical condition with potential ventricular muscle injury is acute myocardial infarction. The *T* wave can be elevated or depressed in the presence of current or previous cardiac ischemia.

The *QT* interval represents ventricular depolarization and repolarization. It is measured from the beginning of the *QRS* complex to the end of the *T* wave. The *QT* interval is usually less than 0.40 second in length, depending on heart rate. The *QT* interval is less than half the R–R interval. As heart rate increases, the *QT* interval shortens. If the heart rate decreases, the *QT* interval lengthens.

Nursing Care of a Patient Who Requires Cardiac Monitoring

Cardiac monitoring is used whenever it is necessary to continuously monitor a patient's heart rate and rhythm. Although there are many types of monitors, all systems use three basic components: an oscilloscope display system, a monitoring cable, and electrodes.

Electrical impulses sent out from the heart are detectable on the skin throughout the body. The components of an ECG monitoring are shown in Figure 14–5. **Electrodes** are small adhesive

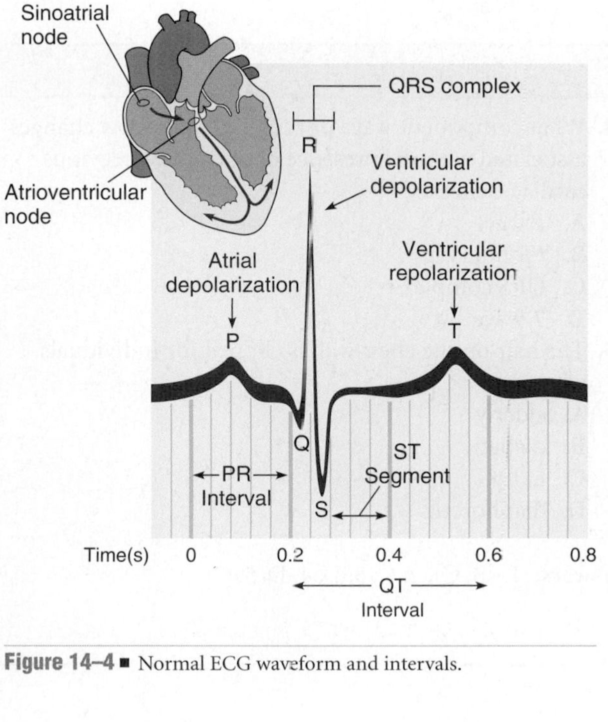

Figure 14–4 ■ Normal ECG waveform and intervals.

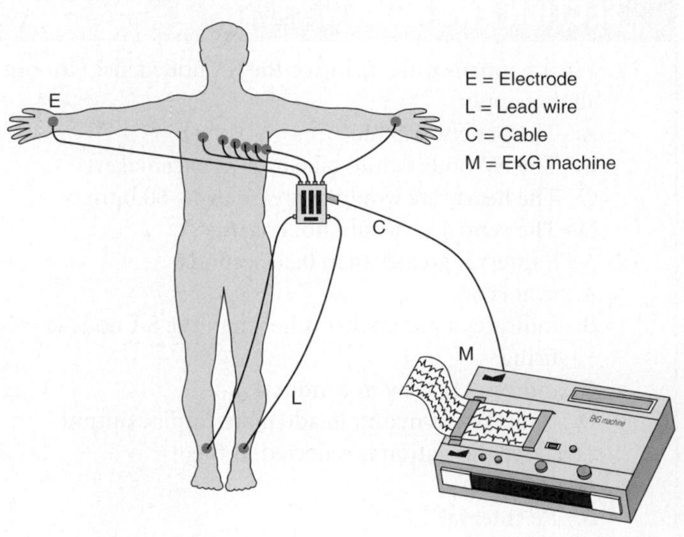

Figure 14–5 ■ Components of ECG Monitoring. Ellis, K. M. (2002) *EKG Plain and Simple* (2nd ed.) Upper Saddle River, NJ: Pearson./Prentice Hall.

patches with conducting gel placed on the skin. Electrodes pick up the impulses and send them thought the **lead** wires to a cable on the ECG machine. These lead wires are usually color coded in order to be user friendly.

High-acuity patients may require continuous ECG monitoring. These patients are attached to five-lead cables (Fig. 14–6). Leads are electrographic pictures of the heart. A five-lead ECG would provide five different views of the heart's electrical activity. The leads are attached to a remote receiver (telemetry). The ECG is sent to a central terminal in the high-acuity unit where the rhythms are observed.

All cardiac monitors use lead systems to record cardiac electrical activity. A lead system is composed of three electrodes: one positive, one negative, and one ground. Each lead system looks at cardiac depolarization from a different location and thus produces *P* waves, *QRS*, and *T wave* complexes of varying configuration.

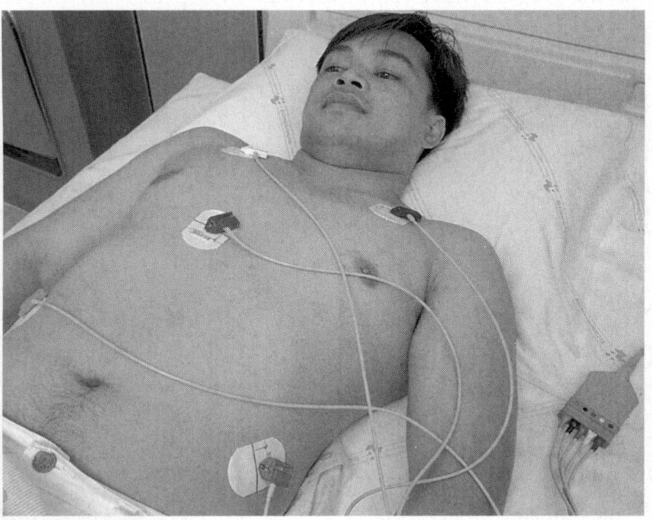

Figure 14–6 ■ Placement of electrodes.

Although a minimum of three electrodes is required, often five electrodes are used, either to monitor two leads simultaneously or to allow selection of different leads. Accurate lead placement is essential for accurate cardiac monitoring. Lead placement is verified at the beginning of each shift.

There are several nursing actions for a patient requiring cardiac monitoring. The patient's skin must be prepared before attaching the ECG electrodes. Electrode site preparation includes clipping excessive hair and cleansing oily skin with alcohol (AACN 2008a). This will help ensure a good connection. Sites are rotated every 24 to 48 hours to prevent skin breakdown. It is important to clean gel residue from previous sites and document skin condition under the pads. The sensitivity knob of the cardiac monitor may need to be adjusted to view complexes. Alarms on the monitor are set typically at 20 bpm higher and lower than the patient's baseline rates. The alarms are left on and audible to the nurse. An ECG strip is recorded and placed in the nursing record on a regular basis per unit protocol, when the cardiac rhythm changes, or with any change in patient condition. Each strip is analyzed using the eight-step process outlined in Section Three.

Assuring patient safety during ECG monitoring is imperative. Frayed wires and/or electrical outlet damage can cause electricity to go directly to the patient. Always check for frayed wires or components before performing an ECG.

Patients need to know why they require cardiac monitoring. They need reassurance that they are protected from electric shocks from the equipment. Patients and families should also be informed that the alarms can sound as a result of patient movement and other factors, in addition to cardiac abnormalities.

SECTION TWO REVIEW

1. What happens if the firing of the SA node fails? (choose all that apply)
   - **A.** The patient will die.
   - **B.** The AV node would take over as pacemaker.
   - **C.** The heart rate would decrease to 40-60 bpm.
   - **D.** The ventricles would not contract.
2. A *PR* interval greater than 0.20 seconds
   - **A.** is normal
   - **B.** indicates a pacemaker other than the SA node is firing
   - **C.** indicates a delay in conduction
   - **D.** is too fast to maintain adequate cardiac output
3. Atrial repolarization is reflected in the
   - **A.** *P* wave
   - **B.** *PR* interval
   - **C.** *T* wave
   - **D.** *QRS* complex
4. What component wave of the ECG may show changes associated with the presence of current or previous cardiac ischemia?
   - **A.** *P* wave
   - **B.** *PR* interval
   - **C.** *QRS* complex
   - **D.** *T* wave
5. The hair on the chest wall is clipped for individuals who are
   - **A.** elderly
   - **B.** diabetic
   - **C.** hairy
   - **D.** diaphoretic

Answers: 1. (B, C), 2. C, 3. D, 4. D, 5. C

SECTION THREE: Interpretation Guidelines

At the completion of this section, the learner will be able to identify a system for interpreting ECG patterns.

The ECG is printed on graph paper (Fig. 14–7). Each small block of the graph paper is equal to 1 mm, or 0.04 seconds, on the horizontal axis. The horizontal axis of the graph paper represents time. The vertical axis of the graph paper represents voltage. Each small block is equivalent to 1 mm (0.1 mV) on the vertical axis. Each large box is 5 mm (0.5 mV). For the purposes of basic ECG interpretation, time is the most important factor to consider. Because each small block equals 0.04 seconds, a large block, composed of five small blocks, equals 0.20 seconds. Five large blocks represent 1 second. There are eight steps to follow when interpreting an ECG:

1. Measure the heart rate.
2. Examine the R–R interval.
3. Examine the *P* wave.
4. Measure the *PR* interval.
5. Determine if each *P* wave is followed by a *QRS* complex.
6. Examine and measure the *QRS* complex.
7. Examine and measure the QT interval.
8. Diagnose the rhythm.

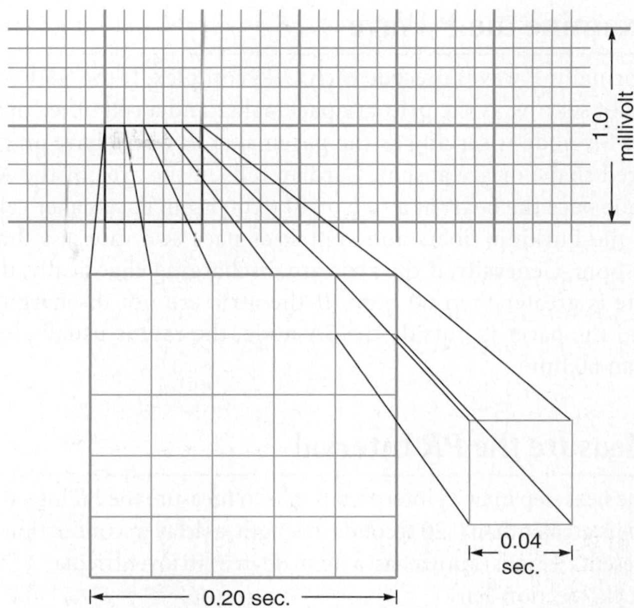

Figure 14–7 ■ ECG paper is a graph divided into millimeter squares. Time is measured on the horizontal axis. With a paper speed of 25 mm/sec, each small (millimeter) box equals 0.04 seconds and each larger (5-mm) box equals 0.2 seconds. The amplitude of any wave is measured on the vertical axis in millimeters.

Measure the Heart Rate

There are two methods commonly used to determine heart rate by visual examination of an ECG strip. Using the first method, the number of 0.20-seconds boxes are counted between two *R* waves and divided into 300. This method is used only when the rate is regular. The second method is based on a 6-second rhythm strip. This method can be utilized with either a regular or irregular rhythm. ECG paper is marked at the top margin in 3-second intervals. *QRS* complexes in a 6-second strip (30 large blocks) are multiplied by 10 to get the heart rate per minute ($6 \times 10 = 60$ seconds). Figure 14–8 demonstrates this method of rate calculation.

Examine the R–R Interval

Next, the *R* waves are examined. If the *R* waves appear in regular intervals (are constant), the rhythm is a regular rhythm. If the *R* waves do not occur in a regular pattern, a dysrhythmia is present.

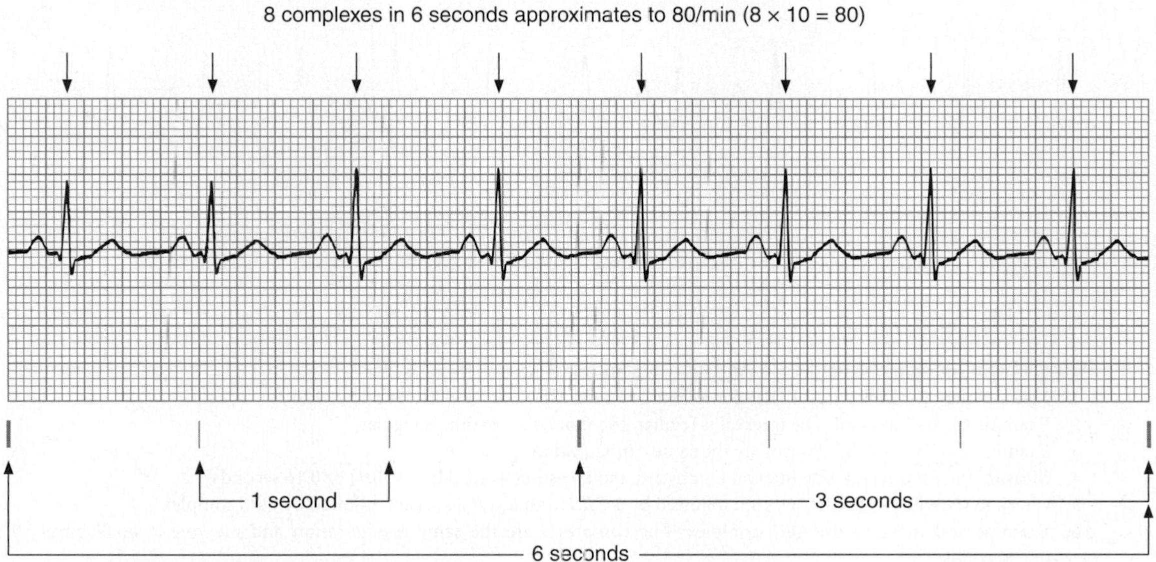

Figure 14–8 ■ Calculation of heart rate.

Examine the *P* Wave

Normally, *P* waves precede each *QRS* complex. If the SA node is not serving as the primary pacemaker and a cell other than the SA node is serving as the pacemaker, *P* waves have an altered shape or are absent. Cardiac cells in the area of the AV node pace the heart at a rate of 40 to 60 bpm. Pacemaker cells in the Purkinje fibers and ventricles pace at a rate less than 40 bpm. Generally, if the atria are discharging chaotically, the rate is greater than 60 bpm. If the atria are not discharging and the pacer is outside the SA node, the rate is usually less than 60 bpm.

Measure the *PR* Interval

The next step in ECG interpretation is to measure the *PR* interval. If it is greater than 0.20 seconds in length, a delay in conduction is present. This is known as a first degree atrioventricular (AV) block. (Section Ten).

P Waves Precede Each *QRS*

Next, determine if each *P* wave is followed by a *QRS* complex. If *P* waves are present but they are not followed consistently by a *QRS* complex, a second- or third-degree heart block (Section Ten) is present.

Examine and Measure the *QRS* Complex

The next step involves examination of the *QRS* complexes. The complex should be 0.12 seconds or less in length unless there is a delay in the impulse reaching the ventricles. A widened *QRS* complex means delayed conduction through the bundle branches (bundle branch block), abnormal conduction within the ventricles, or early activation of the ventricles through a bypass route.

Measure the QT Interval

The *QT* interval reflects the duration of ventricular depolarization. The *QT* interval is measured from the beginning of the *Q* wave to the end of the *T* wave. The *QT* interval lengthens with **bradycardia** and shortens with **tachycardia.** The interval should be correct for heart rate (*QTc*) by using the formula:

$$QTc = QT/\text{square root of the R-R interval}$$

A *QTc* greater than 0.50 seconds is considered to be dangerously prolonged (AACN 2008b). AACN (2008b) recommends *QT* intervals should be assessed for high-risk patients. *QT* intervals should be monitored in patients with low serum potassium or magnesium levels, new onset of bradycardia, patients who overdose on prodysrhythmic drugs, and patients on medications known to prolong QT intervals (such as Quinidine, procainamide, etc.; Section Eleven).

Diagnose the Rhythm

There are various different rhythms and/or ectopic heart beats that may be present in high-acuity patients. These rhythms are discussed in greater detail in Sections Five through Ten. Some rhythms have deleterious hemodynamic consequences while others are benign. Knowledge of basic ECG rhythm interpretation allows the nurse to quickly identify any potential life-threatening cardiac conduction abnormalities and take appropriate action.

Figure 14–9 illustrates the application of the principles discussed in this section. This should provide a consistent and comprehensive approach to ECG interpretation. If the heart rate is 60-100 bpm, R-R intervals are regular, *P* waves look alike, PR interval is less than 0.20 seconds, every *P* wave is followed by a *QRS*, *QRS* is less than 0.12 seconds, QT interval is less than half the R-R interval, then the rhythm is interpreted as normal sinus rhythm.

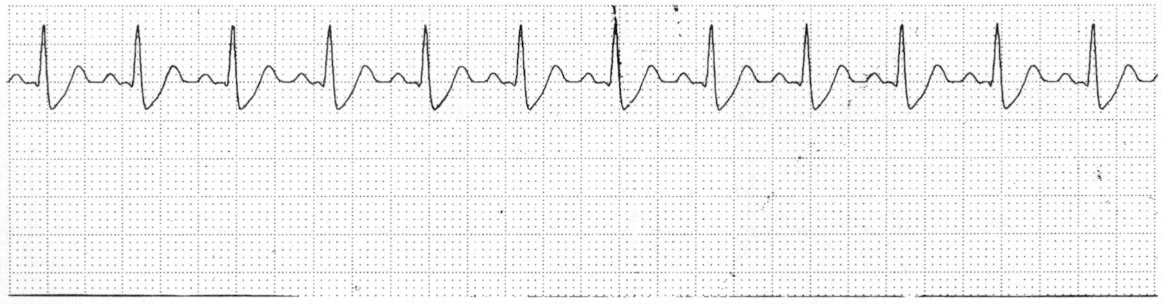

Figure 14–9 ■ Interpretation of ECG using eight-step process.

1. Measure the rate. There are 12 *QRS* complexes in 6 seconds: 12 × 10 = Heart rate of 120.
2. Examine the R-R interval. The interval is regular; therefore, the rhythm is regular.
3. Examine the *P* wave. The *P* waves are the same configuration.
4. Measure the *PR* interval. The interval is constant and measures 4 small boxes (0.4) or 0.16 seconds.
5. Check to see whether the *P* waves are followed by a *QRS* complex: *P* waves are followed by *QRS* complex.
6. Examine and measure the *QRS* complex: The complexes are the same configuration and measure 2 small boxes (0.04) or 0.08 seconds.
7. Measure the *QT* interval. The interval measures at 7 small boxes or 0.28 seconds.
8. Rhythm diagnosis is Sinus Tachycardia.

ECG INTERPRETATION EXERCISE

1. Identify the *P* wave, QRS complex, and *T* wave

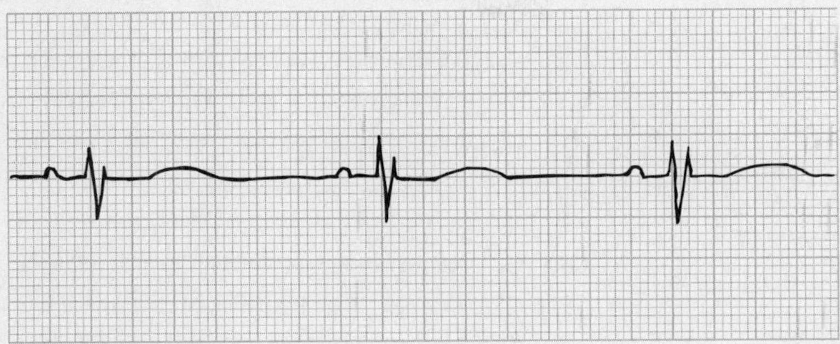

2. Measure the PR interval, QRS complex and QT interval

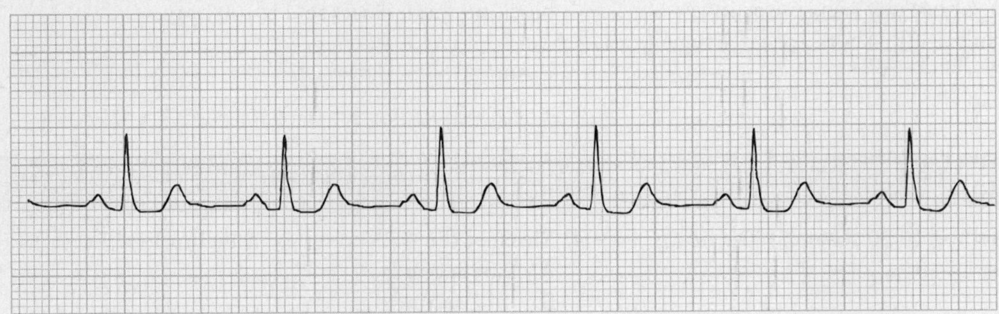

3. Measure the PR interval, QRS complex, and AT interval

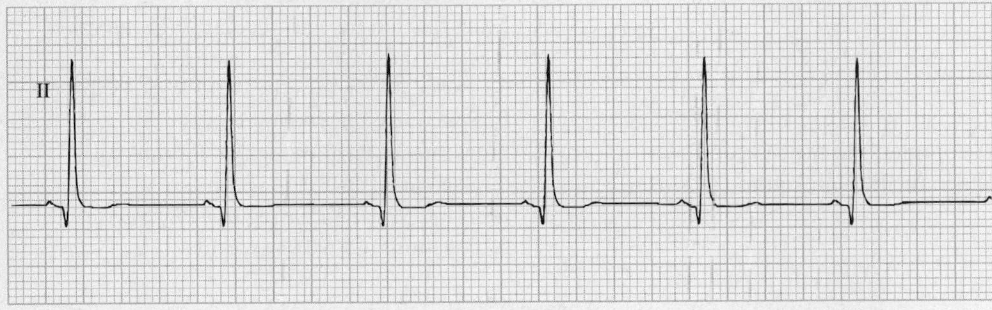

4. Calculate the heart rate

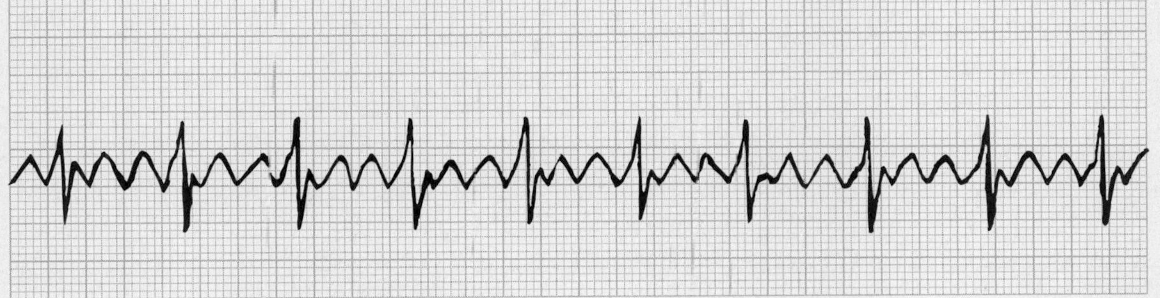

(continued)

(continued)

ECG Interpretation Exercise Answers:

1\.

P T P T P T
QRS QRS QRS

2. *PR* 0.20 seconds, *QRS* 0.08 seconds, *QT* 0.36 seconds
3. *PR* 0.08 seconds, *QRS* 0.12 seconds, *QT* 0.36 seconds
4. This is a regular rhythm. Chose any two consecutive *QRS* complexes and calculate HR. There are three big blocks (14 little blocks) between *QRSs*. Divide 300 by 3 for the big block method and 1500 by 15 for the little block method. Heart rate is 100 bpm.

SECTION THREE REVIEW

1. Using the large-block method (0.20 seconds), the heart rate in the ECG in Figure 14–10 is
   A. 35 bpm
   B. 30 bpm
   C. 40 bpm
   D. 45 bpm
2. Measure the *PR* interval in Figure 14–10.
   A. 0.04 seconds
   B. 0.12 seconds
   C. 0.20 seconds
   D. 0.28 seconds
3. Using the number of *QRS* complexes in the 6-second strip method, the heart rate in the ECG in Figure 14–11 is
   A. 120 bpm
   B. 140 bpm
   C. 130 bpm
   D. 70 bpm
4. Measure the *QRS* complex in Figure 14–11.
   A. 0.08 seconds
   B. 0.12 seconds
   C. 0.20 seconds
   D. 0.28 seconds
5. Which of the following criteria is representative of the patient in normal sinus rhythm?
   A. heart rate 64; rhythm regular; *PR* interval 0.24 seconds; *QRS* 0.12 seconds
   B. heart rate 88, rhythm regular; *PR* interval 0.18 seconds; *QRS* 0.06 seconds
   C. heart rate 54, rhythm regular, *PR* interval 0.16 seconds; *QRS* 0.14 seconds
   D. heart rate 92; rhythm irregular; *PR* interval 0.16 seconds; *QRS* 0.04 seconds

Answers: 1. B, 2. C, 3. A, 4. A, 5. B

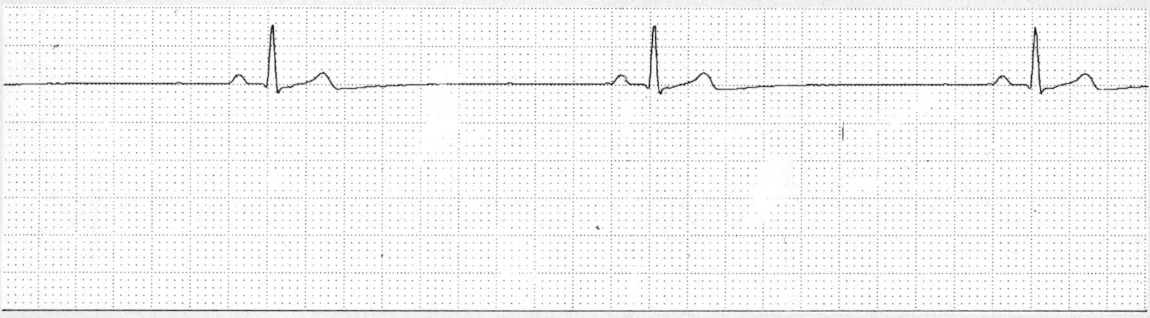

Figure 14–10 ■ Section Three Review: Review Questions 1 & 2.

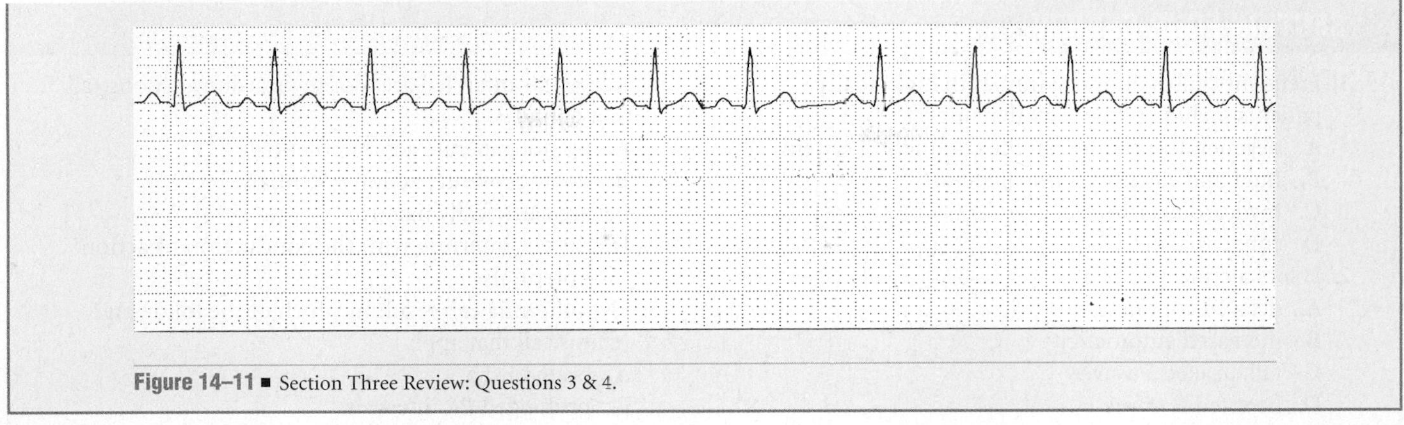

Figure 14–11 ■ Section Three Review: Questions 3 & 4.

SECTION FOUR: Risk Factors for Development of Dysrhythmias

At the completion of this section, the learner will be able to identify factors that place a person at risk for developing dysrhythmias.

Dysrhythmias are abnormal heart rhythms. There are many causes of dysrhythmias. They are not necessarily pathologic. They can occur in healthy as well as diseased hearts. Frequent causes of dysrhythmias in the high-acuity patient include congenital defects, degenerative changes in the conduction system, fluid and electrolyte imbalances, myocardial ischemia and infarction and the effects of drug ingestion (White-Winters, 2005). The major complication associated with dysrhythmias is their negative impact on myocardial contractility.

Electrolyte Abnormalities

High-acuity patients with electrolyte abnormalities are at an increased risk of developing dysrhythmias. Hypokalemia causes the resting membrane potential to become more negative (hyperpolarized). This means that it takes a greater stimulus to reach threshold for excitation and open the sodium channels. Therefore, the *PR* interval is longer, and the *T* wave is flat. The *QT* interval lengthens. An extra wave follows the *T* wave (*U* wave). Bradydysrhythmias and conduction blocks are common. Premature ventricular contractions (PVCs) can occur. On the opposite spectrum, hyperkalemia causes the resting membrane potential to become more positive (hypopolarized) which decreases excitability. Tall, peaked *T* waves are present. The *QT* interval shortens. Eventually the cell becomes too positive to respond and depolarize, and **asystole** (no heartbeat) occurs. Before asystole, the *PR* interval lengthens, and the *QRS* complex widens.

Other electrolyte imbalances can potentiate the development of dysrhythmias. Increased levels of calcium strengthen contractility and shorten ventricular repolarization, shortening the *QT* interval. Hypocalcemia prolongs the *QT* interval (Jacobson, 2000). Decreased levels of magnesium increase the irritability of the nervous system and can produce dysrhythmias. Prominent *U* waves and a flattening of the *T* wave can occur, as well as prolongation of the *QT* interval (Jacobson, 2000). Increased levels of magnesium can produce a prolonged *PR* interval; wide *QRS* complexes; bradycardia; and tall, peaked *T* waves.

Fluid Volume Abnormalities

Fluid volume status is a risk factor for dysrhythmias. Tachydysrhythmias, rapid abnormal rhythms, are noted in patients with a fluid volume deficit. The heart rate increases in response to a diminished stroke volume. Fluid volume overload can result in ventricular enlargement and decreased contractility. Premature beats, cardiac conduction blocks, and abnormalities in heart rate can appear in response to excess fluid volume.

Hypoxemia

Hypoxemia and myocardial ischemia are risk factors for the development of dysrhythmias. During periods of decreased myocardial tissue perfusion, injured or infracted areas of cardiac muscle become electrically inactive and they do not conduct or generate action potentials. Other areas of the myocardium become overly excitable. These different levels of membrane excitability set the stage for development of dysrhythmias and conduction defects (Porth, 2005). Specific ECG changes associated with myocardial ischemia and infarction are discussed in detail in Module 17, Alterations in Myocardial Tissue Perfusion.

Altered Body Temperature

Alterations in body temperature are risk factors for the development of dysrhythmias. Hypothermia decreases the electrical activity of the heart. Thus, **bradycardia** (rate of less than 60 bpm), prolongation of the *PR* and *QT* intervals, and wide *QRS* complexes may occur. Hyperthermia increases electrical activity of the heart. Heart rate increases about 10 bpm for each degree Fahrenheit (18 bpm per degree Celsius) up to about 105° F (40.5° C); beyond this, the heart rate may decreased because of progressive debility of the heart muscle as a result of fever (Guyton, 2006).

SECTION FOUR REVIEW

1. Frequent causes of dysrhythmias in high-acuity patients include (choose all that apply)
   - A. degenerative changes in the conduction system
   - B. fluid and electrolyte imbalances
   - C. myocardial ischemia
   - D. congential defects
2. Hypokalemia results in
   - A. delayed conduction
   - B. increased automaticity
   - C. tall, peaked *T* waves
   - D. inverted *P* waves
3. Hypocalcemia results in
   - A. decreased sodium influx into the cell
   - B. delayed repolarization
   - C. prolonged *QT* interval
   - D. spontaneous conduction
4. Injured or infarcted areas of myocardium (choose all that apply)
   - A. do not generate action potentials
   - B. do not conduct action potentials
   - C. are electrically inactive
   - D. do not interfere with the conduction of action potentials
5. Hypothermia can result in which of the following? (choose all that apply)
   - A. bradycardia
   - B. prolonged *PR* intervals
   - C. prolonged *QT* intervals
   - D. tall, peaked *T* waves

Answers: 1. (A, B, C, D), 2. A, 3. C, 4. (A, B, C), 5. (A, B, C)

SECTION FIVE: Sinus Dysrhythmias

At the completion of this section, the learner will be able to identify common dysrhythmias arising from the SA node and describe the treatment of these dysrhythmias.

Sinus Bradycardia

Sinus bradycardia is defined as a heart rate less than 60 bpm and originates from the SA node, as evidenced by a regular *P* wave preceding each *QRS* complex. The only abnormality noted in this rhythm is the rate. This rhythm can be present in athletes because they have strong cardiac muscle contractions; therefore, a slower heart rate can still maintain an efficient CO. Sinus bradycardia is not treated unless the person experiences symptoms of decreased CO, such as syncope, hypotension, and angina. If the rate drops too low, the chance of ectopic (abnormal) pacemakers firing increases. Lethal ventricular dysrhythmias can result. Symptomatic sinus bradycardia is treated by administering atropine because it blocks the parasympathetic innervation to the SA node, allowing normal sympathetic innervation to gain control and increase SA node firing. Sinus bradycardia is illustrated in Figure 14–12.

Sinus Tachycardia

Sinus **tachycardia** has a rapid rate, from 100 to 150 bpm. There are no other abnormal characteristics associated with this rhythm. The rapid rate results from sympathetic nervous stimulation. This stimulation can be in response to fear, increased activity, hypermetabolic states (such as fever), pain, and decreased CO as a result of hypovolemia or ventricular failure. Sinus tachycardia can produce angina if the CO decreases to the point of reducing coronary circulation or if myocardial oxygen demand is increased without an increase in coronary circulation. Treatment is aimed at relieving the cause of increased

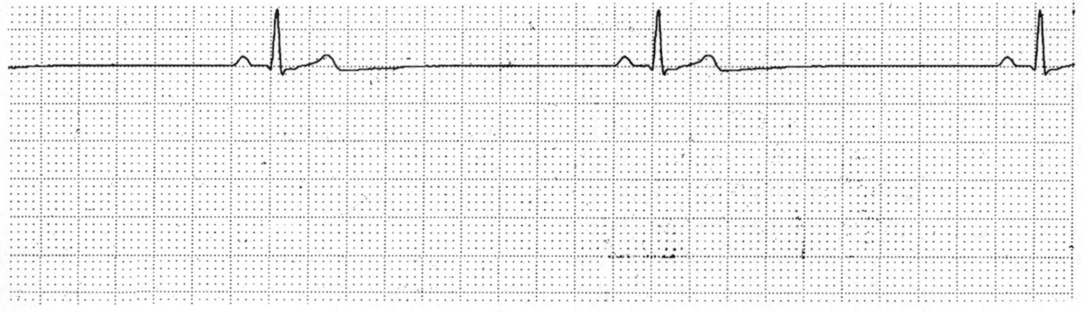

Figure 14–12 ■ Sinus bradycardia

1. Rate = 30
2. R-R interval: regular
3. *P* wave has same configuration
4. *PR* interval = 0.20
5. *P* wave precedes *QRS*: yes
6. *QRS* complex = 0.08
7. *QT* interval = 0.36

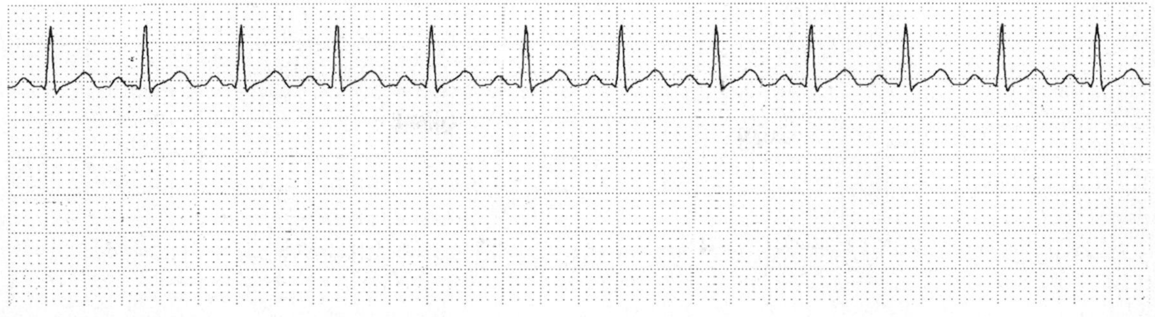

Figure 14–13 ■ Sinus Tachycardia

1. Rate = 120
2. R-R interval: regular
3. *P* wave has same configuration
4. *PR* interval = 0.14–0.16
5. *P* wave precedes *QRS*: yes
6. *QRS* complex = 0.06–0.08
7. *QT* interval = 0.28

(From Beasley, B. M. [2003]. *A Practical Approach* (2nd ed.). Upper Saddle River, NJ: Pearson/Prentice Hall.)

sympathetic stimulation. Nursing measures may include imagery, distraction, and promoting a calm environment, as well as drug therapy. Drugs used include sedatives, tranquilizers, antianxiety agents, analgesics, and antipyretics.

An ECG tracing of sinus tachycardia is presented in Figure 14–13.

In cases of sinus node dysfunction, atrial conduction becomes less effective, and "rescue" rhythms originating elsewhere in the atria occur to maintain cardiac output (e.g., atrial flutter and atrial fibrillation; see Section Six). Ultimately, a pacemaker may be required (see Section Twelve).

The nurse assesses the patient for signs of decreasing level of consciousness, hypotension, and angina. When these symptoms occur, the dysrhythmia is treated. Table 14–2 compares sinus dysrhythmias.

TABLE 14–2 Sinus Dysrhythmias: ECG Characteristics and Treatment Strategies

RHYTHM	CHARACTERISTIC	SYMPTOMATIC TREATMENT STRATEGIES
Sinus bradycardia	Rate less than 60 bpm	Atropine/Pacemaker
Sinus tachycardia	Rate greater than 100 bpm and less than 150 bpm	Antianxiety measures Pain relief measures Antipyretics Oxygen Calcium channel blockers Beta-blocking agents Fluids Vagal nerve stimulus (cough/bear down) Carotid artery massage

ECG INTERPRETATION EXERCISE

1.

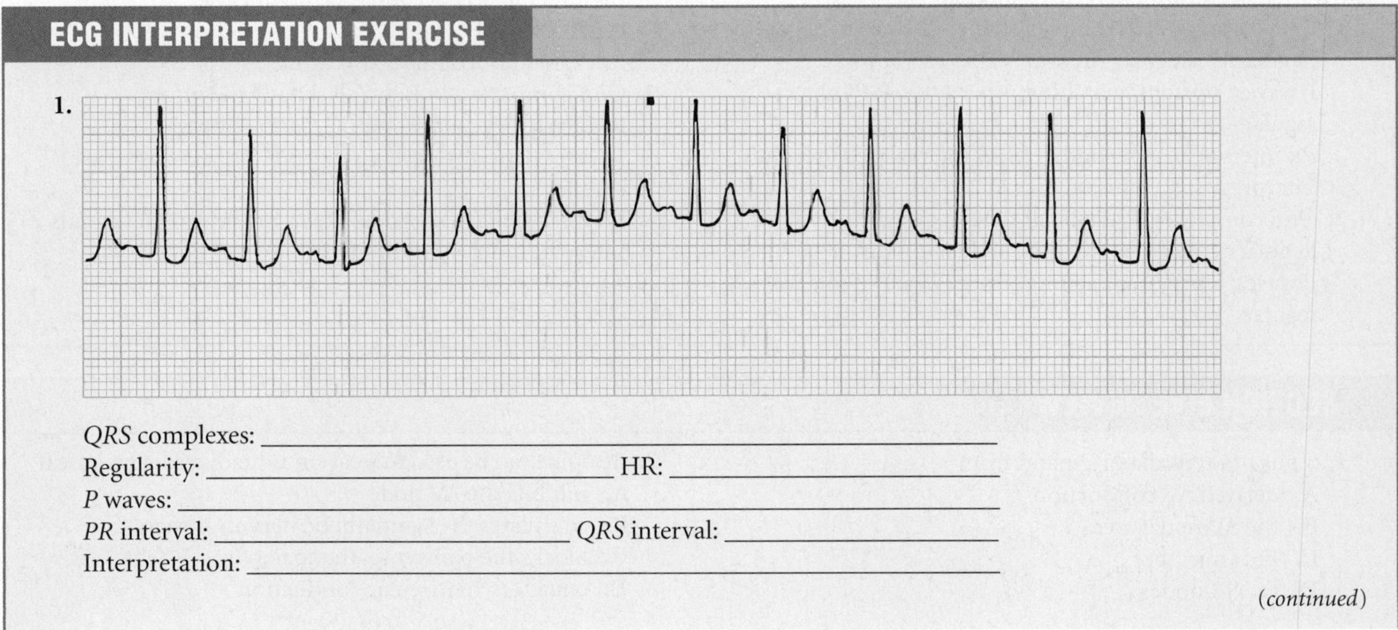

QRS complexes: ______

Regularity: ______ HR: ______

P waves: ______

PR interval: ______ *QRS* interval: ______

Interpretation: ______

(*continued*)

(continued)

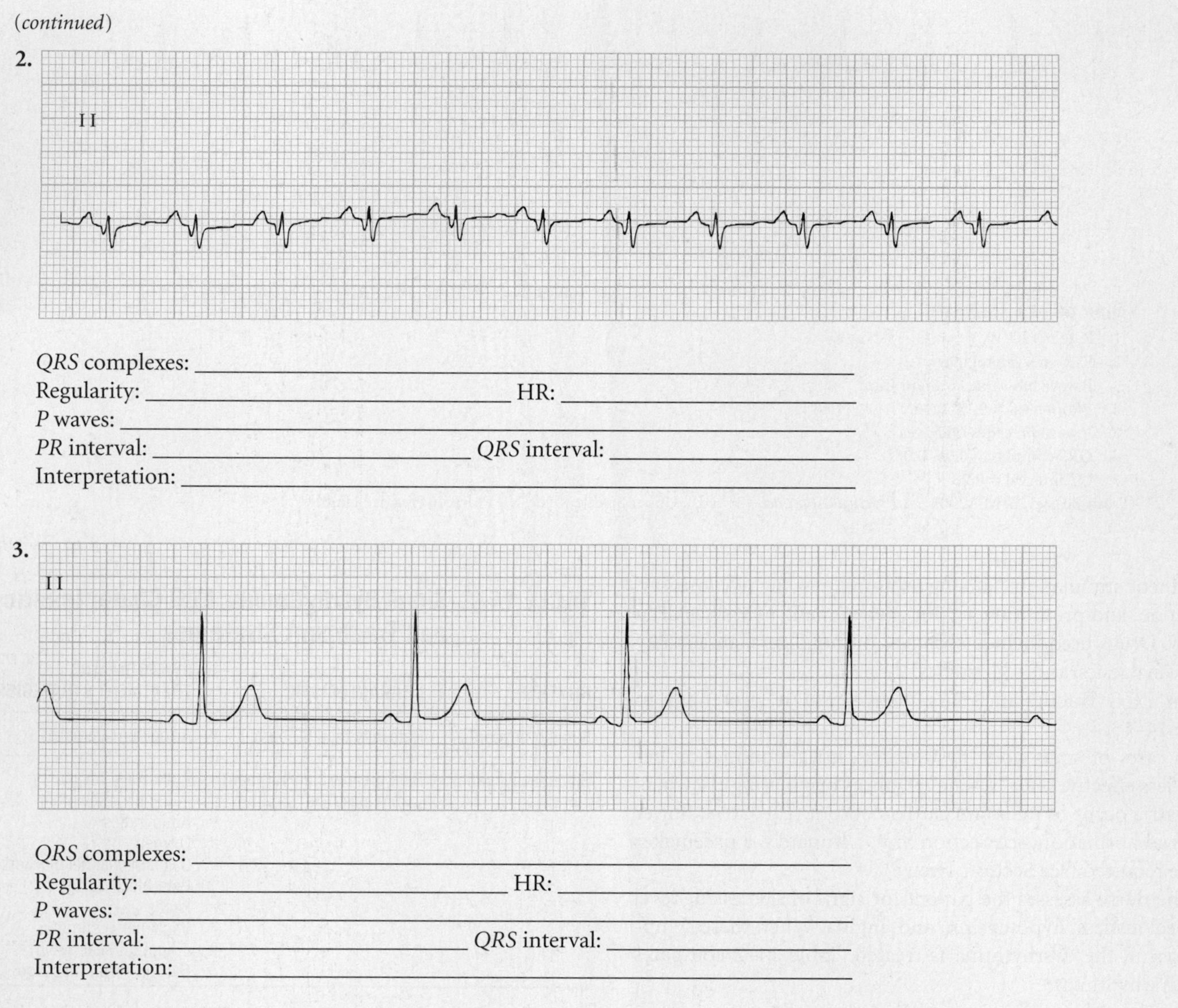

2.

QRS complexes: ______________________

Regularity: ______________ HR: ______________

P waves: ______________________

PR interval: ______________ *QRS* interval: ______________

Interpretation: ______________________

3.

QRS complexes: ______________________

Regularity: ______________ HR: ______________

P waves: ______________________

PR interval: ______________ *QRS* interval: ______________

Interpretation: ______________________

ECG Interpretation Exercise Answers:

1. *QRS* complexes: Present, all shaped the same
   Regularity: Regular rhythm HR: 125 bpm
   P waves: Upright, matching, 1 per *QRS*, P-P interval regular
   PR interval: 0.14 seconds *QRS* interval: 0.08 seconds
   Interpretation: Sinus tachycardia
2. *QRS* complexes: Present, all shaped the same
   Regularity: Regular rhythm HR: 115 bpm
   P waves: Upright, matching, 1 per *QRS*, P-P interval regular
   PR interval: 0.12 seconds *QRS* interval: 0.10 seconds
   Interpretation: Sinus tachycardia
3. *QRS* complexes: Present, all shaped the same
   Regularity: Regular rhythm HR: 47 bpm
   P waves: Upright, matching, 1 per *QRS*, P-P interval regular
   PR interval: 0.16 seconds *QRS* interval: 0.08 seconds
   Interpretation: Sinus bradycardia

SECTION FIVE REVIEW

1. Sinus bradycardia originates from
   A. delayed AV conduction
   B. the AV nodal area
   C. Purkinje fibers
   D. the SA node
2. Atropine can be used to treat sinus bradycardia because it
   A. inhibits the AV node
   B. stimulates the sympathetic nervous system
   C. blocks the parasympathetic nervous system
   D. enhances ventricular conduction

3. Sinus tachycardia results from all of the following EXCEPT
   A. parasympathetic stimulation
   B. anxiety
   C. pain
   D. fever
4. What interventions are used to treat symptomatic sinus tachycardia?
   A. imagery
   B. promoting a calm environment
   C. defibrillation
   D. A and B
5. Decreasing levels of consciousness associated with sinus dysrhythmias indicates
   A. decreased ventricular contractility
   B. decreased cardiac output
   C. increased atrial filling
   D. decreased AV conduction

Answers: 1. D, 2. C, 3. A, 4. D, 5. B

SECTION SIX: Atrial Dysrhythmias

At the completion of this section, the learner will be able to identify basic atrial dysrhythmias and describe appropriate treatment.

Common atrial dysrhythmias include supraventricular tachycardia (SVT), atrial flutter, and atrial fibrillation (AFib). Each of these dysrhythmias is characterized by a rapid atrial rate. A rapid ventricular response can occur as a result of the rapid atrial rate and when this happens, the patient can be symptomatic. Symptoms can include a fluttering sensation in the chest, dyspnea, lightheadedness, or angina. The rapid heart rate decreases ventricular filling time and stroke volume.

Supraventricular Tachycardia

Supraventricular tachycardia (SVT) has a rate between 150 and 250 bpm. The rhythm is regular, but *P* waves are not distinguishable because they are buried in the preceding *T* wave (Fig. 14–14). The *QRS* complex appears normal because ventricular conduction is not affected. Normal *QRS* complexes indicate that the **ectopic pacemaker** is located above the ventricles. SVT can be treated with Valsalva's maneuver or adenosine. Adenosine temporarily inhibits AV node conduction and blocks reentry of impulses from the ventricles. Consequently, heart rate decreases and conduction of impulses through the AV node slows. Adenosine has a very short half-life (approximately 10 seconds). A brief period of asystole (up to 15 seconds) is common after rapid administration. Side effects include facial flushing, dyspnea, and chest pressure. Calcium channel blocking agents (i.e., diltiazem) are used to prevent the influx of calcium into the cell and to prevent depolarization. Verapamil, digitalis preparations, or beta blockers can also be used. In cases in which the patient is experiencing distress or is unresponsive to drug therapy, electric cardioversion is used to rapidly correct the dysrhythmia (Section Eleven).

Atrial Flutter

Atrial flutter has a faster rate than SVT. The atrial rate is greater than 250 bpm. The ventricular rate depends on the number of impulses that pass through the AV node. The ventricular rate can be irregular if some of the impulses are blocked. The atrial oscillations appear as sawtooth or flutter waves. A fast ventricular rate decreases SV in the absence of digitalis toxicity. Cardioversion is the preferred method of treating this dysrhythmia. Calcium channel blockers,

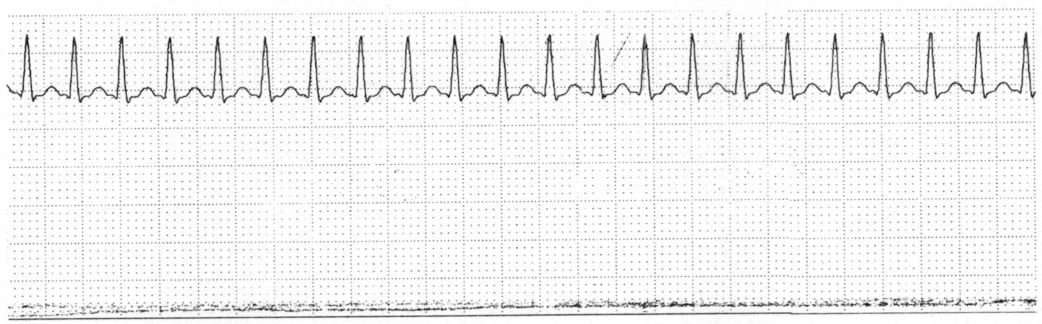

Figure 14–14 ■ Supraventricular tachycardia

1. Rate = 250
2. R-R interval: regular
3. *P* wave: difficult to distinguish
4. *PR* interval: cannot calculate
5. *P* wave precedes each *QRS*: cannot identify
6. *QRS* complex = 0.06
7. *QT* interval = 0.20

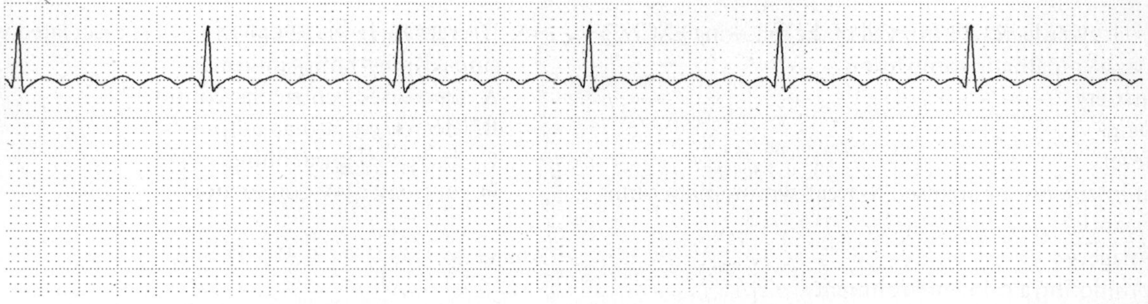

Figure 14–15 ■ Atrial flutter.

1. Rate: artrial = 250 ventricular = 60
2. R-R interval: regular
3. *P* wave: cannot distinguish, flutter wave present
4. *PR* interval = cannot calculate
5. *P* wave precedes *QRS*: cannot identify
6. *QRS* complex = 0.06
7. *QT* interval = cannot be determined

beta-blocking agents, and digitalis preparations may be used (Section Eleven). Atrial flutter is described by the number of atrial oscillations (*f waves*) between each *QRS* complex (Fig. 14–15).

Atrial Fibrillation

Atrial fibrillation (AFib) is the most common sustained arrhythmia and is found in more than 2 million patients in the United States, with increase risk of developing in the elderly population (Futterman & Lemberg (2005). AFib is a condition in which the atria are contracting so fast that they are unable to refill before contraction. Therefore, the ventricles are inadequately filled and SV is diminished by approximately 25 percent. The atria are not able to empty completely because of the fast rate of depolarization. Blood that remains in the atria is prone to forming clots, which increases the risk of thrombotic stroke. AFib has an irregular ventricular response (Figure 14–16). The *QRS* complexes are normal in appearance but occur at irregular intervals. This is manifested clinically as a difference between the apical heart rate and the peripheral pulse rate because the SV is inadequate with some beats to produce a peripheral pulse. The atria can be discharging at a rate greater than 400 bpm. Absent *P* waves and irregular *QRS* intervals are characteristic of this dysrhythmia.

Control of the ventricular rate is important in AFib. Drugs that are particularly effective in controlling ventricular rate are amiodarone, digoxin, beta-adrenergic blocking agents, and calcium channel blocking agents. Conversion of the AFib to a normal sinus rhythm improves hemodynamics. In some cases, AFib is resistant to conversion by either method. AFib is not treated if it is of long-standing duration and does not produce symptoms. A significant risk factor, however, is the formation of clots in the fibrillating atria, thereby increasing the risk of stroke and pulmonary embolism in the patient. Generally, patients in AFib require anticoagulation such as warfarin therapy.

Table 14–3 summarizes the ECG characteristics and treatment strategies for the atrial dysrhythmias

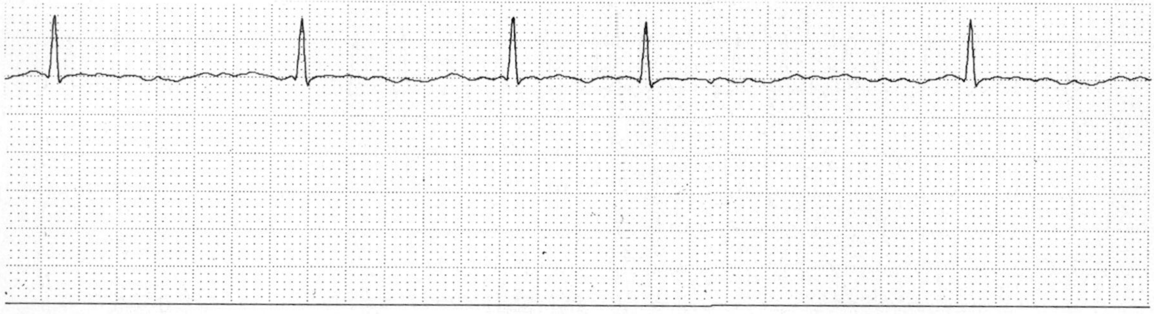

Figure 14–16 ■ Atrial fibrillation.

1. Rate: artrial: unable to calculate, ventricular = 50
2. R-R interval: irregular
3. *P* wave: undistinguishable
4. *PR* interval: cannot calculate
5. *P* wave precedes each *QRS*: cannot identify
6. *QRS* complex = 0.06
7. *QT* interval = cannot be determined

TABLE 14–3 Atrial Dysrhythmias: ECG Characteristics and Treatment Strategies

RHYTHM	CHARACTERISTIC	TREATMENT STRATEGIES
Supraventricular tachycardia	*P* waves not distinguishable R–R interval regular Atrial rate 150 to 250 bpm	Adenosine Vagal maneuvers Beta-blocking agents Calcium channel blocking agents Cardioversion
Atrial flutter	R–R interval may be regular or irregular Atrial rate may be up to 350 bpm Sawtoothed waves	Cardioversion Digitalis
Atrial fibrillation	R–R interval irregular Atrial rate greater than 350 bpm	Digitalis Amiodarone Cardioversion Beta-blocking agents Calcium channel blocking agents *Note: If atrial fibrillation duration greater than 48 hours, anticoagulation must be considered before rhythm conversion is attempted to avoid clot dislodgement from the atria.

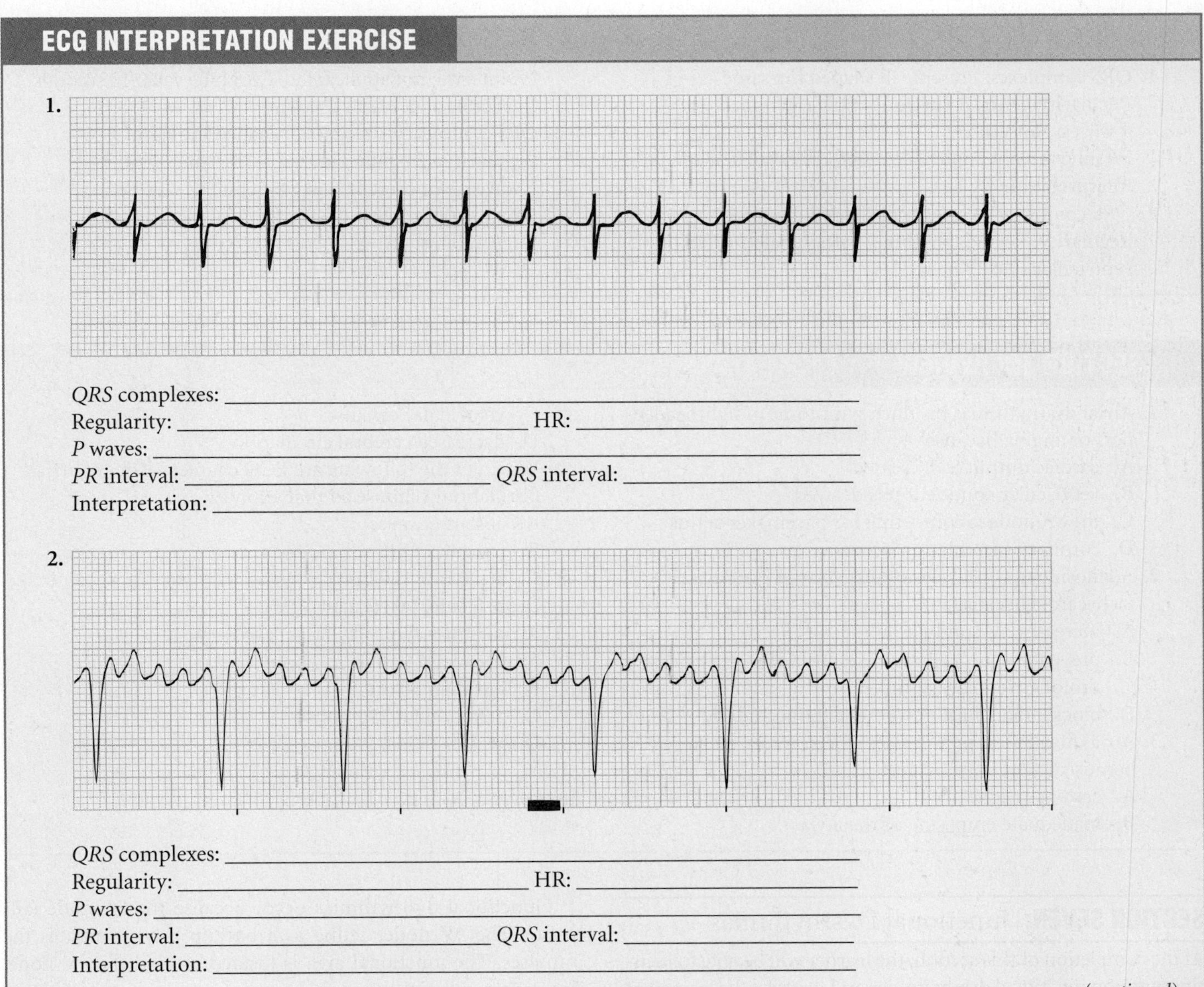

ECG INTERPRETATION EXERCISE

1.

QRS complexes: ____________________

Regularity: ____________________ HR: ____________________

P waves: ____________________

PR interval: ____________________ *QRS* interval: ____________________

Interpretation: ____________________

2.

QRS complexes: ____________________

Regularity: ____________________ HR: ____________________

P waves: ____________________

PR interval: ____________________ *QRS* interval: ____________________

Interpretation: ____________________

(continued)

(continued)

3.

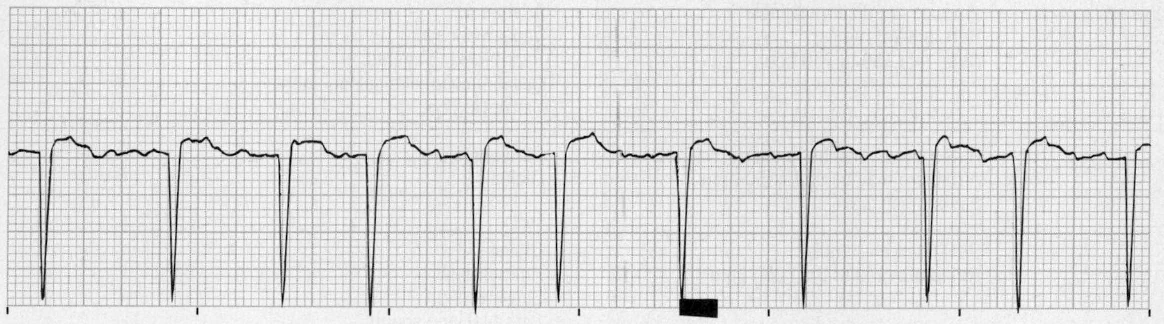

QRS complexes: ______________________________
Regularity: ______________ HR: ______________
P waves: ______________________________
PR interval: ______________ *QRS* interval: ______________
Interpretation: ______________________________

ECG Interpretation Exercise Answers:

1. *QRS* complexes: Present, all shaped the same
   Regularity: Regular rhythm HR: 150 bpm
   P waves: Not visible
   PR interval: not applicable *QRS* interval: 0.08 seconds
   Interpretation: SVT
2. *QRS* complexes: Present, all shaped the same
   Regularity: Regular rhythm HR: Atrial rate 375 bpm, ventricular rate 79 bpm
   P waves: Not present, flutter waves present
   PR interval: not applicable *QRS* interval: 0.10 seconds
   Interpretation: Atrial Flutter
3. *QRS* complexes: Present, all shaped the same
   Regularity: irregular rhythm HR: 88-137 bpm
   P waves: Not present, wavy baseline
   PR Not applicable *QRS* interval: 0.08 seconds
   Interpretation: AFib

SECTION SIX REVIEW

1. Atrial dysrhythmias produce symptoms of lightheadedness or angina because
   A. cardiac output is decreased
   B. ventricular conduction is delayed
   C. the SA node is competing for pacemaker status
   D. coronary vasodilation occurs
2. Adenosine may be used to treat supraventricular tachycardia because it
   A. increases AV conduction
   B. prevents reentry of impulses from the ventricles
   C. prolongs repolarization
   D. blocks potassium movement extracellularly
3. Atrial fibrillation predisposes a person to a stroke because it produces
   A. cardiac fatigue
   B. inadequate emptying of the atria
   C. ventricular exhaustion
   D. decreased cerebral circulation
4. Which of the following are ECG characteristics of atrial fibrillation? (choose all that apply)
   A. absent *P* waves
   B. irregular *QRS*
   C. atrial rate 150 bpm
   D. R-R interval regular
5. Atrial flutter typically has an atrial rate
   A. between 150 and 250 bpm
   B. less than 60 bpm
   C. greater than 250 bpm
   D. greater than 400 bpm

Answers: 1. A, 2. B, 3. B, 4. (A, B), 5. C

SECTION SEVEN: Junctional Dysrhythmias

At the completion of this section, the learner will be able to identify common junctional dysrhythmias and describe the treatment of these dysrhythmias.

Junctional dysrhythmias occur because the SA node fails to fire. The AV node, acting as a backup mode, initiates the impulses. The junctional area is located around the AV node. Pacemaker cells in this area have an intrinsic rate of 40 to 60 bpm. After the pacemaker cell discharges, it spreads upward

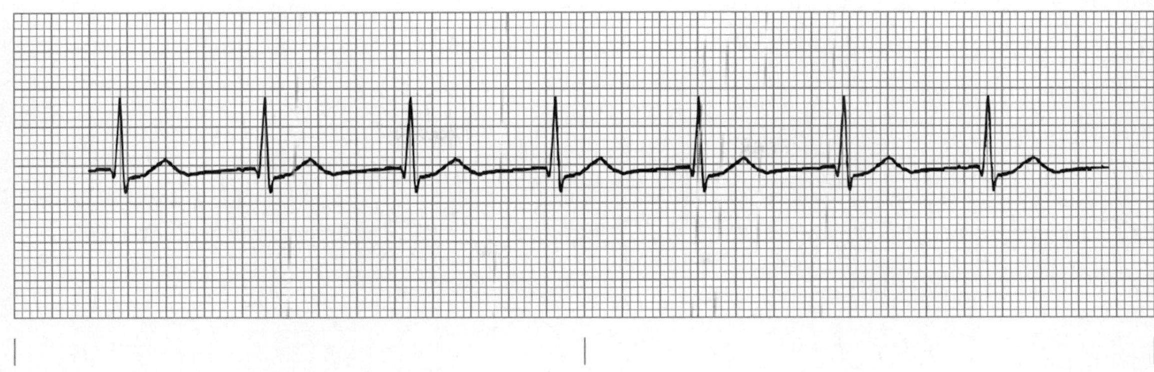

Figure 14–17 ■ Accelerated junctional rhythm.

to depolarize the atria and downward to depolarize the ventricles. Because the ventricles usually are depolarized in a downward fashion, the *QRS* complex appears normal. The atria are depolarized in an abnormal manner so the *P* wave can be inverted. The timing of the *P* wave is abnormal. It may precede the *QRS* complex, but the *PR* interval is shorter than 0.12 seconds. The *P* wave can be buried in the *QRS* complex and be indistinguishable or it can follow the *QRS* complex.

Junctional Tachycardia

The term *junctional tachycardia* refers to a junctional rhythm with a rate greater than 100 bpm. If the rate of the rhythm is between 60 and 100 bpm, it is called an *accelerated junctional rhythm* (illustrated in Fig. 14–17).

Digitalis decreases the automaticity of the AV node and slows conduction between the SA and AV node; therefore, digitalis toxicity can precipitate junctional rhythms. The dysrhythmia is treated by withholding the medication. Usually, the patient can tolerate junctional rhythms; however, if the patient experiences symptoms of decreased CO because the rate is too slow, atropine is administered. A pacemaker may be inserted as a protective measure in case the junction fails or if the patient is symptomatic.

Table 14–4 compares the ECG characteristics and treatment strategies for junctional dysrhythmias.

TABLE 14–4 Junctional Dysrhythmias: ECG Characteristics and Treatment Strategies

RHYTHM	CHARACTERISTIC	TREATMENT STRATEGIES
Junctional rhythm	Rate 40 to 60 bpm Inverted or absent *P* waves	May not be treated if patient is asymptomatic Atropine Pacemaker insertion
Junctional tachycardia (Accelerated Junctional Rhythm)	Rate greater than 100 bpm Inverted or absent *P* waves	May not be treated if patient is asymptomatic Pacemaker insertion Withhold digitalis if associated with digitalis toxicity

ECG INTERPRETATION EXERCISE

1.

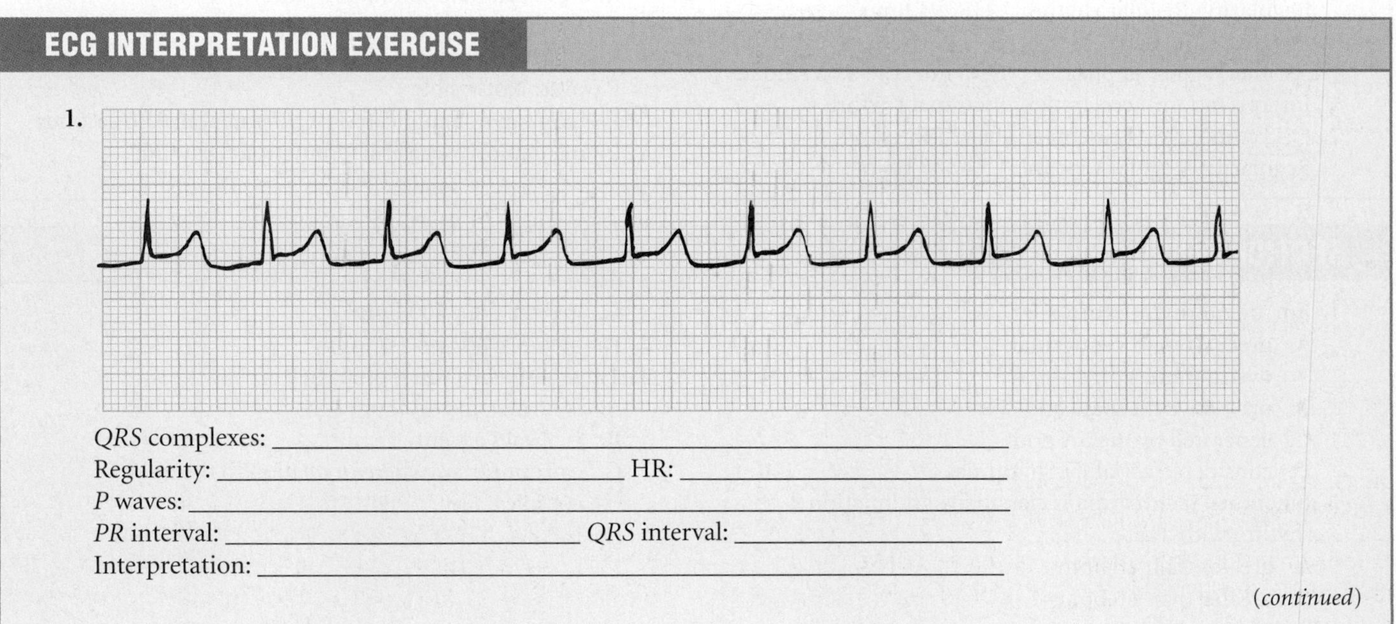

QRS complexes: ____________________

Regularity: ____________________ HR: ____________________

P waves: ____________________

PR interval: ____________________ *QRS* interval: ____________________

Interpretation: ____________________

(continued)

(continued)

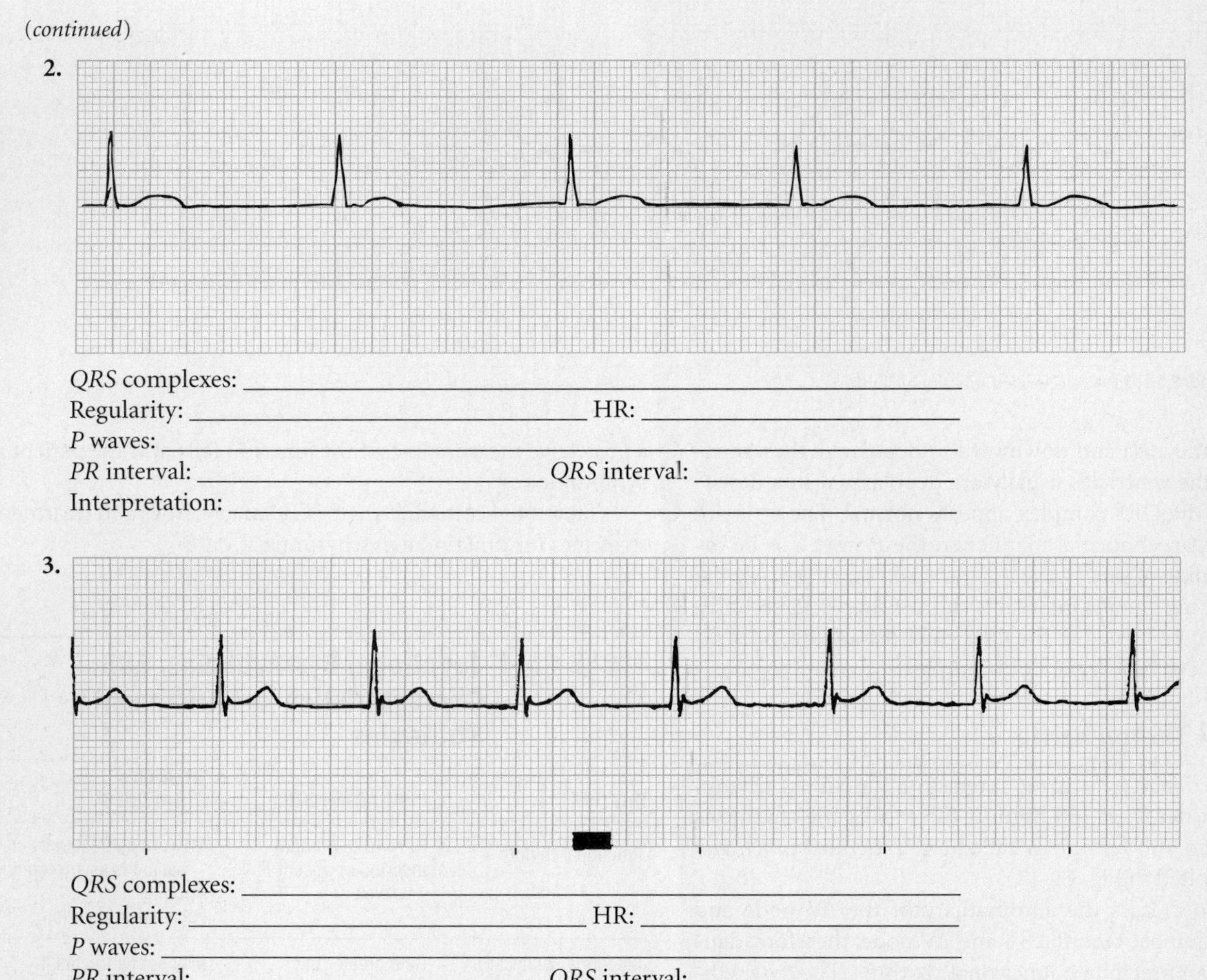

2.

QRS complexes: ______________________

Regularity: ______________ HR: ______________

P waves: ______________________

PR interval: ______________ *QRS* interval: ______________

Interpretation: ______________________

3.

QRS complexes: ______________________

Regularity: ______________ HR: ______________

P waves: ______________________

PR interval: ______________ *QRS* interval: ______________

Interpretation: ______________________

ECG Interpretation Exercise Answers:

1. *QRS* complexes: Present, all shaped the same
   Regularity: Regular rhythm HR: 94 bpm
   P waves: Not visible
   PR interval: not applicable *QRS* interval: 0.08 seconds
   Interpretation: Accelerated junctional rhythm
2. *QRS* complexes: Present, all shaped the same
   Regularity: Regular rhythm HR: 48 bpm
   P waves: Not visible
   PR interval: not applicable *QRS* interval: 0.08 seconds
   Interpretation: Junctional rhythm
3. *QRS* complexes: Present, all shaped the same
   Regularity: Regular rhythm HR: 72 bpm
   P waves: Not visible
   PR interval: not applicable *QRS* interval: 0.10 seconds
   Interpretation: Accelerated junctional rhythm

SECTION SEVEN REVIEW

1. Junctional rhythms are
   - **A.** precursors to ventricular dysrhythmias
   - **B.** protective mechanisms
   - **C.** generated by the SA node
   - **D.** considered atrial dysrhythmias
2. Junctional tachycardia is classified as a junctional rhythm with a rate
   - **A.** greater than 40 bpm
   - **B.** greater than 60 bpm
   - **C.** greater than 100 bpm
   - **D.** between 60 and 100 bpm
3. The *P* wave in a junctional rhythm
   - **A.** is bizarre in configuration
   - **B.** is always absent
   - **C.** can appear anywhere in relation to the *QRS* complex
   - **D.** is flat

4. An accelerated junctional rhythm has a rate of
   A. less than 60 bpm
   B. 60 to 100 bpm
   C. 100 to 120 bpm
   D. greater than 150 bpm

5. Interventions for junctional rhythms may include (choose all that apply)
   A. administration of digitalis
   B. atropine
   C. a pacemaker
   D. cardioversion

Answers: 1. B, 2. C, 3. C, 4. B, 5. B, C

SECTION EIGHT: Premature Contractions

At the completion of this section, the learner will be able to compare and contrast atrial and ventricular premature beats, identify their origin, and describe the treatment of these premature beats.

Premature heart beats originate from an excitable focus outside of the normal SA node pacemaker (an ectopic pacemaker). Premature heart beats are a relatively common phenomenon and in healthy people they are benign. In the presence of cardiovascular disease, however, ectopic pacemakers can trigger potentially life-threatening cardiac dysrhythmias. Premature heart beats are usually caused by enhanced automaticity of cardiac cells resulting from a stimulus such as caffeine, nicotine, alcohol, or stress. In patients with cardiovascular disease, the most dangerous cause is cardiac ischemia.

Premature Atrial Contractions

Premature atrial contractions (PACs) originate from one (**unifocal**) or more (**multifocal**) ectopic pacemakers located in the atria. A *P* wave is visible, unless it is hidden in the preceding *T* wave. The premature *P* wave may look different from the normal *P* wave, depending on the location of the originating impulse. The underlying rhythm is usually regular with the PAC causing a brief irregularity. There is a characteristic short pause following a PAC called a *noncompensatory pause* (i.e., the R-R interval from the *R* wave preceding the PAC to the *R* wave following the PAC is less than two regular R-R intervals measured on the underlying regular rhythm). PAC's are generally benign, however they may serve as an early warning for the development of atrial dysrhythmias (A-fib, A-flutter, SVT) and therefore, they warrant continued close observation of the patient. Figure 14–18 shows an example of a PAC.

Premature Ventricular Contractions

Premature ventricular contractions (PVCs) are premature ventricular beats that originate in an irritable ventricle before the next sinus beat is due. Since the electrical stimulus is originating outside of the atria, there is no *P* wave preceding the PVC. The wave form of a PVC is usually large (higher voltage on ECG monitor and wider than 0.12 seconds). The wave form is also bizarre appearing and is generally in the opposite direction of the person's usual *QRS* complex. There is a characteristic full *compensatory pause* (i.e., the R-R interval from the *R* wave preceding the PVC to the *R* wave following the PVC is equal to two regular R-R intervals of the underlying rhythm). Unifocal PVCs (Fig. 14–19) originate from same location so their configuration is the same. Multifocal PVCs (Fig. 14–20), however, originate from two or more locations and therefore have different configurations. Ventricular diastole following a PVC is too brief, therefore ineffective and does not contribute significantly to cardiac output.

Certain circumstances warrant close observation of PVCs because they are associated with development of ventricular

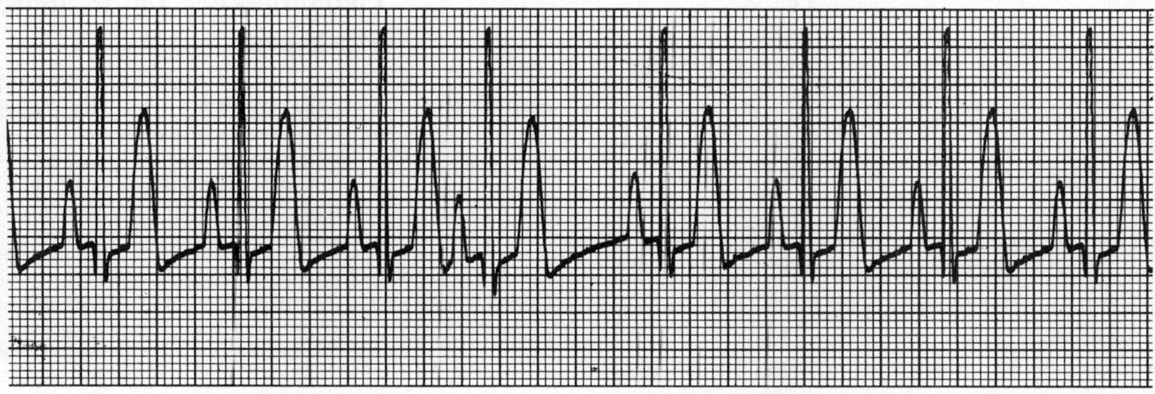

Figure 14–18 ■ Premature atrial contractions. Note the PAC that occurs following the third *QRS* complex. This is followed by a normal appearing *QRS* and a short (noncompensatory) pause.

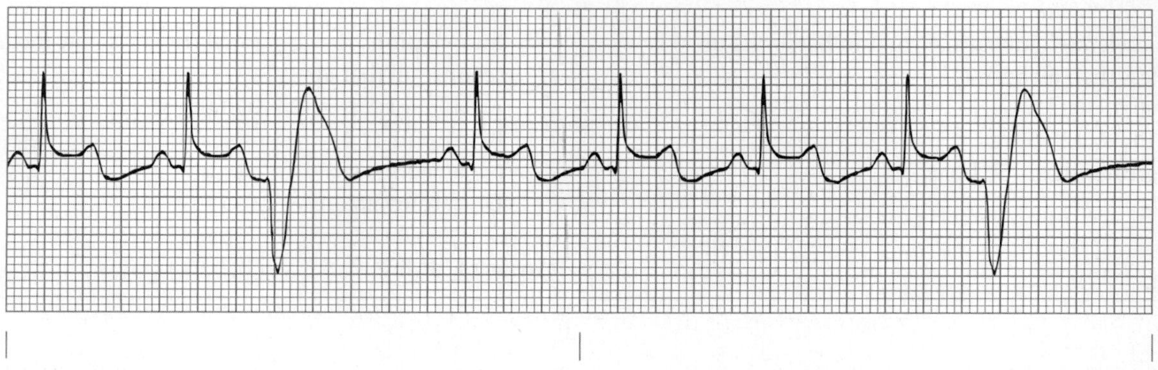

Figure 14–19 ■ Unifocal PVCs. Note that the two PVCs are bizarre in appearance and the wave forms are in opposite directions of the underlying *QRS* complexes.

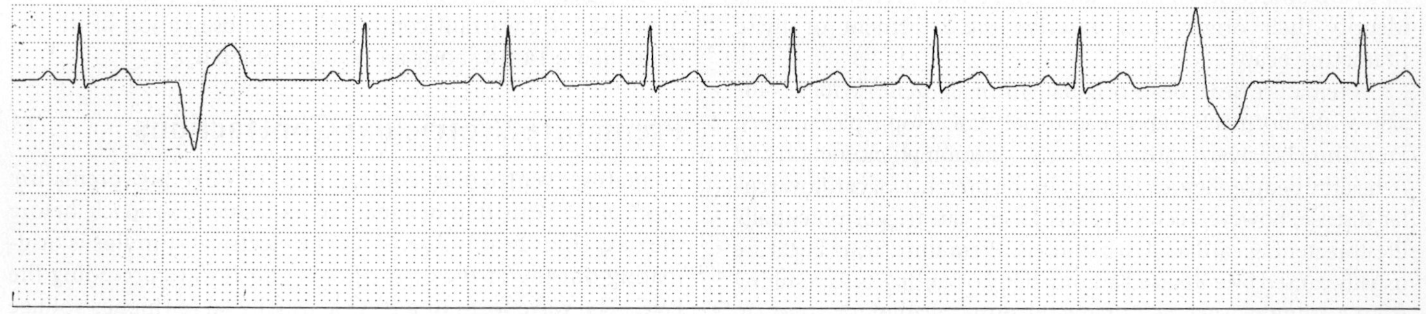

Figure 14–20 ■ Multifocal PVC's. [*Note:* Strip is longer than 6 seconds = 37 (0.20) boxes.] Note the differences in PVC configurations.

TABLE 14–5 Circumstances that Warrant Close Observation of Premature Ventricular Contractions

- More than six PVCs per minute
- PVCs occurring together (couplet)
- Multifocal PVCs (from more than one ectopic focus)
- A run of ventricular tachycardia (more than three PVCs in a row)
- R-on-T phenomenon (PVC that occurs on the down-stroke of the *T* wave preceding the PVC. The down-stroke of the *T* wave is a relative refractory or vulnerable period whereby a strong enough stimulus can excite the heart and trigger VT or VF).

tachycardia (VT) and ventricular fibrillation (VF). These circumstances are listed in Table 14–5.

The nurse assesses and describes the patient's underlying cardiac rhythm and the type of PVC (unifocal versus multifocal). The timing of the PVCs is described if they occur in a repeatable pattern. For example, **bigeminy** is a pattern of one normal SA node–initiated beat followed by one PVC (Fig. 14–21). **Trigeminy** is a pattern of two normal beats followed by one PVC (Fig. 14–22).

A major responsibility of the nurse is to assess the patient for factors that contribute to the development of PVCs. Electrolyte balance, particularly a low potassium and/ or magnesium, should be evaluated as potential causes of the myocardial irritability. Hypoxemia can contribute to the development of PVCs. Occasional PVCs do not require treatment. If the potassium is low, supplemental potassium is given. Hypoxemia is corrected with supplemental oxygen. Amiodarone is most commonly administered if frequent PVCs occur in the setting of myocardial ischemia or if the patient is symptomatic (hypotension).

Table 14–6 compares ECG characteristics and treatment strategies for premature atrial and ventricular beats.

TABLE 14–6 Premature Contractions: ECG Characteristics and Treatment Strategies

CONTRACTION	CHARACTERISTIC	TREATMENT STRATEGIES
Premature atrial contraction	*PR* interval may be normal or prolonged *QRS* normal	May not be treated if patient is asymptomatic Reduce caffeine, alcohol intake Beta-blocking agents
Premature ventricular contraction	*PR* interval absent in premature beat *QRS* greater than 0.12 second(s)	May not be treated if patient is asymptomatic Reduce caffeine intake Decrease stress Amiodarone Correct low electrolyte levels

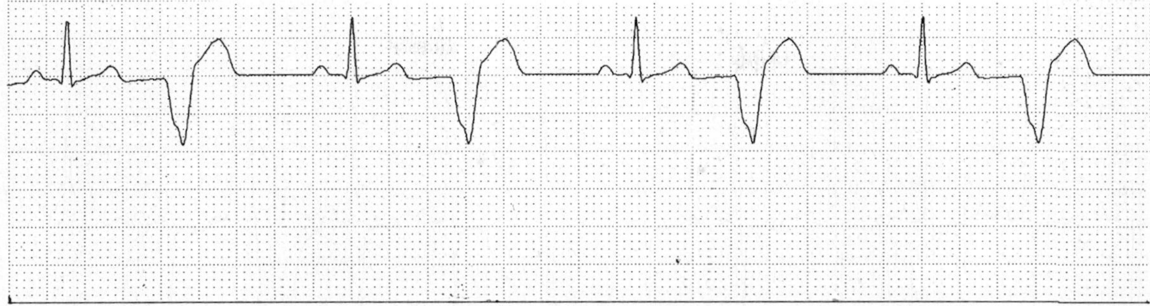

Figure 14–21 ■ Ventricular bigeminy. Note that the heart rate is actually 40 bpm since PVCs do not contribute to the cardiac output.

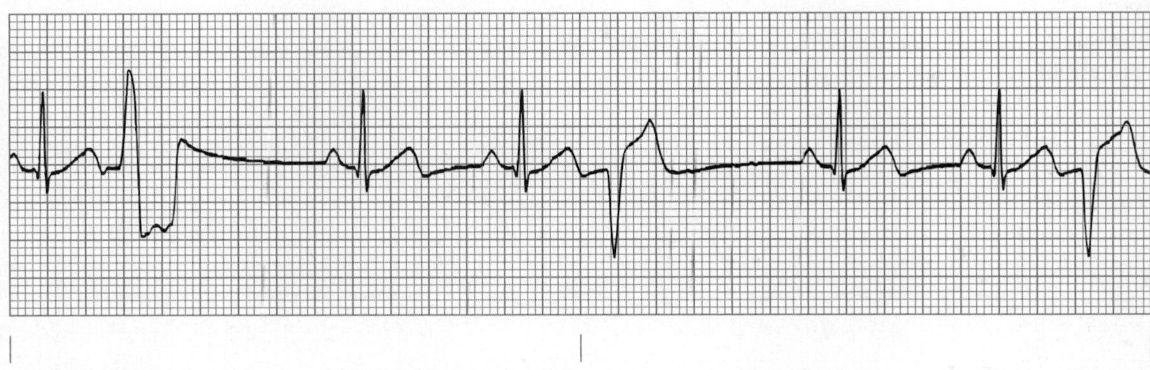

Figure 14–22 ■ Ventricular trigeminy with multifocal PVCs.

ECG INTERPRETATION EXERCISE

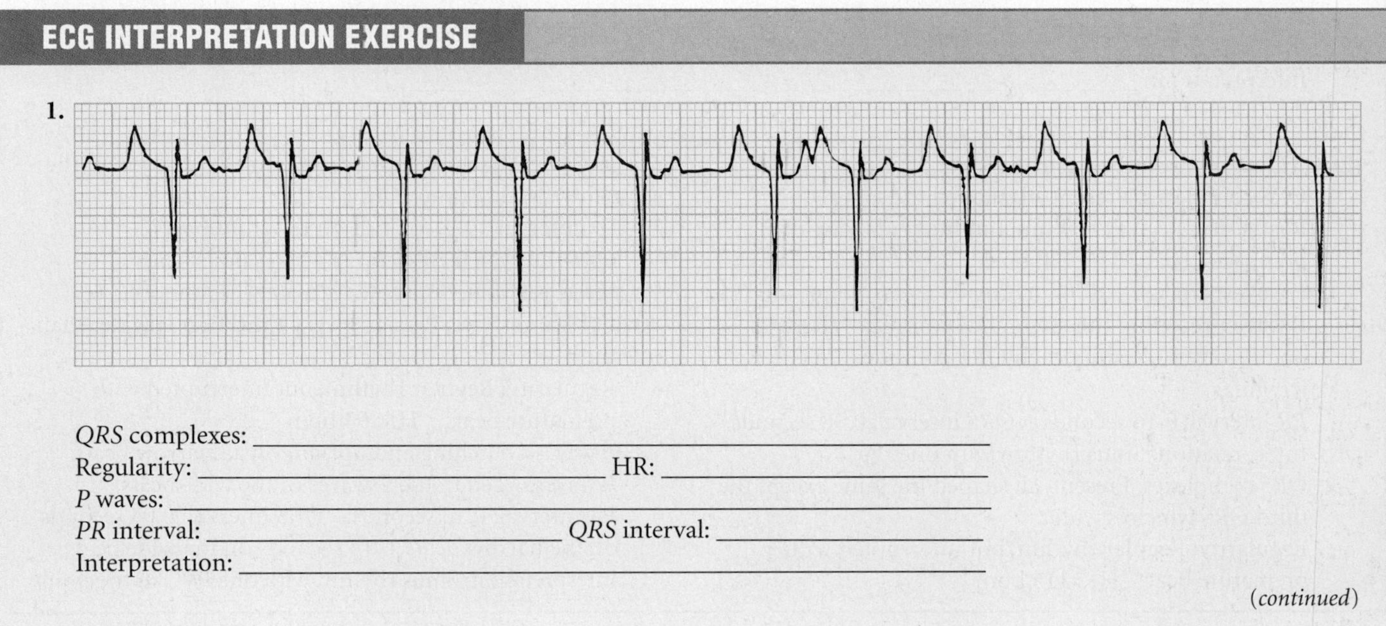

1.

QRS complexes: ____________________

Regularity: ____________________ HR: ____________________

P waves: ____________________

PR interval: ____________________ *QRS* interval: ____________________

Interpretation: ____________________

(continued)

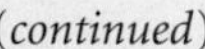

(*continued*)

2.

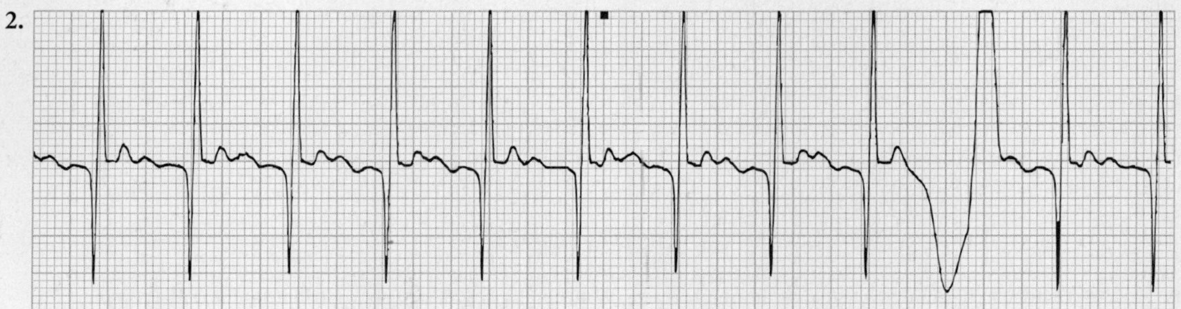

QRS complexes: ____________________
Regularity: ____________________ HR: ____________________
P waves: ____________________
PR interval: ____________________ *QRS* interval: ____________________
Interpretation: ____________________

3.

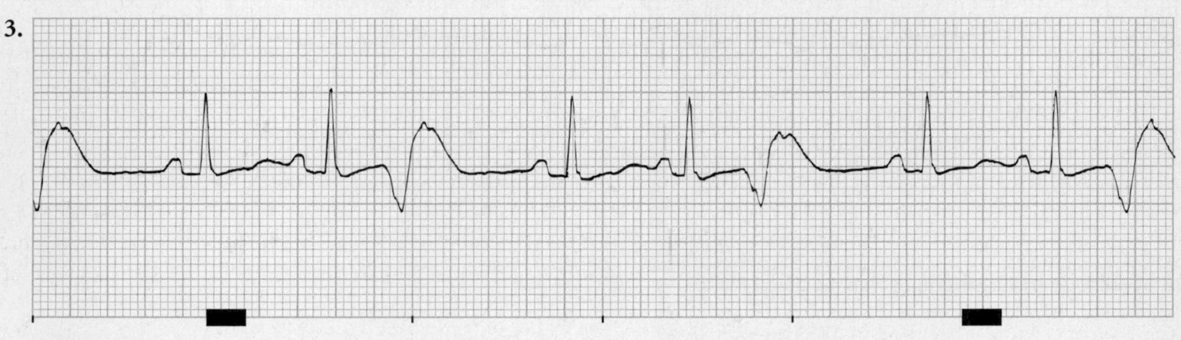

QRS complexes: ____________________
Regularity: ____________________ HR: ____________________
P waves: ____________________
PR interval: ____________________ *QRS* interval: ____________________
Interpretation: ____________________

ECG Interpretation Exercise Answers:

1. *QRS* complexes: Present, all shaped the same
   Regularity: Regular rhythm, but interrupted with a premature beat HR:100 bpm
   P waves: Upright, all matching except for a premature *P* wave preceding the sixth *QRS* complex. There is one *P* wave preceding each *QRS* complex, P-P irregular
   PR interval: 0.16 seconds *QRS* interval: 0.08 seconds
   Interpretation: Sinus rhythm with one PAC
2. *QRS* complexes: Present, all shaped the same except the third *QRS* which is wider.
   Regularity: Regular rhythm, but interrupted with a premature beat HR: 115 bpm
   P waves: Matching and upright on all beats except the third which has no *P* wave.
   PR interval: 0.12 seconds on the sinus beats
   QRS interval: 0.10 seconds on the sinus beats
   Interpretation: Sinus tachycardia with one PVC
3. *QRS* complexes: Present, every third beat is wider than the rest
   Regularity: Regular rhythm, but interrupted with premature beats HR: 94 bpm
   P waves: Matching and upright on all narrow beats. *P* waves noted in the *T* waves of the wide beats.
   PR interval: 0.16 seconds *QRS* interval: 0.06 seconds on the narrow beats, 0.14 seconds on the wide beats
   Interpretation: Sinus rhythm with one PVC in trigeminy

SECTION EIGHT REVIEW

1. Which of the following statements best describes premature beats?
   - **A.** They originate anywhere along the cardiac conduction pathway.
   - **B.** They originate in the atria.
   - **C.** They originate in the ventricles.
   - **D.** They originate in the junctional (AV nodal) area.
2. Which of the following is/are characteristic of PACs? (choose all that apply)
   - **A.** There is a premature ventricular contraction.
   - **B.** There is a premature *P* wave.
   - **C.** The underlying rhythm is irregular.
   - **D.** There is a noncompensatory pause.
3. PVCs are frequently associated with
   - **A.** hyponatremia
   - **B.** hypocalcemia
   - **C.** hypoglycemia
   - **D.** hypokalemia
4. In PVCs, the *QRS* complex is
   - **A.** greater than 0.12 seconds
   - **B.** negatively deflected
   - **C.** isoelectric
   - **D.** preceded by a *T* wave
5. PVCs that warrant close observation include
   - **A.** 3 PVC's per minute
   - **B.** unifocal PVCs
   - **C.** more than 3 PVCs in a row
   - **D.** a PVC associated with caffeine use

Answers: 1. A, 2. B, 3. D, 4. A, 5. C

SECTION NINE: Ventricular Dysrhythmias

At the completion of this section, the learner will be able to identify common ventricular dysrhythmias and describe treatment of these dysrhythmias.

Ventricular dysrhythmias can be life-threatening. Inadequate ventricular ejection produces inadequate SV. If prolonged, oxygen delivery to the body's tissues is compromised, producing ischemia, organ failure and cell death. Two common ventricular dysrhythmias are ventricular tachycardia and ventricular fibrillation.

Ventricular Tachycardia

Ventricular tachycardia (VT) is classified as three or more consecutive PVCs occurring at a rapid rate, usually greater than 100 bpm. Although the SA node continues to fire, ectopic pacemakers in the ventricles fire spontaneously and bear no relationship to the SA node–initiated impulse. *P* waves are not identifiable because they are buried in the *QRS* complexes. The R–R interval is often regular, and the *QRS* complex is greater than 0.12 seconds. Short runs of VT (less than 30 seconds) generally can be tolerated. A danger of VT is that it may deteriorate into ventricular fibrillation. Patients can be alert while experiencing VT, and a carotid pulse can be present; however, as CO diminishes, a loss of consciousness may occur. Synchronized cardioversion may be used to convert the rhythm. When pulseless, defibrillation is used. Pharmacological treatment of VT includes amiodarone, lidocaine, and magnesium (AHA, 2006). Figure 14–23 is an example of VT.

Ventricular Fibrillation

Ventricular fibrillation is the most common cause of sudden death. The ECG pattern is chaotic. It is impossible to identify any *PQRST* waves, and the rhythm is grossly irregular (Fig. 14–24). The patient will be unresponsive, without a pulse, and requires emergency treatment and advanced cardiopulmonary resuscitation. Defibrillation is the treatment of choice and is used beginning with 120 J and progressing up to 360 J (dependent on type of defibrillator) (AHA, 2006). In public settings (airports, malls, etc.), an Automated External Defibrillator (AED) may be available to treat an individual

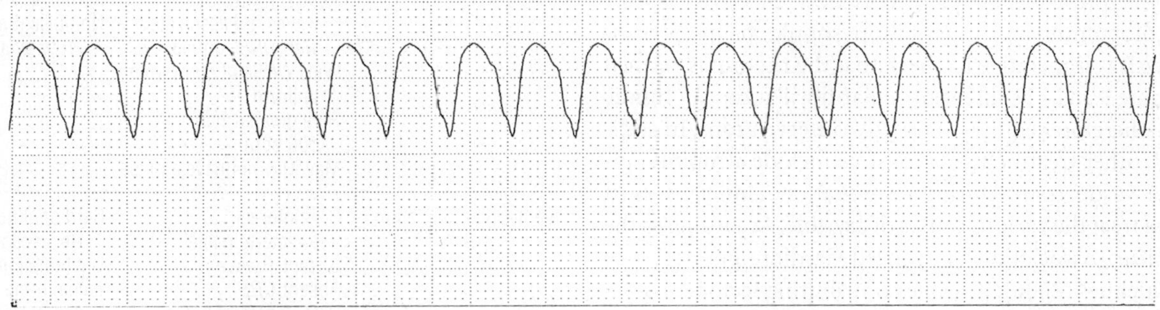

Figure 14–23 ■ Ventricular tachycardia.

1. Rate: atrial: unable to calculate
   ventricular = 180
2. R-R interval: regular
3. *P* wave: undistinguishable
4. *PR* interval: none
5. *P* wave precedes each *QRS*: no
6. *QRS* complex = 0.28

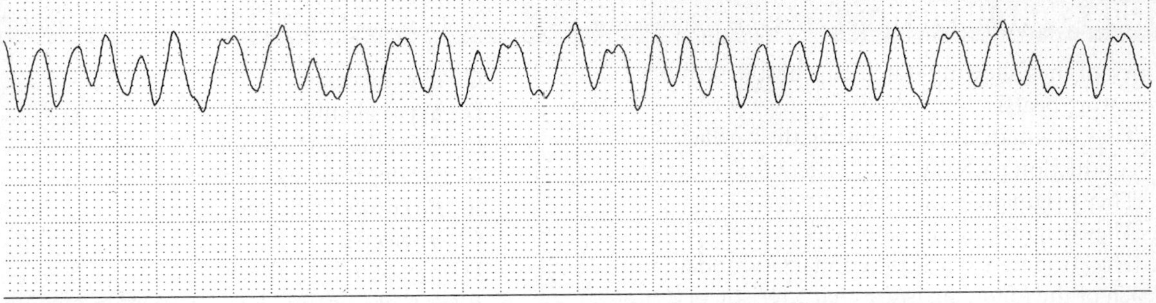

Figure 14–24 ▪ Ventricular fibrillation

1. Rate: atrial: none
   Ventricular: none
2. R-R interval: undeterminable
3. *P* wave: none
4. *PR* interval: none
5. *P* wave precedes each *QRS*: no
6. *QRS* complex: none

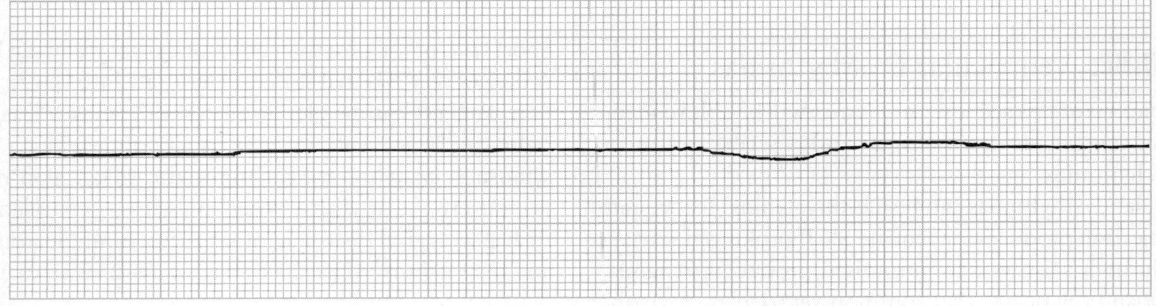

Figure 14–25 ▪ Asystole. (Ellis KM (2002). *EKG Plain and Simple*. Upper Saddle River, NJ: Prentice Hall).

experiencing sudden cardiac arrest. Pharmacotherapy includes a bolus of vasopressin or epinephrine. If the patient remains pulseless, CPR and attempts at defibrillation continue. For persistent or recurrent pulseless ventricular tachycardia or fibrillation, amiodarone, lidocaine, and magnesium are used. Once the patient has converted from ventricular fibrillation and has a pulse, a continuous infusion of the last drug used to convert the rhythm is initiated. Myocardial infarction and premature ventricular beats can precede the development of ventricular fibrillation.

Asystole represents complete cessation of electrical impulses. Cardiopulmonary resuscitation should be performed immediately. It is imperative to check that the rhythm is verified in two separate leads – as fine ventricular fibrillation can mimic asystole and therefore requires alternative interventions. In addition to CPR, other treatments for asystole include atropine, epinephrine, or vasopressin. During resuscitation, clinicians must consider and treat the various causes of asystole. According to the American Heart Association's Advanced Cardiopulmonary Life Support guidelines (2006), possible contributing factors of asystole include hypovolemia, hypoxemia, electrolyte imbalances (acidosis, potassium), hypoglycemia, hypothermia, various toxins, cardiac tamponade, tension pneumothorax, pulmonary or coronary thrombosis, and trauma. Often, despite rigorous efforts, asystole is a terminal rhythm. Figure 14–25 is an example of asystole.

Table 14–7 compares ECG characteristics and treatment strategies for ventricular dysrhythmias.

TABLE 14–7 Ventricular Dysrhythmias: ECG Characteristics and Treatment Strategies

RHYTHM	CHARACTERISTIC	TREATMENT STRATEGIES
Ventricular tachycardia	R–R interval usually regular, but can be irregular Absent *P* waves or *P* waves not associated with *QRS* complex Wide *QRS* but somewhat uniform Rate greater than 100 bpm May/May not have a pulse	Amiodarone Lidocaine Magnesium Cardioversion No pulse: Same treatment strategy as VF
Ventricular fibrillation	R–R interval undeterminable Absent *P* wave Absent *QRS* Rate undeterminable Chaotic waveform No pulse present	Cardiopulmonary Resuscitation Defibrillation Epinephrine Vasopressin Amiodarone Lidocaine
Asystole	Complete absence of electrical impulses	CPR Epinephrine Vasopressin Atropine Search for and treat possible causes

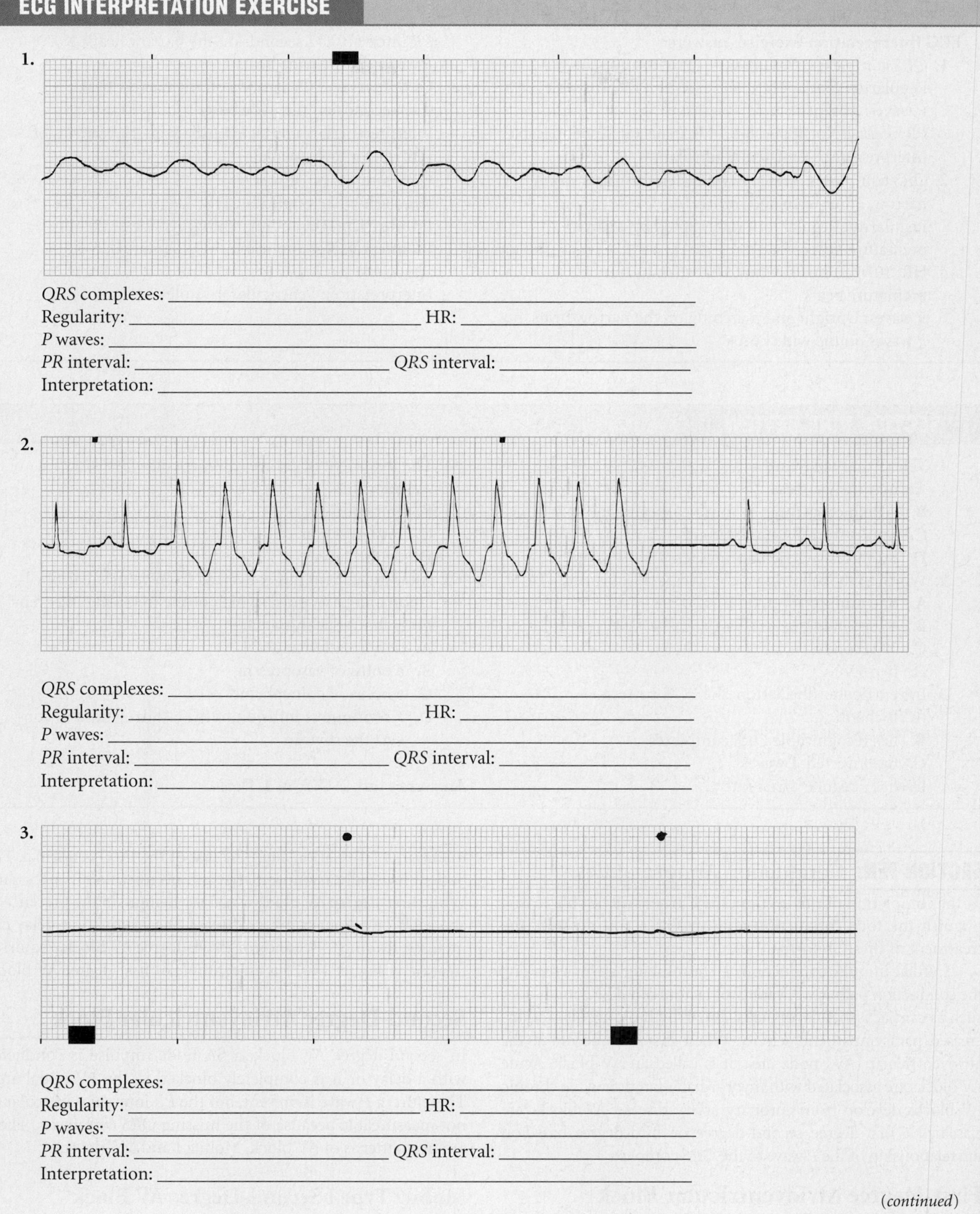
ECG INTERPRETATION EXERCISE
1.
QRS complexes: ______
Regularity: ______ HR: ______
P waves: ______
PR interval: ______ QRS interval: ______
Interpretation: ______
2.
QRS complexes: ______
Regularity: ______ HR: ______
P waves: ______
PR interval: ______ QRS interval: ______
Interpretation: ______
3.
QRS complexes: ______
Regularity: ______ HR: ______
P waves: ______
PR interval: ______ QRS interval: ______
Interpretation: ______
(continued)

(*continued*)

ECG Interpretation Exercise Answers:

1. *QRS* complexes: Absent, wavy baseline present
   Regularity: Not applicable HR: Not measureable
   P waves: Absent
   PR interval: Not applicable *QRS* interval: Not applicable
   Interpretation: Ventricular fibrillation
2. *QRS* complexes: Present, two different shapes (some narrow, other wide and bizarre).
   Regularity: Regular, but interrupted by a run of premature beats
   HR: 107 in sinus rhythm, 187 when in run of premature beats
   P waves: Upright and matching on the narrow beats, no *P* waves on the wide beats
   PR interval: 0.12 seconds on the narrow beats; No *P* waves on the wide beats
   QRS interval: 0.06 seconds on the narrow beats, 0.12 seconds on the wide beats
   Interpretation: Sinus tachycardia with 11 beat run of ventricular tachycardia
3. *QRS* complexes: Absent
   Regularity: Not applicable HR: 0
   P waves: Upright and matching, atrial rate 26 bpm
   PR interval: Not applicable *QRS* interval: Not applicable
   Interpretation: Ventricular asystole

SECTION NINE REVIEW

1. Ventricular tachycardia
   A. may be harmless
   B. is defined as three or more consecutive PVCs
   C. results from SA node fatigue
   D. produces ventricular rates less than 100 bpm
2. Which of the following is considered a "short run" of VT?
   A. one minute
   B. 45 seconds
   C. 30 seconds
   D. two PVCs
3. In ventricular fibrillation, the ECG pattern
   A. is chaotic
   B. has recognizable *QRS* complexes
   C. has inverted *T* waves
   D. has a regular atrial rate
4. The treatment of choice in ventricular fibrillation is
   A. lidocaine
   B. epinephrine
   C. cardioversion
   D. defibrillation
5. After the patient has converted from ventricular fibrillation and has a pulse, which of the following interventions should be initiated?
   A. defibrillation at 360 J
   B. a bolus of vasopressin
   C. a bolus of epinephrine
   D. a continuous infusion of the last drug used to convert the rhythm

Answers: 1. B, 2. C, 3. A, 4. D, 5. D

SECTION TEN: Conduction Abnormalities

At the completion of this section, the learner will be able to distinguish the four conduction abnormalities and describe the treatment of these abnormalities.

Cardiac impulse conduction can be inhibited anywhere along the conduction pathway. A variety of factors can slow conduction, such as cardiac ischemia, digitalis, antiarrhythmic agents, and increased parasympathetic activity. When the delay occurs at the atrioventricular (AV) node area, it is called an AV block. Acute AV blocks are associated with myocardial infarction while chronic AV blocks develop from coronary artery disease. AV blocks are classified as first-degree, second-degree, or third-degree, based on the relationship of the *P* wave to the *QRS* complex.

First-Degree Atrioventricular Block

A first-degree AV block is denoted by a prolonged *PR* interval (greater than 0.20 seconds). There is a delay in conduction through the AV node; however, the *P* wave and *QRS* complex maintain a 1:1 relationship. The rest of the ECG is normal. The patient is usually asymptomatic, and no treatment is necessary. While first-degree AV block is usually benign, in the presence of acute MI or coronary artery disease, the conduction delay can increase, leading to second- or third-degree AV block, requiring treatment. Figure 14–26 is an example of first-degree AV block.

Second-Degree Atrioventricular Block

In second-degree AV block, a SA node impulse is conducted with a delay or it is completely blocked in the AV nodal area. Therefore, a *P* wave is present, but the *PR* interval is irregular or not measureable because of the missing *QRS* complexes. There are two patterns of AV block, Mobitz I and Mobitz II.

Mobitz Type I Second-Degree AV Block (Wenckebach)

In Mobitz type I, the *PR* interval lengthens progressively before the dropping *QRS* complex.

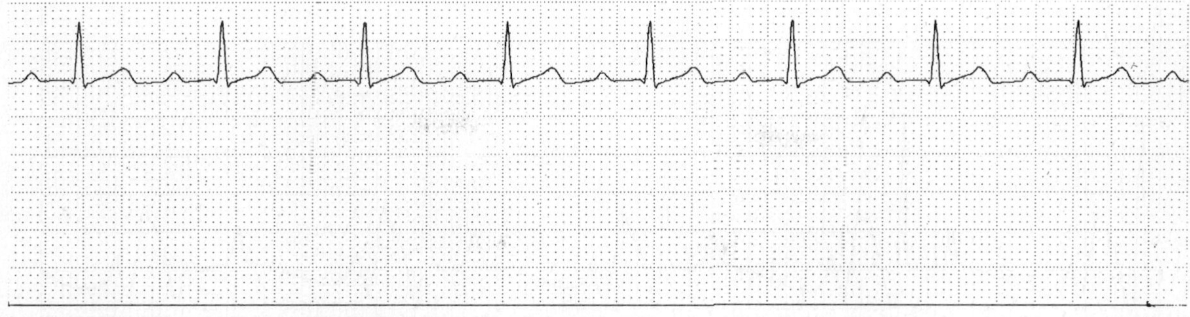

Figure 14–26 ■ First degree AV block. Note the prolonged *PR* interval and the 1:1 relationship between the *P* waves and *QRS* complexes.

Mobitz Type II Second-Degree AV Block

In Mobitz type II second-degree AV block, the *PR* intervals are of constant duration before dropping the *QRS* complex. *QRS* complexes are wide because the block is usually lower in the conduction system (bundles). This type of AV block is less common but is considered more serious because it is associated with third-degree AV block and asystole.

Management of Second-Degree AV Block

The nurse determines the ventricular rate (number of *QRS* complexes) of the rhythm and the frequency of dropped beats. Angina, light-headedness, and dyspnea can occur because of decreased cardiac output. In the case of type I second-degree AV block, if the rate is below 60 bpm and the patient is asymptomatic, no treatment is initiated. The patient is observed. A patient with type II second-degree AV block, whether symptomatic or asymptomatic, will likely receive a pacemaker. The point at which the pacemaker is inserted may vary because symptoms are initially managed with medications. Regardless of the type of second-degree block, if the patient experiences symptoms, atropine is administered. Dopamine or epinephrine is used in severe symptomatic bradycardia. A temporary (transvenous/ transcutaneous) pacemaker may be inserted for symptomatic patients with type I second-degree AV block. Transcutaneous pacing is extremely effective. If bradycardia is severe and the patient is unstable, transcutaneous pacing is performed immediately. Figure 14–27 is an example of type I second-degree AV block, and Figure 14–28 is an example of type II second-degree AV block.

Third-Degree (Complete) Atrioventricular Block

Third-degree (complete) AV block requires emergency treatment because the atria and ventricles are contracting independently. Thus, cardiac output is greatly diminished because of inadequate filling of the ventricles. Impulses are not conducted through the AV node. The atria and ventricles fire at a regular rate, but they do not function as a single unit. The *P–P* wave interval is regular, as is the R–R wave interval, but the *PR* interval varies. There is no relationship between the *P* wave and the *QRS* complex because the atria and the ventricles are paced by a separate pacemaker. The *QRS* complex is usually wide because of the ventricular origin of the stimulus. Complete heart block is usually associated with myocardial infarction. In rare cases, the ventricular rate is fast enough to maintain cardiac output, and symptoms are less severe. Usually, the patient experiences an alteration in mental status and syncope. Complete heart block can progress to ventricular fibrillation. Treatment of complete heart block is the same as that for type II second-degree heart block. If symptomatic, the patient is administered atropine, dopamine, or epinephrine. External pacing and transvenous pacing may also be used. Figure 14–29 is an example of complete heart block.

Bundle Branch Block

A bundle branch block (BBB) results from an impairment in conduction through the bundle of His branches. Once the impulse enters the ventricles, its conduction through the right and left bundle branches can be impaired. The impulse

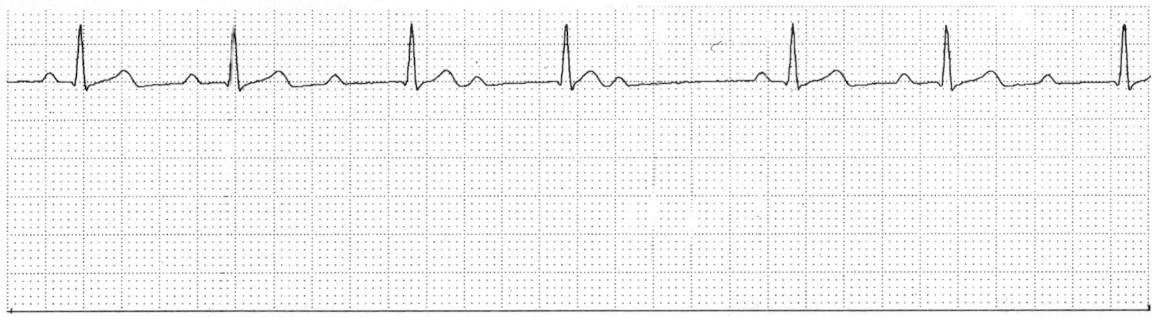

Figure 14–27 ■ Type I second degree block. Note the regularity of the *P-P* intervals and increasing *P-R* intervals that end in a nonconducted (dropped) *QRS*.

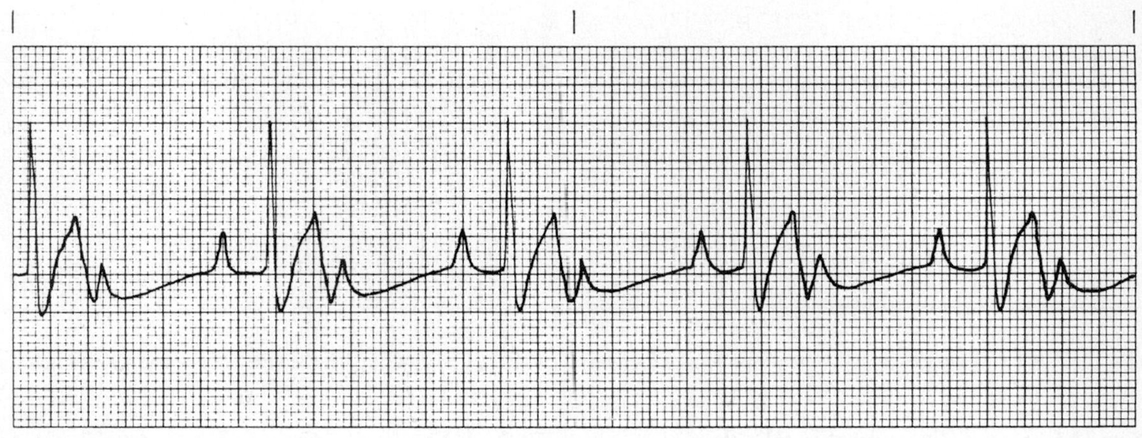

Figure 14–28 ■ Type II second degree block. Note the *P-P* interval regularity and that every other *P* wave is nonconducted (a 2:1 block). The conducted *P* waves have a stable *P-R* interval.

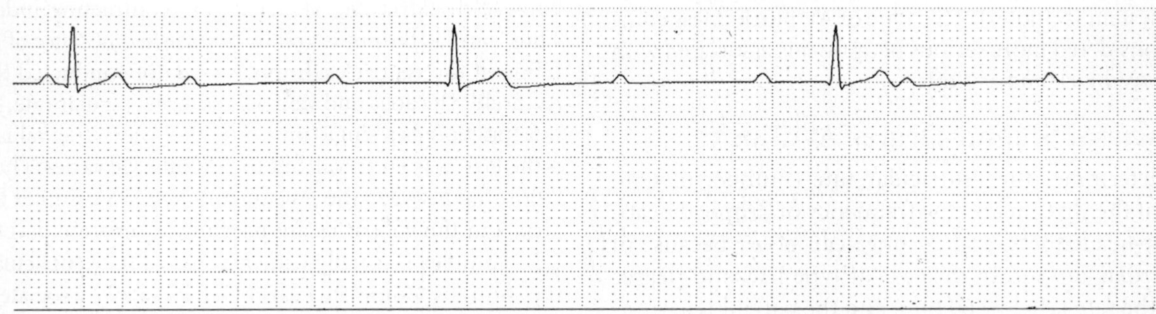

Figure 14–29 ■ Third-degree (complete) heart block. Note that the P-P and R-R intervals are regular but have no relationship to each other.

travels slowly through the blocked side; thus, one ventricle depolarizes faster than the other. On the ECG, the *QRS* complex is prolonged (greater than 0.12 seconds) and its appearance varies, depending on the affected side (right or left). A 12-Lead ECG is necessary to determine which side the block is occurring. Treatment is not necessary except in the case of a new onset left BBB in which the patient may be experiencing a myocardial infarction.

Table 14–8 summarizes the ECG characteristics and treatment strategies of AV blocks.

TABLE 14–8 Atrioventricular (AV) Blocks: ECG Characteristics and Treatment Strategies

BLOCK	CHARACTERISTICS	TREATMENT STRATEGIES
First degree	*PR* interval greater than 0.20 seconds R–R interval is regular	Usually not treated unless patient is symptomatic Possibly medication related (i.e. digitalis)
Second degree, Mobitz type I	Atrial rate is greater than ventricular rate R–R interval is irregular *PR* interval gradually lengthens until a *P* wave is blocked (no *QRS* follows the *P* wave)	Withhold digitalis if associated with digitalis toxicity Atropine Dopamine Epinephrine Transcutaneous pacemaker Permanent pacemaker insertion
Second degree, Mobitz type II	Atrial rate is greater than ventricular rate No consistent pattern to the blocking of the *P* wave When present, PR interval is consistent R–R interval usually irregular	Atropine Dopamine Epinephrine Transcutaneous pacemaker Permanent pacemaker insertion
Third degree, complete	*PR* interval varies R–R interval regular *QRS* may be widened	Atropine Dopamine Epinephrine Transcutaneous pacemaker Permanent pacemaker insertion

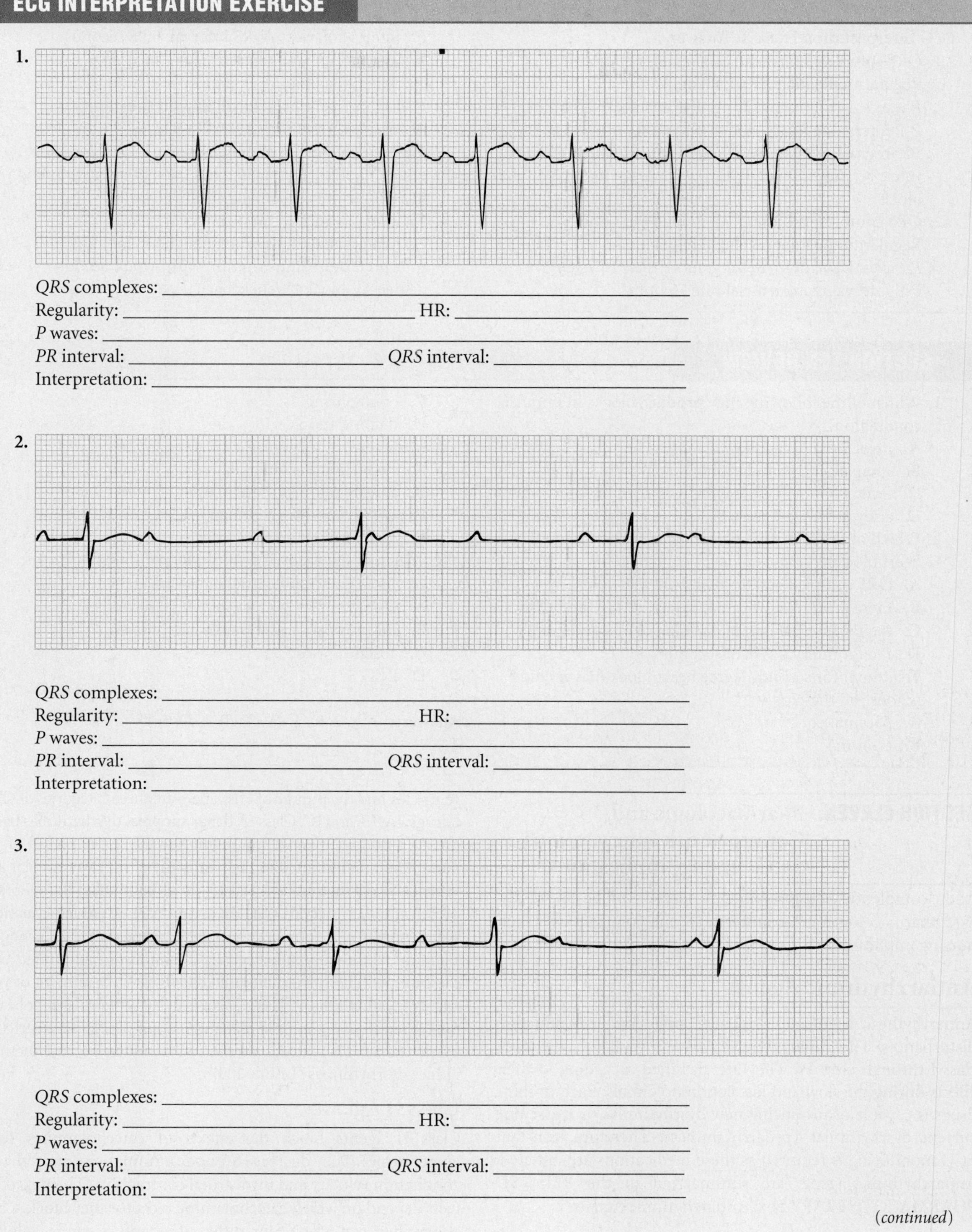

ECG INTERPRETATION EXERCISE

1.

QRS complexes: ______________________________
Regularity: ______________________ HR: ______________________
P waves: ______________________________
PR interval: ______________________ *QRS* interval: ______________________
Interpretation: ______________________________

2.

QRS complexes: ______________________________
Regularity: ______________________ HR: ______________________
P waves: ______________________________
PR interval: ______________________ *QRS* interval: ______________________
Interpretation: ______________________________

3.

QRS complexes: ______________________________
Regularity: ______________________ HR: ______________________
P waves: ______________________________
PR interval: ______________________ *QRS* interval: ______________________
Interpretation: ______________________________

(*continued*)

(continued)

ECG Interpretation Exercise Answers:

1. *QRS* complexes: Present, all shaped the same
   Regularity: Regular HR: 88 bpm
   P waves: Upright, matching, 1 to each *QRS* complex, P-P interval regular
   PR interval: 0.24 seconds *QRS* interval: 0.10 seconds
   Interpretation: Sinus rhythm with first-degree AV block
2. *QRS* complexes: Present, all shaped the same
   Regularity: Regular HR: 30 bpm
   P waves: Upright, matching, more than 1 per *QRS*; P-P interval regular, atrial rate 75 bpm
   PR interval: Varies *QRS* interval: 0.08 seconds
   Interpretation: Sinus rhythm with third-degree AV block
3. *QRS* complexes: Present, all shaped the same
   Regularity: Irregular HR: 37-68 bpm
   P waves: Upright, matching, 1 to each *QRS* complex except the fifth *QRS* which has two *P* waves preceding it; P-P interval regular, atrial rate 60 bpm
   PR interval: Varies, prolongs progressively
   QRS interval: 0.08 seconds
   Interpretation: Sinus rhythm with Type I Second-degree AV block (Wenckebach)

SECTION TEN REVIEW

1. Which of the following may produce blocks in impulse conduction?
   A. myocardial ischemia
   B. sympathetic stimulation
   C. fever
   D. antipyretic agents
2. Which of the following characterize first-degree AV heart block?
   A. *QRS* complex greater than 0.20 seconds
   B. there is no relationship between *P* wave and QRS
   C. the *PR* interval is greater than 0.20 seconds
   D. the *PR* interval is 0.12 seconds
3. Treatment for second-degree heart block may include (choose all that apply)
   A. pacemaker
   B. atropine
   C. epinephrine
   D. defibrillation
4. Complete heart block is characterized by
   A. a constant *PR* interval
   B. a heart rate less than 50 bpm
   C. *QRS* complexes less than 0.12 seconds
   D. regular *P–P* and R–R intervals
5. Which of the following would help differentiate a left versus a right bundle branch block?
   A. *QRS* complex greater than 0.12 seconds
   B. *PR* interval greater than 0.12 seconds
   C. absent *P* wave
   D. ECG

Answers: 1. A, 2. C, 3. (A, B, C), 4. D, 5. D

SECTION ELEVEN: Pharmacologic and Countershock Interventions and Nursing Implications

At the completion of this section, the learner will be able to discuss pharmacologic and countershock interventions and their nursing implications.

Antiarrhythmic Agents

Antiarrhythmic agents are used in treating cardiac conduction disturbances. The antiarrhythmics have several subcategories, class I through class IV. They are classified according to their effects during the slow and fast action potentials. Each of these drugs is capable of producing new dysrhythmias or worsening current dysrhythmias (proarrhythmics). Therefore, constant ECG monitoring is required as these medications are initiated. Antiarrhythmic agents are summarized in the RELATED PHARMACOTHERAPY box: Antiarrhythmic Agents.

Class I Agents

Class I drugs are fast sodium channel blockers. By blocking these channels, these drugs slow impulse conduction through the atria, ventricles, and the Bundle of His. There are three categories of Class I drugs: IA, IB, and IC. Class IA drugs suppress dysrhythmias by reducing automaticity and prolonging the refractory period of the heart. They are indicated in the treatment of supraventricular and ventricular dysrhythmias. Class IA drugs can widen the *QRS* and prolong the *QT* intervals. Class IB drugs decrease refractory periods but do not affect automaticity to a great extent, therefore having no significant ECG effects. In fact, repolarization is accelerated with these agents. These drugs are used chiefly in the treatment of ventricular dysrhythmias. Class IC agents delay ventricular repolarization. They are used as a maintenance therapy for supraventricular dysrhythmias. These drugs are used with caution because they can induce dysrhythmias (Lehne, 2007).

Class II Agents

Class II agents block the effects of catecholamines (e.g., epinephrine). They decrease SA node automaticity and slow AV conduction velocity and myocardial contractility. Their exact effects depend on which catecholamine receptor they block. Catecholamines can affect four different receptors: $alpha_1$, $alpha_2$, $beta_1$, and $beta_2$. For example, phentolamine (Regitine) is an alpha-blocking agent; therefore, it produces peripheral vasodilation. However, most of the agents used to treat dysrhythmias

RELATED PHARMACOTHERAPY: Antiarrhythmic Agents

Class IA Sodium Channel Blockers

Quinidine (Apo-Quinidine), Procainamide (Procanbid), Disopyramide (Norpace, NAPAmide)

Action and Uses

Slow conduction and impulses in the atria, ventricles and bundle of His

Major Side Effects

May widen *QRS* complex, prolong *QT* interval, induce heart block

Nursing Implications

Monitor cardiac rhythm and immediately report the following: widening of *QRS* complex, changes in *QT* interval, disappearance of *P* waves, sudden onset of or increase in ectopic ventricular beats.

Monitor blood pressure closely.

Class IB Sodium Channel Blockers

Lidocaine (Xylocaine), Mexiletine (Mexitil), Phenytoin (Dilantin)

Action and Uses

Suppresses automaticity in bundle of His, Purkinje fibers and elevated electrical stimulation thresholds of ventricles during diastole

Major Side Effects

Difficulty breathing or swallowing, convulsions, respiratory depression, neurotoxicity (drowsiness, dizziness, confusion), cardiovascular collapse

Nursing Implications

Stop infusion if ECG indicates excessive cardiac depression (prolongation of *PR* interval or *QRS* complex) and the appearance of dysrhythmias.

Monitor blood pressure and ECG continuously.

Assess respiratory and neurologic status.

Monitor serum blood levels.

Class IC Sodium Channel Blockers

Flecainide (Tambocor)

Action and Uses

Slows conduction velocity throughout myocardial conduction system; increases ventricular refractoriness.

Major Side Effects

Dizziness, nausea, dysrhythmias

Nursing Implications

Correct serum potassium levels prior to administration

Monitor serum blood levels.

Class II: Beta Blockers

Propranolol (Inderal), Esmolol (Brevibloc), Acebutolol (Sectral, Monitan)

Action and Uses

Reduces automaticity in the SA node and slow conduction in the AV node. Blocks sympathetically mediated increases in cardiac rate and blood pressure as the drug binds to beta-1 receptors in cardiac muscle.

Major Side Effects

Anaphylactic reactions, Stevens-Johnson syndrome, laryngospasm, bronchoconstriction, bradycardia

Nursing Implications

Monitor vital signs before and after administration.

Monitor for hypotension during initial titration phase and when increasing dosage.

Class III: Potassium Channel Blockers

Amiodarone (Cordarone, Pacerone), Bretylium, Sotalol (Betapace), Ibutilide (Corvert), Dofetilide (Tikosyn)

Action and Uses

Acts on cardiac tissue to prolong duration of action potential refractory period without affect resting membrane potential. Used for treatment of life-threatening ventricular dysrhythmias, supraventricular dysrhythmias, atrial fibrillation.

Major Side Effects

Dizziness, hypotension, sinus arrest

Nursing Implications

Correct serum potassium and magnesium levels prior to initiation of drug.

Monitor for hypotension during initial titration phase and when increasing dosage. Slow infusion if significant bradycardia or hypotension occurs.

Sustained monitoring is essential due to long half-life.

Class IV: Calcium Channels Blockers

Verapamil (Calan), Diltiazem (Cardizem)

Digitalis glycosides (Lanoxin)

Endogenous nucleoside (Adenosine, Adenocard)

Action and Uses

Reduces automaticity in the SA node and slows conduction in the AV node

Major Side Effects

Hypotension, AV block

Nursing Implications

Correct serum potassium and magnesium levels prior to initiation of drug.

Incidence of adverse events is highest during IV administration in older adults and patients with impaired kidney function.

Monitor serum drug levels (digoxin).

in this category are beta-blocking agents. Thus, they decrease cardiac stimulation and may produce vasodilation and bronchoconstriction. Drugs in this category are used in treating tachydysrhythmias. These drugs are not to be used in patients with severe congestive heart failure, significant bradycardia, and second-degree or higher heart blocks because of decreased cardiac stimulation. They are contraindicated in asthma because of bronchoconstriction. Because class II drugs decrease the heart rate, the heart rate may be unable to increase to maintain CO in some situations, such as exercise. In cases of cardiac arrest, the heart may be less sensitive to sympathomimetic drugs (i.e., epinephrine) because of the beta-blocking effect.

Class III Agents

Class III agents block potassium channels, thereby delaying repolarization and prolonging the refractory period. A prolonged *QT* interval is likely to develop. They increase the fibrillation threshold (making the cell more resistant). They are indicated in the treatment of atrial and ventricular dysrhythmias. Sotalol is an agent in this category. Amiodarone, another class III agent, is a first-line medication for VT and VF resistant to defibrillation.

Class IV Agents

Class IV agents are calcium channel blockers. These drugs block the entry of calcium through the cell membranes, thereby decreasing depolarization. Automaticity in the SA is reduced, AV note conduction is slowed, and overall decrease in myocardial contractility is produced with class IV agents. Verapamil and Diltiazem are calcium channel blockers commonly used for treating supraventricular tachydysrhythmias.

Adenosine and Digoxin do not fit within the major classes. Both of these drugs reduce AV node automaticity and slow AV conduction. While Digoxin can be used to treat supraventricular tachycardia, atrial fibrillation, and atrial flutter, Adenosine is only beneficial in supraventricular tachycardia.

Prior to administration of any antiarrhythmic agent, the nurse assesses the following baseline data: vital signs; ECG interpretation using the seven-step process; and a physical assessment of the cardiac, respiratory, and neurologic systems. These data are monitored during drug administration. An infusion pump is used when these drugs are administered by the IV route. The patient should be instructed to report dizziness, palpitations, skin rashes, or wheezing. It must be noted that while the goal of these drugs is to suppress or convert dysrhythmias, virtually all antiarrhythmic drugs also have prodysrhythmic effects. Essentially, the drugs can worsen existing dysrhythmias and precipitate new ones.

Countershock

Cardioversion delivers electrical current that is synchronized with the patient's heart rhythm. It is used to treat SVT that is resistant to medication, atrial fibrillation or atrial flutter, and ventricular tachycardia in an unstable patient. The unstable patient may have hypotension; dyspnea or complain of chest pain. The patient may also have symptoms suggestive of heart failure, myocardial ischemia, or infarction. Analgesia is often provided before the electric shock. A synchronizer button is pushed on the defibrillator machine, which allows the machine to discharge after the *R* wave and before the downstroke of the *T* wave. Initially, low voltages are delivered, depending on the size of the patient, and the type of defibrillator used (monophasic or biphasic). Cardioversion is repeated using higher voltages if it is unsuccessful at lower voltages.

Emerging Evidence

- Cardiac resynchronization therapy in patients with systolic heart failure improves exercise capacity, functional status and quality of life *(De Marco et al., 2008)*.
- A prolonged QRS duration is common in patients with reduced left ventricular ejection fraction who are hospitalized for heart failure and is an independent predictor of high post discharge morbidity and mortality *(Wang, Maggioni, Konstam et al., 2008)*.
- At two weeks post-discharge after recent diagnosis of atrial fibrillation, self-management education provided during hospitalization did not appear to be retained. Factors such as short length of stay, complexity of information, learning styles, and personal meaning of the illness may influence knowledge retention *(McCabe, Schad, Hampton et al., 2008)*.

The nurse assists with cardioversion by obtaining an ECG strip prior to, during, and after the procedure. Informed consent is obtained and IV access is confirmed before the procedure. If hemodynamically stable, the patient will likely be given a sedative, or be placed under conscious sedation prior to treatment to minimize discomfort. Any serum electrolyte abnormalities are reported to the physician (especially calcium, magnesium, and potassium). Oxygen and all metallic objects are removed from the patient. Conductive pads are placed on the chest below the right clavicle to the right of the sternum, and in the midaxillary line on the left. After the procedure, the nurse assesses for complications, including emboli (especially cerebral), respiratory depression, skin burns, and dysrhythmias. An ECG strip should be obtained after the procedure and

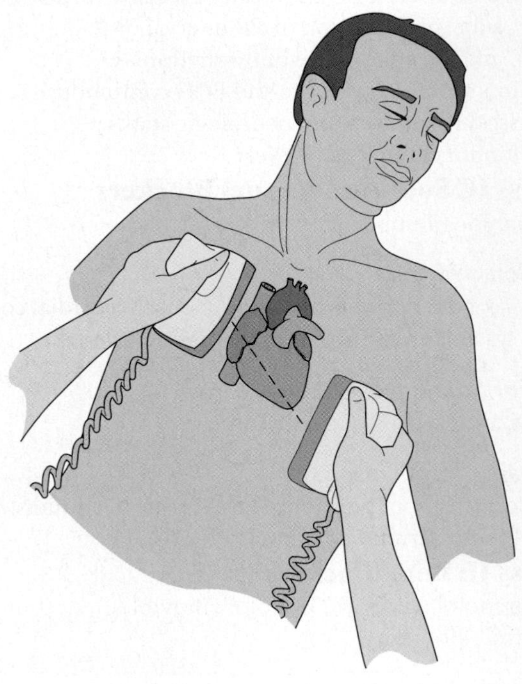

Figure 14–30 ■ Placement of paddles for defibrillation.

placed in the medical record along with documentation of the specific treatments administered.

Defibrillation is an emergency procedure used to treat ventricular tachycardia in an unresponsive patient and ventricular fibrillation. Defibrillation is an unsynchronized electric shock that usually administers a larger number of joules (J) than cardioversion (up to 360 J); once again depending on the type of defibrillator used. With defibrillation, conductive paste or gel pads are applied on the chest wall at the apex and base of the heart (Fig. 14–30). A continuous ECG recording is obtained during the procedure. Only those health care providers with advanced cardiac life support certification can deliver defibrillation therapy. The person delivering the current announces "All clear!" prior to dispensing the electrical current to ensure that no one is touching the patient or the bed. CPR is immediately resumed after the shock. When an IV line is available, pharmacological interventions take place. After five cycles of CPR, the pulse and rhythm are checked. If indicated, electric shock and pharmacological therapy continues (AHA, 2006).

ECG INTERPRETATION EXERCISE

1.

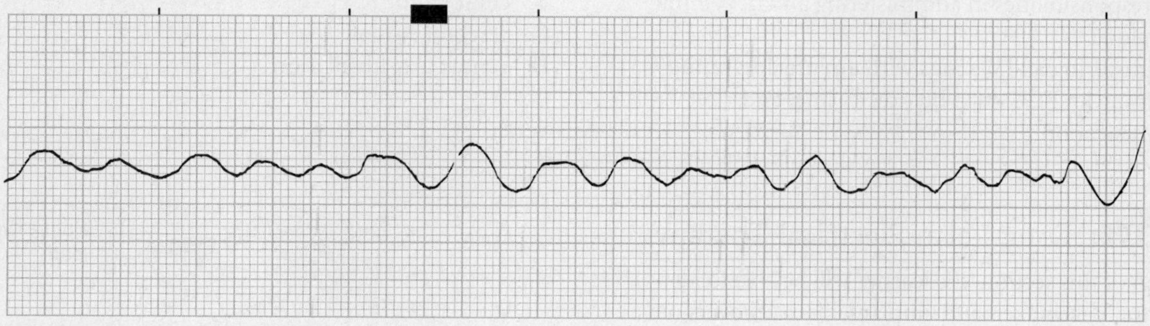

QRS complexes: ____________________

Regularity: ____________________ HR: ____________________

P waves: ____________________

PR interval: ____________________ *QRS* interval: ____________________

Interpretation: ____________________

2.

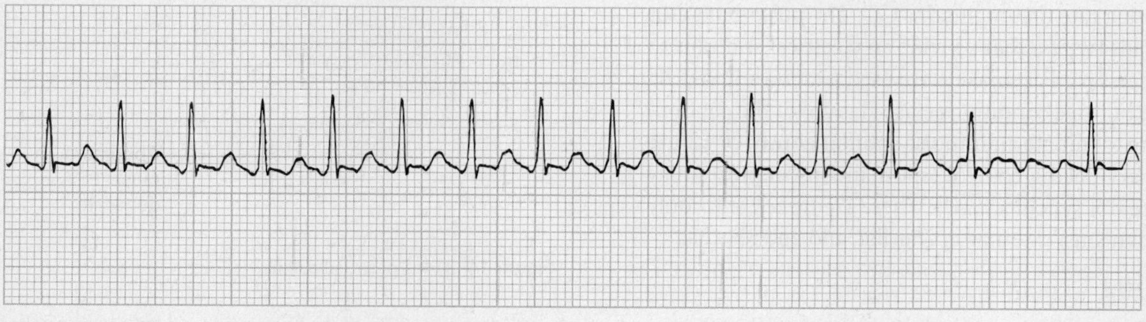

QRS complexes: ____________________

Regularity: ____________________ HR: ____________________

P waves: ____________________

PR interval: ____________________ *QRS* interval: ____________________

Interpretation: ____________________

3. Which of the above rhythms would be treated with cardioversion?

ECG Interpretation Exercise Answers:

1. *QRS* complexes: absent, wavy baseline present
Regularity: Not applicable HR: Not measureable
P waves: Absent
PR interval: Not applicable *QRS* interval: Not applicable
Interpretation: Ventricular fibrillation

2. *QRS* complexes: present, all same shape
Regularity: Regular, but interrupted by a pause
HR: Atrial rate 300 bpm, ventricular rate 98-158 bpm
P waves: None present, flutter waves present
PR interval: Not applicable *QRS* interval: 0.08 seconds
Interpretation: Atrial flutter

3. Rhythm Strip 11.2, atrial flutter

SECTION ELEVEN REVIEW

1. Beta blockers (class II agents) may produce which of the following side effects?
   A. weight gain
   B. hypokalemia
   C. wheezing
   D. hives
2. The difference between cardioversion and defibrillation is
   A. defibrillation uses a lower amount of joules
   B. cardioversion is synchronized
   C. defibrillation cannot be repeated
   D. cardioversion is used only to treat atrial dysrhythmias
3. Nursing responsibilities in administering antiarrhythmic agents include
   A. administering all IV drugs with an infusion pump
   B. obtaining an ECG strip before, during, and after administration
   C. obtaining vital signs before, during, and after administration
   D. all of the above
4. Which of the following classes of antiarrhythmics is a fast sodium channel blocker?
   A. class I
   B. class II
   C. class III
   D. class IV
5. Which of the following is a complication of cardioversion?
   A. nausea
   B. chest pain
   C. cerebral emboli
   D. ventricular fibrillation

Answers: 1. C, 2. B, 3. D, 4. A, 5. C

SECTION TWELVE: Long-Term Electrical Therapy

At the completion of this section, the learner will be able to identify indications for pacemaker and implantable cardioversion/defibrillation therapy, types of devices, and nursing implications for the patient receiving these therapies.

Pacemakers

A pacemaker is a pulse generator used to provide an electrical stimulus to the heart when the heart fails to conduct or generate impulses on its own at a rate that maintains CO. The pulse generator is connected to leads (wires) that provide an electrical stimulus to the heart when necessary. Pacemakers are used in addition to drug therapy when one of three conditions exists: failure of the conduction system, failure to initiate an impulse spontaneously, or failure to maintain primary pacing control (spontaneous impulses may occur, but they are not synchronized). There are three commonly used pacing mechanisms: external, epicardial, and endocardial.

External Pacing

External pacing is a temporary measure. It delivers electric impulses to the myocardium transthoracically through two electrode pads placed anteriorly and posteriorly on the chest. However, during periods of hypoxia and acidosis, the myocardium is less responsive to external pacing. This type of pacing may be a painful experience for the patient, who should therefore be medicated accordingly. When caring for a patient receiving external pacing, the nurse notes the date and time external pacing is initiated, as well as pacing rate, mode, and the amount of current needed for capture. An ECG strip is obtained and analyzed before, during, and after the procedure. The presence of an adequate pulse and blood pressure demonstrates mechanical capture (the ability of the heart to respond to the electrical impulse).

Permanent Implanted Pacemakers

Permanent pacemakers use an internal pulse generator. This generator is located in a subcutaneous tissue pocket in the chest or abdominal wall. The leads are sewn directly into the heart (epicardial pacing; Fig. 14–31) or passed transvenously into the heart (endocardial pacing; Fig. 14–32). Epicardial pacers are inserted during open heart surgery; electrodes are placed directly on the surface of the heart. Endocardial pacers are usually inserted through the subclavian, jugular, or femoral veins into the right ventricle, where they are lodged.

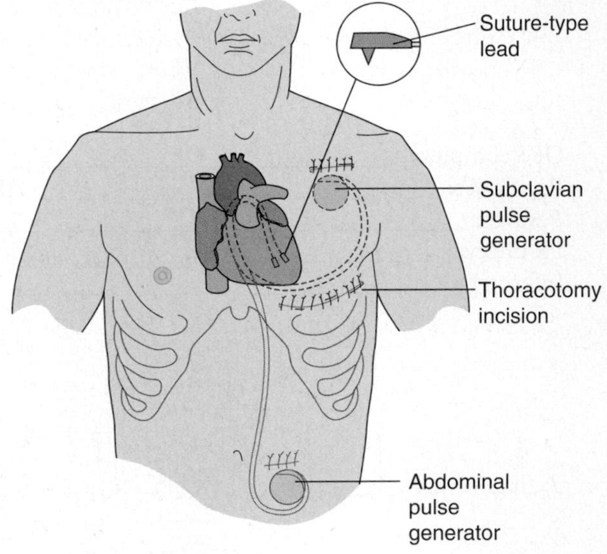

Figure 14–31 ■ Epicardial pacing.

Types of Pacing

Pacemakers are programmed to pace different areas of the heart at specific time intervals and in response to a level of stimulation. Most pacemakers are designed to pace the ventricles. In this case, a spike will occur before the *QRS* complex (Fig. 14–33). This method of pacing is used when transmission of impulses from the atria is blocked (i.e., complete heart block; see Section Ten). The atria can also be paced. A spike will appear before the *P* wave (Fig. 14–34). This method of pacing is used with sinus node disease. AV sequential pacing is used to synchronize heart depolarization in order to maintain CO. In this type of pacing, both the atria and the

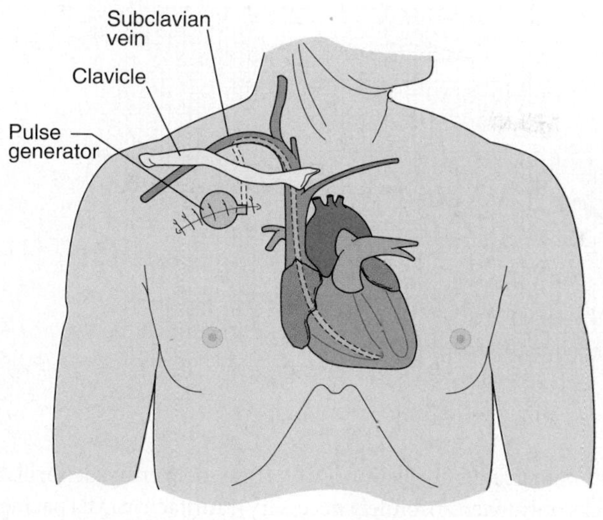

Figure 14–32 ■ Endocardial pacing.

ventricles are paced (dual chamber). Spikes appear before the *P* wave and the *QRS* complex (Fig. 14–35). Another use of pacemakers is in heart failure. Since 2001, cardiac resynchronization therapy (CRT) has been a promising treatment for patients suffering from left ventricular dysfunction. In combination with optimum pharmacotherapy, several studies have shown a significant decrease in morbidity and mortality among patients with heart failure and the use of CRT (McAlister et al., 2007).

A pacemaker can be programmed to function in the inhibited mode, where a pacing impulse is initiated only when an intrinsic beat is not sensed. If it is programmed in a triggered mode, it fires an impulse in response to sensing electrical activity (e.g., ventricular fibrillation). A double function pacemaker reacts to both inhibition and triggering.

Pacing Problems

The number of times the pacemaker fires is determined by the sensitivity setting of the pacemaker. If the sensitivity is low, the pacemaker does not sense the patient's cardiac electrical activity and will pace more frequently. If the sensitivity is high, the pacemaker is better able to sense the patient's cardiac electrical activity and is inhibited from firing. Most are set on demand, with a high-sensitivity setting. A paced beat occurs only when the patient's atria or ventricles fail to discharge. Fixed-rate pacing is used only with individuals whose inherent rhythm is exceedingly slow. If the pacemaker competes with the patient's own impulse generation, the term **failure to sense** is used (Fig. 14–36). This is a potentially dangerous situation because the pacemaker can discharge an impulse during the relative refractory or supranormal periods of ventricular repolarization, precipitating ventricular fibrillation. The term **failure to capture** is used to describe the situation in which the pacemaker initiates an impulse but the stimulus is not strong enough to produce depolarization. A pacing spike is present, but *P* waves or *QRS* complexes or both are absent (Fig. 14–37). For sensing and capturing to occur, the pulse generator must have adequate battery function, the leads must be firmly attached to the pacemaker and the myocardium, and the lead wires must be intact.

Pacemaker Classification

Pacemakers are classified according to a uniform system that is universally used to describe how the device functions according to where the pacing leads are and the mode of pacing. Pacemaker code is written using a five-letter format, using no more letters

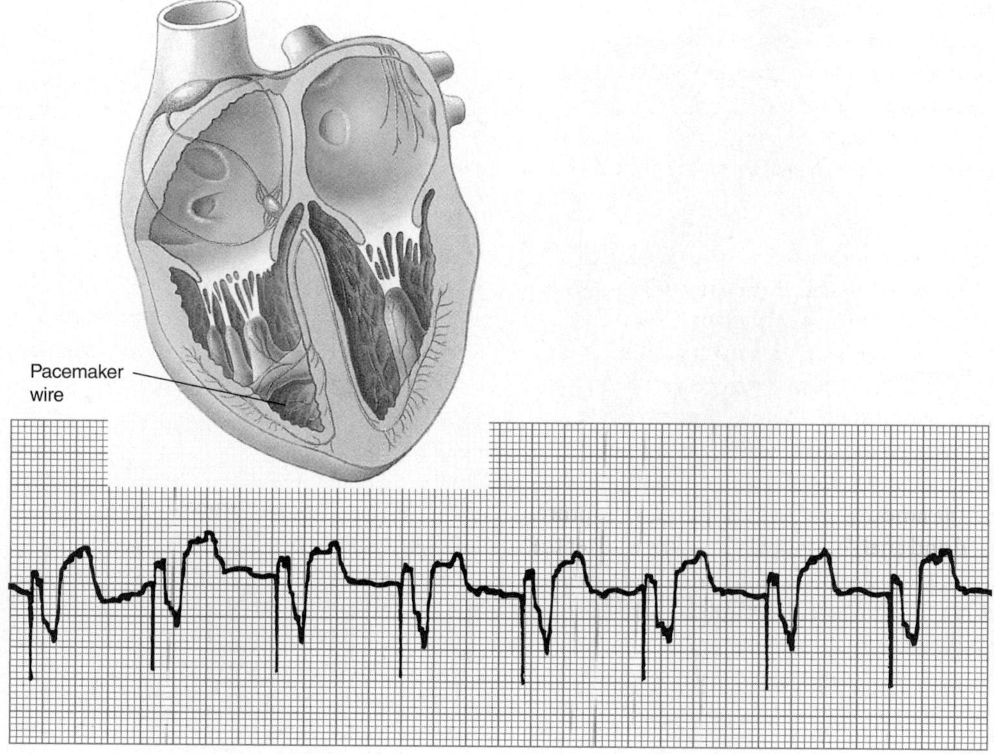

Figure 14–33 ■ Ventricular pacemaker spikes occur before the *QRS*.

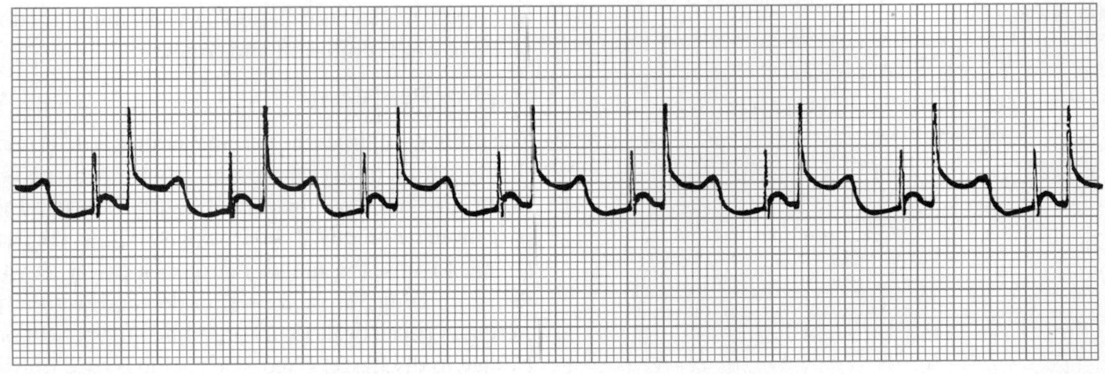

Figure 14–34 ■ Atrial pacemaker spikes occur before the *P* wave.

than necessary (Table 14–9). A DDD pacemaker is a dual-chamber pacemaker that is able to pace and sense. A DDDR pacemaker is rate responsive, which means that it can detect the metabolic need for rate adjustment (e.g., during exercise) and adjust accordingly if the native pacemaker fails to achieve this rate.

Implantable Cardioverter/Defibrillator

An implantable cardioverter/defibrillator (ICD) is placed in patients who have had prior aborted sudden cardiac death or proven sustained ventricular tachycardia. It also may be placed prophylactically in high-risk groups, such as those with various forms of cardiomyopathy. The device is a fully implantable, battery-operated system designed to recognize and terminate ventricular tachyarrhythmias that can cause sudden death. The device discharges to override the ectopic ventricular pacemaker. The most recent ICDs are capable of distinguishing ventricular tachycardia (VT) from ventricular fibrillation (VF) (thus delivering defibrillation shocks only when absolutely necessary); antitachycardia pacing (to treat VT without resorting to cardioversion shocks unless necessary); providing backup bradycardia pacing (eliminating the need for a standard pacemaker); and storing cardiac events so that they can be retrieved for analyzing the patient's response to treatment. Generator longevity depends on how often the device's features are used but generally is at least four years.

Implantation of the ICD is accomplished percutaneously through the subclavian or cephalic vein. The lead is positioned in the heart transvenously and the generator is implanted subcutaneously in the upper chest. Once in place the device is programmed and tested using electrophysiologic studies. In essence, VF is intentionally induced in a controlled environment. The ICD is set to deliver shocks at the rate necessary to convert the VF to a sinus rhythm.

If the ICD malfunctions, it may be necessary to deactivate the device by applying a special magnet over the ICD. The

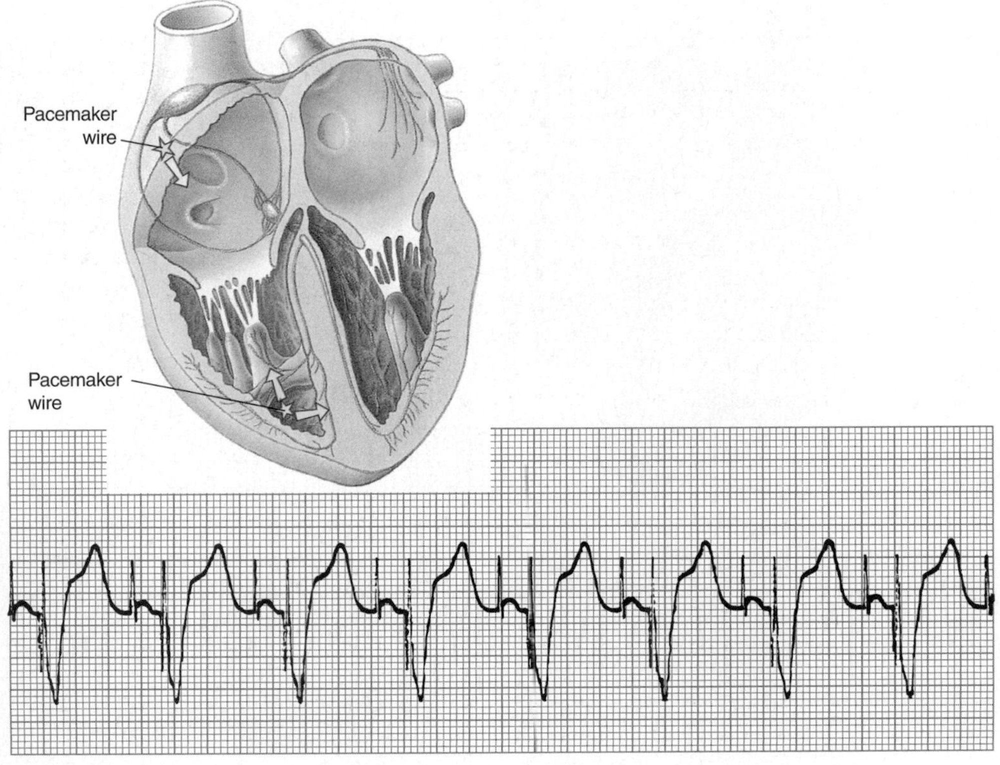

Figure 14–35 ■ AV sequential pacing: both atria and ventricles are paced.

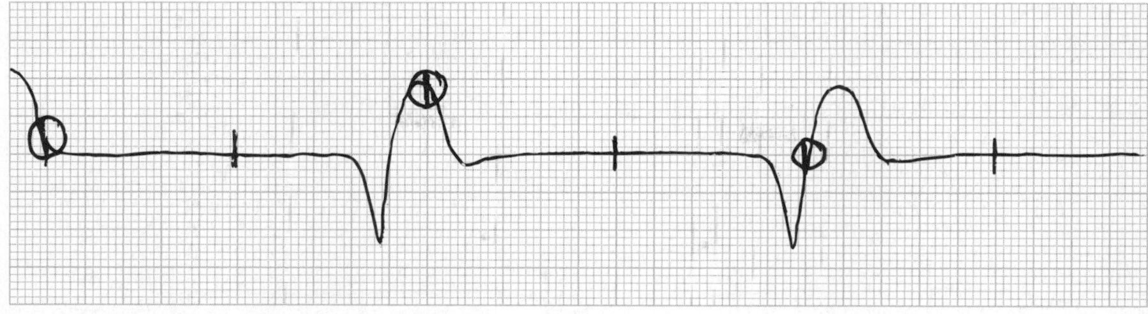

Figure 14–36 ■ Failure to sense.

nurse must be familiar with the correct procedure for deactivating the device. If the ICD malfunctions, or if the heart does not respond to shocks delivered, life-support measures are initiated. During cardiopulmonary resuscitation (CPR), the rescuer can feel a mild shock (similar to a static electricity shock) if the device fires. External defibrillation is performed using anterior– posterior paddle placement. If temporary external pacing is required, the ICD is deactivated.

Patients who need an ICD require extensive training. Patients must understand the difference between heart attack and cardiac arrest. The ICD does not prevent a myocardial infarction, but it does prevent cardiac arrest. The patient is taught that the ICD can "reorganize" his or her heart rhythm as well as stimulate the heart (pacemaker action is available on most recent models). Patients are encouraged to keep a diary of shocks received, activities before and after treatment, symptoms, and response after shock. They should contact their cardiologist when they receive a shock.

Patients with ICDs must adhere to restrictions and limitations, for example, individuals may be restricted from driving in some states. Patients are advised that magnetic fields can deactivate the device and must be avoided. These patients should not receive diathermy treatment, magnetic resonance imaging, or lithotripsy. Arc welders and large industrial motors should be avoided. Cellular phones can interfere with the operation of all defibrillators if held closer than 6 inches from the pulse generator.

An automatic external defibrillator (AED) may be used by some medical and nursing service personnel and lay persons to treat ventricular tachycardia and ventricular fibrillation. AED use is taught to the general public as well, and devices can be found in public places (airports, malls) and even purchased for personal use. The ECG pattern is detected through large patches placed on the patient's chest. If a lethal dysrhythmia is detected, the AED discharges to defibrillate the patient. Once turned on, the device will instruct the user on proper operation of the AED.

Caring for a patient with a pacemaker or ICD requires specialized nursing care, including preparing the patient for insertion of an endocardial pacemaker or applying an external pacing device correctly. The ECG pattern is monitored to determine if the pacemaker is pacing at the correct rate (demand versus fixed), capturing with each impulse, and sensing the patient's own rhythm. Additionally, the nurse assesses the threshold (minimal amount of output required to initiate depolarization) of the pacemaker. The learner is referred to the literature associated with each pacing and defibrillation device to determine the correct method of checking the threshold for that device. It is helpful if patients with histories of dysrhythmias carry copies of their most recent ECGs. Patients are encouraged to obtain MedicAlert bracelets to identify themselves as having pacemakers or ICDs. The type of device, manufacturer, and model number should be readily available.

TABLE 14–9 Generic Pacemaker Code

LETTER CHAMBER PACED	SECOND LETTER CHAMBER SENSED	THIRD LETTER PACEMAKER RESPONSE	FOURTH LETTER PROGRAMMABLE FUNCTIONS	FIFTH LETTER ANTI-TACHYCARDIA FUNCTIONS
Atrium	Atrium	Triggered	Programmable	Pacing
Ventricle	Ventricle	Inhibited	Multiprogrammable	Shock
Dual	Dual	Double	Communication	Dual
$\alpha \times 5$	α	α	Rate modulated	α

Key: α = None

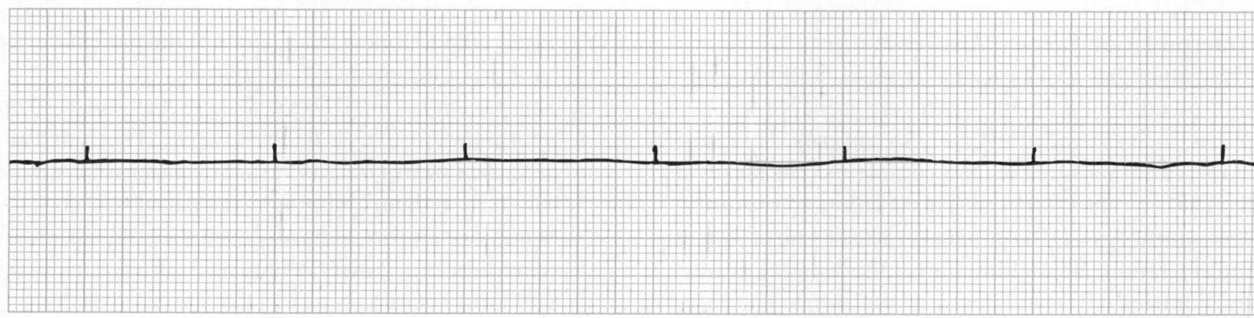

Figure 14–37 ■ Failure to capture.

ECG INTERPRETATION EXERCISE

Directions: In the ECG rhythm strips below, identify the pacemaker malfunction, if any.

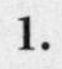

1.

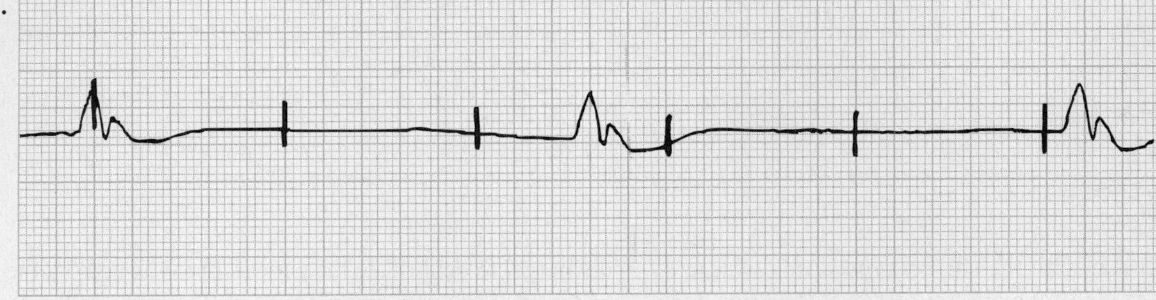

This patient has a ______________ pacemaker set at a rate of ______________ bpm.
Interpretation: ____

2.

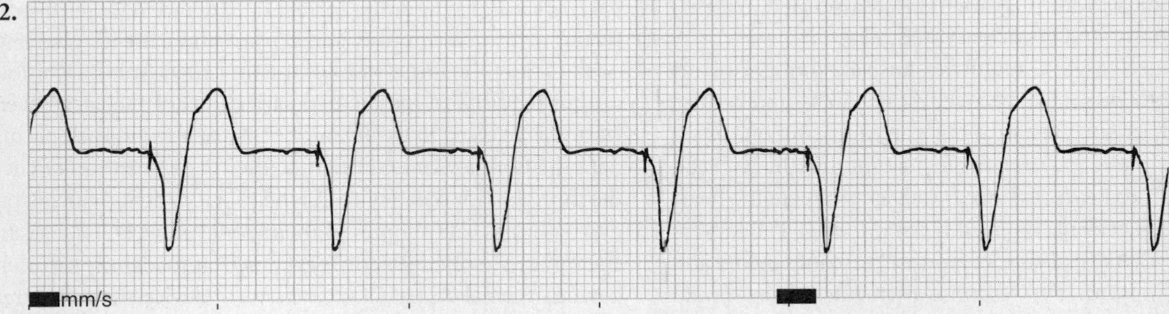

This patient has a ______________ pacemaker set at a rate of ______________ bpm.
Interpretation: ____

3.

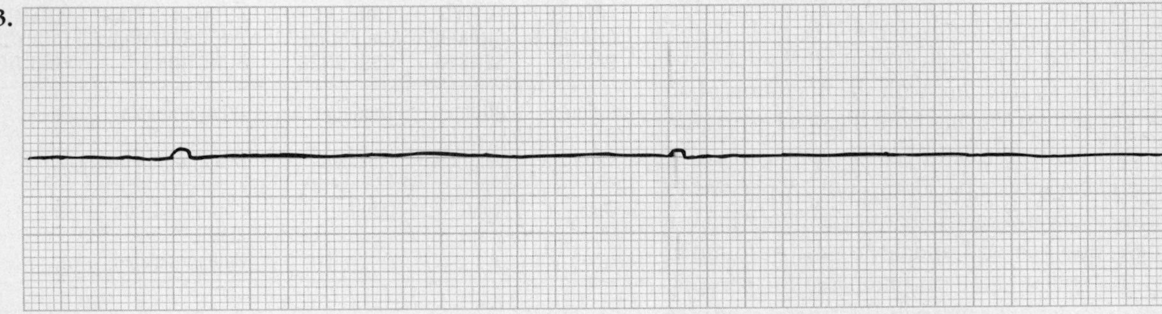

This patient has a ______________ pacemaker set at a rate of ______________ bpm.
Interpretation: ____

ECG Interpretation Exercise Answers:

1. This patient has a VVI pacemaker set at a rate of 60 bpm. Interpretation: Pacemaker spikes are at inappropriate places, such as inside the first *QRS* complex. This pacemaker is not sensing the *QRS* complexes. The spikes are regular at a rate of 60 bpm. This is failure to capture.
2. This patient has a DDD pacemaker set at a rate of 72 bpm. Interpretation: No malfunction at this time. Note the small intrinsic *P* waves preceding each *QRS*. The pacemaker senses them and tracks them, providing the paced *QRS* to follow those Ps since the patient does not have his or her own *QRS* complexes.
3. This patient has a DDD pacemaker set at rate of 70 bpm. Interpretation: This is failure to sense. There are two intrinsic *P* waves on this strip. The pacemaker should have sensed them and provided a paced *QRS* to follow. In addition, it should have sensed the atria and then the ventricles, as necessary, at it programmed rate of 70. But it did not and therefore, there are no visible pacemaker spikes.

SECTION TWELVE REVIEW

1. An epicardial pacing device is
   A. placed through the subclavian vein
   B. applied to the chest wall
   C. inserted in open heart surgery
   D. used exclusively for AV sequential pacing
2. Failure to sense means
   A. The pacing device is turned off.
   B. Depolarization is not occurring.
   C. The patient is tachycardic.
   D. The pacing device is competing with the patient's own rhythm.
3. Failure to capture means
   A. Depolarization does not occur after a pacer-generated impulse.
   B. Atria and ventricles are not contracting in a synchronous manner.
   C. The pacing device needs to be replaced.
   D. The patient will require cardioversion.
4. When a pacemaker is functioning in an inhibited mode
   A. A pacing impulse is generated when an intrinsic beat is not sensed.
   B. It fires an impulse in response to sensing electrical activity.
   C. The SA node is overriding the pacing rate.
   D. The device is malfunctioning.
5. When should patients with an ICD device contact their HCP?
   A. when they get the flu
   B. when they have a fever
   C. when they go out of the country
   D. when they receive a shock

Answers: 1. C, 2. D, 3. A, 4. A, 5. D

POSTTEST

1. The nurse cares for a patient who has hypoxemia. The nurse knows that the patient is at risk to develop dysrhythmias as a result of:
   A. early depolarization
   B. early repolarization
   C. prolonged absolute refractory period
   D. prolonged plateau phase
2. Which of the following electrolyte abnormalities can interfere with myocardial function? (choose all that apply)
   A. hyperkalemia
   B. hypokalemia
   C. hypernatremia
   D. hyponatremia
3. The nurse should intervene if which of the following is observed on ECG?
   A. There is a *P* wave before the *QRS*.
   B. The *PR* interval is 0.25 seconds.
   C. The *QRS* is spiked in appearance.
   D. The *QRS* segment is less than 0.10 seconds.
4. A patient is scheduled to receive ECG monitoring. In preparing the patient for this procedure, what intervention should the nurse implement first?
   A. Check for frayed wires on the leads.
   B. Place the electrodes on the patient.
   C. Connect the lead wires to the electrodes.
   D. Turn the alarms off.
5. The nurse should intervene if which of the following is observed? (choose all that apply)
   A. R-R intervals are regular.
   B. *PR* interval is 0.30 seconds.
   C. *P* waves precede *QRS* complexes.
   D. *QRS* interval is 0.20 seconds.
6. When interpreting an ECG, the nurse notes the following: HR 75 bpm, R-R intervals are regular, each *P* wave looks alike, the *PR* interval is 0.15 seconds, each *P* wave is followed by a *QRS*, the *QRS* complex is 0.10 seconds, the *QT* interval is half the R-R interval. The nurse should interpret this as:
   A. a dysrhythmia
   B. sinus bradycardia
   C. normal sinus rhythm
   D. heart block
7. A patient's morning potassium is 2.0 mEq/L. As a result, the nurse identified which nursing diagnosis as a priority?
   A. alteration in fluid volume (deficit)
   B. altered nutrition (less than) body requirements
   C. decreased cardiac output
   D. altered urinary elimination
8. The nurse receives report for the shift. Which of the following patients should the nurse see first?
   A. patient with hyperkalemia, prolonged PR interval, wide *QRS* complex
   B. patient with fluid volume deficit, HR 100, rate regular
   C. patient with temperature 100° F
   D. patient with history of myocardial infarction 10 years ago
9. A patient has sinus dysrhythmias. The nurse should intervene if which of the following is observed? (choose all that apply)
   A. dizziness
   B. hypotension
   C. angina
   D. fever

10. A patient receives atropine for symptomatic sinus bradycardia. Which outcome indicates to the nurse that this drug is having the desired effect?
A. decrease in heart rate
B. increase in heart rate
C. dry mouth
D. constipation

11. A patient takes digitalis. What would necessitate holding this patient's usual morning dose?
A. sinus bradycardia, rate 60 bpm
B. sinus tachycardia, rate 100 bpm
C. junctional dysrhythmia
D. atrial fibrillation

12. A patient develops a dysrhythmia. The rate is 50 bpm. *P* waves are inverted. The *PR* interval is 0.10 seconds. *QRS* complex is normal. What nursing measure is essential for this patient?
A. Assess for symptoms of decreased CO.
B. Call the code team.
C. Prepare the patient for cardioversion.
D. Ask the patient to cough or bear down.

13. A patient is diagnosed with a junctional dysrhythmia. The nurse knows that the etiology of this dysrhythmia is due to
A. failure of the SA node to fire
B. failure of the AV node to fire
C. failure of the atria to contract
D. failure of the ventricles to contract

14. The patient takes digitalis (digoxin). Development of which of the following dysrhythmias would necessitate holding the patient's usual morning dose?
A. sinus tachycardia
B. normal sinus rhythm
C. junctional dysrhythmia
D. atrial fibrillation, rate 80 bpm

15. A patient develops PAC's. He is having 3-4 of these beats per minute. What is the best initial action by the nurse?
A. Assess the patient's blood pressure.
B. Prepare the patient for cardioversion.
C. Prepare the patient for defibrillation.
D. Continue to monitor and observe the patient.

16. A patient is having PVC's. Which of the following circumstances would warrant the nurse to notify the HCP? (choose all that apply)
A. more than six PVCs per minute
B. PVC couplets
C. more than 3 PVCs in a row
D. R or T phenomena

17. A patient is having frequent episodes of a dysrhythmia. There are three PVC's in a row. There are no identifiable *P* waves, the R-R interval is regular and the *QRS* complex is 0.20 seconds. The nurse would interpret this rhythm as:
A. bigeminy
B. trigeminy
C. ventricular tachycardia
D. ventricular fibrillation

18. The patient has developed a dysrhythmia. There are no identifiable *P* waves, *QRS* complexes or *T* waves. The patient is unresponsive and does not have a pulse. What intervention should the nurse implement first?
A. Initiate CPR.
B. Continue to monitor and observe.
C. Apply oxygen.
D. Prepare the patient for cardioversion

19. A patient has a new onset of second degree heart block and hypotension. Which treatment should the nurse anticipate implementing?
A. no treatment at this time
B. cardioversion
C. defibrillation
D. insertion of a transcutaneous pacemaker

20. The nurse interprets an ECG rhythm strip. The following are noted: Rate 80 bpm. *P* waves precede each *QRS*, *PR* interval is 0.28 seconds. *QRS* is 0.08 seconds. The nurse would interpret this rhythm as:
A. normal sinus rhythm
B. first degree AV block
C. type I second degree block
D. left bundle branch block

21. The nurse knows that widening of the *QRS* complex is a side effect commonly associated with which of the patient's current medications?
A. quinidine
B. lidocaine
C. glecainide
D. propranolol

22. Which outcome on the ECG should the nurse use to evaluate the efficacy of cardioversion?
A. atrial fibrillation
B. atrial flutter
C. ventricular tachycardia
D. normal sinus rhythm

23. A patient has a pacemaker. Which assessment data warrants immediate intervention by the nurse?
A. A pacing spike appears before the *P* and *QRS*.
B. A paced beat occurs only when the patient's ventricle fails to discharge.
C. A pacing spike is present but *P* waves are absent.
D. A pacing spike is followed by a *P* wave.

24. A patient has an ICD inserted. Which information is most important for the nurse to provide this patient?
A. There are no driving restrictions.
B. Magnetic fields do not interfere with the device.
C. Cellular phones do not interfere with their operation.
D. The patient should be instructed to obtain a MedicAlert bracelet.

Posttest answers with rationale are found on MyNursingKit.

REFERENCES

AACN (American Association of Critical Care Nurses) (2008a). AACN Practice Alert: Dysrhythmia Monitoring. www.aacn.org./WD/Practice/Docs/Dysrhythmia_Monitoring_04-2008.pdf. Accessed July 14, 2008.

AACN (American Association of Critical Care Nurses) (2008b). AACN Practice Alert: Dysrhythmia Monitoring Educational PowerPoint Presentation. www.aacn.org./WD/Practice/Content/practicealerts.pcms?menu=practice. Accessed July 14, 2008.

AHA (American Heart Association). (2006). *Advanced Cardiovascular Life Support, Professional Provider Manual.* Dallas, Texas.

DeMarco, T., Wolfel, E., Feldman, A. M., et al. (2008). Impact of cardiac resynchronization therapy on exercise performance, functional capacity, and quality of life in systolic heart failure with QRS prolongation: COMPANION trial sub-study. *Journal of Cardiac Failure, 14*(1), 9–18.

Ellis, K. M. (2007). *EKG: Plain and simple* (2nd ed.). Upper Saddle River, N.J.: Pearson Prentice Hall.

Futterman, L. G. & Lemberg, L. (2005). Cariology Casebook: A. Fib. *American Journal of Critical Care, 14*(5), 438–440.

Guyton, A. C. & Hall, J. E. (2006). Cardiac arrhythmias and their electrocardiographic interpretation. In, Guyton, A. C. & Hall, J. E. (eds.). *Textbook of Medical Physiology.* Philadelphia: Elsevier-Saunders, pp. 147–157

Lehne, R. A. (2007). *Pharmacology for nursing care* (6th ed.) St. Louis: Saunders Elsevier.

McCabe, P. J., Schad, S., Hampton, A., et al., (2008). Knowledge and self-management behaviors of patients with recently detected atrial fibrillation. *Heart & Lung, 37*(2), 79–90.

McAlister, F. A., Ezekowitz, J, Hooton, N., et al. (2007). Cardiac resynchronization therapy for patients with left ventricular systolic dysfunction. *JAMA, 297*(22), 2502–2514.

Porth, C. M. (2005). Disorders of cardiac function. In, Porth, C. M. (Ed). *Pathophysiology: Concepts of altered health states.* (7th ed.). Philadelphia: Lippincott, Williams, Wilkens, pp. 535–579.

Wang, N. C., Maggioni, A. P., Konstam, M. A., et al. (2008). Clinical implications of QRS duration in patients hospitalized with worsening heart failure and reduced left ventricular ejection fraction. *JAMA* 299(22), 2656–2666.

White-Winters, J. M. (2005). Cardiac conduction and rhythm disorders. In, Porth, C. M. (Ed). *Pathophysiology: Concepts of altered health states.* (7th ed.). Philadelphia: Lippincott, Williams, Wilkens, pp. 581–599.

MODULE

15 Alterations in Cardiac Output

Nancy Munro

OBJECTIVES Following completion of this module, the learner will be able to

1. Describe heart valve disease, including
   - The pathophysiologic mechanisms of cardiac valve dysfunction (valvular stenosis, valvular regurgitation, and infective endocarditis)
   - Cardiac murmurs that occur with valve dysfunction
   - Nursing interventions for patients with valvular dysfunction
2. Describe heart failure, including:
   - The pathophysiologic and compensatory mechanisms that occur during heart failure
   - The pharmacologic therapies used in the collaborative management of heart failure
3. Explain hypertension, including:
   - The ranges of systolic and diastolic blood pressure for prehypertension, stage 1 hypertension, and stage 2 hypertension
   - The pathophysiologic mechanisms that contribute to hypertension
   - Collaborative and nursing interventions for the patient with hypertension

The cardiac system plays a pivotal role in pumping and transporting oxygen to tissues. As with any other organ, the heart is composed of various components that must work congruently in order to function optimally. Conceptually, the cardiac system is a sophisticated "plumbing system" where the heart is the pump that has valves to direct blood flow into the "pipes" (the vascular system). Pump, valve, or pipe dysfunction can lead to alterations in cardiac output. This module addresses these alterations in cardiac output, which include pump dysfunction (heart failure and cardiomyopathy), valve dysfunction (stenosis and regurgitation), and "pipe" dysfunction (hypertension).

This self-study module is divided into three sections. Section One discusses valvular heart disease and infective endocarditis. Section Two reviews heart failure and cardiomyopathy and Section Three discusses hypertension. For each section the clinical manifestations, pathophysiologic mechanisms, collaborative management, and nursing interventions are presented. All Section Reviews include answers. It is suggested that the learner review those concepts answered incorrectly in the review questions before proceeding to the next section.

PRETEST

1. With mitral stenosis, the following hemodynamic changes occur:
   A. Left atrial pressure increases and left ventricular diastolic pressure decreases.
   B. Left atrial pressure increases and pulmonary artery pressures increase.
   C. Left atrial pressure decreases and left ventricular diastolic pressure decreases.
   D. Left atrial pressure and left ventricular diastolic pressures do not change.
2. Aortic regurgitation is caused primarily by
   A. rheumatic heart disease
   B. myocardial infarction
   C. ventricular hypertrophy
   D. chronic renal disease
3. Subacute infective endocarditis is commonly caused by
   A. *Staphylococcus aureus*
   B. *Pseudomonas aeruginosa*
   C. *Candida albicans*
   D. *Streptococcus viridans*
4. A compensatory mechanism that plays a major role in sodium and water retention in heart failure is
   A. the parasympathetic nervous system
   B. the sympathetic nervous system
   C. the renin–angiotensin–aldosterone system
   D. reflex tachycardia

5. Mr. P. has been diagnosed with heart failure. He is asymptomatic. Which of the following drugs would most likely be used to manage his condition?
   A. ACE inhibitor
   B. beta blocker
   C. digitalis
   D. A and B
6. Patients in heart failure present with the following signs and symptoms:
   A. fatigue
   B. orthopnea
   C. dyspnea
   D. all of the above
7. Prehypertension is defined as
   A. SBP less than 150 mm Hg or DBP less than 80 mm Hg
   B. SBP greater than 160 mm Hg or DBP greater than 100 mm Hg
   C. SBP between 140 and 159 mm Hg or DBP between 90 and 99 mm Hg
   D. SBP of 150 to 139 mm Hg and DBP of 80 to 89 mm Hg
8. Nursing interventions for the hypertensive patient include
   A. lifestyle modifications
   B. education about medications
   C. education about monitoring blood pressure
   D. all of the above
9. Target organ damage from hypertension occurs to which of the following organs?
   A. eyes
   B. kidneys
   C. peripheral vasculature
   D. all of the above

Pretest answers are found on MyNursingKit.

SECTION ONE: Valvular Heart Disease

At the completion of this section, the learner will be able to describe heart valve disease, including the pathophysiologic mechanisms of cardiac valve dysfunction (valvular stenosis, valvular regurgitation, and infective endocarditis); cardiac murmurs that occur with valve dysfunction; and nursing interventions for patients with valvular dysfunction.

Structure and Function of Cardiac Valves

There are four heart valves, which are thin, paperlike structures that allow forward blood flow, prevent **regurgitation** (or backward flow of blood), and open and close in response to changes in pressure gradients (Fig. 15–1). When the pressure is higher in the preceding chamber, the valve opens. When the gradient reverses, the valve closes. The flimsy structure of the valves enables them to perform these functions easily. The tricuspid and mitral valves are referred to as the atrioventricular (AV) valves. They direct blood flow from the atria to ventricles. The pulmonic and aortic valves are referred to as the semilunar valves. They direct blood flow from the ventricle into the circulation.

During mid-to-late diastole when the ventricles are filling, the AV valves are open and the semilunar valves are closed (Fig. 15–2A)

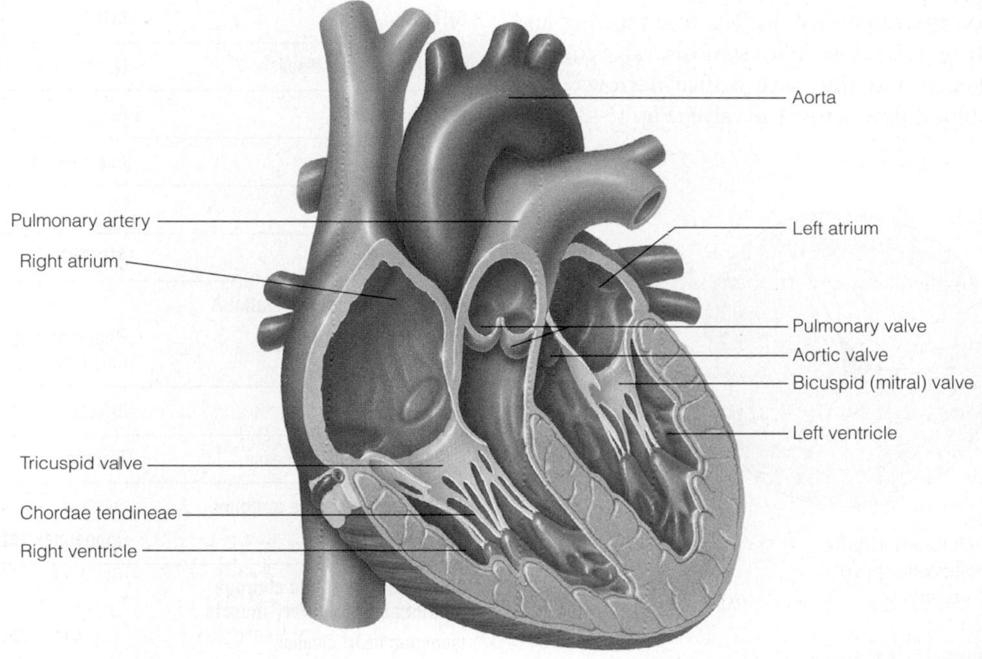

Figure 15–1 ■ The four chambers and four heart valves.

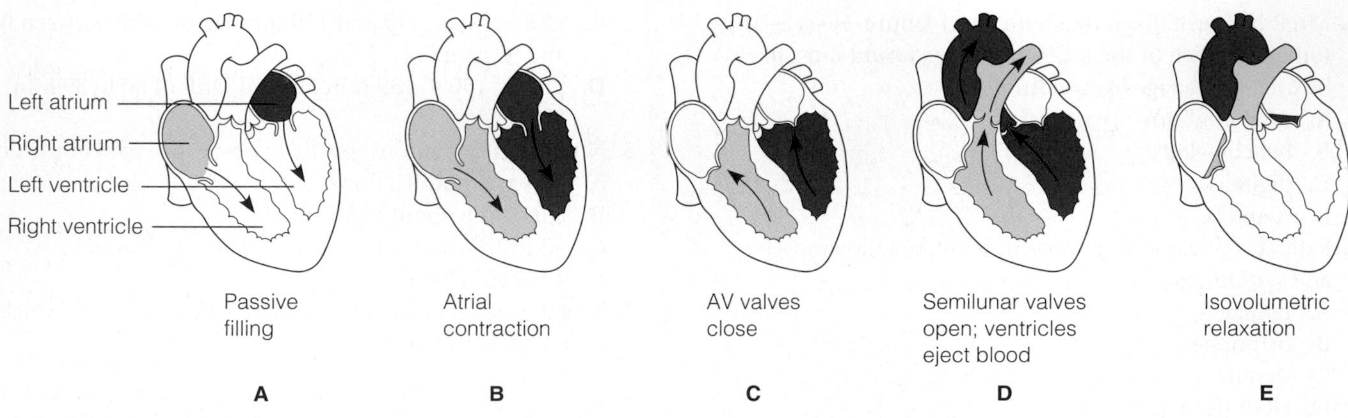

Figure 15–2 ■ Opening and closing of the heart valves during the cardiac cycle.

As pressure in the atria rises above pressure in the ventricles, the AV valves open and blood rushes into the ventricles. At the end of diastole, the atria contract to eject about 20 percent more volume into the ventricles (Fig. 15–2B). In early systole all valves are closed, the pressure within the ventricles is high and the ventricles begin to contract (Fig. 15–2C). Finally, the semilunar valves open and the ventricles eject the blood (Fig. 15–2D). After the ventricles eject their volume, all valves are closed and there is a period of isovolumetric relaxation (Fig. 15–2E). The opening and closing of the valves during the cardiac cycle allows for forward unidirectional movement of blood through the four chambers of the heart. When valve dysfunction occurs, this forward unidirectional movement of blood flow through the heart is affected. The two major categories for valvular dysfunction are stenosis and regurgitation.

Valve Stenosis

Stenosis of a valve occurs when valve leaflets fuse together and the valve cannot fully open or close. With stenosis, valve components become thickened and the valve orifice narrows. This causes resistance of blood flow across the valve (Fig. 15–3). The chamber before the valve is exposed to an increased afterload because flow through the valve is more difficult. The blood from that chamber "backs up" to the preceding chamber. Stenosis of a valve may be caused by calcification, congenital factors, or rheumatic fever (Otto & Bonow, 2008). Risk factors for the development of stenosis are listed in Table 15–1.

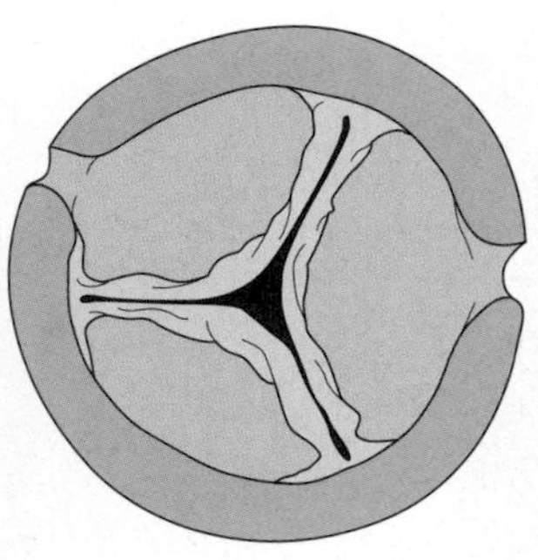

Figure 15–3 ■ Stenosis of a heart valve. Thickened and stenotic valve leaflets.

Mitral Valve Stenosis

Mitral stenosis (MS) is a narrowing of the mitral valve orifice that obstructs blood flow from the left atrium into the left ventricle

TABLE 15–1 Risk Factors for the Development of Valve Disorders

Stenosis	
MITRAL	**AORTIC**
Rheumatic heart disease	Congenital
Female gender	Acquired
	Age-related
Regurgitation	
MITRAL	**AORTIC**
Abnormalities of the leaflets	
Rheumatic heart disease	Rheumatic heart disease Calcification
Infective endocarditis	Infective endocarditis
Collagen–vascular disease	Trauma
Abnormalities of the annulus	
Cardiomyopathy	Congenital (less common)
Abnormalities of the chordae tendineae or papillary muscle	
Ischemic heart disease	
Mitral valve prolapse	

during diastole. It is predominantly caused by rheumatic fever and occurs more frequently in women (Otto & Bonow, 2008). Left atrial (LA) pressure increases with MS and eventually causes an increase in pulmonary artery (PA) pressure and pulmonary vascular resistance (PVR) (Fig. 15–4). Cardiac output (CO) can be normal with mild MS, but as the MS becomes more severe, CO decreases. With severe MS, an increase in PVR causes the right ventricle (RV) and right atrium (RA) to fail. Left ventricular (LV) diastolic pressure also increases because the pressure gradient across the valve is higher.

An important factor to consider with MS is heart rate (HR). Recall from Module 12, Determinants and Assessment of Cardiac Output that during ventricular diastole the ventricle relaxes and fills. If a patient with MS experiences a sudden increase in HR, diastolic filling time is shortened. This results in a substantial decrease in CO and an increase in LA pressure. Elevated LA pressures lead to LA dilatation and changes in the LA electrical refractory period, which may precipitate atrial fibrillation. A vicious cycle occurs if the HR is not controlled.

Aortic Valve Stenosis

Aortic stenosis (AS) is a condition in which the aortic valve is narrowed and blood flow is obstructed from the LV into the aorta during systole. It is caused by congenital or acquired conditions, such as rheumatic heart disease and aging. Through the aging process, degenerative calcifications occur.

In aortic stenosis, the valvular orifice narrows, increases the pressure gradient between the LV and aorta, and causes a "back-up phenomenon." The LV end-diastolic pressure increases and the LV hypertrophies (Fig. 15–5). LA contractility increases to eject volume against higher LV pressures. However, in the event of a loss of an effective atrial contraction, such as that which occurs with atrial fibrillation (see Module 14, Assessment of Cardiac Rhythm), immediate decompensation can occur (Otto & Bonow, 2008).

Valvular Regurgitation

Insufficient or incompetent valves that do not close completely are called regurgitant valves (Fig. 15–6). This allows regurgitation of blood through the valve and back into the chamber that

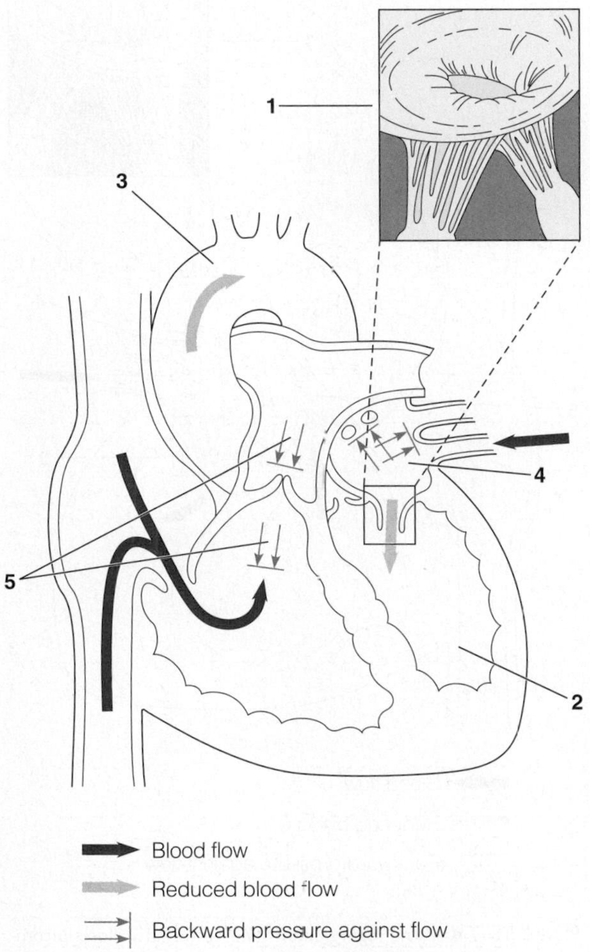

Figure 15–4 ■ Mitral stenosis. Narrowing of the mitral valve orifice (1) reduces blood volume to left ventricle (2) reducing cardiac output (3) Rising pressure in the left atrium (4) causes left atrial hypertrophy and pulmonary congestion. Increased pressure in pulmonary vessels (5) causes hypertrophy of the right ventricle and right atrium.

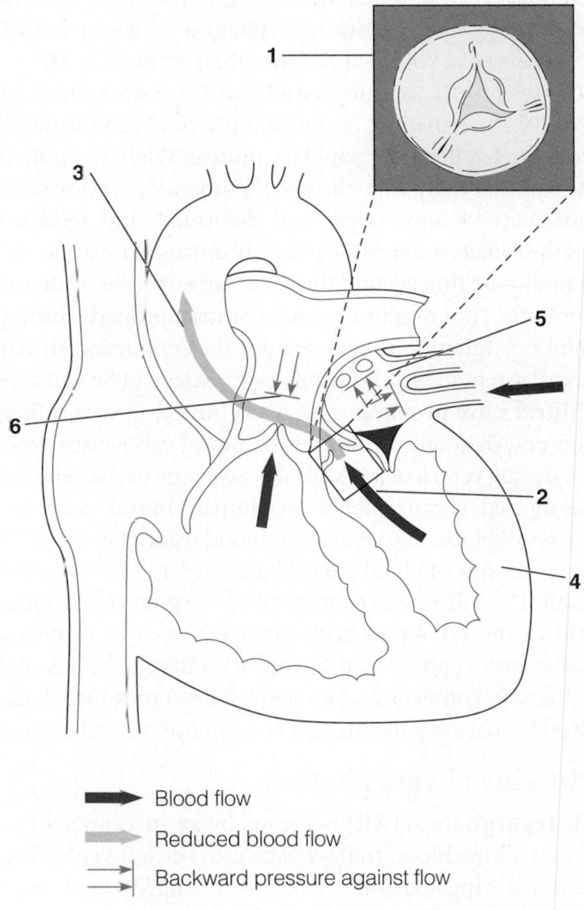

Figure 15–5 ■ Aortic stenosis. The narrowed aortic valve orifice (1) decreases the left ventricular ejection fraction during systole (2) and cardiac output (3) The left ventricle hypertrophies (4) Incomplete emptying of the left atrium (5) causes backward pressure through pulmonary veins and pulmonary hypertension. Elevated pulmonary artery pressure (6) causes right ventricular strain.

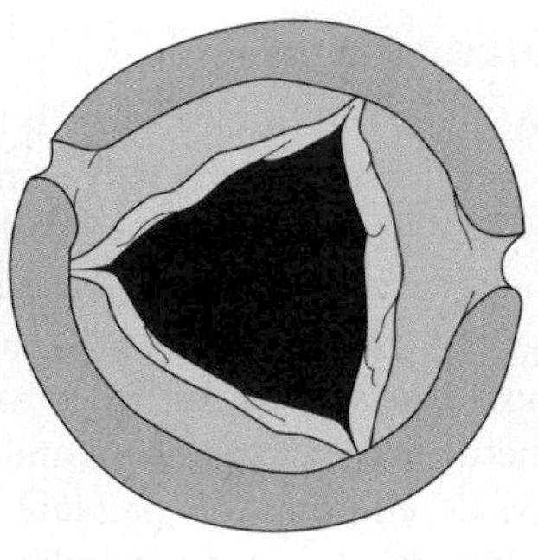

Figure 15–6 ■ An incompetent or regurgitant valve. Retracted fibrosed valve openings.

the blood just left. Risk factors for the development of regurgitant valves are summarized in Table 15–1.

Mitral Valve Regurgitation

Mitral regurgitation (MR) occurs when the mitral valve does not completely close and allows blood to flow back into the LA during systole. This causes regurgitation of a portion of the ventricular stroke volume (SV) into the LA (Fig. 15–7).

Causes of MR are categorized into (1) abnormalities of the leaflets, (2) abnormalities of the annulus, or (3) abnormalities of the chordae tendineae or papillary muscle. When the leaflets are abnormal (especially with chronic rheumatic heart disease), they shorten, become more rigid and deformed, and retract. This causes the leaflets not to close properly during ventricular systole. The annulus or ring around the valve can either be dilated, calcified, or both. The annulus does not constrict properly during systole and regurgitation occurs. Finally, the supporting structures, the chordae tendineae, and papillary muscles can be damaged.

Mitral valve prolapse is a type of mitral valve insufficiency that occurs when one or both of the mitral valve cusps flow into the LA during ventricular systole. Excess tissue in the valve leaflets and elongated chordae tendineae impair mitral valve closure during systole and some ventricular blood regurgitates (Fig. 15–8). The large volume of blood ejected backward into the LA over time causes the LV to dilate and hypertrophy in response to the increased preload of the LA. In an acute situation, such as a myocardial infarction and rupture of the papillary muscle, the LA and LV cannot acutely compensate. Elevated left heart pressures "back up" to the pulmonary vasculature and acute pulmonary edema occurs.

Aortic Valve Regurgitation

Aortic regurgitation (AR) is caused by an incompetent aortic valve that allows blood to flow back into the left ventricle from the aorta during diastole. It occurs primarily as a result of rheumatic heart disease. The leaflets' structures are altered because of infiltration of fibrous tissue. The fibrous tissue causes the leaflets to retract and, therefore, they do not completely close during systole.

With aortic regurgitation, regurgitation of part of the ventricular stroke volume back into the left ventricle leads to ventricular hypertrophy (Fig. 15–9). This is structurally different than the hypertrophy that develops with aortic stenosis. The hypertrophy associated with AR is more severe and significantly decreases SV (Otto & Bonow, 2008).

Infective Endocarditis

When valves have structural abnormalities, it increases their susceptibility to infection. **Infective endocarditis (IE)** is a disease caused by a microbial infection of the endothelial lining of the heart. The process starts with damage to the endothelium of a valve. Damage may be the result of congenital diseases (e.g., rheumatic heart disease) or iatrogenic (with the introduction of intracardiac catheters or other devices). The disrupted surface of the endothelium attracts platelets that adhere to the surface and starts the development of nonbacterial thrombi. The next phase of IE is the introduction of bacteria in the blood through portals of entry, such as wounds, biopsy sites, pacemakers, intravenous and arterial catheters,

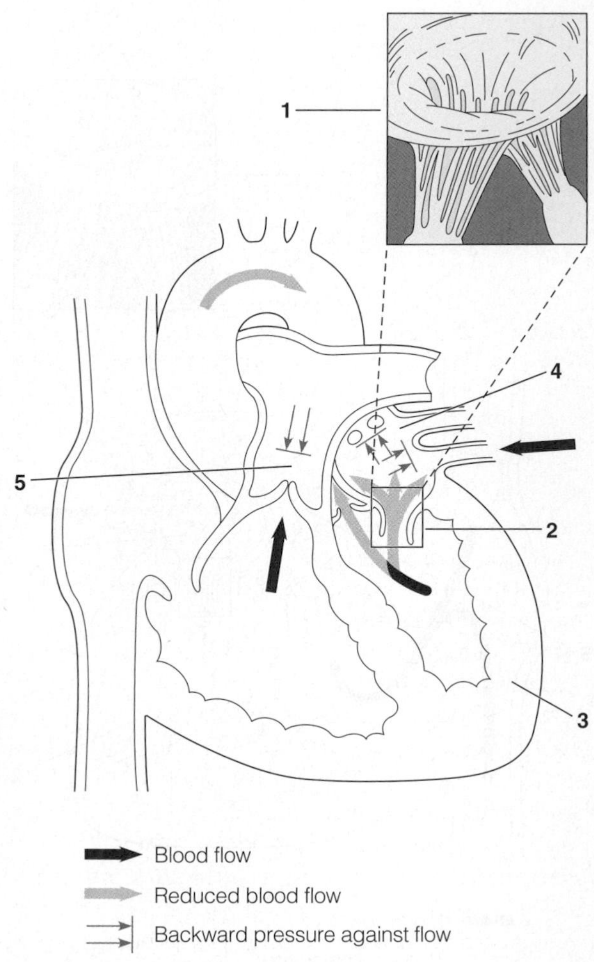

Figure 15–7 ■ Mitral regurgitation. The mitral valve closes incompletely (1), allowing blood to regurgitate during systole from the left ventricle to the left atrium (2). Cardiac output falls, to compensate, the left ventricle hypertrophies (3). Rising left atrial pressure (4) causes left atrial hypertrophy and pulmonary congestion. Elevated pulmonary artery pressure (5) causes slight enlargement of the right ventricle.

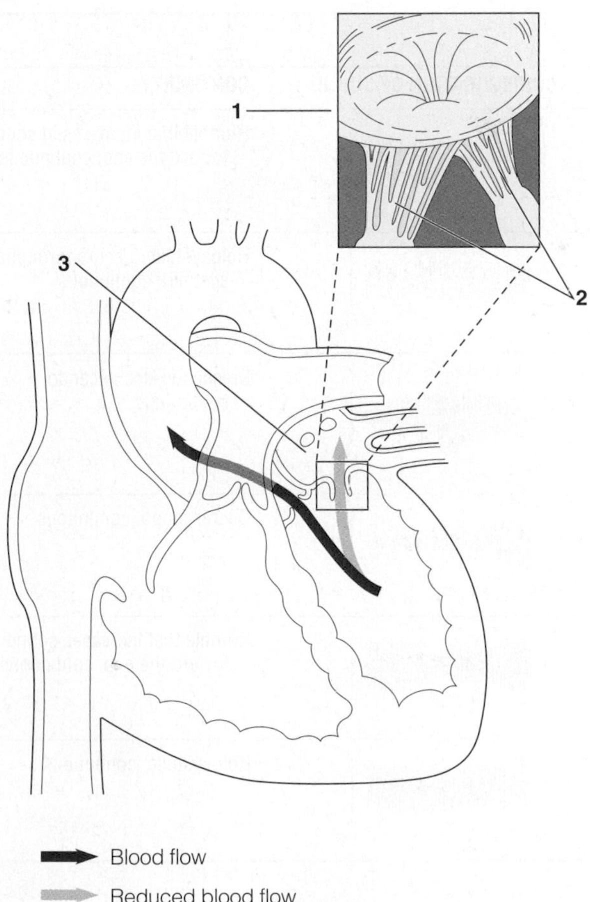

Figure 15–8 ■ Mitral valve prolapse. Excess tissue in the valve leaflets (1) and elongated chordae tendineae (2) impair mitral valve closure during systole. Some ventricular blood regurgitates into the left atrium (3).

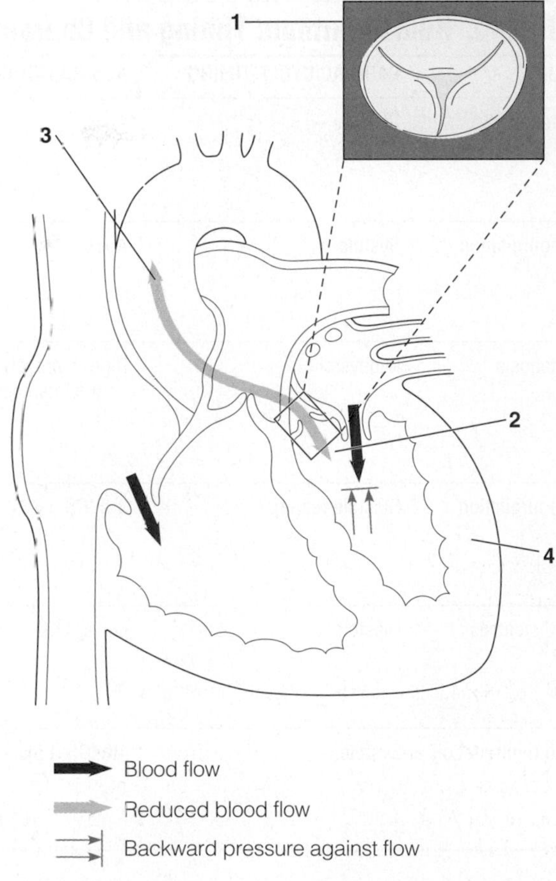

Figure 15–9 ■ Aortic regurgitation. The cusps of the aortic valve widen and fail to close during diastole (1). Blood regurgitates from the aorta into the left ventricle (2), increasing left ventricular volume and decreasing cardiac output (3). The left ventricle dilates and hypertrophies (4) in response to the increase in blood volume and work load.

urinary catheters, or through other invasive mechanisms, such as dental or gastrointestinal (colonoscopy) procedures. After bacteria enter the blood, they settle on the thrombi on the heart valve. The infected thrombi enlarge with time and increases valve dysfunction (Haldar & O'Gara, 2008).

Some groups of patients are more susceptible to this infection, including those with preexisting heart disease, children, the elderly, intravenous drug abusers, patients infected with human immunodeficiency virus, patients after cardiac surgery, and patients who require hemodialysis. These patients have weakened local and systemic defense mechanisms that are unable to destroy the bacteria and stop the infectious process. The course of the disease can develop over months (subacute), or it can be very rapid, developing within a few days (acute). There are several bacteria that can cause infective endocarditis but the more common species are *streptococci* (*alpha-hemolytic* or *viridans*) and *staphylococcus aureus*. The *streptococci viridans* is found in the oropharyngeal and gastrointestinal flora and is a low-grade pathogen that is usually responsible for subacute endocarditis. *Staphylococcus aureus* is a more virulent organism and is the leading cause of acute bacterial endocarditis (Haldar & O'Gara, 2008). Although all heart valves can be affected by this disease, aortic stenosis and mitral regurgitation most commonly occur as a result of infective endocarditis.

The treatment goal for infective endocarditis is appropriate and aggressive administration of antibiotics over the course of several weeks. Timely administration of antibiotics is imperative so that adequate levels can be maintained and resistance of bacteria to antibiotics can be reduced. If valvular dysfunction is severe, valve replacement may be required. In high-risk patient populations, antibiotic prophylaxis is suggested prior to procedures that may introduce bacteria. This practice is still followed although there is little evidence to support this intervention (Haldar & O'Gara, 2008).

Assessment and Diagnosis

The assessment process starts with a thorough physical assessment. Because turbulent blood flow is the result of valvular dysfunction, auscultation of the heart can reveal a murmur. The key to understanding the timing of murmurs in the cardiac cycle is to think about the valve position in relation to ventricular systole or diastole. Table 15–2 includes a summary of heart murmurs, their timing in the cardiac cycle, and characteristics.

TABLE 15–2 Heart Murmurs Timing and Characteristics

MURMUR	CARDIAC CYCLE TIMING	AUSCULTATION SITE	CONFIGURATION OF SOUND	CONTINUITY
Mitral stenosis	Diastole	Apical	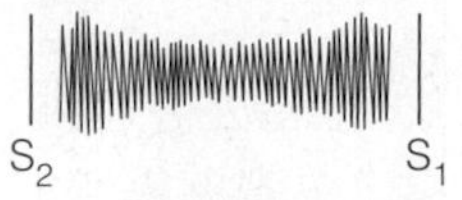 S_2 S_1	Rumble that increases in sound toward the end, continuous
Mitral regurgitation	Systole	Apex	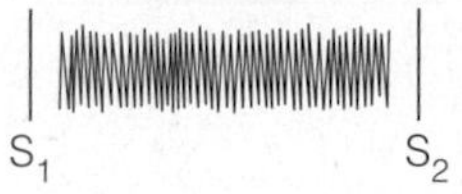 S_1 S_2	Holosystolic (occurs throughout systole), continuous
Aortic stenosis	Midsystolic	Right sternal border (RSB) 2nd intercostal space (ICS)	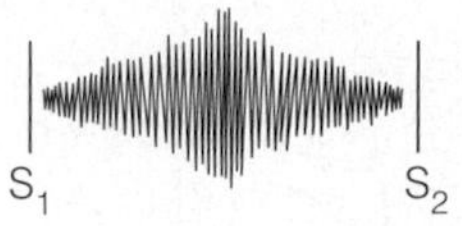 S_1 S_2	Crescendo-decrescendo, continuous
Aortic regurgitation	Diastole (early)	3rd ICS, LSB	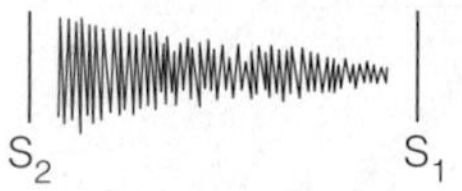 S_2 S_1	Decrescendo, continuous
Tricuspid stenosis	Diastole	Lower LSB	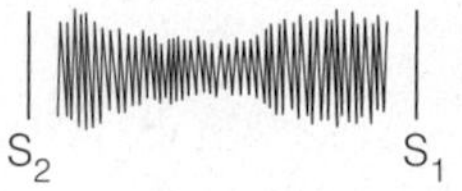 S_2 S_1	Rumble that increases sound toward the end, continuous
Tricuspid regurgitation	Systole	4th ICS, LSB	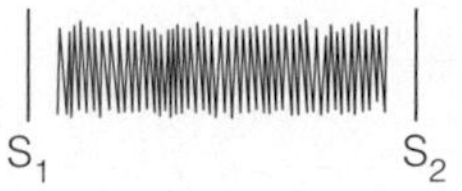 S_1 S_2	Holosystolic, continuous

The mitral valve is open during ventricular diastole, so the murmur of mitral stenosis occurs during diastole. The aortic valve is open during ventricular systole, so the murmur of aortic stenosis occurs during systole.

The opposite timing for murmurs applies for regurgitation. The mitral valve is closed during systole, so the murmur of mitral regurgitation occurs during systole. The aortic valve is closed during diastole, so the murmur of aortic regurgitation occurs during diastole.

With aortic stenosis, angina can occur because of possible disturbance of blood flow through the coronary arteries since the opening of these arteries is located close to the aortic valve. One symptom specific to aortic stenosis includes syncope on exertion as a result of decreased cerebral perfusion. If valvular dysfunction is critical, the patient can experience heart failure or pulmonary edema. Dyspnea, tachypnea, crackles in the lungs, tachycardia, and chest pain can be present. A chest X-ray may reveal pulmonary edema or an enlarged left atrium.

Another assessment tool that is helpful in the diagnosis of valvular disease is an echocardiogram. The **echocardiogram** is noninvasive technology that allows visualization of the valves as well as the size, thickness, and function of the atria and ventricles. Abnormal findings in the echocardiogram can be confirmed by cardiac catheterization. During this procedure, the valves can be thoroughly examined, and intracardiac pressures and pressure gradients across the chambers can be measured.

Collaborative Management

Patients who are asymptomatic with a valvular dysfunction usually do not require medical intervention. As the dysfunction becomes more severe, heart rate is controlled with drugs such as beta blockers (BB), calcium channel blockers (CCB), and digoxin. Examples of these drugs are listed in Table 15–3. The major therapeutic goal is to maintain normal sinus rhythm and avoid atrial fibrillation. If atrial fibrillation does occur, immediate treatment with cardioversion may be required. If heart failure (HF) occurs, diuretics and sodium and fluid restriction may be required. With regurgitation, afterload reduction is very important. Reducing afterload lessens the degree of regurgitation and significantly improves symptoms. Angiotensin-converting enzyme (ACE) inhibitors are particularly effective for afterload reduction and controlling hypertension.

Surgical intervention is required if valvular dysfunction is severe. The valve is replaced with either a tissue or mechanical, artificial valve. Mechanical valves last longer, but anticoagulation is required because the foreign material causes clot formation. The type of valve used depends on patient age and tolerance of anticoagulation. Anticoagulation is also required if chronic atrial fibrillation is present. A new intervention for aortic stenosis is percutaneous aortic valve replacement. This procedure is performed by an interventional cardiologist in the cardiac catheterization laboratory and is an alternative therapy for the elderly patient (Lauck et al, 2008). The stent

TABLE 15–3 Brief Listing of Common Drugs by Classes

THIAZIDE DIURETICS	LOOP DIURETICS	ACE INHIBITORS	ANGIOTENSIN RECEPTOR BLOCKERS	BETA BLOCKERS	CALCIUM CHANNEL BLOCKERS
Chlorothiazide (Diuril)	Bumetanide (Bumex)	Captopril (Capoten)	Losartan (Cozaar)	Atenolol (Tenormin)	Diltiazem (Cardizem)
Metolazone (Zaroxolyn)	Furosemide (Lasix)	Enalapril (Vasotec)	Valsartan (Diovan)	Metoprolol (Lopressor)	Verapamil (Calan)
		Lisinopril (Zestril, Prinivil)	Irbesartan (Avapro)	Nadolol (Corgard)	
		Ramipril (Altace)		Propranolol (Inderal)	

valve is placed over a valvuloplasty balloon which is then inserted into the aortic valve using an arterial retrograde approach. The balloon is inflated and the stent valve is deployed in the valve area. These artificial valve patients also require anticoagulation to maintain proper valve function (Lauck et al, 2008). Care of this patient population is similar to the percutaneous cardiac interventional patient (see Module 16, Alterations in Myocardial Tissue Perfusion). Advancement in surgical and medical management has decreased mortality and improved quality of life in patients with valvular disease.

Nursing Management

Nursing diagnoses for a patient with a valve disorder may include decreased cardiac output, activity intolerance, fatigue, risk for infection, ineffective protection, and ineffective health maintenance. Nursing priorities include assessing and maintaining cardiac output, assessing for side effects of the disorder, preventing complications, administering pharmacologic therapies, and providing patient education.

All valve disorders affect ventricular filling or emptying and result in decreased cardiac output. Vital signs are carefully monitored. Hypotension and tachycardia indicate decreased cardiac output. If a pulmonary artery catheter is present, hemodynamic findings may include decreased cardiac output and elevated pulmonary artery wedge pressure and right atrial pressure. These findings are associated with pulmonary congestion. Auscultation of heart sounds is performed regularly. Atrial fibrillation may be averted by aggressive repletion of potassium and magnesium as needed and administration of antiarrhythmics as prescribed.

Failure of the heart to function as a pump results in decreased oxygen delivery to tissues and impaired tissue perfusion. An early sign of valve disease is dyspnea with exertion. The nurse monitors the patient's vital signs before and during activities. A change of heart rate of more than 20 beats per minute (bpm) or change in blood pressure of more than 20 mm Hg indicates activity intolerance. Other signs of activity intolerance include shortness of breath, chest pain, fatigue, diaphoresis, dizziness, or syncope. Activities and self-care activities are gradually increased. Rest periods between activities help the patient and decreases oxygen demand of the heart. Using a shower chair during bathing saves valuable energy. A physical therapy consult is initiated to help the patient regain and maintain physical strength. Asymptomatic patients are counseled about exercise tolerance, the importance of compliance with medications, and the need for periodic exams with their health care provider to monitor valve function.

Discharge planning includes education about the importance of monitoring blood pressure and heart rate. Because a therapeutic goal is to maintain a regular heart rate, the nurse educates the patient and family about monitoring pulse rate. They are observed for proper technique. Patient education includes information about medications, including mechanism of action and possible side effects.

Ineffective protection can occur as a result of anticoagulation therapy. The most common drugs used for anticoagulation are heparin, aspirin, clopidogrel, and warfarin (Table 15–4). The patient is at risk for bleeding. Therefore, vigilant assessment is necessary of serum coagulation studies, such as prothrombin time (PT), international normalized ratio (INR), and partial thromboplastin time (PTT) as well as hemoglobin and hematocrit. When heparin is used, the PTT is the laboratory parameter used to guide therapy. If the patient is on warfarin (Coumadin), an INR goal is set. The nurse must be cognizant of this INR goal. Aspirin may also be prescribed. Patients receiving anticoagulant therapy are monitored for signs of bleeding, such as unexplained bruises, bleeding gums, and blood in stools. Patients who go home on anticoagulant therapy must receive patient education about monitoring for signs of bleeding, the need for drawing blood samples, taking the medication in the

TABLE 15–4 Common Drugs Used for Anticoagulation

DRUG	ACTION
Aspirin	Inhibits the production of thromboxane A_2 which promotes platelet aggregation
Clopidogrel (Plavix)	Inhibits adenosine diphosphate binding to platelet receptors
Warfarin (Coumadin)	Antagonist to Vitamin K
Heparin	Inactivates thrombin by binding to antithrombin III

evening, and avoiding foods that have a high vitamin K content, such as bananas and citrus fruits.

Although this intervention is controversial, patients with artificial or abnormal valves may require antibiotic prophylaxis when undergoing certain procedures, such as dental work or endoscopies. They are encouraged to wear emergency identification tags about this condition.

SECTION ONE REVIEW

1. If a patient is on Coumadin, which lab value guides the therapeutic goal?
   A. activated clotting time
   B. thrombin time
   C. partial thromboplastin time
   D. INR
2. When a patient has mitral stenosis, the abnormal heart sound would be
   A. diastolic murmur
   B. systolic murmur
   C. S_3
   D. S_4
3. A condition in which the orifice of the mitral valve has narrowed and blood flow is obstructed during diastole is called
   A. mitral stenosis
   B. mitral regurgitation
   C. aortic stenosis
   D. infective endocarditis
4. Which of the following patients are susceptible to infective endocarditis?
   A. patients with preexisting heart disease
   B. patients with human immunodeficiency virus
   C. patients that require hemodialysis
   D. all of the above
5. When a patient has mitral regurgitation, the abnormal heart sound is
   A. diastolic murmur
   B. systolic murmur
   C. S_3
   D. S_4

Answers: 1. D, 2. A, 3. A, 4. D, 5. B

SECTION TWO: Heart Failure

At the completion of this section, the learner will be able to describe heart failure, including the pathophysiologic and compensatory mechanisms that occur during heart failure; and the pharmacologic therapies used in the collaborative management of heart failure.

Heart failure (HF), a major health problem in our society today, is a clinical syndrome that results from any structural or functional cardiac disorder that decreases the ability of the ventricle to fill or eject.

Clinical manifestations of heart failure include dyspnea and fatigue that limit exercise tolerance, and fluid retention that leads to pulmonary congestion and peripheral edema. Because not all patients have fluid volume excess at the time of evaluation, the term *heart failure* is considered a better description of this condition than the older term *congestive heart failure* (Hunt et al., 2005). Symptoms of patients with HF are a result of impairment of left ventricular function.

The New York Heart Association (NYHA) developed a classification of HF based on functional limitations. There are four classes (Francis et al., 2008):

- Class I includes patients with cardiac disease but without resulting limitations of physical activity.
- Class II includes patients with cardiac disease resulting in slight limitations of physical activity.
- Class III includes patients with cardiac disease resulting in marked limitations of physical activity.
- Class IV includes patients with cardiac disease resulting in inability to carry on any physical activity without discomfort.

There are two categories of heart failure: (1) **systolic dysfunction**, characterized by an ejection fraction (EF) less than 40 percent and (2) **diastolic dysfunction**, characterized by an impairment of ventricular relaxation (Hunt et al., 2005). In two thirds of patients with HF, the cause of the syndrome is coronary artery disease; and in one third of HF patients it is caused by a cardiomyopathy.

Heart failure is a progressive disease and causes cardiac remodeling. The left ventricle dilates, hypertrophies, and becomes more spherical. The mechanism that causes HF is not clearly understood. Current theories support its development as the result of a sequence of events. Heart failure begins with a primary event that results in a loss of myocardium or excessive overload on the muscle. Many conditions can trigger heart failure, as summarized in Table 15–5.

Whatever the cause, some cardiomyocytes are destroyed, whereas other cells try to adapt by increasing their size and elongating. The cardiac muscle hypertrophies in order to sustain the

TABLE 15–5 Conditions That Trigger Heart Failure

Hypertension	Rheumatic fever
Diabetes	Exposure to cardiotoxic agents (some chemotherapies)
Hypercholesteremia	Illicit drug use
Coronary artery disease	Alcohol abuse
Valvular heart disease	
Peripheral vascular disease	

increased workload. When the muscle can no longer maintain that workload, the left ventricle dilates in order to maintain stroke volume even though the ejection fraction has decreased. Compensatory neurohormonal mechanisms help achieve this adaptive response.

Sodium and water retention occurs in an effort to increase preload and cardiac output. The renin–angiotensin system stimulates aldosterone release and increases sodium retention. As cardiac output decreases, the sympathetic nervous system releases norepinephrine and vasopressin to increase blood pressure, heart rate, and contractility. All these mechanisms help with short-term adaptation but have untoward long-term effects. A chronic increase in afterload eventually causes a decrease in cardiac output. A lower cardiac output leads to pulmonary congestion and peripheral edema. Prolonged increases in adrenergic activity lead to dysrhythmias, increased cardiac cellular activity, increased energy utilization, and cell death (Francis et al., 2008).

Recall from Module 12, Determinants and Assessment of Cardiac Output the counterregulatory hormones atrial natriuretic peptide (ANP) and B-type natriuretic peptide (BNP) are released in response to distention of heart chambers. ANP is released in response to atrial distention and BNP is released in response to ventricular distention. Both hormones cause vasodilation and induce natriuresis (loss of sodium).

Assessment and Diagnosis

A careful history and physical examination provide important information. Heart failure has multisystem effects (Fig. 15–10). Dyspnea, orthopnea, and paroxysmal nocturnal dyspnea (PND) are classic respiratory symptoms of patients with HF. **Orthopnea** is the sensation of shortness of breath in the supine position, whereas PND is sudden dyspnea at night that may awaken patients. Fatigue is another hallmark symptom. Jugular vein distention is a sign of fluid volume excess. Peripheral edema may also be present as a sign of fluid volume excess, although it can result from noncardiac causes. Crackles are an unreliable sign of heart failure. Most patients with chronic HF do not have crackles. A third heart sound (S_3) is an important assessment finding.

The single most useful diagnostic test for heart failure is the two-dimensional echocardiogram with Doppler flow studies. With these studies, an ejection fraction (EF) is obtained and pericardial, valvular, or myocardial dysfunction is visualized (Hunt et al., 2005). A chest X-ray gives an estimate of heart size and pulmonary congestion. A 15-lead electrocardiogram (ECG) can demonstrate myocardial infarction, ventricular hypertrophy, or dysrhythmia. However, the chest X-ray and electrocardiogram do not provide specific information to make the diagnosis of heart failure. Cardiac catheterization may also be needed to provide further information about coronary artery or valvular disease. B-type natriuretic peptide (BNP) can be useful if the diagnosis of heart failure is uncertain (Hunt et al., 2005).

It is important to remember that heart failure is a syndrome with many presentations, including decreased exercise tolerance, fluid retention, or symptoms of another cardiac or noncardiac disorder (Hunt et al., 2005).

Collaborative Management

The American College of Cardiologists and the American Heart Association established evidence-based guidelines for the management of HF (Hunt et al., 2005). Therapy is divided into four categories:

- Stage A includes patients at high risk for developing heart failure without structural heart disease or heart failure symptoms.
- Stage B includes patients with structural heart disease who have not developed heart failure symptoms.
- Stage C includes patients with structural heart disease with prior or current heart failure symptoms.
- Stage D includes patients with refractory heart failure requiring specialized interventions.

The focus of treatment for patients at high risk for heart failure is to control risk factors. Management of hypertension, diabetes, and hyperlipidemia reduces the risk of developing heart failure. Counseling patients on the hazards of recreational substances, such as tobacco, alcohol, and illicit drugs, provides a strong impetus for patients to reduce the use of these agents. There is no evidence that controlling dietary sodium intake and exercise helps prevent heart failure, but these habits can promote general health.

First-line drug management for heart failure usually includes an ACE inhibitor and a beta-blocker (see the RELATED PHARMACOTHERAPY box later in this module). This regimen controls the neurohormonal and sympathetic compensatory responses and decreases the occurrence of heart failure. Once patients display symptoms of heart failure, a combination of four types of drugs are used: diuretics, ACE inhibitors, beta-blockers, and ionotropic agents (Hunt et al., 2005).

Furosemide (Lasix) is the most common diuretic used. If two diuretics are needed to obtain the desired response, the two drugs used typically act on different sections of the nephron. For example, furosemide, a loop diuretic, acts on the loop of Henle, and metolazone (Zaroxolyn), a thiazide diuretic, works on blocking sodium reabsorption at the proximal tubule (Brunton et al, 2006). Diuretic resistance can occur and can be averted by doubling the dose or using continuous infusion (Moser, 2009).

ACE inhibitors are commonly administered. However, there are important contraindications to the use of ACE inhibitors of which nurses must be aware. Contraindications include previous severe adverse reactions to ACE inhibitors, serum creatinine greater than 3 mg/dL, systolic blood pressure less than 80 mm Hg, and serum potassium levels greater than 5.5 mEq/L (Hunt et al., 2005). Beta blockers may be administered to patients who do not have fluid retention. There are BBs that are used in HF including carvedilol (Coreg) which are now in controlled release form so that they can be dosed once daily. Aldosterone antagonists such as spironolactone (Aldactone) may be used if the patient with HF has adequate renal function and a normal potassium level. However, simultaneous use with higher doses of ACE inhibitors should be avoided due to compromise of renal function (Hunt et al., 2005). Close monitoring of potassium levels is required.

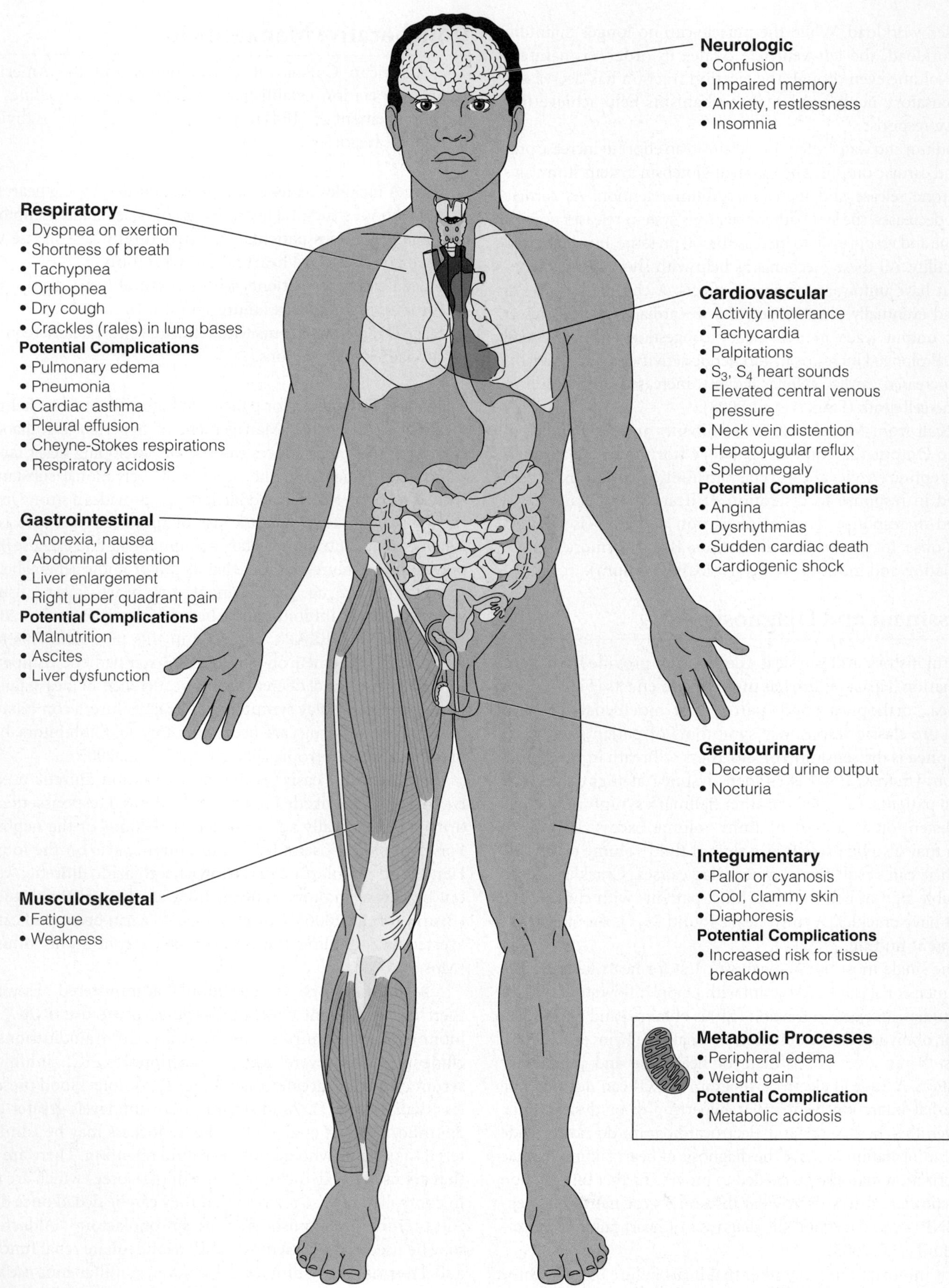

Figure 15–10 ■ Multisystem effect of heart failure.

Emerging Evidence

- Patients with heart failure who have better control of physical symptoms, those who work, are older and less anxious at baseline report better health-related quality of life. These results suggest that interventions that improve psychological status may improve physical symptoms and health related quality of life in patients with heart failure *(Heo, Doering, Widener et al., 2008)*.
- In patients hospitalized with heart failure, animal assisted therapy improved cardiopulmonary pressures (decreased systolic pulmonary artery pressures and pulmonary artery wedge pressures), decreased neurohormonal levels (epinephrine, norepinephrine) and decreased anxiety than patients who did not receive animal assisted therapy *(Cole, Gawlinski, Steers, et al., 2007)*.
- In older adults with stable heart failure, fatigue is a persistent symptom. Fatigue intensity is associated with lower quality of life, perceived health, and satisfaction with life *(Stephen, 2008)*.

Angiotensin receptor blockade (ARB) may be used for patients who cannot tolerate an ACE inhibitor because of a side effect or allergic reaction (Hunt et al., 2005). The ARB drugs can have similar clinical results as the ACE inhibitors. Figure 15–11 depicts how ARBs and ACE inhibitors work to block the renin–angiotensin–aldosterone system. ARBs do not have some of the adverse effects that are associated with ACE inhibitors, such as cough.

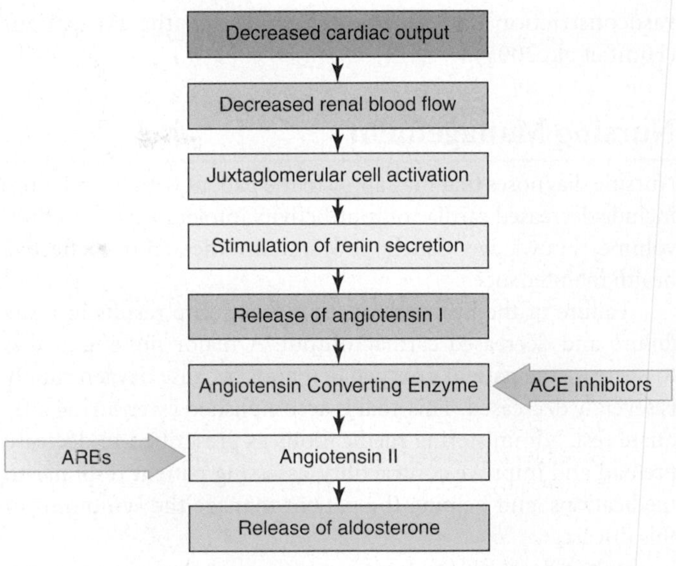

Figure 15–11 ■ ACE inhibitors and ARBs block the renin-angiotensin-aldosterone system.

Drugs classes that should be avoided in HF include antiarrhythmics due to their cardio-depressant effects. Amiodarone and dofetilide have not demonstrated adverse effects on survival (Hunt et al., 2005). Non steroidal anti-inflammatory agents cause sodium retention and peripheral

RELATED PHARMACOTHERAPY: Agents for Treatment of Heart Failure and Hypertension

Beta Adrenergic Blocking Agents

Carvedilol (Coreg, Kredex)

Action and Uses

Selective alpha activity and nonselective beta-adrenergic blocking agents which both lower blood pressure. Alpha-1 blocking causes peripheral vasodilation and decreased peripheral vascular resistance. Decreases myocardial oxygen demand and lowers cardiac workload. Used in the management of hypertension and heart failure.

Major Side Effects

Dizziness

Nursing Implications

Monitor for lessoning of signs and symptoms of heart failure and improved blood pressure control

Monitor for orthostatic hypotension

Monitor liver function tests

Monitor digoxin levels with concurrent use; plasma digoxin concentration levels may increase

Educate patients to report any dizziness, faintness

Angiotensin Converting Enzyme Inhibitors

Captopril (Capoten)

Action and Uses

Lowers blood pressure by inhibition of angiotensin converting enzyme. Interrupts conversion of angiotensin I to angiotensin II, a potent vasoconstrictor. Lowers peripheral vascular resistance by vasodilation. Used in hypertension and heart failure to decrease dyspnea and improve exercise tolerance.

Major Side Effects

Angioedema

Agranulocytosis

Maculopapular rash

Nursing Implications

Monitor blood pressure closely, especially after the first dose. Hypotension may occur 1-3 hours after the first dose. Advise the patient to remain on bedrest for 3 hours after the initial dose.

Two weeks of therapy may be required before full therapeutic effect is achieved.

Mild skin eruptions may occur during first 4 weeks of therapy.

Angiotensin II Receptor Antagonists

Losartan (Cozaar)

Action and Uses

Selectively blocks the binding of angiotensin II to the angiotensin I receptors in vascular smooth muscle. Used for hypertension (produces vasodilation) and inhibition of aldosterone effects on sodium and water.

Major Side Effects

Headaches

Nursing Implications

Monitor blood pressure; notify HCP for hypotension, patient complaints of dizziness or faintness.

vasoconstriction and should be avoided in the HF patient (Hunt et al., 2005).

Nursing Management

Nursing diagnoses that may apply to the patient with heart failure include decreased cardiac output, activity intolerance, excess fluid volume, knowledge deficit: low-sodium diet, and ineffective health maintenance.

Failure of the heart to function as a pump results in heart failure and decreased cardiac output. A major nursing goal is to decrease the patient's oxygen demands because oxygen supply is severely decreased. This goal is accomplished by ensuring adequate rest, administering medications as prescribed to decrease preload and improve contractility, assessing patient response to medications, and helping the patient manage the symptoms of this disease.

As the heart fails to function as a pump, less oxygen is delivered to tissues and ineffective tissue perfusion results. Many of the nursing interventions listed for the patient with valve disease are pertinent for the patient with heart failure. Nursing assessments focus on astute observation of the patient for signs of decompensation. Vital signs are monitored for signs of decreased cardiac output. Palpation of the apical pulse can be located to the left of the midclavicular line because of left ventricular enlargement. Heart sounds are auscultated regularly. An early sign of heart failure is an S_3 heart sound. Lung sounds are monitored for the development of crackles. Cardiac rhythm, exercise tolerance, and renal function are assessed for early signs of deterioration.

Continuous telemetry monitoring is recommended for patients in the high-acuity setting because BBs, digitalis, and other medications affect heart rate. Because digitalis and beta blockers slow the heart rate, patients are instructed on how to correctly take their pulse and when to call the health care provider if pulse parameters are violated.

The patient with heart failure may have activity intolerance and fatigue from a couple of sources. First, the disease process itself causes fatigue because of decreased oxygen delivery to peripheral tissues. Fluid volume excess in the lungs interferes with pulmonary gas exchange. BBs cause fatigue, a significant side effect that often causes patients to discontinue taking the drug. It is important for patients to know that the fatigue may disappear after the first several weeks of therapy. The patient is encouraged to rest between activities and to gradually increase activities. The nurse monitors the patient's activity tolerance. This includes taking vital signs before, during, and after an activity.

Because fatigue is one of the major symptoms of heart failure, proper sleep and sleeping habits are very important to maintain quality of life. The nurse recognizes that these patients have sleep disturbances and obtains a brief sleep history, ensuring that other causes of sleep disturbances, such as depression or sleep apnea, are ruled out. The hospital environment is optimized to promote sleep using relaxation techniques, sleep protocols, and a quiet environment. Sleep disturbances are treated by (1) reviewing good sleep habits; (2) considering alternative practices, such as relaxation, or cognitive or behavioral therapy; or (3) suggesting structured changes in sleep habits. Family focused care is another helpful intervention that can be implemented to maintain compliance with the health care regimen.

Careful monitoring of fluid status is important for patients with heart failure. The initial assessment of the patient population should include accurate measurement of height and weight, orthostatic blood pressure changes and calculation of body mass index (Hunt et al., 2005). Fluid status determination using jugular vein distension, breath sounds and the degree of peripheral and central edema should be monitored (Hunt et al., 2005). Diuretics can deplete circulating volume and cause hypovolemia, as well as potassium and magnesium deficits. These electrolytes are replaced either by oral/IV supplements or food source supplementation. Potassium depletion is further exacerbated if digitalis is used with a diuretic. A decreased urine output can indicate a significant decrease in cardiac output and renal perfusion. Monitoring weight trends is also very important in controlling fluid retention. Obtaining and recording daily weights is vital. Typically, a weight gain of 2.2 pounds (1 kg) equates to fluid retention of a liter. For discharge planning, the patient is given tools for recording daily weights and advised to call a health care provider if he or she gains 3 or more pounds (1.4 kg) in 24 hours.

Nursing interventions focus on patient education in an effort to improve patient compliance with the prescribed drug regimen. Drug therapy is a major component of management of this condition. One of the most important concepts for patients to understand is the difference between a drug side effect and a drug allergy. A **drug allergy** refers to some display of anaphylactic shock, such as a rash, airway compromise (edema of the tongue or larynx), or hypotension. A **drug side effect** is a reaction to some action of the drug other than anaphylaxis. A patient may say that he or she has an allergy to a drug but it is really a side effect. For example, a patient thinks that he or she has an allergy to ACE inhibitors because they cause a cough. Cough is really a side effect of ACE inhibitors, not an allergy. Coughing is the result of the release of kinins that cause coughing with prolonged therapy (Hunt et al., 2005). It would be unfortunate for this patient to not reap the benefits of ACE inhibitors because of incorrect information.

It is also important to understand any financial constraints that the patient may have in order to ensure that he or she is able to obtain needed drugs.

Cardiomyopathy

End-stage heart failure is referred to as **cardiomyopathy** and is classified class IV heart failure. At this stage, symptoms of heart failure occur at rest and the patient cannot perform activities of daily living.

The disease progression is diffuse and affects all heart chambers, although it may be more extensive in one chamber than others. Cardiomyopathies are classified into three categories according to clinical and structural findings: dilated cardiomyopathy, hypertrophic cardiomyopathy, and constrictive cardiomyopathy. The causes, pathophysiology, manifestations, and management of each of these cardiomyopathies are summarized in Table 15–6.

TABLE 15–6 Classifications of Cardiomyopathy

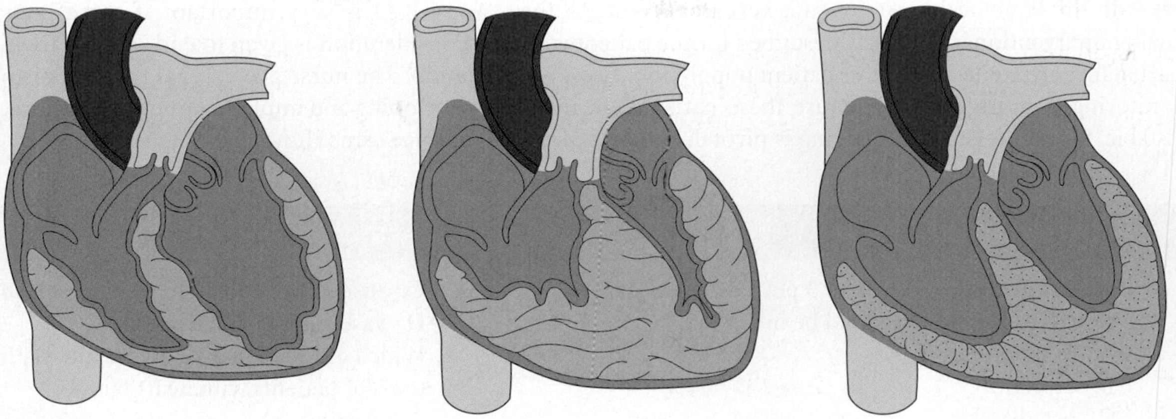

	DILATED	HYPERTROPHIC	RESTRICTIVE
Causes	Usually idiopathic; may be secondary to chronic alcoholism or myocarditis	Hereditary; may be secondary to chronic hypertension	Usually secondary to amyloidosis, radiation, or myocardial fibrosis
Pathophysiology	Scarring and atrophy of myocardial cells Thickening of ventricular wall Dilation of heart chambers Impaired ventricular pumping Increased end-diastolic and end-systolic volumes Mural thrombi common	Hypertrophy of ventricular muscle mass Small left ventricular volume Septal hypertrophy may obstruct left ventricular outflow Left atrial dilation	Excess rigidity of ventricular walls restricts filling Myocardial contractility remains relatively normal
Manifestations	Heart failure Cardiomegaly Dysrhythmias S_3 and S_4 gallop; murmur of mitral regurgitation	Dyspnea, anginal pain, syncope Left ventricular hypertrophy Dysrhythmias Loud S_4 Sudden death	Dyspnea, fatigue Right-sided heart failure Mild to moderate cardiomegaly S_3 and S_4 Mitral regurgitation murmur
Management	Management of heart failure Implantable cardioverter-defibrillator (ICD) as needed Cardiac transplantation	Beta blockers Calcium channel blockers Antidysrhythmic agents ICD, dual-chamber pacing Surgical excision of part of the entricular septum	Management of heart failure Exercise restriction

Dilated cardiomyopathy is associated with left ventricular dilation and decreased ejection fraction (EF). **Hypertrophic cardiomyopathy** is associated with left ventricular hypertrophy that decreases the ability of the chamber to relax (diastolic dysfunction). **Constrictive cardiomyopathy** is associated with normal left ventricular size, slightly depressed EF, and a marked decrease in cardiac muscle compliance. Depending on the type of cardiomyopathy, collaborative management may differ, but the same general principles of heart failure treatment continue.

Control of volume overload is aggressive. A loop diuretic and a second diuretic are usually needed. ACE inhibitors or beta blockers are used cautiously. Typically, these patients are very unstable. Patients with refractory heart failure may also require intermittent hospitalization for infusion of positive ionotropic medications (such as dobutamine or milrinone) and vasodilators (such as nitroprusside or nitroglycerin) (Hunt et al., 2005). These drugs improve contractility and decrease afterload. Another newer drug that may be used is nesiritide (Natrecor). This drug, given as an IV infusion, mimics brain natriuretic peptide and is given to enhance diuresis.

Other interventions have demonstrated some improvement in symptoms and are being used more frequently. Fast cardiac rhythms that quickly cause decompensation are controlled with an automatic implantable cardioverter/defibrillator (AICD). Biventricular pacing is another intervention that improves both right and left ventricular electrical activity and enhances ventricular mechanical performance.

Surgical intervention may include mitral valve replacement to decrease LV dilatation (Hunt et al., 2005). Removal of a hypertrophied left ventricle, known as the Batista procedure, is another surgical option. Cardiomyoplasty is a procedure that uses muscle or other material to "wrap" the heart, thereby mechanically increasing the contractility of the heart muscle. Final surgical interventions that may be considered are placement of ventricular assist devices (VAD) and cardiac transplantation. These interventions are reserved for when heart failure has become unresponsive to conventional medical treatment (Hunt et al., 2005).

Patient and family education is ongoing. Continuity of care with the same health care team is very important. All the nursing interventions previously described for the patient with heart failure are applicable to this patient population. However, monitoring is more intense because these patients are more unstable. Blood pressure monitoring is pivotal. Subtle changes in mental status indicate a change in cerebral perfusion and the physician is notified immediately. Renal function is monitored because of diuresis and decreased renal perfusion as a result of decreased cardiac output. Patient education about pacing or AICD is very important if these interventions are used. Consideration is given to end-of-life care in this patient population. The nurse plays a vital role in assisting these patients in developing and implementing advance directives and the use of hospice care (Hunt et al., 2005).

SECTION TWO REVIEW

1. Weight gain of greater than 3 pounds might dictate which drug category would be increased
   A. ACE inhibitor
   B. diuretic
   C. beta blocker
   D. digitalis
2. Mr. M. has a blood pressure of 75/45 mm Hg. You are the nurse and it is time to administer his ACE inhibitor. Which nursing action is MOST appropriate?
   A. Give the drug immediately; it will improve his blood pressure.
   B. Wait one hour and recheck the blood pressure.
   C. Notify the physician and ask if the dose should be held.
   D. Discuss the issue with your colleague.
3. ANP and BNP cause
   A. myocardial infarction
   B. hypertension
   C. vasoconstriction and fluid retention
   D. vasodilation and diuresis
4. Which of the following are classic respiratory symptoms of patients with heart failure?
   A. dyspnea
   B. orthopnea
   C. paroxysmal nocturnal dyspnea
   D. all of the above
5. Normal left ventricle size, slightly depressed ejection fraction (EF), and a marked decrease in compliance of cardiac muscle describes
   A. constrictive cardiomyopathy
   B. dilated cardiomyopathy
   C. hypertrophic cardiomyopathy
   D. stage II heart failure

Answers: 1. B, 2. C, 3. D, 4. D, 5. A

SECTION THREE: Hypertension

At the completion of this section, the learner will be able to explain hypertension, including the ranges of systolic and diastolic blood pressure for prehypertension, stage 1 hypertension, and stage 2 hypertension; the pathophysiologic mechanisms that contribute to hypertension; and collaborative and nursing interventions for the patient with hypertension.

The focus on hypertension and its early detection, prevention, and treatment is a top priority in health care because hypertension contributes to an increased risk of heart attack, heart failure, stroke, and kidney disease. Hypertension can be found in the young as well as the elderly, and frequently patients do not have symptoms. Risk factors for the development of hypertension have been identified (Table 15–7).

TABLE 15–7 Risk Factors for the Development of Hypertension

Hypertension
Cigarette smoking
Obesity
Physical inactivity
Hyperlipemia
Diabetes mellitus
Estimated glomerular filtration rate less than 60 mL/min
Age (older than 55 for men; 65 for women)
Family history of premature cardiovascular disease
Obstructive sleep apnea

Parameters for hypertension are defined in the *Seventh Report of the Joint National Committee on Prevention, Detection, Evaluation and Treatment of High Blood Pressure* (Chobanian, 2003) for adults over 18 years. In this report, normal blood pressure is defined as a systolic blood pressure (SBP) less than 150 mm Hg and a diastolic blood pressure (DBP) less than 80 mm Hg. A new category for blood pressure classification, **prehypertension** assists with earlier identification of those at risk for developing hypertension. Prehypertension is defined as a SBP of 150 to 139 mm Hg and DBP of 80 to 89 mm Hg. Definitions of the classifications of blood pressure, as summarized by Chobanian (2003), are listed in Table 15–8.

Although a lot of research has focused on identifying the cause of hypertension, the exact cause has not been identified

TABLE 15–8 Classification of Blood Pressure

BLOOD PRESSURE CLASSIFICATION	SYSTOLIC BLOOD PRESSURE (mm Hg)	DIASTOLIC BLOOD PRESSURE (mm Hg)
Normal	Less than 150	Less than 80
Prehypertension	150 to 139	80 to 89
Stage 1 hypertension	140 to 159	90 to 99
Stage 2 hypertension	160 or greater	100 or greater

(Victor & Kaplan, 2008). Neurohormonal mechanisms appear to be key to the development of hypertension. The sympathetic nervous system plays a major role by releasing catecholamines that result in increased heart rate and vasoconstriction. The renin–angiotensin system also influences the development of hypertension by secreting aldosterone to promote sodium and water retention. Hyperinsulinemia and insulin resistance may contribute to the development of hypertension. Although the mechanism is not clear, peripheral tissues do not use insulin. Insulin may act as a vasopressor. Nitric oxide, produced by endothelial cells, normally causes vasodilation; however, with hypertension, it appears that nitric oxide release is inhibited (Victor & Kaplan, 2008). Endothelin-1, a factor produced by endothelial cells, has significant vasoconstrictor properties and appears to contribute to the development of hypertension (Victor & Kaplan, 2008). Another mechanism that is thought to increase the stiffness of the vascular wall with aging is the accumulation of advanced glycation end-products which form abnormal cross-links with vascular wall collagen and increase compliance (Williams, 2008).

Assessment and Diagnosis

The diagnosis of hypertension is based on measurement of blood pressure. Measurements are done on both arms and obtained on at least two different occasions before the diagnosis is made. The issue of blood pressure measurement must also consider self measurement and its accuracy (Williams, 2008). Masked hypertension, defined as elevated blood pressure reading at home but a normal office measurement, has been identified with the advent of self measurement (Williams, 2008). Once hypertension has been identified, the patient is assessed for identifiable causes, possible lifestyle changes, and for the presence of target organ damage. **Target organ damage** refers to dysfunction that occurs in organs affected by high blood pressure. Cardiovascular consequences of hypertension can include LV hypertrophy, angina or myocardial infarction, heart failure, stroke, and peripheral arterial disease. Target organ damage may also include renal dysfunction and retinopathy.

Patient assessment is focused on detection or limitation of target organ involvement. An initial physical examination includes ophthalmoscopic visualization of the optic fundi; auscultation of the carotid, abdominal, and femoral arteries; assessment of lower extremities for pulses and edema; a thorough exam of the heart, lungs, and abdomen (for enlarged kidneys); and a neurologic assessment.

Before initiating therapy, routine laboratory assessment includes an electrocardiogram; urinalysis; and serum evaluations of glucose, hematocrit, potassium, creatinine, calcium, and lipid profiles. Once hypertension has been diagnosed, further testing may be indicated.

Collaborative Management

The ultimate goal of therapy is to lower the systolic blood pressure (SBP). Diastolic blood pressure usually decreases before SBP. Management centers on pharmacologic agents and lifestyle changes. For patients who are overweight or obese, the dietary approaches to stop hypertension (DASH) eating plan is implemented. This plan consists of a diet rich in calcium and potassium, sodium reduction (especially in children), physical activity, and moderation of alcohol consumption. If these interventions do not achieve the target blood pressure, pharmacologic treatment is initiated.

Pharmacologic treatment is evidence-based and includes the use of several classes of drugs previously described in this module, including ACE inhibitors, angiotensin receptor blockers (ARB), beta blockers (BBs), calcium channel blockers (CCBs), and thiazide-type diuretics. Thiazide diuretics are the basis of antihypertensive therapy. These diuretics are used either alone or in combination with another drug for initial therapy. For stage 1 hypertension, thiazide diuretics are most commonly prescribed. For stage 2 hypertension, a two-drug combination is usually needed (a thiazide diuretic and an ACE inhibitor, ARB, BB, or CCB). Direct renin inhibitors are a new class of drugs to treat hypertension. Aliskiren is a potent renin inhibitor and has a long half-life that is favorable for once daily dosing. The recommended daily dose is 300 mg and the only significant side effect is diarrhea (Williams, 2008). There is also some evidence that suggests that statins (lipid lowering drugs) may also decrease blood pressure (Strazzullo, 2007).

Hypertension along with certain comorbidities requires special consideration. In patients with ischemic heart disease, beta blockers and ACE inhibitors are the first drugs of choice. Patients with heart failure also attain good blood pressure control with beta blockers and ACE inhibitors unless they become symptomatic, in which case aldosterone blockers and loop diuretics are recommended. Diabetic hypertension responds better to ACE inhibitors or angiotensin receptor blockers. However, ACE inhibitors should not be used as first line therapy for African-Americans. Chronic kidney disease is treated aggressively and may require three or more types of drugs.

Nursing Management

Nursing diagnoses that may be appropriate for the patient with hypertension include altered peripheral tissue perfusion, excess fluid volume, ineffective health maintenance, and risk for noncompliance.

Nursing management of patients with hypertension starts with accurate blood pressure measurement. The patient should be in a sitting or supine position for five minutes with the arm supported at heart level. An appropriately sized cuff is one that has at least 80 percent of the cuff bladder encircling the arm. Measurements are taken in both arms in an initial screening. In the acute care setting, noninvasive blood pressure machines are commonly used. All the same techniques in obtaining accurate blood pressure measurement are applied when using these machines. All blood pressure equipment is properly calibrated and checked at regular intervals. Patients and family are also instructed on how blood pressure is measured at home.

Patient education is a major component in nursing the management of this patient population and increases compliance with treatment plan. Patients and families need significant training to manage this chronic condition. The nurse assists the patient to develop a medication administration schedule to assist with compliance. It is essential the patient and/or caregivers learn about medications, their actions, and side effects. An example is the importance of understanding drugs that block the sympathetic nervous system (angiotensin receptor blockers, beta blockers). These medications cause orthostatic hypotension. The nurse instructs the patient to slowly rise from a supine position. The family must follow through on instructions like these after the patient has been discharged.

Diuretics cause potassium and magnesium depletion. Patients receiving diuretics have these serum electrolytes monitored on a regular basis. Patients must know how to correctly take their pulse. Dietary restrictions of fluid and salt are part of routine patient education. Exercise programs are introduced using the expertise of other disciplines, such as physical therapy.

SECTION THREE REVIEW

Mr. G. is an 85-year-old man with a medical history of diabetes mellitus, hypertension, and coronary artery disease. He had coronary artery bypass surgery 10 years ago. He is now admitted for increasing fatigue and shortness of breath with minimal exertion. His blood pressure is 160/150 mm Hg. His serum creatinine is 2.3 mg/dL.

The following questions pertain to this scenario.

1. Which of the following risk factors does Mr. G. have for the development of hypertension?
   A. diabetes mellitus
   B. poor renal function
   C. advancing age
   D. all of the above
2. What may be the cause of Mr. G.'s high serum creatinine?
   A. target organ damage
   B. chronic aldosterone secretion
   C. release of endothelin-1
   D. release of nitric oxide
3. Mr. G. needs education about his diet. Which of the following plans would be most beneficial for him?
   A. a diet rich in calcium and potassium
   B. a restricted-sodium-intake diet
   C. a diet rich in vitamin K
   D. A and B
4. To accurately measure Mr. G.'s blood pressure, what cuff size would be appropriate?
   A. any cuff as long as it is an adult cuff
   B. a cuff that has at least 80 percent of the cuff encircling the arm
   C. it would be best to use a noninvasive machine cuff
   D. one that is two thirds the diameter of his arm
5. Patient education for those receiving antihypertensive agents should include information about
   A. orthostatic hypotension
   B. potassium intake
   C. magnesium intake
   D. weight changes

Answers: 1. D, 2. A, 3. D, 4. B, 5. A

POSTTEST

1. The nurse should monitor the patient with aortic valve stenosis for the development of a cardiac dysrhythmia that can cause immediate decompensation. Development of which of the following dysrhythmias would prompt the nurse to call the health care provider?
   A. premature ventricular contractions
   B. premature atrial contractions
   C. atrial fibrillation
   D. sinus bradycardia
2. A patient with infective endocarditis may require antibiotics for
   A. 24 hours
   B. 72 hours
   C. seven to ten days
   D. several weeks

3. Which of the following heart murmurs would be heard between S_1 and S_2? (choose all that apply)
   A. mitral regurgitation
   B. aortic stenosis
   C. mitral stenosis
   D. aortic regurgitation
4. Which of the following nursing diagnoses can apply to the patient with a valve disorder? (choose all that apply)
   A. decreased cardiac output
   B. activity intolerance
   C. fatigue
   D. ineffective protection
5. The nurse notes a patient with mitral valve regurgitation has new orders. The HCP has ordered furosemide and Zaroxolyn. Why would the health care provider order two diuretics for this patient?
   A. The two drugs act on different sections of the nephron.
   B. It is a common mistake and should not be done.
   C. They have different time releases.
   D. They act synergistically.
6. Which of the following are important nursing interventions for patients with heart failure?
   A. monitor weight trends
   B. promote sleep
   C. patient education about drug allergies
   D. patient education about drug side effects
7. Which of the following is the <u>major</u> cause of heart failure?
   A. cardiomyopathy
   B. coronary artery disease
   C. peripheral vascular disease
   D. diabetes
8. Cardiomyopathy can be categorized into what categories? (choose all that apply)
   A. dilated
   B. hypertrophic
   C. constrictive
   D. systolic dysfunction
9. A patient has a BP of 139/85 mm Hg. Which statement is correct about this BP?
   A. This is a normal BP.
   B. This patient has prehypertension.
   C. This patient has stage 1 hypertension.
   D. This patient has stage 2 hypertension.
10. Patient education for patients with on ARBs and BBs should include:
    A. instruction to get up as quickly as possible when rising from supine position
    B. instruction to get up as slowly as possible when rising from supine position
    C. eat foods rich in potassium
    D. do not exercise while taking these medications
11. The ultimate therapeutic goal for the treatment of hypertension is
    A. the ability to exercise without shortness of breath
    B. to lower SBP
    C. to lower DBP
    D. all of the above
12. A 30-year-old patient has a BP of 140/90 mm Hg. What factors could contribute to a person this age to have this BP? (choose all that apply)
    A. This is a normal BP for this age group.
    B. He may be obese.
    C. He may smoke.
    D. He may have obstructive sleep apnea.

Posttest answers with rationale are found on MyNursingKit.

PEARSON
EXPLORE mynursingkit™

MyNursingKit is your one stop for online chapter review materials and resources. Prepare for success with additional NCLEX®-style practice questions, interactive assignments and activities, web links, animations and videos, and more!

Register your access code from the front of your book at **www.mynursingkit.com.**

REFERENCES

Brunton, L., Lazo, J. & Parker, K. (2006). *Goodman and Gillman's the pharmacological basis of therapeutics* (11th ed.). New York: McGraw-Hill Medical Publishing Division.

Chobanian, A. V. (2003). *Seventh report of the Joint National Committee on prevention, detection, evaluation and treatment of high blood pressure.* Washington, DC: National Institutes of Health; National Heart, Lung and Blood Institute.

Cole, K. M., Gawlinski, A., Steers, N., Kotlerman, J. (2007). Animal assisted therapy in patients hospitalized with heart failure. *Am J Crit Care 16*; 575-588.

Francis, G. S., Sonnenblick, E. H. & Wilson Tang, W. H. (2008). Pathophysiology of heart failure. In V. Fuster, R. A. O'Rourke & R. A. Walsh (eds.), *Hurst's the heart* (15th ed.). New York: McGraw-Hill Medical Publishing Division.

Haldar S. M. & O'Gara P. T.(2008). Infective endocarditis. In V. Fuster, R. A. O'Rourke & R. A. Walsh (eds.), *Hurst's the heart* (15th ed.). New York: McGraw-Hill Medical Publishing Division.

Hoe, S., Doering, L. V., Widener, J., Moser, D. K. (2008). Predictors and effect of physical symptom status on health related quality of life in patients with heart failure. *Am J Crit Care 17*; 124-132.

Hunt, S. A., Baker, D. W., Chin, M. H., et al. (2005). ACC/AHA guidelines for the diagnosis and management of chronic heart failure in the adult. *Journal of American College of Cardiology, 46*, 1116-1143.

Kotchen, T. A. (2008). Hypertensive vascular disease. In A. S. Fauci, E. Braunwald, D. L. Kasper et al. (eds.). *Harrison's Principles in Internal Medicine* (17th ed.). New York: McGraw-Hill Medical Publishing

Lauck, S., Mackay M,, Galte, C., et al. (2008). A new option for the treatment of aortic stenosis : Percutaneous aortic valve replacement. *Critical Care Nurse, 28*, 40-51.

Moser, D. K., Riegel, B., Paul, Sara et al. (2009) Heart Failure in Carlson, K. K. (ed.) *Advanced Critical Care Nursing*. St. Louis: Saunders-Elsevier.

Otto, C. M. & Bonow, R. O.. (2008). Valvular heart disease. In P. Libby, R. O. Bonow, D. L. Mann et al. (eds.), *Braunwald's heart disease: a textbook of cardiovascular medicine* (8th ed.). Philadelphia: Saunders-Elsevier

Strazzullo, P., Kerry, S. M., Barbato, A. et al. (2007). Do statins reduce blood pressure? a meta-analysis of randomized, controlled trials. *Hypertension 49*, 792-798.

Stephen, S. A. (2008). Fatigue in older adults with heart failure. *Heart and Lung 37*; 122-131.

Victor, R. G. & Kaplan, N. M. (2008) in P. Libby, R. O. Bonow, D. L. Mann et al. (eds.), *Braunwald's heart disease: a textbook of cardiovascular medicine* (8th ed.). Philadelphia: Saunders-Elsevier

Williams, B. (2008). The year in hypertension. *Journal of the American College of Cardiology 51*, 1803-1817.

MODULE

16 Alterations in Myocardial Tissue Perfusion

Clifford Pyne, Julia King

OBJECTIVES Following completion of this module, the learner will be able to

1. Describe the pathophysiology of atherosclerosis.
2. Identify modifiable and nonmodifiable risk factors for atherosclerosis.
3. List nursing diagnoses appropriate for the patient with risk factors for atherosclerosis.
4. Discuss collaborative interventions to reduce and manage risk factors for atherosclerosis.
5. Describe normal coronary artery anatomy and regulation of coronary perfusion.
6. Identify subjective data associated with coronary artery disease.
7. Differentiate types of angina including stable angina, unstable angina, and variant angina.
8. Discuss the focused physical assessment for a patient who complains of chest pain.
9. Identify electrocardiogram changes associated with myocardial ischemia and myocardial infarction.
10. Identify cardiac markers that, when present in the serum, indicate myocardial muscle damage.
11. Discuss the purpose of three commonly used diagnostic tests available for assessment of myocardial tissue perfusion.
12. Define acute coronary syndromes, unstable angina, and myocardial infarction.
13. List nursing diagnoses appropriate for a patient with an acute coronary syndrome.
14. Discuss initial collaborative management of a patient presenting with chest pain.
15. State the collaborative interventions commonly used to restore myocardial tissue perfusion.
16. Discuss nursing management priorities for patients requiring thrombolytic therapy, percutaneous coronary intervention, and coronary artery bypass surgery.

This self-study module focuses on disease processes that alter myocardial perfusion, signs and symptoms of altered myocardial perfusion, collaborative interventions used in the high-acuity setting to restore myocardial tissue perfusion, and nursing care of patients who require these myocardial tissue reperfusion interventions. The module is composed of seven sections. Section One reviews the pathophysiology of atherosclerosis. Section Two discusses the assessment and management of risk factors for atherosclerosis. Section Three reviews normal coronary tissue perfusion. Section Four presents the signs and symptoms associated with decreased myocardial tissue perfusion. Section Five considers the diagnostic studies used in the evaluation of myocardial tissue perfusion. Section Six presents the acute coronary syndromes. Section Seven reviews collaborative interventions to restore myocardial tissue perfusion, and discusses nursing management priorities for patients who receive myocardial reperfusion therapies. Each section includes a set of review questions to help the learner evaluate his or her understanding of the section's content before moving on to the next section. All Section Reviews include answers. It is suggested that the learner review those concepts answered incorrectly in the review questions before proceeding to the next section.

PRETEST

1. Fatty streaks are
   A. lesions that contain foam cells
   B. flat, thick, yellow lesions that gets progressively bigger
   C. found in children
   D. all of the above

2. The basic lesion associated with atherosclerosis is a(n)
   A. fibrous atheromatous plaque
   B. atheroma
   C. type I lesion
   D. foam cell

3. Which of the following is NOT a modifiable risk factor for atherosclerosis?
   A. hypercholesterolemia
   B. type 2 diabetes
   C. age
   D. hypertension
4. High-density lipoprotein (HDL)
   A. is the major cause of atherosclerosis
   B. contains high-density protein and low amounts of cholesterol
   C. deposits in the intimal lining of arteries
   D. should be less than 100 mg/dL
5. Blood supply to the lateral walls of the left ventricle is from the
   A. left anterior descending artery
   B. left main coronary artery
   C. left circumflex artery
   D. right coronary artery
6. Currents of injury result in
   A. hyperacute *T* waves
   B. *ST* elevation
   C. *T* wave inversion
   D. all of the above
7. A troponin I level is 1.0 mcg/L. This level indicates
   A. significant damage to the left ventricle
   B. a normal level
   C. less than 25 percent cardiac muscle damage
   D. a myocardial infarction has occurred
8. Patients with ischemic *ST* changes and presence of serum cardiac markers are diagnosed as having
   A. unstable angina
   B. stable angina
   C. non-*ST* elevation myocardial infarction (MI)
   D. *ST* elevation
9. Morphine is given for patients with chest pain for all of the following reasons EXCEPT
   A. to increase cardiac output
   B. to cause vasodilation
   C. to decrease myocardial workload
   D. because it has a direct action on pain receptors
10. Postpercutaneous coronary intervention procedures require the patient to remain supine for
    A. 24 hours
    B. 12 hours
    C. 6 hours
    D. 1 hour
11. Which of the following is NOT a sign associated with Beck's triad?
    A. elevated right atrial pressure
    B. hypotension
    C. muffled heart sounds
    D. pulsus paradoxus
12. Blood flow through the coronary arteries is regulated by
    A. the sympathetic nervous system
    B. the parasympathetic nervous system
    C. aortic pressure
    D. calcium
13. Which of the following is the easiest and most cost effective diagnostic test to assist in evaluating the adequacy of myocardial tissue perfusion?
    A. ECG
    B. cardiac markers
    C. exercise stress test
    D. myocardial perfusion imaging
14. Changes in the ______ is the most sensitive electrographic indicator of ischemia and injury to the myocardium.
    A. *PR* interval
    B. *QRS* complex
    C. *ST* segment
    D. *T* wave

Pretest Answers are found on MyNursingKit.

SECTION ONE: Pathophysiology of Atherosclerosis

At the completion of this section, the learner will be able to describe the pathophysiology of atherosclerosis.

Atherosclerosis, commonly referred to as "hardening of the arteries," accounts for a large percentage of deaths as a result of cardiovascular disease (CVD) in the United States and is the primary underlying cause of peripheral artery disease (PAD), coronary artery disease (CAD), and cerebrovascular disease. Atherosclerosis and its associated disorders are pervasive and affect both men and women. Cardiovascular disease is the single largest killer of both men and women in the United States (AHA, 2008).

A normal artery consists of three concentric layers: the innermost layer is the tunica intima, the middle layer is the tunica media, and the outermost layer is the tunica adventitia (Fig. 16–1a).

Atherosclerosis is a chronic inflammatory disorder associated with injury to the intimal lining. It is a progressive disease characterized by formation of plaque in the intimal lining of medium and large arteries, including those in the aorta and its branches, the coronary arteries, and large vessels that supply the brain.

Although the precise mechanisms are unknown, atherosclerosis appears to begin with chronic injury or inflammation to the endothelial cells that line blood vessels. Collectively, all these endothelial cells are called the **endothelium.**

Sources of chronic injury and inflammation may include such things as hypertension, smoking, viruses, and high blood levels of cholesterol and glucose. These factors damage the endothelium causing endothelial cells to separate. This allows monocytes from the bloodstream to enter into the intimal lining and become macrophages. Macrophages release substances that oxidize low-density lipoproteins (LDL) that are toxic to endothelial cells.

This causes further endothelial cell dysfunction. Macrophages engulf LDL and become "foam cells." A group of foam cells becomes the core of a "fatty streak" along the vessel wall (Fig. 16–1a). **Fatty streaks** are flat, thick, yellow lesions that progressively get thicker and bigger, and protrude into the lumen of the artery.

As fatty streaks mature over several decades they begin to develop into another type of atherosclerotic lesion called a **fibrous atheromatous plaque.** This is the basic lesion associated with atherosclerosis. Inside this lesion is an accumulation of lipids, collagen, scar tissue, and vascular smooth muscle cells (Matfin & Porth, 2005) (see Fig. 16–1b). As these lesions grow, they become thicker and more complex. A fibrous cap forms on the top of the lesion. Eventually, they narrow the vessel lumen and reduce blood flow. Reduced blood flow leads to myocardial ischemia, a state where oxygen demand exceeds supply causing chest pain (angina pectoris).

Some of these lesions advance to a more complicated lesion called an **atheroma.** Atheromas are calcified lesions that contain areas of hemorrhage, surface ulcerations, and scar tissue deposits (Matfin & Porth, 2005). Decreased or sluggish blood flow past the lesion can result in the formation of a thrombus on the lesion. The formation of this thrombus is dangerous because not only does it further reduce blood flow but it can occlude the artery or break off to become an embolus.

Histologic Classification of Atheromatous Plaque Progression

Over the last decade new plaque classification systems have been developed. One such classification system divides plaque development into five types of lesions (Fuster, Moreno, Fayad et al., 2005).

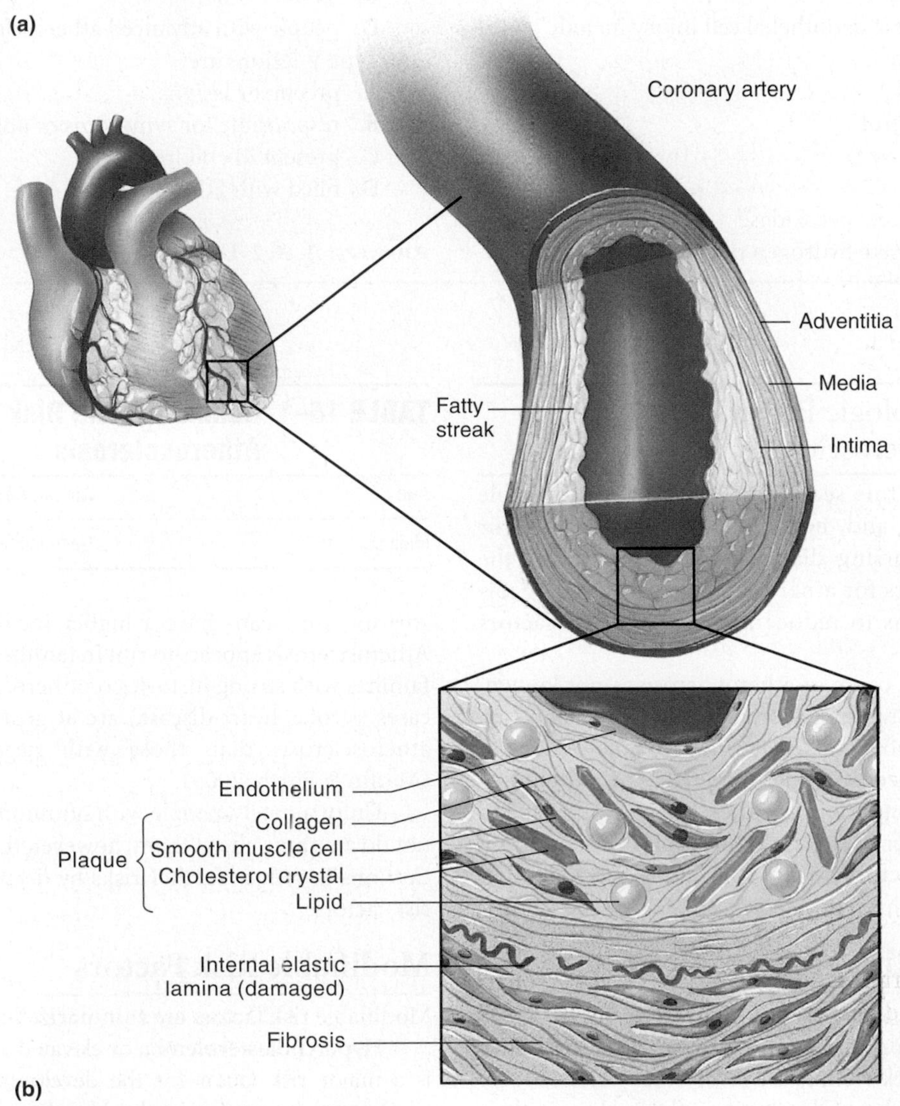

Figure 16–1 ■ The normal artery layers: intima, media, and adventitia. (a) Fatty streaks are lesions in the intimal lining that enlarge and protrude into the lumen of the artery. (b) Plaque consists of cholesterol, phospholipids, collagen and vascular smooth muscle cells.

Type I lesions include lesions that are not visible to the naked eye and precursor lesions that are associated with fatty streaks. Type I lesions, commonly found in children and young adults, tend to be small and nonobstructive and contain lipid droplets, some foam cells, and smooth muscle cells. Type II lesions include more advanced lesions and may be prone to rupture due to the thin nature of their fibrous cap and high lipid content. Types II and III lesions are called precursor lesions. Many of these lesions form during the teenage years. Type III lesions consist of lesions that have eroded, leading to a nonobstructive thrombosis. Type IV lesions consist of complicated lesions with a fixed recurring occlusive thrombosis. These lesions are responsible for the majority of symptoms associated with **acute coronary syndromes (ACS)** (Section Four). Finally, Type V lesions are highly fibrotic and in many cases contain calcium deposits. These lesions are responsible for the majority of angina symptoms and when they rupture, can cause a **myocardial infarction (MI),** the death of cardiac tissue.

SECTION ONE REVIEW

1. Atherosclerosis is a disease associated with injury to
   A. intimal lining of arteries
   B. medial lining of arteries
   C. fibrous atheromatous plaque
   D. macrophages
2. Sources of chronic endothelial cell injury include
   A. hypertension
   B. smoking
   C. high cholesterol
   D. all of the above
3. Foam cells are
   A. cells that secrete peroxidase
   B. cells that secrete hydrogen peroxide
   C. macrophages that have engulfed LDL
   D. endothelial cells with LDL
4. Type I lesions may be present in
   A. children
   B. 20-year-olds
   C. 30-year-olds
   D. people with advanced atherosclerosis
5. Type V lesions are
   A. precursor lesions
   B. responsible for symptoms of angina
   C. present in children
   D. filled with HDL

Answers: 1. A, 2. D, 3. C, 4. A, 5. B

SECTION TWO: Etiologic Factors for Atherosclerosis

At the completion of this section, the learner will be able to identify modifiable and, nonmodifiable risk factors for atherosclerosis, list nursing diagnoses appropriate for the patient with risk factors for atherosclerosis, and discuss collaborative interventions to reduce and manage risk factors for atherosclerosis.

Although the exact cause of atherosclerosis is not known, epidemiologic studies have found certain risk factors that, when present, seem to predispose the development of atherosclerosis. Risk factors are categorized as either modifiable or nonmodifiable. **Modifiable risk factors** include those risk factors that can be altered through either lifestyle modification or medication. **Nonmodifiable risk factors** include those risk factors that, regardless of therapy, cannot be altered.

Nonmodifiable Risk Factors

Nonmodifiable risk factors are summarized in Table 16–1. Increasing age is a nonmodifiable risk factor. More than 50 percent of heart attack victims are 65 or older (AHA, 2008). Men are at a greater risk for developing atherosclerosis than premenopausal women. Estrogen may have some type of protective effect on endothelial cells. After menopause, the risk of atherosclerosis-related diseases increases in women.

TABLE 16–1 Nonmodifiable Risk Factors for Atherosclerosis

Age	African American
Male sex	Genetics

African Americans have a higher incidence of hypertension. Atherosclerosis appears to run in families because persons from families with strong histories of atherosclerotic-associated diseases (stroke, heart disease) are at greater risk for developing atherosclerosis than those with negative family histories (Matfin & Porth, 2005).

Unfortunately, people with nonmodifiable risk factors cannot do anything about them; however, they can take special precautions to reduce further risks by decreasing their modifiable risk factors.

Modifiable Risk Factors

Modifiable risk factors are summarized in Table 16–2.

Hypercholesterolemia, or elevated serum cholesterol levels, is a major risk factor for the development of atherosclerosis. Cholesterol is carried in the bloodstream bound to proteins. When cholesterol is bound to proteins, this combination forms a molecule called a **lipoprotein.** There are different amounts, or densities, of proteins and cholesterol that form lipoprotein

TABLE 16–2 Modifiable Risk Factors for Atherosclerosis

Hypercholesterolemia	Obesity
Elevated LDL levels	Physical inactivity
Type 2 diabetes	Smoking
Metabolic syndrome	Diet
Hypertension	

molecules. Recall from Module 12, Determinants and Assessment of Cardiac Output, when a lipoprotein molecule contains a high amount of cholesterol and low-density protein, it is called a **low-density lipoprotein (LDL).** LDLs, which can be remembered by the mnemonic "less desirable lipoproteins," are commonly referred to as "bad" cholesterol. When a lipoprotein molecule contains a small amount of cholesterol and high-density protein, it is called a **high-density lipoprotein (HDL)**, or "good" cholesterol (to remember this, think of highly desirable lipoproteins). The LDLs accumulate in the intimal lining of arteries and promote formation of atherosclerotic lesions. Recommended levels for serum cholesterol and LDL are listed in Table 16–3.

Other diseases, including type II diabetes, metabolic syndrome, hypertension, and obesity, are additional risk factors for the development of atherosclerosis. Although the exact mechanisms by which these diseases contribute to atherosclerosis is not completely understood, it is theorized that they participate in the chronic injury and inflammation that damages endothelial cells. Hypertension, another modifiable risk factor, is believed to be one of the forces that causes chronic injury to endothelial cells and promotes the development of atherosclerotic lesions. Control of the risk factor diseases with medications and changes in health care behaviors can reduce the risk of developing atherosclerosis and may reduce disease progression (Ridker & Libby, 2008).

Several modifiable risk factors can be altered with lifestyle changes. These include physical inactivity, obesity, smoking, and diet. Components of cigarette smoke cause endothelial damage and vasoconstriction. Obese individuals (body weight greater than 30 percent more than ideal body weight) have higher rates of hypertension, hyperlipidemia, and diabetes. The cardiovascular benefits of exercise are well established. Individuals who engage in regular exercise programs have lower risk of development of cardiovascular diseases related to atherosclerosis.

In addition to the well studied risk factors described above, several novel risk factors for atherosclerosis are beginning to emerge. These risk factors include high-sensitivity **C-reactive protein** (CRP), homocysteine, and fibrinogen. CRP is considered a downstream marker for inflammation and is now considered a major risk factor for cardiovascular disease. CRP levels can be decreased by the use of cholesterol lowering medications (HMG Co-A reductase enzyme inhibitors, commonly referred to as the "statins"). Homocysteine is an amino acid that when elevated, is associated with an elevated risk of premature atherosclerosis. Fibrinogen affects platelet aggregation and has been shown to be a weak predictor of atherosclerosis. As discussed in Module 12, Determinants and Assessment of Cardiac Output, it is now recommended that CRP and, to a lesser extent, homocysteine be included in routine clinical cardiovascular risk screening (Ridker & Libby, 2008).

Collaborative Management of Risk Factor Reduction

Nursing diagnoses may include *imbalanced nutrition: more than body requirements,* and *altered health maintenance.* Aggressive reduction and management of risk factors is crucial to reducing the incidence and progression of atherosclerosis. Identification of risk factors begins with a thorough history. Laboratory testing to assess risk factors may include serum cholesterol and lipid profiles (triglycerides, LDL, HDL levels), fasting glucose, high sensitivity CRP, and homocysteine. Additionally, liver function tests are evaluated so that liver function changes associated with initiation of cholesterol lowering medications can be assessed.

When people stop smoking, the risk of atherosclerotic heart disease is greatly reduced. All people who smoke should be advised to quit. Educational material regarding tobacco cessation programs should be provided. Dietary recommendations to reduce cholesterol and LDL levels are listed in Table 16–4. People who are overweight or obese are encouraged to lose weight through a program that includes diet and exercise. Unless contraindicated, most individuals should participate in at least

TABLE 16–3 Classification of Serum Cholesterol and LDL Values

	TOTAL CHOLESTEROL (mg/dL)	LDL CHOLESTEROL (mg/dL)
Very high		Greater than 190
High	Greater than 240	Greater than 160
Borderline high	200 to 239	130 to 159
Desirable	Under 200	100 to 129
Optimal		Less than 100

As defined by National Cholesterol Education Program (2002).

TABLE 16–4 Dietary Recommendations to Reduce Total Cholesterol and LDL

NUTRIENT	RECOMMENDATION
Total Fat	25 to 35% of total calories
Saturated fat	Less than 7% of total calories
Polysaturated fat	Up to 10% of total calories
Monosaturated fat	Up to 20% of total calories
Cholesterol	Less than 200 mg per day
Carbohydrates	50 to 60% of total calories
Dietary fiber	20 to 30 grams per day
Protein	About 15% of total calories

According to the National Cholesterol Education Program (2002).

30 minutes of moderate-intensity physical activity 5 to 6 days a week.

Control of hypertension is vital to reducing atherosclerosis. Management strategies include a low sodium diet, regular exercise, stress management, and compliance with medication regimens. (Refer to Module 15, Alterations in Cardiac Output, for additional information on hypertension.)

An integral part of reducing atherosclerotic disease progression is drug therapy to reduce serum cholesterol and LDL levels. Drug therapy must be used in combination with a diet that is low in fat and cholesterol. The first-line drugs used are the HMG Co-A enzyme inhibitors, or statins: Lovastatin (Mevacor), Provastatin (Pravachol), Simvastatin (Zocor), Fluvastatin (Lescol), Atorvastatin (Lipitor), and Rosuvastatin (Crestor). These drugs lower LDL by creating more LDL receptors on liver cells. LDL receptors bring in LDL from the blood into liver cells where LDL is further broken down. Other classes of cholesterol reducing drugs include bile acid sequestrants (Cholestyramine [Questran], Colestipol [Colestid], and Colesevelam [Welchol]); fibric acid derivatives (Gemfibrozil [Lopid], Fenofibrate [Tricor], and Clofibrate [Atromid-S]); and Ezetimibe (Zetia), which inhibits absorption of cholesterol at the small intestinal brush border. The RELATED PHARMACOTHERAPY: Antilipidemic Agents box summarizes these agents.

RELATED PHARMACOTHERAPY: Antilipidemic Agents

HMG CO-A Reductase Inhibitors

Lovastatin (Altoprev, Mevacor), Atorvastatin (Lipitor), Provastatin (Pravachol), Simvastatin (Zocor), Fluvastatin (Lescol), Rosuvastatin (Crestor)

Action and Uses

Increases the number of hepatic LDL receptors, thus increasing LDL uptake and catabolism of LDL and increasing HDL blood levels. Used as adjunct to diet to reduce LDL and triglycerides in patients with hypercholesterolemia and to prevent cardiovascular disease in patients with multiple risk factors.

Major Side Effects

Myalgesias
Rhabdomyolysis

Nursing Implications

Lipid levels lower within 2-4 weeks after initiation of therapy or change in dosage.
Assess for muscle pain, tenderness and if present CPK levels may be monitored.
Monitor liver function tests at 6 and 12 weeks after initiation or elevation of dose and periodically thereafter.

Bile Acid Sequestrants

Cholestyramine (Questran), Colestipol (Colestid), and Colesevelam (Welchol)

Action and Uses

Absorbs and combines with intestinal bile acids to form nonabsorbable complex that is excreted in the feces. Lowers LDL levels. Used as adjunct to diet therapy in management of hypercholesterolemia.

Major Side Effects

Constipation, bloating, GI upset

Nursing Implications

Always dissolve powder before administration. Place contents with 120-180 mL preferred liquid. Permit drug to hydrate without stirring 1-2 minutes, then stir until suspension is uniform.
Administer before meals.
Preexisting constipation maybe worsened in the older adult, women, and in those taking greater than 24 gm/day.

Fibrates

Gemfibrozil (Lopid), Fenofibrate (Tricor), and Clofibrate (Atromid-S), Ezetimibe (Zetia)

Action and Uses

Lowers plasma triglycerides by inhibiting their synthesis, reduces VLDL production, increases HDL levels. Used as adjunctive therapy to diet for patients with high triglycerides.

Major Side Effects

Fatigue
Parasthesias
Arrhythmias

Nursing Implications

Assess for muscle pain, tenderness, weakness and if present CPK levels may be monitored.
Monitor patients on type drugs for prolongation of coagulation.

SECTION TWO REVIEW

1. Which of the following is a nonmodifiable risk factor for atherosclerotic disease?
   A. age
   B. smoking
   C. obesity
   D. hypercholesterol

2. A lipoprotein that contains a high amount of cholesterol and a low-density protein is called (a)
   A. high-density lipoprotein
   B. low-density lipoprotein
   C. hypercholesterolemia
   D. lipoprotein A

3. When people stop smoking, the risk of atherosclerotic heart disease
   A. does not change
   B. decreases after 15 years
   C. is greatly reduced
   D. actually is greater
4. Desirable levels of cholesterol are ______ mg/dL and LDL is ______ mg/dL.
   A. greater than 240; greater than 160
   B. 200 to 300; 130 to 159
   C. less than 100; greater than 190
   D. less than 200; 100 to 129
5. Statins work to reduce atherosclerotic disease progression by
   A. increasing LDL receptors on liver cells
   B. increasing HDL concentration
   C. decreasing total body cholesterol
   D. sequestering cholesterol in bile

Answers: 1. A, 2. B, 3. C, 4. D, 5. A

SECTION THREE: Myocardial Tissue Perfusion

At the completion of this section, the learner will be able to describe normal coronary artery anatomy and regulation of coronary perfusion.

Coronary Artery Anatomy

The main coronary arteries lay along the epicardial surface of the heart. There are four primary coronary arteries consisting of the left main coronary artery (LMCA), left anterior descending artery (LAD), left circumflex artery (LCX), and right coronary artery (RCA) (Fig. 16–2). The LAD and the LCX are branches of the LMCA after its bifurcation. The RCA predominantly supplies the right ventricle and atrium and gives rise to the posterior descending artery (PDA). The LAD supplies the anterior aspect of the left ventricle and septum, and the LCX supplies the lateral walls of the left ventricle. As the arteries cross the epicardial surface, small feeder arterioles penetrate the chamber walls giving rise to a dense network of thousands of capillaries per square millimeter called arteriosinusoidal channels. This dense network of capillaries ensures that each myocyte is in contact with a bordering capillary.

There are no connections between the large coronary arteries, but there are collateral channels between the smaller arterioles. Collateral circulation usually develops to compensate for chronic low output heart disease (i.e., heart failure) over a long period of time and is seen in patients with chronic cardiovascular disease. These channels become important when the large arteries occlude, which can cause a myocardial infarction. These collateral channels, if present, can enlarge to provide an alternate route for myocardial tissue perfusion, therefore, decreasing or preventing the myocardial infarction damage.

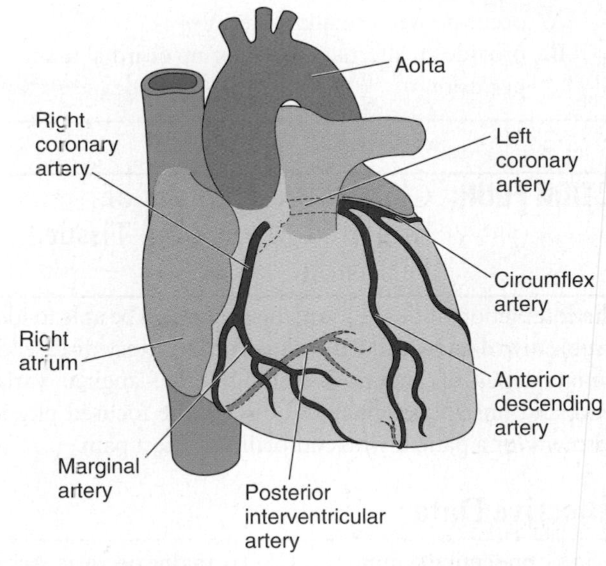

Figure 16–2 ■ Coronary arterial circulation.

Regulation of Coronary Perfusion

Blood flow through the coronary arteries and perfusion of the myocardium is regulated primarily by aortic pressure. The coronary arteries fill with blood after closure of the aortic valve during diastole (resting phase). Coronary blood flow is greatest just after closure of the aortic valve and gradually slows during diastole. One way to evaluate the effectiveness of coronary perfusion is to calculate the coronary perfusion pressure (CPP). The CPP is derived by subtracting the pulmonary artery wedge pressure (PAWP) from the diastolic blood pressure (DBP): (DBP – PAWP). CPP should be maintained above 50 mm Hg to provide adequate blood flow to the myocardium. Autoregulation maintains CPP at a fairly constant level within an aortic pressure range of 40-130 mm Hg. During times of extreme stress this pressure may rise above 140 mm Hg. This is one possible explanation for the increased incidence of plaque rupture during episodes of stress and elevated blood pressure.

SECTION THREE REVIEW

1. There are ______ primary coronary arteries.
   A. two
   B. three
   C. four
   D. five
2. The artery that supplies the right ventricle and right atrium is the
   A. right coronary artery
   B. right descending artery
   C. right circumflex artery
   D. posterior descending artery

(continued)

(continued)

3. Coronary perfusion pressure is calculated as
   - **A.** mean arterial pressure minus right atrial pressure
   - **B.** diastolic blood pressure minus pulmonary artery wedge pressure
   - **C.** mean arterial pressure minus cerebral perfusion pressure
   - **D.** systolic blood pressure minus right atrial pressure
4. Coronary collateral channels
   - **A.** occur between smaller arterioles
   - **B.** provide an alternate route for myocardial tissue perfusion
   - **C.** become important when large arteries occlude
   - **D.** all of the above
5. Mr. T has a blood pressure of 90/50 and a PAWP of 12 mm Hg. What is your interpretation of his CPP?
   - **A.** It is 38 mm Hg and this is an inadequate CPP.
   - **B.** It is 38 mm Hg and this is a normal CPP.
   - **C.** It is 78 mm Hg and this is an inadequate CPP.
   - **D.** It is 50 mm Hg and this is a normal CPP.

Answers: 1. C, 2. A, 3. B, 4. D, 5. A

SECTION FOUR: Clinical Presentation of Impaired Myocardial Tissue Perfusion

At the completion of this section, the reader will be able to identify subjective data associated with coronary artery disease; differentiate types of angina, including stable angina, variant angina, and unstable angina; and discuss the focused physical assessment for a patient who complains of chest pain.

Subjective Data

The classic presenting symptom of CAD is **angina pectoris.** Angina is chest pain that is usually precipitated by exercise and relieved by rest. Angina is caused by an increase in myocardial oxygen demand and a decrease in myocardial oxygen supply as a result of partially occluded coronary arteries. When myocardial cells do not have an adequate oxygen supply for aerobic metabolism, they switch to anaerobic metabolism. The byproduct of anaerobic metabolism is lactate. Lactate, an acid, irritates nerve endings and causes pain.

Patients may describe their angina as tightness, heaviness, or a vise-like sensation in the chest. It may be accompanied by diaphoresis, shortness of breath, and lightheadedness. Patients will often report that the pain radiates to the left arm and hand, jaw, and shoulder. They also may report symptoms of nausea, shortness of breath, or fatigue.

Time is an important variable to consider when assessing a patient complaining of angina symptoms. Temporal questions to consider include the time of onset of the pain, the activity that the patient was participating in when the pain began, and the length of the anginal episodes. Typically, angina begins gradually and peaks over a period of minutes as the precipitating activity continues. Chest pain that lasts several seconds or constant pain over a period of hours is not typical pain associated with altered myocardial tissue perfusion.

Quantifying the level of pain is important because treatment decisions may be based on the initial intensity and the response of the patient to the pain therapy. Patients are asked to describe the pain using a numerical scale of 0 to 10, with 0 indicating no pain and 10 representing pain of maximum intensity.

Symptoms that are suggestive of CAD but do not include angina are called **anginal equivalents.** These symptoms include dyspnea, fatigue, and lightheadedness (dizziness). Patients reporting a history of exertional or resting dyspnea require close scrutiny because these symptoms strongly correlate with CAD.

When assessing a patient presenting with angina symptoms it is helpful to employ the mnemonic PQRST as an assessment tool: precipitating factors (P), quality (Q), radiation and region (R), associated symptoms (S), and timing and treatment strategies (T). This is a systematic way to remember to ask appropriate questions to a patient having chest pain (Table 16–5).

TABLE 16–5 Assessing Chest Pain

PAIN DESCRIPTOR	DESCRIPTION	EXAMPLES
P	Provoked pain Palliative factors	Mowing the lawn, exercise, sexual activity Nitroglycerine, watching TV, or rest/sleep
Q	Quality	Burning, tightness, heaviness, or vise-like sensation in the chest
R	Region of Pain Radiation	Located in center of chest, substernal or left breast Radiates to left arm, hand, jaw, or shoulder
S	Severity Symptoms	Scored from 0-10 Dyspnea, pallor, tachycardia, anxiety, fear, nausea, emesis, diaphoresis, sense of impending doom
T	Time factors	Time of onset, how long does it last, does it come and go? Does it occur in association with something else like eating?

There are three types of angina: stable angina, Prinzmetal's angina, and unstable angina. **Stable angina** is chest pain that is predictable. It occurs with increased physical activity. Often patients know they will get chest pain if they participate in a certain amount of activity. For example, a patient will state, "I get chest pain when I walk three blocks. I know I'm okay at two blocks, but three blocks does it." Stable angina is relieved by rest or nitroglycerin tablets. The typical sequence is activity, chest pain; rest, relief.

Prinzmetal's angina, or **variant angina,** is not common and is a unique form of angina: chest pain that occurs at rest and is not related to physical activity or heart rate. It often occurs at night and may be related to coronary artery spasms. The exact cause of these spasms is not known. **Unstable angina** is chest pain that is not predictable. It occurs with rest or minimal activity and it occurs with increased frequency and severity. Unstable angina requires immediate medical attention.

Not all patients with altered myocardial tissue perfusion have classic anginal chest pain symptoms. Diabetics, women, and elderly patients are more likely to experience anginal equivalents or silent ischemia. Diabetics are especially prone to having silent ischemia and usually present with shortness of air and fatigue. This is due to the microvascular changes associated with diabetes leading to neuropathies and decreased sensitivity to pain. It is important to remember that these changes not only occur in the extremities and eyes (i.e., vision loss), but also the heart. Women are also more likely to experience anginal equivalents. They more often complain of fatigue or upper-arm weakness. Some women with chest pain attribute the pain to heartburn. Older people have a greater incidence of silent ischemia. They often have vague complaints of shortness of air, dizziness, or confusion (Devon et al., 2008)

Objective Data: Physical Assessment

After obtaining the patient's history, a focused physical assessment of the cardiovascular and pulmonary systems is completed. Patients with CAD may or may not exhibit any outward signs of the disease. They may be of normal weight and have normal vital signs. An attempt should be made to correlate subjective data with physical signs.

The vital signs are reviewed for evidence of hypertension and alterations in the heart and respiratory rates. The overall appearance of the patient is noted, taking into account the patient's weight, skin color and tone, posture, and level of functional ability. The skin is examined for evidence of cyanosis and **xanthomas** (cholesterol-filled lesions commonly seen around the eyes). The color and temperature of the extremities are evaluated along with the intensity of the peripheral pulses. Peripheral edema is evaluated and graded according to the severity of pitting identified. Alterations in these findings may indicate peripheral vascular disease (PVD) or left ventricular dysfunction. PVD and left ventricular dysfunction are commonly associated with CAD.

The chest and abdomen are inspected. Heart sounds are auscultated. Any abnormalities in rhythm and rate, any murmurs, rubs, or gallops are reported. Abnormal or additional heart sounds can be associated with left ventricular failure and fluid volume overload caused by an ischemic left ventricle (for more information, see Module 15, Alterations in Cardiac Output). Respirations are assessed for depth and adventitious sounds. The abdomen is auscultated for bowel sounds and the presence of abdominal bruits. The presence of abdominal bruits can be an indication of renal artery stenosis or abdominal aortic aneurysm.

SECTION FOUR REVIEW

1. The classic presenting symptom(s) of CAD is (are)
   A. angina pectoris
   B. chest pain with nausea
   C. elevated lactate with chest pain
   D. nausea, vomiting, heartburn
2. Mr. G. is now unable to walk a block or climb one flight of stairs without getting chest pain. What type of angina pectoris does he have?
   A. stable
   B. variant
   C. unstable
   D. Prinzmetal's
3. Chest pain that is not related to physical activity and often occurs at night is called
   A. unstable angina
   B. Prinzmetal's or variant angina
   C. stable angina
   D. silent myocardial ischemia
4. Xanthomas are
   A. atherosclerotic lesions in the intimal lining of arteries
   B. pockets of cyanosis in nail beds
   C. symptoms of upper arm numbness and weakness
   D. cholesterol filled skin lesions
5. Renal artery stenosis may be evidenced by
   A. abdominal bruits
   B. abdominal distention
   C. decreased urine output
   D. absent bowel sounds

Answers: 1. A, 2. C, 3. B, 4. D, 5. A

SECTION FIVE: Diagnosis of Alterations in Myocardial Tissue Perfusion

At the completion of this section, the reader will be able to identify electrocardiogram changes associated with myocardial ischemia and myocardial infarction; identify cardiac markers that, when present in the serum, indicate myocardial muscle damage; and discuss the purpose of three commonly used diagnostic tests available for assessment of myocardial tissue perfusion.

Electrocardiogram

Several diagnostic tests are available to assist in evaluating the adequacy of myocardial tissue perfusion. The easiest and most cost effective to perform is the 12-lead electrocardiogram (ECG). Thousands of ECGs are performed each year. All patients being evaluated for chest pain have a 12-lead ECG performed to document baseline cardiac rhythm. The ECG aids in the identification of *QRS* or *ST* segment abnormalities indicating ischemia or injury to the myocardium.

The standard ECG includes 12 leads. ECG leads are categorized as limb leads (leads I, II, III), augmented limb leads (aVR, aVL, aVF), and the precordial leads (V_1 through V_6). Each lead overlies a specific area of the myocardium and provides an electrographic snapshot of electrochemical activity taking place at the level of the cell membrane (Pyne, 2004). The basic components of the ECG, as discussed in depth in Module 14, Assessment of Cardiac Rhythm: Basic Electrocardiogram Rhythm Interpretation, are depicted in Figure 16–3.

The *ST* segment represents the early stage of ventricular recovery, and corresponds with the plateau phase of the ventricular action potential. It begins at the end of the *QRS* complex and ends at the beginning of the T wave. As Figure 16–3 also shows, the point where the *S* wave returns to the isoelectric line is described as the J point.

The *T* wave is a graphical representation of ventricular repolarization and should be isoelectric at its conclusion. Changes in the *ST* segment are the most sensitive electrographic indicators of ischemia and injury to the myocardium (Davis, 2005). When blood flow is reduced or occluded to an area of the myocardium, depolarization changes take place. These changes result in a decrease in the resting membrane potential (from a more negative to a less negative value) and a reduction in the action potential. These changes, called "currents of injury," result in *ST* depression, hyperacute *T* waves, *ST* elevation, and *T* wave inversion (Fig. 16–4).

Continuous *ST* segment monitoring provides valuable information for the management of patients at risk for MI, and for those who have experienced MI, undergone revascularization procedures, or require ECG monitoring after noncardiac surgery (Pyne, 2004). Current monitoring technology includes the ability to monitor *ST* segments continuously and by doing so, *ST* segment changes can be identified early and appropriate therapy implemented.

Myocardial regions and their corresponding leads are listed in Table 16–6. The nurse must be familiar with the leads to ensure rapid identification of which area of the myocardium may be ischemic or damaged. This is crucial because treatment options and potential conduction abnormalities differ depending on the myocardial region affected.

Proteins released by necrotic myocytes into the bloodstream are referred to as serum **cardiac markers.** When present in the blood, these markers signify myocardial muscle damage. These markers include the troponins (cTn), creatine phosphokinase (CK), and creatine phosphokinase–myocardial bands (CK-MB). These different markers appear in the blood at

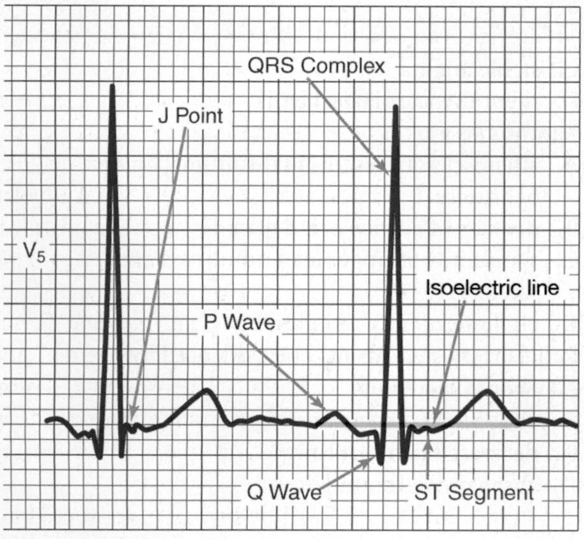

Figure 16–3 ■ Components of a normal ECG.

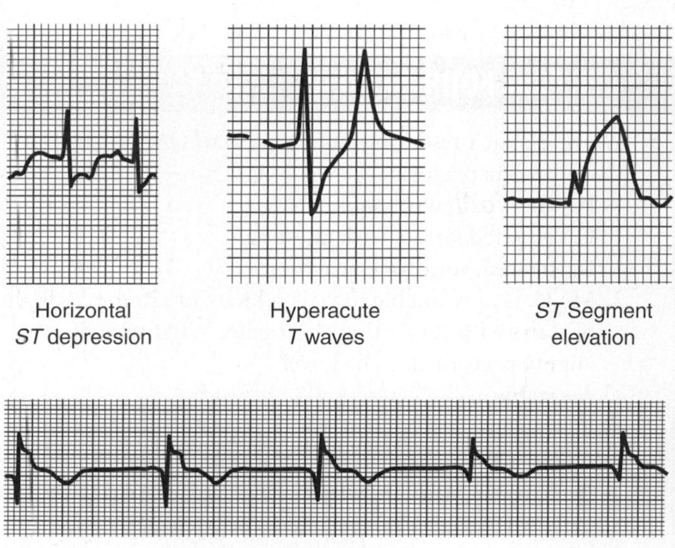

Figure 16–4 ■ ECG ischemia and injury patterns: Horizontal *ST* depression, hyperacute *T* waves, *ST* segment elevation, and *T* wave inversions.

TABLE 16–6 Anatomical Regions of the Myocardium and Their Corresponding Leads

ANATOMICAL REGION	CORONARY ARTERY	ECG LEADS	CLINICAL IMPLICATIONS
Anteroseptal wall	LAD	V_1, V_2, V_3, V_4	Potential for significant muscle damage leading to pump failure and shock. Septal necrosis can lead to prolonged *PR* interval and heart block.
Left lateral wall	LCX	I, aVL, V_5, V_6	Some muscle damage and possible arrhythmias secondary to sinoatrial (SA) nodal dysfunction.
Inferior wall	RCA, LCX	II, III, aVF	Inferior wall infarctions result from occlusion of the RCA in about 80% of the cases and LCX in 20% of the cases. *ST* elevation greater in lead III than II suggests RCA, whereas *ST* elevation greater in lead II than III suggests LCX occlusion.
Right ventricular infarction	RCA	V_{4R}, *ST* elevation in V_1, II, III, aVF	Requires increased preload. Use of nitrates may be contraindicated.
Posterior wall	RCA	Tall *R* wave and *ST* depression in right precordial leads V_1 and V_2. V_7 to V_9 *ST* elevation.	

Adapted from Morton, P. G. (1996). Using the 12-lead ECG to detect ischemia, injury, and infarction. *Critical Care Nurse,* 16(2), 85–95.

different times, and often the higher the marker, the worse the amount of necrotic cardiac muscle damage. Cardiac markers are summarized in Table 16–7.

CK is an enzyme found in the brain, skeletal muscle, and cardiac muscle. Therefore, it is not specific to heart muscle damage when it is present in the blood. The CK-MB is a subset of CK that is specific to cardiac muscle. A level greater than 5 percent is usually considered a positive indicator of cardiac muscle damage. The cardiac muscle troponins, troponin-I (cTnI) and troponin-T (cTnT), are the most specific indicators of cardiac muscle damage. Troponins are proteins that are part of the actin–myocin unit. They are not normally in the blood, unless there is damage to the actin–myocin units of cardiac muscle. Even if there is a small amount of cardiac muscle damage, they appear in the blood.

For most patients who complain of chest pain, cardiac markers are obtained on admission (or when the patient complains of chest pain if already admitted to the hospital). Cardiac markers are redrawn approximately every six hours to evaluate for trends in elevation or decline that signals continued or resolving myocardial damage. Serial levels help determine the extent of myocardial damage.

TABLE 16–7 Cardiac Markers

MARKER	NORMAL LEVEL	ONSET	PEAKS	DURATION
CK	Male: 12 to 80 U/L Female: 10 to 70 U/L	3 to 6 hours	12 to 24 hours	24 to 48 hours
CK-MB	0 to 3%	4 to 8 hours	18 to 24 hours	72 hours
cTnT	Less than 0.2 mcg/L	2 to 4 hours	24 to 36 hours	10 to 14 days
cTnI	Less than 3.1 mcg/L	2 to 4 hours	24 to 36 hours	7 to 10 days

CK = creatine phosphokinase; CK-MB = creatine phosphokinase-myocardial bands; cTnT = Troponin-T; cTnI = Troponin-I.

Exercise Stress Test

The exercise stress test (EST) is one of the most commonly used diagnostic tests available for the assessment of a patient suspected of having CAD. ESTs combine the use of exercise (on a treadmill or bicycle) and continuous ECG monitoring to evaluate the patient's likelihood of having altered myocardial tissue perfusion. Patients with CAD may have a normal ECG at rest when myocardial oxygen supply meets myocardial oxygen demand. However, in some patients when myocardial oxygen demand increases (as with exercise), myocardial oxygen supply is not sufficient to meet this increased demand. This imbalance of myocardial oxygen demand and supply produces altered myocardial tissue perfusion and the resultant ECG changes.

Not all patients can exercise. Patients who cannot exercise may include those with arthritis, amputation, severe peripheral vascular disease, or chronic obstructive pulmonary disease. These patients undergo a pharmacologic stress test. An inotropic drug is given, such as dobutamine, to increase myocardial contractility and workload similar to that which would occur with exercise.

Indications of myocardial ischemia during an EST include the development of angina, *ST* segment depression of 1 mm or more, failure to increase systolic blood pressure to 120 mm Hg or more, or a sustained decrease of 10 mm Hg or more with progressive increase in exercise. EST is less specific in young or middle-aged women than in men.

In preparation for the EST, the patient is instructed not to eat, smoke, or drink beverages containing caffeine for several hours prior to the test. Certain drugs, such as beta blockers, may be held for 24 hours prior to the procedure, and patients are instructed to wear comfortable shoes.

Echocardiography is an imaging technique used to assess the functional structures of the heart using ultrasound waves. Ultrasound waves are applied to the chest wall through a transducer and transect the heart at different planes providing pictures of various cardiac structures. The echocardiogram identifies structural abnormalities of valves, the chamber size of the atria and ventricles, great vessels, and heart wall motion. Echocardiography can be done in conjunction with stress testing or performed at the bedside in the high-acuity unit.

During a stress echocardiogram the patient's ECG is monitored for abnormalities and the myocardial walls are evaluated for ischemia-induced motion abnormalities. Myocardial wall motion abnormalities noted may include **hypokinesis** (decrease in movement), **akinesis** (lack of movement), and **dyskinesis** (movement in the opposite direction).

Myocardial Perfusion Imaging

Radionuclide myocardial perfusion imaging (MPI) is performed by injecting an intravenous nucleotide during peak exercise. Pictures are taken of the myocardial walls with a special type of camera. This procedure is very helpful in identifying specific areas of myocardial ischemia and damage. The perfusion images help differentiate between exertional and resting myocardial perfusion abnormalities. Perfusion is reported as being without defect (normal), a fixed defect, or a reversible defect.

SECTION FIVE REVIEW

1. Changes in the ______ are the most sensitive electrographic indicators of ischemia and injury to the myocardium.
   A. *ST* segment
   B. *U* wave
   C. *QRS* complex
   D. *P* wave
2. *T* wave inversion and *ST* segment depression in two or more contiguous leads are hallmarks of
   A. myocardial infarction
   B. myocardial ischemia
   C. conduction defect
   D. good myocardial tissue perfusion
3. A CK-MB level greater than ______ is indicative of cardiac muscle damage.
   A. 2 percent
   B. 5 percent
   C. 10 percent
   D. 15 percent
4. Mr. B. has an echocardiogram that revealed evidence of hypokinesis in the left ventricle. What is your understanding of how his left ventricle is working?
   A. It is working just fine; these are normal findings.
   B. His left ventricle is not moving at all.
   C. His left ventricle is moving in the opposite direction.
   D. There is a decrease in movement in his left ventricle.
5. An exercise stress test may be ordered to
   A. assess the functional structures of the heart
   B. induce the release of cardiac markers in the blood
   C. evaluate the patient's likelihood of having altered myocardial tissue perfusion
   D. identify specific areas of myocardial ischemia and damage

Answers: 1. A, 2. B, 3. B, 4. D, 5. C

SECTION SIX: Impaired Myocardial Tissue Perfusion, Acute Coronary Syndromes

At the completion of this section, the learner will be able to define acute coronary syndromes, unstable angina, and myocardial infarction; list nursing diagnoses appropriate for a patient with an acute coronary syndrome; and discuss initial collaborative management of a patient presenting with chest pain.

Diagnosis of Acute Coronary Syndromes

Coronary heart disease is commonly divided into two types of disorders: chronic ischemic heart disease and the acute coronary syndromes (ACS). Chronic ischemic heart disease includes stable angina and variant angina (Section Four). ACS represents a continuum of the atherosclerotic disease processes described in Section One and include unstable angina and myocardial infarction.

ACS is characterized by an imbalance between myocardial oxygen supply and demand. As blood flow is reduced, the affected myocardium becomes ischemic, leading to symptoms of angina. Thrombi that partially occlude arteries produce symptoms of unstable angina (**UA**). Total occlusion of the artery results in cell necrosis, release of cardiac markers, and MI distal to the occlusion.

Classification of ACS has changed based on a clearer understanding of plaque disruption and thrombus development. Not all patients with symptoms of chest pain are experiencing an acute MI, but many have a nonocclusive thrombus on preexisting plaque (Anderson et al., 2007). Current guidelines establish the following diagnostic criteria:

1. Patients with ECG changes suggestive of ischemia, but without the presence of serum biomarkers, are diagnosed as UA.
2. Patients with ischemic *ST* segment changes and the presence of elevated serum cardiac markers are diagnosed as having non-*ST* elevation myocardial infarction (**NSTEMI**).
3. Patients with *ST* segment elevation and the presence of elevated serum cardiac markers are diagnosed as having *ST* elevation MI (**STEMI**) (Alpert et al., 2000).

T wave inversion and *ST* segment depression in two or more contiguous leads are hallmarks of myocardial ischemia. In patients suspected of having ACS, symmetrical *T* wave inversion of 2 mm (0.2 mv) or greater strongly suggests acute ischemia. *ST* segments that are depressed from the baseline by 0.5 mm (0.05 mV) or greater and are horizontal or down sloping in two contiguous leads are also suggestive of ischemia. Nonspecific *ST* segment changes can complicate the picture of a patient presenting with symptoms suggestive of ACS. Nonspecific changes are usually defined as *T* wave inversion less than 2 mm or *ST* segment variations of less than 0.05 mV (0.5 mm).

ECG criteria indicative of acute MI include hyperacute *T* waves (early), *ST* segment elevation of 1 mm (0.1 mV) or greater in two contiguous leads, and the presence of new or presumably new left bundle branch block.

Patients presenting with symptoms suggestive of ACS require a rapid assessment and ECG. Chest pain that is suggestive of acute MI typically lasts longer than 20 minutes, but less than 12 hours. Patients may describe the pain as crushing or gripping or they may report chest heaviness and a sense of impending doom. UA is defined as having three possible presentations: symptoms of angina at rest (usually prolonged, greater than 20 minutes), new-onset angina with ordinary physical activity (such as walking one or two blocks), and increasing angina that has become more frequent and longer in duration. Some patients (for example, women, the elderly, and diabetics) may not have chest pain but may present with exertional symptoms of jaw, neck, arm, or epigastric pain; fatigue; nausea; or unexplained worsening of exertional dyspnea.

Other diagnostic and prognostic tools have been developed and are in use for risk stratification (Singh, 2007). The Thrombolysis in Myocardial Infarction (TIMI) score is a well validated, easy to use calculation that predicts risk of death and ischemic events for unstable angina and NSTEMI (Antman et al., 2004).

Initial Collaborative Management

Nursing diagnoses that may be pertinent for the patient with ACS are listed in Table 16–8. Nursing care priorities include relieving chest pain and reducing myocardial oxygen demand. (See NURSING CARE: Angina box) Psychosocial support for the patient and family is important at this time because they are faced with potential mortality.

Medical management of ACS varies depending on the initial 12-lead ECG findings, risk stratification, and evidence of elevated serum cardiac markers. In 2007, the American Heart Association and American College of Cardiology updated guidelines for the management of patients with UA and NSTEMI (Anderson et al., 2007). The current guidelines recommend that an initial ECG be obtained within 10 minutes of presentation to the emergency department (or in the high-acuity unit, an ECG is obtained within 10 minutes of the patient complaining of chest pain). This ECG is used to differentiate patients with *ST* elevation (potential candidates for reperfusion) from UA and NSTEMI. Evidence supports that mortality is decreased and myocardium preserved when this critical treatment decision is made within 30 minutes of the patient's presentation.

Initial management of all patients with chest pain includes rapid triage to immediate care and placement in a treatment area

TABLE 16–8 Nursing Diagnoses for the Patient with ACS

Altered tissue perfusion
Decreased cardiac output
Fatigue
Altered comfort: pain (acute)
Fear
Anxiety
Alterations in family or individual coping
Knowledge deficit
Altered health maintenance
Activity intolerance

established to manage such emergencies. After a 12-lead ECG is obtained, acetylsalicylic acid (**ASA** [aspirin]) is administered. Oxygen by nasal cannula is applied and intravenous (**IV**) access is obtained. Administration of ASA has been shown to significantly reduce mortality and non-fatal MI by 50 percent in patients with ACS and begins to decrease platelet aggregation and clot formation by blocking thromboxane A_2 within 10 minutes after oral administration (Van Horn & Maniu, 2007). Supplemental oxygen raises the partial pressure of oxygen in the blood supplying more oxygen to the ischemic myocardium. At the time that IV access is obtained, blood is drawn for serum cardiac markers. Nitroglycerin may be administered sublingually for ongoing chest pain. Intravenous nitroglycerin may be given for the first 24 to 48 hours. Nitroglycerin, a direct vasodilator, decreases ischemic pain by decreasing preload and, subsequently, myocardial oxygen demand. If chest pain is not relieved with nitroglycerin, morphine IV is given. Morphine decreases pain through direct action on pain receptors, decreases anxiety, and causes vasodilation to further decrease myocardial workload. Morphine is administered intravenously in small doses (2 to 4 mg) and repeated every five minutes until chest pain is relieved. Repeated doses of morphine require the nurse to monitor the patient for respiratory depression. Use of a pulse oximeter aids in detection of impaired oxygenation associated with morphine administration.

If the preliminary ECG is normal or nondiagnostic (meaning there are no specific changes), the patient may be monitored in a chest pain unit. Here, serial serum cardiac markers and ECGs are obtained every six hours. The patient is "ruled out" for an MI if subsequent ECGs and serum cardiac markers remain unchanged for 12 to 24 hours. Most patients will undergo some form of noninvasive testing (stress test or noninvasive cardiac imaging) prior to discharge.

In addition to the therapies described here, patients with UA and NSTEMI are admitted to cardiac high-acuity units where they receive continuous ECG monitoring (telemetry). ECG monitoring with continuous *ST* segment monitoring technology is particularly helpful in monitoring these patients.

Early pharmaceutical management should include beta blockers unless contraindicated. Beta blockers are administered to block catecholamine stimulation, decrease myocardial oxygen demand (with goal heart rate of 50-60 bpm), which increases the time of diastole (rest) and allows more time for coronary artery and myocardial perfusion. Beta blockers have been shown to have significant reduction in mortality and morbidity (Van Horn & Maniu, 2007). Commonly used beta blockers include metoprolol and esmolol.

Pharmaceutical management may include an antithrombin regimen including unfractionated heparin (**UH**) or low molecular weight heparin (**LMWH**), glycoprotein (**GP**) IIb/IIIa inhibitors, and, in many cases, thienopyridines (clopidogrel). Heparin exerts its effect by increasing the effect of antithrombin. This results in inactivation of factors IIa, IXa, and Xa of the coagulation cascade. Heparin is given as an initial bolus dose followed by a continuous infusion. Serum activated partial thromboplastin time (**aPTT**) is monitored at 6, 12, and 24 hours until the aPTT is maintained at 2 to 2.5 times the normal reference value. Patients are monitored for evidence of bleeding. Incidence of cerebral bleeding increases with an aPTT greater than 2.5 times normal; therefore, elevated aPTTs are reported to the physician and the heparin dose is appropriately adjusted (Van Horn & Maniu, 2007).

LMWH (enoxaparin) has also demonstrated excellent efficacy when used in conjunction with ASA in patients with UA and NSTEMI. Advantages to the use of LMWH include its subcutaneous administration, safety, and its ability to be administered without aPTT monitoring. Enoxaparin is dosed at 1 mg/kg every 12 hours in patients with UA or NSTEMI for up to eight days.

In addition to ASA, thienopyridines may be administered to patients with ACS. Clopidogrel blocks platelet aggregation and is recommended for patients with UA and NSTEMI.

GP IIb/IIIa inhibitors are selective antagonists of the IIb/IIIa receptor expressed on the surface of activated platelets. Once activated, this receptor binds with fibrinogen resulting in platelet aggregation. GP IIb/IIIa inhibitors are indicated in patients with UA and NSTEMI. Currently available GP IIb/IIIa inhibitors include abciximab (Reopro), tirofiban (Aggrastat), and eptifibatide (Integrelin). GP IIb/IIIa inhibitors are typically administered as a bolus dose followed by an infusion for 18 to 24 hours. Adverse side effects include bleeding and thrombocytopenia. Complete blood counts are monitored at regular intervals and the patients are monitored for signs of bleeding.

NURSING CARE: Angina

Expected Patient Outcomes and Related Interventions

Outcome: Optimize myocardial tissue perfusion

Assess and compare to established norms, patient baselines, and trends

Assess pain and compare to patient's baseline. Assess for nausea, vomiting, anginal equivalents.

Perform focused physical assessment including vital signs, heart sounds, lung sounds, peripheral pulses, skin color and temperature; physical appearance during pain (shortness of air, diaphoresis).

Obtain 12-lead ECG if ordered.

Administer related drug therapy and monitor for therapeutic and nontherapeutic effects

Nitrates (nitroglycerin)

Oxygen

Related Nursing Diagnoses

Ineffective Tissue Perfusion: Cardiac

Acute Pain

SECTION SIX REVIEW

1. Patients with ECG changes suggestive of ischemia, but without the presence of serum biomarkers, are diagnosed as having
   A. unstable angina
   B. non *ST* elevation myocardial infarction
   C. *ST* elevation myocardial infarction
   D. stable angina
2. ECGs indicative of an acute MI include all of the following EXCEPT
   A. hyperacute *T* waves
   B. *ST* segment elevation
   C. presence of new left bundle branch block
   D. loss of *P* waves
3. Current guidelines recommend that an ECG is obtained within ______ of the complaint of chest pain in the high-acuity unit.
   A. 1 minute
   B. 10 minutes
   C. 30 minutes
   D. 1 hour
4. After an initial ECG is obtained, what is the first drug that is usually administered?
   A. oxygen
   B. nitroglycerin
   C. aspirin
   D. morphine
5. A patient is ruled out for MI if
   A. ECG and cardiac markers remain unchanged for 12 to 24 hours
   B. chest pain subsides within 30 minutes
   C. there are no *ST* changes on the ECG
   D. serum cardiac markers return to normal after six hours

Answers: 1. A, 2. D, 3. B, 4. C, 5. A

SECTION SEVEN: Collaborative Interventions to Restore Myocardial Tissue Perfusion

At the completion of this section, the learner will be able to state the collaborative interventions commonly used to restore myocardial tissue perfusion; and discuss nursing management priorities for patients requiring thrombolytic therapy, percutaneous coronary intervention, and coronary artery bypass surgery.

Reperfusion

As noted in Section Six, patients with chest pain, *ST* elevation greater than or equal to 1 mm (1 mv) in two contiguous leads, or new bundle branch blocks in the absence of ECG cofounders are diagnosed with STEMI. Patients with STEMI have a high likelihood that a thrombus is the cause of the infarct. As discussed in Section Six, the initial collaborative management of patients presenting with STEMI includes rapid triage, administration of oxygen, ASA, nitroglycerin, analgesics, beta blockers, and antithrombins (e.g., UH). The goal of these interventions is to promote reperfusion of the affected artery within 30 minutes.

Rapid reperfusion of the affected artery reduces the amount of damage to the myocardium and preserves ventricular function. Maximum damage occurs approximately six hours after the initial occlusion. The amount of damage depends on the artery occluded and the location of the thrombus. Survival and quality of life are significantly improved if the function of the left ventricle is preserved. Left ventricular (**LV**) function is typically gauged by measuring the LV **ejection fraction (EF).** EF is the ratio of blood ejected from the left ventricle with each beat. Normal is greater than 50 percent. EFs between 40 and 50 percent are considered mildly depressed, and LV dysfunction (e.g. heart failure) is defined by an EF of less than 40 percent.

Interventions to restore myocardial tissue perfusion include administration of thrombolytic therapy, percutaneous coronary intervention, and coronary artery bypass surgery.

Thrombolytic Therapy

Thrombolytic therapy includes the use of drugs that break up blood clots. These drugs activate the fibrinolytic system to dissolve the blood clot and restore blood flow to the obstructed artery. This actually changes the course of an MI by reducing the area of infarction, decreasing mortality and the likelihood that the patient will develop Q waves on an ECG, and increasing the likelihood that LV function will be preserved (Knokle, Simon, & Schafer, 2008).

Candidates for thrombolytic therapy include those whose time of onset of symptoms was less than 12 hours. Contraindications are typically categorized as absolute or relative based on the degree of bleeding risk. Table 16–9 summarizes contraindications to thrombolytic therapy. The learner should be aware that the literature is not conclusive regarding contraindications or their classification as absolute or relative. Risks and benefits must be carefully weighed. Where the risks outweigh the benefit of thrombolytic therapy, other reperfusion therapies should be considered.

TABLE 16–9 Contraindications to Thrombolytic Therapy*

Absolute
Active internal bleeding
Cardiovascular: Acute myocardial infarction resulting from dissected aortic aneurysm, severe uncontrolled hypertension
CNS: Aneurysm, AV malformation, neoplasm, or previous hemorrhagic stroke within the past year or CNS surgery or trauma within two months
Known predisposition for bleeding
Previous hypersensitivity response to thrombolytics
Relative
Age: Older than 75
Cardiovascular: High risk for cardiac thrombosis, hypertension, subacute bacterial endocarditis, current oral anticoagulant therapy
Conditions that have been associated with increased risk for bleeding
End-stage diseases
History of stroke (brain attack)
Pregnancy
Recent major surgery, trauma (to include CPR), GI bleed or active ulcer disease
Terminal cancer

CNS=Central nervous system, INR=International normalized ratio, PT=Prothrombin time

*Each thrombolytic agent provides product-specific contraindications information and consensus on absolute and relative contraindications have not been established for thrombolytic agents.

Data from Gahart & Nazareno, 2005.

Nursing responsibilities for the patient receiving thrombolytics include monitoring for evidence of bleeding, hemodynamic instability, reperfusion, and reocclusion. The risk for intracranial hemorrhage (ICH) is relatively low but increases in patients older than 65 years of age, those with low body weight, hypertension, and females. The first 24 hours after fibrinolytic administration holds the highest risk for intracranial hemorrhage. Routine neurologic checks are performed to detect evidence of a change in the level of consciousness. Change in level of consciousness is a very sensitive indicator of increased intracranial pressure secondary to intracranial hemorrhage (refer to Module 20, Determinants and Assessment of Cerebral Tissue Perfusion). IV sites and wounds are monitored closely for evidence of bleeding, and pressure dressings may be required at IV removal sites. Hemodynamic instability may be an indication of hemorrhage or allergic reaction.

Thrombolysis and reperfusion of the affected myocardium is indicated by resolution of *ST* segment elevation, pain resolution, and the occurrence of reperfusion arrhythmias, such as premature ventricular complexes or ventricular tachycardia. Antiarrhythmics, such as amiodarone, are necessary for sustained ventricular arrhythmias that influence hemodynamic stability. Continuous *ST* segment monitoring is useful in this setting to identify evidence of reperfusion. Reocclusion remains a problem with thrombolytics and occurs in 5 to 20 percent of patients. Reocclusion is indicated by reoccurrence of chest pain and *ST* segment elevation. Reocclusion most commonly occurs within the first 24 hours. Intravenous heparin, low molecular weight heparins, and GP IIb/IIIa inhibitor can be administered after thrombolytics or in combination with thrombolytics to minimize the incidence of reocclusion. The dose of thrombolytics should be reduced by 50 percent to reduce the risk of intercranial hemorrhage (Cannon, 2006).

Patients not eligible for revascularization will typically be admitted to a high-acuity cardiac unit for observation and continued medical management. Patients who are not eligible for revascularization include those who are of advanced age and are accompanied by significant comorbidities (e.g., end-stage renal failure, severe chronic obstructive pulmonary disease, advanced cancer, and significant LV dysfunction). In these patients, the risks of the procedure outweigh the potential benefit. Patients admitted to the high-acuity unit may require short-term support with an intraaortic balloon counter pulsation device or inotropic support for cardiogenic shock (Module 18, Alterations in Oxygen Delivery and Consumption: Shock States). Vital signs and fluid balance are closely monitored. Continuous ECG monitoring allows for prompt treatment of dysrhythmias.

Percutaneous Coronary Intervention

Primary **percutaneous coronary intervention (PCI)** is the procedure of choice for patients with STEMI. PCI is especially useful for patients who are elderly, not candidates for thrombolytics, or those who have experienced reocclusion after receiving thrombolytic therapy. Guidelines recommend that hospitals performing PCI as a primary therapy in STEMI use experienced interventional cardiologists and operate within a multidisciplinary institutional infrastructure for support and response to emergencies that include balloon dilation within 90 minutes of diagnosis, documented quality assurance programs with clinical success rates, an emergency bypass surgery rate less than 2 percent, and a risk-adjusted mortality rate less than 7 percent (Smith et al., 2005).

Patients considered for PCI receive all the appropriate therapies used in the management of STEMI with the exception of thrombolytics. Thrombolytics are not necessary in the setting of acute PCI because their intended purpose is to lyse the thrombus. LMWH such as enoxaparin may be administered prior to PCI but it is not yet clear if it affords the same level of anticoagulation benefit as heparin. Clopidogrel may be administered in the catheterization lab once the need for emergent coronary artery bypass surgery is ruled out. PCI is performed in an angiography lab (Fig. 16–5) under the direction of an interventional cardiologist specially trained to perform this procedure.

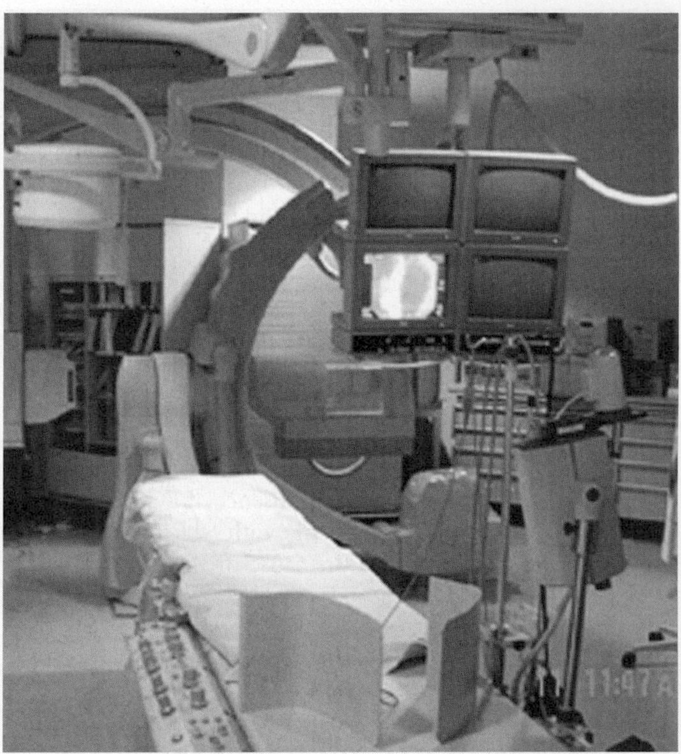

Figure 16–5 ■ Angiography lab.

Preparing the Patient for PCI

Prior to the procedure, nursing responsibilities include continued monitoring of the patient's vital signs, timely medication administration, and patient and family education. Many institutions use standardized heart catheterization videos to instruct on the procedure and answer questions. A witnessed consent should be verified and placed in the chart. Some institutional protocols may include clipping of hair in the patient's groin area. Bilateral groin clippings are recommended in the event that the cardiologist is unable to access the femoral artery from either side. The patient should have nothing to eat or drink after midnight and the time of the patient's last meal is assessed and documented. Renal function is assessed (blood urea nitrogen and serum creatinine). Renal function can be altered by contrast dye used during the procedure. Patients with renal insufficiency may receive N-acetylcysteine (mucomyst) prior to and after the procedure to decrease the renal toxic effects of contrast dye. Patients with IV contrast allergy or allergies to shellfish are premedicated with benadryl and corticosteroids to help prevent allergic reactions to the contrast dye. Diabetic patients who have taken their oral medications may require finger stick glucose checks during the procedure. Diabetic patients should not have oral hypoglycemic agents (such as metformin) or metformin containing products the day before, morning of, or for 48 hours after the procedure as it may cause renal failure in combination with IV contrast used in PCI. Oral anticoagulants (Warfarin) should also be stopped prior to PCI. Patients should void prior to being transported to the catheterization lab and women may require a Foley catheter.

PCI Procedure

The procedure typically involves the insertion of an introducer catheter into the femoral or radial artery. Guiding catheters, similar to those shown in Figure 16–6, are inserted through the introducer and the target vessel is engaged. The coronary anatomy is assessed using fluoroscopy, and the offending thrombus is located. Figure 16–7 shows how a thrombus looks using fluoroscopy.

A key decision at this point is whether the occlusion can be removed and a balloon angioplasty performed safely or whether the patient needs to be transported to the operating room for emergent bypass surgery. Indications for surgery include severe left main coronary artery (LMCA) disease, LMCA equivalent disease, and three or more proximal coronary artery obstructions.

After the decision has been made to proceed with the intervention, the cardiologist crosses the occlusion with a guidewire and removes the thrombus. A thrombectomy device such as the Angiojet™ (Possis Corporation, 2006) may be used to remove the thrombus. The Angiojet™ uses a catheter and high-pressure saline jets to create a vacuum effect that removes the thrombus. The lesion is then predilated with an angioplasty balloon (Fig. 16–8).

Following the angioplasty, a coronary stent (a meshed hollow tube) is placed at the point of the blockage to maintain coronary artery patency. Figure 16-9 illustrates this procedure.

Bare metal stents are commonly used for PCI procedures and have significantly reduced the potential for acute closure and restenosis of the dilated coronary artery. Restenosis rates averaging 30 to 50 percent with plain balloon angioplasty have now been reduced to 5-15 percent with the use of stents (King et al., 2008). Additionally, stents have decreased the need for emergent bypass surgery resulting from failed angioplasty attempts. New metal stents are available with special coatings that help decrease further the likelihood of restenosis. Drug-eluting stents (DES) are coated with a polymer coating containing either the drug paclitaxel (Taxus stent) or sirolimus (Cypher stent). These medications are released slowly over several months suppressing endothelial growth and the likelihood of restenosis. In order to reduce the likelihood of thrombus formation patients who receive DES must remain on Plavix for a minimum of one year after implantation (King et al., 2008).

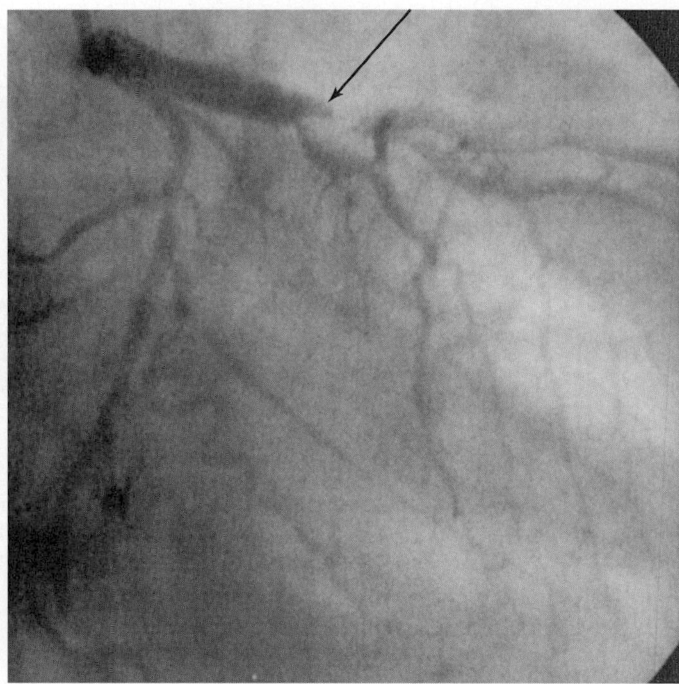

Figure 16–7 ■ Thrombus identified by fluoroscopy during PCI.

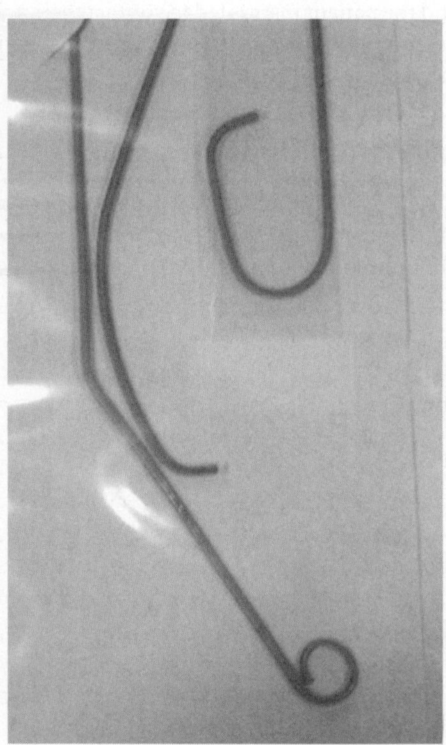

Figure 16–6 ■ Guiding catheters used in coronary angiography.

The catheters, guidewires, and introducer are removed and the patient is prepared for transport to a recovery area. Depending on the location of the insertion site, either direct pressure or closure devices are used to achieve homeostasis at the insertion site. Examples of currently available closure devices include the Angioseal™ and Perclose® devices. The Angio-seal™ device uses an anchoring device and a collagen plug to achieve arterial homeostasis and the Perclose® device uses sutures. Homeostasis of radial artery insertion sites is achieved using direct pressure with a hemoband. The advantage of closure devices is the ability to allow the patient to ambulate within three hours after the procedure (Abbott Laboratories, 2007; St. Jude Medical, 2005).

Care of the Patient Post-PCI

Postprocedure management of the PCI patient includes monitoring frequent vital signs, the ECG, and assessing the access site for pain, swelling or bleeding. Routine blood work typically includes complete blood count, chemistry panel, and coagulation studies. IV infusions may include a GP IIb/IIIa inhibitor and crystalloid solutions. GP IIb/IIIa inhibitors are continued for a minimum of 18 hours post-PCI unless contraindicated. Clopidogrel and ASA may be ordered. IV hydration continues

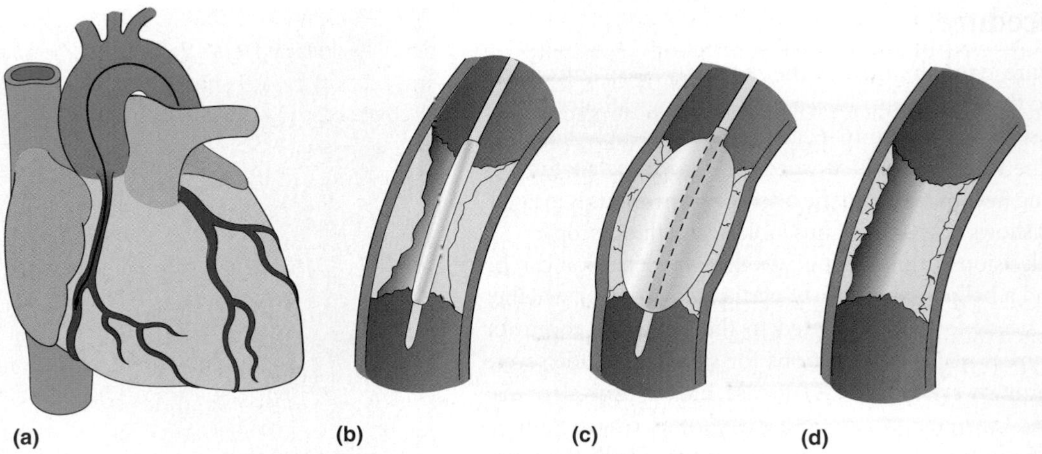

Figure 16–8 ■ Balloon angioplasty. (a) The balloon catheter is threaded into the affected coronary artery. (b) The balloon is positioned directly at the site of the lesion. (c) The balloon is inflated, compressing the lesion against the artery wall. (d) The balloon is deflated and catheter removed, leaving a patent artery.

until just prior to discharge if the patient is to go home the same day. If the patient is admitted to a high-acuity unit, IV hydration may continue for another 10 to 12 hours.

Patients whose access site was sealed using a closure device (i.e., Perclose® or Angio-Seal™) must remain flat for approximately 30 minutes. After this time, the head of the bed may be elevated to 30 degrees followed by ambulation in approximately four hours. Access sites closed with direct pressure require that the patient remain supine for approximately six hours with the affected leg straight. Palpation of pedal pulses and observation of the access site are important nursing assessments that are made frequently after the procedure.

The most common postprocedure complications include chest pain, hypotension, and bleeding at the access site. Chest pain shortly after PCI can indicate acute closure. If the patient complains of chest pain, the nurse obtains vital signs, an ECG, and notifies the cardiologist. Acute closure requires the patient to return to the catheterization lab. Hypotension can be caused by bleeding at the access site, retroperitoneal bleeding, or delayed IV contrast reaction. Patients are instructed to notify the nurse if they feel wetness or warmth around the affected leg, are dizzy or lightheaded, or experience backache. If the patient becomes hypotensive, tachycardic, or experiences an unexplained vagal episode, bleeding may be present and the cardiologist is notified immediately. A computed tomography scan is required if a retroperitoneal bleed is suspected.

Patient and family education is important prior to discharge and will include activity limitations, such as when to shower, drive, lifting, exercise, and taking care of the access site. Also, medication instruction is paramount so that the patient/family understands the importance of taking medications as prescribed. The patient should be given a wallet card with information about the stent they had placed and instructed to keep it with them at all times. Signs and symptoms that are cause for concern should be discussed and the patient instructed to contact their nearest emergency room or licensed care provider if they occur. Contact phone numbers should be provided.

Coronary Artery Bypass Surgery

Coronary artery bypass graft (CABG) has been performed in the United States since the late 1960s. Advances in surgical technique, cardiopulmonary bypass (CPB), conduit selection, and

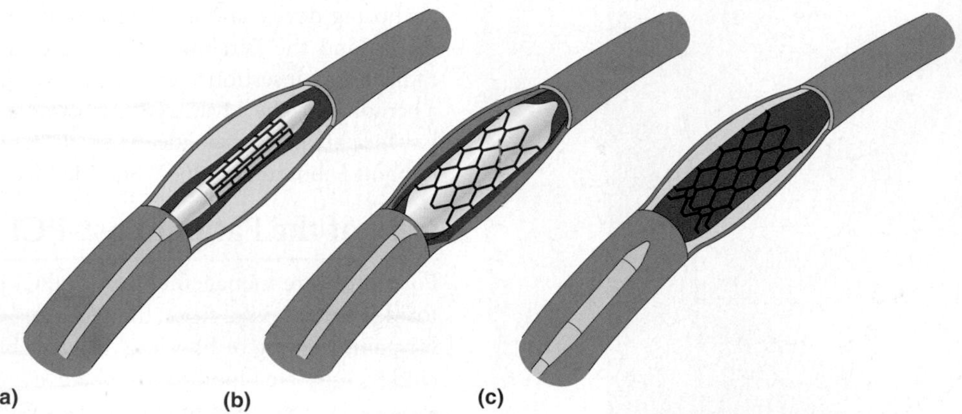

Figure 16–9 ■ Placement of the balloon expandable intraccronary stent. (a) and (b) The balloon catheter with the stent is threaded into the affected coronary artery. The stent is positioned across the blockage and expanded. (c) The balloon is deflated and removed, leaving the stent in place.

cardioplegic solutions have improved their outcomes and made the procedure available to a broader selection of patients. In elective CABG surgery, operative mortality ranges between 1 and 4 percent, depending on patient selection, surgeon experience, and comorbidities. Operative mortality increases with advanced age, an EF less than 30 percent, female sex, diminished renal function, and when done as a result of failed PCI. Emergent CABG mortality rates are very high if cardiogenic shock is present or cardiac arrest occurs.

In the setting of ACS, CABG is performed after angiography has determined the anatomy of the coronary arteries and location of culprit lesions. Indications for CABG include severe left main coronary artery (LMCA) disease, LMCA equivalent disease, and three or more proximal artery obstructions. Additionally, CABG may be performed as a rescue procedure for acute restenosis or rupture of a coronary artery. Additional factors that influence the suitability of a patient for bypass include the size of the native coronary artery, muscle viability, left ventricular function, and extent of disease distal to the stenotic lesion. The primary goal of CABG surgery performed under emergency conditions is prompt restoration of blood flow to the ischemic portion of the myocardium.

CPB is a technique used during surgery whereby blood is directed from the vascular system and circulated through a system of reservoirs and pumps (Fig. 16–10). The system that performs this function is referred to as extracorporeal circulation. Blood that filters through the bypass system undergoes oxygenation, filtration, and cooling, and is returned to the systemic circulation. Moderate hypothermia is achieved by cooling the patient's temperature to approximately 28 to 32°C. This cooling process helps protect target organs and the myocardium from damage.

Monitoring of the bypass machine is under the control of a specially trained technician called a **perfusionist.** The perfusionist monitors the CPB machine and administers heparin and other medications to maintain anticoagulation and hemodynamic stability. CPB is exclusively used for heart surgery. Factors associated with bypass that influence the patient's postoperative course include hypothermia, hemodilution, catecholamine release, hormone release, and platelet damage.

Bypass of the coronary artery lesion is performed under general anesthesia using blood vessels from the right or left internal mammary artery (RIMA, LIMA), saphenous vein grafts (SVG), or a combination of both (Fig. 16–11).

The grafts are harvested from either the anterior chest wall (in the case of IMA grafts) or the saphenous veins of the legs. Many surgeons prefer the use of IMA grafts (depending on lesion location) because of the higher patency rates and increased longevity of the IMA grafts (10 to 15 years). Alternate (but not commonly used) graft conduits include the gastroepiploic artery, inferior gastric artery, and radial artery. Great care is taken during the harvesting of the grafts to prevent injury to the vessel.

CABG surgery is classically performed through a median sternotomy incision. In order to reduce the risk of myocardial ischemia the heart is infused with cold cardioplegia solution, which inhibits membrane depolarization and action potential propagation. This produces a temporary diastolic arrest (stopping the heart) that allows the surgeon to perform the delicate grafting procedure. The distal anastomoses are performed first so that cardioplegia solution may be infused into the vein graft. The proximal aortic anastomoses are performed as rewarming of the patient begins. The aortic cross clamps are removed and

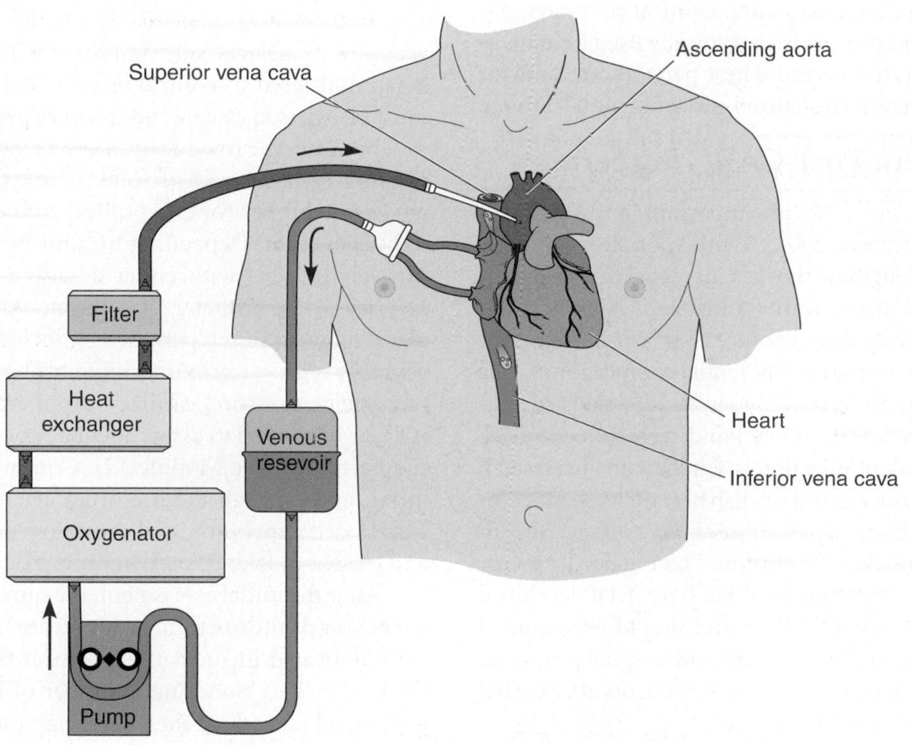

Figure 16–10 ■ A diagrammatic representation of cardiopulmonary bypass.

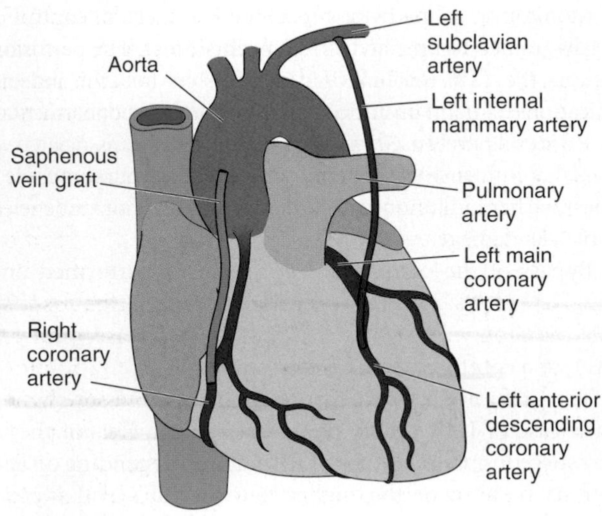

Figure 16–11 ■ Coronary artery bypass grafting using the internal mammary artery and a saphenous vein graft.

the rewarming process is completed. Once rewarming has taken place and the heart begins beating, the anastomoses sites are checked for leaks and final preparations are made for completion of the procedure. Epicardial pacing wires and mediastinal chest tubes are inserted. The sternotomy incision is closed using stainless steel wires after homeostasis is achieved. Usually five or six wire sutures secure the sternum prior to skin closure.

Dedicated surgery teams that include surgeons, anesthesiologists, perfusionists, nurses, and operating room and intensive care unit (ICU) staffs are available at most hospitals that provide bypass surgery. This team approach provides the best outcomes for patients undergoing this procedure. Clinical pathways, patient care guidelines, and protocols are typically used to manage patients in the postoperative period. These patients are cared for by nurses who have received specialized education and training.

Care of the Patient Post-CABG Surgery

Evidence-based nursing outcomes are important in this group of patients (Idemoto & Kresevic, 2007). While mortality from this surgery has decreased, length of stay has increased due to the increased survivability of those with multisystem complications who would have previously died. Because of this, it is important for the nurse to be knowledgeable of potential complications. The patient post CABG is at an increased risk for infections such as ventilator-associated pneumonia (VAP) and central line or incisional infections. The risk of infection is significantly increased if patients have poor glucose control or diabetes. Increased risk for pressure ulcers exsists from decreased mobility; other risks include postoperative delirium or confusion. There are order sets or "bundles" (for example, VAP bundles) that have been developed to prevent some of these complications and should be instituted per Institute for Healthcare Improvement and hospital protocols. Nursing diagnoses that may be pertinent for patients after CABG surgery are listed in Table 16–10.

TABLE 16–10 Nursing Diagnoses for Patients Who Have Had CABG Surgery

Decreased cardiac output
Altered tissue perfusion
Alterations in fluid volume
Altered comfort: pain
Ineffective airway clearance
Potential for infection
Activity intolerance
Sleep pattern disturbances
Knowledge deficit

Management during the immediate postoperative period is aimed at optimizing cardiac output/tissue perfusion and preventing and treating lethal complications. Frequently this period is guided by unit protocols and guidelines. Nursing responsibilities include frequent and ongoing physical assessments of cardiopulmonary status, vital signs, strict intake and output, ECG rhythms and level of consciousness. Ongoing physical assessments also include the gastrointestinal and renal systems.

On arrival in the ICU, a nursing priority is to confirm a patent airway by assessing endotracheal tube placement and auscultating breath sounds. Ventilator settings are usually verified by a respiratory therapist. Ventilation management includes pulmonary hygiene, turning the patient every two hours, and suctioning. If there are no pulmonary complications postoperatively, the patient is extubated within a few hours of surgery.

Postoperative analgesia is usually accomplished with IV propofol or dextromedetomidine HCL. Benzodiazepines may be administered to control anxiety and level of consciousness must be assessed during the recovery period.

Because the mediastinum was opened during surgery, negative intrathoracic pressure is restored through the use of mediastinal tubes (or chest tubes) connected to wall suction or to bulb suction. Depending on unit protocol, patients will return to the ICU with either a central venous line or a pulmonary artery catheter. If a pulmonary artery catheter is in place, hemodynamic parameters, including continuous mixed venous oxygen saturation, right atrial pressure, pulmonary artery wedge pressure, cardiac output (CO), and cardiac index (CI), are obtained to assess adequacy of cardiac output and tissue perfusion (see Module 12). Continuous blood pressure is monitored through the use of an arterial catheter. A tube for gastric decompression and a urinary catheter may be present and output must be closely monitored.

After the initial assessment, the nurse receives a report from a member of the operating room team. Key information that is communicated includes the length of time the patient was on CPB, estimated blood loss, number of bypass grafts that were performed and where these were harvested from, current medications, and blood products received. All medications infusing by IV route are assessed for accuracy.

A 12-lead ECG and chest X-ray are obtained shortly after arrival at the ICU. Initial postoperative laboratory tests are obtained, (complete blood count, coagulation studies, and electrolytes including calcium, magnesium and phosphorus). Vital signs are taken frequently initially to ensure that hemodynamic instability is detected early and treated promptly. Temperature is monitored to ensure the patient's temperature returns to normal.

The nurse must be vigilant in detecting problems in the postoperative period, the most common being hypovolemia from postoperative bleeding, diuresis, and vasodilation (Katz, 2007). During the initial postoperative period, the patient is typically rewarmed to a temperature of 37°C using a warming blanket. Care must be taken to avoid excessive peripheral rewarming, which can lead to vasodilation and cardiac decomposition. Vital signs and central temperature are closely monitored during the rewarming phase to avoid potential complications.

Additional problems that can occur include low cardiac output (CO), hypotension or hypertension, electrolyte imbalances, and postoperative arrhythmias (Katz, 2007). Hypovolemia and vasodilatation lead to inadequate preload and low CO. Diuresis (greater than 2 to 3 liters/hour) can be significant during the initial postoperative period. Patients undergoing bypass surgery typically gain several kilograms of body weight as a result of fluid shifts (third spacing) and neurohormonal activation. Prior to being taken off the bypass pump, the perfusionist may administer a diuretic. Aggressive volume resuscitation is the first step and usually occurs in the first six to eight hours of arrival to ICU (Katz, 2007).

Low CO exists when the cardiac index (CI) is less than 2.0 L/min/m^2. Clinical manifestations of low CO include cool, clammy extremities, tachycardia, decreased urine output: and diminished pulses. Hypovolemia associated with bleeding may result from disruption of an anastomosis site or coagulopathies. Chest tube drainage is monitored frequently for evidence of excessive bleeding that may require reexploration. Chest tube drainage greater than 300 to 500 mL/h for the first hour or greater than 200 to 300 mL/h during the second hour should be reported to the health care provider (Marolda & Finkelmeier, 2000). If coagulation abnormalities are present, they are promptly corrected by administering blood products. There are usually institutional protocols for electrolyte replacement for potassium, calcium and magnesium.

Decreased CO in spite of increased preload may indicate impaired cardiac function. Impaired cardiac function can result from preexisting heart failure, perioperative MI, reperfusion injuries, or cardiac tamponade. Inotropic medications are used to treat impaired ventricular function and when fluid resuscitation fails. Norepinephrine is most commonly used (Katz, 2007). Other vasoactive medications may include vasopressin, dopamine, dobutamine, epinephrine, and milrinone. All should be used with caution as they increase myocardial workload through inotropic properties (increase heart rate) and increased oxygen consumption.

Continuous ECG monitoring is required for postoperative dysrhythmias. Common causes are related to electrolyte disturbances (diuretic use, fluid volume shifts, volume repletion), myocardial ischemia, decreased CO and medications (Katz, 2007). Usually, an external pacer is in place and settings for capture and sensitivity should be verified. Atrial fibrillation is the most common dysrhythmia (Katz, 2007). Ventricular dysrhythmias are treated per ACLS guidelines. Amiodarone has replaced lidocaine as first-line treatment for ventricular dysrhythmias (AHA, 2005).

Cardiac tamponade is a life-threatening postoperative complication. Cardiac tamponade is caused by bleeding into the nonflexible sac around the heart. The accumulating pressure around the heart increases intracardiac pressures, impairs ventricular filling, and decreases CO. **Pulsus paradoxus** is one of the classic signs of cardiac tamponade. This is an exaggerated decrease (greater than 10 mm Hg) of the systolic blood pressure during inspiration. **Beck's triad,** which includes elevated right atrial pressure, hypotension, and muffled heart sounds, may be present. Treatment of cardiac tamponade requires the physician to open the chest incision to drain the blood by a procedure called pericardiocentesis (Module 17, Determinants and Assessments of Oxygen Delivery and Oxygen Consumption). Many ICUs require that wire cutters, chest trays, and staple removers are readily available for this purpose.

Elevated systemic vascular resistance and cardiac dysrhythmias can also exacerbate low CO states. If systemic vascular resistance is elevated, this represents increased afterload for the heart. Vasodilators, such as nitroglycerin and sodium nitroprusside, are used to decrease afterload. Caution must be taken to ensure that adequate preload exists prior to administration of vasodilators to avoid unexpected hypotension.

Within 24 hours of surgery, most patients are extubated. The pulmonary artery catheter, nasogastric tube, and Foley catheter are removed. Patient-controlled analgesia is initiated. The patient receives aggressive pulmonary hygiene, including coughing and deep breathing exercises with incentive spirometry. Patients begin preparation for getting out of bed by dangling their feet over the edge of the bed. Patients may get out of bed to sit in a chair. Diet is advanced as tolerated. At this time, if they are stable, patients are transferred from the ICU to a cardiac high-acuity unit.

Emerging Evidence

- Women with acute coronary syndrome report higher intensity of four symptoms than men. These symptoms include indigestion, palpitations, numbness in the hands, and unusual fatigue (*DeVon, Ryan, Ochs et al., 2008*).
- At initial presentation for coronary angiography, patients report high levels of uncertainty about illness and low levels of perceived control and these markedly reduce health-related quality-of-life outcomes for at least one year (*Eastwood, Doering, Roper et al., 2008*).
- In a survey of 247 nurses from 41 states, 92.1 percent of respondents reported that atrial epicardial pacing wires were left in place after cardiac surgery, 10.2 percent stated they recorded atrial electrograms often, and more than 30 percent had never recorded one. Development of institutional standards, protocols, and education programs are needed for safe and effective use of atrial electrograms (*Miller & Drew, 2007*).
- Cognitive performance improves after coronary artery bypass graft surgery. Patients on average improve in attention/concentration, verbal fluency, and logical/verbal memory. Patients with more education (high school and beyond) performed better in each test (*Dupuis, Kennedy, Lindquist et al., 2006*).

Discharge planning is multidisciplinary and includes health care team members from physical therapy, occupational therapy, and nutritional support. Patient recovery, discharge planning, along with patient and family education continues until the patient is discharged, usually five to seven days after surgery. Cardiac rehabilitation is coordinated for after discharge.

Education is a priority in this phase and has become increasing difficult due to the decreased length of stay after transfer from the ICU. However, psychological support, and individualized patient and family education remains a priority. Videotapes/DVDs show promise in educating about survival skills of coughing and deep breathing, relaxation, and self-care after discharge (Idemoto & Kresevic, 2007). Nurses should use their experience to develop individualized patient goals, based on established protocols, which assist the patient to smoothly transition through the various stages of the postoperative period.

SECTION SEVEN REVIEW

1. The goals of thrombolytic therapy include all of the following EXCEPT
   A. reducing the area of infarction
   B. decreasing the likelihood of developing *Q* waves on ECG
   C. increasing the likelihood that LV function will be preserved
   D. containing the clot in a localized area
2. Which of the following signs may indicate that reocclusion has occurred after thrombolytic therapy?
   A. hypotension
   B. chest pain
   C. *ST* segment depression
   D. change in level of consciousness
3. The advantage of using closure devices post-PCI is that
   A. patients can ambulate within three hours
   B. they are associated with less bleeding
   C. they require less nursing time
   D. they are associated with lower rates of occlusion
4. Which of the following assessments is made frequently after PCI?
   A. PTT levels
   B. *ST* segment measurements
   C. palpation of pedal pulses
   D. Glascow Coma Scale
5. All of the following blood vessels can be used for CABG surgery EXCEPT
   A. left internal mammary artery
   B. right internal mammary artery
   C. saphenous vein
   D. jugular vein
6. Patients who have CABG surgery will require a chest tube
   A. only if the lungs are injured during the operative procedure
   B. to drain blood from the mediastinum
   C. to keep pressure off the heart
   D. for at least a week
7. Which of the following is NOT a sign of cardiac tamponade?
   A. high peak pressures on the ventilator
   B. elevated right atrial pressures
   C. muffled heart sounds
   D. pulsus paradoxus

Answers: 1. D, 2. B, 3. A, 4. C, 5. D, 6. B, 7. A

POSTTEST

1. Atherosclerosis is an inflammatory disorder caused by chronic injury or inflammation to the endothelium. Sources of injury include (choose all that apply)
   A. hypotension
   B. smoking
   C. hypercholesterolemia
   D. hypoglycemia
2. Which of the following lesions are responsible for the majority of angina symptoms and when they rupture can cause MI?
   A. Type II lesions
   B. Type III lesions
   C. Type IV lesions
   D. Type V lesions
3. The nurse is developing a teaching handout for patients with hypercholesterolemia. Which patient has the greatest risk for developing atherosclerosis?
   A. LDL less than 100 mg/dL
   B. LDL 120 mg/dL
   C. total cholesterol 210 mg/dL; LDL 140 mg/dL
   D. total cholesterol 250 mg/dL; LDL 170 mg/dL
4. A patient has atherosclerosis. He is placed on a HMG Co-A Enzyme Inhibitor, atorvastatin (Lipitor). Which outcome indicates to the nurse that the drug is having the desired effect? (choose all that apply)
   A. reduction of LDL levels
   B. reduction of HDL levels
   C. reduction of CRP levels
   D. normal glucose levels
5. A patient has a coronary angiogram and reveals a complete occlusion of the right coronary artery. The nurse understands that the patient is at greatest risk for which of the following problems?
   A. right ventricular MI
   B. MI in the anterior aspect of the left ventricle

C. MI in the lateral wall of the left ventricle
D. development of collateral circulation

6. The nurse is monitoring a patient's coronary perfusion pressures. Which of the following findings should prompt the nurse to contact the health care provider immediately? (choose all that apply)
A. CPP 30 mg Hg
B. CPP 40 mm Hg
C. CPP 60 mm Hg
D. CPP 70 mm Hg

7. How do patients with stable angina usually present in the initial stages of this disease?
A. Chest pain occurs at rest and is not related to physical activity.
B. Chest pain occurs at rest or with minimal activity.
C. Chest pain occurs with activity and is relieved by rest.
D. Chest pain is not relieved with nitroglycerine tablets.

8. A 60-year-old female was just diagnosed with stable angina. Which information is most important for the nurse to provide this patient?
A. Contact your health care provider if you experience tightness in the chest.
B. You may not experience crushing chest pain. Your symptoms may also include fatigue, upper arm weakness, or heartburn. If these occur, contact your health care provider.
C. Contact your health care provider when rest relieves your chest pain.
D. Contact your health care provider when nitroglycerine relieves your chest pain.

9. The patient with an MI is receiving continuous *ST* segment monitoring. The nurse notes a 2 mm *ST* segment depression from baseline. What initial action should the nurse take?
A. Assess the patient and call the licensed care provider.
B. Continue to monitor the patient; this is a normal finding.
C. Administer nitroglycerine as ordered.
D. Adjust the sensitivity of the alarms.

10. A patient with a recent MI asks the nurse why he has to have his blood drawn so many times per day. What explanation is best for the nurse to provide this patient?
A. We are evaluating if you need more oxygen in your blood.
B. I can give you some medication to help with your anxiety.
C. We are evaluating the damage to and recovery of your heart muscle.
D. There must be some mistake. I will call the licensed care provider.

11. A patient with ACS complains of angina at rest (greater than 20 minutes) and increasing angina that has become more frequent and longer in duration. What intervention or action by the nurse is the best response? (choose all that apply)
A. Call the licensed care provider.
B. Perform a rapid physical assessment.
C. Obtain an ECG.
D. Instruct the patient to call the nurse if symptoms persist for the next 20 minutes.

12. The nurse knows that thrombocytopenia is a side effect commonly associated with which of the patient's current medications?
A. ASA
B. heparin
C. Clopidogrel
D. GP IIb/IIIa receptor inhibitors

13. A patient with a MI is admitted to the high-acuity unit. He has an order to initiate thrombolytic therapy. Which of the following statements obtained during the history requires the nurse to contact the health care provider about this order?
A. I have hemophilia A.
B. I have end-stage renal disease.
C. I have peptic ulcer disease.
D. I have hypertension.

14. A patient has just had a PCI. The nurse should intervene if which of the following is assessed? (choose all that apply)
A. chest pain
B. hypotension
C. there is bleeding at the access site
D. the patient complains of dizziness

15. A patient has just been admitted to the ICU after CABG surgery. Which nursing diagnosis has priority in the initial hours after surgery?
A. knowledge deficit
B. sleep pattern disturbances
C. activity intolerance
D. decreased cardiac output

Posttest answers with rationale are found on MyNursingKit.

REFERENCES

Abbott Laboratories. (2007). Perclose AT: suture-mediated Closure system, instructions for use [brochure]. Redwood City, CA: Abbott Vascular Inc., Author.

American Heart Association (2005, November 28). Part 7.2: Management of cardiac arrest. Retrieved January 27, 2008, from http://circ.ahajournals.org/cgi/content/full/112/24_suppl/IV-58.

AHA (American Heart Association). (2008). Heart disease and stroke statistics-2008 update. Dallas: American Heart Association.

Alpert, J. S., Thygesen, K., Antman, E., & Bassand, J. P. (2000). Myocardial infarction redefined—a consensus document of The Joint European Society of Cardiology/American College of Cardiology Committee for the redefinition of myocardial infarction. *Journal of American College of Cardiology, 36*(3), 959–969.

Anderson, J. L., Adams, D. D., Antman, E. M., Bridges, C. R., Calliff, R. M., & Casey, D. E. Jr., et al., (2007). ACC/AHA 2007 guidelines for the management of patients with unstable angina/non-ST-elevation myocardial infarction - executive summary. *Journal of the American College of Cardiology, 50*(7), 652–726.

Antman, E. M., Anbe, D. T., Armstrong, P. W., Bates, E. R., Green, L. A., Hand, M., et al. (2004). ACC/AHA guidelines for the management of patients with ST segment myocardial infarction: a report of the American College of Cardiology/American Heart Association task force on practice guidelines (Committee to revise the 1999 Guidelines for the Management of Patients with Acute Myocardial Infarction). Available at: http://www.acc.org/clinical/guideline/stemi/index.pdf. Accessed January 20, 2008.

Antman, E. M., Cohen, M., Bernink, P. J., McCabe, C. H., Horacek, T., & Papuchis, G. et al. (2000). The TIMI risk score for unstable angina/non-ST elevation MI. *JAMA, 284*(7), 835–842.

Campeau, L. (1976). Grading of angina pectoris. *Circulation, 54,* S22–S23.

Cannon, C. P. (2006). Evolving management of ST-segment elevation myocardial infarction: Update on recent data. *The American Journal of Cardiology, 98*(12A), 10Q–21Q.

Conover, M. B. (2003). *Electrocardiography.* Baltimore, MD: C.V. Mosby.

Davis, D. (2005). *Quick and accurate12-lead ECG interpretation* (4th ed.). Philadelphia: Lippincott Williams & Wilkins.

DeVon, H. A., Ryan, C. J., Ochs, A. L., Shapiro, M. (2008). Symptoms across the continuum of acute coronary syndromes: differences between women and men. *American Journal of Critical Care, 17,* 14–25.

Dupuis, G., Kennedy, E., Linquist, R., Barton, F. B., Terrin, M. L., Hoogwerf, B., et al. (2006). Coronary artery bypass graft surgery and cognitive performance. *American Journal of Critical Care, 15,* 471–479.

Eastwood, J., Doering, L., Roper, J., Hays, R. D. (2008). Uncertainty and health-related quality of life one year after coronary angiography. *American Journal of Critical Care, 17,* 232–245.

Fuster, V., Moreno, P. R., Fayad, Z. A., Corti, R., & Badimon, J. J. (2005). Atherothrombosis and High risk Plaque, Part I: Evolving Concepts. *Journal of the American College of Cardiology, 46*(6),937–954.

Gahart, B. L., & Nazareno, A. R. (2005). *Intravenous medications* (21st ed.) St. Louis: Elsevier/Mosby.

Genentech. Tenecteplase. Accessed April 1, 2005. Available online at: http://www.gene.com/gene/products/information/cardiovascular/tnkase/index.jsp.

Gotto, A. M., & Pownall, H. J. (2003). Atherosclerosis: overview and histologic classification of lesions. In A. M. Gotto & H. J. Pownall (eds.), *Manual of lipid disorders* (pp. 68–79). Philadelphia: Lippincott Williams & Wilkins.

Idemoto, B. K., & Kresevic, D. M. (2007). Emerging nurse-sensitive outcomes and evidence based practice in postoperative cardiac patients. *Critical Care Nursing Clinics of North America, 19,* 371–384.

Katz, E.A. (2007). Pharmacologic management of the postoperative cardiac surgery patient. Critical Care Nursing Clinics of North America, 19, 487-496.

King III, S. B., Smith, S. C., Hirshfeld, J. W., Jacobs, A. K., Morrison, D. A., & Williams, D. O. (2008). 2007 focused update of the ACC/AHA/SCAI 2005 guideline update for percutaneous coronary intervention. *Journal of the American College of Cardiology, 51*(2), 172–209.

Konkle, B. A., Simon, D. & Schafer, A. I. (2008) Hemostasis, thrombosis, fibrinolysis, and cardiovascular disease. In Peter Libby M. D., Robert Bonow M. D., Douglas Mann M. D. & Douglas Zipes M. D. (eds.), *Braunwald's heart disease* (8th ed., pp. 2049-2075).Philadelphia: Saunders Elsevier.

Matfin, G., & Porth, C. M. (2005). Disorders of blood flow in the systemic circulation. In C. M. Porth (ed.), *Pathophysiology: concepts of altered health states* (7th ed., pp. 474–503). Philadelphia: Lippincott Williams & Wilkins.

Miller, J. N. & Drew, B. J. (2007). Atrial electrograms after cardiac surgery: survey of clinical practice. *American Journal of Critical Care, 16,* 350–359.

National Cholesterol Education Program. (2002). Third report of the National Cholesterol Education Progam (NCEP). Expert panel in detection, education, and treatment of high blood cholesterol in adults: final Report. Bethesda, MD: National Institutes of Health.

Possis Cooperation. (2006). Technical manual pertaining to the Angiojet thrombectomy device [brochure]. Available at: http://www.possis.com. Accessed July 3, 2008.

Pyne, C. C. (2004). Classification of acute coronary syndromes using the 12-lead electrocar diogram as a guide. *AACN Clinical Issues, 15,* 558–567.

Punjasawadwong, Y., Boonjeungmonkol, N., & Phongchiewboon, A. (2007). *Bispectral index for improving anesthetic delivery and postoperative recovery.* Retrieved January 27. 2008, from Cochrane Database of Systematic Reviews 2007, Issue 4, Art. no.: CD 003843. DOI: 10.1002/14651858.CD003843.pub2.

Ridker, P. M., & Libby, P. (2008) Risk factors for atherothrombotic disease. In Peter Libby M. D., Robert Bonow M. D., Douglas Mann M. D. & Douglas Zipes M. D. (eds.), *Braunwald's heart disease* (8th ed., pp. 1004-1022).Philadelphia: Saunders Elsevier.

Singh, M. (2007). Risk stratification following acute myocardial infarction. *The Medical Clinics of North America, 91 (4),* 603–616.

Smith, S. C., Jr., Feldman, T. E., Hirshfeld, J. W., Jr., Jacobs, A. D., Kern, M. J., & King, S. B., et al., (2005). ACC/AHA/SCAI 2005 guideline update for percutaneous coronary intervention: a report of the American College of Cardiology/American Heart Association Task Force on Practice Guidelines (ACC/AHA/SCAI Writing Committee to Update the 2001 Guidelines for Percutaneous Coronary Intervention). American Heart Association Web Site. Available at: http://www.americanheart.org. *American College of Cardiology Foundation.*

St.Jude Medical. The angio-seal vascular closure device VIP [brochure]. St. Jude Medical.

The Joint European Society of Cardiology/American College of Cardiology Committee. (2000). Myocardial infarction redefined: a consensus document of the Joint European Society of Cardiology/American College of Cardiology committee for the redefinition of myocardial infarction. *Journal of the American College of Cardiology, 36*(3), 959–969.

Van Horn, S. E., Jr., & Maniu, C. V. (2007). Management of non-ST-segment elevation myocardial infarction. *The Medical Clinics of North America, 91*(4), 683–700.

MODULE

17 Determinants and Assessment of Oxygen Delivery and Oxygen Consumption

Karen L. Johnson

OBJECTIVES Following completion of this module, the learner will be able to

1. Explain the concept of oxygenation.
2. Discuss pulmonary gas exchange.
3. Describe the physiologic components of oxygen delivery.
4. Describe oxygen consumption in terms of aerobic and anaerobic metabolism.
5. Define pathophysiologic conditions that result in impaired oxygenation.
6. Identify techniques to assess oxygenation status in relation to pulmonary gas exchange, oxygen delivery, and oxygen consumption.

This self-study module focuses on the physiologic as well as the pathophysiologic processes involved in oxygenation. The module is composed of six sections. Section One considers the underlying general principles involved in the oxygenation process. Sections Two through Four review the processes of pulmonary gas exchange, oxygen delivery, and oxygen consumption. In Section Five, definitions of clinical conditions that occur as a result of impaired oxygenation are presented. Section Six reviews oxygenation assessment techniques. Each section includes a set of review questions to help the learner evaluate his or her understanding of the section's content before moving on to the next section. All Section Reviews include answers. It is suggested that the learner review those concepts answered incorrectly in the review questions before proceeding to the next section.

PRETEST

1. Oxygenation is
   A. a concept that involves multisystem coordination of the intake, delivery, and use of oxygen for energy
   B. a process that occurs in the lungs
   C. a process that involves the transportation of oxygen to cells
   D. a process that depends on ventilation, diffusion, and perfusion
2. Gas exchange depends on
   A. ventilation and diffusion
   B. ventilation, diffusion, and perfusion
   C. oxygen content in the alveoli
   D. oxygen diffusion across alveolar–capillary membranes
3. Oxygen delivery is affected by
   A. hemoglobin and the oxygen content of arterial blood
   B. cardiac output, autoregulation, and the oxygen content of arterial blood
   C. cardiac output, autoregulation, and autonomic nervous system input
   D. cardiac output, autoregulation, autonomic nervous system input, and oxygen content of arterial blood
4. Ninety-seven percent of oxygen carried to tissues is
   A. dissolved in the plasma
   B. carried as oxyhemoglobin
   C. unavailable for cellular use
   D. delivered to cells by the heart
5. The most effective mechanism of oxygen consumption occurs by
   A. aerobic metabolism
   B. anaerobic metabolism
   C. producing two ATP molecules, lactate and pyruvate
   D. oxygen extraction
6. Completion of a nursing assessment would have what impact on oxygen consumption?
   A. none
   B. increase consumption by 10 percent
   C. increase consumption by 20 percent
   D. increase consumption by 30 percent
7. Impaired oxygenation can result in
   A. hypoxemia and hypoxia
   B. hypoxemia, hypoxia, and dysoxia
   C. hypoxemia, hypoxia, dysoxia, and shock states
   D. hypoxemia, hypoxia, dysoxia, shock states, and multiple organ dysfunction

8. Hypoxemia is defined as
   A. PaO_2 less than 60 mm Hg
   B. $PaCO_2$ greater than 50 mm Hg
   C. inadequate amount of oxygen in arterial blood
   D. hemoglobin less than 10 mg/dL
9. Clinical assessment of oxygenation includes assessment of
   A. arterial blood gases
   B. the cardiovascular and pulmonary systems
   C. pulmonary gas exchange and oxygen delivery
   D. pulmonary gas exchange, oxygen delivery, and oxygen consumption
10. An indirect assessment of oxygen consumption is made using
    A. mixed venous oxygen saturation
    B. arterial blood gases
    C. serum hemoglobin levels
    D. serum adenosine triphosphate levels

Pretest answers are found on MyNursingKit.

SECTION ONE: Oxygenation

At the completion of this section, the learner will be able to explain the concept of oxygenation.

Oxygenation is a concept of multisystem integration and coordination in the intake, delivery, and use of oxygen for energy metabolism. Oxygenation cannot be understood solely by understanding the pulmonary system or the cardiovascular system. Oxygenation involves the integration and coordination of pulmonary, cardiovascular, neurologic, hematologic, and metabolic processes.

Unlike the heart, which has intrinsic rhythmic properties to work independently, the respiratory system requires continuous input from the nervous system. Depending on various internal and external stimuli, the nervous system regulates the respiratory system to meet identified body needs for oxygen. Oxygen is brought into the internal environment via the respiratory system during the process of ventilation. Oxygen crosses alveolar–capillary membranes by diffusion, combines with hemoglobin, and is transported via the pulmonary vein to the left side of the heart. The heart pumps oxygenated blood into the vascular system where it is transported to cells. Oxygenated blood then leaves the capillaries by diffusion and enters cells. Depending on cellular energy requirements, each cell extracts the amount of oxygen it needs to fulfill its metabolic requirements. Cells use oxygen to convert food substrates into energy. Carbon dioxide and "unused" oxygen are carried to the right side of the heart and back to the lungs for elimination and reuse.

The concept of oxygenation involves three physiologic components for the intake, delivery, and use of oxygen for energy: pulmonary gas exchange, oxygen delivery, and oxygen consumption, as summarized in Figure 17–1. Adequacy of oxygenation depends on the integration of these physiologic components. **Pulmonary gas exchange** involves the intake of oxygen from the

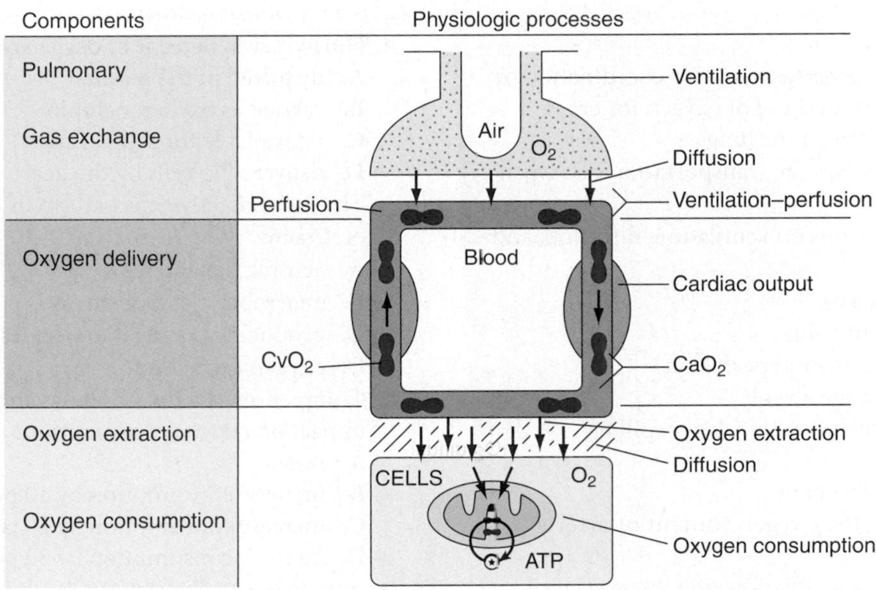

Figure 17–1 ■ Johnson's Conceptual model of oxygenation depicts oxygenation as a process involving the intake, delivery, and use of oxygen for energy metabolism. (Adapted, with permission, from Taylor, C.R., & Weibel, E.R. [1981]. *Design of the mammalian respiratory system, Respiration Physiology, 41* [p. 2]. Copyright © 1981 by Elsevier Science.)

external environment into the internal environment and is carried out by the processes of ventilation, diffusion, and perfusion. **Oxygen delivery** (DO_2) is the process of transportation of oxygen to cells and is dependent on cardiac output (CO), hemoglobin saturation with oxygen, and the partial pressure of oxygen in arterial blood (PaO_2). **Oxygen consumption** (VO_2) involves the use of oxygen at the cellular level to generate energy for cells to use to perform their specific functions. Impaired oxygenation can result from impaired pulmonary gas exchange, decreased oxygen delivery, or impaired oxygen consumption.

SECTION ONE REVIEW

1. Oxygenation is
   A. a process that occurs in the pulmonary system
   B. a process that involves ventilation, diffusion, and perfusion
   C. a process that involves the transportation of oxygen to cells
   D. a concept that specifies that the intake, delivery, and use of oxygen requires multisystem integration and coordination
2. Which of the following are the physiologic processes involved with oxygenation?
   A. pulmonary gas exchange, oxygen delivery, and oxygen consumption
   B. diffusion, ventilation, and perfusion
   C. cardiac output and hemoglobin saturation with oxygen
   D. the pulmonary and cardiovascular systems
3. Pulmonary gas exchange is carried out by which of the following?
   A. inspiration of oxygen by the process of ventilation
   B. expiration of carbon dioxide by the process of diffusion
   C. ventilation, diffusion, and perfusion
   D. ventilation, oxygen consumption, and perfusion
4. Oxygen consumption
   A. depends on cardiac output and hemoglobin saturation with oxygen
   B. involves the use of oxygen to generate energy
   C. involves the intake of oxygen from the external environment
   D. is the process of transporting oxygen to cells

Answers: 1. D, 2. A, 3. C, 4. B

SECTION TWO: Pulmonary Gas Exchange

At the completion of this section, the learner will be able to discuss pulmonary gas exchange. For more detailed information, please refer to Module 9, Determinants and Assessment of Pulmonary Gas Exchange. An understanding of FiO_2, PAO_2, PaO_2, and PvO_2 is necessary to fully comprehend the following section.

The initial component of oxygenation involves pulmonary gas exchange. Pulmonary gas exchange involves the inspiration and delivery of oxygen from the external environment to the alveoli and diffusion across the alveolar–capillary membrane, where oxygen combines with hemoglobin in the pulmonary capillaries. Adequate blood flow must exist to "carry away" the oxygenated blood to the left side of the heart and the systemic circulation. These functions are carried out by physiologic processes involving ventilation, diffusion, and perfusion (Fig. 17–2).

Ventilation is the movement of air to and from the atmosphere and the alveoli. It involves the actual work of breathing

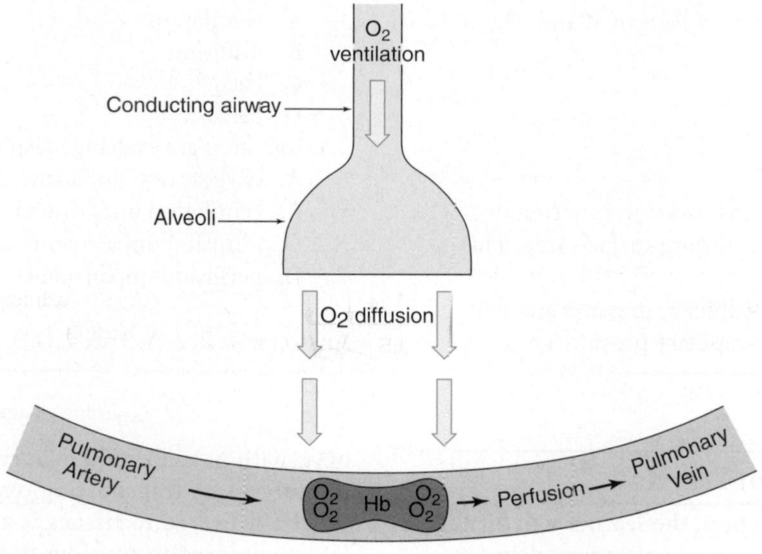

Figure 17–2 ■ Initial process of oxygenation: pulmonary gas exchange.

and requires adequate functioning of the ventilatory muscles, thorax, lungs, conducting airways, and nervous system. Decreased functioning of any one of these systems can affect ventilation and impair oxygenation.

Diffusion is the movement of gas across a pressure gradient from an area of high concentration to one of low concentration. Diffusion is the mechanism by which oxygen moves across the alveoli and into the pulmonary capillary. There are three factors that affect diffusion across the alveolar–capillary membrane: pressure gradient, surface area, and thickness. The greater the difference between alveolar oxygen and pulmonary capillary oxygen pressures, the greater the diffusion of oxygen from the alveoli to the pulmonary capillaries. The greater the available alveolar–capillary membrane surface area, the greater the amount of oxygen that can diffuse across it. Many conditions can cause a significant reduction in functional surface area. The thickness of the alveolar–capillary membrane affects diffusion of oxygen from the alveoli to the pulmonary capillary. Conditions that increase the thickness of the alveolar–capillary membrane can decrease diffusion.

The third component of gas exchange involves perfusion. Three factors affect perfusion: hemoglobin (Hb) concentration, affinity of oxygen to Hb, and blood flow. When oxygen diffuses across the alveolar–capillary membrane, it combines with hemoglobin in the pulmonary capillary and is carried to the left side of the heart. Certain factors affect the affinity of oxygen to hemoglobin, including body temperature; acid–base balance; 2, 3 diphosphoglycerate (2, 3 DPG); and CO_2. (Refer to Module 9, Determinants and Assessment of Pulmonary Gas Exchange, for factors that affect the oxyhemoglobin dissociation curve.) Perfusion of alveoli has an effect on oxygenation. A decrease in blood flow through the pulmonary vasculature results in an imbalance between ventilation and perfusion. Any disease or condition that impairs pulmonary perfusion impairs pulmonary gas exchange. Some conditions and diseases that affect oxygenation as a result of impaired gas exchange are summarized in Table 17–1.

TABLE 17–1 Conditions That Impair Pulmonary Gas Exchange

Ventilation Impairment
Inspiratory muscle weakness or trauma (Guillian-Barré, spinal cord injury)
Decreased level of consciousness
Obstruction or trauma to airways, lung, thorax (flail chest, mucous plug)
Restrictive pulmonary disorders
Diffusion Impairment
Decrease in alveolar–capillary membrane surface area (atelectasis, lung tumors, pneumonia)
Increase in alveolar–capillary membrane thickness (acute respiratory distress syndrome, pulmonary edema, pneumonia)
Decreased pressure gradient for oxygen (↓ FiO_2)
Perfusion Impairment
Decreased Hb (anemia, carbon monoxide poisoning)
Decreased perfusion (↓ cardiac output, hemorrhage, pulmonary embolism)
Pulmonary vasoconstriction (pulmonary hypertension, hypoxemia)

SECTION TWO REVIEW

1. Which of the following conditions has an effect on ventilation?
   A. low hemoglobin levels
   B. upper airway obstruction
   C. pulmonary embolism
   D. hypovolemic shock
2. A PAO_2 of 100 mm Hg and a PaO_2 of 40 mm Hg would
   A. facilitate diffusion
   B. decrease diffusion
   C. decrease ventilation
   D. facilitate perfusion
3. Atelectasis results in a decrease in functional alveolar– capillary membrane surface area. This results in a(n)
   A. increased alveolar–capillary pressure gradient
   B. decreased alveolar–capillary pressure gradient
   C. decrease in oxygen diffusion across alveolar–capillary membranes
   D. increase in oxygen diffusion across alveolar–capillary membranes
4. Anemia affects which component of the gas exchange process?
   A. ventilation
   B. diffusion
   C. PaO_2
   D. perfusion
5. Impaired gas exchange results in
   A. oxygenation impairment
   B. ventilation impairment
   C. diffusion impairment
   D. perfusion impairment

Answers: 1. B, 2. A, 3. C, 4. D, 5. A

SECTION THREE: Oxygen Delivery

At the completion of this section, the learner will be able to describe the physiologic components of oxygen delivery.

As you will recall, the initial component of oxygenation is pulmonary gas exchange. The second component of oxygenation is oxygen delivery. Oxygen delivery involves the process of transporting oxygen to cells. The amount of oxygen delivered to tissues is approximately 1,000 mL/min. (When indexed to consider body surface area, oxygen delivery is approximately 600 mL/min/m^2.) Factors that affect oxygen delivery include cardiac output (CO), autoregulation, oxygen content of arterial blood (CaO_2), and autonomic nervous system innervation.

Cardiac output (CO) is the amount of blood pumped by the heart each minute (see Module 12, Determinants and Assessment of Cardiac Output). The greater the cardiac output, the greater the amount of oxygen delivered to the tissues per minute. Conversely, conditions that cause a decrease in cardiac output result in a decrease in the amount of oxygen delivered to tissues per minute.

Under normal circumstances, the volume of oxygenated blood pumped by the heart is proportional to the body's demands. When tissues require more oxygen, heart rate will increase in an attempt to augment cardiac output in the delivery of more oxygenated blood. Tissues have the ability to regulate their own blood supply by dilating or constricting local blood vessels through the mechanism of **autoregulation.** Tissues have varying energy requirements and use autoregulation to meet their metabolic demands. When the body is at rest, not all tissue capillaries are open at the same time. Increased metabolic rate (e.g., during exercise) and arterial hypoxemia (decreased PaO_2) open more tissue capillaries, thereby allowing more oxygen to be extracted by tissue beds. Autoregulation serves to protect tissues by controlling blood flow and oxygen delivery in response to individual tissue needs.

Oxygen is carried in arterial blood in two forms: It can be combined with hemoglobin or it can be dissolved in the plasma. The content of oxygen in arterial blood (CaO_2) depends on the amount of Hb available to carry oxygen, the amount of oxygen carried in the blood in the "nondissolved" form (PaO_2), and the saturation of hemoglobin with oxygen (SaO_2). Normal CaO_2 is 20 mL/100 mL. Almost 97 percent of all oxygen delivered to cells is in the form of oxyhemoglobin (HbO_2), and the remaining 3 percent is delivered partially dissolved in plasma.

Each molecule of hemoglobin has the ability to carry four oxygen molecules. When hemoglobin is fully saturated with oxygen, oxyhemoglobin is formed. Each hemoglobin molecule can be thought of as a bus that carries four oxygen passengers to tissues. The measurement of SaO_2 by arterial blood gas (ABG) analysis is a measurement of the ratio of oxygenated hemoglobin to total hemoglobin (see Module 9, Determinants and Assessment of Pulmonary Gas Exchange). For example, if the SaO_2 is 95 percent, it can be interpreted that 95 percent of all the available seats on the "hemoglobin bus" are occupied by oxygen. Because the majority of oxygen is carried to tissues by hemoglobin, any condition or disease that decreases hemoglobin content will severely decrease the amount of oxygen carried to tissues.

Many conditions impair oxygen delivery. High-acuity patients are particularly at risk for impaired oxygen delivery as a result of decrease in heart function, such as that occurring with arrythmias or heart failure. An uncompensated decrease in cardiac output, hemoglobin, or SaO_2 can significantly reduce oxygen delivery. Patients who have what may appear to be clinically insignificant decreases in all three factors can have a significant decrease in oxygen delivery when they are considered together.

The autonomic nervous system exerts partial control of oxygen delivery through excitatory or inhibitory effects on the heart, lungs, and blood vessels. Specific cell receptors present in the cardiovascular and respiratory systems, when stimulated, result in a target cell response. The types of cell receptors and their physiologic responses are summarized in Table 17–2.

TABLE 17–2 Alpha, Beta, and Dopaminergic Receptor Stimulation and Physiologic Response

RECEPTOR	LOCATION	RESPONSE
Alpha	Vessels of intestines, kidneys, muscles, skin	Vasoconstriction of arterioles
$Beta_1$	Heart	Increase in heart rate, conduction, and contraction
$Beta_2$	Bronchial and vascular smooth muscles	Bronchodilation Vasoconstriction of arterioles
Dopaminergic	Renal vasculature Mesenteric vasculature	Increased renal blood flow Increased mesenteric blood flow

SECTION THREE REVIEW

1. Oxygen delivery is the
   A. amount of oxygen in arterial blood
   B. process of transporting oxygen to cells
   C. process of utilizing oxygen for energy
   D. amount of blood pumped by the heart per minute
2. Factors that affect oxygen delivery include
   A. ventilation, diffusion, and perfusion
   B. cardiac output, hemoglobin concentration, and ventilation
   C. cardiac output, autoregulation, and oxygen content of arterial blood
   D. cardiac output, autoregulation, oxygen content of arterial blood, and autonomic nervous system innervation
3. A patient who has suffered a myocardial infarction is at risk for impaired oxygenation primarily related to
   A. overactive autoregulation
   B. impaired autonomic nervous system innervation
   C. decreased cardiac output
   D. decreased oxygen content of arterial blood

(continued)

(continued)

4. 97 percent of all oxygen delivered to cells
   - **A.** is in the form of oxyhemoglobin
   - **B.** is dissolved in plasma
   - **C.** is carried as PaO_2
   - **D.** is carried as HCO_3

5. Administration of a drug that stimulates $beta_1$ receptors
   - **A.** decreases blood pressure
   - **B.** increases heart rate
   - **C.** increases renal blood flow
   - **D.** decreases afterload

Answers: 1. B, 2. D, 3. C, 4. A, 5. B

SECTION FOUR: Oxygen Consumption

At the completion of this section, the learner will be able to describe oxygen consumption in terms of aerobic and anaerobic metabolism.

The third component of oxygenation is oxygen consumption. **Oxygen consumption** (VO_2) (Fig. 17–3) is the process by which cells use oxygen to generate energy. Oxygen enables the energy contained in food to be converted into a usable form of energy. Ingested carbohydrates, fats, and proteins are broken down into substrates that are converted in the Krebs cycle into energy in the form of adenosine triphosphate (ATP). This process is called **aerobic metabolism** (Fig. 17–4). The purpose of forming ATP is to create intracellular energy stores. When energy is needed, ATP is broken down and energy is released. Aerobic metabolism results in the creation of 36 molecules of ATP. Cells use ATP molecules as their energy source to perform all their necessary functions. Without the ATP energy stores, cellular processes break down and cells cannot function. The primary value of oxygen is its ability to develop ATP.

As a "backup" mechanism, cells have the ability to generate energy in the absence of oxygen by the process of **anaerobic metabolism** (Fig. 17–5). When anaerobic metabolism is used, carbohydrates are broken down to generate ATP. Carbohydrates are the only food substrates that can be broken down to generate ATP without the use of oxygen. Anaerobic metabolism produces only two ATP molecules and produces the byproducts pyruvate and lactate. When cells use anaerobic metabolism, lactate (an acid) accumulates in the body and results in lactic acidosis. The acidic environment alters cellular structure and greatly impairs cellular function. Anaerobic metabolism is less efficient than aerobic metabolism and results in some potentially harmful byproducts. Table 17–3 compares aerobic and anaerobic metabolism.

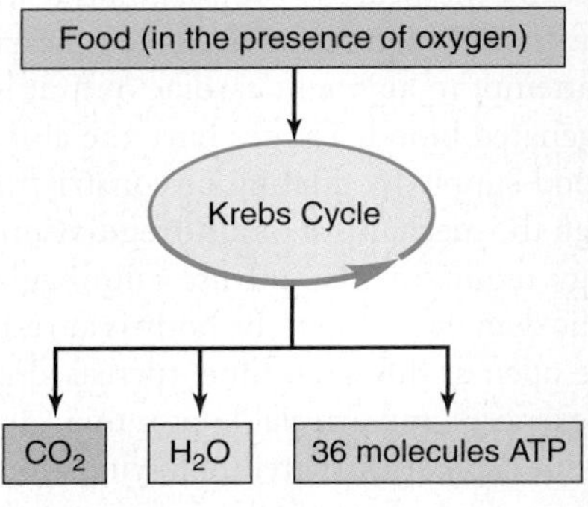

Figure 17–4 ■ Aerobic metabolism.

The process by which cells take oxygen from the blood is called **oxygen extraction.** Normal DO_2 is approximately 1,000 mL/min, and approximately 250 mL of this oxygen is required by tissue metabolic processes (VO_2); therefore, the usual oxygen extraction is 25 percent. Under normal circumstances, oxygen is loosely attached to hemoglobin so that oxygen is readily released from the hemoglobin. The degree to which hemoglobin releases oxygen is called **affinity.** The affinity of oxygen to hemoglobin is determined by the oxyhemoglobin dissociation curve (see Module 9, Determinants and Assessment of Pulmonary Gas Exchange). Release of oxygen from hemoglobin at the cellular level depends on the relationship demonstrated in the oxyhemoglobin dissociation curve. A shift of the curve to the right results in decreased affinity of hemoglobin for oxygen. This decreased affinity increases the release of oxygen and is beneficial for tissue oxygenation. For example, a shift to the right occurs when there is an increase in body temperature. Increased body temperature increases metabolic rate and a greater need for oxygen. A shift to the left increases the capacity of hemoglobin to carry oxygen but decreases unloading of oxygen to tissues. Oxygen dissociates

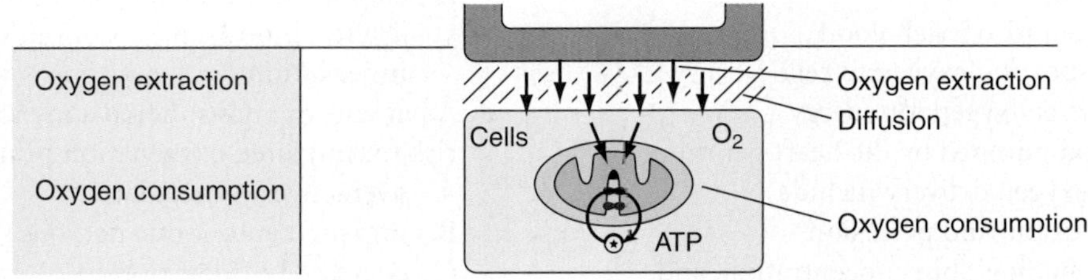

Figure 17–3 ■ Oxygen consumption: Cells extract and use oxygen to generate energy. (Adapted, with permission, from Taylor, C.R., & Weibel, E.R. [1981]. *Design of the mammalian respiratory system, Respiration Physiology, 41* [p. 2]. Copyright © 1981 by Elsevier Science.)

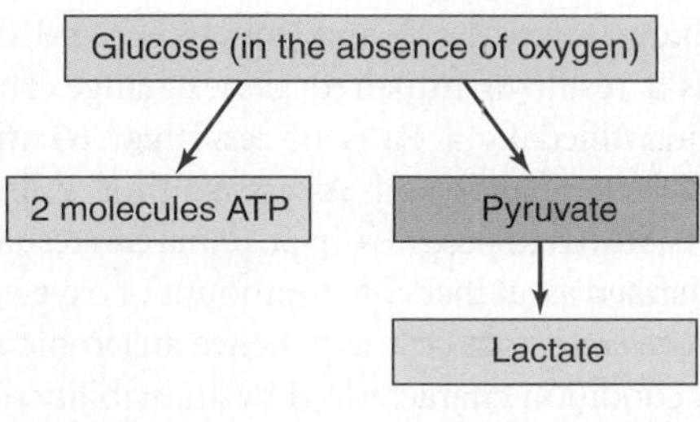

Figure 17–5 ■ Anaerobic metabolism.

from hemoglobin in response to local tissue oxygen demands. When cells have increased energy demands, they extract more oxygen from the blood. For example, during exercise, muscle cells extract more oxygen than they do when at rest.

The amount of oxygen actually used (or "consumed") by cells is normally 250 mL/min. When indexed to body surface area, oxygen consumption is 110 to 130 mL/min/m^2.

Numerous conditions alter the oxygen consumption of high-acuity patients (Table 17–4). Coexisting conditions can have an additive effect on oxygen consumption. For example, a patient with a fever, infection, and increased work of breathing can have oxygen consumption two times the resting oxygen consumption.

Routine nursing care increases oxygen consumption in critically ill patients (Swinamer et al., 1987). Table 17–5 lists some routine activities that increase oxygen consumption.

TABLE 17–3 Aerobic Versus Anaerobic Metabolism

AEROBIC METABOLISM	ANAEROBIC METABOLISM
Generation of energy through the use of oxygen	Generation of energy in the absence of oxygen
Carbohydrates, fats, proteins broken down into substrates	Carboyhydrates broken down into substrates
Produces 36 ATP molecules	Produces 2 ATP molecules, lactate, and pyruvate
Generates large amount of energy	Generates small amount of energy

TABLE 17–4 Conditions That Alter Oxygen Consumption

Increase O_2 consumption	Hyperventilation, hyperthermia, trauma, sepsis, anxiety, stress, hyperthyroidism, increased muscle activity
Decrease O_2 consumption	Hypoventilation, hypothermia, sedation, neuromuscular blocking agents, anesthesia, hypothyroidism, inactivity

TABLE 17–5 Activities That Increase Oxygen Consumption

ACTIVITY	APPROXIMATE INCREASE ABOVE RESTING OXYGEN CONSUMPTION (%)
Nursing assessment	10
Repositioning patient	30
Dressing change	10
Bed bath	20
Weighing patient on sling bed scale	40
Visitors	18
Restlessness/agitation	18

SECTION FOUR REVIEW

1. A continuous supply of oxygen is
   - **A.** not necessary because oxygen is stored in cells
   - **B.** required for adequate ATP synthesis
   - **C.** dependent on the amount of blood ejected from the left ventricle
   - **D.** dependent on adequate supplies of hemoglobin
2. A blood sample for a newly admitted trauma patient reveals a high level of lactate. This is indicative of
   - **A.** adequate oxygen delivery
   - **B.** anaerobic metabolism
   - **C.** adequate oxygen consumption
   - **D.** aerobic metabolism
3. Which of the following conditions increases oxygen consumption?
   - **A.** hypoventilation
   - **B.** sedation
   - **C.** bedrest
   - **D.** temperature of 102°F
4. All of the following statements are true EXCEPT
   - **A.** Aerobic metabolism produces 36 molecules of ATP.
   - **B.** Aerobic metabolism generates a small amount of energy.
   - **C.** Anaerobic metabolism produces 2 ATP molecules.
   - **D.** Anaerobic metabolism generates energy in the absence of oxygen.

Answers: 1. B, 2. B, 3. D, 4. B

SECTION FIVE: Impaired Oxygenation

At the completion of this section, the learner will be able to define pathophysiologic conditions that result in impaired oxygenation.

Sections Two through Four of this module reviewed the three physiologic components of oxygenation: pulmonary gas exchange, oxygen delivery, and oxygen consumption. Any condition or disease that affects one or more of these components will result in impaired oxygenation (e.g., acute respiratory distress syndrome, anemia, hyperventilation). These conditions represent a "continuum" of oxygen disturbances. Life-threatening oxygenation impairments usually involve deficiencies of all three components of oxygenation.

Matching of ventilation to perfusion is essential for gas exchange; otherwise, impaired oxygenation occurs. Conditions such as pulmonary embolus or pneumothorax can produce ventilation–perfusion mismatching. The mismatching of ventilation to perfusion is a common cause of hypoxemia. **Hypoxemia** is a condition characterized by an inadequate amount of oxygen in the blood as a result of impaired gas exchange. Hypoxemia is frequently quantified as a PaO_2 of less than 60 mm Hg (see Module 9, Determinants and Assessment of Pulmonary Gas Exchange). If allowed to progress, hypoxemia can result in hypoxia. **Hypoxia** is defined as an inadequate amount of oxygen available at the cellular level such that cells experience anaerobic metabolism. **Dysoxia** is a condition characterized by an inability of the cells to use oxygen properly despite adequate levels of oxygen delivery.

If left untreated, hypoxemia, hypoxia, or dysoxia can lead to more life-threatening oxygenation impairments, including shock states and multiple organ dysfunction syndrome (MODS). Shock states are characterized by an imbalance of oxygen supply and demand (see Module 18, Alterations in Oxygen Delivery and Oxygen Consumption: Shock States). MODS is characterized by a continuing impairment of oxygenation, mediated by the inflammatory process (refer to Module 19, Alterations in Tissue Perfusion: Multiple Organ Dysfunction Syndrome).

SECTION FIVE REVIEW

1. Hypoxemia is defined as
   A. an inadequate amount of oxygen in the blood
   B. an inadequate amount of oxygen available at the cellular level
   C. $PaCO_2$ of less than 50 mm Hg
   D. an imbalance of oxygen supply and demand
2. Hypoxia is defined as
   A. an inadequate amount of oxygen in the blood
   B. an inadequate amount of oxygen available at the cellular level
   C. $PaCO_2$ of less than 50 mm Hg
   D. the inability of cells to use oxygen properly
3. Dysoxia is defined as
   A. an inadequate amount of oxygen in the blood
   B. an inadequate amount of oxygen available at the cellular level
   C. $PaCO_2$ of less than 50 mm Hg
   D. the inability of cells to use oxygen properly
4. Shock states are characterized by
   A. an inadequate amount of oxygen in the blood
   B. an inadequate amount of oxygen available at the cellular level
   C. $PaCO_2$ of less than 50 mm Hg
   D. an imbalance of oxygen supply and demand
5. MODS is characterized by
   A. continuing hypoxemia
   B. continuing hypoxia
   C. continuing impairment of oxygenation mediated by the inflammatory response
   D. continuing dysoxia mediated by the inflammatory response

Answers: 1. A, 2. B, 3. D, 4. D, 5. C

SECTION SIX: Assessment of Oxygenation

At the completion of this section, the learner will be able to identify techniques to assess oxygenation status in relation to pulmonary gas exchange, oxygen delivery, and oxygen consumption.

Monitoring oxygenation is an important component of a nursing assessment. Accurate assessment and treatment of oxygenation disturbances may determine whether or not patients survive. Identification of impaired oxygenation requires an understanding of the three components of oxygenation: pulmonary gas exchange, oxygen delivery, and oxygen consumption. Each of these three components of oxygenation may vary independently in response to pathophysiologic conditions and therapeutic interventions. Therefore, it is necessary to accurately assess all three components of oxygenation.

There are two goals in the assessment of oxygenation: (1) to determine overall adequacy of oxygenation and (2) to determine which component of oxygenation dysfunction should be manipulated. Oxygenation can be assessed using direct and indirect assessment techniques.

Pulmonary Gas Exchange

Assessment of gas exchange must include techniques to assess ventilation, diffusion, and perfusion. Techniques to assess for pulmonary gas exchange are summarized in Table 17–6.

Auscultation of the lungs is a common and easy assessment technique to assess ventilation. The key physiologic disturbance that auscultation detects is a change in airflow. Often there are no adventitious breath sounds or changes in chest radiographs during early stages of alteration in pulmonary gas exchange (Smyth, 2005). However, when changes do occur it is important for the nurse to convey the assessment accurately, using correct terminology. Crackles should be used to describe a discontinuous

TABLE 17–6 Assessment of Pulmonary Gas Exchange

ABG (PaO_2, $PaCO_2$)
Auscultation
End-tidal CO_2
Assessment of respiratory muscle efficiency (V_T, $M\dot{V}$, $A\dot{V}$, RR, VC, pulmonary function tests)
Calculation of intrapulmonary shunt (Qs/Qt)
PaO_2/FIO_2 ratio

sound and wheeze should be used to describe a continuous sound. Ventilation is the only mechanism of eliminating carbon dioxide. Therefore, assessment of $PaCO_2$ provides valuable information about this physiologic process. Ventilatory failure is commonly defined as a $PaCO_2$ greater than 50 mm Hg. Carbon dioxide can also be assessed using end-tidal CO_2 measurements whereby a sensor is placed at the end of the endotracheal tube to measure the amount of exhaled CO_2.

Assessment of respiratory muscle efficiency is accomplished by pulmonary function tests (see Module 9) and includes measurements of tidal volume (V_T), minute ventilation ($M\dot{V}$), alveolar ventilation ($A\dot{V}$), respiratory rate (RR), and vital capacity (VC).

The rapid shallow breathing index is an accurate predictor of how well a patient is tolerating weaning from mechanical ventilation. The ratio is expressed as the frequency of respiration (bpm) divided by the tidal volume (liters) as measured during spontaneous unsupported respiration. It is an accurate predictor of weaning failure if the result is greater than 105 and success if the result is less than 105 (Lingren & Ames, 2005).

Calculation of intrapulmonary shunt can be made for patients who have peripheral arterial and pulmonary artery catheters in place. Intrapulmonary shunt (Qs/Qt) is the proportion of blood that flows past alveoli without participating in gas exchange. An elevated intrapulmonary shunt indicates a large proportion of blood is flowing past alveoli without participating in gas exchange. Elevated intrapulmonary shunt can be attributed to either a diffusion impairment or abnormalities in the ventilation to perfusion ratio. Data needed to calculate Qs/Qt are obtained by drawing simultaneous mixed venous and arterial blood gases. It is a complex formula to calculate, although most bedside monitoring systems in the ICU have the capability to calculate Qs/Qt once mixed venous and arterial blood gas data are available. Normal intrapulmonary shunt is less than 5 percent. A Qs/Qt of 30 percent would mean that 30 percent of blood is flowing past alveoli without participating in gas exchange.

Because Qs/Qt requires simultaneous mixed venous and arterial blood gases, simpler, less cumbersome formulas for the determination of intrapulmonary shunt are often used. The simplest formula to estimate intrapulmonary shunt is the PaO_2/FIO_2 ratio. A normal value is more than 286, with a value less than 200 suggesting a large intrapulmonary shunt. For example, a patient with a PaO_2 of 80 mm Hg on 40 percent FIO_2 (80/0.40) = 200.

Oxygen Delivery

Assessment of oxygen delivery must include the components of oxygen delivery, including cardiac output, Hb, SaO_2, and PaO_2.

Physical assessment of oxygen delivery is difficult because oxygen is a colorless, odorless gas. Physical assessments of oxygen delivery can be made using skin color and temperature assessments and capillary refill. *Cyanosis,* a term used to describe bluish skin discoloration, is difficult to use because of subjectivity. Cool extremities indicate poor perfusion. Capillary refill may be a useful assessment parameter in children, but is not as useful in elderly patients (Johnson, 2004). Restlessness, confusion, rapid heart rate and tachypnea may be early signs of inadequate oxygen delivery (Smyth, 2005).

Direct measurement of PaO_2, SaO_2, and hemoglobin can be made with an ABG. Although PaO_2 minimally contributes to oxygen delivery (less than 3 percent of all oxygen delivered to tissues), it is still used in the evaluation of oxygen delivery. Arterial oxygen saturation, the ratio of oxygenated hemoglobin to total hemoglobin, can be measured by ABG (SaO_2) or by pulse oximetry (SpO_2). Pulse oximetry is used for continous noninvasive measurement of arterial oxygenation saturation. Pulse oximetry is recommended for any patient at risk for hypoxemia because desaturation is detected earlier by pulse oximetry than by clinical observation (Grap, 2002).

Cardiac output can be assessed directly or indirectly. An indirect assessment of cardiac output would include an evaluation of heart rate and stroke volume, including the components of preload and afterload (see Module 12, Determinants and Assessment of Cardiac Output). Direct measurement of cardiac output can be made using a pulmonary artery catheter. Cardiac output measurements can be made using thermodilution techniques or by the use of a special pulmonary artery catheter that measures cardiac output continuously (see Module 13, Assessment of Hemodynamic Status: Hemodynamic Monitoring). Oxygen delivery (DO_2) can also be calculated for these patients. Calculation of oxygen delivery requires a cardiac output measurement, serum hemoglobin analysis, and ABG analysis for SaO_2 and PaO_2. Oxygen delivery can be calculated as the product of cardiac output and oxygen content of arterial blood as follows:

$$DO_2 = (CO \times [Hb \times 1.34 \times SaO_2] + [PaO_2 \times 0.003]) \times 10^*$$

*10 is a conversion factor

Oxygen Consumption

Assessment of oxygen consumption must include techniques that assess the availability and use of oxygen at the cellular level. Direct assessment of oxygen consumption in the clinical setting is currently not possible. There are no physical assessment parameters that can be used to evaluate oxygen consumption. Traditional means of assessing oxygenation (ABGs, cardiac output, etc.) do not reflect oxygen availability at the cellular level. Future technologies will focus on measuring oxygenation at the cellular level.

Current methods of assessing oxygen consumption are limited to indirect measurement techniques including measurement of serum lactate levels, base deficit, and mixed venous oxygen saturation monitoring.

Under conditions of inadequate oxygen delivery, cells convert from aerobic metabolism to anaerobic metabolism. The

Emerging Evidence

- Practice guidelines suggest timely assessment of oxygenation and timely administration of antibiotics in patients who present to the ER with community acquired pneumonia. In this study, the investigators found that postponing oxygenation assessment (pulse oximetry or ABG) greater than one hour was associated with significantly longer time to initiation of antibiotics (median six hours). A delay in assessment of oxygenation greater than three hours was associated with an increased risk of death (relative risk 2.24, 95 percent confidence interval 1.17 – 4.30) (*Blot, Rodriquez, Sole-Violan, 2007*).
- Hypoxia is common after acute stroke. These investigators were interested in whether there are differences in oxygenation between daytime and nighttime after stroke. They found that all indicators of oxygenation were significantly worse at night than during the day. Because daytime and nighttime results were strongly correlated, borderline hypoxia during the day is strongly predictive of overt hypoxia at night (*Ali, Cheek, Sills, 2007*).
- These investigators assessed whether SaO_2/FIO_2 ratio could be substituted for PaO_2/FIO_2 ratio for the assessment of oxygenation. They found a SaO_2/FIO_2 ratio of 235 corresponded to a PaO_2/FIO_2 ratio of 200; SaO_2/FIO_2 ratio of 315 corresponded to a PaO_2/FIO_2 ratio of 300. The SaO_2/FIO_2 ratio threshold values of 235 and 315 resulted in 85 percent sensitivity and 85 percent specificity and 91 percent sensitivity and 56 percent specificity, respectively, for the PaO_2/FIO_2 ratio of 200 and 300. This study demonstrated that SaO_2/FIO_2 ratio correlates with PaO_2/FIO_2 ratio (*Rice, Wheeler, Bernard, et al., 2007*).

byproduct of anaerobic metabolism is lactate. Normal serum lactate levels are less than 2 mMol/L. The underlying cause of high serum lactate levels may be inadequate oxygen delivery to meet cellular oxygen needs. Serum lactate levels, evaluated using serial measurements (for example, every four to eight hours), can be used as an indicator of improving or worsening oxygen delivery in relation to oxygen consumption. Serum lactate levels must be interpreted with caution in patients with liver or renal disease and alcohol intoxication (Johnson, 2004).

Base deficit is defined as the amount of base (mMol) required to titrate 1 L of arterial blood to a normal pH. It is calculated from an ABG. Normal base deficit is +2 mMol to –2 mMol. It is used as an approximation of acidosis. A base deficit results from an imbalance between oxygen delivery and oxygen consumption, which results in a lactic acidosis secondary to anaerobic metabolism. Positive values reflect metabolic alkalosis and negative reflect metabolic acidosis. Base deficit can be classified as mild (–2 to –5 mMol), moderate (–6 to –14 mMol), and severe (greater than –15 mMol). Administration of sodium bicarbonate, hypothermia, and hypocapnea can affect base deficit (Johnson, 2004).

Mixed venous oxygen saturation (SvO_2) reflects the balance between oxygen supply and oxygen demand. Measuring SpO_2 provides information about the oxygen saturation of arterial blood. Measuring SvO_2 provides information about the oxygen saturation of venous blood. Monitoring both of these parameters allows clinicians to make an assessment about the amount of oxygen delivered to tissues and the amount of oxygen returned from tissues.

When the supply of oxygen to the tissues is sufficient, tissues extract the amount of oxygen needed for their metabolic processes. Each organ system requires a different amount of oxygen. The kidneys actually have a relatively low demand for oxygen because much of their function uses passive transport. The oxygen saturation of the venous blood leaving the kidney averages 74 percent. Conversely, the heart requires a large amount of oxygen for its work. The oxygen saturation of blood leaving the coronary circulation averages only 30 percent. Each body part extracts a certain percentage of the oxygen depending on the metabolic rate of that organ system. The venous blood from all organ systems is transported to the right heart. The venous blood from all body systems is considered "mixed" when it has reached the pulmonary artery. The saturation of this mixed venous blood (SvO_2) represents an average of the venous saturation of blood from all parts of the body. Normal mixed venous oxygen saturation is 60 to 80 percent.

If the oxygen delivery to tissues is adequate for tissue demands, oxygen saturation of the blood in the pulmonary artery will be 60 to 80 percent. The SvO_2 provides information about the adequacy of CO. The patient's blood gases and CO may be within normal limits, but if the SvO_2 is below 60 percent, oxygen delivery is inadequate for tissue oxygen demands. A low SvO_2 means that less oxygen is returning to the right heart; the cells are not getting enough oxygen to meet their needs. Conversely, a low CO of 3.0 L/min in a postoperative patient may not be of concern if the patient's SvO_2 is between 60 and 80 percent. These patients are hypothermic, sedated, intubated, and mechanically ventilated so their tissue oxygen demands are very low. A normal SvO_2 indicates that oxygen delivery is adequate for tissue oxygen demands. Causes of decreased and increased SvO_2 are summarized in Table 17–7.

TABLE 17–7 Causes of Decreased and Increased SvO_2

Decreased SvO_2	Increased SvO_2[a]
1. Decreased oxygen supply	1. Increased oxygen supply
Decreased cardiac output	Increased cardiac output
Heart failure	Inotropic drugs
Hypovolemia	Intraaortic balloon pump
Dysrhythmias	Afterload reduction
Cardiac depressants (i.e., beta blockers)	Early septic shock
Decreased oxygen saturation	Increased oxygen saturation
Respiratory failure	Increased FiO_2 (inspired oxygen)
Pulmonary infiltrates	Improvement in lung problem
Suctioning	Increased hemoglobin
Ventilator disconnection	Blood transfusion
Decreased hemoglobin	2. Decreased oxygen demand
Anemia	Hypothermia
Hemorrhage	Fever reduction
2. Increased oxygen consumption	Sepsis (late stages)
Hyperthermia	Paralysis
Seizures	Pain relief
Shivering	Anesthesia
Pain	
Increased work of breathing	
Increased metabolic rate	
Exercise	
Agitation	

[a]A wedged pulmonary artery catheter may result in a falsely elevated SvO_2.

To illustrate how Svo_2 monitoring can be used to assess oxygen consumption, consider the following patient example. Mr. X. has an Sao_2 of 100 percent and an Svo_2 of 75 percent. Mr. Z has an Sao_2 of 98 percent and an Svo_2 of 40 percent. Mr. X.'s Sao_2 indicates that the oxygen content of arterial blood is fully saturated and that the oxygen saturation of the blood returning to the right side of the heart is 75 percent. If 100 percent was delivered and 75 percent was returned, it appears that the cells extracted 25 percent of the oxygen they received. This is a normal oxygen extraction. Mr. X. appears to have a normal oxygen supply and demand balance. Now consider Mr. Z.'s values. The Svo_2 value is below normal. This is interpreted as a decrease in oxygen delivery compared with oxygen demand. Thus, more oxygen is extracted at the cellular level. The alteration in this Svo_2 value does not indicate which of the determinants of oxygen delivery has changed but implies an oxygenation impairment. The nurse should then assess for changes in cardiac output, Sao_2, and hemoglobin, or for conditions that cause an increase in oxygen consumption (e.g., fever). (Conditions that increase oxygen consumption were discussed in Section Four of this module.)

Svo_2 can be measured intermittently by blood gas analysis of a mixed venous blood sample drawn from the distal port of a pulmonary artery catheter. Svo_2 can be measured continuously through the use of a special fiber-optic pulmonary artery catheter. A fiber-optic filament in the catheter emits a constant beam of light on the red blood cells flowing past it in the pulmonary artery. The amount of emitted light reflected back to the computer through a receiving fiber-optic depends on the oxygen saturation of the red blood cells flowing past it. The computer uses this information to determine the oxygen saturation of mixed venous blood. A digital readout of the Svo_2 is updated several times each minute. Trends in Svo_2 can be used to assess patient tolerance to interventions.

SECTION SIX REVIEW

1. The "gold standard" for the assessment of oxygen delivery is
   A. Pao_2
   B. cardiac output
   C. Svo_2
   D. auscultation
2. Direct measurement of oxygen consumption
   A. is made using Svo_2 monitoring
   B. is made using transcutaneous oxygen measurements
   C. is not clinically possible
   D. can be calculated as the product of cardiac output and oxygen content of arterial blood
3. A patient has the following values: Sao_2 100 percent and Svo_2 55 percent. Which one of the following assessments would be helpful in determining the source of the oxygenation imbalance?
   A. auscultating lung fields
   B. taking temperature
   C. drawing an arterial blood gas
   D. measuring preload
4. Calculation of oxygen delivery requires all of the following EXCEPT
   A. cardiac output measurement
   B. serum hemoglobin analysis
   C. ABG analysis
   D. measurement of blood pressure

Answers: 1. B, 2. C, 3. B, 4. D

POSTTEST

1. The concept of oxygenation involves
   A. pulmonary gas exchange, oxygen delivery, and oxygen consumption
   B. integration of the pulmonary and cardiovascular systems
   C. ventilation, diffusion, and perfusion
   D. oxygen extraction and oxygen consumption
2. Oxygen delivery is dependent upon (choose all that apply)
   A. CO
   B. Sao_2
   C. Pao_2
   D. $Paco_2$
3. Your patient's postoperative hemoglobin is 6 mg/dL. What impact would this have on the initial component of oxygenation?
   A. none
   B. ventilation impairment
   C. diffusion impairment
   D. perfusion impairment

4. A pulmonary embolism would result in impaired gas exchange as a result of
A. ventilation impairment
B. diffusion impairment
C. perfusion impairment
D. decreased oxygen content of arterial blood

5. Which of the following contributes minimally to oxygen delivery?
A. Pa_{O_2}—50 mm Hg
B. Sa_{O_2}—70 percent
C. CO—3 L/min
D. Hb—6 mg/dL

6. Which of the following conditions can significantly impair oxygen delivery? (choose all that apply)
A. dysrhythmias
B. heart failure
C. decreased Sa_{O_2}
D. decreased Pa_{O_2}

Mr. B. is admitted with a diagnosis of pneumonia. His data on admission are as follows:

ABG:	Pa_{O_2} 45, Pa_{CO_2} 50, Sa_{O_2} 70 percent, pH 7.30, HCO_3 28
Lactate:	8 mMol/L
Hb:	10 mg/dL
CO:	3 L/min
Sv_{O_2}:	60 percent

Questions 7, 8, and 9 pertain to Mr. B.

7. Based on the preceding data, Mr. B. has impaired oxygen consumption as evidenced by
A. Pa_{O_2} of 45, Pa_{CO_2} of 50
B. Pa_{CO_2} of 50, Sa_{O_2} of 70 percent
C. lactate 8 mMol/L and Sv_{O_2} of 60 percent
D. Hb 10 mg/dL and CO of 3 L/min

8. Based on the data on Mr. B., you determine that Mr. B. has
A. multiple organ dysfunction syndrome
B. shock
C. hypoxemia and hypoxia
D. dysoxia

9. Based on the data on Mr. B., calculate the oxygen delivery.
A. 282 mL/min
B. 28,142 mL/min
C. 125 mL/min
D. 243 mL/min

10. Which of the following would decrease oxygen consumption?
A. administration of an antibiotic
B. preoperative anxiety
C. nursing assessment
D. administration of a sedative

11. The clinical condition characterized by inadequate oxygen in arterial blood is
A. hypoxia
B. hypoxemia
C. dysoxia
D. shock

12. Which of the following represents the most complete oxygenation assessment?
A. arterial blood gas, auscultation, and calculation of intrapulmonary shunt
B. auscultation of lung fields, measurement of cardiac output, and Sv_{O_2}
C. cardiac output, serum measurement of hemoglobin, Sa_{O_2}, and Pa_{O_2}
D. serum lactate level, Sv_{O_2}, and arterial blood gas

Posttest answers with rationale are found on MyNursingKit.

REFERENCES

Ali, K., Cheek, E., Sills, S. (2007). Day-night differences in oxygenation saturation and frequency of desaturations in the first 24 hours after acute stroke. *J Stroke & Cerebrovasc Dis, 16*, 239–244.

Blot, S. I., Rodriquez, A., Sole-Violan, J. (2007). Effects of delayed oxygenation assessment on time to antibiotics and mortality in patients with severe community acquired pneumonia. *Crit Care Med, 35*, 2509–2515.

Grap, M. J. (2002). Protocols for practice: Pulse oximetry. *Critical Care Nurse, 22*, 69–76.

Johnson, K. L. (2004). Diagnostic measures to evaluate oxygenation in critically ill adults. implications and limitations. *AACN Clinical Issues, 15*, 506–524.

Lindgren, V. A., & Ames, N. J. (2005). Caring for patients on mechanical ventilation. *AJN* 105(5), 50–60.

Marklew, A. (2006). Body positioning and its effect on oxygenation: A literature review. *Nursing in Critical Care, 11*(1), 16–22.

Rice, T. W., Wheeler, A. P., & Bernard, G. R. (2007). Comparison of the SpO_2/FiO_2 ratio and the PaO_2/FiO_2 ratio in patients with acute lung injury or ARDS. *Chest, 132*, 410–417.

Smyth, M. (2005). Acute respiratory failure: failure in oxygenation. *AJN* 105(5), 72GG – 72OO.

Swinamer, D. L., Phang, P. T., Jones, R. L., Grace, M., & King, E. G. (1987). Twenty-four hour energy expenditure in critically ill patients. *Crit Care Med, 15*, 637–643.

MODULE

18 Alterations in Oxygen Delivery and Oxygen Consumption: Shock States

Kiersten Henry, Karen L. Johnson

OBJECTIVES Following completion of this module, the learner will be able to

1. Describe the mechanism of impaired oxygenation for each of the four functional classifications of shock states.
2. Describe the compensatory mechanisms that occur in response to shock states.
3. Discuss the clinical manifestations of each of the four functional shock states.
4. State the medical and nursing interventions used in the treatment of shock states that optimize oxygen delivery and decrease oxygen consumption.

This self-study module is composed of four sections. Section One describes the mechanisms of impaired oxygenation for each of four functional classifications of shock. Section Two reviews the compensatory mechanisms that occur in response to shock states. In Section Three, clinical manifestations for each of the four functional shock states are given. Section Four describes medical and nursing interventions that optimize oxygen delivery and decrease oxygen consumption. Each section includes a set of review questions to help the learner evaluate his or her understanding of the section's content before moving on to the next section. All Section Reviews include answers. It is suggested that the learner review those concepts answered incorrectly in the review questions before proceeding to the next section.

PRETEST

1. Which of the following is common to all shock states?
   A. blood pressure of 90 mm Hg, heart rate greater than 100 beats per minute
   B. loss of blood volume
   C. decreased oxygen delivery with decreased oxygen consumption
   D. inadequate oxygen delivery to meet cellular oxygen demands
2. Which of the following shock states have similar pathologic mechanisms?
   A. neurogenic and septic shocks
   B. anaphylactic and cardiogenic shocks
   C. left ventricular myocardial infarction and cardiac tamponade
   D. carbon monoxide poisoning and cardiac tamponade
3. Which of the following is NOT one of the sympathetic nervous system's fight-or-flight responses?
   A. increased heart rate
   B. dilation of pupils
   C. increased respiratory rate
   D. increased intestinal peristalsis
4. Which of the following is a potent vasoconstrictor?
   A. renin
   B. aldosterone
   C. angiotensin II
   D. antidiuretic hormone (ADH)
5. In neurogenic shock, signs and symptoms are related to
   A. loss of spinal fluid
   B. damaged parasympathetic cells
   C. loss of hypothalamic control
   D. loss of sympathetic innervation
6. Shock states result from
   A. an imbalance of oxygen delivery and oxygen consumption
   B. an increase in oxygen delivery and oxygen consumption
   C. a decrease in oxygen delivery and oxygen consumption
   D. inadequate blood pressure, heart rate, and urine output
7. Transport shock states are the result of
   A. an increase in vessel diameter
   B. a dysfunctional or inadequate amount of hemoglobin
   C. a barrier to flow of oxygenated blood
   D. failure of the heart to adequately pump blood

8. All of the following are stages of shock EXCEPT
   A. initial
   B. compensatory
   C. noncompensatory
   D. progressive
9. A systemic response to infection that includes a temperature greater than 38°C and a heart rate greater than 90 beats per minute characterizes
   A. sepsis
   B. severe sepsis
   C. septic shock
   D. septic syndrome
10. All of the following may be used in the treatment of cardiogenic shock EXCEPT
    A. a ventricular assist device
    B. an intraaortic balloon pump
    C. a cardiac transplantation
    D. isoproterenol

Pretest answers are found on MyNursingKit.

SECTION ONE: Functional Classifications of Shock States

At the completion of this section, the learner will be able to describe the mechanism of impaired oxygenation for each of the four functional classifications of shock states.

The major function of the cardiovascular system is to deliver blood, oxygen, and nutrients to the cells, tissues, and organs of the body and to remove metabolic wastes. When this fails to occur, a state of shock develops; however, defining shock is trickier than defining other disease entities. It is difficult to agree on one concise definition because **shock** is a syndrome, a complex of signs and symptoms that describe a sequence of changes that occur when tissue oxygen supply does not meet oxygen demand. The relationship between oxygen supply (delivery) and oxygen demand (consumption) serves as the conceptual framework for shock in this module.

Common to all shock states is inadequate oxygen delivery to meet cellular oxygen demand. Traditionally, shock states have been classified according to their etiology (e.g., septic shock, hemorrhagic shock, neurogenic shock). Shock may also be categorized into functional shock states. Several functional classifications have been used. For our purposes in this module, shock is classified into four categories: hypovolemic, transport, obstructive, and cardiogenic (Clochesy, 1988). This classification system groups shock states not according to the cause of the shock state but according to similar pathophysiologic mechanisms responsible for impaired oxygenation.

Hypovolemic shock states have impaired oxygenation because of inadequate cardiac output (CO) as a result of decreased intravascular volume. **Transport shock** states have impaired oxygenation because of a diminished supply of hemoglobin (Hb) in which to carry oxygen to tissues. **Obstructive shock** states have impaired oxygenation because of a mechanical barrier to blood flow. **Cardiogenic shock** states have impaired oxygenation because the heart fails to function as a pump to deliver oxygenated blood. The functional states, causes, and mechanisms of impaired oxygen delivery are summarized in Table 18–1.

Hypovolemic Shock States

Hypovolemic shock can result from two conditions: either the fluid volume in the circulation has decreased, or the size of the intravascular compartment has increased in proportion to fluid volume. When either or both of these conditions exist, venous return to the right atrium decreases. This reduces ventricular filling pressure, stroke volume, cardiac output, and blood pressure (Baldwin et al., 2006).

TABLE 18–1 Functional States of Shock, Causes, and Pathologic Mechanisms

FUNCTIONAL STATE	ETIOLOGY	MECHANISM OF IMPAIRED O_2 DELIVERY
Hypovolemic	Fluid volume loss (dehydration, burn injuries, third spacing) Vasodilation (neurogenic shock, anaphylactic shock, septic shock)	Loss of intravascular volume Increase in vessel diameter due to loss of sympathetic tone, histamine release, endotoxin release
Transport	Diminished supply of Hb to carry O_2 (anemia, hemorrhage, carbon monoxide poisoning)	Dysfunction or inadequate amount of Hb to bind with O_2
Obstructive	Mechanical barriers to blood flow (pulmonary embolism, tension pneumothorax, cardiac tamponade)	Barrier to flow of oxygenated blood due to Pulmonary artery blocked Great vessels kinked Ventricles unable to fill or eject blood volume
Cardiogenic	Heart fails to function as a pump (myocardial infarction, dysrhythmias)	Ischemic muscles fail to contract Irregular rate/rhythm causes heart to fail its function as a pump

Compiled from Clochesy, J. M. (ed.) (1988). *Essentials of critical care nursing* (p. 127). Rockville, MD: Aspen Publishing.

Loss of intravascular volume can be caused by loss of blood volume (hemorrhage), loss of intravascular fluid from the skin (as with dehydration or burns), loss of fluid from persistent vomiting or diarrhea, or loss of fluid from the intravascular compartment to interstitial spaces (third spacing). A diminished fluid volume leads to a decreased cardiac output (CO), resulting in impaired oxygen delivery.

When the size of the intravascular compartment has increased in proportion to the amount of fluid in the intravascular compartment, the body interprets this as a state of hypovolemia. Blood volume may be normal, but the intravascular space has increased without a proportional increase in blood volume. Vasodilation causes the intravascular compartment to increase without a corresponding increase in volume. Vasodilation can occur with neurogenic shock, anaphylactic shock, and septic shock.

Neurogenic shock may occur with a spinal cord injury. When there is injury to the spinal cord above the midthoracic region, impulses from the sympathetic nervous system cannot reach the arterioles. The loss of sympathetic innervation prohibits vasoconstriction of blood vessels, but blood vessels continue to receive parasympathetic innervation, allowing vasodilation. Blood then pools in the dilated peripheral venous system. The right heart receives an inadequate venous return, and cardiac output decreases. The lack of sympathetic innervation also causes a decreased heart rate, further reducing the CO. As CO decreases, delivery of oxygen-carrying blood decreases (Guly et al., 2008).

Anaphylactic shock occurs in response to a severe allergic reaction to such things as foods (peanuts, fish, eggs, milk), drugs (nonsteroidal anti-inflammatory drugs, aspirin, antibiotics, anesthetic agents, blood products), insect venoms, and latex (Lieberman et al., 2005). Massive amounts of vasoactive substances (e.g., histamine and kinins) are released from mast cells (Fig. 18–1). This causes vasodilation and increases capillary permeability. Vasodilation increases the size of the intravascular compartment. Increased capillary permeability allows fluid to move from intravascular to interstitial spaces. As fluid is lost from the vascular compartment, a relative hypovolemia develops. The net consequences of combined massive vasodilation and increased capillary permeability are a decrease in venous return, decrease in CO, and a decrease in oxygen delivery.

Septic shock is a systemic response to invading microorganisms of all types: gram-positive and gram-negative bacteria, fungi, or viruses. The systemic response to infection triggers a complex series of cellular and humoral events (Fig. 18–2). These organisms release endotoxins that invade the bloodstream and stimulate the release of cytokines (such as tumor necrosis factor

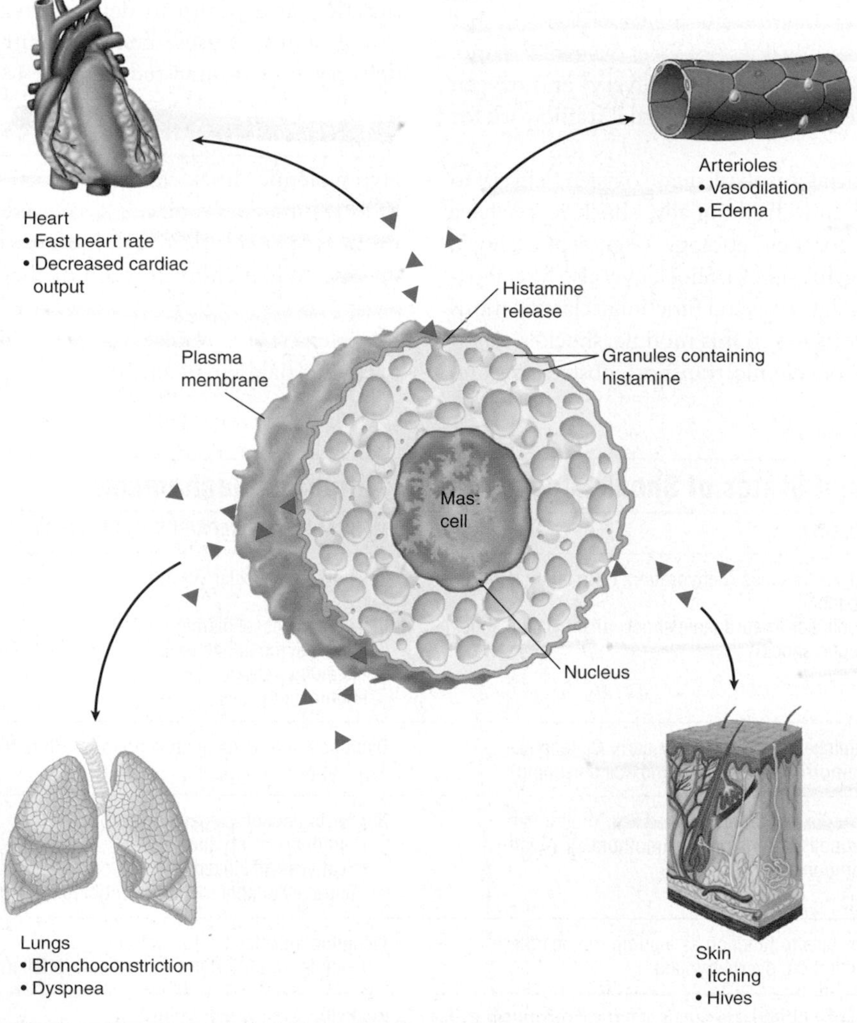

Figure 18–1 ■ Pathophysiologic response to anaphylaxis.

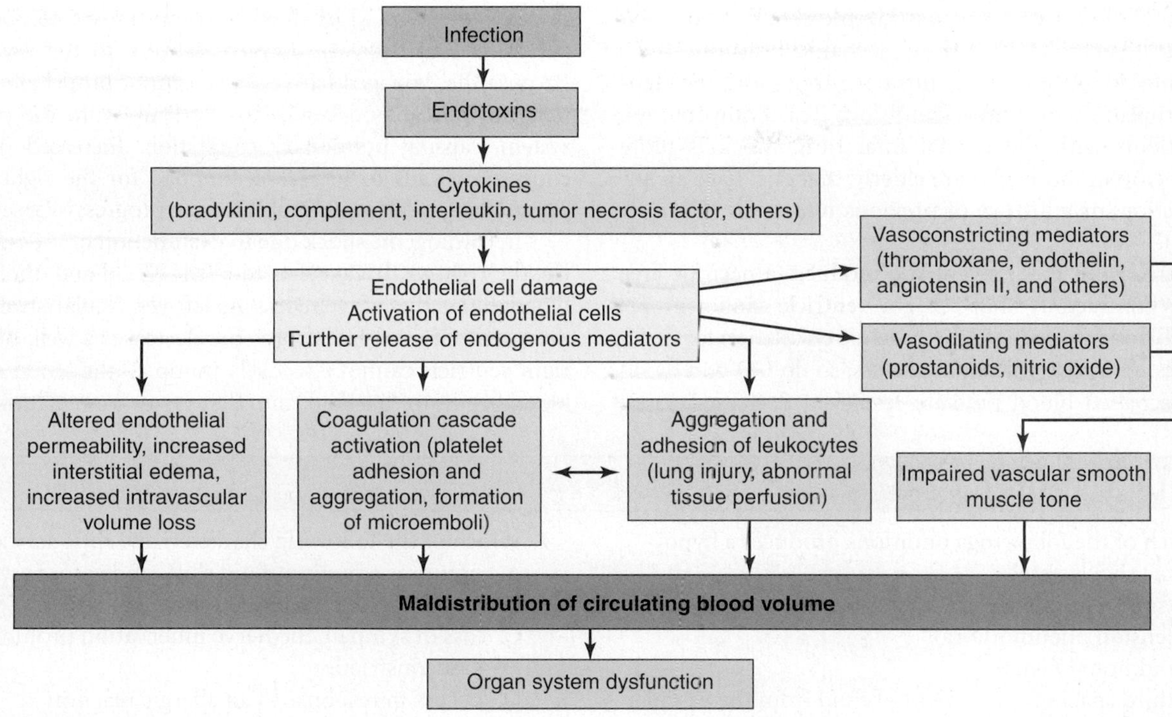

Figure 18–2 ■ Pathophysiology of septic shock.

and interleukins). These substances produce vasodilation and increased capillary permeability. This reduces venous return, and cardiac output decreases. A second fluid alteration that occurs with septic shock is a maldistribution of circulating blood volume. Some organs receive more blood than needed as a result of vasodilation, while other organs (skin, lungs, kidneys) do not receive the blood needed. Altered fluid volume related to vasodilation, increased capillary permeability, and maldistribution of circulating volume characterize septic shock.

Transport Shock States

The common pathologic mechanism in transport shock states is a diminished supply of Hb to carry O_2 to tissues. Recall that Hb is referred to as the "bus" that carries O_2 molecules to tissues. Anemia and hemorrhage are characterized by a decrease in red blood cells and Hb for O_2 to bind to.

Carbon monoxide toxicity represents another form of transport shock state. Carbon monoxide is a colorless, odorless gas that, when inhaled, rapidly binds to Hb to form carboxyhemoglobin. The Hb bus seats are occupied by carbon monoxide, which has a much stronger affinity for hemoglobin than O_2. This leaves no room for O_2 to blind to Hb, and oxygen cannot be transported to tissues. The presence of carbon monoxide interferes with the release of O_2 from Hb and also interferes with the cell's ability to use O_2 properly (Wolf et al., 2008). A state of shock occurs as the transport of O_2 to tissues is severely limited.

Obstructive Shock States

Obstructive shock states occur as a result of a mechanical barrier to blood flow that blocks O_2 delivery to tissues. Obstructive shock states can be caused by pulmonary embolism, tension pneumothorax, or cardiac tamponade.

Pulmonary embolism can range from clinically unimportant thromboembolism to massive embolism with sudden death. Hypercoagulability leads to formation of thrombi in the deep veins of the legs, pelvis, or arms. The thrombi dislodge and embolize to the pulmonary arteries. Pulmonary arteries become partially obstructed, which results in an increase in alveolar dead space and a ventilation–perfusion mismatch, which impairs gas exchange. Obstruction of the pulmonary arteries by emboli also results in increased pulmonary vascular resistance. As right ventricular afterload increases, right ventricular dysfunction can occur. Shock states in response to a pulmonary embolism can result from inadequate systemic O_2 delivery because of impaired gas exchange and cardiac dysfunction.

A tension pneumothorax occurs when air enters the pleural space during inspiration but cannot leave during expiration. The progressive accumulation of air within the thoracic cavity leads to a shift of the mediastinal structures and compression of the opposite lung. The increased pleural pressure impedes venous return and serves as a barrier to O_2 delivery.

Cardiac tamponade is caused by bleeding into a nonflexible pericardial sac. The accumulating pressure around the heart impairs ventricular filling and decreases CO.

Cardiogenic Shock States

Cardiogenic shock states occur as a result of impaired O_2 delivery due to cardiac dysfunction. Dysfunction of either the right or left ventricle can lead to cardiogenic shock. However, the most common cause of cardiogenic shock is an extensive myocardial infarction (MI), particularly in the anterior portion of the left ventricle (Josephson, 2008). Failure can occur when the right ventricle fails to pump the volume of blood it receives or when the left ventricle fails to pump oxygenated blood into the systemic circulation. Causes of cardiogenic shock include extensive acute myocardial infarction, mechanical complications (papillary muscle rupture, acute mitral regurgitation, ventricular septal rupture), or other conditions (cardiomyopathy). Among patients with myocardial infarction, shock is more likely to develop in those who are elderly, diabetic, have an anterior infarction, or a history of previous infarction (Gurm & Bates, 2007).

An infarction in the left ventricle produces a necrotic area that impairs contractility and CO. The ventricle cannot propel oxygenated blood forward into the systemic circulation for delivery to tissues. As stroke volume decreases, so do CO and blood pressure. Decreased blood pressure results in decreased aortic diastolic pressure which further compromises coronary artery perfusion and decreases oxygen delivery to the myocardium. Because the damaged left ventricle cannot propel all of its contents forward, blood begins to "back up" into the pulmonary system, causing pulmonary congestion. Increased pulmonary congestion leads to increased afterload for the right ventricle. These changes can occur rapidly or can progress over several days.

In cardiogenic shock due to dysfunction of the right ventricle, the right ventricle ejects too little blood and, therefore, less blood enters the left ventricle. As left ventricular stroke volume decreases, CO and blood pressure decrease as well. Because the right ventricle cannot effectively pump all the blood it receives, blood begins to "back up" into the systemic circulation.

SECTION ONE REVIEW

1. Which of the following conditions produces a hypovolemic shock state?
   - **A.** carbon monoxide poisoning
   - **B.** tension pneumothorax
   - **C.** pulmonary emboli
   - **D.** third spacing (movement of fluid from the vascular to the interstitial space)
2. Which of the following conditions can produce a transport shock state?
   - **A.** carbon monoxide poisoning
   - **B.** dehydration
   - **C.** cardiac tamponade
   - **D.** anaphylactic shock
3. Which of the following conditions can produce an obstructive shock state?
   - **A.** myocardial infarction
   - **B.** anemia
   - **C.** pulmonary emboli
   - **D.** sepsis
4. Which of the following characterizes septic shock?
   - **A.** occurs as a result of fluid shifts and vasoconstriction
   - **B.** endotoxins in the blood release cytokines
   - **C.** loss of sympathetic nerve innervation prohibits vasoconstriction
   - **D.** occurs in response to an allergic reaction
5. Which of the following characterizes cardiogenic shock?
   - **A.** increasing stroke volume in the face of decreasing cardiac output
   - **B.** the heart fails to function as a pump
   - **C.** increasing stroke volume in the face of increasing cardiac output
   - **D.** hypovolemic shock as the result of a massive myocardial infarction

Answers: 1. D, 2. A, 3. C, 4. B, 5. B

SECTION TWO: Physiologic Response to Shock

At the completion of this section, the learner will be able to describe the compensatory mechanisms that occur in response to shock states.

Shock occurs when O_2 delivery does not support tissue O_2 demands. In an attempt to stabilize this life-threatening situation, a pattern of responses, or compensatory mechanisms, occurs.

Compensation in Shock

Complex neuroendocrine responses are triggered to overcome ineffective circulating blood volume. Low-pressure stretch receptors in the right atrium sense a decrease in circulating blood volume when there is a decrease in venous return to the right atrium. Baroreceptors in the aorta and carotid arteries sense a decrease in blood volume and CO. Carotid body chemoreceptors sense alterations in pH and partial pressure of arterial carbon dioxide ($Paco_2$). The baroreceptors and chemoreceptors alert the hypothalamus to activate the sympathetic nervous system's fight-or-flight response. This system releases a massive amount of norepinephrine, epinephrine and cortisol, which produce several compensatory mechanisms (Table 18–2). The beneficial effects of these mechanisms are an increase in venous return, an increase in CO, and an increase in O_2 delivery.

In response to shock states, the endocrine system is activated to increase oxygen delivery by increasing blood volume (Fig. 18–3). The hypothalamus releases adrenocorticotropic hormone (ACTH), which activates the adrenals to secrete aldosterone. Aldosterone causes sodium and water retention, attempting to increase the blood volume and blood pressure. Sodium and water retention stimulates the release of antidiuretic hormone (ADH), which increases reabsorption of water in the kidney tubules and increases blood volume. These hormones are released to preserve blood volume and conserve the amount of fluid the kidneys excrete.

CO must be augmented in shock to ensure adequate tissue perfusion. CO is proportional to venous return. To increase venous return, sodium and water are retained by aldosterone and ADH. In addition to these hormones, another mechanism, the renin–angiotensin–aldosterone system, is activated to increase

TABLE 18–2 Sympathetic Nervous System's Fight-or-Flight-Response

PHYSIOLOGIC RESPONSE	PHYSIOLOGIC RATIONALE
Increased heart rate	For rapid delivery of needed oxygen
Increased respiratory rate	To receive more oxygen and correct acidosis
Increased glycolysis, gluconeogenesis, mobilization of free fatty acids	To increase availability of glucose for energy
Decreased urine output	To conserve fluid volume, return more blood volume to cardiovascular system to increase volume and blood pressure
Decreased blood flow to internal organs (e.g., kidneys, gastrointestinal tract, liver)	To allow more blood flow to more vital organs (e.g., heart and lungs)
Decreased intestinal peristalsis	Shunting of blood to vital organs, no need for digestion as body energy is redirected to lifesaving measures
Cool skin	Alpha receptors produce peripheral vasoconstriction to shunt blood to more vital organs
Diaphoresis	To release heat as a by-product of metabolism

blood volume and venous return. As a result of decreased blood flow to the kidneys, the juxtaglomerular cells in the kidneys excrete renin. Renin catalyzes angiotensinogen in the liver, which then converts to angiotensin I in the circulation. Once in the lungs, angiotensin I converts to angiotensin II, which is a potent vasoconstrictor. The vasoconstriction produced by angiotensin II increases blood pressure by increasing afterload. Angiotensin II stimulates the release of aldosterone. The renin–angiotensin–aldosterone system is depicted in Figure 18–4. The net effects of these hormonal mechanisms are increased blood pressure through vasoconstriction and increased venous return through retention of sodium and water, and decreased urine output.

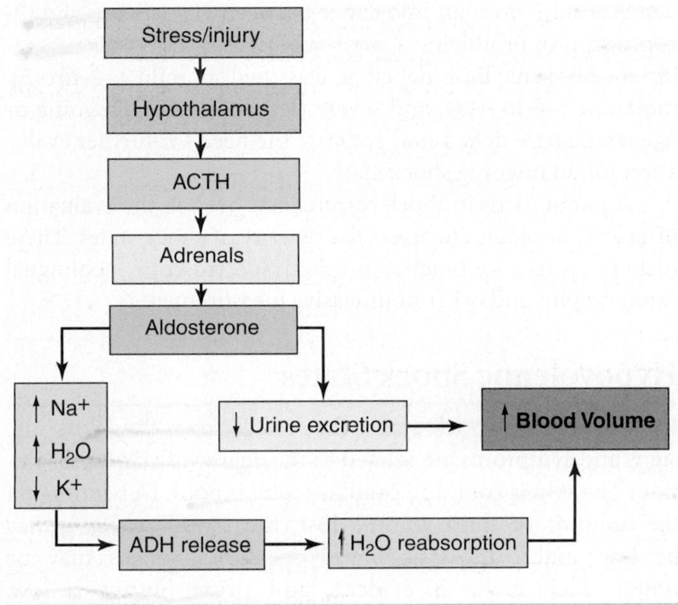

Figure 18–3 ■ ACTH, aldosterone, and ADH release.

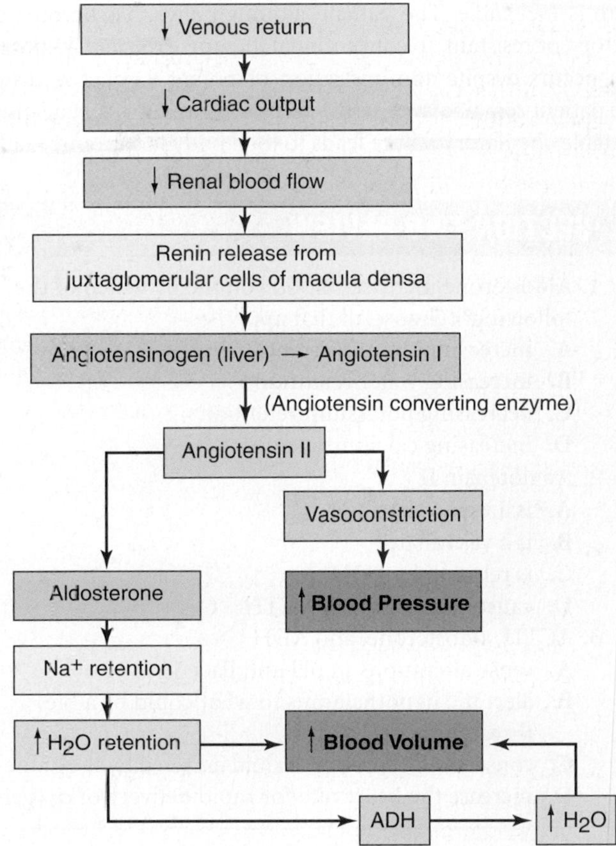

Figure 18–4 ■ Renin-angiotensin-aldosterone system.

Compensatory mechanisms that occur in response to shock are designed to restore O_2 delivery by augmenting CO, redistributing blood flow, and restoring blood volume.

Progression of Shock

There are four stages of shock: initial, compensatory, progressive, and refractory. This applies to all classifications of shock states. In the *initial stage,* decreased CO and decreased tissue perfusion are evident. Decreased O_2 delivery to cells results in anaerobic metabolism and lactic acidosis. In the *compensatory stage,* neuroendocrine responses are activated to restore CO and O_2 delivery. Clinical signs and symptoms are evident.

When compensatory mechanisms cannot restore homeostasis and if prompt and proper treatment has not been instituted, the third stage of shock can occur. *Progressive shock* results in major dysfunction of many organs. The continued low blood flow, poor tissue perfusion, inadequate O_2 delivery, and buildup of metabolic wastes over time lead to multiple organ dysfunction syndrome, or MODS (See Module 19, Alterations in Tissue Perfusion: Multiple Organ Dysfunction Syndrome).

The final stage of shock is the *refractory stage.* In this stage, the shock state is so profound and cell destruction is so severe that death is inevitable. The patient, although alive, has become refractory, or resistant, to conventional therapy. Profound hypotension occurs despite administration of potent vasoactive drugs. The patient remains hypoxemic despite O_2 therapy. A state of intractable circulatory failure leads to total body failure and death.

Not every patient progresses through all four stages. Often, the progression from one stage to the next is not obvious. If the shock state is assessed early and appropriate treatment is instituted, the progression of shock is halted, the O_2 supply-and-demand balance is restored, and the patient recovers.

SECTION TWO REVIEW

1. Aldosterone increases blood volume by which of the following? (choose all that apply)
   - **A.** increasing sodium retention
   - **B.** increasing water retention
   - **C.** decreasing potassium retention
   - **D.** increasing calcium retention
2. Angiotensin II
   - **A.** is a vasoconstrictor
   - **B.** is a vasodilator
   - **C.** is released by ADH
   - **D.** causes the release of ACTH
3. ACTH, aldosterone, and ADH
   - **A.** sense alterations in pH and $PaCO_2$
   - **B.** alert the hypothalamus to what could be a life-threatening situation
   - **C.** conserve the amount of fluid excreted by the kidneys
   - **D.** increase the heart rate for rapid delivery of oxygen
4. Norepinephrine produces which of the following compensatory (fight-or-flight response) mechanisms?
   - **A.** decreased blood pressure
   - **B.** increased intestinal peristalsis
   - **C.** increased glycolysis
   - **D.** decreased heart rate
5. Unresolved low blood flow, poor tissue perfusion, and inadequate oxygen delivery eventually cause
   - **A.** multisystem organ dysfunction
   - **B.** the hypothalamus to release ACTH
   - **C.** the release of renin from renal cells
   - **D.** decreased urine output

Answers: 1. (A, B, C), 2. A, 3. C, 4. C, 5. A

SECTION THREE: Clinical Findings Associated with Shock States

At the completion of this section, the learner will be able to list the clinical manifestations of each of the four functional shock states.

Clinical manifestations of all shock states are the result of inadequate O_2 delivery and the activation of compensatory mechanisms (Fig. 18–5).

Traditional parameters used to assess shock include blood pressure, heart rate, mentation, and urine output. However, these signs often underestimate the degree of physiologic abnormalities. Blood pressure is hard to assess because it is so individualized. A blood pressure of 90/60 mm Hg may be normotensive for one patient but hypotensive for another patient. There are many factors that cause tachycardia, including anxiety, pain, arrhythmia, and fever. Mentation may be hard to assess because of the presence of head injury, alcohol, drugs, or chronic diseases (e.g., Alzheimer's). Several factors may produce a false sense of security when adequate urine output is present. These can include the neuroendocrine response to shock, hyperglycemia, and diabetes insipidus. Research is ongoing, but evidence is mounting that shock states persist despite normalization of blood pressure, heart rate, and urine output.

Serum lactate levels can be used as an indirect measure of impaired oxygenation and shock. Normal serum lactate levels are less than 2 mMol/L. However, during shock states when there is impaired O_2 delivery to meet cellular O_2 demand, anaerobic metabolism occurs (see Module 17, Determinants and Assessment of Oxygen Delivery and Oxygen Consumption). The by-product of this is lactate. Hyperlactatemia can produce metabolic acidosis. Lactate levels indicate the degree of hypoperfusion. Patients whose lactate levels return to normal within 24 hours have increased survival rates and decreased occurrence of organ dysfunction (Dunne et al., 2005).

Base deficit is the amount of base required to titrate 1 L of arterial blood to a normal pH. It is calculated from an arterial blood gas. Normal base deficit is +2 mMol to –2 mMol. A base deficit results from an imbalance between O_2 delivery and O_2 consumption producing a lactic acidosis secondary to anaerobic metabolism. Base deficit is classified as mild (–2 to –5), moderate (–6 to –14), and severe (less than –15). Ongoing or worsening base deficit may indicate the need for further evaluation for an ongoing shock state.

A major focus in shock research has been in the evaluation of new technologies to assess the severity of shock states. These include gastric tonometry, infrared spectroscopy, sublingual capnography, and other noninvasive measurements.

Hypovolemic Shock States

In hypovolemic shock states that result from fluid loss, the signs and symptoms are related to the degree of volume depletion. The skin is cool, and capillary refill is poor. Depending on the amount of fluid volume lost, the blood pressure may be low, and orthostatic blood pressure changes may be noted. Tachycardia is evident, and urine output is low. Hemodynamically, as less volume is returned to the right

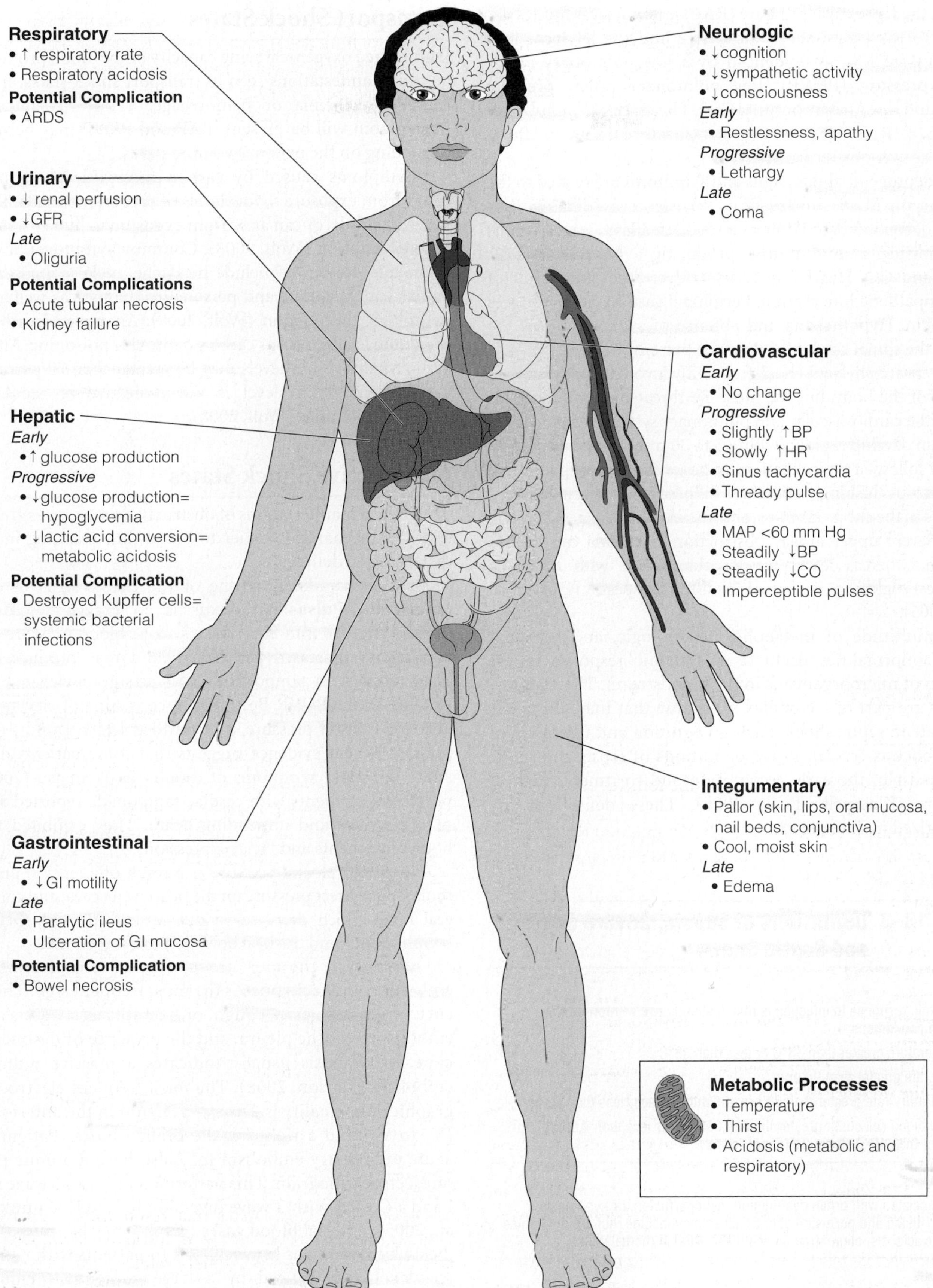

Figure 18–5 ■ Multisystem effects of shock.

atrium, the right atrial pressure (RAP) is low. As less fluid is delivered to the pulmonary vasculature and the left ventricle, pressures are low, as evidenced by a low pulmonary artery wedge pressure (PAWP), low pulmonary artery pressure (PAP), and low cardiac output (CO). The systemic vascular resistance (SVR) is elevated as vasoconstriction occurs in efforts to increase venous return and CO.

In neurogenic shock, signs and symptoms are related to the loss of sympathetic innervation. Persistent vasodilation produces a decreased SVR. Pooling of blood in dilated vessels results in diminished venous return, producing a lower RAP, PAP, PAWP, and CO. Heart rate (HR) is decreased as a result of parasympathetic innervation. Peripheral vasodilation produces warm skin. Hypothermia and absence of sweating below the level of the spinal cord injury may be present.

Severe anaphylactic shock frequently involves multiple organ systems of the body, but the most life threatening are those involving the cardiovascular and pulmonary systems. Anaphylactic shock can develop rapidly (within 5 to 30 min) or slowly (6 to 12 hrs) but follows a typical pattern of generalized itching followed by cutaneous flushing, urticaria, a fullness in the throat, anxiety, tightness in the chest, faintness, and loss of consciousness (Brown, 2005). Severe upper airway obstruction by edema can lead to asphyxia, whereas lower airway obstruction with wheezing and chest tightness is caused by bronchospasm (Lieberman et al., 2005).

A multitude of metabolic, hematologic, and hemodynamic abnormalities occur as a systemic response to the invasion of microorganisms in the bloodstream. These abnormalities are part of a complex syndrome that may ultimately culminate in septic shock. Early recognition and treatment of septic shock is crucial. Broad definitions of sepsis and septic shock assist in the early recognition and treatment of these disorders (Kleinpell et al., 2006). These definitions are summarized in Table 18–3.

TABLE 18–3 Definitions of Sepsis, Severe Sepsis, and Septic Shock

Sepsis

The systemic response to infection is manifested by two or more of the following conditions:

1. Temperature greater than 38°C or less than 36°C
2. Heart rate greater than 90 bpm
3. Respiratory rate greater than 20 breaths/min or $Paco_2$ less than 32 mm Hg
4. White blood cell count greater than 12,000/mL or less than 4,000/mL or greater than 10% immature (band) forms

Severe sepsis

Sepsis associated with organ dysfunction, hypoperfusion, or hypotension. Hypoperfusion and perfusion abnormalities may include, but are not limited to, lactic acidosis, oliguria, or an acute alteration in mental status.

Septic shock

Sepsis associated with hypotension despite adequate fluid resuscitation along with the presence of perfusion abnormalities that may include, but are not limited to, lactic acidosis, oliguria, or an acute alteration in mental status.

Transport Shock States

Diminished oxygen-carrying capacity of the blood produces the clinical manifestations seen in transport shock states. In shock caused by anemia or hemorrhage, a low hematocrit and hemoglobin will be present. RAP and PAWP may be normal, depending on the patient's volume status.

Symptoms caused by carbon monoxide poisoning can result from exposure to low levels of carbon monoxide for prolonged periods, or can arise from exposure to higher levels for a shorter duration (Wolf, 2008). Common symptoms of carbon monoxide poisoning include headache, malaise, nausea, difficulties with memory, and personality changes, as well as gross neurologic dysfunction (Wolf, 2008). An elevated carboxyhemoglobin level confirms carbon monoxide poisoning. Although carboxyhemoglobin levels may be greater than 70 percent, the carboxyhemoglobin level is not indicative of the level of neurological injury (Wolf, 2008).

Obstructive Shock States

The clinical manifestations of obstructive shock states are the result of a mechanical barrier to blood flow resulting in inadequate oxygen delivery.

Pulsus paradoxus is one of the classic signs of cardiac tamponade. **Pulsus paradoxus** is an exaggerated decrease (greater than 10 mm Hg) of the systolic blood pressure during inspiration. Increased pericardial fluid may produce distant heart sounds. In tamponade, RAP usually is elevated and is equaled by the PAWP. Beck's triad, consisting of elevated RAP, decreased blood pressure, and muffled heart sounds, may be present. Recent evidence suggests that some patients demonstrate signs and symptoms of dysphoria. Ikematsu (2007) reported that patients with cardiac tamponade reported feelings of restlessness and impending death. They exhibited restless body movements and facial expressions.

Increased pleural pressure as a result of a tension pneumothorax puts direct pressure on the heart, vena cava, and contralateral lung, which decrease venous return and CO. Decreased breath sounds and tracheal deviation may be present.

Dyspnea is the most frequent symptom of pulmonary embolism, and tachypnea is the most frequent sign. The presence of pleuritic pain, cough, or hemoptysis suggests a small embolism near the pleura, and the presence of dyspnea, syncope, or cyanosis usually indicates a massive pulmonary embolism (Tapson, 2008). The most frequent electrocardiographic abnormality is *T* wave inversion in the anterior leads (V_1 to V_3) and a right bundle branch block. Patients with acute pulmonary embolism may also have a unique pattern on electrocardiogram. This pattern includes an *S* wave in lead I and a *Q* wave with *T* wave inversion in lead II (Punukollu et al., 2005). Arterial blood gases (ABGs) may be normal or indicate hypoxemia or hypercapnia. In patients with right ventricular failure caused by a large pulmonary embolism, echocardiography will show right ventricular enlargement and pulmonary hypertension. Perfusion lung scans, pulmonary angiography, spiral CT of the chest with contrast, or transthoracic echocardiography may be used in the diagnostic workup.

Cardiogenic Shock States

Clinical manifestations produced in cardiogenic shock states depend on whether heart failure is on the left or the right side of the heart.

Left ventricular failure produces clinical manifestations associated with hypoperfusion and pulmonary congestion, including dyspnea, bilateral crackles, and distant heart sounds, and third or fourth heart sounds are usually present (Gurm & Bates, 2007). The hemodynamic profile of cardiogenic shock includes an elevated PAWP (greater than 15 mm Hg), a low cardiac index (less than 1.8 L/min/m^2 without inotropic support, or less than 2.2 L/min/m^2 with inotropic support), and sustained hypotension (systolic blood pressure less than 90 mm Hg or mean blood pressure 30 mm Hg lower than baseline) (Reynolds & Hochman, 2008).

Clinical manifestations of right ventricular failure are associated with systemic venous congestion. Peripheral edema may be evident. Lung sounds will be clear unless there is also left ventricular dysfunction (Gurm & Bates, 2007). A split-second heart sound may be heard. This sound, produced by delayed closure of the tricuspid valve, indicates a distended right ventricle. The hemodynamic profile of right ventricular failure includes elevated RAPs in the presence of normal or low PAWP. This elevated RAP may cause the intraventricular septum to shift, impairing the filling of the left ventricle (Reynolds & Hochman, 2008).

SECTION THREE REVIEW

1. The signs and symptoms of anaphylactic shock are
   A. related to the loss of sympathetic tone
   B. related to the release of chemical mediators
   C. decreased SVR, PAWP, and increased temperature
   D. decreased RAP, increased CO, and increased temperature
2. A low Hct and Hb will be present in shock caused by
   A. a pulmonary embolism
   B. cardiac tamponade
   C. anemia
   D. right ventricular failure
3. Mr. G. was involved in a motor vehicle crash. He sustained a spinal cord injury. Which of the following are clinical manifestations of a spinal cord injury?
   A. increased heart rate, SVR, and RAP
   B. decreased heart rate, decreased SVR, and increased RAP
   C. increased heart rate, increased SVR, and decreased RAP
   D. decreased heart rate, SVR, and RAP
4. Mr. T. has hypovolemic shock. Which of the following clinical manifestations would be present?
   A. decreased SVR, decreased CO
   B. increased SVR, decreased CO
   C. decreased SVR, increased CO
   D. increased SVR, increased CO
5. Which of the following would characterize right-sided heart failure?
   A. RAP will be high and much higher than PAWP.
   B. RAP will be low.
   C. PAWP will be high and much higher than RAP.
   D. RAP and PAWP will be greatly elevated.

Answers: 1. B, 2. C, 3. D, 4. B, 5. A

SECTION FOUR: Treatment of Shock

At the completion of this section, the learner will be able to state the medical and nursing interventions used in the treatment of shock states that optimize oxygen delivery and decrease **oxygen consumption**—that is, the amount of oxygen used by the body. The primary goals of treatment are to identify and treat the underlying cause of shock, optimize oxygen delivery, and decrease oxygen consumption.

Interventions to Optimize Oxygen Delivery

Supplemental oxygen may be administered in an attempt to improve oxygen delivery to hypoxic tissues. For patients who are conscious, spontaneously breathing, and have adequate arterial blood gases, oxygen delivered by nasal cannula or mask may be all that is necessary. In the unconscious patient or in the patient demonstrating respiratory distress, intubation and mechanical ventilation may be required.

Administration of IV fluids assists in restoring optimal tissue perfusion by restoring preload and increasing the cardiac output component of oxygen delivery. The fluid best suited for shock states remains controversial. Usually, a combination of crystalloids and colloids is administered. Crystalloid solutions (e.g., lactated Ringer's solution) restore interstitial and intravascular fluid volumes, and increase preload and cardiac output. Administration of colloids enhances the blood's oxygen-carrying capacity. Colloids have oncotic capabilities not inherent in crystalloids. Packed red blood cells are usually given to provide adequate hemoglobin concentration and to increase oxygen-carrying capacity. Blood may be given with crystalloids to maintain adequate circulatory volume. Inotropic medications may be necessary if volume administration is not sufficient to improve oxygenation.

Positive inotropic drugs increase contractility by stimulating the beta$_1$ receptors in the heart. Increased contraction results in increased stroke volume as the ventricles eject more completely. Inotropic drugs that increase cardiac output and enhance tissue perfusion include dopamine, dobutamine, and milrinone. Dopamine has both alpha- and beta receptor effects.

RELATED PHARMACOTHERAPY: Positive Inotropic Agents

Beta Adrenergic Agonist
Dobutamine (Dobutrex)

Action and Uses
Acts on $beta_1$ receptors in the heart to increase inotropic activity (increase contractility) and increase conduction through AV node (increase HR).

Major Adverse Effects
Angina
Increased myocardial workload
Tachycardia

Nursing Implications
- Monitor ECG and BP closely while patient receives this drug.
- Administer via infusion pump.
- Marked hypertension and tachycardia, and appearance of dysrhythmias are usually reversed by promptly decreasing the dose.

Phosphodiesterase Inhibitor
Milrinone (Primacor)

Action and Uses
Inhibits cyclic AMP phosphodiesterase in cardiac and smooth muscle, thereby increasing myocardial contractility (increased CO) and causing vasodilation (decreased PAWP, decreased SVR). Little chronotropic activity, therefore does not significantly increase myocardial oxygen demand or increase HR.

Major Adverse Effects
Ventricular dysrhythmias
Hypotension

Nursing Implications
- Monitor ECG and BP closely while patient receives this drug.
- Administer via infusion pump.
- In presence of significant hypotension, stop infusion, notify HCP.

In moderate doses (greater than 5 mcg/kg/min), $beta_1$ receptors are activated, and cardiac output increases. Larger doses (greater than 10 mcg/kg/min) stimulate alpha receptors and increase blood pressure. Dobutamine selectively acts on $beta_1$ receptors to increase contractility and CO. Dobutamine also decreases SVR. Milrinone is a phosphodiesterase inhibitor that increases contractility, reduces SVR, and results in improved cardiac output. All inotropic drugs must be used with caution because they increase myocardial oxygen consumption (see RELATED PHARMACOTHERAPY: Positive Inotropic Agents box).

Vasoactive drugs act on the smooth muscle layer of blood vessels and affect preload and afterload (Module 15, Alterations in Cardiac Output). These drugs are either vasoconstrictors or vasodilators. Vasoconstrictors, or vasopressors, mimic the sympathetic nervous system to increase blood flow to vital organs by increasing blood pressure and cardiac output. Vasopressors include epinephrine, norepinephrine, dopamine, and vasopressin. These drugs increase SVR and blood pressure and should be given only when the patient's volume status is adequate (as reflected by RAP or PAWP or both). See RELATED PHARMACOTHERAPY: Vasoconstricting Agents box for additional information.

Afterload-reducing (vasodilating) drugs improve cardiac output and oxygen delivery. Peripheral arterial vasodilators (nitroprusside, nitroglycerine) decrease SVR. When afterload is decreased, stroke volume is improved. The ventricles have less resistance to overcome and eject blood with less force. These drugs decrease preload as well as afterload and therefore should be used with caution when treating shock. Afterload-reducing drugs should be given only to patients who have adequate fluid volume. The patient must be monitored carefully so that the blood pressure does not become so low that reflex tachycardia occurs and coronary perfusion suffers.

RELATED PHARMACOTHERAPY: Vasoconstricting Agents

Selective Alpha Adrenergic Agents
Phenylephrine (Neo-synephrine)

Action and Uses
Sympathomimetic agent that acts directly on alpha adrenergic receptors to cause peripheral vasoconstriction (increase BP). Has some $beta_1$ activity at high doses.

Major Adverse Effects
Ventricular dysrhythmias

Nursing Implications
- Monitor BP closely while patient receives this drug. Titrate dose to target BP as ordered by HCP. Give at lowest dose possible to maintain BP.
- Administer via infusion pump.
- If administering drug via peripheral IV site, monitor site closely for infiltration. If infiltration does occur, stop infusion and call HCP immediately (infiltration can cause ischemia and necrosis of tissue).
- Avoid abrupt withdrawal; when drug is discontinued, infusion rate is slowed gradually.

NonSelective Alpha Adrenergic Agents
Norepinephrine (Levaterenol, Levophed, Noradrenaline)

Action and Uses
Sympathomimetic agent that acts directly on alpha adrenergic receptors to cause peripheral vasoconstriction (increase BP). Has moderate $beta_1$ inotropic activity (increase contractility).

Major Adverse Effects

Ventricular dysrhythmias
Increased myocardial workload
Hepatic or renal necrosis

Nursing Implications

Monitor BP closely while patient receives this drug. Titrate dose to target BP as ordered by HCP. Give at lowest dose possible to maintain BP.

Administer via infusion pump.

If administering drug via peripheral IV site, monitor site closely for infiltration. If infiltration does occur, stop infusion and call HCP immediately (infiltration can cause ischemia and necrosis of tissue).

Avoid abrupt withdrawal; when drug is discontinued, infusion rate is slowed gradually.

NonSelective Alpha Adrenergic Agents

Dopamine

Action and Uses

Has dose-dependent pharmacologic effects. At doses less than 5 mcg/kg/minute, dopaminergic receptors are activated leading to vasodilation in renal and mesenteric vascular beds. At doses of 5-10 mcg/kg/minute, the $beta_1$ adrenergic effects predominate resulting in increased myocardial contractility and increased heart rate. At doses greater than 10 mcg/kg/minute, alpha-adrenergic effects predominate leading to arterial vasoconstriction (increased BP).

Major Adverse Effects

Tachycardia (particularly at higher doses)
Dysrhythmias
Hypotension

Nursing Implications

Notify HCP of decreased urine output in absence of hypotension, increasing tachycardia, dysrhythmias, or signs of peripheral ischemia (pallor, cyanosis, mottling, coldness).

Monitor lung sounds in patients with pulmonary congestion or edema because of its vasoconstrictive properties, it can increase venous return to right side of the heart and can worsen pulmonary edema.

Administer via infusion pump.

If administering drug via peripheral IV site, monitor site closely for infiltration. If infiltration does occur, stop infusion and call HCP immediately (infiltration can cause ischemia and necrosis of tissue).

Avoid abrupt withdrawal; when drug is discontinued, infusion rate is slowed gradually.

In most circumstances, a combination of drugs may be advantageous. Combining an inotropic drug with a vasodilating drug can maximize oxygen delivery by increasing contractility and decreasing afterload. Sympathomimetic drugs are temporary agents because they do not treat the underlying cause of shock. They have a relatively short duration of action and can be easily titrated to the patient's rapidly changing condition.

Placing the patient in Trendelenburg position is a controversial intervention used for the treatment of hypotension. Trendelenburg position may displace blood from the systemic venules and small veins into the right heart and increase stroke volume. However, Trendelenburg position may also increase afterload to the left ventricle and decrease stroke volume. Further research is needed to evaluate the effects of Trendelenburg position on stroke volume and blood pressure (Bridges & Jarquin-Valdivia, 2005).

The patient's response to treatment must be assessed frequently for signs of improved oxygen delivery. Signs of improved oxygen delivery include improvements in cardiac index, urine output, and mean arterial pressure (Module 12, Determinants and Assessment of Cardiac Output).

Interventions to Decrease Oxygen Consumption

In addition to optimizing oxygen delivery, interventions also should include measures to decrease oxygen consumption. Interventions to decrease oxygen consumption should be directed toward decreasing total body work, decreasing pain and anxiety, and decreasing temperature (see Module 12, Determinants and Assessment of Cardiac Output).

Decreasing total body work is an attempt to decrease oxygen demands of all tissues. Hyperventilation occurs in an effort to increase oxygen delivery to meet demands, but this requires a great deal of effort, and the patient can rapidly develop respiratory distress. Ventilation is ensured with intubation and mechanical ventilation. Mechanical ventilation also decreases the respiratory muscle oxygen demands. Decreasing oxygen consumption of voluntary muscles can be achieved with neuromuscular blocking agents such as pancuronium (Pavulon) or vecuronium (Norcuron). These drugs eliminate unnecessary muscle activity and allow oxygen to be redirected for use in involuntary muscles, such as the heart. Neuromuscular blockade is not ideal for long-term management of the mechanically ventilated patients, and should be utilized when other methods of sedation and analgesia are not adequate. These agents have been shown to increase the time to extubation and the incidence of muscle wasting in high-acuity patients (Arroliga et al., 2005). For patients in which chemical paralysis is not desirable (e.g., patients with head injury), the use of propofol (Diprovan) may be ideal. Propofol quickly induces deep sedation and has a short half-life. When the drug is discontinued, the patient is arousable within minutes and an evaluation of mental status can be performed. When the drug is resumed, deep sedation is induced.

Pain and anxiety stimulate the sympathetic nervous system to release catecholamines. Catecholamines increase metabolic rate and oxygen consumption. Measures are taken to minimize pain and anxiety. Appropriate analgesics and anxiolytics are administered.

Hyperthermia increases metabolic demands and oxygen requirements. This is controlled with antipyretic drugs, such as acetaminophen, or physical cooling measures, such as a fan or cooling blanket.

Interventions to optimize oxygen delivery and minimize oxygen consumption are used for all patients in shock. Individualized interventions are initiated to treat the underlying cause of shock. These interventions are described briefly in the remainder of this section.

Hypovolemic Shock States

The treatment goal for hypovolemic shock states is to restore fluid volume. In hypovolemic shock, the source of the fluid loss is identified and controlled. Additional intravenous fluids (crystalloid or colloid) are administered. Assess for an improvement in heart rate, blood pressure, and urine output. If no response is noted, additional fluids may be administered.

The treatment goals for neurogenic shock are to maintain stability of the spine and optimize oxygen delivery (see Module 23, Alteration in Sensory Perceptual Function: Acute Spinal Cord Injury). Because of unopposed parasympathetic innervation, patients with complete, cervical spinal cord injuries have hypotension and bradycardia. Preload is restored with IV fluids or vasopressors. A slight bradycardia requires close monitoring. If a marked bradycardia occurs, medications to increase heart rate may be given.

The immediate goals for treatment of anaphylactic shock are to maintain an airway and to support blood pressure. Oxygen may be administered, with mechanical ventilation as needed. Epinephrine (subcutaneous or intravenous routes) may be given to restore vascular tone and blood pressure. Hypotension is treated with IV fluids to restore intravascular volume. Antihistamines (diphenhydramine), H_2 histamine antagonists (ranitidine), bronchodilators (inhaled or IV), and steroids may be used. These agents are considered second-line, as epinephrine is the first medication that should be administered to a patient with anaphylactic shock (Lieberman et al., 2005).

"Surviving Sepsis Campaign Guidelines," management guidelines for severe sepsis and septic shock, were developed to improve outcomes. These multi-disciplinary guidelines provide evidence-based recommendations for the care of patients with severe sepsis and septic shock (Dellinger et al., 2008). A summary of the guidelines is presented in the following paragraphs; however, the reader is encouraged to review the full set of guidelines written by Dellinger and colleagues (2008) or to visit the Surviving Sepsis Campaign website (http://www.survivingsepsis.org).

A nursing priority should be to administer antibiotics within one hour after a HCP initiates the order (Dellinger et al., 2008). Initial fluid resuscitation (using colloid or crystalloids) is given until the RAP is 8–12 mm Hg, mean arterial pressure (MAP) greater than 65 mm Hg, urine output greater than 0.5 mL/kg/hr, or central venous oxygen saturation is greater than 70 percent. Administration of blood products and/or dobutamine may be required to achieve these goals. Fluids may be given at a rate of 500–1000 mL for crystalloids or 300–500 mL for colloids over 30 minutes; these doses may be repeated based on response of increases in urine output and blood pressure. The rate of fluid administration should be decreased if the RAP increases without hemodynamic improvement. Red blood cell transfusion is given only when Hb is less than 7 g/dL.

The initial priority in managing septic shock is to maintain a reasonable MAP and CO while the source of infection is identified and treated (Hollinger, 2007). When fluid administration fails to restore adequate MAP and organ perfusion, vasoconstricting agents are usually initiated. Vasopressors (norepinephrine or dopamine administered through a central line) may be administered to restore blood pressure even when hypovolemia has not yet been completely corrected. All patients receiving vasopressors should have an arterial catheter in place to monitor blood pressure. In shock states, the measurement of MAP using a blood pressure cuff may be inaccurate, therefore MAP should be measured by an arterial catheter (Hollenberg, 2007). Vasopressin may be used to treat hypotension that does not respond to norepinephrine or dopamine. The goal of fluid resuscitation or vasopressor therapy in shock is a MAP greater than 65 mm Hg (Dellinger et al, 2008). Corticosteroids may be considered for patients with septic shock who, despite adequate fluid replacement, require vasopressor therapy to maintain adequate blood pressure. Historically, low-dose dopamine was used to increase renal perfusion and urine output. However, this practice is no longer recommended.

A sedation protocol should be in place for patients requiring mechanical ventilation. Neuromuscular blockade is discouraged, but in the instance that it is required for more than a few hours, the depth of blockade is determined using train-of-four monitoring. Blood glucose levels are maintained to less than 150 mg/dL with continuous IV insulin infusion. Nutritional support should be provided using the enteral route. Prevention of deep vein thrombosis is accomplished with the administration of either low-dose unfractionated heparin or low-molecular weight heparin. Prevention of stress ulcer formation is accomplished with the administration of H_2 receptor inhibitors. Communication with the patient and family must include realistic treatment goals and likely outcomes. Decisions to limit or withdraw support may be in the patient's best interest so the information must be clearly presented and carefully considered.

Research into the pathophysiologic processes involved in sepsis and septic shock has highlighted the role of the coagulation

Emerging Evidence

- During the first six hours of initial resuscitation of sepsis-induced hypoperfusion, the following parameters should be used as treatment goals: RAP 8 to 12 mm Hg; MAP greater than 65 mm Hg; urine output greater than 0.5 mL/kg/hr; SvO_2 greater than 70 percent *(Dellinger et al., 2008)*.
- To optimize identification of causative organisms of sepsis, at least two blood cultures should be obtained with at least one drawn percutaneously and one drawn through each vascular access device unless the device was recently (less than 48 hours) inserted. Other cultures (wound, sputum, urine) should be obtained as clinically indicated *(Dellinger et al., 2008)*.
- Intravenous antibiotics should be started within the first hour of diagnosis of severe sepsis after appropriate cultures have been obtained *(Dellinger et al., 2008)*.
- Following stabilization of patients with severe sepsis, blood glucose should be maintained less than 150 mg/dL by the use of a continuous insulin infusion. Serum blood glucose should be monitored every one to two hours initially; once the serum glucose stabilizes, serum glucose should be monitored every four hours *(Dellinger et al., 2008)*.

cascade. A key feature of this pathophysiology is microscopic clots that occlude blood flow to organs. Under normal circumstances, these clots are degraded by the body's fibrinolytic system. However, during septic shock, activated protein C (APC), a key component of fibrinolysis, is consumed at such a rate that clot dissolution is impeded. APC not only plays a role in the coagulation cascade but it also has anti-inflammatory properties (Russell, 2006). Repletion of the stores of APC shows promise in the treatment of septic shock (Bernard et al., 2004).

Drotrecogin alfa is a recombinant APC that can be administered IV. Patients with multiple organ dysfunction who receive drotrecogin alfa have a higher recovery rate from septic shock than those patients not receiving the drug. Those patients with sepsis who have a low risk of death (single organ failure) have not been shown to benefit from APC administration (Abraham et al., 2005). Patients at high risk of bleeding should not be treated with APC because bleeding is the most frequent and serious adverse event induced by this drug. For patients receiving intravenous APC, the infusion should be stopped for two hours prior to any invasive procedure.

Transport Shock States

The treatment goal for transport shock states is to restore the oxygen-carrying capacity of red blood cells. For the treatment of anemia or hemorrhage, packed red blood cells may be administered in an effort to provide an adequate Hb concentration.

The treatment for carbon monoxide poisoning consists of the administration of high-fractional concentrations of supplemental oxygen. Data indicate that early, aggressive hyperbaric oxygen therapy may decrease the negative sequelae of carbon monoxide poisoning. Serial carboxyhemoglobin levels should be monitored to evaluate patient response to treatment.

Obstructive Shock States

The treatment goal for obstructive shock states is to remove the mechanical barrier to blood flow. For a tension pneumothorax, trapped air is decompressed by a physician with the insertion of a 14-gauge needle or a chest tube (Fig. 18–6). Needle pericardiocentesis may decompress the pericardium for cardiac tamponade. This decompression should improve the heart's pumping ability. If not, a thoracotomy may be required to surgically control and decompress the tamponade.

The cornerstone of management for pulmonary embolism is heparin because it prevents additional thrombi from forming and permits fibrinolysis to dissolve some of the clot (Tapson, 2008). Inferior vena cava filters may be used in the presence of active hemorrhage, contraindications to anticoagulation, or recurrent pulmonary embolism despite intensive prolonged anticoagulation (Tapson, 2008). The use of thrombolytic therapy or surgical embolectomy may be necessary in the face of hemodynamic instability and shock (Tapson, 2008).

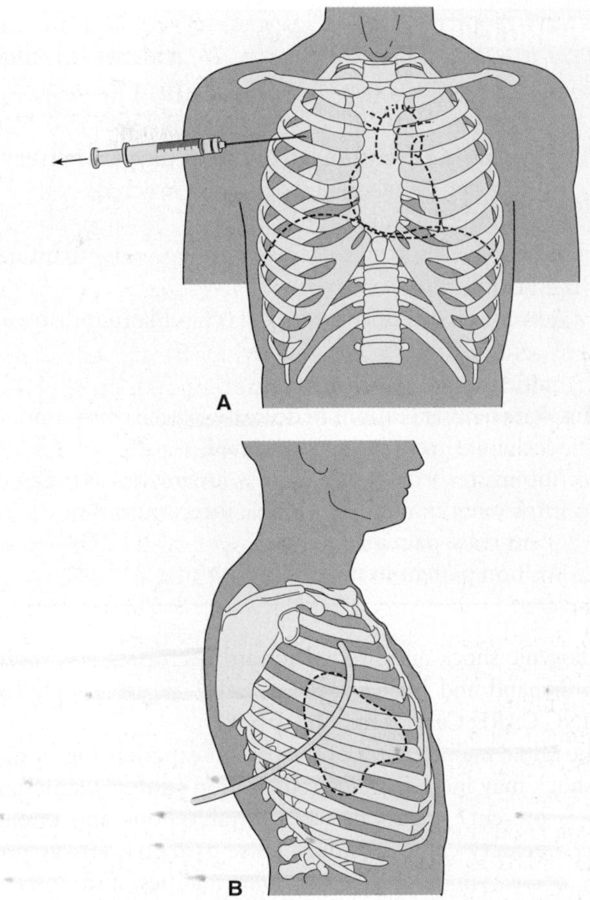

Figure 18–6 ■ A needle thoracostomy may be used in the emergency treatment of a tension pneumothrax. A, A large gauge needle is introduced, and air and fluid are aspirated. B, Alternatively, a chest tube may be inserted and connected to a chest drainage system.

Cardiogenic Shock States

The specific treatment for cardiogenic shock is based on the cardiac abnormality and whether the shock is caused by left-sided or right-sided heart failure. Nursing and medical interventions for patients

NURSING CARE: Cardiogenic Shock

Expected Patient Outcomes and Related Interventions

Outcome: Optimize cardiac output

Assess and compare to established norms, patient baselines and trends.

Assess for clinical manifestations of left ventricular failure including dyspnea, bilateral crackles, distant heart sounds, third or fourth sounds, elevated PAWP, low CI, sustained systolic hypotension.

Assess for clinical manifestations of right ventricular failure including peripheral edema, split S_2 heart

(continued)

NURSING CARE *(continued)*

sounds, elevated RAP in the presence of normal or low PAWP.

Implement interventions to optimize oxygen delivery.
- Administer supplemental oxygen as ordered.
- Administer IV fluids as ordered.
- Administer inotropic agents as ordered (Dobutamine [Dobutrex]).
- Administer afterload-reducing (vasodilating) drugs as ordered.
- Implement IABP as ordered.

Implement interventions to decrease oxygen consumption.
- Mechanical ventilation as ordered.
- Administer sedative, analgesics, anxiolytics as ordered.
- Implement nonpharmacologic interventions to decrease pain and anxiety.
- Position patient to maximize comfort.
- Provide calm, quiet environment.
- Offer support to decrease anxiety.

Administer related drug therapy and monitor for therapeutic and non therapeutic effects.
- Diuretics (e.g. furosemide [Lasix])
- Vasodilators (e.g. nitroprusside [Nipride])
- Inotropic agents (e.g. phosphodiesterase inhibitors [Primacor])
- Thrombolytic therapy

Related nursing diagnoses
- Ineffective cardiopulmonary tissue perfusion related to acute myocardial ischemia
- Decreased cardiac output related to altered contractility
- Decreased cardiac output related to altered heart rate

in cardiogenic shock are directed toward decreasing myocardial oxygen demand and improving myocardial oxygen supply (see NURSING CARE: Cardiogenic Shock box).

The initial management of the patient experiencing cardiogenic shock may include fluid resuscitation (unless pulmonary edema is present), placement of central venous and arterial catheters, urinary catheterization, pulse oximetry, airway protection, correction of electrolyte abnormalities, and relief of pain and anxiety (Gurm & Bates, 2007).

Inotropic agents may be used in patients with normovolemia but inadequate tissue perfusion. Dobutamine can be used to improve myocardial contractility and increase cardiac output (Topalian et al., 2008). Dobutamine is used only if the MAP is adequate or it may be combined with a vasopressor (Josephson, 2008). Hemodynamic monitoring using a pulmonary artery catheter permits serial measurements of CO, which allows titration of inotropic and vasopressor drugs to the minimum dose required to achieve therapeutic goals. Diuretics may be used to treat pulmonary congestion. Vasodilators may be used (after blood pressure has been stabilized) to decrease both preload and afterload. Further treatment may include thrombolytic therapy, an intraaortic balloon pump, and revascularization (angioplasty or coronary artery bypass surgery).

Although aspirin has not been specifically studied in the setting of cardiogenic shock, its benefits are well documented to support its administration in patients who develop cardiogenic shock (Menon et al., 2006). Patients in cardiogenic shock have a high concentration of fibrinogen, therefore the administration of heparin helps to prevent further clot formation and maintain coronary perfusion once it is established (Josephson et al., 2008). Glycoprotein IIa/IIIb inhibitors may be used, especially if the patient had a non-*ST* segment elevation MI. Thrombolytic therapy reduces mortality rates in patients with acute MI, however, the benefits of this therapy in patients with cardiogenic shock are less certain. Thrombolytic therapy can reduce the likelihood of developing cardiogenic shock after initial presentation (Topalian et al., 2008).

Patients in cardiogenic shock can experience a deterioration in mentation due to decreased CO and therefore may require mechanical ventilation to protect their airway and to provide and adequate oxygen supply.

An intraaortic balloon pump (IABP) reduces afterload and augments coronary perfusion, which increase cardiac output and improve coronary blood flow. The IABP has a 40 mL balloon mounted on a catheter which is inserted into the femoral artery and advanced until it is in the descending thoracic aorta. The IABP is synchronized with the patient's heart rate. During ventricular diastole, the balloon inflates (Fig. 18–7). With the balloon inflated, the blood distal to the balloon is forced back toward the aortic valve. This supplies the coronary arteries with additional oxygenated blood to meet myocardial oxygen needs. Before ventricular systole, the balloon deflates, which decreases pressure in the aorta. This makes it easier for the left ventricle to contract and eject its stroke volume. In hospitals without direct angioplasty

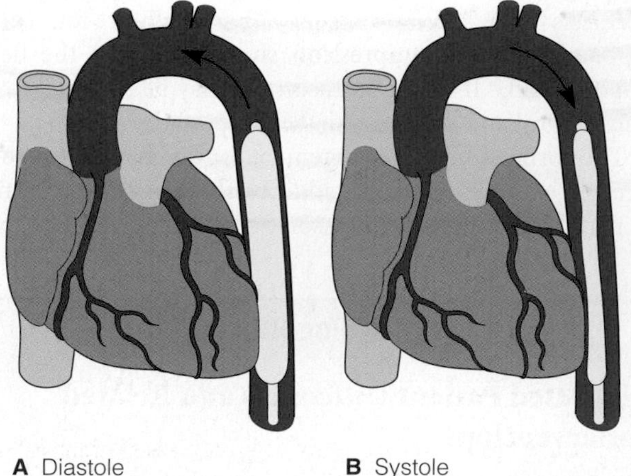

Figure 18–7 ■ The intraaortic balloon pump. A, When inflated during diastole, the balloon supports cerebral, renal, and coronary artery perfusion. B, The balloon deflates during systole, so cardiac output is unimpeded.

capabilities, stabilization with IABP and thrombolysis followed by transfer to a tertiary care facility may be the best treatment option (Reid & Cottrell, 2005). Stabilization with the IABP is only temporary. It does not reestablish coronary blood flow but does allow stabilization until a definitive therapy can be instituted.

Mechanical revascularization for patients in cardiogenic shock caused by MI can be performed. Direct percutaneous transluminal coronary angioplasty (PTCA) may be used to improve wall motion in the infarct area and increase perfusion of the infarct zone. In patients with cardiogenic shock who have either left main coronary artery or three vessel coronary disease, coronary artery bypass surgery may be performed (Reid & Cottrell, 2005).

In the case of patients who present with advanced cardiogenic shock refractory to IABP and PTCA or bypass surgery, the use of left ventricular assist devices (LVAD) may be the only other option. There are three potential uses for LVADs. First, the LVAD may be used as a short-term mechanism to rest the injured myocardium, after which point it is removed from the patient (Birks et al., 2006). If the myocardium does not recover, the LVAD may be left in as a bridge to cardiac transplantation (Topalian et al., 2008). Finally, in those patients who are not suitable candidates for transplant, there are some LVADs approved for permanent use (Topalian et al., 2008). The major risks of LVADs include infection, stroke, dysrhythmias, bleeding, and device malfunction (Leeper, 2006).

SECTION FOUR REVIEW

You have been assigned to provide nursing care to Mr. J., a 74-year-old male with a diagnosis of septic shock. During the change-of-shift report, you are given the following information:

- Vital signs: blood pressure 70/42 mm Hg, pulse 140 bpm sinus tachycardia, respirations 38/minute, temperature 103°F
- Ventilator settings: SIMV 10, FiO_2 40 percent, tidal volume 350 mL, PEEP 5 cm H_2O
- Recent laboratory results: ABGs: pH 7.25, $PaCO_2$ 30, PaO_2 60, HCO_3 18, base deficit 8, Hct 27 percent, Hb 8 g/dL, Na 140 mEq/L, K 4.5 mEq/L
- Hemodynamic readings: MAP 51 mm Hg, RAP 3 mm Hg, PAP 18/8 mm Hg, PAWP 8 mm Hg, CO 4 L/min, SVR 356 dynes/sec/m^2
- IV fluids: D_5 and 1/2 NS plus 20 mEq KCl at 100 mL/hr
- Urine output past 8 hours: 160 mL/hr

As you walk to Mr. J.'s bedside, you note that he is pale and restless. He is lying in the semi-Fowler's position. Answer the following questions based on the information provided about Mr. J.

1. Which of the following would best increase Mr. J.'s cardiac output and restore preload?
   A. acetominophen
   B. O_2 therapy by nasal cannula
   C. low-dose dopamine
   D. located Ringer's Solution at 200 mL/hr
2. Which of the following indicate that Mr. J.'s oxygen delivery is improving?
   A. pH 7.40
   B. RAP 1 mm Hg
   C. Hct 27 percent
   D. respiratory rate of 38/min
3. Which of the following indicates Mr. J. has increased oxygen consumption?
   A. sinus tachycardia
   B. temperature 103°F
   C. respirations 38/min
   D. all of the above
4. Mr. J. may require vasopressors. Which of the following may be administered?
   A. norepinephrine
   B. dopamine
   C. dobutamine
   D. A and B are correct
5. The physician orders an antibiotic. The nurse must administer this drug within ______ hour(s) of the written order.
   A. one
   B. two
   C. four
   D. eight

Answers: 1. D, 2. A, 3. D, 4. D, 5. A

POSTTEST

1. A patient has neurogenic shock. Which assessment findings is this patient likely to exhibit? (choose all that apply)
   A. hypertension
   B. hypotension
   C. increased HR
   D. decreased HR
2. A patient presents with a five-day history of nausea, vomiting, diarrhea, and fever. He has not been able to take fluids by mouth. The nurse understands that this patient is at greatest risk for which of the following problems?
   A. cardiogenic shock
   B. transport shock

C. obstructive shock
D. hypovolemic shock

3. The nurse cares for a patient who presents to the ER with anaphylactic shock. Which vital sign should the nurse take first?
A. BP
B. temperature
C. pulse
D. assessment of pain

4. A patient has cardiogenic shock and now requires dialysis. The patient's wife asks the nurse why his kidneys are not working. Which of the following is the best explanation?
A. He has probably had poor functioning kidneys for a long time.
B. He is going into a stage of multiple organ failure.
C. It's the body's way of increasing oxygen to other tissues such as the heart and brain.
D. We don't fully understand why this is happening.

5. A patient with hypovolemic shock is given 2 liters of lactated Ringers IV solution. Which outcome indicates to the nurse that the fluid is having the desired effect? (choose all that apply)
A. patient is now normotensive
B. patient is now in normal sinus rhythm
C. patient has a urine output of 10 mL/kg/minute
D. patient is alert, oriented

6. How do patients in refractory shock present?
A. profound hypotension despite administration of potent vasoactive drugs
B. hypotension that responds to fluid therapy
C. tachycardia and decreased urine output
D. hypoxemia despite oxygen therapy

7. A patient has hypovolemic shock as a result of massive gastrointestinal bleeding. The patient is given fluids and vasopressors. Which outcome indicates to the nurse that these treatments are having the desired effects?
A. base deficit – 6 mMol
B. lactate levels are decreasing from admission levels
C. urine output is normal
D. blood pressure is 90/60 mm Hg

8. A patient is assessed to have a low right atrial pressure, low pulmonary artery wedge pressure and low CO. The systemic vascular resistance is elevated. The nurse identifies which nursing diagnosis is the priority?
A. impaired gas exchange
B. altered tissue perfusion
C. alterations in fluid volume (excess)
D. altered urinary elimination

9. A patient has just returned to the ICU from having coronary artery bypass surgery. The nurse notes the patient's blood pressure drops during inspiration and goes back up on expiration. His BP is 90/60 mm Hg on expiration and 70/40 mm Hg on inspiration. What intervention should the nurse implement first?
A. Increase the dopamine to maintain BP at 90/60 mm Hg.
B. Suction the patient.
C. Assess the patency of the IV catheter.
D. Call the HCP.

10. It is important for the nurse to question which of the following orders by the HCP?
A. Administer dopamine 5 mcg/kg/min to keep MAP greater than 80 mm Hg.
B. Administer dopamine 15 mcg/kg/min to keep MAP greater than 80 mm Hg.
C. Administer dopamine 10 mcg/kg/min to keep CO greater than 4 L/hr.
D. Administer dobutamine 10 mcg/kg/min to keep CO greater than 4 L/hr.

11. A patient has septic shock. The HCP initiates an order for Vancomycin. According to the Surviving Sepsis Guidelines, the nurse should administer this drug within ______hour(s) from the time the order was initiated.
A. one
B. two
C. four
D. six

12. A patient with septic shock is receiving activated protein-C. When planning care for this patient, which diagnosis has priority?
A. potential for infection
B. altered nutrition, less than body requirements
C. potential for injury
D. ineffective thermoregulation

Posttest answers with rationale are found on MyNursingKit.

REFERENCES

Abraham, E., Laterre, P. F., Garg, R., et al. (2005). Drotrecogin alpha (activated) for adults with severe sepsis and low risk of death. *New England Journal of Medicine, 353,* 1332–1341.

Arroliga, A., Frutos-Vivar, F., Hall, J., et al. (2005). Use of sedatives and neuromuscular blockers in a a cohort of patients receiving mechanical ventilation. *Chest, 128,* 496–506.

Baldwin, K. M., Cheek, D. J., & Morris, S. E. (2006). Shock, multiple organ dysfunction syndrome, and burns in adults. In McCance, K. L, & Huether, S. E. (eds.) *Pathophysiology: the biologic basis for disease in adults and children,* 5th ed. St. Louis: Elsevier Mosby.

Bernard, G. B., Margolis, B. D., Shanies, H. M., et al. (2004). Extended evaluation of recombinant human activated protein C United States trial (EHNHANCE US). *CHEST, 125,* 2206–2216.

Birks, E. J., Tansley, P. D., Hardy, J., et al. (2006). Left ventricular assist device and drug therapy for the reversal of heart failure. *New England Journal of Medicine, 355,* 1873–1884.

Bridges, N., & Jarquin-Valdivia, A. A. (2005). Use of the Trendelenburg position as the resuscitation position: To T or not to T? *American Journal of Critical Care, 14,* 364–368.

Brown, S. G. A. (2005). Cardiovascular aspects of anaphylaxis: implications for treatment and diagnosis. *Current Opinion in Allergy and Clinical Immunology, 5,* 359–364.

Clochesy, J. M. (ed.). (1998). *Essentials of critical care nursing* (p.127). Rockville, MD: Aspen Publishing.

Dellinger, R. P., Levy, M. M., Carlet, J. M., et al. (2008). Surviving sepsis campaign: international guidelines for management of severe sepsis and septic shock: 2008. *Intensive Care Medicine, 34,* 17–60.

Dunne, J. R., Tracy, J. K., Scalea, T. M., & Napolitano, L. M. (2005). Lactate and base deficit in trauma: does alcohol or drug use impair their predictive accuracy? *Journal of Trauma Injury, Infection, and Critical Care, 58: 959–966.*

Guly, H. R., Bouamra, O., & Lecky, F. E. (2008). The incidence of neurogenic shock in patients with isolated spinal cord injury in the emergency department. *Resuscitation, 76,* 57–62.

Gurm, H. S., & Bates, E. R. (2007). Cardiogenic shock complicating myocardial infarction. *Critical Care Clinics, 23,* 759–777.

Hollenberg, S. M. (2007). Vasopressor support in septic shock. *Chest* 132(5), 1678–1687.

Ikematsu, Y. (2007). Incidence and characteristics of dysphoria in patients with cardiac tamponade. *Heart & Lung, 36(6),* 440–449.

Josephson, L. (2008). Cardiogenic shock. *Dimensions in Crit Care Nursing, 27(4),* 160–170.

Kleinpell, R. M., Graves, B. T., & Ackerman, M. H. (2006). Incidence, pathogenesis, and management of sepsis. *AACN Advanced Critical Care, 17(4),* 385–393.

Leeper, B. (2006). Advanced cardiovascular concepts. In Chulay, M. & Burns, S. M. (eds): *AACN Essentials of Critical Care Nursing.* New York: McGraw Hill.

Lieberman P., Kemp, S. F., Oppenheimer, J., et al. (2005). The diagnosis and management of anaphylaxis: an updated practice parameter. *Journal of Allergy and Clinical Immunology, 115,* S483–523.

Menon, V., & Honcheman, J. S. (2006). Treatment and prognosis of cardiogenic shock complicating acute myocardial infarction. *UpToDate,* August 27, 2006.

Punukollu, G., Gowda, R. M., Vasavada, B. C., & Khan, I. A. (2006). Role of electrocardiography in identifying right ventricular dysfunction in acute pulmonary embolism. *American Journal of Cardiology, 96,* 450–452.

Reid, M. B., & Cottrell, D. (2005). Nursing care of patients receiving intra-aortic balloon counterpulsation. *Critical Care Nurse, 25(5),* 40–49.

Reynolds, H. R., & Hochman, J. S. (2008). Cardiogenic shock: current concepts and improving outcomes. *Circulation, 117,* 686–697.

Russell, J. A. (2006). Management of sepsis. *New England Journal of Medicine, 355,* 1699–713.

Tapson, V. F. (2008). Acute pulmonary embolism. *New England Journal of Medicine, 358,* 1037–1052.

Topalian, S., Ginsberg, F., & Parrillo, J. E. (2008). Cardiogenic shock. *Critical Care Medicine, 36,* S66–74.

Wolf, S. J., Lovanas, E. J., Sloan, E. P., & Jagoda, A. S. (2008). Clinical policy: critical issues in the management of adult patients presenting to the emergency department with acute carbon monoxide poisoning. *Annals of Emergency Medicine, 51,* 138–152.

MODULE

19 Alterations in Tissue Perfusion: Multiple Organ Dysfunction Syndrome

Karen L. Johnson

OBJECTIVES

Following completion of this module, the learner will be able to

1. State the physiologic changes that occur during the local inflammatory process.
2. Contrast the physiologic changes that occur with the local inflammatory response with those that occur with the systemic inflammatory response syndrome (SIRS).
3. Discuss four pathophysiologic changes that occur with multiple organ dysfunction syndrome.
4. Identify the seven most common organ systems that fail as a result of the SIRS process.
5. Describe the collaborative management of the patient with multiple organ dysfunction syndrome.

Multiple organ dysfunction syndrome (MODS) is characterized by the progressive dysfunction of two or more organ systems. The clinical course of MODS typically results in prolonged hospital stays, during which potentially enormous resources are utilized. Despite the expenditure of significant time, resources, and technology, the mortality rate from MODS remains high. Through identification of risk factors and timely interventions, nurses can have an important role in detecting and preventing this highly lethal cascade of events.

This self-study module is divided into five sections. Section One describes the local inflammatory response to injury. Section Two discusses how the local response can progress to pathophysiologic changes associated with a systemic inflammatory response. This is followed by Section Three, the progression to MODS. As pathophysiologic changes continue, organ involvement and dysfunction can occur remote from the initial site of injury, as discussed in Section Four. Nursing management of the patient with MODS is presented in Section Five.

Each section includes a set of review questions to help the learner evaluate his or her understanding of the section's content before moving on to the next section. All Section Reviews include answers. It is suggested that the learner review those concepts answered incorrectly in the review questions before proceeding to the next section.

PRETEST

1. Which of the following elicit the inflammatory response?
   A. mediators
   B. endotoxin
   C. bacteria
   D. heat
2. Which of the following cells are most important in the inflammatory process?
   A. neutrophils
   B. mast cells
   C. epithelial cells
   D. endothelial cells
3. Systemic inflammatory response syndrome (SIRS) can be characterized by the following (choose all that apply)
   A. temperature greater than 38°C (100°F)
   B. heart rate less than 80 beats per minute
   C. white blood cells greater than 12,000 cells/mm^3
   D. immature bands (greater than 10 percent)
4. A theory has emerged that suggests the SIRS response is rapidly followed by
   A. death
   B. septic shock
   C. mixed antagonistic response syndrome
   D. compensatory anti-inflammatory response syndrome
5. MODS is a progressive dysfunction of at least
   A. one organ
   B. two organ systems
   C. three organ systems
   D. four organ systems
6. Two forms of MODS are
   A. initial and progressive
   B. progressive and refractory
   C. local and systemic
   D. primary and secondary

7. Which of the following is essential to prevent mortality in MODS?
   A. early recognition and management
   B. strict aseptic technique
   C. preventing febrile states
   D. strict handwashing

8. Jaundice and coagulopathy characterize
   A. renal failure
   B. hematologic failure
   C. liver failure
   D. MODS

Pretest answers are found on MyNursingKit.

SECTION ONE: The Endothelial Cell and Local Inflammatory Response

At the completion of this section, the learner will be able to state the physiologic changes that occur during the local inflammatory process.

An initiating event, such as an injury, invading organism, or ischemia, can trigger inflammation. The goal of a local inflammatory process is to limit the extent of injury and promote healing. Normally, the inflammatory process is contained within a local environment by a complex system of checks and balances. Mediators elicit the inflammatory response. **Mediators** are bioactive substances that stimulate physiologic changes in cells. They are released from endothelial cells.

Endothelial cells are not simply cells that line the inside of all blood vessels; they have many important functions (Table 19–1). They are very active cells that are constantly sensing and responding to alterations in the local cell environment. Endothelial cells "cross talk" to other cells including erythrocytes, platelets, leukocytes, and vascular smooth muscle cells (Abraham & Singer, 2007). They are activated by alterations in the local environment, such as minor trauma to blood vessels, transient bacteria, and stress. Endothelial cell activation is a normal adaptive response under physiologic conditions, but it also occurs in response to pathophysiologic conditions. When bacteria invade local tissues, endothelial cells are activated and release mediators. These mediators stimulate the inflammatory process, recruit white blood cells to the area, and promote localized clotting to contain the infection. During this process, endothelial cells undergo necrosis and **apoptosis,** or programmed cell death, as tissues are repaired.

The endothelium orchestrates this local physiologic response by promoting the adhesion and transmigration of white blood cells, altering local vasomotor tone, increasing permeability, inducing thrombin generation and fibrin formation, and triggering apoptosis. Normally, local and systemic negative feedback mechanisms maintain the response at local sites and dampen the response at more remote sites. Inflammation-induced activation of coagulation, deposition of fibrin, and inhibition of fibrinolysis is instrumental in containing the inflammatory activity to the site of infection (Boos, Goon, & Lip, 2006).

How endothelial cells respond to alterations in the environment differ, according to the host genetics, age, gender, nature of the pathogen, and location of the vascular bed. Endothelial cells can undergo intracellular structural changes in their cell membranes, cytoplasm, or nucleus. However, they more commonly undergo functional changes that include shifts in intracellular homeostatic balance, adhesion of certain cells (particularly white blood cells) to their cell membrane, altered vasomotor tone regulation, loss of barrier function, and apoptosis. The most important endothelial function is probably the regulation of permeability (Abraham & Singer, 2007).

Containment of the localized inflammatory response limits further damage to the host and preserves the integrity of uninvolved endothelial cells. When the host response generalizes, it escapes the well-developed local checks and balances, resulting in an unregulated inflammatory response with widespread involvement of endothelial cells and a more generalized activation of inflammation and coagulation. This type of generalized response can lead to systemic inflammatory response syndrome (SIRS) and multiple organ dysfunction syndrome (MODS), which are discussed in the next sections.

TABLE 19–1 Functions of Endothelial Cells

Mediate vasomotor tone
Maintain vessel wall integrity
Control cellular and nutrient "traffic"
Regulate inflammatory and anti-inflammatory mediators
Participate in generating new blood vessels
Undergo apoptosis

SECTION ONE REVIEW

1. A local inflammatory response can be initiated by which of the following? (choose all that apply)
   A. injury
   B. ischemia
   C. bacteria
   D. biologically active mediators

2. Mediators stimulate the local inflammatory response. They are released from activated
   A. platelets
   B. endothelial cells
   C. epithelial cells
   D. bacteria

(continued)

(continued)

3. The endothelium orchestrates the local inflammatory response by which of the following? (choose all that apply)
   A. decreasing capillary permeability
   B. promoting adhesion of white blood cells
   C. altering local vasomotor tone
   D. inducing thrombin generation
4. Endothelial cells "cross talk" to (choose all that apply)
   A. erythrocytes
   B. platelets
   C. leukocytes
   D. vascular smooth muscle cells
5. One of the most important functions of endothelial cells is regulation of
   A. inflammation
   B. immunity
   C. permeability
   D. coagulation

Answers: 1. (A, B, C), 2. B, 3. (B, C, D), 4. (A, B, C, D) 5. C

SECTION TWO: Systemic Inflammatory Response Syndrome

At the completion of this section, the learner will be able to contrast the physiologic changes that occur with the local inflammatory response with those that occur with the systemic inflammatory response syndrome.

As discussed in Section One, localized inflammation is a physiologic defense mechanism that occurs in response to an injury, ischemia, or an invading pathogen. Containment of the localized inflammatory response limits further damage to the host and preserves the integrity of uninvolved endothelial cells. This response must be tightly controlled by the body at the local injury site or the response becomes overly activated, leading to an exaggerated, systemic response. When the local inflammatory response becomes generalized, a dysregulated inflammatory response occurs with widespread endothelial cell involvement and a more generalized activation of inflammation and coagulation.

Systemic inflammatory response syndrome (SIRS) is a term used to describe a condition in which there is a systemic (rather than local) inflammatory process. The initiating event may be caused by infection, trauma, major surgery, acute pancreatitis, or burns. This systemic response is manifested by two or more conditions as listed in Table 19–2 (American College of Chest Physicians & Society of Critical Care Medicine, 1992).

The term SIRS recognizes that in critical illness, clinical inflammation can arise from infectious and noninfectious stimuli. SIRS denotes systemic inflammation regardless of its cause. When the cause of SIRS is infection, the process is termed **sepsis.** The term *MODS* indicates that this complication is variable in what specific organ systems are involved and in the magnitude of physiologic derangement that occurs.

Some patients with infection, trauma, or surgery will have only mild SIRS and minor organ dysfunction that resolves rapidly, whereas others exhibit a massive inflammatory reaction and die from profound shock. As summarized in Table 19–3, a number of patient-related and treatment related risk factors for the development of SIRS have been identified (Kohl & Deutschman, 2006).

The frequent association of MODS with sepsis, SIRS, acute respiratory distress syndrome (ARDS), and other inflammatory processes suggests there is a link to the complex pathophysiologic processes that are characteristic of SIRS. A theory has emerged that suggests that the SIRS response is rapidly followed in most patients by a compensatory anti-inflammatory response syndrome (CARS). CARS occurs in an attempt to limit SIRS. The balance between proinflammatory (SIRS) and anti-inflammatory (CARS) has been referred to as the mixed antagonistic response syndrome (MARS). The balance is difficult to achieve and typically either proinflammatory or anti-inflammatory responses predominate. When there are excessive proinflammatory responses, organ dysfunction is likely to occur. When there is excessive anti-inflammatory response, the patient is at risk for secondary or opportunistic infections, which serve as additional insults to trigger the SIRS response (Abraham & Singer, 2007).

TABLE 19–2 Definition of SIRS

Two or more of the following:
Temperature greater than 38°C or less than 36°C
Heart rate greater than 90 beats per min
Respiratory rate greater than 20 breaths/min or $Paco_2$ less than 32 mm Hg
White blood cell count greater than 12,000/mm^3 or less than 4,000/mm^3, or greater than 10% immature (band) forms

TABLE 19–3 Risk Factors for Developing SIRS

PATIENT-RELATED	TREATMENT-RELATED
Age greater than 65	Inadequate or delayed resuscitation
Baseline organ dysfunction	Persistent inflammation or infectious focus
Alcohol abuse	Immunosuppression (steroids, chemotherapy, transplant, asplenia)
Malnutrition	
Immunosuppression (cancer, AIDS)	
Mechanical ventilation	

SECTION TWO REVIEW

1. Which of the following may cause SIRS? (choose all that apply)
   - A. obesity
   - B. infection
   - C. trauma
   - D. major surgery
2. Your patient is assessed to have the following: temperature 39.5°C, heart rate 110 beats per minute, respiratory rate 12/min, WBC 15,000 cells/mm^3 with greater than 10 percent bands. This patient may have which of the following?
   - A. MODS
   - B. bacteremia
   - C. SIRS
   - D. a local inflammatory response
3. The pathogenesis of SIRS is
   - A. not associated with MODS
   - B. associated with MODS
   - C. occurs in an attempt to limit CARS
   - D. associated with an excessive anti-inflammatory response
4. Which of the following are risk factors for developing SIRS? (choose all that apply)
   - A. age greater than 65
   - B. alcohol abuse
   - C. inadequate resuscitation
   - D. mechanical ventilation
5. When there is an excessive anti-inflammatory response, the patient is at risk for
   - A. MARS
   - B. SIRS
   - C. CARS
   - D. opportunistic infections

Answers: 1. (B, C, D) 2. C, 3. B, 4. (A, B, C) 5. D

SECTION THREE: Multiple Organ Dysfunction Syndrome

At the completion of this section, the learner will be able to discuss four pathophysiologic changes that occur with MODS.

Multiple organ dysfunction syndrome (MODS), a complication of critical illness, is characterized by progressive (but potentially reversible) dysfunction of two or more organ systems and develops after an acute life-threatening disruption of systemic body homeostasis. MODS, the most common cause of death among patients requiring care in an ICU, is the clinical manifestation of a dysregulated inflammatory response (Fink & Delude, 2005). Physiologic derangements of MODS occur as the result of an insult that initiates the inflammatory response. Although infection is the most common insult, numerous other stimuli have been implicated and are recognized as being risk factors for developing MODS. The pathophysiology of MODS is complex and not completely understood. It appears that MODS is the result of uncontrolled systemic infection.

MODS appears to follow two distinct pathways (Fig. 19–1). **Primary MODS** occurs as the direct consequence of an initiating event. It occurs early and may be the direct consequence of injury, hemorrhage, or hypoxemia. Early MODS tends to occur in the first 72 hours of admission and late MODS occurs after that (Lausevic et al., 2008). Primary MODS is thought to be the result of inadequate oxygen delivery to cells and a failure of the microcirculation to remove metabolic end products. As progressively more cells die, organ dysfunction and failure occur. Acute tubular necrosis is an example of primary MODS. **Secondary MODS** is an event that occurs later in the patient's course, often weeks after the initial acute insult, and is thought to be secondary to SIRS. The initial insult is thought to prime the inflammatory response and a second insult reactivates it at an exaggerated level.

Risk factors for primary and secondary MODS have been identified. Risk factors for primary MODS include severity of injury, shock, or SIRS; and risk factors for secondary MODS include infection, transfusion, and multiple surgical operations. Advancing age and preexisting medical conditions have also been identified as host factors for MODS (Table 19–4).

The pathophysiology of MODS is complex. Literally hundreds of biochemical and cellular abnormalities have been described. There appear to be four prominent explanations for the pathologic changes that occur with MODS, including (1) uncontrolled systemic inflammation, (2) tissue hypoxia, (3) unregulated apoptosis, and (4) microvascular coagulopathy.

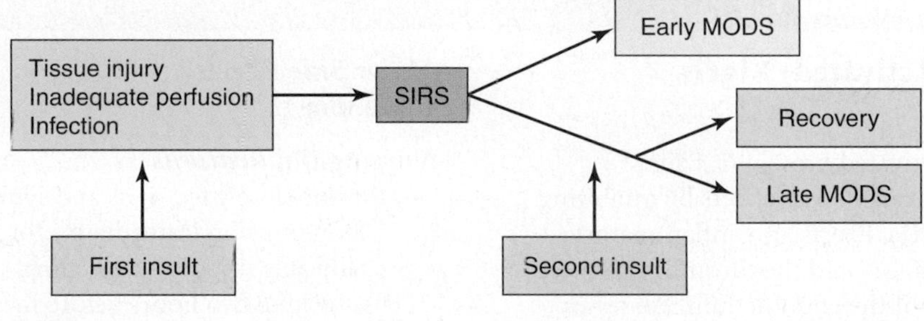

Figure 19–1 ■ MODS pathways.

TABLE 19–4 Advancing Age and MODS

Those over 45 years of age have two to three times greater likelihood of developing MODS
Advancing age affects all organ systems
Worse outcome in elderly is attributed to presence of preexisting conditions (cirrhosis, ischemic heart disease, COPD, diabetes)
Advancing age decreases functional reserve and impairs stress response

Uncontrolled Systemic Inflammation

Clinical evidence of systemic inflammation is evident in almost all patients with MODS. A large number of proinflammatory mediators have been implicated in initiating and potentiating a systemic inflammatory response, but the mechanisms through which these mediators induce organ injury are not clear. During sepsis, early activation of immune cells (monocytes, macrophages, lymphocytes, neutrophils) is followed by down regulation of their activity that leads to a state of immune deficiency and increased risk of superinfection (Abraham & Singer, 2007). Proinflammatory mediators can increase capillary permeability resulting in edema in organs such as the lungs (ARDS) or brain (altered sensorium). Proinflammatory mediators cause the release of nitric oxide from endothelial cells, which results in vasodilation. Neutrophils induce the release of oxygen radicals and proteolytic enzymes. Neutrophils also potentiate increased vascular permeability.

Tissue Hypoxia

Decreased oxygen delivery or reduced cellular use of oxygen inhibits normal cell function. Current theories on the pathophysiology of MODS indicate that the common pathway to organ dysfunction is cellular hypoxia. Even though the patient may appear clinically to have adequate oxygenation, regional tissue hypoxia may occur, particularly in the intestinal tract and brain. Tissue hypoxia may result from derangements in the cellular use of oxygen in the face of adequate oxygen delivery, a pathologic state termed **cytopathic hypoxia.**

As a result of cytopathic hypoxia, a state of metabolic shutdown occurs because of an inadequate supply of energy to power the various cellular processes (Singer, 2005). As cells receive less oxygen for adenosine triphosphate (ATP) production, cells cannot perform protein synthesis or maintain function of sodium-potassium pumps. When this failure is widespread and severe, organ function is compromised.

Unregulated Apoptosis

The controlled process of cellular death is called apoptosis. Derangements in the normal expression of apoptosis appear to be important in MODS. There appears to be an increase in apoptosis in some cell types (lymphocytes, gut epithelial cells) and delayed apoptosis with others (neutrophils). In addition, excessive apoptosis occurs in certain organ systems, such as the liver, kidney, and heart.

Microvascular Coagulopathy

The coagulopathy associated with MODS is biologically complex and intertwined with normal physiologic processes. The mechanisms that regulate inflammation are linked with those that control coagulation. Microvascular thrombosis is an important factor in the development of MODS.

Coagulation is initiated through tissue factor on the endothelial cell membrane. Tissue factor is released in response to the presence of endotoxin, or inflammatory cytokines. Tissue factor activates factor VII of the extrinsic pathway of the coagulation cascade. The end result of the coagulation cascade is the formation of fibrin clots. The fibrin clot plays a critical role in hemostasis and localizing microorganisms. However, these microvascular clots impede blood flow and oxygen delivery to cells. This leads to the release of further inflammatory mediators. Anticoagulation mechanisms, such as those mediated by activated protein C, are impaired. Protein C is activated in the presence of thrombin that is bound to thrombomodulin. Activated protein C acts as a feedback messenger to inhibit further thrombin generation. In addition to its antithrombotic properties, activated protein C has anti-inflammatory and profibrinolytic properties (see RELATED PHARMACOTHERAPY box: Activated Protein C). Clinical studies indicate that administration of activated protein C improves outcomes of patients with sepsis (see Module 18, Alterations in Oxygen Delivery and Consumption: Shock States). Drotrecogin alpha (activated), a recombinant form of human activated protein C, has been shown to decrease markers of coagulation and inflammation (Bernard et al., 2001).

RELATED PHARMACOTHERAPY: Activated Protein C

Drotrecogin Alfa (Activated) Xigris

Action and Uses

Recombinant form of activated protein C. Exerts antithrombotic and anticoagulation effects by inhibiting clotting factor Va and VIIIa. Exerts anti-inflammatory effect by inhibiting mediators and the thrombin-induced inflammatory responses of the endothelium. Possesses profibrinolytic and anti-inflammatory properties. Reduces mortality in patients with sepsis and evidence of MODS.

Major Side Effects

Bleeding

Nursing Implications

Monitor closely for signs and symptoms of hemorrhage. Stop infusion immediately for signs and symptoms of clinically important bleeding.

Discontinue two hours before invasive procedures.

Monitor prothrombin time closely.

SECTION THREE REVIEW

1. MODS is characterized by the dysfunction of how many organ systems?
   A. one
   B. two or more
   C. three or more
   D. four or more
2. Primary MODS can occur in response to
   A. the insult itself
   B. secondary complications
   C. an exaggerated SIRS
   D. septic shock
3. Advancing age is a risk factor for developing MODS because the elderly
   A. don't have money to pay for services
   B. don't take antibiotics as prescribed
   C. have decreased functional reserve
   D. have increased functional reserve
4. Early MODS tends to occur within ______ hours of admission.
   A. 12
   B. 24
   C. 48
   D. 72
5. Which of the following occur as a result of cytopathic hypoxia?
   A. metabolic shutdown
   B. apoptosis
   C. uncontrolled systemic inflammation
   D. tissue hypoxia

Answers: 1. B, 2. A, 3. C, 4. D, 5. A

SECTION FOUR: Organ Involvement and Failure

At the completion of this section, the learner will be able to identify the seven most common organ systems that fail as a result of the SIRS process.

As the pathophysiologic changes continue, organ dysfunction continues as well. Organ dysfunction can occur far from the initial injury site as a result of SIRS. Mediators enable organ-to-organ interaction. There appears to be "cross talk" between organs. The lungs and kidneys are particularly vulnerable to distant organ injury. This may be due to leakage of mediators from an injury site into the systemic circulation. Examples include translocation of endotoxin from the gut into the portal circulation and leakage of proinflammatory mediators from the lung into the circulation (Abraham & Singer, 2007). Organ ischemia and cellular damage perpetuate SIRS, which perpetuates MODS. A vicious cycle develops. As each additional organ fails, mortality escalates.

Several different scoring systems and assessment tools have been proposed for the use of quantifying the extent of organ system dysfunction, but to date there has not been uniform acceptance of one tool over another. Most of the tools use an assessment of six major organ systems: respiratory, cardiovascular, neurologic, renal, hepatic, and hematologic. Evaluation of disease severity involves assessment of several major organ systems for common indications of dysfunction in those organs. One of the most common tools used is the Sequential Organ Failure Assessment (SOFA) score (Table 19–5). The main purpose of the SOFA score is to describe the sequence of complications, not to predict mortality. The scores can be calculated daily

TABLE 19–5 Sequential Organ Failure Assessment (SOFA) Score

ORGAN FAILURE	VARIABLE	SCORE 0	SCORE 1	SCORE 2	SCORE 3	SCORE 4
Respiratory	Pa_{CO_2}/Fi_{O_2}	≥400	<400	<300	<200 on MV	<100 on MV
Hematology	Platelets, 10^9/L	≥150	<150	<100	<50	<20
Liver	Bilirubin, mg/dL	<1.2	1.2-1.9	2.0-5.9	6.0-11.9	>12.0
Cardiovascular	MAP, mm Hg	≥70	<70			
	Dopamine, mcg/kg/min			≤5	>5	>15
	Dobutamine, mcg/kg/min			Any dose		
	Epinephrine, mcg/kg/min				≤0.1	>0.1
	Norepinephrine, mcg/kg/min				≤0.1	>0.1
Central Nervous System	GCS	15	13-14	10-12	6-9	<6
Renal	Creatinine, mg/dL	<1.2	1.2-1.9	2.0-3.4	3.5-4.9	≥5.0
	Urine Output, mL/day	≥500			<500	<200

Pa_{O_2} = partial pressure of arterial oxygen; Fi_{O_2} = Fraction of inspired oxygen; GCS = Glasgow Coma Scale; MAP = mean arterial pressure; MV = mechanical ventilation
Data from Ferreira, F. L., Bota, D. P., Bross, A. et al. (2001). Serial evaluation of SOFA score to predict outcome in critically ill patients. *JAMA, 266*; 1754–1758.

to provide an assessment of the patient's ICU course, the effects of therapeutic interventions, and help gain an understanding of what ICU-acquired organ dysfunction is (Afessa, Gajic, & Keegan, 2007).

The lungs are usually the first to show signs of dysfunction, and respiratory failure rapidly progresses to ARDS. The respiratory system is the main organ system affected in MODS. Many conditions have been associated with ARDS either as a direct result of injury to the lung or as a result of a pulmonary response to a systemic insult. The most common direct, nonsurgical cause of ARDS is pneumonia. ARDS risk factors in the surgical patient and trauma patient include sepsis, major trauma, multiple transfusions, aspiration of gastric contents, pulmonary contusion, pneumonia, and smoke inhalation. The lungs are particularly at risk for dysfunction when there is a loss of the alveolar epithelial barrier. The alveolar epithelium usually forms a tight barrier so that even small molecules and electrolytes can't pass. The epithelium also produces surfactant to maintain normal stability and remove excess alveolar fluid. Loss of the alveolar epithelial barrier, as in sepsis, allows leakage of proteins to and from the lungs, and decreased rate of fluid clearance and alveolar collapse (Matthay, Robriquet, & Fang, 2005).

The cardiovascular dysfunction of MODS includes abnormalities of cardiac function (hypotension unresponsive to fluid administration, dysrhythmias) and abnormalities of peripheral vascular function (increased capillary permeability, edema, alterations in regional blood flow). Cardiovascular failure has been defined as a product of heart rate and the difference between mean arterial pressure and right atrial pressure (HR × [MAP-RAP]). This formula, called the pressure adjusted heart rate (PAR), is analogous to the PaO_2/FiO_2 ratio with ARDS and is used as a measure of cardiovascular dysfunction in MODS. Increasing values of the PAR reflect worsening cardiovascular function.

Neurologic dysfunction is manifested in MODS as alterations in level of consciousness, confusion, and psychosis. There are many potential causes but the pathogenesis of these neurologic changes are controversial. They may occur as a result of hypoperfusion, microvascular coagulopathy, or cerebral ischemia. Peripheral nervous system dysfunction presents as peripheral neuropathy and includes debility, muscle weakness, and atrophy. Risk factors include prolonged sedation or therapeutic paralysis and bedrest, aminoglycoside therapy, malnutrition, electrolyte abnormalities, and muscle deconditioning from disuse and lack of exercise. Despite its limitations in the sedated and mechanically ventilated patient, the Glasgow Coma Scale is the most widely used measure of neurologic function.

The development of acute renal failure is multifactorial and can occur as the result of toxic or ischemic insults to renal tubular cells. Renal dysfunction tends to develop later in the course of MODS. Loss of renal function is evidenced by a rise in serum levels of substances normally excreted by the kidneys including creatinine, nitrogen, potassium, and drug metabolites. Regardless of the serum creatinine level, mortality appears to be lower when urine output is greater than 400 mL/day in an average sized adult.

Hepatic failure involves progressive dysfunction in liver functions. Abnormalities of its synthesizing functions include low serum albumin, fibrinogen, and other clotting factors. Liver dysfunction typically manifests as high levels of serum bilirubin.

Gastrointestinal (GI) bleeding from acute stress ulceration of the stomach is not as common as it used to be. There are no reliable measures of GI function in MODS. There is subjective evidence of GI dysfunction with the development of an ileus or intolerance to enteral tube feedings (lack of absorption or diarrhea).

The most common hematologic dysfunction in MODS is thrombocytopenia secondary to increased consumption, sequestration of platelets in the vasculature, and impaired thrombopoesis as a result of bone marrow suppression. In its most severe form, the hematologic dysfunction of MODS is disseminated intravascular coagulation (DIC). DIC is characterized by widespread intravascular clotting with bleeding secondary to consumption of coagulation factors.

SECTION FOUR REVIEW

1. Respiratory dysfunction is characterized by
   - **A.** a high $PaCO_2$ with a high PaO_2
   - **B.** excessive secretions
   - **C.** rapid Kassmaul-like breathing
   - **D.** a decrease in PaO_2/FiO_2 ratio
2. Which of the following reflects worsening cardiovascular function?
   - **A.** a high cardiac output
   - **B.** increasing PAR values
   - **C.** increasing PaO_2/FiO_2
   - **D.** tachycardia
3. A lower mortality in renal failure with MODS occurs when
   - **A.** urine output is greater than 400 mL/day
   - **B.** serum creatinine is greater than 4.0 mg/dL
   - **C.** neurologic function is maintained
   - **D.** hemodialysis is delayed until absolutely necessary
4. The most severe manifestation of hematologic dysfunction is
   - **A.** anemia
   - **B.** thrombocytopenia
   - **C.** DIC
   - **D.** jaundice
5. Loss of the alveolar epithelial barrier allows (choose all that apply)
   - **A.** leakage of proteins to the lungs
   - **B.** leakage of proteins from the lungs
   - **C.** alveolar collapse
   - **D.** decreased rate of fluid clearance

Answers: 1. D, 2. B, 3. A, 4. C, 5. (A, B, C, D)

SECTION FIVE: Nursing Management of MODS

At the completion of this section, the learner will be able to describe the collaborative management of the patient with MODS.

An awareness of the natural progression of SIRS to MODS may help the nurse to identify patients at risk and prevent the progression of SIRS to MODS. Awareness of SIRS and MODS criteria can help nurses promote early diagnosis and treatment. Early recognition and management of MODS is essential to prevent escalating mortality rates. A number of nursing measures can be used to assess and monitor patients for MODS.

Continuous monitoring of clinical and physiologic parameters, early recognition of changes, and appropriate interventions are cornerstone to the management of patients with MODS (Singh & Evans, 2006). These parameters include monitoring of electrocardiograms, temperature, arterial and mixed venous oxygen saturation, central venous pressure, lactate and cardiac output. Nursing assessments are crucial to early identification of patients who may be progressing from SIRS to MODS. There is no definitive treatment for MODS. Current management of patients with MODS is focused on supporting organ function (See NURSING CARE: MODS box).

Patients at risk for primary and secondary MODS should be identified (Section Three). The nurse should monitor vital signs indicative of SIRS including hypo/hyperthermia, tachycardia, tachypnea, and hypotension. Signs of organ dysfunction should be identified early. Hypotension may be present as a result of external loss of fluids and internal fluid shifts, vasodilation and loss of normal vascular tone. Although cardiac output may be elevated, myocardial function is often depressed (Abraham & Singer, 2007). Early correction of hypotension and tissue hypoperfusion has a major impact on survival.

Considerable attention has been paid to the role of hyperglycemia in the pathogenesis of MODS since the finding that intensive insulin therapy with tight glycemic control resulted in decreased mortality and prevention of MODS (Van den Berghe, Wouters, & Weekers, 2001). High glucose levels are toxic to hepatocytes, neurons, renal tubular cells, endothelial cells and immune cells. Maintaining adherence to ICU tight glycemic control protocols is an important nursing intervention to help prevent MODS.

Nurses play a vital role in preventing, recognizing, and managing patients with sepsis. Prevention of sepsis includes enforcement of infection control measures and measures to prevent nosocomial infections, including oral care, proper positioning (elevated head of bed during mechanical ventilation), turning, skin care, invasive catheter care, and wound care.

In addition to providing comprehensive treatment of sepsis, including organ system support for patients with MODS, monitoring and reporting responses to therapies are essential aspects of nursing care. There is increasing evidence that many current treatments may interfere with the body's attempt to correct MODS and these therapies may actually have detrimental consequences (Singer & Glynne, 2005). Examples include sedatives, antibiotics, blood transfusions, inotropes, and mechanical ventilation (Singer, 2007).

Emerging Evidence

- Intensive renal support in critically ill patients with acute renal failure did not decrease mortality, improve recovery of kidney function, or reduce the rate of nonrenal organ failure as compared with less-intensive renal therapy involving a defined dose of intermittent hemodialysis three times a week and continuous renal replacement therapy at 20 mL/kg/hour (*Veterans Administration/National Institutes of Health, 2008*).
- Pathophysiological processes in the first few days after traumatic injury are important for the development of MODS. The most important parameters associated with the development of MODS were serum interleukin-6 concentration of the first day of hospitalization and the number of positive SIRS criteria on the fourth day of hospitalization (*Lausevic, Lausevic, Stankovic et al., 2008*).
- In medical records with sepsis, early enteral feeding with glutamine, vitamins C and E, beta-carotene, selenium, zinc, and butyrate resulted in a significantly faster recovery of organ function (*Beale, Sherry, Lei et al., 2008*).

NURSING CARE: MODS

Expected Patient Outcomes and Related Interventions

Outcome: Optimize pulmonary gas exchange

Assess and compare to established norms, patient baselines and trends.

Parameters and calculate SOFA score.

Respiratory rate, breath sounds, tidal volumes, peak and plateau pressures, assess for dyspnea or evidence of increased work of breathing (use of accessory muscles).

Temperature.

Pulse oximetry and end-tidal CO_2 if ordered.

Arterial blood gases.

Obtain sputum cultures as ordered.

Obtain timely and accurate serum antibiotic peak and trough levels as ordered.

Implement interventions to optimize pulmonary gas exchange.

Mechanical ventilation settings and parameters as ordered.

Elevate head of bed at least 30 degrees.

Decrease patient oxygen needs by promoting rest, comfort and relief of pain and anxiety.

Position patient to improve diaphragm excursion.

Perform tracheal suctioning as needed.

Administer fluids as ordered to prevent dehydration of secretions.

(*continued*)

NURSING CARE *(continued)*

Administer related drug therapy and monitor for therapeutic and nontherapeutic effects.
IV antibiotics
Beta-adrenergic agents that promote bronchodilation
Related nursing diagnoses
Impaired gas exchange
Ineffective breathing patterns
Ineffective airway clearance

Outcome: Optimize tissue perfusion

Assess and compare to established norms, patient baselines and trends.
Peripheral perfusion, capillary refill, skin temperature/color, peripheral pulses.
Mean arterial pressure, pressure adjusted heart rate, hemodynamic parameters (CVP, PAWP, CO), lactate, arterial and mixed venous oxygen saturation.
Monitor ECG.
Implement interventions to optimize tissue perfusion.
Administer supplemental oxygen as ordered.
Administer IV fluids as ordered.
Implement interventions to decrease oxygen consumption.
Mechanical ventilation as ordered.
Administer sedative, analgesics, anxiolytics as ordered.
Implement nonpharmacologic interventions to decrease pain and anxiety.
Position patient to maximize comfort.
Provide calm, quiet environment.
Offer support to decrease anxiety.
Administer related drug therapy and monitor for therapeutic and nontherapeutic effects.
Administer inotropic agents as ordered (Dobutamine [Dobutrex]).
Administer vasoconstricting agents as ordered (Norepinephrine [Levophed]).
Administer activated protein-C as ordered.
Related nursing diagnoses
Altered tissue perfusion
Decreased cardiac output
Activity intolerance

SECTION FIVE REVIEW

1. Which of the following is essential to preventing mortality in MODS?
   A. early recognition and management of MODS
   B. administration of acetaminophen for febrile episodes
   C. prompt administration of aminoglycosides as ordered
   D. knowing how to operate a dialysis machine
2. Vital signs indicative of SIRS include which of the following? (choose all that apply)
   A. hypothermia
   B. tachycardia
   C. hypertension
   D. tachypnea
3. Continuous monitoring of patients with MODS should include (choose all that apply)
   A. electrocardiogram
   B. temperature
   C. mixed venous oxygen saturation
   D. lactate
4. Which of the following is true about cardiac function in MODS? (choose all that apply)
   A. cardiac output is elevated
   B. myocytes undergo necrosis
   C. myocardial function is depressed
   D. myocytes undergo apoptosis
5. Which of the following has been shown to contribute to MODS? (choose all that apply)
   A. sedatives
   B. antibiotics
   C. mechanical ventilation
   D. blood transfusions

Answers: 1. A, 2. (A, B, D) 3. (A, B, C, D) 4. (A, C) 5. (A, B, C, D)

POSTTEST

1. The goal of local inflammation is to
   A. produce heat
   B. produce swelling
   C. kill bacteria
   D. limit the extent of injury and promote healing
2. Endogenous substances that stimulate physiologic and pathophysiologic changes are called
   A. endotoxins
   B. mediators
   C. white blood cells
   D. neurotransmitters
3. SIRS is an exaggerated systemic response to
   A. bacteria
   B. sepsis
   C. local inflammation
   D. endotoxins

4. Which of the following is a major etiologic factor in the development of MODS? (choose all that apply)
   A. advancing age
   B. malnutrition
   C. immunosuppresion
   D. delayed resuscitation
5. A patient has a temperature of 35.5°C, heart rate 120 bpm, and a white blood cell count of 3,000/mm^3. This patient may have which of the following?
   A. MODS
   B. bacteremia
   C. SIRS
   D. a local inflammatory response
6. Secondary MODS occurs in response to
   A. sepsis
   B. SIRS
   C. renal failure
   D. cardiac arrest
7. Prominent explanations for the pathologic changes that occur with MODS include (choose all that apply)
   A. uncontrolled systemic circulation
   B. tissue hypoxia
   C. unregulated apoptosis
   D. microvascular coagulation
8. Calculate the SOFA score for a patient with a PaO_2/FiO_2 of 100 when on mechanical ventilation, platelets 18 x 10^9/L, bilirubin 12.5 mg/dL, MAP less than 70 mm Hg on norepinephrine 0.2 mcg/kg/min, GCS 5, creatinine 5.0 mg/dL and urine output 198 mL/day.
   A. 7
   B. 17
   C. 29
   D. 45
9. Which of the following is true about definitive treatment for MODS? (choose all that apply)
   A. there is no definitive treatment for MODS
   B. current management is focused on supporting organ function
   C. continuous renal replacement therapy must be used for patients with MODS
   D. mechanical ventilation must be used for patients with MODS
10. High glucose levels are toxic to (choose all that apply)
   A. heart muscle
   B. adipose tissue
   C. endothelial cells
   D. renal tubular cells

Posttest answers with rationale are found on MyNursingKit.

REFERENCES

Abraham E., & Singer, M. (2007). Mechanisms of sepsis-induced organ dysfunction. *Crit Care Med 35*(10), 2408–2416.

Afessa B., Gajic O., Keegan, M. T. (2007). Severity of illness and organ failure assessment in adult intensive care units. *Crit Care Clin 23*:639–658.

American College of Chest Physicians & Society of Critical Care Medicine. (1992). The AACP/SCCM consensus conference on sepsis and organ failure. *Chest 101,* 1481–1483.

Beale, B. J., Sherry, T., Lei, K., et al. (2008). Early enteral supplementation with key pharmaconutrients improves SOFA score in critically ill patients with sepsis: Outcome of a randomized, controlled, double blind study. *Crit Care Med 36*(1), 131–144.

Bernard, G. R., Ely, E. W., Wright, T. J., et al. (2001). Safety and dose relationship of recombinant human activated protein C for coagulopathy in severe sepsis. *Critl Care Med 29*: 2051–2059.

Boos, C. J., Goon, P. K., Lip, G. Y. (2006). The endothelium, inflammation, and coagulation in sepsis. *Clin Pharmacol Ther 79*: 20–22.

Fink, M. P. & Delude, R. L. (2005). Epithelial barrier dysfunction: A unifying theme to explain the pathogenesis of multiple organ dysfunction at the cellular level. *Crit Care Clinics 21*:177–196.

Kohl, B. A., & Deutschman, C. S. (2006). The inflammatory response to surgery and trauma. *Curr Opinion in Crit Care 12*:325–332.

Kuiper, J. W., Groeneveld J., Slutsky, A. S. et al., (2005). Mechanical ventilation and acute renal failure. *Crit Care Med 33:* 1408–1415.

Lausevic, Z., Lausevic, M., Stankovic, J. T., et al. (2008). Predicting multiple organ failure in patients with severe trauma. *Can J Surg 51*(2):97–102.

Matthay, M. A., Robriquet, L., Fang, X. (2005). Alveolar epithelium: role of lung fluid balance and acute lung injury. *Proc Am Thorac Soc 2*:206–213.

Singer, M. & Glynne, P. (2007). Treating critical illness: the importance of first doing no harm. *PLOS Med 2*:e167.

Singer, M. (2005). Metabolic failure. *Crit Care Med 33* (12 Suppl):S539–S542.

Singh, S. & Evans, T. W. (2006). Organ dysfunction during sepsis. *Intens Care Med 32*:349–360.

Van den Berghe, G., Wouters, P., Weekers, F., et al. (2001). Intensive insulin therapy in critically ill patients. *New Engl J Med 345*:1359–1367.

Veterans Administration/National Institute of Health Acute Renal Failure Trial Network. (2008). Intensity of renal support in critically ill patients with acute kidney injury. *New Eng J Med 359*:7–20.

Vincent, J. L., Moreno R., Takala, J., et al. (1996). The SOFA score to describe organ dysfunction/failure: On behalf of the working group on sepsis related problems of the European Society of Intensive Care Medicine. *Intens Care Med 22*(7):707–710.

MODULE

20 Determinants and Assessment of Cerebral Tissue Perfusion

Melanie Hardin-Pierce, Karen L. Johnson

OBJECTIVES Following completion of this module, the learner will be able to

1. Explain selected anatomy and physiology of cerebral tissue perfusion.
2. Describe the components of intracranial pressure (ICP) including the Monro-Kellie hypothesis.
3. Calculate a cerebral perfusion pressure based on mean arterial pressure and intracranial pressure.
4. Describe decreased intracranial adaptive capacity, including causes and effects of increases in brain volume, cerebral blood volume, and CSF volume.
5. Assess cerebral tissue perfusion.
6. Describe procedures used in diagnosing brain injury.
7. Discuss the management of decreased cerebral tissue perfusion.

This self-study module focuses on the physiologic and pathophysiologic processes involved in cerebral tissue perfusion. This module is composed of seven sections, beginning with a brief review of anatomy and physiology pertinent to cerebral tissue perfusion. Section Two reviews pathophysiologic mechanisms that increase intracranial pressure. Section Three discusses how cerebral perfusion pressure is measured in the high-acuity setting. Section Four summarizes the causes and effects of decreased intracranial adaptive capacity. Section Five presents a wide variety of clinical assessment tools available to assess for impaired cerebral tissue perfusion and decreased intracranial adaptive capacity. Section Six provides an overview of the diagnostic procedures used for brain injury. Finally, Section Seven identifies collaborative interventions used to optimize cerebral tissue perfusion and improve intracranial adaptive capacity across medical diagnoses. Each section includes a set of review questions to help the learner evaluate his or her understanding of the section's content before moving on to the next section. All Section Reviews include answers. It is suggested that the learner review those concepts answered incorrectly in the review questions before proceeding to the next section.

PRETEST

1. Cerebral blood vessels dilate in response to
   A. increased serum oxygen
   B. increased serum carbon dioxide
   C. systemic hypertension
   D. decreased serum carbon dioxide
2. Pressure regulation is an autoregulatory mechanism whereby cerebral blood vessels constrict in response to
   A. systemic hypertension
   B. hypercarbia
   C. systemic hypotension
   D. hypoxia
3. Cerebral blood flow decreases with
   A. cerebral edema
   B. low cardiac output
   C. cerebral vasoconstriction
   D. all of the above
4. The Monro–Kellie hypothesis states that volume increases in the adult intracranial vault
   A. are initially well tolerated through compensatory mechanisms
   B. are tolerated well because of the flexibility of the cranial vault
   C. can be compensated for only by cerebrospinal fluid buffering techniques
   D. usually result in death because the vault is unable to accommodate increases in volume
5. Which of the following components of intracranial volume is displaced most easily and rapidly?
   A. brain volume
   B. cerebral blood volume
   C. CSF
   D. cranium

6. Flexion of the neck may cause elevations in intracranial volume by
   A. causing a decrease in venous outflow
   B. causing an increase in venous return
   C. causing cerebral vasodilation
   D. increasing venous outflow
7. What is the cerebral perfusion pressure if mean arterial pressure (MAP) = 95 mm Hg and intracranial pressure (ICP) = 15 mm Hg?
   A. 65 mm Hg
   B. 80 mm Hg
   C. 110 mm Hg
   D. 125 mm Hg
8. Normal cerebral perfusion pressure is
   A. highly individualized
   B. 50 to 80 mm Hg
   C. 80 to 100 mm Hg
   D. 100 to 120 mm Hg
9. Cerebral perfusion decreases when
   A. ICP is high
   B. MAP is low
   C. ICP is the same as MAP
   D. all of the above
10. Cerebral edema is caused by
   A. an increase in cerebral blood volume
   B. an increase in brain volume
   C. an increase in CSF
   D. an increase in ICP
11. An accumulation of CSF is called
   A. herniation
   B. hydrocephalus
   C. cerebral edema
   D. intracranial hypertension
12. An increase in brain volume can result in
   A. herniation
   B. cerebral vasodilation
   C. autoregulation
   D. hydrocephalus
13. Your patient responds to stimuli and the Glasgow Coma Scale (GSC) is 15. What would be your initial assessment and your next action?
   A. Level of responsiveness is intact; vital signs would be the next logical step.
   B. Level of responsiveness is most probably not intact; an in-depth neurological assessment is required.
   C. You are unable to completely evaluate the level of responsiveness and need more clinical data.
   D. The patient demonstrates no cognitive deficits; pupillary assessment would be the next logical step.
14. The most important component of the neurologic assessment is
   A. vital signs
   B. level of consciousness
   C. pupillary reactions
   D. protective reflexes
15. A unilaterally dilated pupil is indicative of
   A. atropine or atropine-like drugs
   B. a brainstem lesion
   C. opioid overdose
   D. cranial nerve lesion
16. The Glasgow Coma Scale assesses
   A. cognition
   B. speech patterns
   C. arousal
   D. problem-solving abilities
17. Mean arterial pressure should be maintained at more than ______ mm Hg to keep the cerebral perfusion pressure greater than ______ mm Hg.
   A. 90; 70
   B. 100; 80
   C. 50; 40
   D. 40; 80
18. A patient with a GCS less than ______ must have the airway secured.
   A. 9
   B. 10
   C. 13
   D. 15
19. Current guidelines recommend hyperventilation may be used to reduce ICP. What is the optimal range of $PaCO_2$?
   A. less than 25 mm Hg
   B. less than 35 mm Hg
   C. 35 to 45 mm Hg
   D. 45 to 55 mm Hg
20. Which of the following drugs may be used FIRST to reduce ICP?
   A. loop diuretics
   B. neuromuscular blocking agents
   C. barbiturates
   D. analgesics

Pretest answers are found on MyNursingKit.

SECTION ONE: Selective Anatomy and Physiology of Cerebral Tissue Perfusion

At the completion of this section, the learner will be able to explain selected anatomy and physiology of cerebral tissue perfusion (CPP).

Arterial Circulation

Cerebral arteries are structurally different from other arteries. They are thinner and more delicate and are, therefore, more susceptible to rupture with hypertension. The brain is supplied by two major pairs of arteries: the right and left internal carotid arteries and the right and left vertebral arteries (Fig. 20–1). Together their branches unite within the brain to form the **circle of Willis** a connecting junction that provides collateral blood flow to either side of the brain. The internal carotids supply the retinas and the anterior two thirds of the cerebral hemispheres via its branches: the middle cerebrals, the anterior cerebral, and the anterior and posterior communicating arteries. The middle cerebral arteries are the largest branches of the internal carotids. They supply almost the entire lateral surface of the frontal, parietal, and temporal lobes; the underlying white matter; and the basal ganglia. These are the arteries most frequently involved with strokes. The anterior communicating artery connects the anterior cerebral arteries; and the posterior communicating arteries join the posterior cerebral arteries (PCAs) to complete the circle of Willis. The circle of Willis is protective because it is the primary collateral pathway when major cerebral vessels are occluded. For example, if the carotid artery is occluded, collateral flow may still be possible via the posterior communicating or anterior cerebral arteries to ischemic brain areas.

The vertebrobasilar system supplies the posterior portion of the cerebrum, cerebellum, and brainstem. The vertebral arteries originate from the subclavian arteries, enter the cranium, and, at the pontine-medullary level, join to form the single basilar artery. The vertebral arteries supply the lateral medulla and a portion of the cerebellum. The basilar artery supplies the pons and cerebellum. It divides at the junction of the pons and midbrain into the PCAs. The PCAs supply the midbrain, diencephalon (hypothalamus, subthalamus, thalamus), and inferior portion of the cerebrum. These major arteries are called conducting arteries and their small branches, called penetrating arteries, penetrate into the depths of the brain. Penetrating arteries are frequently involved in small lacunar or ministrokes.

Venous Circulation

The venous circulation is a low-pressure system, as compared with the arterial circulation, which is a high-pressure, high-resistance system. Craniospinal veins are valveless and drain by gravity, an important characteristic to remember when positioning patients with increased **intracranial pressure** (ICP). The dura mater contains venous sinuses that collect blood from the cerebral, meningeal, and diploic veins of the cranium and empty it into the internal jugular veins. These veins drain the cerebral hemispheres and to a lesser degree the brainstem and cerebellum. When intracranial pressure (ICP) increases, venous outflow from the brain decreases because the low pressure veins are compressed.

Cerebral Oxygenation

The brain requires a continuous supply of glucose, oxygen, and substrates for energy because it cannot store oxygen, and its glucose reserves last for only a few minutes. Cerebral metabolism varies regionally, with some areas of the brain being more metabolically active than others at any given time. **Cerebral blood flow (CBF)**, or blood flow to the brain, varies regionally as well. The brain attempts to meet metabolic demands by locally increasing or decreasing CBF as needed. This localized matching of CBF with metabolism is achieved through the process of cerebral pressure **autoregulation.** Autoregulation enables cerebral arterioles to alter their blood flow within an average systemic arterial pressure limit (60 to 130 mm Hg in adults), to promote a constant blood supply to the brain regardless of systemic blood pressure fluctuations. When systemic blood pressure increases, cerebral arterioles constrict; when systemic blood pressure decreases, cerebral arterioles dilate, ensuring adequate cerebral perfusion. When CBF is inadequate to meet the brain's metabolic needs, a state of mismatching occurs, and ischemia results. Because the brain is unable to store oxygen or glucose, aerobic metabolism can no longer be supported and the brain

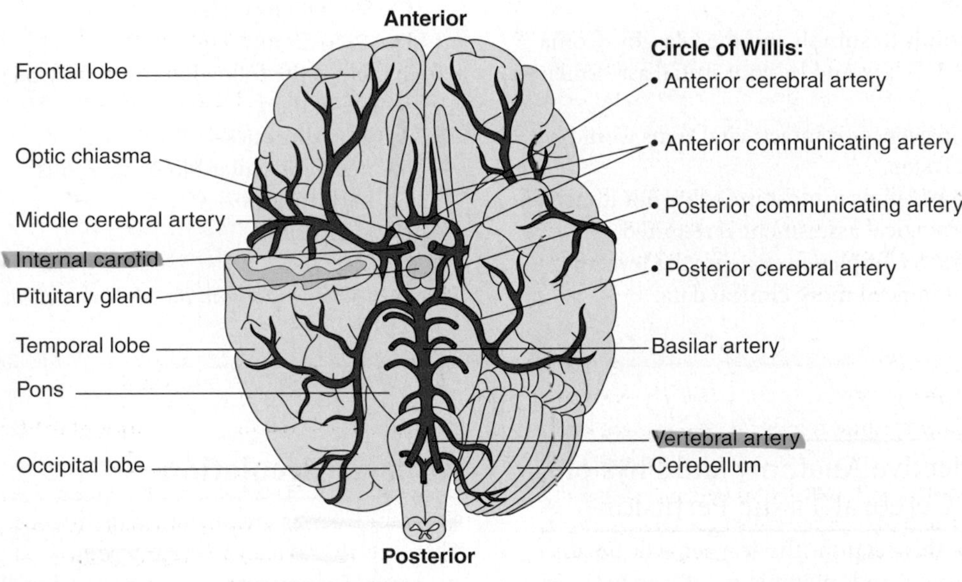

Figure 20–1 ■ Major arteries serving the brain and the Circle of Willis.

is forced to switch to anaerobic metabolism. The end product of anaerobic metabolism is lactate. Lactate accumulates in brain tissue, resulting in cerebral acidosis. Cerebral acidosis upsets the state of equilibrium in the cranial vault.

The brain, through autoregulation, has the ability to maintain constant CBF with changes in body metabolism and in situations of altered acid–base balance. An increase in body metabolic rate (such as with fever or pain) increases CBF, whereas a decrease in body metabolic rate (as with sedation, paralysis, or hypothermia) decreases CBF. Conditions that cause alkalosis (such as hypocapnia) produce cerebral vasoconstriction and a reduction of CBF. Conditions that cause acidosis (e.g., elevated lactate levels, retention of CO_2, and ischemia) produce cerebral vasodilation with an increase in CBF.

Because of the brain's attempt to match CBF with cerebral metabolism, CBF is an important variable when addressing cerebral oxygenation. Cerebral hypoxia occurs when CBF is too low to support cerebral metabolism. CBF decreases with cerebral edema, low cardiac output, or vasoconstriction. When CBF is higher than the metabolic needs of the brain, a state of **hyperemia** exists, also known as *luxury perfusion*. Patients with this condition have progressive vasodilation, increased CBF, and eventual loss of autoregulation, all of which contribute to increased ICP. Both cerebral hypoxia and hyperemia have been described as pathophysiologic changes that occur following brain injury. Maintaining adequate cerebral oxygenation is of the utmost importance to support aerobic metabolism. Every effort should be made to avoid episodes of cerebral hypoxia or hypotension.

SECTION ONE REVIEW

1. Which of the following is protective because it is the primary collateral pathway when major cerebral vessels are occluded?
   A. Circle of Willis
   B. left internal carotid artery
   C. right internal carotid artery
   D. middle cerebral artery
2. Cerebral arteries are more prone to rupture during hypertension because
   A. there are so many of them
   B. they have autoregulation
   C. they are thin and delicate
   D. they are not protected by skeletal muscles
3. Which of the following are TRUE statements about the venous circulation of the brain?
   A. Craniospinal veins are valveless.
   B. Craniospinal veins drain by gravity.
   C. The venous circulation is a low-pressure system.
   D. All of the above.
4. The localized matching of CBF with cerebral metabolism occurs through
   A. autoregulation
   B. anaerobic metabolism
   C. luxury perfusion
   D. cerebrospinal fluid

Answers: 1. A, 2. C, 3. D, 4. A

SECTION TWO: Intracranial Pressure

At the completion of this section, the learner will be able to describe the components of intracranial pressure including the Monro-Kellie hypothesis.

The intracranial vault is a rigid container within a limited space. The contents of the intracranial vault include the brain, cerebral blood volume, and cerebrospinal fluid. The volume of each component remains relatively stable (brain 80 percent; blood 12 percent; and CSF 8 percent) (LeMone & Burke, 2008). The **Monro–Kellie hypothesis** states that a change in volume of any one of these components must be accompanied by a reciprocal change in one or both of the other components. If this reciprocal change is not accomplished, the result is an increase in ICP (Barker, 2008).

Brain Volume

The brain volume is mainly water, and the majority of the water is intracellular. The brain volume remains constant through the **blood–brain barrier.** The blood–brain barrier, a network of cells and membranes in the brain capillaries, controls brain volume by regulating the solutes and water that attempt to cross it and enter the cerebral circulation. This barrier is selective in terms of membrane permeability and molecular size of the substance attempting to enter the cerebral circulation. It is permeable to water, oxygen, lipid-soluble compounds, and carbon dioxide and slightly permeable to the electrolytes. Most drugs do not cross the blood–brain barrier. This barrier is physically disrupted by trauma or functionally impaired by metabolic abnormalities, such as drug overdoses. Disruption of the barrier results in increased brain volume. Fluid escapes from the intravascular space to the interstitial space of brain tissue, resulting in cerebral edema. According to the Monro–Kellie hypothesis, there is only so much room in the cranial vault and an increase in brain volume necessitates a decrease in either cerebral blood volume or CSF volume. (Under normal conditions, the brain cannot decrease its own size or displace itself.) With the increase in brain volume, CSF or cerebral blood volume decreases to maintain normal ICP. If this does not occur, ICP continues to increase.

Cerebral Blood Volume

Cerebral blood volume is the amount of blood in the cranial vault at any point in time. Cerebral blood volume is maintained at a constant level through cerebral blood flow (CBF). Recall from Section One that CBF is normally controlled by the process of pressure and chemical autoregulation. Conditions that affect cerebral blood flow and therefore cerebral blood volume are summarized in Table 20–1.

TABLE 20–1 Conditions That Affect Cerebral Blood Flow and Cerebral Blood Volume

INCREASED CBF AND CBV	DECREASED CBF AND CBV
Systemic hypotension	Systemic hypertension
Increase in body metabolic rate (fever, pain)	Decrease in body metabolic rate (sedation, paralysis, hypothermia)
Systemic acidosis (hypercapnia, ischemia)	Systemic alkalosis (hypocapnia) Cerebral edema Low cardiac output
Cerebral vasodilation	Cerebral vasoconstriction

CBF=cerebral blood flow, CBV=cerebral blood volume.

Cerebrospinal Fluid

Cerebrospinal fluid (CSF) is the third component of intracranial volume. CSF circulates in the subarachnoid spaces and spinal cord and is reabsorbed into the venous system. Approximately 10 percent of the total intracranial volume is CSF, which accounts for about 150 mL of CSF at any given time. The functions of CSF are to (1) cushion and support the brain and spinal cord; (2) maintain a stable chemical milieu for the central nervous system; and (3) excrete toxic wastes, such as carbon dioxide, lactate, and hydrogen ions (LeMone & Burke, 2008). The normal adult CSF pressure varies from 5 to 13 mm Hg, or 50 to 200 cm H_2O (Barker, 2008). Cerebrospinal fluid is similar to plasma content but has greater amounts of sodium, chloride, and magnesium. Potassium, glucose, and protein are lower in CSF than in plasma. This information is used to interpret CSF test results.

Of the three components in the cranial vault, CSF is displaced most easily and rapidly into the external jugular veins. This explains why a flexed neck or tight endotracheal tube ties obstruct CSF outflow and increase ICP.

Intracranial Pressure

The combination of the three intracranial compartment volumes forms the total intracranial volume and intracranial pressure (ICP). ICP is measured in the CSF and is defined as the pressure exerted by the CSF within the ventricles of the brain.

Normal ICP ranges from 0 to 15 mm Hg. ICP greater than 15 mm Hg in adults and 10 for more than 5 minutes is considered abnormally elevated. Transient elevations in ICP greater than 10 to 15 mm Hg because of coughing or suctioning are normal if not sustained. ICP is dynamic. It fluctuates constantly in response to changes in respiratory rate, body position, and such activities as coughing and sneezing. Whereas ICP is a fluctuating phenomenon, intracranial volume is kept relatively stable and constant by reciprocal compensation, the principle outlined in the Monro–Kellie hypothesis. By decreasing the volume of one or more of the other brain components, the total brain volume remains fixed.

$$\textit{CSF volume} + \textit{Blood volume} + \textit{Brain volume} = 1700 \textit{ to } 1900 \textit{ mL}$$

As this principle states, reciprocal compensation can occur in any one of the three compartments. The three intracranial components are kept in dynamic equilibrium (Barker, 2008; LeMone & Burke, 2008). When ICP approaches 30 mm Hg, the components can no longer adapt to increases in volume. At this point, compliance is lost and ICP increases. This is considered a decompensated state where normal autoregulation has failed (Marik, 2002; Powers & Schulman, 2009). Table 20–2 illustrates the causes of increased intracranial pressure.

TABLE 20–2 Causes of Increased Intracranial Pressure

Cranial Surgery
Blood clot/hematomas Pneumocephalus (air) Cerebral edema
Increased CBF
Increased BP Increased $Paco_2$ Decreased Pao_2 Vasodilator drugs (nitroprusside, nitroglycerine)
Increased intrathoracic pressure
Coughing Straining (Valsalva) Suctioning PEEP
Decreased cerebral venous drainage
Supine position with head of bed flat Neck flexion/rotation

SECTION TWO REVIEW

1. According to the Monro–Kellie hypothesis, an increase in one intracranial compartment must be accompanied by a reciprocal
   - **A.** decrease in another compartment
   - **B.** increase in the blood–brain barrier
   - **C.** decrease in the blood–brain barrier
   - **D.** increase in another compartment
2. Which mechanism controls brain volume?
   - **A.** cerebral blood flow
   - **B.** displacement of CSF
   - **C.** blood–brain barrier
   - **D.** vasoconstriction

3. ICP remains relatively stable and, under normal conditions, it is usually less than
   A. 5 mm Hg
   B. 15 mm Hg
   C. 30 mm Hg
   D. 50 mm Hg
4. Normal adult CSF pressure in the supine position is
   A. 1 to 5 mm Hg
   B. 5 to 13 mm Hg
   C. 13 to 20 mm Hg
   D. 50 to 200 mm Hg
5. Which of the following is a cause of increased ICP?
   A. decreased cerebral blood flow
   B. decreased CSF production
   C. increased cerebral venous drainage
   D. increased intrathoracic pressure

Answers: 1. A, 2. C, 3. B, 4. B, 5. D

SECTION THREE: Cerebral Perfusion Pressure

At the completion of this section, the learner will be able to calculate a cerebral perfusion pressure based on mean arterial pressure and intracranial pressure.

Cerebral perfusion pressure (CPP) depends on cerebral blood flow (as discussed in Section One) and intracranial pressure (as discussed in Section Two). CPP is defined as the pressure gradient necessary to supply adequate amounts of blood to the brain. It is the difference between mean arterial pressure (MAP) and ICP. The formula to calculate MAP is: MAP = [systolic BP + 2(diastolic BP)]/3. CPP is calculated using the following formula: CPP = MAP – ICP.

The normal CPP is 80 to 100 mm Hg. CPP must be greater than 70 mm Hg to ensure adequate cerebral oxygenation (Powers & Schulman, 2009; Bullock & Povlishock, 2007). Pressures above or below this will result in a loss of autoregulation and inadequate cerebral tissue oxygenation. Cerebral perfusion is decreased when ICP is high or MAP is low. Cerebral perfusion increases when ICP is low or MAP is high. If the ICP rises to the level of MAP, brain perfusion ceases and brain death results.

Calculate the CPP for the following scenario: The ICP is 10 mm Hg and the blood pressure is 120/80 mm Hg. The calculation of CPP is as follows:

$$CPP = MAP - ICP$$
$$MAP = SBP + 2(DBP)/3$$

Answer:
The MAP is 93(120 + 2(80) = 280/3 = 93). The CPP in this situation would be 83(93 − 10 = 83). CPP is within normal range. Decreased CPP requires prompt recognition and treatment. Interventions for patients with decreased CPP include mechanisms to increase MAP and reduce ICP. Section Five discusses assessment of CPP and ICP. Section Seven reviews interventions used to optimize CPP in the high-acuity patient.

SECTION THREE REVIEW

1. CPP depends on all of the following (choose all that apply)
   A. cerebral blood volume
   B. brain volume
   C. CSF volume
   D. cerebral medullary regulation
2. CPP must be greater than ______ mm Hg to ensure adequate cerebral oxygenation.
   A. 70
   B. 60
   C. 50
   D. 40
3. Your patient's MAP is 80 mm Hg and the ICP is 15 mm Hg. What is the cerebral perfusion pressure?
   A. 50 mm Hg
   B. 65 mm Hg
   C. 95 mm Hg
   D. 110 mm Hg
4. Interventions for patients with decreased CPP include mechanisms to (choose all that apply)
   A. increase MAP
   B. increase ICP
   C. decrease ICP
   D. decrease MAP

Answers: 1. (A, B, C), 2. A, 3. B, 4. (A, C)

SECTION FOUR: Decreased Intracranial Adaptive Capacity

At the completion of this section, the reader will be able to describe decreased intracranial adaptive capacity, including causes and effects of increases in brain volume, cerebral blood volume, and CSF volume.

When intracranial mechanisms fail to compensate for increases in intracranial volume, intracranial pressure (ICP) increases. The nursing diagnosis for this condition is *decreased intracranial adaptive capacity.* Several conditions can cause an elevation in ICP: (1) an increase in brain volume (e.g., cerebral edema, space-occupying lesions such as hematoma), (2) an increase in cerebral blood volume (e.g., hypercapnia, hypoxia), or (3) an increase in CSF. Increasing ICP impairs cerebral perfusion and oxygenation of brain cells. **Intracranial hypertension** is a sustained elevation in ICP and is potentially life threatening.

Increase in Brain Volume

Space-occupying lesions and cerebral edema are the primary processes that increase brain volume. Space-occupying lesions may be due to tumors, abscesses, hemorrhages, and hematomas. Cerebral edema is caused by an abnormal accumulation of fluid that increases brain tissue volume. It may occur in a localized area of the brain or it may occur throughout a more generalized area of the brain. Cerebral edema may occur after any type of insult to the head, including trauma, surgery, brain anoxia, or ischemia. Cerebral edema does not impair brain function until the edema increases ICP. When ICP increases due to cerebral edema, cerebral perfusion decreases. The effect of increased brain volume depends on the rate of development. Slower-growing lesions, such as a chronic hematoma or slow-growing tumor, may be tolerated for a longer time period than an acute subdural hematoma, which develops at a faster rate.

A mass or edema that progresses and is uncompensated eventually results in a shifting of brain tissue, or **herniation,** and carries a grave prognosis. This process displaces brain tissue and exerts pressure or traction on cerebral structures. Herniation syndromes are described based on the end stage of the herniation (Table 20–3) and are depicted in Figure 20–2.

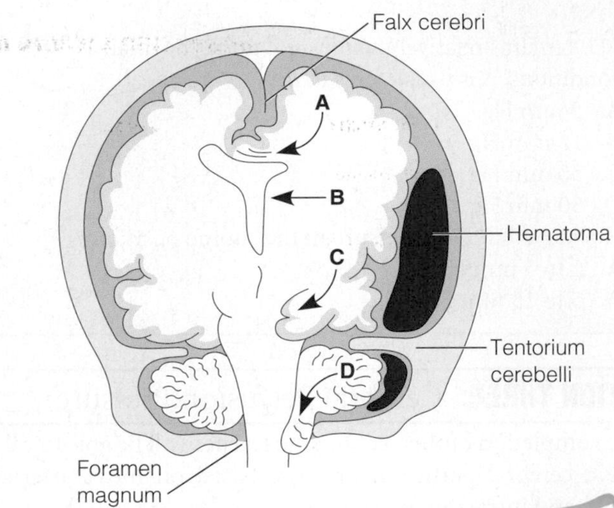

Figure 20–2 ■ Forms of brain herniation due to intracranial hypertension. A, Cingulate herniation occurs when the cingulate gyrus is compressed under the falx cerebri. B, Central herniation occurs when a centrally located lesion compresses central and midbrain structures. C, Lateral herniation occurs when a lesion at the side of the brain compresses the uncus or hippocampal gyrus. D, Infratentorial herniation occurs when the cerebellar tonsils are forced downward, compressing the medulla and top of the spinal cord.

Cerebral Blood Volume

Any systemic process that affects blood levels of carbon dioxide affects CBF, CPP, and cerebral blood volume. Therefore, conditions that produce hypercapnia and hypoxemia result in cerebral vasodilation and increased blood volume. These conditions may include chronic respiratory insufficiency, inadequate ventilation, hypoventilation, sedation by drugs, and insufficient supplemental oxygen. Cerebral blood volume increases with any process that impedes venous outflow. This includes anything that impedes jugular vein drainage, such as head/neck rotation or flexion, or endotracheal tube ties that are too tight or circumferential around the head and neck, Valsalva's maneuver, and use of positive end-expiratory pressure (PEEP). A third cause of increased blood volume is loss of autoregulation. This regulatory mechanism becomes ineffective in states of ischemia, sustained elevations in ICP, and sustained states of hyperemia. When autoregulation is lost, the cerebral blood vessels passively dilate, and produce further increases in cerebral blood volume and ICP.

Cerebrospinal Fluid

Cerebrospinal Fluid (CSF) volume increases with increased production, obstructed circulation, or decreased absorption. This is a condition termed **hydrocephalus.** Obstruction to CSF can be caused by mass lesions or infection. Decreased absorption can result from a subarachnoid hemorrhage or meningitis. Hydrocephalus may be treated in one of two ways. If it is considered to be a permanent condition, a surgical shunt is placed; if it is considered temporary, a ventricular drain is inserted for intermittent or continuous drainage of CSF.

Table 20–4 summarizes the causes and effects of increased brain volume, cerebral blood volume, and CSF. Keep in mind that uncompensated increases in brain or blood volume or CSF, if not treated, can result in herniation.

TABLE 20–3 Four Herniation Syndromes

Cingulate herniation	Lateral shift of brain tissue, usually as the result of a lesion in one of the cerebral hemispheres
Central or transtentorial herniation	Downward shift of one or both cerebral hemispheres, usually because of lesions in the frontal or parietal lobes
Uncal or lateral transtentorial herniation	Lateral and downward shift of brain tissue, usually the temporal lobe, as a result of lesions located most laterally, such as the middle fossa in the temporal lobe; this type of herniation causes compression of the oculomotor nerve, or cranial nerve III, evidenced by the classic sign of a unilaterally dilated pupil
Tonsillar herniation	Downward shift of brain tissue through the foramen magnum, which results in compression of the medulla and upper cervical spinal cord

TABLE 20–4 Causes and Effects of Increases in Brain Volume, Cerebral Blood Volume, and CSF

COMPONENT	CAUSE	EFFECT
Brain volume	Space-occupying lesions Cerebral edema	Herniation
Blood volume	Hypercapnia Hypoxemia Loss of autoregulation Venous outflow obstruction	Cerebral vasodilation Passive cerebral vessels Increased cerebral blood volume
CSF	Obstruction Decreased absorption Increased production	Hydrocephalus

SECTION FOUR REVIEW

1. Which of the following conditions is NOT associated with increased intracranial volume?
   A. subdural hematoma
   B. hypotension
   C. subarachnoid hemorrhage
   D. meningioma
2. Which of the following is NOT a direct cause of increased CSF?
   A. meningitis
   B. hypoglycemia
   C. subarachnoid hemorrhage
   D. brain tumor
3. ICP can be increased by anything that
   A. increases intracranial volume
   B. results in high compliance
   C. results in low elastance
   D. decreases carbon dioxide levels
4. Accumulation of CSF results in
   A. herniation
   B. cerebral dilation
   C. hydrocephalus
   D. seizures
5. A downward shift of brain tissue through the foramen magnum which results in compression of the medulla and upper cervical spinal cord is called a(n)
   A. cingulate herniation
   B. uncal transtentorial herniation
   C. lateral transtentorial herniation
   D. tonsillar herniation

Answers: 1. B, 2. B, 3. A, 4. C, 5. D

SECTION FIVE: Assessment of Cerebral Tissue Perfusion

At the completion of this section, the learner will be able to assess cerebral tissue perfusion.

Decreased cerebral perfusion pressure (CPP) requires prompt recognition. This section reviews assessment techniques used for and abnormal findings associated with decreased cerebral tissue perfusion and decreased intracranial adaptive capacity. The first part of this section reviews pertinent physical assessment findings the high-acuity nurse must know in caring for patients with impaired cerebral tissue perfusion. The types of systems used for ICP monitoring and nursing care for patients undergoing this monitoring are discussed. The last part of this section explains some common systems for monitoring brain tissue oxygenation.

Level of Consciousness

Level of **consciousness** is the most important component of the neurologic assessment in the high-acuity patient. These assessments must be performed and documented in a reliable and consistent manner to provide an accurate transfer of information from clinician to clinician. Often a change in level of consciousness is the first sign of neurologic deterioration. In the high-acuity environment, assessment of level of consciousness is part of the recurring systems assessments made by the nurse. The common etiologies for impaired consciousness are:

Alcohol	Trauma
Epilepsy	Infection
Insulin	Psychological
Opiates	Poisons
Urates (renal failure)	Shock

Components of Consciousness

There are two components of consciousness: arousal (alertness) and content (awareness).

Arousal. The term **arousal** refers to the component of consciousness concerned with an individual's ability to respond to environmental stimuli, such as opening the eyes to speech or turning the head toward a noise. Assessment of the arousal component of consciousness involves an evaluation of the

TABLE 20–5 Terms Used to Describe Level of Consciousness

Full consciousness	Alert; oriented to time, place, and person; comprehends spoken and written words
Confusion	Unable to think rapidly and clearly; easily bewildered, with poor memory and short attention span; misinterprets stimuli; judgment is impaired
Disorientation	Not aware of or not oriented to time, place, or person
Obtundation	Lethargic, somnolent; responsiveness to verbal or tactile stimuli but quickly drifts back to sleep
Stupor	Generally unresponsive; may be briefly aroused by vigorous, repeated, or painful stimuli; may shrink away from or grab at the source of stimuli
Semicomatose	Does not move spontaneously; unresponsive to stimuli, although vigorous or painful stimuli may result in stirring, moaning, or withdrawal from the stimuli, without actual arousal
Coma	Unarousable; will not stir or moan in response to any stimulus; may exhibit nonpurposeful response (slight movement) of area stimulated but makes no attempt to withdraw
Deep coma	Completely unarousable and unresponsive to any kind of stimulus, including pain; absence of brainstem reflexes, corneal, pupillary, and pharyngeal reflexes and tendon and plantar reflexes

From LeMone, P. & Burke, K. (2008), *Medical-Surgical Nursing: Critical Thinking in Client Care,* 4th ed. Upper Saddle River, NJ: Pearson/Prentice Hall Health, p. 1529.

reticular activating system. Conditions that affect arousal do so by directly or indirectly depressing the brainstem structures and the reticular activating system. These conditions result in immediate loss of consciousness and produce coma. Any condition that impairs arousal will naturally impair content as well. Processes that impair arousal include mass lesions that destroy brainstem structures, compression of the brainstem by herniation, or any process that involves the brainstem and the cerebral hemispheres that are sufficient to produce a depressed level of consciousness. Table 20–5 lists the various labels or terms used to describe levels of consciousness (LOC). Labels like *comatose, lethargic,* and *stuporous* lend themselves to subjective interpretation so should be interpreted with caution.

The Glasgow Coma Scale (GCS) is the most frequently used assessment tool to identify changes in arousal. The scale assesses eye opening, verbal response, and best motor response to stimuli (Table 20–6). The best possible score is 15 and the lowest score is 3. A score less than 7 is consistent with a significant alteration in level of consciousness (coma state). Any deterioration in the GCS score is significant and requires immediate physician notification to allow for early intervention and prevention of further neurologic compromise. Certain patient conditions prevent the use of the GCS. Patients with periorbital edema who are unable to open their eyes receive an eye opening response score of 1, which may or may not be valid. Motor deficits, such as hemiparesis or paraplegia, may be overlooked because the motor response scored is the best response elicited. Finally, it is impossible to evaluate a verbal response for patients who are intubated or have a tracheostomy; they also receive a score of 1, which may not be valid (Blissett, 2009). There may also be some limitations in the pediatric population.

The first step is to determine what stimulus arouses the patient. First, address the patient by his name. If he does not

TABLE 20–6 Glasgow Coma Scale

CATEGORY	SCORE	RESPONSE
Eye opening	4	Spontaneous—eyes open spontaneously without stimulation
	3	To speech—eyes open with verbal stimulation but not necessarily to command
	2	To pain—eyes open with noxious stimuli
	1	None—no eye opening regardless of stimulation
Verbal response	5	Oriented—accurate information about person, place, time, reason for hospitalization, and personal data
	4	Confused—answers not appropriate to question but correct use of language
	3	Inappropriate words—disorganized, random speech, no sustained conversation
	2	Incomprehensible sounds—moans, groans, and mumbles incomprehensibly
	1	None—no verbalization despite stimulation
Best motor response	6	Obeys commands—performs simple tasks, response on command; able to repeat performance
	5	Localizes to pain—organized attempt to localize and remove painful stimuli
	4	Withdraws from pain—withdraws extremity from source of painful stimuli
	3	Abnormal flexion—decorticate posturing spontaneously or in response to noxious stimuli
	2	Extension—decerebrate posturing spontaneously or in response to noxious stimuli
	1	None—no response to noxious stimuli; flaccid

respond, shake his arm or shoulder gently. If no response is elicited, proceed from light pain to deeper pain in an attempt to elicit a response. If it is determined that a patient cannot comprehend and/or follow a simple command, the use of noxious stimuli is necessary to determine the patient's best motor response. There are a variety of ways to administer painful or noxious stimuli, some acceptable, others not. It is important to vary the means of eliciting a response, to document the type of stimuli, location, and duration of time it was applied to illicit the response. If it becomes necessary to apply the stimulus for a longer period of time, a potential deterioration of the patient's neurological status should be suspected and appropriate actions taken.

Central stimulation involves applying pain stimulus to the central portion or trunk of the body to produce an overall body response. This type of stimulation tests the ability of the brain to respond to a noxious stimulus. Examples of central noxious stimulation include:

1. trapezius pinch – administered by squeezing or pinching the trapezius muscle
2. sternal rub – administered by applying firm pressure with an open hand to the sternum in a rubbing motion
3. supraorbital pressure – administered by pressing the thumb under the upper part of the ocular orbit; should be avoided in patients with facial fractures, frontal craniotomies, or glaucoma

Peripheral stimulation is delivered distally in the extremities (e.g., nail bed pressure). Response to this type of stimulus means that a functioning spinal cord exists or that the lesion is not complete.

Always start with the least noxious stimulus and proceed to a more intense stimulus or increase the amount of time the stimulus is applied: for example, shaking the arm, applying nail bed pressure, applying the trapezius pinch. This assesses two things: Is the patient responsive to verbal stimuli? If not, does the patient exhibit purposeful movement? Purposeful movement, such as removing the stimulus or withdrawing from the stimulus, indicates functioning of sensory pathways. Abnormal posturing in response to a noxious stimulus indicates a dysfunction of either the cerebral hemispheres or the brainstem. **Decorticate posturing** (abnormal flexion) indicates cerebral hemispheric dysfunction. In response to painful stimuli, the upper arms move up toward the chest with the elbows, wrists, and fingers. Flexed legs extend with internal rotation and the feet flex (as shown in Fig. 20–3A). **Decerebrate posturing** (abnormal extension) indicates brainstem dysfunction and is a more ominous sign. With decerebrate posturing, the neck extends, the jaw clenches, arms pronate and extend straight out, and the feet plantar flex (see Fig. 20–3B). Patients may exhibit a "combination" of posturing, with components of both decerebrate and decorticate, depending on the level of the injury.

Content. Assessment of the content (cognitive) component of consciousness is an evaluation of the cerebral hemispheres. **Content,** a higher level of functioning than arousal, centers on

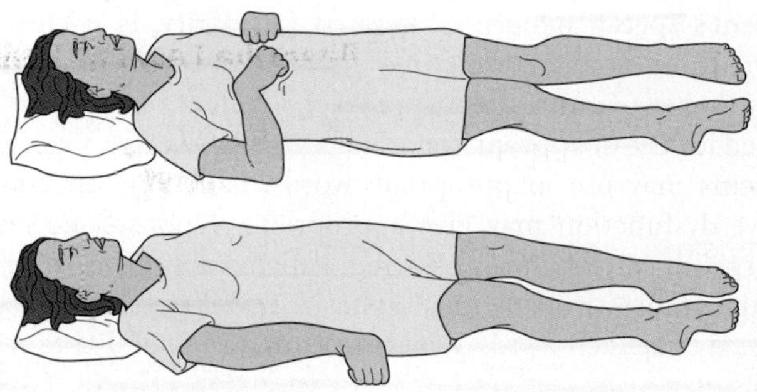

Figure 20–3a and b ■ Decorticate and decerebrate posturing. A, Decorticate (abnormal flexion)-upper arms move upward to the chest; elbows, wrists, and fingers flex; legs extend with internal rotation; feet flex. B, Decerebrate (abnormal extension)-neck is extended with jaw clenched; arms pronate and extend straight out; feet are plantar flexed.

the patient's orientation to time, place, and person. Content is sometimes referred to as awareness. The patient should respond to questions appropriately; any sign of disorientation may be the first indication of neurologic deterioration. Conditions that impair content do so by widely affecting the cerebral hemispheres. Alterations in content are manifested by cognitive deficits such as memory impairment, disorientation, impaired problem-solving abilities, and attentional deficits. The degree of cognitive deficit is related to the location and size of the lesion. Lesions that affect small areas of the hemispheres usually do not produce a significant depression in the level of consciousness. Hemispheric strokes and small intracerebral hematomas and contusions result in localized deficits. Conditions that diffusely affect the hemispheres cause a significant depression in the level of consciousness and may result in coma. Anoxia, ischemia, metabolic alterations, poisons, drugs, and psychiatric disturbances cause diffuse cerebral hemispheric dysfunction (LeMone & Burke, 2008).

The content of consciousness is assessed by noting behavior. The patient should be assessed for orientation and should know his or her name, the date, and where she or he is. The patient is considered disoriented if unable to answer the questions correctly. Testing for orientation also assesses short-term memory. Orientation can be assessed only if the patient is able to respond verbally. After assessing orientation, the ability to follow commands is assessed. Ask the patient to perform such acts as sticking out the tongue or holding up two fingers. This not only helps determine whether the patient is awake enough to respond but also whether he or she is aware enough to interpret and carry out the commands. Next, behavioral changes are assessed by noting any restlessness, irritability, or combativeness. Such behavioral indicators can be caused by hypoxia, hypoglycemia, drug use, pain, or increased ICP. It is part of a nurse's role to notice and evaluate clues that may point to causes for changes in behavior. The last component of content that is assessed is verbal response. Assessment of speech provides information about the function of the relationship between the speech centers in the cerebrum and the cranial nerves, and can help localize the area of dysfunction. The patient's speech pattern is assessed for clarity. Is it clear or slurred and garbled? This may indicate drug use, metabolic disturbance, or cranial nerve injuries. Content of speech is assessed for use of appropriate or inappropriate words. Confused patients may use inappropriate words. Patients with cranial nerve dysfunction may give appropriate responses; however, the speech pattern may be slurred. Patients may experience receptive, expressive, or global aphasia. Inability to understand written or spoken words is **receptive aphasia.** Inability to write or use language appropriately is **expressive aphasia. Global aphasia** includes the inability to use or understand language (LeMone & Burke, 2008).

In-Depth Clinical Assessment

Beyond the assessment of arousal and content, a more in-depth neurological assessment includes assessments of pupillary and oculomotor reactions, vital signs, and cranial nerve reflexes.

Pupillary and Oculomotor Reactions

Pupillary reactions provide information about the location of lesions. Pupils are assessed for size, symmetry, shape, and reaction to light. Pupil size is assessed using a standard pupil gauge (Fig. 20–4). Pupils should be equal in size. Abnormal pupil responses are shown in Figure 20–5. Nonreactive pupils in the midposition indicate damage to the midbrain (Fig. 20–5A). Pupils that are nonreactive to light and pinpoint indicate a pons lesion or opiate drug overdose (Fig. 20–5B). Pupils that are small but reactive to light may indicate a bilateral injury to the thalamus or hypothalamus or metabolic coma (Fig. 20–5C). A unilaterally dilated and fixed pupil may indicate compression of the oculomotor nerve (cranial nerve III) (Fig. 20–5D). Pupil changes are on the same side (ipsilateral) as the lesion. When both pupils are dilated and nonreactive (fixed), emergency action is required. This may be caused by severe anoxia or ischemia. Remember that certain drugs (atropine, epinephrine) can dilate the pupils (Fig. 20–5E).

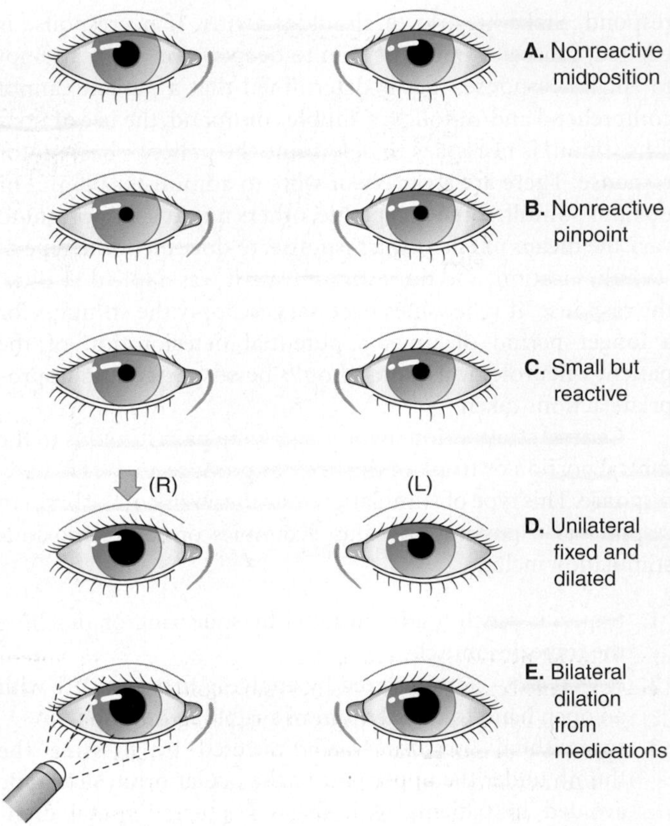

Figure 20–5 ■ Pathophysiology.

Oculomotor Responses

Two reflexes used to determine brainstem integrity are the oculovestibular (caloric) and oculocephalic (doll's eyes) reflexes. Both reflexes involve cranial nerves III (oculomotor), IV (trochlear), VI (abducens), and VIII (acoustic). In the awake patient, it is easy to test these cranial nerves by asking the patient to perform a full range of eye movements. Asking the patient to look upward, downward, outward, inward, medially upward and outward, and laterally upward and outward demonstrates the full range of eye motion, also known as extraocular eye movements. Deficits in eye movements indicate a cranial nerve dysfunction of one or more of the previously mentioned cranial nerves. However, in the unresponsive patient, voluntary eye movement is lost and the patient is unable to perform extraocular eye movements. In this case, oculocephalic and oculovestibular responses are tested to evaluate eye movements.

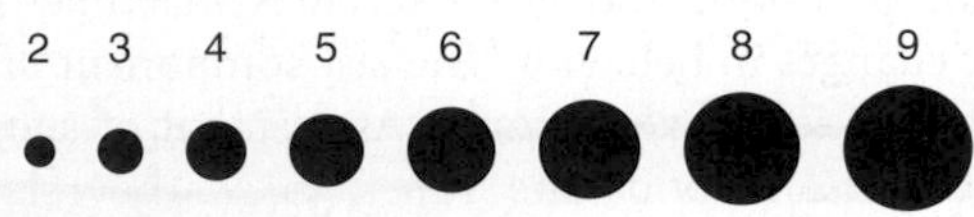

Figure 20–4 ■ Pupil gauge in millimeters.

In deteriorating levels of consciousness, spontaneous eye movements may be lost. Under normal conditions, both eyes move spontaneously in the same direction. Injury to the midbrain and pons impairs normal movement. **Doll's eye movements** (oculocephalic reflex) are reflexive movements of the eyes in the opposite direction of head rotation. This reflex is tested by holding the patient's eyes open and briskly turning the head from side to side, pausing at each side. If the patient has an intact brainstem, the examiner sees conjugate eye movement opposite to the side the head is turned, known as "full doll's eyes" (Fig. 20–6). In cases of brainstem injury, the eyes will remain fixed in the midposition as the head is turned, and doll's eyes are absent. This test is contraindicated in patients whose cervical spine has not been cleared of injury.

Another reflex, oculovestibular reflex (cold caloric test) may be performed when determining brainstem function. Instilling cold water into the ear canal causes **nystagmus** (lateral tonic deviation of the eyes) toward the stimulus. This reflex is lost when brainstem function is lost. The oculovestibular reflex is a more sensitive indicator of brainstem function

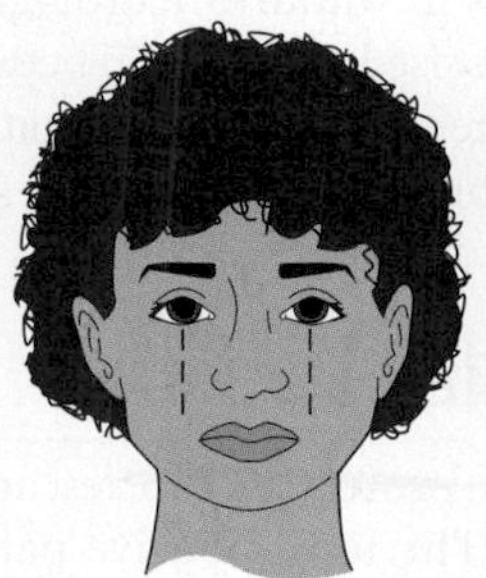

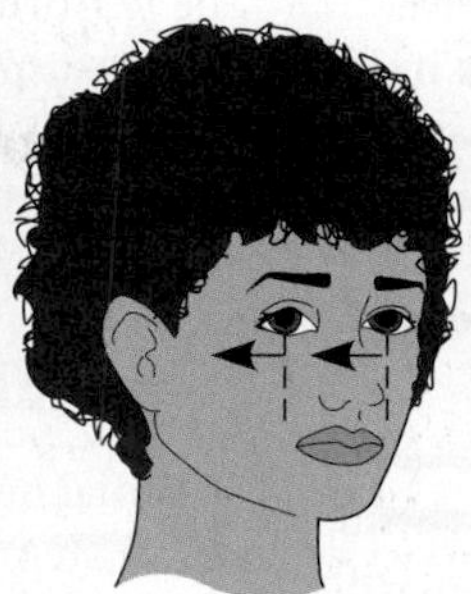

Doll's eyes absent:
Eyes do not move
in relation to head.
Direction of vision follows
head to left.

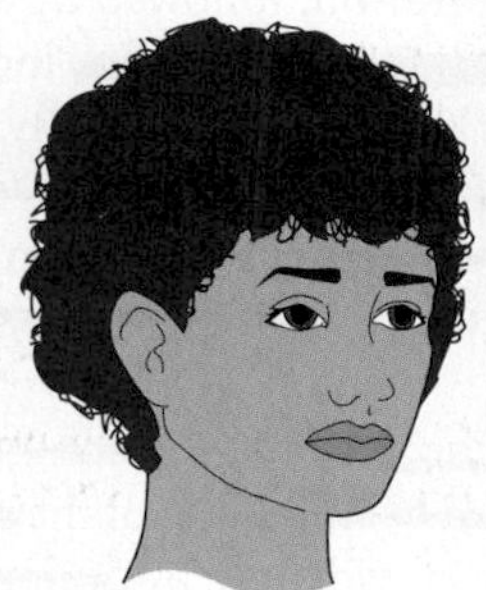

Figure 20–6 ■ Doll's eye movements characteristic of altered LOC.

and central nervous system injury. Patients with an absent oculocephalic reflex may have a normal oculovestibular reflex. Therefore, testing for the oculovestibular reflex always follows testing for the oculocephalic reflex. Testing the oculovestibular reflex is contraindicated if CSF or purulent drainage is leaking from the ear, or if there is perforation or a tear of the tympanic membrane.

Results of oculocephalic or oculovestibular testing are interpreted with caution because pharmacologic agents such as ototoxic drugs, neuromuscular blockers, and ethyl alcohol depress these reflexes.

Vital Signs

Routine parameters assessed in the high-acuity patient include respiratory rate and pattern, heart rate and rhythm, pulse oximetry, blood pressure, and temperature. Because the brainstem influences the cardiovascular and respiratory systems, changes in vital signs may indicate neurologic deterioration.

Respiratory pattern provides valuable information because it is correlated with the anatomic level of dysfunction. Respiratory rhythm and pattern are controlled by the medulla. Respirations are assessed for rate and rhythm and are counted for one full minute before stimulating the patient. Common abnormal respiratory patterns observed in neurologically impaired patients are discussed in the following paragraphs and depicted in Table 20–7. As a nurse, remember that it is more important to describe the pattern than to try to fit the patient's respiratory pattern into a category. If the patient is mechanically ventilated, it is difficult to observe these patterns, and it would be extremely detrimental to the patient to remove ventilatory support for the purpose of assessing abnormal patterns. Deteriorating respiratory patterns are as follows:

- *Cheyne–Stokes* pattern indicates a bilateral lesion in the cerebral hemispheres, cerebellum, midbrain or, in rare circumstances, upper pons, and may be caused by cerebral infarction or metabolic diseases. This respiratory pattern

TABLE 20–7 Abnormal Respiratory Patterns

PATTERN	DESCRIPTION
Cheyne-Stokes respirations	A regular crescendo–decrescendo pattern with increasing then decreasing rate and depth of respirations followed by a period of apnea
Central neurogenic hyperventilation	A sustained pattern of rapid, regular, deep respirations (hyperpnea)
Apneustic breathing	Prolonged inspiration with a pause at full inspiration followed by expiration and a possible pause following expiration
Cluster breathing	Clusters of several breaths with irregular periods of apnea between clusters
Ataxic respirations	Respirations that are completely irregular in pattern and depth with irregular periods of apnea

is evidenced by a rhythmic waxing and waning in the depth of the respiration, followed by a period of apnea.

- *Central neurogenic hyperventilation* indicates a lesion in the low midbrain or upper pons and may be caused by infarction or ischemia of the midbrain or pons, anoxia, or tumors of the midbrain. This pattern is evidenced by respirations increased in depth, rapid (greater than 24), and regular.
- *Apneustic breathing* indicates a lesion in the mid or low pons that may be caused by infarction of the pons or severe meningitis. This pattern is evidenced by prolonged inspiration, with a pause at the point where the respiration is at its peak, lasting for two to three seconds. This may alternate with an expiratory pause.
- *Cluster breathing* indicates a lesion in the low pons or upper medulla that may be caused by a tumor or infarction of the medulla. This pattern is described as clusters of irregular breathing with periods of apnea that occur at irregular intervals.
- *Ataxic breathing* indicates a lesion in the medulla that may be caused by a cerebellar or pons bleed, tumors of the cerebrum, or severe meningitis. These respirations are completely irregular, with deep and shallow random breaths and pauses.

Remember that abnormal respiratory patterns also may be initiated by conditions such as acid-base and electrolyte imbalances, anxiety, pulmonary disease, or drugs, especially narcotics and anesthetic agents that depress the respiratory center.

The pulse is assessed for rate, rhythm, and quality. Increased heart rate may indicate poor cerebral oxygenation. Decreased heart rate is present in the late stages of increased ICP.

The medulla regulates blood pressure based on input from chemoreceptors and baroreceptors. Mean arterial pressure must be maintained at a sufficient level to produce adequate cerebral tissue perfusion when ICP is elevated. Cerebral trauma is rarely associated with hypotension; quite the contrary, cerebral trauma produces systemic hypertension. An important response to ischemia, known as the **Cushing's triad** is a classic syndrome of increased ICP characterized by a specific change in vital signs evidenced by (1) an increase in systolic blood pressure, (2) a decrease in diastolic blood pressure, and (3) bradycardia. This response is activated when ICP rises to a point where it equals or exceeds MAP. Signs of a widening pulse pressure should alert the vigilant nurse of this complication (impending brain herniation) in the setting of severe intracranial hypertension.

The center for temperature regulation is in the hypothalamus. Injury to or dysfunction of the hypothalamus produces alterations in body temperature. Hypothermia occurs as a result of spinal shock, metabolic coma, drug overdose (especially depressants), and destructive lesions of the brainstem or hypothalamus. Hyperthermia occurs as a result of CNS infection, subarachnoid hemorrhage, hypothalamic lesions, or hemorrhage of the hypothalamus or brainstem. Temperature fluctuates widely and often exceeds 106°F. Hyperthermia is treated promptly because of the increased metabolic demands placed on the body and brain.

An abbreviated neurological assessment (Table 20–8) can be performed on patients in whom a neurological impairment is not suspected or diagnosised as well as in between more comprehensive neuro assessments. Other manifestations of progressive deterioration in brain function are summarized in Table 20–9.

Cranial Nerve Reflexes

Cranial nerve reflexes are protective reflexes, and they indicate brainstem functioning. The unresponsive patient is assessed for these reflexes and if they are absent or decreased, measures must be taken to protect the patient from injury. The protective reflexes include (1) corneal reflex (blink), (2) gag reflex, (3) swallow reflex, and (4) cough reflex. The corneal reflex is assessed by touching the cornea, from the side, with a sterile wisp of cotton. The eye blinks rapidly if the reflex is intact. The gag reflex is assessed by touching the posterior tongue with a tongue blade. If intact, the patient gags. The cough and gag reflexes can also be assessed while suctioning the intubated patient.

ICP monitoring provides continuous data regarding the pressure within the cranial vault. The primary reasons for ICP monitoring are to assist in calculating and maintaining adequate CPP and to permit early detection and treatment of increased ICP (LeMone & Burke, 2008; Barker, 2008; Powers & Schulman, 2009). Continuous monitoring allows titration of therapies to maintain adequate tissue perfusion and thereby prevent ischemia. It enables the identification of impending brain herniation secondary to escalating ICP, determines the need for and impact of therapies, and predicts outcome. Patient selection is an important decision because not all patients with altered cerebral tissue perfusion require or are appropriate candidates for ICP monitoring. Current guidelines recommend that ICP monitoring may be appropriate for two situations: (1) patients with a GSC of 8 or less who also have abnormal findings on a head CT scan; or (2) patients with evidence of altered cerebral tissue perfusion, but who have a normal head CT scan, and have two or more of the following: age greater than 40 years, unilateral or bilateral motor posturing, or systolic blood pressure less than 90 mm Hg (Bullock & Povlishock, 2007; Barker, 2008; Helmy, Vizcaychipi & Gupta, 2007).

TABLE 20–8 Abbreviated Neurologic Assessment (for clients in whom a neurologic impairment is not suspected)

1. Assess LOC (response to auditory and/or tactile stimulus).
2. Obtain VS (BP, P, R).
3. Check pupillary response to light.
4. Assess strength of hand grip and movement of extremities bilaterally.
5. Determine ability to sense touch/pain in extremities.

LeMone, P. & Burke, K. (2008). *Medical Surgical Nursing: Critical Thinking in Client Care*, 4th ed. Upper Saddle River, NJ: Prentice Hall, p. 1518.

TABLE 20–9 Manifestations of Progressive Deterioration in Brain Function

LEVEL OF CONSCIOUSNESS	PUPILLARY RESPONSE	OCULOMOTOR RESPONSES	MOTOR RESPONSES	BREATHING
Alert, oriented to time, place, person	Equal, round, reactive to light	Eyes move as head turns	Purposeful movements; responds to commands	Regular rate, pattern
Responds to verbal stimuli; episodes of confusion, restlessness	Equal, round, reactive to light progressing to small, reactive	Caloric testing produces nystagmus	Purposeful movement in response to pain	Yawning, sighing
Requires continuous stimulation to rouse	Small reactive progressing to slowing response to light (sluggish)	Roving eye movements	Decorticate posturing	Cheyne–Stokes
Reflexive posturing to pain stimulus	Ipsilateral dilation; fixed (nonreactive)	Roving or no eye movements	Decerebrate posturing	Central neurologic hyperventilation
No response to stimuli	Bilateral dilation and fixation	No spontaneous eye movements; eyes fixed in midposition with doll's eye No eye movements to cold caloric testing	Flaccidity	Cluster or ataxic breathing; apnea

Data from Lemone & Burke (2008).

Types of ICP Monitoring Devices

Intracranial pressure (ICP) monitoring is classified by the anatomic placement of the device. Basic monitoring systems include intraventricular catheters, subarachnoid screws, intraparenchymal catheters, and epidural probes (Fig. 20–7). Each system has advantages and disadvantages for monitoring ICP (Table 20–10).

Intraventricular monitoring, the gold standard for ICP monitoring, is used for both diagnostic and therapeutic purposes. This type of monitoring involves placing an intraventricular catheter (IVC) into the anterior horn of the lateral ventricle, preferably in the nondominant hemisphere. Diagnostically, it is the most reliable of the monitoring devices and provides precise and consistent waveforms. Therapeutically, cerebrospinal fluid (CSF) can be drained from the intraventricular cavity, thereby decreasing the CSF compartment and reducing ICP. Drainage of CSF can be continuous or intermittent. Continuous drainage is an open system whereby CSF automatically drains when the ICP exceeds a certain point. This point is determined by how high or low the drainage bag is placed above the foramen of Munro, which is the anatomic landmark for the lateral ventricle. Usually, this landmark is at the top of the external ear. Intermittent drainage is a closed system that is opened for periodic drainage when the ICP exceeds a certain point, to be stipulated by the physician, but usually in the range of 20 to 25 mm Hg (Powers & Schulman, 2009; Barker, 2008; Blank-Reid, McClelland & Santora, 2008; Bullock & Povlishock, 2007). The IVC has several advantages. Because it is placed directly into the ventricle, it provides direct measurement of ICP and allows for drainage of CSF. However, the IVC is not risk-free. It is the most invasive of the monitoring types and, therefore, carries the risk of infection. Because it is introduced directly into brain tissue, the risk of bleeding and destruction of neurons are factors that must be considered. Contraindications for placement of an IVC include patients with coagulopathies, small or collapsed ventricles, or severe generalized cerebral edema.

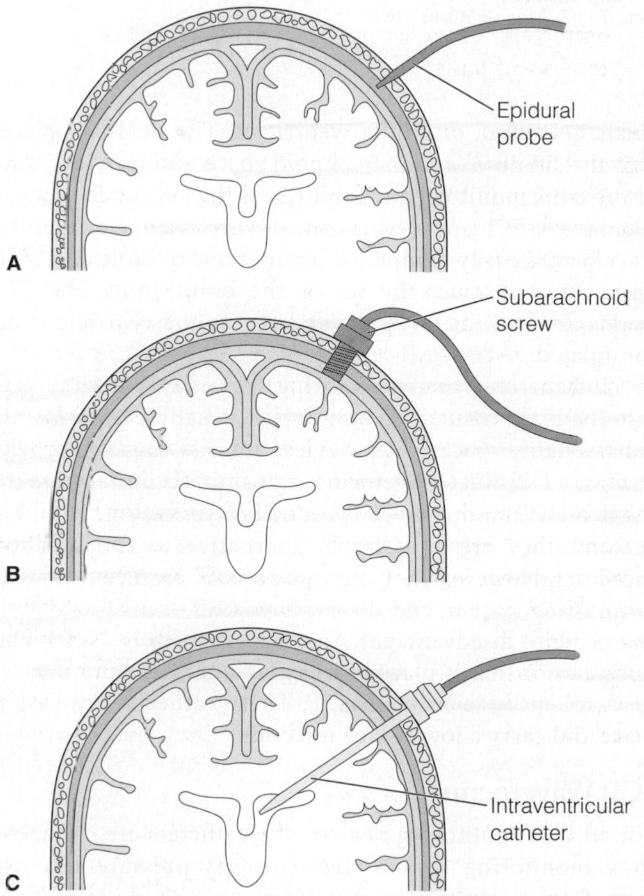

Figure 20–7 ■ Types of intracranial pressure monitoring. A, Epidural probe. B, Subarachnoid screw. C, Intraventricular catheter.

An alternative to the IVC is the subarachnoid bolt or screw. This type of monitoring device is used in patients with

TABLE 20–10 Comparison of Monitoring Sites

SITE	ADVANTAGES	DISADVANTAGES
Intraventricular	Gold standard Allows for therapeutic intervention by drainage of CSF Direct measurement of CSF pressure Highly accurate	Most invasive; carries high risk for hemorrhage, infection Contraindicated with coagulopathies, or small, misshaped, or collapsed ventricles
Subarachnoid	Less invasive Easy placement Low risk of infection Useful if ventricles cannot be cannulated Able to sample CSF	Unable to drain CSF May become obstructed with bone or tissue Not as accurate as time progresses Needs frequent recalibration Unreliable at high ICPs
Intraparenchymal	Easy placement Low risk of infection Highly accurate	Unable to drain CSF Requires separate monitoring system Catheter fragile; may kink Cannot zero once in place Risk of hemorrhage, infection
Epidural probe	Easy placement Low risk of infection	Unable to drain CSF Cannot zero once in place Accuracy is variable

Data from LeMone & Burke, 2008.

small, collapsed, or shifted ventricles. The device is placed into the subdural or subarachnoid space and provides some of the same monitoring capabilities as the IVC, such as measurement of ICP and evaluation of waveforms, although the waveform is easily dampened because bits of bone and brain tissue may obstruct the tip of the bolt. Unlike the IVC, drainage of CSF is not possible because the ventricle is not cannulated.

Intraparenchymal monitoring devices are placed directly into the brain tissue via a bolt device, usually 1 cm below the subarachnoid space. These devices are easy to place, provide sharp and distinct waveforms, transmit accurate measurement of ICP, and carry a lower risk of infection. For these reasons, they are a desirable alternative to subarachnoid monitors. However, they are more costly, require a separate monitoring system, and do not have CSF drainage capabilities (a major disadvantage). An epidural probe is a small fiber optic sensor that is placed through a burr hole and into the epidural space to monitor ICP. These catheters are easy to place and carry a low risk of infection.

ICP Waveforms

For all ICP monitoring devices, the catheters are connected to a monitoring system that converts pressure impulses (waveforms) into an electronic display on a bedside monitor, very much like hemodynamic monitoring. The waveform comes from pulsations that are transmitted in the brain from intracranial arteries and veins. The nurse must be able to recognize normal waveform patterns and identify dangerous signs and trends that indicate increased ICP. There are three peaks within each ICP waveform (Fig. 20–8). The first peak is P1 which is referred to as the percussion wave. It has a sharp peak and it originates from pulsations of the choroid plexus. The second peak, P2, reflects the compliance of brain tissue. If P2 is as high or higher than P1, a situation of decreased compliance is present. The third wave, P3, is the dicrotic wave.

There are three types of ICP pressure waveform patterns: A waves, B waves, and C waves (Fig. 20–9). A waves, or plateau waves, are clinically significant. They typically occur when ICP is elevated. They are spikes of sharp increases in ICP that may be sustained in a plateau fashion for up to 20 minutes. Signs of

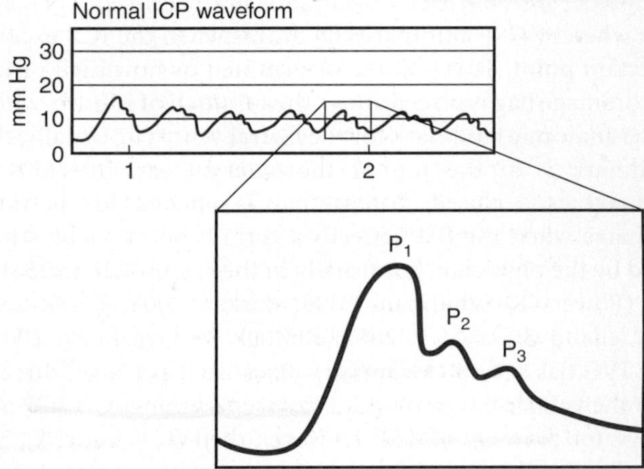

Figure 20–8 ■ Three points within each ICP waveform. P1, percussion wave; P2, reflects brain compliance, P3, dicrotic wave. Normally P1 is the highest.

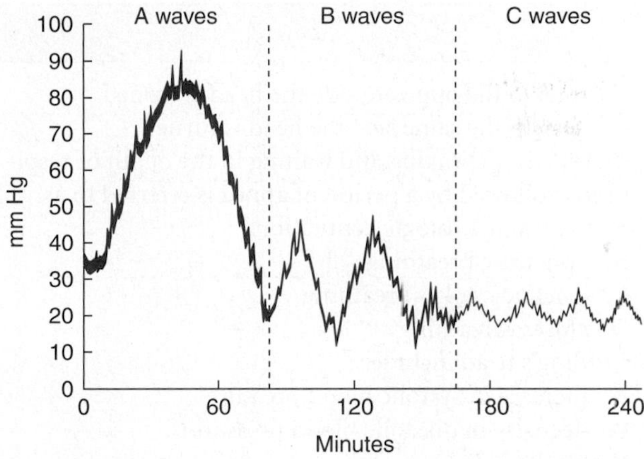

Figure 20–9 ■ A waves, spikes of sharp increases in ICP, are clinically significant; signs of neurologic deterioration may be present. B waves are oscillating waves that are normal except when elevated above 15 mm Hg. C waves are small rhythmic waves that are normal.

neurologic deterioration may be seen with these waves (decreasing level of consciousness, pupillary changes, posturing). Plateau waves are significant, especially when the elevation in ICP decreases cerebral perfusion pressure (CPP). B waves often precede A waves. These waves are sharp oscillating waves. They occur every 30 seconds to two minutes. They are normal except when B waves elevate to an amplitude of greater than 15 mm Hg. This represents a state of low intracranial compliance. C waves are small rhythmic waves. They occur every 5 to 8 minutes and are normal. They vary with respiration and blood pressure (Barker, 2008).

Jugular Bulb Oximetry

Monitoring ICP and CPP provides an indirect assessment of cerebral tissue perfusion, but they do not indicate the adequacy of cerebral oxygenation. Measurement of cerebral oxygen saturation via jugular bulb oximetry (Sjo_2) is used to assess the relationship between cerebral oxygen supply and demand. These catheters are similar to other mechanisms to monitor oxygenation, such as pulse oximetry (Spo_2) and systemic mixed venous oxygen saturation (Svo_2). Sjo_2 monitoring permits continuous measurement of cerebral venous oxygen saturation. The amount of oxygen extracted by cerebral tissue is reflected in the difference between the percentage of oxygen delivered to cerebral tissue (Sao_2 or Spo_2) and the percentage returning from cerebral tissue (Sjo_2). Therefore, cerebral oxygen extraction (CEO_2) is $Spo_2 - Sjo_2$. Normal CEO_2 is 30 percent. If the brain is receiving less oxygen than it needs, it extracts more oxygen from the cerebral circulation and Sjo_2 is lower. If CBF is higher than the brain requires, less oxygen will be extracted and the Sjo_2 is higher. This information helps to determine therapies and interventions to improve cerebral oxygenation. The major advantage of using Sjo_2 monitoring over simple ICP or CPP monitoring is that it can help determine if a given CPP is sufficient to satisfy cerebral metabolic demand.

Normal Sjo_2 is 60 to 80 percent. Sjo_2 less than 55 percent or CEO_2 greater than 40 percent reflect a state of oligemia; Sjo_2 greater than 75 percent or CEO_2 less than 24 percent reflect a state of hyperemia or death of brain cells (dead tissue does not extract oxygen). If either hypoxia or hyperemia persists for more than 15 minutes, notify the physician (Kidd & Criddle, 2001; Blank-Reid, Kaplan & Santora, 2008).

The difference in the content of oxygen delivered to cerebral tissue and the content returned from cerebral tissue is calculated using the following formula:

$$\text{Cerebral } Pao_2 - Pvo_2 = [(Sao_2 - Sjo_2) \times 1.34 \times Hgb/100]$$

Normal cerebral $Pao_2 - Pvo_2$ is 4 to 8 mL/dL. A narrow cerebral $Pao_2 - Pvo_2$ (less than 4 mL/dL) is associated with hyperemia, whereas a wide cerebral $Pao_2 - Pvo_2$ (greater than 9 mL/dL) is associated with oligemia.

The Sjo_2 catheter is inserted by a physician in a similar manner to that of a central venous catheter. The fiber optic catheter is usually inserted into the right internal jugular vein because this vein drains a greater proportion of blood from the sagittal sinus than the left internal jugular and readings are more representative of global (versus local) brain oxygenation (Blissett, 2009; Kidd & Criddle, 2001). After placement has been confirmed, the catheter is connected to a saline solution at a rate of 3 to 5 mL/hr. No other fluids or medications should be infused through this catheter. Further nursing care priorities for patients receiving this type of monitoring are reviewed in Section Seven.

Arterio-jugular venous difference of oxygen (Avj_{DO2}) is calculated by subtracting the content of jugular venous oxygen from the arterial oxygen content (McQuillan & Mitchell, 2002). This provides an overall picture of cerebral blood flow and oxygen consumption. Normal Avj_{DO2} ranges from 4.5 to 8.5 mL/dL. Elevations can be due to an inadequate CBF or decreased oxygen consumption. Decreased values reflect an excessive oxygen delivery over oxygen demand (McQuillan & Mitchell, 2002).

Brain Tissue Oxygen Monitoring

Brain tissue oxygen monitoring ($PbtO_2$) provides continuous measurement of local brain tissue oxygen partial pressure. Normal $PbtO_2$ is greater than 20 mm Hg. A $PbtO_2$ of 15 mm Hg is accepted as the critical lower limit in patients with traumatic brain injury (TBI) (Bader, March & Littlejohns, 2002; Blissett, 2009). Brain tissue extracts oxygen from the hemoglobin into the brain tissue and is measured as partial pressure. Recommendation for placement of the brain tissue oxygen catheter is in the frontal white matter, 2 to 3 cm below the dura. A CT scan is recommended to verify correct placement (Dings, Meixenberger & Amscher, 1996; Blissett, 2009; van den Brink, 2000).

SECTION FIVE REVIEW

1. Findings from an initial assessment of a patient are as follows: Patient is awake; eyes are open and focusing; patient responds appropriately to verbal commands. Based on these findings, you could determine that
   A. The state of arousal is intact, but not content.
   B. The state of content is intact, but not arousal.
   C. Arousal is intact; not enough data have been gathered to assess content completely.
   D. Content is intact; not enough data have been gathered to assess arousal.
2. The Glasgow Coma Scale assesses
   A. cranial nerves
   B. arousal
   C. abstract thinking
   D. awareness
3. The Glasgow Coma Scale is useful because it
   A. is standardized
   B. evaluates the ability to interpret stimuli
   C. is subjective
   D. evaluates vital signs and pupil reactivity
4. A decorticate motor response indicates
   A. brainstem dysfunction
   B. the patient is close to death
   C. cerebral hemispheric dysfunction
   D. arousal is intact
5. Pupils that are bilaterally pinpoint and nonreactive to light indicate
   A. unilateral brain lesion
   B. metabolic coma
   C. herniation
   D. lesion in the pons
6. In cases of brainstem injury, doll's eye movements will
   A. remain fixed in the midposition as the head is turned
   B. conjugate opposite to the side the head is turned
   C. turn to the opposite side the head is turned
   D. turn to the same side the head is turned
7. The rhythmic waxing and waning in the depth of respiration followed by a period of apnea is referred to as
   A. central neurologic ventilation
   B. apneustic breathing
   C. Cheyne–Stokes breathing
   D. cluster breathing
8. Cushing's triad includes
   A. increase in systolic blood pressure
   B. decrease in diastolic blood pressure
   C. bradycardia
   D. all of the above
9. Which of the following ICP monitoring systems is the most accurate and reliable, and allows for drainage of CSF?
   A. intraventricular catheters
   B. intraparenchymal catheters
   C. subarachnoid bolt
   D. epidural catheters
10. Which of the following ICP waveforms occur when ICP is elevated and are considered to be clinically significant?
   A. P_1 waves
   B. *A* waves
   C. P_2 waves
   D. *B* waves
11. SjO_2 less than 55 percent or CEO_2 greater than 40 percent indicates
   A. adequate cerebral oxygenation
   B. hyperemia
   C. oligemia
   D. death of brain cells

Answers: 1. C, 2. B, 3. A, 4. C, 5. D, 6. A, 7. C, 8. D, 9. A, 10. B, 11. C

SECTION SIX: Diagnostic Procedures

At the completion of this section, the learner will be able to describe procedures used in diagnosing brain injury.

Prompt and proper treatment of neurologic dysfunction is based on accurate and timely diagnosis. A variety of diagnostic tests are available. Some of the more commonly performed diagnostic tests will be reviewed.

Computed Tomography Scanning

Computerized tomography (CT) of the head is useful for detecting primary injuries, such as skull fractures, hematomas, and contusions; secondary injuries such as herniation, edema, and shifting of brain tissue secondary to swelling; and abscesses and tumors. The CT scan remains the initial procedure of choice in acute head injury because it is noninvasive, produces rapid results, is safe and painless, and reduces the need for more invasive procedures, such as angiograms. CT scans may be done with IV contrast to enhance visualization of vascular structures.

A xenon-enhanced CT can measure CBF quantitatively. It is able to quantify the uptake and clearance of xenon gas, which is administered by inhalation or intravenously (Kirkness, 2009).

Magnetic Resonance Imaging

A magnetic resonance imaging (MRI) is superior to CT scanning. As with CT scanning, MRI can determine the anatomic location of a lesion. Additionally, MRI allows examination of the tissue itself, providing more anatomic detail than CT scanning. Therefore, detecting white matter shearing, infarction, and ischemic tissue is possible. MRI has the ability to detect pathologic processes at an earlier stage than is possible with a CT, and is therefore the procedure of choice for early diagnosis of cerebral infarction and brain tumors. MRI is the preferred diagnostic study for cervical spine imaging and evaluation of spinal cord injury. However, MRI has limitations that CT does not. Removal of all metal from the patient's body is essential because the MRI is a powerful magnet. Most dental fillings, prostheses, and internal clips do not prevent the patient from having an MRI, but specific questions and concerns must be directed to the neuroradiologist. Obtaining an MRI takes longer than a CT, and MRI provides a poor image of bone tissue. Therefore, a CT remains the procedure of choice when time is a factor, as with the unstable trauma patient or in the detection of spinal fractures (Kirchness, 2009).

Tomography

Diagnostic procedures using tomography involve IV injection and tracking of radionucleotides to evaluate cerebral blood flow. Two types are available: positron emission tomography (PET) and single photon emission computed tomography (SPECT). PET uses paired radiation sensitive detectors, whereas SPECT uses unpaired detectors. PET costs more than SPECT. The CT is preferred in the acute setting. These techniques are helpful in determining changes in CBF and metabolism during recovery. Areas of brain dysfunction and ischemia may be detected by these techniques that are not detected by CT and are helpful when determining prognosis following TBI (Iaia & Barker, 2008).

Transcranial Doppler

Transcranial Doppler (TCD) is a noninvasive tool for measuring cerebral blood velocity in branches of the Circle of Willis. TCD is governed by the underlying principle that velocity depends on the pressure gradient between the two ends of a vessel, the radius of the vessel, and blood viscosity. Therefore, changes in velocity may reflect either changes in CBF or in the diameter of a vessel. Diameter and flow do not always change in concert, so interpretation must be cautious. Low velocity may reflect low flow or arterial dilation; high velocity may indicate high flow or vessel constriction. TCD is ideal for use in the high-acuity environment because it is noninvasive and uses portable equipment. TCD is often used to monitor for cerebral vasospasm, intracranial lesions poststroke, and to detect cerebral blood flow changes associated with elevated ICP. TCD may be used during evaluation and determination of brain death.

Evoked Potentials

Evoked potentials are recordings of cerebral electrical impulses generated in response to visual, auditory, or somatosensory stimuli. Stimulation of the visual or auditory sensory organs or the peripheral nerves evokes an electrophysiologic response that is extracted from continuous electroencephalography (EEG) monitoring. Evoked potentials are used to detect lesions in the cerebral cortex or ascending pathways of the spinal cord, brainstem, and thalamus. This test is so sensitive that it detects lesions that cannot be detected with other clinical or laboratory tests. Visually evoked potentials are elicited by a flashing light or changing geometric pattern that stimulates the visual center in the occipital lobe. The delay, known as the degree of latency, correlates with disease severity. These are used to diagnose multiple sclerosis and Parkinson's disease; and lesions of the optic nerve, optic tract visual center, and eye. Auditorily evoked potentials are elicited by transmitting transient sounds, such as clicking noises, through earphones. They are useful to detect lesions in the central auditory pathway of the brainstem, identify lesions that result in hearing disorders, and assist in the diagnosis of acoustic tumors. Somatosensory-evoked potentials are elicited by the application of a peripheral stimulus. The response to this stimulus and the degree of latency is measured. These are used in the evaluation of spinal cord injury, to monitor spinal cord function during surgery and treatment of multiple sclerosis, and to assist in the evaluation of the location and extent of brain dysfunction after head injury. Testing for evoked potentials does not require an alert cooperative patient and is not affected by anesthesia or sedation. Evoked potentials may be useful in predicting coma outcome. They are also especially useful during therapeutically induced comas (such as barbiturate coma) because the sensory pathways are not affected by barbiturates.

Electroencephalography

Electroencephalography (EEG) allows recording of the electrical activity of the brain using electrodes attached to the scalp. Abnormal voltage fluctuations indicate seizures or space-occupying lesions, cerebral infarct, altered consciousness, and brain death. For this test, electrodes are placed on the patient's head. Electrical impulses are detected and transferred to a device that interprets and converts the impulses into waveforms. Absence of electrical activity provides evidence for clinical determination of brain death. An EEG may detect seizure activity in the brain when seizures are not clinically apparent. However, abnormal EEG findings do not identify the cause of the abnormality. It is important to note that significant pathology can be present even in the face of a normal EEG. Continuous EEG may be used in some high-acuity units to monitor ICP, seizure activity, and cerebral ischemia.

Cerebral Angiography

Cerebral angiography involves the injection of contrast material into arteries to visualize intra- and extracranial circulation. An angiogram traces blood flow through the cerebrovascular circulation and allows visualization of the size and patency of these vessels. Results can diagnose arteriovenous (AV) malformations, aneurysms, carotid artery disease, vasospasm, and venous thrombosis. Although angiography is useful in the evaluation of cerebral vasculature, a major complication of the procedure is stroke caused by the dislodgement of an atherosclerotic plaque.

Magnetic Resonance Angiography

Magnetic resonance angiography (MRA) combines MRI with angiography for noninvasive visualization of cerebral vasculature. MRA is useful in the evaluation of carotid artery disease and in the identification of intracranial aneurysms. MRA can be done with or without contrast.

Lumbar Puncture

For the lumbar puncture (LP) procedure, a needle is placed into the subarachnoid space, usually at the L4–L5 interspace or less commonly the L3-L4 interspace. CSF is removed for laboratory analysis for the presence of blood or infection. Medications may also be administered by this route. This procedure is contraindicated in patients with increased ICP. Complications of LP include herniation of the brainstem, infection, and headache.

SECTION SIX REVIEW

1. CT, rather than MRI, scanning would be the procedure of choice for detecting
   - **A.** white matter shearing
   - **B.** the early stages of brain tumors
   - **C.** cerebral infarction
   - **D.** spinal or skull fractures
2. PET scanning is useful for evaluating
   - **A.** cerebral blood flow
   - **B.** spinal fractures
   - **C.** skull fractures
   - **D.** anatomic location of a brain tumor
3. Evoked potentials
   - **A.** is an invasive procedure
   - **B.** is useful for imaging cellular metabolism
   - **C.** is used in clinical research only
   - **D.** evaluates a sensory response to a stimulus
4. Brain tissue oxygen monitoring ($PbtO_2$) measures
   - **A.** generalized oxygen tension of gray matter
   - **B.** brain regional oxygen partial pressure
   - **C.** global brain oxygenation
   - **D.** regional cerebral electrical impulses

Answers: 1. D, 2. A, 3. D, 4. B

SECTION SEVEN: Management of Decreased Cerebral Tissue Perfusion

At the completion of this section, the learner will be able discuss the management of decreased cerebral tissue perfusion.

Decreased cerebral tissue perfusion requires prompt recognition and treatment. Treatment is aimed at reducing one or more of the components of the cranial vault: blood volume, brain tissue volume, or CSF. A major goal is to identify and eliminate the cause of an elevation in these components. Interventions for patients with decreased cerebral tissue perfusion include mechanisms to increase MAP and reduce ICP.

Optimizing Cerebral Perfusion Pressure and Oxygenation

Because CPP controls CBF, CPP is optimized by controlling blood pressure and temperature and promoting venous return. MAP is maintained at levels greater than 90 mm Hg so as to keep CPP greater than 70 mm Hg (Bullock & Povlishock, 2007; March & Madden, 2009). Pressures outside this range result in loss of autoregulation and inadequate CPP. CPP is maintained at 70 to 80 mm Hg with IV fluids to achieve euvolemia or slight hypervolemia to ensure adequate cerebral tissue perfusion. IV therapy and vasoactive agents enhance CPP and facilitate the delivery of oxygen to cerebral tissue (Powers & Schulman, 2008; March & Madden, 2009; Bullock & Povlishock, 2007).

Temperature control is important because hyperthermia raises cerebral metabolism. Under conditions of increased cerebral metabolic rate, cerebral blood flow increases to meet tissue metabolic demands. To avoid an increased metabolic rate, hyperthermia must be prevented. Antipyretics and cooling blankets help to control body temperature. Severe injury/ischemia to the hypothalamus impairs thermoregulation and causes neurogenic (or central) fever, which does not respond to antipyretics (Bullock & Povlishock, 2007).

Induced hypothermia therapy has been studied over the years with mixed reactions. Cardiovascular complications such as dysrhythmias and impaired coagulation have been associated with this therapy. In 2000, it was reported that there was an improved neurologic outcome at 6 months following TBI (Marion, 2000). In a follow up study, the beneficial effects with regard to the GCS were limited to patients with a GCS score of less than 8 and to patients younger than 45 years of age (Marion, 2000). Further data are needed to define the role of hypothermia in the management of traumatic brain injury.

Nursing care can promote venous return using body positioning. Unless the patient has a cervical spine injury, the head of the bed is elevated at least 30 degrees. This position avoids jugular compression, promotes venous drainage, and facilitates control of ICP. However, this practice has been questioned recently because it may place some patients at risk for cerebral ischemia caused by a decrease in CPP. Therefore, the recent trend is to individualize head position based on nursing judgment. The nurse must assess the patient's response to position changes and determine which position maximizes CPP and minimizes ICP. Neck flexion, lateral head rotation, and hip flexion of greater than 90 degrees should be avoided because these positions cause venous congestion in the intracranial and abdominal compartments, which can increase ICP. The patient's body is turned as a unit; head, neck, trunk, and lower extremities are turned in unison to avoid head and neck rotation. Patients who are alert are assisted to move up in the bed. Asking patients to help by pushing with their legs initiates Valsalva's maneuver, which increases intrathoracic pressure and impedes venous return (Bullock & Povlishock, 2007).

Cerebral blood flow is an important variable to monitor with cerebral oxygenation, but more importantly, one must assess whether CBF matches cerebral metabolism. This can be determined by calculating cerebral PaO_2–PvO_2.

Maintaining Ventilation

A patient with a GCS less than 9 who cannot maintain an airway or who remains hypoxemic must have an airway secured (Bullock & Povlishock, 2007). Hypoxia and hypercapnia are better controlled with mechanical ventilation. Hyperventilation reduces $PaCO_2$. A reduction in $PaCO_2$ produces vasoconstriction. Hyperventilation has been used to produce vasoconstriction of cerebral blood vessels. Standard practice for many years included using hyperventilation to keep the $PaCO_2$ less than 25 mm Hg. However, studies indicate that blood flow is compromised during the first 24 hours after injury/ischemia (Gopinath et al., 1999; Van den Brink et al., 2000). Current guidelines recommend that hyperventilation (to keep $PaCO_2$ less than or equal to 35 mm Hg) should be avoided during the first 24 hours because reduced blood flow compromises cerebral perfusion (Bullock & Povlishock, 2007). Furthermore, long-term hyperventilation ($PaCO_2$ less than or equal to 25 mm Hg) during the first 5 days (in the absence of increased ICP) should be avoided (Bullock & Povlishock, 2007). Patients are best maintained within a normal $PaCO_2$ range (35 to 45 mm Hg) because the level at which irreversible ischemia occurs has not been determined but the deleterious effects of continued hyperventilation are well documented (Littlejohns & Bader, 2001). Hyperventilation may be necessary for brief periods of time during acute neurologic deterioration, but only after all other options have been instituted. If hyperventilation is instituted, monitoring of cerebral blood flow and jugular bulb oxygen saturation may be helpful in detecting periods of reduced cerebral tissue perfusion (Bullock & Povlishock, 2007).

TABLE 20–11 Clinical Management of Head Injury

Intubation with avoidance of mechanical hyperventilation unless intracranial hypertension becomes refractory to other therapies
Optimization of oxygenation to maintain $PaO_2 > 100$ mm Hg
Diuresis using osmotic and/or loop diuretics
Control of cerebral metabolic rate with sedation, anticonvulsant, antipyretic therapies
Maintenance of SBP > 90 mm Hg
Fluid resuscitation to attain and maintain normal fluid balance

Data from Bullock & Povlishock, 2007.

Table 20–11 summarizes the clinical management of the patient with a brain injury.

Pharmacologic Therapy

Drug therapy is initiated for most patients with increased ICP to decrease intracranial volume, either by decreasing brain volume, decreasing CSF production, or decreasing the metabolic rate. Drug therapy includes osmotic diuretics, sedatives and paralytics, and barbiturates.

Nursing Care of Patients Receiving ICP or SjO_2 Monitoring

The focus of nursing care of the patient with an ICP monitoring device is on prevention of complications and maintenance of system integrity. Complications include those related to insertion, such as hemorrhage or hematoma formation; overdrainage of CSF; and infection, particularly with the IVC device. Patients with coagulopathies are at higher risk for hemorrhage or hematoma formation. Because a hemorrhage or hematoma is a space-occupying lesion, the patient's neurologic status must be carefully monitored before, during, and after insertion of the ICP monitoring device to detect neurologic deterioration. If an intraventricular device is inserted, the color of the CSF must be carefully observed. Pink-tinged or bloody CSF is an indication of bleeding.

The determination of when to drain CSF is important. Current guidelines recommend that ICP treatment is initiated at upper thresholds of 20 to 25 mm Hg. Interpretation and treatment is corroborated by frequent clinical examinations and CPP monitoring (Bullock & Povlishock, 2007). Clinical assessment and overall hemodynamic status are considered when the physician selects the appropriate ICP at which to initiate treatment (Littlejohns & Bader, 2001; Powers & Schulman, 2009). It is imperative that the nurse clarify with the physician and receive orders that specify the ICP at which CSF drainage is initiated and terminated.

Overdrainage of CSF is a major complication of an intraventricular device, particularly an open system. To prevent overdrainage, the nurse observes unit standards for CSF drainage; accurately measures and positions the CSF drainage bag using the correct landmarks; and securely fastens the drainage bag at the prescribed level. Systems that are closed and periodically opened for therapeutic drainage require nursing interventions that are sound and clinically based. For this type of system, drainage is instituted when the ICP is consistently elevated. The keyword is *consistent,* rather than transient. Many factors transiently increase ICP including environmental stimuli, patient positioning, and nursing care activities. Once these stimuli are eliminated ICP may decrease to an acceptable level. If ICP remains elevated for several minutes, the appropriate nursing action is to institute CSF drainage.

The risk of infection is the greatest concern. Factors associated with infection are duration of ICP monitoring and type of device and system used. Sterile techniques must be absolutely observed during insertion of the ICP monitoring device. For fluid-filled systems, system integrity must be maintained. All connection points are checked to ensure that they are tight. Because fluid-filled systems require routine zero referencing and calibration, the risk of introducing pathogens into the system is increased. Care must be taken to rezero and recalibrate in an aseptic manner. The insertion site is inspected for signs of infection. The appearance of the insertion site and duration (in days) of the monitoring device placement is documented.

Troubleshooting and Maintenance of System Integrity

One of the most important nursing interventions is to gather, document, and report accurate data. Medical and nursing interventions are based on these data. Instituting interventions for data that are inaccurate negatively impact patient outcomes. It is the nurse's responsibility to ensure that ICP monitoring systems are intact and that data are accurate (Table 20–12). Accuracy is affected by a dampened, absent, or distorted waveform. Any interference, such as air bubbles within the system; kinked tubing; loose connections; or catheter occlusion from blood, brain, or bone tissue, produces a dampened waveform and inaccurate ICP readings. Technical malfunction within the external system also produces inaccurate data. Fiber optic cables are delicate and easily broken. If this occurs, the device must be removed and a new device inserted. Additionally, the internal transducer cannot be recalibrated. If significant drift is suspected and the data are suspect, the device must be replaced. When caring for patients with ICP monitoring technology, the nurse must have a clear understanding of the benefits and limitations of the system used, troubleshooting scenarios, and support from the manufacturer when needed (Littlejohns & Bader, 2001; March & Madden, 2009).

Just as with ICP monitoring, it is the nurse's responsibility to ensure data obtained from SjO_2 catheters are also accurate. A major limitation of these data is they are not reliable. Troubleshooting strategies, offered by March & Madden (2009), are summarized in Table 20–13.

Providing a Safe and Protective Environment

The following nursing interventions are for patients with impaired content and are directed at protecting the patient from injury, reorienting, and creating a calm, safe environment. Patients with cognitive deficits become easily confused with external stimuli. Noise is kept to a minimum, information is presented simply and calmly, and the number of visitors at one time is limited. Keeping a dim light on at night and frequent checking by the nurse controls confusion caused by misperception of stimuli. Patients with cognitive deficits often attempt to get out of bed and may pull out IV lines and catheters. Interventions, such as keeping the bed in a low position, using side rails, and frequent checks, keep the patient safe from harm. Frequent reorientation decreases confusion and disorientation.

TABLE 20–12 Troubleshooting System Integrity with ICP Monitors

PROBLEM	POTENTIAL SOURCE	ACTION
Dampened, absent, or distorted waveform	Catheter occlusion by blood, brain, or bone tissue Air bubbles in system Loose connections Recalibration and zero referencing needed Kinked catheter or tubing Technical problem with transducer/pressure module Fiber optic cables broken Dislodgement of catheter	Systematically assess for problems Remove air from system Tighten all connections Recalibrate and zero Examine tubing for kinks Replace transducer or pressure module Replace fiber optic device Replace monitoring device
ICP values suspect	Recalibration and zero referencing needed Incorrect placement of catheter or transducer	Recalibrate and zero if fluid-filled system, replace device if fiber optic Verify correct placement of external transducer
Leakage of fluid from tubing	Loosened connections	Tighten all connections

TABLE 20–13 Troubleshooting System Integrity with SjO_2 Monitoring

PROBLEM	ACTION
Low light intensity	Monitor light intensity status indicator Flush catheter with 2 to 3 mL saline to remove debris from catheter tip Reposition patient's head to move catheter to area of more blood flow Notify physician if the light intensity monitor reading remains low
Questionable accuracy of reading	Upon catheter insertion and every 8 to 12 hours, confirm accuracy of catheter by sending a sample of mixed venous blood obtained from the SjO_2 catheter to the lab for analysis If SjO_2 readings are low, but light intensity indicator is within normal range, verify accuracy with a lab analysis A difference of more than 4% between oximetric readings and the results of blood gas analysis indicates the need to recalibrate the monitor

Emerging Evidence

- Hyperventilation exacerbates cerebral ischemia and compromises oxygen metabolism following closed head injury. Such ischemia is underestimated by common bedside monitoring tools and may represent a significant mechanism of avoidable neuronal injury following head trauma (*Coles, Fryer, Coleman et al., 2007).*
- Using a nutritional algorithm focused on enteral nutrition, but including parenteral nutrition as a supplement, it is possible to improve the delivery of clinical nutrition in the intensive care unit patients (*Wøien & Bjørk,* 2006).
- Energy expenditure following traumatic brain injury is highly variable, and the use of standard factors to estimate the energy needs of individual patients may not be accurate. The administration of paralyzing agents, sedatives, or barbiturates reduced metabolic rate by approximately 12-32 percent. Propranolol and morphine are associated with smaller decreases in energy expenditure. Factors that do not appear to augment the hypermetabolic response include the administration of steroids and method of feeding (enteral vs. parenteral). It is unclear if elevated temperature, the presence of extracranial injury, or the severity of injury further exacerbates hypermetabolism (*Foley, Marshall, Pikul, Salter & Teasell, 2009).*

SECTION SEVEN REVIEW

1. Interventions to increase cerebral perfusion pressure includes those that (choose all that apply)
A. increase MAP
B. increase temperature
C. decrease heart rate
D. decrease ICP

2. Nursing interventions for patients with impaired content center around
A. protection from injury
B. maintaining the airway
C. control of cerebral perfusion pressure
D. drug therapy

3. A patient's ICP is 22 mm Hg for more than 5 minutes. Your first action would be to
A. recalibrate and zero the internal transducer
B. immediately drain CSF until the desired ICP is obtained
C. notify the physician immediately
D. eliminate all stimuli and reposition the patient

Answers: 1. (A, D), 2. A, 3. D

POSTTEST

1. Hypoxemia and hypercapnia cause
   A. cerebral vasodilation
   B. decreased ICP
   C. cerebral vasoconstriction
   D. decreased CBF
2. Keeping the head and neck in alignment results in
   A. decreased venous outflow from the head
   B. increased venous outflow from the head
   C. increased intrathoracic pressure
   D. increased intraabdominal pressure
3. As a compensatory mechanism, pressure regulation acts by constricting cerebral blood vessels in response to
   A. elevated blood levels of oxygen
   B. decreased blood levels of oxygen
   C. elevated systemic blood pressure
   D. decreased systemic blood pressure
4. The principle that explains reciprocal mechanisms involved in increased ICP is
   A. Monro–Kellie hypothesis
   B. cerebral perfusion formula
   C. autoregulation
   D. chemical regulation
5. When ICP increases, CSF is displaced into the
   A. external jugular veins
   B. blood–brain barrier
   C. spinal cord
   D. medulla
6. The blood–brain barrier is permeable to which of the following? (choose all that apply)
   A. water
   B. oxygen
   C. lipid soluble compounds
   D. most drugs
7. Your patient's MAP is 100 mm Hg and ICP is 10 mm Hg. What is the CPP?
   A. 80 mm Hg
   B. 90 mm Hg
   C. 110 mm Hg
   D. 120 mm Hg
8. Cerebral perfusion pressure at or below ______ mm Hg will result in a loss of autoregulation and inadequate cerebral oxygenation.
   A. 70 mm Hg
   B. 60 mm Hg
   C. 50 mm Hg
   D. 40 mm Hg
9. What happens when ICP and MAP are equal?
   A. nothing; this is normal
   B. cerebral vasodilation
   C. CSF is displaced
   D. brain perfusion ceases
10. Which of the following disorders can produce an elevation in ICP?
    A. cerebral edema
    B. cerebral hematoma
    C. hydrocephalus
    D. all of the above
11. The net effect of a prolonged increase in ICP is
    A. impaired cerebral tissue perfusion
    B. cerebral vasodilation
    C. cerebral edema
    D. hydrocephalus
12. How does hypercapnia affect ICP?
    A. It impedes venous outflow.
    B. It impairs autoregulation.
    C. It results in cerebral vasodilation and increased blood volume.
    D. It increases CSF production and increases ICP.
13. Decorticate posturing is
    A. abnormal flexion and indicates cerebral hemispheric dysfunction
    B. abnormal extension and indicates brainstem dysfunction
    C. an ominous sign
    D. when the arms are pronated and extended
14. Which of the following GCS scores is consistent with coma?
    A. 8
    B. 10
    C. 12
    D. 15
15. Cushing's triad is evidenced by
    A. increase in systolic pressure
    B. decrease in diastolic pressure
    C. bradycardia
    D. all of the above
16. Which of the following methods is the most accurate measure of ICP?
    A. lumbar puncture
    B. intraventricular catheters
    C. epidural probe
    D. subarachnoid screw
17. Normal SjO_2 is
    A. 25 to 35 percent
    B. 40 to 60 percent
    C. 60 to 80 percent
    D. greater than 90 percent
18. Which of the following can be used in high-acuity units to monitor ICP, seizure activity, and cerebral ischemia?
    A. CT scan
    B. MRI
    C. PET
    D. Continuous EEG
19. Which of the following measures may be instituted to maintain CPP at 70 to 80 mm Hg?
    A. IV fluid
    B. dopamine
    C. phenylephrine
    D. all of the above

20. When should hyperventilation be instituted to decrease ICP?
  A. during the first 24 hours in ICU
  B. during the first 5 days in ICU
  C. when the $PaCO_2$ is 35 to 45 mm Hg
  D. for brief periods of time during acute neurologic deterioration

21. When administering mannitol to a patient, the nurse should monitor which of the following lab tests?
  A. serum osmolality
  B. urine sodium
  C. serum calcium
  D. serum potassium

22. Continuous EEG monitoring is useful for patients who receive
  A. mannitol
  B. high-dose barbiturates
  C. propofol
  D. neuromuscular blocking agents

Posttest answers with rationale are found on MyNursingKit.

EXPLORE PEARSON mynursingkit™

MyNursingKit is your one stop for online chapter review materials and resources. Prepare for success with additional NCLEX®-style practice questions, interactive assignments and activities, web links, animations and videos, and more!

Register your access code from the front of your book at **www.mynursingkit.com.**

REFERENCES

Alderson, P., & Roberts, I. (2005). Corticosteroids for acute traumatic brain injury. *Cochrane Database Systemic Review, 4,* CD000196;PMID:10796701.

Bader, M. K., March, K. S., & Littlejohns, L. (2002). *Cerebral oxygenation: how do we manage it and how will the patient benefit from targeted therapy?* Preconference Workshop, National Teaching Institute and Critical Care Exposition, Atlanta, Ga.

Barker, E. (2008). Intracranial pressure and monitoring. In E. Barker (ed.) *Neuroscience nursing: a spectrum of care* (3rd ed.). St. Louis: Mosby/Elsevier, Chapter 10, 305–309.

Barker, E. (2008). The adult neurologic assessment. In E. Barker (ed). *Neuroscience nursing: a spectrum of care* (3rd ed.). St. Louis: Mosby/Elsevier, Chapter 2, 57.

Blank-Reid, C., McClelland, R., & Santora, T. (2008). Neuroscience critical care management. In E. Barker (ed). *Neuroscience nursing: a spectrum of care* (3rd ed.) St. Louis; Mosby: Elsevier, 278–304.

Blank-Reid, C., McClelland, R., & Santora, T. (2008). Neurotrauma: traumatic brain injury. In E. Barker (ed.) *Neuroscience nursing: a spectrum of care* (3rd ed.). St. Louis: Mosby/Elsevier, 337–367.

Blissitt, P. A. (2009). Brain oxygen monitoring. In L. R. Littlejohns & M. K. Bader (eds.), *AACN-AANN protocols for practice: monitoring technologies in critically ill neuroscience patients.* Sudbury, MA: Jones & Bartlett Publishers.

Blissitt, P. A. (2009). Cerebrovascular disorders. In K. K. Carlson (ed.), *AACN's advanced critical care nursing.* St. Louis: Saunders/ Elsevier, 576–636.

Bullock, M. R. & Povlishock, J. T (eds). (2007). Guidelines for the management of severe traumatic brain injury. (3rd ed.). *Journal of Neurotrauma, 24*(suppl 1); pp. 1–95. Accessed at www.braintrauma.org. Retrieved August 1, 2008.

Coles, J. P., Fryer, T. D., Coleman, M. R. et al (2007). Hyperventilation following head injury: effect on ischemic burden and cerebral oxidative metabolism. *Critical Care Medicine*:35(2):663–4.

Cooper, P. R. et al. (1979). Dexamethasone and severe head injury. a prospective double-blind study. *Journal of Neurosurgery, 51,* 307–316.

CRASH TRIAL Collaborators. (2004). Effect of intravenous corticosteroids on death within 14 days, 10008 adults with clinically significant head injury (MRC CRASH trial): Randomized placebo-controlled trial. *Lancet,* 364, 1321–1328.

Dearden, N. M., et al. (1986). Effect of high-dose dexamethasone on outcome from severe head injury. *Journal of Neurosurgery,* 6481–88.

Dings, J., Meixenberger, J., Amscher, K. B., et al. (1996).Brain tissue pO_2 in relation to cerebral perfusion pressure, TCD findings and TCD-CO_2–reactivity after severe head injury. *Acta Neurochirurgica, 138*(4), 425–34.

Foley, N., Marshall, S., Pikul, J., Salter, K., Teasell, R. J. (2009). Hypermetabolism following moderate to severe traumatic acute brain injury: a systematic review. *Journal of Neurotrauma, PMID:19118457.*

Gopinath, S. P., Valadka, A. B., Uzura, M., & Robertson, C. S. (1999). Comparison of jugular venous oxygen saturation and brain tissue Po_2 as monitors of cerebral ischemia after head injury. *Critical Care Medicine, 27,* 2337–2345.

Helmy, A., Vizcaychipi, M., Gupta, A. K. (2007). Traumatic brain injury: intensive care management. *Journal of Neurotrauma,* (1): 32–42.

Iaia, A., & Barker, E. (2008). Neurodiagnostic studies. In E. Barker (ed.), *Neuroscience nursing: a spectrum of care* (3rd ed.). St. Louis: Mosby/ Elsevier, 104.

Kidd, K. C., & Criddle, L. (2001). Using jugular venous catheters in patients with traumatic brain injury. *Critical Care Nurse, 21*(6), 16–24.

Kirkness, C. (2009). Cerebral blood flow monitoring. In L. R. Littlejohns & M. K. Bader (eds.), *AACN-AANN protocols for practice: monitoring technologies in critically ill neuroscience patients.* Sudbury, MA:Jones & Bartlett, 145–168.

LeMone, P. & Burke, K. (2008). *Medical-surgical nursing: critical thinking in client care,* 4th ed. Upper Saddle River, NJ: Prentice Hall.

Littlejohns, L. R., & Bader, M. K. (2001). Guidelines for the management of severe head injury: clinical applications and changes in practice. *Critical Care Nurse, 21*(6), 48–65.

March, K., & Madden, L. (2009). Intracranial Pressure Management. In L.R. Littlejohns & M.K. Bader (eds.), *AACN-AANN protocols for practice: monitoring technologies in critically ill neuroscience patients.* Sudbury, MA: Jones & Bartlett, 35–60.

Marik, P., Varon, J., & Trask, T. (2002). Management of head trauma. *Chest, 122*(2), 699–711.

Marion, D. (2000). Hypothermia in severe head injury. *European Journal of Anesthesiology, 17*(suppl 18):45–46.

McQuillan, K. A., & Mitchell, P. H. (2002). Traumatic brain injuries. In K. A. McQuillan, K. T. Von Rueden, & M. B. Harsock, et al. (dds.), *Trauma nursing* (3rd ed.). Philadelphia: Saunders.

Powers, J. & Schulman, C. S. (2009). Head injury and dysfunction. In K. K. Carlson (ed.), *Advanced Critical Care Nursing.* St. Louis: Saunders/Elsevier, 529–575.

Saul, T. G., et al. (1981). Steroids in severe head injury: a prospective randomized clinical trial. *Journal of Neurosurgery, 54,* 596–600.

Van den Brink, W. A., van Santbrink, M., Steyerberg, E. W., et al. (2000). Brain oxygen tension in severe head injury. *Neurosurgery, 46,* 868–878.

Wøien, H., and Bjørk, I. T. (2006). Nutrition of the critically ill patient and effects of implementing a nutritional support algorithm in ICU. *J Clin Nurs.* 15(2):168–77.

MODULE

21 Alteration in Cerebral Tissue Perfusion: Acute Brain Attack

Melanie G. Hardin-Pierce, Karen L. Johnson, Theresa M. Glessner

OBJECTIVES Following completion of this module, the learner will be able to

1. Define stroke and discuss the major classifications of stroke.
2. Explain the pathophysiology of stroke.
3. Identify the modifiable and nonmodifiable risk factors for stroke.
4. List the manifestations of stroke and explain the rationale of various diagnostic tests used in the evaluation of stroke.
5. Describe the implications of the medications used to treat patients who have had strokes and discuss the rationale for surgical interventions for management of stroke.
6. Discuss priority nursing interventions for the patient with an acute brain attack.

This self-study module is composed of six sections. Section One defines stroke and discusses the two major classifications of stroke (ischemic and hemorrhagic). Section Two explains the pathophysiology of stroke. Section Three presents the modifiable and nonmodifiable risk factors for stroke. Section Four presents the manifestations of stroke and the rationale for various diagnostic tests used in the evaluation of stroke. Section Five presents the medical management of stroke including pharmacological and surgical interventions as well as the nursing diagnoses and management of the patient postoperatively. Section Six discusses the nursing challenges in caring for a patient with an acute brain attack in the acute phase. All Section Reviews include answers. It is suggested that the learner review those concepts answered incorrectly in the review questions before proceeding to the next section.

PRETEST

1. Stroke is an important cerebral vascular disorder because it
   A. is the second-leading cause of adult disability in North America
   B. is the third-leading cause of adult death in North America
   C. claims approximately 100,000 new victims each year in the United States
   D. is responsible for 500,000 deaths in the United States each year
2. The highest incidence of stroke is caused by
   A. atherothrombosis
   B. emboli
   C. primary intracerebral hemorrhage
   D. subarachnoid hemorrhage
3. A transient ischemic attack (TIA) is a(n)
   A. completed stroke
   B. stroke that extends beyond 24 hours but is reversible
   C. episode of focal neurologic deficit that resolves in a short period of time
   D. stroke that evolves over several days,
4. The penumbra is
   A. caused by excessive intracellular sodium
   B. a band of minimally perfused cells around an infarcted region of cells
   C. a central core of dead or dying cells
   D. a region in the brain that controls speech
5. The most important modifiable risk factor for stroke is
   A. diabetes mellitus
   B. cardiac disease
   C. hypertension
   D. drug abuse
6. Mr. Dixon, age 65, is an African American with a history of atrial fibrillation. His blood pressure is 180/100 mm Hg. He weighs 200 pounds and is 5 feet 5 inches tall. His blood cholesterol is 290 mg/dL; he has drinking binges on weekends, and for the past 30 years has smoked one pack of cigarettes per day. How many modifiable stroke risk factors does Mr. Dixon have?
   A. 2
   B. 4
   C. 6
   D. 8

7. The most common manifestation of stroke is
   A. seizures
   B. loss of vision in one eye
   C. numbness and weakness involving the face and arm
   D. a sudden loss of memory
8. In the acute care phase, a focused neurologic assessment for the patient with a stroke should include tests for
   A. dysphagia
   B. hemianopsia
   C. hemiparesis
   D. all of the above
9. Computerized tomography should be performed as soon as possible after the patient presents to the emergency department because
   A. it improves patient outcome
   B. it can differentiate hemorrhagic from ischemic stroke
   C. if the patient loses consciousness, the test is invalid
   D. none of the above
10. Tissue plasminogen activator should be given within
    A. three hours of onset of ischemic stroke
    B. three hours of onset of hemorrhagic stroke
    C. 24 hours of onset of ischemic stroke
    D. 24 hours of onset of hemorrhagic stroke
11. Which of the following interventional procedures has been successfully used to reverse neurologic deficits caused by atherosclerotic lesions of the cerebral arteries?
    A. aneurysm clipping
    B. embolization by arteriography
    C. cerebral angioplasty
    D. anticoagulant therapy
12. Which of the following statements is TRUE about seizures in the patient who has had a stroke?
    A. They commonly occur after the first month.
    B. They occur regularly and frequently after a stroke.
    C. Because of the high incidence of poststroke seizures, anticonvulsant therapy is necessary.
    D. Seizures are most likely to occur in the first 24 hours after a stroke.
13. Surgical management of hemorrhagic strokes may include all of the following EXCEPT
    A. evacuation of the hematoma
    B. craniotomy
    C. aneurysm clipping
    D. carotid endarterectomy
14. Patients with subarachnoid hemorrhage are at risk for developing hyponatremia as a result of
    A. syndrome of inappropriate ADH secretion
    B. too much IV fluid given in the emergency department
    C. low sodium diets
    D. infusion of sodium chloride IV solutions
15. Which of the following characterize upper motor neuron lesions?
    A. muscle spasticity
    B. muscle hypertonicity
    C. abnormally brisk reflexes
    D. all of the above
16. Which of the following is a TRUE statement about drooling after a stroke?
    A. Drooling rarely occurs after a stroke.
    B. Drooling signifies significant cerebellar dysfunction.
    C. Drooling is a clue that there may be swallowing problems.
    D. Drooling is a normal finding in all high-acuity patients.
17. The term used to describe flaccid bladder is
    A. detrusor hyporeflexia
    B. detrusor hyperreflexia
    C. detrusor-sphincter dyssynergy
    D. none of the above
18. Which of the following interventions would be appropriate for the patient with diplopia?
    A. Initiate aspiration precautions.
    B. Support the affected extremity during turning.
    C. Apply an eye patch to one eye.
    D. Talk loudly and slowly to the patient.
19. Agnosia is
    A. the inability to recognize familiar sensory information
    B. a sign of Alzheimer's disease
    C. a sign of impending stroke
    D. the inability to swallow
20. Which of the following strategies should the nurse use to reinforce a positive body image after a stroke?
    A. Use the terms *good side* and *bad side.*
    B. Use the terms *affected side* and *unaffected side.*
    C. Do not let the patient see himself or herself in the mirror.
    D. Do not mention the hemiplegic extremities when a patient has hemiplegic neglect syndrome.

Pretest answers are found on MyNursingKit.

SECTION ONE: Definition and Classifications of Strokes

At the completion of this section, the learner will be able to define stroke and discuss the major classifications of stroke.

Stroke is an acute neurologic deficit that occurs when impaired blood flow to a localized area of the brain results in injury to brain tissue. The term *brain attack* has been advocated to raise awareness of the need for rapid emergency treatment, similar to that with heart attack. Stroke is the third-leading cause of death in the United States and a leading cause of serious long-term disability (AHA, 2005).

Major Classifications of Stroke

Strokes are commonly classified by cause as either ischemic or hemorrhagic (see Fig. 21–1). Ischemic strokes occur when blood supply to a part of the brain is suddenly interrupted

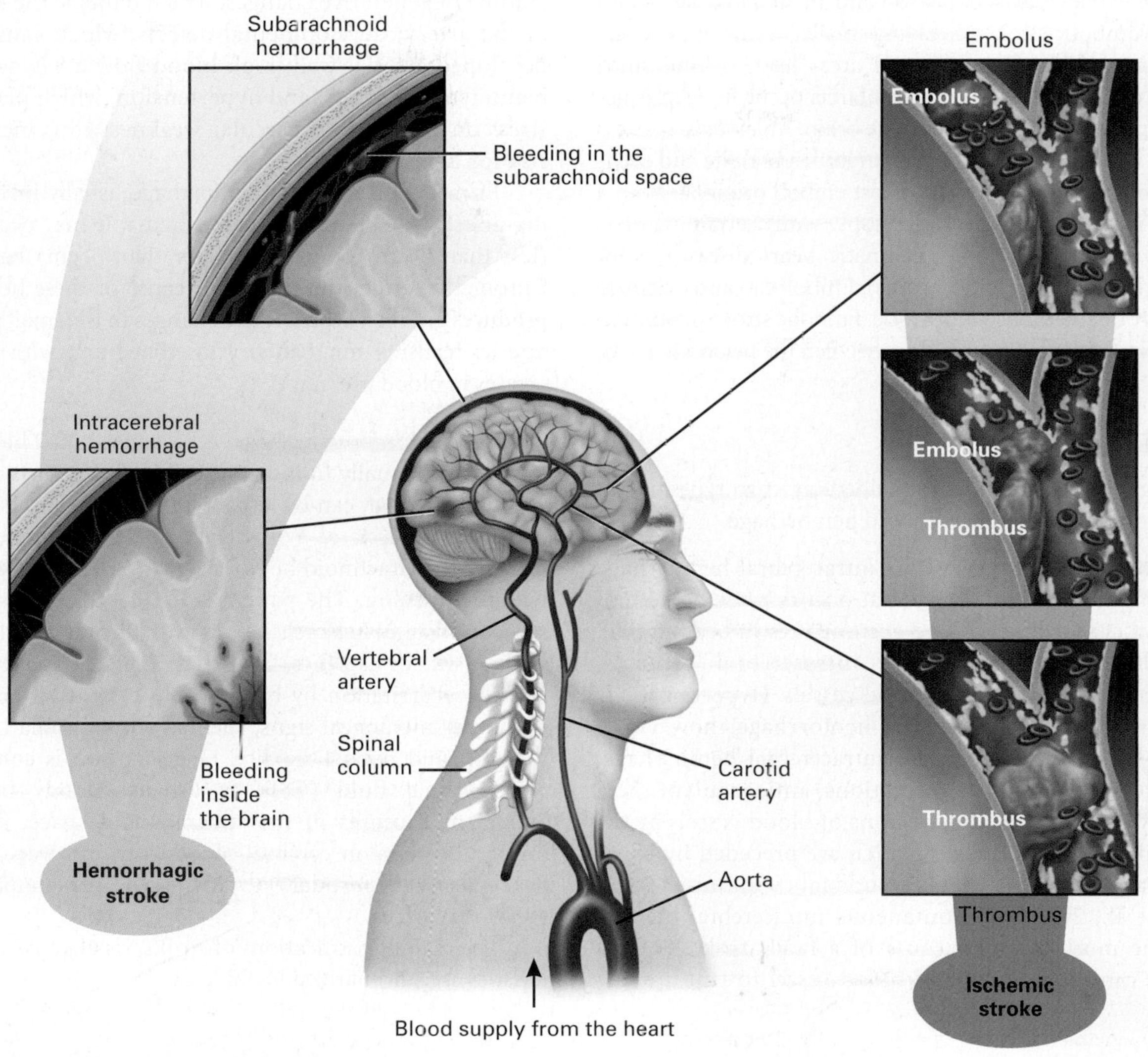

Figure 21–1 ■ Causes of Stroke: Hemorrhagic and Ischemic.

(thrombus or embolus). Hemorrhagic strokes occur when there is bleeding into brain tissue or cranial vault, such as that which occurs with head injury, aneurysms, arteriovenous malformations, or hypertension.

Ischemic Strokes

Ischemic strokes are caused by an interruption of cerebral blood flow by a thrombus or embolus. Interruption of cerebral blood flow can result in **transient ischemic attacks (TIAs).** TIAs are episodes of focal neurologic deficits that usually resolve in a few minutes or hours but are always completely resolved within 24 hours (Adams et al., 2008). A stroke may be preceded by a TIA similar to angina in a heart attack. Clinically, the patient may present with sudden unilateral dimness or partial loss of vision in one eye, weakness, numbness, tingling, severe headache, speechlessness, or unexplained dizziness. The symptoms are produced by inadequate perfusion to the brain. Inadequate perfusion can be caused by carotid stenosis (from atherosclerotic disease) or microemboli (from atherosclerotic plaques in major extracranial vessels). TIAs are warnings of an impending stroke and require immediate referral for treatment. The highest incidence for stroke occurs within the first few weeks after the TIA. The more frequently the TIAs occur, the higher the probability of stroke.

Atherosclerosis of cerebral arteries is the most common cause of ischemic stroke (Sharma, et al, 2005). Deposits of atherosclerotic plaque narrow vessel lumens and decrease cerebral blood flow. Plaque deposits in the intimal lining of arteries cause the internal elastic media to thin, weaken, expose the collagen layer, and create a "hole" in the vessel lining. Platelets become activated to adhere and aggregate in the tissue defect to "plug" the hole. Formation of a platelet plug initiates the coagulation cascade, which results in the formation of a stable fibrin clot. This clot may remain at the site, eventually getting large enough to completely occlude the vessel, or it may break off and become an embolus.

Thrombotic strokes are more common in older persons and are frequently accompanied by evidence of atherosclerotic plaque deposits in the coronary (heart) or peripheral vasculature.

Thrombotic strokes may occur at rest and are not associated with activity. Thrombotic strokes involving smaller vessels are referred to as *lacunar infarcts.* The infarcted areas leave behind small cavities (lacunae, or lakes). Lacunar infarcts occur in deep penetrating arteries in a single region of the brain. An *embolic stroke* is caused by a blood clot that travels from its original site and eventually becomes lodged in a vessel. Most emboli originate from a thrombus in the heart that develops with certain cardiac conditions (atrial fibrillation, rheumatic heart disease, recent myocardial infarction, or endocarditis). Emboli can also originate from rupture of atherosclerotic plaque. Embolic strokes, common in younger individuals, occur suddenly when the person is awake and active.

Hemorrhagic Strokes

Hemorrhagic strokes are further divided into two types, intracerebral hemorrhage or subarachnoid hemorrhage.

Intracerebral hemorrhage. The intracerebral hemorrhage is a type of hemorrhagic stroke that occurs when a cerebral blood vessel ruptures and blood accumulates in brain tissue. This results in compression of intracerebral contents, edema, and spasm of adjacent blood vessels. Hypertension is a common cause of intracerebral hemorrhage; however, a variety of factors can also cause intracerebral hemorrhage, including arteriovenous malformations, anticoagulant therapy, aneurysms, trauma, and erosions of blood vessels by tumors. Unlike ischemic strokes, which are preceded by TIAs, intracerebral hemorrhage appears suddenly without warning (Sharma et al., 2005). A spontaneous intracerebral hemorrhage is the most common cause of a fatal stroke. Several conditions can cause a cerebral blood vessel to rupture, including degenerative changes, which damage the elastic layer of the artery; developmental defects, which cause a poorly developed arterial wall; high blood flow areas, which cause hemodynamic stress; and hypertension, which places greater stress on any areas of vascular weakness thus increasing the risk for hemorrhage.

Primary intracerebral hemorrhage usually involves bleeding directly into the brain parenchyma; it may occur as small (less than 3 cm) or large (greater than 3 cm) hemorrhages. Chronic hypertension, the major cause of these hemorrhages, produces gradual, degenerative changes in the small penetrating arteries, causing microaneurysms that burst with sudden increases in blood pressure.

Subarachnoid hemorrhage. Leakage of blood from **aneurysms,** usually found at arterial bifurcations where blood velocity is higher, can be lethal with rupture and is usually located in the circle of Willis (Fig. 21–2). This type of stroke, usually a subarachnoid hemorrhage (SAH), develops suddenly without warning. The patient often complains of a sudden, severe unilateral headache—"the worst headache of my life"—neck pain or stiffness (**nuchal rigidity**) and vomiting. Meningeal irritation by blood produces the severe headache and other meningeal signs, such as photophobia (intolerance to light) and nuchal rigidity. Hypertension is common. The cerebrospinal fluid (CSF) is usually bloody because the aneurysm ruptures in the subarachnoid space. Following a SAH, a decrease in cerebral blood flow and transient loss of consciousness secondary to increased intracranial pressure (ICP) may occur.

The major classifications of stroke, risk factors, and characteristics are summarized in Table 21–1.

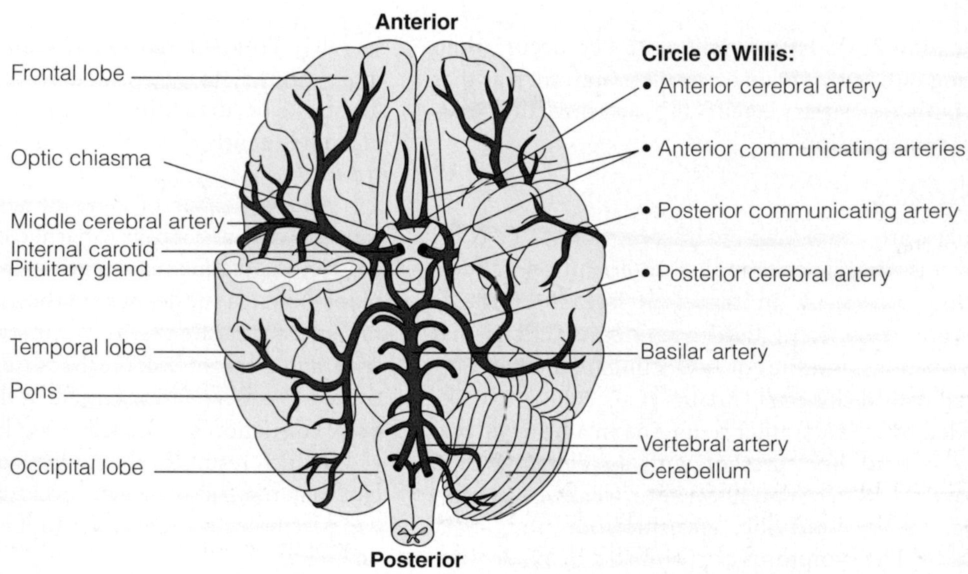

Figure 21–2 ■ Major arteries serving the circle of Willis.

TYPE OF STROKE	AGE	RISK FACTORS	CHARACTERISTICS
Ischemic Stroke			
Thrombotic	Older adults	Hypertension, smoking, high cholesterol, diabetes mellitus, atherosclerosis	May have TIAs Develop during sleep or on awakening May have mild headaches Predictable locations and symptoms Intermittent attacks and progression
Embolic	Adults of all ages	Cardiac abnormalities: Atrial fibrillation, valvular heart disease, carotid plaque or thrombosis	No warning, sudden attack Symptoms vary with attack Usually occur during daytime
Hemorrhagic Stroke			
Subarachnoid hemorrhage	Young, middle-aged adults	Ruptured aneurysms Arteriovenous malformations Trauma	Usually no warning, sudden attack Very severe headache, nausea/vomiting, photophobia Hypertension Decreasing level of consciousness Bloody CSF, nuchal rigidity
Intracerebral hemorrhage	Adults of all ages	Chronic hypertension Aneurysms Anticoagulant therapy Trauma Brain tumors Arteriovenous malformations	Usually no warning Gradual development Headache, nausea/vomiting, photophobia Hypertension Decreased level of consciousness Motor-sensory deficit of face, arm, leg

SECTION ONE REVIEW

1. Mrs. Davis, age 33, had a brief (3-min) episode of heaviness in her right arm and inability to speak. Symptoms disappeared and function returned to normal. The category of brain attack she most likely experienced is a(n)
   - A. subarachnoid hemorrhage
   - B. transient ischemia attack
   - C. intracerebral hemorrhage
   - D. lacunar stroke
2. Which of the following are the major classifications of stroke?
   - A. subarachnoid and intracranial hemorrhage
   - B. thrombotic and embolic
   - C. ischemic and hemorrhagic
   - D. TIA and embolic
3. The most common cause of ischemic stroke is
   - A. hypertension
   - B. subarachnoid hemorrhage
   - C. trauma
   - D. atherosclerosis
4. Which of the following conditions are associated with emboli formation?
   - A. myocardial infarction
   - B. atrial fibrillation
   - C. endocarditis
   - D. all of the above
5. Which of the following appears suddenly and without warning?
   - A. subarachnoid hemorrhage
   - B. ischemic strokes
   - C. TIAs
   - D. all strokes appear without warning

Answers: 1. B, 2. C, 3. D, 4. D, 5. A

SECTION TWO: Pathophysiology of Stroke

At the completion of this section, the learner will be able to explain the pathophysiology of stroke.

Recall from Section One that a stroke is characterized by neurologic deficits that occur when cerebral blood flow is diminished as a result of ischemic or hemorrhagic cerebral vascular events. The majority of strokes result from ischemic infarction and inadequate blood flow (Sacco et al., 2006). Atherosclerosis of cerebral arteries is a process similar to that found in cardiovascular arteries. Atherosclerosis and plaque formation result in narrowing or occlusion of arteries. The process of atherosclerosis results in plaque formation, which enhances platelet aggregation. Formation of a blood clot superimposed on atherosclerotic plaque causes significant stenosis of cerebral arteries. The most common site for the atherosclerotic process to occur is at the bifurcation of the common carotid artery. An embolism results in a stroke when a clot, plaque, or platelet plug breaks off an atherosclerotic lesion, enters the circulation, and blocks an artery.

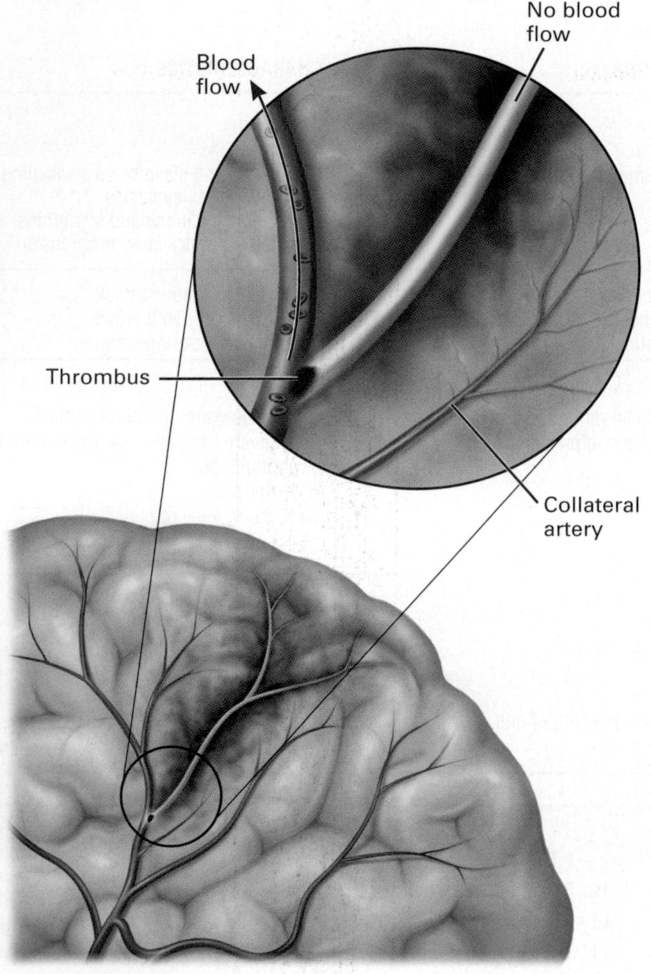

Figure 21–3 ■ Ischemia, infarction, and collateral flow. Brain tissues distal to a rupture, thrombus, or embolus receive little or no perfusion and become ischemic and eventually infarct. When a thrombus forms slowly, collateral arteries may form to perfuse or partially perfuse the ischemic area of the brain.

Diminished blood flow impairs oxygen delivery to neurons. Cerebral ischemia can be focal (localized) or global (widespread). Global ischemia is associated with a lack of collateral blood flow and irreversible brain damage (within minutes). With focal ischemia, some degree of collateral circulation remains, which allows for the survival of neurons and for reversal of neuronal damage after periods of ischemia. Focal ischemia is treatable because of the potential for recovery. Figure 21–3 provides an illustration of brain tissue distal to the stroke event.

Impaired oxygen delivery results in impaired cellular function because the cells do not have enough oxygen to generate energy. Without oxygen, the cellular sodium–potassium pumps fail. This results in increased intracellular concentrations of sodium, chloride, and calcium. Accumulation of these intracellular electrolytes is toxic to intracellular structures, particularly the mitochondria. Severe or prolonged ischemia leads to cellular death.

In the evolution of a stroke there are usually two zones of affected neurons. In the central zone are neurons that are infarcted (dead). They do not function and do not regain function. Surrounding the infarcted zone is a zone of neurons that are minimally perfused but not totally ischemic. This zone of neurons is called the **penumbra** (Fig. 21–4). Although these neurons still function, they are somewhat impaired. They remain viable and are capable of responding to therapy within a certain time frame. If perfusion to neurons in the penumbra is reestablished, many of the cells recover function. If perfusion is not reestablished, neurons in the penumbra die and the core of the nonfunctional neurons enlarges. Therefore, the fundamental goal of medical management is to restore cerebral blood flow and limit the size and extension of the infarcted zone.

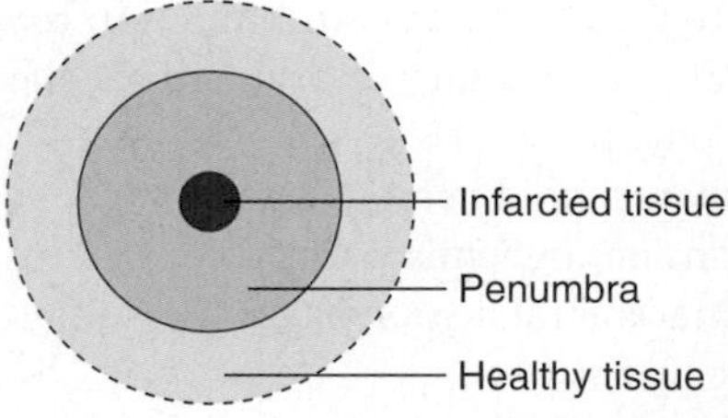

Figure 21–4 ■ Ischemic penumbra. Surrounding the infarcted zone is the penumbra. In this zone are neurons that are minimally perfused but still viable and capable of responding to therapy. The goal of medical management is to limit the size of the infarct zone and reestablish perfusion to neurons in the penumbra zone.

SECTION TWO REVIEW

1. Impaired cerebral oxygen delivery results in
   A. failure of sodium–potassium pumps
   B. aerobic metabolism
   C. immediate cell death
   D. none of the above
2. The penumbra is defined as the
   A. infarct zone
   B. zone of neurons that are minimally perfused
   C. zone of healthy neurons
   D. danger zone
3. The fundamental goal of medical management during cerebral ischemia is to
   A. limit sodium–potassium pumps
   B. promote anaerobic metabolism
   C. restore cerebral perfusion
   D. prevent clot formation

Answers: 1. A, 2. B, 3. C

SECTION THREE: Risk Factors for Stroke

At the completion of this section, the learner will be able to explain the modifiable and nonmodifiable risk factors for stroke.

Prevention of stroke is heavily dependent on the identification and modification of risk factors. These risk factors, categorized as modifiable or nonmodifiable, are summarized in Table 21–2.

Modifiable Risk Factors

Hypertension is an important modifiable risk factor for stroke and is implicated in both ischemic and hemorrhagic strokes. Both systolic and diastolic hypertensions (greater than 140/95) are risk factors (JNC, 2003). Reduction of both systolic and diastolic pressures in hypertensive individuals reduces stroke risk by 30–40 percent (Sacco et al., 2006). Hypotension, particularly in the elderly, may be a significant risk factor if the hypotensive episode is sudden and profound as may happen with the use of powerful antihypertensive agents, myocardial infarction, or bleeding. Dehydration also may dangerously lower blood pressure and decrease perfusion in the elderly, who already have an age-related decline in cerebral blood flow.

Cardiac disease is another important modifiable risk factor for stroke. Individuals with cardiac disease such as coronary heart disease, heart failure, left ventricular hypertrophy, or dysrhythmias (specifically atrial fibrillation) have more than twice the stroke risk compared with those without cardiac disease (Sacco et al., 2006). Therefore, cardiovascular risk reduction must be implemented to reduce the risk of coronary heart disease and, in turn, risk of stroke. This involves treating hyperlipidemia with antilipemic therapy, such as; HMG-CoA; reductase inhibitor (statin) to reduce risk for atherosclerosis.

Diabetes mellitus is a risk factor for ischemic stroke involving large and small vessels. An individual with a previous stroke has a high risk of developing a recurrent stroke. Dyslipidemia is a risk factor for atherosclerosis in both the coronary and cerebral vascular beds. Hypercholesterolemia is, therefore, another modifiable risk factor for stroke. Multiple studies have shown that lipid-lowering drugs (statins) reduce risk of stroke in those with coronary artery disease and elevated total or low-density lipoprotein cholesterol (Adams et al., 2008)

Cigarette smoking causes increased fibrinogen and platelet aggregation, as well as a reduction in high-density lipoproteins (Sacco, 2006). Cessation of smoking rapidly reduces the risk of vascular mortality (e.g., stroke) (Kenfield, Stampfer, Rosner & Colditz, 2008).

TABLE 21–2 Risk Factors for Stroke

MODIFIABLE	NONMODIFIABLE
Hypertension and hypotension	Age
Cardiac disease	Gender
Dysrhythmias (atrial fibrillation)	Race/ethnicity
Coagulopathies	Genetic factors
Diabetes mellitus	Prior stroke or heart attack
Drug abuse Cigarette smoking Excessive alcohol consumption Cocaine	
Physical inactivity	
Hypercholesterolemia	

Nonmodifiable Risk Factors

Nonmodifiable factors for stroke include age, gender, race, and genetic factors. Age is the single most important nonmodifiable risk factor for stroke; for each successive decade after 55 years, the stroke rate more than doubles (AHA, 2003). Men have a greater risk than women. African Americans, particularly males, have more hypertensive disease and more strokes than other races. Obesity, smoking, and diabetes mellitus are more prevalent among African Americans, which may account for their higher incidence of strokes (Sacco et al., 2006). Aging women sustain a large burden for stroke. While estrogen replacement therapy appears to have benefits for preventing stroke in animal studies, recent clinical trials do not support the use of estrogen replacement therapy for the prevention of vascular disease in humans (Sharma, 2005). Although the specific gene has not been identified, there appears to be a genetic predisposition to stroke in women.

Despite our knowledge of the importance of reducing risk factors for stroke, control of these factors is still inadequate because of poor patient compliance and adherence to behavior modifications, as well as decreased detection and treatment by health care providers. Further reductions in the risk of stroke require improvements in the ability to identify, modify, and manage cerebral vascular risk factors (Sacco et al., 2006).

SECTION THREE REVIEW

1. The most important modifiable risk factor for stroke is
   - **A.** age
   - **B.** hypertension
   - **C.** atrial fibrillation
   - **D.** diabetes mellitus

2. Which of the following modifiable risk factors are associated with increased risk of stroke?
   - **A.** cigarette smoking
   - **B.** heavy use of alcohol
   - **C.** physical inactivity
   - **D.** all of the above

(continued)

(continued)

3. The single most common nonmodifiable risk factor for stroke is
   A. advancing age
   B. race
   C. diabetes
   D. family history of stroke

Answers: 1. B, 2. D, 3. A

SECTION FOUR: Assessment and Diagnosis of Stroke

At the completion of this section, the learner will be able to list the manifestations of stroke and explain the rationale of various diagnostic tests used in the evaluation of stroke.

Assessment of Stroke

Manifestations of stroke vary according to the cerebral artery involved. About one third of patients who are having a stroke are aware of the symptoms; however, most bystanders are not knowledgeable about the signs of stroke (AHA, 2003). The most common manifestation is numbness and weakness of the face and arm. Other manifestations may include difficulties with balance or speech and loss of vision in one eye. Symptoms are usually sudden at onset and one sided. The specific stroke signs depend on the specific vascular territory compromised as summarized in Table 21–3.

Manifestations that occur rapidly but progress slowly are typically associated with thrombotic strokes. Manifestations that appear suddenly and cause immediate neurologic deficits are typically associated with embolic strokes. The manifestations of hemorrhagic stroke appear suddenly and depend on the location of the hemorrhage but may include headache, nausea/vomiting, seizures, **hemiplegia** (Fig. 21–5), and loss of consciousness.

A patient thought to be having a stroke requires prompt triage. Accurate diagnosis is based on a complete history and a thorough physical assessment with a focused neurologic exam. The goal of the exam is to quickly determine whether the stroke is ischemic or hemorrhagic because each requires different medical interventions. Important information to elicit includes any reports of recent medical or neurologic events (hemorrhage, surgery, trauma, myocardial infarction, or stroke) and medication history (antiplatelet or anticoagulant drugs). Particular attention is given to vital signs. An irregular heart rhythm may indicate atrial fibrillation. Hypertension increases the likelihood for intracranial hemorrhage. The focused neurologic assessment is key and includes tests for **dysphagia, hemianopsia** (Fig. 21–6), **hemiparesis,** and other signs of focal injury (Sacco et al., 2006).

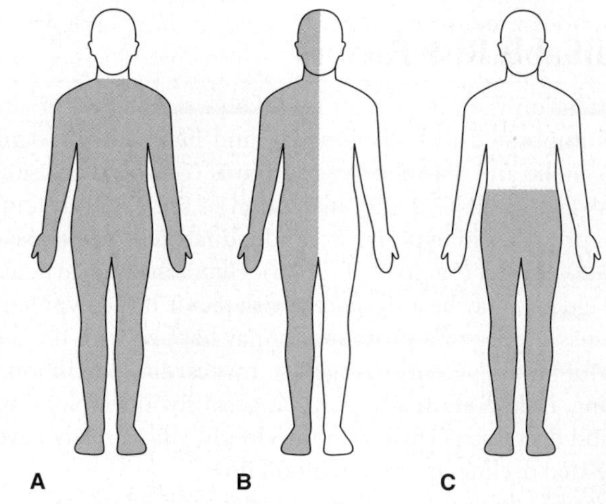

Figure 21–5 ■ Types of paralysis. **A.** Quadriplegia is complete or partial paralysis of the upper extremities and complete paralysis of the lower part of the body. **B.** Hemiplegia is paralysis of one-half of the body when it is divided along the median sagittal plane. **C.** Paraplegia is paralysis of the lower part of the body.

TABLE 21–3 Signs and Symptoms of Stroke Related to Vascular Territory Compromised

VASCULAR TERRITORY COMPROMISED	SIGNS AND SYMPTOMS
Carotid ischemia	Monocular vision loss Aphasia (dominant hemisphere) Hemineglect (nondominant hemisphere) Contralateral sensory or motor loss
Vertebrobasilar ischemia	Ataxia Diplopia Hemianopsia Vertigo Cranial nerve defects Contralateral hemiplegia Sensory deficits

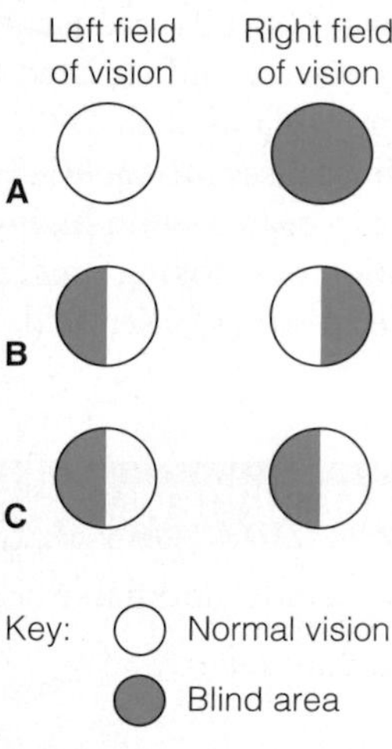

Figure 21–6 ■ Abnormal visual fields. **A.** Normal left field of visions with loss of vision in right field. **B.** Loss of vision in temporal half of both fields (bitemporal hemianopsia). **C.** Loss of vision in nasal field of right eye and temporal field of left eye (homonymous hemianopsia).

A focused clinical assessment of the patient is important to establish a baseline and to assist in diagnosis and prognosis in terms of survival and functional recovery. When a stroke is suspected, the ABCs (airway, breathing, and circulation) are assessed. Impaired airway clearance may result from hemiplegia, dysphagia, a weak cough reflex, and immobility. This places the patient at high risk for hypoxemia, pneumonia, and aspiration. Continuous monitoring of breath sounds, breathing patterns, oxygen saturation, skin color, and arterial blood gases (ABGs) is important. The patient's ability to handle secretions is assessed. Intubation and mechanical ventilation are required for the patient who is comatose and has evidence of increased ICP. The patient may present with ineffective breathing patterns because of decreased level of responsiveness, aspiration, loss of protective reflexes, or a decrease in respiratory movements on the affected side. With inadequate ventilation, hypercapnia occurs, causing cerebral vasodilation. This, however, diverts blood from the penumbra and contributes to an extension of the infarct. To prevent **hypercapnia,** the nurse monitors rate and rhythm of breathing, ABGs, and level of consciousness. Cardiovascular assessment includes frequent monitoring of vital signs (particularly blood pressure and heart rate) until the patient is stable. The heart rhythm is assessed for dysrhythmias. Peripheral and carotid pulses are palpated. Continuous telemetry identifies abnormal cardiac rhythms.

There are several key physical assessment findings in a patient who has had a stroke that the nurse must recognize. If the patient is awake, the probability of a hemispheric stroke is high. Ptosis of the eyelid and cranial nerve III (oculomotor) involvement suggest a posterior stroke may have occurred. Contralateral hemiparesis involving the face and limbs is indicative of a hemispheric (anterior or carotid) stroke. Assessment of extremity position and handgrips, arm drifts, and leg pushes for strength are imperative. The tone (**flaccidity** or **spasticity**) of the extremities is noted. Speech is assessed for coherency, content, and fluency. Orientation and the ability to follow commands is assessed. Loss of consciousness raises suspicion of a posterior (vertebrobasilar) stroke or a bilateral hemispheric stroke. During the physical assessment, sensitivity to cognitive and perceptual–visual–spatial deficits and patient behavior manifesting as neglect or poor judgment choices is a key in assessment findings. Cranial nerve abnormalities (III to XII) reflect brainstem involvement or a vertebrobasilar stroke. Cranial nerve assessment helps to establish a baseline against which to compare the patient's progress. Figure 21–7 illustrates many of the common general findings associated with stroke.

The National Institutes of Health Stroke Scale is widely used in the United States to assess neurologic outcome and degree of recovery (Table 21–4). The complete questionnaire with

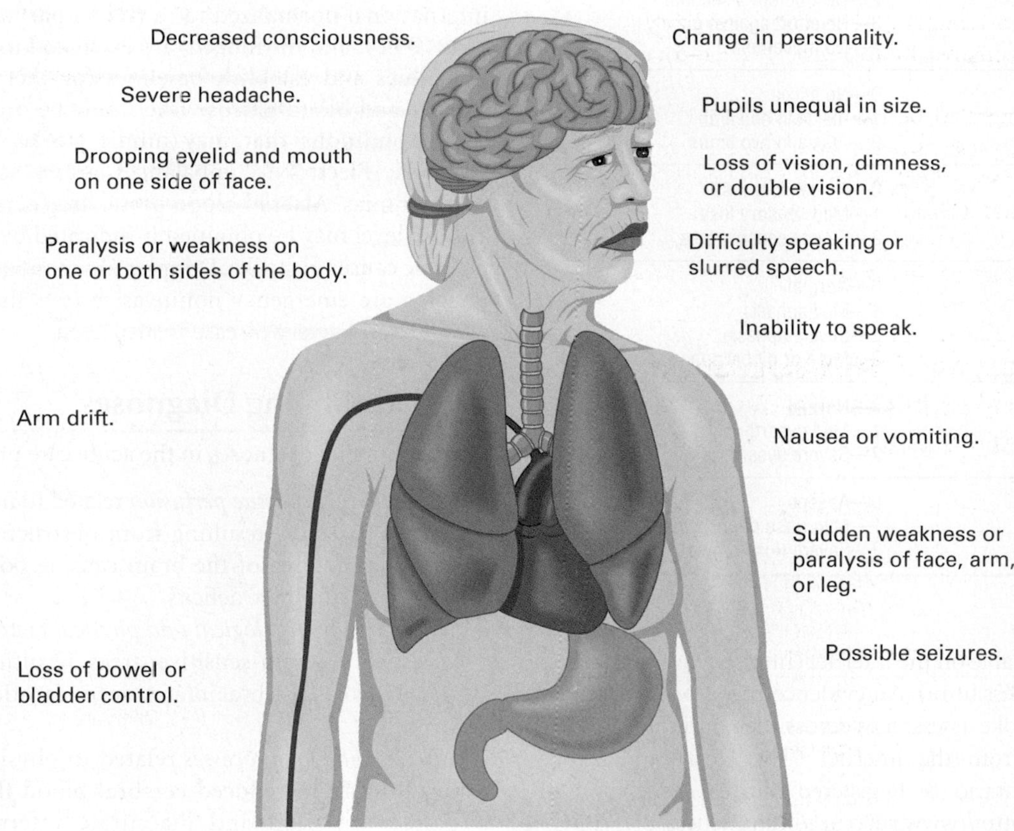

Figure 21–7 ■ General manifestations of stroke.

TABLE 21–4 National Institutes of Health Stroke Scale

TITLE	RESPONSES AND SCORES
Level of consciousness	0—Alert 1—Drowsy 2—Obtunded 3—Coma/unresponsive
Orientation questions (two)	0—Answers both correctly 1—Answers one correctly
Response to commands (two)	0—Performs both tasks correctly 1—Performs one task correctly
Gaze	0—Normal horizontal movements 1—Complete gaze palsy
Visual fields	0—No visual field defect 1—Partial hemianopsia 2—Complete hemianopsia 3—Bilateral hemianopsia
Facial movement	0—Normal 1—Minor facial weakness 2—Partial facial weakness 3—Complete unilateral palsy
Motor function (arm) a. Left b. Right	0—No drift 1—Drift before 5 seconds 2—Falls before 5 seconds 3—No effort against gravity 4—No movement
Motor function (leg) a. Left b. Right	0—No drift 1—Drift before 5 seconds 2—Falls before 5 seconds 3—No effort against gravity 4—No movement
Limb ataxia	0—No ataxia 1—Ataxia in one limb 2—Ataxia in two limbs
Sensory	0—No sensory loss 1—Mild sensory loss 2—Severe sensory loss
Language	0—Normal 1—Mild aphasia 2—Severe aphasia 3—Mute or global aphasia
Articulation	0—Normal 1—Mild dysarthria 2—Severe dysarthria
Extinction or inattention	0—Absent 1—Mild (loss of one sensory modality) 2—Severe (loss of two modalities)

instructions is available on the internet (http://www.strokecenter.org/trials/scales/nihss.html). An evidence-based practice guideline that guides stroke assessment across the continuum of care can be accessed from the internet (The Heart and Stroke Foundation of Ontario & Registered Nurses Association of Ontario. (2005). http://www.rnao.org/bestpractices/PDF/BPG_Stroke_Assessment.pdf.

TABLE 21–5 Scans and Angiography Used in Diagnosis of Acute Stroke

TESTS	PURPOSE
Computerized tomography (CT) scan of brain	Differentiate hemorrhagic from ischemic cause
Special CT scans (Transcranial and extracranial contrast enhanced or single-photon-emission)	Establish the anatomical regions and structures involved; determine the cause of infarction
Cerebral vessel arteriography	Evaluate vessel structures, vasospasm, or stenosis
Magnetic resonance imaging (MRI) with angiography	Diagnose brain lesions

Diagnostic Tests and Procedures

A variety of tests and procedures are performed as soon as possible after arrival of the patient to the ED to determine the exact nature of the stroke. Table 21–5 lists some of the more common scans and angiography tests used for diagnosing strokes. Lumbar puncture may be performed to detect blood in the cerebrospinal fluid if subarachnoid hemorrhage (SAH) is suspected but not confirmed by CT scan. Transesophageal echocardiography detects cardiac and aortic causes of embolism. A 12-lead ECG is performed because cardiac abnormalities are prevalent among patients with stroke. A complete blood count, including platelets, prothrombin time (PT), international normalized ratio (INR), partial thromboplastin time (PTT), and fibrinogen, are evaluated to detect any coagulopathies and establish baselines for therapy. Serum electrolytes and blood glucose levels may be ordered to rule out other conditions that may mimic stroke, including hypoglycemia. Electrolyte imbalances are a source of cardiac dysrhythmias. Arterial blood gases, drug screen, and a serum alcohol level may be obtained if indicated by history to detect possible causes of stroke. Doppler ultrasonography and duplex imaging are emergency noninvasive tests that are conducted when carotid artery disease is suspected.

Related Nursing Diagnoses

Priority nursing diagnoses in the acute care phase include

- *Altered cerebral tissue perfusion* related to interruption of arterial blood flow resulting from obstruction or rupture of vessels in an area of the brain causing possible increase in ICP and neurologic deficits
- *Pain related to biological and physical* factors of pressure or irritation to pain-sensitive areas resulting from hemorrhagic stroke, cerebral infarction, or carotid artery occlusive stroke
- *Altered thought processes* related to physiological changes resulting from reduced cerebral blood flow, causing impaired sensation and inaccurate interpretation of the environment

SECTION FOUR REVIEW

1. The most common manifestation of stroke is
   - A. numbness and weakness of the face and arm
   - B. monocular vision loss
   - C. aphasia
   - D. hemineglect
2. Headache, nausea, vomiting, and seizures are common manifestations of
   - A. thrombotic strokes
   - B. embolic strokes
   - C. hemorrhagic strokes
   - D. TIAs
3. Which of the following may be used to detect cardiac and aortic causes of embolism?
   - A. CT scan
   - B. MRI
   - C. transesophageal echocardiography
   - D. lumbar puncture
4. Sensory deficits are common symptoms of strokes that involve
   - A. cartoid ischemia
   - B. middle cerebral artery ischemia
   - C. vertebrobasilar ischemia
   - D. Circle of Willis ischemia

Answers: 1. A, 2. C, 3. C, 4. C

SECTION FIVE: Medical and Nursing Management

At the completion of this section, the learner will be able to describe the implications of the medications used to treat patients who have had strokes and discuss the rationale for medical and surgical interventions for management of stroke.

Medical Management of Strokes

Because most strokes are caused by an occlusion of a cerebral vessel, improvement and restoration of perfusion to the ischemic area is imperative. The concept of the penumbra is fundamental in treating ischemic strokes. Although a core of infarcted tissue is not salvageable, adjacent dysfunctional tissue is salvageable if circulation is promptly restored (Adams et al., 2008). Patients with acute ischemic stroke presenting to the emergency department within 48 hours of the onset of symptoms are given aspirin (50 to 325 mg/day) to reduce stroke mortality and decrease morbidity, provided contraindications, such as allergy and gastrointestinal bleeding, are absent and the patient has not or will not be treated with tissue plasminogen activator (Jauch, Kissela & Stettler, 2007).

Intravenous tissue plasminogen activator (rtPA) is strongly recommended for carefully selected patients who can be treated within three hours of onset of ischemic stroke (Adams et al., 2008). The patient who receives this medication is usually admitted to an intensive care unit or stroke unit. A small dose is given as a bolus, and is followed by an IV infusion of the drug over an hour. During and after the infusion, the nurse performs frequent neurological assessments and evaluates the patient's blood pressure. The schedule for both of these assessments is every 15 minutes for the first two hours, every 30 minutes for the next six hours, and then every hour for 24 hours after treatment (Adams et al., 2008). During the infusion, if the patient develops nausea, vomiting, severe headache, or acute hypertension, the infusion is discontinued and the physician is notified immediately. Antihypertensive medications are given as required. The placement of nasogastric tubes, bladder catheters, or intra-arterial catheters should be delayed (Adams et al., 2008).

Emerging Evidence

- Treatment of stroke patients with extended-release (ER) niacin, alone or in combination with statins, should be considered in stroke patients with atherosclerotic mechanisms with low serum HDL-C levels *(Keener & Sanossian, 2008)*.
- Evidence-based guidelines suggest that stroke patients should be screened for dysphagia before oral intake. Investigators validated a three-part (swallow, cough, and vocal quality) dysphagia screening tool to identify patients who are able to swallow and eat from a safe menu until a formal evaluation by a speech therapist (ST) can be done. RN-performed screenings were compared with independent screenings performed on the same patient within one hour by a speech therapist. Eighty-three paired screenings were completed, with 94 percent agreement between the RNs and the STs *(Weinhardt, Hazelette, & Barrett et al., 2008)*.
- Investigators conducted a prospective randomized controlled trial of 500 cases to determine the optimal time-window for surgical treatment of spontaneous intracerebral hemorrhage (ICH). The study yielded conclusive evidence that the early stage (within 7-24 hours) was the optimal time-window for surgical intervention of spontaneous ICH *(Wang, Wu & Mao et al., 2008)*.

The use of anticoagulant medications (heparin, low molecular weight heparin, or antiplatelet agents) for acute stroke care has been the subject of much debate. For many years, early anticoagulation was used frequently in the treatment of ischemic stroke. This practice has changed substantially because evidence has shown it has not been effective (Albers et al., 2008). The administration of anticoagulants is currently contraindicated during the first 24 hours following treatment with rtPA (Adams et al., 2008). Administration of these medications increases the risk of serious bleeding complications. (See RELATED PHARMACOTHERAPY box: Agents Used in the Treatment of Stroke) Much is known about the benefits of aspirin and antiplatelet drugs in patients with acute myocardial ischemia, but less is known about the use of these drugs in patients with cerebral ischemia. Recent research has evaluated the use of these antiplatelet drugs in the setting of acute

TABLE 21–6 Current Recommendations of Antiplatelet Therapy and Ischemic Strokes

Aspirin should be given as soon as possible after onset of stroke symptoms for most patients.
The administration of aspirin, as an adjunct therapy, within 24 hours of the use of thrombolytic agents is NOT recommended.
Aspirin should NOT be used as a substitute for other acute interventions (rtPA) for the treatment of acute ischemic stroke.
No recommendation can be made about the urgent administration of other antiplatelet aggregating agents.

stroke and additional research is in progress. Current recommendations, as summarized by Adams and colleagues (2008), are summarized in Table 21–6.

Seizures are most likely to occur within 24 hours of stroke; however, there is no evidence to support the use of prophylactic administration of anticonvulsants after stroke (Adams et al., 2008).

Cerebral angioplasty has been successfully used to reverse neurological deficits caused by atherosclerotic lesions in the cerebral arteries. This technique uses a balloon catheter to mechanically dilate vessels. Microballoon catheters are introduced via the femoral artery and directed to the major arteries at the base of the brain. Vascular stenting is an alternative to angioplasty. There are currently many different types of stents in various stages of clinical use and approval by the Federal Drug Administration, although additional clinical trials must be completed before widespread use can be recommended. Cerebral angiography carries the risks of intracerebral hemorrhage, injury to the vessel wall, and distal embolization. Following cerebral angioplasty or stenting, nursing assessments for neurologic and vital sign changes are done frequently until the patient is neurologically stable.

Surgical Management of Strokes

Cerebellar lesions are critical because a hemorrhage or infarction can rapidly become life-threatening by compromising the brainstem. Emergency surgery is indicated for cerebellar infarction or hemorrhage with clinical evidence of brainstem compression and increased ICP, such as decreasing level of

RELATED PHARMACOTHERAPY: Agents Used in the Treatment of Stroke

Thrombolytic Agent

Recombinant tissue plasminogen activator (Alteplase)

Action and Uses

Acute ischemic stroke or thrombotic stroke rt-PA therapy converts plasminogen to plasmin leading to breakdown of fibrin clots.

Major Adverse Effects

Bleeding, anaphylaxis, cardiac dysrhythmias

Nursing Implications

Because of the increased risk for life-threatening intracranial bleeding, a head CT without contrast should be obtained before administration along with baseline labs (CBC, PT and PTT, fibrinogen, type and screen for blood).

Heparin, warfarin, and aspirin should not be co-administered for 24 hours following administration of this agent.

Venipunctures and invasive line placement should be avoided for 24 hours also.

Anticonvulsant

Phenytoin (Dilantin)
Fosphenytoin (Cerebyx)
Lorazepam (Ativan)

Action and Uses

Prevent or treat seizures

Anticonvulsant agents, in general, stabilize cell membranes thereby increasing the seizure threshold and reducing electrical discharges in the motor cortex.

Major Adverse Effects

Hypotension, bradycardia, tissue irritation (phenytoin), respiratory depression

Nursing Implications

Phenytoin - Administer slowly, no faster than 50 mg/min to avoid hypotension and bradycardia; administer with in-line filter. Monitor serum drug levels (therapeutic is 10-20 mcg/ml); avoid peripheral IV injection of phenytoin or administration with other drugs.

Fosphenytoin - May administer via peripheral route as it is less irritating to tissues; may cause less hypotension and bradycardia than phenytoin.

Lorazepam – May cause decreased level of consciousness and respiratory depression.

Antihypertensive

Hydralazine (Apresoline)
Labetalol (Trandate)
Nicardipine (Cardene)
Nifedipine (Procardia)

Action and Uses

Reduces BP by directly dilating arterioles (hydralazine).
Reduces BP by blocking alpha1, beta1, and beta 2-adrenergic receptors (labetalol).
Reduces BP by calcium channel blocking properties resulting in depression of cardiac and vascular smooth muscle (nicardipine and nifedipine).

Major Adverse Effects

Hypotension, tachycardia, dizziness, headache, lupus (hydralazine), bradycardia, bronchospasm (labetalol)

Nursing Implications

Labetalol - Avoid using in patients with asthma, AV heart block and bradycardia.

Nifedipine and nicardipine- Do not abruptly discontinue this medication as it may result in cardiac ischemia and chest pain.

Monitor for hypotension; avoid sublingual route due to increased risk of hypotension.

Anticoagulant

Enoxaparin (Lovenox) (low molecular weight)
Heparin
Warfarin (Coumadin)

Action and Uses

Prevention of deep vein thrombosis (Enoxaparin and heparin) Management of DVT and pulmonary embolism; prevention of new emboli associated with carotid or vertebral dissections, prosthetic heart valve replacements and atrial fibrillation by interfering with vitamin K dependent clotting factor synthesis (warfarin).

Major Adverse Effects

Bleeding, thrombocytopenia

Nursing Implications

Enoxaparin – Monitor for bleeding and thrombocytopenia.

Heparin – Monitor for bleeding, thrombocytopenia; trend aPTT levels and have protamine sulfate available as an antidote.

Warfarin – Not used in the acute phase of stroke management; PT/INR must be monitored; monitor for bleeding; requires intensive education regarding drug-food interactions and need for monitoring.

Antiplatelet

Acetylsalicylic acid (aspirin)
Clopidogrel (Plavix)
Dipyridamole (Persantine)
Ticlopidine (Ticlid)

Action and Uses

Antiplatelet aggregation; prolongs bleeding time, thereby reducing atherosclerotic events in high-risk patients.

Major Adverse Effects

Bleeding, particularly in the gastrointestinal tract.; GI irritation, thrombocytopenia, rash

Nursing Implications

Aspirin – Monitor for gastric irritation; use enteric coated varieties and take with food.

Clopidogrel – Monitor for gastrointestinal distress, heartburn, nausea, and bleeding; Avoid administering with aspirin.

Dipyridamole – Monitor for bleeding and thrombocytopenia.

Ticlopidine- Monitor for gastrointestinal distress, heartburn, nausea; monitor for neutropenia, anemia, and thrombocytopenia, particularly during the first three months of therapy.

Data obtained from Wilson, B. A., Shannon, M. T., Shields, K. M., and Stang, C. L. (2008). *Nurse's Drug Guide.* Upper Saddle River, NJ: Pearson/Prentice Hall.

consciousness, restlessness, or cranial nerve palsies. The size of the hemorrhage or infarction is a critical variable in medical management. Patients with large hemorrhages or infarctions are more likely to have brainstem compression and an urgent need for surgery.

Bleeding into the subarachnoid space, such as that which occurs with a ruptured aneurysm, requires immediate medical attention. Treatment, however, depends on the severity of neurological symptoms. Persons with no neurological deficits may require cerebral arteriography and early surgery. The surgical procedure, performed within 72 hours of the bleed, is known as an "aneurysm clipping" and involves opening the cranium (craniotomy) and inserting a metal clip around the aneurysm to prevent rebleeding. Postoperative complications include cerebral vasospasm. Vasospasm decreases perfusion to brain tissue. Vasospasm is prevented and treated with "triple H therapy": hypervolemia, hypertension, and hemodilution. This combination of therapies is used to augment cerebral perfusion pressure (CPP) by raising systolic blood pressure, cardiac output, and intravascular volume to increase cerebral blood flow and minimize cerebral ischemia. Triple H therapy is maintained for the first two to three days postoperatively.

For ischemic cerebrovascular disease, surgery may be performed to prevent recurring cerebral infarcts and TIAs. This procedure is done to remove the source of the occlusion and to increase cerebral blood flow to the ischemic area. A carotid endarterectomy (Fig. 21–8) is a surgical procedure performed to remove atherosclerotic plaque. This involves the removal of exposed occlusive atherosclerotic plaque from the carotid artery. Postoperative nursing care for the patient who has a carotid endarterectomy is summarized in Table 21–7.

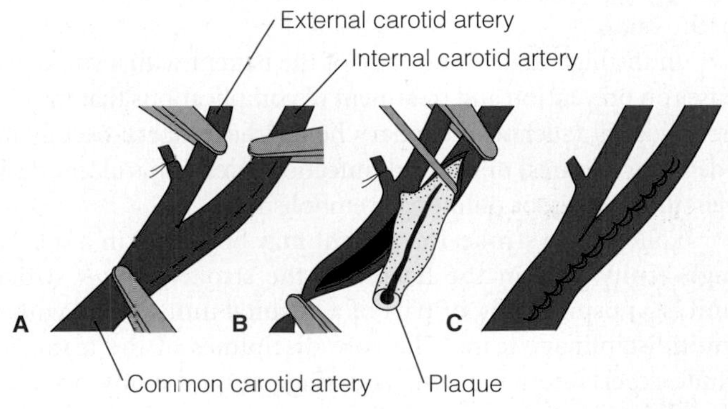

Figure 21–8 ■ Carotid endarterectomy. **A.** The occluded area is clamped off and an incision is made in the artery. **B.** Plaque is removed from the inner layer of the artery. **C.** To restore blood flow through the artery, the artery is sutured, or a graft is completed.

TABLE 21–7 Caring for the Patient after Carotid Endarterectomy

NURSING INTERVENTION	RATIONALE
Position patient on the nonoperative side, with head of bed elevated 30 degrees	Elevation reduces operative site edema
Maintain head and neck alignment; avoid rotating, flexing, or hyperextending head	Proper alignment prevents additional tension or pressure on the operative side and facilitates blood flow
Support the head during position change (teach patient to do the same)	Support prevents additional tension/stress on operative side; tension/stress may cause bleeding and hematoma formation
Nursing assessments focus on early identification of complications, including hemorrhage, respiratory distress, cranial nerve impairment, and alterations in blood pressure	The most common cause of respiratory problems is pressure on the trachea from hematoma formation Cranial nerves may be stretched during surgery, leading to temporary deficits in cranial nerve function; assess for facial drooping, tongue deviation, hoarseness, dysphagia, or loss of facial sensation Patients who have this procedure are at risk for developing unstable blood pressure as a result of denervation of the carotid sinus

SECTION FIVE REVIEW

1. Which of the following is fundamental to the current approach to the treatment of ischemic strokes?
   A. ischemic penumbra
   B. infarcted area
   C. cerebral edema
   D. cerebral perfusion pressure
2. During administration of rtPA, neurological assessments initially should be made every
   A. 12 hours
   B. six hours
   C. hour
   D. 15 minutes
3. Which of the following statements is FALSE about aspirin administration in cerebral ischemia?
   A. It should be given within 24 hours of thrombolytic agents.
   B. It should not be given within 24 hours of thrombolytic agents.
   C. It should not be used as a substitute for rtPA.
   D. Less is known about the use of this drug with cerebral ischemia.

Answers: 1. A, 2. D, 3. A

SECTION SIX: Brain Attack: Nursing Challenges in the Acute Phase

At the completion of this section, the learner will be able to discuss priority nursing interventions for the patient with acute brain attack.

In the high-acuity unit, care of the patient with a stroke focuses on prevention and treatment of complications that may be neurological (such as secondary hemorrhage, space-occupying edema, or seizures) or medical (infections, decubitus ulcers, deep vein thrombosis, or pulmonary embolism).

Following a stroke, the patient may be placed in a special high-acuity unit in the hospital—the stroke unit. A stroke unit is a hospital unit, or part of a hospital unit, staffed with a multidisciplinary team. The core disciplines of the team include experts from medicine, nursing, physiotherapy, occupational therapy, speech and language therapy, and social work. The acute stroke unit admits patients quickly and continues treatment for several days, until transfer to a rehabilitation or nursing facility, or to the patient's home.

Alteration in Tissue Perfusion

Altered tissue perfusion related to interruption of flow and venous stasis from inactivity is a priority nursing diagnosis for patients in the acute phase after a stroke. A serious threat to the hemiplegic stroke patient is a deep vein thrombosis (DVT), which may lead to pulmonary embolus. Stroke patients are at high risk for DVT because of hemiplegia, loss of vasomotor tone, venous stasis, and edema in the paralyzed, flaccid limbs; and immobility. Dehydration places the patient at high risk for DVT. Hemiplegia or hemiparesis decreases muscle pump action for return of venous blood to the heart. Poor positioning (one extremity lying on another) or sitting for long periods in a chair can precipitate or exacerbate DVT formation. Subcutaneous unfractionated heparin, low-molecular-weight heparin, and heparinoids may be given for DVT prophylaxis for at-risk patients with ischemic stroke as well as other nonpharmacologic measures, such as sequential compression devices, to prevent DVT (Albers et al., 2008).

Impaired Physical Mobility

Impaired physical mobility is related to motor and sensory deficits, particularly hemiplegia and impaired balance, changes in postural tone, and disinhibition of primitive reflex activity. Rehabilitation begins early after a stroke in an effort to increase independence. A multidisciplinary effort is required for maximum rehabilitation potential (Broderick & Hacke, 2002). Physical therapists assess motor function, plan exercise programs, and provide splints to prevent contractures. Occupational therapists assess the patient, provide a plan of therapy, and evaluate sensory and cognitive problems that interfere with functional independence. The physiatrist is a physician responsible for diagnosing and treating rehabilitative problems, such as spasticity and **subluxation.**

Following a stroke, cerebral shock may occur, causing hypotonicity or flaccid hemiplegia. During cerebral shock, a state of temporary disruption of neural transmission and integration processes occurs. When a stroke causes hemiplegia, initially the patient's affected limbs are flaccid; later, tone is palpated in affected limb muscles and spasticity begins, with some resistance to movement. Spasticity results when reflex activity is released from cerebral inhibition after damage to the motor system. This spasticity is associated with an upper motor neuron lesion because the frontal cortex (motor centers) and/or corticospinal (voluntary motor) tracts are interrupted. Muscle spasticity, hypertonicity, resistance to passive stretch in joints, and abnormally brisk reflexes characterize upper motor neuron lesions. Depending on the stroke site, the patient can present with mild hemiparesis to severe hemiplegia, quadriplegia, ataxia, or involuntary movements.

Poststroke spasticity (excessive muscle tone) affects the antigravity muscles. In the lower limbs, these are the knee extensors and plantar flexors of the foot. In the upper limbs, these are the elbow flexors and wrist and finger flexors. The patient assumes a spastic "hemiparetic posture," with the neck and trunk tilted toward the hemiparetic side; the shoulder pulled down and back; the elbow, wrist, and fingers flexed; and the arm adducted. The lower limb is extended, with the hip internally rotated and adducted, and the foot plantar is flexed with supination, inversion, and flexed toes. Because flexor muscles are stronger in the arms and extensors stronger in the legs, the patient is prone to flexion contractures in the upper extremity and extension contractures in the lower extremities.

Maintaining functional abilities in the acute phase after stroke is an important component of patient care. Active and/or passive range of motion (ROM) exercises performed at least three or four times a day help prevent contractures. Proper body alignment is also important to prevent contractures. The patient is placed in positions that neutralize the abnormal hemiparetic posture. When lying supine, the head and spine are straight and the entire affected arm is elevated on pillows with the hand and fingers extended in a functional position, preferably with the palm up. A folded towel is placed under the affected shoulder so that both shoulders are symmetrical. A firm roll along the lateral aspect of the hip and thigh neutralizes the tendency of the affected leg to rotate externally. If positioned on the affected side, the patient's body is rotated slightly less than 90 degrees to rest on the shoulder blade rather than directly on the shoulder, to avoid the body's weight on the paralyzed arm or leg. The affected arm is extended perpendicular to the body, and the leg slightly flexed (Fig. 21–9). When positioned on the unaffected side, the patient's body is rotated more than 90 degrees with the affected shoulder forward, extremities beyond midline, the affected arm extended and elevated on pillows, and the affected leg functionally flexed and elevated on pillows. When eating in the upright position, the affected arm is elevated on a pillow to maintain proper body alignment. During turning, avoid pulling on the affected arm because this may produce subluxation of the shoulder joint. Tennis shoes help to prevent contractures in the flaccid stage but tend to stimulate more spasticity in the hyperreflexic stages. Hard rolls or inflatable splints are used to maintain functional hand and arm position and are applied, particularly at night. Correct positioning by abduction and external rotation of the shoulder prevents shoulder pain.

Ambulation and Activities of Daily Living

The patient is ready to ambulate when there is evidence of leg strength, some balance, and **proprioception.** Muscle tone is assessed regularly, and the patient is not asked to do an activity with the disabled limb until muscle tone is restored. Traditional slings are avoided because they reinforce the abnormal posture of the spastic flexed arm and adduction, and promote shoulder contractures. The affected arm is supported with pillows and handled gently to avoid subluxation of the shoulder joint.

Potential Alteration in Nutrition

Dysphagia, absent or diminished gag reflexes, facial paralysis, perceptual and cognitive deficits, hemiplegia (particularly affecting the dominant hand), an inability to perform bilateral hand tasks, and immobility all contribute to undernutrition. Absent gag reflexes and facial paralysis limit chewing and swallowing movements and increase the risk for aspiration. Perceptual deficits, such as impaired depth perception, agnosia, apraxia, hemianopsia, or neglect, may produce injury during eating.

The hypermetabolic stress response initiated by the brain attack results in hyperglycemia as well as decreased intake. Thus, metabolic demands become greater at a time when oral intake is often acutely restricted. Clinically, the patient may manifest a decrease in serum protein leading to a compromised immune state, weight loss, muscle weakness and atrophy, increased risk of pressure ulcers, higher morbidity and mortality, and a prolonged hospital stay. In well-nourished patients, nutritional support is started if no oral intake is anticipated for greater than five days. If the patient is malnourished on admission, as defined by a greater than 10 percent weight loss before critical illness, nutritional support is initiated promptly (Blissett, 2009).

The patient is assessed for the ability to bring food to the mouth, handle utensils, see all the food on the tray, and successfully chew and swallow food and liquids, with no pocketing in the affected cheek. Early and rapid evaluation of swallowing is done as soon as possible (Sacco et al., 2006). In addition, the patient is assessed for (1) cognitive ability to feed self, (2) drooling (a clue to swallowing problems) or difficulty swallowing liquids or foods, (3) continuous clearing of the throat or coughing while eating, and (4) appropriate positioning during eating. Dysphagia, or difficulty in swallowing, is usually caused

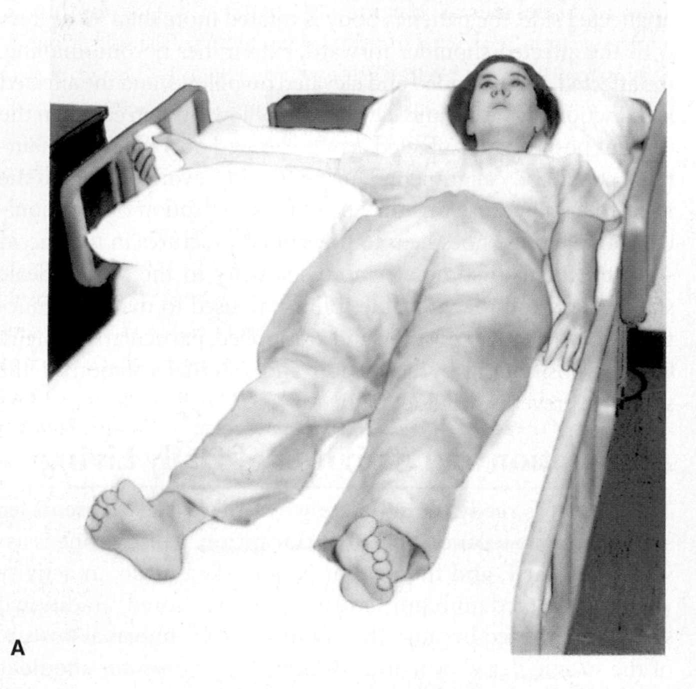

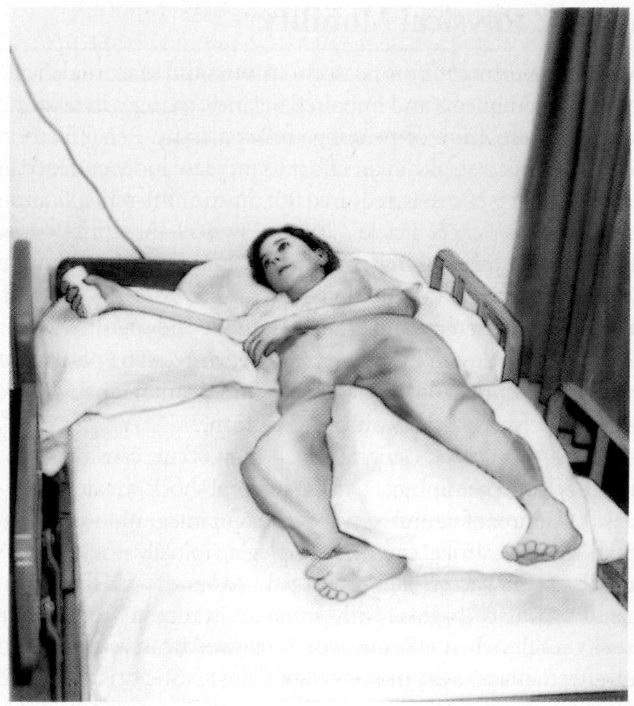

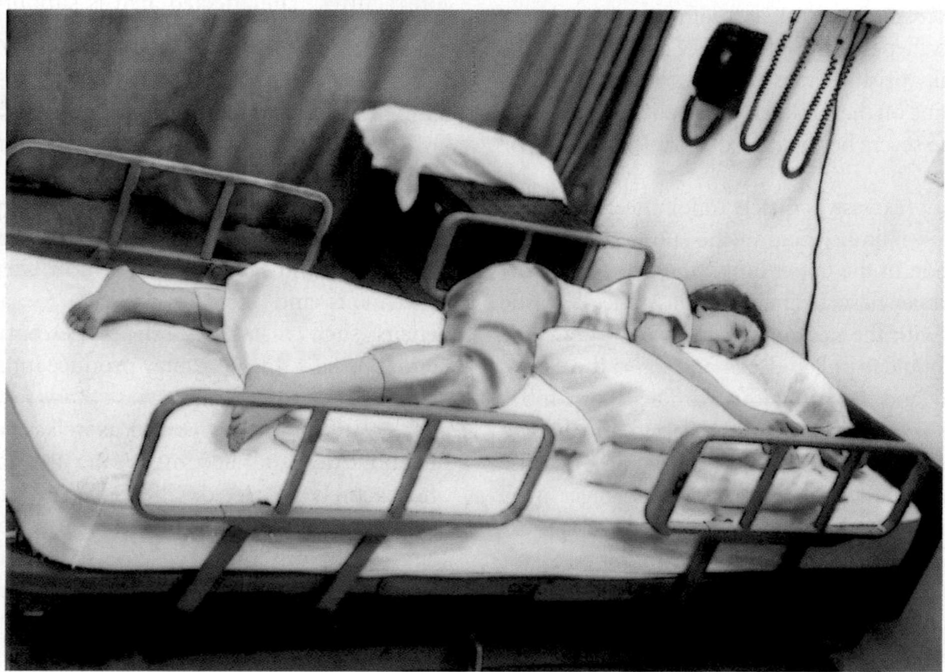

Figure 21–9 ■ Positioning the stroke patient. **A.** Lying on back. **B.** Lying on affected side. **C.** Lying on unaffected side.

by lesions involving cranial nerves V (trigeminal), VII (facial), IX (glossopharyngeal), X (vagus), XI (accessory), and XII (hypoglossal). Dysphagia is suspected when these signs appear: food put in the mouth causes the patient to choke, drool, have poor lip closure, engage in food pocketing, or have asymmetry of the mouth or a protruded tongue; food in the back of the throat causes the patient to choke, aspirate or have nasal regurgitation, become weak, or develop a hoarse voice; and food passing through the esophagus causes the patient to regurgitate (Blissett, 2009; LeMone & Burke, 2008).

Alteration in Elimination

Alteration in elimination may be related to impaired mobility, cognitive impairment, aphasia, and preexisting elimination problems. Urinary elimination problems most frequently encountered in the stroke patient are as follows:

- Detrusor muscle hyporeflexia (flaccid bladder)
- Detrusor muscle hyperreflexia (uninhibited or spastic bladder)
- Detrusor muscle–sphincter dyssynergy (unsynchronized detrusor and sphincter muscles producing urinary retention)

Patients with detrusor hyporeflexia have large-capacity, flaccid bladders with overflow incontinence. An indwelling urinary catheter should be inserted as soon as possible after the stroke with intake and output monitoring. After the acute phase of the injury has passed, the indwelling urinary catheter is removed and an intermittent catheterization program is implemented (every four hours) to ensure that the urine volume does not exceed 400 mL. For patients with bladder hyperreflexia, a voiding schedule is established with the patient and family based on previous patterns of voiding. When possible, diapers and long term indwelling urinary catheter use should be avoided. Refer to Table 21–8 for a description of neurogenic bladder types.

Constipation is common after stroke, probably because of age-related hypotonicity of the bowel, a decrease in roughage and fluid intake, immobility and the inability to communicate the need to defecate. To promote adequate bowel elimination, a convenient pattern is established after assessing former and current bowel patterns. Information related to fluids and foods that normally elicit bowel movements and patient preferences in roughage foods is elicited. Constipation should be avoided because straining during defecation can elevate the blood pressure. Stool softeners and suppositories are used to establish a regular pattern, as well as gastrointestinal reflexes when establishing an optimal toileting time (e.g., after meals). Daily assessment and outcome criteria are established for bowel elimination based on the individual's pattern.

Sensory Alterations

Sensation and skin integrity may be altered in the stroke patient related to loss of the sense of touch, pressure, temperature and sensation; or motor or vascular tone loss. Lesions in the parietal cortex or its afferent pathways produce a loss of primary sensations or **paresthesias** placing the patient at risk for burns, bruises, and other forms of injury. Impaired tactile sensation affects motor activity because sensory feedback is limited. It also affects perception because sensory information needed for interpretation and integration is limited. Loss of proprioception or position sense may lead to falls. Loss of vision and hearing can cause injury, social isolation, and impaired learning. A care priority in these patients is to protect them from injury.

The nurse protects the cornea by patching the eye and administering prescribed artificial tears or lubricants to prevent drying and corneal ulceration. For the diplopic patient, an eye patch applied to one eye and alternated every three to four hours while the patient is awake permits a clear image. Avoiding extremes in heat and cold to desensitized areas is also important to prevent injury. Gentle handling of patients when transferring from bed to wheelchair, and teaching the patient and family environmental hazards to avoid in the home are essential aspects of care for patients with altered sensation. It is important to inform both patient and family that when transferring from bed to wheelchair, the neglected or hemiplegic part must be supported and protected.

In the acute stages of stroke, the patient is prone to develop pressure ulcers because of sensory, motor, or vascular tone loss as well as incontinence, parietal neglect, and spasticity. The patient with a hemisensory deficit or hemiplegia cannot change positions. In addition, if nutrition is poor, the skin tissue is likely to break down in the immobile patient. Perceptual deficits compound the problem, particularly parietal neglect, when portions of the body are ignored.

To protect the patient from injury and to maintain skin integrity in hemiplegics or those who are experiencing neglect or

TABLE 21–8 Neurogenic Bladder Types in the Acute Stroke Patient

BLADDER TYPE	FEATURES	LESION SITE	EFFECTS ON PATIENT	NURSING APPROACH
Detrusor hyporeflexia	Flaccid (large capacity)	Above the pons	Overflow incontinence Distended bladder High urine residual volumes	Monitor intake and output Observe for overdistention Intermittent catheterization Keep urine volume less than 400 mL
Detrusor hyperreflexia (uninhibited)	Spastic (small capacity)	Cerebral cortex, internal capsule, basal ganglia	Urinary frequency, urgency Bladder contractions/spasms Nocturia Low-volume voidings Incontinence (unable to reach toilet in time)	Voiding schedule every two hours or longer Monitor intake, output Encourage fluids Limit caffeine and evening fluids Upright position to void
Detrusor–sphincter dyssynergy (uncoordinated)	Spastic bladder and external sphincter that contract simultaneously (small capacity)	Pons, and pathways between pons and above sacral spinal cord	Small, frequent, or no voids Sensation of bladder fullness Dribbling, overflow incontinence High urine residual volumes Dysuria	Antispasmodics may be prescribed Consistent fluid intake Time voiding schedule Possibly intermittent catheterization within five minutes of voiding Observe for overdistention symptoms Keep residuals less than 75 mL Monitor intake, output

denial, the patient and family must be alerted to the deficit and hazards related to the deficit. This includes teaching them to inspect the skin with mirrors; to observe the skin for adequate capillary refill, pallor, and hyperemia; and to avoid pressure on the area should any of these appear. The patient is repositioned at least every two hours and the skin is inspected with each reposition. The turning schedule is revised based on patient tolerance and skin integrity.

Perceptual hemineglect is a disorder of attention causing an inability to integrate and use perceptions in the contralateral side or space. The patient fails to respond to stimuli presented to the side contralateral to the brain lesion; therefore, that side is ignored but can be used if attention is drawn to it. Right brain damage produces this syndrome. Hemineglect is seen alone or in combination with **anosognosia** and left homonymous hemianopsia (hemineglect syndrome).

Patients with hemineglect syndrome can be assisted by increasing the awareness of their surroundings and by alleviating apprehension as to the source of the problem. When homonymous hemianopsia is present, initially the patient is compensated for and approached from the unaffected side, positioned so that the intact visual field is toward the action, personal items are arranged within the field of vision, and taught to scan the environment by turning the head vertically and horizontally. As the patient's apprehension decreases, the patient is stimulated by placing personal items toward the affected side to encourage awareness of and attention to that side. This is accomplished by positioning so that the eyes are facing the affected side and by teaching the patient to handle, position, exercise, bathe, and dress the affected extremities with the patient's unaffected arm. Denial of illness usually resolves as the patient recovers.

Agnosia is a cortical impairment that results in the inability to recognize or interpret familiar sensory information although there is no impairment of sensory input or dementia. The agnosias can be tactile, visual, or auditory (Table 21–9). Tactile agnosia (astereognosia) is the inability to recognize objects by touch although tactile sensation is present. Visual agnosia is the inability to recognize or name familiar objects or faces although visual acuity is intact (e.g., the patient is unable to recognize utensils, toothbrush, clothes, or photographs). Auditory agnosia is the inability to recognize familiar sounds, such as a doorbell, telephone, horn, gun, or siren. When assessing for agnosias, the patient is asked to name objects and cite their purpose. The patient is asked to identify objects in the hands or to identify sounds, music, or songs with his or her eyes closed. When deficits are found, a referral is made to an occupational therapist (OT) who evaluates and establishes a rehabilitative program.

Apraxia is the inability to carry out a purposeful movement although movement, coordination, and sensation are intact. There are several types of apraxias summarized in Table 21–10. To assess for motor apraxia, the nurse observes the ability to initiate responses to motor commands, such as "Brush your teeth … comb your hair … put on your gown." The nurse notes the patient's ability to do spontaneous simple acts. Ideational apraxia is assessed by observing the patient's ability to perform spontaneous acts or acts on command, such as writing. The patient with ideational apraxia is unable to conceptualize the act and cannot perform a spontaneous act. Asking the patient to copy or draw a clock or daisy, or to build three-dimensional designs, such as a house or block, are requests used to assess the patient with constructional apraxia. Asking the patient to put on or remove a shirt, gown, or robe assesses dressing apraxia.

The effectiveness of therapy for ideomotor and ideational apraxia is uncertain. For ideomotor and ideational apraxia, the components of a motor sequence leading up to the entire activity need to be broken down and taught in simple terms, speaking slowly with clear directions. The patient with dressing apraxia is assisted by the use of labels to distinguish right and left, back from front, right and wrong side, or by color-coding garments. For all apraxic patients, repetition, consistency, avoidance of distractions, and visual motor coordination exercises are useful.

Impaired Communication

Patients with left hemispheric dysfunction caused by middle cerebral artery involvement experience **aphasic dysphasia** if the speech centers or their pathways are involved in the lesion. Aphasia/dysphasia is a disorder of linguistic processing in which there is a disruption of translating thought to language. Literally, **aphasia** means a total inability to understand or formulate language. Language comprehension, speech expression, or writing ability may be lost. Dysphasia refers to difficulty with comprehending, speaking, or writing.

In Wernicke's aphasia, the patient receives auditory impulses but is unable to comprehend them. It is a receptive aphasia characterized by fluent, well-articulated speech with intact tone but

TABLE 21–9 Agnosias

TYPE	DEFICIT
Tactile	Inability to recognize objects by touch
Visual	Inability to recognize or name familiar objects or faces
Auditory	Inability to recognize familiar sounds

TABLE 21–10 Apraxias

TYPE	LESION SITE
Motor	Memory deficit for motor sequences affecting only upper limbs, although muscle and sensory function are intact
Ideomotor	Inability to perform a motor act on command even though the patient understands the act and has muscle and sensory function; can perform spontaneous, simple, isolated acts but not complex acts, such as writing or dressing
Ideational	Inability to perform activities automatically or on command
Constructional	Inability to copy, draw, or construct designs in two or three dimensions on command or spontaneously
Dressing	Inability to dress self because of a disorder in body schema, unilateral neglect, and/or spatial relations

inappropriate speech content that is unintelligible because of poor word choices. The patient makes up new words. Reading and speech comprehension, repetition of speech, and naming of objects is impaired. The patient is unable to write coherently. Motor deficits are seldom seen in these patients because the lesion is in the left temporal lobe. The goal of therapy for patients with Wernicke's aphasia is to develop an awareness of the language problem and to increase comprehension. Removing extraneous sounds and distractions, such as the television or radio, assist in getting the person's attention. The patient and nurse use nonverbal behavior to enhance communication. Keeping the conversation on one defined subject with one question at a time and avoiding multiple choices when communicating is helpful.

Broca's aphasia is an expressive aphasia characterized by nonfluent, telegraphic speech with outbursts of profanity, uninhibited speech, and word-finding difficulty, which reflects impaired memory for language. The patient uses nouns or phrases with pauses between words, and lacks grammar. An awareness of speech errors is present and speech production is labored and frustrating. A poor capacity for repetition and difficulty naming objects exists although recognition of objects is present. Oddly, these patients can sing fluently because musical ability is intact in the nondominant hemisphere. Comprehension is usually intact and responses are appropriate. Reading comprehension is variable and writing ability is impaired, possibly because an associated right hemiparesis or hemiplegia is often found in these patients since Broca's area is located adjacent to the primary motor centers in the frontal lobe. The goal for the patient with Broca's aphasia is to establish reliable language output to express needs. This may be accomplished initially by asking the patient "yes–no" questions.

Global aphasia is a combination of Broca's and Wernicke's aphasia with an almost complete loss of comprehension and expression of speech. The lesion involves the frontal and temporal lobes. The patient has nonfluent speech and an inability to express his or her ideas in speech or writing. The goal for the patient with global aphasia is to improve the ability to communicate. The patient is taught to enhance communication with nonverbal gestures and facial expressions. The measures cited for both Wernicke's and Broca's aphasias are applicable with these patients as well.

Dysarthria is an impairment of the muscles that control speech. Hemispheric or brainstem strokes produce dysarthria, which is characterized by slurred, muffled, or indistinct speech. Uncoordinated, slow, monotone speech results if the basal ganglia or cerebellum are involved. Language comprehension and formulation are intact unless the patient also has aphasia. The goal of therapy is to strengthen the speech muscles in order to speak more clearly and fluently. Encouraging the patient to enunciate one word at a time, particularly consonants, and increasing voice volume when it is low helps.

High Risk for Ineffective Patient and Family Coping

Patients and their families are faced with multiple psychosocial stressors. The potential for ineffective coping is related to abrupt change in lifestyle, loss of roles, dependency, and economic insecurity. The inability to cope with abrupt and severe changes in body function or image, lifestyle changes, fears of becoming a burden on the family, dependency, and economic insecurity with loss of the breadwinner role provide ample and valid reasons for ineffective coping. In addition, the family may have to assume new roles as care providers and relinquish jobs and salaries. They may be overwhelmed with medical bills or faced with nursing home placement of their loved one and subsequent guilt. Fears of another stroke as well as inability to care for the patient at home create more stress. Dominant hemispheric stroke patients, in addition, are prone to severe depression because of their awareness of their deficits.

Other causes for ineffective coping are the emotional and cognitive impairments following a stroke. Emotional lability with inappropriate crying, laughing, or euphoria, or socially inappropriate behavior with an inability to interpret social cues of communication, creates stress for both the patient and family. Uninhibited behavior with outbursts of profanities or abrupt or impulsive behavior provides additional sources of stress. Confusion and bewilderment may compound the problem. In terms of impaired cognition, there may be delayed processing, diminished learning and reasoning ability, and a short attention span. Memory deficits vary with the hemispheric involvement. If the nondominant hemisphere is involved, a memory deficit for performance may be seen; if the dominant hemisphere is involved, a memory deficit for language, word-finding difficulty, and naming problems surface. In addition, there are hemispheric differences in judgment. Patients with lesions in the left hemisphere are slow and cautious, and underestimate their abilities. In contrast, patients with right hemispheric lesions may be prone to injury because they overestimate their abilities.

To assist the patient in coping effectively, he or she is provided with appropriate information to alleviate fears and strengthen support systems. Clergy, friends, and family support groups may help assist the patient in coping and may provide comfort for both the patient and the family. Informing the patient that most recovery takes up to six months (and some, even longer) may be helpful in preventing unrealistic expectations for recovery.

If inappropriate crying or laughter occurs, divert the patient's attention from the behavior to stop it. Provide feedback in a matter-of-fact way when behavior is inappropriate. Avoid nagging, angry, or punitive responses. Be patient and gently slow down impulsive behavior.

A positive body image is reinforced when one focuses on the function that is left and not on that which is lost. Speak positively about the remainder of body functions. Use terms such as *affected* and *unaffected* rather than *good* and *bad* side. Reinforce independence early by involving the patient in decisions about care. Teach the family to do the same related to family roles and care.

For the patient and family, multidisciplinary referrals may be necessary. Social workers, home health nurses, dieticians, occupational therapists, physiatrists, support groups, and voluntary and governmental agencies (e.g., Medicare) provide assistance. The American Heart Association and the National Stroke Association provide free and low-cost literature on stroke care developed by experts. These referral groups and services are essential for the functional recovery and provide invaluable assistance in restoring the patient to a functional or complete recovery. Priority nursing interventions for the patient with acute brain attack are summarized in the NURSING CARE box, The Patient with Acute Brain Attack.

NURSING CARE: The Patient with Acute Brain Attack

Expected Patient Outcomes and Related Interventions

Outcome 1:Prevent secondary brain injury and preserve neurologic function

Assess and compare to established norms, patient baselines, and trends

Surveillance of BP, HR, hemodynamic and cardiac stability
Seizure precautions
ICP (< 20 mm Hg); CPP (60-70 mm Hg)
Cerebral oxygenation ($SjvO_2$ at 55-75 mg/dl; $PbtO_2$ 20-24 mm Hg)
Changes in mental status and LOC, restlessness, drowsiness, lethargy, inability to follow commands, reflexes, and strength

Administer related drug therapy and monitor for therapeutic and nontherapeutic effects

Seizure prophylaxis
Diuretics, hypertonic saline, and sedation
Intravenous hydration – dextrose 5 percent or 0.9 percent normal saline – initial rate 150-200 mL/hr

Related nursing diagnoses

Alteration in cerebral tissue perfusion and autoregulation

Outcome 2: Optimize oxygenation

Assess and compare to established norms, patient baselines, and trends

PaO_2, SaO_2, SpO_2, P_{ETCO_2}

Administer related drug therapy and monitor for therapeutic and non-therapeutic effects

Oxygen to maintain $SaO_2 > 92$ percent
DVT prophylaxis
Sequential pneumatic compression devices

Interventions to enhance oxygenation

Keep head of the bed at 30 degrees
Frequent oral care – plaque removal, moisturize mucous membranes to reduce bacterial load in the mouth so as to decrease risk for pneumonia

Related nursing diagnoses

Alteration in pulmonary function: gas exchange

Outcome 3: Hemodynamic and cardiac rhythm stability will be achieved and maintained

Assess and compare to established norms, patient baselines, and trends

BP, HR, hemodynamic parameters from a pulmonary artery catheter (Swan Ganz) such as PAP, PCWP, CVP, CO/CI
Systemic vascular resistance
Electrolyte levels
CK-MB, troponin levels

Administer related drug therapy and monitor for therapeutic and nontherapeutic effects

Administer medications per established ACLS protocols as needed for rate/rhythm disturbances:
Amiodarone, Diltiazem, Adenosine, beta blockers

Investigate and reverse underlying cause of crisis

Related nursing diagnoses

Tissue perfusion/hemodynamic dysfunction

Outcome 4: Prevention, rapid diagnosis and treatment of infections

Assess and compare to established norms, patient baselines, and trends

Monitor for infection and fever
WBC count
Culture and sensitivity results
Observe for signs of infection in patients considered to be at increased risk: those with invasive lines, incisions, and those who require mechanical ventilation.

Administer related drug therapy and monitor for therapeutic and nontherapeutic effects

Antibiotic therapy as ordered

Related nursing diagnoses

Potential for infection
Altered body temperature: hyperthermia

Outcome 5: Achieve fluid and electrolyte balance

Assess and compare to established norms, patient baselines, and trends

Intake and output status
Electrolyte levels
Daily weights, CVP, and PCWP
Chest X-rays
Lung sounds

Administer related drug therapy and monitor for therapeutic and nontherapeutic effects

Electrolytes: potassium, calcium, phosphorous, sodium

Related nursing diagnosis

Alteration in fluid and electrolyte balance

Outcome 6: Avoid malnutrition, complications from stress ulcer or gastrointestinal bleeding

Assess and compare to established norms, patient baselines, and trends

Serum glucose levels
Indices of nutrition: C-reactive protein, albumin, pre-albumin
Ability to swallow
Coughing with eating or drinking is indicative of dysphagia

Administer balanced nutritional and medication regimen and monitor therapeutic and nontherapeutic effects

Start nutrition as soon as possible
obtain consult for study to assess intake ability to swallow on admit and prior to initiating PO intake
Avoid dextrose-containing IV fluids
Administer GI/ulcer prophylaxis (H_2 blockers, proton pump inhibitors)
Monitor for coughing with eating or drinking as this may be indicative of dysphagia.

Related nursing diagnoses:
Impaired nutritional status
Risk for aspiration

Outcome 7: Skin, mucous membrane integrity, and optimal joint mobility will be maintained.

Assess and compare to established norms, patient baselines, and trends
Skin and mucous membranes

Interventions to maintain skin integrity
Maintain a clean and dry environment
Utilize pressure reducing surfaces

Prevent loss of joint mobility or musculoskeletal deformity
Reposition every two hours
Physical therapy and occupational therapy consults should be ordered as soon as the patient has stabilized
Prevent contractures (foot and wrist drop)
Use protective padding, surfaces as needed
Mobilize the patient and/or get them out of the bed and into a chair as soon as stable

Related nursing diagnoses
Impaired musculoskeletal function
Impaired skin integrity

Outcome 8: Gastrointestinal and urinary elimination will be maintained, and complications will be prevented.

Assess and compare to established norms, patient baselines, and trends
Urine and stool output
Function and effect of nephrotoxic agents
Neurogenic bowel and bladder complications – incomplete emptying, incontinence, retention, diarrhea or constipation

Interventions to promote elimination and prevent complications
Monitor and treat urinary tract infection – remove indwelling urinary catheter as soon as the patient is able to participate
Fluids, fiber and activity stimulate intestinal motility
Establishing a regular daily time for bowel movements in the upright position and in privacy promote normal bowel elimination

Administer related drug therapy and monitor for therapeutic and nontherapeutic effects
Stool softeners and/or fiber therapy
Antidiarrhea medications

Related nursing diagnosis
Impaired bowel and bladder function

Data from Blissett, P. (2009).

SECTION SIX REVIEW

1. Correct positioning of the hemiplegic patient is described in which of the following statements?
   A. Unaffected side: the patient's body is at 90 degrees with the affected arm flexed and elevated on a pillow.
   B. Supine: the head is midline and in neutral position with the arms at the side.
   C. Affected side: the patient's body is rotated laterally less than 90 degrees with the affected arm extended and elevated on pillows and the affected leg slightly flexed on pillows.
   D. Affected side: the patient's body is at 90 degrees with a pillow between the legs and the arm extended and elevated on pillows.
2. Causes of undernutrition in stroke patients include (choose all that apply)
   A. dysphagia
   B. hemiplegia
   C. perceptual deficits
   D. hypometabolic state
3. Which of the following is true of elimination problems in acute stroke patients?
   A. Bowel incontinence is common.
   B. Indwelling urinary catheters are useful for patients with hyperreflexic bladders.
   C. Incontinence is usually stress-related.
   D. Scheduled voiding programs can promote continence.
4. Which of the following is true regarding the hemineglect syndrome seen in stroke patients?
   A. It usually occurs in dominant strokes.
   B. It is accompanied by left homonymous hemianopsia.
   C. The patient is paralyzed on one side of his or her body.
   D. The patient has insight into the cause of the impairment.
5. M. B. age 30, had an embolic stroke involving her left frontal and parietal lobes. She follows commands, has difficulty naming objects, blurts out profanities on occasion, and speaks in words and phrases in nonfluent speech. Her communication impairment most likely is
   A. Wernicke's aphasia
   B. global aphasia
   C. Broca's aphasia
   D. dysarthria
6. Which of the following is not a potential stressor for patients with acute brain attacks?
   A. changes in body image
   B. independence
   C. fears of becoming a burden to the family
   D. role modification

Answers: 1. C, 2. (A, B, C), 3. D, 4. B, 5. C, 6. B

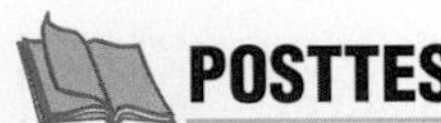

POSTTEST

1. Which of the following statements is true about stroke?
   A. Stroke is an acute neurologic deficit.
   B. Stroke occurs in a localized area of the brain.
   C. Stroke occurs as a result of impaired blood flow.
   D. all of the above
2. W. J. is a 79-year-old man who presents to the emergency department with the following symptoms: partial loss of vision in one eye, along with numbness, tingling, and weakness of the left arm. These symptoms usually last 15 to 30 minutes and then go away. W. J. most likely has
   A. a cerebellar brain tumor
   B. hyponatremia
   C. TIAs
   D. subarachnoid hemorrhage
3. Which of the following cardiac conditions places patients at risk for developing an embolic stroke?
   A. carotid stenosis
   B. recent myocardial infarction
   C. ventricular hypertrophy
   D. pulmonary artery stenosis
4. A penumbra is defined as
   A. an infarct to brain cells
   B. a band of minimally perfused brain cells
   C. an aura that precedes onset of stroke
   D. an inability to recognize familiar objects
5. Impaired oxygen delivery to brain cells results in
   A. intracellular accumulation of sodium
   B. failure of the sodium–potassium pump
   C. mitochondrial injury
   D. all of the above

J. C. is an 82-year-old African American man with a history of hypertension, type 1 diabetes, and a stroke (two years ago). He is a smoker and admits to leading a very sedentary life-style.

6. How many modifiable risk factors for stroke does J. C. have?
   A. one
   B. two
   C. three
   D. four
7. How many nonmodifiable risk factors for stroke does J. C. have?
   A. two
   B. four
   C. six
   D. eight
8. What is the role of lipid-lowering drugs (statins) in preventing strokes?
   A. They prevent heart disease, not stroke.
   B. They must be instituted at the first sign of a TIA.
   C. They may reduce the risk of ischemic strokes.
   D. They are actually harmful to patients at high risk for stroke.
9. P. E. is a 79-year-old female who presents to the emergency department with monocular vision loss, aphasia, and hemineglect. These signs and symptoms are typical of patients with
   A. carotid ischemia
   B. vertebrobasilar ischemia
   C. cranial nerve defects
   D. subarachnoid hemorrhage
10. To evaluate contralateral hemiparesis, the nurse would
    A. have the patient swallow
    B. ask the patient, "Who is the president of the United States?"
    C. examine the flaccidity and spasticity of bilateral extremities
    D. give the patient the Snellen eye chart for a vision examination
11. One of the first priorities in the evaluation of a patient who has had a stroke is to determine whether the stroke was caused by ischemia or hemorrhage. Which of the following diagnostic tests helps to differentiate these causes?
    A. lumbar puncture
    B. electrocardiogram
    C. transcranial doppler ultrasonography
    D. CT scan
12. T. P. is receiving an infusion of rtPA for treatment of acute ischemic stroke. In which of the following situations would it be most appropriate to emergently discontinue the infusion?
    A. if the patient develops a severe headache, acute hypertension, and vomiting
    B. if the patient's blood pressure elevates to 180/100
    C. if the patient required placement of a nasogastric tube
    D. if the patient developed atrial fibrillation
13. Which of the following is a FALSE statement about aspirin administration?
    A. It should be given within 24 hours of thrombolytic therapy.
    B. It should not be given within 24 hours of thrombolytic therapy.
    C. It should not be used as a substitute for rtPA.
    D. Less is known about the use of aspirin with cerebral ischemia.
14. A carotid endarterectomy is a surgical procedure to remove
    A. an embolism
    B. atherosclerotic plaque
    C. a carotid artery
    D. a subarachnoid hemorrhage
15. The patient with SAH is at risk for developing which of the following complications?
    A. cerebral vasospasm
    B. hypertension
    C. respiratory arrest
    D. cor pulmonale

16. The type of incontinence in acute stroke patients that is due to bladder capacity being small is produced by
- **A.** bladder hyperreflexia (spasticity)
- **B.** bladder hyporeflexia (flaccidity)
- **C.** detrusor–sphincter dyssynergy
- **D.** stress

Mrs. J., age 40, is an acute stroke patient with hemiplegia and parietal neglect following a stroke.

17. She is at risk for decubitus ulcers for all of the following reasons EXCEPT
- **A.** She has a loss of vasomotor tone.
- **B.** She ignores her left side.
- **C.** She has venous stasis of her affected limbs.
- **D.** She has dysphagia.

18. The nurse assists Mrs. J. by
- **A.** teaching her to inspect her skin for pallor or redness with a mirror
- **B.** turning her every four hours
- **C.** avoiding reference to her neglected side
- **D.** massaging her legs every four hours

19. Which of the following assessments would not be used in the assessment of M. C., age 30, for visual–perceptual deficits following an acute stroke?
- **A.** Ask her to draw a clock.
- **B.** Observe her dietary tray after meals.
- **C.** Ask her to read a page.
- **D.** Ask her to sing a song.

Posttest answers with rationale are found on MyNursingKit.

REFERENCES

Adams, R. J., Chimowitz, M. I., Alpert, J. S., et al. (2008). Coronary risk evaluation in patients with transient ischemic attack and ischemic stroke. *Circulation, 108,* 1278–1290.

AHA (American Heart Association),(2003). Heart and stroke facts, American Heart Association. Retrieved December 19, 2008 from http://www.americanheart.org/downloadable/heart/1056719919740HSFacts2003text.pdf.

AHA (American Heart Association), (2005). Heart disease and stroke statistics – 2005 update. Retrieved December 19, 2008, from http://www.americanheart.org/downloadable/heart/1105390918119HDSStats2005Update.pdf.

Albers, G. W., Amarenco, P., Easton, J. D., Sacco, R. L., and Teal, P. (2008). Antithrombotic and thrombolytic therapy for ischemic stroke: American college of chest physicians evidence-based clinical practice guidelines (8th ed.). *Chest, 133* (6 suppl- June 2008), 630.

Blissett, P. (2009). Cerebrovascular disorders. In Karen K. Carlson (ed.) *Advanced Critical Care Nursing,* 610–611. St. Louis: AACN and Saunders-Elsevier.

Heart and Stroke Foundation of Ontario & Registered Nurses Association of Ontario, (2005). *Stroke assessment across the continuum of care.* Toronto, Canada: Heart and Stroke Foundation of Ontario, Registered Nurses Association of Ontario. Retrieved December 8, 2008, from http://www.rnao.org/bestpractices/PDF/BPG_Stroke_Assessment.pdf.

Jauch, E. C., Kissela, B., & Stettler, B. (2007). Acute stroke management. Retrieved December 19, 2008 from http://emedicine.medscape.com/article/1159752.

JNC. 2003. Prevention, detection, evaluation, and treatment of high blood pressure (JNC 7). National Heart Lung and Blood Institute. Retrieved December 19, 2008 from http://www.nhlbi.nih.gov/guidelines/hypertension/.

Kenfield, S., Stampfer, M., Rosner, B., Colditz, G. (2008). Smoking and smoking cessation in relation to mortality in women. *JAMA, 299*(17), 2037–2047.

Keener, A. & Sanossian, N. (2008). Niacin for stroke prevention: evidence and rationale. *Rehabil Nurs,33*(6): 247–52.

LeMone, P. and Burke, K. (2008). Nursing care of clients with cerebrovascular and spinal cord disorders. In P. LeMone and K. Burke, *Medical-Surgical Nursing: Critical Thinking in Client Care* (4th ed.) 1578–1594. Upper Saddle River, NJ: Pearson/ Prentice Hall.

Sacco, R. L., & Boden-Albala, B. (2006). Stroke risk factors: identification and modification. In M. Fisher (ed.), *Stroke therapy* (2nd ed., 1–17). Boston: Butterworth, Heinemann.

Sharma, M., Clark, H., Armour, T., Stotts, G., Cote, R., Hill. M., Demchuck, A., Moher, D., Garrity, C., Yazdi, F., Lumely-Leger, K., Murdock, M., Sampson, M., Barrowman, N., & Lewin, G. (2005) Acute Stroke: Evaluation and Treatment. www.ahrq.gov., 127.

Wang, Y. F., Wu, J. S., Mao, Y., et al. (2008). The optimal time-window for surgical treatment of spontaneous intracerebral hemorrhage: result of a prospective randomized controlled trial of 500 cases. *Stroke,* December [E-pub ahead of print].

Weinhardt, J., Hazelett, S., Barrett, D., et al. (2008). Accuracy of a bedside dysphagia screening: a comparison of registered nurses and speech therapists. *Acta Neurochir Supplement, 105*:141s.

MODULE

22 Alteration in Sensory Perceptual Function: Acute Head Injury

Melanie G. Hardin-Pierce, Adam DaDeppo

OBJECTIVES Following the completion of this module, the learner will be able to

1. Describe focal and diffuse brain injuries including general management.
2. Explain the pathophysiology and interventions related to secondary brain injury.
3. Discuss the management of traumatic brain injury.
4. Identify complications and interventions associated with traumatic brain injury.

This module focuses on traumatic brain injury (TBI) including: the mechanisms of injury, pathophysiological changes that accompany such injuries, and of the medical and nursing care high-acuity patients with these injuries require. The module is composed of four sections. Section One introduces the reader to mechanisms of injury and skull fractures associated with head trauma. Section Two discusses the different types of primary brain injury and the medical and nursing interventions used to treat these injuries. Section Three reviews the pathophysiology and consequences of traumatic brain injury and how secondary brain injury can be prevented. Section Four discusses complications associated with traumatic brain injury, medical and nursing interventions, and introduces the reader to the criteria used to diagnose brain death. All Section Reviews include answers. It is suggested that the learner review those concepts answered incorrectly in the review questions before proceeding to the next section.

PRETEST

1. Which of the following are mechanisms of closed-head injury associated with trauma to the head? (choose all that apply)
   A. rotational
   B. diffuse
   C. acceleration/deceleration
   D. penetrating
2. Which of the following skull fractures are most commonly associated with an increased risk of infection?
   A. linear
   B. open
   C. basilar
   D. depressed
3. Battle's sign, raccoon eyes, and otorrhea are all common physical assessment findings associated with
   A. linear fractures
   B. depressed skull fractures
   C. open skull fractures
   D. basilar skull fractures
4. Which of the following are examples of focal brain injury? (choose all that apply)
   A. concussion
   B. subdural hematoma
   C. subarachnoid hemorrhage
   D. epidural hematoma
5. Which focal brain injury has acute, subacute, and chronic stages?
   A. subdural hematoma
   B. intracerebral hematoma
   C. epidural hematoma
   D. subarachnoid hematoma
6. Which of the following are causes of secondary brain injury? (choose all that apply)
   A. ischemia
   B. cerebral swelling
   C. axonal shearing
   D. inflammation
7. Which of the following are nursing interventions to prevent secondary injury? (choose all that apply)
   A. completing multiple patient care activities at once to decrease patient stimulation
   B. maintaining neck alignment
   C. keeping the patient's hip flexion at less than 90 degrees
   D. preoxygenating patients prior to suctioning
8. Diabetes insipidus is the result of
   A. increased production of antidiuretic hormone
   B. decreased production of antidiuretic hormone
   C. elevated blood glucose
   D. hypoglycemia

9. Treatment of SIADH includes
A. fluid restriction
B. fluid resuscitation
C. replacement of sodium with salt tabs and intravenous saline
D. administration of vasopressin

10. Cushing's triad includes which of the following? (choose all that apply)
A. tachycardia
B. hypertension
C. bradycardia
D. irregular breathing pattern

Pretest Answers are found on MyNursingKit.

SECTION ONE: Mechanisms of Injury and Skull Fractures

At the completion of this section, the learner will be able to discuss the mechanisms of brain injury and skull fractures.

Traumatic brain injury (TBI), often referred to as a closed-head injury (CHI), is a brain insult that results from a mechanical disruption of brain tissue from an external impact or injury to the head (Lovasik, 2001; Dawodu, 2008). Approximately 1.4 million to 1.5 million Americans sustain a TBI annually. Of these, 50,000 deaths occur and 235,000 require hospitalization with high-acuity nursing care (Langlois, 2003; Lovesik, 2001). The cost to society is more than $30 billion annually. Approximately 80,000 to 90,000 people will sustain permanent disabilities from their injury (CDC, 2004). These figures do not include those treated in primary care settings. An estimated 25 percent of patients with TBI do not receive medical attention (Alderson, 2005; Powers & Schulman, 2009).

Mechanisms of Injury

Traumatic brain injury is a diagnosis with a wide-ranging degree of severity. In its simplest form, closed-head injury is represented by **concussion.** At the other end of the spectrum is severe traumatic brain injury, which occurs with **epidural hematoma** and **diffuse axonal injury,** both of which are associated with high mortality. Understanding the mechanism of injury associated with TBI is essential to assessing and managing patients with these injuries. There are three primary mechanisms of injury associated with TBI: acceleration/deceleration, rotational, and penetrating.

Acceleration/Deceleration Injury

The most common mechanism of TBI is the result of acceleration and deceleration forces. *Acceleration injury* occurs when the stationary brain is suddenly and rapidly moved in one direction along a linear path (Fig. 22–1). This type of injury is seen in victims of assault who have been hit in the head with a fist or bat. The sudden acceleration causes brain injury at the site of impact. *Deceleration injury* occurs when the brain stops rapidly in the cranial vault. As the skull ceases movement, the brain continues to move until it hits the skull. The force of deceleration causes injury at the site of impact with the skull. An example of this is the victim of a fall. The rapid deceleration of the person's head hitting the ground results in a deceleration injury of the brain as it hits the bony wall of the cranium. Acceleration and deceleration injuries can occur together, as can be seen in a coup–contrecoup injury. Coup (acceleration) injury affects the cerebral tissue directly under the point of impact. Contrecoup (deceleration) injury occurs in a line directly opposite the point of impact.

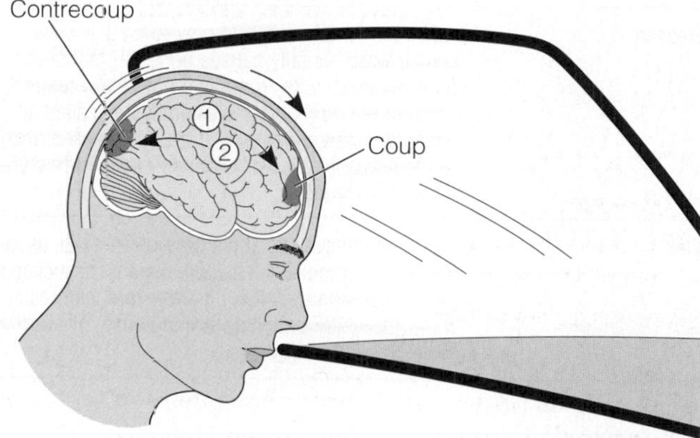

Figure 22–1 ▪ Coup-contrecoup head injury. 1) Following the initial (acceleration) injury (coup), 2) the brain rebounds within the skull and sustains additional (deceleration) injury (contrecoup) in the opposite part of the brain.

Rotational Injury

Rotational injury occurs when the force impacting the head transfers energy to the brain in a nonlinear fashion, resulting in shearing forces being exerted throughout the brain. An example of this type of mechanism is in boxing. When a boxer is punched in the side of the head, the force causes rapid rotational movement of the head and its contents, which causes tearing of the axons in the brain.

Pentrating Injury

Penetrating injury occurs when a foreign object invades the brain. The penetrating object may be a bullet, knife, or a falling object. The penetrating object may pass completely through the brain and exit on the opposite side or it may bounce around the cranium causing multiple areas of injury. In addition to the obvious injury, some projectiles, such as bullets, may cause additional injury from shock waves transmitted throughout the brain.

Skull Fractures

Table 22–1 shows the four types of skull fractures that can occur with injury to the head: linear, depressed, open, and basilar skull fractures. All types indicate substantial force has been absorbed by the skull and underlying brain tissue injury may be present (See Fig. 22–2 Types of Skull Fractures).

TABLE 22–1 Types of Skull Fractures

TYPE	DESCRIPTION
Linear	A simple fracture involving the entire bony thickness without bone movement; considered the most benign type of skull fracture; associated with low-velocity blunt trauma; usually requires no interventions
Open	A fracture in which the scalp has been lacerated, creating a communication between the skull and the outside environment; in the presence of a depressed skull fracture the dura may be torn, exposing the brain to possible contamination
Depressed	A fracture in which a high-energy force depresses the skull inward; usually causes bone fragmentation (comminuted) with fragments potentially tearing through the dura and into brain tissue; called an "open depressed fracture" if the scalp is lacerated to the bone or called a "closed depressed fracture" if the scalp is intact
Basilar	A fracture that develops at the base of the skull; usually located in temporal or occipital regions; associated with a high-energy force; if dura is torn, can result in rhinorrhea (CSF draining from the nose) or otorrhea (CSF draining from the ear)

Linear Skull Fracture

Linear skull fractures are associated with minor traumatic injury. They are not typically obvious to the naked eye and are usually discovered during a head computerized tomography (CT) scan. Linear skull fractures are not life-threatening and are allowed to heal over time without surgical intervention.

Depressed Skull Fracture

As the force of impact increases, depressed skull fractures may occur. Depressed skull fractures may be visible and palpable. The fracture itself may tear the underlying meninges of the brain and extend into brain tissue. Clearly, with such force to cause the skull to lose its shape, the probability of substantial cerebral injury is high. Medical interventions include surgical repair of the fracture and meninges and the evacuation of any hematomas beneath the fracture. Nursing interventions focus on frequent neurological assessments and pain management. The nurse must be cautious when administering pain medications to patients with head injuries. The presence of narcotics may obscure the neurological exam and make it difficult during an assessment to differentiate changes in mental status as a result of the actual injury from changes caused by the narcotic.

Open Skull Fracture

Open skull fractures are skull fractures accompanied by a scalp laceration. These fractures are of particular concern because of the risk of infection associated with exposure of the dura to a contaminated environment. Medical interventions include surgical repair and debridement of the contaminated wound. Nursing care is focused on neurological assessment, pain management, and administration of antibiotics to prevent infection.

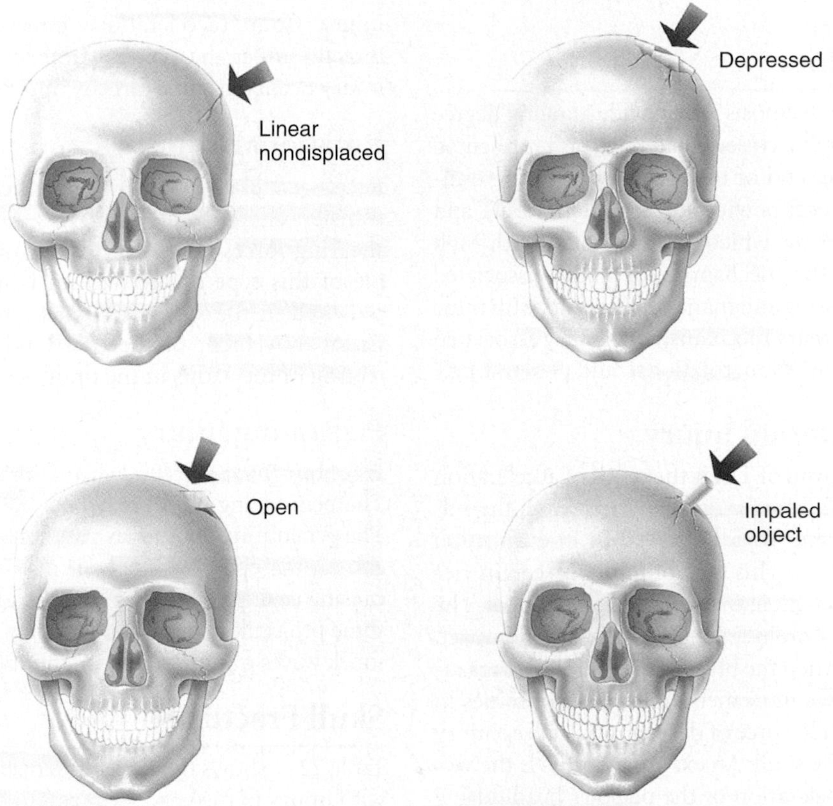

Figure 22–2 ■ Types of skull fractures. This figure was published in *Medical-Surgical Nursing,* by Lewis, S., Heitkemper, M., et al., *Assessment and management of clinical problems,* p. 1482, Copyright Elsevier, (2007).

Basilar Skull Fracture

Basilar skull fractures, another common sequelae of high-impact head injury, are fractures of one of the bones that make up the base of the skull. Assessment findings associated with a basilar skull fracture may include the presence of periorbital ecchymosis ("raccoon eyes"), mastoid ecchymosis ("Battle's sign"), otorrhea, rhinorrhea, or facial nerve paralysis. Careful physical assessment of drainage from the nares and ear canals must be performed to detect the presence of cerebral spinal fluid (CSF) drainage. CSF drainage indicates the meninges are torn. CSF may leak through the nose (**rhinorrhea**) or through the ear (**otorrhea**). Any drainage from the ear or nose should be tested for the presence of glucose with a glucose reagent strip. Clear drainage that tests positive for glucose indicates the fluid is CSF. Figure 22–3 illustrates major signs of basilar skull fracture.

Medical management of basilar skull fracture includes allowing the CSF to drain and the dura to close on its own. If the injury does not heal within the first one to two weeks postinjury, surgical repair may be necessary. Nursing priorities include neurological assessment, pain management, and monitoring the patient for signs and symptoms of infection associated with the disrupted meningeal layer. All dressings should be changed with aseptic technique in an effort to reduce the possibility of an infection. Sterile cotton gauzes are placed in the ear or under the nose. Dressings are changed when wet because moisture facilitates the movement of microorganisms and predisposes the patient to infection.

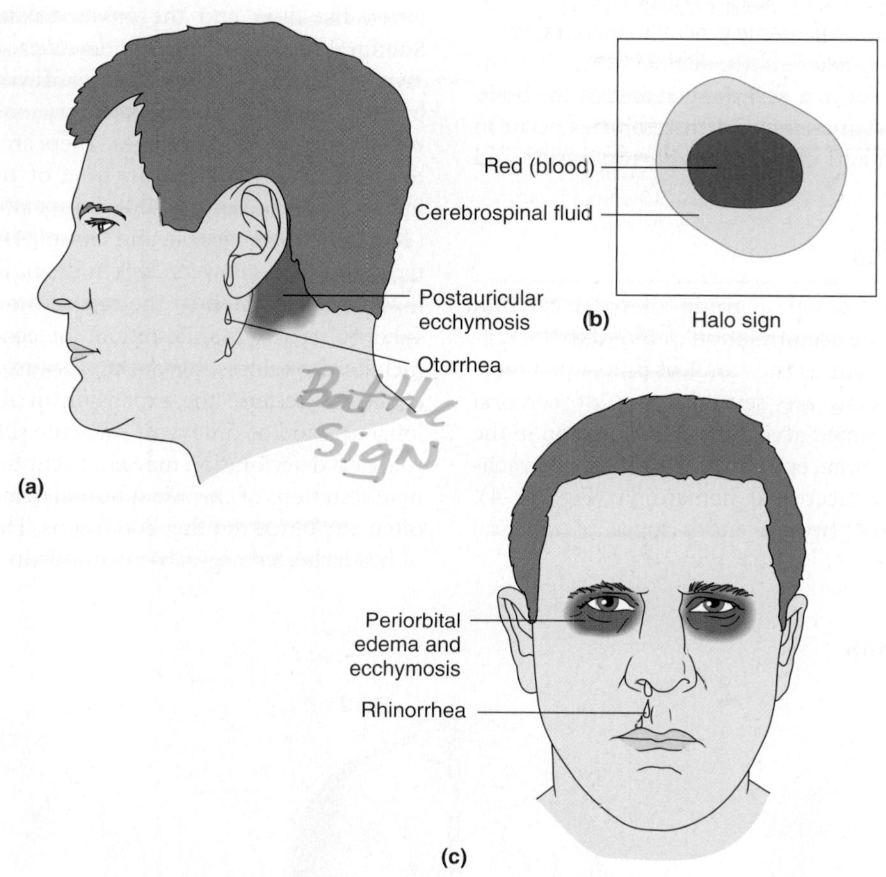

Figure 22–3 ■ Signs of basilar skull fracture. (a) Battle sign. (b) Halo sign. (c) Raccoon eyes. American Spinal Injury Association: International Standards for Neurological Classification of Spinal Cord Injury Teaching Package, revised, 2005, Atlanta, GA.

SECTION ONE REVIEW

1. Acceleration/deceleration injuries are the result of impact following
   - **A.** rotational movement of the brain in the skull
   - **B.** penetrating trauma
   - **C.** linear movement of the brain in the skull
   - **D.** none of the above

2. Which of the following mechanisms of injury commonly results in the tearing of axons in the brain?
   - **A.** rotational injury
   - **B.** acceleration injury
   - **C.** deceleration injury
   - **D.** penetrating injury

(*continued*)

(*continued*)

3. The administration of narcotics to a patient with a traumatic brain injury
   A. will make the pain worse
   B. may mask neurological changes in the patient
   C. allows the injury to heal quicker
   D. is a priority nursing intervention

4. Raccoon eyes are an assessment finding typically associated with what type of skull fracture?
   A. linear fractures
   B. depressed fractures
   C. open fractures
   D. basilar fractures

Answers: 1. C, 2. A, 3. B, 4. D

SECTION TWO: Focal and Diffuse Brain Injuries

At the completion of this section, the learner will be able to describe focal and diffuse brain injuries including general management.

Traumatic brain injury takes on two distinct forms: focal or diffuse. **Focal injuries** occur in a well-defined area of the brain and may be the result of hematomas. **Diffuse injuries** occur in several areas of the brain and may occur with concussion and diffuse axonal injury.

Focal Head Injuries

Cerebral hematomas represent a group of focal cerebral injuries associated with the accumulation of blood in the cranial vault. Hematomas occur as the result of injury to a cerebral vein or artery. There are several types of cerebral hematomas and each is named according to its location in the cranium: subdural hematoma, epidural hematoma, subarachnoid hematoma, and intracerebral hematoma (Fig. 22–4). With high-impact injury, two or more types of cerebral hematomas may occur.

Subdural Hematoma

Subdural hematoma (SDH) is the accumulation of blood between the dura and the arachnoid layers of the meninges. Subdural hematoma usually develops secondary to venous injury. This results in a slower onset of symptoms. It is categorized by the time between when the injury took place and the development of neurological changes. There are three categories of subdural hematoma, based on time of onset of manifestations, including acute (less than 48 hours after the injury), subacute (48 hours to two weeks), and chronic (more than two weeks after the injury) (Powers & Schulman, 2009). Assessment findings are determined by the rate of blood accumulation in the subdural space. Manifestations of acute subdural hematoma include drowsiness, headache, confusion, slowed thinking, or agitation. Because the expansion of the hematoma is over a longer period of time with subacute subdural hematoma, neurological deterioration may not occur for days or weeks. Clinical manifestations of chronic subdural hematoma are vague and are often attributed to other conditions. The patient may complain of headache, lethargy, absent-mindedness, and vomiting. Other

CRANIAL HEMATOMAS

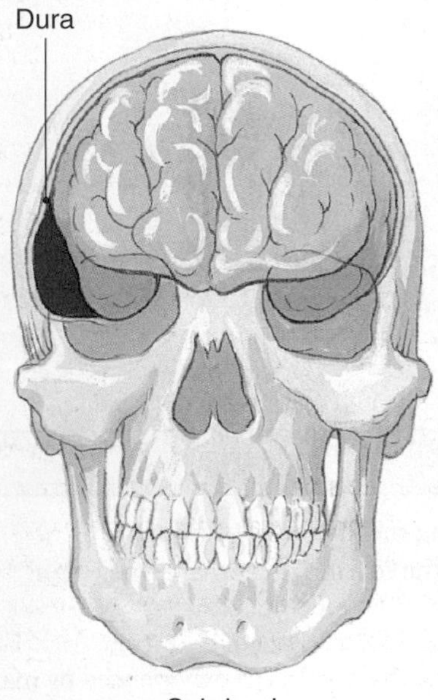

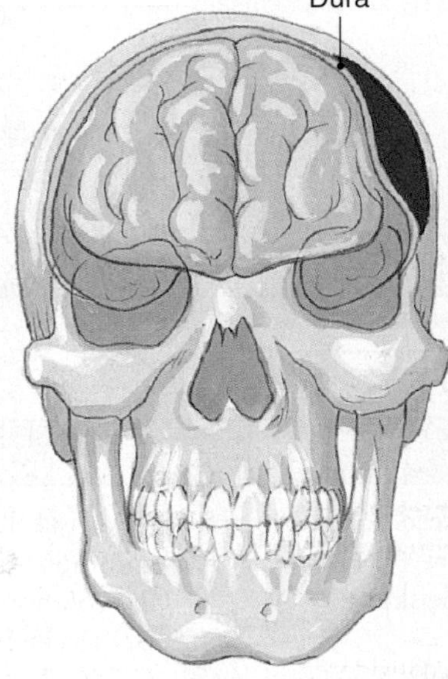

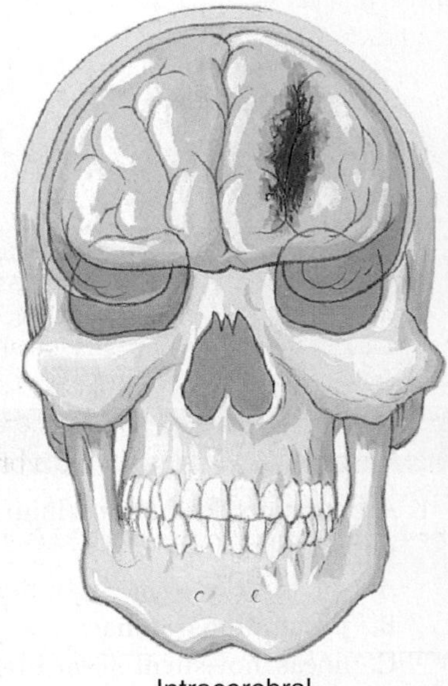

Figure 22–4 ■ Three types of hematomas. Epidural, subdural, and intracerebral.

more serious symptoms may be present, including seizures, stiff neck, pupil changes, or hemiparesis (Blank-Reid, McClelland & Santora, 2008).

Medical management of SDH involves surgical evacuation of the hematoma and possible placement of a subdural drain, which may remain in place for a few days postoperatively. Nursing priorities for SDH include monitoring level of consciousness and performing regular and frequent focused neurological assessments (Powers & Schulman, 2009).

Epidural Hematoma

An **epidural hematoma (EDH)** occurs in the space between the dura mater and the skull. High impact to the temporal areas of the brain can induce an epidural hematoma. When the force of the impact is transferred to the brain, small arteries are sheared. This results in an accumulation of blood between the skull and the dura mater. People with these injuries may have a brief loss of consciousness immediately following the injury, followed by an episode of being alert and oriented, and then a loss of consciousness again. This scenario is the classical presentation of epidural hematoma, but it is important to remember that not all patients with epidural hematoma will present with these symptoms. A fixed and dilated pupil on the same side as the impact area may be present. Because an artery is most often the source of the hematoma, the rapid accumulation of blood makes it essential to identify and treat these injuries quickly before intracranial pressure reaches a critical point causing brain herniation.

Medical management of the epidural hematoma involves surgical evacuation of the hematoma with possible placement of an intracranial pressure (ICP) monitor. These patients may be admitted to the ICU for frequent neurological checks and ICP monitoring. Nursing care associated with epidural hematoma focuses on diligent neurological assessment. The nurse must look for sudden changes in level of consciousness and for the presence of a fixed and dilated pupil on the side of injury. These findings suggest bleeding has recurred and represents an emergent medical situation.

Intracerebral Hematoma

Intracerebral hematoma (ICH) is the accumulation of blood in the parenchyma of brain tissue rather than between the meninges. Intracerebral hematomas result from uncontrolled hypertension, ruptured aneurysm, or trauma with a high-impact blow to the head. Manifestations vary according to the location of the hematoma and may include headache along with decreasing level of consciousness, dilation of one pupil, and hemiplegia. Surgical evacuation of an intracerebral hematoma is usually not possible because the hematoma is deep within brain tissue. Medical management includes management of intracranial pressure and cerebral perfusion pressure (CPP) (Powers & Schulman, 2009).

Contusion

A **contusion** refers to a bruising of soft tissue and is considered a moderate-to-severe injury. It is commonly seen in traumatic brain injury that may begin local but become more diffuse over time. A contusion causes macroscopic tissue and vessel damage that is detectable through CT or MRI scanning; however, the MRI is the more sensitive test. Contusions are associated with longer periods of unconsciousness and a more guarded prognosis, depending on the severity of injury. The Glasgow Coma Scale (GCS) is useful in determining the severity of the injury. While a concussion causes only mild alterations in level of consciousness (GCS of 13-15), a contusion is associated with more significant alterations, moderate injury (GCS = 9-12) or severe injury (GCS = 3-8) (Morales, Diaz-Daza, Hlatky, & Hayman, 2007).

Diffuse Head Injuries

Diffuse head injuries are those that involve the brain more globally and include concussion, diffuse axonal injury, and subarachnoid hemorrhage.

Concussion

Concussion classified as mild traumatic brain injury (MTBI), is caused by blunt trauma to the head. Cerebral damage is at the microscopic level and not detectable through radiographic or other testing. Signs of concussion include a transient period of unconsciousness (lasting up to 20 minutes) and a Glasgow Coma Scale score of 13 to 15; however and signs of neurological deficits (e.g., unilateral weakness, pupillary abnormalities) are usually absent (Blank-Reid et al., 2008). Although the term MTBI implies a relatively benign injury, the injury can have devastating effects including the inability to function at preinjury levels. On presentation to the emergency department the patient may report having amnesia about the event that caused the injury. The patient may report headache, dizziness, vertigo, nausea, vomiting, slurred speech, or confusion. Patients who report any of these symptoms will require a CT scan of the head for further evaluation. Almost half of patients with concussion develop postconcussive syndromes that include symptoms similar to those on presentation to the emergency department. These symptoms may continue for three months or more after injury (Blank-Reid et al., 2008; Freeborn, 2004).

Diffuse Axonal Injury

Diffuse axonal injury (DAI) occurs when shearing forces disrupt the structure of neurons and their nearby blood vessels; however, DAI may be present without bleeding, making it difficult to visualize on CT or MRI. It typically results from high-speed acceleration/deceleration injury that occurs with motor vehicle crashes. The mechanism of injury involves a rotational (twisting motion) movement of the brain within the skull that causes widespread shearing of axons in the white matter. The severity of injury can range from mild to severe. Although DAI is difficult to assess on a CT scan, the presence of multiple small hemorrhages is strongly suggestive. The use of MRI may provide a more conclusive diagnosis. The outcome of the patient with DAI is unpredictable. Mild DAI can result in a comatose state lasting hours-to-days followed by recovery with minimal residual neurological damage. Mild DAI may contribute to postconcussive syndrome experienced by many patients following a brain concussion. In more severe DAI the prognosis is poor and may include: prolonged coma, death, or a persistent vegetative state (Powers & Schulman, 2009).

Subarachnoid Hemorrhage

Subarachnoid hemorrhage (SAH) is the accumulation of blood/hematoma between the arachnoid layer of the meninges and the brain. Additional accumulation of blood results in blood leaking into the cerebrospinal fluid. The bleeding associated with SAH can be focal with little consequence, or it can be massive and diffuse with subsequent intracranial hypotension. Patients with this type of hematoma may manifest nuchal rigidity (neck stiffness) (Powers & Schulman, 2009). A severe headache is also a common finding, often described as the worse headache the person has ever experienced. Subarachnoid hemorrhage is presented in more detail in Module 21, Alteration in Cerebral Tissue Perfusion: Acute Brain Attack.

Management of Diffuse Head Injuries

Diffuse head injuries are not limited to a localized area, which can make them more difficult to detect and treat. Depending upon the severity of the injury, the patient's recovery can be unpredictable (Powers & Schulman, 2009). Management in the acute care phase includes diligent and frequent neurological assessments and pain management. When moderate-to-severe injury is present (e.g., contusion or DAI) management may include interventions to lower ICP, increase cerebral perfusion pressure, and stabilize vital signs, which all contribute to an improved outcome (Helmy et al., 2007; Zenati, 2002; Littlejohns & Bader, 2005; Butcher et al., 2007). Discharge planning must begin early because many patients require rehabilitation services. Management of traumatic brain injury is presented in more detail in the next section.

SECTION TWO REVIEW

1. A brief loss of consciousness followed by a period of being alert and oriented, and then a loss of consciousness again, is a typical presentation for which of the following?
   A. subdural hematoma
   B. epidural hematoma
   C. intracranial hematoma
   D. subarachnoid hemorrhage
2. Accumulation of blood within the parenchyma of brain tissue is called a (n)
   A. intracerebral hematoma
   B. subarachnoid hemorrhage
   C. epidural hematoma
   D. subdural hematoma
3. Management of intracerebral hematoma may include
   A. anticoagulation
   B. maintaining mean arterial pressure ≤ 70 mm Hg
   C. emergent surgical evacuation
   D. maximizing cerebral perfusion pressure (CPP)
4. Presence of dizziness, headache, and confusion for long periods of time after concussion is
   A. always expected
   B. known as postconcussive syndrome
   C. caused by taking too much pain medication
   D. the result of something other than the concussion

Answers: 1. B, 2. A, 3. D, 4. B

SECTION THREE: Management of Traumatic Brain Injury

At the completion of this section, the learner will be able to discuss the management of traumatic brain injury.

This section focuses on interventions specific to traumatic brain injury. Section Seven of Module 20, Determinants and Assessment of Cerebral Tissue perfusion provides additional information on the management of decreased cerebral tissue perfusion as it applies across diagnoses.

Primary and Secondary Brain injury

Primary injury occurs when neurons sustain direct injury from the offending event (for example, a person's head striking the dashboard resulting in DAI during a motor vehicle crash). The primary injury in this case is the shearing of the axons. Primary injury is immediate and often irreversible damage.

Secondary injury occurs in response to the primary injury. There are four causes of secondary injury: ischemia, neuronal death, cerebral swelling, and inflammation (Littlejohns & Bader, 2005 Helmy et al., 2007; Powers & Schulman, 2009). Collaborative interventions are directed at preventing these causes of secondary injury in order to maximize positive patient outcomes. Many of the traditional methods to prevent secondary injury target the reduction of intracranial pressure (ICP) and the improvement of cerebral perfusion pressure (CPP), thus minimizing ischemic injury to the brain. The Brain Trauma Foundation guidelines (2007) recommend maintaining a CPP greater than 60 mm Hg to reduce secondary injury. Medical interventions, such as osmotic diuretics, hypertonic saline, hypothermia, and, at times, hyperventilation, is used alone or in combination to help achieve this recommended CPP. Ongoing research on the assessment and management of secondary brain injuries includes new methods for measuring cerebral perfusion, new drugs that reduce cerebral swelling and ischemia, drugs that limit the release of inflammatory mediators and cell death, and surgical interventions to treat intractable intracerebral hypertension.

The advent of cerebral tissue oxygen monitoring is reshaping current thoughts on management of brain injury. Clinicians now have the ability to measure local brain tissue oxygen content ($PbtO_2$). The measurement of this new parameter is achieved using a fiber optic monitoring device, which is inserted into the white matter of the brain (Littlejohns et al., 2005; Blissitt, 2009). $PbtO_2$ levels less than 15 mm Hg have been associated with poor outcomes including death (Littlejohns et al., 2005; Blissitt, 2009);

therefore, current practice recommends maintaining $PbtO_2$ levels greater than 20 mm Hg (Littlejohns et al., 2005 Blissitt, 2009).

Treatment of Traumatic Brain Injury

The first goal in treating TBI is to limit the primary ischemic tissue injury by aggressive prevention and treatment of hypoxia and hypotension. This is accomplished with supplemental oxygen and mechanical ventilation to maintain PaO_2 greater than 60 mm Hg and $PaCO_2$ between 35 and 40 mm Hg. Systolic blood pressure should be maintained at greater than 90 mm Hg with fluids and vasopressors. Fluids and vasopressors are given to enhance cerebral perfusion pressure and cerebral blood flow, preventing ischemic etiologies of increased intracranial pressure. Cerebral perfusion pressure should be maintained at greater than or equal to 60 mm Hg. As with all aggressive fluid resuscitation, the patient is at risk of developing pulmonary complications such as pulmonary edema (Brain Trauma Foundation Guidelines, 2007).

Leveled Approach to Intracranial Pressure Management

Treatment and management of elevated intracranial pressure (ICP) involves a leveled approach (Table 22–2). Sustained elevations in ICP of 20 mm Hg or higher for more than 5-10 minutes should be treated. Table 22–3 provides a summary of intracranial parameters for treatment of traumatic brain injury.

Level One Interventions. First-level interventions to reduce elevated ICP include patient positioning strategies to prevent constriction of venous outflow from the brain. Patients should be positioned with the head of the bed elevated 30 to 45 degrees, avoiding hyperextension, flexion, or rotation of the head and neck. Reverse Trendelenburg's position may be helpful as well to ensure that there is no constriction of jugular veins from endotracheal tube tape, ties or cervical collars. Hyperthermia increases cerebral metabolic needs, so fever should be treated. Abdominal distention, agitation and increased levels of PEEP also increase ICP by increasing intrathoracic pressure and reducing venous outflow. Reducing environmental stimulation, providing pain control, and sedation for agitation are additional measures to optimize cerebral oxygenation by decreasing cerebral metabolic demand. It is best to use short acting agents for sedation along with daily wake-ups for opportunities to assess neurological status and to avoid over sedation.

TABLE 22–2 Leveled Approach for Treatment of Elevated ICP

LEVEL	TREATMENT APPROACH
One	Pain and sedation medications Maintain normothermia Patient positioning with head-of-bed elevation and midline neck alignment
Two	Consideration of external ventricular drainage Hyperosmolar therapy Mechanical ventilation maintaining PaO_2 greater than 60 mm Hg and $PaCO_2$ 35–40 mm Hg
Three	Neuromuscular blockade Mild hyperventilation Mild hypothermia
Four	Barbiturate coma Decompression craniotomy

Data from Brain Injury Foundation (2007). Guidelines for the management of severe traumatic brain injury. *Journal of Neurotrauma, 24, supplement 1: 1–95.*

TABLE 22–3 Intracranial Parameters for Treatment of Traumatic Brain Injury

PARAMETER	RECOMMENDATION	SUPPORTIVE THERAPY
ABG:		
PaO_2	Greater than 60 mm Hg	Oxygen therapy with mechanical ventilation as needed
$PaCO_2$	Keep between 35–40 mm Hg	
Blood pressure	Systolic pressure greater than 90 mm Hg	IV fluids and vasopressors as needed
Cerebral perfusion pressure (CPP)	Greater than 60 mm Hg	IV fluids and vasopressor therapy as needed
Intracranial pressure (ICP)	Less than 20 mm Hg	Treat ICP of 20 mm Hg or greater that is sustained for more than 5–10 minutes See Table 22-2: Leveled approach for treatment of elevated ICP

Level Two Interventions. Level two interventions to reduce elevated intracranial pressure (ICP), optimize cerebral perfusion pressure (CPP), and prevent secondary injury include cerebrospinal fluid drainage, hyperosmolar therapy, and maintenance of normal $PaCO_2$ levels with mechanical ventilation. Drainage of cerebrospinal fluid (CSF) requires placement of an intraventricular catheter (IVC). The IVC allows direct monitoring of the ICP and the color and amount of CSF. It allows for therapeutic drainage of CSF to reduce ICP.

Hyperosmolar therapy consists of osmotic diuretics such as mannitol (Osmitrol) given as a 20 percent solution in bolus doses of 0.25 to 1g/kg. Mannitol draws fluid from the intracellular and interstitial spaces into the vascular compartment, reducing blood viscosity resulting in improved cerebral blood flow (Wilson, Shannon, & Shields, 2008). Mannitol can cause a rebound reverse osmosis and draw fluid into the brain if serum osmolarity becomes greater than 320 mOsm/L. Furosemide (Lasix) is a loop diuretic that can be administered cautiously during acute phase of TBI. Administration of diuretics must be monitored carefully because it can contribute to dehydration, precipitating a decrease in CPP. The goal for volume maintenance should be to keep the patient in a euvolemic state to optimize cerebral perfusion. Volume replacement strategies should include fluid boluses, fluid replacements, and albumin administration. Intravenous fluids are usually isotonic and low in glucose to prevent gradient shifts across the blood-brain barrier in the TBI patient (Stacey, 2009).

Hypertonic saline has been shown to prevent secondary injury. Hypertonic saline has several effects on injured brain tissue. It causes reduction of cerebral edema by creating an osmotic gradient that promotes passage of intracellular fluid from swollen neuronal cells into the blood vessels. Hypertonic saline also possesses hemodynamic, vasoregulatory, and anti-inflammatory properties that help reduce secondary injury (Doyle et al., 2001; Cooper, 2004; Tyagi, Donaldson, Loftus, & Jallo, 2007; Brain Trauma Foundation, 2007). Nurses caring for patients receiving hypertonic saline must pay careful attention to the patient's serum sodium levels and serum osmolality because extreme elevations in these values may result in neurological injury and renal failure.

Level Three Interventions. Level three interventions to reduce intracranial pressure (ICP) include neuromuscular blockade, mild hyperventilation, and mild hypothermia. Neuromuscular blockade may be necessary to facilitate mechanical ventilation and prevent coughing, posturing, and severe agitation that increases ICP. Controlled hyperventilation may be necessary to manage elevated ICP that is refractory to lower level strategies. Hyperventilation reduces ICP by causing cerebrovascular vasoconstriction that reduces cerebral blood flow. Studies have shown that aggressive hyperventilation actually causes over constriction of the cerebral blood vessels, severely compromising blood flow to the point of causing ischemia. Current research based recommendations from the National Brain Trauma Foundation (2007) suggest maintaining $Paco_2$ levels in the low-normal range ($Paco_2$ of 35-40 mm Hg). Hyperthermia impairs metabolism, disrupts the blood-brain barrier, and increases release of inflammatory cytokines, free radicals which contribute to secondary injury. It remains controversial as to whether induced hypothermia improves outcomes in traumatic brain injury. However, there is ample research evidence to demonstrate that preventing hyperthermia and maintaining normothermia can help prevent increased ICP (Bullock, 2000; Bullock, Chestnut, & Clifton, 2001).

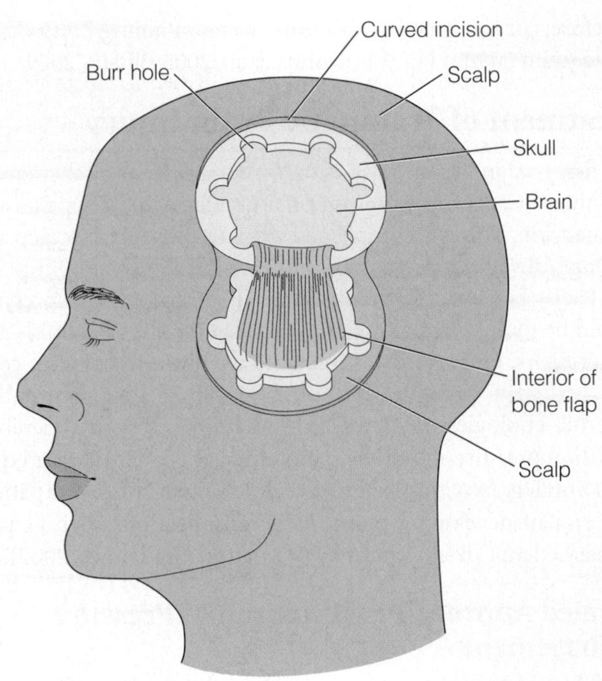

Figure 22–5 ■ Craniotomy. In a craniotomy, a portion of the skull and overlying scalp is removed to allow access to the brain.

Level Four Interventions. Level four interventions to reduce intracranial hypertension include medical interventions for the treatment of severe, refractory intracranial hypertension that does not respond to conventional therapeutic measures. Treatment of increased intracranial pressure (ICP) refractory to all other medical interventions may include the use of high-dose barbiturates. This intervention induces a comatose state and significantly decreases cerebral oxygen requirements (Powers & Schulman, 2009). Surgical intervention for the treatment refractory increased of ICP may include decompressive craniotomy (Nortje & Menon, 2004; Jaeger et al., 2003). Decompressive craniotomy is a surgical procedure

RELATED PHARMACOTHERAPY: Agents Used to Treat Traumatic Brain Injury

Osmotic Diuretic

Mannitol (Osmitrol)

Action and Uses

Reduces ICP by inducing diuresis

Mannitol creates an osmotic gradient across the BBB and increases serum osmolality. It pulls fluid out of brain cells shifting it into the blood.

Major Adverse Effects

Hypotension, fluid, and electrolyte imbalance, especially hyponatremia, hypokalemia, pulmonary edema, rebound increase in ICP

Nursing Implications

Monitor closely serum and urine electrolytes and kidney function.

Measure intake and output.

Monitor vital signs closely and ICP.

Sedative/Hypnotic and Sedative

Propofol (Diprivan)

Midazolam (Versed)

Lorazepam (Ativan)

Action and Uses

Rapid onset sedative-hypnotic used in maintenance of sedation. Sedatives reduce restlessness and agitation; all decrease metabolic rate and oxygen consumption.

Major Adverse Effects

Most common: dizziness, headache, hypotension, respiratory depression, CNS depression

Nursing Implications

- Monitor hemodynamic status and assess for dose-related hypotension.
- Observe seizure precautions.
- Pain may occur at insertion site.
- Monitor for hypoglycemia with Propofol.
- Monitor for excessive sedation and respiratory depression.
- Use lowest, most effective dosing.
- Obtain baseline respiratory and pupillary assessment data prior to initiation.

Pain Medication

Morphine or Fentanyl

Action and Uses

Narcotic analgesic

Major Adverse Effects

Most common: hypotension and respiratory failure, nausea and vomiting, constipation

Nursing Implications

- Monitor for respiratory depression and hypotension,
- Monitor for excessive sedation; use lowest, most effective dosing,
- Obtain baseline respiratory rate, depth and rhythm, and size of pupils before administering the drug.
- Record relief of pain.
- Cautious use of opiods–may obscure neurological changes

Hypertonic Saline

Action and Uses

Diuresis through action of atrial natriuretic peptide; restores resting membrane potential and cell volume; inhibits inflammation

Major Adverse Effects

Electrolyte abnormalities

Nursing Implications

Monitor serum sodium and osmolality, and renal function

DDAVP

Desmopressin

Action and Uses

Reduces urine output and osmolality in patients with central diabetes insipidus by increasing reabsorption of water by kidney collecting tubules.

Major Adverse Events

Dose related transient headache, dizziness, rhinitis, nausea, abdominal cramps, heartburn, facial flushing, shortness of air, pain/swelling at injection site

Nursing Implications

Monitor intake and output.
Daily weights.
Assess for edema from severe water retention.
Monitor BP.
Monitor urine and plasma osmolality.

Barbiturates

Thiopental
Pentobarbital

Action and Uses

Induces coma to control ICP/prevent seizures; lowers cerebral metabolism and CBF; stabilizes cell membranes

Major Adverse Events

Most common: hypotension with rapid infusion; respiratory depression

Nursing Implications

- BP and CPP may fall with loading dose.
- Requires complex monitoring, nursing and medical care.
- Requires the patient to be mechanically ventilated.

Neuromuscular Blocking Agents

Pancuronium (Pavulon)
Atracurium (Tracrium)
Vecuronium (Norcuron)

Action and Uses

Reduces skeletal muscle activity, metabolic rate, and oxygen consumption.

Major Adverse Effects

Causes total skeletal muscle paralysis. Always used with sedatives and mechanical ventilation.

Nursing Implications

- Assess cardiovascular and respiratory status continuously.
- Observe patient closely for residual muscle weakness and signs of respiratory distress during recovery period.
- Monitor BP and vital signs.
- Peripheral nerve stimulator may be uses to assess the effects of pancuronium and to monitor restoration of neuromuscular function.

Anticonvulsants

Phenytoin (Dilantin)
Fosphenytoin (Cerebyx)
Lorazepam (Ativan)
Levetiracetam (Keppra)

Action and Uses

In general, these agents stabilize cell membranes; prevent and control seizure activity in patients who are at high risk for seizures.

Major Adverse Effects

May cause hypotension. Serial measurements of serum drug levels are required to assess therapeutic dosing.

Nursing Implications

- Continuously monitor vital signs during IV infusion, and for an hour afterward.
- Monitor for respiratory depression and hypotension.
- Continuous cardiac monitoring is recommended.
- Monitor serum drug levels.
- Monitor and trend CBC, hematocrit, hemoglobin, glucose, calcium, and liver function tests.

where a portion of skull is removed to allow more space for the injured brain to expand during the acute phase of injury (Fig. 22–5). By opening the cranial vault, ICP is reduced and ischemia prevented. Not all patients are candidates for this form of aggressive treatment. The RESCUEicp study (Randomized Evaluation of Surgery with Craniotomy for Uncontrolled Elevation of Intra-Cranial Pressure) is a multicenter trial that is ongoing and may answer questions about risks and benefits of this procedure (Nortje & Menon, 2004). The role of corticosteroids is not recommended for improving outcomes in severe TBI (Brain Trauma Foundation Guidelines, 2007; CRASH trial, 2004).

The box RELATED PHARMACOTHERAPY: Agents Used to Treat Traumatic Brain Injury summarizes common drugs for treatment of TBI.

Nursing Interventions

Nursing interventions to reduce secondary injury focus on preventing complications associated with traumatic brain injury and normalizing intracranial pressure (ICP). Astute

NURSING CARE: The patient with acute traumatic brain injury

Expected Patient Outcomes and Related Interventions

Outcome 1: Treat/manage intracranial hypertension

Assess and compare to established norms, patient baselines, and trends.

Monitor for signs and symptoms of intracranial compromise.

ICP greater than 20 mm Hg, CPP less than 60 mm Hg

Vital signs: MAP less than 90 mm Hg; bradycardia, sudden onset of hypertension; deteriorating breathing pattern

Pupils: abnormal pupil changes (e.g., pinpoint and sluggish; unequal; fixed and dilated)

IO: Fluid balance excess or fluid balance deficit; serum osmolality greater than 320 mOsm

Interventions to maintain normal intracranial pressure and prevent cerebral metabolic rate

Maintain fluid balance.

Intravenous fluid therapy, vasopressor therapy, or diuretic therapy as needed

Monitor for manifestations of fluid volume excess or deficit.

Facilitate venous drainage from the head.

Elevate head of the bed 30 degrees; neutral body positioning.

Control seizure activity.

Monitor for development of seizures; protect patient from injury.

Prevent overstimulation.

Observe closely for the effect of interventions on ICP; careful timing of activities and rest based on patient's tolerance; dark, quiet environment as needed; control/limit noxious stimuli.

Control body temperature.

Prevent hyperthermia - Monitor temperature, cooling blanket, tepid baths

Hypothermia therapy (e.g., cooling blanket); prevent shivering

Administer related drug therapy and monitor for therapeutic and nontherapeutic effects.

Antipyretic agent as needed to control fevers

Diuretic therapy (e.g., mannitol) to decrease ICP

Sedation, analgesics, neuromuscular blockade agents to control agitation, and movements that drive up ICP; barbiturate coma if other interventions are insufficient

Anticonvulsant agents to control seizure activity

Related nursing diagnoses

Activity intolerance

Altered body temperature

Altered cerebral tissue perfusion

Potential for injury

Outcome 2: Optimize oxygenation

Assess and compare to established norms, patient baselines, and trends.

Monitor for manifestations of inadequate cerebral oxygenation.

Unstable breathing pattern

ABG: PaO_2 less than 60 mm Hg, $PaCO_2$ less than 35 or greater than 45, SaO_2 less than 92 percent

Hemoglobin (Hgb) less than 10g, hematocrit (Hct) less than 32 percent

Interventions to optimize cerebral oxygenation

Administer oxygen at 2-4 L/min per nasal cannula; endotracheal intubation and mechanical ventilation if needed

Packed red blood cells to maintain adequate Hgb and Hct – monitor for therapeutic and nontherapeutic effects

Prevent pneumonia through aggressive pulmonary toilet, elevate head of bed 30 degrees, frequent oral care, turn every two hours.

Decrease cerebral metabolic rate (refer to Outcome 1)

Related nursing diagnoses

Altered cerebral tissue perfusion

Ineffective breathing pattern

Potential for infection

Outcome 3: Prevent complications of Immobility

Assess and compare to established norms, patient baselines, and trends.

Monitor for signs and symptoms of complications of immobility.

Deep vein thrombosis: Swelling, redness or warmth of lower extremity

Contractures: Increased resistance to passive range of motion

Interventions to prevent complications of immobility

Deep vein thrombosis: Anticoagulant therapy if appropriate; antiembolism stockings

Contractures: Passive range of motion exercises, neutral body and limb positioning; physical therapy

Turn every 2 hours, log role if spinal cord injury is present

Early ambulation if feasible

Related nursing diagnoses

Impaired physical mobility

Ineffective tissue perfusion

Pain

Risk for impaired skin integrity

nursing assessments are required, especially during routine care, such as bathing and suctioning, to evaluate the patient's response to interventions. Although relatively benign in nature, simply touching the patient to wash the face can be enough stimulation to elevate ICP and compromise cerebral blood flow and oxygenation. In order to avoid unnecessary elevations of ICP, nursing activities are spaced apart to allow recovery time for the patient (LeMone & Burke, 2008; Albano et al., 2005). The patient's neck is kept in proper neutral alignment (no flexion or rotation) and hip flexion is kept at less than 90 degrees to allow for proper venous return and prevention of elevated ICP. Elevating the head of the bed to 30 degrees reduces ICP without compromising CPP and may decrease the risk of pneumonia (Marik et al., 2002; Meixensberger, Baunach & Amschler, 1997; Bullock, 2000). Because hyperthermia increases cerebral metabolic rate and increases cerebral oxygen requirements, antipyretics or cooling measures are used to reduce body temperature. Finally, when suctioning patients, the nurse preoxygenates the patient and limits passage time of the suction catheter to 10 seconds or less (LeJeune & Howard-Fain, 2002; Chulay, 2005). The nurse plays an instrumental role in monitoring for the therapeutic and nontherapeutic effects of the various fluid and drug therapies.

There are a number of interventions that prevent ischemia of neuronal tissue. Although not all have been scientifically proven to provide long-term benefits, the importance of monitoring the patient and providing the best possible medical and nursing care improves outcomes in this population. The box NURSING CARE: The Patient with Traumatic Brain Injury summarizes major nursing management.

Emerging Evidence

- TBI patients on clopidogrel may have increased long-term disability and fatal consequences when compared with patients who are not on this drug or on other anticoagulants. Patients on clopidogrel should be advised of safety when engaging in potentially dangerous activities to avoid the consequences of TBI *(Wong, Lurie, & Wong, 2008).*
- The incidence and onset time of pneumonia for patients with severe traumatic brain injury (TBI) in the early phase of rehabilitation and the parameters associated with the risk of pneumonia among 173 patients with severe TBI: 27 percent had pneumonia at transfer from the intensive care unit. Pneumonia developed in only 12 percent of the participants during rehabilitation. Patients with a low level of consciousness and patients with a tracheostomy tube or feeding tube had a higher likelihood of pneumonia *(Hansen, Larsen, & Engberg, 2008).*
- The incidence of post traumatic cerebral infarction (PTCI) in patients with severe TBI is higher after severe brain injury than previously thought. PTCI has a significant impact on mortality and length of stay. The presence of a blunt cerebral vascular injury, the need for craniotomy, or treatment with factor VIIa are risk factors for PTCI. Recognition of this secondary brain insult and the associated risk factors may help identify the group at risk and tailor management of patients with severe TBI *(Tawil, Stein, Mirvis, & Scalea, 2008).*
- A systematic review was conducted to determine the prevalence of chronic pain as an underdiagnosed consequence of TBI and to review the interaction between chronic pain and severity of TBI as well as the characteristics of pain after TBI among civilians and combatants. Investigators concluded that chronic pain is a common complication of TBI. It is independent of psychologic disorders such as PTSD and depression and is common even among patients with apparently minor injuries to the brain *(Nampiaparampil, 2008).*

SECTION THREE REVIEW

1. A nursing intervention to reduce secondary injury is
   A. maintaining CPP less than 60 mm Hg
   B. spacing out patient care activities
   C. vigorous suctioning of the patient
   D. keeping the patient flat at all times

2. Secondary injury is caused by
   A. hypoxia and ischemia
   B. cerebral swelling
   C. inflammation of cerebral tissue
   D. all of the above

(continued)

(continued)

3. Decompressive craniotomy
   A. is appropriate for all patients with secondary injury
   B. is used to treat intractable ICP elevation in some patients
   C. will reduce CPP
   D. will increase ICP

4. Hypertonic saline:
   A. increases ICP
   B. decreases CPP
   C. increases cellular swelling
   D. decreases cellular inflammation

Answers: 1. B, 2. D, 3. B, 4. D

SECTION FOUR: Complications Associated with Traumatic Brain Injury

At the completion of this section, the learner will be able to identify complications and interventions associated with traumatic brain injury.

A significant number of complications occur as a result of traumatic brain injury. Complications that commonly occur in high-acuity patients with traumatic brain injury include diabetes insipidus, syndrome of inappropriate antidiuretic hormone, cerebral salt wasting, seizures, brain herniation, and brain death.

Diabetes Insipidus

Diabetes insipidus (DI) is a condition associated with improper water balance. Water balance is maintained in the body in part because of the secretion of antidiuretic hormone (ADH) by the posterior pituitary gland. DI is characterized by polyuria and polydipsia resulting from either inadequate ADH secretion (central or neurogenic DI) or from a decreased renal response to ADH (nephrogenic DI). Normally ADH is secreted to prevent diuresis and loss of urine in times of physiologic stress (such as hypotension). However, traumatic brain injury (TBI) may result in pressure on (or damage to) the pituitary gland and loss of ADH secretion. Loss of ADH secretion results in polyuria. Any patient with traumatic brain injury and increased intracranial pressure is at risk of developing DI.

The time of onset for diabetes insipidus (DI) is 5 to 10 days following the initial injury (Barker, 2008). The earliest signs of DI include large amounts of pale, clear "waterlike" urine and hypotension. The classic diagnostic profile of DI includes the production of large amounts (greater than 200 mL/hr) of dilute (specific gravity less than 1.005) urine with an associated increase in serum sodium (greater than 145 mEq/L). Treatment of DI involves aggressive replacement of intravascular volume with intravenous (IV) fluids and the administration of synthetic antidiuretic hormone (ADH). Administration of ADH may be either in the form of a vasopressin infusion or desmopressin (DDAVP) either IV, subcutaneous, or intranasal (Holcomb, 2002; Barker, 2008; Wilson et al., 2008). Indications of improvement are decreased urine output and increased specific gravity.

Syndrome of Inappropriate Antidiuresis Hormone

Syndrome of inappropriate antidiuretic hormone (SIADH) increases total body water because excess antidiuretic hormone (ADH) secretion results in retention of water. The classic profile of SIADH includes the production of small amounts (less than 400 mL/day) of concentrated (specific gravity greater than 1.020) urine with an associated decrease in serum sodium (dilutional hyponatremia). The presence of this hypoosmolar state results in cellular swelling, systemically and intracerebrally (Barker, 2008; Yanko & Mitcho, 2001). Cerebral swelling increases intracranial pressure and leads to secondary injury. Treatment of SIADH involves restricting fluid intake to prevent further dilution of the serum (Palmer, 2000; Powers & Schulman, 2009). Nursing interventions for the patient with SIADH include monitoring intake and output, neurologic status, and enforcement of fluid restriction.

Cerebral Salt Wasting

Cerebral salt wasting (CSW) is similar to SIADH because patients present with low serum sodium and a low serum and urine osmolality. However, whereas SIADH represents a state of fluid overload, CSW is a state of hypovolemia. The mechanism of CSW is not well understood, but the end result is the loss of sodium into the urine causing water to follow. It is important to differentiate CSW from SIADH because restricting fluid in the CSW patient, who is already volume depleted, can lead to disastrous results. The patient with CSW is treated with salt replacement via IV saline and oral salt tablets. Cerebral salt wasting tends to correct itself over the course of 3 to 4 weeks (Palmer, 2000; Barker, 2008). In more severe cases, hypertonic saline and fludrocortisones (Florinef) may be used (Powers & Schulman, 2009). Table 22–4 provides a comparison of diabetes insipidus, syndrome of inappropriate ADH and cerebral salt wasting.

TABLE 22–4 Summary of DI, SIADH, and CSW

COMPLICATION	PATHOPHYSIOLOGY	URINE OUTPUT	SPECIFIC GRAVITY	SERUM SODIUM
DI	No ADH secretion leads to fluid volume deficit	Diuresis	Low	High
SIADH	Excess ADH secretion leads to fluid volume excess	Oliguria	High	Low
CSW	Mechanism unknown leads to fluid volume deficit	Diuresis	Low	Low

Seizure Activity

Seizure activity is a complication of traumatic brain injury with an incidence of 22 percent and as high as 50 percent in penetrating injuries (Bayir, H., Clark, R.S., Kochanek, P.M. (2003). Posttraumatic seizures are classified as early (occurring within seven days of the injury) or late (occurring more than seven days after the injury). Early-onset seizures may cause increased intracranial pressure, hypoxia, and increased metabolic demands increasing the severity of secondary injury. Early seizures should be managed with intravenous lorazepam (Ativan) 0.1mg/kg up to 10 mg. Lorazepam can be followed by phenytoin (Dilantin) or fosphenytoin (Cerebyx) loading dose. The loading dose for phenytoin is 15 to 20 mg/kg IV at 50 mg/minute followed by a maintenance dose of 100 mg every six to eight hours. The loading dose for fosphenytoin is 15 to 20 mg/kg IV at 150 mg/min followed by a maintenance dose of 4 to 6 mg/kg/day (Wilson et al., 2008). The goals of treatment should be to keep the patient safe, timely administration of anticonvulsant drugs, and attention to airway, breathing, and circulation (Chang & Lowenstein, 2003).

Brain Herniation

Brain herniation is a catastrophic complication of traumatic brain injury caused by increased intracranial pressure. Pressure within the confines of the rigid intracranial vault increases as the space occupying the skull becomes filled with edematous brain tissue, an accumulation of blood, or a combination of both. As space becomes tight, the brain tissue shifts from its normal position in the cranial vault to an area of less pressure. The direction in which the brain herniates depends on the type and location of injury. Two common types of herniation are cingulate and central (Fig. 22–6). Cingulate herniation occurs when one hemisphere of the brain is forced across the falx cerebri (the portion of the dura separating the hemispheres) into the space occupied by the contralateral (opposite) hemisphere. This usually occurs as a result of accumulation of blood on one side of the brain as seen with subarachnoid hemorrhage. Central herniation occurs when cerebral swelling forces both hemispheres to be displaced downward across the tentorium (the separation between the cerebrum and the cerebellum and medulla).

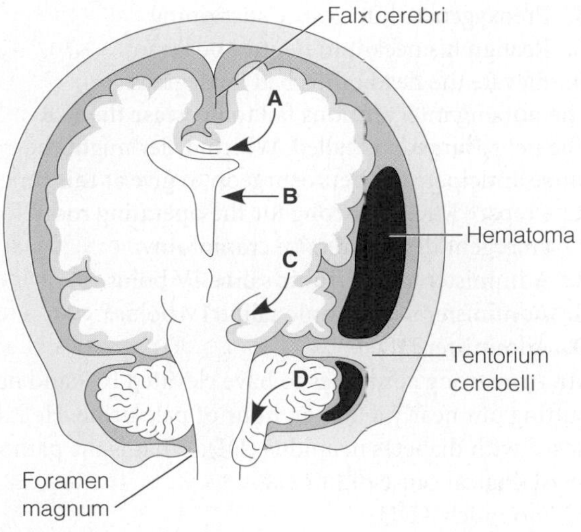

Figure 22–6 ■ Types of brain herniation. A, Cingulate herniation occurs when the cingulate gyrus is compressed under the falx cerebri. B, central herniation occurs when a centrally located lesion compresses central and midbrain structures.

Herniation of either type is devastating as increased pressure is placed on the medulla where basic functions needed to sustain life are located. When herniation is occurring, the nurse will see drastic deterioration patterns in the patient's neurologic status and vital signs. The classic vital sign changes are called *Cushing's triad,* which consists of bradycardia, severe systolic hypertension with a widened pulse pressure, and irregular breathing. Another important sign of herniation is the classic pupillary pattern of development of unequal pupils with sluggish or no reaction to light followed by bilateral fixed, fully dilated pupils. Management of herniation requires emergent interventions to relieve the intracranial pressure, which may include emergency craniotomy. Prevention of herniation is key to improving outcomes through close monitoring and control of intracranial pressure.

Brain Death

Brain death is an irreversible cessation of all brain function, including brainstem function. The evolution of traumatic brain injury to brain death can be both long and, at times, unexpected. Some patients may arrive in the ICU for something as simple as frequent neurological exams following a seemingly mild or moderate brain injury and then decline rapidly as a missed or new injury develops. Other patients may survive for weeks as health care providers battle increased ICP and associated injuries, only to succumb to total cerebral infarction. Brain death is suspected when there is no evidence of brainstem function for up to 24 hours in a patient with a normal temperature who is not under any influence of depressant drugs, paralytics, or alcohol. Signs of impending death include loss of the body's ability to maintain adequate blood pressure, profound bradycardia, and loss of basic neurological functioning (e.g., fixed and dilated pupils and absence of reflexes).

The diagnosis of brain death is made using several different methods. Ultimately, the physician must be able to document coma, absence of brainstem reflexes, and apnea (Sullivan & Severance-Lossin, 2005). Spontaneous respiratory effort is absent (apnea is present). The apnea test is performed by taking the patient off the ventilator, allowing the $Pa{CO_2}$ to rise above 60 mm Hg. If the brainstem is functional, this high level of $Pa{CO_2}$ should stimulate respiration. Pupils are fixed and dilated. Ocular responses to head turning and cold caloric stimulation are absent. The electroencephalogram demonstrates absence of brain activity with flat (isoelectric) waves. An angiogram reveals no cerebral blood flow. Motor and reflex movements are absent. However, it is also not unusual for the body to continue to exhibit signs of movement even after brain death has been established. The movements represent spinal reflexes only, and their significance must be explained to family members. The nurse caring for the brain-dead patient needs to be able to provide support to the family with emotional reassurance and to provide a spiritual advisor on request.

SECTION FOUR REVIEW

1. Treatment of diabetes insipidus (DI) includes
   A. massive fluid resuscitation
   B. fluid restriction
   C. administration of vasopressin
   D. A and C
2. Syndrome of inappropriate ADH (SIADH) is treated with
   A. fluid restriction
   B. fluid resuscitation
   C. salt restriction
   D. potassium replacement
3. Cerebral salt wasting (CSW) is treated with
   A. fluid restriction
   B. administration of vasopressin
   C. salt restriction
   D. salt replacement
4. The single most important indicator(s) of progression of brain injury is/are
   A. change in mental status exam
   B. changes in vital signs
   C. elevation of ICP
   D. reduced CPP
5. Early onset seizures occur within ______ days of the TBI; and should be managed with ______ and/or ______ or ______

Answers: 1. D, 2. A, 3. D, 4. A, 5. Seven; IV Lorazepam; phenytoin or fosphenytoin

POSTTEST

The Posttest questions all relate to the following case scenario. Mr. Armstrong is admitted to the emergency department following an assault with a baseball bat.

1. An MRI shows the presence of DAI. What is the most likely mechanism of injury for Mr. Armstrong?
   A. acceleration
   B. deceleration
   C. rotational
   D. penetrating
2. Mr. Armstrong's Glasgow Coma Scale decreases by one point and he develops a fixed and dilated pupil. Which of the following interventions would you do FIRST?
   A. Reassess the patient in 15 minutes.
   B. Call the physician immediately.
   C. Prepare the patient for a CT scan.
   D. Inform the family of these changes.
3. You notice the presence of clear fluid draining from Mr. Armstrong's ears and nose. It is found to be CSF. With what type of skull fracture is CSF drainage most commonly associated?
   A. linear
   B. open skull fracture
   C. depressed skull fracture
   D. basilar skull fracture
4. Several hours after admission to the unit, you walk into Mr. Armstrong's room and find he is lethargic, confused, mumbling his speech, and very difficult to arouse. What may be the cause(s) of these changes in his level of consciousness?
   A. decreased ICP
   B. worsening brain injury
   C. Mr. Armstrong is simply tired.
   D. oversedation
5. Mr. Armstrong is rushed to a CT scan where it is revealed he has an expanding epidural hematoma. He is taken to the OR to have it evacuated and returns to the ICU ventilated and with an intraventricular catheter in place. What is the minimal cerebral perfusion pressure (CPP) he should have?
   A. greater than 50 mm Hg
   B. greater than 60 mm Hg
   C. greater than 70 mm Hg
   D. greater than 80 mm Hg
6. Mr. Armstrong's ICP increases. Before calling the neurosurgeon you decide to try to decrease the ICP with nursing interventions. Which of the following interventions will decrease his ICP? (choose all that apply)
   A. Keep him supine with the head of bed flat.
   B. Preoxygenate him before suctioning.
   C. Realign his neck into neutral position.
   D. Elevate the head of his bed 30 degrees.
7. The nursing interventions fail to decrease the ICP. The neurosurgeon is called. Which order might the nurse anticipate the neurosurgeon to give at this time?
   A. Prepare Mr. Armstrong for the operating room for emergent decompressive craniotomy.
   B. Administer a hypertonic saline IV bolus.
   C. Administer a hypotonic saline IV bolus.
   D. Administer DDAVP.
8. Mr. Armstrong continues to have elevated ICP and now is putting out nearly a liter an hour of pale urine. He is diagnosed with diabetes insipidus (DI). What is the pathophysiological cause of DI?
   A. too much ADH
   B. too much circulating DDAVP
   C. retention of sodium
   D. not enough ADH

9. Mr. Armstrong develops an abrupt hypertension, bradycardia, and an irregular breathing pattern. These signs are indicative of
A. pain
B. anxiety
C. impending herniation
D. brain death

10. Which of the following is NOT a criterion for brain death?
A. spontaneous breathing
B. apnea
C. presence of coma
D. loss of brainstem reflexes

Posttest answers with rationale are found on MyNursingKit.

REFERENCES

Albano, C., Comandante, L., Nolan, S. (2005). Innovations in the management of cerebral injury. *Critical Care Nursing Quarterly, 28,* (2): 135–149.

Alderson, P., & Roberts, I. (2005). Corticosteroids for acute traumatic brain injury. *Cochrane Database Systematic Reviews,* 4. CD000196; PMID: 10796701.

Barker, E. (2008). *Neuroscience nursing: a spectrum of care.* St. Louis: Mosby-Elsevier, 175–179.

Bayir, H., Clark, R. S., Kochanek, P. M. (2003). Promising strategies to minimize secondary brain injury after head trauma. *Critical Care Medicine, 31*(1 supplement): 5112–5117.

Blank-Reid, C., McClelland,R., & Santora, T. (2008). Neurotrauma: traumatic brain injury. In E. Barker (ed.) *Neuroscience nursing: a spectrum of care* (3rd ed.). St. Louis: Mosby Elsevier, 337–367.

Blissitt, P. (2009). Brain oxygen monitoring. In AACN-AANN, *Protocols for practice: monitoring technologies in critically ill neuroscience patients,* 103–106.

Brain Trauma Foundation. (2007). Guidelines for the management of severe traumatic brain injury. *Journal of Neurotrauma, 24*(supplement 1): 1–95. Can be accessed at www.braintrauma.org.

Bullock, R. (2000). Intracranial pressure treatment threshold. *Journal Neurotrauma, 17,*493–495.

Bullock, R., Chestnut, R, & Clifton, G. (2001). Management and prognosis of severe traumatic brain injury. *Journal Neurotrauma, 17*(6–7), 451–627.

Butcher, I., Maas, A. I., Lu, J., Marmasou, A., et al (2007). Prognostic value of admission blood pressure in traumatic brain injury: results of the IIMPACT study. *Journal of Neurotrauma, 24*(2): 294–302.

Chang, B. S., Lowenstein, D. H. (2003). Practice parameter: antiepileptic drug prophylaxis in severe traumatic brain injury. *Neurology, 60,* 10–16.

Chulay, M. (2005). Suctioning: endotracheal or tracheostomy tube. In D. J. Lynn-McHale Weigand & K. K. Carlson (eds.) *AACN procedure manual for critical care,* 5th ed. St Louis: Elsevier Saunders, 62–70.

Cooper, D. (2004). Prehospital hypertonic saline resuscitation of patients with hypotension and severe traumatic brain injury: a randomized controlled trial. *Journal of American Medical Association, 291,* 1350–1357.

CRASH Trial. (2004). Effect of intravenous corticosteroids on death within 14 days, 10,008 adults with clinically significant head injury (MRC CRASH trial): randomized placebo controlled trial. *Lancet, 364,* pp. 1321–1328.

Dawodu, S. T. (2008). Traumatic brain injury: definition, epidemiology, pathophysiology. *Emedicine fromWebMD.* Retrieved February 28, 2009 from http://emedicine.medscape.com/article/326510-overview.

Doyle, J. A., Davis, D. P., & Hoyt, D. B. (2001). The use of hypertonic saline in the treatment of traumatic brain injury. *Journal of Trauma Injury Infection and Personal Care, 50,* 367–383.

Freeborn, K. (2004). Neurotrauma – the role of the nurse practitioner in traumatic brain injury. *Topics in Emergency Medicine, 26*(3), 225–288.

Hansen, T. S., Larsen, K., Engberg, A. W. (2008). The association of functional oral intake and pneumonia in patients with severe traumatic brain injury. *Arch Phys Med Rehabil, 89*(11), 2114–2120.

Helmy, A. Vizcaychipi, M., Gupta, A. K., (2007). Traumatic brain injury: intensive care management. *Journal of Neurotrauma, 99*(1): 32–42.

Holcomb, S. S. (2002). Diabetes insipidus. *Dimensions of Critical Care Nursing, 21,* 94–97.

Jaeger, M., Soehle, M., & Meixensberger, J. (2003). Effects of decompressive craniectomy on brain tissue oxygen in patients with intracranial hypertension. *Journal of Neurology, Neurosurgery, and Psychiatry, 74,* 513–515.

Langlois, J. A., Kegler, S. R., Butler, J. A., et al. (2003). Traumatic brain injury-related hospital discharges. Results from a 14-state surveillance system, 1197. *MMWR* 52(4):1–20.

LeJeune, G. M., & Howard-Fain, T. (2002). Nursing assessment and management of patients with head injuries. *Dimensions of Critical Care Nursing, 21,* 226–227.

LeMone, P. & Burke, K. M. (2008). Nursing care of clients with intracranial disorders. In *Medical-surgical nursing: critical thinking in client care,* 4th ed. Upper Saddle River, NJ: Prentice Hall, 1535–1562.

Littlejohns, L. R., Bader, M. K. (2005). Prevention of secondary brain injury: targeting technology. *AACN Clinical Issues, 16*(4), 501–514.

Lovasik, D., Kerr, M. E., & Alexander, S. (2001). Traumatic brain injury research: a review of clinical studies. *Critical Care Nursing Quarterly, 23*(4), 23–41.

Marik, P. E., Varon, J., & Trask, T. (2002). Management of head trauma. *Chest, 122,* 699–711.

Meixensberger, J., Baunch, S., Amschler, J. et al. (1997). Influence of body position on tissue PO2, cerebral perfusion pressure, and intracranial pressure in patients with acute brain injury. *Journal of Neurology Research, 19*(3): 249–253.

Morales, D., Diaz-Daza, O., Hlatky, R., & Hayman, L. (2007). Brain, Contusion. eMedicine from WebMD. Retrieved March 2, 2009 from http://emedicine.medscape.com/article/337782-overview.

Nortje, J. & Menon, D. K. (2004). Traumatic brain injury: physiology, mechanisms, and outcome. *Current Opinion Neurology, 17,* 711–718.

Palmer, B. F. (2000). Hyponatremia in a neurosurgical patient: syndrome of inappropriate antidiuretic hormone secretion versus cerebral salt wasting. *Nephrology Dialysis Transplantation, 15,* 262–268.

Powers, J. & Schulman, C. S. (2009). Head injury and dysfunction. In K. K. Carlson (ed.), *Advanced critical care nursing.*St. Louis: Saunders Elsevier, 529–575.

Sullivan, J., & Severance-Lossin, L., (2005). Determination of death. In D. J. L-M Weigand & K. K. Carlson (eds.), *AACN procedure manual for critical care.* (5th ed.). St Louis: Elsevier Saunders, 1174–1182.

Tawil, I., Stein, D. M., Mirvis, S. E., & Scalea, T. M. (2008). Posttraumatic cerebral infarction: incidence, outcome, and risk factors. *J Trauma, 64*(4), 849–853.

Tyagi, R. Donaldson, K., Loftus, C. M., Jallo, J. (2007). Hypertonic saline: a clinical review. *Journal of Neurotrauma, 30*(4): 277–289.

Wilson, B., Shannon, M., Shields, K. (2008). *Nurses Drug Guide.* Upper Saddle River, NJ: Prentice Hall.

Wong, D. K., Lurie, F., & Wong, L. L. (2008). The effects of clopidogrel on elderly traumatic brain injured patients. *Journal of Trauma, 65*(6), 1303–1308.

Yanko, J. R., & Mitcho, K. (2001). Acute care management of severe traumatic brain injuries. *Critical Care Nurse Quarterly, 23*(4), 1–23.

Zenati, M. S. (2002). A brief episode of hypotension increases mortality in critically ill trauma patients. *Journal of Trauma, 53,* 232–237.

MODULE

23 Alteration in Sensory Perceptual Function: Acute Spinal Cord Injury

Grace Nolde-Lopez, Melanie G. Hardin-Pierce, Karen L. Johnson

OBJECTIVES Following completion of this module, the learner will be able to

1. Explain anatomic features of the spinal cord and vertebrae, including unstable spinal cord injury.
2. Discuss spinal cord injury, including types of injury and primary and secondary injury.
3. Describe physical assessment techniques and diagnostic tests frequently used to identify the type and severity of spinal cord injury.
4. Discuss stabilization techniques used for spinal cord injuries.
5. Identify priority nursing assessments and interventions for the patient with a spinal cord injury in the acute care phase of recovery.

This self-study module focuses on patients with the sensory perceptual disorder, acute spinal cord injury. Successful completion of this module will help the reader prepare to care for patients with this disorder in a high-acuity environment.

The module is composed of five sections. Section One reviews the spinal cord anatomy and physiology. Section Two discusses the mechanisms of injury to the spinal cord and the sequelae of those injuries on sensory and motor function. Section Three explains the diagnostic procedures used in the evaluation of spinal cord injury and the key nursing assessments that must be made for patients with spinal cord injuries. Section Four introduces the reader to the surgical and manual stabilization techniques used in spinal cord injuries and the nursing implications of these therapeutic modalities. Section Five identifies the important nursing interventions and assessments for care of the patient with a spinal cord injury in the acute care phase. Each section includes a set of review questions to help the learner evaluate his or her understanding of the section's content before moving on to the next section. All Section Reviews include answers. It is suggested that the learner review those concepts answered incorrectly in the review questions before proceeding to the next section.

PRETEST

1. M. W. has a stable C5 spinal cord injury. Which of the following statements is true about this injury?
   - **A.** The vertebrae are unable to support the injured area.
   - **B.** The vertebral and ligamentous structures are able to support and protect the injured area.
   - **C.** Two of the columns are damaged.
   - **D.** Ligamentous structures are unable to support the injured area.
2. In order to bear weight, vertebral bodies
   - **A.** increase in size as they descend
   - **B.** decrease in size as they descend
   - **C.** consist of a body and an arch
   - **D.** are fused to one another
3. Which region of the spinal cord is most susceptible to injury?
   - **A.** cervical
   - **B.** thoracic
   - **C.** lumbar
   - **D.** sacral
4. Diving accidents typically result in damage to which region of the spinal cord?
   - **A.** cervical
   - **B.** thoracic
   - **C.** lumbar
   - **D.** sacral
5. Secondary injury to the spinal cord occurs from
   - **A.** improper movement of the patient
   - **B.** the forces producing a closed-head injury
   - **C.** biochemical processes that destroy neurons
   - **D.** small hemorrhages in spinal gray matter
6. The presence of perineal reflexes indicate
   - **A.** priapism
   - **B.** intact bulbocavernosus reflex
   - **C.** upper motor neuron injury
   - **D.** bowel and bladder training may be feasible

7. Swimmer's position X-ray may be used to diagnose
   A. a spinal cord tumor
   B. C7-T1 injuries
   C. C1-C2 injuries
   D. vascular disruptions to the cord
8. Sensation that begins at or above the nipple line is associated with which dermatome?
   A. C5
   B. C7
   C. T4
   D. L1
9. Gardner-Wells tongs are inserted to stabilize a cervical spine. This device requires which of the following? (choose all that apply)
   A. screws implanted in the skull
   B. weights
   C. part of the head to be shaved
   D. bone grafting
10. Timely spinal alignment and stability
    A. maximizes cord recovery
    B. minimizes additional damage
    C. prevents late deformity
    D. all of the above
11. Which of the following statements would you use to prepare a patient with a SCI for placement of Gardner-Wells tongs?
    A. "A wrench will be placed on your chest."
    B. "Two screws will be implanted in your skull."
    C. "You will feel pressure but not pain."
    D. "Four pins will be inserted into your skull."
12. The rehabilitation potential of a person with an L1–L5 injury is
    A. independent eating, independent bathing, independent mobility with the use of knee, ankle, and foot orthoses
    B. independent eating, independent bathing, electric wheelchair
    C. independent eating, minor assistance with bathing, manual wheelchair
    D. independent eating, independent bathing, manual wheelchair
13. Autonomic dysreflexia is a health emergency because
    A. airway spasm occurs
    B. severe vasoconstriction occurs
    C. spasticity produces joint immobility
    D. hypoxia results from regurgitation
14. Suctioning may produce which of the following in the SCI patient?
    A. airway spasm
    B. bradycardia
    C. hypertension
    D. vomiting

Pretest answers are found on MyNursingKit.

SECTION ONE: Spinal Cord Anatomy and Physiology

At the completion of this section, the learner will be able to explain anatomic features of the spinal cord and vertebrae, including unstable spinal cord injury.

Spinal Cord Anatomy

The spine is composed of 33 individual and fused vertebrae. There are 7 cervical (C), 12 thoracic (T), and 5 lumbar (L) vertebrae. The sacral and coccygeal vertebrae are fused in the adult. Each vertebra consists of a body (anterior) and an arch (posterior). The arch section is composed of two pedicles that attach the arch to the body and two laminae that form the roof of the arch. The spinous process is located at the rear of the vertebrae. In order to bear additional weight, vertebral bodies increase in size as they descend.

As illustrated in Figure 23–1, the spine is conceptualized as having three columns: an anterior column that includes the anterior part of the vertebral body, a middle column that houses the posterior wall of the vertebral body, and a posterior column that includes the vertebral arch. If two or more of these columns are damaged, the injury is considered to be unstable. **Unstable spinal injury** exists when the vertebral and ligamentous structures are unable to support and protect the injured area.

The spinal cord runs through the center of the vertebral column through the spinal canal. It starts at the foramen magnum ofthe brain and ends at the first or second lumbar vertebra (Fig. 23–2). In the cervical region, the cord receives afferent impulses from the upper and lower extremities. The distal end of the cord contains reflex centers for bowel, bladder, and sexual function. The C1–C7 spinal nerves exit above the correspondingly numbered vertebrae. The C8 spinal nerve exits below the C7 vertebrae. The spinal nerves of T1 and below exit below the correspondingly numbered vertebrae. The spinal nerves join complex networks after leaving the cord to innervate parts of the body.

The main blood supply to the spinal cord is provided by the anterior spinal artery and the posterior spinal arteries. Any disruption in this vascular supply may damage the cord without direct physical trauma.

Neuronal Function

The spinal cord consists of an outer region of white matter and an inner region of gray matter. The gray matter helps transmit motor activity from the brain to the body. It also serves as a "relay" station for sensory messages from the body to the brain. In the first thoracic through the second lumbar section of the cord, the gray matter gives rise to the sympathetic nervous system. Activation of the thoracic section gray matter stimulates the sympathetic nervous system to increase perfusion and ventilation, and decrease elimination and digestion.

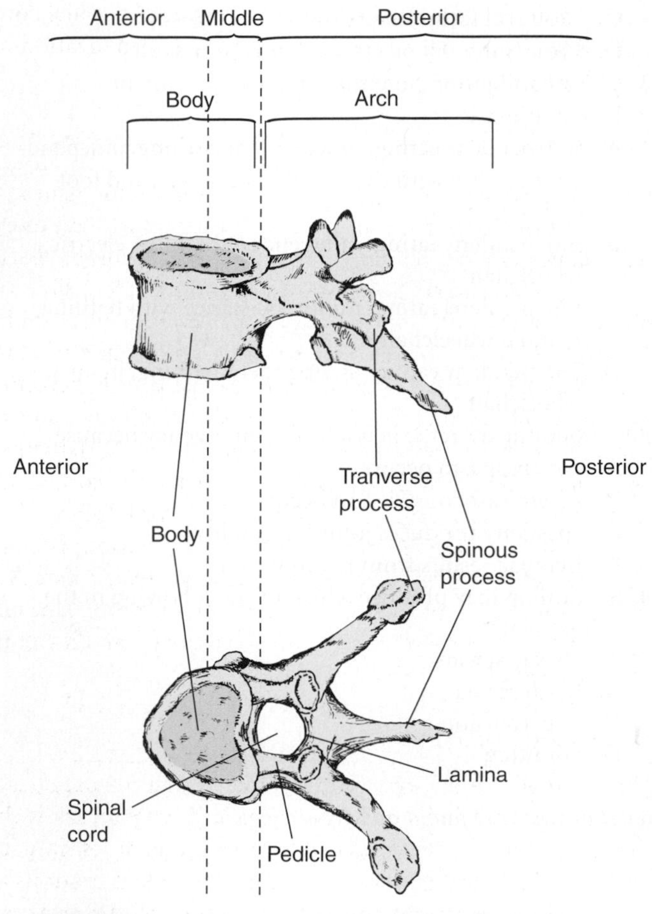

Figure 23–1 ■ A lateral view and cross-section of a vertebra.

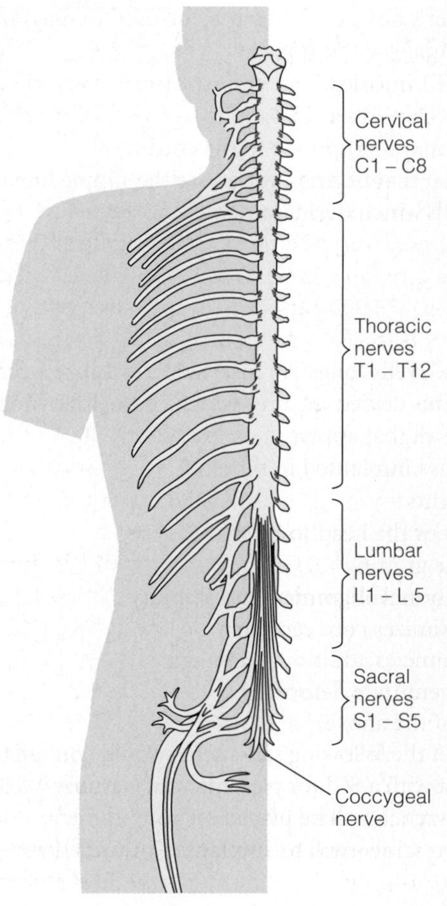

Figure 23–2 ■ Distribution of spinal nerves.

The white matter of the spinal cord consists of insulated nerve fibers that function as transmission cables (tracts). The three major tracts are the corticospinal, spinothalamic, and posterior column tracts for touch, vibration, and position sense, respectively. The corticospinal tract originates in the brain and crosses over in the brainstem to innervate the opposite side of the body. It transmits motor activity. The spinothalamic tract originates in the spinal cord, where it crosses over within two segments of entry into the cord and ascends to the thalamus in the brain. It transmits pain and temperature. The posterior horn contains axons from the peripheral sensory neurons.

The parasympathetic nervous system originates in a group of neurons located in the brainstem and in another group located between the second and fourth sacral segments of the cord. Parasympathetic stimulation produces specific responses that assist elimination and digestion, among other functions. Damage to specific regions of the cord may produce alterations in either sympathetic or parasympathetic function.

SECTION ONE REVIEW

1. JR has been diagnosed with an unstable spinal injury. This means
   - **A.** she has injured the reflex center for bowel function
   - **B.** the vertebral structures are unable to support the injured area
   - **C.** multiple spinal fractures are present
   - **D.** the main blood supply to the spinal cord is disrupted
2. The spinal cord is located in the
   - **A.** spinal canal
   - **B.** spinous process
   - **C.** plexus
   - **D.** body of vertebrae
3. The end of the spinal cord contains reflex centers for
   - **A.** bowel function
   - **B.** bladder function
   - **C.** sexual function
   - **D.** all of the above
4. Activation of the thoracic section gray matter stimulates the
   - **A.** sympathetic nervous system
   - **B.** parasympathetic nervous system
   - **C.** brainstem
   - **D.** spinothalamic tract

Answers: 1. B, 2. A, 3. D, 4. A

SECTION TWO: Spinal Cord Injury

At the completion of this section, the learner will be able to discuss spinal cord injury, including types of injury and primary and secondary injury.

Approximately 40 cases per million population or 11,000 individuals in the United States sustain a permanent spinal cord injury (SCI) each year (National SCI Statistical Center, 2007). The number of people in the United States living with a SCI is approximately 253,000 persons. The most frequent neurological level of injury is incomplete tetraplegia (34.1 percent), followed by complete paraplegia (23 percent) and complete tetraplegia (18.5 percent) (National SCI Statistical Center, 2007). Motor vehicle crashes account for 46.9 percent of SCI cases, next is falls, then acts of violence (primarily gunshot wounds), last is sports activities. The proportion of injuries due to sports has decreased over time while the proportion of injuries due to falls have increased (National SCI Statistical Center, 2007). Pneumonia, pulmonary emboli, and septicemia are the most frequent causes of death. Prognosis is poorest for individuals over the age of 50 with complete lesions at the time of injury. For severely injured persons, mortality rates are significantly higher during the first year after injury than in following years.

Spinal cord injury may be described as **complete spinal cord injury** (loss of all voluntary motor and sensory function below the level of injury) caused by damage to the entire level of the spinal cord or **incomplete spinal cord injury** (preservation of some sensory or motor function below the level of injury because of partial damage to the spinal cord). The patient will also be told his or her American Spinal Injury Association (ASIA) classification level (see Fig. 23–3). The injury is identified by vertebral level. For example, a C5 ASIA B classification SCI is at the fifth cervical vertebrae with some sensation preserved below the level of the injury, and minimum sensation around the rectum (S4-S5). About 60 percent of patients admitted to high-acuity units have incomplete SCI and 59 percent of these develop significant recovery of function. Less than 1 percent of persons experience complete neurologic recovery by hospital discharge (National SCI Statistical Center, 2007).

Complete Spinal Cord Injury

Complete spinal cord injury results in one of two conditions: paraplegia or tetraplegia.) **Paraplegia** is the result of injury to the thoracolumbar region (T2 to L1) causing loss of motor and sensory function of the lower extremities. Upper extremity function remains intact. **Tetraplegia** (also referred to as **quadriplegia**) is the result of injury to cervical or thoracic regions (C1 to T1). Muscle function depends on the specific segments involved but impaired function of the arms, trunk, legs, and pelvic organs may occur. Figure 23–4 compares the extent of paralysis with level of injury.

Incomplete Spinal Cord Injury

Types of incomplete spinal cord injuries are described in Table 23–1. Note that with these syndromes each has evidence of partially interrupted motor and sensory pathways. The alterations in function that occur as the result of a spinal cord injury vary greatly depending on the amount and location of tissue damage, and the level of injury.

Upper and Lower Motor Neuron Injuries

Spinal cord injury damages upper or lower motor neurons. Motor neurons are functional units that carry motor impulses. *Upper motor neurons* are located in the cerebral cortex, thalamus, brainstem, and corticospinal tracts and are responsible for voluntary movement. Damage to an upper motor neuron pathway results in loss of cerebral control over reflex activity below the lesion level. Upper motor neurons may become hyperactive to local stimuli, producing **spastic paralysis** (the inability to carry out a skilled movement). *Lower motor neurons* originate in the spinal cord and form spinal nerves outside the cord. They transmit from target organs to the spinal cord, where they synapse with another lower motor neuron to transmit back to the same target organ. Lower motor neurons create reflex arcs and involuntary responses. Damage to lower motor neurons produces **flaccid paralysis** (loss of both voluntary and involuntary movement).

Mechanisms of Injury

Like traumatic brain injuries, spinal cord injuries occur as a result of primary and secondary injury. **Primary injury** is the neurologic damage that occurs at the moment of impact. Primary spinal cord injuries are caused by violent motions of the head and trunk, fracture or dislocation of the vertebral column, and blunt or penetrating trauma. **Secondary injury** occurs as a result of vascular injury to the cord from arterial or venous disruption causing bleeding, edema, and hypoxia of the spinal cord. Secondary injury refers to the complex biochemical processes that occur within minutes of injury and can last for days to weeks. Secondary processes include edema, ischemia, inflammation, excitotoxicity, disturbances to ionic homeostasis, excessive cytokine release, and damage to axons and myelin from calpain activation, which causes a cellular influx of calcium resulting in apoptosis (programmed cell death) (Fehlings & Baptiste, 2005; Blissitt, 2009).

Primary Spinal Cord Injuries

Primary injury to the spinal cord occurs when excessive force is applied to the spinal cord. Mechanisms of injury include hyperflexion, hyperextension, rotation, and axial loading.

Hyperflexion Injury

Hyperflexion injury is most often caused by a sudden deceleration of the motion of the head (e.g., head-on collision). This forcible bending forward dislocates anterior vertebrae, tears posterior ligaments, and compresses the cord (Fig. 23–5A). The spinal column is unstable because torn posterior muscles and ligaments cannot support the spinal column. As shown in Figure 23–1, recall from Section One that the vertebral column is composed of three structural columns; anterior, middle and posterior. An unstable spine occurs when loss of integrity occurs in two of the three columns.

MUSCLE GRADING

0 total paralysis

1 palpable or visible contraction

2 active movement, full range of motion, gravity eliminated

3 active movement, full range of motion, against gravity

4 active movement, full range of motion, against gravity and provides some resistance

5 active movement, full range of motion, against gravity and provides normal resistance

5* muscle able to exert, in examiner's judgement, sufficient resistance to be considered normal if identifiable inhibiting factors were not present

NT not testable. Patient unable to reliably exert effort or muscle unavailable for testing due to factors such as immobilization, pain on effort or contracture.

ASIA IMPAIRMENT SCALE

☐ **A = Complete**: No motor or sensory function is preserved in the sacral segments S4-S5.

☐ **B = Incomplete:** Sensory but not motor function is preserved below the neurological level and includes the sacral segments S4-S5.

☐ **C = Incomplete:** Motor function is preserved below the neurological level, and more than half of key muscles below the neurological level have a muscle grade less than 3.

☐ **D = Incomplete:** Motor function is preserved below the neurological level, and at least half of key muscles below the neurological level have a muscle grade of 3 or more.

☐ **E = Normal:** Motor and sensory function are normal.

CLINICAL SYNDROMES (OPTIONAL)

☐ Central Cord
☐ Brown-Sequard
☐ Anterior Cord
☐ Conus Medullaris
☐ Cauda Equina

STEPS IN CLASSIFICATION

The following order is recommended in determining the classification of individuals with SCI.

1. Determine sensory levels for right and left sides.
2. Determine motor levels for right and left sides.
   Note: in regions where there is no myotome to test, the motor level is presumed to be the same as the sensory level.
3. Determine the single neurological level.
   This is the lowest segment where motor and sensory function is normal on both sides, and is the most cephalad of the sensory and motor levels determined in steps 1 and 2.
4. Determine whether the injury is Complete or Incomplete (sacral sparing).
   If voluntary anal contraction = **No** *AND all S4-5 sensory scores =* **0** *AND any anal sensation =* **No**, *then injury is COMPLETE. Otherwise injury is incomplete.*
5. Determine ASIA Impairment Scale (AIS) Grade:

Is injury <u>Complete</u>? If **YES**, AIS=A Record ZPP
(For ZPP record lowest dermatome or myotome on each side with some (non-zero score) preservation)

NO ↓

Is injury motor <u>incomplete</u>? If **NO**, AIS=B
(Yes=voluntary anal contraction OR motor function more than three levels below the motor level on a given side.)

YES ↓

Are <u>at least</u> half of the key muscles below the (single) <u>neurological</u> level graded 3 or better?

NO ↓ AIS=C

YES ↓ AIS=D

If sensation and motor function is normal in all segments, AIS=E
Note: AIS E is used in follow up testing when an individual with a documented SCI has recovered normal function. If at initial testing no deficits are found, the individual is neurologically intact; the ASIA Impairment Scale does not apply.

Figure 23–3 ▪ ASIA Impairment Scale. With permission from the American Spinal Injury Association ASIA.

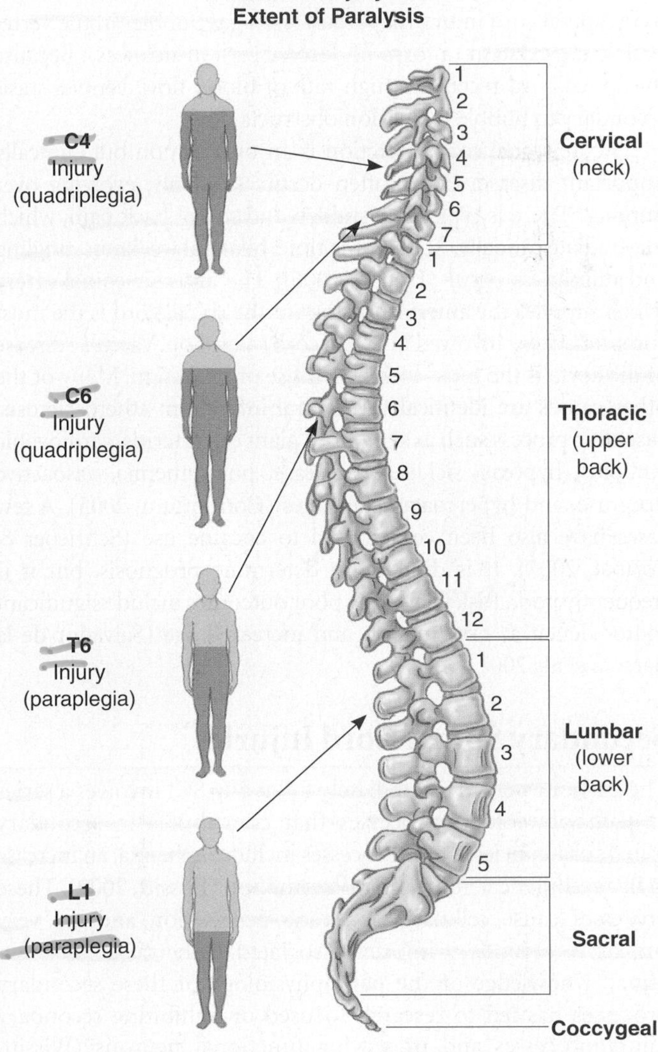

Figure 23–4 ■ Spinal injury levels.

TABLE 23–1 Incomplete Spinal Cord Injury Syndromes

SYNDROME	FUNCTIONS LOST	FUNCTIONS PRESENT
Anterior cord	Motor, pain, temperature, touch, paralysis below the level of injury	Proprioception, vibration, and pressure sense
Brown–Séquard	Loss of voluntary motor movement on same side as injury; loss of pain, temperature, sensation on the opposite side (below the level of injury)	Side of the body with the best motor control has little or no sensation
Central cord	Motor, sensory deficit in upper extremities, often spastic; variable paralysis of lower extremities	Motor, sensory pathways in lower extremities; some bladder, bowel function
Posterior cord	Proprioception, vibration sensation below the level of injury	Motor function, sense of pain and light touch

Hyperextension Injury

Hyperextension injuries are caused by a forward and backward motion of the head (e.g. rear-end collisions). With this injury, the anterior ligaments are torn and the spinal cord is stretched (Fig. 23–5B). A mild form of hyperextension injury is the whiplash injury. Rotation injury is caused by severe rotation of the neck causing a tearing of the posterior ligaments and rotation of the spinal column (e.g. nonbelted person in a car hit broadside).

Axial Loading Injury

Axial loading injury, or compression fracture, is caused by a vertical force along the spinal cord. This vertical force fractures vertebral bodies that send bony fragments into the spinal cord (Fig. 23–5C). Compression fractures typically occur with diving into shallow water or jumping from tall heights and landing on the feet or buttocks.

Cervical Injuries

The cervical region is the most vulnerable region of the spine because of its poor stability. Complete cord injuries at the C1 or C2 level are often fatal. Hyperflexion injuries of the cervical spine, especially C5 to C6, are associated with rapid deceleration. C4 and C5 damage frequently occurs from diving accidents.

Thoracic and Lumbar Injuries

Great force is needed to produce T1 through T10 injuries because of the stability of the rib cage. The most common site of thoracic spinal injury is located at the T12–L1 junction. Flexion may occur with compression of the anterior aspects of the vertebrae. A fall onto the upper back can produce flexion along with rotation. Thoracic region injuries may result from vertical compression forces experienced during a fall onto the buttocks or feet. A patient with calcaneus fractures of the feet should be suspected of having thoracic vertebral or cord damage. The same forces producing thoracic injuries may be responsible for lumbar injuries. Violent flexion of the lumbar spine may occur with wearing a lap belt without a shoulder restraint (e.g., middle passenger in the rear seat) in a motor vehicle crash.

Nontraumatic Etiologies

Several conditions may produce narrowing of the spinal canal and subsequent SCI. Degenerative changes as a result of osteoarthritis in the spine predispose a person to hyperextension injuries. Ankylosing spondylitis (calcification of ligaments and soft tissue) and rheumatoid arthritis (inflammation causing osteoporosis and decreased mobility) are two precipitating causes of SCI. Space-occupying lesions (abscesses and solid tumors) may produce spinal cord compression. Lymphoma and multiple myeloma are two oncologic conditions associated with bone metastases. The first sign of spinal cord compression from tumor growth is usually a constant, dull back pain aggravated by coughing or sneezing. Leg weakness, urinary retention, and sexual dysfunction may also develop.

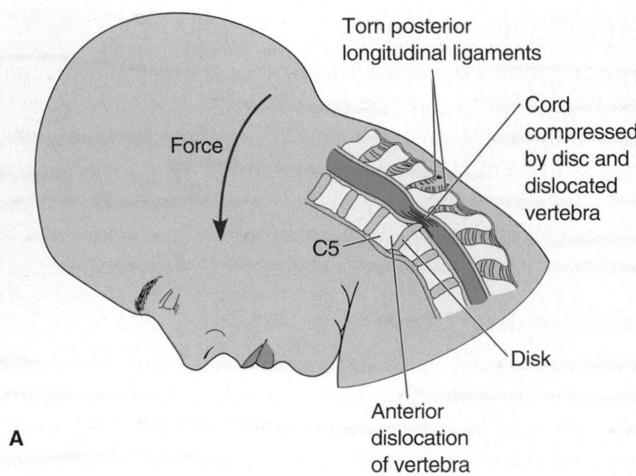

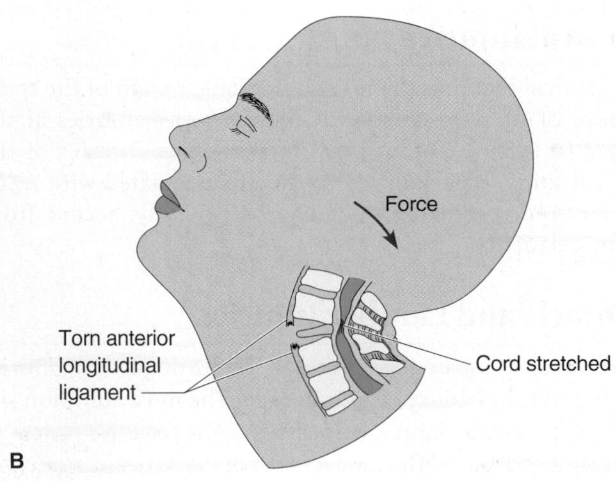

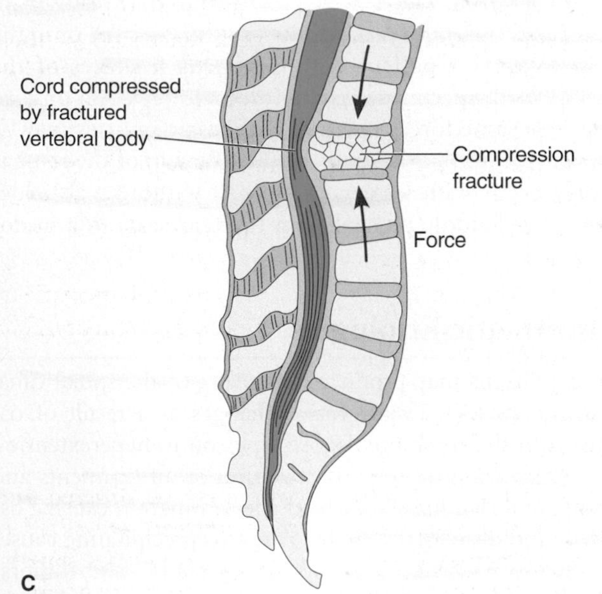

Figure 23–5 ▪ Mechanism of spinal cord injury.

In some regions where deep sea diving is a recreational activity, spinal cord injury may result from gas bubbles in the vertebral venous system (a form of decompression sickness). Because the spinal cord receives a high rate of blood flow, venous stasis secondary to bubble formation obstructs flow.

Acute spinal cord infarction is an uncommon but clinically important disease. Onset often occurs suddenly, evolving over minutes. There is typically a sudden and severe back pain, which may radiate caudally. At the same time, bilateral weakness, tingling and numbness occur (Hogan, 2006). The anterior spinal artery which supplies the anterior portion of the spinal cord is the most common artery involved in spinal cord infarction. Vascular disease of the aorta is the most common cause of infarction. Many of the other causes are identical to cerebral infarction: atherosclerosis, vasculitic process such as syphilitica giant cell arteritis, cardiogenic embolus, hypoxia, sickle cell disease, polycythemia, vasoactive drug use, and hypercoagulable states (Continuum, 2005). A few cases have also been contributed to cocaine use (Schrieber & Formal, 2007). It is difficult to determine prognosis, but it is frequently poor. Risk factors for poor outcomes include significant motor deficit at presentation and increased age (Salvador de la Barrera et al., 2001).

Secondary Spinal Cord Injuries

The 24-hour period immediately following SCI involves a series of pathophysiologic processes that contributes to secondary spinal cord injuries. These processes include: ischemia, an increase in intracellular calcium, and inflammation (Blissitt, 2009). These processes cause cellular membrane destruction and are very similar to secondary injuries associated with traumatic brain injury. Knowledge of the pathophysiology of these secondary processes has led to research focused on inhibiting secondary injury processes and preserving functional neurons (Blissitt, 2009; Dubendorf, 1999).

Ischemia

Blood flow to the spinal cord decreases immediately on injury as a result of hypotension and vasospasm-induced thrombosis. Thrombi in the microcirculation impede blood flow. Elevated interstitial pressure related to edema further impairs perfusion to the cord. Vasoconstrictive substances, such as norepinephrine, are released postinjury, contributing to decreased circulation and cellular perfusion. The zone of ischemia can spread if perfusion to the cord is not restored.

Elevated Intracellular Calcium

Calcium ions accumulate in injured cells, causing a breakdown of intracellular protein and phospholipids. Demyelination and destruction of the cell membranes occur when these substances are broken down. The breakdown of phospholipids releases fatty acids. The fatty acids produce arachidonic acid, which ultimately produces leukotrienes and prostaglandins, mediators in the inflammatory process. Eicosanoids, prostaglandins, and mediators contribute to cellular membrane damage. Once the cell membrane is damaged, neuronal death occurs.

Inflammatory Processes

Leukocytes infiltrate the injured area immediately postinjury. The inflammatory process is another factor in edema formation, further decreasing blood supply to the injured area. As the cord swells within the bony vertebrae, edema moves up and down the cord. A patient may exhibit symptoms as a result of the edema and not the initial injury. For example, a patient with a C4 injury may have edema up to the C2 level. Because edema can extend the level of injury for several cord segments above and below the affected level, the extent of injury may not be determined for several days, until after the cord edema has resolved.

SECTION TWO REVIEW

1. D. W. has been diagnosed with anterior cord syndrome. This syndrome represents
   - **A.** an upper motor neuron problem
   - **B.** a lower motor neuron problem
   - **C.** the best prognosis for recovery
   - **D.** an incomplete cord syndrome
2. Damage to upper motor neurons can produce
   - **A.** quadriplegia
   - **B.** spastic paralysis
   - **C.** flaccid paralysis
   - **D.** paraplegia
3. Whiplash is a mild form of which of the following primary injuries to the spinal cord?
   - **A.** hyperflexion
   - **B.** axial loading
   - **C.** hyperextension
   - **D.** rotation
4. Which region of the spine is most vulnerable to injury?
   - **A.** cervical
   - **B.** thoracic
   - **C.** lumbar
   - **D.** sacral
5. The events contributing to secondary injury of the spinal cord include which of the following? (choose all that apply)
   - **A.** ischemia
   - **B.** increased intracellular calcium
   - **C.** hypertension
   - **D.** inflammation

Answers: 1. D, 2. B, 3. C, 4. A, 5. (A, B, D)

SECTION THREE: Assessment and Diagnosis of Spinal Cord Injury

At the completion of this section, the learner will be able to describe physical assessment techniques and diagnostic tests frequently used to identify the type and severity of spinal cord injury.

The diagnosis of spinal cord injury (SCI) begins with a detailed history of events surrounding the incident, radiographic studies of the spine, and an assessment of sensory and motor function. Frequently, diagnostic testing of the SCI patient is completed in the emergency department. In situations in which SCI is suspected later in the hospitalization, diagnostic testing may be initiated in the high-acuity setting. Therefore, the nurse should be aware of the types of tests ordered and the information they provide in order to prepare the patient and family. Spinal cord injury is frequently associated with traumatic brain injury. Therefore, the health care professional assumes that an unconscious patient has an SCI until it is ruled out. SCI should also be suspected in a patient with maxillofacial injury and clavicle or upper rib fractures.

Patients with acute cervical SCI are admitted to an ICU for close monitoring of cardiac, respiratory, and hemodynamic function (Hadley, Walters & Grabb, 2002; Blissitt, 2009; Royster, 2004).

Radiographs

Radiographic assessment documents the level of injury and provides information regarding the stability of the cord injury. As soon as the patient is stabilized (airway, breathing, and circulation), X-rays of the spine are obtained. Not everyone with a potential neck injury needs an X-ray, only those who have changes in level of consciousness as a result of injury, alcohol, or drugs who cannot complain of neck tenderness or those who complain of neck tenderness and have some obvious symptoms (American Association of Neurological Surgeons, 2002; Royster, 2004). Anterior and posterior views of the spine may be ordered. An X-ray that is taken with the patient's mouth open is needed to visualize C1-2 and the odontoid process. Another specialized view or position, called the swimmer's position, is needed to visualize C7 to T1. To obtain this view, the physician or specially trained nurse pulls the patient's shoulders downward toward the foot of the bed (Hickey, 2003; Royster, 2004).

Computed Tomography Scan

A computed tomography (CT) scan may be ordered after completion of X-rays if the spine is not well visualized or there are suspicious findings. A CT scan provides superior visualization of bony structures of the spine and identifies spinal fractures. The CT scan is more accurate for detecting posterior and central column injuries as well as cord impingement. If radiopaque contrast is used, the nurse must question the patient about dye and seafood allergies and any underlying kidney disease.

Magnetic Resonance Imaging

Magnetic resonance imaging (MRI) identifies injuries to the spinal cord, ligaments, and disks. It is also used to detect tumors, inflammation, infection, degenerative disorders, and vascular disruptions in the spinal cord and brain. Noninvasive fields and radiofrequency waves are used to align protons (hydrogen atoms) in tissue. The computer reconstructs signals from the resonance or vibration of protons into video images based on signal intensity in order to diagnose specific lesions or abnormalities. MRI has greater sensitivity than CT for contusions, hematomas, and edema (Richardson, 2009).

Angiography

Because of the proximity of the cervical spine and vertebral arteries, routine screening should be used in patients with complex cervical spine fractures involving subluxation, extension into the foramen transversarium, or upper C1 to C3 fractures (Cothren, Moore, E., Biffl, W., Ciesla, D., et al., 2003). Angiography remains the standard test. An alternative noninvasive diagnostic test for vertebral artery injury is magnetic resonance angiography (Ren, Wang & Zhang, 2006). As with the MRI, magnetic resonance angiography (MRA) is a noninvasive test using magnetic fields sensitive to proton movement. For MRA, the focus is on proton oscillations within the bloodstream that are magnetically manipulated for signal alteration and creation of desired video images. A limitation of MRA is that it may not differentiate spasm or small disruption of the intima from other conditions.

Somatosensory-Evoked Potentials

Somatosensory-evoked potentials (SEPs) are used to establish a functional prognosis after resolution of spinal cord edema. In an extremity below the level of injury, a peripheral nerve is stimulated. The response of the cerebral cortex to this stimulation (evoked potential) is recorded using scalp electrodes. In complete SCI, SEPs are absent because the stimulus is not transmitted to the cortex.

Physical Assessment

Accurate assessment of motor, sensory, and reflex function is important for several reasons: to assist in diagnosis of the lesion, to provide a baseline with which to compare effectiveness of treatment, and to determine realistic functional goals. The American Spinal Injury Association (ASIA) Standard Neurological Classification of SCI assessment form is used to document sensory and motor function (Fig. 23–6). This scale remains the most frequently used tool to evaluate both acute and long-term progress (Barker & Saulino, 2002; Blissitt, 2009). Serial neurologic exams are performed hourly for at least the first 24 hours after SCI (Hedger, 2002; Royster, 2004).

Motor Assessment

Motor strength varies based on preinjury characteristics including gender, fitness level, and age. Voluntary movement requires both upper and lower motor neuron activity. Motor activity is assessed for strength. The examiner begins at the head and moves toward the toes (Blissitt, 2009). Initially, the examiner starts with eliminating gravity (for example, the wrist is propped on a pillow and placed through flexion and extension). Next, movement against gravity is assessed (pillow removed and the arm dangles off the bed during flexion and extension). Finally, the patient's range of movement against resistance (examiner's hand) is noted. Each side is evaluated and compared. Flexion and extension of the joints are assessed (Johnson, Mowery & Bergman, 2008).

Sensory Assessment

The most important data to collect in the sensory examination is the exact point on the patient where normal sensation is present. The sensory assessment begins by moving from the lower to upper body regions because it is easier for the patient to recognize the onset of a sensory stimulus rather than cessation of a stimulus (Blissitt, 2009).

Sensation is tested along dermatomes. A **dermatome** is a section of the body innervated by a particular spinal (or cranial) nerve (Fig. 23–7). A cotton swab is used to assess sensation (spinothalamic tract function). A pin prick is used to assess pain (posterior column function). The patient's eyes are closed. The examination begins distal and moves proximal (that is, up to the neurologically intact area). Position sense (**proprioception**) is tested by moving the big toes and thumbs up and down and asking the patient to confirm the direction. The areas where sensation and pain are present are marked and dated on a dermatome diagram similar to that shown in Figure 23–6. Table 23–2 shows the relationship between nerve root and innervated area.

Reflex Activity

The presence of deep tendon reflexes (Table 23–3) below the level of injury indicates an incomplete lesion. The presence of perineal reflexes indicates that bowel and bladder training may be feasible. **Priapism** (persistent penile erection) may be present in males. The anal wink reflex is initiated by a pin prick in the perianal area. A visual external anal sphincter contraction will occur if the reflex is present. The bulbocavernosus reflex is initiated by placing a gloved finger in the patient's rectum and tugging on the penis or the clitoris. The rectal sphincter will contract if the reflex is present. The presence of the anal wink and bulbocavernosus reflexes indicate that the injury is an upper motor neuron injury.

Assessing for Shock States

The autonomic nervous system functions to maintain homeostasis within the body. With trauma to the spinal cord autonomic dysfunction develops. The degree of dysfunction varies by level and severity of injury. Autonomic dysfunction is more extensive when the level of injury is higher. Following severe cord trauma, two major types of shock commonly develop, spinal shock and neurogenic shock. It is important for the nurse to be able to rapidly recognize and differentiate these two potentially life threatening problems.

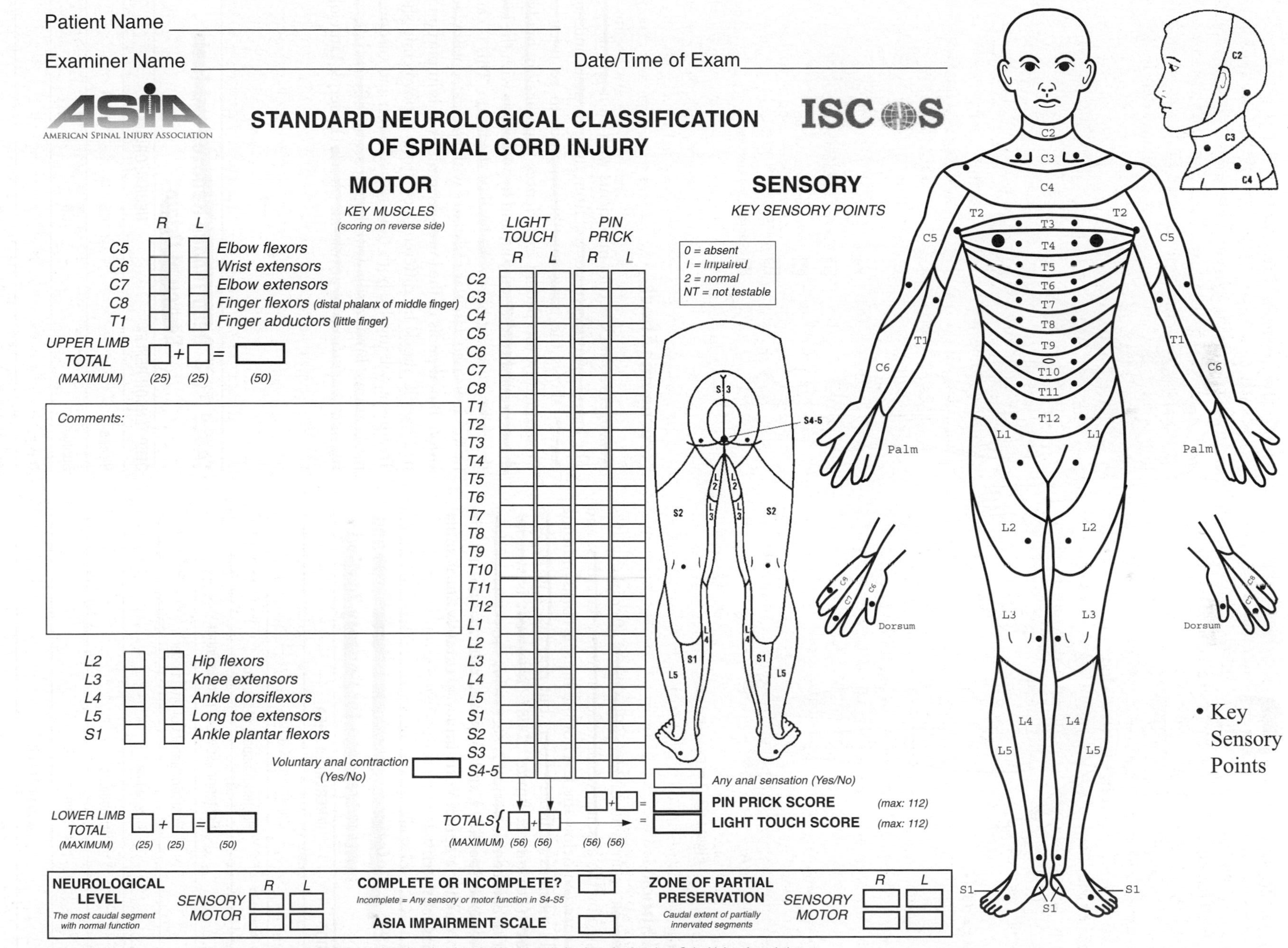

Patient Name ______________________

Examiner Name ______________________ Date/Time of Exam ______________________

ASIA
AMERICAN SPINAL INJURY ASSOCIATION

STANDARD NEUROLOGICAL CLASSIFICATION OF SPINAL CORD INJURY

ISCoS

MOTOR

KEY MUSCLES
(scoring on reverse side)

	R	L	
C5			Elbow flexors
C6			Wrist extensors
C7			Elbow extensors
C8			Finger flexors (distal phalanx of middle finger)
T1			Finger abductors (little finger)

UPPER LIMB TOTAL ☐ + ☐ = ☐
(MAXIMUM) (25) (25) (50)

Comments:

	R	L	
L2			Hip flexors
L3			Knee extensors
L4			Ankle dorsiflexors
L5			Long toe extensors
S1			Ankle plantar flexors

Voluntary anal contraction (Yes/No) ☐

LOWER LIMB TOTAL ☐ + ☐ = ☐
(MAXIMUM) (25) (25) (50)

SENSORY

KEY SENSORY POINTS

	LIGHT TOUCH R	LIGHT TOUCH L	PIN PRICK R	PIN PRICK L
C2				
C3				
C4				
C5				
C6				
C7				
C8				
T1				
T2				
T3				
T4				
T5				
T6				
T7				
T8				
T9				
T10				
T11				
T12				
L1				
L2				
L3				
L4				
L5				
S1				
S2				
S3				
S4-5				

TOTALS ☐ + ☐ ☐ + ☐
(MAXIMUM) (56) (56) (56) (56)

0 = absent
1 = impaired
2 = normal
NT = not testable

☐ Any anal sensation (Yes/No)

☐ **PIN PRICK SCORE** (max: 112)

☐ **LIGHT TOUCH SCORE** (max: 112)

NEUROLOGICAL LEVEL
The most caudal segment with normal function

	R	L
SENSORY		
MOTOR		

COMPLETE OR INCOMPLETE? ☐
Incomplete = Any sensory or motor function in S4-S5

ASIA IMPAIRMENT SCALE ☐

ZONE OF PARTIAL PRESERVATION
Caudal extent of partially innervated segments

	R	L
SENSORY		
MOTOR		

This form may be copied freely but should not be altered without permission from the American Spinal Injury Association.

Figure 23–6 ■ Standard neurological classification of spinal cord injury (2006 Revision). With permission from American Spinal Injury Association (2006). (ASIA)

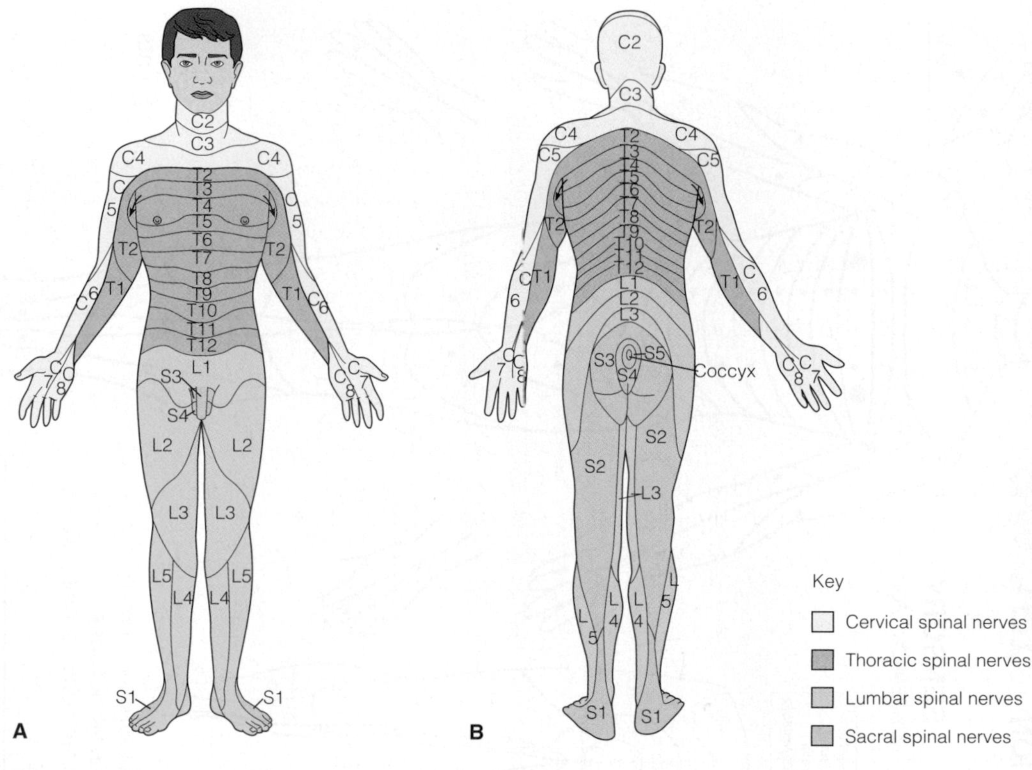

Figure 23–7 ■ Dermatomes.

Spinal Shock

Spinal shock occurs within 30 to 60 minutes after injury. It is manifested by the absence of all reflex activity, flaccidity, and loss of sensation below the level of the injury. This syndrome generally subsides within 24 hours but may last 7 to 20 days postinjury (LeMone & Burke, 2008). Treatment is symptomatic. The end of this period is seen with the return of deep tendon reflexes, spasticity, and increased muscle tone. It is difficult to classify a spinal cord injury accurately until spinal shock has resolved.

TABLE 23–2 Relationship between Nerve Root and Innervated Area for Sensory Testing

NERVE ROOT	INNERVATED AREA
	Upper lateral arm
C6	Posterior aspect of thumb
C7	Posterior aspect of middle finger
C8	Posterior aspect of little finger
T4	Nipple line
T10	Umbilicus
L1	Groin
L2	Anterior thigh
S1	Sole of the foot
S3, S4, S5	Perianal

Neurogenic Shock

Neurogenic shock occurs in patients with an injury above T6. The loss of sympathetic control from the brainstem and higher centers allows the parasympathetic output to go unchecked. Consequently, the patient experiences hypotension, bradycardia, decreased cardiac output, and hypothermia with the loss of the ability to sweat below the level of the lesion. This is caused by the decreased vascular resistance with associated vascular dilation. Blood pools in the lower extremities. It is important that neurogenic shock be differentiated from hypovolemic shock. Treatment will involve both fluid resuscitation and vasopressor medications. Bradycardia with hypotension differentiates neurogenic shock from hypovolemic shock (Bader & Littlejohns, 2004).

TABLE 23–3 Deep Tendon Reflexes and Their Source of Origin

DEEP TENDON REFLEX	NEURAL ORIGIN
Biceps	C5
Supinator	C6
Triceps	C7
Knee (patellar)	L3
Ankle (Achilles)	S1

SECTION THREE REVIEW

1. MF has been admitted with a diagnosis of a possible C7 compression injury. A CT scan with contrast of the cervical spine is ordered for MF The nurse should
   A. remove all metal objects
   B. supply in-line mobilization of the neck
   C. ask if MF is allergic to seafood or radiopaque dye
   D. prep MF's neck with povidone–iodine solution
2. Two days later a SEP test is used to help establish a functional prognosis. M.F. did not have any SEPs during the test. This means
   A. the SCI is complete
   B. the SCI is unstable
   C. an upper motor neuron lesion is present
   D. a lower motor neuron injury is present
3. Which of the following scales is the most frequently used tool to evaluate acute and long-term progress after SCI?
   A. Glasgow Coma Scale
   B. NIH scale
   C. ASIA Standard Neurological Classification
   D. CT scan
4. The exact point on the patient where normal sensation is present is assessed with
   A. dermatomes testing
   B. MRI
   C. proprioception
   D. SEPs
5. Hypotension, bradycardia, and flaccid paralysis are signs of
   A. priapism
   B. autonomic dysreflexia
   C. neurogenic shock
   D. spinal shock

Answers: 1. C, 2. A, 3. C, 4. A, 5. D

SECTION FOUR: Stabilization and Management of Spinal Cord Injury in the Acute Care Phase

At the completion of this section, the learner will be able to discuss stabilization techniques used for spinal cord injuries.

Stabilization of the Spinal Cord

Timely spinal cord alignment and stabilization maximize cord recovery, minimize additional damage, and prevent late deformity. The spinal cord is stabilized using surgical or manual techniques. Stabilization in the high-acuity unit includes bedrest with log rolling maneuvers, and a hard cervical collar until the spine has been stabilized with surgery or traction.

Surgical Stabilization

There is great controversy concerning the need for surgical stabilization of SCI. There are currently no standards regarding timing of decompression in acute SCI. But there is emerging evidence that surgery within 24 hours of the injury may reduce length of intensive care unit stay, and reduce postinjury medical complications (Fehlings & Perrin, 2006).

A recent large multicenter study presented at the American Association of Neurological Surgeons showed early decompression surgery significantly improves outcomes and reduces complication rates. One year, results from the Surgical Treatment of Acute Spinal Cord Injury Study (STASCIS) showed 24 percent of patients who received decompressive surgery within 24 hours of their injury experienced a 2-grade or greater improvement on the ASIA Impairment Scale, compared with 4 percent of those in the delayed-treatment group (Cassels, 2008).

Spinal segments are fused during surgery and spinal canal decompression is accomplished. Rods are inserted to stabilize thoracic spinal injuries. External traction may be required postoperatively. Special braces, such as the Jewett orthosis, may be used postoperatively to maintain hyperextension when the patient is not supine. Surgery is reserved for patients not sufficiently aligned with manual stabilization.

Manual Stabilization

The spinal cord may be immobilized through the use of manual fixation devices including tongs, halos, and braces.

Skull Tongs

Tong devices, such as Gardner-Wells or Vinke cervical tongs, may be used initially to reduce a fracture (Fig. 23–8). Screws

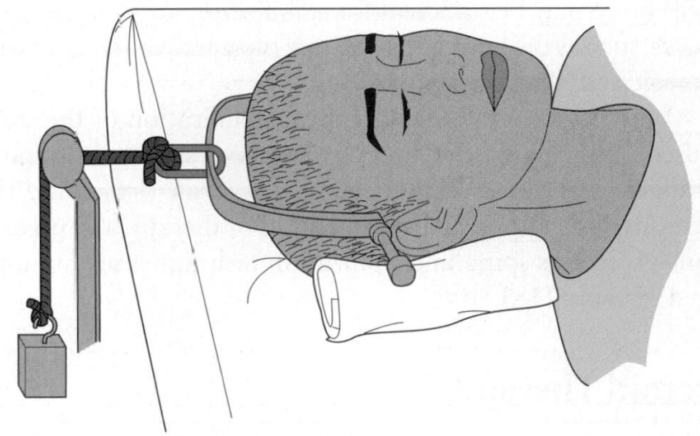

Figure 23–8 ■ Cervical traction may be applied by several methods, including Gardner-Wells tongs.

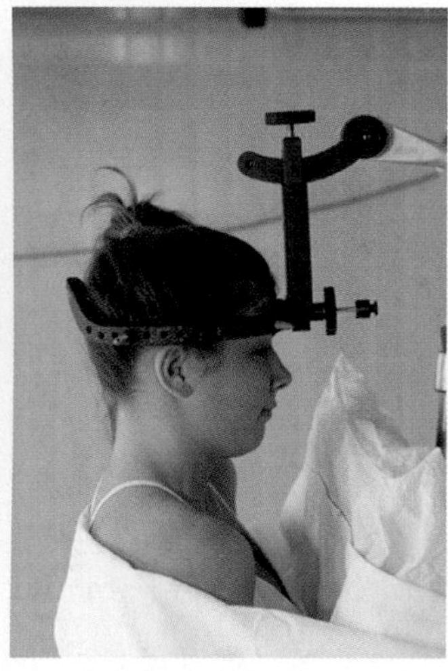

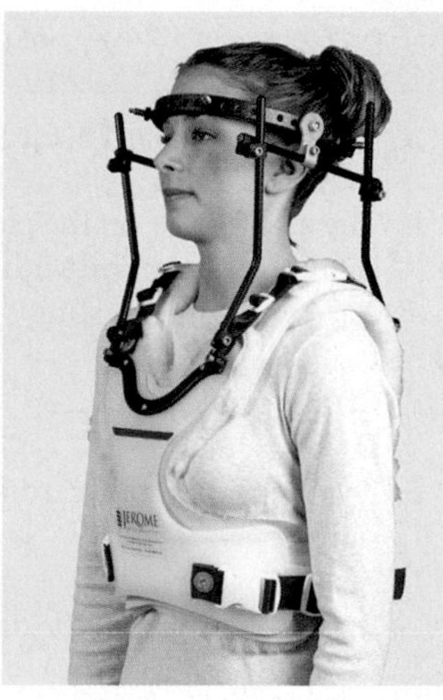

Figure 23–9 ■ Examples of traction or external fixation devices. The image on the right shows a halo device with vest.

are implanted into the patient's skull a few centimeters above the ear using a local anesthetic. The patient feels pressure but usually, not pain. Sequential weights are added to these devices. Ten pounds of traction is applied if an injury but no fracture is present. If a fracture is present, 5 pounds per interspace beginning with C1 to the level of lesion is applied. Muscle relaxants promote the efficacy of the traction.

Halo Device

The halo device is an external fixation device (Fig. 23–9). It keeps the spine aligned and prevents flexion, extension, and rotational movement of the head and neck, and allows for early mobilization. The device is secured with four pins inserted in the skull—two in the frontal lobe and two in the occipital bone. The halo ring is attached to a rigid plastic vest. Patients in these devices require special nursing interventions, which are summarized in Table 23–4.

TABLE 23–4 Caring for the Patient in a Halo Vest

INTERVENTION	RATIONALE
1. Tape a halo vest wrench on the front of the vest.	The fixation device must be taken off to remove the vest to expose the chest in the event CPR is required.
2. Inspect pins and traction bars for loose pins.	It is a nursing responsibility to maintain the integrity of the external system.
3. Do not pull the vest's struts to move or position the patient.	This can disrupt the integrity of the device and potentially damage the cord.
4. Assess motor function and sensation every two to four hours.	Early identification of neurologic deficits can be made.
5. Perform pin care per unit protocol and monitor pin sites for signs of infection.	Organisms can enter through the pin insertion sites.
6. Turn every two hours, inspect skin around vest edges.	Prevent skin breakdown. Prevent stasis complications.
7. Skin care.	Clean skin under vest with a moist cloth. Use a pillow case to pull through vest from top to bottom to remove dead skin and debris and to monitor for any wound drainage.

Braces

A hard cervical collar and a molded plastic body jacket (clam shell) brace may be sufficient for stabilization of some injuries. Braces, such as the Jewett orthosis, are most frequently used with thoracic and lumbar spine injuries.

Whether surgical or mechanical stabilization of the spine is used, the goals are the same: to align and stabilize the spine, minimize additional damage, and prevent late deformity. The methods, indications, goals and lengths of therapy, and precautions of various spine immobilization techniques are summarized in Table 23–5.

Steroid Therapy

Methylprednisolone, administered post-SCI, may decrease free fatty acid production, inhibit phospholipid breakdown, and reduce infiltration of leukocytes (Hickey, 2003 Johnson, Mowery, and Bergman, 2008). By these actions, secondary injury to the spinal cord is prevented because blood flow to the cord is improved and mediators of the inflammatory process are not released. Studies have shown that patients who receive methylprednisolone after SCI have a reduction in secondary injury to the spinal cord and that methylprednisolone has a profound effect on functional level (Tierney, McPhee & Papadakis, 2005). National Acute Spinal Cord Injury studies suggest that secondary injury may be diminished if methylprednisolone is initiated within eight hours of injury with an initial bolus of 30 mg/kg, followed by a continuous infusion of 5.4 mg/kg/hr over 24 to 48 hours (Bracken, 2002).

Currently, considerable controversy exists on the use of methylprednisolone for the management of spinal cord injury in the acute care phase. The use of this therapy must be weighed against its potential adverse reactions including gastric ulceration, electrolyte imbalances, and delayed wound healing (American Association of Neurological Surgeons, 2002: Johnson, Mowrey, and Bergman, 2008). Both the neurosurgical guidelines and the Consortium of Spinal Cord Medicine clinical practice guidelines consider the use of high-dose methylprednisolone to be a treatment option, rather than a standard (Wuermser, Ho & Chiodo, 2007).

TABLE 23–5 Methods, Indications, Goals and Lengths of Therapy, and Precautions of Various Spine Immobilization Techniques

METHODS	INDICATIONS	GOAL OF THERAPY	LENGTH OF THERAPY	PRECAUTIONS
Cervical spine (c-spine)				
Hard cervical collar (short term)—Philadelphia collar and Stiff-neck collar	Prehospital immobilization Uncleared c-spine	Preevaluation, presumptive	Less than 48 hours	Ensure good collar fit Skin care Decubitus ulcers
Hard cervical collar (long term)—Miami-J collar and Aspen collar	Stable c-spine fracture Ligamentous injury	Hasten healing, diminish pain	8–12 weeks	Ensure good collar fit Worn continuously—provide second collar for washing Meticulous skin care
Soft cervical collar	Cervical strain, whiplash	Symptom management	Varies, depending on symptom severity	Limit use to avoid dependence (e.g., nighttime, riding in car only)
Cervical traction				
Gardner-Wells tongs	Unstable malaligned c-spine fracture, dislocation, or ligamentous injury	Cervical reduction Bridge to operative therapy	Varies	Pin site care and assessment Reposition patient every two hours
Halo vest	Unstable c-spine fracture, dislocation, or ligamentous injury	Definitive cervical immobilization	8–12 weeks	Pin site assessment and care Decubitus ulcers beneath vest
Four poster or Yale brace	Stable c-spine injuries or adjunct to surgery for unstable c-spine injuries	Hasten healing, diminish pain	8–12 weeks	
Thoracic or lumbar spine				
Hyperextension cast and thoraco–lumbar support orthotic (clam shell or tortoise shell brace)	Stable thoracic or lumbar spine column fractures; anterior compression fracture with <40% loss of height; burst fractures with no neurologic deficit, <50% vertebral body involvement, <30% canal compromise, angulation <20 degree	Hasten healing, diminish pain After spinal decompressive and stabilization surgery for support and comfort	8–12 weeks	Requires custom fit Meticulous skin care
Elastic thoraco–lumbar supports	Minor compression fractures or transverse process fractures Lumbar strain	Symptom management	Varies, depending on symptom severity	

From Logan © 1999, *Principles of Practice for the Acute Care Nurse Practitioner.* Upper Saddle River, NJ: Prentice Hall Inc. Reprinted by permission of Prentice Hall Inc.

SECTION FOUR REVIEW

1. BR is admitted to the unit with an unstable T2 SCI. The physician will place cervical traction in six hours. What is a priority nursing intervention?
   A. Administer pain medications as ordered.
   B. Place a hard cervical collar and perform log rolling maneuvers.
   C. Shave and prep BR's head.
   D. Place a wrench at BR's bedside.
2. The best advantage to surgical stabilization is that it
   A. decreases complications attributed to immobility
   B. secures the spine better than cervical tongs
   C. is cheaper
   D. is available to all patients with SCI
3. Which of the following is a priority nursing intervention for the patient with a halo vest?
   A. Place an appropriate wrench on or near the patient.
   B. Maintain the hard neck collar.
   C. Log roll the patient.
   D. Add sequential weights.
4. Which of the following statements is TRUE about the use of methylprednisolone for SCI?
   A. It must be given to all patients within six hours of injury.
   B. It is now considered to be contraindicated in all patients with SCI.
   C. It is considered to be a treatment option.
   D. High doses are better than low doses.

Answers: 1. B, 2. A, 3. A, 4. C

SECTION FIVE: High-Acuity Nursing Care of the Patient with a Spinal Cord Injury

At the completion of this section, the learner will be able to identify priority nursing assessments and interventions for the patient with a spinal cord injury in the acute care phase of recovery.

Impaired Gas Exchange, Ineffective Breathing Patterns

As with any high-acuity patient, the nurse begins the patient assessment using the ABCs. The patient's airway and breathing may be compromised, particularly with a cervical cord injury. Patients with C1-C2 injuries will require mechanical ventilation because of loss of phrenic nerve innervation to the diaphragm. Those with injuries to C3-C5 will have varying degrees of diaphragm paralysis and need some ventilatory support. They may be able to be weaned from mechanical ventilation. Injuries below C6 have varying degrees of impaired intercostal and abdominal muscle function. Patients with these injuries experience compromise in respiratory protective reflexes, including coughing and sneezing.

Patients with SCI, especially cervical injuries, have a high incidence of pulmonary complications, including pneumonia, atelectasis, and respiratory failure; and respiratory failure is the leading cause of death in patients with SCI (Lanig & Peterson, 2000; LeMone & Burke, 2008). According to Cook (2003), the goals of respiratory management in the patient with SCI are to (1) prevent secondary neural damage, (2) prevent hypoxemia, (3) prevent and treat atelectasis, (4) maximize alveolar ventilation, and (5) maximize pulmonary hygiene for impaired cough and secretion clearance. Patients with SCI require close monitoring of respiratory drive, ventilation, ability to cough, pulse oximetry, and arterial blood gases (Johnson, Mowrey & Bergman, 2008).

The respiratory management goals are achieved through aggressive respiratory therapy, and careful monitoring to identify and promptly treat actual and potential respiratory problems. Humidified oxygen is administered via nasal cannula or face mask. The patient is taught to use an incentive spirometer and assisted with "quad" coughing. Quad coughing is the use of pillows to push against the abdomen to increase intra-abdominal pressure to cough. When assisted coughing is used, bronchodilators and mucolytics are beneficial in mobilizing secretions to gain maximal benefit from the cough (Lanig & Peterson, 2000; LeMone & Burke 2008; Johnson, Mowrey & Bergman, 2008).

Recommendations from the Consortium for Spinal Cord Medicine Respiratory Management (2005) include obtaining initial laboratory assessments (ABGs, CBC, coagulation profile, comprehensive metabolic profile, cardiac enzyme profile, urinalysis, and toxicology screen). Respiratory function testing should be carried out on a periodic basis to monitor lung compliance, volumes, respiratory muscle strength, and need for mechanical ventilation. Respiratory care should include aggressive interventions to prevent and treat atelectasis, pneumonia, and aspiration.

Chest physiotherapy may be performed depending on the patient's ability to tolerate this procedure and the level and extent of injury. The decision to suction the patient should be based on assessment findings because this procedure may stimulate the vasovagal response and lead to bradycardia. Mobilization of secretions is best obtained with frequent turning and position changes. However, this may not be possible because of the patient's injury and the use of traction devices. The nurse should collaborate with the health care team to determine if the use of a specialized bed is warranted for the patient with a spinal cord injury.

Decreased Cardiac Output

The patient with SCI is at high risk for developing decreased cardiac output related to orthostatic hypotension, spinal and neurogenic shock, venous pooling, emboli, and bradycardia. In the acute care phase, invasive and noninvasive monitoring may be used to closely monitor cardiac output. Cardiac monitoring allows for early detection of bradycardia which is a constant threat because of unopposed vagal stimulation of the heart. Patients with a SCI are at risk for developing bradycardia and even asystole during endotracheal tube manipulation, suctioning, or insertion of a nasogastric tube (Blissitt, 2009). Atropine should be at the bedside at all times (Hedger, 2002). All sensitive patients should be premedicated with atropine before high-risk procedures (Karlet, 2001).

Techniques to monitor cardiac preload may be required. Judicious use of IV fluids is required when treating hypotension because too much fluid can precipitate pulmonary edema. Inotropic and/or vasopressor support may be required to maintain adequate cardiac output and tissue perfusion. In patients with SCI, it may be difficult to keep the systolic blood pressure over 90 mm Hg. Therefore, the aim of therapy is to maintain adequate tissue perfusion, not an absolute blood pressure (Gunnarsson & Fehlings, 2003; Karlet, 2001). However, a systolic blood pressure less than 90 mm Hg is detrimental because it causes hypoperfusion to the cord and, therefore, current guidelines recommend that MAP should be maintained 85 to 90 mm Hg for the first seven days post-SCI (American Association of Neurological Surgeons, 2002).

Altered Urinary Elimination and Constipation

The degree of bladder dysfunction depends on the location and completeness of the SCI. Spinal cord injury removes the ability of the pontine micturition center and higher centers in the brain to inhibit, control, or coordinate the activity (Siroky, 2002). Patients with complete quadriplegia are typically unaware of bladder activity except through ancillary clues (sweating, chills). For the first few days post-SCI, an indwelling urinary catheter is used. After this initial phase, the catheter is removed and an intermittent catheterization schedule may be used. Overdistension of the bladder must be prevented. After the acute care phase, the patient is taught self-catheterization. Constipation and fecal impaction are major problems (Johnson, Mowrey, and Bergman, 2008).

Cervical or high thoracic injuries cause reflex bowel—the patient does not feel the urge to defecate, but the anal–rectal reflex remains intact (Gibson, 2003). A bowel care program is employed including laxatives and stool softeners and appropriate fluid and fiber intake. A bowel training program to regulate fecal elimination is instituted using chemical and mechanical stimulation. A suppository is used for chemical stimulation. Mechanical methods in bowel care are digital stimulation and manual evacuation (for lower motor neuron injuries). Digital stimulation is a technique that increases peristalsis and relaxes the external anal sphincter. It is performed by gently inserting a gloved, lubricated finger into the rectum and slowly rotating the finger in a circular motion. Rotation is continued until relaxation of the bowel wall is felt, flatus passes, stool passes, or internal sphincter contracts. Digital stimulation is repeated every five to ten minutes until stool evacuation is complete (Consortium for Spinal Cord Medicine, 1998). This intervention should be scheduled on a regular basis in patients with lower motor neuron injuries (Johnson, Mowrey, and Bergman, 2008).

Ineffective Thermoregulation

Interruption in communication between the spinal cord and the hypothalamus results in loss of temperature control (**poikilothermia**). This condition is dangerous because the patient's body temperature depends on the temperature of the environment. Hyperthermia then becomes a problem because loss of sympathetic control of the sweat glands below the level of the lesion prohibits sweating as temperature rises. The patient may need to be kept warm with passive warming devices. However, when these devices are used, the patient is monitored carefully to avoid thermal injury to insensitive skin (Blissitt, 2009; Karlet, 2001).

Imbalanced Nutrition

In the initial phase of recovery, paralytic ileus is common. A nasogastric tube prevents gastric distention. A nutrition consult is initiated as soon as possible to help ensure the patient's nutritional needs are met. In the acute care phase, patients with SCI are hypermetabolic (American Association of Neurological Surgeons, 2002; Johnson, Mowrey, and Bergman, 2008). They are at risk for receiving less nutrition than their bodies' requirements because of interruption of bowel innervation, limited ability to feed self, anorexia from lack of taste sensation, and depression. The type of diet patients receive depends on their level of consciousness and the severity of associated injuries. Nursing care includes monitoring intake, changes in the patient's weight, assessing electrolyte balance, and administering total parenteral nutrition or enteral feedings as ordered. In some cases, dysphagia is problematic. Thickening food to allow formation of a food bolus is helpful.

Self-Care Deficits

Baseline and ongoing motor, sensory, and reflex assessment provide information about the patient's neurological progress. Rehabilitative goals are set and independence (to the degree possible) of the patient encouraged early. Bowel and bladder routines are initiated and ambulation supported as necessary. Table 23–6 outlines functional goals appropriate for the patient, based on level of SCI.

Preventing Complications

Complications associated with SCI (Fig. 23–10) can be classified into three broad categories related to changes in mobility, perfusion, and reflex activity.

Complications Related to a Change in Mobility

Skin Integrity. Several factors contribute to skin breakdown in the patient with a SCI. Sensory and motor impairment results in areas of the skin being subjected to prolonged periods of pressure. The patient is unable to feel the discomfort or pain from pressure and is unable to change position independently. In addition to the usual areas of pressure development (sacrum, heels) the patient's ears, ankles, and occipital area of the head need to be assessed for early indications of the development of pressure ulcers. Moisture exposure from bladder or bowel incontinence, or sweating, also contributes to pressure ulcer formation. Frequent positioning, specialized beds, and foot and heel protectors help minimize this risk. Routine daily to twice daily inspection of all skin is important to identify areas at risk of breakdown.

Decreased Joint Mobility. This complication is preventable. The tendency to remain in one position for extended periods is greater when one is dependent on someone else to initiate movement. Spasticity may contribute to this problem by exaggerating responses to movement. Spasms can be used positively to enable use of some assistive devices. Deformity and contracture develop if joint mobility is not maintained through range of motion.

Thromboembolism. Venous thromboembolic disease (deep vein thrombosis [DVT] and pulmonary embolism [PE]) is a leading cause of mortality and morbidity following acute SCI. The major factors predisposing persons with acute SCI to venous thromboembolism include venostasis due to failure of the venous muscle pump with paralysis and a transient hypercoagulable state. Alterations in hemostasis seen after acute

TABLE 23–6 Functional Status Based on Level of SCI

LEVEL	EATING	DRESSING	BATHING	BOWEL/BLADDER	MOBILITY
C1–C4	Dependent	Dependent	Dependent	Dependent	Electric wheelchair with breath, head, or shoulder controls; requires ventilatory support (partial or full)
C5	Independent with aids	Major assistance with aids	Wheelchair shower with major assistance	Major assistance with aids	Electric wheelchair with adapted hand controls
C6	Independent with aids	Minor assistance with aids	Independent in wheelchair shower	Independent with aids	Independent in manual wheelchair with hand controls; can use some manual wheelchair types
C7	Independent	Independent with aids	Independent wheelchair shower or tub with bath board	Independent with aids	Independent in manual wheelchair with hand controls
C8–T1	Independent	Independent	Independent in tub with bath boards	Independent with aids	Independent in manual wheelchair
T2–T12	Independent	Independent	Independent	Independent with aids	Independent in manual wheelchair
L1–L5	Independent	Independent	Independent	Independent	Optional use of knee, ankle, or foot orthoses
S1–S5	Independent	Independent	Independent	Independent	Independent with or without ankle or foot orthoses

SCI include reduced fibrinolytic activity and increased blood factor VIII activity despite normal values on routine coagulation measures (Consortium for Spinal Cord Medicine, 1999; Blissitt, 2009; Geerts, 2004).

The Consortium for Spinal Cord Medicine has the following recommendations in their Prevention of Thromboembolism Clinical Practice Guidelines (1999). Whenever possible, compression hose or pneumatic devices should be applied to the legs of all patients for the first two weeks following injury. During every nursing shift, compression devices should be inspected for proper placement and underlying skin conditions. Anticoagulant prophylaxis should be initiated within 72 hours after SCI, provided there is no active bleeding or coagulopathy. Anticoagulants should be continued for 12 weeks or until discharge from rehabilitation for those with complete motor injury and other risk factors, and for eight weeks in patients with uncomplicated complete motor injuries. Vena cava filter placement is indicated in SCI patients who have failed anticoagulant prophylaxis or who have a contraindication to anticoagulation. Nursing staff should be aware of the signs and symptoms of DVT and should perform physical assessment to detect this complication. The American Association of Neurological Surgeons (2002) also recommends low molecular weight heparin or adjusted dose heparin, and pneumatic compression stockings.

Heterotopic Ossification. Ectopic bone formation (overgrowth of bone) occurs below the level of the SCI, further restricting joint mobility. The cause of this phenomenon is unknown. Patients can develop the same symptoms as DVT.

Complications Related to Abnormal Perfusion

Autonomic Dysreflexia. **Autonomic dysreflexia,** a potentially life-threatening complication, occurs when a stimulus triggers excessive sympathetic nervous system activation below the level of the SCI. Systemic vasoconstriction results, producing sweating, anxiety, headache, blurred vision, and hypertension. The most serious danger of autonomic dysreflexia is severe hypertension (systolic blood pressure greater than 200 mm Hg), which can trigger cerebral hemorrhage and stroke, myocardial infarction, or seizures. The parasympathetic nervous system compensates for this reaction by producing massive vasodilation above the level of the lesion and bradycardia (heart rate less than 40 beats per minute). However, this compensation is inadequate because it affects only the neurologically intact section of the body, whereas the sympathetic reaction affects the total body. This phenomenon occurs after spinal shock has resolved, usually within the first six months of injury. However, autonomic dysreflexia remains a potential problem throughout the patient's life. Therefore, both family and patient are taught how to recognize and treat the condition. It is more prevalent in lesions at and above T6. Numerous factors produce autonomic dysreflexia; the most frequent factors are summarized in Table 23–7. While the search for the stimulus that triggered the sympathetic response is conducted, antihypertensive agents are administered. Bladder distention and or spasm are the most frequent cause of autonomic dysreflexia. Medications to manage hypertension associated with-autonomic dysreflexia include nifedipine (Procardia), nitroglycerine (Nitrostat sublingual tablets or Nitrol topical ointment). Refer to the box RELATED PHARMACOTHERAPY: Agents Used for Treating Traumatic Spinal Cord Injury.

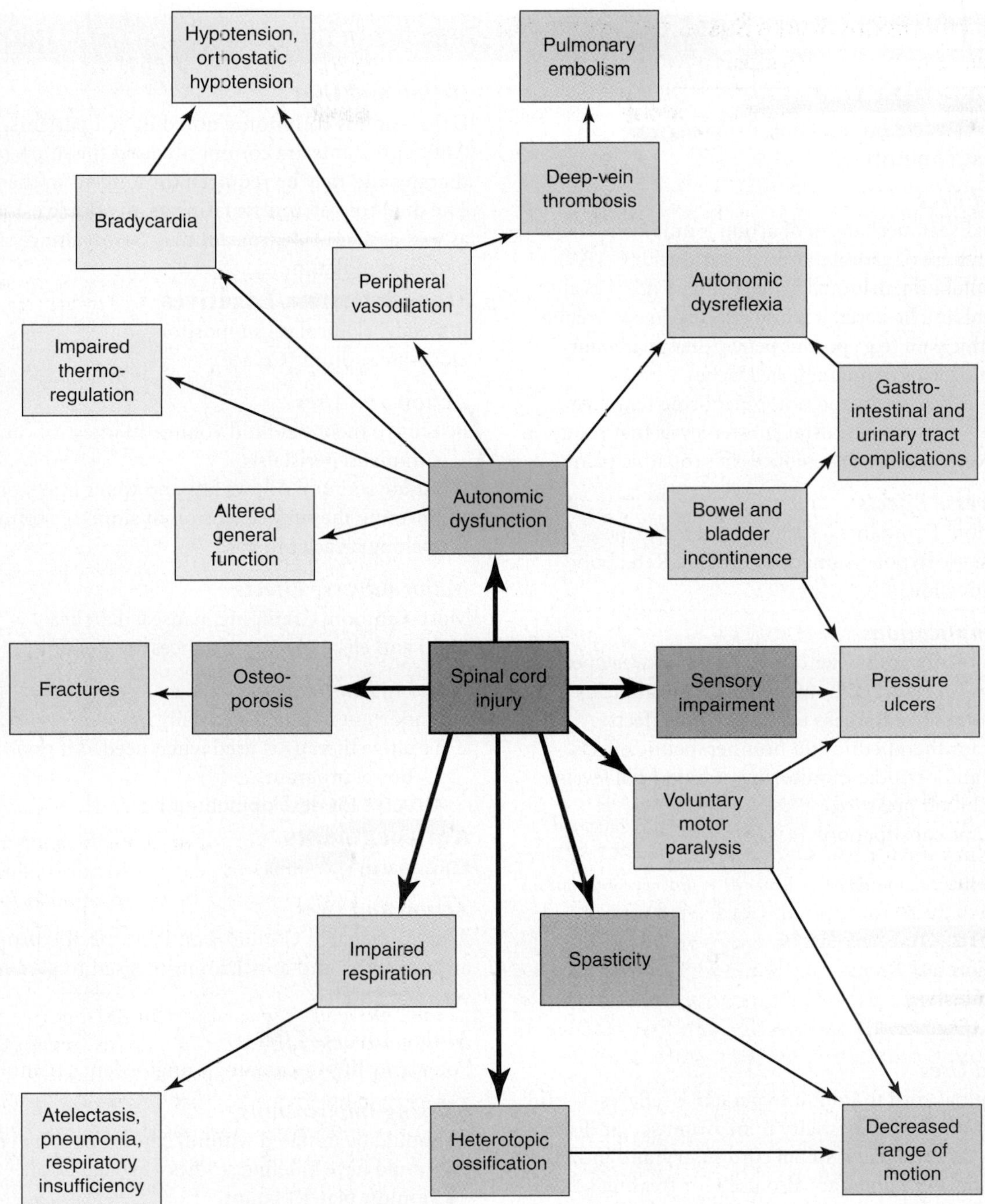

Figure 23–10 ■ Schematic representation of the physical effects of spinal cord injury. From Somers, Martha Freeman, *Spinal Cord Injury: Functional Rehabilitation*, 1st, © 1992. Electronically reproduced by permission of Pearson Education, Inc., Upper Saddle River, New Jersey.

TABLE 23–7 Factors That Produce Autonomic Dysreflexia

- Bladder distention/spasm
- Bowel impaction
- Stimulation of anal reflex
- Labor
- Temperature change
- Ingrown toenails
- Tight, irritating clothes
- Urinary tract infection
- Decubitus ulcer
- Pain

Orthostatic Hypotension. Chronic peripheral vasodilation causes orthostatic hypotension, particularly for patients with injuries at T6 or above (Gibson, 2003). This factor in combination with a quick position change results in a loss of consciousness. Therefore, initial attempts to mobilize the patient are done slowly. Gradually raise the head of bed, and assess patient tolerance to these position changes. Feet are dangled on the side of the bed prior to movement out of bed to a chair, abdominal binder and compression hose are applied. Medications to reduce orthostatic hypotension include ephedrine and midodrine.

RELATED PHARMACOTHERAPY: Agents Used for Treating Acute Traumatic Spinal Cord Injury

Neuropathic Pain Analgesics*
Gabapentin (Neurontin) and pregabalin (Lyrica)
Amitriptyline (Amitril)

Action and Uses

Gabapentin: Exact mechanism of action is unknown. It may increase release of gamma-aminobutyric acid (GABA) thereby inhibiting neuronal firing. Primary use is as an anticonvulsant; however, it is also effective in controlling neuropathic pain (e.g., postherpetic pain, spinal injury pain, some forms of migraine headache),

Amitriptyline: Serotonin and norepinephrine reuptake inhibitor – restores neurotransmitter levels that results in antidepressant effect; also reduces neuropathic pain

Major Adverse Effects

Most common: Drowsiness, fatigue; Other: dizziness, sedation, orthostatic hypotension, constipation. Rare: bone marrow depression

Nursing Implications

Do not stop abruptly – withdraw over one-week period.
Space dose at least two hours when taking antacids.
May require several weeks to achieve full effects.
Monitor for therapeutic and nontherapeutic effects.
Baseline and periodic monitoring of blood cell levels.
Monitor blood pressure.
Monitor for constipation.

*Opioid analgesia (e.g., morphine or fentanyl) is ordered for nonneuropathic pain.

Skeletal Muscle Relaxants
Baclofen (Lioresal)
Diazepam (Valium)
Dantrolene (Dantrium)

Action and Uses

Act in the spinal cord to inhibit hyperactive reflexes. Useful in treatment of muscle spasticity in neuromuscular disorders such as cerebral palsy, spinal cord injury, and multiple sclerosis. Benzodiazepines are also used for treating anxiety and sleep problems in spinal cord injured patients.

Major Adverse Effects

Most common: Drowsiness

Nursing Implications

Cautious use in presence of hepatic or renal dysfunction
Interacts with other drugs that depress CNS, including alcohol
Can increase serum glucose, AST, and alkaline phosphatase levels
Should not be stopped suddenly – results in withdrawal symptoms that can be severe

Antidepressants
Amitriptyline (as previously described)
Others

Action and Uses

Depression is commonly noted in SCI patients. Antidepressants are commonly used for short-term therapy and may be required for long-term therapy. The dual role of amitriptyline as an effective analgesic as well as an antidepressant may be advantageous in this patient population.

Stool Softeners/Laxatives
Bisacodyl (Dulcolax) suppository
Docusate sodium (Colace)

Action and Uses

Bisacodyl: Increases fluid volume in intestines and stimulates peristalsis

Docusate sodium: Allows fats and water into stool through lowering the surface tension of stool this softens stool, making it easier to pass

Major Adverse Effects

Most common: Cramping, nausea, diarrhea
Fluid and electrolyte imbalances are possible

Nursing Implications

Important to establish a daily bowel program.
Laxative therapy is used when needed if poor results on bowel program.
Observe for development of ileus.

Anticoagulants
Enoxaparin (Lovenox)

Action and Uses

A LMW heparin Contains antithrombotic properties – antifactor Xa and antithrombin. Used to prevent deep vein thrombosis.

Major Adverse Effects

Potentially life-threatening – angioedema, hemorrhage

Nursing Implications

Should be initiated within 72 hours of spinal cord injury.
Should have baseline studies of coagulation.
Monitor platelet count.
Monitor for bleeding.

Anti-inflammatory
Methylprednisolone (Solu-Medrol)

Action and Uses

A synthetic corticosteroid with strong anti inflammatory action. Used for reducing inflammation and edema in spinal cord injury

Major Adverse Effects

No major common SE for short-term use

Nursing Implications

For acute nonpenetrating SCI within eight hours of trauma but not recommended for SCI over eight hours after injury nor for penetrating SCI

Blood Pressure Agents Antihypotensives
Ephedrine (Efedron)
Midodrine (ProAmatine)
Antihypertensives
Nifedipine (Procardia)
Nitroglycerine

Action and Uses

Antihypotensives: Stimulates the sympathetic nervous system, thereby increasing contractility and cardiac output. Used when nonpharmacologic therapies are not successful in controlling orthostatic hypotension in patients with spinal cord injury.

Antihypertensives: Through various mechanisms cause vasodilation that results in decreased blood pressure. Use in SCI is as a treatment for autonomic dysreflexia to rapidly reduce blood pressure.

Major Adverse Effects

Antihypotensives: Tachycardia, hypertension, tremors, nervousness, and restlessness

Antihypertensives: Dizziness, hypotension, flushing, diarrhea, headache

Nursing Implications

Antihypotensives: Give 45 minutes to one hour before raising head of the bed or assuming a sitting position. Midodrine: Dose may need to be adjusted for renal dysfunction

Antihypertensives: Nifedipine - Capsules must be opened so that liquid contents come into direct contact with oral mucosa for rapid onset of action (one to five minutes) Sublingual – onset is one to three minutes liquid contents come into direct contact with oral mucosa for rapid onset of action (one to five minutes)

Monitor blood pressure and heart rate

Find and relieve cause of dysreflexia episode

Complications Related to Abnormal Reflex Activity

Bladder Dysfunction. In the recent past, renal disease was the leading cause of morbidity and mortality in individuals with SCI (National Spinal Cord Injury Statistical Center, 2007). Recent improvements in treatments for infection, bladder surveillance and management techniques have helped to improve outcomes. Goals of bladder management are bladder drainage, low-pressure urine storage, and voiding without urinary leakage, over-distention or incontinence. A proper bladder management program may prevent urinary tract infection, bladder wall damage, over distention, vesicoureteral reflux, and development of renal stones (Perkash & Giroux, 1993). Incontinence, reflux, development of renal stones, and neuronal obstruction also increase the risk for UTI.

Bladder function is dependent on level of injury. Because of the effects of spinal shock and the usual need for aggressive fluid replacement immediately after SCI, patients with acute SCI are best managed with an indwelling urinary catheter. It is best to facilitate a catheter-free status as soon as reflex activity returns, the patient is medically stable, and urine output averages two liters in 24 hours. At this point, the catheter should be discontinued and a bladder management program initiated (Burns, Rivas, and Ditunno, 2001). Most injuries above the T12 level will result in an upper motor neuron (hyperreflexic or spastic) bladder dysfunction. Intermittent catheterization is the management technique of choice in this type of bladder (Burns et al., 2001; Chua, Tow & Tan, 2006).

Intermittent catheterization when compared to indwelling catheters reduces the risk of infection and is the preferred method of bladder drainage in this patient population, but it too is associated with risks, including urethral trauma, urethral strictures, and hematuria (Siroky, 2002). Hydrophilic-coated catheters have been shown to result in a lower rate of urinary tract infections compared to uncoated catheters (Ridder et al., 2005). The use of condom catheters in male patients is associated with infection rates similar to intermittent catheterization, but this method does not guarantee proper drainage of the bladder and may itself be the source of obstruction (Siroky, 2002). Although changing the catheter daily is standard practice, there is no evidence to support this practice. Chronic use of the same drainage bag predisposes colonization of the drainage bag and retrograde introduction of bacteria into the anterior urethra (Siroky, 2002). UTIs are often preceded by colonization of bowel bacteria on genitalia, perineum, and the urethra; therefore, strategies to prevent UTIs must include good perineal hygiene (Siroky, 2002).

Bladder spasticity may lead to problems such as leaking between catheterizations or leaking around the indwelling catheters. Anticholinergic (antispasticity) agents may be required to prevent leaking (refer to the RELATED PHARMACOTHERAPY box for more information).

Bowel Dysfunction. The bowel is innervated by the sacral segments of the spinal cord. Normal bowel function is preserved in incomplete SCI above the sacral level. In complete SCI, or during spinal shock, the bowel is flaccid or areflexic. With resolution of spinal shock, the bowel in a SCI above the sacrum (an upper motor neuron lesion), will become reflexic. The presence of this reflex activity facilitates bowel evacuation. Bowel training typically begins with bisacodyl (Dulcolax) suppository and/or digital stimulation. If the SCI is a lower motor neuron lesion (below the sacral level), then the bowel will remain areflexic, and retention of stool becomes a problem. In this case stool softeners and suppositories are indicated, although less effective than with SCI above the sacrum. Manual removal of stool may be necessary (Blissitt, 2009). Anticholinergic agents, vitamins, iron supplements, and opioids increase the risk of constipation, ileus, and fecal impaction in the patient with SCI (Gibson, 2003).

Sexual Dysfunction. Although it may not be a priority in the acute care phase post-SCI, the patient or partner may ask questions about sexual function after an injury to the spinal cord. Sexual function is still possible for all patients with SCI. Men may have reflexogenic erections, but very few men are able to ejaculate (Gibson, 2003; Johnson, Mowrey & Bergman, 2008). Fatherhood is a possibility because ejaculation can be stimulated and the sperm used to inseminate the partner. Men should be referred at some point to an urologist for information on new erectile and fertility treatments.

Approximately 50 to 70 percent of women with SCI are able to have an orgasm (Gibson, 2003). Menses may be disrupted for several months postinjury, but after menses return, pregnancy is still possible. The major risk these pregnant women face is autonomic dysreflexia that can occur during labor and delivery (Johnson, Mowrey & Bergman, 2008).

Psychosocial Issues

Spinal cord injury changes the independent individual into a more dependent person. In the initial acute care phases, patients with SCI experience severe dependency, profound distress, and social isolation (Lohne, 2001; Livneh & Martz, 2005). Nursing research has demonstrated these patients often have feelings of despair that may dominate feelings of hope (Lohne & Severinsson, 2004). Therefore, patients tend to focus on the present concrete daily routines to avoid the unpleasant sensations of disappointment and uncertainty about the future (Lohne & Severinsson, 2004). Adaptation depends on personality, coping styles, and life experiences. Self-esteem, body image, and role performance are affected. Emotions may include fear of death, fear of living, anger, denial, and hopelessness. Educational level, employment status, income, and social support systems are factors associated with postinjury quality of life. The nurse encourages verbalization of feelings, and encourages the patient to take an active role in self-care activities and health care decisions. The family is included in these discussions. Referral to a local support group or professional counseling is also helpful (Livneh & Martz, 2005).

Neuropathic Pain

Neuropathic pain (referred to as phantom or central pain) is frequently experienced. This pain is described as a burning, stabbing, shooting, aching, numbness and/or tingling, or electric shock-like pain that occurs at or just above the level of injury or may be experienced at or below the level of injury. Around 40 percent of SCI patients develop persistent neuropathic pain (Baastrup, et al., 2008). Gabapentin (Neurontin) has shown promising results and is considered a first line treatment for neuropathic pain (Levendoglu, Ogun, Ozerbil et al., 2004). Antiepileptics and antidepressants are the most common treatments prescribed for treatment of neuropathic pain. Gabapentin, pregabalin, and amitriptyline can significantly reduce neuropathic pain following SCI (Baastrup et al., 2008). Serotonin noradrenalin reuptake inhibitors as well as steroids may also be used to treat patients with SCI neuropathic also pain (Baastrup et al., 2008).

The box, NURSING CARE: The Patient with Acute Spinal Cord Injury, summarizes nursing care appropriate in the acute care phase for the patient with a spinal cord injury.

Emerging Evidence

- In a small study investigating patterns of residence in adults with tetraplegia, major factors that influenced place of residence included: money, accessibility, insurance, intimate relationships, personal assistants, and information *(Bergmark, Winograd & Koopman, 2008).*
- In a retrospective study involving SCI patient with cervical level injuries, neurological outcomes were better in patients with cord edema when compared to patients with cord hemorrhage or contusion. MRI was found to be invaluable for evaluation of cervical SCI *(Mahmood, Kadavigere, Ramesh, & Rao, 2008).*
- In an analysis of approximately 16,800 patients with SCI who had spinal fracture fixation performed, the best outcomes (fewer complications and requiring fewer resources) were seen in patients who had the fixation procedure within three days of injury *(Kerwin, Tepas, Schinco, Devin et al., 2008).*
- Use of cranberry extract tablets for six months to prevent urinary tract infection (UTI) was found to reduce incidence of UTI for SCI patients who have a neurogenic bladder. The study found that patient with the highest GFR benefited the most from use of cranberry tablets *(Hess, Hess, Sullivan, Nee & Yalla, 2008).*

NURSING CARE: The Patient with Acute Spinal Cord Injury

Expected Patient Outcomes and Related Interventions

Outcome 1: Maintain pulmonary oxygenation and ventilation.

Assess and compare to established norms, patient baselines, and trends.

Monitor for signs of pulmonary dysfunction.
ABGs, breath sounds, respiratory pattern and rate
Temperature, sputum color and consistency, pulmonary function tests, pulse oximetry

Interventions to maintain pulmonary oxygenation and ventilation

Quad assist cough
Suction as needed
Deep breathe, incentive spirometer
Reposition every two hours
Elevate head of bed 30 degrees
Intake and output (for adequate hydration)

Administer related drug therapy and monitor for therapeutic and nontherapeutic effects.

Administer oxygen therapy as ordered.

Related nursing diagnoses

Ineffective airway clearance; impaired gas exchange; ineffective breathing patterns R/T diaphragm muscle paralysis

Outcome 2: Optimize cardiac output

Assess and compare to established norms, patient baselines, and trends.

Monitor for signs of decreased cardiac output.

Heart rate and rhythm, mentation, blood pressure (Keep systolic BP > 90 mm Hg)

Extremities for warmth, capillary refill, pulses

Intake and output balance

Interventions to maintain cardiac output

Continuous cardiac monitoring

Slowly elevate head of bed to prevent orthostatic hypotension.

Administer related drug therapy and monitor for therapeutic and nontherapeutic effects.

Intravenous fluids as ordered

Vasopressors as ordered

Related nursing diagnoses

Decreased cardiac output R/T impaired vasomotor tone

Outcome 3: Maintain normal elimination

Assess and compare to established norms, patient baselines, and trends.

Monitor for signs altered urinary and bowel elimination.

Intake and output balance

Residual urine after voiding (< 400 mL residual is desired)

Bowel elimination pattern (regular pattern, soft stool desired)

Interventions to maintain normal urine and bowel elimination

Begin intermittent urinary catheterization when intake is less than 2 L/day.

Record bowel movements.

Adhere to bowel elimination schedule.

Administer related drug therapy and monitor for therapeutic and nontherapeutic effects.

Administer stool softeners as ordered.

Related nursing diagnoses

Impaired urinary elimination R/T impaired reflex function

Impaired bowel elimination R/T impaired reflex function

Outcome 4: Maintain normal skin integrity

Assess and compare to established norms, patient baselines, and trends.

Monitor for signs altered skin integrity.

Redness, edema, skin breakdown especially over pressure points (e.g., elbows, coccyx, heels, lateral malleolus)

Interventions to maintain normal skin integrity

Determine need for specialized bed (based on hospital policy).

Turn every two hours; log roll if appropriate.

Inspect bed for foreign objects.

Remove wrinkles from bedding underneath patient.

Maintain body in neutral position.

Related nursing diagnoses

Risk for impaired skin integrity R/T decreased mobility, impaired bowel/bladder function

Outcome 5: Free from thrombus formation and pulmonary embolus

Assess and compare to established norms, patient baselines, and trends.

Monitor for signs of deep vein thrombosis (DVT) and pulmonary embolus (PE).

DVT: swelling, redness, warmth in legs; fever.

PE: Sudden shortness of breath, decreased Spo_2, pain on breathing, bloody secretions

Interventions to prevent DVT and PE

Compression devices on lower limbs (for at least the first two weeks post injury)

Keep well hydrated.

Administer related drug therapy and monitor for therapeutic and nontherapeutic effects.

Administer low-molecular weight heparin as ordered.

Related nursing diagnoses

Impaired physical mobility R/T loss of neurologic function below C4 level

Outcome 6: Maintain normal nutritional state

Assess and compare to established norms, patient baselines, and trends.

Monitor for signs of altered nutrition.

Weight and muscle mass loss

Serum albumin and prealbumin

Development of ileus

GI bleeding (stress ulcer)

Interventions to maintain nutritional state

Early nutrition consult

Feeding tube as ordered

Administer tube feedings as ordered; check for proper tube tip placement.

Administer related drug therapy and monitor for therapeutic and nontherapeutic effects.

Administer histamine blocking agent or proton pump inhibitor as ordered.

Related nursing diagnoses

Altered nutrition: less than body requirement R/T hypermetabolic processes, NPO status

Outcome 7: Free from infection

Assess and compare to established norms, patient baselines, and trends.

Monitor for signs infection.

Fevers

Urine color and clarity

Skin and mucous membranes

Sputum color and consistency, lung sounds

(*continued*)

NURSING CARE (continued)

Interventions to maintain normal skin integrity
Careful cleaning of urinary catheter and meatus with soap and water
Related nursing diagnoses
Potential for infection

Outcome 8: Minimize anxiety of patient and family
Assess and compare to established norms, patient baselines, and trends.
Monitor for signs of anxiety.
Expressions of anxiety, concerns

Interventions to maintain normal skin integruty
Provide psychological support to patient and family
Make appropriate referrals (e.g., social worker, chaplain)
Related nursing diagnoses
Anxiety
Grieving
Impaired adjustment

SECTION FIVE REVIEW

1. Which of the following SCIs require long-term mechanical ventilation?
   - A. C1-C2
   - B. C6-C7
   - C. T1-T5
   - D. All patients with SCI require long-term mechanical ventilation.
2. The main cause of complications or deaths post-SCI are related to
   - A. sepsis
   - B. respiratory complications
   - C. autonomic dysreflexia
   - D. bradycardia
3. A patient is admitted to your unit with a C8 SCI. Which of the following statements is true about recovery after this injury?
   - A. The patient will be independent with eating.
   - B. The patient will be independent with dressing.
   - C. The patient will be independent in a manual wheelchair.
   - D. All of the above
4. Which of the following signs indicate autonomic dysreflexia?
   - A. heart rate 60 beats per minute
   - B. blood pressure 220/120
   - C. priapism
   - D. poikilothermia
5. To prevent orthostatic hypotension, the nurse
   - A. gradually increases the head of bed
   - B. administers dopamine PRN as ordered
   - C. administers antihypertensives PRN as ordered
   - D. prevents constipation
6. AB has a T1 SCI. His wife asks you if they will ever have sexual relations again. What is the most appropriate response?
   - A. He will never be able to have an erection.
   - B. He can have an erection, but he will be infertile.
   - C. Sexual function is still possible.
   - D. They will never have sexual relations again.

Answers: 1. A, 2. B, 3. D, 4. B, 5. A, 6. C

POSTTEST

1. A diagnosis of unstable SCI is made based on
   - A. disruption of two or more of the spinal columns
   - B. degree of sensory involvement
   - C. presence of associated hemodynamic changes
   - D. degree of flaccid paralysis present
2. The corticospinal tract originates in the brain and innervates the
   - A. peripheral sensory neurons
   - B. opposite side of the body
   - C. parasympathetic nervous system
   - D. sympathetic nervous system
3. A lower motor neuron lesion results in
   - A. permanent loss of bladder function
   - B. flaccid paralysis
   - C. contralateral motor effects
   - D. spastic paralysis
4. Which of the following is an example of an incomplete spinal cord injury?
   - A. paraplegia
   - B. quadriplegia
   - C. tetraplegia
   - D. Brown-Sequard syndrome
5. A sudden deceleration of the head in a head-on collision can produce which of the following injuries to the spinal cord?
   - A. hyperflexion
   - B. hyperextension
   - C. rotation
   - D. axial loading

6. Which of the following radiographic tests may be needed to diagnose a ligament injury?
   A. lateral X-ray
   B. CT scan
   C. MRI
   D. SEP
7. Moving the big toe up and down and asking the patient to confirm the direction assesses
   A. priapism
   B. proprioception
   C. dermatomes
   D. sensation
8. A spinal cord injury cannot be accurately classified until the resolution of
   A. spinal shock
   B. neurogenic shock
   C. autonomic dysreflexia
   D. priapism
9. Which of the following is NOT an external fixation device used for stabilizing a SCI?
   A. halo device
   B. Gardner-Wells tongs
   C. Vinke cervical tongs
   D. cervical rods
10. Which of the following is an external fixation device that is secured with four pins inserted into the skull?
   A. Gardner-Wells tongs
   B. halo device
   C. clam shell
   D. Jewett orthosis
11. Which of the following interventions is contraindicated for the patient in a halo vest?
   A. Pull the vest's struts to move the patient up in bed.
   B. Inspect the pins for security.
   C. Perform pin care per unit protocol.
   D. Turn the patient every two hours.
12. The patient with a SCI is at risk for developing decreased cardiac output related to
   A. orthostatic hypertension
   B. neurogenic shock
   C. venous pooling
   D. all of the above
13. Which of the following statements accurately describes autonomic dysreflexia?
   A. It is a spastic disorder limiting mobility.
   B. It is a cardiovascular problem produced by decreased cardiac output secondary to bradycardia.
   C. It is a vasoconstrictive problem produced by excessive sympathetic nervous system stimulation.
   D. It is a parasympathetic nervous system problem resulting from unopposed vasodilation.
14. When assessing a patient's ability to cope with a SCI, which of the following is the most important factor to assess?
   A. income
   B. education
   C. age
   D. social support system

Posttest answers with rationale are found on MyNursingKit.

REFERENCES

American Association of Neurological Surgeons. (2002). Guidelines for the management of acute cervical spine injury. *Neurosurgery, 50*(3, suppl), S1–S84.

Bader, M. K. & Littlejohns, L. R. (2004). *AANN core curriculum for neuroscience nursing,* 4th ed. St. Louis: Saunders/Elsevier.

Barker, E., & Saulino, M. (2002). First ever guidelines for spinal cord injury. *RN, 65*(10), 32–37.

Baastrup, C. & Finnerup, N. (2008). Pharmacological management of neuropathic pain following spinal cord injury. *CNS Drugs, 22*(6), 455–475.

Bergmark, B. A., Winograd, C. H., Koopman, C. (2008). Residence and quality of life determinants for adults with tetraplegia of traumatic spinal cord injury etiology. *SPINAL CORD, 46*(10), 684–689.

Blissitt, P. A. (2009). Spinal cord injury. In K. K. Carlson (ed.). *AACN's advanced critical care nursing.* St. Louis: Saunders/Elsevier, 637–665.

Bracken, M. B. (2002). Steroids for acute spinal cord injury. *Cochrane Database Systematic Review, 3,* CDOO1046.

Cassels, C. (2008). STASCIS: early surgery in spinal cord injury improves outcomes, lowers complications. Proceedings of the American Association of Neurological Surgeons (AANS) 76th Annual Meeting, Chicago, IL. *Medscape Today,* Retrieved June 20, 2008 from www.medscape.com/viewarticle/573672.

Consortium for Spinal Cord Medicine. (1998). Clinical practice guideline: neurogenic bowel management in adults with spinal cord injury. *Paralyzed Veterans of America.* Retrieved March 5, 2009 from http://www.pva.org/site/News2?page=NewsArticle&id=7651.

Consortium for Spinal Cord Medicine (1999). Clinical Practice Guideline: Prevention of thromboembolism in spinal cord injury, 2d ed. *Paralyzed Veterans of America.* Retrieved March 5, 2009 from http://www.pva.org/site/News2?page=NewsArticle&id=7659.

Consortium for Spinal Cord Medicine. (2005). Clinical practice guidelines: respiratory management following spinal cord injury. *Paralyzed Veterans of America.* Accessed 3/5/09 at http://www.pva.org/site/News2?page=NewsArticle&id=7645.

Continuum. (2005). Lifelong learning in neurology. *Spinal Cord Disorders, 11*(3): 87–96.

Cook, N. (2003). Respiratory care in spinal cord injury with associated traumatic brain injury: bridging the gap in critical care nursing interventions. *Intensive & Critical Care Nursing, 19*(3), 143–53.

Cothren, C., Moore, E., Biffl, W., Ciesla, D., et al. (2003). Cervical spine fracture patterns predictive of blunt vertebral artery injury. *Journal of Trauma-Injury Infection & Critical Care, 55*(5), 811–813.

Dubendorf, P. (1999). Spinal cord injury pathophysiology. *Critical Care Nurse Quarterly, 22*(2), 31–39.

Fehlings, M. and Perrin, R. (2006). The timing of surgical intervention in the treatment of spinal cord injury: a systematic review of recent clinical evidence. *Spine. 31*(11), supplement, S28–S35.

Fehlings, M., & Baptiste, D. (2005). Current status of clinical trials for acute spinal cord injury. *Injury, International Journal Care Injured, 36,* (Supple), S-B113-S-B122.

Geerts, W. H. (2004). Prevention of venous thromboembolism: the seventh AACP conference on antithrombotic and thrombolytic therapy. *CHEST, 126*(3 Suppl). 338S–400S.

Gibson, K. L. (2003). Caring for a patient who lives with a spinal cord injury. *Nursing, 33*(7), 36–41.

Gunnarsson, R., & Fehlings, M. (2003). Acute neurosurgical management of traumatic brain injury and spinal cord injury. *Current Opinions in Neurology, 16*(6), 717–723.

Hadley, M. N., Walters, B. C., Grabb, P. A., et al. (2002). Guidelines for management of acute cervical spine and spinal cord injuries. In Disorders of the Spine and Peripheral Nerves, of the American Association of Neurological Surgeons, of the Congress of Neurological Surgeons. Retrieved June 9, 2008 from www.spineuniverse.com/pdf/traumaguide/.

Hedger, A. (2002). Action stat: spinal cord injury. *Nursing, 32*(12), 96.

Hess, M. J., Hess, P. E., Sullivan, M. R., Nee, M., & Yalla, S. V. (2008). Evaluation of cranberry tablets for the prevention of urinary tract infections in spinal cord injured patients with neurogenic bladder. *SPINAL CORD, 46*(9), 622–626.

Hickey, J. V. (2003). *Neurological and neurosurgical nursing.* Philadelphia: Lippincott Williams & Wilkins.

Hogan, E. (2006). Spinal cord infarction. *Emedicine.* Updated March 29, 2006. Retrieved May 12, 2008 from http://emedicine.medscape.com/article/1164217-overview.

Johnson, K., Mowrey, K., Bergman, M. (2008). Neurotrauma: spinal injury. In E. Barker (ed.), *Neuroscience nursing: a spectrum of care* (3rd ed.). St. Louis: Mosby/Elsevier, 368–401.

Karlet, M. C. (2001). Acute management of the patient with spinal cord injury. *International Journal of Trauma Nursing, 7*(2), 43–8.

Kerwin, A. J., Tepas, J. J., Schinco, M. A., Devin, T., et al. (2008). Best practice determination of timing of spinal fracture fixation as defined by analysis of the National Trauma Data Bank. *J TRAUMA, 65*(4), 824–831.

Lanig, I. S., & Peterson, W. (2000). The respiratory system in spinal cord injury. *Physical Medicine and Rehabilitation Clinics of North America, 11*(1), 29–43.

LeMone, P. & Burke, K. (2008). Medical surgical nursing: critical thinking in client care, (4th ed.). Upper Saddle River, NJ: Pearson Prentice Hall, 1597–1606.

Levendoglu, F., Ogun, C., Ozerbil, O., et al. (2004). Gabapentin is a first line drug for the treatment of neuropathic pain in spinal cord injury. *Spine, 29*(7), 743–751.

Livneh, H. & Martz, E. (2005). Psychosocial adaptation to spinal cord injury: a dimensional perspective. *Psychological Reports, 97*(2), 577–586.

Lohne, V. (2001). Hope in spinal cord injury patients: A literature review related to nursing. *Journal of Neuroscience Nursing, 33*(6). 317–326.

Lohne, V., & Severinsson, E. (2004). Hope during the first few months after acute spinal cord injury. *Journal of Advanced Nursing, 47,* 279–286.

Mahmood, N. S., Kadavigere, R., Ramesh, A. K., & Rao, V. R. (2008). Magnetic resonance imaging in acute cervical spinal cord injury: a correlative study on spinal cord changes and 1 month motor recovery. *SPINAL CORD, 46*(12), 791–797.

National Spinal Cord Injury Statistical Center. (2007). Facts and figures at a glance. Retrieved June 25, 2008 from http://images.main.uab.edu/spinalcord/pdffiles/Facts08.pdf.

Ren, X., Wang, W., Zhang, X., et al. (2006). The comparative study of magnetic resonance angiography diagnosis and pathology of blunt vertebral artery injury. *Spine, 31*(18), 2124–2129.

Richardson, J. (2009). Special neurologic patient populations. In K. K. Carlson (ed.), *AACN's advanced critical care nursing.* St. Louis: Saunders/ Elsevier, 682.

Ridder, D., Everaert, K., Garcia Fernandez, L., et al. (2005). Intermittent catheterization with hydrophilic-coated catheters reduces the risk of clinical urinary tract infection in spinal cord injured patients: a prospective randomized parallel comparative trial. *European Urology, 48,* 991–995.

Royster, R. (2004). Critical care in the acute spinal cord injury. *Topics Spinal Cord Injury Rehabilitation, 9*(3), 11–31.

Salvador de la Barrera, S., Barca-buyp, A., Montoto-Marques, A., et al. (2001). Spinal cord infarction: prognosis and recovery in a series of 36 patients. *Spinal Cord, 30,* 520–525.

Siroky, M. B. (2002). Pathogenesis of bacteriuria and infection in the spinal cord injured patient. *American Journal of Medicine, 113,* 67S–79S.

Tierney, L. McPhee, S., and Papadakis, M. (Eds.). (2005). *Current Medical Diagnosis & Treatment* (43rd ed.). Stamford, CT: Appleton & Lange.

Wilson, B. A., Shannon, M. T., Shields, K. M., Stang, C. L. (2008). *Nurse's drug guide.* Upper Saddle River, NJ: Prentice Hall.

Wuermser, L., Ho, C., Chiodo, A., et al. (2007). Spinal cord injury medicine & acute care management of traumatic and nontraumatic injury. *Archives Physical Medical Rehabilitation, 88* (supplement 1), S55–S61.

MODULE

24 Sensory Motor Complications of Acute Illness

Melanie G. Hardin-Pierce

OBJECTIVES Following completion of this module, the learner will be able to

1. Explain disorders of mentation and consciousness common to acute and critical illness.
2. Describe characteristics and management of delirium and coma.
3. Explain disorders of movement that occur with acute and critical illness.
   - Polyneuropathy
   - Myopathy
   - Neuromuscular blockade
   - Related muscle weakness
4. Describe characteristics and management of common seizure complications associated with acute and critical illness.

This self-study module focuses on assessment and management of the high-acuity patient who experiences disruption of normal mentation, consciousness, and movement. This module is composed of four sections. Section One begins with an overview of sensory motor conditions common to the acute and critically ill patient including disorders of mentation and consciousness. Section Two describes characteristics and management of delirium and coma. Section Three reviews disorders of movement and includes a review of neuromuscular syndromes, including critical illness polyneuropathy (CIP), critical illness myopathy (CIM), and prolonged weakness associated with neuromuscular blockade. Section Four reviews seizure complications of acute and critical illness. All Section Reviews include answers. It is suggested that the learner review those concepts answered incorrectly in the review questions before proceeding to the next section.

PRETEST

1. Disorders of mentation that are common in the critically ill population are
   A. delirium and altered level of consciousness
   B. myopathy and polyneuropathy
   C. neuromuscular weakness
   D. anxiety and pain
2. Arousal and awareness are components of
   A. delirium
   B. anxiety
   C. consciousness
   D. sensory perception
3. Delirium may contribute to which of the following?
   A. long-term cognitive impairments
   B. chronic depressive symptoms
   C. increased intracranial pressure
   D. acute coronary vasospasm
4. Delirium is a (an) ______ confusional state for acute or critically ill patients.
   A. chronic
   B. acute
   C. prolonged
   D. temporary
5. An acute axonal sensory-motor condition with loss of pain, temperature, and vibration sensory abilities that mainly affects the lower limb nerves is known as
   A. critical illness polyneuropathy
   B. critical illness myopathy
   C. neuromuscular blockade
   D. acute ICU psychosis
6. Neuromuscular blocking agents are associated with the development of
   A. CIP
   B. delirium
   C. hyperreflexia
   D. CIM
7. The time period surrounding a seizure when the patient is likely to have impaired mentation and sensorium is which of the following?
   A. the period just before the seizure
   B. the postictal period following seizure activity

C. the period of time when the seizure is taking place
D. all of the above

8. The type of seizure that is characterized by a brief loss of motor tone where the patient may fall is known as which of the following?
A. generalized tonic/clonic seizure
B. absence seizure
C. atonic seizure
D. petit mal seizure

Pretest answers are found on MyNursingKit.

SECTION ONE: Decreased Level of Consciousness, Abnormal Mentation, and Anxiety

At the completion of this section, the learner will be able to explain disorders of mentation and consciousness common to acute and critical illness.

Decreased levels of consciousness and abnormal mentation are common and often early signs of serious illness. Abnormalities in mentation occur in 80 percent of ventilator-dependent patients. Mentation disorders are associated with increased mortality, increased number of days requiring mechanical ventilation, and longer lengths of stay in the hospital and intensive care unit (ICU) (Ely, Shintani & Truman, et al., 2004; Stevens & Bardwaj, 2006). Even with these consequences, impaired mentation is often unrecognized and not treated. Altered consciousness and delirium are two disorders of mentation that are common in critically ill patients. Alterations in mentation can range from subtle decreases in level of consciousness to coma.

Normal **mentation,** or mental activity, is characterized by an awareness of self and surroundings. The patient knows his/her name and is aware of the present surroundings. These patients have the ability to accurately perceive what is experienced in terms of sensory input and orientation to environment. Patients who are normally mentating have the ability to store and retrieve information. They are able to demonstrate memory, judgment and reasoning in that they are able to process data to generate more meaningful information.

Mental processes include consciousness (wakefulness and responsiveness) and **cognition** (the ability to reason and mentate). For the purposes of this discussion, disorders of mentation will be classified as alterations in the level of consciousness and alterations in cognitive ability.

The two components of consciousness are **arousal** (wakefulness) and **awareness** (responsiveness). Normal consciousness ranges from an unaroused and unaware state (sleep) to an aroused and aware state (wakefulness). Abnormal states of consciousness may be similarly classified where coma and brain death are both consistent with an unaroused and unaware state of consciousness. Coma is characterized by the absence of arousal and awareness and may be reversible. Brain death is similar to coma in that the individual is in an unarousable and unaware mental state but irreversible and associated with cessation of brain function, ending in death. Delirium and dementia are conditions where arousal is associated with varying degrees of awareness.

There are many causes of cognitive dysfunction or impaired mentation in patients who have not sustained a head injury. (refer to Table 24–1). The causes involve global brain disorders caused by multiple factors that may be infectious, ischemic, drug-related, or metabolic. Ischemic stroke has been found to be the most frequent cause of impaired mentation on admission to an ICU. Septic encephalopathy has been reported by researchers to be the most common cause of abnormal mentation that develops after admission to the ICU (Marino, 2007).

Anxiety and Insomnia

Anxiety and **insomnia** are contributing factors to the development of cognitive dysfunction and altered mentation. Anxiety and insomnia may be attributed to a variety of underlying medical or psychiatric disorders, and symptoms may be exacerbated by hospitalization for acute or critical

TABLE 24–1 Causes of Impaired Cognitive Function in Acute and Critically Ill Patients

Ischemic, thrombotic, or hemorrhagic stroke
Drug or alcohol withdrawal
Insomnia
Anxiety
Thiamine deficiency
Toxins
Water intoxication
Hyperthyroid or hypothyroid
Medications
Central line infection
Heart failure
Hypoxia, hypercapnia (e.g., ARDS, pneumonia)
Hyper- or hypotension
Adrenal insufficiency
Renal failure
Liver failure
Sepsis
Hyper- or hyponatremia
Hypercalcemia
Hypophosphatemia
Fat embolism

illness. Possible causes of insomnia to consider include mood and anxiety disorders, substance abuse disorders, common medications (i.e., beta blockers, steroids, bronchodilators, etc.), sleep apnea, hyperthyroidism, and **nocturnal myoclonus.** Anxiety may be seen in certain anxiety disorders, depression, substance abuse disorders, hyperthyroidism, and complex partial seizures (Thoelke & Gutjahr, 2007).

Treatment for insomnia, anxiety, or both includes the administration of benzodiazepines. Therapy should be started at the lowest recommended dosage with intermittent dosing schedules. In the elderly, it is important to remember that toxicity can occur in the presence of malnutrition, advanced age, hepatic disease, and the concomitant use of alcohol, other CNS depressants, isoniazid, and cimetidine. Also, realize that certain benzodiazepines with a longer half-life may contribute to an accumulation of active metabolites in the elderly or those with liver disease. This accumulation can contribute to the development of prolonged sedation, delirium, psychomotor impairment, and respiratory depression. Tolerance and dependence may develop after two to four weeks of therapy, resulting in a withdrawal syndrome. Seizures and delirium are more likely to occur with sudden discontinuation of benzodiazepines. Flumazenil, a benzodiazepine antagonist, may be administered for overdose. Caution should be observed when administering flumazenil to patient with a known history of seizures (Thoelke & Gutjahr, 2007).

SECTION ONE REVIEW

1. Seizures and delirium may occur with sudden discontinuation of
   - **A.** opiate narcotics
   - **B.** benzodiazepines
   - **C.** calcium channel blockers
   - **D.** neuromuscular blocking agents
2. Alterations in mentation refer to a patient's inability to
   - **A.** withdraw from pain
   - **B.** cough and gag
   - **C.** localize to noxious stimuli
   - **D.** recognize surroundings
3. Disorders of mentation that are common in the critically ill population are
   - **A.** delirium and altered level of consciousness
   - **B.** myopathy and polyneuropathy
   - **C.** neuromuscular weakness
   - **D.** anxiety and pain
4. Components of consciousness consist of
   - **A.** involuntary reflex activity
   - **B.** arousal and awareness
   - **C.** ability to perceive pain stimulus
   - **D.** pupillary reactivity
5. Conditions that can increase the risk of benzodiazepine toxicity include
   - **A.** diabetes
   - **B.** obesity
   - **C.** coronary artery disease
   - **D.** advanced age

Answers: 1. B, 2. D, 3. A, 4. B, 5. D

SECTION TWO: Delirium in Acute and Critically Ill Patients

At the completion of this section, the learner will be able to describe the characteristics and management of delirium and coma; differentiate delirium from dementia; and describe valid assessment and management strategies.

Delirium

Delirium is the most common cognitive disorder in acute and critically ill patients. Delirium is considered one of six leading causes of preventable injury in those older than 65 years old. Delirium develops in 20 to 50 percent of ICU patients not receiving mechanical ventilation, and in 60-80 percent of patients receiving mechanical ventilation. This problem is predictive of a threefold-higher reintubation rate and can add as many as 10 additional days to a patients hospital stay. Delirium in ICU is associated with higher in-hospital mortality (Ely, Shintani, Truman et al, 2004; Ouimet, Kavanagh, Gottfried, et al, 2007). Studies show that delirium risks are cumulative in that for each additional day spent in delirium there is a 20 percent increase in the risk of prolonged hospitalization and a 10 percent increase in risk of death. Between 10 and 24 percent of patients experience persistent delirium that may be related to long-term cognitive impairment (Marcantonio, Simon, Bergman et al, 2003).

Delirium is an acute confusional cognitive disorder characterized by attention deficits, fluctuating mental status, and either disordered thinking or an altered level of consciousness that develops over a short period of time (hours to days) and fluctuates over time (Pun & Ely, 2007). The hallmark of delirium is its acute onset and/or fluctuating clinical course. This hallmark also distinguishes it from dementia. Delirium is a dynamic state that is characterized by both hypo- and hyperactive behaviors. It is common for patients to oscillate frequently between these two behaviors (Gunther, Jackson, & Ely, 2007; Peterson, Pun, Dittus et al., 2006). Although there are multiple pathophysiologic causes that are thought to be involved in the development of delirium, most are thought to be related to imbalances in neurotransmitters that modulate cognition, behavior, and mood. The current consensus is to consistently use the unifying term *delirium* and to categorize as either *hyperactive, hypoactive, or mixed delirium.* Hyperactive delirium, often referred to as ICU psychosis, is less common than hypoactive delirium and is associated with a better overall prognosis (Marino, 2007). It is characterized by agitation, restlessness, and it is common for these patients to "pick" at their monitoring, feeding, or intravenous devices. There is a tendency to consider delirium as a state of agitation. There also exists a hypoactive form of delirium characterized by lethargy rather than agitation, withdrawal, flat affect, apathy, and decreased responsiveness. This type of delirium is often referred to as encephalopathy. Hypoactive delirium is the most common form of delirium, especially in the elderly, and is a source of missed diagnoses of delirium in many patients. In fact, it is estimated that hypoactive delirium is the most common form, is more deleterious for the patient in the long term, and remains unrecognized in 66 to 84 percent of hospitalized patients (Marino, 2007; Pun & Ely, 2007 Peterson, Pun, Dittus et al., 2006). The data do not support the common notion that hyperactive delirium is more common, it is likely that this perception is due to the fact that these patients attract more attention due to their agitation and increased activity. It is important that nurses assess for hypoactive delirium because of its worse prognosis.

Septic encephalopathy is a type of delirium that results from a noncentral nervous system infection or sepsis in 50-70 percent of ICU patients. The encephalopathy can be an early sign of a septicemia signaling that something is wrong, especially in the elderly population (Papadopoulos, 2002). Sepsis itself is a major infection-induced syndrome that promotes failure of vital organs such as lung, brain, liver and kidney. Studies have demonstrated that both neuromuscular and cognitive dysfunction can result from sepsis, systemic inflammatory response syndrome (SIRS) and multiple organ failure (Young, et al., 1990; Bolton et al., 1993; Lacomis et al., 2000; Stevens & Pronovost, 2006). Septic encephalopathy is just one term that is used to describe these disturbances. Others include coma, delirium, acute confusional state, organic brain syndrome, acute organic reaction, cerebral insufficiency, brain failure, and ICU psychosis. Septic encephalopathy, like hepatic encephalopathy is an etiology-specific terms used when there is a strong suspicion of the causative mechanism. It has been proposed that many of these disorders are clinical expressions of a pathophysiologic spectrum of events collectively defined as critical-illness associated cognitive dysfunction (Stevens & Nyquist, 2007). A process that contributes to the development of septic encephalopathy is increased permeability of the blood-brain barrier resulting in cerebral edema. Inflammatory mediators can cross the blood-brain barrier and impair brain function. Like hepatic encephalopathy, amino acids and ammonia cross the blood-brain barrier and cause inflammation to the brain tissue. Also, cerebral blood flow is decreased to about 60 percent of normal which can cause cerebral ischemia (Stevens & Pronovost, 2006). There appears to be multiple mechanisms by which septic encephalopathy may develop, and the systemic inflammatory response to sepsis, rather than the infection itself seems to be the cause. Septic encephalopathy is considered by some to be one of the components of a more widespread multiorgan injury associated with the systemic inflammatory response syndrome (Meyer & Hall, 2006; Petzold et al., 2005; Stevens & Nyquist, 2007).

Delirium vs. Dementia

Dementia is characterized by slow, insidious onset of memory impairment that follows a long-term, progressive course over a period of months to years. It is irreversible, chronic in nature, and progressive. Delirium and dementia are distinct mental disorders that are easily confused because of two overlapping clinical characteristics including attention deficits and abnormal thinking (refer to Figure 24–1). As noted above, the features of delirium that are not present in dementia are its acute onset and/or fluctuating course (Marino, 2007). They often can and do coexist together. As many as two-thirds of hospitalized patients with dementia can have a superimposed delirium, and the delirium can provoke further mental and functional decline and deterioration of the dementia (Inouye, 2006; Fick, 2002).

Delirium may be caused by multiple conditions. Table 24–2 lists risk factors for the development of delirium. Infectious or septic, ischemic, drug-related, or metabolic encephalopathy can cause delirium. Medications are perhaps the most prevalent modifiable risk factor for delirium in acute or critically ill patients, but especially in the elderly population (Ouimet, Kavanagh, Gottfried, et al., 2007). Opioid narcotics (morphine and fentanyl) and benzodiazepines (midazolam and lorazepam) are linked to the development of delirium (Ouimet, et al., 2007; Pandharipande, et al., 2006). Refer to

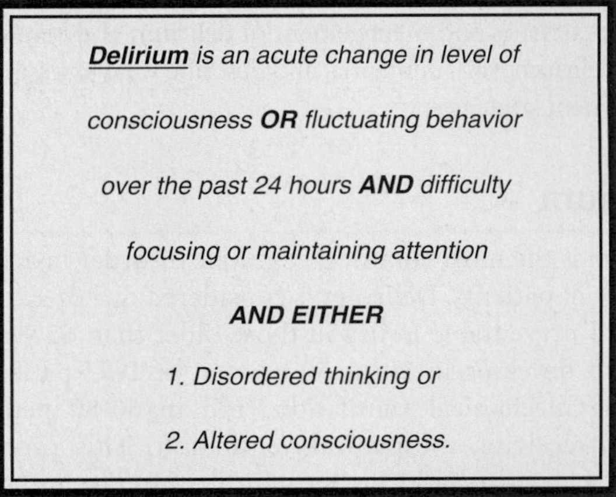

Figure 24–1 ■ Clinical characteristics of delirium.

TABLE 24–2 Risk Factors for the Development of Delirium

Primary risk factor: Preexisting cognitive impairment (e.g., dementia)
Other risk factors:
- Older age
- Presence of acute systemic illnesses
- Medical comorbid diseases
- Use of benzodiazepines
- Sleep deprivation/loss of circadian rhythm
- Metabolic disturbances

Table 24–3 to review medications associated with the development of delirium.

Sleep deprivation or loss of circadian rhythm is another potentially modifiable risk factor for the development of delirium. This is a common problem in the critically ill due to excessive noise and lighting, patient care activities, metabolic consequences of critical illness, mechanical ventilation, and sedative and analgesic medications (Gabor et al., 2003). Sleep deprivation has been linked with decreased protein synthesis, impaired cellular immunity, and metabolism that result in both cardiopulmonary and cognitive problems (Gabor et al., 2003).

Dementia, advanced age, comorbidity, and depression are other risk factors that may predispose patients to the development of delirium (McNicoll et al., 2003). Additionally, preexisting hypertension, smoking, alcoholism, increased severity of illness scores, hypoxia, metabolic disturbances, electrolyte imbalances, withdrawal syndromes, acute infection, seizures, dehydration, hyperthermia, head trauma, vascular disorders, impaired vision or hearing, and immobilization are precipitating factors for delirium (Pun & Ely, 2007).

TABLE 24–3 Medications Associated with the Development of Delirium in Critically Ill Patients

Alcohol	Digitalis
Amiodarone	Isoniazid
Amphoteracin B	Lidocaine, bupivacaine
Aminoglycosides	Metaclopramide
ACE inhibitors	Metronidazole
Atropine	NSAIDs
Benzodiazepines	Opioids
Beta blockers	Phenytoin
Cimetidine	Penicillin
Corticosteroids	Quinidine
Cephalosporines	Ranitidine
Cocaine	Trimethoprim-sulfamethoxazole

Assessment and Management of Delirium

The management and prevention of delirium should focus on identifying and treating the underlying cause. Assessment for delirium should occur early into a patient's hospitalization; as critical care course. Delirium can develop within 24 hours of admission. Early detection and treatment are necessary if adverse effects of delirium are to be avoided. Patients who are mechanically ventilated are often sedated, making assessment particularly challenging. Early monitoring for delirium along with daily goals for sedation and analgesia are essential to create a treatment plan that effectively manages pain and sedation while avoiding over use of agents that are known to cause delirium. A validated tool for monitoring and assessing delirium is the Confusion Assessment Method for the ICU, known as the CAM-ICU. The CAM-ICU has been validated and found to be reliable in mechanically ventilated patients (Jacobi et al., 2002).

Prevention should be the major goal of care although no established protocol exists. Interventions are classified as physiologic, environmental, patient safety, and pharmacologic. Physiologic measures include identifying those at risk for delirium, early diagnosis and treatment. Correction of dehydration, metabolic disturbances, and oxygenation imbalances are important physiologic interventions. Environmental interventions include early mobilization, adequate sleep/rest, and providing patients with eyeglasses and hearing aids when appropriate. Encouraging family/significant other visitation, placing patients near a window, providing for TV or radio stimulation and maintaining normal day/night light variations help the patient to remain oriented, rested and free of delirium.

Pharmacologic interventions for delirium include using neuroleptics or benzodiazepines to manage symptoms. It is important to review and treat all metabolic and electrolyte imbalances and organ dysfunction. Also, current medications should be reviewed regularly for possible triggers to the development of delirium. Benzodiazepines and opioids, often used in the acute care setting to treat pain and anxiety, may worsen the patient's cognitive state or may increase agitation, contributing to delirium. While an appropriate dose of opioids may be needed to treat pain, the challenge is to determine the optimal dose for analgesia without aggravating the delirious state of the patient. Pharmacologic strategies center on either of the following: (1) optimizing the quantity and type of sedative and analgesic medications delivered to patients, or (2) instituting currently recommended medications such as antipsychotics. Haloperidol has been recommended for behavioral management of agitation and hallucinations, and is recommended by the Society of Critical Care Medicine as the preferred agent for the treatment of delirium based on case study and anecdotal reports (Jacobi et al., 2002; Pun & Wesley, 2007). Risperidone (Risperidol) is an alternative to Haldol. Table 24–4 summarizes the management of delirium. The drug management for treatment of delirium is summarized in the Delirium section of the RELATED PHARMACOTHERAPY box.

TABLE 24–4 Summary of Management Principles for Delirium

- Monitor delirium regularly using a valid, reliable tool (CAM-ICU) with daily discussion of delirium assessment scores
- Identify patients with risk factors for new onset or persistent delirium
- Daily review of sedation and analgesia therapy
- Implement strategies for tight titration of all sedative and analgesic medications including daily sedation vacation
- Consider the use of antipsychotic medication (Haloperidol)

Data from Pun, B. T., & Ely, E. W. (2007). *The importance of diagnosing and managing ICU delirium.* Chest, 132:624–636.

Coma is persistent unarousability lasting for more than six hours, and implies extensive brain injury (Marino, 2007). Common causes of coma are cardiac arrest, stroke, or intracerebral hemorrhage. Coma is rarely permanent, but less than 10 percent of patients survive coma without some kind of significant disability. For ICU patients with persistent coma, the outcome is grim (Ely, Shintani, Truman et al., 2004). Outcomes of coma include full recovery with no long-term residual effects, recovery with residual damage that may include learning deficits, emotional instability, or impaired cognition/judgment. More severe outcomes include persistent vegetative state or brain death.

Emerging Evidence

- Practice and perceptions of delirium assessment vary widely among critical care nurses despite the presence of institutional sedation guidelines that promote delirium assessment *(American Journal of Critical Care.* 2008; 17:555–566).
- The Society of Critical Care Medicine practice guidelines recommend patients be routinely screened at least once every 12 hours for delirium using a validated screening tool. The Confusion Assessment Method for the Intensive care Unit [CAM-ICU]) has been developed specifically for the detection of delirium in nonverbal ICU patients by nonpsychiatric personnel The CAM-ICU has been found to have good validity and reliability for assessment of delirium in critically ill patients. Ely et al. (2001). Evaluation of delirium in critically ill patients: validation of the Confusion Assessment Method for the Intensive Care Unit (CAM-ICU) *Critical Care Medicine, 29*(7):13770–1379).
- Four postoperative factors, hematocrit less than 30 percent, cardiogenic shock, hypoalbuminemia, and acute infection, were significant, independent predictors of postoperative delirium in a cardiovascular intensive care unit (Chang, Y., Tsai, Y., Lin, P. (2008). Prevalence and risk factors for postoperative delirium in a cardiovascular intensive care unit. *American Journal of Critical Care, 17*(6): 567–575).

SECTION TWO REVIEW

1. Delirium is a preventable complication.
   A. True
   B. False
2. Studies show that for each day spent in a delirious state, the risk of mortality increases by ______ percent
   A. 25 percent
   B. 20 percent
   C. 15 percent
   D. 10 percent
3. Hypoactive delirium is more common in
   A. the perioperative period
   B. the female population
   C. the elderly population
   D. the noncritically ill population
4. Which of the following patients is least likely to develop delirium?
   A. a patient with numerous comorbid illnesses
   B. a patient who is receiving IV midazolam continuous infusion
   C. a patient with preexisting cognitive impairments
   D. a patient who is young

Answers: 1. True, 2. D, 3. C, 4. D

SECTION THREE: Disorders of Movement

At the completion of this section, the reader will be able to describe sensory motor disorders of movement that are common in high-acuity patients.

Neuromuscular Weakness Syndromes

Neuromuscular weakness disorders can produce severe and life-threatening complications that can impair function and quality of life following acute or critical care illness. Critical illness polyneuropathy and myopathy are complications of acute and critical illness that are associated with progressive and uncontrolled systemic inflammation such as that which occurs with systemic inflammatory response syndrome (SIRS), severe sepsis, and multiorgan failure. These neuromuscular weakness disorders are relatively common, and often go undetected because they are overshadowed by the more prominent clinical manifestations of the inciting conditions.

Critical Illness Polyneuropathy and Myopathy

Both critical illness **polyneuropathy** (CIP) and critical illness **myopathy** (CIM) are complications of clinical conditions that involve progressive and uncontrolled systemic inflammation, and can occur together. Patients with weakness acquired in the intensive care unit are often sedated and mechanically ventilated. Accurate sensory and motor examinations are often difficult to accomplish in these patients making it difficult to get an accurate measure of the incidence and prevalence of CIP and CIM. Some estimates published in the scientific literature note as many as 70 percent of patients with SIRS or sepsis and multiple organ failure will have evidence of polyneuropathy or myopathy, and that often both disorders occur together in the same patient (Bolton, 2005). CIP is most likely to develop in severely ill patients who have both systemic inflammatory response syndrome and an elevated score on the Acute Physiology and Chronic Health Evaluation III, a scoring system used to assess mortality risk in ICU patients (DeLetter et al., 2001). The onset of CIP can occur as early as three days after the diagnosis of sepsis or SIRS (van Mook, 2002). CIP and MIP have also been associated with prolonged mechanical ventilation, malnutrition, coagulopathies, high dose corticosteroids, the use of certain antibiotics (aminoglycosides such as gentamicin), use of neuromuscular blocking agents most notably pancuronium bromide, and electrolyte disturbances, and elevated glucose levels (Bolton, 2005; Schweickert & Hall, 2007). CIP and MIP are thought to be due to microcirculatory dysfunction or hyperinflammation that may cause damage to the motor neuron integrity (Latronico et al., 2005). Despite variability in reports of incidence of CIP and CIM, after a review of the research evidence, Pandit and Agrawal (2006) report that both are present in 52-57 percent of patients in the ICU for seven days or more and in 68-100 percent of patients with sepsis or SIRS, making this a significant event in the illness trajectory for patients who require high-acuity nursing care.

CIP is an acute axonal sensory-motor polyneuropathy that mainly affects the lower limb nerves. It is often preceded by septic encephalopathy and is followed by difficulty in weaning from the ventilator. In these patients, a symptom of CIP is when a painful stimulus such as nail bed pressure is applied, the patient may demonstrate facial grimacing but have reduced or absent movement of the affected limbs. There seems to be distal loss of pain, temperature, and vibration sensory abilities even in alert patients. Deep tendon reflexes are preserved in CIP. Autonomic function is preserved which helps to distinguish this condition from other weakness syndromes such as **Guillain-Barré syndrome.** Onset of CIP is variable, occurring from two days to a few weeks after the onset of the inciting illness (Marino, 2007). Electrodiagnostc testing (with nerve conduction studies and **electromyograms**) are necessary to diagnose this disorder. There is no specific treatment, and prevention by anticipation of this complication and prompt treatment of the predisposing condition is the plan of care. Van den Berg, (2001) found that tight glucose control with intensive insulin therapy can reduce the incidence of critical illness polyneuropathy by 44 percent. Complete recovery is expected in 50 percent of cases (van Mook, 2002). Recovery can be complete within a few weeks in milder cases, but can take months in more severe cases (Marino, 2007).

CIM is a spectrum of muscle disorders that present with diffuse weakness, depressed deep tendon reflexes, and mildly elevated creatine kinase levels (Lacomis, 2002; Bolton, 2005). **Electrodiagnostic testing** reveals a myopathy, and muscle biopsy reveals atrophy with loss of the thick myosin filaments (Lacomis 2002; Bolton, 2005). CIM is associated with status asthmaticus in approximately one third of these patients. This association is thought to be more prevalent in patients who receive high dose corticosteroid therapy. Also, neuromuscular blocking agent use is associated with CIM. Like CIP, there is no specific treatment for CIM, and most patients with this disorder make a full recovery within a few months. CIM, like CIP prolongs mechanical ventilation, and increases complications of immobility in high-acuity patients. Pulmonary complications are particularly problematic for patients with CIP and CIM. Pulmonary consequences of progressive neuromuscular weakness include decreased respiratory muscle strength, impaired cough and ability to clear secretions, increased risk of infection and airway obstruction, atelectasis and progressive hypoxemia, alveolar hypoventilation, and hypercapnia. Management of these complications includes careful observation of oxygenation and ventilator status, chest physiotherapy, tracheal intubation, supplemental oxygen, mechanical ventilation, and PEEP. As the neuromuscular weakness progresses, atelectasis and hypoxemia become prominent, followed by alveolar hypoventilation and progressive CO_2 retention. Hypoxemia is often a late finding (Marino, 2007). Early intubation and mechanical ventilation before the occurrence of respiratory failure is indicated.

Neuromuscular Blockade and Paralysis

It is common to administer neuromuscular blockade to induce paralysis in mechanically ventilated patients whose agitation interferes with ventilation or increases oxygen consumption. Neuromuscular blocking agents (NMB) are used only when analgesia and sedation have not been effective, or when needed to facilitate treatment. They may be indicated for patients who are mechanically ventilated, for those with tetanus, or for patients with increased intracranial pressure (ICP). The goal of neuromuscular blockade is to maximize oxygenation and ventilation by control of ineffective breathing patterns. NMB agents work by binding to nicotinic acetylcholine receptors on the postsynaptic side of the neuromuscular junction. Depolarizing neuromuscular blocking agents act just like acetylcholine, producing a sustained postsynaptic depolarization that blocks subsequent muscle contraction. Nondepolarizing agents act by competitively inhibiting acetylcholine-induced postsynaptic depolarization.

Nondepolarizing neuromuscular blocking agents that are used in the critical care setting are Pancuronium (Pavulon), cisatracurium (Nimbex), vecuronium (Norcuron), and rocuronium (Zemuron). Pancuronium is the longest acting nondepolarizing neuromuscular blocker. It has a tendency to accumulate with prolonged use and is associated with significant tachycardia. If used, it is best to give it by intermittent boluses to help to prevent accumulation of the drug. Dosage must be reduced in the presence of both renal and hepatic failure (Marino, 2007). Rocuronium (Zemuron) has a more rapid onset of action without the cardiovascular side effects, causing less tachycardia. Rocuronium dosage should be reduced in patients with hepatic failure as it is mostly eliminated in the bile. Cisatracurium (Nimbex) is a newer version of atracurium (Tracrium), both nondepolarizing agents that have fallen out of favor due to their side effects of neuroexcitation and excessive histamine release. Cisatracurium is preferred because it does not cause histamine release or cardiac depression, and it produces fewer active metabolites that cause neuroexcitation. Also, its clinical effect is not prolonged by hepatic or renal failure. Succinylcholine (Anectine) is a depolarizing neuromuscular blocking agent that is used infrequently in the ICU for prolonged neuromuscular blocking purposes. It is used more for rapid sequence endotracheal intubation where paralysis is very short-term and not prolonged. This agent is a ultrashort acting paralytic that has an onset of action of 60 seconds, with an effect lasting for about five minutes. Side effects of succinylcholine include life-threatening hyperkalemia, making it an unwise choice for use in prolonged paralysis. Neuromuscular blockade agents are summarized in the RELATED PHARMACOTHERAPY box.

The use of neuromuscular blockade to induce paralysis is associated with some serious complications and should be used with caution. These complications include prolonged muscle weakness after the drug is discontinued, which may be due to residual drug effect with accumulation of active metabolites and delayed clearance, or a synergistic effect that occurs when the agents are given with corticosteroids or aminoglycosides. Aminoglycosides, antibiotics, hypothermia, hyperkalemia, and hypercalcemia potentiate the effects of neuromuscular blocking agents. Prolonged muscle weakness is associated with elevated serum creatine kinase levels, muscle fiber atrophy, and muscle fiber necrosis (Loyola, 2003; Marini & Wheeler, 2006). Neuromuscular blockade should be avoided in any patient who is receiving prolonged corticosteroid therapy as this increases the risk for prolonged weakness. Another complication of neuromuscular blockade is immobility. Complications of immobility include deep vein thrombosis, pulmonary embolism, atelectasis, and pneumonia (Marino, 2007).

When administering neuromuscular blocking agents, the nurse should monitor the level of paralysis or neuromuscular blockade by applying a "train of four" series of low-frequency (2 Hz) electrical impulses (current strength 50-90 milliamps) to the ulnar nerve at the forearm, and observe for adduction of the thumb. If there is an absence of thumb adduction, the level of neuromuscular blockade is excessive. The drug infusion is titrated to achieve one or two thumb twitches out of the four electrical impulses (Marino, 2007). Another method used to monitor the level of neuromuscular blockade is continuous airway pressure monitoring (CAPM), which uses a transducer cable, high-pressure tubing, and a transducer to display continuous airway pressures. CAPM can identify spontaneous diaphragmatic effort before any other signs of neurologic activity can be detected in patients with neuromuscular blockade. When continuous or prolonged neuromuscular blockade is indicated (occurs for more than 48 hours), the infusion should be stopped daily to assess for its continued need (Loyola, 2003). When excessive neuromuscular blockade has been identified, or when there is no longer a need for the therapy, paralysis from nondepolarizing agents can be reversed with administration of an anticholinesterace agent such as physostigmine (Antilirium) (Siedlecki, 2009).

Nursing management during prolonged neuromuscular blockade also consists of protecting the airway, maintaining adequate ventilation, monitoring cardiac rhythm and blood pressure, treating pain and anxiety, protecting eyes, and maintaining skin integrity (Siedlecki, 2009). All patients who receive neuromuscular blockade should receive prophylactic eye care, physical activity including range of motion exercises; and deep vein thrombosis (DVT) prophylaxis. Prophylactic eye care consists of keeping the eyes closed and covered with a soft eye pad, and includes use of eye lubricants or artificial tears. Skin should be observed for potential areas of breakdown, with frequent repositioning, and consideration of pressure-reducing mattresses/surfaces. Continuous rotation therapy with specialty beds that provide lateral rotation along with passive range of motion are strategies to prevent complications of immobility. Neuromuscular blockade does not provide sedation/amnesia, nor does it provide analgesia. Paralysis from neuromuscular blockade can be expected to be anxiety provoking because the sensation of paralysis can be frightening for the patient who is cognitively aware. It is important to administer adequate sedation and/or analgesia simultaneously with neuromuscular blockade to prevent anxiety and manage pain.

SECTION THREE REVIEW

1. Polyneuropathy and myopathy never occur simultaneously in the acutely or critically ill patient.
   - A. True
   - B. False
2. Both CIP and CIM are complications of which clinical condition?
   - a. type II diabetes
   - b. chronic hypertension
   - c. systemic inflammation or infection
   - d. multiple organ dysfunction syndrome
   - A. a and b
   - B. b and c
   - C. c and d
   - D. a and d

3. CIM is characterized by
   a. preserved autonomic function
   b. elevated creatine kinase
   c. preserved deep tendon reflexes
   d. depressed or absent deep tendon reflexes
   A. a and b
   B. c and d
   C. b and d
   D. a and d
4. Risk factors for the development of both CIP and CIM include
   a. administration of vasopressor agents
   b. administration of high dose corticosteroids
   c. administration of antibiotics
   d. administration of aminoglycosides
   A. a and b
   B. b and c
   C. c and d
   D. b and d

Answers: 1. False, 2. C, 3. C, 4. D

SECTION FOUR: Seizure Complications in High-Acuity Patients

At the completion of this section, the learner will be able to describe the characteristics and management of common seizure complications associated with high-acuity illness.

New onset **seizures** are another sensory motor complication that can occur in critically ill patients. The incidence of new onset seizures in ICU patients is 0.8 percent to 3.5 percent (Marino, 2007). Seizures are manifested by muscle contractions characterized as tonic, atonic, clonic, or myoclonic. In a generalized tonic-clonic seizure, the tonic phase is characterized by a sudden loss of consciousness and sharp tonic muscle contractions, where muscles become rigid, arms and legs extend and the jaw is clenched. The clonic phase is characterized by alternating contraction and relaxation of the muscles in all of the extremities along with hyperventilation. The eyes often roll back and there is increased lacrimation. Figure 24–2 shows tonic-clonic seizures, formerly referred to as grand mal. Seizures can also be accompanied by automatisms such as lip smacking or chewing. The postictal period refers to the time immediately following a seizure which can be characterized by transient impairment of mentation and sensorium. Generalized seizures arise from electrical activity that involves the entire cerebral cortex. These kinds of seizures may not be accompanied by muscle contractions. Atonic seizures cause a brief loss of motor tone that can cause the patient to fall. Absence seizures (petitmal) are brief, lasting less than ten seconds and are associated with less prominent changes in muscle tone. Generalized tonic-clonic seizures have an initial tonic phase that is associated with apnea and cyanosis. The tonic phase is followed by a clonic phase where the airway may become lost and respirations are labored (Marino, 2007).

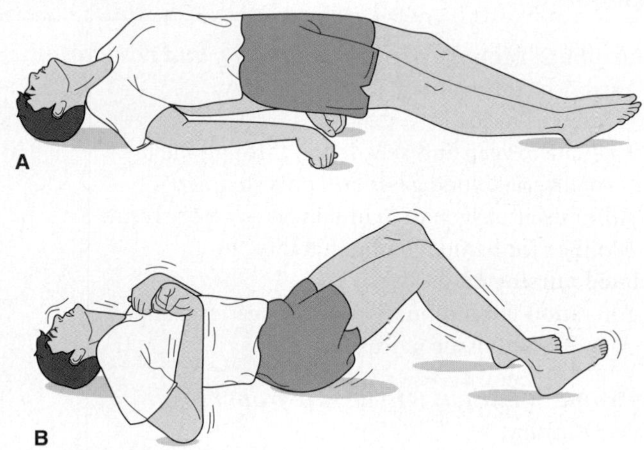

Figure 24–2 ■ Tonic-clonic seizures. **A**, Tonic phase. **B**, Clonic phase.

Status epilepticus refers to seizures that are continuous for more than 30 minutes or seizures that recur without a recovery of consciousness. Mortality is highest in this type of seizure activity because the patient is unable to breathe, making this a medical emergency. New onset seizures can be the result of a drug intoxication, **drug withdrawal** (alcohol, sedative or opioid), infections, head trauma, ischemic injury of the brain, space-occupying lesions of the brain, or systemic metabolic derangements that can occur with hepatic or renal failure, sepsis, hypoglycemia, hyponatremia, or hypocalcemia. Toxic levels of certain drugs can cause seizures. Also, withdrawal from some drugs can precipitate seizure activity. The drugs that may cause seizure activity in critically ill patients are listed in Table 24–5. The adverse effects of generalized seizures include hypertension, lactic acidosis, hyperthermia, respiratory compromise, pulmonary aspiration or edema, rhabdomyolysis, self-injury, and irreversible neurological damage, especially if the seizure lasts for more than 30 minutes (Marino, 2007).

TABLE 24–5 Drugs Associated with New Onset Seizures

INTOXICATION –these drugs can precipitate seizure activity due to toxicity or hypersensitivity	Amphetamines, ciprofloxacin, cocaine, Imipenum, isoniazid, lidocaine, Meperidine, penicillins, phenocyclidine, theophylline, tricyclic antidepressants
WITHDRAWAL of these drugs can precipitate seizure activity	Barbituates, benzodiazepines, ethanol, opiates

Marino, P. L. (2007). *The ICU Book* (3rd ed.). Philadelphia, PA: Lippincott Williams & Wilkins.

Management of Acute Onset Seizures

It is important to identify any correctible etiology of the seizure and treat appropriately (i.e. correct electrolyte imbalance). If the seizure stops and the cause(s) is/are corrected, antiseizure medication may not be needed. However, if a tonic-clonic seizure lasts for longer than five to ten minutes, drug management will be needed because the risk for permanent neurological injury or refractory seizures increases the longer that they persist. Intravenous benzodiazepines (lorazepam, diazepam) are effective in stopping the seizure 65-80 percent of the time (Marino, 2007). Lorazepam in a dose of 0.1 mg/kg IV is the treatment of choice over diazepam 0.15 mg/kg IV because it lasts longer, so that recurrent seizures are less likely to occur. Intravenous phenytoins should be administered with diazepam or if the seizure is persistent despite lorazepam administration. Fosphenytoin (Cerebryx) is preferred over phenytoin (Dilantin) because it can be delivered faster (maximum infusion rate of 150 mg/min), and thus produce more rapid suppression of seizures. Fosphenytoin does not contain propylene glycol which can cause cardiovascular depression. Fosphenytoin is compatible with dextrose solutions and if infiltrated into the skin, it will not cause skin necrosis as seen with phenytoin. Phenytoin is administered at a dose of 20 mg/kg in adults and 15 mg/kg for elderly with a maximum infusion rate of 50 mg/min, therefore, has a slower onset of action than fosphenytoin. Phenytoin administration can be associated with hypotension due to cardiac suppression from the propylene glycol that it contains. Phenytoin cannot be administered in dextrose containing solutions and if infiltration occurs, it will cause tissue vesication and necrosis (Marino, 2007; Myers, 2008). Fosphenytoin may be given IM.

If seizures continue to persist despite administration of benzodiazepines, fosphenytoin or phenytoin, administration of one or more of the following is needed: phenobarbital (20 mg/kg @ 50 mg/min); propofol (3–5 mg/kg load, then 1–15 mg/kg/hr); midazolam (0.2 mg/kg load, then 0.05–2 mg/kg/hr); or pentobarbital (5–15 mg/kg load, then 0.5–10 mg/kg/hr). If propofol, midazolam or pentobarbital are used, then intubation and mechanical ventilation is required, as these drugs will suppress respiratory drive (Marino, 2007; Myers, 2008).

Nursing care for patients who suffer acute onset seizures in the acute care setting includes observing the injection site frequently during administration of phenytoin to prevent infiltration. Vital signs need to be continuously monitored during IV infusion and for an hour afterward. Watch for respiratory depression, hypotension, arrhythmias, or further neurologic compromise such as decreased level of consciousness during IV administration of medications. Observe for signs and symptoms of an allergic reaction such as rash or itching, burning or tingling or glucose intolerance in diabetics. Table 24–6 summarizes the interventions for assessment and management of acute onset seizures. In order to prevent seizures, nurses must be vigilant in monitoring for and identifying any of the previously mentioned etiologies of acute onset seizures in acutely or critically ill patients. A summary of caring for the patient with seizures is found in the following NURSING CARE box.

The RELATED PHARMACOTHERAPY box provides a summary of actions and nursing considerations for the common medications used in the treatment of seizures.

TABLE 24–6 Interventions for Assessment and Management of Acute Onset Seizure Activity

Initial Interventions

- Roll patient onto side to minimize risk of aspiration.
- Remove constricting clothing or items that might cause injury from around patient.
- Assess airway, breathing, and circulation.
  1. Administer oxygen, monitor cardiac rhythm, and vital signs; monitor for respiratory depression.
  2. Establish IV line with normal saline solution.
  3. Measure bedside (fingerstick) glucose; ABG, CBC, electrolytes, calcium, and magnesium levels.
  4. Administer benzodiazepines intravenously (lorazepam, diazepam); and antiepileptic medication (fosphenytoin, phenytoin).
  5. If airway is lost or the seizure is persistent, intubate and consider the administration of propofol, midazolam or pentobarbital.

NURSING CARE: Care for Patients Who Experience Seizures

Expected Patient Outcomes and Related Interventions

Outcome 1: Cessation of seizure activity

Administer anticonvulsant pharmacologic therapy.

Monitor BP, HR, hemodynamic, and cardiac stability.

Monitor for therapeutic and nontherapeutic effects of drug therapy.

Assess for changes in mental status and LOC, restlessness, drowsiness, lethargy, inability to follow commands, reflexes, and strength.

Related nursing diagnoses

Alteration in cerebral tissue perfusion

Impaired breathing pattern

Outcome 2: Manage airway, breathing, and circulation

Establish and maintain a patent airway.

Suction as needed.

Evaluate oxygen and ventilation through the use of arterial blood gases and pulse oximetry.

Administer oxygen to maintain $SaO_2 \geq 92$ percent.

Monitor for hemodynamic stability.

Related nursing diagnoses

Alteration in pulmonary function: gas exchange

Alteration in tissue perfusion

Outcome 3: Patient will be safe from harm

Prevent injury.

Pad side rails of bed.

Have oxygen and suction source readily available.

Monitor continuously for seizure activity.
Have resuscitation equipment available.
Keep area clear of sharp objects.

During and immediately following a seizure:

During a seizure, place patient in a side-lying position to facilitate drainage of secretions.
Maintain an open airway using head-tilt/chin-lift maneuver.
Administer oxygen and suction airway as needed.
Intubate with prolonged seizure activity.
Administer IV fluids or vasoactive medications to offset the effects of continued seizure activity or anticonvulsant drugs.
Monitor temperature closely, treat hyperthermia with passive cooling or antipyretic.
Monitor serum glucose, pH, lactic acid, creatine kinase, or myoglobin levels.
Do not force anything into the patient's mouth during a seizure.
Allow the patient to sleep following seizure activity.
Following a seizure, assess for injury, including the oral cavity.
Document the duration and characteristics of the seizure activity as well as the postictal status of the patient.

RELATED PHARMACOTHERAPY: Common Medications for Delirium, Seizures, and Neuromuscular Blockade

Delirium

Antipsychotic Agent
Haldolperidol (Haldol)

Action and Uses
Blocks dopamine receptors; used in the treatment of delirium, psychotic disorders, agitation; has antiemetic effects.

Major Adverse Effects
Tardive dyskinesia, neuroleptic malignant syndrome, agranulocytosis, laryngospasm, hyperthermia

Nursing Implications
Monitor for therapeutic effect.
Monitor for neuroleptic malignant syndrome especially in those patients who take lithium or who have hypertension; discontinue the drug if symptoms occur.
Monitor for parkinsonium and tardive dyskinesia especially with higher doses and long term therapy.
Monitor for extrapyramidal reactions; these symptoms are usually dose related.
Monitor WBC when on prolonged therapy and seizure activity.

Status epilepticus

Benzodiazepines
Lorazepam (Ativan)
Diazepam (Valium)
Midazolam (Versed)

Action and Uses
Ativan- is the initial drug of choice for most status epilepticus episodes. Does not cause accumulation of active metabolites; less respiratory depression than with diazepam; effects last four to six hours.

Diazepam has a very rapid onset of action (10-20 seconds after IV administration).

Midazolam has the quickest onset of action; can be given IM.

Major Adverse Effects
Hypotension, respiratory depression, confusion, insertion site redness

Action and Uses
Sedation; used to treat acute onset seizure activity, not intended as seizure prevention

Nursing Implications
Monitor respiratory rate, BP (avoid hypotension).
Monitor for arrhythmias.
Avoid extravasations.
Obese patients may have prolonged half-life with IV infusion.
Monitor for overdose symptoms (somnolence, confusion, sedation, diminished reflexes, coma, hypotension, and respiratory depression).

Neuromuscular Blockers

Cistracurium (Nimbex)
Atracurium (Tracrium)
Vecuronium (Norcuron)

Action and Uses
Nondepolarizing skeletal muscle relaxant; paralytic agent
Used for chemical paralysis to optimize mechanical ventilation, treat seizures

Nursing Implications
Patient requires mechanical ventilation.
Monitor for respiratory depression.
Have personnel and equipment ready for endotracheal intubation.
Monitor degree of paralysis using train of four; administer at lowest possible doses.
Monitor BP, pulse; avoid hypotension.
Administer with a sedative and/or opiate as NM blockade does not treat anxiety or relieve pain.

Data from Wilson, B., Shannon, M., Shields, K., et al. (2008). *Nurse's drug guide.* Upper Saddle River, NJ: Prentice Hall.

SECTION FOUR REVIEW

1. The tonic phase of a seizure is characterized by which of the following characteristics?
   a. loss of consciousness
   b. extension and rigidity of extremities
   c. alternating contraction and relaxation of muscles
   d. hyperventilation
      A. a and b
      B. b and c
      C. c and d
      D. a and d
2. In a generalized tonic/clonic seizure, when is it most common for the patient to lose their airway?
   A. the clonic phase
   B. the tonic phase
   C. the postictal phase
   D. Patients rarely lose their airway with this type of seizure.
3. Intravenous phenytoin must be administered in which type of solution?
   A. 10 percent dextrose and water
   B. 5 percent dextrose and water
   C. 0.09 percent normal saline solution
   D. 25 percent dextrose and water
4. Which anti-seizure medication is preferred because it has less cardiovascular depression side effects?
   A. diazepam (Valium)
   B. lorazepam (Ativan)
   C. phenytoin (Dilantin)
   D. fosphenytoin (Cerebryx)

Answers: 1. A., 2. A, 3. C, 4. D

POSTTEST

1. Treatment of insomnia and anxiety includes
   A. opiate narcotics
   B. benzodiazepines
   C. antidepressants
   D. neuromuscular blockers
2. Cognitive dysfunction can be caused by
   A. sepsis
   B. anemia
   C. pain
   D. depression
3. Common clinical characteristics of both dementia and delirium are
   a. attention deficits
   b. abnormal thinking
   c. acute onset
   d. chronic onset
      A. a and c
      B. b and d
      C. a and b
      D. b and c
4. A modifiable risk factor for the development of delirium is
   A. sleep deprivation
   B. high dose diuretic administration
   C. bedrest
   D. open visiting hours
5. Which of the following is associated with a reduced incidence of critical illness polyneuropathy?
   A. tight glucose control
   B. administration of neuromuscular blocking agent
   C. avoiding sedatives
   D. administration of aminoglycosides
6. Complications from progressive neuromuscular weakness include
   A. complications of immobility
   B. acute renal failure
   C. glucose intolerance
   D. rhabdomyolysis
7. Which of the following is an example of a depolarizing neuromuscular blocking agent?
   A. succinylcholine (Anectine)
   B. cisatracurium (Nimbex)
   C. pancuronium (Pavulon)
   D. vecuronium (Norcuron)
8. When a patient is receiving NMBs, it is important to administer which of the following?
   A. only depolarizing NMB agents
   B. high dose corticosteroid agents
   C. sedatives and/or analgesia agents
   D. physostigmine (Antilirium)
9. You are the nurse who discovers a patient having a seizure. What is the initial action the nurse should take?
   A. Roll the patient onto his or her side to reduce the risk of aspiration.
   B. Intubate the patient immediately.
   C. Administer pentobarbitol.
   D. Establish IV line with dextrose containing solution for medication administration.

10. If seizure activity persists despite the administration of both benzodiazepine and antiepileptic medications, what should be considered?
   A. Administer insulin.
   B. Intubate and administer propofol, midazolam, or pentobarbitol.
   C. Remove the patient's restrictive clothing.
   D. Administer a neuromuscular blocking agent.

Posttest answers with rationale are found on MyNursingKit.

REFERENCES

Bolton, C. F., Young, G. B., Zochodne, D. W. (1993). Neurological changes during severe sepsis. *Annals Neurology, 33*:94–100.

Bolton, C. F. (2005). Neuromuscular manifestations of critical illness. *Muscle Nerve, 32*:140–163.

DeLetter, M. Schmitz, P., Visser, L., et al. (2001). Risk factors for the development of polyneuropathy and myopathy in critically ill patients. *Crit Care Med, 29*:2281–2296.

Ely, E. W., Shintani, A., Truman, B., et al. (2004). Delirium as a predictor of mortality in mechanically ventilated patients in the intensive care unit. *JAMA, 291*:1753–1762.

Fick, D. M., Agostini, J. V., Inouye, S. K. (2002). Delirium superimposed on dementia: a systematic review. *J Am Geriatr Soc, 50*:1723–1732.

Gabor, J. Y., Cooper, A. B., Crombach, S. A., et al. (2003). Contributions of the intensive care unit environment to sleep disruption in mechanically ventilated patients and healthy subjects. *Am J Respir Crit Care Med,167*:708888–715.

Gunther, M. L., Jackson, J. C., & Ely, E. W. (2007). The cognitive consequences of critical illness: Practical recommendations for screening and assessment. *Crit Care Med, 23*:491–506.

Inouye, S. K. (2006). Delirium in older persons. *N. Engl J Med, 354*:1157–1165.

Jacobi, J., Frasur, G. L., Coursin, D. B., et al. (2002). Clinical practice guidelines for the sustained use of sedatives and analgesics in the critically ill adult. *Crit Care Med, 30*:119–141.

Lacomis, D., Zochodne, D.W., & Bird, S.J. (2000). Critical illness myopathy. *Muscle Nerve, 23*:1785–1788.

Lacomis, D. (2002). Critical illness myopathy. *Curr Theumatol Rep, 4*:403–408.

Latronico, N., Peli, E., & Botteri, M. (2005). Critical illness myopathy and neuropathy. *Current Opinion in Crit Care, 11*:126–132.

Loyola, R., & Dreher, H. M. (2003). Management of pharmacologically induced neuromuscular blockade using peripheral nerve stimulation. *Dimensions Crit Care Nurs, 22*(4):157–164.

Marini, J. J., & Wheeler, A. P. (2006). *Critical care medicine: the essentials (3rd ed)*. Philadelphia: Lippincott Williams & Wilkins, 280–290.

Marino, P. L. (2007). *The ICU Book* (3rd ed.). Philadelphia, PA: Lippincott Williams & Wilkins.

Meyer, N. J., & Hall, J. B. (2006). Bench-to-bedside review: brain dysfunction in critically ill patients: the intensive care unit and beyond. *Crit Care, 10*(4):223.

Myers, C. M. (2008). Seizure disorders. In T. W. Barkley & C. M. Myers (eds.) *Practice guidelines for acute care nurse practitioners*, 2d ed. St. Louis: Saunders Elsevier, 72–81.

McNicoll, L., Pisani, M. A., Zhang, Y., et al. (2003). Delirium in the intensive care unit: occurrence and clinical course in older patients. *J Am Geriatr Soc, 51*:591–598.

Ouimet, S., & Kavanagh, B. P., Gottfried, S. B., et al. (2007). Incidence, risk factors and consequences of ICU delirium. *Intensive Care Med, 33*:66–73.

Pandharipande, P. P., Shintani, A., Peterson, J., et al. (2006). Lorazepam is an independent risk factor for transitioning to delirium in intensive care unit patients. *Anesthesiology,* 104:21–26.

Pandit, L., & Agrawal, A. (2006). Neuromuscular disorders in critical illness. *Clinical Neurology and Neurosurgery, 108*:621–627.

Papadopoulos, M. C., Davies, D. C., Moss, R. F., et al. (2002). Pathophysiology of septic encephalopathy: a review. *Crit Care Med, 28*:3019–3024.

Petzold, A., Downie, P., & Smith, M. (2005). Critical illness brain syndrome (CIBS): an underestimated entity? *Crit Care Med, 33*(6):1464.

Peterson, J. F., Pun, B. T., Dittus, R. S. et al. (2006). Delirium and its motoric sub-types: a study of 614 critically ill patients. *J. A. Geriatr Soc,54*(3):479–484.

Pun, B. T., & Ely, E. W. (2007). The importance of diagnosing and managing ICU delirium. *Chest, 132*:624–636.

Schweickert, W. D., & Hall, J. (2007). ICU-acquired weakness. *Chest, 131*:1541–1549.

Siedlecki, S. L. (2009). Pain and sedation. In K. K.Carlson (ed.), *AACN advanced critical care nursing.* St. Louis: Saunders Elsevier.

Stevens, R. D., & Bardwaj, A. (2006). An approach to the comatose patient. *Crit Care Med, 34*:31–41.

Stevens, R. D. & Nyquist, P. A. (2007). Coma, delirium, and cognitive dysfunction in critical illness. *Crit Care Clin, 22*:787–804.

Stevens, R. D. & Provonost, P. J. (2006). The spectrum of encephalopathy in critical illness. *Semin Neurol, 264*):440–451.

Thoelke, M. & Gutjahr, C. (2007). Acute inpatient care. In D. H. Cooper, A. J. Krainik, S. J. Lubner, & H. E. L. Reno (eds.). *The Washington manual of medical therapeutics, 32nd ed.* St. Louis: Lippincott, Williams & Wilkins, 12–14.

van den Berg, G., Wouters, P., Weekers, F., et al. (2001). Intensive insulin therapy in critically ill patients. *New Engl J Med, 345*:1359–1367.

Van Mook, W., Hulsewe-Evers, R. (2002). Critical illness polyneuropathy. *Current opinion critical care, 8*:302–310.

Data from Wilson, B., Shannon, M., Shields, K., et al. (2008). *Nurse's drug guide.* Upper Saddle River, NJ: Prentice Hall.

MODULE

25 Determinants and Assessment of Fluid and Electrolyte Balance

Karen L. Johnson

OBJECTIVES Following completion of this module, the learner will be able to

1. Discuss the distribution of body fluids.
2. Describe the regulation of fluid balance.
3. Identify normal serum electrolyte values.
4. Compare and contrast physiologic regulation of the following electrolytes: sodium, chloride, calcium, potassium, magnesium, and phosphorus/phosphate.
5. State the components of an assessment of fluid and electrolyte balance in the high-acuity patient.
6. List four important questions to ask during the nursing history that relate to fluid and electrolyte assessment.
7. Recognize vital sign changes that indicate an alteration in fluid and electrolyte balance.
8. Discuss elements of physical assessment that indicate an alteration in fluid and electrolyte balance.
9. Identify hemodynamic and laboratory parameters that indicate an alteration in fluid and electrolyte balance.

Maintenance of fluid and electrolyte balance is a major goal in improving the outcomes of high-acuity patients with complex health problems. Nurses monitor high-acuity patients for actual or potential alterations in fluid and electrolyte balance. This requires the nurse to have an understanding of the physiologic mechanisms that maintain fluid and electrolyte balance. Nursing observations are then interpreted within the context of the patient's history and pathophysiologic condition to determine if an alteration in fluid and electrolyte balance exists, and if so, to what degree. The high-acuity nurse uses critical thinking skills to determine the appropriate nursing action; this includes determining when a health care provider must be notified.

The module is divided into four sections. Section One reviews body fluid composition and distribution. Sections Two and Three describe physiologic mechanisms that regulate fluid and electrolyte balance. Section Four delineates important parameters that contribute to a complete assessment of the high-acuity patient and the presence of actual or potential alterations in fluid and electrolyte balance. Each section includes a set of review questions to assist the learner in evaluating his or her understanding of the section's content before moving on to the next section. All Section Reviews include answers. It is suggested that the learner review those concepts answered incorrectly in the review questions before proceeding to the next section.

PRETEST

1. Two thirds of total body fluid is in which of the following compartments?
   A. intracellular
   B. extracellular
   C. intravascular
   D. interstitial
2. Which of the following is the pressure exerted by plasma proteins as they flow through the capillary to draw fluid into the capillary?
   A. capillary hydrostatic pressure
   B. capillary colloidal osmotic pressure
   C. tissue hydrostatic pressure
   D. glomerular filtration pressure
3. Which of the following is the primary regulator of water intake?
   A. nervous system
   B. endocrine system
   C. renal system
   D. hypothalamus
4. The sympathetic nervous system responds to decreased volume by producing
   A. antidiuretic hormone (ADH)
   B. adrenocorticotropic hormone (ACTH)
   C. vasoconstriction
   D. aldosterone

5. When the hypothalamus senses a decrease in serum sodium or potassium, it responds by stimulating the pituitary to release
   A. renin
   B. aldosterone
   C. ADH
   D. ACTH
6. The normal range of serum magnesium is
   A. 1.3 to 2.1 mEq/L
   B. 3.5 to 5.3 mEq/L
   C. 4.5 to 5.5 mEq/L
   D. 135 to 145 mEq/L
7. Calcium is absorbed in the intestines under the influence of
   A. phosphorus
   B. vitamin D
   C. sodium
   D. vitamin C
8. Which of the following electrolytes are found predominantly in the extracellular fluid?
   A. potassium
   B. magnesium
   C. phosphate
   D. sodium
9. A low serum osmolality may suggest
   A. fluid volume deficit
   B. fluid volume overload
   C. dehydration
   D. isotonic balance
10. The most common cause of edema resulting from increased capillary hydrostatic pressure is
   A. liver failure
   B. heart failure
   C. immune reactions
   D. burn injury
11. Nursing assessment data found in the patient with fluid volume excess would include
   A. low pulmonary artery wedge pressure (PAWP)
   B. increased hematocrit
   C. moist crackles
   D. decreased blood pressure
12. Signs and symptoms of hypernatremia include
   A. diarrhea
   B. muscle twitching
   C. stomach cramps
   D. decreased muscle tone
13. Hyponatremia is associated with which of the following symptoms?
   A. edema
   B. hyperreflexia
   C. lethargy
   D. restlessness
14. Hypocalcemia is associated with which of the following clinical findings?
   A. tingling and numbness
   B. constipation
   C. lethargy
   D. shortened *QT* interval
15. Hypophosphatemia is associated with which of the following conditions?
   A. malnourished state
   B. metabolic alkalosis
   C. hypocalcemia
   D. hyperthyroidism

Pretest answers are found on MyNursingKit.

SECTION ONE: Body Fluid Composition and Distribution

At the completion of this section, the learner will be able to discuss the distribution of body fluid.

Body Fluid Composition

Body fluids compose about 60 percent of the body weight in the average adult male and about 50 percent in the average female. The composition of body fluids is primarily water with various electrolytes, glucose, urea, and creatinine. These fluids provide both an internal and external environment for the cells, playing crucial roles as a medium for metabolic reactions, a cushion to protect body parts from injury, and an influence on regulation of body heat.

Total body water content is affected by age, gender, and body fat content. The percentage of body water decreases with advancing age. Greater percentages of body fluids are found in individuals with a small body surface area; thus, infants have a larger fluid reserve. Infants, however, are predisposed to serious, rapid fluid volume deficit because of their limited ability to concentrate urine, their proportionately greater ratio of surface area to volume, and their higher metabolic rate. The elderly patient's fluid balance is affected by alterations in thirst and nutritional intake, diminished renal function, chronic illness, and medications. The elderly are predisposed to developing fluid volume deficit related to decreased muscle mass, increased fat stores, and a reduction in percentage of body fluids. Fat cells contain little water; therefore, obese individuals have considerably less fluid. Women tend to have more body fat than men, so they have less body fluid.

Fluid Compartments

Body fluids are primarily found in two compartments: the **intracellular** compartment (within the cells) and the **extracellular** compartment (all other body fluids) (Fig. 25–1). Extracellular fluid is further divided into intravascular fluid (plasma), interstitial fluid (fluid that lies between cells or tissues), and transcellular fluid (cerebral spinal fluid, peritoneal fluid, synovial fluid). Table 25–1 summarizes water distribution in the adult.

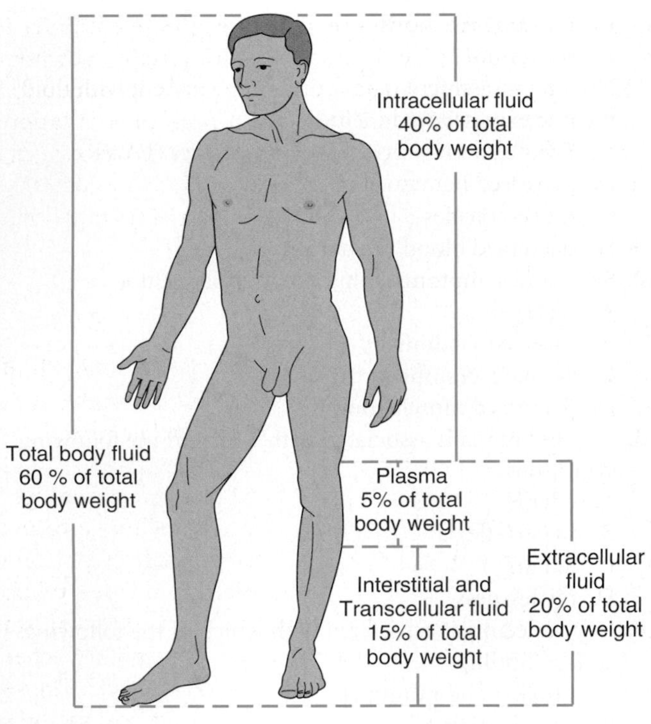

Figure 25–1 ■ Water distribution in the adult body.

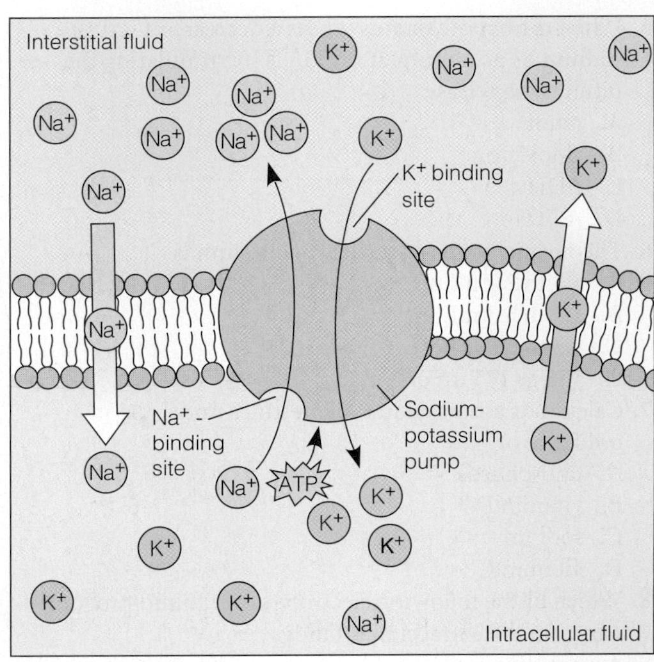

Figure 25–2 ■ The sodium-potassium pump. Sodium and potassium ions are moved across the cell membranes against their concentration gradients. This active transport process is fueled by energy from ATP.

Intracellular Compartment

The intracellular fluids (ICFs) are rich in potassium, phosphate, and protein and contain moderate amounts of magnesium and sulfate ions. Intracellular fluids provide the cells with nutrients and assist in cellular metabolism. ICF volume is regulated by several important mechanisms. First, the presence of intracellular proteins attracts fluid into the cells. Second, negatively charged ions within the cells attract positively charged ions, such as sodium (Na) and potassium (K), which draws fluid into the cells. Without the counterregulating forces provided by the Na+/K+ pump, the cells would rupture and die. The Na+/K+ pump is located in the cell membrane (Fig. 25–2). The pump requires adenosine triphosphate (ATP) for energy to actively move Na+ from the cell into the ECF and to move K+ into the cell. Because water is attracted to Na+ ions, more water accumulates in the extracellular compartment and ICF balance is maintained. Certain pathologic situations interfere with the functioning of the pump, including hypoxia. When the pump fails, Na+ accumulates inside the cell which causes retention of Na+ and water inside the cell and accumulation of K+ outside the cell.

TABLE 25–1 Water Distribution in the Body (Adult)[a]

COMPARTMENTS/ SUBCOMPARTMENTS	% BODY WEIGHT	VOLUME (LITERS)
Intracellular	40	25
Extracellular		
Interstitial	14	11
Plasma	5	3
Transcellular	1	2
TOTAL	60	41

[a] Approximate

Extracellular Compartment

All body fluid outside of the cells exists in the extracellular compartment and is referred to as extracellular fluid (ECF). Plasma is the fluid portion of the blood and is composed of water (about 90 percent), plasma proteins (about 7 percent), and other substances. Interstitial fluid functions as a transport medium for shuttling nutrients, gases, waste products, and other substances between the blood and the body cells. It also acts as a backup fluid reservoir that can rapidly provide fluid during situations in which there is vascular fluid loss (e.g., hemorrhage). The interstitial compartment contains a sponge-like substance called *tissue gel* that helps distribute interstitial fluid evenly. The gel is held together with collagen fibers. Tissue gel exerts force against the capillaries, which helps maintain fluids inside the capillaries. It also keeps free water from accumulating in the interstitial spaces. Transcellular fluid normally comprises about 1 percent of total ECF. It is located in the gastrointestinal and respiratory tracts, sweat glands, cerebrospinal fluid (CSF), and other tissues.

Movement of Fluids

To understand intercompartmental fluid movement, it is crucial to first understand the concepts of osmosis and osmolality. The principle of **osmosis** explains the net diffusion or movement of water across the cell membrane (Fig. 25–3).

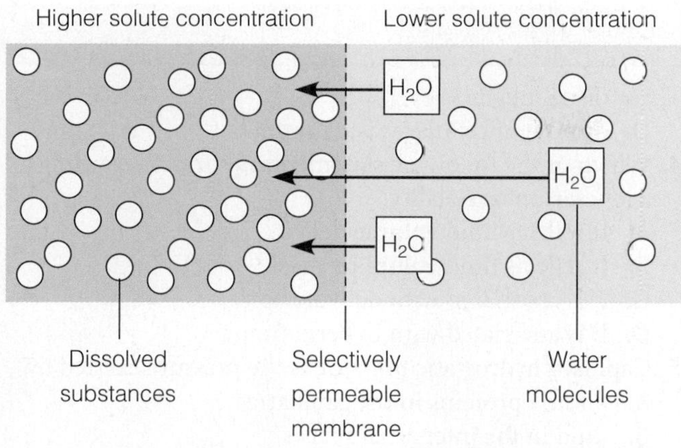

Figure 25–3 ■ Osmosis. Fluid moves across a semipermeable membrane from an area of low concentration to area of high concentration.

Water moves across a semipermeable (or selectively permeable) cell membrane from an area of lesser concentration of solutes to an area of greater concentration of solutes. Water is pulled into the compartment in the same way as a sponge soaks up a spill (David, 2007). Osmosis is a passive process, requiring no expenditure of energy. Its purpose is to maintain fluid equilibrium between the fluid compartments. Water moves freely between the various fluid compartments; therefore, an alteration in one compartment produces a shift in body fluids in another compartment.

Osmolality refers to the concentration of solute in body water and reflects a patient's hydration status. The **osmolarity** of a solution is the solute (or particle) concentration per volume of water. Although osmolality is the correct term to use when referring to body fluids, osmolarity is often used because it is another way to measure concentration. However, instead of representing the number of particles per liter of water, osmolarity instead represents the number of particles per liter of solution. Measurement of the serum osmolality can be used as an approximation of the extracellular fluid volume. Serum osmolality may be increased or decreased in various diseases. Hyperglycemia, diabetes insipidus, and hypernatremia produce an increased serum osmolality, whereas syndrome of inappropriate antidiuretic hormone (SIADH) and certain antidiuretic hormone (ADH)-secreting carcinomas of the lung can produce a low serum osmolality (Goertz, 2006). The clinical manifestations of decreased serum osmolality (fluid volume excess) are similar to those of hyponatremia and those of increased serum osmolality (fluid volume deficit) are similar to those of hypernatremia.

Starling Forces

Through the processes of osmosis and diffusion, body fluids move freely between the interstitial and intravascular compartments. There are four forces, called *Starling forces*, that control this movement (Fig. 25–4). The forces include capillary hydrostatic pressure, capillary colloidal osmotic pressure, tissue hydrostatic pressure, and tissue fluid pressure. *Capillary hydrostatic pressure* is the pressure exerted by fluid moving through the capillaries to push fluid out of the capillary into the interstitial space. The majority of this movement occurs at the arterial end of the capillary, where the hydrostatic pressure is greatest (30 to 40 mm Hg). The venous end of the capillary has a much lower hydrostatic pressure (10 to 15 mm Hg), and fluid is reabsorbed back into the capillary at this end. *Capillary colloidal osmotic pressure* is the pressure exerted by plasma proteins as they flow through the capillary to draw fluid into the capillary. *Interstitial fluid pressure* is the pressure exerted by fluid in the interstitial space that pushes against the capillaries, opposing shifts of fluid out of the capillaries. *Tissue hydrostatic pressure* is pressure exerted by the small amount of proteins located in the interstitial space, which attracts fluid out of the capillaries and into the interstitium. As can be seen, the opposing forces found in the capillaries and the interstitial spaces cause fluids to shift in and out of the capillaries, maintaining fluid balance between compartments and preventing excess fluid buildup in the interstitial spaces. In high-acuity patients, these forces can become unbalanced, causing abnormal fluid shifts or trapping of intravascular fluid into the interstitium, otherwise known as third spacing.

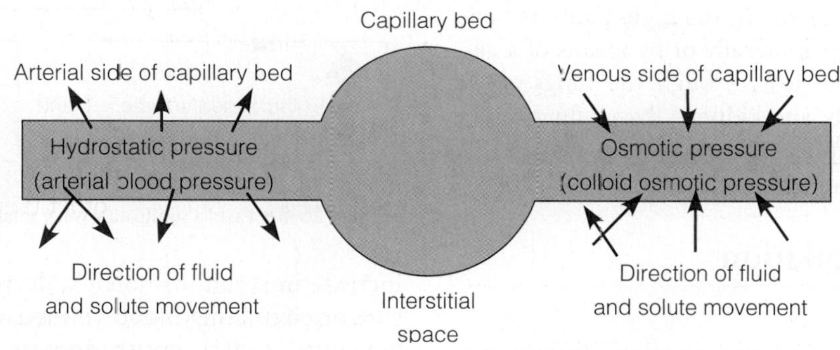

Figure 25–4 ■ Starling forces maintain fluid balance between intravascular and interstitial spaces.

SECTION ONE REVIEW

1. Two thirds of total body fluid is in which of the following compartments?
   A. intracellular
   B. extracellular
   C. intravascular
   D. interstitial
2. Patients with advancing age are predisposed to develop fluid volume deficit related to (choose all that apply)
   A. decreased muscle mass
   B. increased fat stores
   C. decrease in percent of body fluids
   D. alterations in thirst
3. The major function of tissue gel in the interstitial compartment is to
   A. shift fluid out of capillaries
   B. provide a source of electrolytes
   C. distribute fluid evenly
   D. dispose of cellular waste products
4. Which of the following statements is correct regarding a low serum osmolality?
   A. It reflects fluid volume deficit.
   B. It reflects fluid volume excess.
   C. It is associated with dehydration.
   D. It is associated with hypernatremia.
5. Capillary hydrostatic pressure is the pressure exerted by
   A. plasma proteins in the capillaries
   B. fluid in the interstitial spaces
   C. plasma proteins in the interstitial spaces
   D. fluid moving through the capillaries

Answers: 1. A, 2. (A, B, C, D), 3. C, 4. B, 5. D

SECTION TWO: Regulation of Fluid Balance

At the completion of this section, the learner will be able to describe the regulation of fluid balance.

Routes of Gains and Losses

The two main mechanisms in the body that regulate and maintain body water homeostasis include thirst (prompting fluid intake) and excretion of body water via the kidneys (promoting fluid output) (Haskal, 2007). Under normal situations, most fluids are gained by drinking and eating through the **thirst** mechanism. Thirst is the awareness of the desire to drink and plays an important role in maintaining fluid and electrolyte balance. It is the primary regulator of water intake. When blood volume decreases or when serum osmolarity increases, the thirst center in the hypothalamus is stimulated (Fig. 25–5).

The thirst center helps regulate sodium balance. Hypernatremia increases serum osmolarity and stimulates osmoreceptors in the hypothalamus to initiate the thirst mechanism. Unfortunately many high-acuity patients have altered levels of consciousness and therefore do not experience the thirst mechanism. This is why hypernatremia is a common electrolyte imbalance in high-acuity patients. In the high-acuity patient, fluids may be administered parenterally or by means of a gastrointestinal tube. Fluids are lost through the lungs, sweat glands, gastrointestinal fluids, and kidneys. Excess fluid can be lost during periods of tachypnea, fever, vomiting, diarrhea, or any condition that affects kidney function.

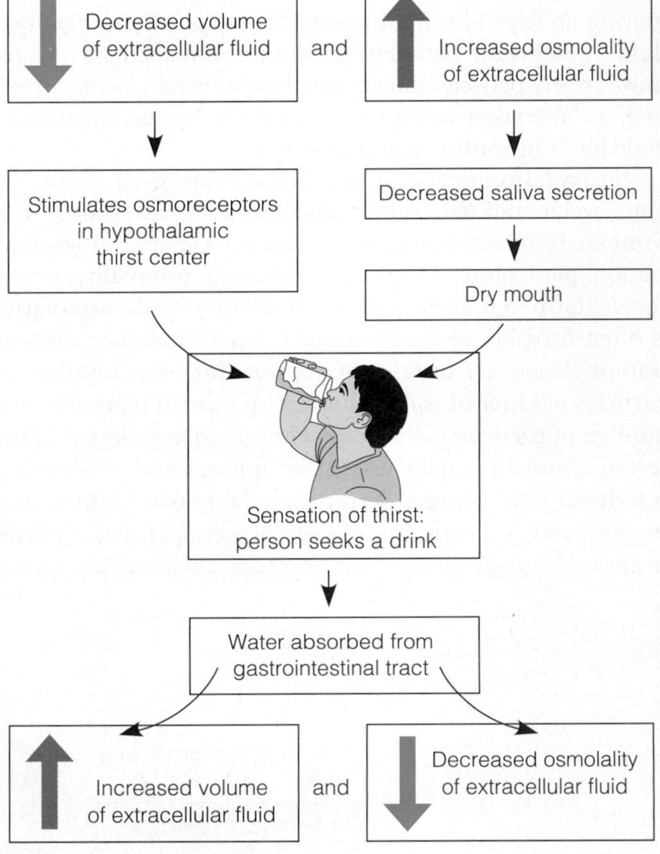

Figure 25–5 ■ Factors stimulating water intake through the thirst mechanism.

Nervous System Regulation

Hypothalamus

The lateral area of the hypothalamus regulates body water, especially thirst and renal excretion of excess water. Cells located in the hypothalamus are sensitive to body fluid concentration (serum osmolality). Thirst is activated by an increase in serum osmolality, decreased arterial blood pressure or circulating blood volume, increased secretion of angiotensin II, and mouth dryness. Thirst is decreased by a lower-than-normal serum osmolality, decreased angiotensin II, increased circulating blood volume or arterial blood pressure, and distention of the stomach. When thirst is triggered, the conscious person responds by drinking fluids. Clinical conditions that decrease the sense of thirst or the individual's ability to respond to thirst can decrease the circulating extracellular volume. Remember, the unconscious or high-acuity patient often cannot respond to thirst signals. For this reason, in the clinical setting, the nurse needs to closely evaluate the patient's fluid status using objective data obtained through physical assessment, and urine and serum lab analysis data.

Arterial Baroreceptors

Arterial **baroreceptors** (pressure receptors) located in the arch of the aorta and carotid sinus detect arterial pressure changes. When baroreceptors sense a decrease in arterial blood pressure, they send a signal to the autonomic nervous system. The sympathetic nervous system responds to this signal by causing peripheral vasoconstriction. Vasoconstriction of renal arteries decreases glomerular filtration, which reduces urine output in an attempt to increase circulating blood volume. The baroreceptors trigger opposite actions if they detect increased arterial blood pressure, causing vasodilation.

Endocrine Regulation

Adrenocorticotropic Hormone

The renal and endocrine systems work synergistically to regulate blood volume. When the hypothalamus senses a decrease in serum sodium or an increase in serum potassium, it sends a signal to the pituitary to release adrenocorticotropic hormone (ACTH). In response, the ACTH stimulates the adrenal cortex to release aldosterone. Aldosterone is the most potent of the mineralocorticoids and is sometimes referred to as the salt-regulating hormone. It regulates water balance by facilitating sodium reabsorption in the renal distal tubules, the collecting tubules, and collecting duct. As sodium is reabsorbed, potassium is excreted by the kidneys. The sodium reabsorption increases circulating blood volume by increasing water reabsorption. In this way, circulating blood volume and arterial blood pressure increase.

Antidiuretic Hormone

When the hypothalamus detects a change in the concentration of body fluid, it also sends a message to the posterior pituitary to either decrease or increase the release of antidiuretic hormone (ADH), which is also called vasopressin. For example, when serum osmolality increases, ADH increases permeability of the renal distal tubules and collecting ducts, allowing a large volume of water to be reabsorbed. This results in expansion of the ECF, decreases serum osmolality, and improves arterial blood pressure and perfusion. (The ADH-regulating mechanism is further described in Module 18, Alteration in Oxygen Delivery and Oxygen Consumption: Shock States.)

Renin–Angiotensin-Aldosterone System

When sodium concentration in the ECF is decreased or blood flow through the kidneys is diminished, the kidneys release renin, a protein enzyme. In response to a drop in arterial blood pressure, renin acts on a plasma protein (renin substrate) to release angiotensin I. Angiotensin I ultimately converts to angiotensin II, a powerful vasoconstrictor. Angiotensin II stimulates the release of aldosterone from the adrenal cortex which causes retention of sodium and water by the kidneys. The combination of actions results in a rapid increase in blood pressure, which improves perfusion. The renin, aldosterone, and ADH mechanisms are three endocrine responses to decreased circulating blood volume. (The renin-angiotensin-aldosterone system is further described in Module 18, Alteration in Oxygen Delivery and Oxygen Consumption: Shock States.)

SECTION TWO REVIEW

1. Which of the following is the primary regulator of water intake?
   A. nervous system
   B. endocrine system
   C. renal system
   D. hypothalamus
2. The sympathetic nervous system responds to decreased volume by producing
   A. ADH
   B. ACTH
   C. vasoconstriction
   D. aldosterone
3. When the hypothalamus senses a decrease in serum sodium or potassium, it responds by stimulating the pituitary to release
   A. ACTH
   B. ADH
   C. aldosterone
   D. renin
4. When the hypothalamus senses a change in serum osmolality, it stimulates the posterior pituitary to release
   A. renin
   B. aldosterone
   C. ADH
   D. ACTH
5. Angiotensin II is a powerful
   A. diuretic
   B. vasoconstrictor
   C. thirst trigger
   D. sodium waster

Answers: 1. D, 2. C, 3. A, 4. C, 5. B

SECTION THREE: Regulation of Electrolyte Balance

At the completion of this section, the learner will be able to identify normal serum electrolyte values and compare and contrast physiologic regulation of the following electrolytes: sodium, chloride, calcium, potassium, magnesium, phosphorus/ phosphate.

Electrolytes, Cations, Anions

Electrolytes are electrically charged microsolutes found in body fluids. There are two types of electrolytes: **cations** (positively charged ions) and **anions** (negatively charged ions). Electrolytes play a vital role in many physiologic activities, including enzyme activities, muscle contraction, and metabolism. There are three major extracellular electrolytes—sodium (Na), chloride (Cl), and calcium (Ca)—and three major intracellular electrolytes—potassium (K), magnesium (Mg), and phosphorus (PO_4). The cortical distal nephron is the segment devoted to the fine regulation of electrolyte balance (Capasso, 2006).

Regulation of Sodium Balance

Sodium, the most abundant cation in the extracellular fluid, is responsible for shifts in body water and the amount of water retained or excreted by the kidneys. It is required for normal transmission of impulses across muscle and nerve cells through the sodium pump mechanism. It helps maintain acid–base balance by combining with chloride or bicarbonate to increase or decrease serum pH. Serum sodium is maintained within normal limits by two important mechanisms: glomerular filtration rate which affects the number of sodium ions that pass from the glomerular capillaries into the renal tubules and the release of aldosterone by the adrenal glands which increases the reabsorption of sodium (Haskal, 2007).

Sodium and Water Balance

Changes in sodium levels alter water balance; thus, the clinical manifestations of sodium alterations also reflect symptoms of water imbalance. Because water is drawn to sodium, an excess sodium level in the extracellular fluid pulls water from the intracellular spaces. This results in shrinking of the intracellular fluid compartment and expansion of the extracellular compartment. Such expansion may precipitate congestive heart failure and pulmonary edema in patients whose renal or cardiovascular systems cannot tolerate such fluid shifts.

When serum levels of sodium are low, water moves from an area of low-sodium concentration (extracellular) to an area of high-sodium concentration (intracellular). This causes excess volume in the intracellular compartment and fluid volume deficit in the extracellular compartment.

The amount of sodium in the diet varies widely because the supply is abundant in many (particularly processed) foods. When sodium intake is excessive, fluid volume in the intravascular compartment increases. In response, the kidneys increase urinary excretion of sodium through enhanced filtering from the blood; inhibition of ADH prevents reabsorption of sodium by the kidneys; and aldosterone release is suppressed, enhancing urinary excretion of sodium. When sodium intake is excessively low, plasma volume is decreased. The kidneys sense the decreased volume, triggering the renin–angiotensin–aldosterone system, which causes increased sodium reabsorption, thus decreasing urine output and increasing fluid volume.

TABLE 25–2 Serum Electrolytes and Osmolality Normal Ranges

ELECTROLYTE	NORMAL RANGE
Sodium (Na^+)	135–145 mEq/L (or mmol/L)
Chloride (Cl^-)	98–106 mEq/L (or mmol/L)
Calcium (Ca^{++})	2.1–2.6 mmol/L (8.5–10 mg/dL)
Potassium (K^+)	3.5–5.0 mEq/L (or mmol/L)
Magnesium (Mg^{++})	1.3–2.1 mEq/L (1.6–2.6 mg/dL)
Phosphate (PO_4^-)	1.7–2.6 mEq/L (2.5–4.5 mg/dL)
Serum osmolality	275–295 mOsm/kg

Regulation of Chloride Balance

Chloride (Cl^-) is the most abundant anion in the ECF. Chloride works with sodium in regulation of body fluids by its influence on osmotic pressures within the interstitial and intravascular compartments. Serum chloride levels tend to closely follow sodium levels because chloride normally follows sodium in the body. Aldosterone regulates chloride levels indirectly by stimulating reabsorption of sodium in the kidney. Chloride assists in maintaining the resting membrane potential of cells and, with sodium, maintains osmolality of the extracellular fluid space.

The extracellular fluid acid–base status requires a balance between the total number of anions and cations within the fluid. Thus, the major cation (sodium) must be in balance with the two major extracellular anions (chloride and bicarbonate). To regulate this balance, chloride and bicarbonate maintain an inverse relationship, competing for sodium ions. For example, if a patient receives an excessive dose of sodium bicarbonate to treat metabolic acidosis, the presence of excess bicarbonate ions in the serum results in the excretion of chloride ions, precipitating hypochloremia.

Regulation of Calcium Balance

Almost all of the body's calcium is located within bone, with a small amount existing in the ECF and soft tissues. Calcium is required for blood coagulation, neuromuscular contraction, enzymatic activities, and bone integrity.

Calcium regulation is under the influence of parathyroid hormone (PTH), calcitonin, and calcitriol. Serum calcium levels are maintained by calcium excretion from the kidneys, absorption of calcium from the gastrointestinal tract, and mobilization of calcium from the bone. Calcium is absorbed in the intestines only under the influence of vitamin D, which is activated in the kidneys. It is reabsorbed in the proximal renal tubules after being filtered by the glomerulus and is excreted by the kidneys. Renal disease prevents activation of vitamin D, thus reducing the body's ability to absorb calcium.

Calcitonin and parathyroid hormone work in opposition to regulate calcium levels. When calcium levels are low, PTH is released by the parathyroid gland, stimulating the conversion of calcitriol (the active form of vitamin D), which causes the small intestines to absorb more calcium. PTH also stimulates release of calcium from bony tissues into the blood. When calcium levels are high, PTH secretion is suppressed as calcitonin is secreted by the thyroid, thereby inhibiting the release of calcium from bone into the blood.

Serum calcium can be measured in two different ways: as total calcium and as ionized calcium. These measurements evaluate body calcium in two different states:

Total Calcium. Total calcium reflects calcium bound to proteins (primarily albumin) in the serum. Total calcium levels are influenced by the patient's nutritional state. Therefore, if a patient's serum albumin level is low (e.g., from malnutrition, liver dysfunction), serum calcium levels will also be low. For every increase in albumin of 1.0 mg/dL, there is a 0.8 mg/dL increase in calcium concentration (Miller & Graham, 2006). A formula can be used to correct calcium based on serum albumin levels:

$$\text{Corrected Ca} = (4.0\text{ g/dL} - \text{plasma albumin}) \times 0.8 + \text{serum Ca}$$

Ionized Calcium. Approximately 50 percent of serum calcium exists in an ionized state. Ionized calcium represents the calcium that is used in the physiologic activities and is crucial for neuromuscular activity. The concentration of ionized calcium is inversely proportional to the albumin concentration (Miller & Graham, 2006). The lower the serum albumin, the higher the plasma ionized calcium. Ionized calcium levels, rather than total calcium, should be monitored in high-acuity patients (Miller & Graham, 2006).

Regulation of Potassium Balance

Potassium is the major intracellular cation, with almost all potassium being located within the cells. Proper distribution between the intracellular and extracellular fluid compartments as well as effective excretion is tightly controlled to maintain potassium homeostasis in the blood. Shifts between extra- and intracellular fluid are important because they respond rapidly and are responsible for the prevention of harmful fluctuations of extracellular potassium (Giebisch, Krapf & Wagner, 2007).

Although the concentration in the plasma is small, monitoring serum potassium is very important because the body is intolerant of abnormal serum levels. Potassium is readily found in many foods; thus, we normally consume sufficient quantities of potassium to meet daily requirements. Excess potassium is eliminated in the urine by the kidneys, and about 40 mEq/L of potassium is excreted daily in the urine.

Potassium is vital in maintaining normal cardiac and neuromuscular function because it affects muscle contraction. Potassium also influences nerve impulse conduction; therefore, abnormal serum potassium levels can produce potentially lethal cardiac conduction abnormalities, which could result in cardiac arrest. Potassium is vital to carbohydrate metabolism and plays an important role in normal cell membrane function. It is important in maintaining acid–base balance because hydrogen ions exchange with potassium ions.

Abnormal serum potassium levels are the most common electrolyte abnormality in high-acuity patients with nearly 20 percent having a level below 3.6 mEq/L (Miller & Graham, 2006). Pathophysiologic loss of serum potassium includes GI potassium loss that may be due to diarrhea, hyperaldosteronism, and prescribed drugs (such as diuretics). Causes of hyperkalemia include metabolic acidosis, insulin deficiency and hyperglycemia, tissue catabolism (rhabdomyolysis), renal tubular acidosis, tumor lysis syndrome secondary to chemotherapy, and beta-adrenergic blockade (Miller & Graham, 2006).

Elevated serum potassium levels are associated with renal failure because of the inability of the kidney to excrete potassium as a result of decreased glomerular filtration rate. Additionally, when metabolic acidosis is present, potassium shifts from the intracellular compartment to the extracellular space in exchange for hydrogen, in an effort to maintain extracellular acid-base balance (Broscious & Castagnola, 2006).

Regulation of Magnesium Balance

Magnesium is an intracellular electrolyte with a distribution similar to potassium. Magnesium ensures sodium and potassium transportation across cell membranes. It is needed for activation of certain enzymes required for normal protein and carbohydrate metabolism. Magnesium is crucial to many biochemical reactions and plays a significant role in nerve cell conduction. It is important in transmitting CNS messages and maintaining neuromuscular activity.

Magnesium is predominantly excreted in feces, but a small amount is excreted in the urine. The kidneys, however, have a remarkable ability to conserve magnesium. Magnesium balance is closely related to potassium and calcium balance.

Hypomagnesemia can occur as a result of GI and renal losses. GI losses may be due to chronic diarrhea, small bowel bypass surgery, malabsorption or pancreatitis (Miller & Graham, 2006). Hypermagnesemia is common in patients with impaired renal function or in those who have received large doses of magnesium. Renal excretion is the only regulatory mechanism for plasma magnesium. In high-acuity patients with renal dysfunction, medications such as laxatives and antacids may cause hypermagnesemia even at therapeutic doses (Miller & Graham, 2006).

Regulation of Phosphorus/Phosphate

Phosphorus is an intracellular mineral commonly found in many foods. In the body, it predominantly exists as phosphate (PO_4). Phosphorus plays an essential part in the development of teeth and bones. It is vital for normal neuromuscular function and is required for energy in the production ATP. It also contributes to protein, fat, and carbohydrate metabolism and assists in the maintenance of acid–base balance.

The serum phosphate level is under the influence of PTH and maintains an inverse relationship to calcium. The kidneys are essential to phosphorus regulation through reabsorption and excretion. When glomerular filtration decreases, phosphorus reabsorption increases, causing an elevation in serum levels. As glomerular filtration increases, phosphorus reabsorption diminishes allowing more phosphorus to be excreted by the kidneys, and reducing serum phosphate levels. Age-related changes in parathyroid function, along with decreased intake and impaired intestinal absorption, make mild hypophosphatemia common in the elderly high-acuity patient.

SECTION THREE REVIEW

1. A major function of Na^+ is
   - A. carbohydrate metabolism
   - B. tissue oxygenation
   - C. blood coagulation
   - D. fluid balance
2. Chloride levels closely follow the levels of which electrolyte?
   - A. K^+
   - B. Na^+
   - C. Ca^{++}
   - D. Mg^+
3. Calcium is absorbed in the intestines under the influence of
   - A. phosphorus
   - B. vitamin D
   - C. sodium
   - D. vitamin C
4. Hyperkalemia can be caused by
   - A. renal failure
   - B. diuretics
   - C. metabolic acidosis
   - D. severe diarrhea
5. Magnesium plays a role in which physiologic functions? (choose all that apply)
   - A. Na^+ and K^+ transport
   - B. nerve cell conduction
   - C. fluid regulation
   - D. energy transfer

Answers: 1. D, 2. B, 3. B, 4. A, 5. (A, B, D)

SECTION FOUR: Assessment of Fluid and Electrolyte Balance

At the completion of this section the learner will be able to state the components of an assessment of fluid and electrolyte balance in the high-acuity patient, list four important questions to ask during the nursing history that relate to fluid and electrolyte assessment, and recognize vital sign changes that indicate an alteration in fluid and electrolyte balance. The learner will also be able to discuss elements of physical assessment that indicate an alteration in fluid and electrolyte balance and identify hemodynamic and laboratory parameters that indicate an alteration in fluid and electrolyte balance.

History

A nursing history is an essential component of an assessment of fluid and electrolyte balance in the high-acuity patient. The following questions should be asked:

- Does the patient have an injury or disease process that can alter fluid and electrolyte balance? Examples may include nausea, vomiting, diarrhea, surgery, placement of a nasogastric tube, diaphoresis, or hyperventilation.
- Is the patient receiving any medications that can alter fluid and electrolyte balance? Examples may include diuretics, laxatives, nonsteroidal anti-inflammatory agents, glucocorticoids, or aminoglycosides.
- Does the patient have dietary restrictions that can alter fluid and electrolyte balance? Examples may include NPO, low-sodium diet restrictions, nausea, loss of appetite, or tube feedings.
- How does the total intake of fluids compare with the total output of fluids? If there an imbalance, what is the imbalance and how long has this imbalance existed?

Vital Signs

Temperature. Elevated temperature can result in excess loss of water and sodium through diaphoresis. Fever also increases basal metabolic rate. Excess water is made and excreted through tachypnea.

Pulse. Tachycardia is associated with decreased intravascular volume and hypomagnesemia and hypokalemia. Conversely, bradycardia can be associated with elevated serum levels of these electrolytes. Alterations in these electrolytes can also produce cardiac dysrhythmias (See Module 14, Assessment of Cardiac Rhythm: Basic ECG Rhythm Interpretation.)

Respirations. Alterations in potassium balance and/or low magnesium levels can cause weakness of respiratory muscles. Dyspnea with mild exertion or dyspnea at night may indicate pooling of fluid in the lungs. Severe acid-base disorders also can affect breathing patterns.

Blood Pressure. Blood pressure and pulse together provide valuable information about a patient's fluid volume status. Orthostatic vital sign measurement can be used to assess for dehydration, blood loss and the effects of antihypertensive medications. **Orthostatic hypotension** is defined as a drop in blood pressure of more than 20 mmHg or an increased in pulse greater than 20 bpm when going from a lying to sitting or sitting to standing position.

Physical Assessment

Inspection. Inspection can reveal important data about the patient's fluid volume status. The patient's eyes may appear to be sunken if a fluid volume deficit is present. A round swollen face may indicate fluid volume overload, such as that which occurs with patients who take steroids ("moon face"). The mouth should be inspected to determine if the oral tissues appear dry. If the patient is breathing through the mouth, fluids are lost through hyperventilation. The patient's tongue should also be checked to see if it appears dry. Additional furrows may be a sign of fluid volume deficit.

Assessment of jugular venous pressure is an important parameter to assess for fluid volume status (Fig. 25–6). Changes in fluid volume are reflected by changes in neck vein filling and can be used as an indicator of central venous pressure. The jugular vein on the right should be assessed because it is in close proximity to the right atrium.

Hand veins provide important data on volume status. Place the patient's hand in a dependent position and observe for venous distention. Hypovolemia may be present if venous filling takes longer than five seconds. Distention should disappear within five seconds when the hand is elevated. Distention that does not clear within five seconds may indicate hypervolemia.

Palpation. Tissue turgor is assessed by pinching the skin on the forehead, sternum or inner aspects of the thigh. In a patient with fluid volume deficit, the skin flattens more slowly after the pinch is released. Patients with advancing age, however, have reduced skin turgor as a result of less elastic tissue. Therefore, this assessment is not used as diagnostic in the elderly. Tissue turgor also varies with race and nutritional status.

Capillary refill. Decreased capillary refill may be present in patients with hypovolemia, vasoconstriction of peripheral vessels, decreased cardiac output, anemia, cold temperatures, or cigarette smoking.

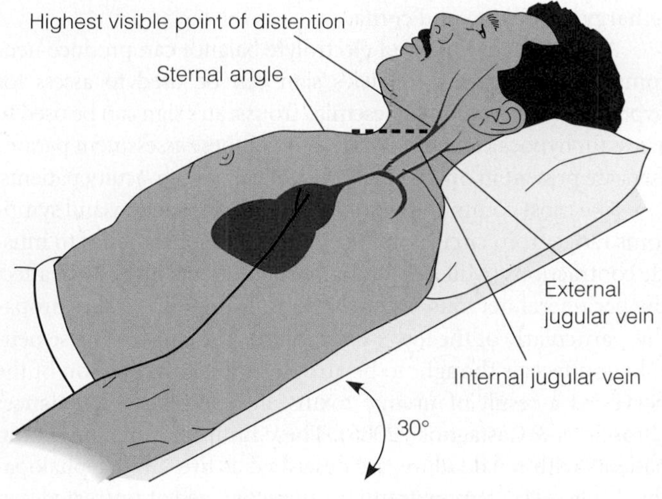

Figure 25–6 ■ Assessing jugular venous pressure.

Edema. **Edema** is an excess accumulation of fluid in interstitial spaces. If a hemodynamically significant volume of fluid escapes from the intravascular compartment into the interstitial or transcellular spaces, the high-acuity patient is at high risk for developing clinical manifestations consistent with hypovolemia or hypovolemic shock. (Hypovolemia and hypovolemic shock are discussed in detail in Module 18, Alterations in Oxygen Delivery and Oxygen Consumption: Shock States.) Edema and third spacing can be described in terms of certain characteristics, including location, whether it is pitting or nonpitting, and amount of fluid weight gain.

Location. Determining whether the edema is localized or generalized provides important clues as to its possible origin because pathologic conditions are usually associated with one or the other. Generalized edema is present all over the body and is primarily seen in the presence of decreased plasma proteins resulting from severe protein malnutrition. Localized edema results from a more localized pathologic condition, such as local inflammation and infection; however, generalized edema develops secondary to a localized process that has expanded, causing widespread damage to the capillary endothelium and generalized edema. Examples of severe conditions in which this form of secondary generalized edema can occur are septic and anaphylactic shock.

Localized edema is confined to areas in which the causative condition is affecting the capillaries or lymph tissues (e.g., the area of inflammation, obstruction, or high capillary hydrostatic pressure). The edema associated with congestive heart failure is considered localized because it is confined to the gravity-dependent body areas (e.g., feet, lower legs, and sacrum). Pulmonary edema caused by left-sided heart failure is localized edema created by increased capillary hydrostatic pressure in the lungs as a result of elevated left heart pressures.

The exact clinical manifestations associated with edema and third spacing depend on their location. For example, a patient with pulmonary edema or pleural effusion is at risk for developing pulmonary gas exchange problems, usually hypoxemia. A patient with cerebral edema is at risk for cerebral herniation, which is a life-threatening complication that clinically presents as a rapid deterioration of the patient's level of consciousness, visual, motor, and respiratory status. Edema around a joint reduces range of motion or immobilizes the joint. Severe edema can compress capillary blood flow, causing tissue ischemia and pain. A patient with ascites may develop problems with gas exchange as fluid in the peritoneal cavity begins to displace the diaphragm upward or impede diaphragmatic movement. A patient with pericardial effusion may develop signs of circulatory shock in the presence of cardiac tamponade.

Pitting or Nonpitting Edema. Pitting edema develops when the accumulation of fluid exceeds what can be absorbed by the interstitial tissue gel. Firm pressure applied to the edematous area displaces the interstitial fluid, causing a temporary pitting (Fig. 25–7). It can be measured on a scale of 1 to 4 based on the depth and the length of time it takes for the indentation to disappear.

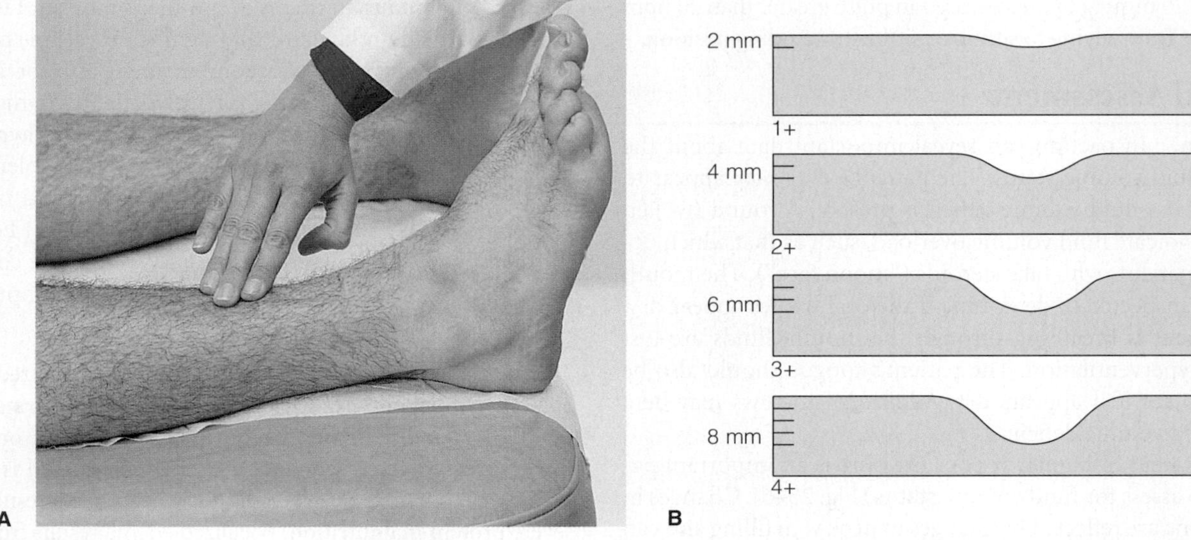

Figure 25–7 ■ Evaluation of edema. **A,** Palpating for edema over the tibia. **B,** Four-point scale for grading edema.

- +1: 2 mm indentation, disappears rapidly
- +2: 4 mm indentation, disappears in 10 to 15 seconds
- +3: 6 mm indentation, disappears within 1 to 2 minutes
- +4: 8 mm indentation, disappears in 2 to 5 minutes

Body Weight. In the adult, peripheral edema develops when 5 L or more of fluid have accumulated in the interstitial spaces, and pitting edema develops with an accumulation of 10 L or more of interstitial fluid. Clinically, a weight gain or loss of 1 kg (2.2 lbs) represents a fluid gain or loss of about 1 L. Evaluating daily weight trends provides valuable information on fluid status.

Assessment of third-spaced fluids is more difficult because the serous cavities are deep structures, particularly the pericardial sac and pleural cavity. A thorough evaluation is necessary and may include a comprehensive physical examination, chest or abdominal radiography, electrocardiogram, echocardiogram, and others. Ascites can involve fluid shifts that are hemodynamically significant. For this reason, close evaluation of arterial blood pressure and serum albumin is important. In addition, daily weights and abdominal girth measurements provide valuable trending data.

Auscultation

Auscultation of the heart may reveal a third or fourth heart sound in patients with fluid volume overload. Tachycardia and hypotension may indicate fluid volume deficit. A pericardial friction rub may be heard and is a sign of an accumulation of fluid in the pericardial sac around the heart, a condition known as **pericarditis.** This is a complication that can occur in patients with renal failure.

Auscultation of the lungs provide extremely valuable information to determine the presence of pulmonary edema. Pulmonary edema results from a shifting of fluid from the vascular space into the pulmonary interstitium. Crackles indicate fluid volume overload (See Module 9, Determinants and Assessment of Pulmonary Gas Exchange.)

Percussion

Pain upon percussion of the flank area may indicate a urinary tract infection that has extended into the kidneys. Percussion of the abdomen can provide information about fluid volume status, particularly in patients with ascites. **Ascites** is an abnormal accumulation of fluid in the peritoneal cavity. Patients with renal failure may have ascites as a result of increased capillary hydrostatic pressure and fluid volume excess. Patients with liver failure may have ascites as a result of decreased intravascular oncotic pressure as a result of decreased serum albumin. Patients with liver failure and ascites have decreased intravascular volume and actually have fluid volume deficit.

Neuromuscular Assessment

Changes in mental status may be due to alterations in fluid and electrolyte balance. Disorientation may occur with acidosis. Alterations in sodium, magnesium and calcium can produce a variety of mental status changes including apprehension, lethargy, confusion and coma.

Alterations in fluid and electrolyte balance can produce neuromuscular changes. Chvostek's sign can be used to assess for hypocalcemia or hypomagnesemia. Trousseau's sign can be used to assess for hypocalcemia. However, both of these assessment parameters are present in only a small percentage of high-acuity patients.

The most common sign of hypocalcemia is tetany and symptoms range from circumoral numbness and paresthesias to muscle contractions (Miller & Graham, 2006). Renal failure can affect the peripheral nervous system and result in peripheral neuropathy, particularly of the lower extremities. The cause of these neurologic effects is thought to be atrophy and demyelination of the nerves as a result of uremic toxins and electrolyte imbalances (Broscious & Castagnola, 2006). These findings, when present in patients with renal failure, are described as uremic encephalopathy. Acute severe hyponatremia, if unrecognized or untreated, can cause irreversible neurological damage or death (Haskal, 2007).

Hemodynamic Monitoring

Hemodynamic monitoring of fluid volume status in high-acuity patients is common, and includes measurements such as central venous pressure (CVP), pulmonary artery wedge pressure (PAWP), cardiac output (CO), cardiac index (CI), and mean arterial pressure (MAP). For a full discussion of these parameters, see Module 13, Assessment of Hemodynamic Status: Hemodynamic Monitoring.

The CVP represents the filling pressure of the right atrium and is a measure of right ventricular preload. Fluid volume deficit is associated with a low CVP, whereas fluid volume excess is associated with a high CVP. The PAWP represents the left atrial pressure and left ventricular pressure at end-diastole. This represents blood volume in the left ventricle, or left ventricular preload. As left ventricular preload increases, PAWP increases and visa versa. CO and CI demonstrate the ejection volume of the heart. When CO and CI are low, the patient may have fluid volume deficit and conversely, when CO and CI are high , the patient may have fluid volume excess; however, cardiac pump failure can occur as a result of fluid volume excess in which case the CO and CI decrease (See Module 15, Alterations in Cardiac Output.).

Laboratory Assessment

Blood Urea Nitrogen. Blood urea nitrogen (BUN) is a byproduct of protein metabolism. Normal BUN values are 9-20 mg/dL. With renal dysfunction and a decrease in glomerular filtration rate (GFR), there is decreased excretion of BUN and therefore an increase in serum BUN levels. However, BUN can increase in the presence of normal kidney function (Bagshaw & Gibney, 2008). Conditions that elevate BUN in the presence of normal kidney function are summarized in Table 25–3. Therefore, BUN levels must be interpreted with caution.

Serum Creatinine. Creatinine (Cr) is an amino acid compound located in skeletal muscle and subsequently is metabolized in the liver. It is released at a relatively constant rate, is freely filtered by the glomerulus and is not reabsorbed or metabolized by the kidney (Bagshaw & Gibney, 2008). The normal range of serum creatinine is 0.6 to 1.5 mg/dL. Creatinine is affected by fewer conditions than is BUN and is therefore a better indicator of renal function. Cr levels increase in states of renal dysfunction.

TABLE 25–3 Conditions That Elevate BUN in the Presence of Normal Kidney Function

Hypovolemia
Excessive Protein Intake
Excessive Protein Catabolism (Examples: starvation, poor nutrition, trauma, surgery)
GI Bleeding
Hematoma Reabsorption
Drugs (Examples: tetracycline, steroids)

Serum BUN to Cr Ratio. The normal ratio of BUN to Cr is 10:1. A change in the ratio can identify the etiology of renal dysfunction. If the ratio is greater than 10:1, the BUN is elevated and the likely etiology is hypovolemia. If both BUN and Cr are elevated and the ratio remains 10:1, then the etiology is likely renal tubuole dysfunction.

Serum Osmolality. Osmolality is expressed in milliosmoles (mOsm), with normal serum osmolality in an adult being 280 to 300 mOsm/kg. Serum values of less than 240 mOsm/kg or more than 320 mOsm/kg are considered critically abnormal. A low serum osmolality suggests fluid volume excess or hemodilution, meaning there is more fluid than solute in the serum. A high serum osmolality suggests fluid volume deficit or hemoconcentration, meaning there is less fluid than solute in the serum. The following formula can be used to calculate serum osmolality:

$$\text{Serum Osm/L} = (\text{serum Na} \times 2) + \frac{\text{BUN}}{3} + \frac{\text{Glucose}}{18}$$

For example: Given that a patient's sodium (Na) is 140 mEq/L, blood urea nitrogen (BUN) is 20 mg/dL, glucose is 250 mg/dL, using the preceding formula, it can be calculated that the serum osmolality is 301 Osm/L. This indicates that there are more particles than fluid in this patient's serum. This osmolality is slightly high, which suggests fluid volume deficit.

Clinically, serum osmolality can be used to determine the need for fluid replacement in the high-acuity patient.

Anion Gap. The anion gap is a calculation of the difference between the cations (sodium, potassium) and anions (chloride and bicarbonate) as shown in the formula below:

$$Na^+ - (Cl^- + HCO_3^-)$$

Normal anion gap is 1-12 mEq/L. The anion gap can be used to determine the cause of metabolic acidosis. Normally the kidney conserves HCO_3^- and excretes H^+. In conditions where the glomeruli are damaged, metabolic acids (such as phosphoric and sulfuric acid) are retained, causing a widening of the gap. An increased anion gap reflects decreased excretion or increased production of acid products. Anion gap is increased with renal failure because of decreased bicarbonate reabsorption and retention of acids.

Serum Albumin. Albumin is synthesized in the liver and it represents the majority of the proteins carried in the blood. Normal blood levels are 3.5 to 5.5 g/dL. As discussed in Section One, albumin is responsible for maintaining intravascular oncotic pressure. The most common cause of decreased plasma albumin levels is related to the inflammatory process. With inflammatory processes, there are four potential causative factors including hemodilution, loss of extravascular volume, increased consumption by cells locally, and decreased synthesis (Hankins, 2006).

Evaluation of Urine

Urine Volume. Evaluating urine output via an indwelling catheter is standard practice and routinely measured in high-acuity patients; however, urine output in general lacks sensitivity

Emerging Evidence

- Due to significant alterations in fluid balance after tube feedings, close attention to recording of fluid balance such as intake/output measurements, body weights and simple bedside assessments is needed to detect fluid imbalances and other serious complications at an early stage in enteral tube feedings (*Oh & Seo, 2007*).
- Cystatin C is an endogenous cysteine proteinase inhibitor that holds many ideal features for use as a surrogate marker of kidney function and GFR. A reduction in GFR correlates well with a rise in serum cystatin C level and performs comparably or superior to that of serum Cr for discrimination of normal from impaired kidney function (*Villa, Jimenez, Soriano et al., 2005*).

and specificity as a marker of kidney function (Bagshaw & Gibney, 2008). It is not a function of the kidneys to make urine. The kidneys produce urine as a byproduct of regulating fluid and electrolyte balance in the body. Therefore, it can be misleading to evaluate kidney function strictly by the volume of urine output. Under normal conditions, a low urine volume suggests fluid volume deficit and a high urine volume suggests fluid volume excess. That said, Table 25–4 summarizes a number of conditions that alter the volume of urine output.

Urine Concentration. Urinary specific gravity (SG) measures the ability of the kidneys to concentrate urine. It is a measurement of the density, or weight of urine compared to distilled water. Distilled water has a SG of 1.000. Normal urine SG is 1.003-1.030. Decreased urine SG indicates concentrated urine which can occur with fluid volume deficit or glomerular disease (such as diabetic nephropathy). However, urine SG can be elevated out of proportion to the actual concentration in the presence of high urine concentrations of glucose, albumin, or radiocontrast dyes. Therefore, it is more accurate to measure urine osmolality in patients with glycosuria, proteinuria, or recent administration of radiocontrast dyes. Urine osmolality can be directly measured. This measurement is more accurate than urine SG as an indicator of the kidney's ability to concentrate urine (Goertz, 2006). Normal urine osmolality is 300-1200 mOsm/L. Urine osmolality increases during fluid volume deficit as the kidneys hold onto water (urine output decreases). Urine osmolality decreases during fluid volume excess as the kidneys excrete more water (urine output increases).

TABLE 25–4 Conditions That Alter the Volume of Urine Output

Volume Status	Decreased cardiac output decreases renal blood flow, decreases glomerular filtration rate, decreased urine output.
Hormones	Renin-angiotensin-aldosterone system Antidiuretic hormone (See Module 18, Alterations in Oxygen Delivery and Oxygen Consumption: Shock States)
Solute Load	Urine volume is increased in conditions where there is increased solute load such as hyperglycemia, alcohol, elevated protein or nitrogenous waste products)
Decreased concentrating ability of the kidneys	Urine volume increases when the kidneys lose their ability to concentrate urine

Electrolytes. Measurement of urine electrolytes is often made though collection of a 24-hour urine specimen. One of the most common urinary electrolytes assessed is sodium. Urinary sodium is helpful in assessing volume status, hyponatremia, acute renal failure, and dietary compliance with patients on sodium-restricted diets. Urine sodium levels are low in patients who have fluid volume deficit as the kidneys retain sodium to increased intravascular volume. Urine sodium levels increases with renal disease, osmotic diuresis, and hypoaldosteronism.

Assessment of excretion of sodium in the presence of oliguria gives insight into the cause of oliguria. The fractional excretion of sodium (FeNa) is calculated as:

$$\text{FeNa} = (\text{urine Na}/\text{plasma Na})/(\text{urine Cr}/\text{plasma Cr})$$

A FeNa less than 1 percent denotes fluid volume deficit. In this situation, oliguria is due to fluid volume deficit as the kidneys try to restore intravascular volume by retaining sodium and water. FeNa greater than 1 percent denotes oliguria and loss of sodium which can occur with renal failure. Although this seems physiologically sensible, in clinical practice the diagnostic accuracy is poor, and its value has been questioned (Bagshaw and Gibney, 2008). There are conditions that affect the accuracy of FeNa including the administration of diuretics, radiocontrast dyes, and adrenal insufficiency.

Urinalysis. Urinalysis involves simple observation and separate measurements using commercially available dipsticks. Urine pH is usually 5.0. Urine is generally acidic as a result of net acid excretion. Alkaline urine may be present in patients on a vegetarian diet, when there is an infection, or acute tubular acidosis. Glucose maybe present during pregnancy and diabetes mellitus. Proteinuria occurs in the presence of glomerular basement membrane disease. The most common protein lost in the urine is albumin. Heme can be present in the urine and can indicate the presence of hemoglobin, myoglobin or red blood cells. Urine sediment is an important component in the assessment of renal disease. The sediment describes the cellular components present in the urine. These can include red blood cells, white blood cells, tubular cells, transitional cells, and squamous epithelial cells.

Creatinine Clearance. Creatinine clearance (CrCl) provides information about kidney function. It is the amount of creatinine secreted in the urine and the amount of Cr in the blood over a 24-hour period. CrCl is the most widely used measure for estimating GFR (Bagshaw & Gibney, 2008). As renal function decreases, CrCl decreases. CrCl is estimated by use of the Cockcroft-Gault formula as listed below:

$$\text{CrCl} = \frac{(140 - \text{age})(\text{weight in kg})(0.85\text{ for women})}{72 \times \text{serum Cr (mg/dL)}}$$

CrCl can also be calculated after obtaining a 24-hour urine sample using the formula below:

$$\text{CrCl} = \frac{\text{Urine Cr} \times \text{volume}}{\text{Plasma Cr}}$$

SECTION FOUR REVIEW

1. Elevated temperature can cause fluid volume deficit through which process? (choose all that apply)
   A. diaphoresis
   B. tachypnea
   C. vasoconstriction
   D. diarrhea
2. In performing a physical assessment it is noted that the patient has pitting edema around the ankles with 4 mm indentation that disappears within 10 seconds. This should be documented as
   A. +1 pitting edema
   B. +2 pitting edema
   C. +3 pitting edema
   D. +4 pitting edema
3. The normal BUN to Cr ratio is
   A. 1:1
   B. 1:5
   C. 5:1
   D. 10:1
4. An increased anion gap reflects
   A. increased serum osmolality
   B. increased renal excretion of sodium
   C. decreased excretion or increased production of acids
   D. inability of the kidneys to concentrate urine
5. A urinalysis reveals a high urine osmolality. What assessment is most accurate?
   A. hypoglycemia
   B. fluid volume deficit
   C. fluid volume excess
   D. hyponatremia

Answers 1. A, B, 2. B, 3. D, 4. C, 5. B

POSTTEST

The following Posttest is constructed in a case study format. A patient is presented, and questions are asked based on available data. New data are presented as the case study progresses.

Donald R., 75-years-old, was admitted to the hospital with severe dyspnea. He has a history of chronic alcohol abuse and cirrhosis. On admission, the nurse assesses the following: Thin, chronically ill-appearing male. Blood pressure 108/62 mm Hg; pulse 118/min; RR 26/min; temperature 97.8°F (36.6°C). He has 3+ pitting generalized edema. His abdomen is distended and tight. He has orthopnea and complains of shortness of breath. Mr. R. states that he has been confined to his chair or couch for the past two weeks because of his breathing difficulty and general weakness.

1. Mr. R.'s age and poor physical condition place him at risk for development of
   A. Alzheimer's disease
   B. dehydration
   C. acute renal failure
   D. congestive heart failure
2. Mr. R.'s edema is an example of fluid located in which space?
   A. intracellular
   B. intravascular
   C. interstitial
   D. transcellular
3. Assuming Mr. R.'s abdominal distention is ascites, the shift of intravascular fluid into his peritoneal cavity is referred to as
   A. third spacing
   B. heart failure
   C. edema
   D. peritonitis
4. As Mr. R.'s blood pressure decreases, the baroreceptors will trigger
   A. renal vasodilation
   B. decreased heart rate
   C. suppression of ACTH release
   D. peripheral vasoconstriction

Mr. R.'s urine output has been 25 mL/hr for the past two hours. His most current serum osmolality is 315 mOsm/L. He is complaining of extreme thirst.

5. Based on the available data, his urine output and serum osmolality are most likely the result of
   A. renal failure
   B. peripheral edema
   C. suppressed ADH release
   D. intravascular fluid deficit
6. His thirst is activated by
   A. hemodilution
   B. release of aldosterone
   C. increased osmolality
   D. ADH release

Mr. R. has a serum albumin drawn. The results show a significantly low albumin level.

7. A low serum albumin directly alters the Starling forces in which way?
   A. Fluids escape out of the capillaries.
   B. Fluids are drawn into the capillaries.
   C. Fluids escape out of the interstitial spaces.
   D. Fluids are drawn into the interstitial spaces.

It is decided that Mr. R. requires intravenous fluids. Mr. R. has received a large volume of IV fluids. His serum electrolytes are drawn. The results are

Sodium: 128 mEq/L
Chloride: 90 mEq/L
Total calcium: 5.8 mEq/L
Potassium: 5.2 mEq/L
Magnesium: 2.7 mEq/L
Phosphate: 1.5 mEq/L

8. Mr. R.'s serum sodium can cause body water to shift from the
A. extracellular into the intravascular compartment
B. interstitial into the intravascular compartment
C. extracellular into the intracellular compartment
D. intracellular into the extracellular compartment

9. Mr. R.'s total calcium level is 4.0 mEq/L. This level is most likely caused by his
A. renal status
B. nutritional status
C. chloride status
D. immobilized status

10. Should Mr. R.'s serum potassium level approach 7 mEq/L, the nurse would be MOST concerned about changes in which body system?
A. cardiovascular
B. respiratory
C. neurologic
D. renal

11. Mr. R. has hypomagnesemia. This can be caused by (choose all that apply)
A. hypercalcemia
B. chronic alcoholism
C. starvation
D. acute pancreatitis

Posttest answers with rationale are found on MyNursingKit.

REFERENCES

Bagshaw, S. M., & Gibney, R. T. N. (2008). Conventional markers of kidney function. *Critical Care Medicine 36*(4 Suppl): 5152–5158.

Broscious, S. K. & Castagnola, J. (2006). Chronic kidney disease: acute manifestations and role of critical care nurses. *Critical Care Nurse 26*(4): 17–28.

Capasso, G. (2006). A crucial nephron segment in acid-base and electrolyte transport: The collecting tubule. *Kidney International 70*;1674–1676.

David, L. (2007). IV fluids: do you know what's hanging and why? *RN*, October:35–41.

Giebisch, G. Krapf, R., Wagner, C. (2007). Renal and extrarenal regulation of potassium. *Kidney International 72*:397–410.

Goertz, S. (2006). Gauging fluid balance with osmolality. *Nursing 2006 36*(10), 70–71.

Hankins, J. (2006). The role of albumin in fluid and electrolyte balance. *Journal of Infusion Nursing 29*(5): 260–265.

Haskal, R. (2007). Current issues for nurse practitioners: hyponatremia. *Journal of the American Academy of Nurse Practitioners 19*:563–579.

Miller, W., & Graham, M. G. (2006). Life-threatening electrolyte abnormalities. *Patient Care*, December: 19–27.

Oh, H., & Seo, W. (2007). Alterations in fluid, electrolytes and other serum chemistry values and their relations with enteral feeding in acute brain infarction patients. *Journal of Clinical Nursing 16*:298–307.

Villa, P., Jimenez, M., Soriano, M. C., et al. (2005). Serum cystatin C concentration is a marker of acute renal dysfunction in critically ill patients. *Critical Care 9*(2): R139–143.

MODULE

26 Alterations in Fluid and Electrolyte Balance

Karen L. Johnson

OBJECTIVES Following completion of this module, the learner will be able to

1. Discuss the etiology, manifestations, medical treatment, and nursing care for a patient with fluid volume deficit.
2. Discuss the etiology, manifestations, medical treatment, and nursing care for a patient with fluid volume excess.
3. Discuss the etiology, manifestations, medical treatment, and nursing care for a patient with alterations in sodium balance.
4. Discuss the etiology, manifestations, medical treatment, and nursing care for a patient with alterations in calcium balance.
5. Discuss the etiology, manifestations, medical treatment, and nursing care for a patient with alterations in potassium balance.
6. Discuss the etiology, manifestations, medical treatment, and nursing care for a patient with alterations in magnesium balance.
7. Discuss the etiology, manifestations, medical treatment, and nursing care for a patient with alterations in phosphorus/phosphate balance.

This self-study module is composed of seven sections that present the etiology, manifestations, medical treatment, and nursing care for patients with alterations in fluid and electrolyte balance. Sections One and Two focus on alterations in fluid volume, including fluid volume deficit and fluid volume excess. In Sections Three and Four, imbalances of sodium and calcium are discussed. Sections Five through Seven discuss imbalances of potassium, magnesium, and phosphorus.

Each section includes a set of review questions to assist the learner in evaluating his or her understanding of the section's content before moving on to the next section. All Section Reviews include answers. It is suggested that the learner review those concepts answered incorrectly in the review questions before proceeding to the next section.

PRETEST

1. High-acuity patients are at high risk for fluid volume deficit from insensible fluid losses. Which of the following contribute to insensible fluid loss? (choose all that apply)
   A. diaphoresis
   B. hyperventilation
   C. fever
   D. mechanical ventilation
2. Which of the following intravenous solutions closely approximates serum osmolality?
   A. 0.45 percent normal saline
   B. 5 percent dextrose in normal saline
   C. lactated Ringer's
   D. 3 percent normal saline
3. Nursing assessment data found in the patient with fluid volume excess would include
   A. low pulmonary artery wedge pressure
   B. increased hematocrit
   C. moist crackles
   D. decreased blood pressure
4. Factors that produce fluid volume excess include (choose all that apply)
   A. cirrhosis
   B. cancer
   C. corticosteriods
   D. low sodium intake
5. Signs and symptoms of hypernatremia include
   A. diarrhea
   B. muscle twitching
   C. stomach cramps
   D. decreased muscle tone
6. Hyponatremia is associated with which of the following symptoms?
   A. edema
   B. hyperreflexia
   C. lethargy
   D. restlessness

7. Hypocalcemia is associated with which of the following clinical findings?
   A. tingling and numbness
   B. constipation
   C. lethargy
   D. shortened *QT* interval
8. Treatment for hypercalcemia may include (choose all that apply)
   A. calcium gluconate
   B. calcium carbonate
   C. IV fluids
   D. diuretics
9. The presence of hypokalemia alters renal excretion of potassium in which of the following ways?
   A. Urine output increases.
   B. Potassium excretion increases.
   C. Potassium is reabsorbed.
   D. Potassium excretion does not change.
10. Which of the following lab values is commonly seen with hyperkalemia?
    A. metabolic alkalosis
    B. metabolic acidosis
    C. respiratory alkalosis
    D. respiratory acidosis
11. The symptoms of hypomagnesemia reflect
    A. central nervous system (CNS) hypoactivity
    B. fluid compartment shifts
    C. cardiac depressant effects
    D. neuromuscular and CNS hyperactivity
12. The symptoms of hypermagnesemia include
    A. absent deep tendon reflexes
    B. tremors
    C. ventricular tachycardia
    D. tetany
13. Hypophosphatemia is associated with which of the following conditions?
    A. malnourished state
    B. metabolic alkalosis
    C. hypocalcemia
    D. hyperthyroidism
14. Severe hypophosphatemia is associated with which of the following symptoms?
    A. joint pain
    B. muscle cramping
    C. respiratory arrest
    D. peptic ulcer disease

Pretest answers are found on MyNursingKit.

SECTION ONE: Alterations in Fluid Balance: Fluid Volume Deficit

At the completion of this section, the learner will be able to discuss the etiology, manifestations, medical treatment, and nursing care for patients with fluid volume deficit (hypovolemia).

Etiology

Extracellular fluid (ECF) volume deficit exists when there is **hypovolemia,** an abnormally low volume of body fluid in the intravascular or interstitial compartments. This produces a state of extracellular dehydration associated with serum hyperosmolality that can lead to intracellular dehydration as fluid shifts out of the cells to increase extracellular volume. It is a common and potentially serious problem in the high-acuity patient. Many factors can cause or contribute to development of fluid volume deficit. These factors are summarized in Table 26–1. Depending on the type of fluid loss, fluid volume deficit can occur slowly or rapidly.

Loss of ECF fluid volume can be due to **third spacing.** Third spacing is the shift of fluid from the intravascular compartment into a "third" (transcellular) space—usually a **serous cavity.** Normally, there is no accumulation of serosal fluid in a serous cavity. The cavities usually remain empty because of balanced Starling forces and the presence of a rich lymphatic network. If, however, any of the Starling forces become imbalanced or lymphatic drainage becomes obstructed or inadequate, a significant volume of serous fluid or exudate can rapidly accumulate. As fluid fills the cavity, pressure is exerted on the soft structures in the cavity, which can result in compression of those structures (e.g., cardiac tamponade). Fluids that are sequestered in a third space are unavailable for physiologic use by the body and may accumulate rapidly because of protein-rich contents, which causes increased tissue colloidal osmotic pressure, attracting more fluids. Third spacing may occur in the peritoneal cavity, pleural cavity, and pericardial sac and is associated with underlying problems such as intestinal obstruction, liver or renal failure, and peritonitis. Clinically, third spacing manifests itself as ascites, pericardial and pleural effusions, and other conditions.

TABLE 26–1 Factors That Produce Fluid Volume Deficit

SOURCE OF FLUID LOSS	RELATED FACTORS
Gastrointestinal	Diarrhea, vomiting, nasogastric suction, fistulas
Urinary	Drug therapy (e.g., diuretics), uncontrolled diabetes, diabetes insipidus, diuretic phase of acute tubular necrosis (ATN)
Integumentary	Burns, diaphoresis, increased capillary permeability
Insensible	Hyperventilation, fever, hypermetabolism, tachypnea, mechanical ventilation
Other	Wound drainage

Manifestations

Assessing the high-acuity patient for the presence of fluid volume deficit is an important part of the daily nursing assessment. Figure 26–1 summarizes common clinical assessments.

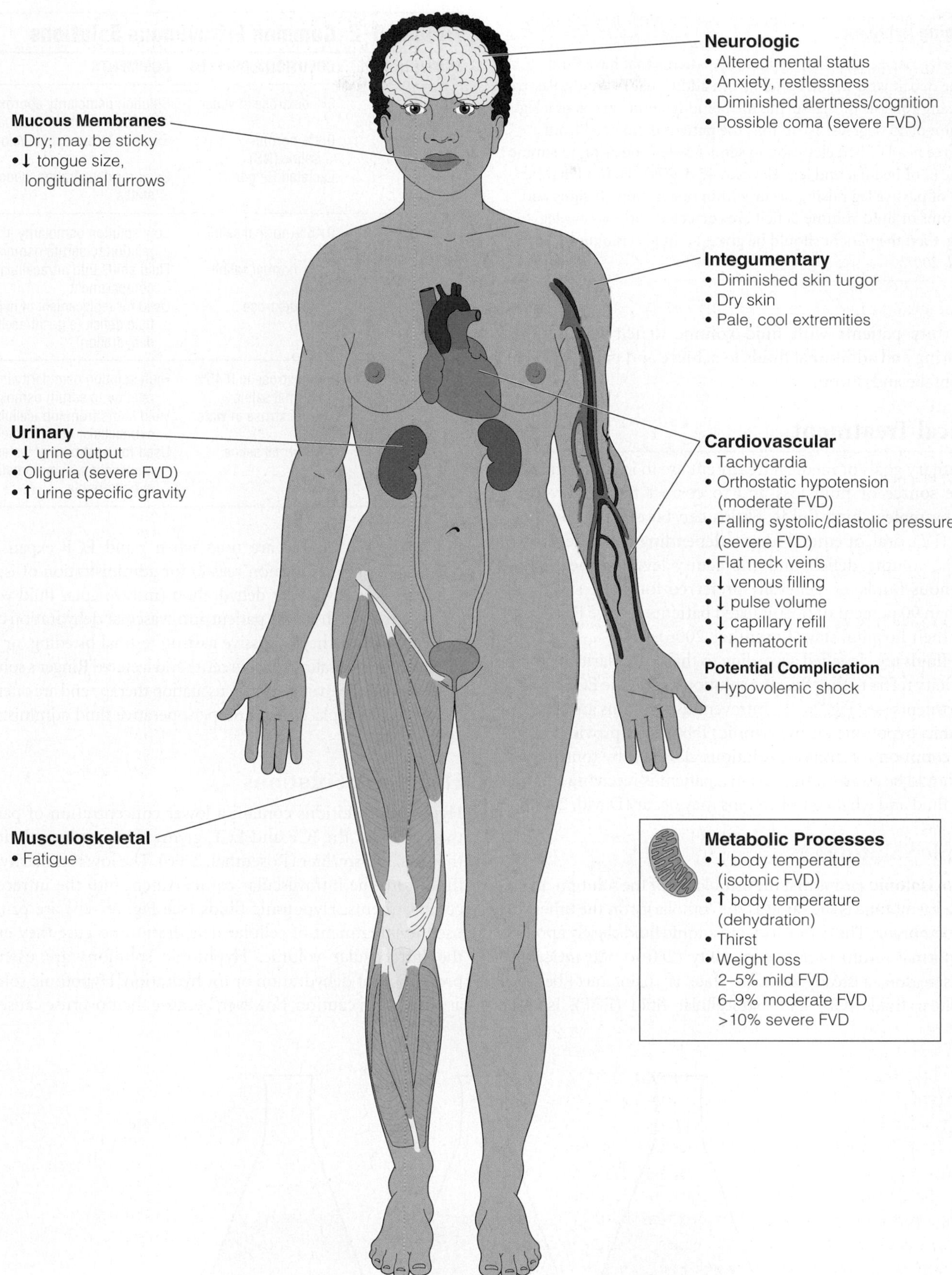

Figure 26–1 ■ Multisystem effects of fluid volume deficit.

Emerging Evidence

- Passive leg raising may help to identify patients that have fluid volume deficit who would benefit from additional IV fluids. Passive leg raising consists of measuring the hemodynamic effects of a leg elevation of 45 degrees. To do this, the patient is changed from a 45 degree head of bed elevation in semi-Fowler's position to supine with head of bed flat and legs elevated 45 degrees. Hemodynamic effects of passive leg raising occur within one minute. If signs and symptoms of fluid volume deficit are corrected with passive leg raising, then the patient should be given IV fluids (*Monnet & Teboul, 2007*).

TABLE 26–2 Common Intravenous Solutions

SOLUTION TYPE	SOLUTION EXAMPLES	COMMENTS
Isotonic	5% dextrose in water	Solution osmolarity approximates the osmolarity of plasma
	0.9% normal saline (NS)	Expands intravascular volume
	Lactated Ringer's	Used for dehydration, shock states
Hypotonic	0.45% normal saline	Low solution osmolarity in relation to serum osmolality
	0.2% normal saline	Fluid shifts into intracellular compartment
	2.5% dextrose	Used for replacement of hypotonic fluid deficit (e.g., intracellular dehydration)
Hypertonic	5% dextrose in 0.45% normal saline	High solution osmolarity in relation to serum osmolality
	10% dextrose in water	Fluid shifts from intracellular to extracellular compartments
	3% normal saline	Used for treatment of water intoxication, symptomatic hyponatremia

High-acuity patients with fluid volume deficit require close monitoring and additional fluids to achieve and maintain a balanced intake and output.

Medical Treatment

The primary goals of medical treatment are to identify and control the source of fluid loss and to correct the fluid volume deficit by replenishing fluids. Fluids can be replaced by intravenous (IV), oral, or enteral routes, depending on the severity of the fluid volume deficit and the acuity level of the patient. Intravenous fluids are generally preferred for acute situations. More than 90 percent of hospitalized patients receive IV therapy during their hospital stay (Rosenthal, 2006).

IV fluids are classified according to their osmolarity or tonicity. **Tonicity** refers to the effect the solution has on the ECF and ICF compartments (see Fig. 26–2). Intravenous solutions are classified as isotonic, hypotonic, or hypertonic. Table 26–2 provides examples of common intravenous solutions classified by tonicity. The nurse should be aware of the reason a patient is receiving a particular IV fluid and what complications may occur (David, 2007).

Isotonic Solutions

The term **isotonic** means that the osmolarity of the solution on one side of a membrane is the same as the osmolarity on the other side of the membrane. The osmolarity of isotonic fluid closely approximates normal serum plasma osmolality (280 to 300 mOsm/L). For this reason, a steady osmolar state is maintained between intracellular fluid (ICF) and extracellular fluid (ECF). Isotonic fluids (see Fig. 26–2a) are used when rapid ECF expansion is needed. The most common reason for administration of isotonic solutions is intravascular dehydration (intravascular fluid volume deficit). In the high-acuity patient, intravascular dehydration can result from hemorrhage, massive gastrointestinal bleeding, or dehydration. Normal saline (0.9 percent) and lactated Ringer's solutions are currently the mainstay of resuscitation therapy and are often used for electrolyte replacement and perioperative fluid administration (David, 2007).

Hypotonic Solutions

Hypotonic solutions contain a lower concentration of particles than exists in the ICF and ECF, giving them an osmolarity less than 280 mOsm/liter (Rosenthal, 2006). The low osmolarity shifts fluid from the intravascular compartment into the intracellular compartments. Hypotonic fluids (see Fig. 26–2b) are primarily used for treatment of cellular dehydration because they expand the intracellular volume. Hypotonic solutions are useful for prevention of dehydration or for hydration. Hypotonic solutions are used with caution, however, because their overuse causes cells

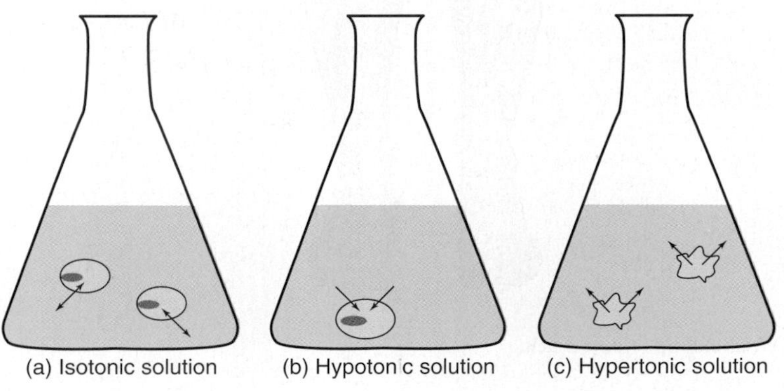

Figure 26–2 ■ Tonicity.

(including blood cells) to expand and burst, resulting in cellular destruction. It is of particular importance to avoid hypotonic solutions in patients with neurological problems, particularly those with increased intracranial pressure. Cellular overexpansion from hypotonic solutions will result in increased intracranial pressure and mental status deterioration.

Hypertonic Solutions

Hypertonic solutions have a high osmolarity (greater than 300 mOsm/liter) because they contain a higher concentration of particles than exists in the ICF and ECF (Rosenthal, 2006). The high osmolarity of the hypertonic solutions shifts fluids from the ICF and ECF into the intravascular compartment, expanding blood volume. Hypertonic solutions (see Fig. 26–2c) are used in the treatment of water intoxication (intracellular fluid volume excess). In the high-acuity patient, water intoxication can be caused by administration of large amounts of electrolyte-free water, overuse of hypotonic solutions (e.g., 0.45 percent sodium chloride), elevated ADH secretion, or renal failure. In addition, overuse of 5 percent dextrose and water (an isotonic solution) can result in water intoxication because of the rapid metabolizing of glucose, which then leaves a hypotonic water solution remaining in the intravascular compartment.

Nursing Care

Nursing diagnoses for patients with fluid volume deficit may include *fluid volume deficit, ineffective tissue perfusion*, and *risk for injury*. Nursing interventions may include measures to decrease vomiting, diarrhea, or fever; increasing oral fluid intake or administration of intravenous solutions; and monitoring of fluid and electrolyte status. Desired patient outcomes include pulse, blood pressure, central venous pressure (CVP), and pulmonary artery wedge pressure (PAWP) within acceptable ranges for the patient; normal serum osmolality; increased urine output with normal specific gravity; improved skin turgor; balanced intake and output; stable weight; moist mucous membranes; hematocrit and blood urea nitrogen (BUN) within acceptable limits; and absence of other dehydration manifestations.

SECTION ONE REVIEW

1. Third spacing of fluids is most commonly located in
   A. joints
   B. a serous cavity
   C. the cranial vault
   D. interstitial fluid
2. Which statement is correct regarding ECF volume deficit?
   A. It can lead to transcellular expansion.
   B. It can lead to intracellular expansion.
   C. It is associated with low serum osmolality.
   D. It is associated with high serum osmolality.
3. Which of the following assessments are consistent with fluid volume deficit? (choose all that apply)
   A. increased PAWP
   B. decreased CVP
   C. orthostatic hypotension
   D. oliguria
4. Which of the following IV solutions is commonly used for patients in a shock state?
   A. lactated Ringer's
   B. 0.45 percent normal saline
   C. 2.5 percent dextrose
   D. 3 percent normal saline
5. Which of the following IV solutions can cause cells to expand, burst, and result in cellular destruction?
   A. isotonic
   B. hypertonic
   C. hypotonic
   D. lactated Ringer's

Answers: 1. B, 2. D, 3. (B, C, D), 4. A, 5. C

SECTION TWO: Alterations in Fluid Balance: Fluid Volume Excess

At the completion of this section, the learner will be able to discuss the etiology, manifestations, medical treatment, and nursing care for a patient with fluid volume excess (FVE, or hypervolemia).

Etiology

Extracellular fluid volume excess, also called fluid overload or **hypervolemia,** produces a state of overhydration in the intravascular compartment and excess fluid in the interstitial compartment (also known as *edema)*. Fluid volume excess results when both water and sodium are retained.

It is associated with fewer contributing factors than are seen with fluid volume deficit. These factors are summarized in Table 26–3.

TABLE 26–3 Factors That Produce Fluid Volume Excess

SOURCE OF FLUID GAIN	RELATED FACTORS
Cardiovascular	Heart failure
Urinary	Renal failure (acute or chronic)
Hepatic	Cirrhosis Liver failure
Other	Cancer Thrombus Peripheral vascular disease Drug therapy (e.g., corticosteroids) High sodium intake Protein malnutrition

Manifestations

ECF volume excess can be generalized or localized. The assessment procedures are essentially the same as those used for assessing for fluid volume deficit. The findings, however, are almost in complete opposition, with the exception of urinary output. A low urine output can be indicative of either a deficit or an excess. For example, a low urine output (less than 30 mL/hr) may be indicative of dehydration or renal failure. Decreased urinary output in the patient with dehydration is actually a protective mechanism for the body to reserve volume. Decreased urinary output in the patient with renal failure, however, causes fluid volume excess. Nursing assessment of the patient for fluid volume excess is summarized in Table 26–4. Altered serum laboratory values may include decreased hematocrit and hemoglobin as a result of plasma dilution from excess ECF.

TABLE 26–4 Nursing Assessment of the Patient with Fluid Volume Excess

ASSESSMENT	DATA
Physical assessment	Mental status changes Weight gain Distended neck veins Periorbital edema, pitting edema over boney prominences Adventitious lung sounds, moist crackles Shortness of breath Generalized or dependent edema
Vital signs	Elevated blood pressure High CVP and PAWP Increased cardiac output
Laboratory data	Decreased hematocrit (dilutional) Low serum osmolality Radiography: pulmonary vascular congestion, pleural effusion, pericardial effusion, ascites Low urine-specific gravity (decreased concentration)

Medical Treatment

The treatment for FVE is aimed at correcting the underlying cause and treating the manifestations. This is accomplished through restriction of sodium and water intake and administration of diuretics. Diuretics inhibit sodium and water reabsorption and increase urine output. Diuretics commonly administered to patients with FVE are summarized in the RELATED PHARMACOTHERAPY box. Each drug works on a different part of the kidney tubule.

Nursing Care

Nursing diagnoses pertinent to patients with FVE may include *fluid volume excess, risk for impaired skin integrity* and *risk for impaired gas exchange.* Nursing interventions may include monitoring adherence to fluid or salt restrictions, administration of diuretics, or dialysis. The desired patient outcomes for intravascular fluid excess include pulse, blood pressure, CVP, and PAWP within acceptable ranges for the patient; lung sounds clear to auscultation; balanced intake and output; weight loss and resolution of edema; and hematocrit and blood urea nitrogen (BUN) within acceptable limits.

RELATED PHARMACOTHERAPY: Diuretics

Loop Diuretics

Furosemide (Fumide, Furomide, Lasix, Luramide)

Action and Uses

Inhibits reabsorption of sodium and chloride in the loop of Henle; decreases edema and intravascular volume.

Major Side Effects

Circulatory collapse
Hypokalemia

Nursing Implications

Monitor vital signs, especially during dosage adjustment.
Monitor for manifestations of hypokalemia.

Thiazide Diuretics

Hydrochlorathiazide (Apo-Hydro, Esidrex, Oretic, HCTZ, Urozide)

Action and Uses

Interferes with absorption of sodium ions across distal renal tubular segment to enhance excretion of sodium, chloride, potassium, bicarbonate, and water. Used in adjunct treatment of edema associated with heart failure, cirrhosis, and renal failure.

Major Side Effects

Hyperglycemia
Hypokalemia

Nursing Implications

Monitor vital signs, especially during dosage adjustment.
Monitor for manifestations of hypokalemia.

Potassium Sparing Diuretics

Spironolactone (Aldactone, Novospiroton)

Action and Uses

Competes with aldosterone for cellular receptor sites in distal renal tubule. Promotes sodium and chloride excretion without loss of potassium. Used for diuresis in cases of refractory edema due to heart failure or cirrhosis.

Major Side Effects

Hyponatremia
Hyperkalemia

Nursing Implications

Monitor serum electrolytes (sodium, potassium) during therapy.

SECTION TWO REVIEW

1. Which of the following factors contribute to FVE? (choose all that apply)
   A. heart failure
   B. renal failure
   C. liver failure
   D. corticosteriods
2. Which of the following assessments are consistent with FVE? (choose all that apply)
   A. weight loss
   B. elevated CVP
   C. elevated PAWP
   D. decreased hematocrit
3. Treatment for FVE may include (choose all that apply)
   A. fluid restriction
   B. protein restriction
   C. carbohydrate restriction
   D. sodium restriction
4. Which of the following drugs works on the distal convoluted tubule?
   A. furosemide
   B. spironolactone
   C. hydrochlorthiazide
   D. loop diuretics
5. Which of the following diuretics can produce hypokalemia? (choose all that apply)
   A. furosemide
   B. hydrochlorthiazide
   C. Aldactone
   D. Lasix

Answers: 1. (A, B, C, D), 2. (B, C, D), 3. (A, D), 4. B, 5. (A, B, D)

SECTION THREE: Alterations in Electrolyte Balance: Sodium

At the completion of this section, the learner will be able to discuss the etiology, manifestations, medical treatment, and nursing care for a patient with alterations in sodium balance (hyponatremia or hypernatremia).

Etiology of Hyponatremia

Hyponatremia occurs when the serum sodium levels fall below 135 mEq/L. It can result from excessive sodium loss, or water gain, which produces a **dilutional effect.**

Excessive Sodium Loss

In high-acuity patients, major sources of sodium loss are through the skin, gastrointestinal tract and kidneys. Gastrointestinal-related losses occur when electrolyte loss is in excess of fluid loss and may result from severe diarrhea, vomiting, or nasogastric suction. Renal loss of sodium is usually a result of diuretic therapy or severe renal dysfunction. Severe diaphoresis can lead to significant loss of sodium through the skin. Excessive sodium loss also results from hyperglycemic osmotic diuresis, as seen with diabetic ketoacidosis (DKA). Persistent sodium excretion can occur with consistent release of antidiuretic hormone (ADH) from the pituitary or ectopic production of ADH. This unregulated production of ADH is associated with the syndrome of inappropriate release of antidiuretic hormone (SIADH), which can result from cerebral trauma, narcotic use, lung cancer, and certain drugs.

Dilutional Effect

Hyponatremia can result from a net gain of water in the ECF compartment. This occurs when water moves into an area without an equivalent increase in sodium. For example, when a patient develops DKA, excessively high-serum glucose levels cause a shift of water from the ICF and other compartments into the intravascular compartment to dilute the glucose and regain equilibrium (Hayes, 2007).

Manifestations

Hyponatremia is associated with early changes in muscle tone because sodium plays a role in transmission of neuromuscular impulses. If sodium levels continue to fall (less than 120 mEq/L), intracellular edema occurs, producing further neurologic deterioration. The clinical manifestations of hypernatremia and hyponatremia are summarized in Table 26–5. The symptoms of hyponatremia usually begin to appear when the serum sodium falls below 125 mEq/L (Haskal, 2007).

Medical Treatment

IV fluids containing sodium must be administered to patients with hyponatremia. Patients with severe hyponatremia may be given hypertonic fluids, such a 3 percent or 5 percent NaCl. Conivaptan hydrochloride (Vaprisol) may be ordered. This drug blocks ADH in the kidneys to cause excretion of water and retention of sodium (Hayes, 2007). Fluid restriction of less than 800 mL/day can raise serum sodium by 1-2 mEq/L per day (Haskal, 2007).

Nursing Care

Nursing diagnoses for patients with hyponatremia may include *risk for imbalanced fluid volume* and *risk for ineffective cerebral perfusion.* If hypertonic fluids are given, the nurse must monitor the patient for pulmonary and cerebral edema due to water retention. Patients with hyponatremia should be monitored for neurologic changes including headache, lethargy, seizures, and coma. The nurse should closely monitor the patient's response to therapy

TABLE 26–5 Manifestations of Hyponatremia (less than 135 mEq/L)

Cardiovascular: hypotension
Neurologic: confusion, headache, lethargy, seizures
Neuromuscular: decreased muscle tone, muscle twitching, tremors
Gastrointestinal: vomiting, diarrhea, cramping

because correcting sodium levels too quickly can cause osmotic demyelination syndrome, leading to dysphagia and death. Generally, serum sodium levels should be increased by no more than 0.5 to 1.0 mEq/L/hour or up to 12 mEq/L in the first 24 hours (Hodges, 2007).

Etiology of Hypernatremia

Serum sodium levels above 145 mEq/L can result from excessive sodium intake or excess water loss. In the high-acuity patient, excessive sodium intake can occur from the overadministration of hypertonic intravenous fluid or sodium bicarbonate, or from overconsumption of dietary sodium. High-serum sodium pulls water from the ICF compartment into the intravascular compartment. The cells shrink and shrivel because of cellular dehydration, whereas the ECF becomes overloaded with water.

Hypernatremia caused by excess water loss can result from renal dysfunction, profuse diaphoresis, or increased adrenocorticotropin hormone (ACTH) secretion (e.g., Cushing's syndrome). Excess fluid loss can also develop from gastrointestinal loss if fluid loss exceeds electrolyte loss (e.g., severe vomiting or diarrhea and excessive nasogastric tube drainage loss). Diabetes insipidus and administration of osmotic diuretics can cause a significant loss of body water without equivalent loss of sodium, which drives up the serum sodium concentration.

Manifestations

The clinical manifestations of hypernatremia are predominantly neurologic because brain cells are especially sensitive to sodium levels. If hypernatremia develops rapidly, cellular shrinkage also contributes to the neurologic symptoms. The clinical manifestations of hypernatremia are summarized in Table 26–6.

TABLE 26–6 Manifestations of Hypernatremia (greater than 145 mEq/L)

Moderate
Confusion, thirst
Severe
Cardiovascular: hypertension, tachycardia Neurologic: restlessness, seizures, coma Neuromuscular: hyperreflexia, muscle twitching Gastrointestinal: nausea and vomiting

Medical Treatment

The primary medical treatment for hypernatremia is water replacement. The fluid volume deficit (FVD) may be corrected with administration of hypotonic IV fluids. Diuretics may also be given to enhance sodium excretion.

Nursing Care

A nursing diagnosis appropriate for patients with hypernatremia is risk for injury. The patient should be monitored for neurologic deterioration. This is especially important when administering water replacement, as changes in serum sodium or osmolality can cause rapid fluid shifts in the brain and result in cerebral edema.

SECTION THREE REVIEW

1. Hyponatremia can be caused by (choose all that apply)
   A. excessive sodium loss
   B. net gain of water in ECF
   C. osmotic diuresis
   D. DKA
2. Hyponatremia is associated with which symptom?
   A. edema
   B. hyperreflexia
   C. lethargy
   D. restlessness
3. Patients with hyponatremia may require IV fluids. Which type of IV fluid is most appropriate?
   A. isotonic
   B. hypotonic
   C. hypertonic
   D. lactated Ringer's
4. Hypernatremia can be caused by (choose all that apply)
   A. renal dysfunction
   B. profuse diuresis
   C. Cushing's syndrome
   D. diabetes insipidus
5. Signs and symptoms of hypernatremia include
   A. diarrhea
   B. muscle twitching
   C. stomach cramps
   D. decreased muscle tone

Answers: 1. (A, B, C, D), 2. C, 3. C, 4. (A, B, C, D), 5. B

SECTION FOUR: Alterations in Electrolyte Balance: Calcium

At the completion of this section, the learner will be able to discuss the etiology, manifestations, medical treatment, and nursing care for a patient with alterations in calcium balance (hypocalcemia or hypercalcemia).

Etiology of Hypocalcemia

Hypocalcemia is defined as a calcium level less than 8.5 mg/dL or an ionized calcium less than 4.2 mg/dL (Miller & Graham, 2006). In the high-acuity patient, common causes of hypocalcemia are hypoparathyroidism from surgery or acute pancreatitis. It is also associated with hypomagnesemia and hyperphosphatemia, which can cause diminished vitamin D synthesis by the kidneys. Hypocalcemia can be induced by the administration of large amounts of stored blood because stored blood is preserved with citrate. Citrate is added to stored blood as a preservative. When blood is administered, the citrate binds with calcium, which lowers ionized calcium. Additional causes of hypocalcemia include other electrolyte imbalances (hyperphosphatemia, hypomagnesemia).

Manifestations

Symptoms generally occur when ionized calcium levels drop below 2.5 mg/dL (Miller & Graham, 2006). Because calcium acts to stabilize neuromuscular cell membranes, when calcium is low, neuromuscular irritability increases. Therefore, hypocalcemia results in neuromuscular excitability, muscle twitching, spasms and tetany. The manifestations associated with hypocalcemia are presented in Table 26–7.

Medical Treatment

Medical management is aimed at correcting the underlying cause and restoring normal calcium balance. Hypocalcemia is treated with IV calcium in the high-acuity patient (See RELATED PHARMACOTHERAPY box: Calcium).

Nursing Care

A nursing diagnosis appropriate for the patient with hypocalcemia is *risk for injury*. Patients with hypocalcemia are at risk for seizures, ECG changes and decreased myocardial contractility. The nurse should monitor the patient for signs and symptoms of decreased cardiac output, bradycardia and ventricular dysrhythmias.

TABLE 26–7 Manifestations of Hypocalcemia (less than 9 mg/dL)

Musculoskeletal: cramps (abdominal and extremities); tingling and numbness; severe: positive Chvostek's or Trousseau's sign, tetany
Neurologic: irritability, reduced cognitive ability, seizures
Cardiovascular: electrocardiographic changes: prolonged QT interval, long ST segment; decreased blood pressure; and myocardial contractility
Skeletal: bone fractures possible
Hematologic: abnormal clotting

Etiology of Hypercalcemia

Hypercalcemia is defined as a serum calcium level above 10.5 mg/dL or ionized calcium greater than 5.2 mg/dL (Miller & Graham, 2006). Hypercalcemia results from mobilization of calcium from bone. Malignancy is a common cause of hypercalcemia, usually through destruction of bone (from bone metastasis). Another malignancy-related mechanism for hypercalcemia is the presence of parathyroid secreting tumors. Malignancies that are most commonly associated with development of hypercalcemia include pulmonary, breast, ovarian, and others. Hypercalcemia also develops from prolonged immobility, hyperparathyroidism, thyrotoxicosis, and thiazide diuretics. Excessive ingestion of vitamin D or calcium and altered renal tubular absorption of calcium also elevate serum calcium levels. Gastrointestinal and renal absorption of calcium decrease the reabsorption of phosphorus; therefore, hypercalcemia accompanies hypophosphatemia because calcium and phosphorus levels shift in opposite directions.

Manifestations

The signs and symptoms of hypercalcemia include decreased neuromuscular excitability, muscle weakness and fatigue. These changes are reflected in dysfunction of the gastrointestinal and musculoskeletal systems. However, serum calcium levels greater than 15 mg/dL may result in complete heart block or cardiac arrest (Miller & Graham, 2006).

The signs and symptoms of hypophosphatemia can accompany hypercalcemia. The manifestations associated with hypercalcemia are presented in Table 26–8.

TABLE 26–8 Manifestations of Hypercalcemia (greater than 11 mg/dL)

Gastrointestinal: anorexia, constipation, peptic ulcer disease
Neurologic: lethargy, depression, fatigue; if severe: confusion, coma
Cardiovascular: cardiac dysrhythmias, heart block, shortened *QT* interval, decreased ST segment
Skeletal: pathologic bone fractures, bone thinning
Other: renal stones

RELATED PHARMACOTHERAPY: Calcium

Loop Diuretics

Calcium chloride; calcium gluconate

Action and Uses

Restores serum calcium levels in acute hypocalcemia, improves myocardial contractility; calcium chloride contains more calcium than does calcium gluconate.

Major Side Effects

Cardiac arrest, hypotension, bradycardia with rapid infusion

Nursing Implications

Monitor ECG and BP closely during administration.
Can be irritating to veins when given in peripheral IV.
Can cause necrosis and sloughing of tissue if extravasation occurs.
Must be administered slowly when given IV.

Medical Treatment

Treatment focuses on correcting the underlying cause and reducing serum calcium levels. Strategies used include the promotion of calcium elimination by the kidneys and reduction of calcium reabsorption from the bone. IV fluids and diuretics may be given to promote elimination of calcium. Other drugs to reduce calcium include bisphosphonates, calcitonin, and sodium phosphate or potassium phosphate.

Nursing Care

Nursing diagnoses appropriate for the patient with hypercalcemia may include risk for injury as a result of a loss of calcium from bones (falls, pathological fractures), decreased mental status and cardiac dysrhythmias.

SECTION FOUR REVIEW

1. The most common causes of hypocalcemia in high-acuity patients include (choose all that apply)
   A. administration of large amounts of stored blood
   B. hypoparathyroidism
   C. acute pancreatitis
   D. malignancy
2. Hypocalcemia ______ neuromuscular excitability.
   A. increases
   B. decreases
3. Rapid infusion of IV calcium can result in (choose all that apply)
   A. tachycardia
   B. hypertension
   C. cardiac arrest
   D. hypotension
4. Hypercalcemia can be caused by (choose all that apply)
   A. bone metastasis
   B. hyperactivity
   C. hypothyroidism
   D. thiazide diuretics
5. An appropriate nursing diagnosis for patients with hypercalcemia is *risk for injury* related to (choose all that apply)
   A. pathological fractures
   B. falls
   C. decreased mental status
   D. cardiac dysrhythmias

Answers: 1. (A, B, C), 2. A, 3. (C, D), 4. (A, D), 5. (A, B, C, D)

SECTION FIVE: Alterations in Electrolyte Balance: Potassium

At the completion of this section, the learner will be able to discuss the etiology, manifestations, medical treatment, and nursing care for a patient with alterations in potassium balance (hypokalemia or hyperkalemia).

Etiology of Hypokalemia

Hypokalemia is defined as a serum potassium level below 3.5 mEq/L. Hypokalemia can result from the following:

- A loss of gastrointestinal secretions (e.g., vomiting, diarrhea, excessive nasogastric suction fluid loss, and fistulas)
- Excessive renal excretion of potassium
- Movement of potassium into the cells (e.g., diabetic ketoacidosis)
- Prolonged fluid administration without potassium supplementation
- Excessive use of potassium-wasting diuretics without adequate potassium supplementation

When hypokalemia occurs, the body does not attempt to retain or reabsorb potassium. The kidneys continue to excrete it regardless of the existing potassium state (Giebisch, Krapf & Wagner, 2007). If allowed to continue, the hypokalemia becomes increasingly severe, causing a steady deterioration in the patient's condition. Because the body does not compensate for potassium loss, it is essential that hypokalemia be rapidly detected and corrected through appropriate potassium supplementation. The body is intolerant of abnormal serum potassium levels. Potassium levels that are less than 2.5 mEq/L or more than 7 mEq/L are critically deranged and can result in cardiac arrest.

Manifestations

Because potassium is important in nerve impulse conduction, muscle contraction, and cell membrane function, the signs and symptoms of imbalances reflect interference with these activities. The clinical manifestations of hypokalemia are summarized in Figure 26–3.

Since potassium affects the transmission of nerve impulses, hypokalemia can result in electrocardiogram (ECG) changes including flattened or inverted *T* waves, the development of *U* waves, and depressed ST segment (see Fig. 26–4). In patients with a history of cardiac disease, even mild to moderate changes in serum potassium can cause cardiac dysrhythmias (Miller & Graham, 2006). In patients receiving digoxin therapy, low serum potassium levels can increase the risk for development of dysrhythmias.

Medical Treatment

Hypokalemia is treated with oral or IV administration of potassium. If the patient is losing large amounts of potassium daily (gastric suction, diuresis), supplemental daily doses may be required.

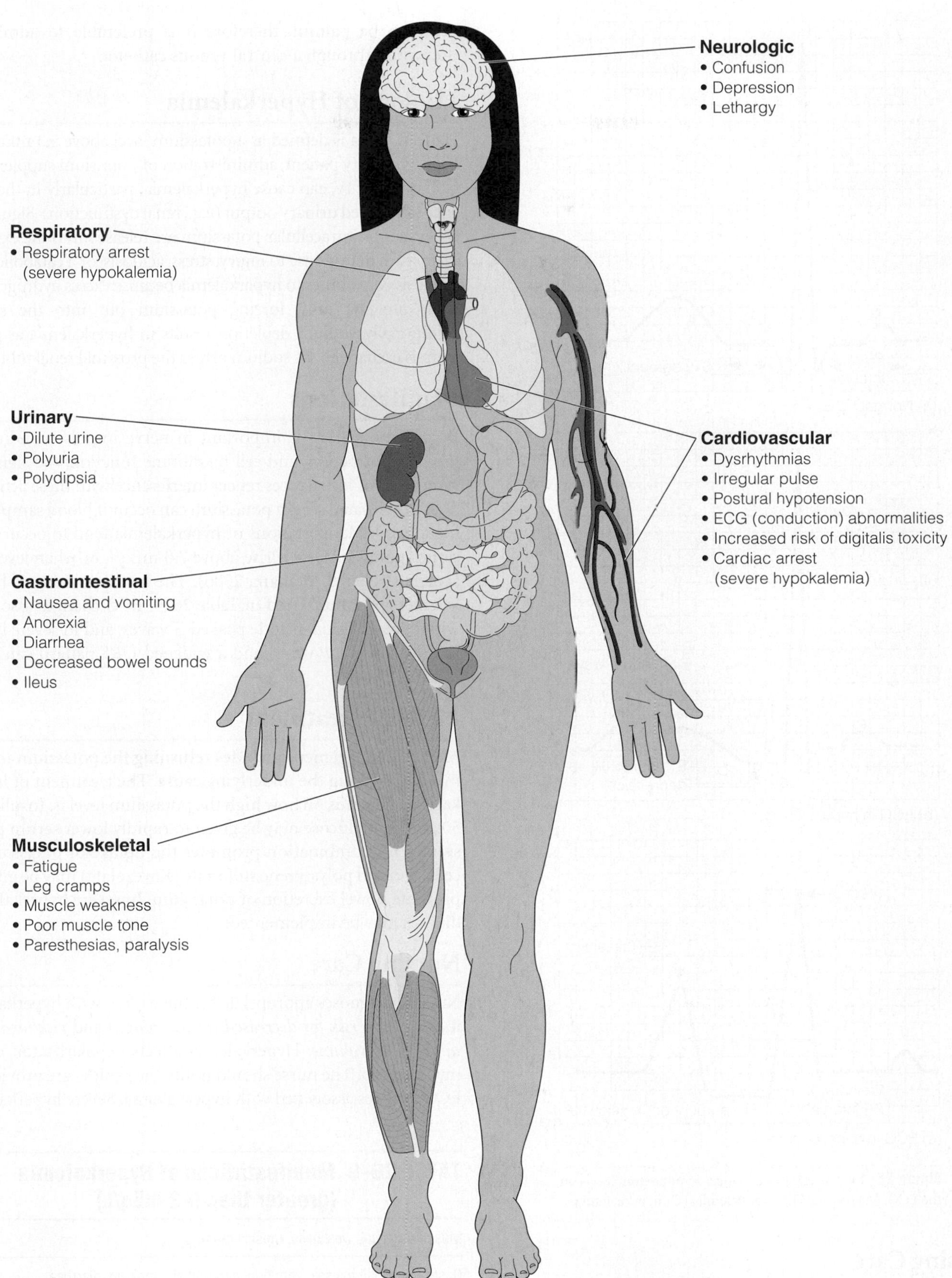

Figure 26–3 ■ Multisystem effects of hypokalemia.

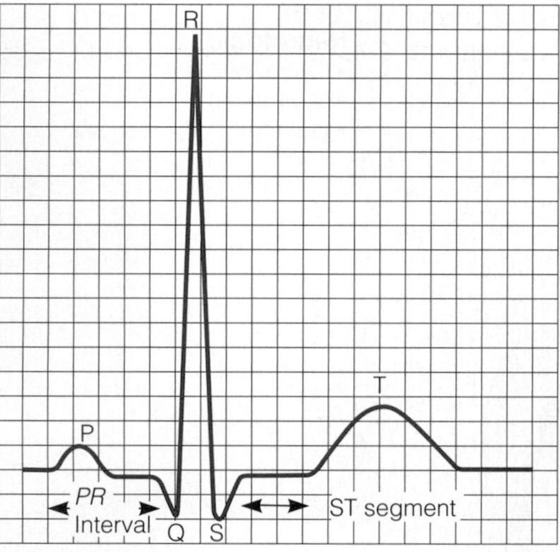

(a) Normal ECG

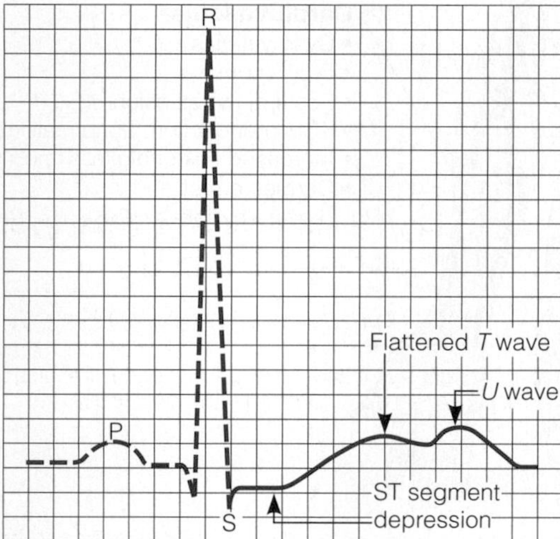

(b) ECG in hypokalemia

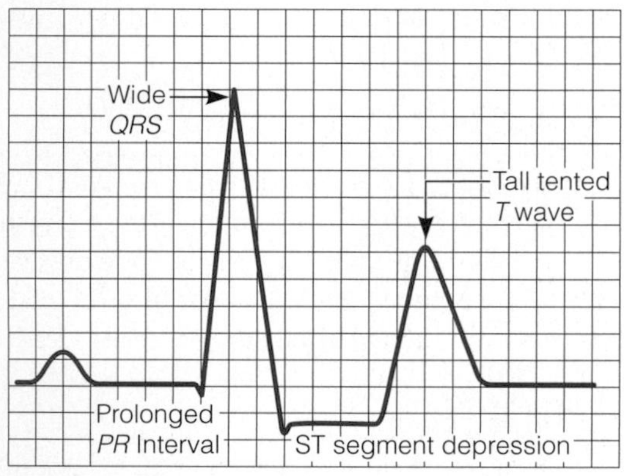

(c) ECG in hyperkalemia

Figure 26–4 ■ The effects of changes in potassium levels on the ECG. (A) normal (B) hypokalemia, (C) hyperkalemia.

Nursing Care

Nursing diagnoses appropriate for the patient with hypokalemia include *decreased cardiac output* and *acute pain.* The patient with hypokalemia should be monitored for dysrhythmias and the development of characteristic ECG changes as identified in Figure 26–4. Administration of potassium through a peripheral vein can be painful, therefore it is preferable to administer potassium through a central venous catheter.

Etiology of Hyperkalemia

Hyperkalemia is defined as a potassium level above 5.3 mEq/L. In the high-acuity patient, administration of potassium supplements, either oral or IV, can cause hyperkalemia, particularly in the presence of reduced urinary output (e.g., renal dysfunction). Significant quantities of intracellular potassium are released into the extracellular space in response to injury, stress, acidosis, or a catabolic state. Acidosis contributes to hyperkalemia because excess hydrogen ions shift into the cells, forcing potassium out into the serum. Additionally, sodium depletion results in hyperkalemia as potassium is exchanged for sodium across the proximal renal tubule.

Manifestations

Because potassium is important in nerve impulse conduction, muscle contraction, and cell membrane function, the signs and symptoms of imbalances reflect interference with these activities. A falsely elevated serum potassium can occur if blood samples are hemolyzed. Manifestations of hyperkalemia tend to occur when serum potassium levels rise above 7.0 mEq/L or when levels rise acutely (Miller & Graham, 2006). The manifestations of hyperkalemia are summarized in Table 26–9. ECG changes associated with hyperkalemia include peaked *T* waves, and in severe hyperkalemia, absent *P* waves and a widened *QRS* pattern can occur (see Fig. 26–4C)

Medical Treatment

Medical management includes returning the potassium to normal and treating the underlying cause. The treatment of hyperkalemia depends on how high the potassium level is. Insulin and 50 grams of glucose may be given to rapidly lower serum potassium. This combination promotes the uptake of potassium by cells. Sodium polystyrene sulfonate (Kayexalate) may be given to promote bowel excretion of potassium. In severe hyperkalemia, dialysis may be implemented.

Nursing Care

Nursing diagnoses appropriate for the patient with hyperkalemia may include *risk for decreased cardiac output* and *risk for imbalanced fluid volume.* Hyperkalemia affects depolarization of the myocardium. The nurse should notify the health care provider of ECG changes associated with hyperkalemia. Severe hyperkalemia

TABLE 26–9 Manifestations of Hyperkalemia (greater than 5.3 mEq/L)

Musculoskeletal: weakness, muscle cramps
Gastrointestinal: nausea, vomiting, abdominal cramping, diarrhea
Cardiovascular: electrocardiographic changes: progression from tachycardia to bradycardia to cardiac arrest is possible; prolonged *PR* interval; flat or absent *P* wave; slurring of *QRS*; tall peaked *T* wave; ST segment depression
Acid–base balance: metabolic acidosis

can result in ventricular defibrillation and cardiac arrest. Renal failure is a major cause of hyperkalemia in high-acuity patients. In the presence of abnormal renal function, the nurse should monitor blood urea nitrogen (BUN) and creatinine (Cr). Monitor the patient's intake and output and report low urine output to the health care provider.

SECTION FIVE REVIEW

1. The presence of hypokalemia alters renal excretion of potassium in which way?
   A. urine output increases
   B. potassium excretion increases
   C. potassium is reabsorbed
   D. potassium excretion does not change
2. For a patient with hypokalemia, the nurse should monitor the ECG for the development of (choose all that apply)
   A. inverted *T* waves
   B. flattened *T* waves
   C. *U* waves
   D. depressed ST segment
3. A common side effect of the administration of potassium in a peripheral IV catheter is
   A. pain
   B. dysrhythmia
   C. diarrhea
   D. tissue necrosis
4. Hyperkalemia can be caused by
   A. renal failure
   B. potassium-wasting diuretics
   C. metabolic alkalosis
   D. severe diarrhea
5. The clinical findings of hyperkalemia include
   A. muscle weakness, *T* wave inversion on ECG
   B. muscle twitching, ST segment depression on ECG
   C. vomiting, peaked *T* wave on ECG
   D. diarrhea, presence of *U* wave on ECG

Answers: 1. D, 2. (A, B, C, D), 3. A, 4. A, 5. C

SECTION SIX: Alterations in Electrolyte Balance: Magnesium

At the completion of this section, the learner will be able to discuss the etiology, manifestations, medical treatment, and nursing care for a patient with alterations in magnesium balance (hypomagnesemia or hypermagnesemia).

Etiology of Hypomagnesemia

Hypomagnesemia is defined as a serum magnesium level of less than 1.3 mEq/L (Miller & Graham, 2006). It can result from decreased intake or decreased absorption of magnesium, or excessive loss through urinary or bowel elimination. Magnesium deficiency can be caused by many disorders, including acute pancreatitis, starvation, malabsorption syndrome, chronic alcoholism, burns, and prolonged hyperalimentation without adequate magnesium replacement. Hypoparathyroidism, with resultant hypocalcemia, can also cause hypomagnesemia because the regulatory mechanisms of magnesium and calcium are closely related.

Manifestations

The signs and symptoms of magnesium and calcium imbalances are similar. Because magnesium is important in maintaining normal CNS and neuromuscular function, magnesium imbalances can cause dysfunction of these activities. Hypomagnesemia is associated with hyperactivity. The clinical manifestations associated with hypomagnesemia are presented in Table 26–10.

Medical Treatment

Medical management is directed at raising serum magnesium levels. Magnesium can also be added to IV fluids if the magnesium deficiency is severe or if neurologic changes or cardiac dysrhythmias occur.

TABLE 26–10 Manifestations of Hypomagnesemia (less than 1.5 mEq/L)

Neuromuscular: tremors, tetany, positive Chvostek's and Trousseau's signs
Cardiovascular: premature ventricular contractions, ventricular tachycardia and/or fibrillation; *T* wave flattening, decreased ST segment

Nursing Care

A nursing diagnosis appropriate for the patient with hypomagnesemia may include *risk for injury*. The nurse should monitor patients with hypomagnesemia for the development of ventricular dysrhythmias.

Etiology of Hypermagnesemia

Hypermagnesemia results when magnesium levels rise above 2.5 mEq/L. This abnormality is rare but can occur with diminished renal excretion as seen in renal dysfunction, or excessive magnesium intake. Consumption of large quantities of magnesium-containing antacids or laxatives can be a source of excessive intake.

Manifestations

The signs and symptoms of magnesium and calcium imbalances are similar. Because magnesium is important in maintaining normal CNS and neuromuscular function, magnesium imbalances can cause dysfunction of these activities. Hypermagnesemia has a depressant effect. The clinical manifestations associated with hypermagnesemia are presented in Table 26–11.

Medical Treatment

The cause of hypermagnesemia should be identified and treated. Medications containing magnesium should be held. The first line treatment for elevated magnesium levels is to give calcium (Miller & Graham, 2006).

TABLE 26–11 Manifestations of Hypermagensemia (greater than 2.5 mEq/L)

Neuromuscular: absent deep tendon reflexes, lethargy, drowsiness
Cardiovascular: hypotension, bradycardia, cardiac arrest; electrocardiogram: prolonged *PR* Intervals, complete heart block, wide *QRS* complex
Respiratory: depression

Nursing Care

Nursing diagnoses appropriate for patients with hypermagnesemia may include *decreased cardiac output* as a result of hypotension, bradycardia and ECG changes.

SECTION SIX REVIEW

1. Magnesium balance is closely related to which other two electrolytes?
   A. potassium and phosphorus
   B. calcium and sodium
   C. sodium and phosphorus
   D. calcium and potassium
2. The symptoms of hypomagnesemia reflect
   A. CNS hypoactivity
   B. fluid compartment shifts
   C. cardiac depressant effects
   D. neuromuscular and CNS hyperactivity
3. Hypermagnesemia is associated with which symptom?
   A. tetany
   B. lethargy
   C. tremors
   D. positive Chvostek's sign
4. Magnesium plays an active part in which physiologic functions? (choose all that apply)
   A. sodium and potassium transport
   B. nerve cell conduction
   C. fluid regulation
   D. transference of energy
5. ECG changes associated with hypermagnesemia include (choose all that apply)
   A. prolonged *PR* Intervals
   B. complete heart block
   C. wide *QRS* complex
   D. inverted *T* waves

Answers: 1. D, 2. D, 3. B, 4. (A, B), 5. (A, B, C)

SECTION SEVEN: Alterations in Electrolyte Balance: Phosphorus/ Phosphate

At the completion of this section, the learner will be able to discuss the etiology, manifestations, medical treatment, and nursing care for a patient with alterations in phosphorus/phosphate balance (hypophosphatemia or hyperphosphatemia).

Etiology of Hypophosphatemia

Hypophosphatemia is defined as a serum phosphorus level below 1.7 mEq/L (2.5 mg/dL). This condition is associated with malnourished states and is a relatively common imbalance in the high-acuity patient. Other conditions that can cause hypophosphatemia include hyperparathyroidism, certain renal tubular defects, metabolic acidosis (including DKA), and disorders that cause hypercalcemia.

Manifestations

Hypophosphatemia depresses cellular function, particularly of the hematologic and cardiovascular systems. This results in symptoms of impaired heart function and poor tissue oxygenation. Because phosphorus is essential in providing energy for ATP, muscle fatigue develops. The clinical manifestations associated with hypophosphatemia are presented in Table 26–12.

TABLE 26–12 Manifestations of Hypophosphatemia (less than 1.7 mEq/L)

Musculoskeletal: weakness, numbness, and tingling; pathologic fractures
Cardiac: diminished myocardial function
Gastrointestinal: nausea and vomiting, anorexia
Neurologic: disorientation, irritability, seizures, coma
Severe hypophosphatemia: severe myocardial, respiratory, and nervous system dysfunction, hemolysis; white blood cell and platelet dysfunction

Medical Treatment

Medical management is directed at treating the underlying cause of the disorder and replacing serum levels. Supplements can be given orally or intravenously, depending on the severity of the serum levels.

Nursing Care

Patients with hypophosphatemia should be monitored for *risk for injury* related to muscle weakness and poor coordination. Weakness of respiratory muscles can result in ineffective breathing patterns.

Etiology of Hyperphosphatemia

Hyperphosphatemia is defined as a serum level above 2.6 mEq/L (4.5 mg/dL). Hyperphosphatemia is less common than hypophosphatemia in the high-acuity patient. It is predominantly associated with chronic renal failure. Other causes include hyperthyroidism, hypoparathyroidism, severe catabolic states, and conditions causing hypocalcemia.

Manifestations

The clinical manifestations associated with hyperphosphatemia are presented in Table 26–13.

Medical Treatment

Treatment of hyperphosphatemia is direct at lowering serum levels. Agents that bind phosphate in the GI tract may be given. Administration of an IV solution with saline promotes renal excretion of phosphate.

TABLE 26–13 Manifestations of Hyperphosphatemia (greater than 2.6 mEq/L)

Musculoskeletal: muscle cramping and weakness
Cardiac: tachycardia
Gastrointestinal: diarrhea, nausea, abdominal cramping

Note: Many other symptoms are those of hypocalcemia.

Nursing Care

Nursing care is directed at monitoring serum lab values and patient response to treatment.

SECTION SEVEN REVIEW

1. Hypophosphatemia is associated with which condition?
   A. malnourished state
   B. metabolic alkalosis
   C. hypocalcemia
   D. hyperthyroidism
2. Severe hypophosphatemia is associated with which symptom?
   A. joint pain
   B. muscle cramping
   C. respiratory arrest
   D. peptic ulcer disease
3. The clinical picture of hyperphosphatemia frequently reflects which other electrolyte abnormality?
   A. hypercalcemia
   B. hypochloremia
   C. hypernatremia
   D. hypocalcemia
4. Severe hyperphosphatemia is associated with which of the following ECG changes?
   A. tachycardia
   B. bradycardia
   C. flattened *T* waves
   D. widened *QRS* complexes
5. IV solutions containing ______ can be given to promote renal excretion of phosphorus.
   A. glucose
   B. saline
   C. potassium
   D. lactate

Answers: 1. A, 2. C, 3. D, 4. A, 5. B

POSTTEST

The following Posttest is constructed in a case study format. A patient is presented, and questions are asked based on available data. New data are presented as the case study progresses.

Donald R., 75-years-old, was admitted to the hospital with severe dyspnea. He has a history of chronic alcohol abuse and cirrhosis. On admission, the nurse assesses the following: Thin, chronically ill-appearing male. Blood pressure, 108/62 mm Hg; pulse, 118/min; RR 26/min; temperature, 97.8°F (36.6°C). 3+ pitting generalized edema is noted. His abdomen is distended and tight. He has orthopnea and complains of shortness of breath. Mr. R. states that he has been confined to his chair or couch for the past two weeks because of his breathing difficulty and general weakness.

It is decided that Mr. R. requires intravenous fluids.

1. Which type of IV solution would be best for treating intravascular fluid deficit?
   A. hypertonic solutions
   B. isotonic solutions
   C. hypotonic solutions
   D. colloid solutions
2. Mr. R. receives an IV fluid to increase his intravascular volume and his arterial blood pressure. The best IV fluid(s) to accomplish this goal is/are (choose all that apply)
   A. lactated Ringer's
   B. 0.45 percent normal saline
   C. 0.9 percent normal saline
   D. 0.2 percent normal saline
3. Mr. R. has evidence of FVE. What factors may have contributed to FVE? (choose all that apply)
   A. age
   B. chronic alcohol abuse
   C. cirrhosis
   D. male gender
4. What assessment findings support FVE? (choose all that apply)
   A. shortness of breath
   B. orthopnea
   C. 3– pitting edema
   D. hypotension, tachycardia

Mr. R. has received a large volume of IV fluids. His serum electrolytes are drawn. The results are

Sodium: 128 mEq/L
Chloride: 90 mEq/L
Total calcium: 8 mg/dL
Potassium: 5.2 mEq/L
Magnesium: 2.7 mEq/L
Phosphate: 1.5 mEq/L

5. Given Mr. R.'s sodium level, the nurse should monitor him for which of the following?
A. hypertension
B. tachycardia
C. prolonged *QT* interval on ECG
D. decreased muscle tone

6. Which of the following may have contributed to Mr. R.'s serum sodium level?
A. rapid administration of IV fluids
B. fever
C. diuretic therapy
D. renal dysfunction

7. Mr. R.'s total calcium level is 8.0 mg/dL. This level is most likely caused by his
A. renal status
B. nutritional status
C. chloride status
D. immobilized status

8. Given Mr. R.'s calcium level, the nurse should monitor the patient for (choose all that apply)
A. decreased cardiac output
B. abnormal clotting
C. constipation
D. pathological fractures

9. Should Mr. R.'s serum potassium level approach 7 mEq/L, the nurse would be MOST concerned about changes in which body system?
A. cardiovascular
B. respiratory
C. neurologic
D. renal

10. ECG changes associated with hypokalemia include (choose all that apply)
A. flattened *T* waves
B. inverted *T* waves
C. development of *U* waves
D. ST segment depression

11. Hypomagnesemia, such as Mr. R. has, can be caused by which of the following problems? (choose all that apply)
A. hypercalcemia
B. chronic alcoholism
C. starvation
D. acute pancreatitis

12. Mr. R. should be monitored for which of the following ECG changes? (choose all that apply)
A. premature ventricular contractions
B. ventricular tachycardia
C. *T* wave flattening
D. inverted *T* waves

13. Mr. R.'s hypophosphatemia can affect his musculoskeletal system in which way?
A. muscle spasm
B. joint pain
C. muscle weakness
D. muscle cramping

14. Given his phosphate level, the nurse should assess Mr. R. for the development of
A. decreased cardiac output
B. tachycardia
C. inverted *T* waves
D. ST depression

Posttest answers with rationale are found on MyNursingKit.

REFERENCES

David, K. (2007). IV fluids: do you know what's hanging and why? *RN*, October, 35–41.

Geibisch, G., Krapf, R., & Wagner, C. (2007). Renal and extrarenal regulation of potassium. *Kidney International, 72*, 397–410.

Haskal, R. (2007). Current issues for nurse practitioners: hyponatremia. *Journal of the American Academy of Nurse Practitioners, 19*, 563–579.

Hayes, D. D. (2007). How to respond to abnormal serum sodium levels. *Nursing*, December, 56hn1–56hn4.

Miller W. & Graham, M. G. (2006). Life-threatening electrolyte abnormalities. *Patient Care*, December, 19–27.

Monnet, X. & Teboul, J. L. (2007). Volume responsiveness. *Current Opinion in Critical Care 13*, 549–553.

Rosenthal, K. (2006). Intravenous fluids: the whys and wherefores. *Nursing 36*(7), 26–27.

MODULE

27 Alteration in Renal Function: Renal Failure

Joan Davenport

OBJECTIVES

Following the completion of this module, the learner will be able to

1. Identify the categories of acute kidney injury as prerenal, intrinsic, or postrenal.
2. Identify assessment findings associated with acute kidney injury.
3. Contrast aspects of various types of renal dialysis used to treat acute kidney injury.
4. Identify nursing priorities and implications for care of the patient with acute kidney injury.
5. Identify and discuss the systematic alterations to health that occur as a result of chronic renal failure.

This self-study module focuses on the disease processes that alter renal function, signs and symptoms of altered renal function, and collaborative interventions used in the high-acuity setting to restore and support renal function. This module is composed of five sections. Section One reviews the pathophysiologic changes that occur in acute kidney injury. Section Two discusses the assessment findings associated with acute kidney injury. Section Three reviews the medical treatment, including the process of renal replacement therapy and Section Four discusses the nursing management of the patient with acute kidney injury. Section Five discusses chronic renal disease and the implications for multiple body systems as this progressive disease eventually leads to a total loss of kidney function. Each section is followed by a set of review questions to help the learner evaluate his or her understanding of the section's content before moving on to the next section. All Section Reviews include answers. It is suggested that the learner review those concepts answered incorrectly in the review questions before proceeding to the next section.

PRETEST

1. Which of the following substances should not be present in a healthy adult's urine?
   A. uric acid
   B. potassium
   C. sodium
   D. glucose
2. A patient is complaining of frequent urination during the night. The term used to describe this voiding pattern is
   A. polyuria
   B. enuresis
   C. nocturia
   D. frequency
3. Which of the following preparations is appropriate for a patient who is to undergo an intravenous pyelogram?
   A. shaving the patient's groin
   B. inserting an indwelling Foley catheter
   C. asking the patient about allergies to iodine
   D. limiting fluid intake in the preceding 12 hours
4. Which of the following electrolyte levels, if elevated and continuing to rise, would be considered a high priority reason for implementing acute renal dialysis?
   A. calcium
   B. potassium
   C. sodium
   D. magnesium
5. Renal ischemia has what effect on renal blood flow?
   A. vasospasm
   B. vasodilation
   C. vasoconstriction
   D. no effect at all
6. Acute kidney injury can precipitate gastrointestinal bleeding as a result of increased levels of
   A. uric acid
   B. creatinine
   C. urea
   D. ammonia

7. The calcium imbalance associated with chronic renal failure is attributed to (choose all that apply)
   A. hyperphosphatemia
   B. hypochloremia
   C. altered vitamin D metabolism
   D. increased gastric absorption of calcium
8. An enlarged prostate gland in an elderly male patient may precipitate which type of acute kidney injury?
   A. prerenal
   B. postrenal
   C. intrinsic
   D. hypertensive
9. The most common complication of peritoneal dialysis is
   A. hemorrhage
   B. confusion
   C. peritonitis
   D. hypokalemia
10. The major cause of death associated with acute kidney injury is
   A. uremic frost
   B. infection
   C. cardiac dysrhythmia
   D. metabolic acidosis

Pretest answers are found on MyNursingKit.

SECTION ONE: Pathophysiology of Renal Failure

At the completion of this section, the learner will be able to identify the categories of acute kidney injury as prerenal, intrinsic or postrenal.

Categories of Renal Failure

Renal failure, a rapidly progressive acute process, can develop in a few hours. However, this acute process can be reversible. This contrasts with a chronic, progressive type of renal failure that often progresses to end-stage renal disease (ESRD) within months to years. Terms used to discuss the components or distinctions in renal failure are listed in Table 27–1.

Acute Kidney Injury

Acute kidney injury, or AKI, and sometimes referred to as *acute renal failure,* is characterized by an abrupt decrease in renal function. There are many causes of abrupt alteration in function, but it is usually identified by **oliguria,** the marked decrease in urine production, and elevations of serum blood urea nitrogen (BUN) and creatinine (Cr). Often these changes take place over a number of hours to days, are associated with a reduction in cardiac output, and are often reversible if identified and treated early. There are no biomarkers capable of detecting kidney injury early in the development of AKI. Therefore, there is a significant interval from the actual time of kidney insult to the clinical detection of AKI (Bagshaw & Bellomo, 2007). When AKI requires treatment with renal replacement therapy (RRT) the mortality rate is 50 to 60 percent (Hoste & Schurgers, 2008).

The term *acute kidney injury* is recommended nomenclature to discuss this broad spectrum of renal insufficiency and it is clear that there is an equally broad range of severity associated with an injury to the kidneys. A consensus conference of the Acute Dialysis Quality Initiative group made recommendations to more clearly define and grade AKI, and suggests the use of a classification system. This system allows a more standardized approach to grading the severity of kidney injury and a clarification of the outcome for the patient (Bellomo et al., 2004), as shown in Table 27–2.

Categories of AKI serve to identify the location of the insult. Prerenal, intrinsic or intrarenal, and postrenal are the descriptors commonly used to aid in understanding the underlying pathophysiology of this condition.

Prerenal Injury

Prerenal injury is kidney dysfunction caused by inadequate renal blood flow, resulting in renal hypoperfusion and renal ischemia. As filtration pressures decline in the face of reduced renal blood flow, the glomerular filtration pressures also fall. Structural damage has not yet occurred and the condition is reversible (Sumnall, 2007).

TABLE 27–1 Definitions of Renal Dysfunction

Azotemia	Increased serum urea levels, frequently associated with increased Cr levels.
Uremia	Increased urea and Cr levels plus associated symptoms of fatigue, anorexia, nausea, vomiting, pruritus, and neurologic changes.
Renal insufficiency	Decline in renal function to approximately 25% of normal.
End-stage renal disease	Decline in renal function to less than 10% of normal.

TABLE 27–2 Rifle Criteria

	GFR CRITERIA	URINARY CRITERIA
Risk	Increased serum Cr by 1.5 times or GFR decreased by more than 25%	Urine output less than 0.5 mL/kg for six hours
Injury	Increased serum Cr by 2 times or GFR decreased by more than 50%	Urine output less than 0.5 mL/kg for 12 hours
Failure	Increased serum Cr by 3 times or GFR decrease by 75% or serum Cr at or above 4 mg/dl	Urine output less than 0.3 mL/kg or anuria for 12 hours
Loss	Complete loss of renal function for at least four weeks	
End-stage kidney disease	Need renal replacement therapy for more than three months	

TABLE 27–3 Common Causes of Acute Prerenal Renal Injury

Excessive fluid loss	Vascular: Hemorrhage Skin: Severe burns Gastrointestinal: Vomiting, diarrhea Renal: Polyuria Endocrine: Diabetes insipidus
Decreased renal perfusion	Decreased Cardiac Output: Heart failure Myocardial infarction Third spacing of fluids
Increased vascular capacity	Shock states
Vascular obstruction	Embolus Dissecting aortic aneurysm Tumor
Drugs that alter renal hemodynamics	Examples include: Angiotensin converting enzyme inhibitors Amphotericin B Angiotensin receptor blockers Cocaine Cyclosporine NSAIDs

Some of the causes of this acute prerenal phenomenon include low cardiac output, renal vasoconstriction or vascular obstruction, and drug-induced alterations in glomerular hemodynamics (Table 27–3). Prerenal injury is also seen in the face of underlying renal insufficiency when a sudden, superimposed stress of a vascular or cardiac nature occurs (Gray, Huether & Forshee, 2006).

Decreased cardiac output from any cause can precipitate prerenal injury. When cardiac output decreases, the kidneys rapidly respond through renal capillary vasoconstriction. This compensation shunts blood away from the kidneys and increases blood supply to other, more critical core organs. In the short term, this adaptive response is helpful to overall system blood flow; however if the low renal blood flow state becomes prolonged, renal tissue ischemia results. This ischemia can then culminate with necrosis of the kidney.

The kidneys are able to tolerate a wide variation in blood flow without causing tissue damage; however, as blood flow falls, so does the glomerular filtration rate (GFR). Both kidneys receive approximately 22 percent of the cardiac output. Since the kidneys constitute less than 0.5 percent of the body weight, it is clear that the kidneys receive relatively more blood flow than other organs (Guyton & Hall, 2006). This greater than expected blood flow to the kidneys supplies enough plasma for the rates of GFR necessary to regulate blood volume and solute concentrations. This demonstrates the expectation that blood flow regulation is closely associated with GFR control and the other regulatory functions of the kidneys.

As cardiac output, blood pressure, and blood flow all decrease, the kidneys' intrinsic compensatory mechanisms fail and ischemic changes occur. The tubules are the most vulnerable to low-flow states because of their relatively high metabolic rate; thus, ischemic tubular epithelial damage occurs first. If the low blood flow state is prolonged, tubular epithelial cell necrosis occurs.

The pressure gradient across renal vasculature is the physiologic measurement of renal blood flow. The pressure gradient, measured as:

$$\frac{\text{(Renal arterial pressure} - \text{Renal venous pressure)}}{\text{Total renal vascular resistance}}$$

For the nurse, it is important to use the blood pressure and urinary output as clinical measures of renal blood flow. It is important to maintain a mean arterial pressure (MAP) of at least 70 mm Hg and an hourly urinary output of 25-30 ml/hour as indicators of adequate GFR.

Vascular obstruction results in reduced renal perfusion distal to the obstruction and is another cause of prerenal renal injury. The obstruction is a localized problem but the effect on the kidney is similar to reduced cardiac output. As blood flow to the kidney diminishes, the GFR falls and the tubular epithelial cells become ischemic.

Drug-induced altered glomerular hemodynamics is a third important cause of prerenal renal injury. Often, a discussion of renal failure includes the many drugs that are nephrotoxic. These drugs cause their damage to the kidney itself (intrinsic failure) but certain drugs alter the hemodynamics of the glomeruli. Nonsteroidal anti-inflammatory drugs (NSAIDs) are often discussed as the exemplar of this type of renal damage. The NSAIDs inhibit the synthesis of prostaglandins. Prostaglandins serve as mediators of glomerular afferent arteriole vasodilation. So, NSAIDs can decrease glomerular capillary pressure. The use of NSAIDs should be restricted in those patients with evidence of reduced renal function. This is particularly true when NSAIDs use is considered in the elderly who often have some degree of preexisting renal insufficiency. Radiographic diagnostic tests may require the use of contrast dyes that can be nephrotoxic. Steps must be taken to minimize nephrotoxicity. The patient should be adequately hydrated with sodium chloride. N-acetylcystine may be given orally or intravenously before contrast administration. N-acetylcystine acts as a free radical scavenger, and counteracts vasoconstriction from contrast agents and indirectly exhibits cyoprotective effects (Hall & Esser, 2008).

Intrinsic Renal Injury

Intrinsic renal injury (or *intrarenal injury)* is caused by problems involving the renal parenchyma (renal tissue) and is categorized further by the primary injury site (e.g., acute tubular necrosis and acute interstitial nephritis) (Table 27–4). There are many conditions that predispose the patient to intrinsic injury, including (but not limited to) renal vasculitis, drug allergy, infection, tumor growth, malignant hypertension, diabetes mellitus, and disseminated intravascular coagulation. It is very important to note clinical events and predisposing factors come together to produce the greatest risk for acute renal injury (Gray, Huether & Forshee, 2006).

Acute tubular necrosis (ATN) refers to necrosis of renal tubule tissue. An operative procedure is the proximate cause in 40-50 percent of cases of ATN, but it is also caused by any destructive process within the renal tubule itself (Sumnall, 2007). Since it is associated with tissue destruction, the incidence of permanent renal damage is high.

TABLE 27–4 Common Causes of Acute Intrinsic (Intrarenal) Renal Injury

Ischemia	Secondary to prerenal failure
Nephrotoxicity	Drugs Aminoglycosides Contrast dyes Ethylene glycol NSAIDs
Rhabdomyolysis	Crush injuries, severe burns, compartment syndrome, severe exertion, seizure activity, certain drug side-effects (HMG Co-A reductase inhibitors for hypercholesterolemia)
Intratubular obstruction	Cellular debris, myoglobin casts, uric acid crystals

Renal tissue ischemia develops as the mean arterial blood pressure falls to the extent that GFR is affected. Renal ischemic damage usually occurs in patches of individual cells or in small clusters of cells in the kidneys. Damage may be mild and reversible if the duration of the ischemia is less than 25 minutes. However, prolonged ischemia usually causes severe, permanent renal damage.

Nephrotoxicity develops from either exogenous or endogenous agents. Common exogenous agents include radiographic contrast dye, aminoglycoside antibiotics, NSAIDS and others. Risk for nephrotoxicity caused by many of these agents can be reduced by keeping the patient well hydrated both before and during treatment and by maintaining an adequate hemodynamic status. Not all agents harm the kidneys to an equal extent. For example, the damage caused by aminoglycoside antibiotics results in mild tubular epithelial sloughing that is usually reversible if the drug is withdrawn promptly. This is in contrast to ethylene glycol (found commonly in antifreeze), which destroys the entire nephron, causing severe irreversible damage.

Rhabdomyolysis and hepatorenal syndrome are causes of endogenous nephrotoxicity. Hepatorenal syndrome is described further in Module 30, Alterations in Hepatic Function. Rhabdomyolysis is a syndrome characterized by excessive muscle breakdown that causes release of muscle cell contents (including electrolytes and myoglobin) in large quantities. In high-acuity settings, the most common cause is severe crush injuries seen in multiple traumatic injuries. The use of HMG-Co-A reductase inhibitor agents to treat hypercholesterolemia may result in intrinsic renal injury because of the release of myoglobin as a side effect of the drug treatment. **Myoglobin** is a ferrous globin complex that is contained in striated muscle and is responsible for the ability of muscle to store oxygen. It also produces the red color in muscle and when released in large quantities, produces urine that is dark red in color. The increased serum myoglobin is both directly and indirectly toxic to the renal tubular cell epithelium. Myoglobin can be measured in both the serum and the urine. The glomerular tubules can become obstructed with cellular debris, myoglobin, hemoglobin casts, or uric acid crystals. These particles block the tubular structure and contribute to intrarenal injury and reduced renal performance.

Postrenal Injury

Postrenal causes of renal injury include any obstruction to the outflow or urine from the kidneys. An obstruction to only one kidney does not necessarily lead to clinical renal failure unless the other kidney is also not functioning or is absent. Bilateral obstruction will precipitate renal injury resulting from backup pressure caused by the increasing volume of urine proximal to the obstruction. Postrenal injury can be caused by obstruction of the bladder, ureters, or urethra. The obstruction can be either mechanical or functional in origin (Table 27–5).

TABLE 27–5 Common Causes of Acute Postrenal Injury

Mechanical causes	Blood clots, calculi, tumors, prostatic hypertrophy, prostate cancer, urethral strictures
Functional causes	Diabetic neuropathy, neurogenic bladder, certain drugs (e.g., parasympatholytics)

SECTION ONE REVIEW

1. Renal injury from hypovolemic shock can be characterized as
   A. prerenal
   B. intrarenal
   C. postrenal
   D. intrinsic
2. Some pharmacologic agents may cause either intrinsic or prerenal dysfunction. An example of a drug category leading to prerenal injury is
   A. antibiotics
   B. cardiac glycosides
   C. nonsteroidal anti-inflammatory drugs
   D. antihypercholesterolemia drugs
3. Which statement reflects the relationship between renal blood flow and glomerular filtration rate (GFR)?
   A. As blood flow decreases, GFR decreases.
   B. As blood flow decreases, GFR increases.
   C. As blood flow increases, GFR decreases.
   D. There is no relationship between blood flow and GFR.
4. A mean arterial pressure below 70 mm Hg may result in
   A. increased renal perfusion and increased GFR
   B. release of autocoids to produce local vasodilation
   C. inadequate renal perfusion pressure
   D. renal artery obstruction
5. Myoglobin release is associated with (choose all that apply)
   A. skeletal muscle damage
   B. intrinsic renal injury
   C. dark red colored urine
   D. increase GFR

Answers: 1. A, 2. C, 3. A, 4. C, 5. (A, B, C)

SECTION TWO: Diagnosis and Clinical Presentation of Acute Kidney Injury

At the completion of this section, the learner will be able to identify assessment findings associated with acute kidney injury.

There are many clinical causes for AKI. Identifying signs of an impending renal problem early on is important so that the adverse effects on the patient are minimized.

Renal Failure (or Success?)

Urinary output is an assessment made routinely and frequently in high-acuity settings. It is not unusual for high-acuity patients to have significant abnormalities in both fluid and electrolyte balance as discussed in Module 26, Alterations in Fluid and Electrolyte Balance. While the amount of urinary output is an important physiologic sign, it is influenced by so many factors that it is vital for the nurse to remember all of the reasons for an altered urine output, including decreased oral intake and excess fluid loss.

Two other routine assessments include BUN and Cr. An increase in both, combined with oliguria or **anuria** (the cessation of urine production), are considered principle features of renal failure. It is important to remember that oliguria and **azotemia** (the buildup of uremic toxins such as urea, uric acid, and creatinine) are features of an expected response by the kidney to changes in extracellular volume or to renal blood flow. Relying on urine output and BUN and Cr levels to guide the diagnosis of renal disease is not sufficient. There are times when these changes actually represent renal health or acute renal success (Kellum, 2008). As intravascular fluid volume is decreased and renal hypoperfusion begins, antidiuretic hormone and aldosterone result in water and sodium conservation and oliguria.

The Focused Renal Assessment

In the high-acuity patient, AKI often has an insidious onset. In spite of considerations of renal success, a decreasing urinary output, increasing azotemia, and electrolyte imbalances (especially hyperkalemia) must be considered. Diagnostic criteria for AKI are 0.3 mg/dL or a greater than 50 percent increase in serum Cr from baseline or a reduction in urine output to less than 0.5 mL/kg/hour over a six-hour interval following adequate volume resuscitation and within a 48-hour window of time (Mehta, Kellum & Shah, 2007).

Health History

Data obtained from the health history can identify risk factors for the development of AKI in the high-acuity patient. These are summarized in Table 27–6.

The Physical Assessment

An assessment of the patient with renal failure requires particular attention to the cardiopulmonary and renal systems to evaluate fluid and hemodynamic status. In addition, the nurse should focus the assessment on monitoring for any manifestations of uremia. Figure 27–1 illustrates the multisystem effects of **uremia.** Uremia is a clinical syndrome that more often accompanies chronic renal failure, but the patient with AKI is likely to develop some manifestations of uremia. The manifestation of fatigue, anorexia, nausea, vomiting, pruritus, and neurologic changes may be difficult to distinguish in the critically ill individual but may be an important sign of a further deterioration of the renal system. It is likely that these symptoms are associated with toxic wastes retention, deficiency states and electrolyte disorders (Gray, Huether & Forshee, 2006).

TABLE 27–6 Risk Factors for the Development of Acute Kidney Injury

Previous history of renal problems
History of hypertension
Proteinuria
History of diabetes mellitus
Recent use of nephrotoxic agents
Recent exposure to heavy metals or organic solvents
Recent hypotensive episode
Presence of tumor or vascular obstruction
Presence of infection

AKI produces multisystem effects that can be recognized to varying degrees dependent upon the severity of the RIFLE classification of the injury and the length of time kidney function is affected. A brief overview of those multisystem effects of prolonged renal failure on various bodily systems follows.

Neurologic Effects. Accumulation of nitrogenous waste products from impaired renal excretion and metabolic acidosis. Both of these situations cause a decrease in mental functioning. As uremic toxins build up in the brain tissue, uremic encephalopathy develops. Accumulation of toxins can slow peripheral nerve conduction and produce peripheral neuropathy. In addition, fluid volume excess caused by renal failure can precipitate cerebral edema, possibly increasing the intracranial pressure and altering the level of consciousness.

Cardiovascular and Pulmonary Effects. Hypertension is a common manifestation of renal failure. It is caused by systemic

Emerging Evidence

- Patients with chronic renal insufficiency have an increased risk of developing hospital-acquired acute kidney injury. Additionally, hypertension, proteinuria, and diabetes mellitus were independent risk factors for AKI (*Hsu et al., 2008*).
- If renal function is affected by contrast dyes, 14–35 percent of patients will require renal replacement therapy, and up to 19 percent of these patients will require long-term dialysis. This is particularly significant in the population of patients with baseline renal insufficiency (*Sinert & Doty, 2007*).
- Sepsis, considered the most common condition precipitating renal dysfunction in the high-acuity patient population, may not be associated with changes in the urinary indices of volume, BUN and Cr in the early stages (*Wan et al., 2006*).

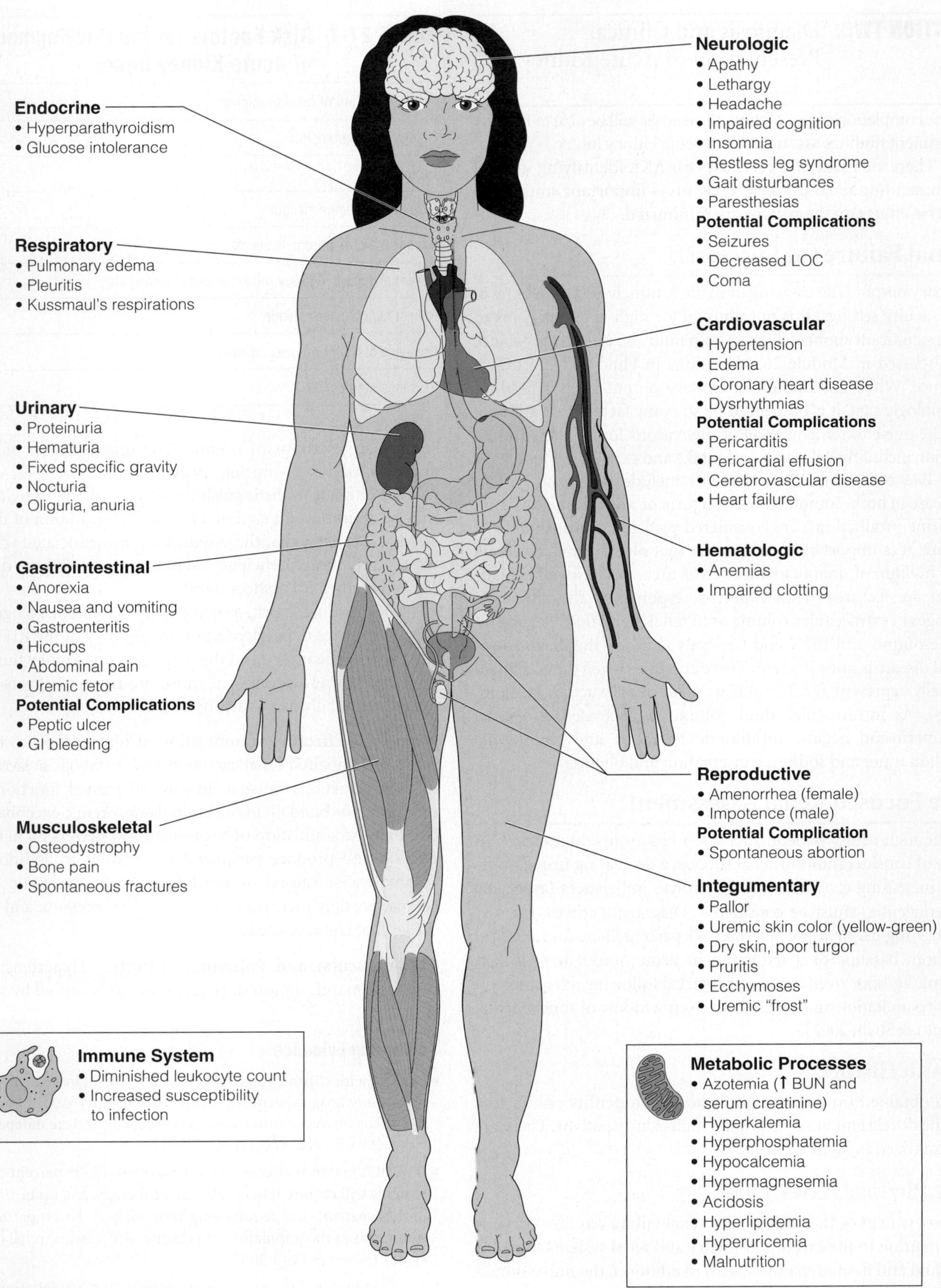

Figure 27–1 ■ Multisystem effects of uremia.

and central fluid volume excess and increased renin production. In the presence of renal ischemia, the renin-angiotensin system is triggered; this results in increased blood pressure and increased renal blood flow. Fluid volume excess and electrolyte imbalances are the basis of most cardiovascular symptoms. The presence of fluid volume excess may cause an exacerbation of heart failure symptoms accompanied by peripheral and pulmonary edema. The inability of the kidneys to adequately excrete hydrogen ions and electrolytes causes them to accumulate in the body. The resulting electrolyte imbalances, most significantly hyperkalemia, can precipitate cardiac dysrhythmias; the accumulation of hydrogen ions often presents a picture of metabolic acidosis for which the respiratory system may compensate with hyperventilation.

Patients with acute renal injury require close monitoring for signs and symptoms of pneumonia. These patients are at increased risk for developing this complication as a result of decreased level of consciousness, weakness, thickened pulmonary secretions, decreased cough reflex, and decreased pulmonary macrophage activity.

Gastrointestinal Effects. Electrolyte imbalances and increasing levels of uremic toxins are the primary contributors to gastrointestinal (GI) manifestations. As urea decomposes in the GI tract, it releases ammonia. Ammonia in the GI tract increases capillary fragility and GI mucosal irritation resulting in small mucosal ulcerations and the potential for pain, decreased appetite, and GI bleeding. Acute renal injury alters GI motility largely as a result of electrolyte imbalances. The patient may develop constipation or diarrhea depending on the GI motility status.

Hematologic Effects. The kidneys produce erythropoietin in response to decreased oxygen delivery to the kidneys. Erythropoietin is necessary for red blood cell (RBC) production and also plays a role in maintaining healthy endothelium, promotes angiogenesis and antiapoptosis. When kidney function deteriorates, RBC production is compromised and the life span of the existing RBCs may decrease. Blood vessels are also at risk for greater injury and the risk of blood clots is increased. Platelet function is impaired by the presence of uremic toxins and the risk of bleeding problems is increased. The combination of hematopoietic factors, GI irritation, and blood loss from hemodialysis all contribute to the development of anemia.

Integumentary Effects. Because the uremic toxins are not excreted by the kidneys, they may accumulate on the skin surface, causing pruritus and dry skin. The patient's skin appears pale and may develop a yellow hue. The yellow skin coloring is different from the jaundice associated with liver disease. The color is duller and does not affect the sclera. Bruising is frequently noted as a result of dysfunctional platelets. Protein wasting seen in renal injury and, most especially in the renal failure patient, may cause thin hair and brittle nails. The development of uremic frost, a late-stage phenomenon of renal failure, is less common in the acute care settings because of earlier more effective management. The term *uremic frost* refers to a fine, white layer of urate crystals that develops on the skin.

Skeletal Effects. Under normal circumstances, more than 85 percent of the calcium is excreted in the feces without being absorbed. The remaining 15 percent is absorbed by the intestines and excreted by the kidneys (Guyton & Hall, 2006). In the presence of kidney injury, the active form of Vitamin D, necessary for calcium absorption is deficient. The result is hypocalcemia, and hyperphosphatemia. In long-term kidney dysfunction, the hypocalcemia results in hyperparathyroidism and significant renal osteodystrophy.

Laboratory Tests

The diagnosis and management of AKI largely depends on laboratory tests that measure uremic toxins and renal excretion. Major laboratory values measuring AKI are summarized in Table 27–7. Note that serum and urine values have an inverse relationship.

BUN and Cr. The diagnosis and management of renal dysfunction largely depend on laboratory assessments measuring uremic toxins and renal excretions. BUN and Cr are the two most important ongoing measurements of renal status. Glomerular filtration and urine-concentrating capacity is reflected by the concentration of urea in the blood. Urea is the major end-product of protein metabolism and is filtered in the glomerulus and eliminated in the urine. Since urea is filtered at the glomerulus, the BUN levels increase as glomerular filtration decreases. The BUN is also affected by the individual's hydration status, level of catabolism, protein intake, and GI bleeding. Because of all of these possible confounding effects on BUN, it is not considered a reliable measure of GFR.

TABLE 27–7 Major Laboratory Values Measuring Kidney Function

LABORATORY TEST	ABNORMAL TREND
Serum	
Blood urea nitrogen	Increased
Creatinine	Increased
Uric acid	Increased
Potassium	Increased
Calcium	Decreased
Chloride	Increased
Phosphorus	Increased
Albumin	Decreased
Urine	
Protein	Increased
Creatinine clearance	Decreased
Urea clearance	Decreased

Cr is the end-product of muscle metabolism and is released into the blood at a constant rate. Cr is larger in size compared to urea and is not reabsorbed back into the blood, but is eliminated at a rate related to the level of renal function. For this reason, it is a more reliable measure of the state of renal health.

The reabsorption of BUN helps to explain the reason that the BUN rises more rapidly than Cr. Under healthy renal conditions, the BUN and Cr maintain a ratio of 10:1 or 15:1. Since BUN increases more quickly, an increase in this ratio to 20:1 may indicate AKI. Since the Cr level is not elevated until approximately 25 percent of the nephrons are nonfunctioning, a rise in the serum Cr is not seen until this level of damage has occurred.

Cr clearance can be calculated according to the formula below. The serum Cr level is compared with the excretion of Cr measured in a volume of urine produced over a specified amount to time. Historically, a 24-hour collection of urine has been used in this analysis but a shorter amount of time has not been shown to be less accurate (Corbett, 2004).

$$\frac{\text{Urine creatinine} \times \text{Urine volume}}{\text{Serum creatinine}} = \text{Creatinine clearance rate}$$

A decrease in the Cr clearance rate indicates a decrease in glomerular function.

Osmolality. The osmolality of urine or of serum is dependent on the number of molecules in the solution. Sodium is the major factor of serum osmolality and urea is the major constituent of urine osmolality. The relationship of urine and blood osmolality is monitored as an indicator of adequate renal function. When renal function is normal, the urine and blood (plasma) osmolality maintains a direct relationship (i.e., as one rises, the other also rises). If renal perfusion becomes diminished, the urine osmolality becomes more elevated than does the blood osmolality and urine specific gravity increases.

Electrolyte Imbalances. Assessment of serum and urine electrolytes provides important information regarding renal status and alerts the nurse to potential complications based on abnormal values (Module 26, Alterations in Fluid and Electrolyte Balance). Electrolyte imbalances cause a wide range of functional problems, particularly in the neurologic, musculoskeletal, cardiovascular, and gastrointestinal systems.

SECTION TWO REVIEW

1. Acute renal success is
   - **A.** a urine output of at least 1 mL/kg/hour
   - **B.** an expected compensatory process resulting in temporary oliguria
   - **C.** a consideration when the urine output remains normal after the use of nephrotoxic agents
   - **D.** associated with a normal serum BUN and Cr level
2. Manifestations of uremia may include any of the following EXCEPT
   - **A.** anorexia
   - **B.** fatigue
   - **C.** fever
   - **D.** pruritus
3. The acidosis associated with renal injury is directly related to
   - **A.** hypoventilation
   - **B.** excessive excretion of bicarbonate ions
   - **C.** decreased cardiac output
   - **D.** accumulation of hydrogen ions
4. Patients with long-term renal dysfunction may develop
   - **A.** hyperparathyroidism
   - **B.** diabetes insipidus
   - **C.** thrombocytosis
   - **D.** hypoparathyroidism
5. Serum osmolality is determined, in large part, by
   - **A.** urea levels
   - **B.** sodium levels
   - **C.** potassium levels
   - **D.** creatinine levels

Answers: 1. B, 2. C, 3. D, 4. A, 5. B

SECTION THREE: Medical Treatment

At the completion of this section, the learner will be able to contrast aspects of various types of renal dialysis used to treat AKI.

Initial interventions focus on prevention of events known to precipitate kidney injury. A prompt response to these episodes to support the bodily systems until renal function stabilizes is of paramount importance. Acute kidney injury is a pathophysiologic complication with the capacity to cause dysfunction of multiple other systems. The four major potential complications routinely addressed are:

- Fluid overload
- Catabolic processes
- Electrolyte/acid-base imbalance
- Infection

Fluid Overload

Fluid overload is the result of two mechanisms: retention of both sodium and water and activation of the renin-angiotensin-aldosterone system. Fluid overload can result in the development of heart failure and pulmonary edema, particularly in those individuals with preexisting cardiac dysfunction. Interventions focus on preventing fluid excess or, if overload is present, restoring optimal fluid balance. This can be accomplished with fluid restriction, diuretic therapy, and renal replacement therapy (RRT).

Fluid Restriction

Fluid replacement is restricted to the sum of measured output (urine, nasogastric (NG) drainage, fistula output) plus an estimate of insensible water loss (about 0.8-1 L per day). The selection of fluid type is dependent upon the electrolyte status of the patient and on the patient's underlying status, as discussed in Module 26, Alterations in Fluid and Electrolyte Balance.

Diuretic Therapy

Diuretics serve to remove excess fluid volume. Surgical patients, patients with sepsis or hypotension may receive large quantities of IV fluids. As these emergency situations are reversed, the excess fluid used during resuscitation may be removed with diuretics if the kidneys do not support diuresis. The forced diuresis is presumed to flush cellular debris from the tubules, reduce difficulties associated with fluid management, limit the extent of damage caused by nephrotoxic drugs and reduce complications from electrolyte disorders (Sumnall, 2007). Diuretic therapy selection may be prescribed in large intermittent doses or by a continuous and titrated intravenous drip with a suitable loop diuretic like furosemide (See Module 26, Alterations in Fluid and Electrolyte Balance, and the RELATED PHARMACOTHERAPY: Diuretics box). Continuous infusion results in improved efficiency and decrease toxicity (Sumnall, 2007).

Catabolic Processes

The high-acuity patient with AKI is often undergoing accelerated catabolic processes as a result of hypermetabolism triggered by high stress levels and increased cortisol secretion, infection, trauma or other acute problems. This increased metabolic activity significantly increases nutritional requirements, particularly protein, and results in increased nitrogenous waste products. These wastes are of particular concern with acutely injured kidneys that are unable to excrete uremic toxins and nitrogen waste, since they accumulate rapidly and produce azotemia. Elevated concentrations of the waste products impair the functions of multiple body systems. The brain (renal encephalopathy) and the gastrointestinal tract (GI bleeding) are at particular risk for serious complications.

Electrolyte/Acid-Base Imbalance

Electrolyte imbalances are a frequent complication associated with acute renal failure. Two electrolytes that require especially close monitoring and management are potassium and sodium.

Hyperkalemia. A pathologic elevation of serum potassium is an ongoing and a potentially lethal complication of AKI. Treatment may include drug therapy or dialysis. Drug therapy may consist of several options. Cation exchange resins (Kayexalate) may be used rectally or orally to bind the potassium and result in its excretion through the GI tract. Sodium bicarbonate, calcium gluconate, insulin, or hypertonic glucose may be ordered to attempt to drive potassium back to the intracellular space and out of the serum. Dialysis may be ordered to control potassium, particularly when the hyperkalemia is accompanied by excess fluid volume.

Sodium. Serum sodium levels vary in the acute renal failure patient and management depends on whether levels are normal, high, or low. The close relationship between sodium and water make it important to control; therefore, values must be monitored closely. Sodium is restricted in the diet and in IV fluids to control fluid excess and prevent dilutional hyponatremia. Maintaining a balance of intake and output helps prevent or control hypernatremia. If renal function is sufficient, diuretic therapy may be ordered to lower sodium levels.

Metabolic Acidosis

Acid-base imbalances can become very severe in AKI, creating disruption of normal cellular functions. The injured kidneys are unable to remove excess hydrogen ions produced normally by metabolic activities and the production and absorption of bicarbonate by the injured renal tubules is reduced. Treatment of metabolic acidosis is accomplished by dialysis, IV fluid administration, and the possible, judicious infusion of bicarbonate. The attempt at compensation to the metabolic acidosis includes the respiratory system and the possibility of hyperventilation. The ongoing medical management utilizing mechanical ventilation may be required.

RELATED PHARMACOTHERAPY: Cation Exchange Agents

Sodium Polystyrene Sulfonate
Kayexalate, SPS Suspection

Action and Uses

Removes potassium from the body by exchanging sodium ions for potassium in the large intestine; potassium containing resin is then excreted in stool. Used to treat hyperkalemia.

Major Adverse Effects

Constipation
Fecal impaction

Nursing Implications

Can be given orally or rectally.
If given rectally, administer at body temperature and introduce by gravity. Urge patient to retain enema at least 30-60 minutes, but as long as possible. Irrigate the colon after the enema solution has been expelled with 1-2 quarts of non-saline containing flush solution.

Infection

Infection is a major cause of death from AKI and is directly related to whether the patient is immunocompromised. The mechanism of immunologic dysfunction is related to a suppression of cell-mediated immune systems, a reduction in the number and function of lymphocytes and diminished phagocytosis (Gray, Huether & Forshee, 2006). Management of strict infection control procedures and of antibiotic therapy is imperative.

Renal Replacement Therapy (RRT)

There are three types of RRT: hemodialysis, peritoneal dialysis, and continuous renal replacement therapy (CRRT).

Early in the course of AKI, diagnostic studies may be performed to define the type of renal injury (e.g., diminished renal function secondary to shock state [prerenal] versus parenchymal tubular damage [intrinsic]. To differentiate between these etiologies, a diuretic challenge may be given, using an osmotic diuretic or furosemide. If the kidneys are able to respond to the diuretic by increasing urinary output, fluid replacement and additional diuretics are given to treat a prerenal type of problem. If, however, there is no response from the diuretic challenge, acute tubular necrosis is seriously considered and RRT becomes a viable treatment option. Patients who experience oliguria for more than four to five days generally require some form of dialysis. RRT has significantly improved the prognosis of patients experiencing intrarenal dysfunction.

RRT is the gold standard to treat renal impairment unresponsive to medications and fluids. RRT utilizes a process of diffusion in which dissolved particles are transported across a semipermeable membrane from one fluid compartment to another. RRT does not correct renal impairment but does serve to correct fluid, electrolyte, and acid-base imbalances and to remove waste products. Indications for immediate need of RRT include hyperkalemia, severe pulmonary edema, metabolic acidosis, and uremia (Sumnall, 2007).

Intermittent hemodialysis (IHD) and continuous renal replacement therapy (CRRT) are two treatment types used in the care of a patient with AKI. Peritoneal dialysis is useful in the care of a patient with chronic renal failure and is discussed in Section Five. Table 27–8 provides a comparison of these three treatment modalities.

Intermittent Hemodialysis (IHD). Hemodialysis requires direct access into the vascular system. For short-term treatment, often the case in the high-acuity patient, a double lumen temporary access catheter may be used. The two most common sites are the subclavian and femoral veins, using a percutaneous insertion approach. For long-term use, an internal arteriovenous fistula, shunt, or graft may be formed surgically. The sites for these devices are usually the lower arm. Figure 27–2 A and B demonstrate the fistula, graft, and temporary venous access.

IHD "cleans" the blood by pumping it out of the patient via the venous access. The blood then passes through a dialyzer, which removes fluid and solutes, returning the filtered blood back to the patient. The semipermeable membrane necessary for diffusion in hemodialysis is penetrable, thin cellophane. The blood comprises the first fluid compartment and the dialysate makes up the second. The semipermeable membrane pores are large enough to allow small substances to pass across (e.g., creatinine,

TABLE 27–8 Comparison of Acute Renal Failure Treatment Modalities

FACTORS	HEMODIALYSIS	CRRT	PERITONEAL DIALYSIS
Indications for use	Acute poisoning Acute/chronic renal failure Transfusion reaction Hepatic coma	Multiple organ dysfunction syndrome Sepsis Acute renal failure Inability to tolerate hemodialysis or peritoneal dialysis	Hemodynamic instability Severe cardiovascular disease Hemodialysis not available Less rapid treatment is appropriate Inadequate vascular access
Disadvantages	Requires vascular access and heparin Restricts activity level	Requires vascular access Slow process Restricts activity level Risk of contamination	Slower than hemodialysis Abdominal discomfort Decreased mobility Risk of peritonitis
Contraindications	Coagulopathy Age extremes Hemodynamic instability	Acute poisoning Hematocrit greater than 45% Inability to anticoagulate Low mean arterial pressure Congestive heart failure	Adhesions of peritoneum or abdomen Peritonitis Recent abdominal surgery
Complications	Infection Decreased cardiac output Cardiac arrhythmias Disequilibrium syndrome[a] Air embolism Disconnection hemorrhage	Infection Bleeding Infiltration Air embolism	Infection Decreased cardiac output Fluid overload Hyperglycemia Metabolic alkalosis Respiratory insufficiency Abdominal pain

[a]Symptoms of disequilibrium syndrome include disorientation, seizures, headache, agitation, and nausea and vomiting.

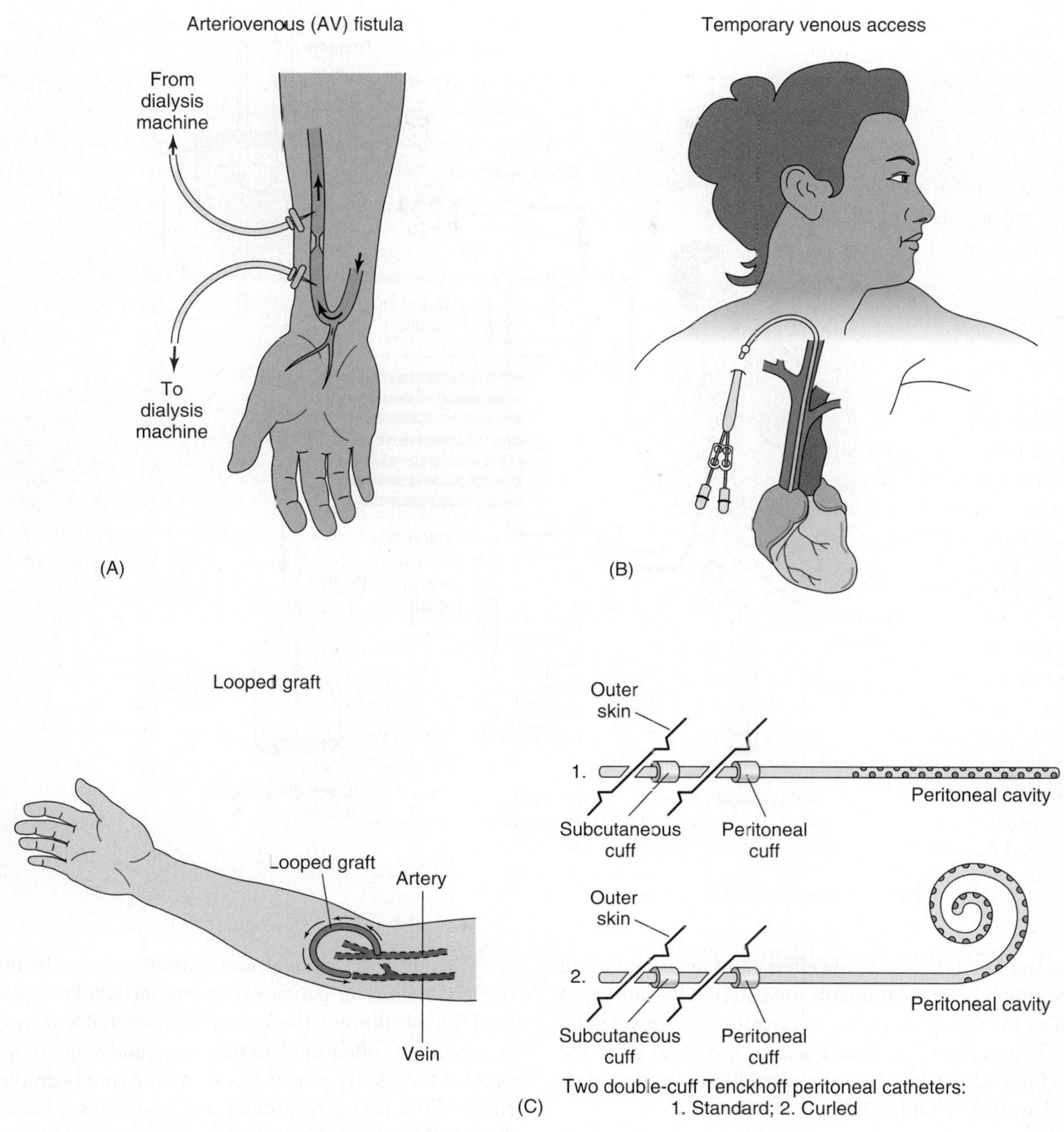

Figure 27–2 ■ Types of renal dialysis access. (A) The arteriovenous (AV) fistula and graft are used for longterm dialysis. (B) A temporary venous access can be placed centrally or into the femoral vein for use in treating acute renal failure. (C) The Tenckhoff catheter is used for peritoneal dialysis and is inserted through the lower abdominal wall. From National Kidney and Urologic Diseases Information Clearing House [NKUDIC]. [2004] National Institute of Diabetes and Digestive and Kidney Diseases. NIH.

urea, uric acid, and water molecules) but too small to allow larger particles to diffuse (e.g. proteins, blood cells, and bacteria). Figure 27–3 illustrates the hemodialysis system.

Diffusion occurs down a concentration gradient because the blood has a higher solute concentration than dialysate. This causes the flow of urea, Cr, and other relatively concentrated solutes to move across the semipermeable membrane (the cellophane) into the dialysate solution without returning to the patient.

Continuous Renal Replacement Therapy (CRRT). When clinical concerns, such as hemodynamic instability, precludes or limits the use of IHD, CRRT is a useful option in the patient with acute kidney injury. CRRT is primarily utilized for patients in the critical care setting because frequent assessments and ongoing monitoring are essential to the success of the treatment. CRRT is actually five different methods used to clear excess fluid alone or fluid plus solutes, electrolytes, Cr, and urea. Table 27–9 differentiates between these five CRRT methods.

Intermittent hemodialysis (IHD) provides more efficient clearance of excess fluid and solutes but is more destabilizing to the patient's hemodynamic and electrolyte status. Because the volume of blood in the extracorporeal circuit at any one time is

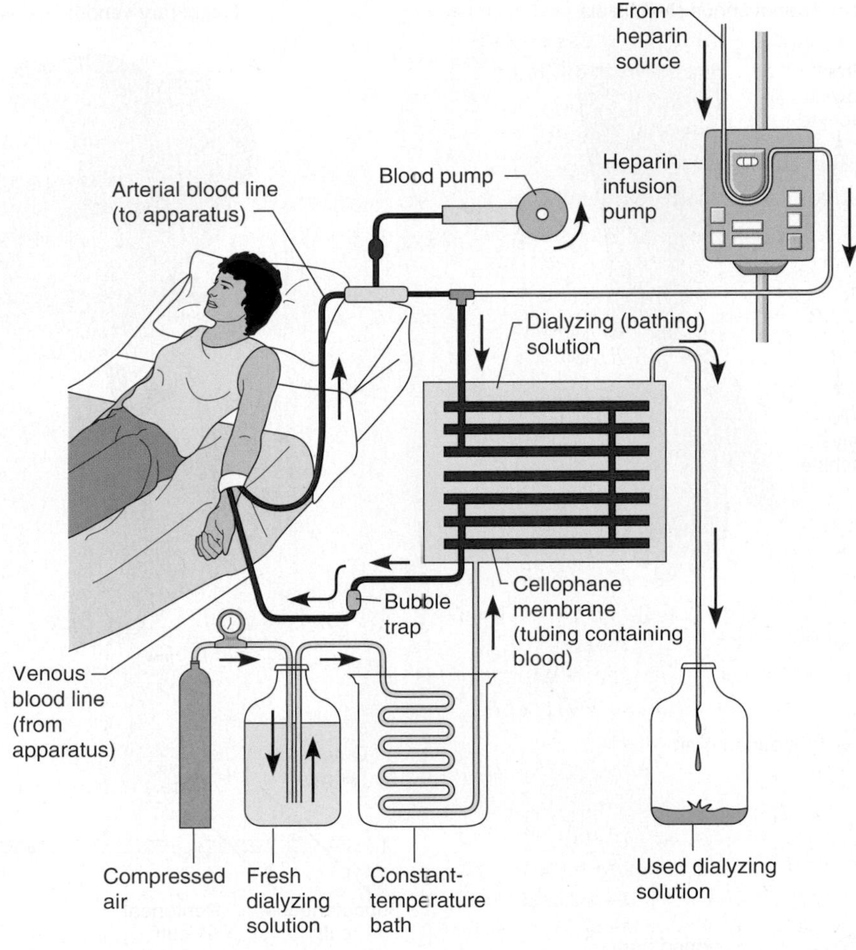

Figure 27–3 ■ Hemodialysis system.

small, it has less hemodynamic side effects and many acutely ill patients are much better candidates for CRRT. The therapy is continuous so the removal of urea, potassium, and other excess electrolytes is more gradual and therefore less drastic for the unstable, acutely ill patient. Potential complications related to CRRT are identified in Table 27–10.

TABLE 27–9 Methods of Continuous Replacement Therapy

SCUF	Uses arteriovenous access and patient's BP to circulate blood through hemofilter; removes fluids.
CAVH	Uses arteriovenous access and patient's BP to circulate blood through hemofilter. Patient receives fluid to maintain filter patency and maintain BP; removes fluids.
CAVH-D	Similar to CAVH plus the infusion pump moves dialysate solution concurrent to blood flow; removes fluids and solutes.
CVVH	Similar to CAVH except a double lumen venous catheter is used for access; removes fluids and solutes.
CVVH-D	Similar to CAVH-D except a double lumen venous catheter is used for access; removes fluids.

The process of continuous arteriovenous hemofiltration (CAVH) utilizes the patient's own arterial blood pressure to move fluid (blood) through the system. Both arterial and venous access are necessary; often the femoral artery and vein are utilized because of the relative ease of access and the vessel size. Blood in the circuit flows past a hemofilter and maintains a lower pressure than the blood circulating past it. This pressure difference facilitates the movement of solutes and water across its semipermeable membrane. The resulting ultrafiltrate drains into a collection apparatus. The level at which the collection device is hung

TABLE 27–10 Potential Complications Related to CRRT

Fluid imbalance
Hemorrhage
Hemofilter occlusion
Infection
Thrombosis
Vascular occlusion

determines the ultrafiltration rate; this rate can also be adjusted by clamping the ultrafiltrate line or by using an infusion control device. Once the blood passes the hemofilter, it is diluted again with a bath of electrolytes, water and glucose, based on the patients underlying lab results. Figure 27–4 illustrates the configuration of continuous arteriovenous hemofiltration (CAVH).

By using a dialysate solution infused into the hemofiltration at the venous or return end of the system continuous arteriovenous hemofiltration-dialysis (CAVH-D) becomes the treatment modality. The dialysate flows in the opposite direction of the blood, which creates a continual diffusion gradient throughout the hemofilter; this gradient facilitates the removal of waste and excess electrolytes while the hydrostatic pressure gradient facilitates volume removal.

Continuous venovenous hemofiltration (CVVH) uses a double-lumen catheter placed in a vein. This eliminates the need for an arterial catheter and the associated risks of this device. Without the arterial pressure to "drive" the system, a small pump propels the blood from one lumen of the catheter through the hemofilter and back into the vein through the second lumen. The pump controls the blood flow and therefore the fluid removal rate.

Continuous venovenous hemofiltration-dialysis (CVVH-D) uses a dialysate solution infused through the hemofilter in the same manner as described in CAVH-D. But like CVVH, an arterial catheter is not used and that risk is eliminated.

Slow continuous ultrafiltration (SCUF) uses the same equipment including both arterial and venous access and, using the patient's blood pressure, circulates blood through the hemofilter. Since the goal of this therapy is to remove fluid only, the patient does not receive any replacement fluid. Since toxins are not removed with SCUF, urea levels and electrolytes are not corrected.

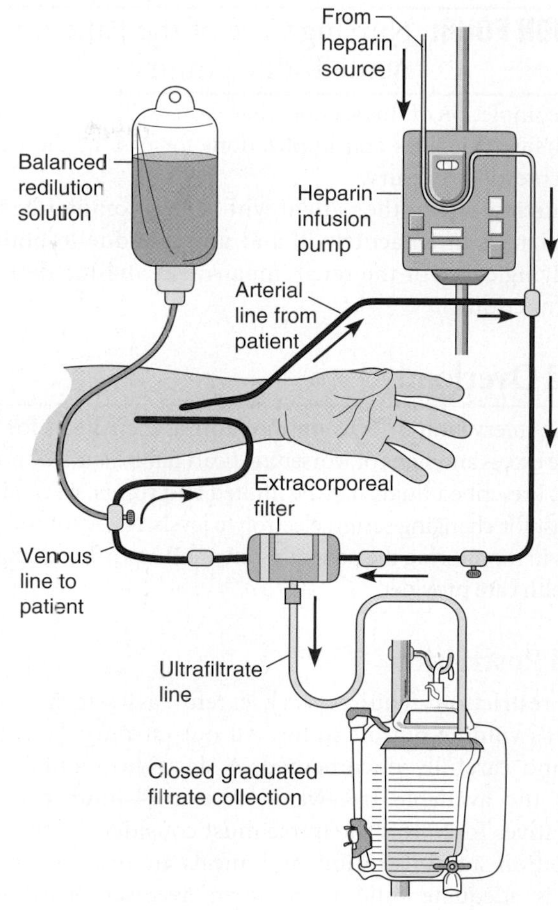

Figure 27–4 ■ Configuration of continuous arteriovenous hemofiltration.

SECTION THREE REVIEW

1. Major complications that are routinely addressed in the patient with acute kidney injury include (choose all that apply)
   A. fluid overload
   B. acid-base imbalance
   C. anabolic processes
   D. infection
2. The catabolic processes that are present in patients with AKI make restriction of ______ an important consideration.
   A. carbohydrates
   B. fats
   C. proteins
   D. essential amino acids
3. The major cause of death from acute kidney injury is
   A. hyperkalemia
   B. metabolic acidosis
   C. fluid volume excess
   D. infection
4. Fluid restriction for the patient with acute kidney injury involves a consideration of
   A. strict nothing by mouth status
   B. insensible water losses plus a match of intake to output
   C. an intake restriction to less than 50 ml hourly
   D. infusion of 0.9 percent NaCl at twice the hourly urine output
5. The major purpose of using dialysis is to
   A. remove proteins from the blood
   B. correct imbalances of fluid and electrolytes
   C. remove drugs from the blood
   D. correct renal dysfunction
6. Assuming that a patient's electrolytes have undergone the typical imbalances associated with acute kidney injury, the dialysate solution will contain low levels of
   A. calcium
   B. chloride
   C. potassium
   D. bicarbonate

Answers: 1. (A, B, D), 2. C, 3. D, 4. B, 5. B, 6. C

SECTION FOUR: Nursing Care of the Patient with Acute Kidney Injury

At the completion of this section, the learner will be able to identify nursing priorities and implications for care of the patient with acute kidney injury.

Nursing care of the patient with AKI is complex because the patient is often acutely ill and unstable due to both the underlying cause of the renal impairment and the deranged renal function.

Fluid Overload

Nursing interventions focus on monitoring the patient for fluid volume excess and signs of worsening heart failure and pulmonary edema. Prescribed fluids may be limited and composition altered to adjust for changing serum electrolyte levels. A key role of nursing lies in monitoring the patient's status and reporting changes to the health care provider.

Fluid Restriction

Fluid restriction requires very careful assessment of the patient's volume output status. All output must be considered and carefully documented. A decision about how to divide the available free-water over a 24-hour period is imperative. To do this the nurse must consider the timing of medication administration and meals in order to ensure there is adequate fluid to perform necessary treatments. Uremic patients may experience extreme thirst; thus oral fluids in small quantities often increase patient comfort. Oral care is also an extremely important intervention to both minimize oral mucosal damage and to increase patient comfort. Using small amounts of ice chips or frozen popsicles can afford greater comfort with less volume. 100 mL volume of ice chips melts to 50 mL of actual fluid volume.

Diuretics

Diuretic therapies are useful to remove volume from patients with AKI. In those patients with some level of kidney function, diuretic therapy may work to reduce excess volume load. The type of diuretic is an important consideration given the patient's needs, symptoms of volume overload, electrolyte, and acid-base status. Furosemide, a frequently prescribed loop-diuretic, may be given in large doses intravenously or by continuous intravenous drip. Intravenous push should not be given faster than 20 mg/minute and continuous infusions should not exceed 4 mg/minute. With large doses of furosemide, a metabolic alkalosis may result. This is contrary to the more usual picture of metabolic acidosis resulting from AKI. Acetazolamide (Diamox), another type of diuretic, is often prescribed in the case of loop-diuretic related alkalosis. Acetazolamide decreases renal bicarbonate reabsorption, thereby increasing bicarbonate loss. Any diuretic therapy requires careful monitoring of urine output and electrolyte studies by the acute care nurse.

Renal Replacement Therapies (RRT)

RRT can be either continuous or intermittent. Regardless of the specific method used (hemodialysis, peritoneal dialysis, or continuous dialysis or ultrafiltration), the nurse must be competent with managing the specialized technology and the necessary education for the patient and their family.

Nursing Diagnoses. Nursing diagnoses that readily apply to fluid overload include:

- *Excess fluid volume*
- *Decreased cardiac output*
- *Altered gas exchange*

Desired Outcomes. The patient will attain:

- Reduced or absence of edema
- Clear or improved lung sounds
- Absence of shortness of breath
- Weight trend toward baseline
- Blood pressure tending toward baseline

Nursing Interventions. Monitor the patient for fluid and volume excess and for evidence of heart failure and electrolyte imbalance associated with these therapies.

Catabolic Processes

The underlying causes of the AKI are often associated with an accelerated metabolism and present unique problems for the high-acuity nurse. A catabolic state requires protein intake; at the same time, the nitrogenous wastes from protein metabolism are not excreted properly and must be carefully monitored.

Nursing Diagnoses. Nursing diagnoses that readily apply to the problem of catabolic processes include:

- *Altered nutrition: less than body requirements*
- *Altered thought processes*
- *Altered bowel elimination: diarrhea*
- *Altered bowel elimination: constipation*
- *Potential complication: GI bleeding*

Desired Outcomes. The patient will attain:

- Weight trending toward baseline
- Serum protein (albumin, prealbumin) trending toward normal ranges
- Nitrogen balance
- Mental status trending toward baseline
- Stools of soft, formed consistency and usual frequency

Nursing Implications. Nursing implications include a focus on adequate nutritional support. The nurse should consider an early nutrition consult to establish estimated nutritional support needs for the patient. The diet should be restricted in protein, sodium, potassium, and fluids, and high in carbohydrates, fats, and essential amino acids.

Nutrition given orally or via enteral feeding routes is preferable to the IV route in order to minimize the risk of infection. If dietary restrictions are not sufficient in maintaining acceptable nitrogenous waste levels (e.g., BUN and Cr), RRT may be initiated.

The patient's weight should be monitored daily with the understanding that rapid weight shifts are probably secondary to fluid excess problems. Serum protein levels should be monitored regularly to evaluate whether the patient's nutritional status is worsening or improving. The patient's mental status needs to be monitored at least every shift to observe for onset of renal encephalopathy. Stool consistency and frequency is monitored and orders are obtained as needed to attain/maintain adequate bowel evacuation patterns.

Electrolyte/Acid-Base Imbalance

Electrolyte imbalance in the patient with AKI is related to both the diminished GFR and to some of the treatments used in an attempt to improve urinary output. The two electrolytes of particular concern are potassium and sodium.

Potassium elevation is a consistent problem with the oliguria of AKI unless potassium intake is limited. Hyperkalemia is considered a clinical emergency since the cardiac dysrhythmias associated with hyperkalemia can lead to cardiac arrest. The nurse must be aware of the electrocardiographic clues of hyperkalemia; a prolonged *QRS* and tall, peaked *T* waves are the typical ECG changes seen with elevated serum potassium. Hypokalemia can be seen in patients with AKI with the use of potassium wasting diuretics.

Sodium levels may be either elevated or reduced in patients with renal insufficiency. More often, the patient with AKI will experience hypernatremia caused by water loss in excess of sodium loss. Alternatively, the use of diuretics prescribed to treat oliguria or a renal dysfunction in which there is sodium wasting in excess of volume loss can produce hyponatremia.

A metabolic acidosis associated with AKI is due to an inability of the kidneys to excrete hydrogen ions and to reabsorb bicarbonate ions. Early in the process of AKI, phosphate buffers are able to correct for acidosis in spite of reduced bicarbonate. As the dysfunction persists and phosphate buffers become unable to compensate, the serum pH will fall and metabolic acidosis will ensue.

Nursing Diagnoses. Nursing diagnoses that readily apply to the problem of electrolyte and acid-base imbalances include:

- *Potential complication: metabolic acidosis*
- *Potential problem: electrolyte imbalance*
- *Potential problem: cardiac dysfunction*
- *Fluid volume excess*

Desired Patient Outcomes. The patient will attain or maintain:

- Serum pH between 7.35 and 7.45
- Serum electrolytes within normal limits
- Normal cardiac rhythm

Nursing Implications. Nursing implications include the need to consistently monitor the patient for clinical manifestations of electrolyte imbalances, especially sodium, potassium, calcium, phosphate, and magnesium. The patient's arterial blood gases are also closely monitored for signs of acidosis. A venous carbon dioxide capacity can be used as a proxy for bicarbonate levels. Sodium chloride may be used to correct for metabolic acidosis but this must be done carefully to minimize the hypernatremic effects. Dialysis may also be initiated to control the effects of acidosis and reduce the hyperkalemia of renal dysfunction.

Infection

The presence of infection may be a precipitate cause of a prerenal AKI because of the hypotension of septic states. In addition, the immunocompromised state associated with significant renal dysfunction increases the likelihood that the patient may acquire a nosocomial infection.

Nursing Diagnosis. A nursing diagnosis that readily applies to the patient with a possible infection is, *high risk for infection.*

Desired Patient Outcomes. The patient will be free of infection as evidenced by:

- All invasive devices removed in a timely fashion
- WBC count within acceptable levels
- Absence of fever
- Negative cultures
- Wounds free of purulent drainage

Nursing Implications. Nursing implications focus on monitoring the patient for signs and symptoms of infection. Scrupulous hand washing is paramount. Major sources of infection in the AKI patient include urinary tract infection, pneumonia, septicemia from vascular catheters, and skin or wound sources. Evidence based practices and care bundles concerning vascular catheter insertion and care, minimizing ventilator associated pneumonias, and sepsis care should be a routine aspect of acute care practices and serve to guide excellent practice. Antibiotic therapy requires dose adjustment based on the severity of renal impairment. If antibiotics are prescribed, the nurse monitors for the therapeutic and nontherapeutic effects of the antimicrobials.

Related Nursing Diagnoses. In addition to the nursing diagnoses previously listed, the patient in AKI frequently meets the clinical criteria for the following:

- *Activity intolerance*
- *High risk for injury*
- *High risk for altered mucous membranes*
- *High risk for altered skin integrity*
- *Altered renal tissue perfusion*
- *Pain*
- *Anxiety*
- *Knowledge deficit*

NURSING CARE: Renal Failure Requiring CRRT

Expected Patient Outcomes and Related Interventions

Outcome 1: Fluid and electrolyte balance

Assess and compare to established normal, patient baselines, and trends.

Fluid – intake and output, weight, mean arterial pressure, breath sounds, jugular veins, extremities, hemodynamic monitoring values

Electrolytes – serum electrolyte levels, especially Na, K. BUN, Cr; Monitor ECG for electrolyte-related changes.

Acid-base balance – arterial blood gases

Assess for dialysis disequilibrium syndrome – headache, nausea, vomiting, altered level of consciousness, hypertension.

Administer related drug therapy and monitor for therapeutic and nontherapeutic effects.

Diuretics (e.g., furosemide [Lasix])

Cation exchange agents (e.g., sodium polystyrene sulfonate [Kayexalate])

Implement fluid restriction as ordered.

Related nursing diagnoses

Excess fluid volume

Decreased cardiac output

Altered gas exchange

Altered urinary elimination

Outcome 2: Patient protected from possible harm

Assess and compare to established normal, patient baselines, and trends.

Coagulation–assess hourly ultrafiltration rate and patency of hemofilter and tubing hourly. Assess serum coagulation studies as ordered. Assess for bleeding at vascular access site or elsewhere.

Infection–assess vascular access device for signs and symptoms of infection, assess white blood cell count, fever, cultures as ordered. Assess peak and trough levels of antibiotics as ordered.

Administer related drug therapy and monitor for therapeutic and nontherapeutic effects.

Anticoagulants as ordered (e.g., heparin)

Antibiotics as ordered. Doses may be adjusted to prevent renal toxicity.

Change hemofilter per unit protocol.

Protect vascular access device from dislodgement.

Related nursing diagnoses:

Potential for injury

Potential for injection

SECTION FOUR REVIEW

1. Hyperkalemia associated with acute kidney injury may lead to
   - **A.** excessive thirst
   - **B.** cardiac arrest
   - **C.** skeletal muscle weakness
   - **D.** dysphagia
2. Dietary protein intake is monitored in patients with renal dysfunction because
   - **A.** dietary sources of protein include excess triglyceride levels
   - **B.** the patient's weight must be controlled and limiting protein is the easiest way to do this
   - **C.** dietary protein intake increases nitrogenous waste products
   - **D.** the nurse should ensure twice the usual protein intake for the patient with AKI
3. A nursing concern when caring for a patient with AKI includes monitoring for acid-base imbalance. The typical acid-base picture for a patient with renal dysfunction is that of
   - **A.** respiratory alkalosis
   - **B.** respiratory acidosis
   - **C.** metabolic alkalosis
   - **D.** metabolic acidosis

Answers: 1. B, 2. C, 3. D

SECTION FIVE: Chronic Renal Failure in the High-Acuity Patient

At the completion of this section, the learner will be able to discuss the implications of caring for a high-acuity patient who has chronic renal failure.

Chronic renal failure, or CRF, is defined as the irreversible loss of renal function and affects nearly all organ systems. Individuals with chronic renal disease progress steadily toward end-stage renal disease (ESRD) (Gray, Huether & Forshee, 2006). CRF is the result of either a primary renal condition in which the kidneys are directly affected (polycystic kidney disease or glomerulonephritis as examples) or is the result of other diseases that produce a long-term renal insult (diabetes or hypertension). Risk factors for ESRD include diabetes mellitus, hypertension, proteinuria, family history, and increasing age (Broscious & Castagnol, 2006).

Pathophysiology of Chronic Renal Failure

The progressive deterioration of kidney function seen in chronic renal failure occurs regardless of the cause of the insult. All forms of renal failure are characterized by a reduction in the GFR, reflecting a corresponding reduction in the number of functional nephrons (Porth, 2005). The kidneys attempt to compensate for renal damage by hyperfiltration (excessive straining of the blood) within the remaining functional nephrons. Over time, hyperfiltration causes further loss of function. Chronic loss of function causes generalized wasting (shrinking in size) and progressive scarring within all parts of the kidneys. In time, overall scarring obscures the site of the initial damage. Yet, it is not until over 70 percent of the normal combined function of both kidneys is lost that most patients begin to experience symptoms of kidney failure.

A few theories are proposed, to account for the differences in the presentation of CRF. These theories serve to clarify why some disorders proceed to renal failure more quickly or with varying presentation features. The first theory, the intact nephron theory, helps to explain why the disease progression is more rapid as the nephron loss progresses. This theory proposes that the compensatory features of renal disease including the maintenance of filtration, reabsorption and secretion occur because the remaining nephrons become hypertrophied and hyperfunctioning. So, as the nephron loss continues and these overworked nephrons fail, the signs and symptoms of disease advance more and more quickly. A second theory, the hyperfiltration hypothesis, explains the pathophysiologic features of CRF. This hypothesis serves to explain how the renal failure progresses in diabetes or hypertension. In these two causes of secondary renal failure, long-term exposure to increased glomerular capillary pressures and increased speed of blood flow result in glomerulosclerosis and continued loss of GFR. In this case, angiotensin-converting enzyme inhibitors or angiotensin-receptor blockers slow the process.

This progressive disease occurs in four stages, each characterized by a further decrease in GFR (Gray, Huether & Forshee, 2006). The stages, as summarized by Porth (2005), are listed in Table 27–11. Stage 1, the *diminished renal reserve,* is characterized by a destruction of nephrons and compensatory hyperfiltration. Often the patient is asymptomatic and the only clinical sign may be an elevated BUN. In this stage, the GFR is reduced to approximately 50 percent of normal function. The second stage, **renal insufficiency,** occurs when the GFR is severely reduced and mild symptoms are present. There remain attempts at compensation from the remaining functional nephrons but it is inadequate to clear the nitrogenous wastes. The BUN and Cr levels are elevated with a normal diet. Further evidence of renal dysfunction is apparent as mild anemia is noted and the patient may experience nocturia because of impaired urine concentration.

The third stage, **renal failure,** occurs as the GFR is reduced below 20 percent. In this stage of CRF, other organ systems are adversely affected. Continued azotemia, metabolic acidosis, worsening anemia, serum potassium and phosphate levels are elevated, and evidence of fluid excess becomes apparent. It is at the third stage that severe alterations in fluid, electrolytes, and acid-base balance occurs, requiring renal dialysis. The fourth and final stage of CRF is **end-stage renal disease** (ESRD).

TABLE 27–11 Stages of Chronic Renal Failure

STAGE	GFR (% OF NORMAL)	ASSOCIATED CLINICAL MANIFESTATIONS
Diminished renal reserve	About 50	*General:* Asymptomatic; at increased risk for nephrotoxicity from drugs and toxins *Renal function laboratory tests:* Normal
Renal insufficiency	20–50	*General:* Onset of hypertension and anemia, development of polyuria ("isosthenuria") *Renal function laboratory tests:* Onset of azotemia
Renal failure	Less than 20	*General:* Onset of renal failure manifestations *Renal function laboratory tests:* Continue to deteriorate
End-stage renal disease	Less than 5	*General:* Worsening of manifestations *Renal function laboratory tests:* Reflect total loss of renal function

Diagnostic Features of CRF

The diagnosis of chronic renal failure is primarily accomplished with laboratory analysis. Renal excretion of Cr is constant in individuals with normally functioning kidneys; the amount released by muscles is essentially equal to the amount excreted in the urine. As GFR declines and Cr excretion decreases, the concentration of Cr in the serum increases reciprocally. Blood urea nitrogen levels also continue to increase as renal failure progresses. However, the relationship of serum urea to the degree of renal dysfunction is not as clearly related as is Cr to renal function. BUN levels vary with the level of hydration and with diet so is a less reliable indicator of renal function.

Urinary output varies as the patient progresses through the stages of CRF. In the first stage, the acute care nurse can expect urine output to be normal as remaining nephrons are able to compensate for the nephrons lost to disease. In the second stage, the inability of the kidneys to concentrate the urine may be indicated by polyuria. As the patient moves into the third stage of CRF, oliguria predominates. Finally, anuria occurs with the near absence of GFR in the final stage or CRF.

Manifestations of CRF

The systemic effects of CRF are wide-ranging and extend from those identified in AKI as illustrated earlier in Figure 27-1. Chronic renal failure is associated with severe fluid and electrolyte aberrations primarily affecting sodium, potassium, calcium and phosphorous. The acid-base imbalance seen in AKI continue as bicarbonate levels stabilize at 15-20 mEq/L and excess hydrogen ions are buffered by anions from bone. These features are summarized in Table 27–12.

Cardiovascular Effects. Hypertension is a common feature of CRF and often progresses to heart failure if untreated. The hypertension is multi-factorial and associated with excess fluid volume

TABLE 27–12 Laboratory Findings Associated with Chronic Renal Failure

LAB FEATURE	CHARACTERISTICS
Cr and BUN	Elevated as CRF progresses with creatinine a more reliable indicator of renal function.
Sodium	May be reduced as normal tubular reabsorption is reduced and urine excretion is increased. As CRF progresses, often hypernatremia predominates.
Potassium	May be at or near normal levels as tubular secretion is increased. As CRF progresses and oliguria occurs, hyperkalemia is a principle feature of CRF and may be life-threatening.
Calcium and phosphate	Reduced renal excretion of phosphate and decreased kidney synthesis of the active form of vitamin D. The reduced vitamin D and elevated phosphate levels bind free calcium causes hypocalcemia and resulting hyperparathyroid activity and bone loss.
Acid-base	Hydrogen ion excretion and bicarbonate reabsorption in the early stage of CRF progresses to metabolic acidosis in later stages.

and sodium derangements but also associated with increased renin production. Altered lipid levels are a feature of early renal failure. In addition, a loss of vessel elasticity associated with atherosclerosis and abnormal calcification of vessel walls (hyperparathyroidism) contribute to macrovascular disease, ischemic heart disease, heart failure, stroke and peripheral vascular disease (Gray, Huether & Forshee, 2006). Pericarditis, associated with uremic toxins or a result of the dialysis treatment causes chest pain, a friction rub, and possible cardiac tamponade.

Hematologic Effects. Chronic anemia associated with a reduced production of the hormone erythropoietin, GI blood loss, and potential blood loss in dialysis treatment is a profound physiologic effect from CRF. There is also an iron deficiency seen in individuals with CRF that contributes to the anemia. There is evidence that elevated uremia renders platelet function impaired and places the patient at risk for unusual bleeding. This coagulopathy is evidenced by easy bruising of the skin, nose bleeds, increased menstrual bleeding, and gastrointestinal bleeding (Porth, 2005).

Gastrointestinal Effects. Nausea, vomiting, and anorexia are often seen in association with the elevated urea levels in patients with CRF and worsen as the disease progresses (Broscious & Castagnola, 2006). The elevated parathyroid hormone levels increase gastric acid production and are associated with complaints of gastric distress and anorexia. In addition, the risk for GI bleeding is increased in this chronically ill population.

Neurologic Effects. Central neurologic symptoms are nonspecific and progressive in the patient with CRF. These symptoms include sleep disorders, memory loss, impaired judgment, muscle cramps, and twitching. These may progress to asterixis, seizures, and coma. These neurologic changes are associated with uremic encephalopathy. Impaired thinking is sometimes referred to as "BUN blunting" (Broscious & Castagnola, 2007). Peripheral neuropathy is also a component of CRF and is evidenced by numbness, tingling, or pain, especially in the lower extremities (Gray, Huether & Forshee, 2006). For those patients receiving hemodialysis, the neurologic risks are compounded with rapidly changing electrolyte and acid-base balance.

Many physiological processes are affected by CRF, as summarized in Table 27–13.

Medical Treatment

Much of the medical treatments associated with the care of the patient with CRF are targeted at the associated symptoms identified earlier in this module. For instance, the anemia of CRF is treated with recombinant human erythropoietin and iron supplementation. Hyperphosphatemia and hypocalcemia are treated with phosphate binding agents (primarily calcium and aluminum hydroxide antacids). The hypertension is treated with potassium-wasting diuretics, angiotensin-converting enzyme inhibitors, and other pharmacologic vasodilator agents. The heart failure may be treated with cardio-selective beta blocking agents.

For the most part, these symptoms and others are also treated with regular dialysis. In addition to hemodialysis, patients with CRF may be treated with peritoneal dialysis, or PD.

Peritoneal Dialysis. In this treatment, the peritoneal cavity is used as the semipermeable membrane to remove waste, excess fluid, and electrolytes from the blood. In PD, a sterile catheter is inserted into the peritoneal cavity and extends out through the abdominal wall (Fig. 27–5). Peritoneal dialysis depends on both diffusion and osmosis. As a prescribed volume and concentration of dialysate solution is instilled through this catheter using strict

TABLE 27–13 Physiologic Processes Affected by Chronic Renal Failure

PROCESSES	CHARACTERISTICS
Sex hormones	Reduced estrogen in females with amenorrhea and inability to maintain pregnancy. In males, reduced testosterone and low sperm levels may result in infertility. Impotence may result from vascular complication of CRF. Reduced libido occurs in both genders.
Immunity	Suppression of cell-mediated responses and antibody production are reduced.
Integumentary	Pale skin from anemia and yellow-brown hue associated with uremia. Dry skin and mucous membranes, decreased perspiration, and pruritus and resultant severe scratching may produce skin breaks.
Carbohydrates, protein & fat metabolism	Catabolic state and negative nitrogen balance, glucose intolerance associated with insulin resistance and reduced HDL, elevated LDL and triglycerides.

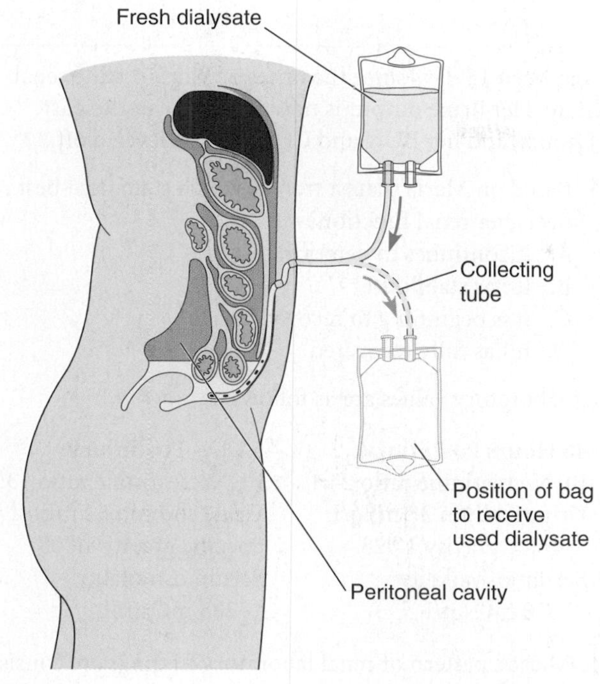

Figure 27–5 ■ Peritoneal dialysis.

aseptic techniques, waste products and excess electrolytes in the blood cross the semipermeable peritoneal membrane into the dialysate. The dialysate fluid "dwells" in the peritoneal space for a prescribed amount of time to maximize this diffusion and is then drained. Osmosis in PD occurs as a high glucose concentration in the dialysate allows water to migrate from the blood and into the peritoneal cavity during the process. This process can be continuous with a prescribed instillation—dwell—drain sequence. It can also be intermittent, perhaps two or three times over the course of a day; or a cycling machine can make the process semiautomatic.

The advantages of peritoneal dialysis include the fact that the patient can perform it on a regular basis, making the fluid and electrolyte shifts less dramatic than with IHD. The PD can be accomplished in the patient's home or ambulatory patients can participate in work or relaxation activities while the process is ongoing. For the hemodynamically unstable patient, it affords a less dramatic alteration in fluid balance, making it a safer alternative than intermittent hemodialysis. Disadvantages include a significant risk for infection from contamination of the peritoneal cavity, respiratory distress associated with the volume of fluid creating pressure against the diaphragm, and significant protein depletion from the blood into the peritoneal cavity and into the dialysate solution.

Nursing Care

The high-acuity patient with CRF enters the hospital setting with significant, preexisting health problems that potentially have altered the majority of body functions because of the multisystem nature of uremic syndrome. Minimally, the acute care nurse can expect the following:

- Dialysis will be required.
- Hypertension is likely.
- Fluid restriction and dietary restrictions of protein, sodium potassium and phosphate will be important.
- Hypoxia associated with anemia will be a focus.
- Increased risk of infection is a concern.

Nursing Diagnoses. As the nurse in a high-acuity setting plans care for the CRF patient, these nursing diagnoses are often considered:

- *Altered fluid and electrolyte balance*
- *Altered nutrition: less than body requirements*
- *Activity intolerance*
- *Risk for infection*
- *Risk for constipation*

SECTION FIVE REVIEW

1. How do the kidneys compensate for significant reductions in GFR?
   A. regeneration of damaged nephrons
   B. hypertrophy of the remaining nephrons
   C. hibernation reflex of the nephrons
   D. There is no compensatory mechanisms to CRF.
2. Hyperparathyroidism of CRF is related to
   A. uremic effects on the parathyroid gland
   B. increased vitamin D absorption from the stomach
   C. increased reabsorption of phosphate by the damaged kidneys
   D. hypermetabolic state created by the chronic disease
3. Peritoneal dialysis works by the processes of
   A. osmosis and diffusion
   B. diffusion and evaporation
   C. glucose metabolism and sodium channel activity
   D. osmosis and temperature regulation
4. With progressive renal failure and loss of 75 percent of the glomerular filtration mechanism, the synthesis of vitamin D_3 is impaired. This contributes to
   A. hypocalcemia and hyperkalemia
   B. hypocalcemia and bone disease
   C. hypercalcemia and hypophosphatemia
   D. hypercalcemia and hyperurecemia
5. The ESRD patient is undergoing peritoneal dialysis and receives too much glucose through the dialysate solution. Which of the following clinical manifestations would the nurse observe?
   A. edema
   B. congestions
   C. dysrhythmia
   D. hypotension

Answers: 1. B, 2. C, 3. A, 4. B, 5. D

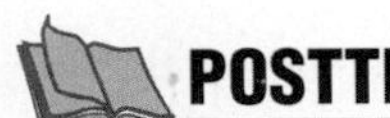

POSTTEST

The following Posttest is constructed in a case study format.

Maria G., a 32-year-old teacher, has been admitted through the emergency department after sustaining multiple injuries in a motor vehicle crash. The emergency medical team relates that when she was found at the scene of the event, she was noted to have an arterial blood pressure of 76/42 mm Hg. It was believed that the ambulance had arrived 20 minutes after the crash. In the emergency department, she was found to have a ruptured spleen and she was prepared immediately for surgery. She has no known history. It has been almost 48 hours since the event. You note that Maria's urine output has been approximately 25 mL for two successive hours.

The following data are now available. It is believed that Maria's blood pressure remained low for at least 30 minutes directly after the crash. The emergency team had difficulty obtaining a vascular access with which to administer fluids. Her daughter has informed you that Maria has no known chronic conditions except for mild arthritis, which she controls with aspirin on a daily basis.

1. Considering Maria's recent history, the origin of her renal problem is most likely?
   A. postrenal
   B. prerenal
   C. intrinsic
   D. perirenal

Five days have passed since the crash. Maria's urine output has fallen to 350 mL over the past 24 hours. She has just received a diuretic challenge, to which she had no response. Her blood pressure is now 165/94 mm Hg.

2. Considering the latest changes, what specifically is Maria most likely developing?
   A. prerenal failure
   B. acute tubular necrosis
   C. postrenal failure
   D. perirenal failure
3. Maria is at high risk for developing renal failure because ischemia occurs when the mean arterial blood pressure drops to below ______ mm Hg for more than 30 minutes.
   A. 60
   B. 70
   C. 80
   D. 90

Maria is now in acute renal failure secondary to acute tubular necrosis. Her urine output has been approximately 350 mL over the past 24 hours, and her creatinine is abnormally elevated. She is confused and drowsy.

4. Assuming that Maria's altered level of consciousness has resulted from her renal failure, it is caused by
   A. accumulated uremic toxins
   B. altered cardiac output
   C. electrolyte imbalances
   D. altered platelet function

It has been 18 days since the onset of Maria's acute renal failure. Her urine output is now 500 mL over the past 24 hours, and her BUN and Cr have both leveled off.

5. Based on Maria's latest trends, which statement best reflects her renal function?
   A. It continues to deteriorate
   B. It has stabilized
   C. It is beginning to recover
   D. It has fully recovered

Her laboratory values are as follows:

48 Hours Postinjury:	5 Days Postinjury:
BUN/creatinine ratio 24:1	BUN/creatinine ratio 13:1
Urine sodium 38 mEq/L	Urine sodium 52 mEq/L
Specific gravity 1.028	Specific gravity 1.008
Serum osmolality 650 mOsm/L	Serum osmolality 285 mOsm/L

6. Maria's pattern of renal laboratory findings are consistent with an initial ______ failure which became a(n) ______ failure.
   A. postrenal, intrinsic
   B. prerenal, postrenal
   C. prerenal, intrinsic
   D. intrinsic, acute tubular necrosis
7. A renal ultrasound is ordered. Which statement is correct regarding ultrasound?
   A. It is an invasive procedure.
   B. It requires use of a contrast dye.
   C. It can be performed at the bedside.
   D. It requires a local anesthetic.

Maria experienced some of the clinical manifestations of uremic syndrome. She was complaining of tingling and numbness of her feet.

8. Maria's symptoms of tingling and numbness were most likely caused by
   A. hyperkalemia
   B. hypocalcemia
   C. stimulated stretch receptors
   D. peripheral neuropathy
9. Skin bruising in acute renal failure is secondary to the effects of
   A. increased erythropoietin
   B. decreased ammonia levels
   C. severe hypocalcemia
   D. excessive uremic toxins
10. Maria's serum phosphate is elevated. Which of the following reasons is most likely the cause?
    A. hypermagnesemia
    B. hypocalcemia
    C. hypomagnesemia
    D. hypercalcemia

11. She is at risk for developing metabolic acidosis primarily as a result of
    A. decreased excretion of potassium
    B. increased excretion of hydrogen ions
    C. increased excretion of potassium
    D. decreased excretion of hydrogen ions
12. Maria is to begin receiving nutritional support. The nurse would anticipate that the preferred route to be used is
    A. oral/GI tract
    B. Hickman catheter
    C. peripheral parenteral nutrition
    D. central venous IV line
13. Maria's nutritional plan will require restriction of
    A. minerals
    B. fats
    C. protein
    D. carbohydrates

It has been decided that Maria needs dialysis. Her present status is as follows. She is hemodynamically stable, and she is eight days postabdominal surgery. She has generalized edema and severe electrolyte abnormalities.

14. Based only on the available data, which type of dialysis is most likely to be ordered for Maria?
    A. hemodialysis
    B. peritoneal dialysis
    C. continuous ultrafiltration
    D. combination of hemodialysis and peritoneal dialysis
15. She is receiving a drug that is highly protein bound while in circulation. What would be the significance of drug protein binding and hemodialysis if this treatment were ordered?
    A. Protein-bound drugs will be released during dialysis.
    B. Protein-bound drugs break down rapidly in the blood.
    C. Protein-bound molecules are too large to dialyze out.
    D. Protein-bound drugs in tissues move into circulation during dialysis.

Posttest answers with rationale are found on MyNursingKit.

REFERENCES

Bagshaw, S. M., & Bellomo, R. (2007). Early diagnosis of acute kidney injury. *Current Opinion in Crit Care 13*, 638–644.

Bellomo, R., Ronco, C., Kellum, J., Mehta, R., Ralevsky, P., & ADQI workgroup. (2004). Acute renal failure-definition, outcome measures, animal models, fluid therapy and information technology needs: The second international consensus conference of the acute dialysis quality initiative (ADQI) group. *Critical Care, 8*, 204–212.

Broscious, S. K., & Castagnola, J. (2006). Chronic kidney disease: acute manifestations and role of the critical care nurse. *Crit Care Nurse 26*(4), 17–28.

Eachempati, S., Wang, J., Hydo, L., Shou, J., & Barie, P. (2007). Acute renal failure in critically ill surgical patients: persistent lethality despite new modes of renal replacement therapy. *The Journal of Trauma, 63*, 987–993.

Gray, M., Huether, S., & Forshee, B. (2006). Alterations of renal and urinary tract function. In K. McCance & S. Huether (eds.), *Pathophysiology: the biological basis for disease in adults and children* (5th ed.). St. Louis, MO: Elsevier Mosby, 1301–1335.

Guyton, A., & Hall, J. (eds.). (2006). *Textbook of medical physiology* (11th ed.). Philadelphia: Elsevier Saunders.

Hall, G. & Esser, E. (2008). Challenges in the care of the patient with acute kidney injury. *J Infusion Nursing 31*(3), 150–156.

Hoste, E., & Schurgers, M. (2008). Epidemiology of acute kidney injury: how big is the problem? *Critical Care Medicine, 36*, S146–151.

Hsu, C., Ordonez, J., Chertow, G., Fan., D. McCulloch, C., & Go, A. (2008). The risk of acute renal failure in patients with chronic kidney disease. *Kidney International, 74*, 101–107.

Kelum, J. (2008). Acute kidney injury. *Critical Care Medicine, 36*, 141–145.

Mehta, R. (2008). From acute renal failure to acute kidney injury: emerging concepts. *Critical Care Medicine, 36*, 1641–1642.

Nagle, P., & Warner, M. (2007). Acute renal failure in a general surgical population: risk profiles, mortality, and opportunities for improvement. *Anesthesiology, 107*, 869–870.

Ostermann, M., & Chang, R. (2007). Acute kidney injury in the intensive care unit according to RIFLE. *Critical Care Medicine, 35*, 1837–1843.

Pannu, N., Klarenbach, S., Wiebe, N. Manns, B., & Tonelli. (2008). Renal replacement therapy in patients with acute renal failure. *JAMA, 299*, 793–805.

Porth, C. (ed.). (2005). Renal failure. In *Pathophysiology: concepts of altered health states* (7th ed.). Philadelphia: Lippincott Williams & Wilkins, 833–850.

Ricci, Z., Cruz, D., & Ronco, C. (2008). The RIFLE criteria and mortality in acute kidney injury: a systematic review. *Kidney International, 73*, 538–546.

Sinert, R. & Doty, C. (2007). Prevention of contrast-induced nephropathy in the emergency department. *Annals of Emergency Medicine, 50*, 335–345.

Sumnall, R. (2007). Fluid management and diuretic therapy in acute renal failure. *Nursing in Critical Care 12*(1), 27–33.

Venkataraman, R., & Kellum, J. (2007). Defining acute renal failure: The RIFLE criteria. *Journal of Intensive Care Medicine, 22*, 187–193.

Wan, L., Bagshaw, S., Langenberg, C., Saotome, T., May, C., & Bellomo, R. (2008). Pathophysiology of septic acute kidney injury: what do we really know? *Critical Care Medicine, 36*, S198–203.

MODULE

28 Determinants and Assessment of Gastrointestinal, Hepatic, and Pancreatic Function

Vicky Turner, Lacey Troutman Buckler, Melanie G. Hardin-Pierce

OBJECTIVES: Following completion of this module, the learner will be able to

1. Identify the anatomic structures of the gastrointestinal tract, liver, and pancreas.
2. Describe the physiologic functions of the gastrointestinal tract, liver, and pancreas.
3. Explain the blood supply and neurologic control of the gastrointestinal tract, liver, and pancreas.
4. Describe the mechanisms that exist within the gastrointestinal tract to protect the integrity of the gut.
5. Discuss the laboratory findings used to evaluate gastrointestinal, liver, and pancreatic function.
6. Explain the diagnostic tests used to evaluate gastrointestinal, liver, and pancreatic function.
7. Describe the components of a focused nursing gastrointestinal database.

This self-study module focuses on the anatomic and physiologic concepts that influence the function of the digestive system, including the gastrointestinal, hepatic, and pancreatic systems. The module is divided into seven sections. Section One presents an overview of the anatomy of the gastrointestinal (GI) system, and accessory organs. Section Two explains the physiology of the GI system and accessory organs. Section Three explains the blood supply and neurologic control of the gastrointestinal tract, liver and pancreas. Section Four describes the mechanisms that exist within the GI tract to protect the integrity of the gut. Section Five presents the laboratory tests used to evaluate gastrointestinal, liver and pancreatic function. Section Six presents the diagnostic tests used to evaluate gastrointestinal, liver and pancreatic function. Section Seven discusses nursing assessment of patients who present with gastrointestinal disorders. All Section Reviews include answers. It is suggested that the learner review those concepts answered incorrectly in the review questions before proceeding to the next section.

PRETEST

1. The primary function of the GI tract is to
   A. metabolize toxic agents
   B. produce clotting factors
   C. provide nutrients needed for metabolism
   D. eliminate carbon dioxide
2. The outermost layer of the GI tract is the
   A. serosa
   B. submucosa
   C. mucosa
   D. peritoneum
3. The functional unit of the liver is called the
   A. hepatocyte
   B. lobule
   C. canaliculi
   D. capsule
4. Bile is secreted by the
   A. terminal bile ducts
   B. quadrate lobe
   C. canaliculi
   D. hepatocytes
5. The functional unit of the pancreas is called the
   A. ampulla of Vater
   B. pancreatic acinus
   C. alpha cell
   D. islets of Langerhans
6. The duct of Wirsung shares the opening into the duodenum with the
   A. acinar cells
   B. duct of Santorini
   C. gallbladder
   D. common bile duct
7. The primary substance in bile is
   A. bile salts
   B. bilirubin
   C. cholesterol
   D. electrolytes

8. The major function of bile salts is to assist with
A. absorption of fat products
B. blood clotting
C. conversion of vitamin D
D. protein synthesis

9. The majority of iron is located in
A. liver
B. bone
C. fat
D. hemoglobin

10. The major byproduct of amino acid deamination is
A. bilirubin
B. ammonia
C. fatty acids
D. glucose

11. The pH of pancreatic juice is
A. highly acidic
B. moderately acidic
C. neutral
D. highly alkaline

12. The pancreas is protected from autodigestion by
A. bicarbonate and water
B. the presence of the hormone secretin
C. protective pancreatic cell wall coverings
D. the production of enzymes in their inactive states

13. Blood flow through the gut, spleen, pancreas, and liver comprise the
A. portal circulation
B. mesenteric circulation
C. splanchnic circulation
D. extrinsic circulation

14. The arterial blood supply to the mesentery and intestines is known as the ______ circulation.
A. mesenteric
B. portocaval
C. visceral
D. aortic

15. Gut-associated lymphoid tissue (GALT) includes
A. thyroid, duodenum, gastric mucosa
B. tonsils, appendix, Peyer's patches
C. adrenal glands, cecum, stomach
D. goblet cells, salivary glands, parietal cells

16. The main aerobic bacteria within the GI tract is
A. *Escherichia coli*
B. *Bacteroides fragilis*
C. *Staphylococcus aureus*
D. beta-hemolytic *streptococcus*

17. Serum enzyme levels are obtained to measure
A. clotting factors
B. organ function
C. cellular injury
D. tissue oxygenation

18. Serum isoenzyme levels often provide better data than parent enzyme levels because they are
A. faster to obtain
B. more tissue specific
C. more plentiful
D. easier to measure

19. Which combination of lactic dehydrogenase (LDH) isoenzymes best reflects hepatic injury?
A. LDH_1 and LDH_2
B. LDH_2 and LDH_3
C. LDH_3 and LDH_4
D. LDH_4 and LDH_5

Pretest answers are found on MyNursingKit.

SECTION ONE: Anatomy of the Gastrointestinal System and Accessory Organs

At the completion of this section, the learner will be able to discuss the anatomy of the gastrointestinal tract, liver and pancreas.

The Gastrointestinal Tract

The anatomy of the gastrointestinal (GI) tract includes the upper and lower digestive systems (Fig. 28–1). The upper portion includes the oral cavity, the teeth and tongue, salivary glands, the pharynx, and the esophagus. The stomach, small and large intestines comprise the lower GI system.

Esophagus

The esophagus is approximately 17.5 inches (45 cm) from the lower incisor teeth. It is a muscular structure with the capacity to contract and release during peristalsis, which facilitates movement of food toward the stomach. The mucosal lining is made up of stratified squamous epithelium and changes to columnar epithelium at or near the gastroesophageal junction. The **lower esophageal sphincter** (LES), also known as the cardiac sphincter, is not formed from a distinct muscle but is a structure with high resting muscle tone at the distal end to prevent gastroesophageal reflux.

Stomach

The stomach is located in the upper left abdominal quadrant. It begins at the terminal end of the esophagus just below the lower esophageal sphincter (LES), where it receives food stuffs from the esophagus. The stomach is divided into three major parts, the fundus, the body, and the antrum (Fig. 28–2). The **fundus** is the area at the top of the stomach, located above the LES, and appears as a bulge that bumps up against the diaphragm. The **body** is the largest part of the stomach, and is located just beneath the fundus and ends at the antrum. The **antrum** is located at the base on the stomach, ending at the pyloric sphincter, which separates the stomach from the

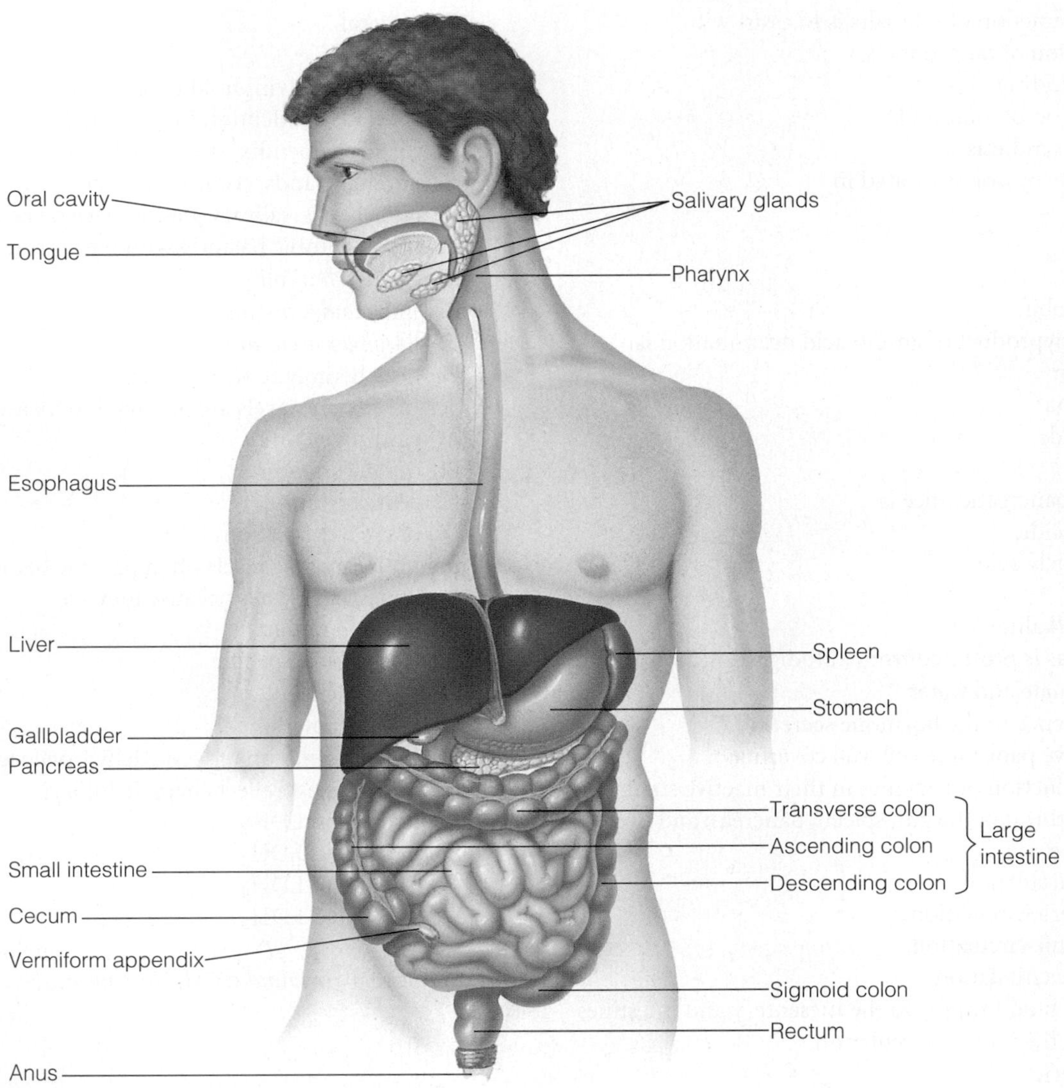

Figure 28–1 ■ Organs of the gastrointestinal tract and accessory digestive organs.

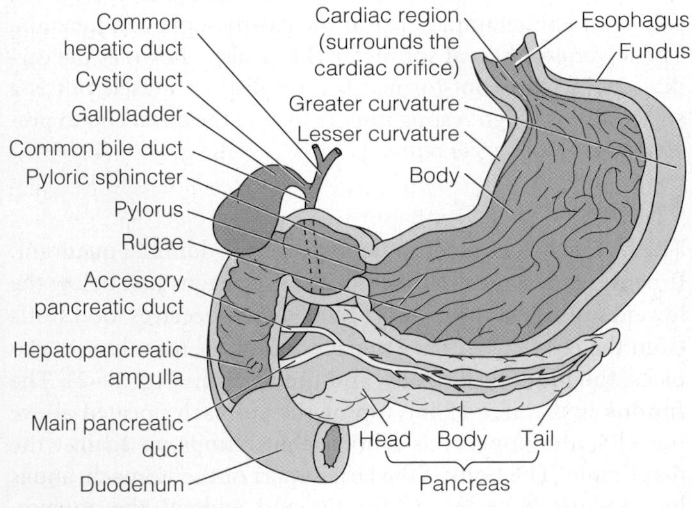

Figure 28–2 ■ The anatomic structures of the stomach, pancreas, and gallbladder.

duodenum. The stomach wall is composed of the innermost lining, the **mucosa;** the **submucosa,** a layer that contains blood and lymphatic vessels; the **muscularis,** a three-layer muscle set; and the **serosa,** the outermost lining (Fig. 28–3). The stomach size is altered based on the volume of contents within it. At rest, it is small, containing only about 50 mL of fluid (Huether, 2008).

Small Intestine

The small intestines are comprised of the duodenum, the jejunum, and the ileum. The small intestines extend from the pylorus of the stomach to the ileocecal valve, with a total length of about 16 to 20 feet (5 to 6 meters) (Huether, 2008). The mucosal and submucosal layers of the small intestines are arranged in folds, and function to slow the passage of chyme through the small intestine to maximize digestion and absorption. Fingerlike projections called **villi** cover the intestinal folds. Each villus is covered with tiny absorptive fingerlike projections called

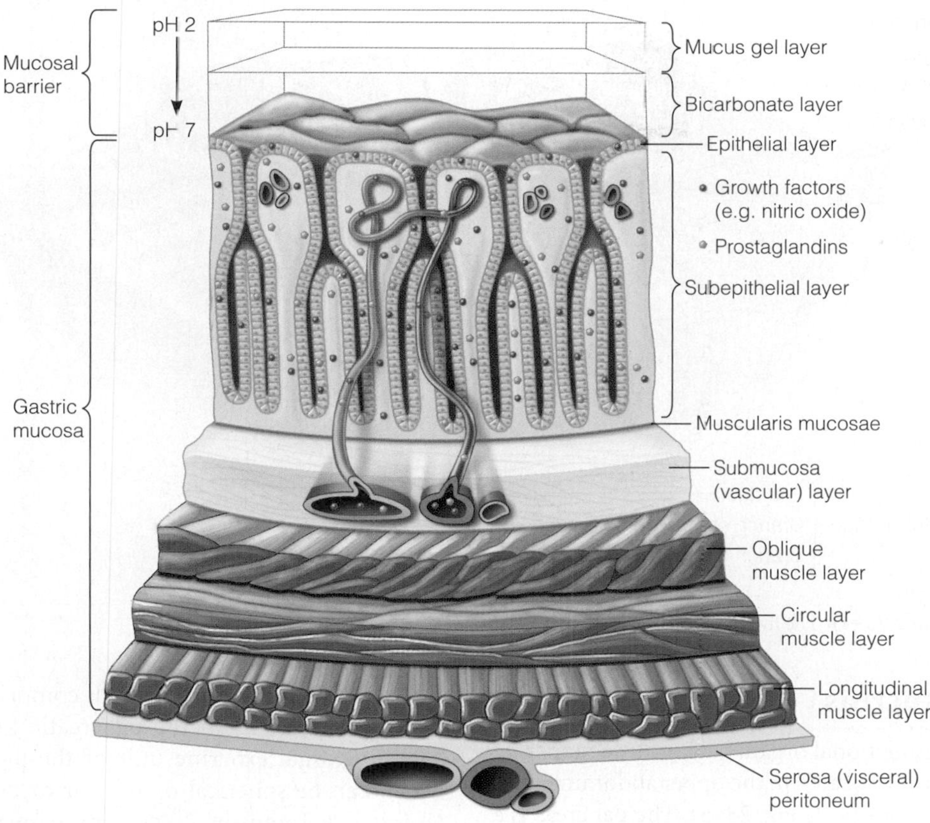

Figure 28–3 ■ Layers of the gut wall and mechanisms for maintaining mucosal integrity.

microvilli and collectively with the villi make up the brush border of the small intestine.

Large Intestine

The large intestine consists of a large, hollow muscular tubular structure that originates at the terminal ileum at the ileocecal valve and extends to the anus. The ileocecal valve prevents backflow of feces from the large to the small intestine. The length of the large intestine is approximately 5 feet (1.5 meters) (Huether, 2008). The large intestine consists of the cecum, colon, and rectum. The colon is further divided into four segments; the ascending, transverse, descending, and sigmoid. The absorption of water and electrolytes is largely completed in the ascending colon. It absorbs approximately one liter of water and electrolytes daily.

When food is consumed, distention of the stomach leads to an immediate increase in colonic contractions, referred to as the **gastrocolic reflex.** The movement of the large intestine is called **haustral churning,** which is slow and causes the intestinal contents to move back and forth in a kneading motion. This churning motion allows time for absorption to occur. As the rectal wall fills with stool, the defecation reflex is initiated.

The Liver

As shown in Figure 28–1, the liver is located in the right upper quadrant of the abdominal cavity and lies directly beneath the diaphragm. The surface anatomy of the liver corresponds to an anterior upper border roughly parallel with the fifth right intercostal space and the lower border that runs obliquely upward from the right ninth to the left eighth costal cartilage. The liver has two major lobes; the right lobe and the left lobe. The lobes are divided by the falciform ligament. The right lobe can be further divided into the caudate and quadrate lobes. The liver is enclosed in the visceral **peritoneum** and covered with a connective tissue structure known as Glisson's capsule. The capsule subdivides into branches called septa that extend into the liver parenchyma to form individual liver lobules. The liver can be divided into eight functionally distinct segments, with each having its own set of blood vessels and bile ducts.

The **lobule** is the functional unit of the liver. It is shaped like a cylinder and surrounds a central vein in a spoke-like fashion (Fig. 28–4). Each lobule is composed of hepatic cellular plates that radiate out of the central vein. The hepatic cells (hepatocytes) secrete **bile** which flows into the bile canaliculi, a small space separating the hepatic cellular plates. From the **canaliculi** the bile flows into terminal bile ducts located in the septa or spaces lying between adjoining lobules. The septa contain the portal venules which provide blood flow from the portal veins. The portal venules supply the blood flow that flows by the hepatic cellular plates and ultimately flows into the central vein of the lobule. The physiologic structure of the lobule allows continuous exposure of blood to the hepatic cells.

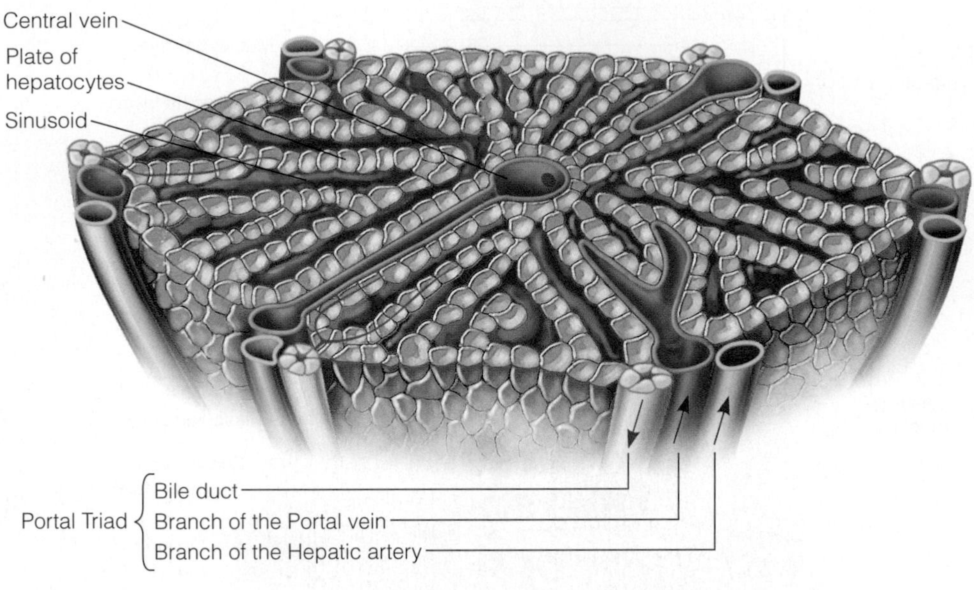

Figure 28–4 ■ The liver lobule.

The Exocrine Pancreas

The pancreas is a multifunctional organ, having both endocrine and exocrine functions. It is located in the upper abdominal cavity, lying in a horizontal position (Fig. 28–5). The pancreas is a soft, elongated, flattened gland 5 to 8 inches (12 to 20 cm) in length (Burdick & Tompson, 2006). In an adult, it normally weighs between 70 and 110 grams. It has three divisions: the head, the body, and the tail. The head lies adjacent to the duodenum, within its curve. The pancreatic body lies directly behind the stomach, and the tail is adjacent to the spleen.

The pancreatic exocrine cells comprise almost the entirety (about 98 percent) of the pancreatic tissue (Sargent, 2006). The functional exocrine unit of the pancreas is the **acinus,** which can be spherical or tubular or even irregular in form (Burdick & Tompson, 2006). The acinus is composed of cells that synthesize, store, and secrete digestive enzymes; and a network of ductal cells that secrete alkaline fluids with important digestive functions. Acini are clustered into larger units called pancreatic lobules. The lobules are separated from each other by septa (see Fig. 28–6).

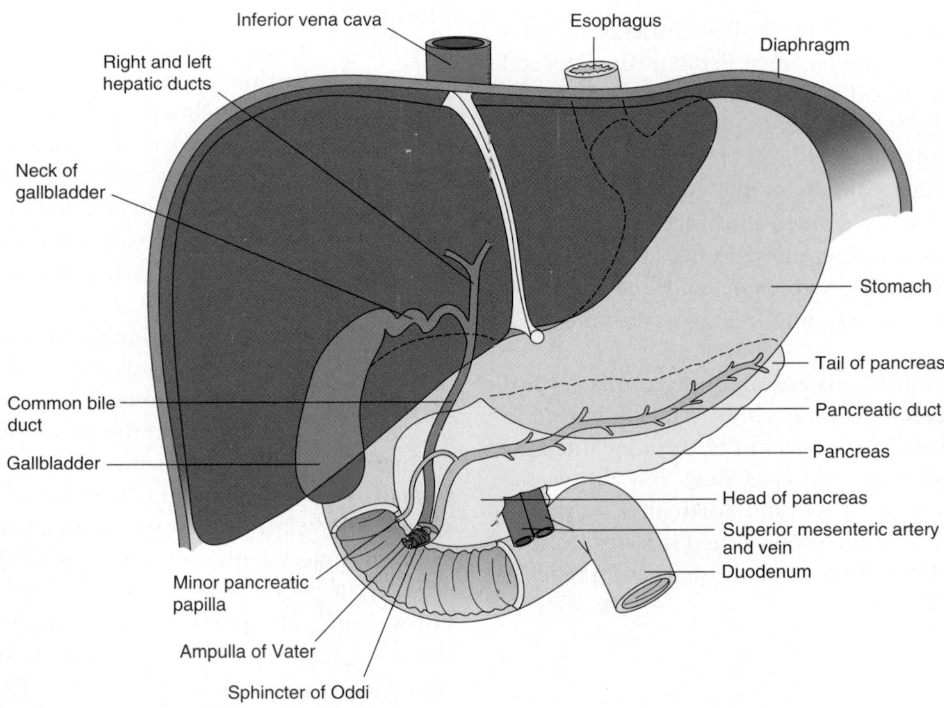

Figure 28–5 ■ The pancreas and pancreatic-biliary system.

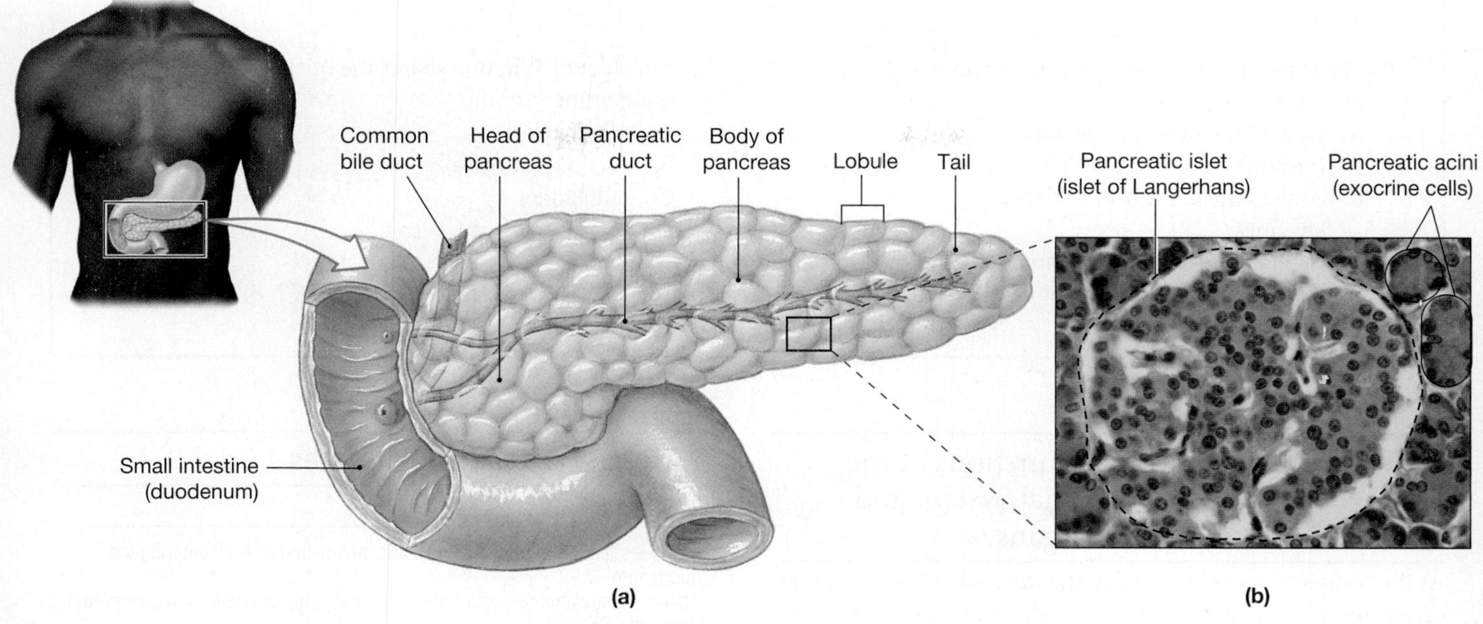

Figure 28–6 ■ The pancreas. (a) Pancreatic anatomic structures. (b) Acinus, the pancreatic functional unit.

Once released, the pancreatic digestive enzymes flow through a ductal system into the duodenum (as shown in Fig. 28–5 and 28-6(a)), through a connecting network of ducts, eventually terminating at the main pancreatic duct, called the **duct of Wirsung.** This duct runs through the center of the organ from head to tail. It joins with the common bile duct, sharing the same opening into the duodenum at the **ampulla of Vater,** which is surrounded by the **sphincter of Oddi.** Located at the junction of the common bile duct and the duodenum, the sphincter of Oddi helps control the rate of pancreatic enzyme and bile flow into the duodenum. An accessory pancreatic duct known as the **duct of Santorini,** exists in approximately 70 percent of the population and generally communicates with the main duct (Fauci et al., 2008).

SECTION ONE REVIEW

1. The largest portion of the stomach is called the gastric
   A. fundus
   B. body
   C. antrum
   D. pyloris
2. The innermost layer of the GI tract which is responsible for secretion of mucus and enzymes is the
   A. submucosa
   B. muscularis
   C. mucosa
   D. mesentery
3. The ______ line(s) the wall of the abdominal cavity.
   A. peritoneum
   B. mucosa
   C. microvilli
   D. brush border
4. The finger-like projections that cover the folds of the small intestine are called
   A. canaliculi
   B. pedicles
   C. villi
   D. septa
5. The functional unit of the liver is called the
   A. hepatocyte
   B. lobule
   C. canaliculi
   D. capsule
6. Bile is secreted by
   A. terminal bile ducts
   B. the quadrate lobe
   C. canaliculi
   D. hepatocytes
7. The functional unit of the exocrine pancreas is called the
   A. lobule
   B. acinus
   C. alpha cell
   D. islets of Langerhans
8. Which structures are part of the pancreatic anatomic structure? (choose all that apply)
   A. body
   B. tail
   C. arm
   D. head

(continued)

(continued)

9. The sphincter of Oddi primarily serves which purpose?
A. control the rate of pancreatic enzyme flow into intestines
B. control the activation of the pancreatic enzymes
C. regulate the level of intestinal secretin
D. regulate the rate of bicarbonate secretion

10. The duct of Wirsung shares the opening into the duodenum with the
A. acinar cells
B. duct of Santorini
C. gallbladder
D. common bile duct

Answers: 1. B, 2. C, 3. A, 4. C, 5. B, 6. D, 7. B, 8. (A, B, D), 9. A, 10. D

SECTION TWO: Physiologic Functions of the Gastrointestinal System and Accessory Organs

At the completion of this section, the learner will be able to describe the physiologic functions of the gastrointestinal tract, liver and pancreas.

The primary function of the gastrointestinal system is to provide the body with nutrients necessary to support and promote cell growth. The mechanisms for digestion include ingestion, digestion, and absorption.

The Stomach

The stomach has a number of functions including food storage, digestion, and propulsion. The stomach receives all food stuffs via the esophagus. In preparation for accepting the food, the gastric wall relaxes through the influences of two hormones, **cholecystokinin** (CCK) and **gastrin.** Once in the stomach, peristaltic waves mix the food material with the digestive juices to form the **chyme,** which is food that is partially broken down by digestive juices (gastric acid and pepsin). While chyme is being formed, it is also being moved through the stomach toward the pyloric sphincter. The peristaltic action facilitates emptying of the chyme into the duodenum where it continues through the gastrointestinal tract for further processing and elimination of waste.

The gastric body is richly supplied with gastric glands that contain **parietal cells** and **chief cells.** Parietal cells secrete **hydrochloric acid** and **intrinsic factor (IF),** and chief cells secrete **pepsinogen. Pepsinogen** is a precursor of pepsin, an enzyme that is necessary for protein digestion. The gastric body also contains cells that secrete histamine when stimulated by acetylcholine or gastrin. The antrum contains **G-cells,** which secrete gastrin. The gastric mucosa is protected from the caustic damaging effects of gastric acid and pepsin by a protective mucus and bicarbonate layer called the mucosal barrier. The health of this barrier is promoted by prostaglandins.

The Small and Large Intestines

The primary function of the small intestine is absorption of nutrients and water. The small intestines secrete hormones that have stimulatory and inhibitory effects that are necessary in the regulation of digestion (see Table 28–1). These hormones include cholecystokinin, secretin, and gastric inhibitory peptide. Cholecystokinin (CCK) is secreted in response to the presence of fat, protein and an acidic pH. The role of CCK is to stimulate secretion of pancreatic digestive enzymes that are necessary for the digestion of fat and protein, to increase contractility of the gallbladder so that bile is released into the duodenum to aid in the absorption of fats, and to inhibit gastric motility in order to slow the digestive process so that absorption can take place.

TABLE 28–1 Intestinal Hormones

HORMONE
Secretin—secreted in response to acidic chyme and alcohol entering the duodenum Action - Stimulates release of bile, pancreatic, bicarbonate, water, and the action of CCK
Cholecystokinin (CCK)—secreted in response to the presence of fat, protein, and acidic chyme in the duodenum Action - Stimulates release of pancreatic digestive enzymes; increases contractility of gallbladder; inhibits gastric motility
Gastric inhibitory peptide (GIP)—secreted in response to carbohydrates and fat Action - Inhibits gastric acid secretion and motility; stimulates insulin secretion

When gastric acid comes into contact with the intestinal mucosa, it stimulates the release of the hormone **secretin.** Secretin further stimulates the release of alkaline pancreatic bicarbonate and water which functions to increase the pH of chyme in the duodenum. This alkalinity of the chyme is important because pancreatic digestive enzymes are active only in an alkaline environment. **Gastric inhibitory peptide** (**GIP**) is a hormone that is secreted in the presence of carbohydrates and fats within the small intestine. It facilitates the digestion of fats and carbohydrates by inhibiting intestinal motility and the secretion of gastric acid. GIP also stimulates insulin secretion. The inhibition of gastric acid contributes to the action of secretin to maintain an alkaline environment which is necessary for pancreatic **proteolytic** enzymes to metabolize proteins and fats.

The primary functions of the large intestine are the completion of water and nutrient absorption; the manufacturing of certain vitamins; the formation of feces; and expulsion of the feces from the body. Digestion that occurs in the large intestine results from bacterial rather than enzymatic action. Normal flora reside in the large intestine that break down dietary cellulose and synthesize folic acid, vitamin K, riboflavin, and nicotinic acid.

Liver Functions

The liver performs a variety of crucial functions, including metabolic, homeostatic, filtering, clotting, and drug and chemical detoxification. Table 28–2 provides a summary of these functions.

Metabolic Functions

The liver plays a crucial role in fat, carbohydrate, and protein metabolism because of its ability to synthesize, convert, degrade, or store these nutritional substances. In addition, the liver is important in maintaining normal levels of fat-soluble vitamins and iron in the body.

Fat Metabolism. The liver is responsible for the synthesis of phospholipids and cholesterol. Through oxidation of fatty acids, the liver can supply the body with massive amounts of energy. The liver is also responsible for the production and excretion of bile. Bile salts, a major component of bile, are necessary for normal digestion. In the intestines, bile salts assist in absorption of fat products, such as fatty acids, cholesterol, and fat-soluble vitamins. Bile salts also assist in the breakdown of fat molecules through a detergent-like action. A second major component of bile is **bilirubin,** a bile pigment (discussed in Section Five).

Carbohydrate Metabolism. The liver plays a major role in maintaining normal blood glucose levels. Glucose is stored in the liver as glycogen, which is converted back into glucose as needed by the body through the process of **glycogenolysis.** The liver is also able to convert amino acids to glucose through the process of **gluconeogenesis.**

Protein Metabolism. Protein metabolism is essential to life. The liver is responsible not only for synthesis of the majority of the body's proteins but it also degrades amino acids for energy use through the process of deamination. The major byproduct of deamination is ammonia, which is toxic to tissues. The liver is responsible for converting ammonia into **urea,** a nontoxic substance. Urea diffuses from the liver into the circulation for urinary excretion. When liver failure occurs, ammonia cannot be converted to urea and levels rapidly build in the blood.

TABLE 28–2 Major Functions of the Liver

GENERAL FUNCTION	COMMENTS
Metabolic	Fat metabolism—massive energy source; produces bile Carbohydrate metabolism—maintains normal blood glucose Protein metabolism—synthesis of proteins and deamination of amino acids; converts ammonia to urea Vitamin and minerals—major role in absorption of fat-soluble vitamins (A, D, E, and K); major storage area for iron
Blood volume reservoir	Able to distend and compress to alter circulating blood volume
Blood filter	Tissue macrophages, Kupffer's cells, purify the blood of bacteria
Blood clotting factors	Produces clotting factors including prothrombin and fibrinogen
Drug metabolism and detoxification	Responsible for metabolism of drugs; is able to deactivate potentially harmful substances and ready them for excretion in a harmless form

Vitamin- and Mineral-Related Functions. Adequate levels of bile are needed for absorption of the fat-soluble vitamins A, D, E, and K. Should the production of bile become deficient, fat absorption decreases and the levels of these vitamins become significantly reduced. The liver requires vitamin K for production of clotting factors. If the level of vitamin K is low, clotting factor production will be reduced. The liver also plays a crucial role in the early steps of the conversion of vitamin D into its active product 1,25-dihydroxycholecalciferol, which helps control the concentration of calcium.

The liver is the major storage center for iron. Approximately 10 percent of iron is bound to ferritin within hepatocytes and is released when iron levels become depleted. Iron is an important part of hemoglobin synthesis; more than half the body's iron is located in hemoglobin. Liver damage (e.g., cirrhosis) can decrease the hepatocytes' ability to store iron, and iron-deficiency anemia can develop if iron stores become depleted.

Blood Volume Reservoir

The liver serves as a reservoir for blood. Its massive vascular bed and its ability to expand and compress provide a large potential overflow receptacle. During periods of high fluid volume states in the right heart, the liver is able to accept approximately one liter of the excess volume by distending, which decreases circulating fluid volume. In periods of fluid volume deficit, the liver is able to compress, shifting blood into the intravascular space, thereby increasing circulating fluid volume.

Blood Filter

Blood flowing through the intestines becomes contaminated with a variety of pathogens. Special fixed macrophages in the liver called **Kupffer's cells** efficiently and rapidly engulf and destroy bacteria, viruses, and other pathogens before the blood moves back into general circulation. The Kupffer's cells, which are located in the sinusoids on endothelial cells, are part of the tissue macrophage system (also called the reticuloendothelial system). This important system consists of mobile macrophages that are able to move freely through the tissues, and fixed macrophages that are attached to tissues. Fixed macrophages, such as the Kupffer's cells, are able to detach from their tissue when stimulated in order to carry out their phagocytic activities. The Kupffer's cells also filter out foreign particles and old cells.

Blood Clotting Factors

The liver is responsible for the formation of most blood clotting factors. Normal formation of clotting factors requires synthesis of vitamin K by the intestines. When vitamin K synthesis is hindered, the formation of clotting factors is inhibited, leading to bleeding tendencies. The liver also produces fibrinogen, a protein that forms fibrin threads and blood clots due to the action of thrombin.

Drug Metabolism and Detoxification

The liver plays a major role in the metabolism of fat-soluble drugs. Through biotransformation, it changes potentially harmful drugs into harmless substances that are then excreted by the kidneys. The liver also has the ability to detoxify harmful endogenous substances.

Exocrine Pancreas Functions

The pancreas is rather unique in that it has both endocrine and exocrine functions. The endocrine functions of the pancreas consist primarily of the secretion of the two major hormones, insulin and glucagon, which maintain glucose homeostasis. An in-depth discussion of the endocrine functions of the pancreas occurs in Module 34, Alterations in Glucose Metabolism. The exocrine functions of the pancreas directly influence the gastrointestinal system and accessory organs.

The pancreas normally secretes approximately 1.5 liters of enzyme fluid daily. These fluids are responsible for digestion of fats, starches and protein. Pancreatic juice is composed of water, bicarbonate, electrolytes (specifically potassium and sodium), and digestive enzymes. In a healthy person, pancreatic juice is clear, colorless, isotonic, protein rich, and alkaline.

There are four major stimuli of pancreatic secretion: gastrin, cholecystokinin (CCK), secretin, and acetylcholine. The acidic pH of the chyme that enters the duodenum from the stomach stimulates mucosal secretion of secretin and CCK by the proximal end of the small intestines. These two hormones are essential in the regulation of intestinal pH; both are regulatory hormones responsive to a negative feedback system. Secretin and CCK are also stimulated by stomach acids, amino acids, and fats, respectively. Gastrin, secretin, and CCK stimulate the pancreatic acinar cells and are responsible for the release of large quantities of pancreatic enzymes. Acetylcholine is secreted by parasympathetic, vagal, and cholinergic nerve endings located throughout the **gut.** Vagal influence stimulates secretion of pancreatic enzymes, which are then placed in temporary storage in the acini, awaiting a transport mechanism to move them into the intestines (Guyton & Hall, 2006).

Release of secretin is stimulated by a drop in pH to less than 4.5. When intestinal pH becomes too acidic, secretin stimulates the pancreas to secrete large quantities of bicarbonate and water. Bicarbonate raises the intestinal pH, which protects the mucosa. Pancreatic enzymes work best within a pH level that is neutral to slightly alkaline (Burdick & Tompson, 2006). The alkaline pH of the small bowel is important for deactivating pepsin, which protects the delicate intestinal mucosa and facilitates normal digestive enzyme processes. In contrast, cholecystokinin is released from gut endocrine cells where fats and proteins enter the intestine. Cholecystokinin uses vagal mechanisms to stimulate acinar cells to release digestive proteolytics (Stevens & Conwell, 2008).

Pancreatic Enzymes

Normal digestion depends on the digestive enzymatic activities of the pancreatic **enzymes** (Table 28–3). Pancreatic digestives enzymes are responsible for the breakdown of proteins (proteolytics), fat (**lipolytics**), and carbohydrates (**amylolytics**).

Pancreatic Self-Protective Properties

The proteolytic pancreatic enzymes (**trypsin, chymotrypsin,** and **elastase**) are responsible for the breakdown of proteins and make up about 90 percent of pancreatic digestive enzymes. The lipolytic pancreatic enzyme, **phospholipase A,** is responsible for breaking down phospholipids into fatty acids. This enzyme may contribute to the development of pulmonary complications (acute respiratory distress syndrome [ARDS]) by decreasing surfactant in the lungs.

Without some protective mechanism, these enzymes are capable of digesting pancreatic and other tissues, a process called **autodigestion.** Under normal circumstances, mechanisms exist to prevent autodigestion. Pancreatic proteolytic enzymes are produced in an inactive, precursor form, remaining inactive while in the pancreas (refer to Table 28–3 for the precursor names). For example, a trypsin inhibitor (secreted by the acinar cells) maintains trypsin in its inactive state while it is present in the pancreatic ducts and cells (Guyton & Hall, 2006).

TABLE 28–3 Major Pancreatic Enzymes

ENZYME	TARGET	PRECURSOR NAME	COMMENTS
Trypsin	Proteins	Trypsinogen	Most abundant proteolytic enzyme; activated in intestinal mucosa by enterokinase or by preexisting trypsin
Elastase	Proteins	Proelastase	Activated by trypsin; breaks down elastic tissue; can break down blood vessel walls
Chymotrypsin	Proteins	Chymotrypsinogen	Activated by trypsin; splits (via hydrolysing) proteins into peptones
Amylase (pancreatic)	Carbohydrates	—	Splits glycogen, starches, and other carbohydrates, with the exception of cellulose, into disaccharides (primarily)
Lipase	Fats	—	Requires bile salts; splits fats into monoglycerides and fatty acids
Phospholipase A	Fats	—	Activated by trypsin or bile salts; splits phospholipids into fatty acids; breaks down cell membranes and is capable of causing pancreatic and fat tissue necrosis, and reduction in lung surfactant levels

SECTION TWO REVIEW

1. The gastric parietal cells secrete
   A. gastrin
   B. pepsinogen
   C. hydrochloric acid
   D. mucus
2. The primary substance in bile is
   A. bile salts
   B. bilirubin
   C. cholesterol
   D. electrolytes
3. The major function of bile salts is to assist with
   A. conversion of vitamin D
   B. blood clotting
   C. breakdown and absorption of fat
   D. protein synthesis
4. The majority of iron is located in
   A. liver
   B. bone
   C. fat
   D. hemoglobin
5. The major byproduct of amino acid deamination is
   A. bilirubin
   B. ammonia
   C. fatty acids
   D. glucose
6. The blood filtering capabilities of the liver are primarily due to the actions of
   A. Kupffer's cells
   B. immunoglobulins
   C. ammonia
   D. bile
7. The pH of pancreatic juice is
   A. acidic
   B. moderately acidic
   C. neutral
   D. alkaline
8. The function of secretin is to
   A. lower the pancreatic pH
   B. stimulate secretion of pancreatic enzymes
   C. directly activate pepsin production
   D. inhibit secretion of pancreatic enzymes
9. The most abundant pancreatic enzyme is
   A. chymotrypsin
   B. lipase
   C. trypsin
   D. elastase
10. The pancreas is protected from autodigestion by
    A. bicarbonate and water
    B. the presence of the hormone secretin
    C. protective pancreatic cell wall coverings
    D. the production of enzymes in their inactive states

Answers: 1. C, 2. A, 3. C, 4. D, 5. B, 6. A, 7. D, 8. B, 9. C, 10. D

SECTION THREE: Blood Supply and Innervation of the Gastrointestinal System

At the completion of this section, the learner will be able to explain the blood supply and neurologic control of the gastrointestinal tract, liver and pancreas.

Blood Supply

Figure 28–4 illustrates the rich blood supply to the liver lobule. The gastrointestinal system receives about one fourth of the resting cardiac output, more than any other organ system. The combination of the portal and mesenteric circulatory systems is called the **splanchnic circulation** (see Fig. 28–7). This system includes blood flow through the gut, spleen, pancreas, and liver.

Arterial Circulation

Arterial blood supply to the intestines is provided by the **mesenteric circulation** (see Fig. 28–8). This begins at the aorta, flowing through the aortic arch to the celiac artery and the inferior and superior mesenteric arteries. Arteries that branch off of the celiac artery supply blood to the stomach, including the left

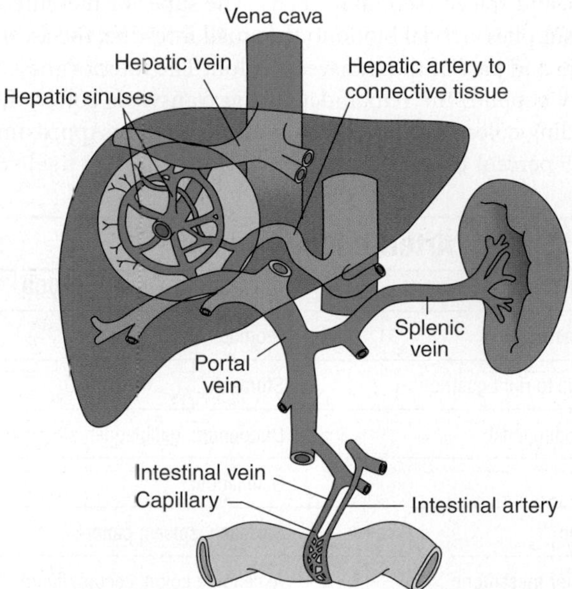

Figure 28–7 ■ Splanchnic circulation. This figure was published in *Textbook of Medical Physiology*, 11th ed., Copyright Elsevier [2006].

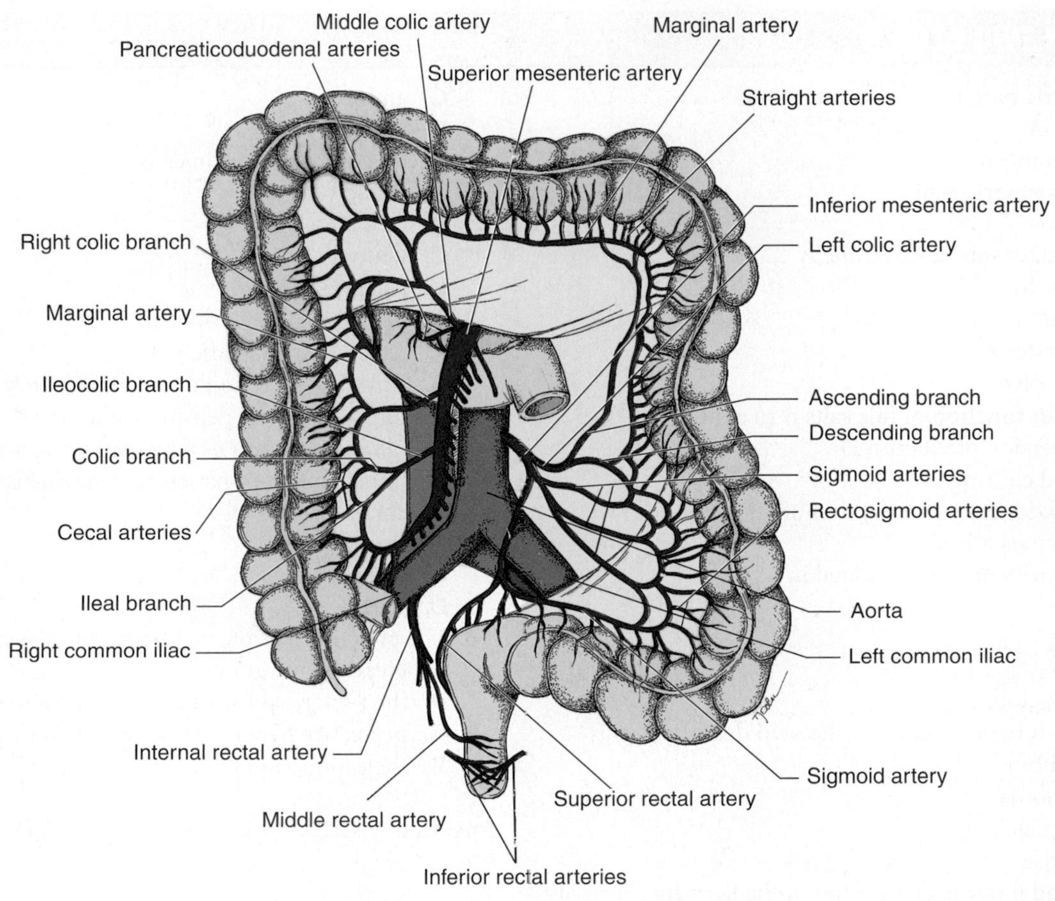

Figure 28–8 ■ Arterial blood supply to the gut.

and right gastric, hepatic, gastroduodenal, and splenic arteries. Arteries that branch off of the larger celiac artery supply the blood to the stomach, esophagus, duodenum, gallbladder, pancreas, and spleen (see Table 28–4). The superior mesenteric artery supplies arterial blood to the small intestine, the ascending colon, and part of the transverse colon. The inferior mesenteric artery supplies the remainder of the transverse colon, the descending colon, sigmoid colon and the rectum. Approximately 10-15 percent of the cardiac output flows through the liver per minute, which is about 1.5 L/min. The volume of blood flowing through the liver is determined by the blood flow through the spleen and the GI tract. The liver is richly supplied with both arterial and venous blood. The arterial blood to the liver is supplied from a branch of the aorta, the hepatic artery.

TABLE 28–4 Arterial Blood Supply

ARTERY	AREA SUPPLIED WITH BLOOD
Left gastric	Stomach and esophagus
Hepatic to right gastric	Stomach
Gastroduodenal	Duodenum, gallbladder, stomach
Cystic	Gallbladder
Splenic	Stomach, spleen, pancreas
Superior mesenteric	Ascending colon, cecum, ileum, jejunum, transverse colon
Inferior mesenteric	Rectum, sigmoid colon, transverse colon

Venous Drainage

The venous blood draining from the GI system organs does not flow directly into the inferior vena cava to return to the heart. Instead, blood that supplies both mesenteric arteries and the celiac artery flows through the hepatic portal system before moving into the vena cava. The hepatic portal system causes blood to shift between capillary beds within the system, such that all blood flows into the liver before moving into the general circulation. This is important because the liver is responsible for regulating and storing nutrients, and handling waste products and toxins that come into the system via the other GI organs (Martini, Bartholomew & Bledsoe, 2008). Table 28–5 lists the portal vein branches and what they drain.

Innervation

The gastrointestinal tract, liver, and pancreas all receive sympathetic nervous system (SNS) innervation via the splanchnic nerves that branch off of the spinal cord at the level of the thoracic segments (Fig 28–9). The splanchnic nerves are routed into several collateral ganglia which, as postganglionic nerves, directly

TABLE 28–5 Portal Vein Branches and Their Drainage Sites

PORTAL VEIN BRANCH	DRAINAGE SITE
Gastric	Esophagus, stomach
Splenic	Duoderum, esophagus, gallbladder, stomach, pancreas
Superior mesenteric	Ascending and transverse colon, small intestine
Inferior mesenteric	Descending and sigmoid colon, rectum

innervate the target mesenteric organs. Activation of the sympathetic nervous system decreases most gastrointestinal system functions to reroute blood to more vital organs during periods of stress. The liver responds to SNS simulation by synthesizing and releasing glucose and breaking down glycogen. Parasympathetic innervation to the **mesentery** comes from cranial nerve ten (CN X), and the vagus nerve. Parasympathetic stimulation of the organs within the gastrointestinal system is responsible for stimulating the normal functions of the GI system, such as processing of food, propulsion of contents through the GI tract, and absorption of nutrients (Martini, Bartholomew & Bledsoe, 2008). In the liver, parasympathetic stimulation results in synthesis of glycogen.

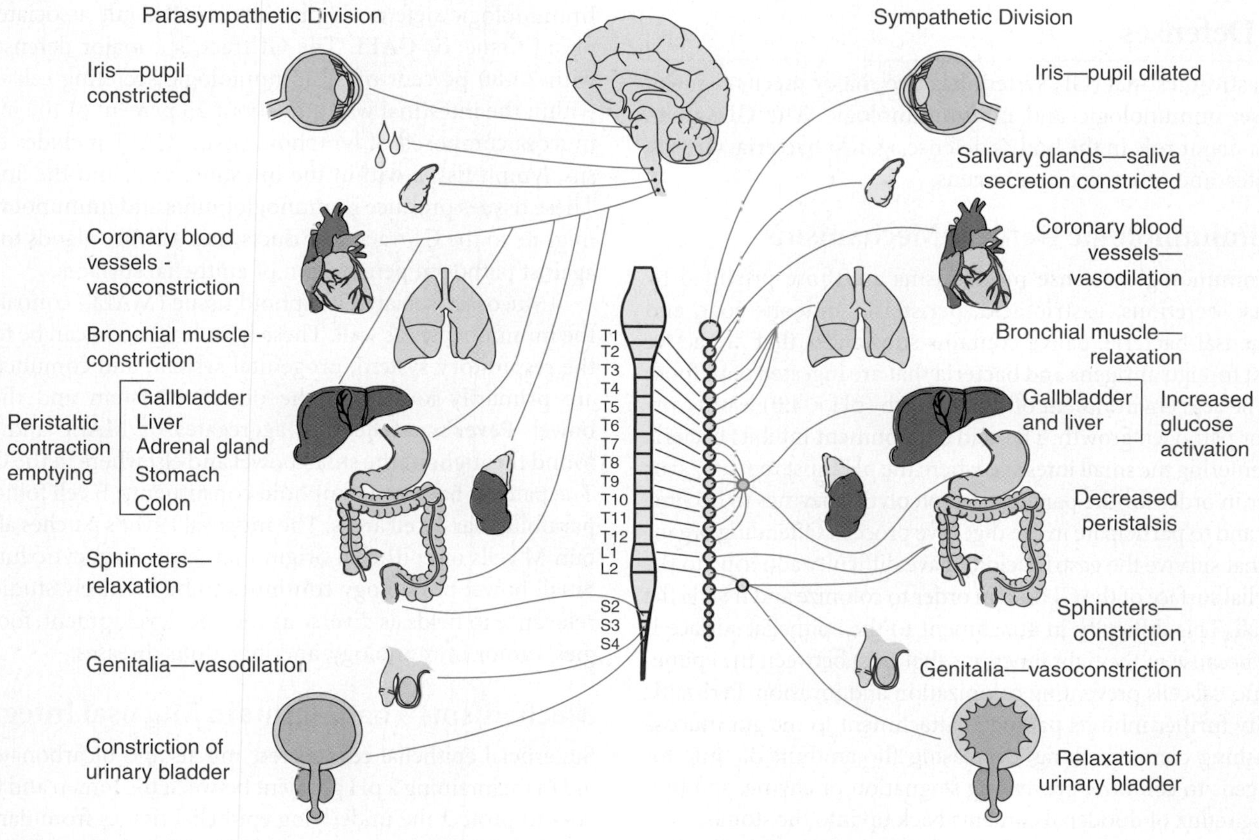

Figure 28–9 ■ Parasympathetic and sympathetic divisions of the autonomic nervous system.

SECTION THREE REVIEW

1. The mesenteric circulation begins its flow at the
   A. celiac artery
   B. hepatic artery
   C. aorta
   D. superior vena cava
2. The blood that supplies the mesenteric and celiac arteries flows through the _______ before moving into the general circulation.
   A. spleen
   B. liver
   C. pancreas
   D. kidneys
3. The blood volume flowing through the liver represents what percentage of cardiac output?
   A. 10-15 percent
   B. 15-20 percent
   C. 20-25 percent
   D. 25-30 percent
4. The GI tract, liver, and pancreas all receive sympathetic nervous system innervation from the
   A. vagus nerve
   B. splanchnic nerves
   C. trigeminal nerves
   D. parasympathetic nerve

(continued)

(continued)

5. An important reason that blood from the digestive system goes through the liver before moving into the general circulation is because
   - A. it needs to drop off bile
   - B. it needs to pick up glucose
   - C. it needs to alter its pH
   - D. it needs to be filtered

Answers: 1. C, 2. B, 3. A, 4. B, 5. D

SECTION FOUR: Gut Defenses

At the completion of this section, the learner will be able to describe the mechanisms that exist within the GI tract to protect the integrity of the gut.

Gut Defenses

The gastrointestinal (GI) system has two major mechanisms of defense: immunologic and nonimmunologic. The GI system plays a major role in the body's defense against bacteria, viruses, parasites, and other toxic pathogens.

Nonimmunologic Defense Mechanisms

Nonimmunologic defense mechanisms are those provided by salivary secretions, gastric acid, peristalsis, mucous coat, and commensal bacteria. Saliva contains substances that are active against foreign antigens and bacteria that are ingested with food.

The acid environment of the stomach (pH < 4.0) is unfavorable for pathogen growth. The acid environment inhibits bacteria from entering the small intestine where the pH must remain 7.0 or greater in order for the pancreatic proteolytic enzymes to become active and to participate in the digestive process. Offending organisms that survive the gastric acidity have difficulty adhering to the epithelial surface of the GI tract in order to colonize and invade the gut wall. This difficulty in attachment to the epithelial surface is partly because of the tight junctions that exist between the epithelial mucosal cells preventing colonization and invasion. Peristaltic motility further inhibits pathogen attachment to the gut mucosa by pushing contents along, decreasing the amount of time for pathogens to colonize, preventing stagnation of chyme, and preventing reflux of duodenal contents back up into the stomach.

The mucosal coating of the GI tract prevents offending pathogens from adhering to the epithelial surface. Goblet cells secrete mucus that provides a protective barrier to potential pathogens.

Commensal bacteria or normal flora reside in the ileum and large intestine and limit proliferation and adherence of potentially harmful bacteria. *Bacteroides fragilis* is the main anaerobic bacteria and *Escherichia coli* are the main aerobic bacteria that prevent overgrowth of other gram-negative and gram-positive bacteria.

Immunologic Defense Mechanisms

Immunologic defense is provided by the gut associated lymphoid tissue, or **GALT.** The GI tract is a major defense organ with 70-80 percent of all immunologic secreting cells located within the intestinal wall and about 25 percent of the intestinal mucosa composed of lymphoid tissue. GALT includes the tonsils, lymph tissue within the intestinal wall, and the appendix. These tissues produce immunoglobulins and immunocytes that migrate to the GI tract, tear ducts, and salivary glands to defend against pathogen penetration of epithelial surfaces.

Mucosa associated lymphoid tissue (MALT) contributes to the immunocytes as well. These lymphoid areas can be found in the respiratory system, urogenital system, and conjunctiva but are primarily located in the digestive system and the small bowel. **Peyer's patches** are aggregates of MALT and can be found throughout the small bowel and elsewhere in the GI tract. The patches have two lymphoid constituents; B cell follicles and parafollicular T cell areas. The mucosal Peyer's patches also contain M cells of epithelial origin that have phagocytic functions. Small bowel physiology continues to be intensely studied with relevance to fields as diverse as vaccine development, food allergies, tumor immunology, and infectious diseases.

Mechanisms That Maintain Mucosal Integrity

Superficial epithelial cells secrete mucus and bicarbonate which aid in maintaining a pH gradient between the lumen and the mucosa to protect the underlying epithelial tissues from damage by gastric acid and pepsin. Mucosal blood flow is also an important mechanism to maintain mucosal integrity. Prostaglandin provides important protection to the mucosal barrier by stimulating secretion of bicarbonate, increasing blood flow to the mucosa, and stimulating mucus secretion (Huether, 2008). Risk factors for disruption of intestinal mucosa include shock, trauma, intestinal obstruction, protein malnutrition, and total parenteral nutrition.

SECTION FOUR REVIEW

1. Commensal bacteria are a part of the gut's
   - A. humoral defense mechanism
   - B. nonimmunologic defense mechanism
   - C. gut-associated lymphatic tissue
   - D. immunologic defense mechanism
2. Peristalsis promotes gastrointestinal health by
   - A. pushing intestinal contents along the GI tract and preventing reflux
   - B. creating an acid environment that is unfavorable to pathogen growth
   - C. secreting substances that are active against foreign antigens
   - D. covering the epithelial surface with mucus
3. The mucosal coating
   - A. maintains an acid environment
   - B. activates protective digestive enzymes

C. provides a physical barrier against invasion by pathogens
D. interferes with bacterial replication

4. Goblet cells secrete
A. gastrin
B. hydrochloric acid
C. secretin
D. mucus

5. The initial nonimmunologic defense mechanism that is active against antigens is provided by
A. salivary secretions
B. intestinal peristalsis
C. *Escherichia coli* bacteria
D. Peyer's patches

Answers: 1. B, 2. A, 3. C, 4. D, 5. A

SECTION FIVE: Laboratory Assessment of Gastrointestinal and Accessory Organ Function

At the completion of this section, the learner will be able to discuss the laboratory tests used to evaluate gastrointestinal, liver, and pancreatic function.

Gastrointestinal

Laboratory tests used to make a differential diagnosis in GI bleeding and acute abdominal pain include electrolytes, end products of metabolism, enzymes, hematology, and arterial blood gases (ABGs). The laboratory studies presented here are summarized in Table 28–6.

Electrolytes

Electrolyte levels that should be monitored with GI dysfunction include calcium, chloride, magnesium, potassium, and sodium. These electrolytes are primarily absorbed by the small intestine. Injury to the small intestines is often reflected in altered serum levels. For example, potassium loss occurs with diarrhea and vomiting.

TABLE 28–6 Laboratory Tests That May Reflect Gastrointestinal Disorders

TEST	NORMAL VALUES	COMMENTS
Electrolytes		
Calcium	Total, 4.5–5.5 mEq/L Ionized, 4.25–5.25mg/dL	In the presence of GI disorders serum electrolyte levels may be reduced or elevated depending on the disorder.
Chloride	95–105 mEq/L	
Magnesium	1.5–2.5 mEq/L	
Potassium	3.5–5.3 mEq/L	
Sodium	135–145 mEq/L	
Chemistry		
Blood urea nitrogen	5–25 mg/dL	Bowel obstruction can cause elevated nitrogen wastes (BUN) without altering creatinine.
Lactic acid	Arterial: 0.5–2.0 mmol/L Venous: 0.5–1.5 mEq/L	Lactic acid is elevated in bowel infarction and metabolic acidosis.
Enzymes		
Alkaline phosphatase	42–136 units/L	Found in bone, intestine, and liver, and released with destruction of those tissues
Amylase	30–170 U/L	Elevated in peptic ulcer disease, intestinal obstruction, mesenteric thrombosis, and after abdominal surgery
Hematologic		
Complete blood count with differential		
Hemoglobin	M: 13.5–17 g/dL F: 12–15 g/dL	Hemoglobin and hematocrit decrease with GI bleeding and malabsorption; with acute blood loss, hematocrit may not decrease for several hours.
Hematocrit	M: 40–54% F: 36–46%	
White blood cells	4,500–10,000/mm^3	White blood cell count elevated with infection, and inflammation
Arterial blood gases		
pH	7.35–7.45	Metabolic acidosis may result from ischemic bowel
$Paco_2$	35–45 mm Hg	
Pao_2	75–100 mm Hg	
Sao_2	> 95%	
HCO_3	24–28 mEq/L	
BE	+2 to −2 mEq/L	
***Helicobacter* antibodies**	Negative	Used to detect *Helicobacter pylori* infection in peptic ulcer disease

Data from Kee, J. (2009). *Prentice Hall handbook of laboratory and diagnostic tests*, 6th ed. Upper Saddle River, NJ: Prentice Hall.

Blood Urea Nitrogen (BUN)

Elevated BUN (greater than 40 mg/dL) in the absence of underlying renal disease, as evidenced by a normal serum creatinine, may indicate significant blood loss (loss of two or more units). Furthermore, an elevated BUN-to-creatinine ratio may occur in upper GI bleeding and volume depletion as a result of hemoconcentration from a fluid volume deficit. Following a GI bleed, old blood may be within the intestines and is digested as it passes through the GI tract, resulting in the production of urea nitrogen as a byproduct of metabolism, thus elevating the BUN. Bowel obstruction can cause increased BUN because stasis of intestinal contents within the intestines allows more digestion to take place, which produces more byproducts of protein metabolism.

Enzymes

Serum enzymes become elevated when tissues are injured. While serum enzymes are relatively nonspecific (they are found in multiple organs and tissues), they are useful in supporting or ruling out a diagnosis. Two enzymes, **alkaline phosphatase** and amylase, are sometimes useful in diagnosing gastrointestinal disorders.

Hematologic Levels

Serum hematocrit (Hct) and hemoglobin (Hgb) may be abnormal in gastrointestinal bleeding; thus, serial measures are most helpful. During acute hemorrhage, however, the hematocrit may not reflect the volume of blood loss. Prior to fluid resuscitation, the hematocrit may be higher than expected as a result of hemoconcentration from volume loss. The hematocrit may fall precipitously after aggressive fluid resuscitation because of hemodilution effects. It takes up to 72 hours for the hematocrit to equilibrate following a sudden loss of blood (Hillman & Hershko, 2006).

Platelets may be increased or decreased with GI bleeding. A prolonged **prothrombin time** (PT) and **partial thromboplastin time** (PTT) can make stabilization of the patient with a GI bleed very challenging. Platelets and clotting factors are also lost with rapid bleeding. It is important to evaluate PT and PTT levels in order to determine requirements for replacement of clotting factors. A decreased mean corpuscular volume (MCV) suggests the possibility of iron-deficiency anemia secondary to chronic GI blood loss. White blood cell (WBC) count elevations suggest an inflammatory or infectious process. This can occur with perforated peptic ulcer, and with ischemic bowel.

Arterial Blood Gases (ABGs)

ABG measures are useful in evaluation of respiratory status and pH deviations. Hypoxemia is an early sign of sepsis. Metabolic acidosis may result from sepsis, ischemic bowel, or peptic ulcer perforation. Decreased oxygen-carrying capacity as a result of blood loss is a common complication from severe upper GI hemorrhage.

Antibodies

Helicobacter antibodies may be detected in the serum of persons with *H. pylori* infection. *H. pylori* infection is associated with peptic ulcer disease.

Assessment of Liver Function

An important part of assessing function of the liver is obtaining a laboratory panel of serum enzymes, proteins, bilirubin, and clotting measures. This panel is often referred to as a liver function panel, or liver function tests (LFTs).

Liver Enzymes

Serum enzymes that are commonly included are **alanine aminotransferase** (ALT), **aspartate aminotransferase** (AST), and alkaline phosphatase (Alk Phos, ALP). These enzymes are not specific to liver cells, so abnormal levels can occur with a variety of other organ disorders. For this reason, **isoenzymes,** which are more specific to the liver, are often measured. These include LDH isoenzymes (LDH_4 and LDH_5), 5'-nucleotidase (5'NT), and gamma glutamyltransferase (GGT). Refer to Table 28–7 for more information on specific enzymes and Table 28–8 for more detailed information on the isoenzymes.

Bilirubin

Bilirubin is the end product of hemoglobin degradation, which occurs in the liver. It is the pigmented portion of heme. Through the oxidation process, heme is turned into bilirubin and is then released into the bloodstream. There are two types of bilirubin: fat-soluble and water-soluble.

TABLE 28–7 Enzyme Studies Measuring Liver Function

ENZYME	NORMAL RANGE	COMMENTS
Alanine aminotransferase (ALT, SGPT)	5–35 units/L	More specific to liver than to other organs. The ratio of AST/ALT usually is greater than one in alcoholic cirrhosis and liver congestion and less than one in acute hepatitis.
Aspartate aminotransferase (AST, SGOT)	0–35 units/L	Rises with damage to kidneys, heart, pancreas, and brain as well as liver
Alkaline phosphatase (Alk Phos)	20–90 units/L	Rises with damage/disease of kidneys and bone as well as liver; a sensitive measure of biliary tract obstruction

Data from Kee, J. (2009), *Prentice Hall handbook of laboratory and diagnostic tests,* 6th ed. Upper Saddle River, NJ: Prentice Hall; and Martin, R., & Hassanein, T. (2009). *Liver dysfunction and failure.* In K. K. Carlson, (ed.) *Advanced Critical Care Nursing.* St. Louis, MO: Saunders/Elsevier, 754–773.

TABLE 28–8 Isoenzymes for Evaluation of Liver Function

ISOENZYME	NORMAL RANGE	COMMENTS
Lactate dehydrogenase isoenzyme 5 (LDH_5)	6–16%	The LDH_5 isoenzyme is much more specific to the liver than the LDH enzyme.
Alkaline phosphatase isoenzyme 1 (ALP_1)	42–136 WI	The ALP_1 is specific to the liver and can increase significantly with liver injury. 5'N when measured with ALP is important in differentiating liver disease from bone disease.
5'nucleotidase (5'N)	Less than 17 U/L	
Gamma glutamyl transferase (GGT)	Males: 9–69 units/L Females: 4–33 units/L	GGT is fairly specific to hepatobiliary tissues; it is, however, also present in pancreatic and renal cells; elevated GGT is present in serum of alcohol abusers.

Data from Kee, J. (2009). *Prentice Hall handbook of laboratory and diagnostic tests,* 6th ed. Upper Saddle River, NJ: Prentice Hall.

Fat-soluble bilirubin has not yet passed through the liver (prehepatic). Prior to undergoing a conversion in the liver, it is called **unconjugated bilirubin.** Once in the liver, bilirubin is first split from albumin molecules by the hepatocytes and then it is conjugated (joined) with glucuronic acid. In this conjugated state, it becomes water-soluble bilirubin and is called **conjugated bilirubin.** In this state, it is transported as bile from the liver into the intestines. From the intestines, most of the bilirubin is excreted through the feces. A small amount is excreted through the urine (**urobilinogen**). Very little conjugated bilirubin remains in the circulation to return to the liver; therefore, when bilirubin is measured, it is primarily the unconjugated (prehepatic) level that is being measured.

Bilirubin is a yellow pigment that provides a yellow cast to its surroundings and is responsible for the brown color of stool. When the normal elimination of bilirubin is obstructed, the yellowish color will be evident in body fluids, the skin, the sclera, and the mucous membranes. This discoloration is referred to as **jaundice.** Jaundice usually is not evident until the total bilirubin level exceeds 3 mg/dl (Kee, 2009).

Bilirubin testing is done by measuring the total bilirubin, the indirect and the direct levels as well as urobilinogen. Conjugated (or "direct") bilirubin (posthepatic, water-soluble) is measured using a direct method because it requires no modifications before being measured. Unconjugated (or "indirect") bilirubin (prehepatic, fat soluble) is measured using an indirect method because it must be altered to a water-soluble state using a solvent before it can be measured. Urobilinogen is measured as a sensitive test for hepatic damage. It may increase before serum bilirubin levels increase. In early hepatitis or mild liver cell damage, the urine urobilinogen level will increase despite an unchanged serum bilirubin level. However, with severe liver failure, the urine urobilinogen level may decrease because less bile will be produced. This test might be ordered along with a urinalysis. Table 28–9 provides a summary of bilirubin laboratory testing.

Clotting Measures

The liver has an important role in maintaining normal coagulation because it produces prothrombin, vitamin K, and other clotting factors essential to the coagulation cascade. If liver function becomes compromised and these substances can no longer be synthesized in adequate quantities, the patient is at increased risk for serious bleeding complications. Two common blood tests used to measure the two coagulation pathways are prothrombin time and partial thromboplastin time.

The prothrombin time (PT) measures the extrinsic coagulation pathway. Prothrombin (factor II of the coagulation cascade) is produced by the liver and is dependent on vitamin K, which is also produced by the intestinal tract. Prolonged prothrombin times may be seen with chronic liver disease (e.g., cirrhosis) or vitamin K deficiency. Normal prothrombin time is 10 to 13 seconds (Kee, 2009). Unfortunately, the traditional measurement of prothrombin time can vary depending on the lab analysis method used. For this reason, the preferred measure of prothrombin time is the

TABLE 28–9 Bilirubin Testing

TYPE	NORMAL VALUES	COMMENTS
Total bilirubin	0.1–1.2 mg/dL	Measures both conjugated and unconjugated bilirubin Elevations seen with biliary obstruction
Indirect (unconjugated)	0.1–1.0 mg/dL	Measures prehepatic, unconjugated bilirubin; elevations associated with viral hepatitis and other disease processes where lysis of red blood cells occurs
Direct (conjugated)	0.1–0.3 mg/dL	Measures posthepatic conjugated bilirubin; elevations associated with multiple intrahepatic and bile duct dysfunctions
Urobilinogen	Negative in freshly voided urine	Measures posthepatic urobilinogen in the urine; elevations associated with early or recovery phase liver cell damage Antibiotics may decrease levels

Data from Kee, J. (2009). *Prentice Hall handbook of laboratory and diagnostic tests,* 6th ed. Upper Saddle River, NJ: Prentice Hall.

international normalized ratio (INR). The normal range of INR is 2.0 to 3.0 (Kee, 2009). INR is particularly recommended for monitoring long-term warfarin therapy once the dose has been stabilized.

Partial thromboplastin time (PTT) measures the intrinsic coagulation pathway. It is more sensitive than the PT in measuring clotting abnormalities in all factors except VII and VIII. Elevations of the PTT are seen with severe liver disease or with heparin administration. Normal values are 60-70 seconds (Kee, 2009). Activated partial thromboplastin time (APTT) is even a more sensitive indicator than PTT in the detection of defects in the clotting factors. APTT differs from PTT in that the reagent contains an activator. Normal APTT is 20 to 35 seconds (Kee, 2009).

Serum Ammonia

Elevations of serum ammonia levels are indicative that the liver is not adequately converting urea to ammonia for proper elimination in the urine. The normal ranges for serum ammonia levels are 15-45 mcg/dl (Kee, 2009). Elevated levels can lead to the development of hepatic encephalopathy, a complication of liver failure.

Serum Albumin

The liver synthesizes albumin and many other proteins; thus, as liver function decreases, protein levels will also decrease. Serum albumin is a good indicator of general protein levels, as the liver synthesizes albumin and many other proteins. The half-life of albumin is relatively long (several weeks) so it is a poor marker of acute hepatic injury but can be an indicator of long-standing illness, malnutrition, or disease. The normal range is 3.5 – 5.0 g/dl (Kee, 2009).

Assessment of Pancreatic Function

A variety of testing methods are used to assess pancreatic function. Each provides the practitioner with different information regarding the function of the pancreas. Tests that directly stimulate the pancreas are the most sensitive.

Pancreatic Enzymes

Pancreatic enzymes can be found in a variety of body fluids. Blood tests are used to evaluate the function of the pancreas. Levels of two pancreatic enzymes, amylase and lipase, can be measured in the serum. Amylase can be detected in the urine, serum, ascitic fluid, pleural fluid, and as an isoenzyme. Amylase is often used as a screening test for pancreatitis in patients with acute abdominal pain or back pain; however there are multiple other causes of elevation of this enzyme. Amylase can be identified in the urine when the serum levels may be normal because renal clearance of the enzyme can be elevated in an acute pancreatic event (Budick & Tompson, 2006). **Lipase** levels in the serum will be elevated if pancreatic inflammation is present. As with amylase, lipase can be elevated for multiple reasons. Lipase is currently the best enzyme to identify acute pancreatitis. A normal value for lipase is 14-280 units/liter (Kee, 2009).

Exocrine Pancreatic Function Testing

Exocrine pancreatic function tests provide the most reliable indication of pancreatic function. The secretin stimulation test measures the ability of the pancreas to respond to secretin. Secretin is a hormone made by the small intestines. Secretin

TABLE 28–10 Measures of Pancreatic Function

LABORATORY TEST	NORMAL VALUES	COMMENTS
Serum		
Amylase	30–170 units/L	In acute pancreatitis, serum levels peak between 4–8 hours after onset, then fall to normal within 48–72 hours; low levels usually indicate pancreatic insufficiency.
Isoamylase P (pancreatic)	30–55%	Elevated in acute pancreatitis
Lipase	14–280 units/L	Elevated only in pancreatitis, markedly in acute cases and with biliary tract disease; remains increased after Amylase returns to normal
Total Calcium Ionized Calcium	8.2–10.2 mg/dL 4.65–5.28 mg/dL	High total calcium levels occur in malignancy of liver, pancreas, and other organs. Ionized calcium is useful in tracking the course of cancer disorders and acute pancreatitis.
Triglycerides	50–250 mg/dL	Patient must fast for 12 hours before specimen is drawn; levels are increased in cirrhosis, diabetes mellitus, hypertension, and hyperlipoproteinemia.
Glucose	65–110 mg/dL [fasting]	Patient must fast for 12 hours before specimen is drawn.
Stool		
Fat	< 6 g/24 hrs	Levels greater than 6 g/24 hour period is suggestive of decreased absorptive ability, and is indicative of pancreatic exocrine insufficiency as in chronic pancreatitis.
Urine		
Amylase	2 hour: 2–34 units 24 hour: 24–408 units	These values are 6–10 hours behind serum values; low levels indicate pancreatic insufficiency.

Data from Kee, J. (2009). *Prentice Hall handbook of laboratory and diagnostic tests*, 6th ed. Upper Saddle River, NJ: Prentice Hall.

stimulates the pancreas to release a fluid that neutralizes stomach acid and aids in digestion. This test may be performed in patients with diseases that affect the pancreas to determine the activity of the pancreas. During the test, a tube is inserted down the throat, into the stomach, then into the upper part of the small intestine. Secretin is administered and the contents of the duodenal secretions are aspirated and analyzed over a period of about two hours. The fecal elastase test is another test of pancreas function. The test measures the levels of elastase, an enzyme found in fluids produced by the pancreas that digests proteins. In this test, a patient's stool sample is analyzed for the presence of elastase (Stevens & Conwell, 2008). Table 28–10 provides a summary of major pancreatic function tests and normal ranges.

SECTION FIVE REVIEW

1. BUN is commonly elevated following a GI bleeding event. Which of the following best explains why this abnormal laboratory measure occurs?
   A. acute renal failure
   B. fluid volume overload
   C. metabolic acidosis
   D. hemoconcentration of the blood
2. BUN elevation (greater than 40 mg/dL), in the absence of underlying renal disease, may suggest
   A. loss of two or more units of blood
   B. impaired circulation to renal tissues
   C. significant fluid volume overload
   D. onset of acute renal failure
3. Bowel obstruction can cause a(n)
   A. elevated AST
   B. elevated BUN
   C. decreased LDH
   D. decreased MCV
4. *H. pylori* infection is associated with
   A. upper GI bleeding
   B. chronic lower GI bleeding
   C. liver disease
   D. peptic ulcer disease
5. ______ may contribute to GI bleeding.
   A. pulmonary disease
   B. hepatic dysfunction
   C. autoimmune complications
   D. connective tissue disease
6. Serum enzyme laboratory levels are obtained to measure
   A. clotting factors
   B. organ function
   C. cellular injury
   D. tissue oxygenation
7. Serum isoenzyme levels often provide better data than parent enzyme levels because they are
   A. faster to obtain
   B. more tissue specific
   C. more plentiful
   D. easier to measure
8. Which combination of LDH isoenzymes best reflects hepatic injury?
   A. LDH_1 and LDH_2
   B. LDH_2 and LDH_3
   C. LDH_3 and LDH_4
   D. LDH_4 and LDH_5
9. Bilirubin is
   A. secreted by hepatocytes
   B. broken down into bile salts
   C. produced primarily in the pancreas
   D. the end product of hemoglobin degradation
10. When a serum bilirubin is obtained, it primarily measures ______ bilirubin.
   A. unconjugated
   B. posthepatic
   C. conjugated
   D. water-soluble
11. Amylase can be detected in which body fluids? (choose all that apply)
   A. blood/serum
   B. urine
   C. cerebral spinal fluid
   D. pleural fluid
12. Which type of pancreatic testing provides the most specific information regarding pancreatic function?
   A. serum enzyme levels
   B. abdominal X-ray
   C. exocrine pancreatic function test
   D. abdominal ultrasound
13. Measurement of serum ______ is often used as a screening test for pancreatitis in patients with acute abdominal pain or back pain.
   A. lipase
   B. elastase
   C. secretin
   D. amylase
14. Elastase, an enzyme found in fluids produced by the pancreas that digests proteins is measured in a ______ sample.
   A. blood
   B. urine
   C. stool
   D. sputum

Answers: 1. D, 2. A, 3. B, 4. D, 5. B, 6. C, 7. B, 8. D, 9. D, 10. A, 11. (A, B, D), 12. C, 13. D, 14. C

SECTION SIX: Diagnostic Tests of Gastrointestinal System and Accessory Organ Function

At the completion of this section, the learner will be able to explain diagnostic tests used to evaluate gastrointestinal, liver and pancreatic function.

Multiple diagnostic studies are used to evaluate the gastrointestinal system and accessory organs. Many of the radiographic studies require a contrast medium; therefore, the patient's allergy status must be known, as severe hypersensitivity reactions can occur in sensitive people.

Diagnosing disorders of the GI system and accessory organs can be challenging because the complex disease status of the high-acuity patient may mask the development of GI or accessory organ complications. Symptoms often are vague initially and may have an insidious onset; thus, early manifestations may be overlooked in the presence of other high priority health concerns. Diagnostic studies, either invasive or noninvasive, are often required to definitively diagnose an acute problem. This section provides a brief overview of some of the major studies used in diagnosing GI and accessory organ disorders.

Radiographic exam or flat plate of the abdomen is helpful in diagnosing intra-abdominal problems such as intestinal obstruction, rupture, masses, abnormal fluid or air levels, and the presence of foreign bodies. An upper GI series with contrast medium is another type of X-ray. It allows visualization of the GI tract in order to diagnose tumors, masses, hernias, obstructions, ulcers, fistulas, or diverticular disease. The patient ingests a contrast material prior to the actual X-ray. The contrast medium allows visualization of any abnormalities. It is important to ask about the client's allergy history prior to administration of the contrast medium in order to prevent serious allergic reactions. Furthermore, it is important to assist the patient in expelling the contrast (barium).

Computed tomography (CT) scan is another test allowing visualization of the abdomen, retroperitoneal structures, masses, abscesses, and abnormal fluid or air levels, which might be visible if perforation has occurred. This noninvasive exam requires the patient to ingest a barium contrast solution prior to the exam. The nurse should provide specific instructions on expelling the barium contrast.

Ultrasound sonography allows visualization of abdominal and retroperitoneal soft tissue structures to diagnose fluid or air pockets, abscesses, masses, and to observe movement (i.e., peristalsis, gastric emptying). This procedure may take place at the patient's bedside. Transducing gel is applied to the skin, and mild pressure is applied with a transducer. Adipose tissue, air, and barium may diminish ultrasound wave transmission.

Magnetic resonance imaging (MRI) scan is used to assess abdominal and retroperitoneal structures for masses, abscesses, and fluid or air pockets. All external metal objects and dental appliances must be removed. Internal metal objects or foreign bodies are a contraindication to MRI. It is very important that the patient lie still for this test; therefore, he or she must be able to cooperate.

A *nuclear scan* allows visualization of organs, gastrointestinal motility, and bleeding. An intravenous contrast medium is administered; therefore, an allergy history should be obtained to reduce the risk of allergic reaction. Nuclear scan is contraindicated in pregnancy, breast-feeding, or recent nuclear exposure. All metal must be removed from these patients also. Nonuniform radioactive uptake in tissues often indicates disease.

Angiography allows visualization of blood flow in selected vascular beds. Obstructed or bleeding vessels can be identified with this test. A contrast medium is administered intravenously; therefore, allergy history is important.

Endoscopy allows inspection of internal surfaces of organs. It includes a series of diagnostic tests for the GI system using a flexible scope with a fiber-optic light and lens system. Removal of tissue for testing (biopsy), as well as some treatments, such as sclerotherapy, suction, and cauterization of bleeding vessels, may be performed during endoscopy of the upper or lower GI tract. Common endoscopic tests are summarized in Table 28–11.

Gastric Tonometry

Gastric tonometry is an invasive monitoring technique that allows the assessment of gut perfusion in critically ill patients. This technique uses a special nasogastric tube with a balloon censure that is inserted into the stomach to measure the carbon dioxide (CO_2) level of the gastric mucosa, which rises when the GI tract is underperfused (Fig. 28–10). Tonometry provides an early warning of reduced gastric perfusion, which can occur when a patient is hypovolemic or in shock. During a period of hypoperfusion, the GI tract is one of the first organ systems to suffer reduced blood flow. A decrease in the delivery of oxygen rich blood to the gut mucosa results in anaerobic metabolism. Tonometry measures the changes in the pH and CO_2 levels of the gut that is indicative of GI tract perfusion. Conditions that alter the intramucosal pH and CO_2 levels include the following: 1) If acid enters and bicarbonate refluxes back into the stomach from the duodenum, 2) if the patient receives enteral feeding that refluxes into the stomach, or 3) if the stomach is continuously aspirated by a sump style nasogastric tube. If any of the aforementioned conditions exist, the gastric tonometry results should be questioned.

Sublingual Capnometry

Sublingual capnometry is a simple, noninvasive technology that provides immediate measures of partial pressure of sublingual carbon dioxide ($P_{sl}CO_2$). It provides an alternative to invasive

TABLE 28–11 Common Endoscopic Tests of the Gastrointestinal System

TEST	PURPOSE	INDICATIONS
Esophagogastroduodenoscopy (EGD)	Visualization of structures from the mouth to the junction of the duodenum and jejunum	Upper GI bleeding
Colonoscopy	Visualization of the large intestine	Lower GI bleeding
Proctoscopy, sigmoidoscopy, proctosigmoidoscopy, anoscopy	Visualization of sigmoid colon and rectal/anal mucosa	Sigmoid, rectal, or anal bleeding

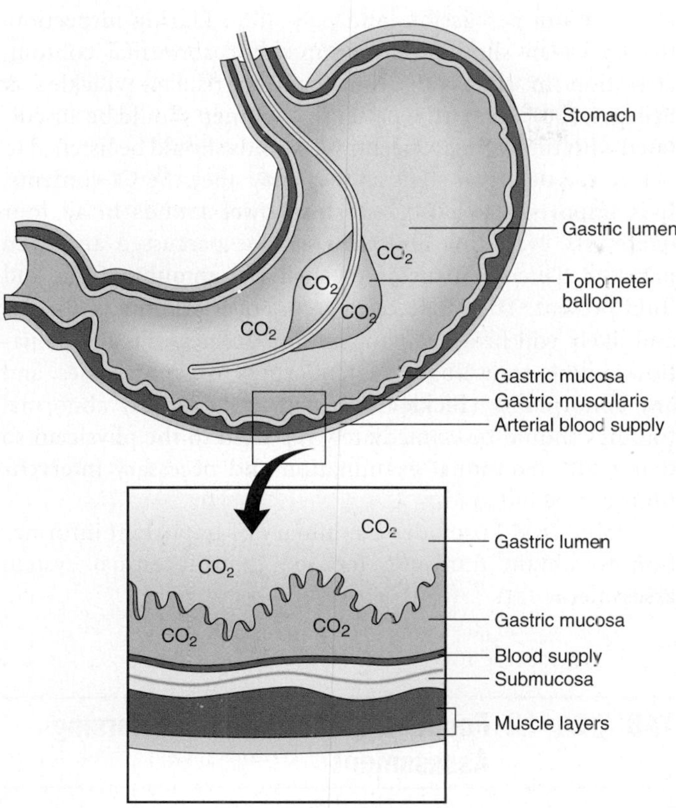

Figure 28–10 ■ Gastric tonometry. A special gastric tube with a balloon on the distal end is inserted into the stomach to measure the CO_2 level of the gastric mucosa. Gastric CO_2 ($PrCO_2$) rises when the mucosa is hypoperfused.

gastric tonometry monitoring for monitoring splanchnic perfusion. It requires a special CO_2 probe to be placed beneath the tongue. Unfortunately, patients often need to be sedated to tolerate both the probe and the endotracheal tube. It provides intermittent measurements that require trending rather than being a continuous measurement of CO_2 trends. The presence of orogastric or nasogastric tubes does not appear to affect the accuracy of the results. With sublingual capnometry, enteral feedings do not need to be stopped to obtain measures. Additional studies in human subjects are necessary, however, before this technology will prove its clinical usefulness (Gallagher, 2009).

Additional Pancreatic Diagnostic Studies

There are multiple studies available to determine if pancreatic structure is intact and functioning properly. Standard abdominal X-ray films are a good starting point for diagnosis; however, many patients with pancreatitis have normal abdominal films. Computed tomography (CT) scans can provide detailed visualization of the pancreas and can also identify other possible causes of elevated pancreatic enzymes. A CT scan can identify complications of pancreatic disease such as fluid around the pancreas, an abscess, or a collection of tissue, fluid, and pancreatic enzymes.

Further investigation of the pancreas to evaluate the pancreatic and bile ducts can be accomplished by magnetic resonance imaging (MRI). This is known as **magnetic resonance cholangiopancreatography (MRCP).** Abdominal ultrasound can provide information regarding swelling, inflammation, calcification, pseudocysts, and lesions of the pancreas. **Endoscopic retrograde cholangiopancreatography (ERCP)** provides visualization of the pancreatic-biliary duct system (Stevens & Conwell, 2008). This test can provide diagnostic data in 60-85 percent of pancreatitis cases. In an ERCP, a health care professional places a tube down the patient's throat, into the stomach, then into the small intestine. Contrast dye is used to help the physician see the structure of the common bile duct, other bile ducts, and the pancreatic duct on an X-ray.

Endoscopic ultrasound is another invasive test where a probe attached to a lighted scope is placed down the patient's throat and into the stomach. Sound waves show images of organs in the abdomen. Endoscopic ultrasound may reveal gallstones and can be helpful in diagnosing severe pancreatitis when an invasive test such as ERCP might make the condition worse. Pancreatic biopsy is the definitive test to be performed when trying to determine whether inflammation is present (Stevens & Conwell, 2008).

SECTION SIX REVIEW

1. A 46-year-old male is admitted to the acute care unit for acute onset of abdominal pain. He has a history of pancreatitis. Which of the following diagnostic tests would be a good starting point for diagnosis of this patient's abdominial pain?
   A. plain abdominal X-ray
   B. magnetic resonance cholangiopancreatography
   C. upper gastrointestinal series with contrast
   D. endoscopic ultrasound
2. Swelling, inflammation, calcification, pseudocysts, and lesions of the pancreas is best identified with the _______ diagnostic test.
   A. magnetic resonance cholangiopancreatography
   B. endoscopic retrograde cholangiopancreatography
   C. gastric tonometry
   D. abdominal ultrasound
3. The test that provides visualization of the pancreatic-biliary duct system is the
   A. endoscopic ultrasound
   B. endoscopic retrograde cholangiopancreatography
   C. magnetic resonance cholangiopancreatography
   D. computed tomography (CT) scans
4. Gastric tonometry and sublingual capnometry are two measures of
   A. CO_2
   B. O_2
   C. pH
   D. hemoglobin saturation

Answers: 1. A, 2. A, 3. B, 4. A

SECTION SEVEN: Gastrointestinal Nursing Assessment

At the completion of this section, the learner will be able to discuss nursing assessment of patients who present with gastrointestinal disorders.

Because of its constant exposure to the environment, the gastrointestinal tract is subjected to toxins, infection with pathogens, and inflammatory processes. It is also susceptible to damage from trauma and insults such as ischemia due to critical illness and systemic diseases. When patients present with gastrointestinal disorders, diagnostic tests for common GI complications require astute nursing assessment and intervention in order to prevent further complications. Acute GI disorders that involve gastrointestinal bleeding, hepatic or pancreatic dysfunction require nursing care that is centered on health promotion, assessment, and identification of priority nursing diagnoses and interventions. Obtaining a thorough database is important upon admission for those clients who present with acute gastrointestinal dysfunction, and provides the foundation upon which collaborative nursing care is based.

Focused Nursing Gastrointestinal System Database

When the patient is admitted to the acute care setting, it is important to obtain a full nursing database to elicit pieces of the patient's history that could aid the diagnostic process and possibly affect the outcome of their hospitalization. As with all patients, a general history should be taken to include past medical history, surgical history, and events leading up to the current admission. The family history should be taken, since many GI disorders are hereditary. A current medication list should be obtained so the critical care nurse and the physician can be aware of the patient's current health status. It is crucial to obtain information directly related to symptoms the patient has been experiencing that have led to this event. If the patient is agreeable, it is often helpful to ask a family member or significant other to assist with the history taking process.

A focused health maintenance history should be taken that focuses on diet and eating patterns, appetite, weight fluctuations, and skin healing problems. Baseline data should be obtained regarding mental status, ability to communicate, and presence of pain. It is also important, with every disease, to discuss with the patient and family their value-belief pattern in order to prepare for future needs.

Patient Abdominal Assessment

A focused abdominal assessment should be completed by the nurse to evaluate the patient who presents with signs of alteration in gastrointestinal, hepatic, or pancreatic function. The steps of abdominal assessment include inspection, auscultation, percussion, and palpation. During inspection, the abdomen should be examined for abnormal contour, alteration in skin, pulsations, and peristalsis (Bickley & Szilagyi, 2007). Next, the patient's abdomen should be auscultated with the stethoscope. Bowel sounds should be listened to before the next two steps as they may alter the GI contents. It is important to auscultate for bowel sounds in all four quadrants. Next, the abdomen can be percussed and then palpated. Percussion helps to elicit the amount of gas and fluid present. The nurse can percuss over all four quadrants and likely will hear tympany and/or dullness. Finally palpation is done to evaluate for tenderness, organs, masses, and any abnormality (Bickley & Szilagyi, 2007). Any abnormal findings should be immediately reported to the physician so that a full abdominal examination and necessary interventions can be initiated.

Table 28–12 provides a summary of important information to obtain during a focused gastrointestinal system assessment.

TABLE 28–12 Focused Gastrointestinal Nursing Assessment

The Nursing History

- Points to elicit include
  - Onset of problem: When did it start, was it gradual or quick, what was the patient doing when it started?
  - Duration of problem: How long does it last, does it come and go?
  - Quality and description of problem: What does the problem feel like (using adjectives)?
  - Severity of problem: How badly does the problem bother the patient?
  - Location of problem: Where is the problem isolated, does it radiate or spread?
  - Precipitating factors: What brought problem on?
  - Alleviating factors: What relieves problem?
  - Associated symptoms: What other symptoms bother the patient?
- Previous medical history
- Family history
- Surgical history
- Current medication list
- Psychosocial factors that affect patient
- Cultural factors that affect patient

The Physical Examination

- Abdominal assessment
  - Ask patient to empty bladder unless patient has Foley catheter.
  - Provide appropriate privacy.
  - Warm hands and stethoscope before use.
  - Inspect abdomen first. Look for contour, shape, masses, bumps, abnormal colors.
  - Auscultate abdomen. Listen in all four quadrants for at least two minutes, note quality and quantity of sounds.
  - Percuss abdomen dullness of tympany will be heard, dullness over solid organs, tympany over air and gas.
  - Palpate abdomen. Include light and deep touch, palpate in all four quadrants.
- General
  - Obtain vital signs and baseline assessment and document in nursing database.
  - Prepare patient and family for further diagnostic testing and medication use.

Emerging Evidence

- In a study of healthy subjects, use of oral nutritional supplement (ONS) containing antioxidants, glutamine, and carbohydrates improved protein balance in the duodenum. The study concluded that further investigation is required to establish the use of ONS in other populations, such as stressed patient *(Coëffier, Claeyssens et al., 2008)*.
- In a secondary analysis of inpatient claims for more than 24,000 oncology patients, gastrointestinal bleeding was found to be the most common postoperative complication (13.2 percent of sample) following surgical removal of solid tumors. GI bleeding was also associated with readmission to the hospital through the emergency department. Investigators concluded that nurses play an important role in early detection of GI bleeding to facilitate early evidence-based management to improve patient outcomes *(Friese & Aiken, 2008)*.
- Gastrointestinal bleeding was one of six adverse events associated with death in the intensive care setting in a study of over 3,600 ICU patients in a prospective observational cohort study. Other common adverse events included infections (e.g., bacteremia, pneumonia, surgical wound), and pneumothorax. The study also found that the adverse events often occur in combination in one patient *(Orgeas, Timsit, Soufir et al., 2008)*.

SECTION SEVEN REVIEW

1. When obtaining a focused GI history, an important question to ask that specifically focuses on precipitating factors of symptoms is:
   - A. When did the symptoms start?
   - B. What brought the problem on?
   - C. What does the problem feel like?
   - D. How long does it last?
2. Just before beginning an abdominal assessment the nurse should
   - A. palpate the abdomen using light touch only
   - B. palpate the abdomen first before inspecting or auscultating
   - C. listen to bowel sounds for at least 30 seconds in each quadrant
   - D. ask the patient to empty his or her bladder unless a Foley catheter is in place

Answers: 1. B, 2. D

POSTTEST

1. The upper GI tract includes (choose all that apply)
   - A. stomach
   - B. esophagus
   - C. salivary glands
   - D. intestines
2. The ______ prevents gastroesophageal reflux.
   - A. upper esophageal sphincter
   - B. lower esophageal sphincter
   - C. gastrocolic sphincter
   - D. ileocecal valve
3. The duodenum, jejunum, and the ileum comprise the
   - A. entire GI tract
   - B. large intestine
   - C. accessory organs
   - D. small intestine
4. Finger-like projections which cover the intestinal folds of the small intestine are called
   - A. microvilli
   - B. goblet cells
   - C. villi
   - D. brush border
5. The absorption of water and electrolytes is largely completed in the ______.
   - A. colon
   - B. rectum
   - C. ileum
   - D. jejunum
6. The brush border is made up of the ______ and ______. (choose all that apply)
   - A. villi
   - B. intestinal folds
   - C. Peyer's patches
   - D. microvilli
7. Blood flow through the gut, spleen, pancreas, and liver comprise the
   - A. portal circulation
   - B. mesenteric circulation
   - C. splanchnic circulation
   - D. extrinsic circulation
8. The primary function of the GI tract is to
   - A. metabolize toxic agents
   - B. produce clotting factors
   - C. provide nutrients needed for metabolism
   - D. eliminate carbon dioxide

9. Arterial blood supply to the mesentery and intestines is known as the ______ circulation.
A. mesenteric
B. portocaval
C. visceral
D. aortic

10. Gut associated lymphoid tissue (GALT) includes
A. thyroid, duodenum, gastric mucosa
B. tonsils, appendix, lymph tissues in the intestinal wall
C. adrenal glands, cecum, stomach
D. goblet cells, salivary glands, parietal cells

11. Venous blood draining from the GI system organs flows directly into the inferior vena cava to return to the heart.
A. True
B. False

12. The normal flora that resides within the large intestine breaks down cellulose and synthesizes
A. hydrochloric acid, vitamin C, calcium, and carbolic acid
B. vitamin E, phosphorous, creatine, and folic acid
C. vitamin K, carbon dioxide, methane, and riboflavin
D. vitamin K, folic acid, riboflavin, and nicotinic acid

13. The ileocecal valve
A. prevents backflow of feces from the large to small intestine
B. prevents backflow of chyme from the duodenum to the stomach
C. allows stomach contents to move into the small intestine
D. allows passage of feces through the rectum

14. The pancreas is protected from autodigestion by
A. bicarbonate and water
B. the presence of the hormone secretin
C. protective pancreatic cell wall coverings
D. the production of enzymes in their inactive states

15. Which laboratory measures are important in evaluating the need for clotting factor replacement?
A. hemoglobin and hematocrit
B. platelet count and hematocrit
C. thrombin time and mean corpuscular volume
D. prothrombin time and partial thromboplastin time

16. The ______ nervous system inhibits GI motility.
A. sympathetic
B. parasympathetic
C. intrinsic
D. enteric

17. Colonoscopy allows for inspection of the
A. duodenal bulb
B. large intestine
C. gastric mucosa
D. small intestine

18. Total bilirubin measures
A. urobilinogen
B. indirect (unconjugated) bilirubin
C. direct (conjugated) bilirubin
D. both indirect and direct bilirubin

19. Bowel infarction and metabolic acidosis is associated with
A. increased lactic acid
B. decreased lactic acid
C. increased hydrochloric acid
D. decreased hydrochloric acid

20. The major pancreatic enzyme responsible for breakdown of protein is
A. secretin
B. amylase
C. trypsin
D. phospholipase

Posttest answers with rationale are found on MyNursingKit.

REFERENCES

Bickley, L. S. & Szilagyi, P. G. (2007). *Bates guide to physical exam and history taking.* (9th ed.). Philadelphia: Lippincott Williams and Williams.

Burdick, J. S. & Tompson, M. (2006). Anatomy, histology, embryology, and developmental anomalies of the pancreas. In M. Feldman, L.S. Friedman, M. H. Sleisenger, & B. F. Scharschmidt (eds.), *Sleisenger and Fordtrans's gastrointestinal and liver disease: pathophysiology, diagnosis, and management* (8th ed.). New York: McGraw Hill, 1174–1184.

Coëffier, M., Claeyssens, S., Lecleire, S., Leblond, J., Coquard, A., Bôle-Feysot, C., Lavoinne, A., Ducrotté, P., & Déchelotte, P. (2008). Combined enteral infusion of glutamine, carbohydrates, and antioxidants modulates gut protein metabolism in humans. *American Journal of Clinical Nutrition, 88*(5), 1284–1290.

Fauci, A. S., Braunwald, E., Kasper, D. L., Hauesr, S. L., Longo, D. L., Jameson, J. L, & Loscalzo, J. (2008). Approach to the Patient with Pancreatic Disease. In *Harrison's principles of internal medicine.* (17th ed.). New York: McGraw Hill, 2001.

Friese, C. R., & Aiken, L. H. (2008). Failure to rescue in the surgical oncology population: implications for nursing and quality improvement. *Oncol Nurs Forum, 35*(5), 779–785.

Gallagher, J. (2009). Shock and end points of resuscitation. In K. K. Carlson, ed. *AACN advanced critical care nursing.* St. Louis: Saunders/Elsevier, 1067–1098.

Huether, S. E. (2008). Structure and function of the digestive system. In S. E. Huether & K .L. McCance, *Understanding pathophysiology* (4th ed.). St. Louis: Mosby/Elsevier, 912–936.

Kee, J. L. (2009). *Prentice Hall Handbook of Laboratory and Diagnostic Tests.* (6th ed.) Upper Saddle River, NJ: Prentice Hall.

Martin, R., & Hassanein, T. (2009). Liver dysfunction and failure. In K. K. Carlson, *Advanced critical care nursing.* St. Louis, MO: Saunders/Elsevier, 754–773.

Martini, F. H., Bartholomew, E. F., & Bledsoe, B. E. (2008). *Anatomy & physiology for emergency care.* (2d ed.) Upper Saddle River, NJ: Pearson.

Orgeas, M. G., Tismit, J. F., Soufir, L., Tafflet, M., Adrie, C., Philippart, F., Zahar, J. R., Clec'h, C, et al. (2008). Impact of adverse events on outcomes in intensive care unit patients. *Crit Care Med, 36*(7), 2041–2047.

Sargent, S. (2006). Pathophysiology, diagnosis, and management of acute pancreatitis. *British Journal of Nursing, 15*(18): 999–1005.

Stevens, T. & Conwell, D. (2008). Pancreatic exocrine function test. *Retrieved March 1, 2008 from Uptodate. online 16.2* http://www.uptodate.com/online/content/topic.do?topicKey=mal_synd/6192&selectedTitle=1&~5&source=search_result.

MODULE

29 Alterations in Gastrointestinal Function

Melanie G. Hardin-Pierce, Tonya L. Appleby, Valerie K. Sabol

OBJECTIVES Following completion of this module, the learner will be able to

1. Describe the incidence and clinical manifestations associated with acute gastrointestinal (GI) bleeding.
2. Discuss the etiology and pathophysiology of acute upper GI bleeding due to ulcers.
3. Discuss the etiology and pathophysiology of acute upper GI bleeding due to stress-related mucosal disease and nonulcer etiologies.
4. Explain the etiology and pathophysiology of acute lower GI bleeding.
5. Describe the etiology, pathophysiology, and management of acute intestinal obstruction and paralytic ileus.
6. Describe the etiology, pathophysiology, and management of intraabdominal hypertension and abdominal compartment syndrome.
7. Describe the nursing diagnosis and management of acute GI bleeding and bowel obstruction.

This self-study module presents the physiologic and pathophysiologic processes involved in acute gastrointestinal (GI) dysfunction and management of the patient with acute GI bleeding, problems in motility, and intestinal ischemia. The module is composed of seven sections. Section One describes the incidence and clinical manifestations of acute GI bleeding. Section Two describes the etiology and pathophysiology of acute upper GI bleeding due to peptic ulcer disease. Section Three describes the etiology and pathophysiology of acute upper GI bleeding due to stress-related mucosal diseases and nonulcer etiologies. Section Four explains the etiology and pathophysiology of acute lower GI bleeding. Section Five describes the etiology, pathophysiology, and management of acute intestinal obstruction and paralytic ileus. Section Six describes the etiology, pathophysiology, and management of intraabdominal hypertension and abdominal compartment syndrome. Finally, Section Seven describes the nursing diagnosis and management of acute GI bleeding and bowel obstruction. All Section Reviews include answers. It is suggested that the learner review those concepts answered incorrectly in the review questions before proceeding to the next section.

PRETEST

1. Which laboratory measures are important in evaluating the need for clotting factor replacement?
   A. hemoglobin and hematocrit
   B. platelet count and hematocrit
   C. thrombin time and mean corpuscular volume
   D. prothrombin time and partial thromboplastin time
2. Elevations in the white blood cell (WBC) count suggests a(n)
   A. inflammatory or infectious process
   B. immunocompromised host
   C. normal nonimmunologic gut defense response
   D. hemoconcentration as a result of fluid volume deficit
3. The appearance of melena is described as
   A. bright red in color from a lower GI tract source
   B. black and tarry in color from an upper GI source
   C. light brown in color from an upper GI source
   D. "coffee ground" in appearance from the colon
4. A patient passes a large amount of loose, maroon-colored stool. When documenting this event, the correct term that applies to this description is
   A. melena
   B. diarrhea
   C. hematochezia
   D. hematemesis
5. Infections associated with peptic ulcer disease include
   A. *Escherichia coli* infection
   B. *Helicobacter pylori*
   C. beta-hemolytic *streptococcus*
   D. *Staphylococcus aureus*
6. Drugs known to disrupt the mucosal barrier are
   A. nonsteroidal anti-inflammatory drugs (NSAIDs)
   B. angiotensin-converting enzyme (ACE) inhibitors
   C. cephalosporins
   D. histamine receptor antagonists

7. The elderly are at increased risk of developing ischemic bowel complications. What is another risk factor for the development of bowel ischemia in this population?
   A. atrial fibrillation
   B. hypertension
   C. immobility
   D. obesity
8. Twenty-five percent of all bleeding from ischemic bowel disease is associated with
   A. recreational drug use
   B. severe malnutrition
   C. anticoagulant use
   D. traumatic injury
9. A good measure of perfusion for the nurse to monitor is
   A. arterial blood gas (ABG)
   B. complete blood count (CBC)
   C. urine output
   D. skin temperature
10. Complications of vasopressin include
   A. hypoglycemia
   B. hypernatremia
   C. decreased coronary blood flow
   D. increased portal pressures
11. Acute paralytic ileus (adynamic ileus) is associated with
   A. adhesions following abdominal surgery
   B. a loss of intestinal peristalsis
   C. volvulus of the intestines
   D. hyperperistalsis of the intestines
12. Medications that are known to contribute to the development of acute paralytic ileus include
   A. ACE inhibitors
   B. aminoglycosides
   C. opioids
   D. beta blockers
13. Fifteen to twenty percent of patients receiving long term NSAID therapy develop ulcers at one time or another.
   A. True
   B. False
14. Although the critical pressure varies between patients, it is generally thought that intra-abdominal hypertension is present when
   A. abdominal pressure reaches 10 to 15 mm Hg
   B. abdominal pressure reaches 5 to 10 mm Hg
   C. abdominal pressure reaches 1 to 5 mm Hg
   D. abdominal pressure reaches 4 to 8 mm Hg
15. Prophylactic measures to prevent the development of peptic ulcers in acutely ill patients include
   A. early enteral feeding and histamine receptor antagonists
   B. surgical resection of all affected mucosa and antacids
   C. total parenteral nutrition and proton pump inhibitors
   D. sclerotherapy and sucralfate
16. Impaired gut perfusion is a risk factor in which of the following conditions?
   A. hypernatremia
   B. diabetes mellitus
   C. hypertension
   D. hypotension

Pretest answers are found on MyNursingKit.

SECTION ONE: Incidence and Clinical Manifestations of Acute GI Bleeding

At the completion of this section, the learner will be able to describe the incidence and clinical manifestations of acute GI bleeding.

Incidence

GI bleeding is a common and major medical problem, despite advances in diagnosis and treatment. The incidence per year of upper GI bleeding is 100 per 100,000 people (Bjorkman, 2007). GI bleeding manifests in one or more of the following clinical scenarios: (1) bleeding is from the upper GI tract; (2) bleeding is from the lower GI tract; (3) bleeding is occult (unknown to the patient); (4) bleeding is obvious but the site (whether it is from the upper or lower GI tract) is obscure (Rockey, 2006). GI bleeding can range in severity from a very slow occult blood loss to a sudden, massive hemorrhage.

The overwhelming majority (75 to 80 percent) of patients with bleeding ulcers stop bleeding spontaneously; but despite progressive advances in diagnosis, the mortality from acute upper GI bleed (UGIB) remains near 4 percent for young patients and as high as 15 percent in the elderly (Bjorkman, 2007).

Etiology and General Manifestations of Upper GI Bleeding

More than 90 percent of upper GI bleeding cases are caused by peptic ulcer, erosive gastritis, Mallory-Weiss tears, or esophagogastric varices (Reicher & Eysselein, 2008). Other etiologies of upper GI bleeding include tumors, arteriovenous malformations, and stress ulcers. Table 29–1 summarizes the causes of upper GI bleeding.

TABLE 29–1 Causes of Upper GI bleeding

ETIOLOGY	OCCURRENCE (PERCENTAGE OF TOTAL UPPER GI BLEED CASES)
Peptic ulcers	50
Gastritis	10-15
Varices	10-15
Esophagitis	15
Mallory-Weiss tear	5–10
Arteriovenous malformation	5

Data from Rockey (2006).

The amount and degree of upper GI bleeding varies. When an ulcer erodes through an artery, the bleeding is profuse. The manifestations of GI bleeding depend on the source, the rate of bleeding, and comorbid disease. Severe GI bleeding may seriously aggravate coronary artery disease, hypertension, diabetes mellitus, pulmonary disease, and renal failure, and it often presents as shock. Lesser degrees of bleeding may present as orthostatic changes in pulse (a change of greater than 10 beats per minute) or blood pressure (a drop of 10 mm Hg or greater) secondary to compensatory mechanisms (Reicher & Eysselein, 2008; Beers et al., 2006). Studies have found that the most common cause of death in GI hemorrhage is the result of exacerbation of the underlying disease rather than intractable hypovolemic shock (Andreoli et al., 2007). However, if unrecognized or treated too late, GI hemorrhage can lead to hypovolemic shock and ultimately death.

Etiology and General Manifestations of Lower GI Bleeding

Lower GI bleeding occurs at a rate of 20 per 100,000 people. Hematochezia, which is the most common presenting symptom, can be described as bloody diarrhea, blood, and/or clots from the rectum. Hematochezia can occur from bleeding anywhere in the GI tract, with 10 percent of patients who present with hematochezia having an upper GI source of bleeding (Bjorkman, 2007). Mortality rates for lower GI bleed (LGIB) is about 5 percent. Most patients with LGIB will resolve spontaneously, but have a 10 percent to 40 percent chance of rebleed. Between 5 to 50 percent of patients will have persistent rebleeding and will require surgical hemostasis (Strate, 2005).

Clinical Manifestations of Upper and Lower GI Bleeding

Gastrointestinal blood loss may be acute (sudden or massive with hypovolemia) or chronic (slow and often unnoticed by the patient). Acute GI bleeding may present in one of several ways:

- **Occult blood**—blood that is present in the GI tract but not really visible. Occult bleeding is often detected by chemical testing of a stool or nasogastric specimen, using a process known as *hemoccult* or *guaiac testing.*
- **Hematemesis**—vomiting of bright red blood or blood that looks like coffee grounds. This bleeding is often brisk and is likely proximal to the ligament of Treitz (considered to be in the upper GI tract).
- **Melena**—black, tarry, foul-smelling stools passed after a GI bleed of usually from an upper GI source. However, a small intestine or right colon bleeding source may also be the cause.
- **Hematochezia**—bright red blood or maroon stool from the rectum, usually the result of lower GI bleeding or massive upper GI bleeding. Ten percent of patients with severe hematochezia have an upper GI source of bleeding.

Chronic GI bleed may exhibit recurrent episodes of melena or hematochezia. Patients may have no signs or symptoms of acute blood loss (occult bleeding), but may present with manifestations associated with anemia, such as fatigue, dyspnea, and low RBC count and hemoglobin (Andreoli et al., 2007).

SECTION ONE REVIEW

1. The section of the GI tract that is involved in an upper GI hemorrhage is
   A. proximal to the ligament of Treitz
   B. proximal to the ileocecal valve
   C. distal to the pyloric sphincter
   D. distal to the duodenal bulb
2. The mortality rate for acute lower GI bleeding is
   A. twice as high as the mortality rate for acute upper GI bleeding
   B. less than the mortality rate for acute upper GI bleeding
   C. the same as the mortality rate for acute upper GI bleeding
   D. slightly higher than the mortality rate for acute upper GI bleeding
3. Characteristics of acute lower GI bleeding include
   A. bleeding commonly of arterial origin
   B. bleeding commonly of venous origin
   C. bleeding massive 80 percent of the time
   D. bleeding always occult
4. A client presents to the emergency department after vomiting bright red blood. The client becomes hypotensive soon after and is admitted into the hospital with GI bleeding. The presentation of this episode of bleeding is
   A. occult
   B. chronic
   C. subacute
   D. acute
5. Patients with occult GI bleeding often present with
   A. nausea and vomiting
   B. mental status changes
   C. headache and abdominal pain
   D. fatigue and syncope
6. Which of the following is a cause of acute upper GI bleeding?
   A. Mallory-Weiss tear
   B. diverticula
   C. ischemic bowel disease
   D. ulcerative colitis

Answers: 1. A, 2. C, 3. B, 4. D, 5. D, 6. A

SECTION TWO: Acute Upper GI Bleeding Due to Ulcers

At the completion of this section, the learner will be able to describe the etiology and pathophysiology of acute upper GI bleeding due to ulcers.

Peptic Ulcer Disease

Peptic ulcer disease (PUD) is the most common cause of upper GI bleeding. Ulcers range in size from several millimeters to several centimeters and are characterized by mucosal damage extending through the **muscularis** mucosae. Peptic ulcers occur in the portion of the GI tract exposed to acid–pepsin secretion, which includes the stomach and the proximal duodenum. Approximately 500,000 people develop PUD in the United States each year. The incidence of PUD is declining, likely as a result of proton pump inhibitors (PPIs) and decreasing rates of *H. pylori* infection. Mortality, as a result of peptic ulcer disease is quite low; however, patients suffer substantial pain as a result of the chronic nature of this disease. Interestingly, peptic ulcer disease is the most common cause of upper GI bleeding in critically ill patients. Peptic ulcer disease accounts for approximately 40 percent of patients admitted to an intensive care unit (ICU) specifically for bleeding and 50 percent of patients who develop upper GI hemorrhage during their stay but are admitted for some other reason (Reicher & Eysselein, 2008).

Risk Factors

Traditional theories on the cause of peptic ulcer disease have focused on acid hypersecretion or the inability of the **mucosa** to secrete mucus for protection. It is now known that acid hypersecretion is not the primary mechanism by which ulceration occurs. Under normal circumstances, a balance exists between hostile and protective mucosal factors (Fig 29–1).The cause of mucosal injury in PUD is usually multifactorial and relates to an imbalance in protective and hostile factors that exist in the stomach and duodenum. The two most common causes of peptic ulcer disease are *H. pylori* infection and nonsteroidal anti-inflammatory drugs (NSAIDs). Both of these factors disrupt the mucosal defense barrier, making it susceptible to the damaging effects of acid. Table 29–2 summarizes the more common alterations in protective and hostile factors.

***H. pylori* Infection.** The bacterium *Helicobacter pylori* (*H. pylori*) is a gram negative rod that can be cultured from the stomachs of approximately 65 percent of patients (Andreoli et al., 2007). *H. pylori* is able to survive and even thrive in the high acid environment of the stomach through its ability to secrete the enzyme urease, which splits urea (which is abundant in gastric secretions) into ammonia and bicarbonate—two strong bases. These bases form an alkaline cloud around the bacterium, protecting it from the low pH gastric environment. The mechanism by which *H. pylori* impairs mucosal integrity is poorly understood. The organism is responsible for the production of cytotoxins and mucolytic enzymes (e.g., protease) that erode the mucous barrier and trigger an inflammatory response, all of which make the mucosa more susceptible to acid damage.

NSAIDs. Fifteen to twenty percent of patients receiving long-term NSAID therapy develop ulcers at one time or another. NSAID-induced ulcers are more common in persons 60 years of age or older (Kethu & Moss, 2008). Other factors that may increase the risk of NSAID-induced ulcers include previous history of peptic ulcer disease, corticosteroid use, and high doses of NSAIDs. Also, the incidence is slightly higher in females (Reicher & Eysselein, 2008). NSAIDs compete with prostaglandin receptor sites in the gastric mucosa. Prostaglandins, particularly prostaglandin E, have been linked to mucosal repair and maintenance of mucosal integrity. When these prostaglandin-supported defense mechanisms are inhibited by the action of NSAIDs, severe inflammation and erosive injury to the gastric mucosa can occur.

Other Risk Factors. Other risk factors include a family history of peptic ulcer disease, the use of aspirin, smoking, and genetic predisposition. Smoking also increases the risk of ulcer recurrence and slows healing (Ramakrishan et al., 2007).

Classification of Ulcers

Ulcers are often classified by how deep into the wall the ulcer has penetrated, and include erosion, acute ulcer, or chronic ulcers

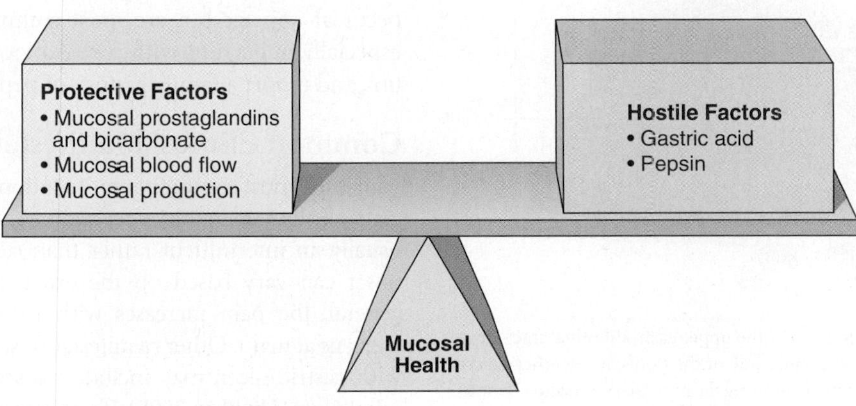

Figure 29–1 ■ Normal balance between protective and hostile factors.

TABLE 29–2 Alterations in Protective and Hostile Factors

FACTORS	ALTERATIONS
Decreased Protective Factors	
Mucosal prostaglandins & bicarbonate	Inhibited by NSAIDs (COX-1 inhibitors)
Mucosal blood flow	Decreased with inhibition of mucosal prostaglandins and severe stress
Mucus production	Decreased with inhibition of mucosal prostaglandins and tissue ischemia
Increased Hostile Factors	
Gastric acid	Corrosive activity when exposed to mucosa; acid hypersecretion may be present
Pepsin	Corrosive activity when exposed to mucosa; promotes clot lysis
H. pylori infection	Invades mucosa, activating cytokines and establishing and maintaining inflammatory response
NSAIDs (COX-1 inhibitors)	Inhibit production of mucosal prostaglandins. Reduced gastric protection: decreased bicarbonate, decreased mucus production, increased acid secretion, decreased blood flow to submucosa[a]
Alcohol	Gastric irritant-stimulates production of gastric acid; direct mucosal injury in large doses. When used with NSAIDs, intensifies injury
Stress	High levels of physiologic stress results in shunting of blood flow from GI tract to more vital organs resulting in reduced blood flow, tissue ischemia, mucosal injury, reperfusion injury, and tissue acidosis ("Curling's ulcers")
Traumatic brain injury and increased intracranial pressure	In patients with increased intracranial pressure, altered vagus nerve stimulation can cause hypersecretion of gastric acid; severe burns also commonly results in hypersecretion ("Cushing's ulcers")

[a]Data from Lehne (2007).

(see Fig 29–2). Erosion is a superficial injury that is confined to the mucosal layer; an acute ulcer has penetrated through the mucosa and **submucosa;** and a chronic ulcer (sometimes called a perforating ulcer) has penetrated into the muscularis layer. A chronic ulcer can perforate through the serosa, exposing the sterile abdominal cavity to GI contents, which can result in peritonitis.

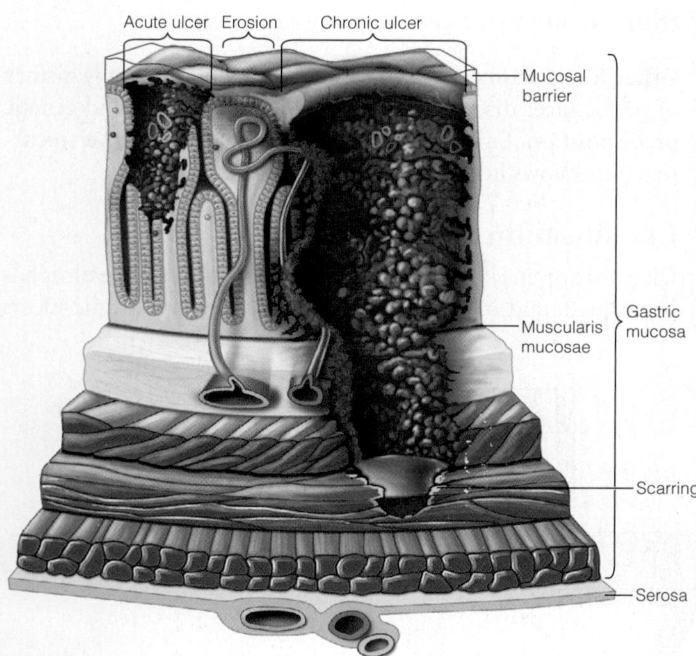

Figure 29–2 ■ Erosion and ulcerations of the upper gastrointestinal tract. Acute and chronic ulcers may penetrate the entire wall of the stomach. Superficial ulcers (erosions) erode the mucosa without penetrating the muscularis mucosae. True ulcers extend through the muscularis mucosae and into deeper layers of the GI wall, damaging blood vessels and potentially penetrating the entire wall.

Types of Peptic Ulcer Disease

There are two types of peptic ulcers based on their location — gastric ulcers (prepyloric) and duodenal ulcers (postpyloric). Figure 29–3 illustrates common sites of peptic ulcers.

Gastric Ulcers. Gastric ulcers affect older adults, largely because of increased long-term NSAID use in this population. Gastric ulcers tend to be chronic, usually involving branches of the left gastric artery, and can produce severe hemorrhage if erosion into the arterial wall occurs.

Duodenal Ulcers. Duodenal ulcers constitute the majority of peptic ulcers (about 75 percent). The most frequent sites for duodenal ulcers are the gastric pylorus and the first portion of the duodenum where the pH is still acidic. Duodenal ulcers can occur at any age but are most common among young adults, especially in persons with type A blood who smoke, abuse alcohol, and report a family history of peptic ulcers.

Common Clinical Manifestations

Pain is the most common manifestation of peptic ulcer disease. It is generally located in the upper abdomen in the epigastric area and is usually an intermittent rather than steady pain. Timing of pain onset can vary based on the exact ulcer location, however, in general, the pain increases within 1–2 hours after eating and worsens at night. Other manifestations, seen more often in patients with gastric ulcer, may include nausea, vomiting, anorexia, and weight loss (Huether, 2008). If a gastric ulcer is located in the pyloric canal (the narrow region of the stomach that opens through the

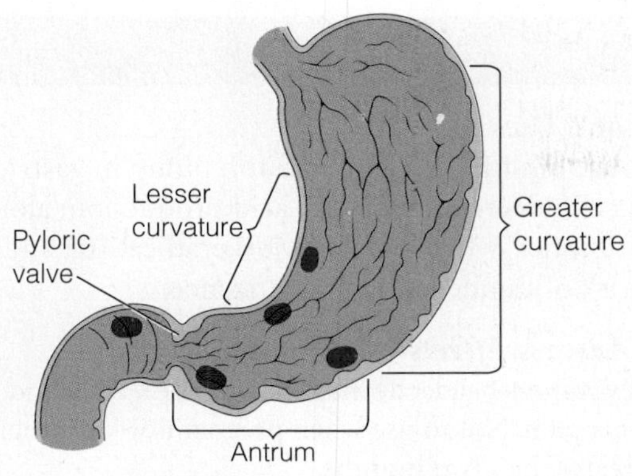

Figure 29–3 ■ Common sites of peptic ulcers.

pylorus into the duodenum), the symptoms are often associated with obstruction (e.g., bloating, nausea, vomiting) (Beers et al., 2006). If GI bleeding is present, it may be hidden (occult) or gross, being evidenced as hematemesis (bloody emesis), melena (tarry stools), or hematochezia (bright blood stools).

Diagnosis and Treatment

Diagnosis of peptic ulcer disease is largely suggested by history and is confirmed by visualization with fiberoptic endoscopy, the diagnostic tool of choice. Barium radiography is contraindicated in acute upper GI bleed, because it interferes with subsequent endoscopy, angiography, or surgery (Bjorkman, 2007). Determination of a duodenal or gastric ulcer by upper endoscopy or radiographic study should be followed by confirmation of *H. pylori* infection. *H. pylori* infection can be definitively diagnosed using endoscopy. Diagnostic tests for the presence of *H. pylori* vary and include serologic testing, carbon-labeled urea breath tests, rapid urease assay (Clotest), and culture or histologic analysis of endoscopic biopsies (Andreoli et al., 2007).

Treatment of peptic ulcer disease involves combination antibiotic therapy (for eradication of *H. pylori*), histamine receptor antagonist agents (H_2RA) as an antisecretory, proton pump inhibitors (PPIs) for acid secretion inhibition, prostaglandins to inhibit acid secretion and enhance mucosal barrier, sucralfate to promote mucosal barrier, and antacids to give symptomatic relief and raise gastric pH. Many high-acuity patients have nasogastric as well as small-bore enteric feeding tubes. The appropriate route of administration for sucralfate and antacids is through the nasogastric tube to allow for direct contact with the gastric mucosa. If the nasogastric tube is attached to suction, it must be interrupted for 30 to 60 minutes. Eliminating foods that cause distress is helpful. Surgery is indicated only to manage severe bleeding and perforation complications of peptic ulcers (Bjorkman, 2007). Drug treatment for peptic ulcer disease is summarized in the RELATED PHARMACOTHERAPY box: Peptic Ulcer Disease. Explain to the patient the importance of completing the entire course of therapy even if symptoms disappear.

RELATED PHARMACOTHERAPY: Peptic Ulcer Disease

H_2 Receptor Blocking Agents
Ranitidine, famotidine, cimetidine

Action and Uses
Reduces gastric acid secretion and increased gastric mucus and bicarbonate production, creating a protective coating on gastric mucosa

Major Adverse Effects
Usually well tolerated. Hypersensitivity is rare but potentially life-threatening.

Nursing Implications
- For intermittent intravenous bolus injection, dilute in normal saline solution or other compatible solution to a concentration not exceeding 2.5 mg/ml. Inject no faster than 4 ml/minute.
- For continuous intravenous infusion in patients with Zollinger-Ellison syndrome, add to dextrose 5 percent in water (D_5W) or other compatible solution; dilute to a concentration not exceeding 2.5 mg/ml, and start infusion at 1 mg/kg/hour.
- Give oral doses with or without food. Give once-daily dose at bedtime.
- Know that intravenous form may be added to total parenteral nutrition solutions.
- Inject intramuscular undiluted deep into large muscle.

Antisecretory Agent
Misoprostol

Action and Uses
Synthetic prostaglandin E analog; replaces prostaglandin lost due to NSAID therapy. Reduces gastric acid secretion and increases gastric mucus and bicarbonate production, creating a protective coating on gastric mucosa. Primary use is in prevention of NSAID-induced peptic ulcer disease.

Major Adverse Effects
Most common: diarrhea, abdominal discomfort
Other important: women - miscarriage, menstrual disorders, postmenopausal bleeding

Nursing Implications
- Assess GI status, report significant adverse reactions
- Instruct patient to take with food.
- Advise patient to report diarrhea, abdominal pain, and menstrual irregularities.
- Tell patient drug may cause spontaneous abortion.
- Caution patient not to take magnesium-containing antacids, which may worsen diarrhea.

Cytoprotective Agent
Sucralfate

(*continued*)

RELATED PHARMACOTHERAPY *(continued)*

Action and Uses

Combines with gastric acid to form protective coating on injured mucosal surface, inhibiting gastric acid secretion, pepsin and bile salts. Action is almost exclusively local. Used for short-term ulcer treatment.

Major Adverse Effects

Most common: constipation

Nursing Implications

Monitor bowel pattern, report severe, ongoing constipation.

Prevention of constipation: unless contraindicated, water intake should be increased to 8-10 glasses per day, increase dietary bulk, increase physical exercise.

Caution patient not to take within 30 minutes of antacids or other drugs.

Antacids

Aluminum carbonate, calcium carbonate, magnesium hydroxide

Action and Uses

Neutralizes excess gastric acid

Major Adverse Effects

Aluminum- and calcium-based: fecal impaction, constipation, abdominal cramping

Magnesium-based: diarrhea, abdominal cramping

Both: metabolic alkalosis

Nursing Implications

Tell patient that taking too much medication can cause systemic problems.

Advise patient to not take with milk and avoid the herb oak bark.

Advise patient that some antacids interfere with action of many common drugs; do not take other oral medications within 30 minutes of taking antacids.

Proton Pump Inhibitors

Esomeprazole (Nexium), omeprazole (Prilosec), pantoprazole (Protonix), lansoprazole (Prevacid), rabeprazole (Aciphex)

Action and Uses

As a group: inhibit activity of proton pump in gastric parietal cells, decreasing gastric acid production; along with antibiotics, will cause *H. pylori* eradication; and reduce risk of duodenal ulcer recurrence.

Major Adverse Effects

Generally minor–headache, nausea, diarrhea, rash, and abdominal pain. Not to use when pregnant or lactating or for greater than two months.

Nursing Implications

General implications include:

Concurrent use with diazepam, phenytoin, CNS depressants, and warfarin may cause increase in blood levels of these drugs.

Give oral forms of medications before meals.

If patient has difficulty swallowing the delayed-release capsule, open it and sprinkle contents onto small amount of soft food, such as applesauce or pudding. Don't crush or let patient chew drug.

When giving oral suspension, empty packet contents into container with two tbsp. water. Stir contents well, and have patient drink immediately. Don't give oral suspension through nasogastric tube.

When putting contents of delayed-release capsule through NG tube, open capsule and mix granules with 40 mL of apple juice. Then rinse tube with additional apple juice to clear.

Advise patient to minimize GI upset by eating frequent servings of food and drinking plenty of fluids.

H. Pylori related antibiotics

Amoxicillin, metronidazole, tetracycline, clarithormycin.

Action and Uses

Eradication of *H. Pylori;* combination theraphy is preferred over single antibiotic therapy related to high risk for development of resistance.

Major Adverse Effects and Nursing Implications

Multiple depending on the combination used. Refer to specific drugs in drug resource of choice.

SECTION TWO REVIEW

1. ______ is the most common cause of upper GI bleeding.
   A. Esophageal varices
   B. Peptic ulcer disease
   C. Arteriovenous malformation
   D. Stress gastritis

2. Peptic ulcers occur in the
   A. stomach and ileum
   B. duodenum and colon
   C. stomach and peritoneum
   D. stomach and duodenum

3. A 35-year-old male is diagnosed with PUD. His father had a gastric ulcer. He smokes one pack of cigarettes per day, takes a diuretic to treat his hypertension, and is obese (310 pounds at 6 feet tall). He takes aspirin every day for his "arthritis." How many risk factors for PUD does this person have?
   A. two
   B. three
   C. four
   D. five

4. Peptic ulcers are caused by
   A. colonization of bacteria within the GI tract
   B. hypersecretion of pancreatic enzymes
   C. underproduction of bicarbonate
   D. disruption of the mucosal barrier

5. Gastric ulcer symptoms
   A. have no relationship to eating
   B. tend to occur 1–2 hours after eating
   C. tend to occur 6–8 hours following eating
   D. follow an inconsistent pattern

Answers: 1. B, 2. D, 3. B, 4. D, 5. B

SECTION THREE: Acute Upper GI Bleeding Due to Nonulcer Etiologies

Stress-Related Mucosal Disease

For many years, the link between critical illness and mucosal injury has been recognized. Stress-related mucosal disease (SRMD) encompasses two types of injury: superficial, diffuse erosions and stress ulcers, which are deeper, discrete lesions. It has been estimated at least 75 percent of critically ill patients have evidence of mucosal injury within the first 24 hours post admission to ICU (Marshall, 2009; Spirt & Stanley, 2006).

Pathophysiology

As presented with peptic ulcer disease, stress-related mucosal disease is believed to be caused by an imbalance in hostile and protective factors in the stomach and duodenum. The high-acuity patient, particularly in the critical care setting, is at significant risk for developing decreased protective factors and increased hostile factors (see Table 29–2). Additional hostile factors that may come to play in the development of SRMD include the presence of bile salts that reflux into the stomach from the duodenum; the generation of free oxygen radicals, and reperfusion injury, which develops in response to tissue hypoxia (Marshall, 2009).

Prevention and Treatment

Early in their ICU stay, it is common practice to initiate prophylactic measures to prevent stress-related mucosal disease (SRMD) in critically ill patients. Drug groups commonly chosen for prophylaxis include histamine-2 receptor blockers, proton pump inhibitors, or possibly sucralfate. If injury occurs, treatment is that of peptic ulcer disease or gastritis.

Acute Erosive or Hemorrhagic Gastritis

Acute gastritis refers to inflammation of the stomach. Acute erosive or hemorrhagic gastritis involves transient inflammation of the gastric mucosa. Common causes of erosive gastritis include NSAIDs, alcohol, and acute stress. Uncommon causes of gastric mucosal erosion include radiation, viral infections, caustic ingestion, and direct trauma (e.g., nasogastric tubes). The role of NSAIDs in precipitating acute gastritis is essentially the same as in peptic ulcer disease. Chronic alcohol ingestion can result in inflammation of the gastric mucosa and the inflammation can progress to erosions and hemorrhage. Episodes of upper GI bleeding as a result of this alcohol-induced gastritis are usually mild. The risk for bleeding significantly increases if a person continues to drink alcohol while on long-term NSAID therapy.

Clinical Manifestations

The most common clinical manifestation of erosive gastritis is upper GI bleeding, which presents as hematemesis, "coffee ground" emesis, bloody aspirate in a patient receiving nasogastric suction, or as melena. Because erosive gastritis involves superficial lesions, bleeding is not as rapid as with a lesion that extends deeper into the mucosa and may erode into a blood vessel. The slow loss of blood can be noted in continuously decreasing hemoglobin and hematocrit levels. Gastritis is often asymptomatic but may cause epigastric pain, nausea, vomiting, and bleeding. GI bleeding as a result of gastritis is usually not severe except in the critically ill. Diagnosis of gastritis is accomplished by direct visualization with endoscopy (Porth, 2007). Diagnosis of gastritis is confirmed by direct endoscopic visualization.

Prevention and Treatment

The incidence of gastritis can usually be decreased or prevented if the gastric pH level is maintained above 4.0. This can be accomplished with the prophylactic administration of histamine receptor antagonists proton pump inhibitors or oral antacids to all at-risk patients to raise the gastric pH above 4.0 (Beers et al., 2006; Lindseth, 2003). Sucralfate, given orally, is also effective in reducing bleeding. Early enteral feeding has been advocated as a means of lowering the incidence of bleeding in acutely ill persons. Treatment is aimed at prophylaxis, but the use of H_2RAs, PPIs, and sucralfate are used for both treatment and prophylaxis (Porth, 2007).

Once significant GI bleeding from gastritis occurs (in about two percent of ICU patients), the mortality rate is more than 60 percent (Reicher & Eysselein, 2008; Beers et al., 2006). Severe bleeding from a localized lesion may be treated with endoscopic sclerotherapy to cauterize the bleeding lesion. Diffusely bleeding lesions may respond to vasopressin administered intravenously or intraarterially into a bleeding vessel. Vasopressin (also known as antidiuretic hormone [ADH]) is a potent stimulator of smooth muscle, particularly those of capillaries and arterioles. It exerts its therapeutic effect in the management of GI bleeding by vasoconstriction of the splanchnic vessels, which reduces blood flow through the bleeding vessel. Vasopressin exerts its vasoconstricting effects systemically; therefore, untoward side effects of abdominal cramping, angina, hypertension, dysrhythmias, and headache may occur. Surgical resection of the involved portions of the stomach is indicated if bleeding does not respond to more conservative treatment.

Conservative treatment for NSAID-induced gastritis includes discontinuation of the drug, reduction to the lowest effective dose, or administration with meals. Patients with persistent gastritis or those who are at increased risk of developing gastric mucosal injury should be treated with sucralfate, histamine receptor antagonists, or with a proton pump inhibitor (e.g., Omeprazole). Misoprostol can be administered along with NSAID therapy to prevent ulcer formation. Misoprostol is a synthetic prostaglandin E analog that replaces the protective prostaglandins consumed with prostaglandin-inhibiting therapies (e.g., NSAIDs). Misoprostol is reserved for use with long-term NSAID therapy in high-risk patients (Ramakrishnan, 2007). If the patient has adequate renal function, switching the patient to a COX-2 inhibitor NSAID may prevent NSAID-induced gastritis. Alcohol-induced gastritis usually responds well to alcohol withdrawal and antiulcer therapy.

Esophageal and Gastric Varices

Upper GI bleeding from esophageal or gastric varices is associated with cirrhosis, portal hypertension, and portal or splenic vein thrombosis. Bleeding from esophagogastric varices is usually massive and occurs without warning. Portal hypertension causes the development of collateral venous pathways, called *varices,* which are located in the esophagus and stomach. Hepatic cirrhosis as a result of alcohol abuse is the most common cause of variceal bleeding in the United States. An in-depth discussion of cirrhosis and esophageal varices is presented in Module 30, Alterations in Hepatic Function.

Mallory-Weiss Tears

A Mallory-Weiss tear is a small laceration in the mucosa at the gastroesophageal junction, although a small percent occur in the esophageal mucosa. Mallory-Weiss tears are commonly thought to be caused by retching or vomiting; however, only about 30 percent of patients report a history of vomiting prior to acute hematemesis (Rockey, 2006). High-risk patients are those with a history of alcohol abuse. Bleeding from a Mallory-Weiss tear often presents with mild-to-massive hematemesis. Bleeding stops spontaneously in 80 to 90 percent of patients and rebleeding is rare (Day, 2009). Diagnosis is confirmed by upper GI endoscopy. If acute intervention is required, endoscopic visualization is performed and coagulation or injection therapies are performed (Day, 2009).

Arteriovenous Malformation

An arteriovenous malformation (AVM), sometimes referred to as an angiodysplasia, is a small, abnormal mucosal or submucosal blood vessel that has a tendency to bleed. Arteriovenous malformations can occur in both the upper GI and the lower GI tracts, but they are most commonly located in the cecal region of the lower GI tract. The cause of arteriovenous malformations is unknown but appears to be genetic. Once GI bleeding from an arteriovenous malformation occurs, recurrent GI bleeding, chronic anemia, or severe acute GI bleeding is the usual clinical course (Strate, 2005). AVM can be associated with chronic renal insufficiency or renal failure, valvular heart disease, specifically aortic stenosis, and congestive heart failure (Esralian & Gralnek, 2005). Upper GI bleeding as a result of an arteriovenous malformation is most commonly diagnosed by upper GI endoscopy. Definitive treatment of the underlying or concomitant conditions (e.g., valvuloplasty or kidney transplantation) can cure bleeding arteriovenous malformations. Endoscopic sclerotherapy is used palliatively because new arteriovenous malformations can continue to develop in high-risk patients (Farrell & Friedman, 2001).

SECTION THREE REVIEW

1. The primary treatment for stress-related mucosal disease (SRMD) is
   A. prophylactic, using antiulcer therapies
   B. flushing the stomach with vasopressin to stop the bleeding
   C. endoscopic visualization with coagulation therapy
   D. reactive, it is treated symptomatically
2. Stress-related mucosal disease (SRMD) begins to develop in most critically ill patients within ______ hours of admission to an ICU.
   A. 12
   B. 24
   C. 36
   D. 48
3. Which drug is often prescribed along with long-term NSAID therapy in high-risk patients to prevent the development of ulcers or SRMD?
   A. neomycin
   B. misoprostol
   C. sucralfate
   D. antacids
4. GI bleeding as a result of a Mallory-Weiss tear often presents with
   A. hematemesis
   B. hematochezia
   C. melena
   D. pain

Answers: 1. A, 2. B, 3. B, 4. A

SECTION FOUR: Acute Lower GI Bleeding

At the completion of this section, the learner will be able to describe the etiology and pathophysiology of acute lower GI bleeding.

The two most common causes of acute lower GI bleeding are diverticulosis and arteriovenous malformations. Other common causes of lower GI bleeding are ischemic colitis, internal hemorrhoids, rectal ulcers, and neoplasms. Lower GI bleeding is anatomically defined as bleeding beyond the ligament of Treitz. Table 29–3 summarizes the most common causes and characteristics of lower GI bleeding. Bleeding stops spontaneously in 80 to 90 percent of patients, with a risk of recurrence in 10 to 40 percent of patients (Strate, 2005). Unlike upper GI bleeding, the majority of lower GI bleeds are slow and intermittent and do not require hospitalization. Less frequent causes of lower GI bleeding include ischemic bowel disease and inflammatory bowel disease. About 10 to 20 percent of the acute lower GI bleeding cases do not resolve spontaneously and, therefore, require high-acuity nursing (Reicher & Eysselein, 2008).

TABLE 29–3 Causes and Characteristics of Lower GI Bleeding

CAUSE	CHARACTERISTICS
Diverticula	Sustained, dark, occasionally massive bleeding throughout the colon
Inflammatory bowel disease (e.g., Crohn's disease, ulcerative colitis, gastroenteritis)	Intermittent bleeding, mixed with frequent bowel movement
Perianal disorders (e.g., hemorrhoids, fissures)	Bright red blood per rectum, intermittent with bowel movements
Carcinoma	Occult bleeding with intermittent melena, right colon tumors
Arteriovenous malformation	Intermittent, both dark and bright red bleeding, clots, coming from cecal area

Data from Cagir & Cirincione (2008).

Diverticular Bleeding

Diverticular disease is the most common etiology of major lower GI bleeding (Cagir & Cirincione, 2008). Diverticula (diverticulum, singular) are small outpouchings (herniations) in the bowel wall caused by weakness in the bowel wall of the descending or sigmoid colon (see Fig. 29–4). Risk factors include age older than 60 and chronic constipation. Complications of diverticular disease include diverticulitis (inflammation/infection) and rupture. Diverticular bleeding occurs in less than 20 percent of people with the disease and is self-limiting in most cases; however, it can also be massive and life-threatening. About 25 percent of these cases rebleed, requiring surgical intervention or angiography with intraarterial infusion of vasopressin (Strate, 2005).

Inflammatory Bowel Disease

Inflammatory bowel diseases (IBDs), which include ulcerative colitis and Crohn's disease, are chronic disorders of the GI tract. They are usually diagnosed by colonoscopy and biopsy. Ulcerative colitis is largely confined to the mucosa and submucosa, but in Crohn's disease, the disease extends through the intestinal wall from mucosa to serosa (Stenson, 2007). Bloody diarrhea is the most common symptom of IBD, and is a major feature of ulcerative colitis. The degree of bleeding is usually light to moderate but it can be massive. Significant bleeding is much more common in patients with ulcerative colitis than Crohn's disease. In very rare instances (about four percent in ulcerative colitis and one to two percent in Crohn's disease), life-threatening bleeding can result when the underlying inflammation ulcerates into adjacent arteries (Cagir & Cirincione, 2008; Reicher & Eysselein, 2008). The treatment of bleeding associated with inflammatory bowel disease is management of the underlying disorder with corticosteroids (Reicher & Eysselein, 2008; Flannery & Tucker, 2002). If the bleeding is uncontrollable by medical means, then surgical resection of the affected portion of the bowel is necessary.

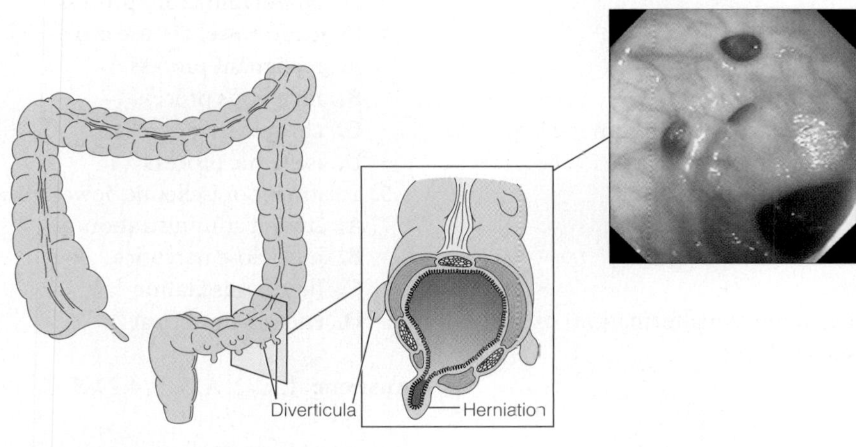

Figure 29–4 ■ Diverticula of the colon.

Neoplasms and Polyps

Colorectal cancers are primarily associated with occult bleeding; however, massive bleeding occurs in 5 to 20 percent of cases (Cagir & Cirincione, 2008). Bleeding from neoplasms is usually slow, chronic, and self-limiting. Only rarely is there acute blood loss of significant proportions from a neoplasm. In these cases, bowel resection and tumor excision are indicated. Bleeding is relatively common following surgical removal of polyps for up to a month following removal.

Arteriovenous Malformations

Bleeding from an arteriovenous malformation is usually slow and chronic, and can be occult. Patients usually present with weakness, fatigue, dyspnea on exertion, and guaiac-positive stools. Bleeding from an arteriovenous malformation is rarely massive. A typical bleeding episode requires less than two to four units of blood and is not associated with hypotension. The elderly have increased risk of severe blood loss from this type of GI bleed. Arteriovenous malformations are angiodysplastic lesions that are usually small, superficial, multiple, and located in the right colon, although lesions can occur throughout the intestinal tract and are often numerous. The cause of an arteriovenous malformation is not clear, but they appear to be associated with cardiac disease, low-flow states, and the aging process. Bleeding occurs from weakened, friable vessel wall lesions caused by chronic tension and dilation of blood vessels most commonly located in the cecal area of the intestine. In cases in which the bleeding does not stop spontaneously, arterial embolization with various agents such as intraarterial infusion of vasopressin or gelatin sponge, microcoils, and polyvinyl alcohol particles are used. Vasopressin can control bleeding in about 91 percent of all cases, but complications such as dysrhythmias, pulmonary edema, hypertension and ischemia range 10 to 20 percent (Green & Rockey, 2005).

Ischemic Bowel Disease

Ischemic bowel disease can be defined as ischemia of the colon resulting from an interruption of the colonic blood supply (Reicher & Eysselein, 2008). It may result from occlusion of a major artery, small-vessel disease, venous obstruction, low-flow states (e.g., cardiogenic shock), or intestinal obstruction. Intestinal ischemia can develop postoperatively following vascular bypass or colon resection with anastomosis. In the elderly, risk factors for developing ischemic bowel disease include atherosclerosis, atrial fibrillation, and hypotension. Older patients are most commonly affected, although younger patients with diabetes, pancreatitis heart disease, sickle cell disease, or systemic lupus erythematosus are also at risk.

Bleeding from ischemic bowel disease is often associated with anticoagulant use (25 percent of all bleeding cases) (Reicher & Eysselein, 2008). The bleeding is usually intermittent, with mixed dark and bright red blood and clots visible from the rectum. Fever and abdominal pain are usually present. Lower GI endoscopy reveals purple discoloration of the bowel, often in the presence of erosion and ulceration. Radiographic X-rays are nonspecific but may reveal abnormal air pockets if perforation is present. Barium contrast studies reveal characteristic "thumbprints," suggesting a necrotic process. Arterial or venous occlusion of the mesenteric vasculature should be suspected and ruled out when ischemia of the bowel is included in the differential diagnosis. Treatment of ischemic bowel disease involves restoration of blood circulation to the intestines and might include fluid resuscitation, optimization of cardiac output, and treatment of any underlying disease. Antibiotics may be required for infections. Resection of the affected bowel may be necessary for fulminant disease or severe bleeding. Patients with ischemic bowel disease often have other medical problems, including multiple organ failure, and therefore have a mortality rate of about 50 percent (Beers et al., 2006).

SECTION FOUR REVIEW

1. Diverticula are found throughout the
   A. stomach
   B. small intestine
   C. colon
   D. GI tract
2. Sustained, dark red lower GI bleeding from the large intestine is a characteristic of a bleeding
   A. diverticula
   B. hemorrhoid
   C. tumor
   D. angiodysplasia
3. Angiodysplasia (arteriovenous malformation) of the lower GI tract is associated with
   A. renal disease
   B. cardiac disease
   C. a high-fat diet
   D. an inflammatory process
4. Ischemic bowel disease is defined as a(n)
   A. malignant process
   B. infectious process
   C. chronic stress process
   D. ischemic process
5. Treatment of ischemic bowel disease may include
   A. steroid administration
   B. high-dose narcotics
   C. fluid resuscitation
   D. enemas until clear

Answers: 1. C, 2. A, 3. B, 4. D, 5. C

SECTION FIVE: Acute Intestinal Obstruction and Paralytic Ileus

At the completion of this section, the learner will be able to describe the etiology, pathophysiology, and management of acute intestinal obstruction and paralytic ileus.

Acute Small-Bowel Obstruction

Obstruction of the small intestine is a common surgical complication, often as a result of the development of adhesions following abdominal surgery. Other causes of obstruction are incarcerated hernias, volvulus, intussusception, adhesions, and tumors (see Fig 29–5). Most obstructions result from actual occlusion of the intestinal lumen (mechanical or physical), resulting in distention and gas and fluid accumulation above the obstruction. When the small bowel is obstructed, distention with gas and fluid occurs proximal to the obstruction. Swallowed air is the major cause of the distention. Bacterial fermentation within the lumen of the intestine produces other gases (methane). Inflammation soon develops and leads to transudation of fluid from the extracellular space into the intestinal lumen and peritoneal cavity. Fluid and electrolytes become trapped within the obstructed bowel and leak out into the **peritoneum,** further disturbing electrolyte and fluid balance. The inflammatory process causes large amounts of fluid and sodium to accumulate within the intestine (mass effect). Fluid losses may be so severe that hypotension results, which can lead to cardiovascular collapse unless the condition is recognized and treated. In severe cases, perforation of the intestinal wall can occur, with spillage of the bowel contents into the peritoneal cavity (Kong & Stamos, 2008).

In severe cases of bowel obstruction, the intestine can become strangulated. **Intestinal strangulation** occurs when the intestine "twists" itself to such an extent that circulation is interrupted. Strangulation can result in necrosis, perforation, and sepsis. Corrective surgery is generally the treatment of choice to prevent ischemic bowel problems. Appropriately treated, simple obstruction has a low mortality rate (less than two percent), whereas strangulation is associated with a high mortality rate (up to 25 percent if surgery is delayed). When the obstruction is located in the colon, it usually stems from a malignant tumor (McQuaid, 2007; Podolsky & Isselbacher, 2001; Kong & Stamos, 2008).

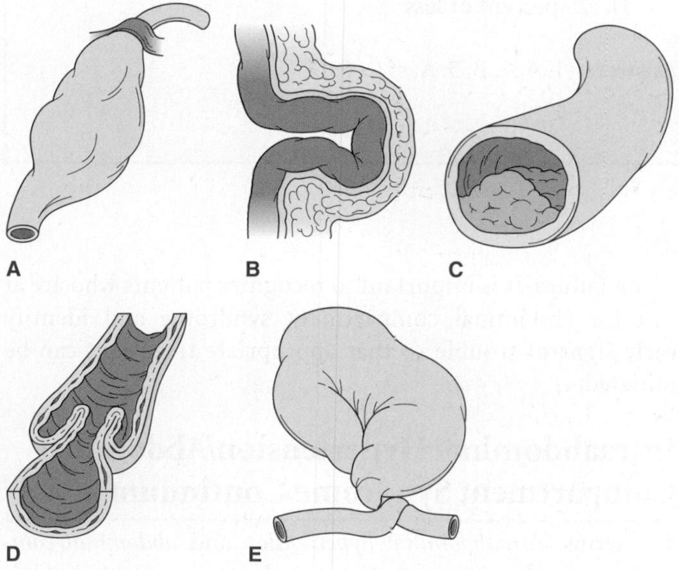

Figure 29–5 ■ Selected causes of mechanical obstruction. A, adhesions; B, incarcerated hernia; C, tumor; D, intussusception; and E, volvulus.

Acute Paralytic Ileus

Paralytic ileus (adynamic ileus) involves bowel obstruction resulting from a loss of intestinal peristalsis in the absence of any mechanical (physical) obstruction commonly seen in hospitalized patients. It can occur anywhere along the GI tract as a complication from trauma, handling of the bowel during surgery, electrolyte disturbances (hypokalemia, hypocalcemia, and hypomagnesemia), intestinal ischemia, peritonitis, and sepsis. In addition, there are multiple medications that reduce gastric motility (e.g., opioids, anticholinergics, and phenothiazines), thus contributing to the development of paralytic ileus. Ogilvie's syndrome involves paralytic ileus of the colon. This is a severe form of ileus that often arises in bedridden patients who have serious systemic illnesses.

Clinical Manifestations

The hallmark clinical manifestation of intestinal obstruction is abdominal distention. Small-bowel obstruction is characterized by cramping and periumbilical pain that occurs in waves, with periods of relative comfort in between the waves of pain. Vomiting, possibly profuse, soon follows the onset of pain and is usually bilious with a large quantity of mucus. Electrolyte imbalances and intraluminal loss of fluids occur, with dehydration soon following. Visible peristaltic waves may be observed on the abdomen, and high-pitched tinkles are auscultated during the painful spasms. The abdomen may be tender to palpation. If rebound tenderness develops, the nurse should observe for signs and symptoms of shock as a result of perforation. Symptoms of colonic paralytic ileus (Ogilvie's syndrome) include abdominal distention and diminished bowel sounds without pain (Kong & Stamos, 2008). Laboratory and radiologic examinations, along with history and physical findings, aid in diagnosing intestinal obstruction.

Laboratory Findings

Hematology, electrolyte, and chemistry studies will reflect inflammation, fluid, and electrolyte imbalances. Mild leukocytosis (greater than 15,000) is common, whereas WBC elevations from 15,000 to 25,000 may occur with strangulation and perforation (Gearhart & Silen, 2007). Serum BUN, creatinine, sodium, and osmolality levels become elevated as fluid and electrolytes leak out of the obstructed bowel and third spacing (translocation of electrolytes and fluid into the intestinal lumen) occurs. Increases in serum amylase levels are common.

Radiologic Findings

Radiology films are taken with the patient in upright, flat, and side-lying positions. Distended bowel loops will reveal air–fluid levels in a "ladderlike" pattern. Distention is more pronounced within the colon in patients with paralytic ileus. Direct visualization and barium studies may help to confirm the diagnosis (Gearhart & Silen, 2007; Kong & Stamos, 2008).

Treatment

It is imperative to identify those patients at risk for developing a bowel obstruction or motility problem. Patients at risk for developing bowel obstruction are the elderly, postoperative, and bedridden, and those with dysfunction of multiple body systems. Initial therapy is directed toward fluid resuscitation and stabilization of the patient. Oral food and fluids are withheld, and a nasogastric tube (Salem-sump) is inserted and attached to low, intermittent suction to relieve vomiting and to decompress abdominal distention. Colonoscopy with decompression is sometimes useful in Ogilvie's syndrome. Isotonic intravenous fluid administration should be used to treat dehydration. Electrolyte losses should be replaced and continually monitored by the nurse. The extent of fluid resuscitation is best guided by the urine output, though in the elderly or those with cardiopulmonary disease, a pulmonary artery catheter (Swan–Ganz) is the best means of determining fluid volume needs. The nurse should closely monitor the patient's urine output using an indwelling urinary drainage catheter. If the patient demonstrates peritoneal signs (board-like abdominal distention with severe pain) and strangulation is suspected, broad spectrum antibiotics should be considered to provide anaerobic and gram-negative coverage. Early surgical consult is advised in high-risk patients. All cases of complete obstruction require surgical resection of the affected bowel (Beers et al., 2006; McQuaid, 2007; Gearhart & Silen, 2007; Kong & Stamos, 2008).

SECTION FIVE REVIEW

1. Common mechanical causes of small-bowel obstruction are
   A. adhesions
   B. myocardial infarction
   C. closed-head injury
   D. inflammatory bowel disease
2. If a patient with a small-bowel obstruction develops rebound tenderness with "boardlike" distention, the nurse should suspect
   A. constipation
   B. perforation
   C. Ogilvie's syndrome
   D. retroperitoneal bleeding
3. ______ accumulates in the bowel proximal to the actual bowel obstruction, resulting in distention.
   A. Fluid
   B. Blood
   C. Stool
   D. Pus
4. Bowel that "twists" itself to such an extent that circulation is interrupted is known as
   A. peritonitis
   B. perforation
   C. strangulation
   D. peristalsis
5. Strangulation is associated with a mortality rate of
   A. less than 2 percent
   B. 50 percent or less
   C. 80 percent or less
   D. 25 percent or less

Answers: 1. A, 2. B, 3. A, 4. C, 5. D

SECTION SIX: Intraabdominal Hypertension and Abdominal Compartment Syndrome

At the completion of this section, the learner will be able to describe the etiology, pathophysiology, assessment, and management of intraabdominal hypertension and abdominal compartment syndrome.

Abdominal compartment syndrome (ACS) is a rare but life-threatening condition resulting from an acute expansion of abdominal contents. Increased abdominal pressure (IAP) causes intraabdominal hypertension (IAH) which impairs blood flow to multiple organs, causing tissue ischemia and organ failure. It is important to recognize patients who are at risk for abdominal compartment syndrome and identify early signs of trouble so that appropriate treatment can be initiated.

Intraabdominal Hypertension/Abdominal Compartment Syndrome Continuum

The terms *intraabdominal hypertension* and *abdominal compartment syndrome* are sometimes used interchangeably, but it is generally accepted that the two represent a continuum of pathophysiologic changes. The critical pressure level varies between patients, but intraabdominal hypertension is present when increased abdominal pressure reaches 10 to 15 mm Hg, whereas abdominal compartment syndrome is defined as intraabdominal hypertension greater than 20 mm Hg, causing end-organ dysfunction that is improved by abdominal decompression (Maxwell & Ivatury, 2008).

Etiology

Intraabdominal hypertension can occur because of a variety of chronic and acute causes, including the accumulation of fluid, pregnancy, blood clots, or third-spacing of fluid into the abdominal cavity. Sudden elevations of increased abdominal pressure are usually associated with abdominal surgery or trauma. Table 29–4 lists disorders that are known to increase the risk for development of intraabdominal hypertension (IAH) and abdominal compartment syndrome (ACS). Patients who are at the most risk for developing IAH and ACS include those with abdominal trauma who are postoperative for repair of the injuries. Because the abdomen functions as a single compartment, an increase in its contents (for example, from fluids accumulation) may cause an elevation in IAP, leading to IAH. Other conditions that place patients at increased risk for developing IAH/ACS include ruptured abdominal aortic aneurysm, bowel obstruction, hemorrhagic pancreatitis, ascites, and intraabdominal neoplasm. Therapies such as intraabdominal packing during surgery, pneumatic antishock garments, and gas insufflation of the abdominal cavity during laparoscopic procedures, are also associated with abdominal compartment syndrome (Maxwell & Ivatury, 2008). In nonsurgical patients the most common cause of IAH/ACS is bowel edema and distention.

TABLE 29–4 Risk Factors for Development of Intraabdominal Hypertension (IAH) and Abdominal Compartment Syndrome (ACS)

Abdominal aortic aneurysm rupture
Abdominal trauma
Acute pancreatitis
Hepatic transplantation
Ileus
Intestinal obstruction
Intraabdominal or retroperitoneal hemorrhage
Massive volume resuscitation
Pregnancy
Severe ascites
Shock states

Multisystem Effects of Intraabdominal Hypertension

Multiple organ systems are affected by intraabdominal hypertension. The gastrointestinal tract is affected first by rising increased abdominal pressure, which compromises perfusion to the intestinal mucosa. The intestinal mucosa becomes ischemic, allowing bacteria to translocate into the bloodstream, predisposing the patient to systemic inflammatory response syndrome (SIRS) and sepsis. Gastrointestinal signs and symptoms of abdominal (SIRS) compartment syndrome include increased gastric carbon dioxide level (measured by **gastric tonometry**), decreased arterial pH, and elevated serum lactic acid. These abnormalities may indicate intestinal ischemia. Table 29–5 provides a summary of the effects of IAH/ACS on major body systems.

TABLE 29–5 Effects of Increased Intraabdominal Pressure/Abdominal Compartment Syndrome on Body Systems

BODY SYSTEM	EFFECTS OF INCREASED INTRA-ABDOMINAL PRESSURE	POTENTIAL OUTCOMES
Cardiovascular	Increased thoracic pressure because of increased pressure on diaphragm	Hemodynamic changes Elevated SVR, CVP, and RAP Tachycardia (compensatory) Decreased CO Hypotension (late sign)
Pulmonary	Decreased lung excursion and expansion because of increased diaphragmatic pressure	Decreased lung compliance Hypercapnia Hypoxemia Elevated PIP
Renal	Decreased renal blood flow because of elevated IAP and decreased CO, which decreases GFR and renal ischemia	Oliguria Azotemia Prerenal failure
Neurologic	Decreased cerebral perfusion pressure (CPP) because of elevated ICP, which results from decreased venous drainage from the head	Increased ICP Altered level of consciousness
Gastrointestinal	Decreased blood flow to abdominal organs which results in tissue hypoxia, conversion to anaerobic metabolism, and generation of free radicals, and lactic acidosis	Small bowel ischemia Translocation of bacteria from gut Sepsis Further increase in intraabdominal pressure Multiple organ dysfunction

SVR=systemic vascular resistance; CVP=central venous pressure; RAP=right atrial pressure; CO=cardiac output; PIP=peak inspiratory pressure; IAP=intraabdominal pressure; GFR=glomerular filtration rate; ICF=intracranial pressure

Measurement of Intraabdominal Pressure

If the patient develops signs of organ system dysfunction and is at risk for the development of IAH or ACS, it is important to consider abdominal compartment syndrome as a complication. The sequelae of abdominal compartment syndrome are often life-threatening, and many clinicians advocate using routine, noninvasive abdominal pressure monitoring for all critically ill patients at risk for developing IAH/ACS. Measurement of transurethral bladder pressure is a valid indirect measure of intra-abdominal pressure (Maxwell & Ivatury, 2008). Although the most accurate and direct technique for measuring increased abdominal pressure would be to insert a catheter directly into the peritoneal cavity, this invasive procedure requires tube placement in the abdomen, increasing the risk of bowel injury or peritoneal contamination.

Alterations in intraabdominal pressure are indirectly reflected by changes in bladder pressure (Maxwell & Ivatury, 2008). When the bladder is filled with approximately 50 to 100 mL of fluid, there is virtually no pressure exerted on the bladder wall, enabling it to act as a passive diaphragm capable of transmitting abdominal pressure without imparting additional pressure from its own musculature. Two methods of measuring intraabdominal pressure using a urinary bladder catheter are the transducer and fluid manometer methods. It is important to ensure that the urinary catheter is draining freely and the bladder is empty for either method. The transducer method uses a conventional cardiac transducer monitoring system, which is connected to the patient's urinary catheter drainage system. Using this method, 60 to 100 mL of saline is injected through a catheter port. The pressure transducer is then connected to the urinary catheter using a 16-gauge needle inserted into the aspiration port at the level of the patient's pubis. The resulting bladder pressure waveform can be viewed on a monitor screen. The fluid manometer method uses the urinary catheter as a manometer. To use this method, 60 to 100 mL of normal saline is instilled into the urinary catheter's aspiration port. The catheter is held at a 90 degree angle to the patient's pelvis, and the height of the fluid in the tubing above the pelvis is measured to determine the pressure reading (Maxwell & Ivatury, 2008) (Fig. 29–6).

Normal bladder pressure is 0 mm Hg. After abdominal surgery, bladder pressures between 0 and 15 mm Hg are not uncommon. Higher pressures indicate the onset of intraabdominal hypertension (the precursor to abdominal compartment syndrome) and may be associated with early organ system pathophysiology (Maxwell & Ivatury, 2008).

Treatment

Grading of the severity of IAH/ACS may be helpful in determining appropriate management (Marshall, 2009). Treatment focuses on decompression and preserving cardiopulmonary and renal function. Interventions vary with the severity of the intraabdominal pressure elevation.

Mild IAH/ACS

For mild intraabdominal hypertension (IAP of 10 to 15 mm Hg), elevating the head of the bed helps to minimize pressure on the diaphragm, allowing maximum lung expansion. Maintaining a state of normovolemia at this time is a management goal

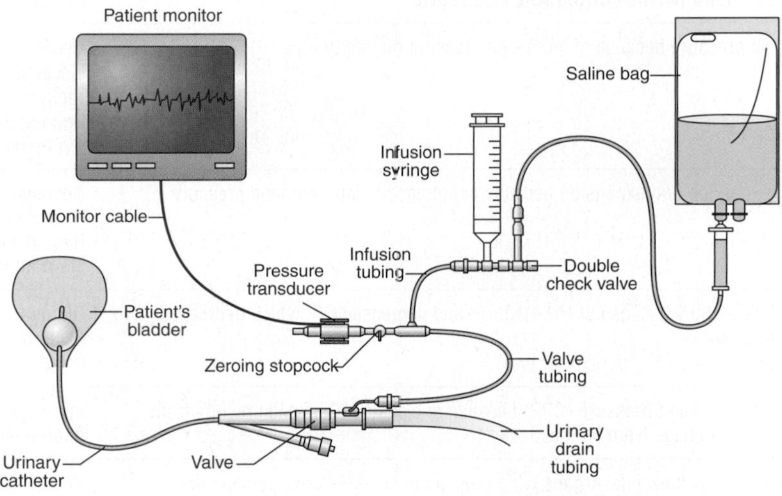

Figure 29–6 ■ Intraabdominal pressure measurement of bladder pressure using a transducer connected to the aspiration port of the patient's urinary catheter drainage system; 60-100 ml of saline is infused through the catheter into the bladder; The bladder pressure is displayed as a waveform on a monitor screen.

(Marshall, 2009). Additionally, assisting the patient to turn, cough, breathe deeply, and use an incentive spirometer will help to improve alveolar ventilation, reduce the risk of atelectasis, and prevent ventilation–perfusion mismatch (shunt) (King, 2004; Cheatham, 2009).

Moderate ACS

If moderate abdominal compartment syndrome develops (IAP of 16 to 25 mm Hg), the patient should be transferred to an intensive care unit for closer monitoring. Sedation or neuromuscular blockade to chemically paralyze and sedate the patient may be indicated. If the patient is hemodynamically unstable (demonstrating, for example, low cardiac output or hypotension), fluid resuscitation may be indicated (Marshall, 2009). It is important to ensure that a surgical service is consulted early in the course of treatment in case surgical decompression using a laparotomy procedure is required. It should be noted that there have been no randomized clinical trials to support the use of routine abdominal decompression through midline laparotomy for treatment of abdominal compartment syndrome.

Severe ACS

Severe abdominal compartment syndrome (IAP greater than 25 mm Hg) requires urgent surgical decompression of the abdominal cavity and may require reexploration of the abdomen (Marshall, 2009). In cases of trauma, the abdomen is sometimes left open after exploratory laparotomy to prevent ACS; however, even with this preventive measure, abdominal pressure may still rise to a dangerous level (Maxwell & Ivatury, 2008).

Surgical decompression of the abdomen, if necessary for severe ACS, involves a risk for hypotension once the abdomen is opened. This hypotension may be caused by reperfusion, and researchers recommend volume resuscitation with fluids containing mannitol and sodium bicarbonate immediately before and during decompression surgery, which may prevent unstable dysrhythmias (Maxwell & Ivatury, 2008).

Complications of ACS

Complications of abdominal compartment syndrome may include reperfusion asystole, which occurs when byproducts from ischemic areas circulate to the heart, causing acidosis-related impairments of electrical activity. Resuscitation equipment and emergency medications should be available in the event asystole occurs. The physician may order an intravenous infusion of sodium bicarbonate and mannitol to prevent this phenomenon.

Pulmonary embolism is a complication that is associated with reperfusion. The nurse should monitor for signs and symptoms of pulmonary embolism, such as dyspnea, pleuritic chest pain, and signs of shock. Oxygen administration, evaluation for and administration of thrombolytic drugs, and anticoagulants may be required if pulmonary embolism occurs.

Nursing Implications

Unless complications occur, abdominal decompression usually improves the patient's condition. If the ACS treatment is effective, end points of therapy will include decreased ventilation pressures, increased oxygenation, and improved cardiovascular and renal function. After surgery, nursing care will consist of maintaining the patient's oxygenation and hemodynamic stability; caring for the abdominal wound; monitoring for infection; and measuring fluid intake and output, including wound drainage, to determine the patient's fluid requirements. The patient may require mechanical ventilation, aggressive volume resuscitation, and vasopressor and inotropic drugs. Management of the patient with ACS is challenging. It is critical for the nurse to recognize the signs of ACS early, so that prompt treatment can be initiated to avoid organ failure and death.

SECTION SIX REVIEW

1. Which patient represents the population with the highest risk of developing abdominal compartment syndrome?
   A. a patient with chronic obstructive pulmonary disease
   B. a patient who is status postmyocardial infarction
   C. a patient who is postoperative for repair of a liver laceration
   D. a patient who is status post-hip replacement
2. Renal effects of increasing intraabdominal hypertension include
   A. increased urine output
   B. increased sodium and water concentration
   C. decreased glomerular filtration rate
   D. decreased renal tubular acidosis
3. Which statement correctly reflects the effects of ACS on preload and cardiac output?
   A. Preload and cardiac output are decreased.
   B. Preload and cardiac output are increased.
   C. Preload and cardiac output are normal.
   D. Preload is increased; cardiac output is decreased.
4. Decreased blood pressure is an early sign of ACS.
   A. True
   B. False

Answers: 1. C, 2. C, 3. A, 4. B

SECTION SEVEN: Management of Acute Gastrointestinal Bleeding

At the completion of this section, the learner will be able to describe the management of acute GI bleeding.

Caring for patients with acute GI bleeding is complex and requires close assessment and monitoring of the patient's condition and progress. Collaborative management of physiological problems and concern for the patient's psychosocial response to the acute illness are priorities for the nurse. Because fear and anxiety often accompany acute GI bleeding, patients and their significant others need information and support during this time. Nurses coordinate plans for the patient's ongoing care based on accurate and ongoing nursing assessment.

Patients who are experiencing acute GI bleeding must be approached in a systematic manner. This approach should be collaborative and include (1) initial assessment, (2) resuscitation, (3) definitive diagnosis, and (4) treatment.

In collaboration with the physician, the nurse's role includes the following

- Assess the severity of blood loss.
- Replace prescribed crystalloids and colloids.
- Assist in determining the cause of the bleeding.
- Plan and implement treatment.
- Manage the ongoing plan of care and monitor progress.
- Provide supportive care and education to the patient and significant others because any bleeding experience is potentially life-threatening.

Initial Assessment

To assess severity of blood loss, the nurse must determine hemodynamic stability. Evidence of instability includes decreased blood pressure or orthostatic hypotension, decreased or altered level of consciousness, and decreased urine output (which is suggestive of fluid volume deficit). Evidence of hemodynamic instability in the presence of hematemesis, hematochezia, or melena should be considered an emergency until proven otherwise, and admission to an intensive care unit (ICU) or intermediate care unit (IMC) is recommended. The following are guidelines for admission to an ICU

1. Clearly documented frank hematemesis
2. Coffee-ground emesis and either melena or hematochezia
3. Hemodynamic instability (hypotension, tachycardia, or orthostatic hypotension)
4. A continued drop in hemoglobin and hematocrit despite aggressive fluid resuscitation
5. A significant unexplained increase in the BUN when GI bleeding is suspected (increased BUN suggests fluid volume deficit or metabolism of blood within the GI tract)

Resuscitation

Resuscitation is the primary goal of early management in the hemodynamically unstable patient and mandates the maintenance of intravascular volume and tissue oxygenation. Blood specimens for type and crossmatching, CBC, PT/PTT, and chemistries should be obtained. Nasal oxygen and pulse oximetry are useful, especially in the elderly or in patients with a history of cardiac or pulmonary disease. Close nursing assessment of the patient's level of consciousness and oxygenation status is important in the acute phase. Endotracheal intubation should be considered for decreased level of consciousness, shock, massive bleeding, or if the patient is unable to protect their own airway. The nurse should have emergency intubation and oxygen equipment ready for use if needed. Vital signs, orthostatic blood pressure changes, and urine output are valuable clinical indicators of perfusion and blood volume. An indwelling catheter should be placed to monitor urine output because this is an indirect measure of perfusion. Central venous pressures or pulmonary capillary wedge pressures are also helpful to monitor volume status.

Volume resuscitation is accomplished with crystalloid (normal saline or lactated Ringer's) at a rate to maintain a systolic blood pressure of higher than 90 mm Hg through at least two large-bore IV lines. If, after two to three liters of crystalloid infusion, the patient remains unstable, an infusion of blood products (packed red cells or whole blood) should be considered. Vasoconstricting drugs (vasopressors) are generally not indicated because hypovolemia is usually the cause of the hypotension. Packed red cells are transfused for massive bleeding to keep the hematocrit higher than 28 to 30 percent. Patients with cardiac or pulmonary disease may require transfusion to a higher hematocrit (higher than 30 percent). Transfusions of whole blood may be considered in massively bleeding patients because they provide increased colloid osmotic pressure, thus decreasing the patient's total fluid requirements. O-negative blood can be used until the patient's blood has been crossmatched. A blood warmer should be considered for rapid fluid or blood administration to prevent hypothermia. Each unit of blood should elevate the hematocrit by three points. Fresh frozen plasma is considered for patients who have a coagulopathy (increased PT or PTT) or who have been on Coumadin therapy. If the patient has thrombocytopenia, platelet transfusion should be considered to maintain the platelet count above 50,000/mm^3 (Andreoli et al., 2007; Beers et al., 2006; Prakash, 2006).

For patients with persistent bleeding, some type of therapeutic intervention is necessary. This intervention can be pharmacotherapy, mechanical (balloon) tamponade (Sengstaken–Blakemore tube), endoscopic therapy (sclerotherapy), or surgery. Once blood volume is restored, the patient is monitored for evidence of further bleeding (e.g., tachycardia, decreased blood pressure, hematemesis, bloody or tarry stools). Specific therapy depends on the bleeding site (refer to previously discussed etiologies of GI bleeding for specific treatments). Table 29–6 provides a summary of interventions for severe GI hemorrhage.

Definitive Diagnosis

Finding the source of the GI bleeding should be undertaken as soon as the patient has been stabilized. Early specialty consultation is essential for patients with GI bleeding. For upper GI

TABLE 29–6 Interventions for Severe GI Hemorrhage with Evidence of Hemodynamic Instability or Persistent Bleeding

INTERVENTION	EFFECTS
Vasopressin	Decreases portal pressure by vasoconstricting splanchnic arteries Untoward effects include decreased coronary blood flow, increased blood pressure
Somatostatin	Decreases portal pressure by vasoconstriction of splanchnic circulation
Octreotide	A synthetic analog of somatostatin; has same action as somatostatin
Mechanical tamponade	Provides tamponade to actively bleeding gastric/esophageal varices (use is restricted to bleeding esophageal or gastric varices)

Data from McQuaid (2007).

bleeding, patients are usually seen by a gastroenterologist and for lower GI bleeding, patients are usually evaluated by a general surgeon. An example of a diagnostic approach to the patient with GI bleeding is provided in Figure 29–7.

Treatments

Endoscopic Interventions

Bleeding peptic ulcers, gastritis, Mallory-Weiss tears, and arteriovenous malformations are often diagnosed and treated with endoscopy. Using a special flexible fiberoptic scope, structures in the GI tract can be viewed directly. A tiny camera provides visualization on a video screen. In some cases, therapeutic interventions to stop bleeding can be performed during the endoscopy. Table 29–7 provides a summary of endoscopic interventions.

Arterial Angiotherapy

Arterial angiography can be used to control massive bleeding from peptic ulcers in patients who are considered to be poor surgical risks. Selective arterial infusion of vasopressin is used to control massive or persistent bleeding in patients who have peptic ulcer disease, stress ulcers, erosive gastritis, Mallory-Weiss tear, and arteriovenous malformation. Selective catheterization of the bleeding artery is required for infusion of vasopressin. Arterial embolization is an alternative to arterial vasopressin where the bleeding vessel is selectively catheterized and a coagulant is placed in the vessel (Beers et al., 2006). Table 29–8 summarizes arterial angiotherapy interventions that may be performed.

Sclerotherapy

Sclerotherapy refers to the use of a chemical (called a sclerosant) to stop the bleeding and harden (sclerose) a blood vessel to prevent rebleeding. It is one alternative to treatment of active bleeding GI vessels, particularly bleeding esophageal varices. The chemicals used are usually sodium tetradecyl sulfate (Sotradecol) or sodium morrhuate (Scleromate). Vital signs

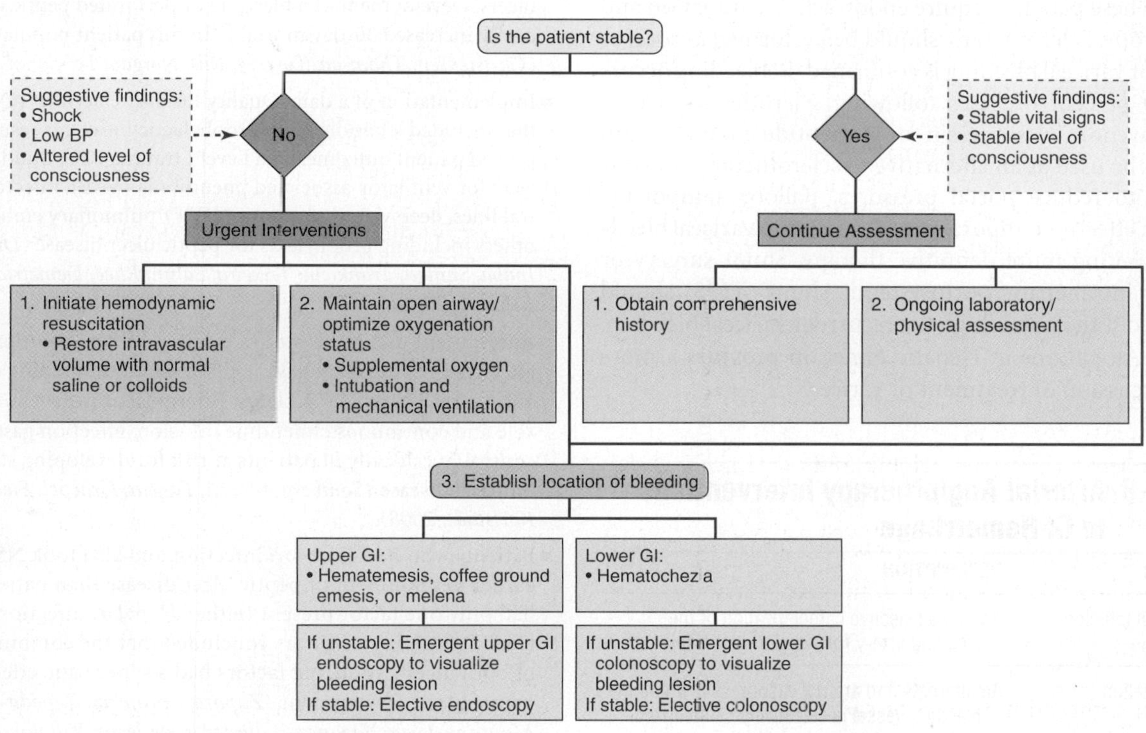

Figure 29–7 ■ Diagnostic approach to the patient with GI bleeding.

TABLE 29–7 Endoscopic Interventions in GI Hemorrhage

INTERVENTION	DESCRIPTION
Endoscopic injection sclerotherapy	Sclerosing agent is injected into bleeding vessel
Endoscopic electrocoagulation	Direct electric current is applied to bleeding lesion = fibrosis
Endoscopic laser therapy	Direct application of heat to coagulate bleeding lesion
Endoscopic heater probe	Direct electric current is applied to coagulate bleeding lesion

Data from McQuaid (2007).

should be taken before and after the procedure. Postprocedure, the patient requires close monitoring for signs of rebleeding and other complications, such as aspiration pneumonia, esophageal scar tissue contraction (which can cause partial obstruction), infection, and esophageal perforation.

Surgery

Surgery is considered for severe hemorrhage or recurrent bleeding when other, less invasive interventions have not been successful or when the patient's condition warrants immediate surgical repair.

Treatments of Specific GI Bleeding Problems

Bleeding from esophageal or gastric varices requires ICU admission. These patients require endotracheal intubation and early endoscopy. Sclerotherapy should be performed as soon as a diagnosis of variceal bleeding is confirmed. Rebleeding occurs in 45 to 50 percent of cases following sclerotherapy (Azer, 2006). Intravenous vasopressin or octreotide (somatostatin analog) may be used as an alternative to sclerotherapy (or concomitantly) to reduce portal pressures. Balloon tamponade therapy is an effective temporary method to stop variceal bleeding while awaiting more definitive therapy. Shunt surgery or transjugular intrahepatic portosystemic shunt (TIPS) should be considered if the risk is high for recurrent variceal bleeding. Module 30, Alterations in Hepatic Function provides a more in-depth discussion of treatment of varices.

TABLE 29–8 Arterial Angiotherapy Interventions in GI Hemorrhage

INTERVENTION	DESCRIPTION
Selective arterial infusion of vasopressin	Requires selective catheterization of the bleeding artery for infusion of vasopressin
Arterial embolization	An alternative to arterial vasopressin where the bleeding vessel is selectively catheterized, and a coagulant is placed in the vessel

Data from Beers (2006); Del Valle (2007); and Prakash (2007).

Bleeding Mallory-Weiss tears that do not stop spontaneously require therapeutic endoscopy or selective arterial angiotherapy, whereas bleeding arteriovenous malformations (AVM) of the colon can be treated with arterial angiotherapy or therapeutic endoscopic procedures. In diverticular bleeding, selective arterial vasopressin is often effective in stopping the bleeding. Selective arterial therapy requires catheterization of the bleeding vessel for infusion of vasopressin. Surgery is needed when the bleeding is severe (Beers et al., 2006; Laine, 2007; McQuaid, 2007).

Management of Shock

A life-threatening complication of acute GI bleeding and bowel infarction is shock (hypovolemic or septic). Key nursing goals for the patient with hypovolemic or septic shock include maintenance of adequate tissue perfusion/oxygenation, prevention of fluid volume deficit related to blood loss and third spacing of fluids, and optimization of hemodynamic status. Regardless of what has caused the shock (GI hemorrhage or sepsis), the nurse must first see that venous access is achieved so that fluid and blood resuscitation therapy can begin. Ensuring adequacy of intravenous infusions remains a nursing priority for the duration of the treatment of shock. In order to maintain adequate gas exchange and tissue perfusion, the nurse should

1. Ensure an open airway and administer supplementary oxygen.
2. Initiate continuous monitoring for cardiac dysrhythmias.

Emerging Evidence

- Patients with COPD are at increased risk for development of peptic ulcers. Development of a bleeding or perforated peptic ulcer significantly increased 30-day mortality in this patient population *(Christensen, Thomsen, Tørring, Riis, Nørgaard & Sørensen, 2008)*.
- Implementation of a daily Quality Rounds Checklist (QRC) tool that included a bundle of 16 prophylactic measures resulted in improved patient outcomes in a Level I trauma ICU. Bundled measures were for ventilator-associated pneumonia (VAP), infections of central lines, deep vein thrombosis (DVT)/pulmonary embolism, and others including prophylaxis for peptic ulcer disease *(DuBose, Inaba, Shiflett, Trankiem, Teixeira, Salim, Rhee, Demetriades & Belzberg, 2008)*.
- Intermittent use of the proton pump inhibitor pantoprazole was effective in controlling gastric pH without developing drug tolerance in high-risk ICU patients. Intermittent intravenous pantoprazole and continuous cimetidine infusion: effect on gastric pH control in critically ill patients at risk for developing stress-related mucosal disease *(Somberg, Morris, Fantus, Graepel, Field, Lynn & Karlstadt, 2008)*.
- Patients who had *H. pylori* infection and also took NSAIDs had earlier development of peptic ulcer disease than patients who had only one factor present (either *H. pylori* infection or NSAID use). Investigators concluded that the combination of both ulcer-producing factors had a synergistic effect on peptic ulcer development *(Zapata-Colindres, Zepeda-Gomez, Mantano-Loza, Vazquez-Ballesteros, de Jesus, Villalobos & Valdovinos-Andraca, 2006)*.

3. Prepare for insertion of a central venous or pulmonary artery catheter and record and monitor cardiac filling pressures once placement has been achieved.
4. Prepare the patient for emergent surgical intervention to control bleeding.

The major nursing assessments and interventions specific to the care of the patient at risk for hypovolemia as a result of GI bleeding are summarized in a pair of boxes titled NURSING CARE: The Patient at Risk for Hypovolemia as a Result of GI Bleeding, and NURSING CARE: The Patient with Acute GI Bleeding. These interventions summarized in these boxes also apply to the patient who is in shock secondary to sepsis.

Related Nursing Diagnoses

Nursing diagnoses that are appropriate for patients diagnosed with GI bleeding, paralytic ileus, and acute intestinal ischemia are listed in Table 29–9.

NURSING CARE: The Patient at Risk for Hypovolemia Due to Acute GI Bleeding

Expected Patient Outcome and Related Interventions

Outcome: The patient will maintain normal fluid volume

Assess and compare to established norms, patient baselines, and trends. Signs and symptoms of shock; vital signs, urine output, hemodynamic measures (PAP, PCWP, CI, CO, SVR, CVP), Sa_{O_2} (oxygen saturation), diminished peripheral pulses, restlessness, agitation, cool, pale, or moist skin
Fluid status: intake and output (urine output, gastric drainage)
Electrolyte levels (may become altered from fluid loss or fluid shifts)
Hemoglobin, hematocrit, RBC, coagulation studies (PT, PTT), renal function (BUN, serum creatinine)
Gastric pH: consult with physician/practitioner about specific pH range and antacid administration
Test gastric drainage, emesis, or stools for occult blood
Adverse reaction to blood products

Institute measures to regain or maintain normal fluid volume.

Consult with physician/practitioner about replacing fluid losses based on assessment findings.
Administer replacement fluids and blood products as directed.

PAP: pulmonary artery pressure; PCWP: pulmonary capillary wedge pressure; CI: cardiac index; CO: cardiac output; SVR: systemic vascular resistance; CVP: central venous pressure; RBC: red blood count; PT: prothrombin time; PTT: partial thromboplastin time; BUN: blood urea nitrogen.

Data from Carpenito-Moyet (2008).

NURSING CARE: The Patient with Gastrointestinal Bleeding

Expected Patient Outcome and Related Interventions

Outcome 1: The patient will maintain hemodynamic stability.

Assess and compare to establish norms, patient baselines, and trends.

Monitor vital signs continuously for changes indicating hypovolemic shock.
  Hypotension, tachycardia
Monitor hemodynamic parameters, including
  Central venous pressure, pulmonary artery wedge pressure, cardiac output, and cardiac index to evaluate the patient's status and response to treatment
Monitor intake and output closely, including all losses from the GI tract.
Check stools and gastric drainage for occult blood.
Serial hemoglobin and hematocrit; notify provider of sudden changes in patient's laboratory findings.
Assess for the extent of blood loss.
Institute continuous cardiac monitoring to evaluate for possible dysrhythmias, myocardial ischemia, or adverse effects of treatment.

Institute measures to regain or maintain hemodynamic stability.

Assist with insertion of central venous or pulmonary artery catheter to evaluate hemodynamic status.
Initiate fluid resuscitation as ordered.
Obtain a type and crossmatch for blood component therapy.
Administer blood component therapy (usually packed red blood cells and fresh frozen plasma) as ordered.

Related nursing diagnoses

Fatigue
Risk for fluid volume deficit
Risk for infection
Knowledge deficit
Tissue perfusion, altered; cardiac

(*continued*)

NURSING CARE (*continued*)

Outcome 2: The patient will maintain adequate oxygenation.

Assess and compare to establish norms, patient baselines, and trends.

- Assess level of consciousness frequently.
- Assess breathing and circulation.
- Monitor cardiac and respiratory status closely.
- Monitor arterial blood gases.

Institute measures to regain or maintain adequate oxygenation.

- Initiate actions to increase oxygen supply.
  - Ensure a patent airway.
  - Administer supplemental oxygen as ordered.
  - Anticipate possible need for endotracheal intubation and mechanical ventilation.
- Initiate actions to decrease oxygen demands.
  - Treat fevers.
  - Keep patient quiet and comfortable.

Related nursing diagnoses

- Risk for aspiration
- Gas exchange, impaired
- Ineffective breathing pattern
- Thought processes, altered
- Tissue perfusion, altered: respiratory

Outcome 3: The patient will exhibit no further signs of bleeding.

Assess and compare to establish norms, patient baselines, and trends.

- Monitor vital signs and hemodynamic status (refer to *Outcome 1*).

Institute measures to regain or maintain adequate oxygenation.

- Assist with or insert NG tube.
- Perform lavage as ordered to clear any blood or clots.
- Administer antisecretory medications as ordered to reduce gastric acid secretion.
- Prepare for possible endoscopic repair or surgery.
- Encourage smoking cessation and avoidance of alcohol.

Related nursing diagnoses

- Anxiety
- Risk for infection
- Actual knowledge deficit
- Pain

TABLE 29–9 Acute GI Problems-Related Nursing Diagnoses

PROBLEM STATEMENT	ETIOLOGIC FACTORS
Gastrointestinal Bleeding	
Fluid volume deficit, risk for	Hypovolemia secondary to blood loss; NPO; vomiting; diarrhea
Tissue perfusion, altered: cerebral, cardiac, respiratory, renal, peripheral, mesenteric	Hypovolemia and decreased oxygenation secondary to anemia, hypotension, shock
Gas exchange, impaired	Hypovolemia, anemia
Anxiety	Fear of bleeding, threat of death
Aspiration, risk for	Hematemesis and potential changes in level of consciousness
Nutrition, less than body requirements, altered	Decreased appet te secondary to bowel irritability; NPO
Pain	Bleeding and discomfort
Diarrhea	Decrease in intestinal transit time secondary to cathartic effects of blood in GI tract
Thought processes, altered	Hypoxia secondary to anemia
Infection, risk for	Immune suppression; intestinal ischemia/infarction secondary to hypotension and shock
Fatigue	Anemia, decreased oxygenation
Knowledge deficit	Precipitating factors; therapeutic procedures/interventions; discharge information
Paralytic Ileus	
Ineffective breathing pattern	Abdominal distention
Fluid volume deficit, actual	Vomiting, distention, electrolyte imbalance, hypovolemia (loss of fluid/electrolytes due to stasis of bowel contents)
Tissue perfusion, risk for, bowel	Decreased oxygenation to tissues secondary to bowel strangulation, perforation, and/or shock

PROBLEM STATEMENT	ETIOLOGIC FACTORS
Infection, risk for	Perforation, strangulation, bowel ischemia → infarction → necrosis → sepsis
Bowel elimination, altered	Absent bowel sounds; NPO; electrolyte loss; constipation
Pain/discomfort, actual	Distention; intestinal angina; perforation
Knowledge deficit, actual	Illness, treatments, procedures, and outcome
Intestinal Ischemia	
Pain/comfort, actual	Intestinal angina; distention; infarction; peritonitis
Infection, risk for	Infarction → necrosis → sepsis
Fluid volume deficit, risk for	Electrolyte imbalance; NPO; vomiting; diarrhea; third spacing; shock if perforation occurs
Knowledge deficit, actual	Illness, treatments, procedures, and outcome

Partial data from Carpenito-Moyet (2008).

SECTION SEVEN REVIEW

1. The first step in the collaborative treatment of a patient who is experiencing an acute GI bleed is
   A. assessment
   B. resuscitation
   C. diagnosis
   D. treatment
2. To assess the severity of blood loss, the nurse should determine
   A. respiratory status
   B. hemodynamic status
   C. level of consciousness
   D. the degree of impairment
3. Signs and symptoms that provide supporting evidence of a fluid volume deficit include
   A. abdominal distention
   B. unchanged level of consciousness
   C. orthostatic hypotension
   D. increased urine output
4. In a patient who has had a GI bleed, an increased BUN suggests fluid volume deficit or
   A. onset of acute renal failure
   B. development of systemic inflammatory response
   C. an acute infectious process
   D. metabolism of blood in the gut
5. Laboratory tests needed in the management of a patient with an acute GI hemorrhage include (choose all that apply)
   A. hourly ABG measurements
   B. blood and urine cultures
   C. type and crossmatch blood for possible transfusion
   D. stool sample for occult blood
6. Volume resuscitation is usually accomplished with
   A. intravenous crystalloid infusion
   B. vasoconstricting drugs
   C. blood transfusion
   D. normal saline via a nasogastric tube
7. A life-threatening complication of acute GI bleeding and bowel infarction is
   A. renal failure
   B. abdominal aorta aneurysm
   C. shock
   D. pancreatitis
8. The nurse caring for a patient with bleeding ulcers. The nursing diagnosis of "Impaired gas exchange" is written. Which etiologic factors most likely relate to this diagnosis?
   A. anemia
   B. decreased appetite
   C. immune suppression
   D. diarrhea

Answers: 1. B, 2. B, 3. C, 4. D, 5. (C, D), 6. A, 7. C, 8. A

POSTTEST

1. ______ may contribute to gastrointestinal bleeding.
   A. Pulmonary disease
   B. Hepatic dysfunction
   C. Autoimmune complications
   D. Cardiac disease
2. In the case of GI bleeding, angiography allows visualization of
   A. vascular beds and flow
   B. GI motility
   C. abscesses
   D. masses

3. All external metal objects must be removed in order for a(n) ______ to be performed.
   A. ultrasound sonography
   B. angiography
   C. CT scan
   D. magnetic resonance imaging (MRI)
4. Occult bleeding is usually
   A. unnoticed by the patient
   B. massive in its presentation
   C. acute in its presentation
   D. bright red in appearance
5. NSAIDs interrupt mucosal integrity by
   A. inhibiting gastric acid production
   B. increasing mucus production
   C. inhibiting prostaglandin function
   D. decreasing bicarbonate secretion
6. After an acute episode of upper GI bleeding, a patient vomits undigested antacids and complains of severe epigastric pain. The nursing assessment reveals an absence of bowel sounds, pulse rate of 134, and shallow respirations of 32 per minute. In addition to calling the physician, the nurse should
   A. keep the client NPO in preparation for surgery
   B. start oxygen per nasal cannula at three to four liters per minute
   C. place the client in the supine position with the legs elevated
   D. ask the client whether any red or black stools have been noted
7. A 45-year-old divorced father of five is diagnosed with a duodenal ulcer. He asks, "Now that I have an ulcer, what comes next?" The nurse's best response would be:
   A. "Most peptic ulcers heal with medical treatment."
   B. "Patients with gastric ulcers experience pain while eating."
   C. "Early surgery is advisable, especially after the first attack."
   D. "If ulcers are untreated, cancer of the stomach can develop."
8. A patient is diagnosed as having a peptic ulcer. When teaching about peptic ulcers, the nurse should instruct the patient to report any stools that appear
   A. frothy
   B. ribbon-shaped
   C. pale or clay-colored
   D. dark brown or black
9. The mortality rate for clients with ischemic bowel disease is
   A. 20 percent
   B. 30 percent
   C. 40 percent
   D. 50 percent
10. ______ is/are the most common symptom(s) of inflammatory bowel disease.
    A. Nausea and vomiting
    B. Bloody diarrhea
    C. Constipation
    D. Abdominal distention
11. The nurse is performing a physical assessment of a patient with ulcerative colitis. The finding most often associated with a serious complication of this disorder would be
    A. decreased bowel sounds
    B. loose, blood-tinged stools
    C. distention of the abdomen
    D. intense abdominal discomfort
12. A 50-year-old female is being treated for esophageal varices and has recently had a banding procedure. The nurse notes that the patient's heart rate is 125 beats per minute (increased from 85). The patient's blood pressure is decreased to 88/40 from 126/62, and the patient is suddenly anxious. These assessment findings can indicate
    A. rebleeding
    B. pain
    C. hypervolemia
    D. hyperglycemia
13. When assessing a patient who has had abdominal surgery, the nurse knows that the first indicator for return of peristalsis would be when the patient
    A. passes flatus
    B. has bowel sounds
    C. tolerates clear liquids
    D. has a bowel movement
14. Initial nursing intervention for a patient with a bowel obstruction includes
    A. rapid initiation of enteral feeding
    B. stat soapsuds enema
    C. insertion of a NG tube for bowel decompression
    D. evacuation by colonoscopy
15. When gut perfusion is compromised, which of the following occurs?
    A. gastric CO_2 level increases
    B. gastric $PrCO_2$ decreases
    C. the $PrCO_2$-$PaCO_2$ gap decreases
    D. GI tract metabolism is anaerobic
16. Interventions that directly improve gut perfusion include
    A. optimizing cardiac output
    B. optimizing hemoglobin levels
    C. administering supplemental oxygen
    D. all of the above
17. An intravenous infusion of ______ before surgical decompression may decrease the occurrence of reperfusion asystole.
    A. epinephrine and furosemide
    B. vasopressin and nitroglycerine
    C. octreotide and calcium chloride
    D. sodium bicarbonate and mannitol

Posttest answers with rationale are found on MyNursingKit.

REFERENCES

Andreoli, T. E., Bennett, J. C., Carpenter, C. C., & Plum, F. (2007). *Cecil's essentials of medicine* (7th ed.). Philadelphia: W. B. Saunders.

Azer, S. A. (2006). Esophageal varices. eMedicine from WebMD. Retrieved November 6, 2008 from http://www.emedicine.com/med/topic745.htm.

Beers, M. H., Porter, R. S., Jones, T. V., Kaplan, J. L., & Berkwits, M. (eds.). (2006). *The Merck manual of diagnosis and therapy* (18th ed.). Whitehouse Station, NJ: Merck Research Laboratories.

Bjorkman, D. J. (2007). Gastrointestinal hemorrhage and occult gastrointestinal bleeding. In L. Goldman & D. Ausiello (eds.), *Goldman: Cecil Medicine* (23rd ed.). Philadelphia: Saunders Elsevier.

Cagir, B. and Cirincione, E. (2008). Lower gastrointestinal bleeding: surgical perspective. eMedicine from WebMD. Retrieved November 5, 2008 from http://www.emedicine.com/Med/topic2818.htm.

Carpenito-Moyet, L. (2008). *Nursing diagnosis: application to clinical practice* (12th ed.). Philadelphia: J. B. Lippincott.

Cheatham, M. (2009). Abdominal compartment syndrome: pathophysiology and definitions. *Scand J Trauma Resusc Emerg Med, 17:10.* Published online March 2, 2009. Retrieved March 15, 2009 from http://www. Pubmedcentral.nih.gov.

Christensen, S., Thomsen, R. W. Tørring, M. L., Riis, A., Nørgaard, M., and Sørensen, H. T. (2008). Impact of COPD on outcome among patients with complicated peptic ulcer. *Chest, 133*(6), 1360-1366.

Day, M. W. (2009). Gastrointestinal bleeding. In K. K. Carlson (ed.) (2009). *AACN advanced critical care nursing.* St. Louis: Saunders/Elsevier, 737-753.

Del Valle, J. (2007). Peptic ulcer disease and related conditions. In E. Braunwald, A. Fauci, D. Kasper, S. Hauser, D. Longo, & J. L. Jameson (eds.), *Harrison's principles of internal medicine* (17th ed.). *CD-ROM version 1.0.* New York: McGraw Hill.

DuBose, J. J., Inaba, K., Shiflett, A., Trankiem, C., Teixeira, P.G., Salim, A., Rhee, P., Demetriades, D., Belzberg, H. (2008). *Journal of Trauma, 64*(1), 22-9.

Farrell, J., & Friedman, L. (2001). Gastrointestinal bleeding in the elderly. *Gastroenterol Clinic North America, 30* (2), 377–407.

Flannery, J., & Tucker, D. (2002). Pharmacologic prophylaxis and treatment of stress ulcers in critically ill patients. *Critical Care Clinics of North America, 14* (1), 39–51.

Gearhart, S. L. & Silen, W. (2007). Acute intestinal obstruction. In E. Braunwald, A. Fauci, D. Kasper, S. Hauser, D. Longo, & J. L. Jameson (eds.), *Harrison's principles of internal medicine* (17th ed.). CD-ROM Version 1.0. New York: McGraw Hill.

Huether, S. E. (2008). Alterations in digestive function. In S. E. Huether, K. L. McCance, V. L. Brashers, and N. S. Rote, *Understanding pathophysiology* (4th ed., 937-984).

Kethu, S. R., and Moss, S. F. (2008). Gastritis and peptic ulcer disease. In R.E. Rakel & E.T. Bope, *Conn's current therapy 2008* (60th ed., not paginated). St. Louis: Saunders/Elsevier. Retrieved 4/20/2009 from http://www./mdconsult.com.

King, J. (2004). Blunt abdominal trauma. In S. D. Melander (ed.), *Case studies in critical care nursing: a guide for application and review.* (2nd ed.). Philadelphia: W. B. Saunders.

Kong, A. P. & Stamos, M. (2008). Acute abdomen. In F. S. Bongard & D. Y. Sue (eds.), *Current critical care diagnosis and treatment* (3rd ed.). New York: Lange.

Laine, L. (2007). Gastrointestinal bleeding. In E. Braunwald, A. Fauci, D. Kasper, S. Hauser, D. Longo, & J. L. Jameson (eds.), *Harrison's principles of internal medicine* (17th ed.). CD-ROM Version 1.0. New York: McGraw Hill.

Lehne, R. A. (2007). Cyclooxygenase inhibitors; Nonsteroidal anti-inflammatory drugs and acetaminophen. In R. A. Lehne, *Pharmacology for nursing care* (6th ed.). St. Louis: Saunders/Elsevier, 809-826.

Lindseth, G. L. (2003). Disorders of the stomach and duodenum. In S. L. Price & L. M. Wilson (eds.), *Pathophysiology: clinical concepts of disease processes* (6th ed). St. Louis: C. V. Mosby, 328.

Maxwell, R. A. & Ivatury, R. R. (2008). Abdominal compartment syndrome. In A. B. Peitzman, M. Rhodes, C. W. Schwab, D. M. Yealy, & T. C. Fabian (eds.), *The trauma manual: trauma and acute care surgery* (3rd ed.). Philadelphia: Lippincott Williams & Wilkins.

McQuaid, K. R. (2007). Alimentary tract. In S. J. McPhee, & M. A. Papadakis, & L. M. Tierney (eds.), *Current medical diagnosis and treatment* (46th ed.). Norwalk, CT: Appleton & Lange.

Prakash, C. (2006). Gastrointestinal bleeding: Principles of diagnosis and management. In R. S. Irwin & J. M. Rippe (Eds.), *Manual of intensive care medicine* (4th ed.). Philadelphia: Lippincott Williams & Wilkins, 421-423.

Prakash, C. (2007). Gastrointestinal diseases: gastrointestinal bleeding. In S. N. Ahya, K. Flood, & S. Paranjothi (eds.), *The Washington manual of medical therapeutics* (30th ed.). Philadelphia: J. B. Lippincott, 352.

Ramakrishnan, K. & Salinas, R. C. (2007). Peptic ulcer disease. *American family physician 76: 1005-12.*

Reicher, S. & Eysselein, V. (2008). Gastrointestinal bleeding. In F. S. Bongard & D. Y. Sue (eds.), *Current critical care diagnosis and treatment* (3rd ed.). New York: Lange.

Rockey, D. C. (2006). Gastrointestinal bleeding. *Gastroenterology Clinics of North America, 34:* 581-588.

Somberg, L., Morris, J. Jr., Fantus, R., Graepel, J., Field, B. G., Lynn, R., & Karlstadt, R. (2008). *Journal of Trauma, 64*(5), 1202-1210.

Strate, L. L. (2005). Lower GI bleeding: epidemiology and diagnosis. *Gastroenterology Clinics of North America, 34: 643-664.*

Zapata-Colindres, J. C., Zepeda-Gomez, S., Mantano-Loza, A., Vazquez-Ballesteros, E., de Jesus, Villalobos, J., & Valdovinos-Andraca, F. (2006). The association of Helicobacter pylori infection and nonsteroidal anti-inflammatory drugs in peptic ulcer disease. *Canadian Journal of Gastroenterology, 20*(4), 277-280.

MODULE

30 Alterations in Hepatic Function

Vicky Turner, Lacey Troutman Buckler, Melanie G. Hardin-Pierce

OBJECTIVES Following completion of this module, the learner will be able to

1. Describe the etiology and clinical manifestations associated with acute hepatitis.
2. Describe the etiology and clinical manifestations associated with acute hepatic dysfunction and failure.
3. Describe the complications of acute hepatic dysfunction.
4. Describe the medical management of the patient with acute hepatic dysfunction.
5. Describe the nursing implications appropriate to management of the patient experiencing acute hepatic dysfunction.

This module presents the pathophysiologic processes involved in acute hepatic dysfunction and management of the patient with acute hepatic failure. The module is composed of five sections. Section One provides an overview of acute hepatitis. Section Two first outlines acute hepatic failure based on causative factors and describes the clinical manifestations of acute hepatic failure. Section Three explains the multisystem complications of hepatic dysfunction. Together, sections Four and Five provide an overview of medical management, therapeutic goals, nursing assessment, and frequently occurring nursing diagnoses. Each section includes a set of review questions to help the learner evaluate his or her understanding of the section's content before moving on to the next section. All Section Reviews include answers. It is suggested that the learner review those concepts answered incorrectly in the review questions before proceeding to the next section.

PRETEST

1. Acute hepatitis is known to be caused by a ______ infection.
   A. bacterial
   B. viral
   C. yeast
   D. fungal
2. The major viral cause of acute and chronic hepatitis and cirrhosis is
   A. human immunodeficiency virus
   B. hepatitis C virus
   C. Epstein–Barr virus
   D. hepatitis B virus
3. Hepatitis A is transmitted primarily through
   A. blood
   B. saliva
   C. stool
   D. respiratory droplet
4. Acute hepatic failure can occur without preexisting liver disease.
   A. True
   B. False
5. Acetaminophen is a major hepatotoxin that is known to cause
   A. fulminant hepatic failure
   B. acute renal failure
   C. acute viral hepatitis
   D. cholestatic hepatitis
6. In the United States, the etiology of cirrhosis of the liver is most commonly the result of
   A. hepatitis A virus
   B. alcohol abuse
   C. hepatitis B virus
   D. Epstein–Barr virus
7. A major cause of ascites is
   A. hyperalbuminemia
   B. low colloid osmotic pressure
   C. acute renal failure
   D. fluid volume overload
8. A major factor contributing to the onset of hepatorenal syndrome is
   A. hepatotoxins
   B. a hypotensive episode
   C. high ammonia levels
   D. portal vein shunting

9. The onset of type 2 hepatorenal syndrome usually occurs in the presence of
A. hepatotoxins
B. a hypotensive episode
C. high ammonia levels
D. severe ascites

10. Dietary management of the patient with acute viral hepatitis would include
A. high protein, low fat
B. low fat, high carbohydrate
C. low carbohydrate, low fat
D. low protein, high fat

11. A patient with acute viral hepatitis will most likely be admitted to the hospital if he or she is experiencing
A. severe fatigue
B. occasional nausea
C. elevated bilirubin
D. hepatic encephalopathy

12. The patient with fulminant hepatic failure will require strict nutritional control of
A. protein
B. fat
C. carbohydrate
D. fiber

Pretest answers are found on MyNursingKit.

SECTION ONE: Acute Hepatitis

At the completion of this section, the learner will be able to describe the etiology and clinical manifestations associated with acute hepatitis.

Acute hepatitis is defined as an inflammatory liver disease that is usually of viral origin but can also result from an acute insult (e.g., ischemia), hepatotoxins, or autoimmune processes. Acute hepatitis involves damage to the hepatocytes, the functional units of the liver, and results in liver injury and possible necrosis. The term *acute* implies that the hepatitis episode has a duration of less than six months. The acute hepatitis episode generally ends with complete resolution of the injured hepatic tissue; in especially severe cases, it can cause rapid liver deterioration ending in liver failure and possibly death. In contrast, chronic hepatitis lasts for more than six months and is characterized by slow, progressive deterioration of hepatic function associated with ongoing hepatic inflammation. Liver function is evaluated using a panel of liver function tests (LFTs) that minimally include specific enzymes, bilirubin, albumin, ammonia, and prothrombin time and partial thromboplastin time. Table 30–1 provides a summary of laboratory tests for

TABLE 30–1 Laboratory Evaluation of Hepatic Function and Abnormal Trends

TEST	NORMAL RANGE	ABNORMAL TREND	COMMENTS
Enzymes			
Alanine aminotransferase (ALT)	5–35 units/mL	All increase	Enzyme elevations are sensitive indicators of hepatic impairment or dysfunction; extreme elevations strongly suggest extensive hepatocellular injury; these enzymes are not specific to the liver, however.
Aspartate aminotransferase (AST)	0–35 units/L		
Alkaline phosphatase (Alk Phos)	20–90 units/L		
Bilirubin			
Total	0.1–1.2 mg/dL	Increased	End product of hemoglobin degradation; increased total bilirubin with decreased direct bilirubin levels suggests hepatic dysfunction. Elevations in direct bilirubin usually indicate a posthepatic biliary problem.
Indirect (unconjugated)	0.1–1.0 mg/dL	Increased	
Direct (conjugated)	0.1–0.3 mg/dL	Decreased	
Albumin	3.5–5.0 g/dL	Decreased	Hypoalbuminemia is seen more commonly in chronic liver disorders such as cirrhosis; other conditions causing decreases include malnutrition, nephrotic syndrome, and other disorders.
Ammonia	15–45 mcg/dL	Increased	Produced by protein metabolism by intestinal bacteria; it is detoxified in liver; elevations develop with liver dysfunction; high levels contribute to mental status changes (e.g., hepatic encephalopathy).
Coagulation:			All of the clotting factors except factor VIII are made exclusively in liver; elevated PT.
Prothrombin time (PT)	10–13 seconds	Prolonged	Five times normal that is refractory to vitamin K is poor prognostic sign of acute viral hepatitis and other liver disorders.
Partial thromboplastin time (PTT)	60–70 seconds	Prolonged	

Normal values from Kee (2009).

monitoring liver function and trends seen in disorders of liver function.

Types of Acute Hepatitis

The major cause of acute hepatitis is viral infection by specific viruses that target hepatocytes. There are five common viruses: hepatitis A (HAV), hepatitis B (HBV), hepatitis C (HCV), hepatitis D (HDV), and hepatitis E (HEV). Other viral sources include cytomegalovirus (CMV), and Epstein–Barr virus (EBV). Less common causes of acute hepatitis include drug toxicity (e.g., acetaminophen, erythromycin, and isoniazid), alcohol abuse, and autoimmune disorders.

Hepatitis A Virus

Hepatitis A (infectious hepatitis, HAV) is transmitted through the fecal–oral route only during acute infection and is most commonly found in children and young adults. HAV is frequently associated with epidemics and is transmitted primarily through contaminated food or water or eating contaminated raw shellfish. There is a high incidence of HAV in underdeveloped countries and the highest rate of this disease is reported in children ages 5–14 years old (Sjögren, 2006). HAV is usually a mild, fairly benign, and self-limiting infection that incurs immunity following acute illness. It is not associated with development of chronic hepatitis. Two vaccines against HAV have been approved in the United States. It is recommended for high-risk populations (e.g., health care and childcare workers, travelers to endemic areas of the world, and persons who are immunosuppressed). Immune globulin should be administered to those with close contacts with HAV as prophylaxis therapy (Deinsteig, 2008).

Hepatitis B Virus

Hepatitis B (serum hepatitis, HBV) is transmitted through contaminated blood serum or body fluids. People who are exposed to contaminated needles or body fluids are at risk for contracting hepatitis B. The at-risk population for HBV is similar to the HIV at-risk group (Table 30–2) and it is considered a significant sexually transmitted disease (STD). There are 1.0 to 1.25 million people in the United States with chronic HBV infection (CDC, 2008). The prevalence of HBV has decreased over the past 15 to 20 years because of increased safe sexual practices in view of the human immunodeficiency virus (HIV) epidemic, as well as the development and wide distribution of HBV vaccine. Hepatitis B is seen in all age groups and it occurs throughout the world and is endemic in many parts of the world; however it is less prevalent in the United States. It is a major cause of acute and chronic hepatitis and cirrhosis as well as a precursor to hepatocellular carcinoma. A vaccine is available to protect at-risk populations from HBV.

Hepatitis C Virus

Hepatitis C (HCV) is a major cause of chronic hepatitis, cirrhosis, and hepatocellular carcinoma. HCV is primarily transmitted through blood and blood products. Major risk factors for developing HCV include blood transfusions prior to 1992, illicit IV drug use, and occupational exposure (see Table 30–3). Additional risk factors include hemodialysis units, as well as tattoos and body piercing performed in nonprofessional settings. In 2006 there were only 802 confirmed cases of hepatitis C while the CDC estimated that approximately 19,000 new cases actually occurred. The disparity between confirmed and estimated cases exists because HCV is an asymptomatic disease in the early stages; therefore, it remains unidentified and underreported (CDC, 2008). The incidence of chronic HCV is approximately 3.2 million people in the United States. The estimated number of new infections per year has declined significantly since the end of its peak in the 1980s (CDC, 2008). HCV has six known genotypes and can be very difficult to treat. It is one of the most common diseases that causes liver cirrhosis and is the leading indication for liver transplantation. There is no vaccine available to prevent hepatitis C.

Hepatitis D Virus

Hepatitis D (HDV), also known as delta virus, is an incomplete virus. To be a viable virus, it requires the surface antigen of the hepatitis B virus (HBsAg) to act as its outer shell. Patients who do not test positive for HBV need not be tested for HDV. It is primarily transmitted through the blood serum and in the United States is primarily found in people with hemophilia, (type of coagulopathy that requires transfusions of specific blood components), and intravenous drug users. There is no vaccine available to prevent hepatitis D.

TABLE 30–2 At-Risk Population for Hepatitis B Virus (HBV)

Illicit drug users and past drug users
Health care workers
Men who have had sex with men
People who require frequent transfusions (e.g., hemophiliac diseases)
People with decreased immunocompetence
Sexual partners of people infected with HBV
Newborns of mothers infected with HBV
Individuals infected with HCV or HIV
Renal dialysis patients
All pregnant women

Data from Sherman (2008) and Deinsteig (2008).

TABLE 30–3 Risk Factors for Hepatitis C

Illicit drug use (injectables)
Cocaine use (intranasal)
Received a transfusion prior to 1992
Tattooing
Birth to a HCV mother
Multiple sexual partners
Occupational exposure (health care workers, daycare workers, etc)
Chronically elevated ALT
HIV
Alcohol abuse
ESRD patients on hemodialysis
Incarceration
Sharing a toothbrush, razor, etc., with an infected person

Data from Deinsteig (2008) and Roth-Kauffman (2008).

Hepatitis E Virus

Hepatitis E (HEV) is similar to HAV in its transmission through the fecal–oral route. Most cases of HEV follow contamination of water supplies in endemic areas of Africa, Asia, India, and Central America. It is rarely encountered in the United States.

Pathophysiologic Basis of Acute Hepatitis

The pathologic effects of acute hepatitis are the same regardless of the causative agent. Acute hepatitis can be divided into three categories based on the severity of the disease: classic hepatitis, submassive hepatic necrosis, and massive hepatic necrosis. Unless complications develop, acute hepatitis is generally considered a reversible disease.

Classic Hepatitis

Classic hepatitis is characterized by a liver that is normal in size and color, or by one that has mild enlargement and edema with bile staining present. Necrosis is localized but inflammation is generalized. The liver tissue structures remain intact throughout the disease process.

Submassive Hepatitis Necrosis

Submassive hepatic necrosis is characterized by more generalized necrosis, with a large number of necrotic hepatocytes. Inflammation is severe and injury leads to the collapse of hepatic tissues with subsequent loss of **lobule** structure. Fibrosis of hepatic tissue may develop during the healing stage.

Massive Hepatic Necrosis

Massive hepatic necrosis is characterized by extensive necrosis with loss of entire lobules. This type of acute hepatitis is associated with the development of fulminant hepatic failure, which is discussed in Section Two of this module.

Clinical Manifestations of Acute Hepatitis

Viral hepatitis is generally associated with a prodromal period in which the patient develops mild-to-moderate flulike symptoms. Classic symptoms of acute hepatitis include anorexia, nausea, vomiting, and severe fatigue. Abdominal pain may be present as well as mild fever, dark urine, and light stools. The urine may become dark one to five days before hyperbilirubinemia causes **jaundice** to be present. Symptoms may precede jaundice usually by one to two weeks (Ghany & Hoofnagle, 2008).

Only about 25 percent of people with acute hepatitis develop jaundice. Based on this manifestation, hepatitis can be divided into anicteric and cholestatic hepatitis. **Anicteric hepatitis** refers to hepatitis with no jaundice. Patients with anicteric hepatitis may have severely compromised liver function that is overlooked because of lack of jaundice. **Cholestatic hepatitis** refers to hepatitis with retention of bile as a result of a biliary obstruction (usually secondary to the inflammatory process). Persons with cholestatic hepatitis usually are severely jaundiced, urine is dark, and feces are clay-colored. Serum bilirubin becomes greatly elevated with obstructive disease. The clinical manifestations of acute viral hepatitis are summarized in Table 30–4.

TABLE 30–4 Clinical Manifestations of Acute Viral Hepatitis

Prodromal period
Flulike symptoms: malaise, headache, anorexia, hyperpyrexia, nausea and vomiting, arthritis, myalgia, abdominal pain
Jaundice
Anicteric hepatitis—no jaundice is present
Cholestatic hepatitis—jaundice that may be severe; dark urine is present several days before jaundice appears; stool is clay-colored; serum bilirubin is 2.0 to 3.0 mg/dL

SECTION ONE REVIEW

1. Acute hepatitis is most commonly caused by
   A. bacterial invasion
   B. viral invasion
   C. yeast invasion
   D. an autoimmune reaction
2. The major cause of acute and chronic hepatitis and cirrhosis is
   A. cytomegalovirus
   B. hepatitis C virus
   C. Epstein–Barr virus
   D. hepatitis B virus
3. Classic hepatitis is characterized by
   A. localized necrosis
   B. a greatly enlarged liver
   C. development of fibrosis
   D. development of fulminant hepatic failure
4. If a patient has anicteric hepatitis, the nurse would expect to see
   A. dark urine
   B. clay-colored stool
   C. normal-colored urine
   D. black stool
5. If a patient has cholestatic hepatitis, the nurse would anticipate serum bilirubin levels to
   A. fall below normal range
   B. remain within normal range
   C. elevate slightly above normal
   D. rise significantly above normal

Answers: 1. B, 2. D, 3. A, 4. C, 5. D

SECTION TWO: Hepatic Failure

At the completion of this section, the learner will be able to describe the etiology and clinical manifestations associated with acute hepatic failure.

The term **hepatic failure** refers to the inability of the liver to perform its normal functions. Acute hepatic failure (AHF) results from one of the three following situations:

1. As a primary disease process in the absence of preexisting hepatic disease such as acute viral hepatitis, autoimmune liver disease, or drug induced liver disease.
2. As a complication of chronic liver disease, cirrhosis.
3. In association with multiple organ failure in the critically ill as in hypoperfusion, or shock.

Regardless of the cause of AHF, many of the clinical manifestations are the same.

Acute Hepatic Failure as a Primary Disease

Although uncommon, acute hepatic failure (AHF) can occur without preexisting liver disease. Four possible etiologies include shock, virulent viral infection, hepatotoxins, and systemic inflammatory response. Acute liver failure is the newest terminology used by the hepatology community. The definition includes evidence of coagulation abnormalities and INR of greater than 1.5, any degree of altered mentation, encephalopathy in a patient without preexisting cirrhosis, and an illness of less than 26 weeks duration. In the US, there are approximately 2,000 cases each year (Polson & Lee, 2005). Mortality is high with the poorest prognosis occurring in patients who are less than 10 years of age or older than 40 years (Sood, 2008).

Shock

The liver is extremely vulnerable to ischemic injury, as are the other splanchnic organs. A sustained hypotensive episode (shock) can result in insufficient oxygenation of liver tissue, which can precipitate ischemic hepatitis. In response to hypoxia, the delicate endothelial lining of the hepatic capillaries becomes damaged and more permeable. Increased permeability allows fluid to leak from the capillaries into the hepatic tissue. As fluid shifts out of the vasculature, microthrombi develop, partly as a result of the high concentration of particulate matter remaining in the vessels. Microthrombi can cause a blockage of blood flow with subsequent tissue ischemia and necrosis distal to the blockages. Though the liver has a large reserve, if tissue destruction exceeds this reserve, acute liver failure will result. Ischemic hepatitis may spontaneously resolve or it may degenerate into acute hepatic failure. The longer the initial hypotensive episode continues, the more severe the liver destruction will be.

Fulminant Hepatic Failure

A particularly severe form of acute hepatic failure is called **fulminant hepatic failure** (**FHF**). Fulminant hepatic failure can result from multiple causes. Two major causes are acute viral infections and hepatotoxins. Hepatitis A and B are the most common viral causes. The most common hepatotoxin precipitating fulminant hepatic failure is acetaminophen. In some cases no cause is found, although an undetected viral etiology is generally suspected. A more extensive listing of known causes of fulminant hepatic failure is presented in Table 30–5.

Definitions of fulminant hepatic failure vary widely. For our purposes, the definition of FHF is based on the following criteria: the level of encephalopathy, the preexisting liver status, and the rate of onset. Fulminant hepatic failure is defined as a form of acute hepatic failure in a patient with no preexisting history of liver disease that develops rapidly (in less than eight weeks) accompanied by encephalopathy. FHF causes rapid, massive deterioration and destruction of liver tissue with widespread hepatocellular necrosis. The result is severe hepatic dysfunction with subsequent development of encephalopathy. FHF is a medical emergency responsible for 2,000 deaths a year in the United States (Fontant, 2006). Survival without liver transplantation is 20 percent.

Acute Hepatic Failure as a Complication of Chronic Liver Disease

The ninth leading cause of death in the United States is cirrhosis. Chronic liver disease and cirrhosis cause 4 percent to 5 percent of deaths in persons 45 to 54 years of age and result in about 30,000 deaths each year (Bataller & Gines, 2007). Cirrhosis is defined as a diffuse process characterized by fibrosis where normal liver structure is converted to abnormal nodules (Garcia-Tsao, 2008). The onset of cirrhosis is insidious and progressive. In the United States, the two most common causes of cirrhosis are alcohol abuse and hepatitis C. Over time, the progressive deterioration of hepatic function becomes sufficient to compromise the normal functioning of the liver.

Acute Hepatic Failure as Part of Multiple Organ Failure

A major body insult, such as sepsis, can set off a systemic inflammatory response that, in turn, leads to a series of physiologic events. This response is called the *systemic inflammatory response syndrome (SIRS)*. When SIRS develops, the normally localized inflammatory response becomes a systemic, malignant process. SIRS results in a single or multiple organ inflammatory insult. In the liver, the inflammatory

TABLE 30–5 Causes of Fulminant Hepatic Failure (FHF)

Viral infections:
Hepatitis A, B, C, and D
Cytomegalovirus (CMV)
Epstein–Barr virus (EBV)
Hepatotoxins:
Acetaminophen
Mushroom toxins
Isoniazid (INH)
Hydrocarbons

TABLE 30–6 Stages of Hepatic Encephalopathy

STAGE[a]	CLINICAL MANIFESTATIONS
I	Awake, apathetic, restless, sleep pattern changes, mental clouding, impaired computational ability, impaired handwriting, subtle intellectual function changes, diminished muscle coordination; electroencephalogram (EEG) shows mild-to-moderate abnormalities
II	Decreased level of consciousness, lethargy, drowsiness, disorientation to time and place, confusion, asterixis, diminished reflexes, slurring of speech; EEG shows moderate-to-severe abnormalities
III	Stupor (arousable), no spontaneous eye opening, hyperactive reflexes, seizures, rigidity, abnormal posturing: decorticate, decerebrate, extensor plantar responses; EEG shows severe abnormalities
IV	Coma (may or may not respond to painful stimuli), seizures, pupillary dilation, flaccidity; EEG shows severe abnormalities

[a]Stage 0 encephalopathy may be used to describe subclinical intellectual impairment.

response sets off a massive release and assault by the liver macrophages (**Kupffer's cells**), causing destruction of liver tissue. The inflammatory response also causes the endothelial lining of the vessels to become more permeable, allowing fluids to leak into the liver parenchyma, and resulting in organ edema and microthrombi. The microthrombi and inflammation eventually lead to the damage of hepatocytes and the blockage of bile flow. When damage becomes severe, hepatic failure ensues.

Clinical Manifestations of Acute Hepatic Failure

The massive tissue destruction caused by AHF produces essentially the same manifestations regardless of its etiology. The clinical manifestations of AHF reflect severe hepatic encephalopathy and multiple metabolic dysfunctions.

Hepatic Encephalopathy

Encephalopathy is the hallmark of acute hepatic failure. **Hepatic encephalopathy**, also called *hepatic coma* or *portosystemic encephalopathy*, is defined as an altered neurologic status caused by a buildup of circulating toxins of hepatic origin (e.g., ammonia). The encephalopathy associated with FHF is frequently associated with hypoglycemia and cerebral edema. Severe cerebral edema with brain herniation is the leading cause of death in FHF. Hepatic encephalopathy has been staged (graded) according to clinical manifestations for clarity (Table 30–6). Hepatic encephalopathy is also considered a complication of AHF and is further discussed in Section Six of this module.

Metabolic Dysfunction

Liver failure develops when more than 60 percent of hepatocytes are injured, reflected in the organ's inability to perform its multiple metabolic functions. Liver failure results in the following metabolically related clinical manifestations

- **Protein metabolic dysfunction.** Ascites, hypoalbuminemia, hepatic encephalopathy, evidence of impaired clotting factors (hemorrhage, epistaxis, purpura)
- **Carbohydrate metabolism dysfunction.** Hypoglycemia
- **Fat metabolism dysfunction.** Nausea and vomiting, anorexia, constipation or diarrhea, prolonged PT

These metabolic dysfunctions are expressed in alterations in body systems, as noted in Table 30–7.

TABLE 30–7 Effects of Hepatic Failure on Body Systems

SYSTEM	CLINICAL MANIFESTATIONS
Neurologic	Stage I to IV encephalopathy
Cardiovascular	Pulmonary edema, hypotension
Gastrointestinal	Nausea and vomiting, constipation or diarrhea, anorexia, ascites
Hematopoietic	Impaired coagulation, prolonged PT
Pulmonary	Tachypnea, crackles

SECTION TWO REVIEW

1. Which of the following statements regarding fulminant hepatic failure is TRUE?
   A. It causes necrosis of liver tissue.
   B. It has a mortality of less than 50 percent.
   C. It is characterized by stage I and II encephalopathy.
   D. It has a slow, insidious onset.

2. A major hepatotoxin that is known to cause fulminant hepatic failure is
   A. acetaminophen
   B. gentamicin
   C. aspirin
   D. cephalosporin

(*continued*)

(continued)

3. In the United States, cirrhosis of the liver is most commonly caused by
   - **A.** hepatitis A virus
   - **B.** alcohol abuse
   - **C.** hepatitis B virus
   - **D.** Epstein–Barr virus
4. Stages III and IV hepatic encephalopathy are characterized by
   - **A.** stupor, coma
   - **B.** lethargy, asterixis
   - **C.** restlessness, slurred speech
   - **D.** sleep pattern changes, drowsiness
5. Hepatic encephalopathy is primarily caused by high levels of
   - **A.** bilirubin
   - **B.** bile
   - **C.** ammonia
   - **D.** blood urea nitrogen (BUN)

Answers: 1. A, 2. A, 3. B, 4. A, 5. C

SECTION THREE: Complications of Hepatic Dysfunction

At the completion of this section, the learner will be able to describe complications of hepatic dysfunction.

The inability of the damaged liver to meet all of the demands placed on it by other systems places the patient at risk for many multisystem complications. The severity of the complications is related to the level of liver dysfunction. The most widely accepted definition of acute liver failure includes evidence of coagulation abnormality, usually an INR of greater than 1.5 and any degree of mental alteration or encephalopathy. Table 30–8 lists the major complications of hepatic dysfunction.

Hepatic Encephalopathy

Recall that hepatic encephalopathy is caused by toxic levels of circulating ammonia, which readily crosses the blood–brain barrier. Normally, the liver rapidly converts ammonia into **urea**, which is then excreted in the urine. When the liver is unable to convert ammonia to urea, toxicity rapidly develops.

TABLE 30–8 Common Complications of Hepatic Failure

- Hepatic encephalopathy
- Portal hypertension
- Esophageal varices
- Ascites
- Infections: sepsis and spontaneous bacterial peritonitis
- Acute renal failure

Contributing Factors

A variety of factors contribute to increased nitrogenous waste, thus contributing to increased ammonia levels

- **Constipation.** Nitrogenous wastes remain in the GI tract longer, providing more opportunity for conversion to ammonia
- **Blood in the GI tract.** As blood in the tract is broken down, ammonia is released
- **Azotemia.** Contributes to the buildup of nitrogenous wastes
- **Dietary protein consumption.** Provides amino acids, thus more ammonia buildup
- **Certain drugs.** Tranquilizers, sedatives, and analgesics remain longer in the body, contributing to neurologic effects

Portal Hypertension

Normal hepatic venous flow meets moderate resistance (8 to 10 mm Hg) when compared with the low resistance level (2 to 8 mm Hg) of the connecting vena cava. When hepatic tissue is injured or destroyed, blood flowing through the damaged areas requires more pressure to maintain organ blood flow. Consequently, increased hepatic capillary resistance occurs in a fashion similar to that which is created in the lungs when they sustain parenchymal damage.

Portal hypertension results from increased resistance within the portal venous system. This is usually caused by cirrhosis, which disrupts the normal lobular structure of the liver. This disruption causes resistance to blood flow into, through, and out of the liver with resultant portal hypertension. Over time, as in chronic hepatic dysfunction, the liver develops a system of collateral circulation that helps to relieve the increase in pressure. These collateral veins are called **varices** and are characterized by their dilated, tortuous appearance. In acute hepatic failure, however, collateral circulation does not have sufficient time to develop, and back flow leads to congestion of other organs in the **splanchnic circulation**. Figure 30–1 illustrates how circulation is affected by portal hypertension.

Esophageal Varices

Esophageal varices are a major complication of portal hypertension. Blood naturally flows through vessels with the least resistance, seeking the easiest path. This diversion of flow is called shunting. The esophageal veins (varices) in the lower portion of the esophagus provide a common collateral flow diversion. Esophageal varices dilate to accept shunted blood. A rapid increase in pressure (e.g., coughing, vomiting, straining) can cause these dilated varices to rupture, precipitating hemorrhage.

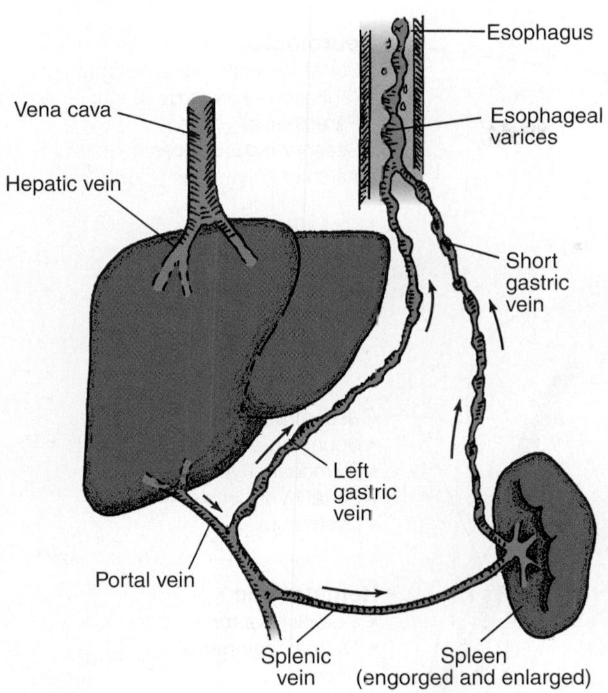

Figure 30–1 ■ Portal hypertension. Damage to liver tissue increases vascular resistance. Venous flow becomes blocked in the liver, causing portal vein pressure to increase. Blood backs up through the splenic vein into the spleen and collateral venous circulation (such as the short and left gastric veins).

Bleeding esophageal varices are considered a medical emergency (Shah & Kamath, 2006).

Ascites

Ascites is defined as an abnormal collection of fluid in the abdominal cavity. Ascites develops during advanced-stage hepatic dysfunction. Two major causes of ascites are decreased colloid osmotic pressure and portal hypertension. Colloid osmotic pressure decreases as a result of a reduction in albumin. Hypoalbuminemia is caused by the inability of the liver to carry out its usual protein metabolism functions. When colloid osmotic pressure becomes too low, fluid shifts from the intravascular compartment into other body compartments (e.g., the intraabdominal cavity). In addition, cirrhotic patients can develop extreme sodium retention by the kidney, which contributes to ascites. Renal salt and water retention leads to over expansion of intravascular volume, causing the shifts of fluids from the intravascular space to the tissues or body compartment spaces including the peritoneum, pericardial space, and the pleura. This leads to an alteration in renal sodium and water excretion related to hypoalbuminemia, hyperaldosteronism, and increased antidiuretic hormone levels (Arguedas & Fallon, 2007).

Hepatorenal Syndrome

Hepatorenal syndrome (HRS) is the complication of end-stage liver disease categorized by functional renal failure in the absence of underlying kidney pathology (Cardenas, 2005). A diagnosis of hepatorenal syndrome should not be made until other types of acute renal failure are ruled out. Common features of HRS include oliguria, hyponatremia, and low urinary sodium (Friedman, 2005). Hepatorenal syndrome can be divided into two subgroups: type 1 and type 2.

Type 1 Hepatorenal Syndrome

Type 1 hepatorenal syndrome (type 1 HRS) is characterized by severe, rapidly progressive renal failure with a doubling of the serum creatinine to a level greater than 2.5 mg/dL or halving of the creatinine clearance to less than 20 mL per minute in less than two weeks (Friedman, 2005; Cardenas, 2005). Type 1 HRS often occurs following a precipitating event that results in a hypotensive episode, such as aggressive diuresis, large volume paracentesis, spontaneous bacterial peritonitis, gastrointestinal bleeding, a major surgical procedure; or acute viral hepatitis superimposed on cirrhosis. Most patients die within two weeks of onset of type 1 HRS (Martin & Hassanein, 2009).

Type 2 Hepatorenal Syndrome

Type 2 hepatorenal syndrome (type 2 HRS) has a slower, chronic, more progressive increase in the serum creatinine level to greater than 1.5 mg/dL or a creatinine clearance of less than 40 mL per minute (Arroyo et al., 2002; Cardena, 2005). Patients with type 2 HRS usually exhibit signs of liver failure and arterial hypotension to a lesser degree than patients with type 1 HRS. Most patients with type 2 HRS have severe ascites refractive to diuresis (Vargas, 2008). Those patients with type 2 HRS are predisposed to the development of type 1 HRS. HRS may be a clinical continuum and not two separate entities. The clinical characteristics of hepatorenal syndrome are presented in Table 30–9.

Figure 30–2 provides a summary of the multisystem effects of cirrhosis.

Infections: Sepsis and Spontaneous Bacterial Peritonitis

Kupffer's cells plays a major role in preventing migration of harmful enteric bacteria to the systemic circulation which can result in sepsis. They are macrophages that engulf bacteria from the blood as it flows through the liver. Also, the liver produces proteins that are necessary to the immune and inflammatory systems. The loss of kupffer's cells in the liver

TABLE 30–9 Clinical Characteristics of Hepatorenal Syndrome

Presence of liver failure
Decreasing glomerular filtration rate (GFR)
Reduced urine sodium (less than 10 mEq/24 hours)
Presence of azotemia (elevated creatinine and blood urea nitrogen)
Oliguria or anuria
High BUN/creatinine ratio

Data from Arguedas & Fallon (2007).

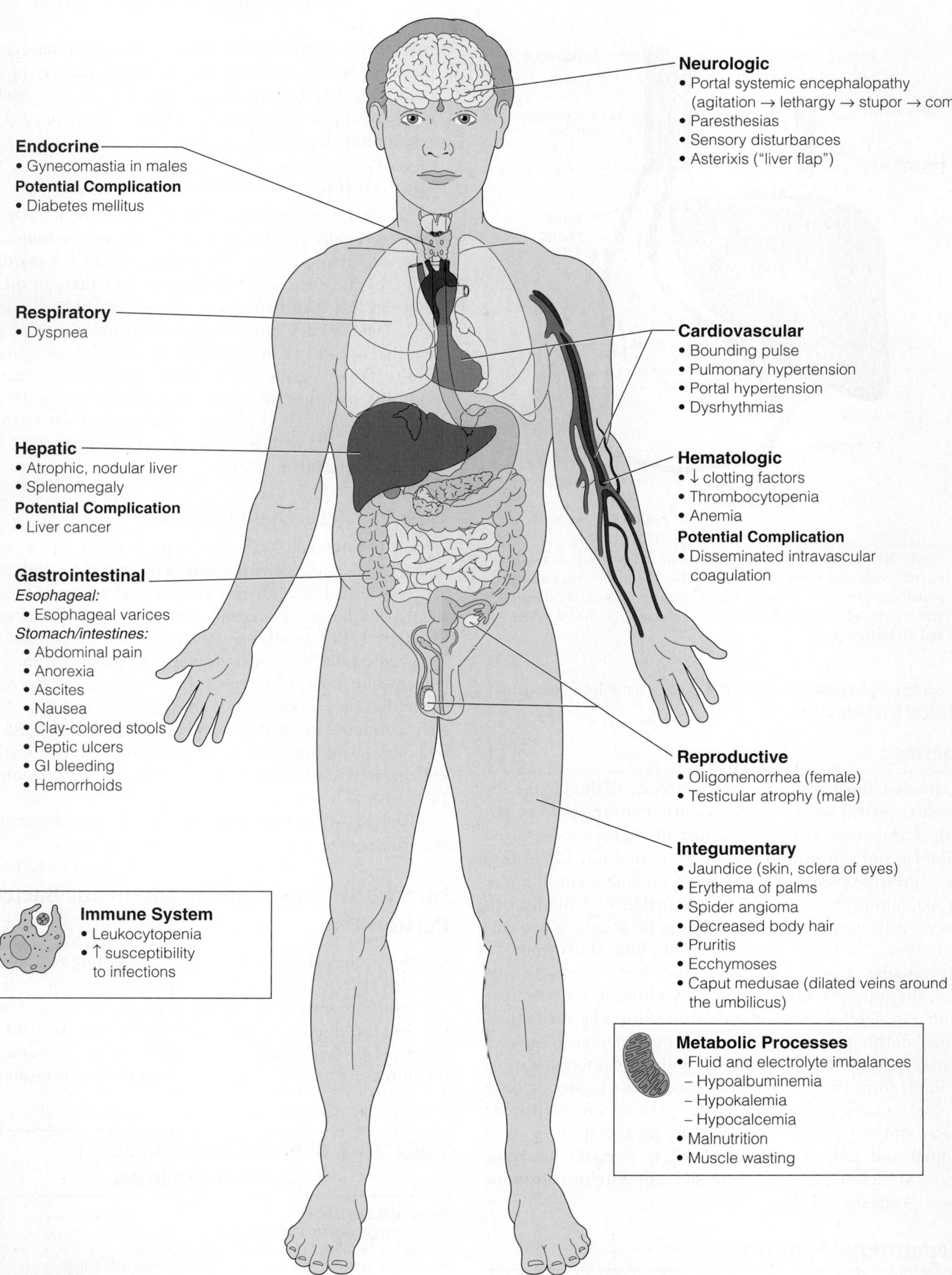

Figure 30–2 ■ Multisystem effects of cirrhosis.

to cleanse the blood as well as loss of protein synthesis places the hepatic failure patient at risk for development of sepsus and SIRS.

The patient with acute hepatic failure is also at risk for development of spontaneous bacterial peritonitis. This form of peritonitis occurs when ascites fluid becomes infected. Bacteria are able to translocate (migrate) into the ascites when the bowel wall loses its integrity as a result of endothelial damage secondary to tissue ischemia or infarct. Intestinal bacteria move across the injured intestinal wall and seed themselves in the ascites fluid. A hypotensive episode is the most common cause of intestinal wall injury in this patient population. The bowel is the primary source of bacteria in both sepsis and spontaneous bacterial peritonitis.

SECTION THREE REVIEW

1. Portal hypertension is caused by
   A. increased vascular resistance
   B. decreased portal vein blood flow
   C. increased hepatic artery volume
   D. decreased hepatic blood flow
2. Esophageal varices dilate in response to
   A. decreased hepatic blood flow
   B. hepatic vasoconstriction
   C. shunted splanchnic blood
   D. increased cardiac output
3. A major cause of ascites is
   A. hyperalbuminemia
   B. low colloid osmotic pressure
   C. hepatorenal syndrome
   D. fluid volume overload
4. A major factor contributing to onset of acute renal failure as a complication of hepatic failure is
   A. hepatotoxins
   B. a hypotensive episode
   C. high ammonia levels
   D. portal vein shunting
5. The onset of type 2 hepatorenal syndrome usually occurs in the presence of
   A. hepatotoxins
   B. a hypotensive episode
   C. high ammonia levels
   D. severe ascites
6. The hepatic failure patient is at risk for spontaneous bacterial peritonitis as a result of
   A. translocation of intestinal bacteria
   B. increased bacterial growth in intestines
   C. secondary hepatic bacterial infection
   D. unknown causes

Answers: 1. A, 2. C, 3. B, 4. B, 5. D, 6. A

SECTION FOUR: Medical Management

At the completion of this section, the learner will be able to describe an overview of the medical management of the patient with hepatic dysfunction. Management of the patient with acute hepatic dysfunction is primarily supportive regardless of the causative agent.

Management of Acute Viral Hepatitis

There is no specific therapy for treatment of viral hepatitis. Table 30–10 summarizes the general focuses for medical management of acute viral hepatitis. Patients with this diagnosis do not necessarily require hospitalization.

Management of Acute Hepatic Failure Complications

Failure of the liver to adequately carry out its many functions has a deleterious effect on multiple body systems. The patient will remain at high risk for complications until the liver has healed adequately to regain its functions. Management is primarily supportive and complications are addressed as they arise. When a complication is identified, management focuses on reversal, reduction, or correction to prevent permanent damage or death. The remainder of this section focuses on major complications that often develop during acute hepatic failure, including hepatic

TABLE 30–10 Supportive Medical Management for Acute Viral Hepatitis

FOCUS	GENERAL MANAGEMENT
Activity/rest	Limit activities based on level of fatigue Require rest based on severity of symptoms
Hydration/nutritional needs	Maintain balanced hydration status Diet: high carbohydrate, low fat; no alcohol intake Nausea management: metoclopramide and hydroxyzine in small doses Vitamin K, if needed
Hospitalization criteria	Hospitalization is indicated if severe nausea and vomiting develops, deteriorating liver function is noted (e.g., hepatic encephalopathy and/or prolonged prothrombin time)

Data from Arguedas & Fallon (2007).

encephalopathy, hypoglycemia, metabolic abnormalities, gastrointestinal hemorrhage, fulminant hepatic failure, cerebral edema, and esophageal varices.

Hepatic Encephalopathy

Management of hepatic encephalopathy centers around four goals, three of which focus on control and elimination of ammonia

- Identify and treat the precipitating factors when possible
- Reduce the amount of ammonia-producing bacteria in the bowel
- Eliminate or reduce generation of ammonia toxins
- Prevent movement of ammonia toxins from the bowel

Identify and Treat the Precipitating Factors. Hepatic encephalopathy can be triggered or worsened by certain precipitating factors (Table 30–11). It is important to rapidly identify and aggressively treat precipitating factors to reduce the severity of the encephalopathy.

Reduce Bacteria in the Bowel. The aminoglycoside neomycin is frequently ordered to suppress ammonia-producing intestinal bacteria. One gram of neomycin administered orally every six to eight hours can maintain long-term suppression for the treatment of hepatic encephalopathy. Neomycin is not well absorbed through the gastrointestinal tract; thus, its effects are primarily local. As with all aminoglycosides, the patient must be monitored for the potential side effects of ototoxicity and nephrotoxicity. Metronidazole (Flagyl) 250 mg administered three or four times a day is as effective as oral neomycin without the risks of ototoxicity or nephrotoxicity. To avoid the development of peripheral neuropathy, treatment with metronidazole should not exceed two weeks (Abou-Assi & Vlahcevic, 2001; Marreno, Martinez & Hyzy, 2003; Martin & Hassanein, 2009).

Gastrointestinal bleeding and constipation can precipitate hepatic encephalopathy. In the event of GI bleeding or constipation, the bowels should be cleansed of all residual blood and stool by administration of enemas. This will prevent further buildup of nitrogenous waste by speeding transit of blood through the bowel (Fitz, 2006).

Eliminate or Reduce Ammonia Toxins. Protein intake must be either eliminated or tightly controlled. There is evidence that controlling protein intake (including the type of protein) rather than eliminating it may be useful in decreasing hepatic encephalopathy. Dietary protein is often limited to 60 grams per day. Vegetable proteins rather than animal proteins may have a beneficial effect because of lower rates of ammonia production (Fitz, 2006).

Prevent Movement of Ammonia Toxins. The synthetic disaccharide, lactulose, may be ordered to help prevent absorption of ammonia from the bowel. Its use began after studies proved colonic bacteria are the main producers of ammonia (Shawcross & Jalan, 2005). The laxative effect of lactulose moves stool through the intestines more rapidly, thus decreasing the amount of ammonia formed before the stool is eliminated. Lactulose also may facilitate trapping of ammonia ions in the intestines for unknown reasons. Lactulose breaks down into lactic acid and other organic acids that may facilitate the ammonia-trapping action. It is also theorized that lactulose may modify the intestinal flora in some manner, thereby causing a reduction in absorption of bacteria through the bowel. Typically, 15 to 30 mL of lactulose is administered four times a day (oral or enema) or adjusted as necessary to attain three to five soft stools per 24 hours (Abou-Assi & Vlahcevic, 2001; Fitz, 2006).

TABLE 30–11 Precipitating Factors Associated with Hepatic Encephalopathy

- Infection
- Elevated protein intake
- Worsening hepatic function
- Constipation
- Azotemia (elevated blood urea nitrogen and creatinine)
- Gastrointestinal bleeding
- Hypovolemia

Hypoglycemia

Liver failure interferes with normal carbohydrate metabolism. Thus, the patient may develop hypoglycemia secondary to decreased gluconeogenesis. Management consists of frequent monitoring of serum glucose levels and close observation for the development of hypoglycemic symptoms, such as slow thinking, slurred speech, nervousness, tachycardia, and cold, clammy skin. Treatment of hypoglycemia may consist of a continuous IV infusion of 10 percent dextrose solution. If the hypoglycemia is severe, 50 percent dextrose may be ordered as immediate treatment.

Metabolic Abnormalities

Electrolyte abnormalities, such as hyponatremia and hypokalemia, are common in patients with liver failure. Hyponatremia results from sodium loss due to diuretic therapy, the hemodilution effect, and sodium restriction. Hypokalemia is caused by diuretic therapy and elevated aldosterone levels, which result from the loss of the liver's ability to metabolize aldosterone. In addition, the renin–angiotensin–aldosterone system is activated by diminished renal blood flow.

Acid–base imbalances are also common occurrences. The acute hepatic failure patient is at risk for developing metabolic acidosis for two major reasons. First, hepatic cellular damage releases lactic acid, which results in lactic acidosis. Second, metabolic acidosis is a complication of acute renal failure, a common sequela of hepatic failure. Respiratory alkalosis may develop from hyperventilation associated with compensatory mechanisms. Treatment of acid–base imbalances consists of correcting the underlying problems and administering bicarbonate if necessary.

Gastrointestinal Hemorrhage

The acute hepatic failure patient is at risk for development of GI hemorrhage for several reasons. One is the stress associated with severe illness, which can precipitate development of stress ulcers. Another is the presence of abnormal clotting factors, which increases the risk for abnormal bleeding. The mortality rate is high for the first episode of GI bleeding and, should the patient survive the first episode, repeated bleeds are common. Therapy generally consists of prevention of stress ulcers using histamine antagonists or antacids, and controlling the coagulopathy through use of vitamin K and blood products. Table 30–12 summarizes the supportive medical management of acute hepatic failure based on common complications.

Fulminant Hepatic Failure

As soon as fulminant hepatic failure (FHF) is suspected, the patient should be transferred to a critical care unit. When feasible, it is also recommended that FHF patients be transferred to medical centers that specialize in FHF management because the patient's survival may often depend on rapid identification and management of multisystem complications. The causative problem of FHF is not usually treatable; therefore, the primary focus of medical management is supportive. Liver transplantation is usually required in patients who do not spontaneously recover from FHF. This requires transfer of the patient to a liver transplant center as soon as

TABLE 30–12 Summary of Supportive Medical Management of Acute Hepatic Failure Complications

COMPLICATION	MANAGEMENT
Hepatic encephalopathy	Correct the precipitating cause, if possible No protein intake, or consider control of protein intake Enema if constipation or gastrointestinal bleeding Lactulose (PO, NG, rectal), 15–30 mL administered every six hours or as necessary to attain three to five soft stools per 24 hours Neomycin, 1–4 g (PO or enema) every six to eight hrs (neomycin should be avoided in patients with FHF because of the risk of nephrotoxicity) Metronidazole 250 mg (PO) three to four times a day Intubate and mechanically ventilate
Hypoglycemia	10% dextrose continuous IV infusion 50% dextrose IV, as required Monitor for low serum glucose and clinical manifestations of hypoglycemia
Metabolic abnormalities	Frequent monitoring of serum electrolytes and pH Correct electrolyte abnormalities Administer bicarbonate, as necessary
Gastrointestinal hemorrhage	Vitamin K Oral antacids or H_2 receptor antagonists (IV to keep gastric pH greater than 5) Fresh frozen plasma, possibly platelets
Cerebral edema	Intracranial pressure monitoring (ICP catheters should be placed in patients with grade IV encephalopathy or with rapidly progressing stage III encephalopathy. (CT scan of the brain should be performed prior to placement) IV mannitol Consider barbiturate-induced coma, if indicated Elevate head of bed 20 to 30 degrees
Hepatorenal syndrome	Liver transplantation Fluid resuscitation May consider transjugular intrahepatic portosystemic (TIPS) shunt Combination of midodrine (a peripheral vasoconstrictor), octreotide (a splanchnic vasoconstrictor), and albumin (an oncotic agent) has been used to successfully treat HRS Fenoldopam IV – if the patient can tolerate Ultrafiltration or continuous hemofiltration - if the patient develops compromised renal function that leads to oliguria, fluids should be removed via these two methods
Spontaneous bacterial peritonitis	Antibiotic therapy Fourth-generation cephalosporin, usually administered for five to seven days (until ascitic fluid cell count is normal)

Data from Arguedas & Fallon (2007); Vargas (2008); and Martin & Hassanein (2009).

TABLE 30–13 Management of the Patient with Esophageal Varices

FOCUS OF TREATMENT	INTERVENTIONS
Control bleeding	**IV vasopressin** Reduces splanchnic blood flow Initial dose of 20 units followed by continuous IV infusion of 0.4–0.6 units per minute **Somatostatin** (or synthetic analog octreotide) Reduces splanchnic blood flow and portal pressure Less systemic vasoconstrictive effects than vasopressin Initial dose of 50 mcg per hour continuous IV infusion **Nitroglycerin** Given with vasopressin to decrease systemic vasoconstrictive effects (i.e., cardiac or mesenteric ischemia) **Fresh frozen plasma** A replacement of clotting factors Platelets may be ordered, although their efficacy is controversial
Aggressive correction of bleeding varices	**Sengstaken-Blakemore** or Minnesota tube placement An inflated balloon that tamponades bleeding varices (see Fig. 30–4) **Portal systemic shunt surgery** Portocaval anastomosis Transjugular intrahepatic shunt (TIPS) (see Fig. 30–5) Distal splenorenal shunt
Preventive therapy	Therapy to reduce portal pressure: Nonselective beta blockers (i.e., propranolol, nadolol) Mononitrates (i.e., isosorbide mononitrate) Elective shunt surgery Endoscopic sclerotherapy Endoscopic variceal banding The varix is isolated and banded, which results in ablation

Data from Argueda & Fallon (2007) and Vargas (2008).

the decision is made. The survival rate of patients with fulminant hepatic failure restricted to medical management is less than 20 percent, whereas the survival rate associated with liver transplantation is greater than 60 percent (Fontant, 2006).

Cerebral Edema

Cerebral edema is an ominous complication of FHF. Its etiology is not fully understood, but may be due to passage of serum toxins and fluid normally cleared by the liver across the blood brain barrier. Its presence significantly reduces the patient's chances of survival. If edema cannot be adequately controlled, intracerebral herniation may result and is generally fatal.

Esophageal Varices

Portal hypertension leads to formation of venous collateral vessels between the portal and systemic circulations. These collateral vessels become dilated, tortuous veins (varices) within the submucosa of the esophagus and stomach. Esophageal varices are unpredictable; they can rupture at any time, placing the patient at high risk for hemorrhage. Management of the patient with bleeding esophageal varices is summarized in Table 30–13.

Multiple drugs are used during the treatment of hepatic dysfunction, as summarized in the RELATED PHARMACOTHERAPY box.

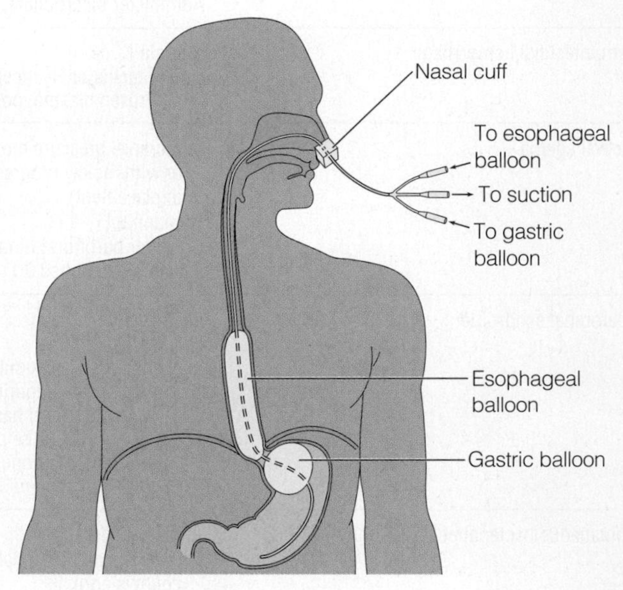

Figure 30–4 ■ Sengstaken-Blakemore tube.

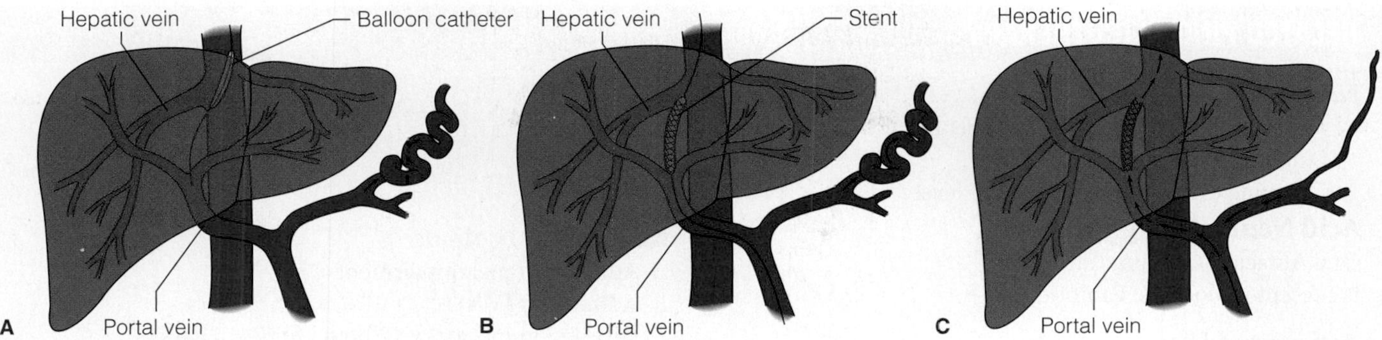

Figure 30–5 ■ Transjugular intrahepatic shunt (TIPS). A, Guided by angiography, a balloon catheter inserted via the jugular vein is advanced to the hepatic veins and through the substance of the liver to create a portacaval (portal vein-to-vena cava) channel. B, A metal stent is positioned into the channel, and expanded by inflating the balloon. C, the stent remains in place after the catheter is removed, creating a shunt for blood to flow directly from the portal vein into the hepatic vein.

RELATED PHARMACOTHERAPY: Agents Used to Treat Hepatic Dysfunction

Ammonia Reducing Agents

Neomycin (Mycifradin)
Metronidazole (Flagyl)

Action and Uses

Neomycin is an aminoglycoside type antibiotic that interferes with bacterial protein synthesis; metronidazole is an amebicide that inhibits DNA synthesis in susceptible organisms. These agents suppress ammonia producing intestinal bacteria to decrease hepatic encephalopathy. Neomycin is not typically used in the presence of hepatic failure but may be used for long term treatment of encephalopathy.

Major Adverse Effects

- Nausea, vomiting, diarrhea
- Stomatitis
- Abdominal cramping
- Neomycin specific: Nephrotoxicity and ototoxicity
- May caused falsely decreased AST/ALT
- Other: Flattening of *T* wave on ECG, impaired coordination

Nursing Implications

- Administered orally
- Monitor renal function (neomycin): Report signs and symptoms of renal dysfunction
- Monitor for overgrowth of *Candida*

Ammonia Detoxicant

Lactulose (Cephulac)

Action and Uses

Lactulose is a hyperosmotic laxative that causes an acidic pH when degraded that promotes NH_3 to NH_4. For treatment of hepatic encephalopathy, it prevents absorption of ammonia from the bowel; moves stool more rapidly decreasing the amount of ammonia formed.

Major Adverse Effects

- Abdominal cramps
- Flatulence, diarrhea

Nursing Implications

- May be administered orally or rectally; drug must be in colon for laxative action to take place
- Monitor intake and output balance

Prevention of Hypoglycemia

Dextrose IV

Actions and Uses

Dextrose IV is used to maintain consistent glucose levels because liver failure interferes with gluconeogenesis

Major Adverse Effects

- Redness, swelling, burning at injection site
- Hyperglycemia

Nursing Implications

- Administered as continuous IV infusion
- Can be given as D10W or D50W
- If administered too quickly can cause nausea

Prevention of Gastrointestinal Hemorrhage

Phytonadione (Vitamin K, AquaMEPHYTON, Mephyton)

Actions and Uses

Vitamin K is useful in correcting abnormal clotting factors. Hepatic patients often have elevated International Normalized Ratio (INR) levels which increases the risk for abnormal bleeding. Vitamin K promotes liver synthesis of clotting factors and therefore controls the coagulopathy of liver failure.

Major Adverse Effects

- Anaphylaxis
- Cyanosis
- Dyspnea
- Hypersensitivity reaction

(*continued*)

RELATED PHARMACOTHERAPY *(continued)*

Nursing Implications

Administer intravenous, subcutaneous, or orally
Dose depends on INR level
Continue to monitor INR and PT level

Acid Neutralizing Agents

Oral Antacids: Calcium Carbonate
H2 receptor blockers: Famotidine

Actions and Uses

These drugs are used as acid neutralizing agents that help to prevent stress ulcers. H2 blockers use competitive inhibition of histamine at the H2 receptors. Both agents help to prevent gastric acid secretion.

Major Adverse Effects

Antacids: headaches, hypophosphatemia, hypercalcemia, constipation, laxative effect, milk-alkai syndrome with high doses
H2 receptor blockers: Agitation, vomiting, AST/ALT increase, agranulocytosis, constipation, diarrhea

Nursing Implications

Use cautiously in renal disease
Give antacids one to two hours after other oral medications
H2 blockers can be given IV or orally. Must give IV if gastric pH level needs to be above 5

Agents to Reduce Bacteria in the Bowel

Fourth-generation cephalosporin (Cefepime)

Actions and Uses

Antibiotics such as Cefepime are used to inhibit bacterial cell wall synthesis. This antibiotic covers gram negative organisms which are often seen in spontaneous bacterial peritonitis. This complication of hepatic failure can be treated aggresively with antibiotics intravenously.

Major Adverse Effects

Positive Coombs test
Thrombocytopenia
Headache
Fever
Nausea
Diarrhea

Nursing Implications

Adjust for renal impairment
Administer IV
Give 1–2 grams every 12 hours for 7–10 days.
Monitor PT (Protime level)
Perform culture and sensitivity prior to giving drug

Agents used to control bleeding esophageal varices

Vasopressin (Pitressin)
Somatostatin
Nitroglycerin

Action and Uses

Vasopressin causes peristalsis by directly stimulating the smooth muscle in the gastrointestinal tract. It therefore inhibits splanchnic blood flow. Somatostatin also reduces splanchnic blood flow, however, it has less vasoconstrictive properties than vasopressin. Nitroglycerin is given in conjunction with vasopressin to decrease systemic vasoconstrictive effects such as cardiac or mesenteric ischemia

Major Adverse Effects

Vasopressin: hypertension, dysrhytmia, uticaria, tremor, diaphoresis, vertigo, fever
Somatostatin: sinus bradycardia, hyperglycemia, diarrhea, flatulence, constipation
Nitroglycerin: hypotension, headache, lightheadness, syncope

Nursing Implications

All three are given intravenously
Monitor vital signs and hemodynamics closely

Data sources: Wilson, Shannon, Shields, & Stand (2008); and Kauch (2009).

Emerging Evidence

- Development of septic shock in patients with preexisting acute liver failure (ALF) is predictive of a poor prognosis. Septic shock in the sample ALF population was associated with hyperlactatemia, elevated renin-angiotensin-aldosterone system activity, and hyperdynamic circulation *(Tsai, Chen, Tian, et al., 2008)*.
- Utilization of a protocol for management of intracerebral pressure (stage III or IV encephalopathy) in patients with fulminant liver failure resulted in improved clinical outcomes. The protocol included intracranial pressure monitoring and a decision protocol for prevention/treatment of intracerebral hypertension and hemostasis. Treatments included IV pentobarbital, hypothermia, hypocapnia, and IV vasopressor and mannitol titration to maintain cerebral perfusion pressure *(Raschke, Curry, Rempe et al., 2008)*.
- The U.S. Acute Liver Failure Study Group consensus recommendations for treatment of acute liver failure (ALF) includes ICU environment; intracranial pressure monitoring (stage III or IV encephalopathy); osmotic therapy for ICP $\geq$ 25 mm Hg using mannitol boluses; possible use of hypertonic saline to maintain high normal serum sodium levels (145–155 mmol/L); and broad-spectrum antibiotics if signs of systemic inflammatory response syndrome (SIRS) or worsening encephalopathy are present. Other recommendations were made for treatment of complications of ALF *(Stravitz, Kramer, & Davern, et al., 2007)*.
- Development of systemic inflammatory response syndrome (SIRS) in patients with fulminant hepatitis B accompanied by fulminant hepatic failure significantly worsens the patient's short-term prognosis and may require liver transplantation *(Miyake, Iwasaki, Terada et al., 2007)*.

SECTION FOUR REVIEW

1. Dietary management of the patient with acute viral hepatitis should include
   A. high protein, low fat
   B. low fat, high carbohydrate
   C. low carbohydrate, low fat
   D. low protein, high fat
2. A patient with acute viral hepatitis will most likely be admitted to the hospital if he or she experiences
   A. severe fatigue
   B. occasional nausea
   C. elevated bilirubin
   D. hepatic encephalopathy
3. The patient with acute hepatic failure will require strict nutritional control of
   A. protein
   B. fat
   C. carbohydrates
   D. fiber
4. The patient with acute hepatic failure would most likely receive which of the following continuous IV infusions based on altered glucose metabolism?
   A. lactated Ringer's
   B. 5 percent dextrose
   C. 10 percent dextrose
   D. normal saline
5. To correct bleeding in the patient with bleeding esophageal varices, the treatment of choice is
   A. sclerotherapy
   B. portosystemic shunt
   C. packed red blood cells
   D. Hespan
6. As a treatment for hepatic encephalopathy, intestinal bacteria levels are suppressed by
   A. lactulose
   B. neomycin
   C. tyrosine
   D. histamine antagonists
7. Acute hepatic failure is associated with development of hyponatremia, which is precipitated by (choose all that apply)
   A. hemodilution
   B. diuretic therapy
   C. sodium restriction
   D. hepatic cell damage

Answers: 1. B, 2. D, 3. A, 4. C, 5. A, 6. B, 7. (A, B, C)

SECTION FIVE: Nursing Implications

At the completion of this section, the learner will be able to describe the nursing implications appropriate to managing care of the patient experiencing acute hepatic dysfunction.

General Goals

Management of acute hepatic dysfunction, particularly during the most active disease stages, is collaborative. Evaluation of hepatic function is performed through laboratory testing and other diagnostic procedures (noninvasive and invasive), which typically require a physician's orders and diagnostic expertise. The two goals that drive the majority of management activities are

1. To determine and correct the underlying cause
2. To support the patient until liver function resumes or until the patient receives a liver transplant

Collaborative interventions to support the patient centers around two goals: (1) promoting stable hemodynamic and ventilatory status and (2) preventing or minimizing secondary complications.

The nurse plays a crucial role in improving patient outcomes by being responsible for bedside assessment and analysis of the patient's status on a continual basis. A major focus of the nursing assessment involves monitoring the patient for the signs and symptoms of multisystem complications. The nurse facilitates the medical diagnostic process by preparing the patient and family for procedures, assisting with procedures, and monitoring the patient's status during and after procedures. The nurse also develops nursing hypotheses and subsequent independent nursing diagnoses based on the patient's response to the illness, rather than the illness itself. The following section provides a description of that part of a comprehensive nursing history and physical assessment, which focuses specifically on hepatic function.

The Focused Nursing Database

On admission, it is crucial that the nurse obtain a comprehensive nursing database. The nurse particularly focuses on data that may have a positive or negative impact on patient outcomes.

The Focused Nursing History

General historical data the nurse should be sure to collect include preexisting medical conditions; surgeries; and recent history information, such as the events leading up to the patient's admission and a description of the patient's symptoms.

Focused Health Maintenance History

When obtaining the health maintenance portion of the history, the nurse should focus on obtaining information regarding

- Diet and eating patterns
- Usual appetite prior to admission
- Weight fluctuations
- History of skin or wound healing problems

Focused Cognitive–Perceptual History

Information regarding the patient's usual mental status, ability to communicate, and presence of discomfort or pain provides important baseline data.

Focused Value–Belief History

Acute hepatic dysfunction may place the patient at significant risk. Information regarding the value–belief patterns of the patient and family can assist the nurse with planning appropriate supportive interventions. Value-belief patterns focus on the philosophical positions held by the patient and family that are used to guide personal decisions and choices. Major concepts include spirituality and quality of life beliefs.

The Focused Nursing Assessment

Assessment of the patient with acute hepatic dysfunction has two major focuses: (1) monitoring for potential complications, a collaborative effort, and (2) monitoring the progress of the independent nursing diagnoses. The following sections present some of the major assessments that may be obtained on an ongoing basis during an acute hepatic dysfunction episode to monitor the patient for potential complications.

Respiratory/Circulatory Assessment

Hepatic failure can significantly alter cardiopulmonary function, primarily through severe third spacing of fluids with subsequent intravascular fluid volume deficit. The nurse must monitor the patient for

- Signs and symptoms of fluid volume deficit
- Edema, which may be peripheral or generalized, or may be present in the form of pulmonary edema
- Diminished or adventitious breath sounds (crackles, in particular)
- Abnormal trends in blood pressure and pulse

Elimination Assessment

The adequacy of renal function is closely monitored because of the risk for development of hepatorenal syndrome. This is accomplished through observation of ordered renal function laboratory tests (e.g., blood urea nitrogen [BUN], creatinine, and urine sodium) and evaluation of renal function by measuring intake and output balance and urinary output volume.

Neurologic Assessment

The patient's neurologic status requires close monitoring throughout the duration of the acute illness because hepatic failure can lead to hepatic encephalopathy and is also known to cause cerebral edema. The clinical manifestations of hepatic encephalopathy are described in Section Three and contributing factors are presented in Section Four. The neurologic assessment should minimally include the following

Focused Cognitive–Perceptual Assessment. The nurse assesses the patient's cognitive-perceptual status using

- **Glasgow Coma Scale (GCS).** The GCS is a useful trending tool that assesses the arousal component of consciousness. An altered level of consciousness is an early finding in hepatic encephalopathy. The GCS specifically addresses eye opening, verbal response, and motor response.

Focused Muscular–Skeletal Assessment. The nurse assesses the patient's

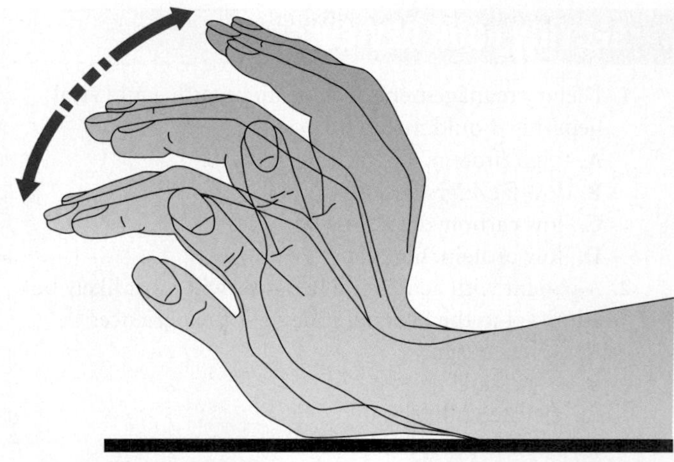

Figure 30–3 ■ Asterixis. Note the downward tremor of the hand on dorsiflexion of the wrist.

- **Coordination.** Coordination becomes increasingly impaired in the early stages of encephalopathy.
- **Reflexes.** Reflexes become hypoactive in the early stages of hepatic encephalopathy and hyperactive in the later stages.
- **Movement.** Asterixis (also called *liver flap* when associated with liver failure; see Fig. 30–3) refers to an involuntary tremor that is particularly noted in the hands but may also be seen in the feet and tongue. It becomes evident at stage II of hepatic encephalopathy.

Focused Neurosensory Assessment. The nurse assesses for the presence of

- **Seizures.** Seizures may develop in the later stages of hepatic encephalopathy.

Gastrointestinal and Integumentary Assessment

Hepatic dysfunction is associated with a variety of GI and integumentary clinical manifestations. The majority of the manifestations result from the accumulation of hepatotoxins, third-spaced body fluids, coagulopathies, decreased protein levels, and complications resulting from portal hypertension.

Focused GI Assessment. The nurse should assess for

- **Nausea and vomiting, anorexia**
- **Presence of diarrhea or constipation**
- **Ascites.** Enlarging abdominal girth; shifting dullness on percussion of the abdomen; abdominal fluid wave; protruding umbilicus. In addition, the patient may develop dyspnea, diminished breath sounds, or the clinical manifestations of fluid volume deficit.
- **Bleeding esophageal varices.** The nurse does not independently evaluate the patient for the existence of varices. Instead, the nurse monitors the patient for active variceal bleeding. This is most directly accomplished by assessing nasogastric fluids for blood. If blood is present, the assessment should also include the volume and characteristics of the blood, as well as close assessment for development of the signs and symptoms of hypovolemic shock.
- **Hepatic tenderness and enlargement on palpation**

Focused Integumentary Assessment. The nurse should assess for

- Jaundice
- Pruritus
- Edema
- Dry, flaky skin
- Poor skin turgor
- Caput medusa (visible veins over the umbilical area caused by congestion and dilation of superficial abdominal wall veins associated with portal vein obstruction)

In addition, the skin can be assessed for several clinical manifestations of problems with coagulation, bleeding, and diminished proteins that usually occur with severe hepatic dysfunction, including

- Evidence of poor wound healing
- Ecchymosis or petechiae
- Bleeding gums
- Pale mucous membranes and nail beds

The Nursing Care Plan

The nursing care plan of the patient experiencing an acute hepatic dysfunction episode usually includes both collaborative problems and independent nursing diagnoses.

Frequently Occurring Collaborative Problems

The following potential complications are commonly associated with hepatic dysfunction (Martin & Hassanein, 2009)

- Hemorrhage (bleeding)
- Metabolic disorders
- Malnutrition
- Drug toxicity
- Renal insufficiency
- Progressive liver degeneration
- Portal hypertension
- Hepatic encephalopathy
- Systemic inflammatory response syndrome
- Infection
- Cerebral edema and herniation

Frequently Occurring Nursing Diagnoses

On completion of the nursing database, the nurse clusters data and develops a set of nursing hypotheses based on the available data. Additional critical data that may either support or eliminate each hypothesis should also be identified and obtained. Once the hypotheses have been established, the nurse is ready to develop a list of nursing diagnoses.

For the patient with acute hepatic dysfunction, a variety of nursing diagnoses frequently occur during the crisis period. The following is a partial list of some of these frequently occurring nursing diagnoses (LeMone, 2008)

- *Ineffective breathing pattern* related to pressure on diaphragm from ascites, weakness, pleural effusion, and thought processes impairment from ammonia toxins
- *Fluid volume deficit* related to reduced intravascular volume, variceal bleeding, and coagulopathy
- *Activity intolerance* related to decreased energy secondary to impaired liver metabolism, tissue hypoxia, and decreased nutritional intake
- *Altered nutrition: Less than body requirements* related to impairment of nutrient absorption and metabolism, decreased nutritional intake, and fat-soluble vitamin malabsorption
- *Altered comfort* related to pruritus secondary to buildup of bile salts and bilirubin pigment
- *Pain: Upper abdominal* related to ascites and enlarged liver
- *Altered thought processes* related to impaired clearance of drugs and ammonia, bleeding, and dehydration
- *High risk for infection* related to leukopenia secondary to hypoproteinemia; and splenic hyperactivity

The box NURSING CARE: The Patient with Hepatic Failure provides a summary of the nursing management.

NURSING CARE: The Patient with Hepatic Failure

Expected Patient Outcomes and Related Interventions

Outcome 1: No evidence of hepatic encephalopathy

Assess and compare to established norms, patient baselines, and trends.

Monitor patient for signs and symptoms of hepatic encephalopathy.

Neurological status: altered mental status, lethargy, drowsiness, abnormal reflexes, asterixis, abnormal posturing, seizures (see Table 30–6 *Stages of Hepatic Encephalopathy,* for detailed information).

Nausea and vomiting

Monitor the results of ordered laboratory tests and report increasingly abnormal trends.

Serum ammonia

Institute measures to reduce serum ammonia levels.

Reduce dietary protein to reduce formation of ammonia.

Nasogastric tube

Administer related drug therapy and monitor for therapeutic and nontherapeutic effects.

Antibiotics to destroy intestinal ammonia-producing bacteria

Lactulose to increase ammonia excretion through the bowel

Related nursing diagnoses

Altered thought processes

Potential for injury

Sensory-perceptual alterations

(*continued*)

NURSING CARE (continued)

Outcome 2: Absence of active bleeding

Assess and compare to established norms, patient baselines, and trends.

Monitor patient for signs and symptoms of bleeding.

Hematemesis, hematochezia

Positive hemoccult test (gastric contents, stool)

Vital signs: increasing or decreasing BP, increasing heart rate

Hemodynamic instability

Monitor the results of ordered laboratory tests and report increasingly abnormal trends.

Hemoglobin and hematocrit

RBC count

PT, PTT, INR

Institute measures to prevent or control bleeding.

Institute bleeding precautions.

Administer related drug therapy and monitor for therapeutic and nontherapeutic effects.

Vitamin K to reverse coagulopathy

IV Vasopressin to stop esophageal bleeding

Related nursing diagnoses

Activity intolerance

Altered tissue perfusion

Decreased cardiac output

Alteration in fluid volume: Deficit

Outcome 3: Improved hepatic function

Assess and compare to established norms, patient baselines, and trends.

Monitor: abdominal girth measurements, jaundice, generalized edema, pruritus

Monitor nutritional status: hypoglycemia, nausea and vomiting, anorexia, constipation or diarrhea, caloric intake

Monitor the results of ordered laboratory tests and report increasingly abnormal trends.

Liver function tests (LFT) including: AST, ALT, alk phos, bilirubin, albumin, LDH, GGT, total protein

Serum or fingerstick glucose

Institute measures to improve liver function.

Nutrition consult

Supportive care

Administer related drug therapy and monitor for therapeutic and nontherapeutic effects.

See RELATED PHARMACOTHERAPY box

Related nursing diagnoses

Alteration in nutrition: less than body requirements

Altered bowel elimination

Alteration in fluid volume: deficit

Outcome 4: Maintains normal renal function

Assess and compare to established norms, patient baselines, and trends.

Monitor patient's renal status: BUN, creatinine, potassium, sodium.

Intake and output[10] notify provider if output less than 0.5 ml/kg/hour.

Institute measures to improve renal function.

Administer intravenous fluids, vasopressor, and oncotic agents.

Administer related drug therapy and monitor for therapeutic and nontherapeutic effects.

See RELATED PHARMACOTHERAPY box

Related nursing diagnoses

Alteration in fluid volume: excess

SECTION FIVE REVIEW

1. A major underlying goal that drives the majority of medical management activities is to
- **A.** promote stable hemodynamic status
- **B.** prevent secondary complications
- **C.** promote stable ventilatory status
- **D.** support the patient until liver function returns

2. Leukopenia secondary to hypoproteinemia and splenic hyperactivity places the patient with acute liver failure for which of the following nursing diagnosis?
- **A.** altered thought processes
- **B.** altered bowel elimination
- **C.** activity intolerance
- **D.** high risk for infection

3. The presence of asterixis indicates that ______ is/are present.
- **A.** involuntary tremor
- **B.** loss of coordination
- **C.** focal seizures
- **D.** skeletal muscle rigidity

4. The nurse notes the presence of ascites. Assessments for the presence of ascites include (choose all that apply)
- **A.** abdominal fluid waves
- **B.** retracting umbilicus
- **C.** shifting abdominal dullness
- **D.** enlarging abdominal girth

5. Dermatologic findings commonly noted in the patient with acute hepatic dysfunction include
- **A.** oily skin
- **B.** generalized rash
- **C.** pruritus
- **D.** shiny skin

Answers: 1. D, 2. D, 3. A, 4. (A, C, D), 5. C

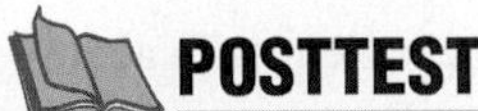

POSTTEST

The following Posttest is constructed in a case study format. Questions are asked based on available data. New data are presented as the case study progresses.

Jerome J., 32-years-old, was admitted seven days ago with a severe drug overdose of acetaminophen. He has been in the medical intensive care unit since admission. Jerome's Glasgow Coma Scale peaked at 15 and during the past 24 hours has steadily decreased. The nurse notifies the physician of the change in neurologic status. Based on their assessment, the medical team suspects liver dysfunction. Jerome has serum enzymes ordered. The results are as follows

ALT = 1,500 units/L
AST = 1,500 units/L
Alk Phos = 140 units/L

1. Jerome's serum enzyme levels indicate that ______ is present.
   A. hepatorenal syndrome
   B. encephalopathy
   C. severe hepatocellular injury
   D. severe cellular injury
2. The physician orders alkaline phosphatase (Alk Phos) isoenzymes for Jerome. Which Alk Phos isoenzyme is considered most hepatobiliary specific?
   A. 5'-nucleotidase
   B. gamma glutamyl transferase (GGT)
   C. ornithine carbamoyl transferase (OCT)
   D. lactic dehydrogenase (LDH) isoenzymes 4 and 5

The nurse notes that Jerome's urine has become dark amber. The quantity was 150 mL in the past hour.

3. Based on the early diagnosis of an acute hepatic dysfunction, the color of Jerome's urine suggests that the nurse can expect
   A. ammonia to decrease
   B. low serum proteins
   C. acute renal failure
   D. jaundice to develop
4. If Jerome is diagnosed as having acute hepatitis, initially he will most likely receive ______ therapy.
   A. antibiotic
   B. antiviral
   C. antifungal
   D. no specific
5. Which type of viral hepatitis is a major cause of chronic hepatitis, cirrhosis, and hepatocellular carcinoma?
   A. hepatitis A
   B. hepatitis B
   C. hepatitis C
   D. hepatitis D
6. If Jerome develops mild hepatic enlargement and edema, with generalized inflammation but localized necrosis, it would be classified as ______ hepatitis.
   A. classic
   B. submassive
   C. massive
   D. anicteric
7. If he has developed cholestatic hepatitis, you would anticipate assessing for
   A. the absence of jaundice
   B. the presence of gallstones
   C. severe jaundice
   D. an inflamed gallbladder
8. Typical prodromal symptoms of the patient developing acute hepatitis include (choose all that apply)
   A. high fever
   B. increased intracranial pressure
   C. nausea and vomiting
   D. arthritis and myalgia
9. If Jerome had developed stage III encephalopathy, you would anticipate a neurologic presentation to include
   A. restlessness, reversal of sleep rhythm
   B. lethargy, drowsiness
   C. disorientation, asterixis
   D. stupor, hyperactive reflexes
10. Based on Jerome's history, he is at risk for developing fulminant hepatic failure based on which cause?
    A. hepatotoxin ingestion
    B. hepatitis virus
    C. multiple organ failure
    D. complication of chronic failure
11. Jerome has no preexisting history of hepatic dysfunction. It is unlikely that he will develop
    A. acute renal failure
    B. esophageal varices
    C. sepsis
    D. acid–base disorders
12. If he develops spontaneous bacterial peritonitis, it is probably caused by
    A. septicemia
    B. translocation of intestinal bacteria
    C. spread of hepatic infective agent
    D. autoimmune reaction
13. Jerome's encephalopathy is worsening. The nurse notes that he has not had a bowel movement in three days. What physician order can the nurse anticipate?
    A. increase dietary protein
    B. neomycin one to two times per day
    C. daily milk of magnesia
    D. lactulose every hour until desired effect
14. The majority of patients experiencing fulminant hepatic failure ultimately require which intervention?
    A. liver transplantation
    B. portosystemic shunt
    C. sclerotherapy
    D. Sengstaken–Blakemore tube
15. The majority of Jerome's plan of care will focus on which underlying goal?
    A. evaluation of renal function
    B. promotion of stable hemodynamic status
    C. support for the patient until liver function resumes
    D. prevention of secondary complications

16. While assessing his integumentary status, the nurse notes visible veins over the umbilical area. In a patient with hepatic dysfunction, this finding is called
A. asterixis
B. ecchymosis
C. ascites
D. caput medusa

17. Based on the typical fluid status of the patient with acute hepatic dysfunction, the most appropriate nursing diagnosis to be added to Jerome's plan of care would be
A. fluid volume deficit
B. fluid volume excess
C. cardiac output: decreased
D. nutrition: more than body requirements

Posttest answers with rationale are found on MyNursingKit.

REFERENCES

Argueda, M. R. & Fallon, M. B. (2007). Cirrhosis of the liver and its complications. In T. E. Andreoli, C. C. J. Carpenter, R. C. Griggs, & J. Loscalzo (eds.), *Cecil essentials of medicine,* (7th ed.). Philadelphia: W. B. Saunders, 454–463.

Abou-Assi, S., & Vlahcevic, Z. R. (2001). Hepatic encephalopathy: Metabolic consequences of cirrhosis often is reversible. *Postgraduate Medicine, 109*(2), 52–70.

Arroyo, V., Guevara, M., & Gines, P. (2002). Hepatorenal syndrome in cirrhosis: pathogenesis and treatment. *Gastroenterology, 122*(6), 1658–1676.

Bataller, R. & Gines, P. (2007). Cirrhosis of the liver. In D. C. Dale & D. D. Federman (eds.), *ACP medicine.* New York: Webmd Corporation.

Cardenas, A. (2005). Hepatorenal syndrome: a dreaded complication of end-stage liver disease. *American Journal of Gastroenterology, 100*:2 460–467.

CDC (Centers for Disease Control). (2006). *Hepatitis C statistics.* Retrieved March 1, 2008 from http://www.cdc.gov/ncidod/diseases/hepatitis/c/fact.htm.

Deinsteig, J. L., (2008). Acute viral hepatitis. In E. Braunwald, A. S. Fauci, D. L.

Kasper, S. T. Hauser, D. L. Longo, & J. L. Jameson (eds.), *Harrison's principles of internal medicine* (18th ed.). New York: McGraw Hill, 1932–1948.

Fitz, J. G. (2006). Hepatic encephalopathy, hepatopulmonary syndromes, hepatorenal syndrome, coagulopathy, and endocrine complications of liver disease. In M. Feldman, L. S. Friedman, M. H. Sleisenger, & B. F. Scharschmidt (eds.), *Sleisenger and Fordtran's gastrointestinal and liver disease: pathophysiology, diagnosis, and management* (8th ed.). Philadelphia: W. B. Saunders, 1966–1986.

Garcia-Tsao, G. (2007). Cirrhosis and its sequelae. In L. Goldman & D. Auseillo (eds.), *Cecil Medicine* (23rd ed.). Philadelphia: Saunders Elsevier, chapter 157.

Ghany, M., & Hoofnagle, J. H. (2008). Approach to the patient with liver disease. In E. Braunwald, A. S. Fauci, D. L. Hauser, S. L. Kasper, S. T. Hauser, D. L. Longo, J. L. Jameson, & Loscalzo, J. (eds.), *Harrison's principles of internal medicine* (17th ed) New York: McGraw Hill, 1918–1922.

Goldberg, E. & Chopra, S. (2008). Overview of the treatment of fulminant hepatic failure. Retrieved March 1, 2008 from Up To Date http://www.uptodate.com/online/content/topic.do?topicKey=hep_dis/13101&view=print.

Kauch, A. M. (2009). *Lippincott nursing drug guide.* Philadelphia: Lippincott Williams & Wilkins.

Kee, J. (2009). *Prentice Hall handbook of laboratory and diagnostic tests* (6th ed.). Upper Saddle River, NJ: Prentice Hall.

Marreno, J., Martinez, F., & Hyzy, R. (2003). Advances in critical care hepatology. *American Journal of Critical Care Medicine, 168*: 1421–1426.

Martin, R. K., & Hassanein, T. (2009). Liver dysfunction and failure. In K. K. Carlson (ed.). *American Association of Critical-Care Nurses Advanced Critical Care Nursing.* St. Louis: Saunders Elsevier, 766.

Roth-Kauffman, M. M. (2008). Hepatitis C infection. *Clinician Reviews, 18*(6): 18–23.

Shah, V. H & Kanam, P. S. (2006). Portal hypertension and variceal bleeding. In M. Feldman, L. S. Friedman, M. H. Sleisenger, & B. F. Scharschmidt (eds.), *Sleisenger and Fordtran's gastrointestinal and liver disease: pathophysiology, diagnosis, and management* (8th ed.). Philadelphia: W. B. Saunders, 1899–1927.

Shawcross, D., & Jalan, D. (2005). Dispelling myths in the treatment of hepatic encephalopathy. *Lancet, 365*(9457): 431–433.

Sherman, C. (2008). Staying up to date on managing hepatitis B. *The Clinical Advisor 11* (5): 17–20.

Sjögren, M. H. (2006). Hepatitis A. In M. Feldman, L. S. Friedman, M. H. Sleisenger, & B. F. Scharschmidt (eds.). *Sleisenger and Fordtran's gastrointestinal and liver disease: pathophysiology, diagnosis, and management* (8th ed.). Philadelphia: W.B. Saunders, 1639–1644.

Sood, G. (2008). Acute liver failure. *eMedicine from WebMD.* Retrieved March 7, 2009 from http://emedicine.medscape.com/article/177354-overview.

Tsai, M., Chen, Y., Lien, J., Tian, Y., Peng, Y., Fang, J., Yang, C., Tang, J., Chu, Y., Chen, P., & Wu, C. (2008). Hemodynamics and metabolic studies on septic shock in patients with acute liver failure. *J CRIT CARE, 23*(4), 468–472.

Vargas, H. I. (2008). Hepatobiliary disease. In F. S. Bongard & D. Y. Sue (eds.), *Current critical care diagnosis and treatment* (3rd ed.). New York: McGraw Hill, 714–723.

Wilson, B., Shannon, M., Shields, K., & Stang, C. (2008). *Prentice Hall nurse's drug guide: 2008.* Upper Saddle River, NJ: Pearson/Prentice Hall.

MODULE

31 Alterations in Pancreatic Function

Zara R. Brenner, Maureen E. Krenzer, Melanie G. Hardin-Pierce

OBJECTIVES Following completion of this module, the learner will be able to

1. Describe the pathophysiologic basis of acute pancreatic dysfunction.
2. Describe medical data used in the diagnosis of acute pancreatic dysfunction.
3. Discuss assessment of the patient with acute pancreatic dysfunction.
4. Explain the complications of acute pancreatitis.
5. Describe the medical management of a patient with acute pancreatitis.
6. Discuss the nursing management for a patient with acute pancreatic dysfunction.

This self-study module focuses on assessment and management of concepts related to the patient with a disruption of normal exocrine pancreatic function. Disruption of normal endocrine pancreatic function is presented in Module 34, Alterations in Glucose Metabolism. The normal anatomy and physiology of the endocrine pancreas is detailed in Module 28, Determinants and Assessment of Gastrointestinal, Hepatic, and Pancreatic Function. It is recommended that normal function be reviewed prior to completing this module. This module is divided into six sections. Section One describes the pathophysiologic basis of pancreatic dysfunction, including etiologic factors. Section Two describes laboratory tests and diagnostic procedures used to diagnose acute pancreatitis. Section Three discusses the nursing assessment of a patient with acute pancreatitis. Section Four offers a brief overview of the major complications associated with acute pancreatitis, and Section Five describes the medical management of a patient with acute pancreatitis. The module closes with Section Six, which presents the nursing management of the patient with acute pancreatitis. Each section includes a set of review questions to help the learner evaluate his or her understanding of the section's content before moving on to the next section. All Section Reviews include answers. It is suggested that the learner review those concepts answered incorrectly in the review questions before proceeding to the next section.

PRETEST

1. Acute pancreatitis is the result of a viral infection.
   A. true
   B. false
2. The primary pathophysiological event that occurs with acute pancreatitis is
   A. hemorrhage
   B. edema
   C. autodigestion
   D. pain
3. Alcohol has which of the following effects on the pancreas?
   A. decreases enzyme secretion
   B. depresses secretion of secretin
   C. inhibits the inflammatory response
   D. causes spasm of the sphincter of Oddi
4. The primary laboratory test used to help make a diagnosis of pancreatitis is serum
   A. amylase and lipase
   B. calcium and magnesium
   C. lactic dehydrogenase (LDH)
   D. elastase and glucose
5. The typical pain associated with acute pancreatitis is characterized as (choose all that apply)
   A. severe
   B. relieved by vomiting
   C. radiating to the back
   D. continuous
6. Shock associated with acute pancreatitis can be caused by (choose all that apply)
   A. necrosis
   B. vasodilation
   C. hemorrhage
   D. third spacing
7. Hypocalcemia is primarily attributed to which of the following pancreatic enzymes?
   A. trypsin
   B. elastase

C. amylase
D. lipase

8. The result of a ruptured pancreatic pseudocyst is
A. peritonitis
B. acute renal failure
C. paralytic ileus
D. septicemia

9. Myocardial depressant factor
A. decreases heart rate
B. decreases cardiac output
C. increases blood pressure
D. increases cardiac output

10. Clinical findings consistent with "peritoneal signs" include (choose all that apply)
A. rebound tenderness
B. rigid abdomen
C. hyperactive bowel sounds
D. leukocytosis

11. Cullen's sign may be noted under which circumstances?
A. acute tubular necrosis (ATN)
B. hemorrhage
C. hypovolemic shock
D. respiratory failure

12. The highest priority in the management of the patient with severe acute pancreatitis is to
A. control pain
B. correct the underlying problem
C. minimize pancreatic stimulation
D. stabilize the hemodynamic status

13. The drug of choice in pain management of the patient with acute pancreatitis is
A. morphine sulfate
B. codeine
C. meperidine (Demerol)
D. ibuprofen

Pretest answers are found on MyNursingKit.

SECTION ONE: Pathophysiologic Basis of Acute Pancreatitis

At the completion of this section, the learner will be able to describe the pathophysiologic basis of acute pancreatitis.

The pancreas is a long, narrow organ located behind the stomach in the upper abdominal cavity. It is unique in that it is actually two organs in one: an exocrine organ secreting powerful digestive enzymes and an endocrine organ producing insulin and glucagon for regulation of glucose. The focus of this module is on the exocrine pancreas and its major pathophysiologic process, acute pancreatitis. Figure 31–1 shows the location of the pancreas with its close proximity to the biliary system. Note that the common bile duct that drains bile from the liver and gallbladder joins with the

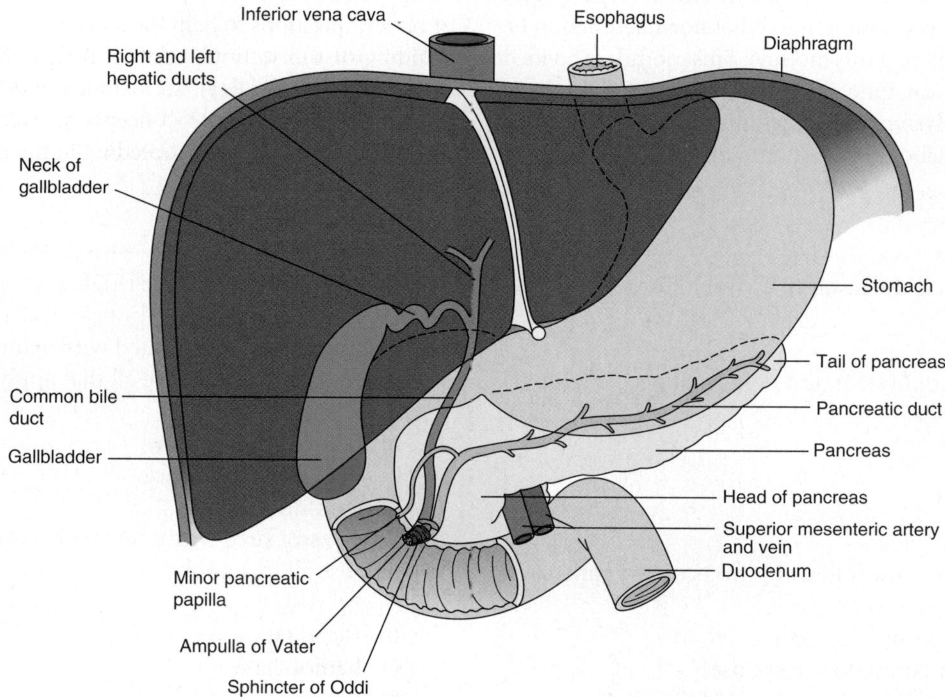

Figure 31–1 ■ The pancreas and pancreaticobiliary system. The head of the pancreas is nestled behind the stomach and adjoins the curve of the duodenum near the pyloric sphincter. The common bile duct draining bile from the gallbladder joins with the pancreatic duct to become the ampulla of Vater which then drains into the intestine through the sphincter of Oddi. Copstead & Banasik (2005). *Pathophysiology, 3e.* St. Louis: Elsevier.

terminal end of the main pancreatic duct to form the ampulla of Vater that empties into the duodenum through the sphincter of Oddi. The common bile duct is an important factor in development of acute pancreatitis.

Pancreatitis is inflammation of the pancreas, which results in autodigestion of the pancreas. It can occur either as an acute or chronic condition. In acute pancreatitis there is a sudden onset of pancreatic inflammation, which progresses to a generalized systemic inflammatory response (SIRS) (Browne, 2006). Acute pancreatitis is characterized by varying degrees of abdominal pain, pancreatic tissue edema, necrosis of pancreatic tissue and, possibly, hemorrhage. The reported incidence worldwide ranges from 5 to 80 persons per 100,000 per year (Sekimoto et al., 2006).

The severity of acute pancreatitis ranges from mild to severe; however, the majority of patients (80 to 90 percent) develop a mild form called interstitial or edematous pancreatitis (Banks et al., 2006; Elfar et al., 2007). In mild acute pancreatitis, there are areas of fat necrosis in and around the pancreas accompanied by interstitial edema and is usually self-limited, resolving within five to seven days. The more severe form of acute pancreatitis, called necrotizing or hemorrhagic pancreatitis (see Fig. 31–2), involves extensive necrosis in and around the pancreas, pancreatic cellular necrosis, and hemorrhage within the pancreas. Severe pancreatitis is associated with local and systemic complications. The mortality rate associated with severe acute pancreatitis is 2.1 to 7.8 percent, which rises to 25 to 30 percent when complications and/or comorbidities are present (Sekimoto et al., 2006). Table 31–1 lists the characteristics of nonhemorrhagic and hemorrhagic acute pancreatitis.

TABLE 31–1 Characteristics of Nonhemorrhagic and Hemorrhagic Acute Pancreatitis

NONHEMORRHAGIC (INTERSTITIAL)	SEVERE HEMORRHAGIC (NECROTIZING)
▪ Short term	▪ Longer duration
▪ Pancreatic edema and swelling	▪ Pancreatic hemorrhage
▪ Little to no necrosis	▪ Extensive fat and tissue necrosis
▪ Localized inflammation	▪ Extrapancreatic invasion of pancreatic enzymes
▪ Reversible	▪ Irreversible damage to pancreas and surrounding tissues
▪ Good prognosis	▪ Poor prognosis—associated with sepsis and multiple organ dysfunction

Etiologies

There are multiple causes of acute pancreatitis. In the United States gallstones and chronic alcohol abuse account for approximately 80-90 percent of cases (Amerine, 2007; Elfar et al., 2007). Gallstone-induced pancreatitis is more common in women and alcohol-induced acute pancreatitis is more common in men. Gallstone-induced pancreatitis is caused by obstruction of the common bile duct by a lodged gallstone. The obstructing gallstone can either obstruct outflow of enzymes from the pancreatic duct or it can cause reflux of bile into the pancreatic duct. Either mechanism is believed to increase pancreatic ductal pressure and permeability with resultant premature activation of pancreatic enzymes (Elfar et al., 2007). Alcohol may induce acute pancreatitis by several mechanisms, including triggering spasms of the sphincter of Oddi resulting in transient obstruction; changing the composition of pancreatic secretions causing the formation of plugs within the pancreas; triggering hyperresponsiveness of monocytes which contributes to increased inflammation; and direct injury to the acinar cells by the alcohol or its metabolites (Szabo et al., 2007).

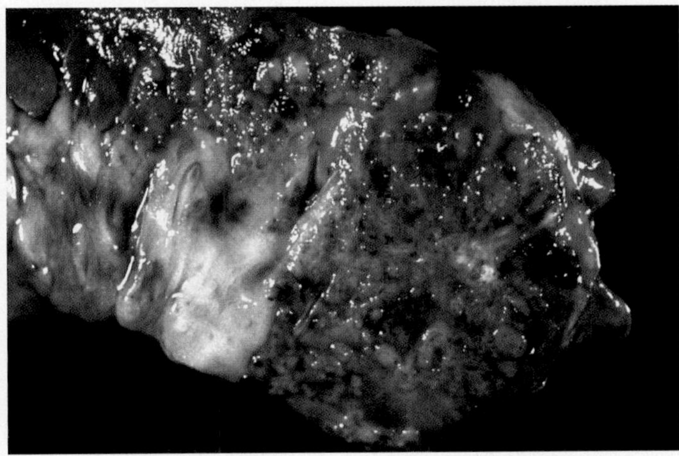

Figure 31–2 ▪ In acute pancreatitis, the pancreas appears edematous and is commonly hemorrhagic. Photo Researchers, Inc.

Medications may induce acute pancreatitis. Hypercalcemia and hypertriglyceridemia are metabolic causes of acute pancreatitis. Idiopathic pancreatitis may develop during pregnancy, administration of total parenteral nutrition, or following major surgery. Acute pancreatitis is one of the major complications of AIDS. Endoscopic manipulation of the ampulla of Vater such as may occur during ERCP (endoscopic retrograde cholangiopancreatography) or EST (endoscopic sphincterotomy) or abdominal trauma may also precipitate acute pancreatitis. Numerous genetic mutations have been identified as causing premature activation of pancreatic precursors (Elfar et al., 2007). Table 31–2 lists the major causes of acute pancreatitis.

TABLE 31–2 Major Causes of Acute Pancreatitis

Alcohol abuse
Biliary disease: Gallstones, microlithiasis, or biliary sludge; common bile duct obstruction
Drugs: Azathioprine, 6-Mercaptopurine, didanosine, dideoxyinosine, ACE-inhibitors, estrogen, furosemide, pantamide, procainamide, sulfonamides, tetracycline, thiazide diuretics, valproic acid, L-asparaginase, salicylates
Hypercalcemia
Hypertriglyceridemia (>1000 mg/dl)
Idiopathic
Infection
 Viral: mumps, coxsackievirus, cytomegalovirus (CMV), HAV, HBV, HIV/AIDS
 Bacterial: *mycoplasma, legionella, salmonella*
 Fungal: *aspergillus, candida albicans*
 Parasitic: *toxoplasma, cryptosporidium*
Inflammatory bowel disease
Pancreas divisum
Peptic ulcer disease
Trauma: blunt or penetrating abdominal trauma; post-ERCP; surgical trauma
Toxins

Pathophysiology

Acute pancreatitis is an inflammatory disease with micro- and macrovascular failure (Cuthbertson & Christophi, 2006). Acute pancreatitis occurs in three stages. First, **trypsin** and other enzymes in the pancreas are prematurely activated. Second is intrapancreatic inflammation. The third phase, extrapancreatic/systemic injury occurs (Banks et al., 2006; Browne, 2006). Regardless of the cause, acute pancreatitis develops when pancreatic enzymes, first trypsin and then the others, become prematurely activated by diverse stimuli within the pancreas. (Banks et al., 2006) This premature activation results in **autodigestion** of the pancreas and surrounding (peripancreatic) tissues. Pathogenesis includes excessive leukocyte stimulation, microcirculatory disorders, gut endothelial barrier dysfunction, bacterial translocation and/or acinar cell necrosis and apoptosis (Liu & Xia, 2006). Intrapancreatic release of trypsin promotes further release of trypsin and activation of the precursors to phospholipase A, elastase, and carboxypeptidase into active enzymes. **Phospholipase A** digests phospholipids on the cell membranes, and **elastase** digests the elastic tissue of vessel walls. As vessel walls sustain increasing damage, both capillary and lymphatic vessels become injured, which results in hemorrhage and edema, respectively. As the damage progresses, more acini are triggered to activate and secrete their digestive enzymes, which further increases autodigestive activities.

As a part of the inflammatory process, kallikrein is activated by trypsin. **Kallikrein** is a basophil mediator of inflammation. It is responsible for causing bradykinin formation. Kallikrein causes vasodilation and increases permeability of blood vessels, pain, and leukocyte invasion. Once kallikrein has been activated, systemic hypotension may lead to shock and multiple organ failure (such as acute respiratory distress syndrome and acute renal failure). Thus, the initial local insult of acute pancreatitis may become a complex multisystem dysfunction disease process.

SECTION ONE REVIEW

1. A common cause of acute pancreatitis is
   A. chronic alcohol abuse
   B. steroid therapy
   C. vascular disease
   D. viral infections
2. Regardless of the etiology of acute pancreatitis, the primary physiologic event is
   A. hemorrhage
   B. edema
   C. autodigestion
   D. pain
3. Premature activation of the pancreatic enzymes ______ and ______ is thought to cause the most pancreatic damage.
   A. trypsin, amylas
   B. lipase, chymotrypsin
   C. phospholipase A, elastase
   D. elastase, amylase
4. Obstruction by gallstones is most commonly seen in which patient population?
   A. persons with diabetes
   B. alcoholic men
   C. those ages 30 to 40
   D. obese women
5. Alcohol affects the pancreas by
   A. decreasing enzyme secretion
   B. depressing secretion of secretin
   C. inhibiting the inflammatory response
   D. causing spasm of sphincter of Oddi

Answers: 1. A, 2. C, 3. C, 4. D, 5. D

SECTION TWO: Diagnosing Acute Pancreatitis

At the completion of this section, the learner will be able to describe medical data used in the diagnosis of acute pancreatitis.

The initial clinical presentation of the patient with acute pancreatitis is similar to that of a variety of other acute abdominal disorders. Diagnosing acute pancreatitis requires data from multiple sources, including laboratory tests and other diagnostic procedures. In addition, the patient history and physical assessment provide valuable information that will support or help rule out a diagnosis of acute pancreatitis. The nursing history and assessment are presented in Section Five of this module.

Generally a diagnosis of acute pancreatitis requires at least two of the following three features: 1) abdominal pain characteristic of acute pancreatitis, 2) serum amylase and /or lipase greater than three times the upper limit of normal, and 3) characteristic findings of acute pancreatitis on computed tomography (CT) scan preferably intravenous contrast enhanced (Banks et al., 2006; AGA Institute, 2007).

Laboratory Assessment of Acute Pancreatitis

Laboratory testing is an important part of monitoring a patient for the development or progression of acute pancreatitis. Enzymes produced by the pancreas escape into the serum and urine when there is damage to the pancreatic parenchyma. The trends in pancreatic enzyme values are closely evaluated as an indication of disease progress. A variety of other laboratory tests may be ordered to further evaluate the pancreatitis as well as the status of any multisystem involvement. A brief description of important laboratory assessments follows.

Pancreatic Enzyme Levels

Measurement of pancreatic enzyme levels is usually obtained from the serum and urine. Cellular enzymes leak into the blood when pancreatic tissue is injured, thereby increasing serum enzyme levels. The most commonly measured pancreatic enzymes are serum **amylase** and **lipase.**

Serum amylase levels rise within 2 to 12 hours in the course of acute pancreatitis and can return to normal within as little as 36 hours (Despins et al., 2005). Serum amylase can increase for a variety of reasons because the enzyme is nonspecific to the pancreas. Altered serum amylase levels, therefore, are examined in the context of other supportive clinical data. Amylase is secreted from both the salivary glands and pancreas, each with a distinct isoenzyme. Measurement of amylase isoenzyme P (P refers to pancreatic) is useful in ruling out nonpancreatic elevations in serum amylase.

Serum lipase level is considered the best pancreatic enzyme parameter (Koizumi et al., 2006). Serum lipase levels rise later than amylase and remain elevated for approximately one to two weeks after serum amylase returns to normal (Despins et al., 2005). Measuring lipase levels provides a longer period for trending values than that provided by serum amylase levels. Serum lipase levels can be elevated by use of opioids or consumption of food within eight hours before the serum level is drawn (Pagana & Pagana, 2007). Elevation of blood amylase and lipase concentration does not necessarily reflect the severity of pancreatitis (Hirota et al., 2006).

An ALT level greater than three times the upper limit of normal has a positive predictive value for acute gallstone pancreatitis (Banks et al., 2006).

Other Laboratory Tests

A variety of laboratory tests may be helpful in evaluating acute pancreatitis and multisystem involvement, particularly the liver and gallbladder. Table 31–3 summarizes some of the major

TABLE 31–3 Differential Laboratory Diagnosis of Acute Pancreatitis

LABORATORY TEST	NORMAL VALUES[a]	TRENDS	TREND VALUES	COMMENTS
Serum				
Amylase	60-120 U/L	↑ ↑	> 500 U/L	Peaks 2–12 hours post onset; may remain elevated 3–5 days; level does not correlate well with severity
Isoamylase P (pancreatic)	30–55%	↑	> 55%	Isoenzyme that is specific to pancreas
Lipase	0-160 U/L	Rapid ↑	> 280 U/L	May remain elevated after amylase returns to normal
Glucose	70–110 mg/dL	Transient ↑	> 180 mg/dL	Secondary to islet cell malfunction; criteria used in absence of preexisting history of hyperglycemia
Calcium	9–10.5 mg/dL	↓	< 7.5 mg/dL	Due to saponification[b] of fat; also attributed to hypoalbuminemia (decreased availability of protein for calcium binding) due to malnutrition especially in alcoholics
White blood cell count	5,000–10,000/mL	↑	> 15,000/mL	Secondary to inflammatory process
Blood urea nitrogen	10–20 mg/dL	↑	> 45 mg/dL	Level remains elevated following correction of fluid volume deficit
Direct bilirubin (posthepatic)	0.1–0.3 mg/dL	↑	> 0.3 mg/dL	Associated with biliary obstruction
LDH	100–190 U/L	↑	> 350 U/L	Associated with biliary obstruction and pancreatitis; LDH4 isoenzyme is found in pancreas and other organs
Serum C-reactive protein	< 1.0 mg/dl or < 10.0 mg/L	↑	>150mg/L at 48 hours	Protein values are useful for severity assessment but may not be reflective within the first 48 to 72 hours
Hematocrit	Male 42–52% Female 37–47%	↑	> 47% on admission or no improvement within first 24 hours	Hemoconcentration caused by dehydration may indicate possible pancreatic necrosis
AST (SGOT)	0–35 U/mL	↑ ↑	> 250 U/mL	May see transient rise in acute pancreatitis; in acute extrahepatic obstruction AST rises quickly to 10 times normal then falls quickly
Serum albumin	3.5–5.0 g/dL	↓	< 3.2 g/dL	Associated with protein deficiency
Pao_2	80–100 mm Hg	↓	< 60 mm Hg	Associated with pulmonary involvement
Stool				
Fat	2–6 g/24 hr	—	> 6 g/24 hr	Steatorrhea; stool is pale or gray, smells foul; caused by deficiency in pancreatic enzymes in bowel

[a]Values may vary slightly according to the laboratory performing the test
[b]Conversion of fat into a soap
Source All normal values are from Pagana, K.D. & Pagana, T.J. (2007). *Mosby's diagnostic and laboratory test reference,* (8th ed.). Philadelphia, PA: Mosby Elsevier. Other sources: Hirota et al., (2006) and Banks et al., (2006).

laboratory tests used in making a differential diagnosis of acute pancreatitis.

Diagnostic Tests

Diagnosis of acute pancreatitis requires data from a variety of sources. Frequently ordered major diagnostic tests include abdominal X-rays, ultrasound, CT scan, endoscopic retrograde cholangiopancreatography (ERCP), magnetic resonance cholangiopancreatography (MRCP), and aspiration biopsy.

Abdominal and Chest Radiography

Radiographs of the abdomen and chest are used to exclude intestinal ileus, perforation, pericardial effusion, and pulmonary disease as causes of abdominal pain. The abdominal radiograph may be used initially as a quick means of revealing abdominal distention as well as gross abdominal abnormalities, such as an ileus. It is limited in its usefulness as a tool for diagnosing organ disorders. Chest films are valuable in revealing pulmonary complications associated with acute pancreatitis, such as atelectasis and pleural effusion.

CT Scan and Ultrasound

A CT scan confirms diagnosis and is used in determination of severity. Dynamic contrast CT helps to distinguish interstitial from necrotizing pancreatitis. The CT scan provides a noninvasive means of viewing the structure of the pancreas, the bile ducts, and the gallbladder. Damaged pancreatic tissue and lesions can be visualized. CT scan is currently considered one of the best tests for assessing pancreatic necrosis, excluding acute pancreatitis, and diagnosing complications and severity of the acute pancreatitis. Ultrasound uses high-frequency sound waves rather than radiation. It provides a "real-time" view of the structure being tested. Ultrasound is particularly valuable in viewing the bile ducts and can identify gallstones more readily than the CT scan. In this way, an ultrasound on admission can assess for gallstones as the etiology of the pain rather than establishing a diagnosis of acute pancreatitis. It may also visualize abnormal findings such as ascites and cholangiectasis (Koizumi et al., 2006). However, abdominal ultrasound is of limited usefulness in visualization of the pancreas because of bowel gas (McPhee et al., 2008). Endoscopic ultrasound (EUS) may be used to evaluate necrotic collections (AGA Institute, 2007).

Cholangiopancreatography

Endoscopic retrograde cholangiopancreatography (ERCP) is an invasive endoscopic test that allows cannulation and direct viewing of the ampulla of Vater, and the pancreatic and bile ducts. It requires injection of a radiographic contrast medium followed by a series of X-rays under fluoroscopy. ERCP is particularly useful in diagnosing obstructions. In addition, the ERCP provides the opportunity for direct removal of mechanical obstructions, such as a gallstone or pancreatic stone, stent placement to provide drainage through a stricture, sphincterotomy, and biopsy (Attasaranya et al., 2007).

Magnetic resonance cholangiopancreatography (MRCP) uses magnetic resonance imaging to produce images used to evaluate the hepatobiliary tree. Because it is noninvasive, and requires no contrast, MRCP has a decreased morbidity when compared to ERCP. MRCP has 81 to 100 percent sensitivity for common bile duct stones (Carroll et al., 2007). The usefulness of MRCP is limited by the inability to intervene with stone extraction, stent insertion, and biopsy or impaired visualization due to peripancreatic fluid collection.

Aspiration Biopsy

Aspiration biopsy involves the removal of a small plug of tissue using a syringe and needle technique. It is useful in diagnosing the severity of pancreatic tissue damage, diagnosing types of lesions, and draining pseudocysts. It is also helpful in distinguishing sterile necrosis from infected necrosis (Banks et al., 2006). Aspiration biopsy can be performed during ultrasound or CT scan, to enable visualization of correct needle placement.

Predicting the Severity of an Acute Pancreatitis Episode

Assessment by a severity scoring system is important for determining treatment and the need for "high-acuity" care. The

TABLE 31–4 Ranson Criteria for Predicting Severity of Acute Pancreatitis

RISK FACTOR	PRESENT AT TIME OF ADMISSION	RISK FACTOR	PRESENT AT TIME INITIAL 48 HOURS
Age	> 55	Hct	Decrease of > 10%
WBC	> 16,000 mm^3	BUN	Rise of > 5 mg/dL
Serum glucose	> 200 mg/dL	Serum calcium	< 8 mg/dL
Serum LDH	> 350 IU/L	Pao_2	< 60 mg/dL
Serum SGOT	> 250 U/dL	Base deficit Estimated fluid sequestration	< 4 mEq/L > 6 L

ASSOCIATED MORTALITY BASED ON NUMBER OF RISK FACTORS:[a]

# Risk Factors	Mortality (%)
< 3	1.0
3–4	16
5–6	40
≥ 7	Near 100

[a]Additional risk factors: respiratory failure with intubation, shock, hypocalcemia, and massive colloid administration (if > 3 of these factors are present, mortality increases to near 65%)

WBC=White blood cells. LDH=lactic dehydrogenase. SGOT=serum glutamic-oxaloacetic transaminase (now called AST). BUN=blood urea nitrogen, Pao_2= Partial pressure of oxygen.

Adapted from Ranson, J. C. (1985). *Risk factors in acute pancreatitis. Hospital Practice, 20*(4), 69–73.

Acute Physiology and Chronic Health Evaluation (APACHE II) scale is useful for assessing severity in the first 24 hours. This scale is used to consider factors such as age, rectal temperature, mean arterial pressure, heart rate, PaO_2, arterial pH, serum potassium, serum sodium, serum creatinine, hematocrit, white blood cell count, Glasgow Coma Scale score, and chronic health status. An APACHE II score that increases during the first 48 hours is strongly suggestive of the development of severe pancreatitis whereas a decrease in the first 48 hours strongly suggests mild pancreatitis (Banks et al., 2006). An APACHE II score of eight or greater correlates with mortality. The Ranson Criteria (Table 31–4) require 48 hours for complete assessment but are commonly used to predict patient outcome, having been shown to be highly accurate (96 percent accuracy) for acute pancreatitis severity. Using these criteria, the following assumptions can be made

- A person who has less than three criteria at the time of admission has a mortality risk of less than 1 to 2 percent.
- A score of three or greater indicates severe acute pancreatitis (Despins et al., 2005; Hirota et al., 2006).
- A person who is admitted with three or four criteria has a mortality risk of 16 percent.
- A person who is admitted with five or six criteria present has a mortality risk of 40 percent.
- A person who is admitted with seven or more criteria present has a 100 percent risk of mortality (Amerine, 2007).
- Obesity is considered a risk factor independent of Ranson criteria for severity in acute pancreatitis and noted to have more systemic and local complications. Obesity (BMI greater than 30), organ failure at admission and pleural effusion and/ or infiltrates at admission are risk factors for severity (Banks et al., 2006). A hematocrit greater than 44 at admission and not decreasing in 24 hours with fluid resuscitation is a good predictor of necrotizing pancreatitis (Banks et al., 2006).

SECTION TWO REVIEW

1. The primary laboratory tests obtained to help make a diagnosis of pancreatitis is serum
   A. amylase and lipase
   B. calcium and glucose
   C. LDH and AST
   D. Hematocrit and BUN
2. Severe acute pancreatitis will most likely have the following effect on serum glucose
   A. severe hypoglycemia
   B. transient hypoglycemia
   C. no effect
   D. transient hyperglycemia
3. According to Ranson Criteria for predicting the risk of mortality in acute pancreatitis patients, a patient who is admitted with five criteria would have a mortality risk of ______ percent.
   A. less than 1
   B. 40
   C. 60
   D. 100

Answers: 1. A, 2. D, 3. B

SECTION THREE: Nursing Assessment of the Patient with Acute Pancreatitis

At the completion of this section, the learner will be able to discuss nursing assessment of the patient with acute pancreatitis.

Pain History and Assessment

Pain is the most consistent complaint associated with acute pancreatitis and is a high-priority assessment. The classic pattern of pain is described as a sudden onset of sharp, knifelike, twisting and deep, upper abdominal (epigastric) pain that frequently radiates to the back, and is often associated with nausea and vomiting. The patient may report some degree of relief by assuming a leaning forward or knee/chest position (Carroll et al., 2007) and may report an increase in pain when doing activities that increase abdominal pressure (e.g., coughing). The pain intensity varies greatly from patient to patient. The pain may be described as vague and mild, or it may be excruciating, unbearable, and refractory to analgesic therapy. The intensity often reflects the degree to which the disease process has extended beyond the confines of the pancreas. If localized, the pain is usually more vague and mild; however, once pancreatic functions infiltrate extrapancreatic tissues (into the peritoneum), the pain becomes well defined and sharp, and the intensity increases significantly. The pain is believed to be a result of edema and distention of the pancreatic capsule, chemical burn of the peritoneum by pancreatic enzymes, and the release of kinin peptides or biliary obstruction. Initially, the patient's complaints of pain intensity may seem out of proportion to other clinical manifestations. The pain intensity does not always correlate with the degree of pancreatic inflammation.

The Focused History and Assessment

The majority of the clinical manifestations of acute pancreatic dysfunction are of GI origin; thus, while taking the nursing history, the nurse should particularly focus on obtaining a complete GI history. Ask the patient about previous symptoms of gallstones, alcohol use, history of hypertriglyceridemia or hypercalcemia, family history of pancreatic disease, drug history (prescription and nonprescription), history of trauma, or the presence of an autoimmune disease. The remainder of this section presents the major signs and symptoms associated with acute pancreatitis.

Gastrointestinal Assessment

The presence of abdominal pain is a major finding in acute pancreatitis. Additional GI clinical manifestations include

- Anorexia
- Upper abdominal tenderness without rigidity
- Abdominal distention
- Nausea and vomiting
- Diarrhea
- Peritoneal signs (noted in severe cases)
  - Diminished or absent bowel sounds (ileus may develop)
  - Increased pain
  - Abdominal rigidity, guarding, rebound tenderness
  - Other: leukocytosis, tachycardia, and fever

Additional Assessments

In addition to the major GI clinical manifestations, a variety of other common or classic signs and symptoms are associated with the disease process.

Integumentary

If the patient has hemorrhagic pancreatitis, two uncommon but classic signs may be observed

1. **Cullen's sign.** A bluish discoloration around the umbilicus
2. **Grey Turner's sign.** A bluish discoloration of the flank region

Other observations that may be noted by skin inspection are jaundice and edema. If the patient develops shock, the skin will become pale, cold, and moist.

Cardiovascular

Cardiac signs and symptoms usually present themselves in conjunction with the complication of shock or the release of **myocardial depressant factor (MDF).** The nurse should observe the patient for the signs and symptoms of hypovolemic shock (tachycardia, hypotension with decreased systemic vascular resistance) and MDF release (decreased cardiac output with increased systemic vascular resistance).

Pulmonary

Respiratory signs and symptoms include those typical of

- Pleural effusion—adventitious breath sounds, particularly crackles (usually left sided)
- Respiratory insufficiency or failure
- Pneumonia

Neurologic

The patient with acute pancreatitis frequently develops an alteration in level of consciousness. The nurse can rapidly trend the state of arousal using the Glasgow Coma Scale (GCS). Common neurologic manifestations include confusion, restlessness, and agitation.

Renal

The patient must be closely monitored for the development of acute tubular necrosis. The urine can also be observed. As increased levels of bile are excreted through the urine, it develops a brownish color and may become foamy.

Hematologic

The nurse should monitor the patient for clinical manifestations of disseminated intravascular coagulation.

Electrolyte Imbalances

Hypocalcemia may develop as a result of fat necrosis because serum calcium migrates to the extravascular space surrounding the pancreas where the fat necrosis is taking place. Two classic signs of hypocalcemia are

1. **Chvostek's sign.** The facial nerve is tapped directly in front of the ear. A positive sign is present when the facial muscles contract on the same side of the face as the tapping (Fig. 31–3A).
2. **Trousseau's sign.** A blood pressure cuff is inflated on the upper arm to a level directly above the patient's systolic blood pressure for two minutes. A positive sign is present when the hand flexes (carpopedal spasm) in response to the test (Fig. 31–3B).

In addition to hypocalcemia, the patient should be monitored for the hypokalemia and hypomagnesemia that may result from GI loss and insufficient intake (Takeda et al., 2006). Detailed information on the clinical manifestations of hypocalcemia, hypokalemia, and hypomagnesemia is available in Module 26, Alterations in Fluid and Electrolyte Balance.

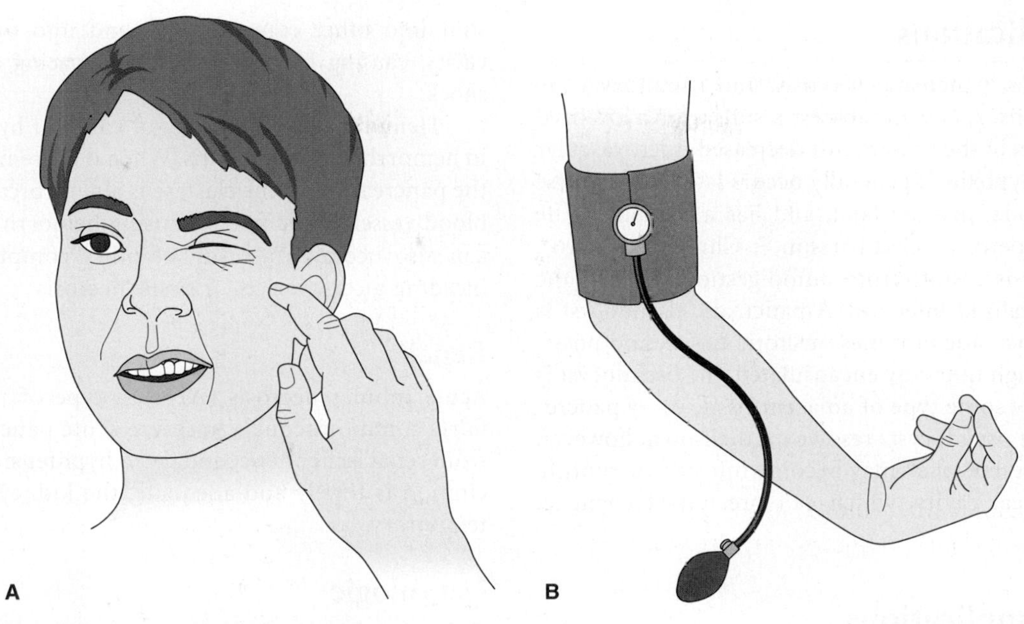

Figure 31–3 ■ A, Positive Chvostek sign. B, Positive Trousseau sign.

SECTION THREE REVIEW

1. The classic pattern of pain typically described by the patient with acute pancreatitis is
   - **A.** dull, diffuse, and poorly defined
   - **B.** sharp and confined to the epigastric area
   - **C.** well defined, dull, localized in the flank area
   - **D.** sharp, knifelike, often radiating to the back
2. The intensity and description of pain associated with acute pancreatitis varies, often based on the
   - **A.** pH of the pancreatic enzymes
   - **B.** degree to which extrapancreatic invasion has occurred
   - **C.** pain threshold of the individual patient
   - **D.** degree of release of myocardial depressant factor (MDF)
3. Peritoneal signs include (choose all that apply)
   - **A.** rebound tenderness
   - **B.** rigid abdomen
   - **C.** hyperactive bowel sounds
   - **D.** leukocytosis
4. Cullen's sign may be noted under which circumstance?
   - **A.** acute tubular necrosis
   - **B.** hemorrhage
   - **C.** hypovolemic shock
   - **D.** respiratory failure
5. The cardiovascular assessment of the patient with acute pancreatitis focuses on monitoring for the development of
   - **A.** hypercapnia
   - **B.** hypertension
   - **C.** cardiac arrhythmias
   - **D.** decreased cardiac output
6. If the pancreatitis is localized, assessment of the abdomen would show (choose all that apply)
   - **A.** tenderness
   - **B.** rigidity
   - **C.** distention
   - **D.** diminished bowel sounds

Answers: 1. D, 2. B, 3. (A, B, D), 4. B, 5. D, 6. (A, C, D)

SECTION FOUR: Complications of Acute Pancreatitis

At the completion of this section, the learner will be able to explain the complications of acute pancreatitis.

Acute pancreatitis is considered a multisystem disease process. Complications are common and may be local and systemic. Both types of complications are mediated by proinflammatory cytokines (Yuan et al., 2007). Obesity is a risk factor for both local and systemic complications and increases the risk of mortality (Martinez et al., 2006). In its most severe form, acute pancreatitis may be complicated by the development of multisystem organ dysfunction syndrome (MODS) which has a mortality rate of 15 to 20 percent (Browne, 2006).

Local Complications

Pancreatic abscess, pancreatic necrosis, and **pseudocyst** are local complications. Pancreatic abscess results from a localized infectious process in the presence of decreased microvascular circulation and hypoxia. It generally occurs late in the course of a severe episode, may be fatal, and has a mortality rate approaching 30 percent (Cuthbertson & Christophi, 2006). Pancreatic necrosis results from autodigestion without the presence of a localized infection. A pancreatic pseudocyst is composed of pancreatic enzymes, necrotic tissue, and possibly blood. Although not truly encapsulated, the pseudocyst is enclosed either by some type of adjacent tissue or by pancreatic tissues. Some pseudocysts resolve on their own; however, while they are present, they may become infected or rupture into the peritoneal cavity, which can precipitate chemical peritonitis.

Systemic Complications

The release of humoral mediators such as **platelet activating factor (PAF),** interleukins, myocardial depressant factor (MDF), neutrophils and the development of systemic inflammatory response syndrome (SIRS) may lead to complications which have the potential to interfere with virtually all of the body's functions. (Liu et al., 2006; Ueda et al., 2007; Yuan et al., 2007)

Pulmonary

Hypoxemia is present in the majority of severe acute pancreatitis patients within the first two days of onset. Respiratory insufficiency and failure are common complications of acute pancreatitis. They are attributed to the release of pancreatic enzyme phospholipase A, which destroys the phospholipid component of surfactant (Browne, 2006). The patient is at risk of developing pneumonia and/or pleural effusion and, in severe cases, acute respiratory distress syndrome (ARDS). Pleural effusions may result from enzyme-induced inflammation of the diaphragm while atelectasis may result from decreased diaphragmatic excursion as a result of abdominal distention or direct injury from exposure to pancreatic enzymes (Browne, 2006).

Cardiovascular

Pancreatic enzymes released into the bloodstream can have devastating effects on the cardiovascular system through the release of myocardial depressant factor (MDF) and hypovolemic shock. MDF is the result of pancreatic autodigestion by proteolytic enzymes and possess a negative inotropic (pumping) effect on heart muscle.

Hypovolemic Shock. Vasoactive substances are released from damaged pancreatic tissue. Trypsin activates the powerful vasodilating circulating enzyme, kallikrein, which forms two plasma kinins (kallidin and bradykinin). These two substances are responsible for vasodilation, decreased systemic vascular resistance, and increased permeability of endothelial linings of vessels. As vessels become more porous, intravascular fluids shift into other compartments and into the retroperitoneal cavity, causing hypovolemia, third spacing and hypovolemic shock.

Hemorrhage is also a major cause of hypovolemic shock in hemorrhagic pancreatitis. When it is prematurely activated, the pancreatic enzyme elastase is able to break down duct and blood vessel elastic fibers, causing hemorrhage. Hemorrhage can also occur as a result of other complications, such as bleeding ulcers, varices or tissue necrosis.

Renal

Acute tubular necrosis (ATN), a type of renal failure, is a fairly common sequela in severe acute pancreatitis. It results from renal ischemia secondary to hypotension. If fluid resuscitation is timely and adequate, the kidney damage may be temporary.

Neurologic

A decreased level of consciousness is a common problem in severe pancreatitis and is related to several potential etiologies, including analgesia and pancreatic encephalopathy. The alleviation of pain associated with acute pancreatitis requires large doses of opioids and possibly sedation. Cerebral function is altered by either of these therapies. The pathogenesis of pancreatic encephalopathy is unclear but is most likely related to multiple factors including both pancreatic and extrapancreatic factors (Zhang & Tian, 2007).

Hematologic

Disseminated intravascular coagulation (DIC) is associated with severe acute pancreatitis. It may be related to early intravascular consumption of factors secondary to circulating pancreatic enzymes, particularly trypsin (Saif, 2005). Table 31–5 summarizes the major systemic complications.

TABLE 31–5 Major Systemic Complications of Acute Pancreatitis

BODY SYSTEM/FUNCTION	COMPLICATIONS
Neurologic	Encephalopathy
Pulmonary	Hypoxia, respiratory failure, pneumonia, pleural effusion, atelectasis, acute respiratory distress syndrome (ARDS)
Cardiovascular	Hemorrhage, hypotension, shock, pericardial effusion, pericardial tamponade
Gastrointestinal	Bleeding, pancreatic pseudocyst
Renal	Acute renal failure
Metabolic	Hyperglycemia, metabolic acidosis, hypocalcemia
Hematologic	Vascular thrombosis, disseminated intravascular coagulation (DIC)
Infectious	Pancreatic abscess, peritonitis, sepsis

SECTION FOUR REVIEW

1. Pancreatic pseudocyst is composed of (choose all that apply)
   A. necrotic tissue
   B. air
   C. blood
   D. pancreatic enzymes
2. If a pseudocyst were to rupture into the peritoneal cavity the patient would most likely develop
   A. septicemia
   B. acute renal failure
   C. paralytic ileus
   D. peritonitis
3. In the acute pancreatitis patient, hypovolemic shock usually results from (choose all that apply)
   A. hemorrhage
   B. third spacing
   C. renal failure
   D. kallikrein release
4. Pulmonary complications are attributed to which of the following pancreatic enzymes?
   A. trypsin
   B. elastase
   C. amylase
   D. phospholipase A
5. The release of MDF by injured pancreatic tissue is believed to have what effect on the heart?
   A. decreases cardiac output
   B. decreases heart rate
   C. increases blood pressure
   D. increases cardiac output

Answers: 1. (A, C, D), 2. D, 3. (A, B, D), 4. D, 5. A

SECTION FIVE: Medical Management

At the completion of this section, the learner will be able to describe the medical management of the patient with acute pancreatitis.

The medical management of the patient with acute pancreatitis may be either supportive or curative but is often a combination of both. Supporting the patient's hemodynamic and oxygenation status is essential while correction of the underlying problem (mechanical obstruction) is undertaken or the underlying problem is allowed to resolve itself (alcohol induced).

Supportive Therapy

Medical management is based on prioritized goals, including stabilizing hemodynamic status, controlling pain, minimizing pancreatic stimulation, correcting the underlying problem, and preventing or treating complications. A summary of general physician orders related to supportive management of the acute pancreatitis patient is listed in Table 31–6.

Goal 1: Stabilize the Patient's Hemodynamic Status

Hypovolemia must be identified and treated aggressively. Hemodynamic stability is accomplished primarily through two types of interventions: fluid resuscitation and inotropic therapy. Fluid resuscitation includes crystalloids, possibly colloids, and plasma expanders. It is essential to closely monitor the patient's hemodynamic status as treatment progresses. Hemodynamic status monitoring might include

- Blood pressure, pulse, and temperature
- Oxygen saturation
- Blood gas analysis for labored respirations or hypotension unrelieved with fluid bolus
- Pulmonary artery pressure
- Pulmonary artery wedge pressure
- Central venous pressure
- Cardiac output, cardiac index

TABLE 31–6 Supportive Therapy for Acute Pancreatitis

TYPE OF SUPPORT	GENERAL PHYSICIAN ORDERS
Fluid resuscitation	May consist of up to 10–20 L of fluid during the first 24 hours, as required Fluids may be crystalloids or colloids If hypoalbuminemic, consider albumin replacement If hemoglobin less than 10 mg/dL, consider blood transfusion Fresh frozen plasma may be ordered for coagulopathy
Inotropic	When hypotension predominates, consider dopamine therapy When poor tissue perfusion predominates, consider dobutamine therapy
Respiratory	If PaO_2 is less than 60 mm Hg in the presence of high oxygen concentration, and/or respiratory rate is greater than 30/min, consider early intubation and mechanical ventilation with sedation and analgesia
Renal	In the presence of impaired renal function timely and adequate fluid resuscitation is essential to prevent permanent damage; some form of dialysis may be required
Nutritional	Once hemodynamic stability has been achieved, total parenteral nutrition (TPN) or nasojejunal enteral feeding is initiated Monitor serum glucose closely, maintaining levels at approximately 150 mg/dL if possible High doses of insulin may be necessary because of severe insulin resistance

Data from Takeda et al., (2006); Banks et al., (2006); and Amerine, (2007).

- Intake and output (hourly), daily weights
- Hematocrit and serum blood urea nitrogen (BUN) levels

Goal 2: Control the Patient's Pain

Acute pancreatitis is extremely painful. Controlling the level of pain is essential for comfort and to decrease secretion of pancreatic enzymes. "Despite the widespread belief that morphine exacerbates pancreatitis by stimulating the sphincter of Oddi, no definitive human study supports this view" (Kingsnorth & O'Reilly, 2006). There is no evidence to suggest an advantage of any particular type of medication (Banks et al., 2006). Fentanyl, morphine, and hydromorphone can increase common bile duct pressure but they remain effective pain relievers for patients with acute pancreatitis (Despins et al., 2005). Meperidine is not considered a drug of choice because of its association with an increased risk for seizures. The risks outweigh the benefits.

Goal 3: Minimize Pancreatic Stimulation

It is important to reduce the stimulation of pancreatic secretion as much as possible. Keeping the GI tract at rest facilitates pancreatic rest and reduces the amount of pancreatic juice secreted. Organ rest needs to continue until serum amylase levels have returned to normal and pain has subsided. In mild pancreatitis, oral intake may be restored in three to seven days and nutritional support is not needed. In more severe cases, this may take up to seven weeks. The physician may order the following

- Initial nothing-by-mouth (NPO) status
- Placement of a nasogastric tube to low-wall suction (in the presence of paralytic ileus and/or frequent vomiting)
- Drug therapy, such as antacids, proton pump inhibitors, or anticholinergics (anticholinergics reduce GI motility)

Patients who are experiencing acute pancreatitis are especially hypermetabolic and hypercatabolic. They have extremely high nutritional demands but are unable to consume nutrients orally for a prolonged period. Nutritional support is essential to improving the patient's outcome. The route of administration remains controversial. Enteral feeding is safer and less expensive and serves to stabilize gut barrier function thereby preventing systemic complications but it may increase pancreatic enzyme synthesis and secretion and the tube is often not tolerated well by the patient (Banks et al., 2006). Conversely, total parenteral nutrition (TPN) is more expensive and carries risks associated with the intravenous central line access. Nutritional support is imperative and should be determined based on individual patient need and tolerance. More studies are needed to determine best practice.

Curative Therapy

Goal 4: Correct the Underlying Problem

Generally, medical interventions are more desirable than surgical ones. Some triggering events, such as binge alcohol abuse, may subside spontaneously if given sufficient rest time using supportive therapy. If the etiology is mechanical, however, the underlying problem can be corrected surgically. For example, if a patient has a biliary obstruction, such as a gallstone, a cholecystectomy may be performed to relieve the obstruction. Certain surgical procedures to relieve obstructions can be performed during an ERCP.

Goal 5: Prevent or Treat Complications

It is imperative that complications be recognized early in their development and then treated aggressively. Close patient monitoring is a crucial part of meeting this goal. Medical interventions are based on correcting or supporting system dysfunctions as they develop. In addition to the various supportive physician orders listed in Table 31–6, the physician may need to order any of the following

- Electrolyte replacement
- Insulin therapy
- Antibiotic therapy
- Antisecretory therapy with octreotide
- Arterial blood gases
- Oxygen therapy
- Pulmonary toilet (e.g., incentive spirometry)
- Radiographic studies
- Cardiac monitoring
- Pulmonary artery flow-directed catheter

CT-guided percutaneous aspiration with Gram stain and culture may be done when infected necrosis is suspected. Surgical debridement may be indicated if the patient develops infected pancreatic necrosis or abscess (Banks et al., 2006). Unfortunately, surgical incisions of pancreatic tissue may lead to the development of pancreatic fistulas, which can result in the entry of pancreatic juice into other tissues, causing further damage and new complications. Pancreatic abscess is treated by percutaneous drainage, surgical drainage, or endoscopic drainage (Banks et al., 2006). Patients with subtotal or total pancreatic necrosis usually require a proton pump inhibitor on a daily basis as the bicarbonate secretion of the pancreas is severely diminished putting the patient at risk for duodenal ulcer (Banks et al., 2006).

Emerging Evidence

- In patients with acute pancreatitis, enteral nutrition was associated with better glucose control than parenteral nutrition *(Petrov & Zagainov, 2007)*.
- In patients with severe acute pancreatitis, prophylactic antibiotics are not an appropriate treatment strategy and should be limited to patients with pancreatic necrosis as seen on CT *(Xiong et al., 2005)*.
- In two recent meta-analyses, prophylactic antibiotics were not found to decrease infected pancreatic necrosis in acute necrotizing pancreatitis *(Bai et al., 2008; and deVries et al., 2007)*.
- When clinically septic intervals are identified in patients with pancreatic necrosis, treatment with antibiotics may be used while investigating the source and then discontinued if the cultures are negative *(Banks et al., 2006)*.
- Potential biologic markers for predicting the severity and prognosis of pancreatitis include trypsinogen activation peptide, C-reactive protein, procalcitonin, phospholipase A2, and interleukin-6 and 8. More studies are needed *(Carroll et al., 2007)*.
- Survivors of acute pancreatitis have a reduced quality of life when studied at two to four years post illness *(Hochman et al., 2006; Symersky et al., 2006)* and a higher Ranson score at presentation may predict those with poorer outcomes in the immediate years post recovery *(Hochman et al., 2006)*.

SECTION FIVE REVIEW

1. The highest priority in management of the patient with severe acute pancreatitis is to
   - **A.** control pain
   - **B.** stabilize hemodynamic status
   - **C.** minimize pancreatic stimulation
   - **D.** correct the underlying problem
2. An appropriate drug for pain management of the patient with acute pancreatitis is
   - **A.** morphine sulfate
   - **B.** codeine
   - **C.** meperidine
   - **D.** ibuprofen
3. Anticholinergics may be ordered for the patient with acute pancreatitis for the primary purpose of
   - **A.** reducing GI motility
   - **B.** reducing pain
   - **C.** increasing pancreatic stimulation
   - **D.** increasing gastric pH
4. The effective management of complications depends on (choose all that apply)
   - **A.** close monitoring
   - **B.** early recognition
   - **C.** aggressive treatment
   - **D.** age of the patient

Answers: 1. B, 2. A, 3. A, 4. (A, B, C)

SECTION SIX: Nursing Care

At the completion of this section, the learner will be able to discuss the nursing care for a patient with acute pancreatic dysfunction.

Frequently Occurring Nursing Diagnoses

On completion of the nursing database, the nurse clusters data and develops a set of nursing hypotheses based on the available data. Additional critical data that may either support or eliminate each hypothesis should also be identified and obtained. Once the hypotheses have been established, the nurse is ready to develop a list of nursing diagnoses based on the patient's response to the illness rather than on the illness itself. Nursing management of the patient experiencing an acute pancreatic dysfunction episode is summarized in the box, NURSING CARE: The Patient with Acute Pancreatitis.

In the patient with acute pancreatic dysfunction, a variety of nursing diagnoses frequently occur. The following is a partial

NURSING CARE: The Patient with Acute Pancreatitis

Expected Patient Outcomes and Related Interventions

Outcome 1: Fluid and Electrolyte Balance

Assess and compare to established norms, patient baselines, and trends.

Intake and output, blood pressure, breath sounds, weights, restlessness

Serum electrolyte levels

Administer related drug therapy and monitor for therapeutic effects.

Intravenous fluids

Electrolyte replacements as ordered

Related nursing diagnoses

Deficient fluid volume

Decreased cardiac output

Ineffective tissue perfusion

Risk for injury

Outcome 2: Pain Control / Relief of Pain

Assess and compare to established norms, patient baselines, and trends.

Level of pain on pain rating scale

Administer related drug therapy and monitor for therapeutic effects.

Analgesics as ordered (refer to RELATED PHARMACOTHERAPY, Agents Used to Control Pain in Acute Pancreatitis, for additional information)

Related interventions

Nothing by mouth (NPO) during acute phase

Assist the patient to use pain rating scale accurately

Careful positioning of patient with head of bed elevated to semi-Fowler position and knees bent may help alleviate pain (Fitzpatrick, 2009)

Related nursing diagnoses

Acute pain

Readiness for enhanced comfort

Anxiety

Outcome 3: Relief of Nausea and Vomiting

Assess and compare to established norms, patient baselines, and trends.

Nausea, vomiting and dry heaves

(continued)

NURSING CARE (*continued*)

Administer related drug therapy and monitor for therapeutic effects.
- Pain medicine
- Antiemetic therapy

Related interventions
- Prevent/relieve gastric distension, nasogastric tube care as needed
- Restrict oral intake, NPO as needed
- Encourage deep slow breathing, change positions slowly, frequent oral hygiene

Related Nursing Diagnoses
- Deficient fluid volume
- Readiness for enhanced comfort

Outcome 4: Optimize Nutrition

Assess and compare to established norms, patient baselines, and trends.
- Weights, serum albumin, prealbumin, serum total protein
- Monitor for ileus formation

Administer related drug therapy and monitor for therapeutic effects.
- Parenteral or enteral feeding as indicated (feeding tube tip should be located below the ligament of Treitz (Fitzpatrick, 2009))
- Antiemetics as needed

Related interventions
- Obtain nutrition consult
- Monitor patient response to each step in diet progression

Related nursing diagnoses
- Altered nutrition: less than body requirements
- Fatigue
- Infection

Outcome 5: Optimize Respiratory Status

Assess and compare to established norms, patient baselines, and trends.
- Respiratory rate, rhythm, and depth; lung sounds; coloring of mucous membranes and skin
- Arterial blood gases; Spo_2

Administer related drug therapy and monitor for therapeutic effects.
- Oxygen therapy as ordered

Related interventions
- Encourage use of incentive spirometer, ambulate as tolerated
- Suction when needed
- Turn every two hours

Related nursing diagnoses
- Ineffective breathing pattern
- Impaired gas exchange
- Risk for infection
- Fatigue

list of some of these nursing diagnoses (Carpenito-Moyet, 2008; Ackley and Ladwig, 2006).

- *Acute pain: Epigastric or abdominal* related to irritation and edema of the inflamed pancreas, localized peritonitis, pancreatic capsule distention, and nasogastric suction (refer to the box RELATED PHARMACOTHERAPY: Agents Used to Control Pain in Acute Pancreatitis)
- *Altered comfort: Nausea and vomiting* related to stimulation of the vomiting center
- *Ineffective breathing pattern* related to abdominal pain, depressant effects of opioid therapy, and decreased lung expansion
- *Deficient fluid volume* related to vomiting, decreased fluid intake, fever, diaphoresis and fluid shifts
- *Imbalanced nutrition: less than body requirements* related to vomiting, anorexia, and impaired digestion secondary to decreased pancreatic enzymes and increased needs as a result of acute illness

RELATED PHARMACOTHERAPY: Agents Used to Control Pain in Acute Pancreatitis

Opioid Analgesics

Morphine
Hydromorphone (Dilaudid)
Fentanyl (Sublimaze)

Actions and Uses

Bind with opiate receptors in the central nervous system, altering the patient's perception of and emotional response to pain.

Major Adverse Effects

- Most common: sedation, constipation, nausea
- Potentially life-threatening: respiratory or cardiac depression/arrest

Nursing Implications

- Monitor: vital signs, respiratory rate and depth, level of sedation, bowel function
- Pain associated with severe acute pancreatitis can be severe and intractable, making pain control difficult to attain
- Meperidine is avoided because of its toxic metabolites with their potentially severe adverse effects (seizures); may be considered if patient is allergic to other opioids.
- Be aware of equianalgesic dosing of these medications
- Reassess patient's response to analgesic within 30 to 60 minutes after administration
- Patient's ability to correctly use a patient controlled analgesia (PCA) mechanism should be closely evaluated before this option is chosen. Critical illness may prevent appropriate use

Data partially taken from Fitzpatrick, E. (2009). Pancreatitis. In K. K. Carlson (ed.), *AACN advanced critical care nursing*. St. Louis: Saunders/Elsevier, 774–791.

- *Anxiety* related to unfamiliar environment; discomfort; lack of understanding of diagnosis, diagnostic tests, and interventions; and fear of death
- *Risk for injury* related to hypoxia, infection, hemorrhage, shock, encephalopathy, acute tubular necrosis
- *Risk for infection* related to pancreatic abscess, peritonitis, sepsis
- *Risk for decreased cardiac output* related to myocardial depressant factor, hypovolemia, vasodilation, and SIRS

Additionally, nursing care of the patient with acute pancreatitis includes frequent focused assessments for the earliest signs and symptoms of the many potential complications identified in Section Six. Any increase in the patient's symptoms or the development of new abnormal findings are immediately communicated in a collaborative manner to other healthcare providers.

Nursing care is also impacted by the cause of the episode of acute pancreatitis. Prevention of future episodes of acute pancreatitis and the development of chronic pancreatitis relies on the continuum of care. Patients whose acute pancreatitis is related to alcohol are referred for alcohol cessation counseling. Patients whose acute pancreatitis is related to gallstones receive surgical consults and may undergo surgery at a subsequent admsission or later in the current admission when the acute episode has resolved. Other causes of pancreatitis often require follow-up after resolution of the acute episode.

SECTION SIX REVIEW

1. Which of the following potential complications is commonly found in the patient with acute pancreatitis? (choose all that apply)
   - **A.** hyperglycemia
   - **B.** sepsis
   - **C.** brain abscess
   - **D.** acute tubular necrosis
   - **E.** liver failure
2. In developing a plan of care for the patient with acute pancreatitis, which nursing diagnosis statement would be correct? *Pain: epigastric or abdominal* related to
   - **A.** gastric distention
   - **B.** pancreatic ischemia
   - **C.** gastric or duodenal wall erosion
   - **D.** localized peritonitis, pancreatic capsule distention
3. Nursing interventions that would directly address the nursing diagnosis *pain: epigastric or abdominal* in a patient in the acute phase of acute pancreatitis would include
   - **A.** offering nothing by mouth
   - **B.** encouraging a soft food diet
   - **C.** monitoring for therapeutic effects of gastric acid reduction
   - **D.** encouraging a patient to assume a prone position to reduce pain

Answers: 1. (A, B, D), 2. D, 3. A

POSTTEST

Ms. J. is 5 feet 4 inches (16.4 m) tall and weighs 161 pounds (73 kg) and gives a history of smoking about one pack per day for 40 years and drinking a glass of wine several days a week with her evening meal. She denies a history of diabetes or heart problems but states having had several "gallbladder attacks" over the past several years.

1. Which type of pancreatitis is Ms. J most likely to have?
   - **A.** acute interstitial
   - **B.** chronic interstitial
   - **C.** acute hemorrhagic
   - **D.** chronic hemorrhagic
2. Which piece of Ms. J.'s history represents the strongest etiologic factor for development of pancreatitis?
   - **A.** smoking history
   - **B.** gallbladder disease
   - **C.** alcohol consumption
   - **D.** obesity
3. If Ms. J. has developed acute interstitial pancreatitis, this form of the disease is typically characterized by
   - **A.** a long duration
   - **B.** fat necrosis
   - **C.** irreversible damage
   - **D.** localized inflammation
4. If her pancreatitis is caused by pancreatic duct obstruction, the obstruction is most likely caused by
   - **A.** a gallstone
   - **B.** edema
   - **C.** a stricture
   - **D.** severe spasms
5. To diagnose Ms. J.'s acute pancreatitis, serial serum lipase levels may be ordered in preference to serum amylase levels because serum lipase
   - **A.** is more accurate
   - **B.** is more specific to pancreatitis
   - **C.** remains elevated for a longer period
   - **D.** requires no special analysis technique
6. It is decided to perform an ERCP on Ms. J. A major advantage of performing an ERCP is that
   - **A.** it is a noninvasive procedure
   - **B.** it can be performed at the bedside
   - **C.** it provides access to the gallbladder and pancreas
   - **D.** mechanical obstructions can be directly removed

7. Ms. J. is complaining of pain. The classic pattern of pain associated with acute pancreatitis has which characteristics?
A. piercing
B. slow onset
C. epigastric
D. sharp

8. Which assessments represent peritoneal signs as a result of extrapancreatic invasion of enzymes?
A. abdominal rigidity
B. hyperactive bowel sounds
C. dulling of abdominal pain
D. onset of bradycardia

9. The nurse assesses Chvostek's sign on Ms. J. This test is conducted by
A. checking for bluish discoloration of umbilicus
B. tapping the facial nerve in front of ear
C. inflating arm with blood pressure cuff
D. checking for flank bluish discoloration

10. Which is the consistent end result of cardiovascular complications associated with acute pancreatitis, no matter what the mechanism?
A. increased systemic vascular resistance
B. increased cardiac output
C. increased pulmonary capillary wedge pressure
D. decreased cardiac output

11. The major pulmonary complications of acute pancreatitis include (choose all that apply)
A. cor pulmonale
B. pleural effusion
C. hypoxia
D. respiratory failure

12. The initial medical management of severe acute pancreatitis focuses on
A. controlling pain
B. minimizing pancreatic stimulation
C. stabilizing hemodynamic status
D. correcting the underlying problem

13. Which drug is the first choice for Ms. J.'s pain management with acute pancreatitis?
A. meperidine
B. morphine
C. NSAIDS
D. codeine

Posttest answers with rationale are found on MyNursingKit.

REFERENCES

Ackley, B. J & Ladwig, G. B. (2008). *Nursing diagnosis handbook*. St. Louis: Mosby/Elsevier.

AGA Institute. (2007). AGA Institute medical position statement on acute pancreatitis. *Gastroenterology, 132*, (5), 2019-2021.

Amerine, A. (2007). Get optimum outcomes for acute pancreatitis patients. *The Nurse Practitioner, 32*, (6) 44-48.

Attasaranya, S., Aziz, A. M., & Lehman, G. A. (2007). Endoscopic management of acute and chronic pancreatitis. *Surgical Clinics of North America, 87*, 1379-1402.

Bai, Y., Gao, J., Zou, D., Li, Z. (2008). Prophylactic antibiotics cannot reduce infected pancreatic necrosis and mortality in acute necrotizing pancreatitis: evidence from a meta-analysis of randomized controlled trials. *American Journal of Gastroenterology, 103*(1), 104-110.

Banks, P. A., Freman, M. L., Practice Parameters Committee of the American College of Gastroenterology. (2006). Practice guidelines in acute pancreatitis. *American Journal of Gastroenterology, 101*, 2379-2400.

Browne, G. W. (2006). Pathophysiology of pulmonary complications of acute pancreatitis. *World Journal of Gastroenterology, 28*, 7087-7096.

Carpenito-Moyet, L. J. (2008). *Handbook of nursing diagnosis* 12th ed. Philadelphia: Lippincott, Williams & Wilkins.

Carroll, J. K., Herrick, B., Gipson, T. (2007). Acute pancreatitis: diagnosis, prognosis, and treatment. *American Family Physician, 75*, (10), 1513-1520.

Cuthbertson, C. M. & Christophi, C. (2006-1). Potential effects of hyperbaric oxygen therapy in acute pancreatitis. *Australia New Zealand Journal of Surgery, 76*, 625-630.

Cuthbertson, C. M. & Christophi, C. (2006-2). Disturbances of the microcirculation in acute pancreatitis. *British Journal of Surgery, 93*, 518-530.

Despins, L. A., Kivlahan, C., & Cox, K. R. (2005). Acute pancreatitis. *American Journal of Nursing, 105*, (11), 54-57.

deVries, A. C., Besselink, M. G., Buskens, E., Ridwan, B. U., Schipper, M. et al. (2007). Randomized controlled trials of antibiotic prophylaxis in severe acute pancreatitis: relationship between methodological quality and outcome. *Pancreatology, 7*, 531-538.

Elfar, M., Gaber, L. W., Sabek, O., Fischer, C. P. & Gaber, A. O. (2007). The inflammatory cascade in acute pancreatitis: relevance to clinical disease. *Surgical Clinics of North America, 87*, 1325-1340.

Hirota, M., Takada, T., Kawarada, Y., Hirata, K., Mayumi, T. et al. (2006). JPN guidelines for the management of acute pancreatitis: severity assessment of acute pancreatitis. *Journal of Hepatobiliary Pancreatic Surgery, 13*, 33-41.

Hochman, D., Louie, B., Bailey, R. (2006). Determination of patient quality of life following severe acute pancreatitis. *Canadian Journal of Surgery, 49*, (2), 101-106.

Kingsnorth, A., O'Reilly, D. (2006). Clinical review acute pancreatitis. *British Medical Journal, 332*, 1072-1076.

Koizumi, M., Takada, T., Kawarada, Y., Hirata, K., Mayumi, T. et al. (2006). JPN guidelines for the management of acute pancreatitis: diagnostic criteria for acute pancreatitis. *Journal of Hepatobiliary Pancreatic Surgery, 13*, 25-32.

Liu, L. R. & Xia, S. H. (2006). Role of platelet-activating factor in pathogenesis of acute pancreatitis. *World Journal of Gastroenterology, 28*, 539-545.

Martinez, J., Johnson, C. D., Sanchez-Paya, J., de Madaria, E., Robles-Diaz, G. & Perez-Mateo, M. (2006). Obesity is a definitive risk factor of severity and mortality in acute pancreatitis: an updated meta-analysis. *Pancreatology, 6*, 206-209.

McPhee, S. J., Papadakis, M. A., Tierney, L. M. (eds.). (2008). *Current medical diagnosis and treatment* 47th ed. New York: McGraw Hill Medical.

Pagana, K. D. & Pagana, T. J. (2007). *Mosby's diagnostic and laboratory test reference,* (8th ed.). Philadelphia: Mosby Elsevier.

Petrov, M. S. & Zagainov, V. E. (2007). Influence of enteral versus parenteral nutrition on blood glucose control in acute pancreatitis: a systematic review. *Clinical Nutrition, 26,* 514–523.

Ranson, J. C. (1985). Risk factors in acute pancreatitis. *Hospital Practice, 20* (4), 69–73.

Saif, M. W. (2005) DIC secondary to acute pancreatitis. *Clinical Laboratory Haematology, 27,* 278–282.

Sekimoto, M., Takada, T., Kawarada, Y., Hirata, K., Mayumi, T., et al. (2006). JPN guidelines for the management of acute pancreatitis: epidemiology, etiology, natural history, and outcome predictors in acute pancreatitis. *Journal of Hepatobiliary Pancreatic Surgery, 13,* 10–24.

Symersky, T., van Hoorn, B., & Masclee, A. A. (2006) The outcome of a long-term follow-up of pancreatic function after recovery from acute pancreatitis. *Journal of the Pancreas, 7,* (4), 447–453.

Szabo, G., Mandrekar, P., Oak, S. & Mayerle, J. (2007). Effect of ethanol on inflammatory responses. *Pancreatology, 7,* 115-123.

Takeda, K., Takada, T., Kawarada, Y., Hirata, K., Mayumi, T., et al. (2006). JPN guidelines for the management of acute pancreatitis: medical management of acute pancreatitis. *Journal of Hepatobiliary Pancreatic Surgery, 13,* 42–47.

Ueda, T., Takeyama, Y., Yasuda, T., Shineki, M., Sawa, H., et al. (2007). Serum interleukin-15 level is a useful predictor of the complications and mortality in severe acute pancreatitis. *Surgery, 142* (3), 319–326.

Xiong, G., Wu, S., Wang, Z. (2006). Role of prophylactic antibiotic administration in severe acute pancreatitis: a meta-analysis. *Medical Principles and Practice, 15,* 106–110.

Yuan, B-S., Zhu, R-M., Braddock, M., Zhang, X-H., Shi, W. & Zheng, M-H. (2007). Interleukin-18: a proinflammatory cytokine that plays an important role in acute pancreatitis. *Informa Healthcare, 11,* 1261–1271.

Zhang, X-P., & Tian, H. (2007). Pathogenesis of pancreatic encephalopathy in severe acute pancreatitis. *Hepatobiliary Pancreatic Disease International, 6,* 134–140.

MODULE

32 Determinants and Assessment of Nutrition and Metabolic Function

Valerie Sabol, Kristine H. L'Ecuyer, Kathleen Dorman Wagner

OBJECTIVES Following completion of this module, the learner will be able to

1. Explain basic normal metabolism concepts, including anabolism and catabolism, aerobic and anaerobic, and energy.
2. Describe the primary functions of carbohydrates, lipids, and proteins as the body's fuel sources.
3. Discuss a focused nutrition nursing history and physical assessment.
4. Describe the laboratory assessment of nutritional and metabolic status.
5. Discuss physiologic studies used to measure nutrition and metabolic status.

Patients in high-acuity areas are vulnerable to significantly altered nutrition and their health status is negatively affected when nutritional needs are not met. Nutritional requirements can be altered by anything that impairs appetite, or interferes with ingestion, metabolism or nutrient absorption; or alters the metabolism of nutrients, such as chronic disease conditions, acute illnesses or surgical interventions. Assessment of nutritional status is performed in order to identify those who are malnourished, and those who are at risk for malnutrition. Nurses play a crucial role in the assessment and management of nutrition in the high-acuity patient.

This module lays the knowledge groundwork for improving your understanding of the various alterations in metabolic function that commonly complicate the recovery of high-acuity patients. The module consists of five sections. Section One provides an overview of normal metabolism. Section Two describes the concept of nutrition, including macronutrients—carbohydrates, proteins, and lipids. Section Three presents a description of a focused nutritional physical assessment. Section Four explains the interpretation of laboratory data pertinent to nutritional assessment of the high-acuity patient. Finally, Section Five discusses physiologic studies commonly used to evaluate the nutritional/metabolic needs of the high-acuity patient. All Section Reviews include answers. It is suggested that the learner review those concepts answered incorrectly in the review questions before proceeding to the next section.

PRETEST

1. Catabolism is best described as
   - A. metabolism occurring in the absence of oxygen
   - B. metabolism occurring in the presence of oxygen
   - C. breakdown of complex nutrients into more basic nutrients
   - D. building of cells and tissues from nutrients
2. A useful serum laboratory test used to evaluate a patient for the presence of anaerobic metabolism is
   - A. total lymphocyte count
   - B. lactic acid
   - C. arterial blood gas
   - D. blood urea nitrogen
3. Which nutrient provides the greatest amount of calories per volume?
   - A. fats
   - B. carbohydrates
   - C. visceral proteins
   - D. somatic proteins
4. Which organ is most dependent on maintenance of normal blood glucose levels?
   - A. heart
   - B. lungs
   - C. kidney
   - D. brain
5. Nitrogen balance assesses the adequacy of
   - A. carbohydrates
   - B. lipids
   - C. protein intake
   - D. calories
6. A BMI of 18 indicates
   - A. malnutrition
   - B. normal weight

C. overweight
D. obesity

7. The total lymphocyte count (TLC) is useful in estimating
A. nitrogen balance
B. iron stores
C. vitamin A, zinc, and magnesium levels
D. immune system function

8. Which laboratory test is an indicator of the patient's daily protein need?
A. albumin
B. BUN
C. hemoglobin
D. UUN

9. Oxygen consumption is a measure of a person's
A. oxygen delivery
B. resting energy expenditure
C. metabolic state
D. anaerobic metabolism

10. The extraction of oxygen by the tissues to meet metabolic needs can be measured using
A. oxygen saturation of arterial blood (SaO_2)
B. oxygen saturation of venous blood ($S\dot{V}O_2$)
C. partial pressure of arterial carbon dioxide ($PaCO_2$)
D. partial pressure of arterial oxygen (PaO_2)

Pretest answers are found on MyNursingKit.

SECTION ONE: Metabolism

At the completion of this section, the learner will be able to explain basic normal metabolism concepts, including anabolism and catabolism, aerobic and anaerobic, and energy.

The energy required to maintain life is generated by chemical processes involving transformation of nutrients and occurring throughout the body. Collectively, these processes are called *metabolism,* which means state of change. Metabolism is further described as anabolic, catabolic, aerobic, or anaerobic.

Anabolism and Catabolism

Anabolism is a constructive metabolic process whereby simple molecules are converted into molecules that are more complex. It involves synthesis of cell components and contributes to tissue building. Anabolic events require energy. **Catabolism** is the process by which complex nutrients and body tissues are broken down into more basic elements such as glucose, fatty acids, and amino acids for the purpose of liberating energy necessary to maintain bodily functions. Anabolism and catabolism are ongoing processes and, under normal circumstances, occur simultaneously to varying degrees. When a person is faced with a serious acute or chronic illness, catabolism may exceed anabolism and sometimes threaten survival. Anabolic and catabolic processes both require enzyme catalysts. Substances acted on by enzymes are called *substrates;* therefore, nutrients are called substrates because enzymatic processes are required for their use as fuel (Pleuss, 2007).

Aerobic and Anaerobic Metabolism

Production of energy is a highly organized process. Nutrients are transformed into energy for immediate use or for storage inside the cell mitochondria for later use. Energy is used or stored in the form of **adenosine triphosphate (ATP)**, which is the major source of energy for all body cells. Energy is generated from two distinct physiologic pathways—aerobic and anaerobic.

Aerobic Metabolism

To form ATP, aerobic metabolism involves either the Krebs (citric acid) cycle or the electron transport chain biochemical sequence of reactions. The cell mitochondria are the sites of aerobic metabolism. When oxygen is adequate, oxidation of nutrients (carbohydrates, lipids, and proteins) occurs in the mitochondria. Pyruvate, which is produced by glycolysis, moves into the mitochondria to be processed in the Krebs (citric acid) cycle, ultimately forming 38 molecules of ATP and end products (carbon dioxide and water). Carbon dioxide and water normally are harmless and easily excreted from the body; however, excess retention of either of these substances can result in acid–base and fluid excess problems. Figure 32–1 shows a simplified concept of the aerobic (oxidative) pathway. The electron transport chain, however, produces even greater amount of ATP. Through a series of catalyzed reactions, hydrogen atoms are oxidized to form hydrogen ions and water. This process releases large amounts of energy, which is used to convert adenosine diphosphate (ADP) to ATP.

Anaerobic Metabolism

Not all cells contain mitochondria, so not all are capable of aerobic metabolism. Cells without mitochondria receive their energy by the oxidation of glucose to pyruvate, which is then converted to ATP. The process of glucose oxidation in the cytoplasm is called

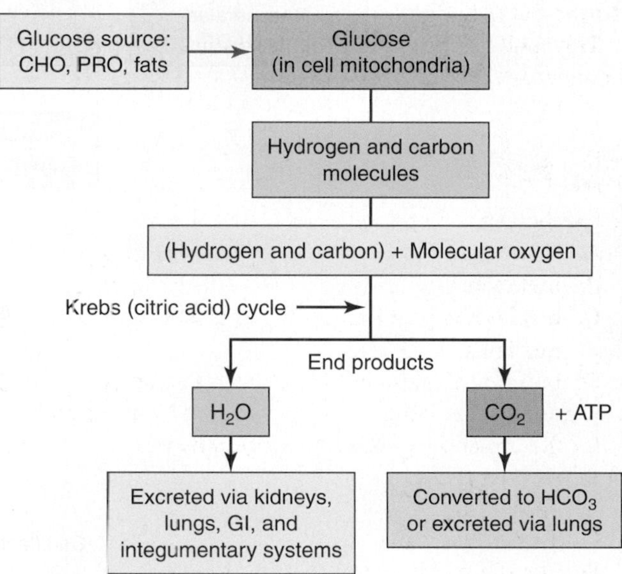

Figure 32–1 ■ Simplified illustration of aerobic (oxidative) pathway. More than 90 percent of metabolism occurs using the aerobic pathway. The end products of water and carbon dioxide are normally eliminated readily from the body.

glycolysis. Under circumstances in which there is decreased or delayed oxygen delivery to the cells (even those containing mitochondria), glycolysis is used for energy production and is referred to as anaerobic metabolism, or the Cori cycle.

Nicotinic acid dehydrogenase (NAD^+), an oxygen-reducing coenzyme, is required for anaerobic glycolysis. Maintaining adequate levels of NAD^+ depends on oxygen. When the supply of oxygen is inadequate, the energy of glucose can be released by the process of anaerobic glycolysis. During the anaerobic process, two ATP molecules are produced, in addition to pyruvate and lactic acid byproducts. Pyruvate is converted to lactic acid by NAD^+, which is then free to participate in further energy synthesis. Most body cells can use lactic acid as an energy source temporarily; however, the brain and nervous system have extremely limited capabilities to extract lactic acid as a fuel source. Figure 32–2 shows a simplified concept of the anaerobic (glycolytic) pathway.

The anaerobic metabolic pathway is inefficient as an energy source but is reversible with the reestablishment of an adequate oxygen supply. Anaerobic metabolism is partially a compensatory mechanism that allows energy production to proceed whenever energy demands exceed the oxygen supply, such as during exercise. Anaerobic metabolism, however, is intended only to be temporary and cannot sustain life indefinitely. High-acuity patients are at increased risk of developing anaerobic metabolism because of periods of severe or sustained decreases in oxygen delivery to the tissues (Pleuss, 2007). Hence, maintaining adequate oxygenation and perfusion is critical for supporting aerobic metabolism.

Elevated serum lactate levels are indicative of inadequate cellular oxygenation. Measuring serum lactic acid level is useful as an indicator of the severity and duration of anaerobic metabolism, such as develops during states of inadequate ventilation and/or perfusion (e.g., shock states, cardiac arrest). A normal serum lactic acid level is less than 2 mmol/L.

Energy

The ability to do work is called **energy**. Heat is generated in the conversion of nutrients to energy. Energy is measured in units called *calories,* which is the amount of energy needed to raise the temperature of 1 gram of water by 1 degree Celsius. Because a calorie is such a minute quantity, energy measurement within the body is usually described in terms of a kilocalorie (1,000 calories). A kilocalorie (kcal) is the amount of energy required to increase the temperature of 1 kg (1,000 g) of water by 1 degree Celsius.

Energy needed by the body is used to maintain ion gradients across cell membranes; approximately one third of all energy generated by the cell mitochondria is utilized to run the **sodium-potassium pump** (Na^+/K^+ pump), an active transport ion gradient

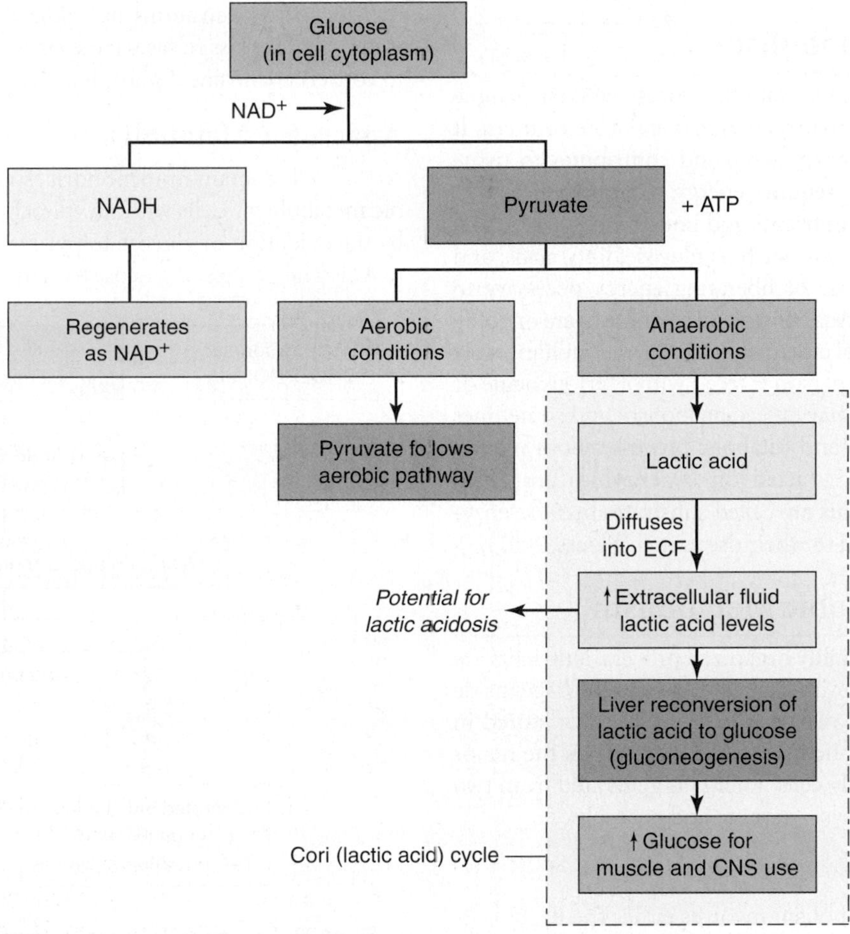

Figure 32–2 ■ Simplified illustration of anaerobic (glycolytic) pathway. The anaerobic pathway is reversible when oxygen becomes available. Severe anaerobic conditions, such as cardiac arrest or shock, can lead to lactic acidosis.

mechanism. The majority of energy needed by the body (about 40 percent) is used to maintain ion gradients across cell membranes. Synthesis of proteins and central nervous system functions each require about 20 percent of the energy expenditure. Other essential functions such as oxidation of nutrients, breathing, and cardiac pumping consume the rest of the energy expenditure. Physical activities require an even greater amount of energy above that required to maintain normal homeostatic mechanisms in a resting state.

SECTION ONE REVIEW

1. Catabolism is best described as
   A. metabolism occurring in the absence of oxygen
   B. metabolism occurring in the presence of oxygen
   C. breakdown of complex nutrients into more basic nutrients
   D. building of cells and tissues from nutrients
2. Which part of the cell is the site of aerobic metabolism?
   A. mitochondria
   B. cell membrane
   C. cytoplasm
   D. nucleus
3. Which lab test is frequently used as an indicator of anaerobic metabolism?
   A. total lymphocyte count
   B. lactic acid
   C. arterial blood gas
   D. blood urea nitrogen
4. High-acuity patients are at risk for significant anaerobic metabolism because of
   A. NPO status
   B. increased energy requirement
   C. severe or sustained decrease in oxygen delivery
   D. fluid volume overload
5. Clinically, energy is usually measured in kilocalories. A kilocalorie is the amount of energy required to increase the temperature of
   A. 1 kg of water by 1 degree Celsius
   B. a person's body by 1 degree Celsius
   C. 1 gram of fat by 1 degree Celsius
   D. a person's body to burn 1 kg of energy

Answers: 1. C, 2. A, 3. B, 4. C, 5. A

SECTION TWO: Nutrition: The Source of Energy

At the completion of this section, the learner will be able to describe the primary functions of carbohydrates, lipids, and proteins as the body's fuel sources.

Nutrition is a complex process by which an organism takes in and uses food substrates for the purpose of providing energy for growth, maintenance, and repair. Nutrition involves ingestion (taking in food), digestion (breaking down food into absorbable substances), absorption (taking up substances from the GI tract into the blood), and metabolism (transformation of substances into energy). **Nutrients** are the elements and compounds necessary for the nutrition process. Nutrients are divided into two basic categories. **Macronutrients** consist of carbohydrates, proteins, and lipids (fats). Vitamins (fat soluble and water soluble), minerals, and trace elements are called **micronutrients.** Adequate intake of both macronutrients and micronutrients is essential to restore health and to promote healing in the high-acuity patient (Pleuss, 2007).

Carbohydrates

Carbohydrates are composed of carbon, hydrogen, and oxygen. Carbohydrates are introduced into the body in various forms of sugars or starches, all of which are ultimately converted into glucose. Carbohydrates are the preferred fuel source for most tissues and are necessary to supply energy for the most basic cellular functions. Heat produced during the oxidation of carbohydrates is used to help maintain body temperature. Excess glucose that is not needed for cellular activities is stored as glycogen in the liver and muscle cells through a process called **gluconeogenesis.** When reserve energy is required, stored glycogen is reconverted to glucose to maintain blood glucose levels within a relatively steady range. During times of physiologic stress, glycogen is metabolized into glucose to provide an immediate energy source. This utilization of glycogen is called **glycogenolysis.** Glucose metabolism is regulated by two pancreatic hormones, insulin (secreted by beta cells) and glucagon (secreted by alpha cells). Insulin is necessary for transport of glucose into cells, and under normal circumstances, ingestion or infusion of glucose causes an increase in insulin release from the beta cells. This process is altered during periods of physiologic stress, leading to hyperglycemia as part of the **metabolic stress response.**

Glucagon, secreted by the alpha cells of the pancreas, is released in response to falling blood glucose levels, stimulating conversion of stored glycogen into glucose. Stored glycogen is also released in response to increased levels of epinephrine, norepinephrine, vasopressin, and angiotensin II, hormones that are released rapidly during physiologic stress. Excess glucose is converted to either glycogen or fatty acids (triglycerides) and stored for later conversion back into glucose when energy is needed. Glycogen stores are depleted rapidly in high-acuity patients who experience intense or prolonged physiologic stress, such as occurs with surgery, trauma, or infection.

Approximately 25 percent of the body's glucose supply is consumed by the brain and nervous system. Although maintenance of blood glucose within a narrow range is essential for preservation of central nervous system (CNS) functioning, it cannot store or synthesize glucose as a fuel source. Instead, the CNS relies primarily on glucose extraction from the bloodstream. The brain can use ketone bodies (derived from fat metabolism) as a fuel source; however, this does not supply enough energy for the brain to maintain its essential cellular functions (Carroll & Curtis, 2007).

Adequate carbohydrate intake prevents proteins from being used as a fuel source. Proteins can provide energy, but this use is not beneficial to overall well-being because proteins are needed primarily for other cellular functions. Carbohydrates supply four kilocalories (kcal) of energy for each gram ingested and normally provide 40 to 60 percent of daily caloric requirements.

Proteins

Proteins are composed of various combinations of amino acids and contain **nitrogen** in addition to carbon, hydrogen, and oxygen. Formation of proteins requires metabolism of carbohydrates and lipids. Proteins serve many complex functions at the cell membrane and are essential for formation and maintenance of all cells, tissues, and organs. Proteins also play a role in many of the body's transport mechanisms, such as transmission of nerve impulses. Proteins are considered building blocks because they contribute to the structure of genes, enzymes, hormones, antibodies, hemoglobin of red blood cells, bone matrix, muscles, and organs. Maintenance of osmotic pressure and appropriate blood pH also depend on an adequate protein supply. Proteins are categorized according to their location in the body.

- *Visceral proteins* - are found within internal organs. Prealbumin, albumin, and transferrin (plasma proteins) are frequently measured in laboratory tests as indicators of protein status as well as overall nutritional status.
- *Somatic proteins* - are found in accessory and skeletal muscles.

Protein synthesis and degradation is an ongoing process. Under usual circumstances, the overall content of proteins in the body is relatively steady; however, under stress conditions, protein catabolism is increased. In the high-acuity patient, inadequate protein intake can quickly lead to **malnutrition**, prolonged wound healing, diminished resistance to infection, and even death. Like carbohydrate metabolism, protein metabolism is influenced by hormones. For example, protein synthesis is enhanced by growth hormone (GH) and diminished by low levels of insulin.

When carbohydrate availability is not adequate to meet the body's energy requirements, proteins are broken down into their amino acid components. Ketoacids, byproducts of amino acid metabolism, can then be further metabolized through the Krebs cycle to produce glucose needed for cellular energy. Proteins supply four kcal of energy per gram. Average, healthy adults require about 15 to 20 percent of their nutrient intake as proteins. This amount increases considerably under conditions of physiologic stress. Protein malnutrition leads to atrophy of the gut mucosa and is a factor in the development of bacterial translocation. Impairment of skin integrity, delayed wound healing, and loss of skeletal muscle mass result from protein malnutrition.

Lipids

Lipids are also referred to as fats. At the cellular level, lipids contribute to the structure of the cell membrane. Lipids are the primary source of energy reserve and are readily stored as triglycerides, phospholipids, and cholesterol for later use as an energy source. A portion of the triglyceride molecule can be used for glucose metabolism. Lipids provide nine kcal of energy per gram, more calories than any other nutrient. Functionally, lipids are similar to carbohydrates because their availability as an energy source can save proteins from being broken down.

As with the other macronutrients, insulin influences lipid synthesis and reserves. Insulin is needed for the transport of glucose into fat cells. Only small quantities of stored fat are found in the circulating blood. Most fat is stored in adipose tissue and the liver. The liver can produce lipids from glucose or amino acids, a process called **lipogenesis**. This occurs when there are more carbohydrates present than required for energy or for glycogen storage in the liver. Under normal conditions, lipogenesis predominates. During stress, lipolytic metabolism predominates, which increases the availability of fatty acids for adenosine triphosphate (ATP) and energy (Guyton & Hall, 2006).

Lipids are a source of essential vitamins and aid the absorption of the fat-soluble vitamins A, D, E, and K. Stored lipids provide insulation for the body in the form of subcutaneous fat and provide structural protection for some organs such as the kidneys. The American Heart Association recommends limiting daily fat intake as follows: no more than seven percent of saturated fat, no more than one percent of trans fat, and less than 300 mg of cholesterol (Lichtenstein et al., 2006) or less than 30 percent of total intake. Fat intake in the United States, however, generally exceeds this recommendation, being approximately 34 percent fat (Dwyer, 2007). Table 32–1 summarizes information on the macronutrients.

TABLE 32–1 Summary of Macronutrients

NUTRIENT	CALORIC VALUE (KCAL/GRAM)	PERCENT OF RECOMMENDED TOTAL DAILY INTAKE	GENERAL FUNCTIONS
Carbohydrates			
Basic unit: glucose	Enteral: 4 Parenteral: 3.4	About 40-60%	■ Maintenance of body temperature ■ Supply energy for basic cell functions
Proteins			
Basic unit: amino acids	4	15–20%	■ Many complex functions at cell membrane ■ Essential for formation and maintenance of all cells, tissues, and organs ■ Contribute to structure of muscles, organs, antibodies, enzymes, and hormones ■ Important role in transport mechanisms ■ Important in maintenance of osmotic pressure and blood pH
Lipids (fats)			
Basic unit: fatty acids	9	No more than 30%	■ Primary source of fuel reserve ■ Body insulation ■ Structural protection for some organs (e.g., kidneys)

SECTION TWO REVIEW

1. An example of a micronutrient is
   A. minerals
   B. carbohydrates
   C. proteins
   D. fats
2. Glucose metabolism is regulated by which two hormones?
   A. epinephrine and norepinephrine
   B. glycogen and glucagon
   C. insulin and vasopressin
   D. glucagon and insulin
3. Which nutrient provides the greatest amount of calories per volume?
   A. carbohydrates
   B. fats
   C. visceral proteins
   D. somatic proteins
4. Which organ is most dependent on maintenance of normal blood glucose levels?
   A. heart
   B. lungs
   C. kidney
   D. brain
5. Maintenance of appropriate osmotic pressure depends on which nutrient?
   A. complex carbohydrates
   B. simple sugars
   C. proteins
   D. fats

Answers: 1. A, 2. D, 3. B, 4. D, 5. C

SECTION THREE: Focused Nutritional History and Physical Assessment

At the completion of this section, the learner will be able to describe a focused nutritional nursing history and physical assessment.

A strong nutritional assessment is an important part of the evaluation of high-acuity patients. History and physical assessment data help identify a patient's current nutrition/metabolic status, provides baseline data with which to compare the effectiveness of therapies, and identify patients who may be at risk for complications related to their nutritional status. Obtaining information regarding nutritional history, as well as current clinical status, risks due to hospitalization, and potential surgeries or treatments, allows the nurse to plan and initiate proper nutritional support.

Malnutrition is a common problem in high-acuity patients that significantly contributes to poor patient outcomes. It is important to quickly identify patients who have preexisting malnutrition and those who are at risk for developing malnutrition in order to set appropriate goals and to help establish proper nutritional support. The influence of an illness or injury on a person's nutritional state is difficult to predict. Some diseases place acutely ill patients at greater risk for malnutrition, such as acute pancreatitis, inflammatory bowel disease, and injuries such as traumas and burns due to their exaggerated metabolic demands (Clark, 2009; Harrington, 2004). The compounding consequences of acute and chronic diseases may contribute to or overlap with the effects of malnutrition, making it difficult to identify any specific source of a patient's nutritional problems.

Medical and Nutritional History

When dealing with the high-acuity patient, the history may be difficult to obtain; it often requires obtaining a patient history from family members. Assessing the patient's nutritional status provides the nurse with information that is essential to the development of a comprehensive nursing care plan. A dietary history is obtained to gain insight into adequacy of nutrition. Usual food intake and food choices are reviewed for caloric density, protein content, and micronutrient concentration. Social, cultural, ethnic, and religious traditions may be considered as they may impact choices, consumption, access, preparation, and storage of food. Social history including a history of smoking, use of illicit drugs or alcohol, dietary supplements, herbal supplements, appetite suppressants and laxatives may provide insight into a patient's nutritional status (Clark, 2009).

General components of the nutritional history include the following

- History of food and fluid intake
- Barriers to normal food consumption
- Alterations in gastrointestinal anatomy and nutrient absorption
- Recent weight changes

The Subjective Global Assessment of Nutritional Status (SGA) (Detsky et al., 1987) is a commonly used tool for assessing nutritional status. It is relatively easy to perform and can be modified based on specific diseases. The assessment includes

- Patient history
  - Weight change
  - Dietary intake change
  - Gastrointestinal symptoms
  - Functional capacity
  - Disease and its relation to nutritional requirements (sorted by levels of stress associated with various diseases)
- Physical findings
  - Basic measurements
  - Edema, including ascites

The final step of the SGA is a three-level rating scale that assigns the patient to a category: well nourished, moderately (or suspected of being) malnourished, or severely malnourished.

Physical Assessment

Many nutrient deficiencies can be revealed by physical exam. General appearance, weight loss or muscle wasting, subcutaneous tissue loss, edema, and even ascites are easily identified and strong indicators of inadequate nutritional status. Objective measurements include a physical exam, anthropometric measurements, assessment of body composition, and laboratory assessment. A careful nutritional physical exam can reveal important clues of nutritional deficiencies. Table 32–2 lists some of the major physical findings that are associated with nutritional deficiencies.

Anthropometric Measurements

Anthropometry is a Greek word meaning the "measure of humans." Anthropometrics is the assessment of height, weight, and waist circumference used to measure the body. Serial measurements of anthropometric measurements are helpful clinically, as they provide evidence of recovery from uncomplicated malnutrition and recovery from illness (Russell & Mueller, 2007; Clark, 2009).

Precise measurements of body composition, including body fat, require technically sophisticated methods, which are not practical in the acute care clinical settings. Still, simple

TABLE 32–2 Physical Findings Associated with Nutritional Deficiencies

BODY SYSTEM	FINDINGS	NURSING IMPLICATIONS
General Survey	▪ Weight loss, muscle wasting, subcutaneous tissue loss ▪ Edema or ascites ▪ Decreased IBW and BMI	Protein-calorie malnutrition (PCM): <90% IBW; or severe malnutrition: <70% IBW Deficits may indicate ineffective feeding
Vital Signs	▪ Increased or decreased temperature ▪ Increased RR and HR ▪ Decreased blood pressure	Increased temperature: increased energy and fluid requirements; decreased temperature: decreased energy demands Elevated vital signs may indicate increased calorie and protein requirements, anemia Decreased BP may indicate dehydration
Skin	▪ Pallor, dermatitis ▪ Petechiae, ecchymosis ▪ Poor wound healing, pressure ulcers ▪ Altered skin turgor, sweat; edema and third spacing	Deficiencies in minerals, vitamins and/or protein Vitamin C or vitamin K deficiency Zinc, Vitamin C, or protein deficiency Altered skin turgor and sweat may indicate poor fluid status; edema indicates accumulation of fluid in tissues May be related to protein malnutrition which leads to decreased capillary osmotic pressure
Nails	▪ Altered shape, color, angle contour, or presence of lesions (e.g., spoon shape; lackluster, dull; poor blanching, pale or mottled)	Deficiencies of iron, protein, or vitamin A or C
Oral Cavity	▪ Dry mucosa, lips, or tongue ▪ Pale mucosa ▪ Missing, chipped, broken teeth, dentures ▪ Spongy, bleeding gums; pale gums	Insufficient hydration Iron, vitamin B_{12}, or folate deficiency (anemia) Problems with chewing Abnormal gums can result from iron deficiency
Pulmonary	▪ Muscle and fat depletion; use of abdominal, rib, or neck muscles with breathing; labored breathing ▪ Pulmonary crackles, rhonchi	Calorie and protein depletion; decreased strength of breathing, decreased reserve. Increased energy requirements for breathing Fluid overload; fluid in the airways
Cardiovascular	▪ Distended neck veins and edema ▪ Pitting edema ▪ Increased heart rate; irregularity in heart rhythm ▪ Presence of S3	Fluid overload Fluid overload, low serum albumin levels, protein malnutrition Consider dehydration; abnormal electrolyte levels Consider fluid overload
Abdomen	▪ Loss of subcutaneous fat; poor muscle tone, wasting; hypoactive or hyperactive bowel sounds ▪ Rounded appearance, or distended	Insufficient calories; nutritional depletion, decreased activity Consider intestinal function in nutritional support route selection Gas distention, obesity; ascites, fluid and sodium imbalances
Kidneys	▪ Dark, concentrated urine; high specific gravity or osmolality ▪ Light, dilute urine; low specific gravity or osmolality	Possible dehydration Possible overhydration
Musculoskeletal	▪ Fat and muscle wasting; swollen, painful joints; altered hand-to-mouth coordination	Protein and calorie deficiency; vitamin C or D deficiencies. Electrolyte alterations can also cause alterations in musculoskeletal function
Neurological	▪ Confusion, irritability, apathy, dementia ▪ Lower body muscle weakness; loss of ankle and knee jerks bilaterally; hyper- or hypoactive reflexes; peripheral neuropathy	Neurological alterations can result from protein, vitamin, and electrolyte deficiencies

Data from Russell & Mueller (2005); Hammond (1999); and Sabol (2004).

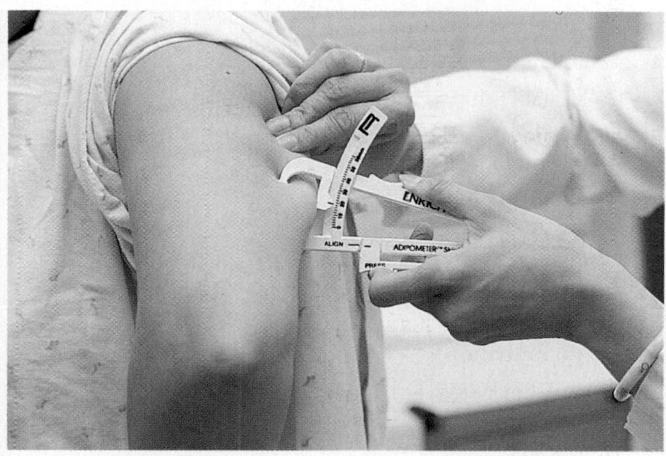

Figure 32–3 ■ Measuring mid-arm circumference with calipers.

measurements of skin-fold thickness, height, and weight can be acquired. Skin calipers are used to obtain an indirect measurement of subcutaneous fat thickness, using the triceps or subscapular region (see Fig. 32–3). Many variables exist in the acute care setting, such as lack of proper training, the presence of wounds, dressings, edema, and other conditions, that make this an imprecise measurement and contribute to the lack of validity and usefulness of the data obtained from the measurements.

Height and Weight

Accurate measurement of height and weight are a cornerstone to assessment of body composition. Height is measured with a measuring rod while the patient is standing upright or lying flat. Under circumstances in which a head-to-toe measurement is not possible, height can also be measured by arm span method, which correlates with height at maturity. The arm span method is obtained by extending both arms out from the body, and measuring the distance between the longest fingertips of each hand (Russell & Mueller, 2007). It is an important measurement as height is used to determine ideal or desirable body weight and is an important factor in determining energy requirements (Russell, & Mueller, 2007; Clark, 2009).

In the high-acuity setting, a precise weight may be difficult to obtain for several reasons. Body water disturbances and electrolyte imbalances are extremely common and cause rapid weight fluctuations. Body weight measurements are usually taken using either a standing weight or a bed or sling weight; however, in the high-acuity patient, use of such scales often does not reflect the patient's true weight. This inaccuracy is partially due to the relative inaccessibility of the patient who is attached to multiple pieces of equipment or tubes; or has dressings, casts, orthopedic pins, or other devices in place. In such cases, weight measurement becomes relative; that is, current weights are compared to previous weights and the patient's "usual" weight, if possible, to identify obvious weight gains or losses. An increase or decrease in weight of as little as two pounds may indicate a gain or loss of up to a liter of fluid.

Ideal Body Weight and Body Mass Index

Once a body weight is obtained, it should be compared to ideal body weight (IBW) and body mass index (BMI). An IBW is the expected weight of an individual based on age, sex, and height. IBW is often determined by the Hamwi rule of thumb method (Hamwi, 1964). In this method, males are given 106 lbs (48 kg) for the first 5 ft of height (1.5 m) and an additional 6 lbs (2.7 kg) for each inch (2.54 cm) over 5 ft. Females are given 100 lbs (45 kg) for the first 5 feet and an additional 5 lbs (2.3 kg) for each inch over 5 ft. Adjustments are made for a large frame by adding 10 percent of body weight, and subtracting 10 percent for a small frame.

A BMI is a widely accepted estimate for obesity, but can also be helpful in the assessment of malnutrition. Generally, a BMI of less than 25 indicates a normal weight, a BMI of 25 to 30 indicates overweight, and a BMI of 30 or more indicates obesity. A BMI over 40 would indicate severe obesity. On the other hand, a BMI of less than 18 indicates malnutrition, and less than 16 indicates severe malnutrition (Russell and Mueller, 2007; Clark, 2009). The BMI calculates body mass by using a formula (see Table 32–3).

TABLE 32–3 Formulas Used to Calculate Body Mass Index (BMI)

Metrics calculation	U.S. customary units calculation
BMI = Wt. (in kg.)/Ht. (in meters^2)	BMI = (Wt. [in lbs.] × 703)/Ht. (in inches^2)

Emerging Evidence

- Abnormally low baseline serum creatinine concentrations are indicative of increased risk of death in the critically ill adult, independent of BMI. Patients with a baseline creatinine of 0.6 or less had a longer length of stay in the ICU environment and increased risk of death *(Cartin-Ceba, Afessa, & Gajic, 2007).*
- In medical and surgical ICU patients admitted with BMIs classifying them as obese, their BMI did not adversely affect survival within the first 12 months following admission. Their BMI was not associated with increased morbidity or mortality and independently predicted survival during the 12 month period. Investigators suggested that being obese may actually have had a protective effect rather than increasing morbidity and mortality *(Peake, Moran et al., 2006).*
- In a review of research literature focusing on nutritional supplement doses and important clinical outcomes, the reviewers concluded that aggressive implementation of enteral nutrition improves clinical outcomes. They also concluded that adding parenteral nutrition either in addition to or in replacement of enteral feedings does not provide significant clinical benefits *(Stapleton, Jones, & Heyland, 2007).*

SECTION THREE REVIEW

1. It is difficult to assess nutritional status and body composition in high-acuity patients because (choose all that apply)
   A. family members are not reliable sources of information
   B. precise weight is difficult to assess
   C. nutritional status is influenced by many factors
   D. fluid and electrolyte imbalances are common
2. Nitrogen balance assesses the adequacy of
   A. carbohydrates
   B. lipids
   C. protein intake
   D. calories
3. An IBW is
   A. the expected body weight
   B. the desired body weight
   C. variable due to the effects of illness
   D. predictive of health outcomes
4. A BMI of 33 indicates
   A. malnutrition
   B. normal weight
   C. overweight
   D. obesity
5. A BMI of 18 indicates
   A. malnutrition
   B. normal weight
   C. overweight
   D. obesity

Answers: 1.(B, C, D), 2. C, 3. A, 4. D, 5. A

SECTION FOUR: Laboratory Assessment of Nutritional/Metabolic Status

At the completion of this section, the learner will be able to discuss the laboratory assessment of nutritional and metabolic status.

A patient's nutritional/metabolic status strongly influences the entire illness experience and outcomes. It is vital, therefore, for the nurse to have a basic understanding of the laboratory tests commonly used to assess the patient's overall metabolic/nutritional status. Common laboratory tests used to assess nutritional/metabolic status include albumin, prealbumin, transferrin, total lymphocyte count (TLC), and serum electrolytes. Serum albumin, prealbumin, and transferrin are indicators of visceral protein status. Abnormally low levels of these plasma proteins indicate that muscle has been catabolized for energy, which can result in serious multisystem complications. Normal values are noted in Table 32–4.

Albumin

The plasma protein, albumin, is the major protein produced in the liver. Over 60 percent of albumin is located in the extravascular space and is crucial for maintenance of intravascular volume because of its influence on blood osmotic pressure. Albumin is frequently measured in high-acuity patients and is often used by clinicians as a primary indicator of overall nutritional status. Low albumin levels coincide with increased occurrence of clinical complications and poor patient outcomes; however, this value must be interpreted cautiously. Albumin has a 15 to 20 day half-life and is heavily influenced by hydration status and hepatocellular injury. These factors make it of little value for assessing acute changes in nutritional status, but it is valuable for tracking long-term changes in protein status. Albumin, therefore, should not be used as an indicator to detect early malnutrition or effectiveness of nutrition support. Abnormally low albumin values may be detected in

TABLE 32–4 Laboratory Assessment of Serum Proteins

PROTEIN	NORMAL	IMPLICATIONS
Albumin	3.5–5.0 g/dL	Less than 3.5 may indicate protein-energy malnutrition Half-life is 15 to 20 days. Changes are slow to correlate with changes in clinical status Albumin can also be affected by hydration status A measure of overall nutrition but not a good measure of ongoing nutritional support When low levels are present, check for edema and ascites
Transferrin	200–430 mcg/dL	Less than 200 indicates protein-energy malnutrition Half-life is eight days Controlled by iron stores depleted iron stores will increase transferrin synthesis Decreased in liver and renal disease, and inflammatory process
Prealbumin	17–40 mg/dL	Less than 17 indicates protein-energy malnutrition Half-life two to three days, assists in monitoring acute changes in nutritional status Should note increase after four to eight days of proper nutrition Decreases in presence of inflammation and postoperatively Low zinc levels impair liver prealbumin synthesis

Data from Kee (2009); Sabol (2004).

patients with liver or renal disease even when protein intake is adequate. In patients who receive fluid resuscitation, serum albumin values are likely to be dilutional and not an accurate indicator of the actual albumin level.

Prealbumin

Transthyretin, better known as prealbumin, is a protein that is extremely helpful in nutritional assessment. Prealbumin is a transport protein that binds retinol-binding protein and thyroxin, a thyroid hormone. The half-life of prealbumin is 48 to 72 hours and is considered a more reliable indicator of acute changes in catabolism than serum albumin. Prealbumin is technically easy and inexpensive to measure in the laboratory and it is not influenced by hydration, renal, or liver status to the same extent as albumin. Periodic monitoring of prealbumin provides an indication of the effectiveness of nutrition support and the overall catabolic state. Prealbumin should increase within four to eight days if a patient is receiving adequate nutritional support.

Transferrin

Transferrin is a plasma protein that binds with and transports iron to cells. Transferrin may be more useful than albumin for tracking responses to nutritional therapies because its half-life is eight to ten days. Accuracy of transferrin as a nutritional indicator depends on the patient's underlying iron level. Use of transferrin as an indicator of adequacy of nutrition in the high-acuity patient may be limited because of other blood-related factors, such as blood loss anemia or blood transfusions.

Nitrogen Balance

In the high-acuity patient, nitrogen balance may be evaluated as an indicator of protein status. One gram of nitrogen is equivalent to 6.25 grams of protein. Simply defined, nitrogen balance is the difference between nitrogen output and nitrogen intake, and is measured by a test called the urine urea nitrogen (UUN) test. Calculation of nitrogen balance first requires collection of a 24-hour urine specimen with an accurate account of urinary output during the collection time. Furthermore, the urine must be chilled, either in a specimen refrigerator or on ice throughout the 24-hour period. Because nitrogen is a component of protein, it also is necessary to know the patient's protein intake during the time of the urine urea nitrogen (UUN) collection. Nitrogen balance is easy to calculate once the UUN is reported by the laboratory. Table 32–5 provides the equations needed to calculate nitrogen balance. Four grams of nitrogen are often added to the UUN test to account for nitrogen losses that are not captured by urine collection alone (e.g., stool, skin, enterocutaneous fistula drainage, excessive wound drainage). The major disadvantage of using the UUN level to assess protein need is that it is not valid in renal failure. Urinary nitrogen output is expected to be low in renal failure because the kidneys are unable to excrete nitrogen wastes. The UUN can be used to calculate the amount of protein needed. For a patient who is stressed and catabolic, the goal of protein administration should be to provide a positive nitrogen balance.

TABLE 32–5 Calculating Nitrogen Balance

Formula: Nitrogen balance = nitrogen in − (nitrogen out + 4 g/day)
Where: Nitrogen in = g of protein received during the 24 hours of UUN collection, divided by the constant 6.25; and nitrogen out = g of protein excreted in the urine as measured by the UUN plus insensible loss, estimated at 4 g

Data from Heimburger (2007).

Vitamin and Mineral Assays

Low serum levels of vitamin A, zinc, and magnesium are common in acutely ill, hospitalized patients. Fat soluble vitamin (A, D, E) and mineral (iron, folic acid) deficiencies should be assessed if a patient has a digestive and/or absorptive disorder. If these or other micronutrient deficiencies are suspected, a variety of serum and red blood cell assays are available to assist with nutritional assessment. Commonly available assays include Vitamin A, Vitamin E, thiamine, folate (serum and red blood cell), Vitamin B_{12}, zinc, magnesium, and phosphorus.

Total Lymphocyte Count

Many cells of the immune system, such as antibodies and lymphocytes, contain a significant amount of protein. Proper functioning of the immune system depends on an adequate total protein level. Measurement of the total lymphocyte count (TLC) provides some quantification of the effect of protein loss on immune system functioning. The total lymphocyte count is an easily obtained indicator of overall immune status and adequacy of protein. This indicator is considered most reliable when white blood cell and lymphocyte counts are relatively stable; therefore, a TLC should be interpreted with caution in the high-acuity patient experiencing **hypermetabolism** or infections.

The total lymphocyte count should be about 20 to 40 percent of the total white blood cell (WBC) count. Although there are many disease states and treatments that affect immunocompetence, poor nutrition is a major contributor to immunosuppression. Malnutrition causes immunosuppression by depressing neutrophil chemotaxis and total lymphocyte count. It also delays hypersensitivity reactivity and may cause complete **anergy** to antigen skin testing. A total lymphocyte count of less than 1,500 mm^3 is indicative of impaired immune functioning. Total lymphocyte count can be calculated using the following formula (Feitelson-Winkler, Gerrior, & Pomp, 1989):

$$\text{TLC} = \frac{\%\ \text{lymphocytes} \times \text{WBC}}{100}$$

Table 32–6 provides a summary of laboratory values pertinent to the nutritional/metabolic assessment of the high-acuity patient.

TABLE 32–6 Laboratory Tests to Assess Nutritional Status

TEST	NORMAL VALUE
Blood urea nitrogen (BUN)	5–25 mg/dL
Serum creatinine	0.5–1.5 mg/dL
Albumin	3.5–5.0 g/dL
Prealbumin (transthyretin)	17–40 mg/mL
Transferrin	200–430 mg/dL

Data from Kee (2009).

Anergy Screen

Cell-mediated immunity is one of the body's defense mechanisms that is most affected by malnutrition. Delayed cutaneous hypersensitivity screening, also referred to as skin testing, is a simple method for evaluating cell-mediated immunity status. A test dose of a known antigen, such as tuberculin, *Candida*, mumps, or *Trichophyton*, is administered intradermally. The individual's ability to respond to this immunologic challenge is evaluated 24 and 48 hours after administration. If cellular immunity is intact, an induration of 2 to 5 mm should be observed at the injection site. If no skin reaction occurs, the patient is considered to be anergic, which means that cellular immunity may have been negatively affected by malnutrition (Porth & Sweeney, 2007).

SECTION FOUR REVIEW

1. A low serum albumin can be caused by which circumstances? (choose all that apply)
   A. liver disease
   B. kidney disease
   C. chronic malnutrition
   D. acute malnutrition
2. Which lab value is the best indicator of current nutritional status?
   A. prealbumin
   B. albumin
   C. transferrin
   D. BUN
3. A urine urea nitrogen (UUN) has been ordered on a patient. The nurse can expect to take which action regarding this order?
   A. no action by the nurse is required
   B. collect the urine over a 24-hour period
   C. obtain a urine specimen by in-and-out catheterization
   D. maintain the urine specimen at room temperature
4. The total lymphocyte count (TLC) is useful in estimating
   A. nitrogen balance
   B. iron stores
   C. vitamin A, zinc, and magnesium levels
   D. immune system function
5. Anergy screening is useful in evaluating
   A. humoral immunity
   B. malnutrition
   C. cell-mediated immunity
   D. nitrogen balance
6. Which laboratory test is an indicator of the patient's daily protein need?
   A. albumin
   B. BUN
   C. hemoglobin
   D. UUN
7. The condition that makes the 24-hour urine urea nitrogen test an invalid indicator of protein breakdown is
   A. diabetes mellitus
   B. liver failure
   C. renal failure
   D. hypercatabolism

Answers: 1. (A, B, C), 2. A, 3. B, 4. D, 5. C, 6. B, 7. C

SECTION FIVE: Physiologic Studies of Nutrition and Metabolic Status

At the completion of this section, the learner will be able to discuss physiologic studies used to measure nutrition and metabolic status.

The goal of nutritional support in the high-acuity patient is maintenance of nutritional status in order to avoid catabolism along with the risk of metabolic stress and its deleterious effects on survival. Accurate estimates of nutritional requirements help prevent complications associated with underfeeding and overfeeding (O'Leary-Kelley, Puntillo, Barr, Stotts, & Douglas, 2005; Clark, 2009). The task of calculating the patient's caloric, protein, and fluid requirements are often accomplished by obtaining a nutritional consultation from a registered dietician or nutritionist. Acute care nurses should be familiar with the intricacies of the process so they may have input into decisions about nutritional plans, and be prepared to implement the nutritional plans created.

A simple estimation of caloric requirements is to calculate 25 kcal/kg/day for a well-nourished, nonstressed individual with a normal albumin level. This individual would have a nitrogen requirement of 0.8 to 1 gram of protein/day. The fluid requirement would be 1 mL of fluid per calorie. Patients in high-acuity settings have additional stressors and disease states, which alter this basic formula, and lead to an increased need for calories, protein, and fluid (Clark, 2009).

Oxygen Consumption and Energy Expenditure

Oxygen consumption ($\dot{V}O_2$) and energy expenditure are indicators of the metabolic state, and can be assessed by various methods. In-depth discussion of energy expenditure is beyond the scope of this module, but a basic understanding of the measurement is beneficial to the nurse caring for the high-acuity patient.

Oxygen consumption and energy expenditure can be measured directly by calorimetry or calculated using the Fick equation. As oxygen consumption cannot occur without energy expenditure, any event or situation that increases cell and tissue oxygen demands will increase energy expenditure accordingly. Fever, shivering, infection, and pain are examples of events that increase metabolic oxygen demands among acutely ill patients. Nurses have a unique opportunity to vigilantly monitor for these events in an effort to minimize the frequency or severity of these occurences.

Calorimetry

Direct calorimetry measures whole body heat production while the individual is isolated in a chamber or a room specifically equipped for this purpose, which makes it highly impractical for clinical application. **Indirect calorimetry** offers a practical approach to bedside measurement of oxygen consumption, nutrient oxidation, and energy expenditure. An indirect calorimeter is also called a "metabolic cart." This portable unit (about the size of a portable cardiac monitor) estimates the resting energy expenditure (REE) by measurement of respiratory gas exchange. An indirect calorimetry measurement procedure takes 15 to 20 minutes, and can be performed on patients receiving mechanical ventilation or breathing room air. Patients receiving oxygen therapy at less than 45 percent will have more accurate results.

Indirect calorimetry measures the amount of inspired oxygen ($\dot{V}O_2$) and the amount of expired carbon dioxide ($\dot{V}CO_2$). From these numbers, the metabolic cart calculates the daily amount of oxygen consumed and carbon dioxide produced, determining energy expenditure. Normal values are established based on gender, height, weight, age, and activity level. Indirect calorimetry is the most accurate method for determining energy requirements. It measures a patient's actual energy expenditure in order to determine precise needs of the patient (Clark, 2009). Therefore, indirect calorimetry allows for individualized nutrition therapy, while it prevents over- or underfeeding (Wooley, 2005; National Guideline Clearing House, 2004).

Respiratory Quotient. The **respiratory quotient (RQ)** is another valuable parameter provided by indirect calorimetry. The RQ is the ratio of carbon dioxide produced to oxygen consumed. The normal value of approximately 0.85 indicates that the individual is using about an equal amount of carbohydrates, fats, and proteins for energy. The greater the amount of glucose being used, the higher the RQ. For example, an RQ above 1.0 indicates that the patient is receiving too much carbohydrate (i.e., overfeeding), and an RQ below 0.70 indicates inadequate nutrition (i.e., underfeeding). Because glucose breaks down to carbon dioxide, excess carbohydrate intake can potentially result in carbon dioxide retention (**hypercapnia**) with subsequent increased work-of-breathing, which can potentially impair weaning from mechanical ventilation.

Fick Equation. Because indirect calorimetry is not available in all facilities, the Fick equation offers an acceptable substitute if the nurse is attentive to drawing the blood over a 30-second time frame while avoiding introduction of air bubbles into the blood specimen. The Fick equation (Table 32–7) requires blood gas analysis of arterial and venous blood. There are two disadvantages of using the Fick method: (1) It represents the oxygen consumption for only one moment in time; and (2) errors in calculation of the cardiac output can occur, which alters the accuracy of the oxygen consumption value obtained.

Oxygen Extraction

While at rest, the amount of oxygen delivered ($\dot{D}O_2$) via arterial blood for consumption by the body's tissues is normally approximately 1,000 mL/min. The tissues extract about 25 percent of this available oxygen, which equates to about 250 mL/m^2/min of oxygen. After gas exchange occurs at the capillary bed, about 750 mL/m^2/min of oxygen is returned to the venous blood, which makes the normal oxygen saturation of venous blood ($S\dot{V}O_2$) about 75 percent. Oxygen consumption can increase considerably in the high-acuity patient; therefore, a higher amount of oxygen may be extracted from arterial blood, which corresponds with a decreased venous oxygen return (or decreased $S\dot{V}O_2$). Monitoring of $S\dot{V}O_2$ can provide important data regarding the amount of additional oxygen extracted from the blood and may help the nurse identify any changes in aerobic or anaerobic metabolic trends. $S\dot{V}O_2$ can be continuously monitored at the bedside using a special thermodilution fiberoptic catheter.

TABLE 32–7 Fick Equation for Oxygen Consumption

Formula: $\dot{V}O_2 = (CaO_2 - CvO_2) \times CO \times 10$
Where: $\dot{V}O_2$ is tissue oxygen uptake; CO is cardiac output; CaO_2 is arterial oxygen content (hemoglobin × 1.34 × arterial oxygen saturation [decimal]); and CvO_2 is mixed venous oxygen content (hemoglobin × 1.34 × venous oxygen saturation [decimal])

Harris–Benedict Equation

There are over 200 equations for predicting energy needs, and many are population-specific. The **Harris–Benedict equation** is one of the more commonly used formulas to calculate resting energy expenditure (REE) (Harris & Benedict, 1919). This formula differentiates gender, and requires knowledge of the patient's height in centimeters, weight in kilograms, and age in years. The Harris–Benedict equation for both genders is as follows:

$$\text{Male: } 66 + (13.7 \times \text{weight [kg]}) + (5.0\ (\text{height [cm]}) - (6.8 \times \text{age})$$

$$\text{Female: } 655 + (9.6 \times \text{weight [kg]}) + (1.8 \times \text{height [cm]}) - (4.7 \times \text{age})$$

The Harris–Benedict equation assumes that the patient is within the range of ideal weight relative to height. Ideal weight for adult males and females is 100 pounds for a height of 5 feet. For males, the weight allowance is 6 pounds for every inch above 5 feet. For females, the ideal weight allowance is 5 pounds for every inch above 5 feet. For patients above their ideal weight, a calculation is made for an adjusted weight to be used in the Harris–Benedict equation. Adjusted weight is obtained from the following calculation:

$$\text{Adjusted weight} = \text{Actual weight} - \text{Ideal weight} \times 0.25 + \text{Ideal weight}$$

Because this prediction does not take into account the metabolic response to injury and illness, stress factors are added to adjust for activity, elevated body temperature, disease processes, surgery, burns, trauma, and sepsis (see Table 32–8) (Long, Schaffel, & Geiger, 1979). The following is an example of use of the Harris–Benedict equation to estimate daily caloric need:

> If a patient with multiple trauma was estimated by the Harris–Benedict equation to have an energy expenditure of 2,000, this figure would be multiplied by 1.1 to 1.5 to obtain an energy expenditure of 2,200 to 3,000. This patient would require 2,200 to 3,000 nonprotein kilocalories per day.

TABLE 32–8 Estimation of Energy Expenditure in Commonly Encountered Conditions: The Harris-Benedict Equation and Stress Factors

COMMON CLINICAL CONDITION	ASSOCIATED STRESS FACTOR
Well-nourished, unstressed	1.0
Maintenance	
▪ mild stress	1.0–1.2
▪ moderate stress	1.4
▪ severe stress	1.6
Surgery	
▪ minor	1.2
▪ major	1.2–1.5
▪ cancer	1.0–1.5
Fever	1.0 (for each ° C above the normal body temperature)
Acute Phase Sepsis	
▪ hypotensive	1.2–1.6
▪ normotensive	1.0–1.4
Recovery Phase of Sepsis	1.0–1.2
Acute Phase Multiple Trauma	
▪ hypotensive	1.2–1.6
▪ normotensive	1.0–1.5
Recovery Phase of Multiple Trauma	1.0–1.2
Burn Injury (before grafting)	
▪ 10% BSA (body surface area)	1.25
▪ 20% BSA	1.5
▪ 30% BSA	1.5
▪ 40% BSA	1.75
▪ Greater than 40% BSA	2.0
Burn Injury (after graft)	1.0–1.4

Data from: Schlichtig, R., & Ayers, T. S. (1988). Nutritional support of the critically ill. *Chicago: Year Book Medical Publishers;* Mann, S., Westenskow, DR, Houtchens, BA. (1985). Measured and predicted caloric expenditure in the acutely ill. *Critical Care Medicine; 13:173-177;* Marino, P. (2007). Metabolic substrate requirements. In Paul Marino (Ed.) *The ICU Book (3rd ed.).* Lippincott Williams & Wilkins, Philadelphia, PA; http://www.adaevidencelibrary.com/evidence.cfm?evidence_summary_id=250450.

SECTION FIVE REVIEW

1. Oxygen consumption is a measure of a person's
   - **A.** oxygen delivery
   - **B.** resting energy expenditure
   - **C.** metabolic state
   - **D.** anaerobic metabolism
2. The most accurate method for determining energy requirements is
   - **A.** calculating 25 kcal/kg/day
   - **B.** the Hamwi method
   - **C.** the Harris-Benedict equation
   - **D.** indirect calorimetry
3. Indirect calorimetry calculates
   - **A.** caloric requirements
   - **B.** resting energy expenditure
   - **C.** resting energy demands
   - **D.** carbon dioxide production
4. The Harris-Benedict equation measures
   - **A.** REE
   - **B.** IBW
   - **C.** BMI
   - **D.** PCM

5. The extraction of oxygen by the tissues to meet metabolic needs can be measured using
   A. oxygen saturation of arterial blood (SaO_2)
   B. oxygen saturation of venous blood ($S\dot{V}O_2$)
   C. partial pressure of arterial carbon dioxide ($PaCO_2$)
   D. partial pressure of arterial oxygen (PaO_2)

Answers: 1. C, 2. D, 3. B, 4. A, 5. B

POSTTEST

Mark M. 34-years-old, was admitted to the trauma ICU three days ago with multiple fractures resulting from a motorcycle crash. He has an open fracture of his right femur, multiple fractures of his right upper arm, and multiple abrasions on the right side of his body. Major surgery was required to repair the femur. Currently Mark has been spiking frequent fevers. He is not receiving any nutritional support at this time.

1. Mark's metabolic state is currently more catabolic than anabolic. This means that his body is
   A. building tissue
   B. breaking down his body tissues
   C. completely focused on healing
   D. turned to anaerobic metabolism
2. When Mark's body is in a state of aerobic metabolism, the end products are normally removed from the body as
   A. pure energy
   B. lactic acid
   C. pyruvate
   D. CO_2 and water
3. Anaerobic metabolism is an abnormal metabolic process.
   A. True
   B. False

CLINICAL UPDATE: Mark's condition has deteriorated and he is having oxygenation problems. It is suspected that Mark is experiencing significant anaerobic metabolism related to his condition.

4. To evaluate him for excessive anaerobic metabolism, the nurse can anticipate that he will have what serum laboratory test drawn?
   A. lactic acid
   B. nicotinic acid dehydrogenase (NAD^+)
   C. pyruvate
   D. glucose
5. Mark's ability to heal his many injuries greatly depends on his nutritional state. Evaluation of his macronutrient status would include which nutrients? (choose all that apply)
   A. minerals
   B. proteins
   C. vitamins
   D. fats
   E. carbohydrates
6. Mark's protein levels are at risk. If he develops low proteins, it will affect his recovery in which ways? (choose all that apply)
   A. impair wound healing
   B. decrease fluid shifts
   C. increase risk for gut bacterial translocation
   D. inhibit immune function
7. Lipids are important for Mark because they are
   A. carbohydrate protective
   B. a source of vitamins C and B
   C. a major basis of the immune system
   D. the primary energy reserve for the body
8. Mark is being weighed daily. In weighing critically ill patients, it is important to remember that in this patient population
   A. weight rapidly decreases
   B. BMI is recalculated daily
   C. obtaining a true body weight is crucial
   D. body water disturbances cause rapid weight fluctuations

CLINICAL UPDATE: Mark is to have his nitrogen balance evaluated in preparation for initiation of nutritional support.

9. Urine urea nitrogen is ordered on Mark. The correct procedure for collecting this specimen includes (choose all that apply)
   A. one-time in-and-out urinary catheterization
   B. 24-hour urine collection time
   C. maintain specimen at room temperature
   D. continuously chill the specimen
10. Mark has nutritional support initiated. To monitor the effects his supplemental nutrition is having on his body, which serum lab test is likely to be periodically monitored to reflect acute nutrition changes?
    A. albumin
    B. prealbumin
    C. nitrogen
    D. total lymphocyte count

CLINICAL UPDATE: Mark's nutritional status is not significantly improving and it is decided to perform a physiologic study.

11. A metabolic cart study is performed at the bedside. This measurement of indirect calorimetry, measures
    A. CO_2 delivery
    B. oxygen wasted
    C. the amount of expired CO_2
    D. cellular metabolism
12. The Harris-Benedict equation uses different formula for males and females.
    A. True
    B. False

Posttest answers with rationale are found on MyNursingKit.

REFERENCES

Carroll, E. W., & Curtis, R. L. (2007). Organization and control of neural function. *Essentials of pathophysiology: concepts of altered health status.* (2d ed.). Philadelphia: Lippincott Williams & Wilkins, 725–758.

Cartin-Ceba, R., Afessa, B., & Gajic, O. (2007). Low baseline serum creatinine concentration predicts mortality in critically ill patients independent of body mass index. *Critical Care Medicine, 35*(10), 2420–2423.

Clark, M. (2009). Nutrition. In K. K. Carlson (ed.). *AACN advanced critical care nursing.* St. Louis: Saunders-Elsevier.

Detsky, A. S., Baker, J. P., Johnston, N., Whittaker, S. (1987). What is subjective global assessment of nutritional status? *Parenteral and Enteral Nutrition, 11*(1). 8–13.

Dwyer, J. (2007). Nutritional requirements and dietary assessment. In E. Brauwald, A. S. Fauci, D. L. Kasper, S. L. Hauser, D. L. Longo, J. L. Jameson, & J. Loscalzo (eds.). *Harrison's principles of internal medicine* (17th ed.). New York: McGraw-Hill, 437–450.

Feitelson-Winkler, M. F., Gerrior, S. A., Pomp, A., & Albina, J. E. (1989). Use of retinol binding protein and prealbumin as indicators of the response to nutrition therapy. *Journal of the American Dietetic Association, 89*, 684–687.

Guyton, A. C & Hall, J. E. (2006). *Textbook of medical physiology* (11th ed.). St. Louis: Elsevier-Saunder.

Hamwi, G. J. (1964). Changing dietary concepts. In T. S. Danowsi (ed.) *Diabetes mellitus: diagnosis and treatment.* New York: American Diabetes Association.

Harrington, L. (2004). Nutrition in critically ill adults: key processes and outcomes. *Critical Care Nursing Clinics of North America, 16*, 459–465.

Harris, J. A., & Benedict, F. G. (1919). *A biometric study of basal metabolism in man.* Publication No. 279. Washington, DC: Carnegie Institute of Washington.

Kee, J. L. (2009). *Prentice Hall handbook of laboratory and diagnostic tests with nursing implications* (6th ed.). Upper Saddle River, NJ: Pearson/Prentice Hall.

Lichtenstein, A. H., Appel, L. J., Brands, M., Carnethon, M., Daniels, S., Franch, H., Franklin, B., Kris-Etherton, P., Harris, W., Howard, B., Karanja, N., Lefevre, M., Rudel, L. Sacks, F., Van Horn, L., Winston, M., Wylie-Rosett, J.(2006). Diet and lifestyle recommendations revision 2006: a scientific statement from the American Heart Association nutrition committee. *Circulation, 114*(1), 82–96.

Long, C., Schaffel, N., & Geiger, J. (1979). Metabolic response to injury and illness: estimation of energy and protein needs from indirect calorimetry and nitrogen balance. *Journal of Parenteral and Enteral Nutrition, 3*, 452.

National Guideline Clearinghouse, (2004). *Metabolic measurement using indirect calorimetry during mechanical ventilation.* Retrieved August 1, 2008 from http://www.guideline.gov.

O'Leary-Kelley, C. M., Puntillo, K. A., Barr, J., Stotts, N., & Douglas, M. K. (2005). Nutritional adequacy in patients receiving mechanical ventilation who are fed enterally. *American Journal of Critical Care, 14*(3), 222–230.

Pesce-Hammond, K. & Wessel, J. (2005). Nutrition assessment and decision making. In R. Merritt (ed.), *The A.S.P.E.N. nutrition support practice manual* (2d ed.). Silver Spring: American Society for Parenteral and Enteral Nutrition, 3–37.

Peake, S. L., Moran, J. L., Ghelani, D. R.; Lloyd, A. J., & Walker, M. J. (2006). The effect of obesity on 12-month survival following admission to intensive care: a prospective study. *Critical Care Medicine, 34*(12), 2929–2939.

Pleuss, J. (2007). Alterations in body nutrition. In C. M. Porth (ed.), *Essentials of pathophysiology: concepts of altered health states* (2d ed.). Philadelphia: Lippincott Williams & Wilkins, 165–178.

Porth, C. M., & Sweeney, K. (2007). Alterations in immune response. In C. M. Porth (ed.), *Essentials of pathophysiology: concepts of altered health states* (2d ed.). Philadelphia: Lippincott Williams & Wilkins. 293–318.

Russell, M. K., & Mueller, C. (2007). Nutrition screening and assessment. In M. M. Gottschlich (ed.) *The A.S.P.E.N. nutrition support core curriculum: a case-based approach – the adult patient.* Silver Spring: American Society of Parenteral and Enteral Nutrition, 163–186.

Sabol, V. K. (2004). Nutritional assessment of the critically ill adult. *AACN Clinical Issues, 15*(4), 595–606.

Stapleton, R. D., Jones, N., & Heyland, D. (2007). Feeding critically ill patients: what is the optimal amount of energy? *Critical Care Medicine, 35*(9) (Suppl.). S535–S540.

Wooley, J. A. (2005). Use of indirect calorimetry in critically ill patients. In R. Merritt (ed.) *The A.S.P.E.N. nutrition support practice manual* (2d ed.). Silver Spring, MD: American Society for Parenteral and Enteral Nutrition, 277–280.

MODULE

33 Alterations in Metabolism

Valerie Sabol, Tonya Appleby, Melanie G. Hardin-Pierce

OBJECTIVES Following completion of this module, the learner will be able to

1. Explain how the physiological stressors of illness and injury affect nutritional needs.
2. Describe the major nutritional alterations associated with specific disease states.
3. Describe enteral nutrition, including the benefits and potential complications, rationale for gastric versus postpyloric feeding, and barriers to providing optimal enteral nutrition to the high-acuity patient.
4. Discuss the parenteral methods used to provide nutrition for the high-acuity patient, including potential complications.

This self-study module focuses on the metabolic responses that occur in the high-acuity patient. The module is composed of four sections. Section One provides an overview of how the physiological stressors of illness and injury affect nutritional needs, including common metabolic alterations encountered in high-acuity patients. Section Two describes the major nutritional alterations associated with specific disease states. Section Three describes the enteral nutrition, including the benefits and potential complications, rationale for gastric versus postpyloric feeding, and barriers to providing optimal enteral nutrition to the high-acuity patient. The last section, Section Four, discusses the parenteral methods used to provide nutrition for the high-acuity patient, including potential complications. Each section includes a set of review questions to help the learner evaluate his or her understanding of the section's content before moving on to the next section. All Section Reviews include answers. It is suggested that the learner review those concepts answered incorrectly in the review questions before proceeding to the next section.

PRETEST

1. The metabolic stress response is the result of
   A. psychologic stress
   B. overexertion from exercise
   C. injured tissue in the body
   D. hyperventilation
2. The two phases of the metabolic stress response are
   A. ebb phase and catabolic phase
   B. ebb phase and flow phase
   C. ebb phase and recovery phase
   D. flow phase and recovery phase
3. Hypermetabolism refers to
   A. an elevated metabolic rate
   B. the breakdown of total body protein
   C. elevated serum insulin levels
   D. increased immunoglobulins
4. Hypercatabolism refers to
   A. an elevated metabolic rate
   B. the breakdown of total body protein
   C. elevated serum insulin levels
   D. increased immunoglobulins
5. Enteral nutrition has many advantages over total parenteral nutrition (TPN), including the fact that it (choose all that apply)
   A. reduces risk for bacterial translocation
   B. provides central venous access
   C. maintains gut morphology and function
   D. is less costly
6. Which nutrient does a person's body use as the "preferred" energy source?
   A. intact proteins
   B. amino acids

C. carbohydrates
D. lipids

7. Feeding tube occlusion is a potential mechanical complication of enteral feedings. Possible causes of occlusion include (choose all that apply)
   A. viscous formulas
   B. lack of proper flushing
   C. food coloring
   D. medications
8. Which condition is a complication associated with gastric enteral tube feeding?
   A. nosocomial pneumonia
   B. bacterial translocation
   C. stress ulcer
   D. metabolic acidosis
9. Total parenteral nutrition is indicated when
   A. adequate amounts of nutrients cannot be delivered through the gastrointestinal tract
   B. the patient is hypermetabolic
   C. bowel sounds are not audible
   D. the hypercatabolic patient is not able to eat for three days
10. Total parenteral nutrition with glucose concentration greater than 10 percent should be administered through a
   A. nasoenteric feeding tube
   B. peripheral vein
   C. surgically placed jejunal feeding tube
   D. central vein
11. Catheter-related sepsis is a potentially lethal complication of total parenteral nutrition and is primarily caused by
   A. a malpositioned catheter or guidewire during the central line insertion
   B. lack of sterility during central line placement and inadequate maintenance of the line
   C. inadvertent puncture or laceration of the subclavian or carotid artery
   D. puncture or laceration of the vein on insertion of the needle/catheter
12. Mechanical complications of TPN consist of (choose all that apply)
   A. air embolism
   B. catheter fracture
   C. pneumothorax
   D. catheter-related sepsis (CRS)
13. What nursing action would you undertake first when a patient receiving tube feeding develops diarrhea?
   A. stop the tube feeding
   B. send a stool specimen for *Clostridium difficile* cytotoxin analysis
   C. check liquid medications for sorbitol content
   D. dilute the tube feeding
14. Nutritional goals for the patient with pulmonary failure include (choose all that apply)
   A. higher sodium content
   B. lower protein content
   C. lower carbohydrate content
   D. higher fat content
15. A high-acuity patient with acute renal failure may experience abnormalities in (choose all that apply)
   A. protein catabolism
   B. fluid and electrolytes
   C. fat absorption and digestion
   D. increased carbon dioxide levels

Pretest answers are found on MyNursingKit.

SECTION ONE: Metabolic Alterations in the High-Acuity Patient

At the completion of this section, the learner will be able to explain how the physiological stressors of illness and injury affect nutritional needs, and will recognize the typical metabolic alterations occurring in the high-acuity ill patient.

Nutrition in the High-Acuity Patient

High-acuity patients may experience high levels of stress and starvation because of their severe illnesses. Both increased stress and a state of starvation significantly alter metabolism. Older adults or those with chronic illness may be in a starvation or semistarvation state at the time of an injury or acute illness. These patients need to be identified rapidly because their already-compromised nutritional/metabolic state complicates any acute disease state they are experiencing. Starvation can also develop in hospitalized patients as a nosocomial problem. Most high-acuity patients have a greatly increased need for nutrients and calories because of the stress response. Patients who receive no nutrients for several days can easily develop starvation. Because many high-acuity patients are unable to take nourishment by mouth as a result of decreased consciousness or treatments, such as intubation or sedation, provision of **nutrition** by alternate means is a nursing priority.

Malnutrition

Malnutrition is defined by ASPEN (2002b, p. 9SA) as "any disorder of nutrition status, including disorders resulting from a deficiency of nutrient intake, impaired nutrient metabolism, or over-nutrition. Inadequate intake can lead to starvation while excessive intake can result in obesity." Both types of malnutrition are disease-promoting conditions. Malnutrition can negatively affect essentially all body systems, as illustrated in Figure 33–1.

Under-Nutrition

It has been estimated that up to 50 percent of hospitalized patients have evidence of malnutrition and a significant number experience considerable weight loss during and after a stay in the intensive care unit. Unintentional weight loss may deplete nutrient reserves and predispose patients to malnutrition. Malnutrition is

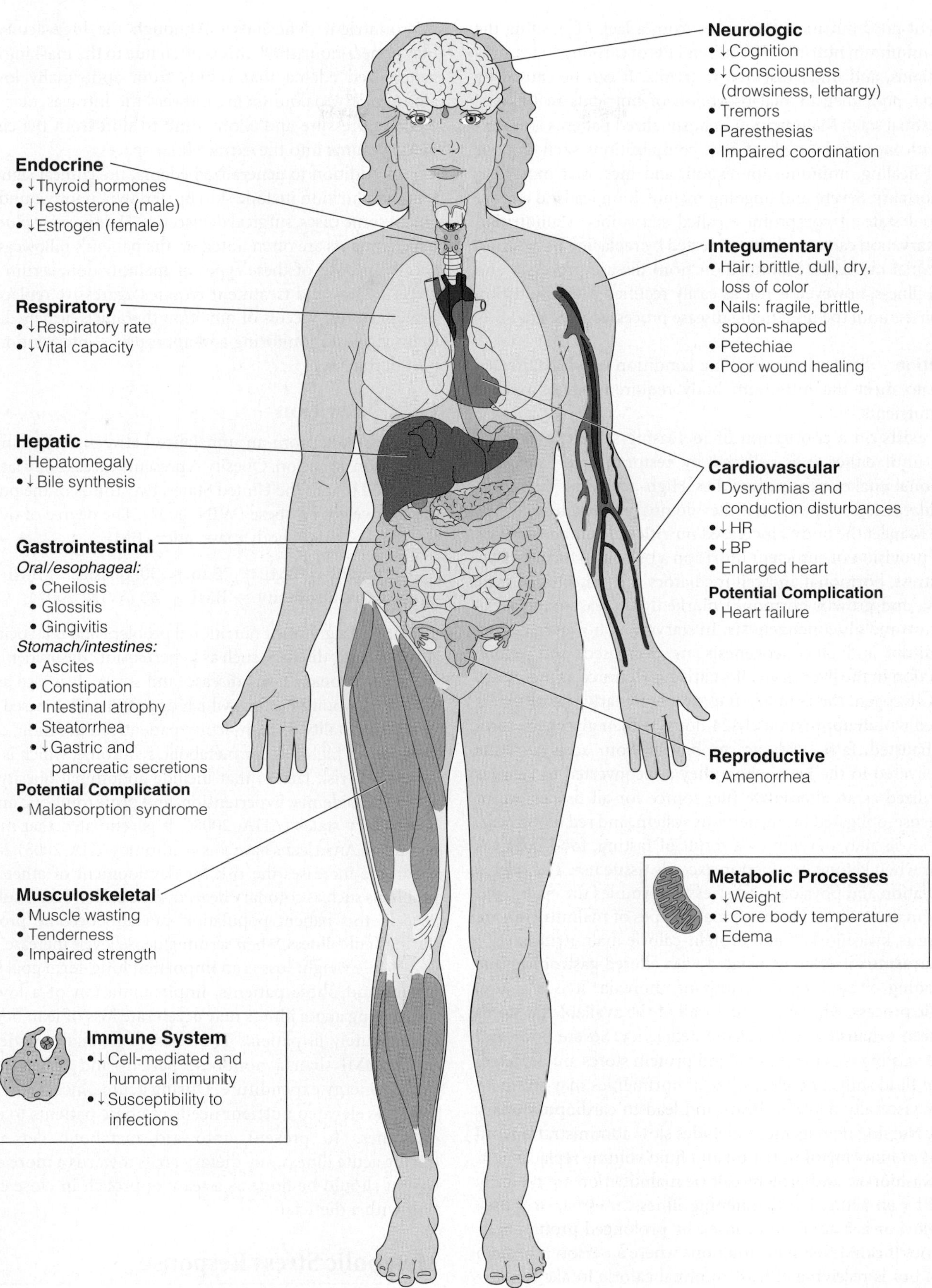

Figure 33–1 ■ Multisystem effects of malnutrition.

a state of poor nutrition that arises from a lack of meeting the body's minimum nutritional requirements of carbohydrates, proteins, lipids, and other essential nutrients. It can be caused by anorexia, poor diet, or malabsorption of nutrients in the gastrointestinal tract. Malnutrition in hospitalized patients is associated with increased length of stay, complications such as poor wound healing, immunosuppression, and increased morbidity and mortality. Severe and ongoing malnutrition leads to a more advanced state of compromise called starvation. Malnutrition from starvation can usually be corrected by replacing body stores of essential nutrients. Malnutrition from disease processes and critical illness, however, is not as easily rectified as malnutrition may persist until the underlying disease process is resolved.

Starvation. Starvation refers to a condition in which there is failure to meet the minimum body requirements of one or more nutrients.

It exists on a continuum of increasing severity that continues until either it is relieved by restoration of adequate nutritional intake or the person dies. High-acuity patients are at particular risk for starvation if they do not receive adequate nutrition to meet the body's increased nutritional demands, which makes provision of sufficient nutrition a priority. During metabolic stress, hormonal and cell mediators (i.e., catecholamines, cortisol, and growth hormone) markedly increase **energy** expenditure and **gluconeogenesis.** In starvation, however, energy expenditure and gluconeogenesis are decreased, and ketone production in the liver as an alternative fuel source, is increased. Stored glycogen, the primary fuel source in early starvation, is depleted within approximately 24 hours. When glycogen stores are exhausted, fatty acids are mobilized from adipose tissue and delivered to the liver, where they are converted to ketones and utilized as an alternative fuel source for all tissues except the glucose-obligated brain, nervous system, and red blood cells. Ketoacidosis may develop as a result of fasting, food deprivation, or when ketone production exceeds tissue use. The degree of starvation and physiological stress determines the extent and type of malnutrition. The three major types of malnutrition are marasmus, kwashiorkor, and protein-calorie malnutrition.

Marasmus is often associated with altered gastrointestinal functioning or prolonged periods of anorexia. It is a severe, **cachetic** process, whereby virtually all of the available fat stores have been exhausted from calorie deficiency. Severe body and muscle wasting is evident as fat and protein stores are depleted. Sudden fluid shifts and electrolyte abnormalities may strain an already viscerally depleted heart and lead to cardiopulmonary failure. Nursing management includes slow administration and vigilant monitoring of nutrition and fluid volume replacement.

Kwashiorkor and protein-calorie malnutrition are typically caused by an acute, life-threatening illness, trauma, or sepsis. **Kwashiorkor** is a condition caused by prolonged protein malnutrition. It can develop in situations where a person is protein starved but is receiving at least minimal calorie intake for survival. It is often described in the context of starving children in developing countries. Protein-calorie malnutrition (a problem of both protein and calories) is more commonly seen in acute and chronic illness due to depletion of fat, muscle wasting, and micronutrient deficiencies. Although the high-acuity patient may appear nourished, this is often due to the masking effects of generalized edema that results from abnormally low serum albumin. Hypoalbuminemia lowers the intravascular colloidal osmotic pressure and allows fluid to shift from the circulating blood volume into the extracellular spaces.

In addition to generalized edema, the clinical signs of protein malnutrition include skin breakdown, poor wound healing, and in some cases, surgical dehiscence. Hair is easily plucked, and hair remnants are often noted on the patient's pillowcase and/or sheets. In both of these types of malnutrition, serum albumin levels are low and treatment requires aggressive replacement of protein stores. Success of nutrition therapy is heavily dependent upon vigilant monitoring and appropriate interventions on the part of nursing.

Over-Nutrition

Obesity results from an imbalance between energy intake and energy consumption. Obesity represents excess body fat, and it is estimated that in the United States, two-thirds of the population are overweight or obese (WIN, 2007). The degree of overweight is leveled based on body mass index (BMI):

> overweight = BMI ≥ 25 to < 30; obesity = BMI ≥ 30; and extreme obesity = BMI ≥ 40 (WIN, 2007).

Obesity is a significant nutritional problem and is associated with many chronic diseases, such as hypertension, dyslipidemia, type 2 diabetes, coronary heart disease, and stroke. It is also associated with poor wound healing, which can result in increased morbidity and mortality in high-acuity patients. In addition, obese patients are at high risk for metabolic syndrome, which is a cluster of medical risk factors that include abdominal obesity, atherogenic dyslipidemia, hypertension, and prothrombotic and proinflammatory states (AHA, 2008). It is estimated that more than 50 million Americans have this syndrome (AHA, 2008). Metabolic syndrome increases the risk for development of atherosclerotic problems such as coronary heart disease and stroke. Insulin resistance in this patient population can also become problematic during acute illness, when serum glucose levels increase.

While weight loss is an important long-term goal for overweight and obese patients, implementation of a low-calorie diet during acute illness may accelerate loss of lean body mass, in an acutely ill patient. The obese high-acuity patient has a higher BMI than a nonobese patient and will have higher resting energy expenditure. During acute illness it is crucial to meet the elevated nutrient needs of obese patients to optimize outcomes. To prevent untoward metabolic derangements during acute illness, any dietary goals towards a more desirable weight should be done as a team approach in close consultation with a dietician.

Metabolic Stress Response

The metabolic responses to physiologic stress, such as surgery, trauma, or infection, are fairly predictable. Two distinct phases of this response have been identified (Cuthertson, 1932) and redefined (Little & Girolami, 1999). The initial phase is called the **ebb phase**, which lasts about 24 hours after the occurrence of tissue injury. The ebb phase is followed by the **flow phase.** The duration of the flow phase is highly variable and is associated with the patient's clinical condition.

Ebb Phase

The individual's metabolic rate is likely to be initially unchanged or slightly decreased during the first 24 hours after injury. Exceptions to this are patients with burns and severe head injury who have a Glasgow Coma Scale score of eight or less. A slightly hypothermic body temperature may be observed secondary to decreased oxygen consumption. Increases in blood glucose and lactate levels are common.

Alterations in both carbohydrate and lipid metabolism are observed in the ebb phase. Glucose production is increased after injury in an attempt to provide energy for wound healing. Increased release of stress hormones, such as epinephrine, glucagon, and cortisol, stimulates conversion of glycogen stores to glucose. Decreased production of insulin along with insulin resistance in peripheral tissues contributes to hyperglycemia following injury.

Controversy exists regarding the utility of providing nutrition during the ebb phase. Arguments that the instillation of nutrients into the GI tract immediately after injury could divert blood flow from the major organs, thereby promoting hemodynamic instability, have not been well supported. Recent studies have observed beneficial effects, such as decreases in the hypermetabolic response, when enteral feeding is initiated within the first 24 hours after injury.

Fat stores are mobilized to contribute to energy needs. As fats are oxidized, fatty acids are produced and contribute to increases in lactate levels. Lactate levels increase as anaerobic metabolism occurs in injured, ischemic tissues. The increasing quantity of lactate is converted to glucose in the liver, thereby increasing hyperglycemia (Pleuss, 2007).

Flow Phase

The onset of the flow phase begins about 24 to 36 hours following the physiologic insult. The flow phase is characterized by increased oxygen and calorie demands to provide for wound healing. Typical symptoms of the flow phase include the onset of tachycardia, tachypnea, increased cardiac output, and fever. **Hypercatabolism** (breakdown of body proteins) is prominent as stored protein is metabolized to help meet the sudden increase in oxygen consumption and energy expenditure. Increased oxygen consumption and energy expenditure along with hypercatabolism comprise the clinical condition known as **hypermetabolism.**

Hyperglycemia is frequently observed after tissue injury. Glucose production is increased in response to increased energy demands. The immediate release of catecholamines at the time of injury stimulates the liver to increase glucose production, and insulin production and utilization are altered. Resistance to insulin in the peripheral tissues contributes to higher levels of blood glucose, but the primary cause of hyperglycemia is increased gluconeogenesis. Administration of insulin may be ineffective in controlling elevated glucose levels during the **metabolic stress response.**

Patient prognosis worsens as hypermetabolism persists. Individuals experiencing tissue trauma (from any etiology) usually have a decreased capacity to take nutrition; therefore, they depend on their caregivers to provide appropriate nutrient intake. Patients with tissue trauma experience a reduced ability to use carbohydrates, proteins, and lipids, another factor that contributes to malnutrition in the high-acuity patient.

The peak of the hypermetabolic response usually occurs three to four days following the initiating event. In the patient without complications, the hypermetabolic stress response usually lasts seven to ten days; however, the hypermetabolic high-acuity patient is rarely without complications. Exacerbation of the hypermetabolic response occurs with repeated episodes of tissue ischemia, localized infections, or septicemia. The metabolic alterations occurring with hypermetabolism and hypercatabolism can be a vicious cycle leading to further clinical deterioration if the patient does not receive adequate metabolic/nutritional support within the first few days of the precipitating event. Table 33–1 provides a synopsis of the metabolic differences between starvation and the hypermetabolic stress response.

Refeeding Syndrome

Refeeding syndrome (**RFS**) refers to a nutritional complication associated with reinitiating nutritional support in a person who is significantly malnourished, particularly if marasmus or kwashiorkor is present. Even though the patient may be in a catabolic state with depleted nutritional stores, many serum electrolytes may remain at a normal steady state because of renal compensatory mechanisms. During periods of starvation, stored fat becomes the body's primary fuel source; however,

TABLE 33–1 Comparison between Starvation and Hypermetabolism

	STARVATION	HYPERMETABOLISM
Metabolic goal	Preservation of lean body mass	Repair of injured tissue
Metabolic rate	Decreased	Increased
Energy needs	Decreased	Increased
Fuel source	Primarily fat (stored glycogen depleted within 24 hours)	Mixed
Protein metabolism	Decreased synthesis Decreased catabolism Decreased ureagenesis Decreased UUN	Decreased synthesis Increased catabolism Increased ureagenesis Increased UUN
Carbohydrate metabolism	Decreased gluconeogenesis (stored glycogen depleted within 24 hours)	Increased gluconeogenesis Hyperglycemia
Fat metabolism	Increased ketones	Increased compared to normal; ketones decreased compared to starvation

once refeeding is initiated with large glucose and protein loads, the pancreas is stimulated to release more insulin. The increased insulin causes an increased uptake of glucose and other electrolytes, such as phosphorus, potassium, and magnesium, into the cells. This causes rapid depletion of serum electrolyte levels, causing hypophosphatemia, hypokalemia, and hypomagnesemia, which, if severe, has the potential to cause life-threatening respiratory and cardiac muscle dysfunction and failure and neurologic symptoms.

Identification of individuals at risk for refeeding syndrome is an important initial step in preventing it. Patients at particular risk for developing RFS include those with cancer, cachexia, HIV/AIDS, chronic alcoholism, severe obesity associated with rapid weight loss, and anorexia nervosa (Clark, 2009). In patients with the potential to develop refeeding syndrome, both initial and frequent evaluation of serum phosphorus, potassium, and magnesium is recommended (Lafrance & Leblanc, 2005; Clark, 2009). It is recommended that nutritional support be advanced slowly and cautiously, only after serum electrolytes have been stabilized. Refeeding should begin slowly; caloric intake should not be greater than 20 kcal/kg of the patient's actual body weight per day (Clark, 2009). Increases of feeding to the target level may need to occur over several days to minimize the sudden and severe electrolyte changes attributable to rapid refeeding in the starved patient.

SECTION ONE REVIEW

1. Which condition is characteristic of the flow phase of the metabolic stress response?
   A. conservation of protein
   B. hypothermia
   C. increased energy expenditure
   D. hypoglycemia
2. Which condition places an individual at risk for refeeding syndrome?
   A. diabetes
   B. NPO status for seven days
   C. excess fat intake
   D. obesity
3. The metabolic rate would be expected to decrease in
   A. flow phase metabolic stress response
   B. hyperthermia
   C. hyperglycemic stress response
   D. starvation
4. During NPO status, the average-sized adult has enough stored carbohydrate to supply energy needs for
   A. one day
   B. one week
   C. 48 hours
   D. three days

Answers: 1. C, 2. B, 3. D, 4. A

SECTION TWO: Nutritional Alterations in Specific Disease States

At the completion of this section, the learner will be able to describe the major nutritional alterations associated with specific disease states.

Dysfunction of any organ results in a relative loss of its ability to maintain metabolic processes and perform its functions. This section provides an overview of some of the major nutritional alterations associated with major organ disorders and includes nutritional implications.

Hepatic Failure

The liver plays a vital role in nutrition and metabolism. Major metabolic functions of the liver include synthesis and excretion of plasma proteins; synthesis of bile acids; conversion of ammonia to urea; storage of fat-soluble vitamins; maintenance of adequate coagulation; and metabolism of carbohydrates, proteins, and lipids.

The liver plays a key role in metabolism of carbohydrates, the body's preferred energy source. The liver converts complex carbohydrates to simple sugars (glucose) that can be used for immediate energy needs or stored for later use. Excess carbohydrate is converted to glycogen and stored in the liver as energy reserves for later use. During times of physiologic stress, when energy needs rapidly accelerate, the liver converts stored glycogen back to glucose. When glycogen stores are depleted, the liver then converts protein and stored fat (triglycerides) to glucose as an energy source.

All plasma proteins, except gamma globulins and immunoglobulins, are produced in the liver. Most of the circulating plasma proteins are also secreted by the liver, including albumin, prealbumin, and transferrin. Decreased serum albumin is a major indicator of severe liver dysfunction; however, with its long half-life of 14 to 21 days, decreased serum albumin is not immediately evident.

The liver is the primary site for lipid synthesis and degradation. Excess carbohydrate is converted to triglycerides by the liver. Triglycerides are then stored in adipose tissue deposits as a reserve energy source. Cholesterol, phospholipids, and lipoproteins, which are also produced by the liver, are necessary for cell wall integrity and transmission of nerve impulses.

Hepatic failure may result from consequences of liver disease, to include but not limited to, cirrhosis, hepatitis, and drug

TABLE 33–2 Metabolic Alterations in Hepatic Failure

FUNCTIONS	ASSOCIATION DISORDERS
Synthesis and storage	Hypoglycemia Hypoalbuminemia Decreased cholesterol production Impaired fat absorption
Metabolic and excretory	Impaired conversion of ammonia to urea Increased steroid hormone production Decreased drug metabolism Hyperbilirubinemia

Data from Porth (2007).

toxicity (e.g., acetaminophen toxicity). Metabolic alterations associated with hepatic failure include disorders of synthesis and storage functions and disorders of metabolic and excretory functions (Porth, 2007). Table 33–2 lists the disorders associated with loss of these metabolic functions. Reduced nutrient intake as a result of general malaise, nausea, vomiting, and/or diarrhea can result in hypercatabolism. Coagulopathy and gastrointestinal varices often complicate feeding tube placement because of the increased potential for bleeding. Progressive malnutrition leads to increased breakdown of skeletal muscle with release of branched-chain amino acids (BCAAs) and aromatic amino acids (AAAs). Excessive uptake of AAA by the central nervous system may contribute to hepatic encephalopathy, a characteristic of late hepatic failure, because the liver is unable to convert aromatic amino acids and ammonia (a byproduct of protein and amino acid metabolism) to urea for excretion in the urine.

Energy expenditure is typically increased in high-acuity patients with hepatic failure; therefore, they require high carbohydrate intake, normal-to-moderate protein intake, but low fat intake. Excessive fat intake contributes to progressive liver dysfunction with accumulation of fatty deposits in the liver cells. Because of the numerous metabolic alterations associated with hepatic failure, overfeeding is just as detrimental as underfeeding. The patient with liver failure particularly benefits from having energy expenditure measured by indirect calorimetry. Severe protein restrictions that were once routinely used to reduce hepatic encephalopathy are no longer considered appropriate since this practice exacerbated protein depletion; however, the appropriate amount and type of protein intake remains controversial. Nutritional products that contain about 50 percent of their protein source as branched-chain amino acids may be beneficial to mental status in some patients. Fluid and electrolyte imbalance and infection contribute to hepatic encephalopathy, and should be corrected before initiating feeding with significant amounts of branched-chain amino acids (Porth, 2007). Table 33–3 provides a summary of the major nutritional derangements associated with liver disease and nutrition-related recommendations.

Pulmonary Failure

Pulmonary failure is the inability of the lungs to maintain adequate pulmonary gas exchange (as evidenced by abnormalities in the respiratory components of arterial blood gases [PaO_2, SaO_2, pH, and $PaCO_2$]). Malnutrition (under-nutrition) is a common problem associated with many chronic pulmonary diseases (e.g., chronic obstructive pulmonary disease, or COPD). When present, malnutrition adversely affects pulmonary structures and functions, which increases work of breathing and can precipitate pulmonary failure. In the absence of adequate calorie and protein intake, the respiratory muscles are catabolized to meet acute energy requirements. As respiratory muscle is consumed, the ability of the patient to properly ventilate becomes impaired, ultimately leading to hypoventilation and pulmonary failure. Hypoventilation results in retention of CO_2 and if allowed to progress, can cause respiratory acidosis. Carbon dioxide is produced by the body as an end-product of

TABLE 33–3 Liver Disease: Summary of Major Nutritional Derangements and Recommendations

MAJOR DERANGEMENTS	RECOMMENDATIONS
Protein-calorie malnutrition Micronutrient deficiencies (especially zinc, vitamins A, D, E, & K) Altered amino acid metabolism (decreased circulating branched-chain amino acids [BCAA] and increased circulating aromatic amino acids [AAA]) In liver disease, the preferred source of calories comes from fat, not carbohydrates Marked insulin resistance is common (especially in cirrhosis)	Perform thorough nutritional assessment (e.g., Subjective Global Assessment [SGA] of Nutritional Status)* Use indirect calorimetry to estimate caloric needs rather than Harris-Benedict equation Monitor: zinc, vitamins A, D, E, and prothrombin time (PT) Administer 1.0 g/kg per day of standard protein Small, frequent meals (four to six each day) to include late evening meal (especially in cirrhosis) For alcohol-induced disease: Consider nitrogen balance maintaining diet (includes standard amino acids and replacement of potassium, phosphate, magnesium, and thiamin) For overt hepatic encephalopathy: ▪ Acute temporary withdrawal from protein ▪ Reverse precipitating cause if possible ▪ Administer therapy to reduce symptoms (e.g., lactulose) ▪ Reintroduce standard protein diet

*Developed by Detsky et al. (1987).
Data from ASPEN (2002a).

metabolism. The greatest quantity of carbon dioxide, however, comes from ingestion of carbohydrates. Therefore, in patients who have problems with CO_2 retention, excessive carbohydrate and overall calorie intake may contribute to increased carbon dioxide levels and pulmonary failure. Malnutrition also decreases the ventilatory drive and the patient's response to hypoxia (ASPEN, 2002a).

The nutritional needs of pulmonary failure patients are similar to other hypermetabolic, hypercatabolic patients. For example, increased work of breathing increases energy expenditure. However, food intake may decline because of cough, dyspnea, fatigue, anorexia, and/or early satiety. Also, protein and iron insufficiency adversely affect the oxygen-carrying capacity of the blood. Phosphorus levels should be closely monitored in patients with impaired gas exchange. Phosphorus is a component of 2,3-diphosphoglycerate (2,3-DPG), which facilitates oxygen transport. Low levels of 2,3-DPG diminishes hemoglobin's ability to release oxygen to the tissues. Elevated levels of 2,3-DPG lowers hemoglobin's affinity for oxygen, thereby contributing to impaired gas exchange. Additionally, low phosphorus may further exacerbate respiratory muscle function at the cellular level. Subsequently, mechanical ventilator weaning should not be attempted until phosphorus stores are restored. As protein deficiency progresses, decreased intravascular colloid osmotic pressure may lead to pulmonary edema and adversely impact ventilation and perfusion.

A carbohydrate intake of about 40-50 percent of total calories is generally recommended for patients with carbon dioxide retention, with the remaining 50-60 percent divided between proteins and lipids (Dwyer, 2007; Dominguez-Cherit, Posadas-Calleja, & Borunda, 2008). Elevations in carbon dioxide may clinically present as an increased respiratory rate, bounding pulse, ruddy face, and drowsiness. Although nitrogen balance, blood urea nitrogen, and creatinine should be monitored frequently to individualize protein dosing, protein intake of 1.0 to 1.5 g/kg/day for patients with stable chronic obstructive pulmonary disease is recommended to prevent loss of lean muscle mass (Baumgartner, 2008; Hogg, Klapholz, & Reid-Hector, 2001). Sodium and fluid restriction may be indicated for patients with pulmonary edema. Table 33–4 summarizes the major nutritional derangements and nutritional recommendations for patients with severe pulmonary disease.

Renal Failure

The main function of the kidneys is to maintain homeostatic balance of fluids, electrolytes and organic solutes (or end waste products of normal metabolism). The majority of solute load consists of nitrogenous wastes that are derived primarily from protein breakdown. Elevation of these waste products is called **azotemia** and results in complex metabolic disturbances. Renal failure is classified as acute or chronic on the basis of presenting symptoms and underlying causes of the problem.

Acute Renal Failure

Acute renal failure (ARF) is characterized by a sudden inability to excrete metabolic waste and is often characterized by **oliguria** (diminished urinary output of less than 500 mL urine in 24 hours), a sudden increase in serum BUN and creatinine levels, and electrolyte abnormalities such as an elevated potassium level. Causes of acute renal failure include decreased blood flow to the kidneys, a disease process within the kidneys, or an obstruction.

Metabolic alterations of acute renal failure include hypercatabolism, hypermetabolism, volume overload, and electrolyte abnormalities. Inadequate nutritional intake, underlying comorbid conditions, and loss of nutrients in the dialysate in patients receiving hemodialysis can contribute to hypermetabolic and hypercatabolic responses. Serum levels of potassium, phosphorus, and magnesium are usually elevated as a result of catabolism of lean body mass and decreased electrolyte excretion by the kidneys. Fluid volume overload is a major concern during the oliguric phase of acute renal failure. Replacement of kidney function during ARF can be carried out by hemodialysis, peritoneal

TABLE 33–4 Pulmonary Disease: Summary of Major Nutritional Derangements and Recommendations

MAJOR DERANGEMENTS	RECOMMENDATIONS
Decreased levels of albumin, transferrin, and prealbumin Weight loss related to increased REE Decreased body mass (fat and nonfat) Decreased ventilatory drive Decreased micronutrients: hypophosphatemia in particular	Perform thorough nutritional assessment (e.g., Subjective Global Assessment [SGA] of Nutritional Status)* Supplemental nutritional support may be of benefit in patients with COPD, pulmonary failure, and acute respiratory distress syndrome (ARDS) Special attention needs to be given to avoiding overfeeding (causes elevated CO_2 levels) Indirect calorimetry may assist in establishing caloric needs Use of fat as a major energy source (lower RQ) may be of benefit Limited carbohydrate intake may be of benefit for reducing CO_2 load If glucose is administered, limit to less than 5 mg/kg per minute to reduce CO_2 load Replace phosphate when hypophosphatemia is present Acute respiratory distress syndrome (ARDS): ■ Use fluid-restricted formulations if restriction is needed ■ Enteral formulas with n-3 fatty acids (e.g., fish oils) may be of benefit

*Developed by Detsky et al. (1987).
Data from ASPEN (2002a).

dialysis, or other forms of continuous hemofiltration in order to correct metabolic acidosis, uremia and eliminate potassium.

Energy and protein needs are determined by hypermetabolic needs, the underlying cause of ARF, and other comorbidities. In patients with mild acute renal failure, 30 to 35 kcal/kg/day is usually sufficient to meet nutritional requirements (Anderson, 2008). Energy needs can be measured by an indirect calorimetry. If unavailable, use of predictive formulas may be beneficial to avoid excessive calorie intake. Protein dosing varies depending on whether the patient is receiving some form of dialysis because large protein loads may necessitate the need for more frequent dialysis. In the absence of dialysis, daily protein intake should be restricted to approximately 0.5 to 0.6 g/kg/day (Anderson, 2008), and in dialyzed patients, daily protein intake can be liberalized to approximately 0.8-2.0 g/kg/day (Wilkins, 2004).

Specialty renal formulas are available, which contain little or no electrolytes and low protein. The protein content is low in most of these formulas so that protein needs to be added to the formula even when the patient is protein restricted. Many patients can be maintained on regular enteral formulas that have lower protein content. Specialty renal formulas may be reserved for use in patients who have elevated electrolytes. Patients with acute renal failure require close monitoring of their fluid and electrolyte status. Nutritional goals will fluctuate relative to changes in the patient's underlying clinical condition and/or utilization of dialysis therapy.

Chronic Renal Failure

Chronic renal failure (CRF) is characterized by a progressive worsening of the kidney's ability to excrete waste products, maintain fluid and electrolyte balance, and produce hormones. Uremia often develops and is the result of increased circulating solute waste in the bloodstream that the kidneys are not able to eliminate. Clinically, uremia presents as malaise, weakness, muscle cramping, itching, nausea, delayed gastric emptying, vomiting, and complaints of a metallic taste in the mouth, which may promote anorexia. Anorexia may also be related to unappetizing and/or restricted renal-specific diets.

Energy needs must be adequate to meet the nutritional needs of a hypermetabolic state in a high-acuity patient. Individuals receiving dialysis will require protein supplementation to adjust for protein losses that occur. The exact nutritional supplementation must be individualized based on multiple factors such as the patient's general condition and nutritional status, stage of renal failure, type and frequency of dialysis, metabolic state, and comorbidities. Table 33–5 provides a summary of major nutritional derangements and nutritional recommendations for renal disease.

Cardiac Failure

Among patients with moderate to severe heart failure, many develop a malnutrition state known as cardiac **cachexia**. Unlike the adipose tissue loss in starvation, cardiac cachexia is characterized by a predominant loss of lean body mass greater than 10 percent. Although it was once believed that the heart was spared from the muscle-wasting effects of malnutrition, cardiac muscle is also affected. Loss of muscle mass in a cachectic heart results in decreased cardiac pumping effectiveness and persistent circulatory failure. As cardiac failure continues, tissues become increasingly deprived of oxygen. This is a form of tissue injury and unless the underlying condition is corrected, the effects of hypermetabolism will further the loss of lean muscle mass.

Nutritional needs of all high-acuity patients with cardiac disease should be closely monitored as the volume associated with nutritional intake can have a negative effect on hemodynamics in some patients. Oxygen consumption increases with food intake. For patients who are able to take food orally, the postprandial elevation of oxygen consumption can be significant enough to cause hemodynamic instability. The presence of food in the gastrointestinal tract results in greater blood flow through the splanchnic circulation. This increased blood volume is obtained by shunting blood from other vital organs, such as the myocardium, kidneys, and/or brain; therefore, among patients who can eat, intake should be limited to

TABLE 33–5 Renal Disease: Summary of Major Nutritional Derangements and Recommendations

MAJOR DERANGEMENTS	RECOMMENDATIONS
Protein-calorie malnutrition Hypermetabolism Accelerated protein breakdown Impaired protein synthesis Altered glucose utilization Impaired lipid metabolism	Perform thorough nutritional assessment (e.g., Subjective Global Assessment [SGA] of Nutritional Status)* Monitor serum albumin, prealbumin Acute renal failure and receiving nutritional support: ■ Provide balanced mix of essential and nonessential amino acids ■ If severely malnourished or hypercatabolic – Protein intake of 1.5 to 1.8 g/kg per day Not on dialysis, may benefit from: ■ Low protein diet (0.6 to 0.8 g/kg per day) ■ Essential amino acid supplementation On dialysis, may benefit from: ■ Maintenance hemodialysis - Protein intake of 1.2 g/kg per day ■ Chronic ambulatory peritoneal dialysis (CAPD) - Protein intake of 1.2 to 1.3 g/kg per day ■ Continuous hemofiltration – Protein intake of more than 1 g/kg per day ■ Supplement: water soluble vitamins (Monitor vitamin A status closely to avoid hypervitaminosis A)

*Developed by Detsky et al. (1987).
Data from ASPEN (2002a).

frequent, small amounts of food. For patients who require enteral or parenteral nutrition support, continuous infusion of the formula may be beneficial to regulate the effects of the nutrients; however, nutrition delivery is generally dictated by individualized tolerance, and, in the case of enteral tube feeding, location of the tip of the feeding tube.

Energy needs of patients with heart failure depend on current weight, activity restrictions, and the severity of their cardiac disease. Calorie restricted diets (i.e., 1,000-1,200 kcal/day) may be beneficial towards helping obese patients with obtaining a more desirable weight, which places less stress on the heart. For undernourished patients with severe heart failure, energy needs may be increased by as much double their resting energy expenditure (REE). In order to achieve nutritional goals, meals should be frequent and in small portions to decrease fatigue and abdominal distention, which may redirect blood flow to the splanchnic circulation and further stress the heart. Anorexia is a frequently observed characteristic in patients with cardiac failure; and dyspnea, fatigue, and unappetizing restricted diets contribute to lack of appetite.

Balanced nutrient intake is important for all patients, but particularly for patients with potential or actual alterations of oxygenation. Hospitalized patients receiving only intravenous glucose have a significant increase in their **respiratory quotient (RQ)**. Recall from Section Five of Module 32, Determinants and Assessment of Nutrition and Metabolic Function, that an RQ value near 1.00 is indicative of significantly increased carbon dioxide production. Fluids are commonly restricted to 500-2000 mL/day, and diuretics commonly used to manage heart failure tend to reduce body stores of potassium, magnesium, and thiamine. Thiamine deficiency leads to vasodilation of the peripheral blood vessels, producing high-output heart failure. Cardiomyopathy has been attributed to selenium deficiency in patients receiving long-term total parenteral nutrition. These deficiencies should be monitored, replaced, or supplemented on a regular basis as these may impair cardiac contractility. Table 33–6 summarizes the major nutritional derangements and nutritional recommendations for cardiac disease.

TABLE 33–6 Cardiac Disease: Summary of Major Nutritional Derangements and Recommendations

MAJOR DERANGEMENTS	RECOMMENDATIONS
Cardiac cachexia	
■ Depleted lean body mass (including heart and other vital organs) – greater than 10% ■ Anorexia ■ Bowel edema with GI hypomotility and nausea ■ Intestinal malabsorption	Perform thorough nutritional assessment (e.g., Subjective Global Assessment [SGA] of Nutritional Status)* Reserve use of parenteral nutrition for cardiac patients with surgical complications that prevent use of GI tract Following cardiac surgery, enteric feedings should not be initiated until hemodynamic stability has been achieved

*Developed by Detsky et al. (1987).
Data from ASPEN (2002a).

Gut Failure

High-acuity patients are at risk for gut ischemia based on how the body reprioritizes blood flow during times of high stress. During such times, blood flow is redirected from the GI tract (low priority) to high priority organs such as the heart and brain. This can lead to decreased splanchnic blood flow, tissue ischemia and possible gut dysfunction or failure. The GI mucosa depends on nutrient delivery, adequate blood flow, and tissue perfusion to remain healthy and prevent atrophy, thereby maintaining the absorptive barrier and immunologic functions of the intestine (Lin & Cohen, 2005). When atrophy develops, the tight junctions between the gastrointestinal enterocytes are lost. This results in decreased barrier functions and increased mucosal permeability, allowing migration of gastrointestinal bacteria into the systemic circulation. This is known as *bacterial translocation* and is now accepted as a major etiology of sepsis in high-acuity patients.

Regional assessment of splanchnic circulation can be performed indirectly by gastric tonometry, which measures the pH and CO_2 levels of the gastric mucosa. Section Six in Module 28, Determinants and Assessment of Gastrointestinal, Hepatic, and Pancreatic Function, describes gastric tonometry in greater detail. The value of the gastric intramucosal P_{CO_2} is obtained by aspiration of a fluid sample via a specially designed nasogastric tube (gastric tonometer). The carbon dioxide (CO_2) level of the gastric mucosa rises when the GI tract is underperfused. Tonometry provides an early warning of reduced gastric perfusion, which can occur when a patient is hypovolemic or in shock. During a period of hypoperfusion, the GI tract is one of the first organ systems to suffer reduced blood flow. A decrease in the delivery of oxygen rich blood to the gut mucosa results in anaerobic metabolism.

The intramucosal pH (pHi) is measured by obtaining an arterial blood gas sample at the same time as a gastric sample. The bicarbonate value of the blood and the P_{CO_2} value of the gastric sample are placed into the Henderson–Hasselbalch equation. The final value is called the intramucosal pH (pHi). If the result is acidic, the assumption is that circulation to the splanchnic organs is compromised. Values of gastric intramucosal pH have been observed to change prior to changes in more traditional assessments of tissue oxygenation, such as oxygen delivery, oxygen consumption, and mixed venous P_{O_2}.

Burns

Burn patients are among those with the highest expected energy, protein, and fluid needs. The extent of the hypermetabolic response is related to the severity of the burn. In severe burn injury, caloric intake is increased to 120 to 150 percent of estimated basal needs (Saffle, 2008). Indirect calorimetry is often standard practice for evaluating actual energy expenditure to optimize feeding. The energy demands of the burn patient are not self-limiting and the hypermetabolic state and increased energy expenditure continues through the recovery and rehabilitative phase.

Increased energy expenditure may persist longer in the burn patient than in patients with other types of tissue injuries. Individualized nutritional and energy requirements are crucial for healing and skin grafting success. As with any extensive wounds, vitamin supplementation is essential for healing and maintenance of overall immune function. Vitamins A, B complex, and C, along with zinc, support wound healing. Standardized protocols for vitamin supplementation are utilized to enhance skin grafting success and to prevent nutritional deficiencies. In burn injuries greater than 20 percent, burn patients have massive fluid shifts due to increased circulating histamine, prostaglandins, and cytokines. These substances increase capillary permeability, causing fluid to shift from the intravascular space to the interstitial space. Fluid resuscitation in the burn patient uses various protocols such as the Parkland and the Consensus Formula. Fluid resuscitation is initiated at the time of burn injury and generally continues for about 48 hours, until fluid shifts stabilize and the patient regains hemodynamic stability. Table 33–7 provides a summary of major nutritional derangements and nutritional recommendations.

Traumatic Brain Injury

Although the brain consumes 20 percent of the body's oxygen supply and 15 percent of the resting cardiac output, it can neither store glucose nor engage in anaerobic metabolism (Porth, 2007). Patients with traumatic brain injury (TBI) are severely hypermetabolic and catabolic due to the massive release of catecholamines (norepinephrine and epinephrine) and cortisol. Increased circulation of these hormones is responsible for conversion of glycogen to glucose for energy. Glucagon acts on the liver to convert amino acids into glucose while stored fat is also converted into glucose. Decreased insulin release from the pancreas combined with rapid conversion of stored nutrients into glucose results in hyperglycemia, which has been identified as a significant predictor of outcome from head injury. Patients with fever, seizure activity, and decerebrate/decorticate muscle posturing have an even higher rate of energy expenditure and oxygen demand often exceeds supply. To compensate, cardiac output is increased along with the amount of oxygen that the brain extracts from the blood. However, if oxygen demand continues to surpass supply, hypoxemia occurs. The brain tries to compensate for the hypoxemia by increasing blood flow and, therefore, oxygen delivery to the brain; however, this compensatory response contributes to the increased intracranial pressure that is the hallmark of head injury. Hypoxemia leads to anaerobic metabolism in the brain tissue. Lactic acid, an end product of anaerobic metabolism, cannot adequately supply the brain's energy needs (Porth, 2007).

The extent of hypermetabolism in head-injured patients is inversely correlated with the Glasgow Coma Score and predictive energy requirement formulas, such as the Harris-Benedict equation, have been known to underestimate energy needs in this patient population. To prevent the deleterious effects of underfeeding, use of indirect calorimetry may be beneficial. Accelerated catabolic rate and increased nitrogen losses associated with traumatic brain injury are particularly notable in the first few days to weeks following the initial injury. The exact mechanism of significant urinary nitrogen losses is unclear. Immobility, decreased nitrogen efficiency, steroid administration, and decreased nutrient intake have all been suggested as causative factors.

Providing adequate energy and protein for a positive nitrogen balance is paramount to successful treatment, and aggressive nutrition support is recommended. Those patients with a decreased level of consciousness or who have a poor cough or gag reflex are at increased risk for pulmonary aspiration. Also, because traumatic brain injured patients are often unable to safely and/or adequately consume oral nutrition, alternative methods such as **enteral nutrition** should be employed. Even though gastrointestinal motility is greatly diminished, absorption of nutrients by the small bowel is usually maintained. Therefore, placement of a postpyloric small-bore feeding tube using a blind approach is often preferred, but success seems to be related to clinician experience and gastric motility. Endoscopic feeding tube placement may be necessary. Enteral feeding during drug-induced coma is efficacious and well tolerated by many patients, thus limiting the need for parenteral nutrition.

TABLE 33–7 Acute Severe Burn Injury: Summary of Major Nutritional Derangements and Recommendations

MAJOR DERANGEMENTS	RECOMMENDATIONS
Severe hypermetabolism and hypercatabolism Weight loss Decreased lean body mass Massive protein and calorie demands Energy expenditure: estimated at 20 to 30% above measured to meet demands Gastric ileus is common	Perform thorough nutritional assessment (e.g., Subjective Global Assessment [SGA] of Nutritional Status)* ■ Emphasis: protein and energy needs ■ Assessment is ongoing Indirect calorimetry may be of use (if feasible) Aggressive nutrition approach ■ Enteral route: initiate EN as soon as is feasible postburn, locate tube postpyloric ■ High-calorie, high-protein supplementation ■ Research does not support routine use of anabolic agents or specific nutrients

*Developed by Detsky et al. (1987).
Data from ASPEN (2002a).

SECTION TWO REVIEW

1. A high-acuity patient with hepatic failure may typically experience (choose all that apply)
   - **A.** breakdown of skeletal muscle protein
   - **B.** diminished fat use
   - **C.** dilutional hyponatremia
   - **D.** increased carbon dioxide levels
2. Nutritional goals for the patient experiencing pulmonary failure includes (choose all that apply)
   - **A.** higher sodium content
   - **B.** lower protein content
   - **C.** lower carbohydrate content
   - **D.** higher fat content
3. A high-acuity patient with acute renal failure may typically experience abnormalities in (choose all that apply)
   - **A.** protein catabolism
   - **B.** fluid and electrolyte levels
   - **C.** metabolic rate
   - **D.** glucose levels
4. The purpose of supplementing nutritional intake with vitamins A, B complex, and C, as well as zinc, is to
   - **A.** promote red blood cell count
   - **B.** promote wound healing
   - **C.** lower BUN level
   - **D.** lower cholesterol

Answers: 1. (A, B, C), 2. (B, C, D), 3. (A, B, C), 4. B

SECTION THREE: Enteral Nutrition

At the completion of this section, the learner will be able to describe enteral nutrition, including the benefits and potential complications, rationale for gastric versus postpyloric feeding, and barriers to providing optimal enteral nutrition to the high-acuity patient.

Criteria for Selection of Enteral Nutrition

Nutrition support should be provided via the enteral route in patients with a functional gastrointestinal tract. Unless there is known traumatic disruption or chronic malabsorptive disease, it is generally assumed that the gastrointestinal tract is capable of absorption of nutrients, fluids, and electrolytes. Patients with a high-acuity illness or injury, who are unable to consume oral nutrition, will require a feeding tube. Selection of the specific type of enteral feeding is based on three criteria: gastrointestinal integrity and function, baseline nutritional status, and illness severity and possible duration. Nursing care is summarized in the box, NURSING CARE: The Patient Receiving Supplemental Enteral Nutrition.

Gastrointestinal Integrity and Function

When assessing a patient's GI function, it is important to first consider if the patient will be able to eat within three to five days. Enteral nutrition should be considered when the patient cannot

NURSING CARE: The Patient Receiving Supplemental Enteral Nutrition

Expected Patient Outcome and Related Interventions

Outcome 1: The patient will achieve adequate nutritional status.

Assess and compare to established norms, patient baselines, and trends.

Type and severity of malnutrition
- Perform Subjective Global Assessment (SGA) of nutritional status or other nutrition-specific assessment.
- Establish baseline values of albumin, prealbumin, transferrin.
- Evaluate nitrogen balance status: obtain urine urea nitrogen (UUN) and 24-hour protein intake.
- Assess vitamin and mineral status (e.g., zinc, iron, magnesium, phosphate, folic acid, vitamins A, D, & E).

Determine the number and type of calories needed to meet nutritional requirements.
- Indirect calorimetry
- Respiratory quotient (RQ)
- Fick method
- Harris-Benedict equation with stress factors included

Monitor intake and output closely, including all losses from the GI tract.

Monitor the patient's response to treatment.
- Daily weights
- Baseline and periodic reassessment of anthropometric measurements
- Periodic reevaluation of prealbumin, albumin, vitamin and mineral status (e.g., zinc, iron, magnesium, phosphate, folic acid, vitamins A, D, & E), WBCs, other

Institute measures to initiate and maintain enteral feedings.
- Insert or assist with insertion of enteral feeding tube.
- If postpyloric route is chosen: administer prokinetic agent(s) as ordered to facilitate passage through pyloric sphincter.
- Assure that feeding tube tip is properly located before initiating feedings.
- Administer enteral nutrition as prescribed.
- Frequently assess for intolerance.

Related nursing diagnoses
- Diarrhea
- Risk for fluid volume deficit
- Imbalanced electrolytes
- Imbalanced nutrition: less than body requirements
- Risk for infection
- Knowledge deficit

Outcome 2: The patient will experience no aspiration.

Assess and compare to established norms, patient baselines, and trends.
- Risks for aspiration
  - Level of consciousness
  - GI tolerance
    - gastric residual volume
    - gastric or abdominal distension
    - gastric or abdominal discomfort
  - Improperly positioned tube

Institute measures to prevent aspiration.
- Position head-of-bed 30 to 45 degrees
- Use pump-assisted feedings rather than gravity-flow[a].
- Verify tube tip placement

Related nursing diagnoses
- Risk for aspiration

Outcome 3: The patient maintains adequate fluid volume.

Assess and compare to established norms, patient baselines, and trends.
- Indications of dehydration (e.g., hypotension, tachycardia, decrease urinary output, and thirst)

Institute measures to maintain adequate fluid volume.
- Identify factors that may cause diarrhea (e.g., bacterial contamination of feeding formula, sorbitol-containing medications, and prokinetic agents).
- Decrease rate of bolus feeding or change to continuous rate to prevent rapid fluid shifts and/or diarrhea.
- Provide high-fiber formula to bulk up stools and prevent diarrhea.
- Check infusion rates for enteral feeding administration, provide free water as prescribed.

Related nursing diagnoses
- Bowel incontinence
- Diarrhea
- Disturbed body image
- Risk for fluid volume deficit
- Actual knowledge deficit
- Risk for infection

[a]Shang, E. & Geiger, N. (2004). Pump-assisted enteral nutrition can prevent aspiration in bedridden percutaneous endoscopic gastrostomy patients. *Journal of Parenteral and Enteral Nutrition, 28(3),* 180–183.

or should not take in food orally, or oral intake is insufficient or unreliable; and if the patient has a functional gastrointestinal tract and access can be safely achieved. If the patient is expected to be unable to eat for this time period or longer, feeding tube placement is recommended. The specific type of feeding tube placed is related to the anticipated time of recovery, the patient's level of consciousness, the patient's comfort, and cost effectiveness.

Illness Severity and Possible Duration

Energy expenditure, calorie, and protein requirements increase with the severity of illness. The hypermetabolism of the metabolic stress response can persist for extended periods in the presence of physiologic complications, such as extensive wounds or sepsis. Advances in the understanding of the metabolic stress response and the immunologic functions of the gut have led to a greater appreciation for the need to provide nutrition support to the high-acuity patient early during the course of illness or injury (Dwyer, 2007).

Timing of Nutrition Support

Providing nutrition early in the course of illness or injury is a treatment priority. Numerous randomized clinical trials among general surgical patients indicate that early provision of enteral nutrition facilitates wound healing. Randomized clinical trials examining the effect of early versus delayed enteral feeding on infectious morbidity in trauma patients have produced contradictory findings. Although studies have shown no significant differences in mortality, meta-analysis supports the benefit of early initial enteral tube feeding in acutely ill patients (Marik & Zaloga, 2001).

Readiness for enteral feeding should not be determined by the presence of bowel sounds. Active bowel sounds have been used as criteria to initiate feeding, but there is no scientific evidence to support this practice. Bowel sounds are a poor indicator of small bowel motility and nutrient absorption, as they are the result of air passing through the intestinal tract. Many interventions prevent the normal passage of air through the GI tract, such as nasogastric suctioning, sedation, and nothing-by-mouth (NPO) status. Therefore, waiting for bowel sounds places the patient at undue risk for malnutrition.

Benefits of Enteral Nutrition

A major benefit of enteral nutrition is that it helps maintain gut barrier function. Reductions in gut barrier function are associated with increased bacterial translocation, systemic inflammatory response syndrome (SIRS), and multiple organ dysfunction

TABLE 33–8 Major Benefits and Contraindications for Enteral Nutrition

Major Benefits

- Helps maintain gut barrier function
- Maintenance of gut immunologic function
- More physiologic than parenteral nutrition
- Possible decrease in severity of metabolic stress response
- More cost effective than parenteral nutrition
- Decreased risk of infectious complications
- Enhanced wound healing

Contraindications

- Absolute contraindication
  - Mechanical obstruction of GI tract
- Relative contraindications
  - Severe hemorrhagic pancreatitis
  - Necrotizing enterocolitis
  - Prolonged ileus
  - Severe, intractable diarrhea
  - Protracted vomiting
  - Enteric high output fistulas
  - Intestinal dysmotility
  - Intestinal ischemia

syndrome (MODS). In animal models, fasting is associated with increased translocation of bacteria from the GI tract into mesenteric lymph nodes, portal circulation, and the peritoneal cavity (Dwyer, 2007). The major benefits and contraindications of enteral nutrition are summarized in Table 33–8.

Although invasive, feeding tube insertion has less inherent risk of mechanical and infectious complications than central venous line insertion for total parenteral nutrition (TPN) administration. The cost of enteral formulas is significantly less than the daily cost of TPN. Even the most expensive specialty enteral formulas do not equal the cost of providing TPN.

Common Contraindications for Enteral Nutrition

Many patients who were once thought to require total parenteral nutrition are now often successfully fed via the enteral route; contraindications to enteral nutrition have diminished as its safety and efficacy has been demonstrated in many types of high-acuity patients. Enteral nutrition can be provided to patients with gastrointestinal fistulas if the tube can be positioned distal to the site of the fistula. Mechanical obstruction is the only absolute contraindication to enteral feedings.

Criteria for Selection of Nutritional Support

Selection of the type of nutritional support is based on three criteria: gastrointestinal (GI) function, baseline nutritional status, and present catabolic state and possible duration.

Gastrointestinal Function

When determining a patient's GI function, the nurse should first assess whether the patient will be able to eat adequate food quantities safely, within two to three days of the initial nutritional assessment. Although nutritional support may not be initially indicated, the nurse should vigilantly monitor for inadequate intake, poor tolerance, or risk of aspiration (if clinically suspect). If the patient is unable or unwilling to ingest sufficient nutrients by mouth and has a relatively functional GI tract, the preferred route of nutritional support is enteral, which requires placement of a feeding tube and provision of an enteral feeding formula that is individualized to meet both energy and protein needs.

Baseline Nutritional Status

Baseline nutritional status is an important determinant for deciding when and what type of nutritional support to initiate. Clinical studies indicate that severely malnourished patients have a greater risk of developing complications and increased mortality. High-acuity patients should be fed as early as possible, particularly if they are malnourished.

Present Catabolic State and Possible Duration

For the high-acuity patient who is highly catabolic (nitrogen loss greater than 15 to 20 g/day), nutritional support should be initiated as soon as possible. The goal is to minimize further breakdown of the skeletal muscle and visceral protein stores. The expected duration of need for enteral feedings helps determine the type of placement. For example, if a patient is expected to require prolonged or permanent enteral feedings, percutaneous or surgical placement may be the best approach.

Types of Enteral Feedings

Numerous enteral formulas are available. Choosing the appropriate formula for the high-acuity patient is based on the energy and protein requirements of the patient, the underlying disease state or organ function, intestinal absorptive and digestive function, and fluid requirements. Commonly used formulas are lactose-free, and nutritionally complete and contain a mixture of carbohydrates, proteins, fats, vitamins, trace elements, and water. When selecting an enteral feeding formula, nutrient requirements, the patient's clinical status, location of the feeding tube tip, gastrointestinal function, cost, and duration must all be considered. Differences lie in how nutrients are structured, their varying osmolality, and range in caloric density, typically 1.0 to 2.0 kcal/mL. Table 33–9 summarizes selected enteral feeding formulas and the patients they are most appropriate for.

Feeding Tube Placement

A number of Silastic or polyurethane, weighted or nonweighted small-bore (8 to 12 Fr) feeding tubes are available. Enteral feeding access can be achieved by a variety of methods that include blind placement of a small-bore feeding tube, radiologic-assisted placement, percutaneous placement of a gastrostomy and/or jejunostomy tube, or surgical placement of a gastrostomy or jejunostomy tube. The small-bore feeding tube is the least invasive and most economical device for delivery of enteral nutrition. This polyurethane weighted or nonweighted tube can be used for gastric or transpyloric feeding.

Successful postpyloric placement of the feeding tube via the nasal or oral cavity often requires advanced clinician skill, special patient positioning and tube design, and use of prokinetic medications to help assist with tube positioning/advancement. Passage of the feeding tube from the stomach into the small

TABLE 33–9 Summary of Selected Enteral Feeding Formulas

TYPE OF FORMULA	COMMENTS	FORMULA CONTENTS	BRAND NAME EXAMPLES
Complete Formulas	Suitable for most patients requiring enteral feedings	■ 1 kcal/mL ■ Protein: approximately 14% total kcal ■ Fat: approximately 30% total kcal ■ Carbohydrates: approximately 60% total kcal ■ Recommended daily intake of all minerals and vitamins is 1,500 mL/day	Compleat, Ensure Isocal Nutren Isolan Sustacal Resource
High-calorie complete	Appropriate for patients on fluid restriction	■ As above; provides 1.5 to 2 kcal/mL	Ensure Plus Sustocal HC Comply Nutren 1.5 Resource Plus Isocal HCN Magnacal TwoCal HN
Complete lactose-free, high residue	Appropriate to prevent/treat diarrhea, constipation	■ Same as complete formulas and also provides fiber	Jevity Profiber Nutren 1.0 with fiber Fiberlan Sustacal with fiber Ultracal Ensure with fiber Fibersource Reabfin
Disease-specific formulas	Appropriate formulas are available for renal failure, respiratory failure, liver failure with hepatic encephalopathy, diabetes	■ Contain essential amino acids, Fat $>$ 50% total kcal, high amounts of branched-chain amino acids	Amin-Aid Travasorb Renal Aminess Pulmocare NutriVent Hepatic-Acid II Travasorb Hepatic Glucerna
Formulas for immune-compromised, systemic inflammatory response syndrome, or for physiological stress states	Appropriate for use in patients with AIDS, burns, trauma, sepsis, SIRS, ARDS	■ Immuno-modulating formulas contain enhanced arginine, omega-3 fatty acids nucleotides, beta carotene, 1-1.3 kcal/mL ■ Formulas for physiologic stress contain increased branched chain amino acids, high protein, or both, 1-1.2 kcal/mL	Immune-modulating formulas include: Impact Immun-Aid Perative Oxepa Physiologic stress formulas include: TraumaCal Streetein

Data from Marino, P. L. (2007). *The ICU book* (3rd ed.) Philadelphia: Lippincott Williams & Wilkins; and Lemone, P. & Burke, K. M. (2008). *Medical-surgical nursing* (4th ed.). Upper Saddle River: Pearson, p. 646, T 22-8.

bowel is associated with upper gastrointestinal motility. Motor function of the upper GI tract is frequently altered in critically ill patients; those on mechanical ventilation; and those with chronic conditions, such as diabetes mellitus, vagotomy, and intestinal pseudoobstruction (Porth, 2007). Repeated attempts to position the feeding tube postpyloric can cause patient discomfort and delay of feeding. Repeated abdominal X-rays to verify tube position and clinician time contribute to increased cost.

Gastric Versus Postpyloric Feeding

One of the ongoing controversies of nutrition support is whether high-acuity patients should be fed by means of intragastric or postpyloric feeding. In situations when repeated blind attempts to place the feeding tube postpyloric delays onset of feeding, it may be beneficial to initiate gastric feeding with a more concentrated formula at a low hourly rate in some patients. Delayed gastric emptying (gastroparesis) associated with critical illness is a primary reason for preference of feeding into the small bowel instead of the stomach. Some clinicians believe that transpyloric feeding decreases the risk of aspiration, but that belief is not supported by the literature. The documented benefits of transpyloric feeding include less interruption of feeding and, therefore, higher nutritional intake; and lower incidence of pneumonia in some groups.

Medications such as histamine type 2 blockers (e.g., cimetidine [Tagamet]) and proton pump inhibitors (e.g., omeprazole [Prilosec]) increase intragastric pH, thereby reducing the protection normally provided by more acidic (lower) gastric pH against bacterial colonization. Aspiration of colonized bacteria is the major mechanism for entry of bacteria into the lungs and contributes to development of nosocomial pneumonia, particularly in mechanically ventilated patients. Other medications that cause relaxation of the lower esophageal sphincter, such as theophylline, dopamine, anticholinergics, calcium channel blockers, and meperidine, also increase aspiration risk.

Complications of Enteral Nutrition

Complications of enteral feedings are classified under five categories: gastrointestinal, nutritional, mechanical, metabolic, and infectious. Table 33–10 lists potential enteral complications,

TABLE 33–10 Complications Associated with Enteral Nutrition

COMPLICATION	POSSIBLE CAUSE	SUGGESTED TREATMENT
Gastrointestinal		
Nausea/vomiting	Hyperosmolar feeding Rapid infusion rate Obstruction Delayed gastric emptying Contaminated solution or infusion set	Start isotonic feeding Start feedings slowly and advance as tolerated Reassess gastrointestinal function Prokinetic agent (metoclopramide, erythromycin) to increase gastric emptying: feed distal to pylorus Hang canned formula for no longer than manufacturer's recommendation; hang prepared formulas no longer than four hours; change container and infusion set every 24 hours; use good handwashing technique before handling formulas
Diarrhea	Antibiotics may alter intestinal flora causing bacteria overgrowth: *Clostridium difficile* infection and pseudomembranous colitis Liquid medications containing sorbitol or other concentrated sugar base have a laxative effect (common cause of diarrhea in patients receiving liquid medications)	Send stool specimens for culture and sensitivity, white blood cell count, ova, parasites, and *Clostridium difficile* cytotoxin. Flexible sigmoidoscopy provides a faster and more reliable diagnosis than stool studies; treatment of choice for *Clostridium difficile* toxin is IV/PO metronidazole (Flagyl) or PO vancomycin; hold any antidiarrheal agents until infectious source is ruled out Crush tablet form of medication if possible
Nutritional		
Malnutrition	Under feeding (delivering less than the prescribed amount of EN) can result in malnutrition; existing malnutrition is also associated with loss of microvilli, villous brush border enzymes, and subsequent reduction in intestinal absorptive surface area	Minimize interruptions to enteral tube feeding delivery; holding enteral feedings for frequent procedure or instillation of medications may prevent patient from receiving energy and protein needs. Minimize high gastric residuals with high caloric, low volume enteral formula and prokinetic agents. Supply elemental diet to improve absorption; elemental diets are for digestive disorders requiring a more easily digested, absorbed diet
Hypoalbuminemia	While not a complication of EN therapy, an existing low serum albumin complicates the effectiveness of and tolerance to EN; a low intravascular osmotic pressure prevents nutrients from being absorbed from the GI tract Protein-losing enteropathy	Poor tolerance is evident in patients with serum albumin less than 2.5 mg/dL; benefit of albumin administration should outweigh cost and potential complications Semielemental formula
Mechanical		
Feeding tube occlusion	Medications lack of proper flushing; viscous formulas	Irrigate feeding tube with 30 to 50 mL warm water every four hours, after medication administration, after checking residuals (gastric) Alternate positive/negative pressure with syringe to dislodge clot Warm water, juices, or colas have been cited as agents to dissolve clots Do not attempt to dislodge clots with stylet; may cause esophageal/gastric mucosal perforations; *prevention* is key
Metabolic		
Hypoglycemia	Sudden cessation of feeding	Provide supplemental glucose
Hyperglycemia	Stress response, diabetic or glucose intolerance	Usually resolves as stress is alleviated; initiate feedings slowly; monitor blood glucose every six hours
Electrolyte imbalance	Dilutional states (dehydration or fluid overload) Excess losses (diarrhea, fistula, nasogastric drainage, ascites) Disease states (renal/liver failure)	Monitor fluid status; monitor electrolytes and replace as needed Replace fluid and electrolytes as needed Provide appropriate organ failure formula
Infectious		
Aspiration pneumonia	High-risk patients include comatose, weak, debilitated Patients with tracheostomies or intubated patients; patients with neuromuscular disorders	Elevate head of bed at least 30 degrees; feed into small bowel distal to pylorus Check for high gastric residuals every 4 hours if feeding into stomach Dye should not be added to enteral feeding as a method of identifying aspiration of gastric contents because not only does it lack sensitivity for identifying aspiration of gastric contents, it has been associated with several adverse events.

possible causes, and suggested treatment. Of note, many clinicians halt feedings inappropriately based on a single high gastric residual volume (GRV) of 400 to 500 mL of enteral feeding formula. Although a single high GRV should raise the suspicion of intolerance, one high value does not necessary indicate feeding failure. Such practices promote malnutrition. Rather, current recommendations for patients with questionable gastrointestinal motility have GRV measurements every four hours during continuous feeding and before initiating intermittent feeding. If the GRV exceeds 200 to 500 mL, careful bedside evaluation is recommended and an algorithmic approach is recommended to reduce aspiration risk (McClave, DeMeo, DeLegge et al., 2002). Even when enteral tube feeding appears to be well tolerated, and GRV is less than 200 mL, evaluation for aspiration risk should be ongoing. Unless there is an institution-specific policy, a common intervention for high GRV involves holding the enteral feeding for one to two hours until the GRV is less than 200 to 250 mL from a nasogastric tube or less than 100 mL from a gastrostomy tube, at which point feedings can be resumed (Kattelmann, Hise, & Russell, 2006). If, however, the patient demonstrates overt signs of regurgitation, vomiting or aspiration, enteral feedings should be held, and the patient should be assessed and reevaluated for alternative strategies to meet nutritional goals. Promotility agents may be useful if high GRVs persist.

Medications

Malnourished patients generally require supplemental vitamins and minerals to restore essential micronutrients. A multivitamin and mineral supplement may be given, or therapy may be tailored to correct specific deficiencies. See the RELATED PHARMACOTHERAPY box for nursing implications of vitamin and mineral supplements.

RELATED PHARMACOTHERAPY: Nursing Implications of Vitamin and Mineral Supplement Administration

Fat-soluble Vitamins

Vitamin A, vitamin D, vitamin E, vitamin K

Action and Uses

The fat-soluble vitamins are absorbed in the gastrointestinal tract. Vitamins A and D are stored in the liver. All fat-soluble vitamins may become toxic if taken in excess amounts.

Major Adverse Effects

Usually well tolerated. Hypersensitivity during parenteral administration is rare but potentially life-threatening.

Nursing Implications

Monitor carefully for hypersensitivity reactions during parenteral administration. Have emergency equipment available.

Administer vitamin A with food.

Avoid administering vitamin K intravenously.

Teach client the importance of eating a well-balanced diet. If indicated, provide a list of foods high in specific vitamins.

Caution that excessive intake of these vitamins may lead to vitamin toxicity.

Water-Soluble Vitamins

Vitamin C (ascorbic acid)

Vitamin B complex: thiamine (B_1), riboflavin (B_2), niacin (nicotinic acid), pyridoxine hydrochloride (B_6), pantothenic acid, and biotin

Action and Uses

These vitamins are used to prevent or treat deficiency problems. If the diet is deficient in one vitamin, it is usually deficient in other vitamins as well; therefore, multivitamin preparations are often administered. Most of these vitamins are well absorbed from the gastrointestinal tract.

Major Adverse Effects

Mostly these drugs are well tolerated; hypersensitivity reactions are rare, but can be life-threatening.

Nursing Implications

Monitor for responses to replacement therapy.

Monitor sensitivity reactions from parenteral administration. Have emergency equipment available.

The recommended daily allowances for the specific vitamin should not be exceeded.

Minerals

Sodium, potassium, magnesium, calcium, copper, fluoride, iodine, zinc, manganese, chromium, selenium

Action and Uses

Minerals are inorganic chemicals that are vital to a variety of physiologic functions. Also called trace elements, these minerals are part of a balanced diet. Recommended daily intakes have not been established for all mineral substances. The dosage of prescribed minerals depends on the specific deficiency, route of administration, and the client's general health.

Major Adverse Effects

Hypersensitivity reactions are rare, but can be life-threatening.

Nursing Implications

All mineral preparations should be diluted prior to administration.

Prior to administration of iodine, assess for history of hypersensitivity to iodine or seafood; if hypersensitive, notify the physician, pharmacist, or nurse practitioner.

Other than fluoride and zinc, administer with or after meals.

Data from Lemone & Burke (2008).

SECTION THREE REVIEW

1. Which condition is associated with intragastric feeding?
   A. nosocomial pneumonia
   B. stress ulcer
   C. accelerated gastric emptying
   D. diarrhea
2. The severely malnourished patient has a greater risk of developing complications and eventual death. These severely malnourished patients should be fed
   A. whenever oral intake is possible
   B. after recovery from the acute illness
   C. as early as possible
   D. never
3. A patient has a relatively functioning gastrointestinal tract but is unable to take adequate nutrients by mouth. What is the best method for administering nutritional support to this patient?
   A. nasoenteric feedings
   B. oral diet
   C. withholding nutrition
   D. TPN
4. Enteral nutrition has many advantages over TPN, including (choose all that apply)
   A. less risk of bacterial translocation
   B. providing central venous access
   C. maintaining gut morphology and function
   D. less costly
5. Enteral feedings are preferably delivered to the ______ via a nasoenteric feeding tube.
   A. oral cavity
   B. gastric mucosa
   C. small bowel
   D. large bowel
6. The categories of potential complications of enteral feedings include (choose all that apply)
   A. gastrointestinal
   B. intravenous
   C. metabolic
   D. mechanical
7. Diarrhea may occur from enteral feedings, but the more common cause is antibiotics. Antibiotics can alter intestinal flora, causing bacterial overgrowth (*Clostridium difficile* infection and pseudomembranous colitis). The suggested treatment includes (choose all that apply)
   A. send stool specimens for testing
   B. perform flexible sigmoidoscopy
   C. administer antidiarrheal agents
   D. administer metronidazole (Flagyl) or vancomycin
8. Possible causes of an occluded feeding include (choose all that apply)
   A. elemental diet
   B. lack of proper flushing
   C. medications
   D. viscous formulas
9. Which one of the following factors is an advantage of transpyloric feeding?
   A. less likely to cause diarrhea
   B. prevents tube feeding aspiration
   C. prevents stress ulcers
   D. patients receive more tube feeding compared to intragastric route

Answers: 1. A, 2. C, 3. A, 4. (A, C, D), 5. C, 6. (A, C, D), 7. (A, B, D), 8. (B, C, D), 9. D

SECTION FOUR: Total Parenteral Nutrition

At the completion of this section, the learner will be able to discuss the parenteral methods used to provide nutrition for the high-acuity patient, including potential complications.

Total parenteral nutrition (TPN) is a nutritionally complete, intravenous-delivered solution composed of macronutrients (carbohydrates, proteins, and lipids), micronutrients (electrolytes, vitamins, trace minerals) and water. Its use is indicated when oral or enteral nutrition is not possible or when absorption or function of the gastrointestinal tract is not sufficient (or unreliable) to meet the nutritional needs of the patient. TPN is contraindicated in those patients with a functioning, usable GI tract capable of absorption of adequate nutrients, when sole dependence is anticipated to be less than five days, when aggressive support is not warranted, and when the risks of TPN outweigh the potential benefits. With the exception of severe hemorrhagic pancreatitis, necrotizing enterocolitis, prolonged ileus, and distal bowel obstruction, some enteral nutrition is recommended in addition to TPN to maintain gut integrity. See the box, NURSING CARE: The Patient Receiving Parenteral Nutrition, for more information.

Delivery of Parenteral Nutrition

Total parenteral nutrition (TPN) with greater than 10 percent glucose is delivered through a central line (Fig. 33–2) to allow higher blood volumes in the larger central veins to rapidly dilute and disperse the solution, which decreases the vessel irritation associated with the increased osmolarity of the solution. Multilumen catheters are commonly used. These catheters allow for one central venous access, with multiple ports for hemodynamic monitoring and fluid/medication delivery without risk of drug incompatibility. If TPN is expected to be needed for more than a few weeks, a more permanent device such as a subcutaneously tunneled Hickman catheter or Port-a-Cath should be placed. A peripherally inserted central catheter (PICC) also allows central venous access for TPN administration. A PICC line is inserted peripherally into the basilic vein and advanced so that the tip of the catheter rests in the superior vena cava. TPN has

NURSING CARE: The Patient Receiving Parenteral Nutrition

Expected Patient Outcomes and Related Interventions

Outcome 1: The patient will achieve adequate nutritional status.

Assess and compare to established norms, patient baselines, and trends.

Type and severity of malnutrition

Perform Subjective Global Assessment (SGA) of nutritional status or other nutrition-specific assessment.

Establish baseline values of albumin, prealbumin, transferrin.

Evaluate nitrogen balance status: obtain urine urea nitrogen (UUN) and 24 hour protein intake

Assess vitamin and mineral status (e.g., zinc, iron, magnesium, phosphate, folic acid, vitamins A, D, & E).

Determine the number and type of calories needed to meet nutritional requirements.

Indirect calorimetry

Respiratory quotient (RQ)

Fick method

Harris-Benedict equation with stress factors included

Monitor intake and output closely, including all losses from the GI tract.

Monitor the patient's response to treatment.

Daily weights

Baseline and periodic reassessment of anthropometric measurements

Periodic reevaluation of prealbumin, albumin, vitamin and mineral status (e.g., zinc, iron, magnesium, phosphate, folic acid, vitamins A, D, & E), WBCs, other

Institute measures to initiate and maintain parenteral nutrition.

Assist with insertion of an central line for TPN (or a peripheral line for PPN).

During line insertion, monitor for signs and symptoms of:

Pneumothorax, catheter fracture

Subclavian/carotid artery puncture, air embolism

Cardiac dysrhythmias

Administer parenteral nutrition as prescribed.

Frequently assess for intolerance and/or infectious, metabolic, or mechanical complications.

Monitor for hyperglycemia, abnormal liver and renal function.

Monitor intake and output closely, including all losses from the GI tract.

Monitor the patient's response to treatment.

Related nursing diagnoses

Risk for fluid volume deficit

Imbalanced electrolytes

Imbalanced nutrition: less than body requirements

Risk for infection

Knowledge deficit

Outcome 2: The patient will maintain normal fluid and electrolyte balance.

Assess and compare to established norms, patient baselines, and trends.

Monitor the patient closely for signs of dehydration and electrolyte imbalance.

Institute measures to maintain fluid and electrolyte balance.

Maintain strict intake and output monitoring, including all emesis and tube drainage

Maintain IV access and administer IV fluids as ordered

Report abnormal electrolytes to provider and replace electrolytes as ordered.

Related nursing diagnoses

Risk for fluid volume

Imbalanced nutrition: less than body requirements

Outcome 3: The patient will experience no catheter-related infection.

Assess and compare to established norms, patient baselines, and trends.

Signs and symptoms of catheter-related sepsis

Sudden onset of fever, rigors or chills that coincide with parenteral infusion

Erythema, swelling, tenderness, or purulent drainage from catheter site

Sudden temperature elevation that resolves on catheter removal

Leukocytosis

Sudden onset of glucose intolerance that may develop up to 12 hours before temperature elevation

Bacteremia/septicemia/septic shock

Institute measures to prevent catheter-related infection.*

Catheter insertion

For central line: insert in subclavian vein; avoid lower extremity insertions.

Meticulous hand hygiene and aseptic technique

Central line insertion – maximal sterile barrier precautions (cap, mask, sterile gown, sterile gloves, sterile drape)

PICC insertion – recommend same as central line placement

Skin antisepsis: either povidone iodine or aqueous chlorhexidine gluconate

Catheter site dressings: either gauze dressings or transparent dressings (transparent dressing can be left in place for duration of catheter insertion)

In-line filters may decrease phlebitis but no clear support for prevention of infection

(*continued*)

NURSING CARE (*continued*)

Consider use of antimicrobial/antiseptic impregnated catheter
Antibiotic/antiseptic ointments at insertion site: povidone-iodine
Catheter replacement:
Peripheral catheters – every 70 to 96 hour intervals (to reduce phlebitis and infection risk)
Central catheters, including PICCs – timing of replacement is controversial for reducing infection (every seven days versus only as needed)

Related nursing diagnoses
Risk for infection

*MMWR. (2002). Guidelines for the prevention of intravascular catheter-related infections. *MMWR, 51*(RR10), CDC, 1–26.

sometimes been referred to as 'hyperalimentation' or 'hyperal'. These terms are not preferred because they incorrectly imply that the patient is receiving more calories, protein, and other nutrients than may be required. TPN solutions are designed to meet the individual energy and protein needs of a patient based on the clinical condition, underlying disease states, and organ function.

Glucose concentrations of 10 percent or less can be delivered as peripheral parenteral nutrition (PPN). PPN is infused into smaller, peripheral veins (e.g., the basilic vein), and is often used for short-term nutrition support (seven to ten days), or as a supplement during transitional phases to enteral or oral nutrition routes. As the osmolarity of parenteral solutions increase, the risk of phlebitis increases; therefore, the osmolarity of PPN solutions are recommended not to exceed 900 mOsm/L (Miller, 2006).

Complications of Total Parenteral Nutrition

Complications from TPN fall under three classifications: infectious, metabolic, and mechanical.

Infectious Complications

Both the solution and the in-dwelling catheter are prime sites for infection because of the high glucose content; any break in the system is a site for infection that can progress to a systemic infection if left unchecked. **Catheter-related sepsis (CRS)** has a 35 percent mortality rate, and hospital stays are reportedly longer and more expensive as a result of complications and associated treatment (Bistrian & Driscoll, 2007). Some of the more common reasons for CRS include lack of sterility during placement of central lines, and inadequate precautions taken during maintenance of the central line and insertion site (e.g., changing tubings, dressings, bags).

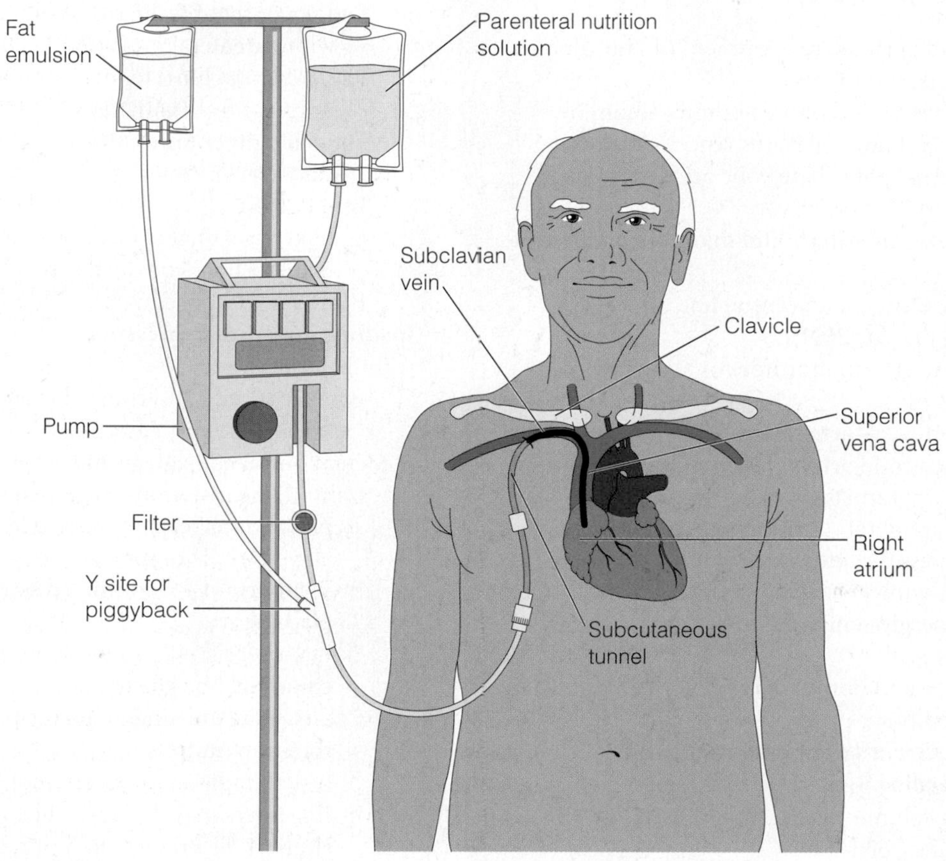

Figure 33–2 ▪ Total parenteral nutrition through a catheter in the right subclavian vein.

Clinical manifestations

The clinical signs and symptoms of catheter-related sepsis include

- sudden onset of fever, rigors, or chills that coincide with parenteral infusion
- erythema, swelling, tenderness, or purulent drainage from the catheter site
- sudden temperature elevation that resolves on catheter removal
- leukocytosis
- sudden glucose intolerance that may occur up to 12 hours before temperature elevation
- bacteremia/septicemia/septic shock

Prevention and Treatment of CRS. To minimize the risk of line infections, one port of multilumen catheters should be dedicated for TPN administration and the catheter requires meticulous care. Although transparent dressings allow for easier observation of the catheter entrance site, they have a tendency to trap moisture, and hence, have a higher incidence of infection than traditional, sterile gauze dressings (Bistrian & Driscoll, 2007). The insertion site should be monitored for signs of leakage, erythema, edema, and inflammation. Chlorhexidine solution has been found to be a more effective local antiseptic than povidine-iodine solutions (Chaiyakunapruk, Veenstra, Lipsky, & Saint, 2002). Additionally, the use of catheters impregnated with either chlorhexidine/silver sulfadiazine or minocycline/rifampin combinations may also reduce the incidence of CRI (MMWR, 2002). Treatment often includes topical and systemic antibiotics, and in many cases, catheter removal.

Metabolic Complications

Metabolic complications of TPN are similar to those of enteral nutrition. Refer to Section Three for metabolic complications, possible causes, and suggested treatment.

Other possible metabolic derangements caused by TPN are hyperglycemia, prerenal azotemia, and hepatic dysfunction.

Hyperglycemia. Hyperglycemia, or elevated blood sugar over 220 mg/dL, commonly occurs in parenteral and enteral nutrition. Elevated glucose levels have been shown to reduce neutrophil chemotaxis and phagocytosis, and may be an independent risk factor for infection. Glycemic control can be achieved by increasing insulin in the TPN solution, by maintaining a continuous insulin drip during TPN administration, or by administering sliding scale insulin subcutaneously at regular intervals.

Prerenal Azotemia. Prerenal azotemia is caused by overaggressive protein administration and is aggravated by underlying dehydration. Presenting signs and symptoms include an elevated serum BUN and serum sodium, and clinical signs of dehydration. If the condition is not corrected, the patient may develop progressive lethargy and possibly coma. Close monitoring of body weight, fluid balance, and adequate protein intake is important in preventing this complication.

Hepatic Dysfunction. Hepatic dysfunction can develop secondary to the macronutrient concentrations in TPN solutions, particularly excessive glucose concentrations. Steatohepatitis (fatty liver), intrahepatic and extrahepatic cholestasis (suppression of bile flow), and cholelithiasis (formation of gallstones) may be reflected in elevated serum liver function tests (including aspartate aminotransferase [AST], amino alanine transferase [ALT], alkaline phosphatase [Alk phos; ALP], and bilirubin levels) during the course of TPN, and usually return to normal spontaneously when the infusion is stopped.

Mechanical Complications

Mechanical complications include pneumothorax, catheter fracture, subclavian/carotid artery puncture, air embolism, and dysrhythmias. All may be a result of the central venous catheter insertion.

Pneumothorax. Pneumothorax, the most common mechanical complication, is caused by the puncture or laceration of the pleura on insertion of the needle/catheter. Air enters into the pleural space, with partial or complete collapse of the lung. Most pneumothoraces produce symptoms, although some are totally asymptomatic. In general, the larger the collapse, the more pronounced the symptoms. Commonly seen are shortness of breath, restlessness, hypoxia, and chest pain radiating to the back. Treatment depends on the severity of the collapse and respiratory compromise. Moderate to large collapse will require a chest tube to restore negative pressure within the chest cavity.

Catheter Fracture. Catheter fracture and occlusion are other mechanical complications that can occur. Fractures or breakage of the catheter can result from reduced pliability over time. Occlusion can occur from lodging of the catheter tip against the vessel wall or from being physiologically "pinched" between the clavicle and first rib. Other occlusions can occur from fibrin buildup, blood or lipid deposition, and drug precipitates. Another type of occlusion, known as "withdrawal occlusion," is an occlusion that allows infusion of a solution but prevents blood withdrawal.

Artery Puncture. Inadvertent puncture or laceration of the subclavian or carotid arteries is indicated by a flashback of arterial blood in the syringe, pulsatile blood flow, bleeding from the catheter site or development of a large hematoma, and hypotension. Treatment involves withdrawing the syringe/catheter and applying direct pressure to the site until bleeding ceases.

Air Embolism. Air embolism may occur whenever the central venous system is open to air. Signs and symptoms vary with the amount of air pulled into the venous system but may include respiratory distress, tachycardia, hypotension, sudden cardiovascular collapse, neurologic deficits, or cardiac arrest. Immediate action is required. Occlude the catheter nearest to the entry site of the skin. Place the patient on the left side and in the Trendelenburg position. This allows an air embolus to float into the right ventricle of the heart, away from the pulmonary artery. Prevention is the key. Always use Luer-Lock or other secure connectors and air-eliminating filters on central line tubings.

Cardiac Dysrhythmias. Dysrhythmias (rhythm irregularities) during central venous insertions are the result of a malpositioned catheter or guidewire. The result may be atrial, junctional, or ventricular dysrhythmias, which may cause decreased cardiac output, decreased blood pressure, or loss of consciousness. Appropriate intervention is to partially withdraw the catheter or guidewire. If the dysrhythmia continues, an antiarrhythmic may be required.

Emerging Evidence

- A comparative study investigated the effectiveness of intravenous (IV) erythromycin alone versus a combination of IV erythromycin and metoclopramide on 75 critically ill, mechanically ventilated medical patients with feeding intolerance. The study concluded that combination therapy was more effective than erythromycin therapy alone in improving feeding tolerance; however, combination therapy had a significantly higher incidence of watery diarrhea unrelated to infections *(Nguyen, Chapman, Fraser, Bryant, Burgstad, & Holloway, 2007)*.
- A prospective study tested a nutritional support algorithm in an intensive care unit to determine whether use of an algorithm would improve the delivery of nutrients to ICU patients. The study results supported the use of an algorithm primarily because it improved physician orders resulting in earlier implementation *(Woien, & Bjork, 2006)*.
- In mechanically, ventilated, critically ill patients, use of morphine and midazolam vs. propofol for sedation were compared in regard to their effect on gastric emptying. The study concluded that use of the combination of morphine and midazolam resulted in slower gastric emptying than sedation with propofol *(Nguyen, Chapman, Fraser, Bryant, Burgstad, Ching, Bellon, & Holloway, 2008*.
- In critically ill patients with feed intolerance, there is a positive correlation between degree of glycemic variation and feed intolerance. The study concluded that improved glucose control through intensive insulin therapy warrants additional study *(Nguyen,Ching, Fraser, Chapman, & Holloway, 2007)*.
- Nurses were surveyed about their EN feeding practices. They reported that they measured gastric residual volumes and managed delayed gastric emptying by decreasing the rate of feeding and using prokinetic agents. Measures such as changing patient position, checking tube placement were less frequently reported. Results suggest that nursing practices associated with the delivery of enteral feedings may contribute to under-feeding in critically ill patients *(Marshall & West, 2006)*.
- Critically ill patients with elevated gastric residual volume during gastric EN have delayed gastric motility. Initiating prokinetic therapy accelerates gastric emptying to resemble that of ICU patients tolerating EN *(Landzinski, Kiser, & Fish, et al., 2008)*.
- A study to evaluate the risk factors of catheter-related blood stream infection (CRBSI) in patients receiving PN revealed the following to reduce incidence of CRBSI: The duration of central venous catheterization should be shortened; the central venous catheter, which is inserted in urgent situations, should be removed as soon as possible and replaced under maximal sterile barrier precautions; and increased attention should be paid to hand hygiene (Yilmas, Kiksal, & Aydin et al., 2007).

SECTION FOUR REVIEW

1. TPN is indicated when
   A. adequate amounts of nutrients can be delivered through the GI tract
   B. adequate amounts of nutrients cannot be delivered through the GI tract
   C. a functioning, usable gastrointestinal tract is capable of absorption of adequate nutrients
   D. aggressive nutritional support is not warranted

2. TPN with a greater than 10 percent glucose should be administered through a
   A. nasoenteric feeding tube
   B. peripheral vein
   C. surgically placed jejunal feeding tube
   D. central vein

3. Which of the following factors can lead to prerenal azotemia in the patient receiving TPN?
   A. excessive protein administration
   B. excessive carbohydrate administration
   C. excessive fluid administration
   D. excessive lipid administration

4. CRS is a potentially lethal complication of TPN and is caused primarily by
   A. a malpositioned catheter or guidewire during the central line insertion
   B. lack of sterility during central line placement and inadequate line maintenance
   C. inadvertent puncture or laceration of the subclavian or carotid artery
   D. puncture or laceration of the vein on insertion of the needle/catheter

5. Hypoglycemia is a potential metabolic complication of TPN and results from
   A. gluconeogenesis
   B. glucose intolerance
   C. sudden cessation of feeding
   D. insulin resistance

6. Mechanical complications of TPN consist of (choose all that apply)
   A. air embolism
   B. hydrothorax
   C. pneumothorax
   D. catheter related sepsis (CRS)

Answers: 1. B, 2. D, 3. A, 4. B, 5. C, 6. (A, B, C)

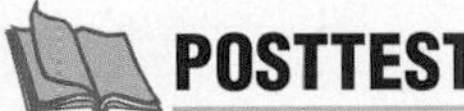

POSTTEST

1. Which one of the following substances is the body's preferred energy source?
   A. proteins
   B. lipids
   C. carbohydrates
   D. amino acids
2. Nutritional goals for the pulmonary failure patient include (choose all that apply)
   A. higher sodium content
   B. lower protein content
   C. lower carbohydrate content
   D. higher fat content
3. For the high-acuity patient with acute renal failure, which of the following nutritional therapies is appropriate for the patient undergoing hemodialysis?
   A. protein intake should be restricted to about 0.5 to 0.8 g/kg/day
   B. protein intake should be liberalized to about 0.8 to 2.0 g/kg/day
   C. carbohydrate intake should be limited to less than 50 percent of total nutrition
   D. lipid intake should not exceed 20 percent of total nutrition
4. A patient has a functioning GI tract but is unable to take adequate nutrients by mouth. What is the BEST method for administering nutritional support to this patient?
   A. nasoenteric feedings
   B. oral diet
   C. withholding nutrition
   D. TPN
5. The primary rationale for postpyloric feeding is that it
   A. prevents aspiration of tube feeding
   B. negates the need for a nasogastric tube
   C. promotes greater amount of nutritional intake in patients likely to have delayed gastric emptying
   D. facilitates bolus feeding
6. TPN is appropriate for use in patients with
   A. liver failure and nausea
   B. nonresectable gastric tumor that prevents passage of enteral feeding tube
   C. chronic pancreatitis
   D. hyperemesis gravidarum
7. When a patient is receiving total parenteral nutrition, it is important for the nurse to assess the
   A. blood for glucose
   B. stool for occult blood
   C. urine for specific gravity
   D. abdomen for bowel sounds
8. The nurse knows that one of the complications of total parenteral nutrition would be
   A. infection
   B. hepatitis
   C. anorexia
   D. dysrhythmias
9. A patient's serum albumin value is 2.8 g/dl. The nurse should evaluate patient teaching as successful when the patient says, "For lunch I am going to have ________."
   A. fruit salad
   B. sliced turkey
   C. spinach salad
   D. clear beef broth
10. Arginine, omega-3 fatty acids nucleotides, and beta carotene are ingredients in which of the following types of enteral formula?
    A. complete lactose-free, high residue
    B. high-calorie complete
    C. complete formulas, without residue
    D. immuno-modulating formulas

Posttest answers with rationale are found on MyNursingKit.

PEARSON

EXPLORE mynursingkit™

MyNursingKit is your one stop for online chapter review materials and resources. Prepare for success with additional NCLEX®-style practice questions, interactive assignments and activities, web links, animations and videos, and more!

Register your access code from the front of your book at **www.mynursingkit.com.**

REFERENCES

American Heart Association. (2008). Metabolic syndrome. Retrieved November 1, 2008 from http://www.americanheart.org/presenter.jhtml?identifier=4756.

Anderson, R. J. (2008). Renal disease and metabolic disorders in the critically ill. In J. E. Parrillo and R. P. Dellinger, *Critical care medicine: principles of diagnosis and management in the adult.* (3rd ed.). Retrieved November 1, 2008 from http://www.mdconsult.com.

ASPEN. (2002a). Specific guidelines for disease – adults. In Board of Directors and The Clinical Guidelines Task Force, guidelines for the use of parenteral and enteral nutrition in adults and pediatric patient. *J Parenter Enteral Nutr* 2002; 26S: 1SA-138SA. Retrieved November 2, 2008 from http://www.nutritioncare.org.

ASPEN. (2002b). Nutrition assessment – adults. In Board of Directors and The Clinical Guidelines Task Force, guidelines for the use of parenteral and enteral nutrition in adults and pediatric patient. *J Parenter Enteral Nutr* 2002; 26S: 1SA-138SA. Retrieved November 2, 2008 from http://www.nutritioncare.org.

Baumgartner, L. (2008). Acute respiratory failure and acute lung injury. In K. K. Carlson (ed.) *AACN advanced critical care nursing.* St. Louis: Saunders/Elsevier.

Bistrian, B. R., & Driscoll, D. F. (2007). Enteral and parenteral nutrition therapy. In E. Brauwald, A. S. Fauci, D. L. Kasper, S. L. Hauser, D. L. Longo, J. L. Jameson, J. Loscalzo (eds.). *Harrison's principles of internal medicine* (17th ed.). New York: McGraw-Hill, 455–462.

Clark, M. (2009). Nutrition. In K. K. Carlson (ed.), *Advanced critical care nursing.* St. Louis: Saunders/Elsevier, 111–129.

Dominguez-Cherit, G., Posadas-Calleja, J. G., & Borunda, D. (2008). Chronic obstructive pulmonary disease. In J. E. Parrillo and R. P. Dellinger, *Critical care medicine: principles of diagnosis and management in the adult.* (3rd ed.). Retrieved November 1, 2008 from http://www.mdconsult.com.

Dwyer, J. (2007). Nutritional requirements and dietary assessment. In E. Brauwald, A. S. Fauci, D. L. Kasper, S. L. Hauser, D. L. Longo, J. L. Jameson, & J. Loscalzo. (eds.). *Harrison's principles of internal medicine* (17th ed.). New York: McGraw-Hill, 437–450.

Hogg, J., Klapholz, A., & Reid-Hector, J. (2001). Pulmonary disease. In Gottschlich, M. M. (ed.). *The science and practice of nutrition support.* Dubuque, Iowa: Kendall/Hunt.

Kattelmann, K. K., Hise, M., Russell, M., et al. (2006). Preliminary evidence for a medical nutrition therapy protocol: enteral feedings for critically ill patients. *Journal of the American Dietetic Association, 106*(8), 1226–1241.

Lafrance, J. P., & Leblanc, M. (2005). Metabolic, electrolytes, and nutritional concerns in critical illness. *Critical Care Clinics, 21*, 305–325.

Landzinski, J., Kiser, T., Fish, D., et al. (2008). Gastric motility function in critically ill patients tolerant vs intolerant to gastric nutrition. *J. Parenteral and Enteral Nutrition, Vol 32,* No 1, 45–50.

Lin, L., & Cohen, N. H. (2005). Early nutritional support for the ICU patient: does it matter? *Contemporary Critical Care, 2*(9), 1–10.

Little, R. A., & Giorlami, A. (1999). Trauma metabolism, ebb and flow revisited. *British Journal of Intensive Care, 9*, 142–146.

Marik, P. E., & Zaloga, G. P. (2001). Early enteral nutrition in acutely ill patients: a systematic review. *Critical Care Medicine, 29*(12), 2264–2270.

Marshall, A. P. & West, S. H. (2006). Enteral feeding in the critically ill: are nursing practices contributing to hypo-caloric feeding? *Intensive and Critical Care Nursing, Vol 22,* Issue 2, 95–105.

McClave, S. A., DeMeo, M. T., DeLegge, M. H., et al. (2002). Northern American summit on aspiration in the critically ill patient: consensus statement. *Journal of Parenteral and Enteral Nutrition, 26*(6), S80–S85.

MMWR (2002). Guidelines for prevention of intravascular catheter-related infections. *MMWR, 51*(RR10); 1-26, CDC. Retrieved November 2, 2008 from http://www.cdc.gov/mmwr/preview/mmwrhtml/rr5110a1.htm.

Nguyen, N. Q., Chapman, J. J., Fraser, R. J., Bryant, L. K., Burgstad, C., Ching, K., Bellon, M., and Holloway, R. H. (2008). The effects of sedation on gastric emptying and intra-gastric meal distribution in critical illness. *Intensive Care Medicine, 34*(3), 454–460.

Nguyen, N. Q., Chapman, M., Fraser, R. J., Bryant, L. K., Burgstad, C., & Holloway, R. H. (2007). Prokinetic therapy for feeding intolerance in critical illness: one drug or two? *Crit Care Med, 35*(11), 2561–2567.

Nguyen, N. Q., Ching, K., Fraser, R., Chapman, M., and Holloway, R. (2007). The relationship between blood glucose control and intolerance to enteral feeding during critical illness. *Intensive Care Medicine, 33*(12), 2085–2092.

Nguyen, N. Q., Chapman, M., Fraser, R. J., Bryant, L. K., Burgstad, C., & Holloway, R. H. (2007). Prokinetic therapy for feeding intolerance in critical illness: one drug or two? *Crit Care Med, 35*(11), 2561–2567.

Nguyen, N. Q., Chapman, M., Fraser, R. J., Bryant, L. K., Burgstad, C., & Holloway, R. H. (2007). Prokinetic therapy for feeding intolerance in critical illness: one drug or two? *Crit Care Med, 35*(11), 2561–2567).

Nguyen, N., Ching, K., Fraser, R., Chapman, M., & Holloway, R. (2007). The relationship between blood glucose control and intolerance to enteral feeding during critical illness. *Intensive Care Medicine, 33*(12), 2085–2092.

Pleuss, J. (2007). Alterations in body nutrition. In C. M. Porth (ed.), *Essentials of pathophysiology: concepts of altered health states* (2d ed.). Philadelphia: Lippincott Williams & Wilkins, 165–178.

Porth, C. M., & Sweeney, K. (2007). Alterations in immune response. In C. M. Porth (ed.), *Essentials of pathophysiology: concepts of altered health states* (2d ed.). Philadelphia: Lippincott Williams & Wilkins. 293–318.

Porth, C. M. (2007). Disorders of hepatic and biliary function. In C. M. Porth (ed.), *Essentials of pathophysiology: concepts of altered health states* (2d ed.). Philadelphia: Lippincott Williams & Wilkins, 631–658.

Saffle, J. R. (2008). Critical care management of the severely burned patient. In J. E. Parrillo and R. P. Dellinger, *Critical care medicine: principles of diagnosis and management in the adult.* (3rd ed.). Retrieved November 1, 2008 from http://www.mdconsult.com.

WIN (Weight-control information service). (2007). National Institutes of Diabetes and Digestive and Kidney Diseases. National Institutes of Health. Retrieved November 1, 2008 from http://www.win.niddk.nih.gov/statistics/index.htm.

Woien, H., and Bjrk, I. T. (2006). Nutrition of the critically ill patient and effects of implementing a nutritional support algorithm in ICU. *Journal of Clinical Nursing, 15*(2), 168–177.

Yilmas, G., Kiksal, I., Aydin, K., et al. (2007). Risk factors of catheter-related bloodstream infections in parenteral nutrition catheterization. *Journal of Parenteral and Enteral Nutrition, Vol. 31,* No. 4, 284–297.

MODULE

34 Alterations in Glucose Metabolism

Kathleen D. Wagner, Theresa M. Glessner, Melanie G. Hardin-Pierce

OBJECTIVES Following completion of this module, the learner will be able to

1. Discuss normal glucose metabolism.
2. Describe the effects of insulin on metabolism.
3. Explain the effects of insulin deficit.
4. Differentiate the two major types of diabetes mellitus.
5. Discuss the pathophysiology, clinical manifestations, and nursing care management of therapy-induced hypoglycemia.
6. Discuss the pathophysiology, clinical manifestations, and nursing care management of diabetic ketoacidosis.
7. Discuss the pathophysiology, clinical manifestations, and nursing care management of hyperglycemic hyperosmolar state.
8. Explain the use of exogenous insulin in the management of the patient with diabetes mellitus.
9. Discuss the acute care nursing implications of chronic diabetic complications.

This self-study module focuses on physiologic processes involved in normal glucose metabolism, as well as the pathophysiologic basis of altered glucose metabolism. The three major diabetic crises are presented. Each is described in terms of pathophysiology, clinical presentation, and management. The module is composed of nine sections. Sections One and Two discuss normal glucose metabolism and the effects of insulin on metabolism. Section Three describes the impact of insulin deficit on metabolism. Section Four provides a brief review of the two major types of diabetes mellitus (type 1 and type 2). Sections Five through Seven discuss the three acute life-threatening consequences of diabetes: therapy-induced hypoglycemia, diabetic ketoacidosis, and hyperglycemic hyperosmolar state. Section Eight reviews exogenous insulin therapy, focusing on types of insulin therapy used during acute illness. Finally, Section Nine presents an overview of chronic diabetic complications and their effects on the nursing management of the acutely ill patient. Each section includes a set of review questions to help the learner evaluate his or her understanding of the section's content before moving on to the next section. All Section Reviews include answers. It is suggested that the learner review those concepts answered incorrectly in the review questions before proceeding to the next section.

PRETEST

1. Insulin promotes use of glucose by
   A. breaking down glucose
   B. assisting glucose into the cells
   C. converting glucose to glycogen
   D. transporting glucose in the blood
2. Which of the following is TRUE regarding the effect of insulin on fat metabolism? It inhibits
   A. synthesis of fatty acids
   B. glucose use by tissues
   C. release of fatty acids
   D. transport of glucose into fat cells
3. When an insulin deficiency exists, the liver responds by converting
   A. fatty acids to glucose
   B. glycogen to glucose
   C. glucagon to glucose
   D. amino acids to glucose
4. Insulin-dependent cells use which of the following nutritional substances FIRST when insulin is not available?
   A. fatty acids
   B. glycogen
   C. glucagon
   D. amino acids
5. The etiology of type 1 diabetes is believed to be
   A. obesity
   B. an autoimmune reaction
   C. a bacterial infection
   D. general pancreatic dysfunction

6. A patient experiencing rapid onset hypoglycemia is most likely to have predominantly ______ symptoms.
   A. cell dysfunction
   B. gastrointestinal
   C. stimulated sympathetic nervous system
   D. stimulated parasympathetic nervous system
7. Central nervous system symptoms associated with hypoglycemia are caused by lack of ______ rather than insulin deficit.
   A. glucose
   B. amino acids
   C. fatty acids
   D. glucagon
8. Clinical manifestations of severe hypoglycemia include
   A. bradycardia
   B. fruity odor of the breath
   C. mental confusion
   D. ketonuria
9. Clinical manifestations of diabetic ketoacidosis include
   A. weight gain
   B. fluid overload
   C. electrolyte depletion
   D. hypoventilation
10. Which of the following statements is correct regarding hyperglycemic hyperosmolar state?
    A. It has a higher mortality rate than diabetic ketoacidosis.
    B. It is most common in young patients with type 1 diabetes.
    C. It causes severe fluid volume overload.
    D. Significant ketosis is present.
11. Exogenous insulin is
    A. used only in the treatment of type 1 diabetes
    B. often used in management of type 2 diabetes during periods of stress
    C. most often derived from animal sources
    D. seldom used in the treatment of hyperglycemic hyperosmolar state
12. Diabetic retinopathy causes blindness as a result of
    A. glucose deposits on the retina
    B. thickening of the retina
    C. destruction of the optic nerve
    D. infarction of retinal tissue
13. Diabetic nephropathy damages the nephrons by causing
    A. glomerulosclerosis
    B. glomerulonephritis
    C. chronic nephritis
    D. renal hypertension

Pretest answers are found on MyNursingKit.

SECTION ONE: Normal Glucose Metabolism

At the completion of this section, the learner will be able to discuss normal glucose metabolism.

Glucose is used by most body cells as an energy source. Some cells (e.g., brain cells) can use only glucose for energy; however, glucose does not cross muscle and fat cell membranes using the same mechanisms, as do most other molecules. It requires a protein carrier, facilitated by insulin, to transport it into these cells. Fat and muscle cells are, therefore, sometimes referred to as **insulin-dependent cells**. After combining with the protein carrier in the cell membrane, glucose is able to diffuse across the membrane into the cell, where the carrier releases it. Supplying the cells with glucose is a complex physiologic task based on important feedback mechanisms for regulating blood glucose levels. This mechanism is primarily controlled by two hormones, insulin and glucagon, with important support by three other hormones, epinephrine, growth hormone, and cortisol. The normal fasting plasma glucose level is 70 to 110 mg/dL (American Diabetes Association, 2008).

Insulin

Insulin is a polypeptide (small protein) produced by the beta cells of the islets of Langerhans in the pancreas. Its underlying role is to lower the blood glucose level, and it sometimes is referred to as the hypoglycemic factor. Insulin plays a crucial part in regulating carbohydrate, fat, and protein metabolism.

Insulin must bind to special insulin receptor proteins in the cell membrane to carry out its functions. Once it is attached to a receptor site, insulin combines with the carrier protein in the cell membrane. The carrier protein, with help from insulin, promotes glucose diffusion across the cell membrane. Insulin's exact role is to enhance the function of the carrier protein.

Glucagon

Glucagon, a small protein, is secreted by alpha cells in the islets of Langerhans in the pancreas. It is the major hormone responsible for raising serum glucose levels and sometimes is referred to as the hyperglycemic factor. Glucagon's effects are in opposition to those of insulin. The stimulus for glucagon release is a decrease in the serum glucose level to a hypoglycemic level (Guvan et al., 2006). Glucagon counterbalances the effects of insulin by converting hepatic **glycogen** (via **glycogenolysis**) into glucose. Once converted, hepatic glucose rapidly moves into the circulation, increasing blood glucose levels. The reciprocal relationship between insulin and glucagon assists in maintaining homeostatic blood glucose levels. Figure 34–1 illustrates how blood glucose levels are regulated by insulin and glucagon.

Epinephrine, Growth Hormone, and Cortisol

When the serum glucose level drops below the normal range, the sympathetic nervous system is stimulated. Consequently, the adrenal glands secrete epinephrine. Epinephrine increases

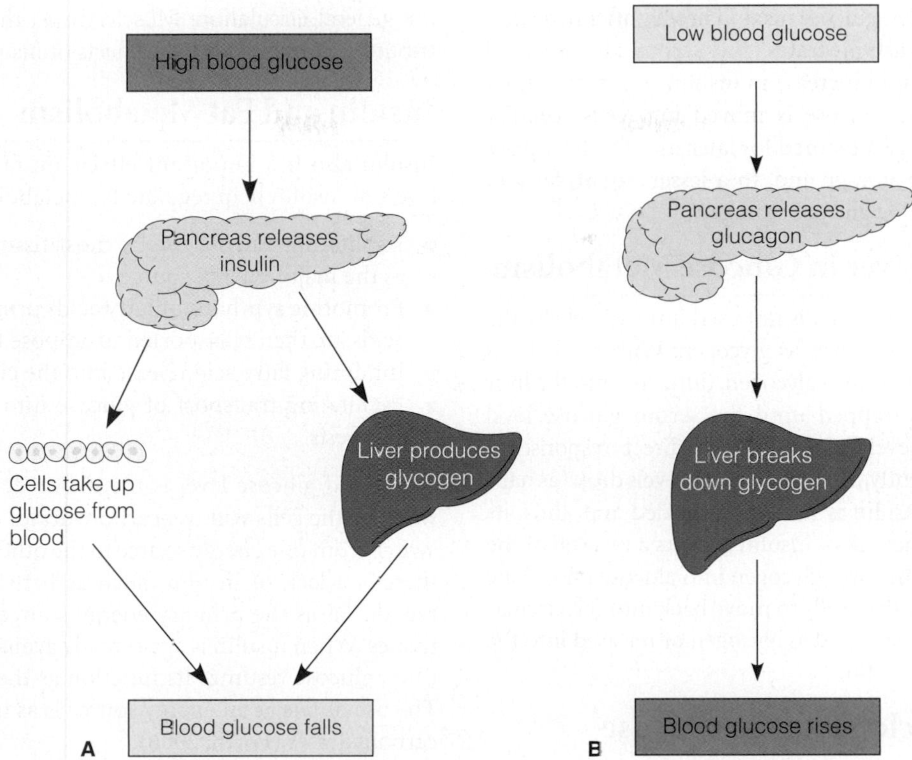

Figure 34–1 ■ Regulation (homeostasis) of blood glucose levels by insulin and glucagon. **A,** High blood glucose is lowered by insulin release. **B,** Low blood glucose is raised by glucagon release.

serum glucose levels in a manner similar to glucagon but to a lesser extent. Pituitary growth hormone and cortisol both respond to prolonged periods of hypoglycemia. They help reestablish a more normal glucose level by decreasing the rate of glucose use by the cells. Growth hormone decreases the body's ability to use carbohydrates, which spares them as an energy source. It facilitates the transport of amino acids into the cells. Oversecretion of growth hormone can lead to glucose intolerance and the development of diabetes (Guvan et al., 2006).

SECTION ONE REVIEW

1. Insulin is produced in the
   A. kidneys
   B. pituitary gland
   C. liver
   D. pancreas
2. Insulin promotes use of glucose by
   A. breaking down glucose
   B. assisting glucose into the cells
   C. converting glucose to glycogen
   D. transporting glucose in the blood
3. Glucagon promotes
   A. decreased use of glucose
   B. conversion of hepatic glycogen
   C. protein synthesis and transport
   D. transport of glucose into the cells
4. Which of the following is TRUE regarding growth hormone?
   A. It decreases cellular use of glucose.
   B. It promotes storage of fat.
   C. It decreases blood glucose levels.
   D. It increases breakdown of glycogen.
5. Release of cortisol
   A. increases mobilization of fats
   B. decreases use of glucose
   C. decreases secretion of insulin
   D. increases breakdown of muscle glycogen

Answers: 1. D, 2. B, 3. B, 4. A, 5. B

SECTION TWO: The Effects of Insulin on Metabolism

At the completion of this section, the learner will be able to describe the effects of insulin on metabolism.

Insulin and Carbohydrate Metabolism

The body depends on adequate levels of glucose to provide energy for normal functioning. **Carbohydrates**, nutritional substances composed of complex and simple sugars, normally provide most of the body's glucose needs. Directly after ingestion and consumption of carbohydrates, the serum glucose level increases, triggering a rapid increase in insulin secretion. Under the influence of insulin, glucose is moved into cells (cellular **uptake**) for immediate use or stored for later use. The liver plays a major role in glucose storage and, to a lesser extent, fat and muscle tissues also provide glucose storage.

Insulin and the Liver in Glucose Metabolism

Directly after a meal, glucose that is not used immediately by the cells is stored rapidly in the liver as glycogen. With the help of insulin, glucose is converted into glycogen, diffusing into the liver cells where it becomes trapped until the serum glucose level becomes low. Insulin levels are altered in direct response to glucose levels. Consequently, as serum glucose levels drop (as happens between meals), insulin is no longer needed and, thus, its level rapidly declines. The lack of insulin triggers a reversal of the process, breaking down the liver glycogen into glucose phosphate and releasing it from the liver cells to move back into the circulation. Thus, glucose may be stored as glycogen or released into the circulation (Guvan et al., 2006).

Insulin and Muscle Tissue in Glucose Metabolism

During normal daily activity, muscle tissue uses fatty acids, not glucose, as its major source of energy. This is because the resting membrane of the muscle does not allow glucose into the cell without the presence of insulin. Insulin levels, however, are very low between meals, thereby requiring use of energy sources other than glucose.

Muscle cells use glucose under two circumstances. First, during heavy exercise, muscle cell membranes become highly permeable to glucose. Second, for several hours after meals, the high level of insulin in the serum enhances transport of glucose into the muscle cells. Muscle cells store available glucose as muscle glycogen for their own use; however, they are unable to convert it back into glucose or transport it back out of the muscle tissue into the general circulation. Muscle tissue, therefore, does not contribute to counteracting the effects of insulin.

Insulin and Fat Metabolism

Insulin also has important effects on fat metabolism. Normal levels of insulin help regulate fat metabolism by

- Facilitating glucose use by most tissues, thereby sparing fat as the major energy source
- Promoting synthesis of fatty acids primarily in the liver; fatty acids are then transported to adipose tissue for storage
- Inhibiting fatty acid release into the circulation
- Facilitating transport of glucose into fat cells for fatty acid synthesis

The blood glucose level is the major determining factor as to whether the cells will use carbohydrates or fats for energy. The switch from one energy source to the other occurs rapidly. When there is a lack of insulin (such as between meals), cells must rely on fat as the primary energy source in insulin-dependent tissues. When insulin is again made available in sufficient quantities, glucose resumes its function as the major energy source. The use of fats as an energy source is as important as the use of carbohydrates (Porth, 2006).

Insulin and Protein Metabolism

Insulin plays an important part in the storage of protein following ingestion of nutrients. Insulin helps regulate protein metabolism by

- Facilitating transport of amino acids across the cell membrane
- Promoting protein **synthesis**
- Decreasing protein **catabolism**

In addition to glucose, amino acids also act as triggers for insulin secretion. Thus, when amino acid levels increase after ingestion of nutrients, insulin is secreted to facilitate cellular uptake, synthesis, and storage of proteins.

SECTION TWO REVIEW

1. Which of the following substances supplies the primary source of cell energy?
   A. fat
   B. protein
   C. carbohydrate
   D. glucagon
2. Cells requiring insulin to facilitate diffusion of glucose into them are called
   A. insulin-dependent
   B. glucose-dependent
   C. glycogen-dependent
   D. carbohydrate-dependent
3. Excess glucose is stored in the
   A. pancreas
   B. muscle tissues
   C. adipose tissues
   D. liver
4. During normal daily activities, muscle cells use which of the following as their major energy source?
   A. glucose
   B. fatty acids
   C. amino acids
   D. glucagon
5. Which of the following is TRUE regarding the effect of insulin on fat metabolism? It inhibits
   A. synthesis of fatty acids
   B. glucose use by tissues
   C. release of fatty acids
   D. transport of glucose into fat cells

Answers: 1. C, 2. A, 3. D, 4. B, 5. C

SECTION THREE: The Effects of Insulin Deficit

At the completion of this section, the learner will be able to explain the impact of insulin deficit on metabolism.

Insulin deficiency results in disordered carbohydrate, protein, and fat metabolism. If carbohydrates are not the major glucose energy source, the liver initiates conversion of glycogen to glucose. The principal metabolic alterations associated with insulin deficiency include (1) impaired cellular uptake and use of glucose, (2) increased extracellular (serum) glucose, (3) increased mobilization of fats, and (4) tissue depletion of protein (Fig. 34–2).

Movement of glucose into insulin-dependent cells occurs in direct proportion to the amount of insulin available. When insulin-dependent tissues are deprived of glucose as a result of either insulin deficiency or insulin resistance, their functional capacities become restricted. Table 34–1 summarizes the effects of insulin deficiency on insulin-dependent tissues.

TABLE 34–1 Effects of Insulin Deficit on Insulin-Dependent Tissues

TISSUES	EFFECTS
Glucose Transport Problems	
Skeletal muscle	Fatigue; decreased strength
Cardiac muscle	Weaker contractions; decreased cardiac output; decreased peripheral circulation
Smooth muscle	Poor bowel tone; decreased vascular tone
Leukocytes	Depressed leukocyte function; impaired inflammatory response
Crystalline lens of eye	Opacity/cataracts
Fibroblasts	Impaired healing
Pituitary gland	Retarded growth; impaired regeneration of tissue; other endocrine problems
Insulin Resistance Problem	
Adipose tissue	Lipolysis; lipidemia; elevated serum ketone levels

Insulin Deficit and Carbohydrate Metabolism

Insulin deficit dramatically alters carbohydrate metabolism. Carbohydrates are the major supplier of simple and complex sugars, producing glucose as the primary energy source. Insulin deficit causes cessation in glucose uptake by insulin-dependent cells and a decrease in glucose use by the cells. The combination of decreased glucose uptake and decreased glucose use causes a rapid buildup of serum glucose, known as hyperglycemia.

In an insulin-poor environment, insulin-dependent cells are actually starving. Though abundant potential energy is available in the form of glucose, it is of no use to the cells. Other sources of energy are used, including fatty acids (the primary backup energy source) and amino acids, once fat reserves are depleted. Clinically, dysfunctional carbohydrate metabolism is evidenced

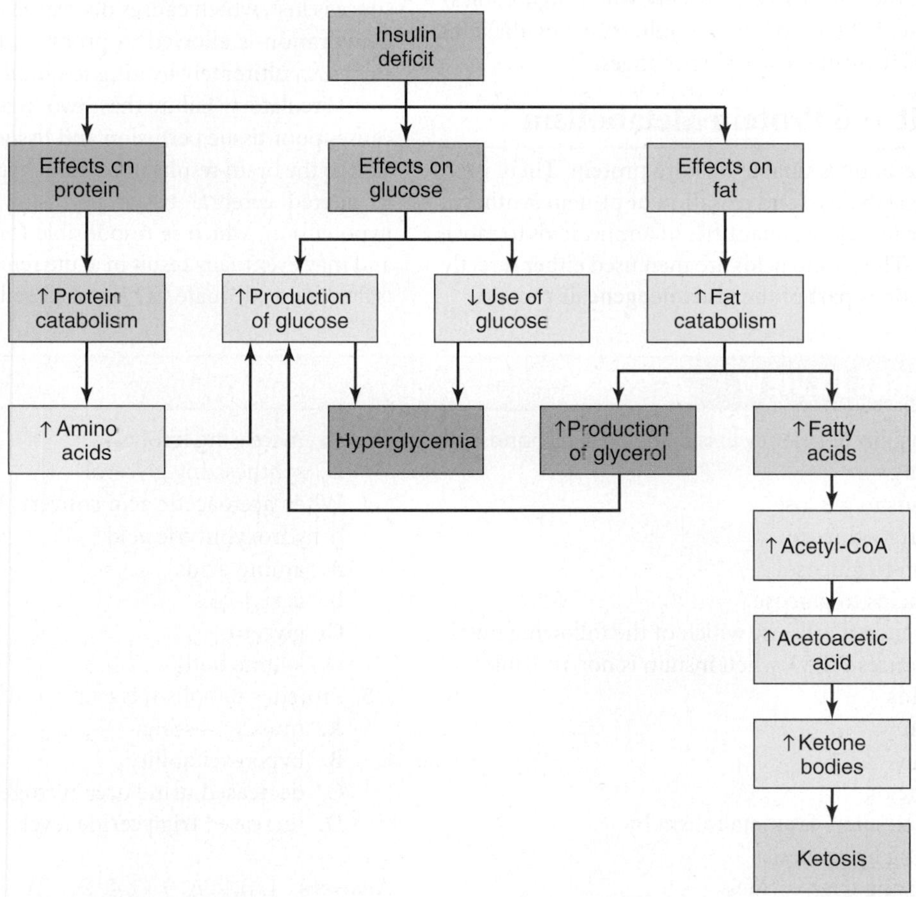

Figure 34–2 ■ Consequences of insulin deficit.

as hyperglycemia. If not controlled, ketosis and **aminoacidemia** may result, each with its own set of complications.

Insulin Deficit and Fat Metabolism

Insulin deficit alters fat metabolism by increasing **lipolysis** (fat breakdown) and decreasing **lipogenesis** (fat formation). The decreased availability of intracellular glucose results in increased breakdown of stored triglycerides by **hormone-sensitive lipase**, causing lipolysis. Free fatty acids become the major energy source for the tissues, with the major exception of the brain. Clinically, this is evidenced as increased blood levels of free fatty acids and glycerol. The liver also converts some of the excess fatty acids into cholesterol and phospholipids. Excess fatty acid breakdown causes increased levels of **acetyl-CoA (acetylcoenzyme A)**, used by the liver for energy. The excess is converted into **acetoacetic acid**. Some of the acetoacetic acid is further converted into **β-hydroxybutyric acid** and **acetone (dimethyl ketone)**. These three substances (acetoacetic acid, β-hydroxybutyric acid, and acetone) move into the circulation as ketone bodies.

Clinically, this sequence of events has both acute and chronic consequences. Acutely, the increased levels of ketone bodies result in **ketosis** and **ketonuria**. When ketosis is extreme, severe **metabolic acidosis** and coma result (e.g., diabetic ketoacidosis). The use of fat as energy is evidenced as a significant increase in plasma lipoproteins (as much as three times normal). In the long term, high levels of lipoproteins are associated with the rapid onset of atherosclerosis, especially when high cholesterol levels are present. Many of the complications of diabetes mellitus are secondary to atherosclerotic changes.

Insulin Deficit and Protein Metabolism

Without insulin, the body is unable to store protein. There is an increase in protein catabolism and cessation of protein synthesis. Protein catabolism causes large quantities of amino acids to move into the circulation. The amino acids are then used either directly as an energy source or as part of the **gluconeogenesis** process.

Clinically, protein catabolism is evidenced by muscle wasting, multiple organ dysfunction, aminoacidemia, and increased urine nitrogen. If nitrogenous wastes accumulate in the body faster than they can be excreted in the urine, the patient will exhibit an altered level of consciousness and mentation. In addition, as gluconeogenesis is initiated, hyperglycemia is further aggravated.

Insulin Deficit and Fluid and Electrolyte Balance

When an insulin deficit exists, the serum glucose level increases, creating increased plasma osmotic pressure. The resulting change in pressure produces a shifting of body fluids from the tissues into the intravascular compartment. This shifting of fluids leads to intracellular dehydration.

As the level of hyperglycemia increases beyond the kidney's ability to reabsorb the extra glucose, **glycosuria** (excretion of glucose in the urine) develops. Urinary excretion of glucose produces an **osmotic diuresis** evidenced as **polyuria** (excessive urination). Osmotic diuresis results in excessive loss of water, potassium, sodium, chloride, and phosphate ions. Loss of these ions further increases both extracellular and intracellular dehydration. Deficits in potassium and sodium are manifested by weakness, fatigue, and other signs and symptoms associated with the specific electrolyte imbalances. As fluid is lost, serum osmolality increases. Dehydration stimulates the hypothalamic thirst center, causing excessive thirst (**polydipsia**). Dehydration also produces hemoconcentration as fluid from the vascular space is lost, which causes decreased cardiac output (CO). If the dehydration is allowed to progress, the CO may become critically low, ultimately leading to circulatory failure.

Circulatory failure has two major consequences. First, it causes poor tissue perfusion and tissue hypoxia. Decreased perfusion to the brain results in cerebral hypoxia and symptoms related to altered cerebral tissue perfusion. Second, it causes severe hypotension, which is responsible for decreased renal perfusion and may eventually result in acute renal failure. Circulatory failure is fatal if an adequate CO is not reestablished in a timely manner.

SECTION THREE REVIEW

1. When an insulin deficiency exists, the liver responds by converting
   A. fatty acids to glucose
   B. glycogen to glucose
   C. glucagon to glucose
   D. amino acids to glucose
2. Insulin-dependent cells use which of the following nutritional substances FIRST when insulin is not available?
   A. fatty acids
   B. glycogen
   C. glucagon
   D. amino acids
3. Insulin deficit alters fat metabolism by
   A. increasing lipogenesis
   B. synthesizing triglycerides
   C. increasing lipolysis
   D. synthesizing glycerol
4. When acetoacetic acid converts to acetone and β-hydroxybutyric acid, ______ is/are formed.
   A. amino acids
   B. acetyl-coA
   C. glycerol
   D. ketone bodies
5. Protein catabolism is evidenced by
   A. muscle wasting
   B. hyperexcitability
   C. decreased urine urea nitrogen
   D. increased triglyceride levels

Answers: 1. B, 2. A, 3. C, 4. D, 5. A

SECTION FOUR: Types of Diabetes Mellitus

At the completion of this section, the learner will be able to differentiate the two major types of diabetes mellitus.

Diabetes mellitus (diabetes) is a complex metabolic disorder in which an individual has either an absolute or relative insulin deficit. It is divided into two major types: type 1 and type 2 diabetes.

Type 1 Diabetes Mellitus

Type 1 diabetes mellitus occurs when there is an absolute lack of endogenous insulin caused by autoimmune beta cell destruction. It can develop at any age but most commonly occurs before the age of 30. The human leukocyte antigen (HLA) genotype, HLA DR-3 or DR-4, is strongly associated with the occurrence of type 1 diabetes mellitus. Viral and chemical agents are also proposed to be triggers for the development of type 1 diabetes mellitus. Regardless of the triggering event, it is believed that an autoimmune reaction destroys the beta cells of the pancreas (American Diabetes Association, 2008).

Type 2 Diabetes Mellitus

Approximately 90 percent of individuals in the United States with diabetes have type 2 diabetes mellitus. Type 2 diabetes mellitus is usually diagnosed after the age of 30 years but is becoming more prevalent in children and adolescents. It is associated with a relative insulin deficiency (less insulin secretion) or insulin resistance rather than a total deficit. The major etiology of type 2 diabetes is progressive pancreatic dysfunction secondary to **hyalinization** of the islets of Langerhans. Over the course of the disease, both the pancreas and the liver develop fatty deposits as a result of high serum lipid levels. They also undergo tissue atrophy, associated with a decrease in size and number of functioning pancreatic and liver cells. Obesity in the presence of hereditary tendencies is considered a major risk factor for development of type 2 diabetes mellitus. Table 34–2 presents a comparison of type 1 and type 2 diabetes mellitus.

Diabetic Crises

Diabetes mellitus is associated with multisystem clinical manifestations. Three acute complications may occur with diabetes: diabetic ketoacidosis (DKA), hyperglycemic hyperosmolar state (HHS), and therapy-induced hypoglycemic coma. DKA and HHS are produced by hyperglycemia, an abnormally high blood glucose level. In contrast, hypoglycemic coma is produced by an abnormally low blood glucose level. Many patients with diabetes are admitted to the hospital for a diagnosis other than their chronic diabetic state; however, the physiologic stress caused by the acute problem may precipitate a diabetic crisis, which further complicates the patient's prognosis.

The Focused History

When a diabetic crisis is suspected, a focused nursing history should be obtained immediately and should include

- Preexisting history of type 1 or type 2 diabetes
- Self-maintenance activities
- Special diet, including adherence with diet
- Insulin or oral antidiabetes agents (type, dosage, adherence to regimen)
- Glucose testing history (blood glucose monitoring, urine testing)
- Exercise and weight loss
- Usual pattern of glucose control (stable versus occasional-to-frequent loss of glucose control)
- Possible precipitating factors (e.g., infection, presence of other physiologic or psychologic stressors, failure to follow diet or drug therapy)
- Preexisting neurologic or vascular complications of diabetes (e.g., decreased kidney function, peripheral or cardiovascular disease)
- Unexplained weight loss of 10 percent or greater.

After the history is obtained, the most appropriate course of action can be determined.

TABLE 34–2 Comparison of the Two Types of Diabetes Mellitus

CHARACTERISTIC	TYPE 1	TYPE 2
Usual age of onset	Younger than 30 years of age	Older than 30 years of age
Rate of onset	Rapid	Slow
Weight status	Not associated with obesity	Commonly associated with obesity
Insulin secretion (beta cell status)	Total loss of beta cells within one year of diagnosis; no insulin secretion	Decrease in size and number of beta cells; decreased insulin secretion
Glucagon secretion (alpha cell status)	Abnormal alpha cell function, but relative excess of glucagon in relation to insulin	Decrease in size and number of alpha cells; glucagon and insulin secretion decreased but often balanced
Ketone status	Ketone prone; high risk for ketoacidosis	Not ketone prone unless under stress; low risk for ketoacidosis
Insulin resistance	Usually only present with elevated glucose levels	Usually present
Insulin supplement status	Insulin dependent	Usually not insulin dependent
Diabetic crises associated with disorder(s)	Diabetic ketoacidosis (DKA); hypoglycemic coma	Hyperglycemic hyperosmolar state (HHS); hypoglycemic coma

SECTION FOUR REVIEW

1. The etiology of type 1 diabetes is believed to be
   - A. obesity
   - B. an autoimmune reaction
   - C. a bacterial infection
   - D. general pancreatic dysfunction
2. By one year after diagnosis of type 1 diabetes, there is ______ percent of functioning beta cells remaining in the pancreas.
   - A. 0
   - B. 10
   - C. 30
   - D. 50
3. Type 2 diabetes is associated with which of the following major risk factors?
   - A. smoking
   - B. viral infection
   - C. obesity
   - D. autoimmune reaction
4. In what way is pancreatic function altered in the patient with type 2 diabetes?
   - A. beta cells become hyalinized
   - B. beta cells become overactive
   - C. alpha cell activity predominates
   - D. alpha cells break down insulin
5. Which of the following statements is TRUE regarding type 2 diabetes mellitus?
   - A. It is less common.
   - B. It has a slower rate of onset.
   - C. It usually occurs at a younger age.
   - D. It is more commonly associated with ketones.

Answers: 1. B, 2. A, 3. C, 4. A, 5. B

SECTION FIVE: Hypoglycemic Coma

At the completion of this section, the learner will be able to discuss the therapy induced diabetic complication, hypoglycemic coma.

Hypoglycemia (abnormally low blood glucose level) is the most common diabetic complication. It may occur with any type of diabetes. Other risk factors include being a female and older age (Smeeks, 2008). Hypoglycemia is triggered by imbalances among exercise, diet, and medication. Onset of symptoms is usually rapid, and, if prolonged, seizures, coma and death may result.

Precipitating Factors

Common precipitating conditions for development of hypoglycemia include

- Excessive administration of insulin or oral antidiabetes agents
  - Patients receiving oral antidiabetes agents (e.g., sulfonylureas) are at highest risk for severe and prolonged symptoms of hypoglycemia because of the extended half-life of these agents
- Consumption of too little food
- High activity levels
- Recent surgery
- Medication related
  - A change in medications
  - Certain medications/drugs (e.g., propranolol) and alcohol, which potentiate the effects of the pharmacologic regimen
- Hormonal changes related to other endocrine disorders
- Renal or hepatic disease
- Stress of any kind

Clinical Presentation

Hypoglycemia occurs from a relative excess of insulin in the blood and results in excessively low blood glucose levels. Hypoglycemia can be defined clinically as a blood glucose level of less than 70 mg/dL or 3.9 mmol/L. The point when hypoglycemic symptoms occur is variable between patients (American Diabetes Association, 2008). Some patients may develop symptoms of hypoglycemia even with a serum glucose of greater than 70 mg/dL, or if the drop in glucose is very rapid. Hypoglycemia becomes symptomatic when there is insufficient glucose available to meet the energy needs of the central nervous system (CNS). A patient's clinical presentation is primarily related to CNS and catecholamine effects.

Central Nervous System Effects

The CNS depends on available glucose for its energy source and is sensitive to insufficient levels of glucose. CNS effects reflect the inability of brain cells to function normally without an adequate energy source. Progressive symptoms include

- Decreased ability to reason and remember (slowed thinking)
- Changing mental status
- Emotional lability
- Headache, dizziness
- Thickened, slurred speech
- Loss of coordination
- Loss of proprioception
- Numbness
- Drowsiness
- Convulsions
- Coma

Catecholamine Effects

The lack of circulating glucose triggers the secretion of stress hormones, subsequently causing production of glucose from alternate body sources, such as hepatic gluconeogenesis. The presence of increased levels of the hormone epinephrine, a catecholamine, triggers a sympathetic response. This stress response accounts for many of the symptoms of hypoglycemia such as

- Anxiety
- Tremors, nervousness
- Cold, clammy skin

- Tachycardia, palpitations
- Hyperventilation
- Tingling in extremities
- Nausea and vomiting
- Hunger
- Diaphoresis

Other Determinants of Hypoglycemic Symptoms

The rate of onset and the patient's age influence the type of symptoms that predominate.

Rapid Onset. When the onset of hypoglycemia is rapid, sympathetic nervous system symptoms often predominate. A significant, rapid drop of blood glucose level stimulates the sympathetic nervous system, which initiates secretion of epinephrine. Epinephrine causes gluconeogenesis in the liver, thereby increasing the serum glucose level. Concurrently, growth hormone and cortisol are secreted to assist in increasing glucose levels by decreasing glucose use by the cells.

Slow Onset. When the onset of hypoglycemia is slow, the symptoms of CNS dysfunction may predominate. Over a period of time, the body is able to adapt to a slow decline in blood glucose. Brain cells are not insulin dependent and take in glucose directly. Central nervous system symptoms, therefore, are caused by lack of available glucose, rather than an insulin deficit. The brain is a high-energy tissue, requiring large amounts of glucose to maintain normal functioning. Without glucose, particularly over a prolonged period, the brain can sustain permanent damage that may be either minor or severe (irreversible coma).

The Influence of Age

The age of the patient has an impact on the clinical presentation of hypoglycemia. Elderly patients tend to have more severe symptoms and may become symptomatic at higher serum glucose levels. CNS symptoms, particularly those relating to altered levels of consciousness, may be misdiagnosed in chronically ill elderly if the onset is very slow. In the elderly, the hypoglycemic symptoms may be masked as worsening dementia.

Medical Interventions

The major goal of interventions is rapid restoration of normal serum glucose levels, which includes treating the underlying cause. The specific type of intervention is based partially on the patient's level of consciousness.

The Conscious Hypoglycemic Patient

Reversal of hypoglycemia in the conscious patient is relatively simple to accomplish. Patients with blood glucose levels less than 70 mg/dL should eat or drink 10 to 15 g of glucose- or carbohydrate-containing foods or beverages. If blood glucose levels are less than 50 mg/dL, 20 to 30 g of glucose or carbohydrate may be needed. Blood glucose levels should be tested 15 to 20 minutes after initiating treatment. If the blood glucose levels remain low, the treatment should be repeated (Manchester & Tracy, 2009)

The Unconscious Hypoglycemic Patient

If a hospitalized adult patient with diabetes becomes hypoglycemic, exhibiting confusion or coma, the following regimen is suggested (American Diabetes Association, 2008; Smeeks, 2008)

1. Evaluate ABCs (airway, breathing, and circulation); initiate intravenous access if not present.
2. Obtain a STAT capillary glucose level prior to initiating therapy. In the absence of equipment to check capillary blood glucose, glucose administration should not be delayed until a blood sample is available, delay in treating severe hypoglycemia may be detrimental to patient outcomes.
3. Administer a 50 mL intravenous (IV) bolus of 50 percent glucose.
4. If 50 percent glucose is not available, administer glucagon 1 mg subcutaneous (SQ), intramuscular (IM), or intravenous (IV).
5. Follow the glucose bolus with a continuous IV glucose infusion (5 to 10 percent) to maintain the plasma glucose at a level greater than 100 mg/dL.

While glucose is the major therapy for treating hypoglycemia, there are several other medications that may be considered, including glucagon and diazoxide. The RELATED PHARMACOTHERAPY box: Agents Used for Treatment of Hypoglycemia, provides a summary of these pharmacologic agents.

RELATED PHARMACOTHERAPY: Agents Used for Treatment of Hypoglycemia

Dextrose

Glucose-D

Action and Uses

When delivered orally, dextrose is rapidly absorbed in the intestine and is taken up and used by tissues. Delivered intravenously, it causes rapid increase in serum glucose levels and provides relief of hypoglycemic states. Dextrose can be used for providing energy and is the primary therapy for treatment of hypoglycemia.

Major Adverse Effects

Hyperglycemia

Nursing Implications

Obtain an initial capillary blood glucose level when possible but do not delay administration if blood glucose cannot be immediately drawn.

Acute treatment of hypoglycemia in an adult is 50 mL of dextrose 50 percent given as an IV bolus on confirmation of hypoglycemia.

Prolonged management in an adult is glucose 10 percent in water delivered via a central line to avoid peripheral vein injury.

Monitor for reversal of hypoglycemia manifestations.

Monitor capillary blood glucose via bedside glucometer.

(*continued*)

RELATED PHARMACOTHERAPY (*continued*)

Glucagon
Glucagen

Action and Uses
A naturally occurring hormone produced by the alpha cells of the pancreas. It increases production of glucose by the liver and relaxes the muscles of the GI tract; used as alternative treatment of hypoglycemia when glucose cannot be administered intravenously.

Major Adverse Effects
Nausea and vomiting
Hypersensitivity reaction

Nursing Implications
Usual dose in an adult is 1 to 2 mg; can be administered subcutaneously, IM, or IV.
Assess for nausea and vomiting during therapy.
Monitor glucose levels via bedside glucometer during and several hours posttreatment.
Monitor for reversal of hypoglycemia manifestations.

Diazoxide
Proglycem

Action and Uses
Diazoxide is primarily an antihypertensive agent. In addition, it suppresses release of insulin; enhances glucose output by the liver while decreasing glucose uptake by cells; may be considered in cases of overdose of oral hypoglycemic agents or rare cases of insulinoma. For treatment of hypoglycemia, it is administered orally.

Major Adverse Effects
Hypotension (IV administration); tachycardia
Fluid and sodium retention possible due to antidiuretic actions; heart failure in patients with cardiac disease
Hyperglycemia (can be markedly high due to overdose)

Nursing Implications
Hyperglycemic effects usually begin within one hour of IV administration and duration is about eight hours.
Monitor for relief of manifestations of hypoglycemia.
Closely monitor blood glucose levels and for manifestations of hyperglycemia. Insulin administration may be required.

SECTION FIVE REVIEW

1. Which of the following statements is TRUE regarding hypoglycemia?
   A. It is defined only in terms of blood glucose levels.
   B. It is defined only in terms of clinical presentation.
   C. It becomes symptomatic only when excessive insulin is present.
   D. It becomes symptomatic at different blood glucose levels.
2. Conditions that increase the risk of hypoglycemia include
   A. dietary fasting
   B. high-fat diet
   C. little exercise
   D. too little insulin
3. Of the following, the clinical presentation of hypoglycemia partially reflects
   A. lack of glucose within the cells
   B. excessive glucose within the cells
   C. stimulation of parasympathetic nervous system
   D. excessive circulating insulin
4. A patient experiencing rapid onset hypoglycemia is most likely to have predominantly ______ symptoms.
   A. cell dysfunction
   B. gastrointestinal
   C. stimulated sympathetic nervous system
   D. stimulated parasympathetic nervous system
5. Central nervous system symptoms associated with hypoglycemia are caused by lack of ______ rather than insulin deficit.
   A. glucose
   B. amino acids
   C. fatty acids
   D. glucagon
6. In the unconscious hypoglycemic patient with a venous access, the treatment of choice is
   A. 50 percent glucose (IV)
   B. 0.5 to 2 mg glucagon (IM)
   C. 10 percent dextrose and water (IV)
   D. 8 ounces of orange juice (orally)

Answers: 1. D, 2. A, 3. A, 4. C, 5. A, 6. A

SECTION SIX: Diabetic Ketoacidosis

At the completion of this section, the learner will be able to describe the diabetic complication, diabetic ketoacidosis.

Diabetic ketoacidosis (DKA) results from an absolute or relative deficiency in insulin. It is a potentially severe, sometimes life-threatening complication characterized by ketosis, acidosis, hyperglycemia, dehydration, and electrolyte imbalances.

Focused Assessment

A rapid assessment of the severity and state of compensation of DKA helps establish management priorities. The signs and symptoms of DKA are multisystemic in nature; thus, a systematic assessment is necessary. Not every patient exhibits all the clinical manifestations of DKA, and confirmation is made by evaluation of appropriate laboratory tests. Table 34–3 summarizes the

TABLE 34–3 Cardinal Characteristics and Specific Signs and Symptoms of Diabetic Ketoacidosis

CHARACTERISTICS	SPECIFIC SIGNS AND SYMPTOMS
Hyperglycemia	Elevated serum glucose (greater than 250 mg/dL) Elevated urine glucose
Metabolic acidosis	Elevated serum and urine ketones Acidotic serum pH (less than 7.30) Acidotic serum HCO_3 (less than 15 mEq/L) Positive high anion gap (greater than 17 mEq/L) Alkalotic serum Pco_2 (less than 35 mm Hg) Elevated respiratory rate and depth (Kussmaul breathing) Fruity odor to breath
Osmotic diuresis	Polyuria Polydipsia Dehydration Hypotension Hemoconcentration Electrolyte abnormalities Azotemia (elevated BUN and creatinine) Elevated serum osmolality (but less than 350 mg/dL)
Compensation	Decreased urine output Increased serum sodium levels Increased blood pressure, pulse, respirations Peripheral vasoconstriction

cardinal signs and their specific associated signs and symptoms. A brief description of the pathophysiologic basis of the cardinal signs of diabetic ketoacidosis follows.

Pathophysiologic Basis of DKA Symptomatology

Hyperglycemia

The origin of **hyperglycemia** is an absolute or relative deficit in insulin, which causes the inability of glucose to move into cells, thus increasing serum glucose levels. Fat from adipose tissue is converted into free fatty acids (FFAs). The FFAs, in turn, are converted to glucose by gluconeogenesis in the liver. The liver also causes glycogenolysis, which converts glycogen to glucose. All these factors contribute to worsening hyperglycemia.

Metabolic Acidosis

Free fatty acids are broken down by the CNS into ketone bodies for energy faster than they can be converted to glucose. Because of the lack of insulin, muscle cells cannot oxidize the ketone bodies sufficiently, causing a buildup of ketone bodies. Increased levels of circulating ketone bodies decreases the pH, and as the pH falls below 7.20, the respiratory center is stimulated to excrete carbonic acid via the lungs in the form of carbon dioxide and water (Kussmaul breathing). Acetone, which is contained in ketone bodies, is excreted through the lungs (ketone breath) and the kidneys (ketonuria). Bicarbonate reserves become overwhelmed and then exhausted by the severity and prolonged state of the acidosis, which causes a drop in serum bicarbonate levels.

Osmotic Diuresis

Elevated serum glucose levels increase intravascular osmotic pressure. The increased pressure draws extravascular fluids into the intravascular compartment. As the levels of glucose and intravascular volume increase, the kidneys respond by dramatically increasing excretion of glucose and urine. This is associated with increased loss of electrolytes, hemoconcentration, and increasing dehydration. Gastrointestinal symptoms associated with DKA may be related to abnormally low electrolyte levels.

Compensatory Mechanisms

The renin–angiotensin–aldosterone system is activated to increase sodium and water reabsorption. Antidiuretic hormone (ADH) is secreted by the posterior pituitary to cause retention of water and sodium. Urine output also is controlled by compensatory vasoconstriction, which limits renal blood flow. The autonomic nervous system is stimulated to secrete catecholamines and glucocorticoids, which results in vasoconstriction; thus increasing the blood pressure and decreasing urine output. Blood pressure, pulse, and respirations are all increased as a result.

Decompensation

The patient with severe DKA can eventually develop failure of compensatory mechanisms. Decompensation represents exhaustion of compensatory mechanisms, which rapidly leads to cardiovascular collapse. The level of consciousness deteriorates and blood pressure and pulse can no longer maintain adequate organ perfusion. The supply of catecholamines becomes exhausted, causing loss of the body's ability to maintain peripheral vasoconstriction. Urine output decreases and ceases as hypoperfusion to the kidneys causes them to fail.

Anion Gap

DKA is only one cause of metabolic acidosis. Measuring **anion gap** is one way to help isolate DKA from some other acidotic conditions. Gaining a basic understanding of the concept of anion gap may facilitate early diagnosis and treatment of DKA.

Metabolic acidosis exists either as normal anion gap acidosis (from loss of bicarbonate ions) or as high anion gap acidosis (from an accumulation of fixed acids in the serum).

Anions are negatively charged particles (e.g., CO_2^-, HCO_3^-, and Cl^-). They are the opposite of cations, or positively charged particles (e.g., Na^+ and K^+). Normally, cations and anions are in balance with each other. Anion gap represents the level of unmeasurable anion excess that exists in the body. Measurement of the anion gap is helpful in differentiating the type of metabolic acidosis present. It is expressed as

$$\text{Anion gap} = (Na^+ + K^+) - (Cl^- + HCO_3^-)$$

Anion gap has a normal range of 10 to 17 mEq/L (Kee, 2005). This normal range is a function of such unmeasured serum anions as phosphates, sulfates, ketones, and lactic acid.

High Anion Gap Acidosis

An anion gap of greater than 17 mEq/L indicates an accumulation of these unmeasured anions and warrants immediate attention.

When metabolic acidosis is caused by elevations in organic acids, the anion gap increases. States such as starvation, lactic acidosis, and DKA cause a high anion gap.

Normal Anion Gap Acidosis

When metabolic acidosis is caused by a loss of bicarbonate (buffer) anions, the anion gap remains normal. This occurs in such states as high chloride intake, renal failure, and diarrhea.

A person admitted with a potential or actual DKA may have an anion gap determination performed. Although anion gap alone is inconclusive for DKA, it is used as adjunctive data in clustering critical cues for differential diagnosis.

Causes of Diabetic Ketoacidosis

DKA is caused by extreme insulin deficiency. Infection is the primary precipitating factor for development of DKA. Illness and infection increase the production of glucocorticoids by the adrenal gland supporting the production of new glucose by the liver (gluconeogenesis). Epinephrine and norepinephrine levels are also increased causing further breakdown of glycogen into glucose (glycogenolysis). Diabetic ketoacidosis is seen most commonly in type 1 diabetics.

Any condition or situation that increases the insulin deficit can precipitate DKA, for example, infection, stroke, myocardial infarction, trauma, alcohol abuse, and drugs. In addition, new-onset type 1 diabetes and omission of exogenous insulin in diagnosed type 1 individuals commonly leads to DKA. In about 20 percent of cases, no specific precipitating event is found.

Stress as a Major Precipitating Factor

An increased level of stress causes further production of stress hormones (e.g., epinephrine, growth hormone, and cortisol). As discussed in Section One, when secreted, these hormones increase blood glucose levels by either increasing conversion of glycogen to glucose or decreasing cellular use of glucose. When the stress is severe, as in a severe acute infection or illness, the increase in glucose can be substantial, precipitating an imbalance in the glucose/insulin relationship.

Severe infection with systemic involvement is typically accompanied by hyperthermia (fever). Hyperthermia increases the metabolic rate, thus greatly increasing cellular need for insulin. Therefore, in the presence of infection, there is both an increased supply and an increased demand for glucose. In such a situation, it would seem that a balance in glucose would exist. This is not the case, however, with type 1 diabetes. A balance can be maintained or regained only when sufficient insulin is present to meet the increased glucose needs of the cells. DKA is precipitated by a relative insulin deficiency in this situation. If insulin dosage is not increased in response, there is insufficient insulin to meet the increased glucose supply as well as the increased metabolic demand.

A similar situation can occur with a patient with type 2 diabetes whose condition normally is controlled by diet, antidiabetes agents, or both. In situations of high stress (infection, trauma, surgery), the level of insulin secretion in the pancreas often is insufficient to meet the increased supply of and demand for glucose; thus, this type of patient clinically develops hyperglycemia, which often requires temporary exogenous insulin therapy. Sliding scale insulin is then administered until the level of physiologic stress is sufficiently reduced and balance is regained between the glucose level and the endogenous insulin supply.

Emerging Evidence

- In patients with diabetes, episodes of severe hypoglycemia (ranging between 58 percent and 73 percent) followed a predictable "signature" pattern of blood glucose fluctuations during the 24 hour period preceding the hypoglycemic episode. The predictability increased with the minimum number of self-monitored blood glucose (SMBG) readings that were obtained (ranging from three to five readings over a 24-hour period). The study used an imminent risk algorithm computing relative changes in the low blood glucose index (LBGI) *(Cox, Gonder, Ritterband et al., 2007)*.
- In adult patients with uncontrolled diabetes, a ß-hydroxybutyrate (betaOHB), of greater than 3.8 mmol/L, can be used for diagnosis of DKA and may be superior as an indicator of DKA when compared to the nonspecific serum HCO_3 levels *(Sheikh-Ali, Karon, Basu et al., 2008)*.
- There was an overall decrease in death rate trends in adult patients with hyperglycemic crises (DKA or HHS) in the United States between 1985 through 2002. The greatest age-related decrease occurred in the older than 62 age group. The smallest race-related decreased occurred in black men *(Wang, Williams, Naravan, & Geiss, 2006)*.

Management of Diabetic Ketoacidosis

The DKA-related treatment goals include

- Correcting fluid and electrolyte imbalances
- Slowly decreasing serum glucose
- Correcting acidosis
- Preventing further complications
- Providing patient education (American Diabetes Association, 2008).

Nursing interventions are based on activities that help the patient meet expected outcomes. They consist of collaborative interventions: (1) activities ordered by the physician or advanced nurse practitioner that require some actions by the nurse and (2) activities that are within the nursing scope of practice (independent nursing orders).

Collaborative Interventions

The American Diabetes Association (2004) has established guidelines for the management of diabetic ketoacidosis; ADA protocol for management of adult patients with DKA is presented in Figure 34–3. These guidelines include:

1. **IV therapy.** The patient's initial management requires rapid rehydration. Osmotic diuresis precipitated by elevated glucose levels severely depletes body fluids. Initial fluid replacement will be with one-half normal (0.45 percent) or normal (0.9 percent) saline. As soon as the serum glucose level is decreased to approximately 250 mg/dL, dextrose (5 percent) may be added to the intravenous fluids. The patient will receive nothing by mouth until the crisis state is resolved.

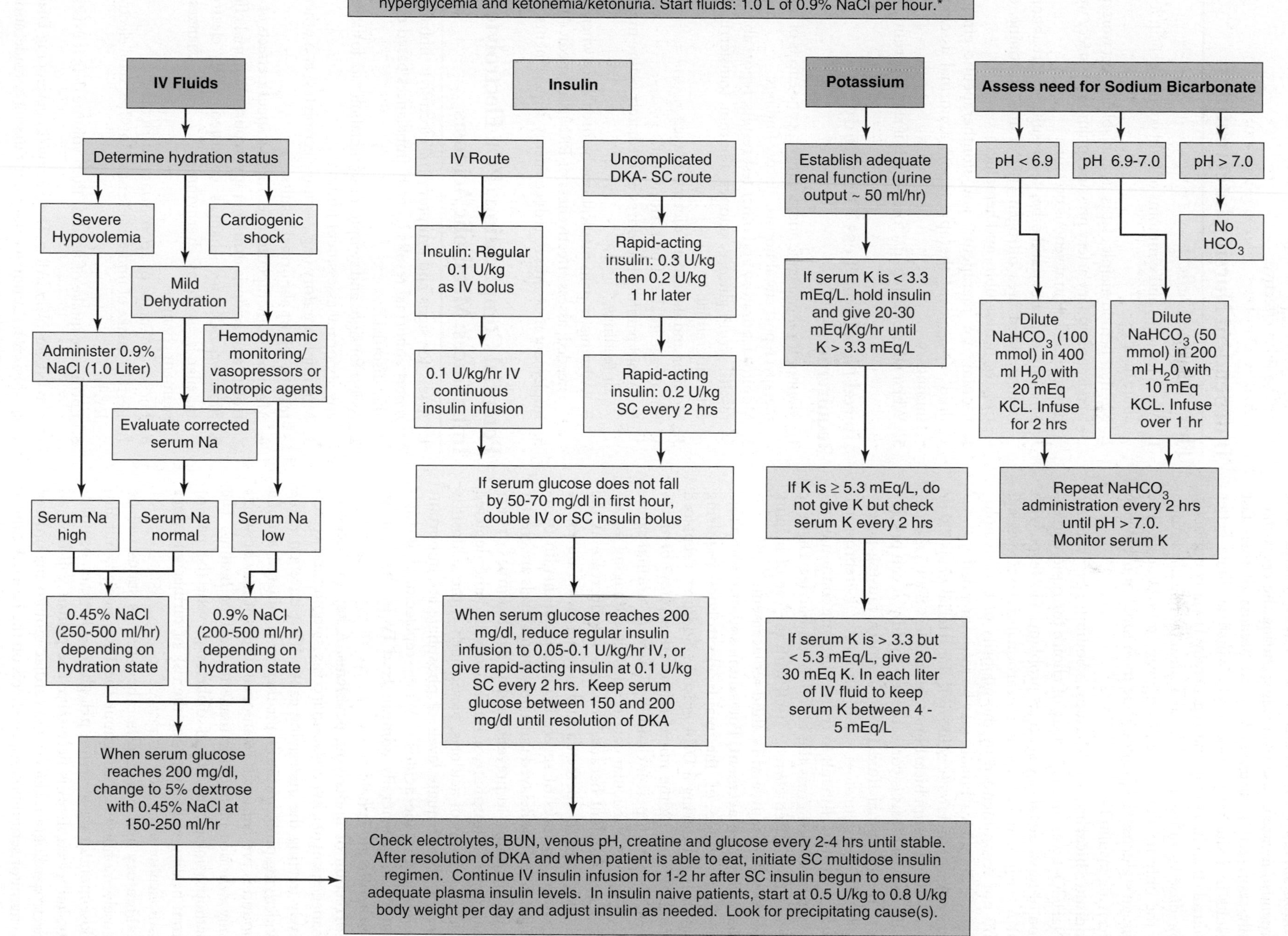

Figure 34–3 ■ ADA Protocol for Management of adult patients with DKA. From American Diabetes Association (ADA). (2006). Protocol for Management of Adult Patient with HHS. Consensus statement: Hyperglycemic crises in adult patients with diabetes.

2. **Insulin therapy.** Correction of the hyperglycemic state depends on careful use of insulin. During the crisis state, only short-acting insulins are used because of their fast results in reducing glucose levels, which facilitate better control. Insulin management generally is via continuous, low-dose IV infusion with regular insulin. Regular insulin is the only insulin that can be given intravenously. The patient's glucose levels should be monitored hourly while receiving insulin IV.
3. **Sodium bicarbonate therapy.** Sodium bicarbonate ($NaHCO_3$) was once the drug of choice for rapid correction of most metabolic acidosis problems. However, with DKA, treatment with sodium bicarbonate is controversial and not recommended by the majority of endocrinologists. Sodium bicarbonate may be recommended with severe cases of metabolic acidosis if the arterial pH is 7.0 or less or if the serum bicarbonate level is less than 5 mEq/L. When ketoacidosis is corrected too rapidly, it can precipitate cerebrospinal fluid (CSF) acidosis, causing potentially severe neurologic complications. Cerebrospinal fluid acidosis is difficult to correct because sodium bicarbonate does not cross the blood–brain barrier. Diabetic ketoacidosis often corrects itself with the use of insulin, electrolyte therapy, and IV fluid replacement.
4. **Electrolyte replacement.** Potassium, sodium, and phosphate are three of the major electrolytes requiring replacement during a DKA episode. Sodium is replaced primarily during the initial rehydration phase of treatment using 0.9 percent and 0.45 percent normal saline IV solutions. Particular care is taken in managing potassium replacement because serum levels decrease as the acidotic state is corrected and normal urine output is regained. In cases of severe hypokalemia, insulin treatment should be delayed until potassium levels are greater than 3.3 mEq/L to prevent cardiac dysrhythmias or cardiac arrest. Phosphate, a buffer, may become depleted during periods of acidosis, particularly if the acidosis is prolonged. Adequate levels of phosphate are important in managing the acidosis. When replacement is warranted, it is generally administered IV in the form of potassium phosphate.
5. **Correction of underlying problems.** A key to successful management of a hyperglycemic crisis is finding and aggressively treating the underlying cause. If an infection is the underlying problem, antibiotic therapy is initiated, and if a wound is present (such as an open ulcer), it may be surgically debrided of necrotic tissue to facilitate healing. The pathophysiologic effects of diabetes prevent the patient from healing well, increasing the risk of further infectious complications.
6. **Laboratory and other tests.** The patient's status will be closely monitored throughout the DKA period. Initially, close monitoring of serum pH, glucose, ketones, osmolality, and electrolytes is necessary. The patient will have an electrocardiogram (ECG) and cardiac monitoring ordered to monitor serum potassium effects on the heart. A culture and gram stain of potentially infected secretions or fluids confirm the type of organism so that IV antibiotic therapy can be most effective.

Independent Nursing Interventions

Fluid Volume Deficit

1. Assess for signs and symptoms of fluid volume deficit; report abnormalities.
2. Monitor hemodynamic status, as available; report worsening trends: pulmonary artery pressure, pulmonary artery wedge pressure, and central venous pressure.
3. Monitor laboratory and other test results; report abnormal results: blood urea nitrogen (BUN) and creatinine, electrolytes, hemoglobin, and hematocrit.
4. Monitor for therapeutic and nontherapeutic effects of fluid replacement therapy; report abnormal assessment findings.
5. When taking oral fluids, force fluids if status permits.

Altered Nutrition: Less Than Body Requirements

1. Monitor for therapeutic and nontherapeutic effects of insulin therapy; report any abnormal glucose findings.
2. Monitor laboratory and other test results; report abnormal results: serum glucose, ketones, albumin, transferrin, CBC with differential.
3. Monitor and document dietary intake.
4. Encourage intake of prescribed diet.
   A. Avoid painful procedures immediately before meals or feedings.
   B. Administer pain medications before meals, when needed; assess effectiveness of PRN pain medications.
5. Implement measures to reduce energy requirements.

Potential Complication (PC): Electrolyte Imbalances: Metabolic Acidosis

1. Assess for signs and symptoms of electrolyte imbalances; report abnormal results (specify imbalances based on specific disorder).
2. Assess for signs and symptoms of metabolic acidosis; report any abnormal assessment findings.
3. Monitor laboratory (e.g., serum electrolytes) and other test results; report abnormal results.
4. Monitor for therapeutic and nontherapeutic effects of electrolyte and acidosis drug therapy; report abnormal effects.
5. Monitor ECG for changes consistent with electrolyte imbalance, such as dysrhythmias, *T* wave changes, *ST* segment changes.
6. Encourage intake of appropriate nutrients.
7. Restrict intake of undesirable nutrients based on electrolyte levels.
8. Encourage intake of fluids if fluid volume deficit exists.

Refer to NURSING CARE: The Patient Experiencing Diabetic Ketoacidosis for a summary of major nursing considerations of patients during the acute phase of DKA.

NURSING CARE: The Patient Experiencing Diabetic Ketoacidosis

Expected Patient Outcomes and Related Interventions*

Outcome 1: Regains normovolemic state

Assess and compare to established norms, patient baseline, and trends.

Arterial blood pressure, heart rate, and rhythm
Hemodynamic status (as available) – cardiac output/cardiac index, CVP, PAP, PAWP
Urine output, intake to output ratio, BUN, and creatinine
Jugular vein status (flat or collapsed)

Interventions to replace fluids

Insert large bore intravenous catheter; central line may be indicated.
Initiate fluid resuscitation with 0.9 percent NaCl based on degree of hypovolemia (see Fig. 34–3, "IV Fluids," in *Protocol for management of adult patients with DKA*).
Urine output should be maintained at greater than 50 mL/hr.

Administer related drug therapy and monitor for therapeutic and nontherapeutic effects.

Possible vasopressor therapy for severe hypovolemia

Related nursing diagnoses

Decreased cardiac output
Fluid volume deficit

Outcome 2: Normalization of glucose and ketones

Assess and compare to established norms, patient baseline, and trends.

Monitor hyperglycemia and ketonemia/ketonuria
Capillary glucose, serum/urine ketones
ABG (monitor pH), anion gap
Kussmaul respirations (elevated rate and depth of breathing)

Interventions to normalize glucose and ketones

Initiate insulin therapy (intravenous route) [uncomplicated DKA may be treated with subcutaneous insulin].

Administer related drug therapy and monitor for therapeutic and nontherapeutic effects.

Insulin therapy (see Fig. 34–3, "Insulin," in *Protocol for management of adult patients with DKA*)

Related nursing diagnoses

Altered nutrition: less than body requirements
Potential complication (PC): ketosis, metabolic acidosis

Outcome 3: Stabilization of electrolytes

Assess and compare to established norms, patient baseline, and trends.

Monitor serum potassium and bicarbonate levels.
Serum electrolytes (focus on potassium and bicarbonate trends)
ABG (monitor pH and bicarbonate)

Interventions to regain electrolyte stability

See Fig. 34–3, "Potassium" and "Assess need for Sodium bicarbonate," in *Protocol for management of adult patients with DKA*).

Administer related drug therapy and monitor for therapeutic and nontherapeutic effects.

Possible potassium replacement
Possible Bicarbonate replacement

Related nursing diagnoses

Potential complication (PC): electrolyte imbalances, metabolic acidosis

Outcome 4: Prevention of future DKA episodes

Assess and compare to established norms, patient baseline, and trends.

Identify etiology of current DKA episode (often infectious process).
Identify learning needs of patient and family regarding diabetes, DKA, and prevention of future occurrences.

Interventions to prevent DKA episodes

Provide diabetes and DKA teaching, based on assessed knowledge deficits.

Related nursing diagnoses

Knowledge deficit

* Note: It is crucial to rapidly identify and treat the underlying cause of DKA to improve patient outcomes.

SECTION SIX REVIEW

1. Which of the following set of laboratory results best reflects diabetic ketoacidosis?
   - **A.** pH 7.28, HCO_3 34 mEq/L, blood glucose 70 mg/dL
   - **B.** pH 7.18, HCO_3 13 mEq/L, blood glucose 100 mg/dL
   - **C.** pH 7.26, HCO_3 14 mEq/L, blood glucose 450 mg/dL
   - **D.** pH 7.38, HCO_3 24 mEq/L, blood glucose 620 mg/dL

2. Typical clinical manifestations of diabetic ketoacidosis include
   - **A.** absence of ketonuria
   - **B.** fluid overload
   - **C.** electrolytes within normal range
   - **D.** progressive dehydration

(*continued*)

(continued)

3. Ketosis results from mobilization of
   A. amino acids
   B. glucagon
   C. glucose
   D. fatty acids
4. A high anion gap acidosis is consistent with which of the following problems?
   A. diarrhea
   B. high intake of chloride
   C. starvation
   D. high intake of sodium
5. A common precipitating factor for development of diabetic ketoacidosis is
   A. a stress-free lifestyle
   B. decreased exercise
   C. infection
   D. food/insulin balance

Answers: 1. C, 2. D, 3. D, 4. C, 5. C

SECTION SEVEN: Hyperglycemic Hyperosmolar State

At the completion of this section, the learner will be able to discuss the diabetic complication, hyperglycemic hyperosmolar state.

Hyperglycemic hyperosmolar state (HHS) is a hyperglycemic complication of diabetes mellitus that results from insulin deficiency or insulin resistance. It is sometimes overlooked and primarily occurs in elderly patients, particularly the sick elderly, with type 2 diabetes. HHS has a higher mortality rate than DKA because of its severe metabolic derangements and the delay in diagnosis. The major precipitating factor for development of HHS is infection. Other precipitating factors include severe diarrhea, severe burns, peritoneal dialysis, myocardial infarction, thiazide usage, and hypertonic feedings.

Pathophysiologic Basis of HHS

The patient with type 2 diabetes produces moderate levels of insulin. In the presence of a precipitating event, the relative lack of insulin in these patients can trigger hyperglycemia by way of acceleration of hepatic gluconeogenesis and decreased peripheral glucose utilization. The result of these events is extreme hyperglycemia (may be in excess of 2,000 mg/dL) while avoiding significant ketoacidosis. Failure to develop significant ketoacidosis is attributed to the production of sufficient insulin to prevent or minimize lipolysis and ketogenesis.

The excess glucose accumulates in the extracellular spaces because it cannot be transported into the cells or metabolized normally, resulting in a progressive increase in osmolality. As extracellular osmolality increases, water is pulled from the intracellular spaces into the extracellular spaces. As the level of hyperglycemia increases and exceeds the renal threshold, osmotic diuresis significantly increases, precipitating progressive dehydration of intracellular and extracellular spaces. Severe dehydration of the intracellular and extracellular spaces results in hyperosmolar coma if the serum osmolality increases to 320 mOsm/L or higher.

Clinical Presentation

DKA and HHS have many similarities; both are associated with

- An absolute or relative insulin deficit
- Hyperosmolality secondary to hyperglycemia and water loss
- Depletion of volume secondary to osmotic diuresis
- Electrolyte abnormalities secondary to the osmotic diuresis
- Altered mental status

TABLE 34–4 Diabetic Ketoacidosis (DKA) and Hyperglycemic Hyperosmolar State (HHS): Comparison of Major Salient Features

FEATURE CONDITIONS	DKA	HHS
Age of patient	Usually less than 40 years old	Usually less than 60 years old
Associated type of diabetes	Primarily type 1	Primarily type 2
Duration of symptoms	Usually less than two days	Usually greater than five days
Plasma glucose level	Greater than 250 mg/dL but less than 600 mg/dL	Usually greater than 600 mg/dL
Sodium concentration	More likely to be normal or low	High, normal, or low
Potassium concentration	High, normal, or low	High, normal, or low
Bicarbonate concentration	Low	Normal
Ketone bodies	High	Small
Arterial pH	Less than 7.30	Greater than 7.30
Serum osmolality	Often less than 320 mOsm/kg (less than 320 mmol/kg)	Usually greater than 320 mOsm/kg (greater than 320 mmol/kg)
Cerebral edema	Often subclinical; occasionally clinical	Subclinical has not been evaluated; rarely clinical
Prognosis	3 to 10% mortality	10 to 20% mortality
Subsequent course	Insulin therapy required in virtually all cases	Insulin therapy not required in many cases
Anion gap	Greater than 12–12	Variable

Data partially from Trachtenbarg, D. E. (2005); and ADA (2006).

There are also many major differences between DKA and HHS that assist the clinician in differentiating the two disorders. Some of the major differences include

- DKA is associated with rapid onset, whereas HHS develops more slowly and insidiously.
- Hyperglycemia is more severe with HHS.
- Hyperosmolality is more severe in HHS, causing profound dehydration.
- Water loss associated with HHS is significantly greater than with DKA.
- HHS is associated with severe neurologic signs (e.g., coma, seizures); in addition, mental status changes may occur over a period of days with HHS.

The clinical features commonly associated with HHS include hyperglycemia, dehydration, absence of significant ketosis, and neurological signs. Table 34–4 presents a comparison of diagnostic criteria for DKA and HHS.

Medical Interventions

Medical goals for management of the patient with HHS are essentially the same as for the patient with DKA. In management of HHS, the first priority is rehydration and restoration of normal electrolyte levels. Other goals include correction of the precipitating event (if possible) and prevention of complications. Fluid replacement needs in the HHS patient are greater than in the DKA patient because of the more profound state of dehydration. Careful monitoring is necessary to prevent complications associated with too rapid rehydration, though complications associated with fluid volume overload during fluid resuscitation of the HHS patient is rare. Because the individual with type 2 diabetes may be sensitive to exogenous insulin, insulin generally is administered in lower doses in treatment of the HHS patient than in the DKA patient. Figure 34–4 provides a protocol for management of HHS in adult clients.

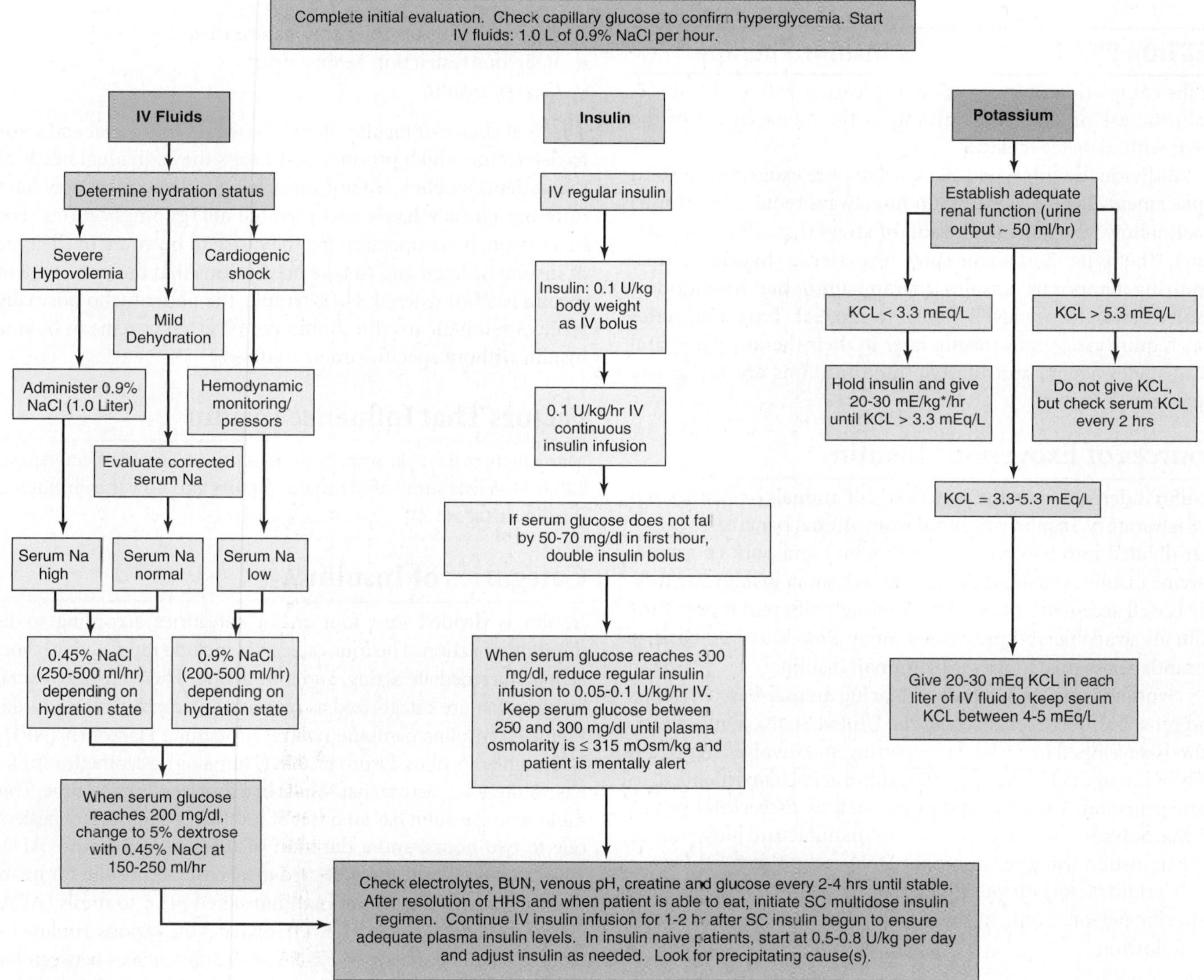

Figure 34–4 ■ ADA Protocol for Management of adult patients with HHS. From American Diabetes Association (ADA). (2006). Protocal for Management of Adult Patient with HHS. Consensus statement: Hyperglycemic crises in adult patients with diabetes. *Diabetes Care, 29*, 2744 [With permission].

SECTION SEVEN REVIEW

1. Which of the following statements is correct regarding HHS?
   A. It has a high mortality rate.
   B. It is most common in type 1 diabetes.
   C. It causes severe fluid volume overload.
   D. Death occurs from severe metabolic acidosis.
2. Common precipitating events causing HHS include which of the following?
   A. hemodialysis
   B. infection
   C. chronic infection
   D. high fat diet
3. HHS does not cause ketosis because
   A. lipolysis does not occur
   B. protein catabolism is occurring
   C. high glucagon levels prevent it
   D. hyperglycemia is not sufficiently severe
4. Which of the following statements regarding the differences between DKA and HHS is correct?
   A. The onset of HHS is faster.
   B. Dehydration is less severe in HHS.
   C. Hyperosmolality is more severe in HHS.
   D. Mental status changes more rapidly in HHS.
5. Which of the following statements is correct regarding insulin management of the patient with HHS?
   A. Insulin management is contraindicated.
   B. The patient usually requires low-dose insulin management.
   C. The type 2 diabetic is resistant to exogenous insulin.
   D. The type 1 diabetic is resistant to exogenous insulin.

Answers: 1. A, 2. B, 3. A, 4. C, 5. B

SECTION EIGHT: Exogenous Insulin Therapy

At the completion of this section, the learner will be able to explain the use of exogenous insulin in the management of the client with diabetes mellitus.

Individuals with type 1 diabetes require exogenous insulin replacement. Type 2 diabetics do not always require exogenous insulin; however, during a period of stress (e.g., illness or surgery), the type 2 diabetic may experience hyperglycemia, requiring temporary insulin therapy until the condition is resolved and glucose levels return to normal. Type 2 diabetics may require exogenous insulin later in their therapy when oral antidiabetes agents and lifestyle modifications are ineffective measures of control.

Sources of Exogenous Insulin

Insulin is derived from the pancreases of animals or synthesized in a laboratory. Insulin produced from animal pancreases is further divided into two types: beef (bovine) and pork (porcine). Porcine insulin is structurally similar to human insulin and usually is well accepted by the body. Although different types of insulin are available and prescribed on an individualized basis, it is standard practice to prescribe human insulin.

Synthetic insulin is rapidly replacing animal-based insulins and is used almost exclusively in the United States. Synthetic insulin is developed in a laboratory setting and involves structural conversion of a substance into the amino acid chains identical to human insulin. Various substances, such as *Escherichia coli* or saccharomyces cerevisiae, are used to manufacture biosynthetic human insulin using recombinant DNA technology.

Certain factors dictate which type of insulin is best suited to a specific person. Some of these factors include the presence of the following

- Insulin allergy
- Insulin resistance
- Adipose tissue atrophy at injection sites
- Religious restriction against pork
- Cost of insulin

The final choice of insulin often is based on using trial and error to determine which product best meets the individual needs of the patient. Insulins are not interchangeable because they have differing efficacy levels and possible allergy implications. For this reason, it is important for the nurse to be aware of the type of insulin ordered and to take precautions that the same type of insulin is administered. For example, the patient who normally receives synthetic insulin should not be given porcine or bovine insulin without specific orders to do so.

Factors That Influence Insulin

Many factors have an impact on insulin dosage or effectiveness. Table 34–5 lists some of the major factors and how they influence insulin dosages.

Categories of Insulin

Insulin is divided into four major categories according to its duration of action. The four categories include rapid acting, short acting, intermediate acting, and long acting. There are also several insulins that are categorized as premixed or combination insulin. Premixed insulins combine neutral protamine Hagedorn (NPH) with regular insulins. Lispro insulin (Humalog), a synthetic insulin, has an altered structure that results in a shortened action time. This rapid-acting insulin has an onset of less than 15 minutes, a peak of one to two hours, and a duration of three to four hours (ADA, 2008). It has become the preferred meal coverage insulin for many diabetics, where the insulin is administered prior to meals (ADA, 2008; Semb, 2004). Table 34–6 differentiates the various insulins according to these categories. Figure 34–5 differentiates between the categories based on the extent and duration of action of the various types of insulin. Typical insulin regimens are shown in Figure 34–6.

TABLE 34–5 Factors Affecting Insulin Dosage

FACTOR	EFFECT
Drug Interactions	
Thiazide diuretics, glucocorticoids, thyroid preparations, nicotine, rifampin	May increase glucose levels and insulin requirements
MAO inhibitors, oral antidiabetes agents, anabolic steroids, salicylates	May reduce glucose levels and insulin requirements
Beta-adrenergic blocking agents	May mask hypoglycemic symptoms
Other	
Exercise	May reduce glucose levels and insulin requirements
Acute illness	Increases blood glucose levels and insulin requirements; often requires sliding-scale insulin administration
Nutritional support	Increases blood glucose levels and insulin requirements; often requires sliding-scale insulin administration

TABLE 34–6 Insulin Preparations

CLASSIFICATION	HUMAN RECOMBINANT INSULINS
Rapid-acting	Aspart (NovoLog) Glulisine (Apidra) Lispro (Humalog)
Regular-acting	Regular (Humulin R) Regular (Novolin R)
Intermediate-acting	NPH (Humulin N) NPH (Novolin N)
Long-acting	Detemir (Levemir) Glargine (Lantus)
Combination therapy (premixed)	NPH/regular 70/30 (Humulin 70/30; Novolin 70/30) Lispro protamine/lispro 75/25 (Humalog Mix 75/25) Aspart protamine/aspart 70/30 (NovoLog Mix 70/30)

Data from ADA. (2008). Insulin. *Diabetes Forecast: 2008 Resource Guide.* RG11–RG14.

Side Effects of Insulin

Administration of too much insulin causes hypoglycemia. The patient is at greatest risk for hypoglycemia during peak action time. It is critical for the nurse to be aware of the type of insulin administered (e.g., rapid acting), when the dose was administered, and what type of nutrition the patient consumed after administration. A person receiving short-acting insulin (e.g., regular insulin) at 8:00 A.M. would peak within two to four hours after subcutaneous administration. This would mean that the risk for hypoglycemia is greatest between the hours of 10:00 A.M. and 12:00 P.M A patient receiving an intermediate-acting insulin (such as NPH) at 8:00 A.M. would peak about 6 to 12 hours later, placing him or her at greatest risk for hypoglycemia between the hours of 2:00 P.M. and 8:00 P.M. Many acutely ill patients require supplemental rapid-acting insulin (regular insulin) as well as their usual intermediate- or long-acting insulin. Mixing types of insulin gives the patient multiple insulin peak periods throughout a 24-hour period. Other factors commonly seen in acutely ill patients, such as prolonged NPO status and nutritional support, all have an impact on glucose levels and insulin needs.

Continuous Low-Dose Intravenous Insulin Infusion

Historically, treatment of DKA in its early stages consisted of administering large doses of insulin (hundreds of units) (Fleckman, 1993). Over time, clinicians found that continuous low-dose IV insulin made regulation easier and provided better control of glucose levels. Other advantages of low-dose IV insulin infusions include fewer complications associated with hypokalemia and hypoglycemia, and rapid rate of insulin dissipation.

During a hyperglycemic crisis, a continuous infusion of regular insulin may be ordered to provide better control of serum insulin levels. When preparing to administer IV insulin, it is important to remember that

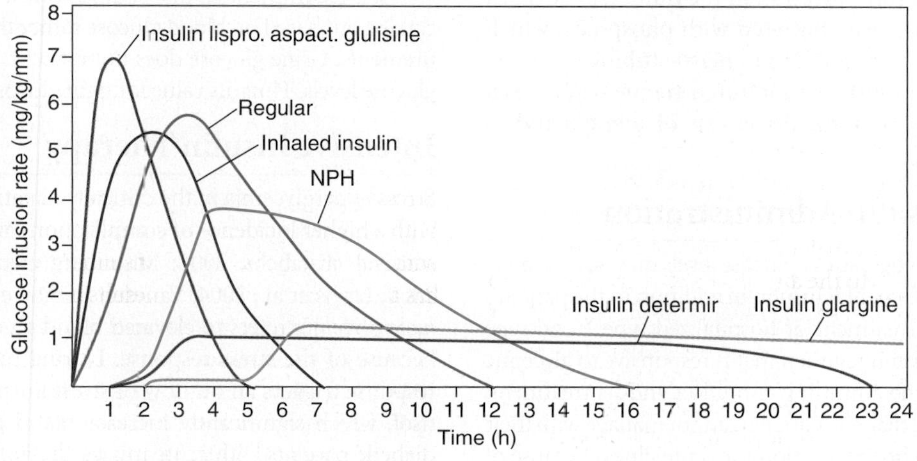

Figure 34–5 ■ Extent and duration of action of various types of insulin as indicated by the glucose infusion rates (mg/kg/min) required to maintain a constant glucose concentration. From Katzung, B. G. [2007]. Basic and clinical pharmacology, (10th ed.), p. 688, New York: McGraw-Hill.

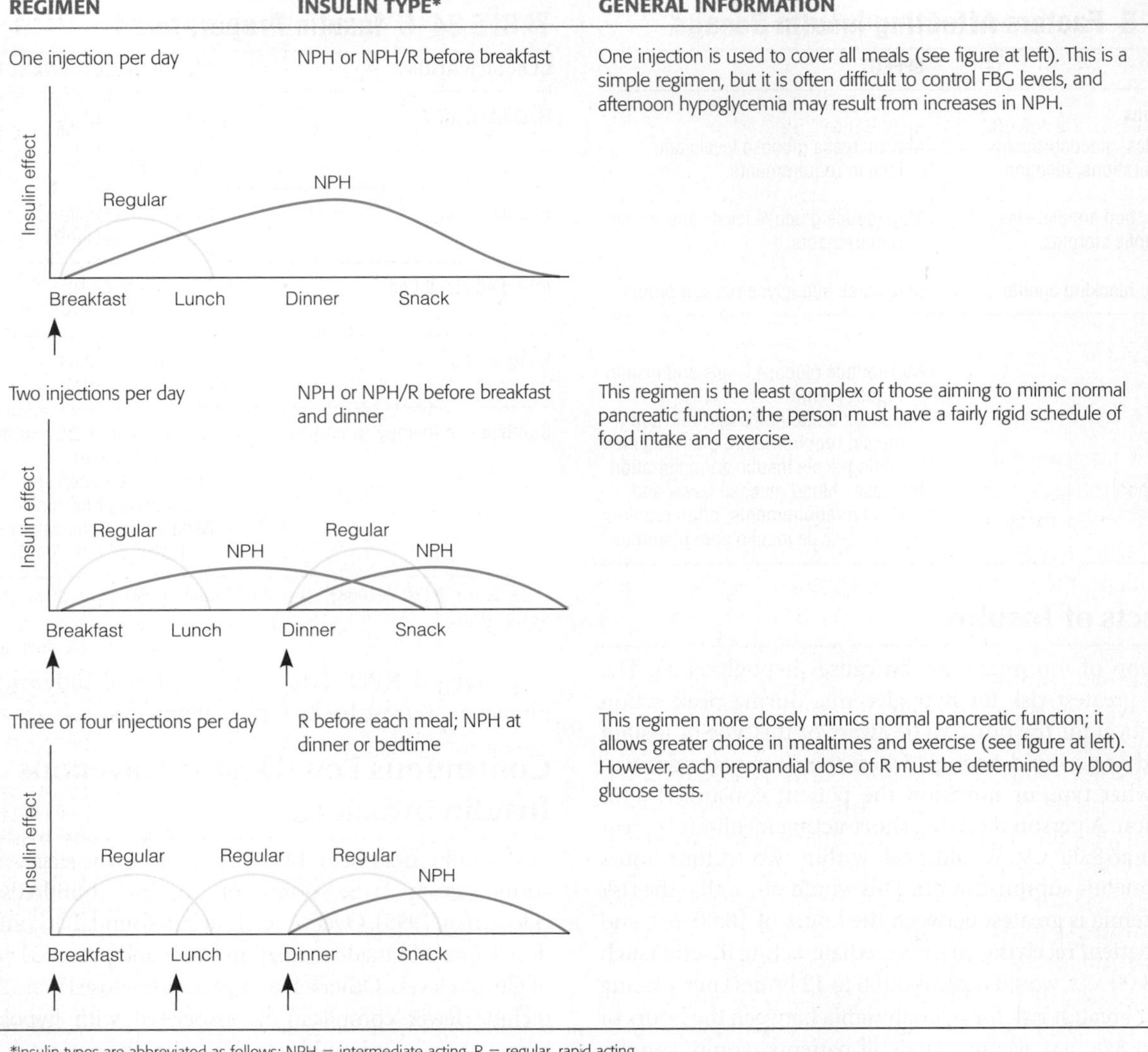

Figure 34–6 ■ Typical insulin regimens.

- Only regular insulin is administered IV.
- Insulin binds to polyvinylchloride in IV bags and tubing, lowering the insulin concentration in the fluid. One form of insulin, Velosulin, has been buffered with phosphate, which prevents the insulin from binding to plastic tubing.
- Blood glucose levels must be monitored frequently, at least hourly, to effectively monitor the effects of therapy and to avoid hypoglycemia.

Sliding-Scale Insulin Administration

During periods of physiologic stress, glucose levels may be extremely unstable, requiring supplemental insulin in addition to the patient's usual insulin coverage. Treatment of hospitalized type 1 and type 2 patients requires an insulin regimen that is responsive to glycemic variation secondary to the admitting condition and its treatment, including surgery. Type 2 diabetic patients cannot manage with their oral medications during hospitalization for acute illness because of the risk of hypoglycemia from not eating and the slower response of these medications to correct hyperglycemia. Consequently, insulin dosage must reflect current blood glucose levels. Orders may be written to titrate the insulin dose to specific glucose levels. This type of insulin regimen is called *sliding-scale insulin* coverage. Table 34–7 provides an example of a sliding-scale insulin order.

It is recommended that sliding-scale insulin administration be carried out based on blood glucose rather than urine glucose measurements. Urine glucose does not reflect hour-by-hour changes in glucose levels. Thus, its value for tight glucose control is diminished.

Intensive Insulin Therapy

Stress hyperglycemia in the critically ill patient has been associated with a higher incidence of complications and decreased long-term survival (Kitabchi, 2006; Malmberg et al., 1999; Capes et al., 2000; Lewis et al., 2004; Van den Berghe et al., 2001, 2003). *Stress hyperglycemia* refers to elevated blood glucose levels that develop because of the stress response. During times of crisis, the stress response triggers an outflow of stress hormones, particularly cortisol, which significantly increase blood glucose levels. In adult diabetic patients with acute myocardial infarctions, the severity of the patient's admission glycometabolic state (measured as Hb A_1c and blood glucose levels) was found to be a significant predictor of mortality, and intensive insulin therapy (continuous intravenous insulin therapy followed by subcutaneous insulin injections for a

TABLE 34–7 Example of Sliding-Scale Insulin Regimen

BLOOD GLUCOSE LEVEL (MG/DL)	REGULAR INSULIN DOSE (SUBCUTANEOUSLY)
200–250	5 units
251–300	10 units
301–350	12 units
351–400	15 units
Greater than 400	Call physician

TABLE 34–8 Example of Insulin Titration Algorithm

BLOOD GLUCOSE LEVEL (MG/DL)	INSULIN RATE (UNITS PER HOUR)	ACTIONS AND FOLLOW-UP PROCEDURES
Admission:		
If > 220	Initiate at four	Initiate insulin infusion and hourly blood glucose checks
If > 110	Initiate at two	Check blood glucose level every hour
Maintenance:		
Rapid reduction of glucose > 5% change	Reduce insulin dose to half	Check blood glucose every 30 minutes.
> 140	Increase by two	
110–140	Increase by one	
Approaching normal	Adjust dose up or down by 0.1 to 0.5 units/hr	
Within normal limits	Maintain current dose	
60–80	Reduce dose adequately (some algorithms stop insulin infusion at this glucose level)	Rate of insulin decrease depends on previous blood glucose level. Check blood glucose every 30 minutes.
40–60	Stop insulin infusion	Assure baseline glucose intake Check blood glucose level every 30 minutes.
< 40	Stop insulin infusion	Assure baseline glucose intake. Give 25 mL dextrose 50% water (D$_{50}$W). Check blood glucose level every 30 minutes.

minimum of three months after the AMI) reduced long-term mortality (Malmberg et al., 1999). Furthermore, stress hyperglycemia can be harmful to high-acuity nondiabetic patients as well as those with diabetes (Capes et al., 2000). Van den Berghe et al. (2001) initiated their landmark investigation involving diabetic and nondiabetic critically ill adult patients. They recommended maintaining tight control of blood glucose levels to 110 mg/dL or less to reduce mortality and morbidity in critically ill patients regardless of whether or not they are diabetics. Several years later, Van den Berghe et al. (2003) further recommended use of an insulin titration algorithm to optimally control hyperglycemia in the critically ill patient population. Currently there is no universally accepted titration algorithm and intensive insulin therapy protocols vary widely. There is growing acceptance of the need to achieve tighter control of blood sugar in individuals who are hospitalized with hyperglycemia, whether they are diagnosed with diabetes, have unrecognized diabetes, or have stress related glucose intolerance (Magee, 2006). Table 34–8 provides an example of an insulin titration algorithm.

Nursing care of the patient receiving intensive insulin therapy includes frequent monitoring of blood glucose levels, titrating the insulin infusion according to the protocol, closely monitoring the patient for development of hypoglycemia as glucose levels approach normal, and intervening rapidly if hypoglycemia occurs to return the patient to a normoglycemic state without complications. Maintaining the blood glucose levels within the normal range is often challenging, particularly if the patient's condition is complex and unstable.

The Somogyi Effect: An Insulin Dosage Problem

Some patients, particularly those who are acutely ill, have wide swings in serum glucose levels from early morning to postprandial serum glucose measurements caused by an excessive insulin dosage. One explanation of this phenomenon is the **Somogyi effect**, triggered by nocturnal hypoglycemia. Hypoglycemia causes release of stress hormones, ultimately increasing serum glucose, which in turn, creates a state of hyperglycemia. Morning urine ketones may be noted as well as an elevated serum glucose caused by catabolic processes. The resulting hyperglycemia, if accompanied by increased insulin dosage, precipitates another episode of hypoglycemia that may be worse than the preceding episode (Fig. 34–7).

Recognition of the presence of the Somogyi effect has important treatment implications. The administration of even more insulin worsens the level of nocturnal hypoglycemia, further aggravating the problem. When the Somogyi effect is suspected, the insulin dosage actually may need to be decreased, or a protein-based snack before bed may be added to the diet to slow down the rebound cycle.

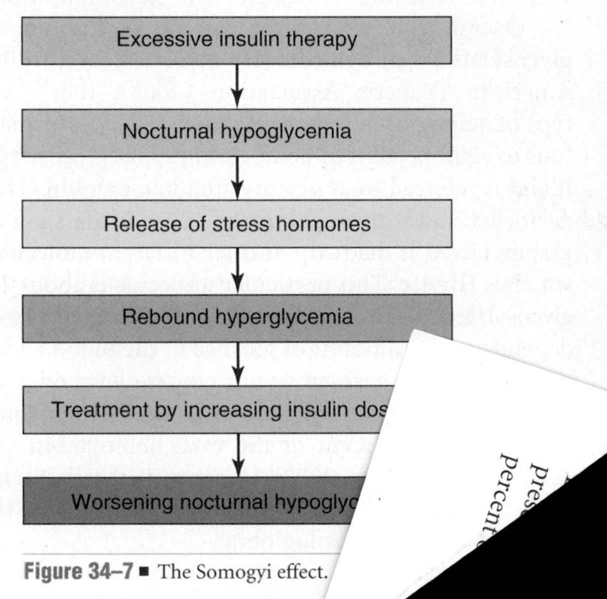

Figure 34–7 ■ The Somogyi effect.

SECTION EIGHT REVIEW

1. Which of the following situations would be MOST likely to necessitate exogenous insulin use in the type 2 diabetic client?
   - **A.** a localized toe infection
   - **B.** a mild common cold
   - **C.** a high fat meal
   - **D.** an episode of delirium
2. Which of the following are sources of insulin? (choose all that apply)
   - **A.** pork
   - **B.** beef
   - **C.** Staphylococcus aureus
   - **D.** Escherichia coli
3. Exogenous insulin is
   - **A.** seldom used in the treatment of HHS
   - **B.** most often derived from animal sources
   - **C.** used only in the treatment of type 1 diabetes
   - **D.** often required in management of type 2 diabetes during stress periods
4. Which of the following are factors that dictate the type of insulin that is best suited for a specific person? (choose all that apply)
   - **A.** a patient's weight
   - **B.** insulin resistance
   - **C.** a patient's allergies
   - **D.** adipose tissue condition
5. Which of the following factors would MOST likely decrease insulin need?
   - **A.** acute illness
   - **B.** steroid therapy
   - **C.** nutritional support
   - **D.** oral antidiabetic agents

Answers: 1. A, 2. (A, B, D), 3. D, 4. (B, C, D), 5. D

SECTION NINE: Acute Care Implications of Chronic Complications

At the completion of this section, the learner will be able to discuss the acute care implications of chronic diabetic complications.

Glucose Control and Complications

Many factors influence acutely ill patient outcomes, such as preexisting chronic diseases. Diabetes is a chronic disease that profoundly affects patient outcomes because of the many acute and chronic complications that can result from it. Though diabetes mellitus is caused by dysfunction of just one organ—the pancreas—it causes dysfunction of virtually all organs. Maintaining long-term glucose control is essential in the prevention or reduction of diabetes-related complications.

Overall glucose control can be monitored using the **glycosylated hemoglobin (Hb A_1c)** test. According to the American Diabetic Association (2008), the predominant type of hemoglobin is hemoglobin A (Hb A). Normally, about four to eight percent of hemoglobin A has glucose attached to it and is referred to as glycosylated hemoglobin (Hb A_1). Hb A_1 forms slowly throughout the 120-day life span of hemoglobin. Hb A_1 is made up of three different molecules, one of which is Hb A_1c. This particular molecule is about 70 percent glycosylated. The amount of glycosylated hemoglobin depends on the amount of glucose in the blood and is a good indicator of the average serum glucose level over a 120-day period. The normal range of glycosylated hemoglobin (Hb A_1c) is 3.9-7.2 percent of the total hemoglobin (American Diabetes Association, 2008). Uncontrolled diabetes mellitus is [illegible]ent if a glycosylated hemoglobin level is more than eight [illegible]f the total hemoglobin.

Chronic Complications

Chronic complications can be divided into three types: peripheral neuropathy, microvascular, and macrovascular. The remainder of this section will present an overview of major long-term complications associated with diabetes mellitus.

Diabetic Peripheral Neuropathies

Peripheral neuropathies are the most common complications of diabetes mellitus. They begin early in the course of the disease, affecting both type 1 and type 2 diabetics. Peripheral neuropathies primarily alter sensory perception. The underlying cause of neuropathies is poorly understood. They may result from thickening of vessel walls that supply peripheral nerves, thus impairing nutrition to the nerves. They may result from a segmental demyelinization that results in slowed or disrupted conduction. There is also some evidence that sorbitol may accumulate in the nerve cells, impairing conduction. Whatever the cause, the result is an alteration in sensory perception.

Neuropathies initially may cause pain or abnormal sensations or both. As nerve degeneration progresses, the patient may experience loss of the ability to discriminate fine touch, a decrease in proprioception, and local anesthesia.

The autonomic nervous system also may be affected. As the myelin sheath undergoes degenerative changes, functions governed by the autonomic nerves are affected adversely. The patient may experience an increase in gut motility and diarrhea, postural hypotension, or other autonomic nervous system–related complications.

The neuropathies experienced by diabetics vary in type, severity, and clinical manifestations. Because of this diversity, it is not possible to predict which neuropathy any individual will develop.

Acute Care Implications

When feasible, patients with diabetes should be assessed for the presence and degree of peripheral neuropathy. The presence of a diminished sense of touch and pain may mask injury or infection. The patient must be protected from injury at all times to prevent damage to affected tissues. The diabetic patient must also be protected from hyperthermic burns. Excessive heat may not be sensed, which increases the risk of burns by heating pads, hyperthermia blankets, and bathing. Some neuropathies are associated with progressive, permanent damage to the neurons. However, others are reversible when good glucose control is maintained.

Microvascular Disease

Microvascular disease is associated with capillary membrane thickening, which causes **microangiopathy** (small blood vessel disease). As the capillary membrane thickens, the tissues become increasingly hypoperfused, and organs become hypoxic and ischemic. Prolonged ischemia eventually causes **infarction** (death of tissue). The degree of microvascular disease may be influenced most by the duration of diabetes rather than the level of glucose control. Two organs at particular risk for microvascular disease secondary to diabetes mellitus are the retina of the eyes (retinopathy) and the kidneys (nephropathy).

Retinopathy

Diabetic retinopathy is responsible for a significant portion of newly diagnosed blindness in the United States. It is caused by an underlying microangiopathy of the retina, leading to retinal microvascular occlusion. Once occlusion exists, the retina undergoes increasing areas of ischemia and infarction, eventually leading to blindness. Damage occurs in two complex stages. Stage I is associated with increased capillary permeability, aneurysm formation, and hemorrhage. Stage II is associated with increasing retinal ischemia and eventual infarction, causing blindness. Diabetic retinopathy is associated with both type 1 and type 2 diabetes.

Acute Care Implications

The acutely ill diabetic patient may have moderate to severe visual impairment. Early assessment of visual status is important, either by questioning the patient directly or by interviewing the family. Medical and nursing management and teaching must be altered to meet the needs of a visually impaired patient. In the high-acuity patient, blindness affects pupillary changes and must be taken into consideration when performing a neurologic assessment. A visually impaired patient in a critical care environment may have more difficulty making sense of distracting noises and equipment surrounding the bedside. Frequent explanation and reorientation may be necessary.

Nephropathy

Diabetic nephropathy is a disease of the glomeruli. The glomerular basement membrane becomes thickened, resulting in intracapillary glomerulosclerosis (hardening and thickening of the glomeruli). Glomeruli become enlarged and eventually are destroyed, ultimately resulting in renal failure. As the degree of renal failure increases, the patient may require a decreased insulin dosage to prevent hypoglycemia. Reduced renal function decreases the ability of the kidneys to metabolize insulin. Insulin not metabolized remains available to facilitate glucose metabolism.

Acute Care Implications

The acutely ill patient with some degree of preexisting renal impairment is at risk for further impairment from hypotensive episodes, nephrotoxic drug therapy, or the multisystemic complications associated with many acute illnesses. Kidney function must be carefully monitored at regular intervals. Drug therapy may need to be altered based on kidney function. Kidney failure, as a disease entity, has its own set of actual and potential complications.

Macrovascular Disease

Macrovascular disease (**macroangiopathy**) refers to atherosclerosis. **Atherosclerosis** is a form of arteriosclerosis (thickening and hardening of arterial walls), characterized by plaque deposits of lipids, fibrous connective tissue, calcium, and other blood substances. Atherosclerosis, by definition, affects only medium and large arteries (excluding arterioles). The cause of rapid development of atherosclerosis in the diabetic patient is described in Section Three.

Macrovascular disease is associated with the development of coronary artery disease, peripheral vascular disease, brain attack (stroke), and increased risk of infection. Type 2 diabetes is more closely associated with macrovascular diseases than type 1 diabetes. Peripheral vascular disease and increased risk of infection have important implications in the care of the acutely ill patient.

Peripheral Vascular Disease

Progressive atherosclerotic changes in peripheral arterial circulation lead to decreasing arterial blood flow to peripheral tissues. As the disease progresses, small arteries become occluded, precipitating a tissue ischemia/infarction sequence of events. In the type 2 diabetic, this is typically noted as small isolated patches of gangrene, particularly on the feet and toes. As circulation becomes increasingly compromised, areas of gangrene become larger, and amputation may be required.

Acute Care Implications

The patient with peripheral vascular disease is at increased risk for complications secondary to poor tissue perfusion and loss of skin integrity. Of particular concern in the acutely ill patient is the development of decubitus ulcers and infection. Development of either of these two problems could potentially lead to gangrene and possible amputation. Careful limb positioning, excellent skin hygiene, and close monitoring of skin integrity are extremely important.

Increased Risk of Infection

The diabetic patient is at high risk for development of infection for a variety of reasons.

1. **Diminished early warning system.** Impaired vision and peripheral neuropathy contribute to the decreased ability of the diabetic patient to perform self-monitoring. Breaks in skin integrity may not be seen or felt because of the underlying disease process.
2. **Tissue hypoxia.** Vascular disease causes tissue hypoxia. When skin integrity is broken, there is a decreased ability to heal, secondary to lack of oxygen. Glycosylated hemoglobin in RBCs decreases release of oxygen to the tissues, thus contributing to hypoxia.
3. **Rapid proliferation of pathogens.** Once inside the body, pathogens rapidly multiply because of increased glucose in body fluids, which acts as an energy source for the pathogens.
4. **Impaired white blood cells.** Diabetes is associated with the development of abnormal white blood cells, particularly phagocytes, and also alters chemotaxis (movement of WBCs to the site of infection).
5. **Impaired circulation.** A diminished blood supply decreases the ability of WBCs to move into the infected area.

Acute Care Implications

The acutely ill diabetic patient is at increased risk for the development of severe, difficult-to-treat infections. Any infection, no matter how minor, may become life-threatening in this population. Close monitoring for infection and rapid, aggressive interventions are needed. Remember that decreased kidney function may be a complicating factor in aggressive antibiotic therapy.

Wound healing also is impaired in the diabetic for several reasons. Impaired tissue perfusion, especially in the distal extremities, interferes with healing in those areas because of lack of circulation and tissue hypoxia. Hyperglycemic states adversely affect wound healing by interfering with collagen concentrations in a wound. Good control of blood glucose significantly facilitates wound healing.

SECTION NINE REVIEW

1. Peripheral neuropathies primarily affect
   A. motor functions
   B. sensory functions
   C. optic functions
   D. vascular functions
2. Microvascular diseases are associated with
   A. deposits of lipoproteins
   B. deposits of calcium products
   C. large blood vessel disease
   D. small blood vessel disease
3. Diabetic retinopathy causes blindness as a result of
   A. glucose deposits on the retina
   B. thickening of the retina
   C. destruction of the optic nerve
   D. infarction of retinal tissue
4. Diabetic nephropathy damages the nephrons by causing
   A. glomerulosclerosis
   B. glomerulonephritis
   C. chronic nephritis
   D. renal hypertension
5. Diabetes-induced atherosclerosis is associated with which of the following complications? (choose all that apply)
   A. peripheral vascular disease
   B. brain attack (stroke)
   C. gastrointestinal ulcers
   D. coronary artery disease
6. Diabetes increases a patient's chance of infection as a result of which of the following?
   A. abnormal white blood cells
   B. abnormal platelet function
   C. slow proliferation of pathogens
   D. decreased body fluid glucose levels

Answers: 1. B, 2. D, 3. D, 4. A, 5. (A, B, D), 6. A

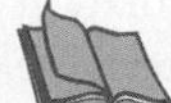

POSTTEST

The following Posttest is constructed in a case study format. A patient is presented. Questions are asked based on available data. New data are presented as the case study progresses.

Connie D is a 44-year-old housewife with a history of diabetes mellitus. She has been admitted to the hospital for reevaluation of insulin dosage. She has been having periods of drowsiness and confusion at home.

1. Connie's brain cells
   A. do not require glucose for energy
   B. require fatty acids as their major energy source
   C. do not require insulin for cellular uptake of glucose
   D. require high levels of insulin for cellular uptake of glucose
2. When Connie's blood glucose drops below normal, the sympathetic nervous system stimulates secretion of which hormone that subsequently causes many of the major manifestations of hypoglycemia?
   A. epinephrine
   B. cortisol
   C. glucagon
   D. growth hormone

3. Which statement best reflects the effect of insulin on glucose metabolism in Connie's liver? Insulin facilitates conversion of _______.
   A. excess amino acids into glucose
   B. excess fatty acids into glycogen
   C. excess glycogen into glucose
   D. excess glucose into glycogen
4. When Connie's blood amino acid levels increase, insulin
   A. facilitates storage of proteins
   B. inhibits synthesis of protein
   C. facilitates protein catabolism
   D. inhibits transport of amino acids into cell

Connie has an absolute insulin deficit.

5. An absolute insulin deficit would affect her carbohydrate metabolism in which of the following ways?
   A. Brain cells rapidly become glucose starved.
   B. Insulin-dependent cells become glucose starved.
   C. Brain cells convert glycogen to glucose directly.
   D. Insulin-dependent cells take in glucose directly.
6. In which way does insulin deficit affect Connie's protein metabolism?
   A. Protein synthesis is increased.
   B. Protein catabolism is halted.
   C. Protein cannot be stored without insulin.
   D. Protein cannot be used as energy without insulin.

Connie's diabetes is characterized by the following. Her mother also had diabetes. Connie was diagnosed with diabetes at the age of 32. She is 5 feet 5 inches (16.5 meters) tall and weighs 173 pounds (78.6 kg). She requires insulin on a daily basis.

7. Which of the preceding data is most suggestive of type 1 diabetes?
   A. Her mother also had diabetes.
   B. She was diagnosed at the age of 32.
   C. She is 5 feet 5 inches (16.5 m) tall and weighs 173 pounds (78.6 kg).
   D. She requires insulin on a daily basis.
8. If Connie had type 2 diabetes, the most common etiologic factors include
   A. viral infection and obesity
   B. obesity and genetic predisposition
   C. immune reaction and viral infection
   D. obesity and autoimmune reaction

During her hospitalization, Connie was kept NPO for eight hours for a particular set of blood tests. She, however, did receive her usual morning insulin dosage. Consequently, Connie experiences symptoms typical of a hypoglycemic episode.

9. Typical clinical manifestations of Connie's hypoglycemia would include which of the following? (choose all that apply)
   A. bradycardia
   B. tremor
   C. diaphoresis
   D. vomiting
10. Common causes of hypoglycemic episodes include
    A. lack of dietary intake
    B. heavy carbohydrate meal
    C. insufficient insulin dose
    D. decreased exercise level

Connie has developed an infection from an ingrown toenail. She currently has a temperature of 100°F (37.8°C) (oral). A rapid assessment reveals the following: opens eyes and groans to mild shaking but closes them immediately after stimulation.

11. What other clinical manifestations would help confirm a diagnosis of diabetic ketoacidosis at this time?
    A. polydipsia
    B. hand tremors
    C. fruity breath odor
    D. shallow respirations
12. Which laboratory result would be most diagnostic of diabetic ketoacidosis?
    A. pH 7.34
    B. anion gap 18 mEq/L
    C. HCO_3 17 mEq/L
    D. $PaCO_2$ 28 mm Hg

It has been decided that Connie's diabetic ketoacidosis was precipitated by her foot infection.

13. Infection can precipitate a diabetic ketoacidosis episode as a result of
    A. stress response
    B. increased insulin resistance
    C. increased glucagon levels
    D. diminished cortisol activity
14. Connie's diabetic ketoacidosis can be differentiated best from hyperglycemic hyperosmolar state (HHS) by measuring
    A. pH
    B. ketones
    C. bicarbonate
    D. blood glucose

Connie is experiencing large swings in her glucose levels throughout the day. The physician orders a larger insulin dose to better control the hyperglycemia. The next day, her hyperglycemia is worse. It is decided that she may be experiencing the Somogyi effect. Connie is confused but conscious.

15. The Somogyi effect is characterized by a rebound phenomenon caused by release of
    A. glucagon
    B. amino acids
    C. fatty acids
    D. stress hormones
16. Considering her status, which of the following interventions would be most appropriate?
    A. five units of regular insulin
    B. glucagon 1.5 mg (IM)
    C. bedtime snack
    D. 50 percent dextrose (IV)

During her diabetic ketoacidosis episode, Connie receives a continuous drip of IV insulin.

17. Important rules to remember in infusing IV insulin include which of the following? (choose all that apply)
   A. Only regular insulin is used IV.
   B. Most insulins bind to plastic bags and tubing.
   C. Obtain urine glucose every hour.
   D. IV doses usually are small.

Upon reviewing Connie's history, you note that she has a long history of peripheral neuropathy, poor vision, and peripheral vascular disease.

18. Connie's peripheral neuropathy is best controlled by
   A. steroid therapy
   B. good glucose control
   C. vitamin supplementation
   D. nothing; there is no slowing the process

19. Connie's vision has become progressively impaired over the duration of her diabetes. Diabetic retinopathy is a result of
   A. glucose deposits on retina
   B. macrovascular occlusion
   C. fatty deposits on retina
   D. microvascular occlusion

20. Connie's peripheral vascular disease may lead to further complications because it causes
   A. tissue ischemia
   B. acute infection
   C. peripheral edema
   D. coronary artery disease

Posttest answers with rationale are found on MyNursingKit.

REFERENCES

American Diabetes Association [ADA]. (2008). Insulin. *Diabetes forecast: 2008 resource guide.* American Diabetic Association, RG11–RG14.

American Diabetes Association [ADA]. (2008). Hyperglycemic crises in patients with diabetes mellitus. *Diabetes Care, 276*(1), S109S94–S117S102.

Capes, S. E., Hunt, D., Malmberg, K., & Gerstein, H. C. (2000). Stress hyperglycemia and increased risk of death after myocardial infarction in patients with and without diabetes: a systematic overview. *The Lancet, 355,* 773–778.

Cox, D. J., Gonder_Frederick, L., Ritterband, L. Clarke, W., & Kovatchev, B. P. (2007). Prediction of severe hypoglycemia. *Diabetes Care, 30*(6). 1370–1373.

Fleckman, A. M. (1993). Diabetic ketoacidosis. *Endocrinology Metabolic Clinics of America, 22*(2), 181–206.

Guvan, S., Kuenzi, J. A., & Matfin, G. (2006). Diabetes mellitus. In C. M. Porth (ed.), *Essentials of pathophysiology.* (2d ed.). Philadelphia: Lippincott Williams & Wilkins, 560–579.

Katzung, B. G. (2007). *Basic and clinical pharmacology,* (10th ed.). New York: McGraw-Hill, 688.

Kee, J. L. (2005). *Laboratory and diagnostic tests with nursing implications,* (7th ed.). Upper Saddle River, NJ: Prentice Hall.

Kitabchi, A. E., Umpierrez, G. E., Murphy, M. B., & Kreisberg, R. A. (2006). Hyperglycemic crises in adult patients with diabetes. *Diabetes Care, 29*(12), 2739–2748.

Lewis, K., Kane-Gill, S., Bobek, M., & Dasta, J. (2004). Intensive insulin therapy for critically ill patients. *The Annals of Pharmacotherapy, 38,* 1243–1251.

Malmberg, K., Norhammar, A., Wedel, H., & Ryden, L. (1999). Glycometabolic state at admission: Important risk marker of mortality in conventionally treated patients with diabetes mellitus and acute myocardial infarction. *Circulation, 99,* 2626–2632.

Manchester, C. S. & Tracy, M. F. (2009). Glycemic control. In K. K. Carlson, *Advanced critical care nursing.* St. Louis: Saunders/Elsevier, 915–938.

Magee, M. (2006). Insulin therapy for intensive glycemic control in hospital patients. *Hospital Physician, 42*(4), 17–27, 38.

Porth, C. M. (2006). *Pathophysiology: Concepts of altered health states,* (8th ed.). Philadelphia: Lippincott, Williams & Wilkins.

Semb, S. (2004). Nursing management: diabetes mellitus. In S. M. Lewis, M. M. Heitkemper, & S. R. Dirksen (eds.), *Medical-surgical nursing: assessment and management of clinical problems,* (6th ed.. St. Louis: C. V. Mosby, 1268–1302.

Sheikh-Ali, M., Karon, B., Basu, A., et al. (2008). Can serum beta-hydroxybutyrate be used to diagnose ketoacidosis? Diabetes Care. Apr 31(4): 643-7.

Trachtenbarg, D. E. (2005). Diabetic ketoacidosis. *American Family Physician, 71,* 1721–1722.

Van den Berghe, G., Wouters, P., Bouillon, R., Weekers, F., Verwaest, C., et al. (2003). Outcome benefit of intensive insulin therapy in the critically ill: Insulin dose versus glycemic control. *Critical Care Medicine, 31*(2), 359–366.

Van den Berghe, G., Wouters, P., Weekers, F., Verwaest, C., Bruyninckx, F., et al. (2001). Intensive insulin therapy in critically ill patients. *New England Journal of Medicine, 324*(19), 1359–1367.

Wang, J., Williams, D. E., Naravan, K. M. V., & Geiss, L. S. (2006). Declining death rates among adults with diabetes, U.S., 1985–2002. *Diabetes Care, 29*(9), 2018–2022.

MODULE

35 Determinants and Assessment of Skin Integrity

Karen L. Johnson

OBJECTIVES Following completion of this module, the learner will be able to

1. Identify anatomic structures and of the skin.
2. State the three phases of wound healing.
3. Describe the events that occur in each phase of wound healing.
4. Define three methods of wound closure.
5. State physiologic and environmental factors that affect wound healing.
6. Identify the common clinical assessments made to evaluate wound healing.

This self-study module is divided into four sections. Section One describes the anatomic structures of the skin. Section Two focuses on physiologic events that occur when an alteration in skin integrity occurs. Section Three discusses the factors that affect wound healing, and Section Four covers clinical assessment of wound healing.

Each section includes a set of review questions to help the learner evaluate his or her understanding of the section's content before moving on to the next section. All Section Reviews include answers. It is suggested that the learner review those concepts answered incorrectly in the review questions before proceeding to the next section.

PRETEST

1. The layer of the skin that contains connective tissue, elastic fibers, blood vessels, and nerves is the
   A. epidermis
   B. dermis
   C. hypodermis
   D. subcutaneous tissue
2. Which of the following is an example of a superficial wound? (choose all that apply)
   A. stage II pressure ulcer
   B. stage IV pressure ulcer
   C. contusion
   D. abrasion
3. Which of the following is not a major event that occurs during the proliferative phase of wound healing?
   A. hemostasis
   B. epithelialization
   C. granulation
   D. collagen cross-linking
4. The four cardinal signs of inflammation occur as a result of
   A. normal chemical and vascular events
   B. an infectious process
   C. bradykinins
   D. an increased number of white blood cells (WBCs)
5. Wounds that have significant contamination or significant tissue loss usually are not sutured. These wounds are left open to heal by the process of
   A. primary intention
   B. secondary intention
   C. delayed primary intention
   D. delayed secondary intention
6. Which of the following factors impair wound healing? (choose all that apply)
   A. edema
   B. stress
   C. carbon dioxide
   D. smoking
7. Which of the following vitamins prevents oxygen free radical related cellular damage? (choose all that apply)
   A. vitamin A
   B. vitamin B
   C. vitamin C
   D. vitamin E

8. Which of the following predispose the patient to a wound infection? (choose all that apply)
   A. susceptible host
   B. compromised wound
   C. infectious organism
   D. diabetes

9. Which of the following terms describes a wound with black thick nonpliable necrotic tissue?
   A. slough
   B. eschar
   C. maceration
   D. exudate

Pretest anwsers are found on MyNursingKit.

SECTION ONE: Anatomy and Physiology of the Skin

At the completion of this section, the learner will be able to identify the anatomic structures of the skin.

The skin is a tough membrane covering the entire body surface. It is the largest organ of the body and is composed of three layers of tissue: the epidermis, the dermis, and the hypodermis or subcutaneous tissue. The **epidermis,** the outermost layer, contains epithelial cells. The middle layer, often referred to as the true skin, is the **dermis**. This layer contains connective tissue and elastic fibers, sensory and motor nerve endings, and a complex network of capillary and lymphatic vessels and muscles. From the dermis arise the appendages of the skin—hair, nails, and sebaceous and sweat glands—which then penetrate the epidermis. The dermis lacks exact boundaries and merges with subcutaneous tissues containing blood vessels, nerves, muscle, and adipose tissue. The anatomy of the skin is depicted in Figure 35–1.

The epidermis contains epithelial tissue responsible for regeneration of the skin. This tissue is composed of cells that rapidly reproduce and regenerate through the process of epithelialization.

The various components of the dermis provide elements to protect and combat foreign materials and regenerate itself after exposure to the external environment. Connective tissue and elastic fibers provide strength and pliability to protect the internal environment. Nutrients are delivered to and cellular wastes are removed by the blood and lymphatic vessels. The nerve endings within the dermis respond to cold, heat, touch, pain, and pressure.

Subcutaneous tissue consists of adipose tissue and fascia. Adipose tissue is highly vascular, loose connective tissue that stores

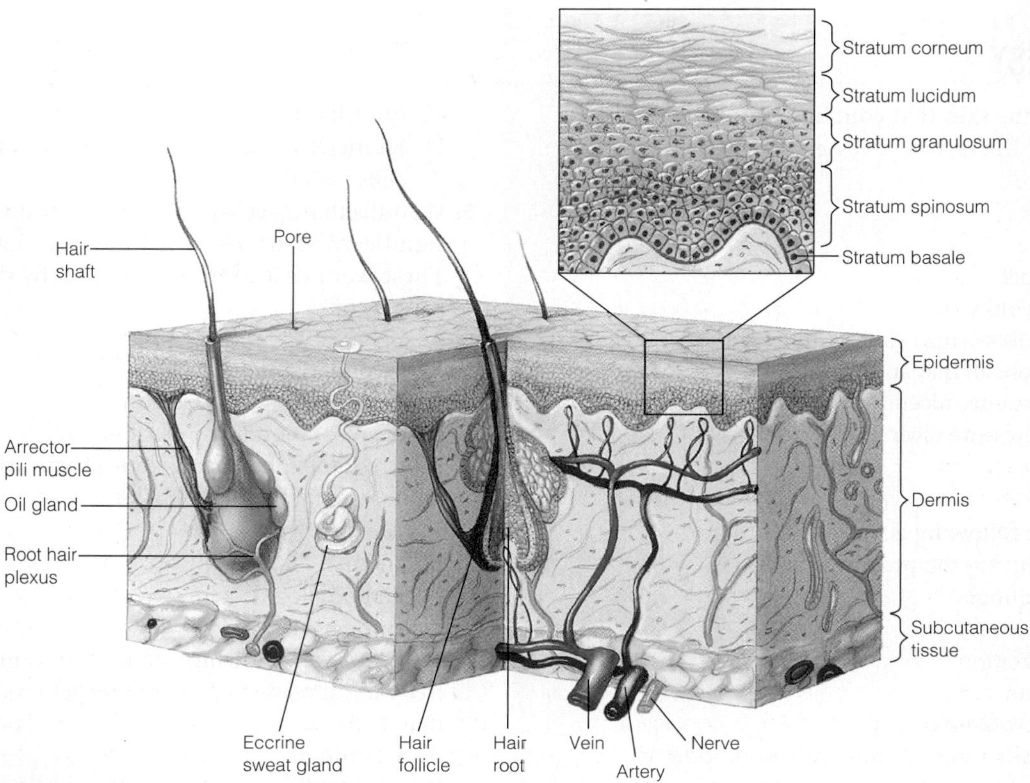

Figure 35–1 ■ Anatomy of the skin. The skin is composed of three layers of tissue: the epidermis, dermis, and hypodermis.

fat, which provides energy, cushioning and insulation. Healthy adipose tissue is white to yellow in color. Darker adipose tissue can be associated with dehydration (Myers, 2008a). Fascia is fibrous connective tissue that separates and surrounds structures.

A wound creates an alteration and disruption of the anatomic and physiologic functions of the skin. A wound can be created intentionally, as with a surgeon's knife; by accidental trauma, such as occurs in a motor vehicle crash; or by chronic forces, such as that which occurs with pressure ulcer formation. It is important for the nurse to know the normal structures of the skin; this familiarity aides in determining the extent of tissue involvement in an open wound. The extent of tissue involvement is typically categorized as **superficial, partial thickness** or **full thickness.** These are described in greater detail in Module 37, Alteration in Skin Integrity: Acute Burn Injury. Superficial wounds affect the epidermis only. An **abrasion** is an example of a superficial wound. An abrasion is a wound to the top layer of the skin that exposes the top layer of the dermis. Abrasions are commonly seen with traumatic injuries such as motor vehicle crashes. **Contusion** is another example of a superficial wound. A contusion is associated with a disruption of blood vessels and extravasation of blood into the skin. Partial thickness wounds involve the epidermis and part of the dermis. A stage II pressure ulcer is an example of a partial thickness wound. In full thickness wounds, the epidermis and entire dermis are injured and the subcutaneous tissue is exposed. An **avulsion** is an example of a full thickness wound.

SECTION ONE REVIEW

1. Which of the following is NOT a layer of the skin?
   A. endothelial cells
   B. epidermis
   C. dermis
   D. subcutaneous tissue
2. The components of the dermis are
   A. epithelial cells, subcutaneous tissue
   B. adipose tissue, subcutaneous tissue
   C. hair, nails, and sebaceous glands
   D. connective tissue, blood, and lymph vessels
3. The "true skin" is the
   A. epidermis
   B. dermis
   C. subcutaneous tissue
   D. fascia
4. Which of the following is a function of adipose tissue? (choose all that apply)
   A. provides energy
   B. provides cushioning
   C. provides insulation
   D. stores water
5. An abrasion is an example of a ______wound.
   A. superficial
   B. partial thickness
   C. full thickness
   D. superficial full thickness

Answers: 1. A, 2. D, 3. B, 4. (A, B, C) 5. A

SECTION TWO: Wound Physiology

At the completion of this section, the learner will be able to state the three phases of wound healing, describe the events that occur in each phase of wound healing, and define the three methods of wound closure.

Acute wounds progress through a predictable series of events that result in a healed wound. In contrast, chronic nonhealing wounds fail to proceed through an orderly and timely healing process (Brown, 2009a). On injury, the body immediately begins the process of restoring its integrity and the physiologic functions of the skin. A basic understanding of the wound healing process helps to assess, diagnose, plan, and evaluate nursing interventions for the patient with altered skin integrity.

From the moment of injury, overlapping physiologic processes work to restore a functional barrier. Wound healing occurs by two methods: regeneration, when lost tissue is replaced with identical tissues, and connective tissue repair, when lost tissue is replaced by scar formation. The method of repair depends on the layers of tissue involved and their ability to regenerate. Superficial dermal and epidermal wounds heal by regeneration. Wounds extending through the dermis heal by scar formation. There are three phases of wound healing: (1) the inflammatory phase, (2) the proliferative phase, and (3) the remodeling/maturation phase.

Inflammatory Phase

The inflammatory phase occurs immediately after injury and lasts several days. This is a critical phase because the wound environment is being prepared for subsequent tissue development. The major events that occur in this phase are hemostasis and removal of cellular debris and bacteria.

Immediately on injury, vascular and cellular events are initiated. Thromboplastin is released from injured cells activating the clotting cascade. Platelets aggregate at the injury site to form a plug to seal a break in the vessel wall. The platelets also liberate growth factors essential in tissue development during the subsequent phase of healing (platelet-derived growth factor, epidermal growth factor, etc.). A great deal of research currently revolves around the activities of these factors and other cytokines. Once hemostasis is achieved, the blood vessels dilate

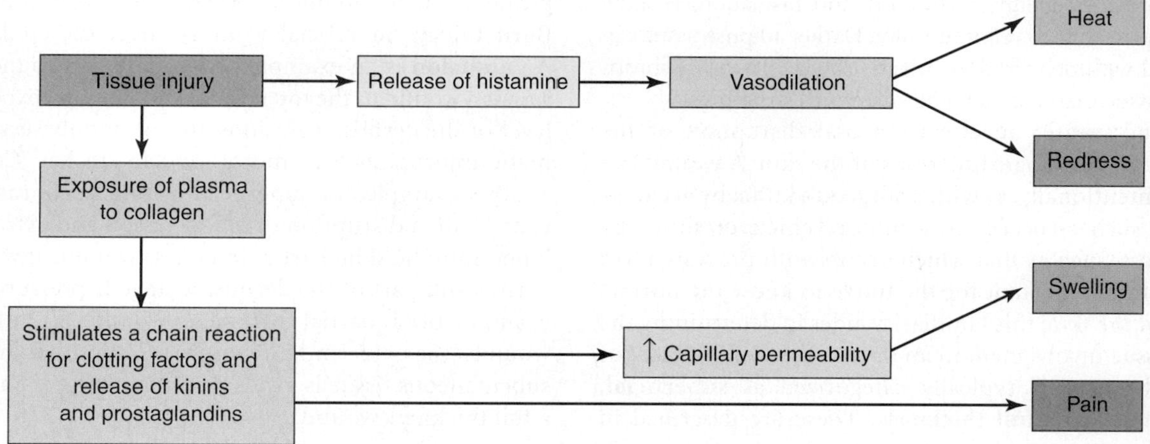

Figure 35–2 ■ Basic inflammatory response produces the four cardinal signs of inflammation. The chemical and vascular events that occur during the reaction phase of wound healing produce the four cardinal signs of inflammation.

to bring needed nutrients, chemical, and white blood cells (WBCs) to the injured area. WBCs quickly adhere to the endothelium and begin to control any bacterial contamination that has gained entry into the wound. Macrophages appear and begin to engulf and remove dead tissue. The chemical and vascular events that occur during the reaction phase of wound healing produce the four cardinal signs of inflammation: heat, redness, swelling, and pain (Fig. 35–2).

An example of a wound in the inflammatory phase of wound healing is shown in Figure 35–3. Inflammation is essential to the healing process. Therefore use of anti-inflammatory drugs to relieve the symptoms should be used cautiously. It is only when the inflammation is excessive or prolonged that negative consequences occur (Myers, 2008b).

Proliferative Phase

The **proliferative phase** begins several days after injury and continues for several weeks. Major processes that occur during this phase are focused on building new tissue to fill the wound space and restoring a functional barrier. The key cell during this phase is the fibroblast, a connective tissue cell that synthesizes and secretes the collagen, proteoglycans, and glycoproteins needed for wound healing (Porth & Sommer, 2009). Major events that occur during this phase include angiogenesis, epithelialization, collagen formation, granulation tissue formation, and contraction.

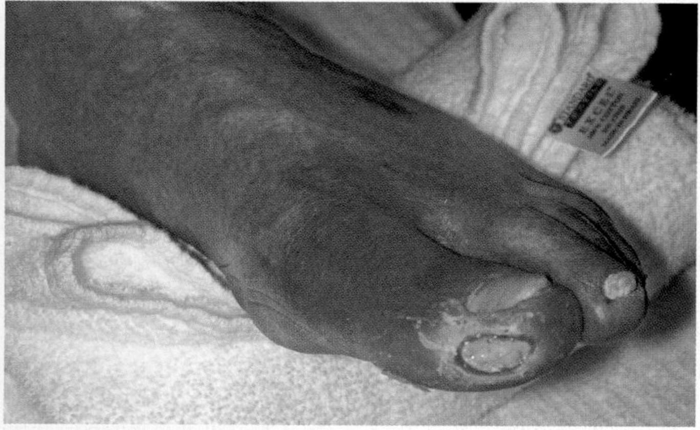

Figure 35–3 ■ Example of a wound in the inflammatory phase of wound healing. The great toe is warm to the touch. Notice the redness and edema surround the great toe. Additionally the patient reports the great toe is tender to the touch.

Angiogenesis is the formation of new blood vessels in order to reestablish perfusion to the wound bed. The process is driven by growth factors, cytokines, and the hypoxic gradient that exists from the healthy tissue near the wound to the center of the wound. Capillary buds arise from venules in close proximity to the wound bed. Capillary formation is then followed by the creation of arterioles, which grow to form a network across the wound and eventually undergo reanastamosis with preexisting vessels. The tissue is fragile and bleeds easily because of the numerous capillary buds (Porth & Sommer, 2009).

Epithelialization involves the migration of epithelial cells across a wound's surface. The cells rapidly undergo mitotic divisions and migrate along fibrin strands to reestablish layers of epithelium in an attempt to cover the defect. A moist environment enhances epithelialization. Epithelial cells cannot spread on a surface laden with debris or bacteria. Therefore, the healing process will be inhibited by the presence of debris or bacteria. The process of epithelialization serves to provide a barrier against the external environment and further bacterial invasion.

The proliferative phase provides strength to the healing wound. The dominant cells of this phase are fibroblasts. Fibroblasts produce **collagen,** the major component of new connective tissue. Fluid collections, hematomas, dead tissue, and foreign materials act as physical barriers that prevent fibroblast penetration. Therefore, one of the primary goals of wound management is removal of these materials. The wound space fills with fiber bundles that enlarge and form a dense collagenous structure (the scar) that binds the tissues firmly together.

As the population of fibroblasts decreases, collagen fibers become dominant in the wound. Collagen cross-linking provides tensile strength to the wound. Collagen requires several nutrients and minerals for its synthesis. Thus, the nutritional status of the patient becomes very important during wound healing. This is discussed in greater detail in Section Three.

At the same time that epithelialization is occurring and collagen is forming, the formation of **granulation tissue** continues. The vascular endothelium proliferates, and a great deal of capillary budding appears. These buds give the new granulation tissue its characteristic pink-red color and appearance. As new granulation tissue fills in the wound, the wound margins begin to contract or pull together, and the surface area of the wound decreases.

Contraction of a wound occurs when the wound margins begin to pull toward the center of the wound to decrease the wound surface area. The amount of wound contraction is determined by the size, shape, and depth of the wound. Linear wounds contract faster than square wounds and circular shaped wounds contract the slowest (Myers, 2008b). Shrinkage of the wound progresses from the wound's edges to heal open defects.

Remodeling/Maturation

Usually by the third week after a disruption in skin integrity, the wound has closed and the remodeling phase begins. **Remodeling/maturation** is the final repair process. This phase can last months to years. Major events of this final phase include increased collagen reorganization and increased tensile strength. The final product of all the events that occur during wound healing is the scar, which has covered the defect and restored the protective barrier against the external environment. Factors affecting the final appearance of the scar include wound tension, body location, and wound closure technique. Even when the wound is completely healed, only about 80 percent of the tensile strength of normal skin is regained and the patient is at risk for recurrent breakdown (Brown, 2009a).

Methods of Wound Closure

Methods of wound closure include primary intention, secondary intention, and tertiary intention (Fig. 35–4). The rate of wound healing differs depending on the method used to close the wound. The method used depends on the amount of tissue damage or loss and the potential for wound infection.

Primary intention refers to closing the wound by mechanical means. This method is used when there is minimal tissue loss and skin edges are well approximated. Clean lacerations and most surgical incisions are closed using primary intention.

Mechanical means used to close wounds include tape, sutures, staples, or glue. Taping with microporous tape (steri-strips) is best used in areas that are not over hairy surfaces or joints. However, these tapes cannot be exposed to water and frequently fall off. Benzoin placed on the skin prior to tape application may prevent the tape from falling off. Suturing is the most common technique to close wounds to heal by primary intention. Absorbable sutures are used to close dermal and subcutaneous layers and nonabsorbable sutures are used for external closure. Staples allow for rapid closure and are typically used on the extremities, torso, or scalp. Tissue glue (Dermabond) can be applied topically along the wound.

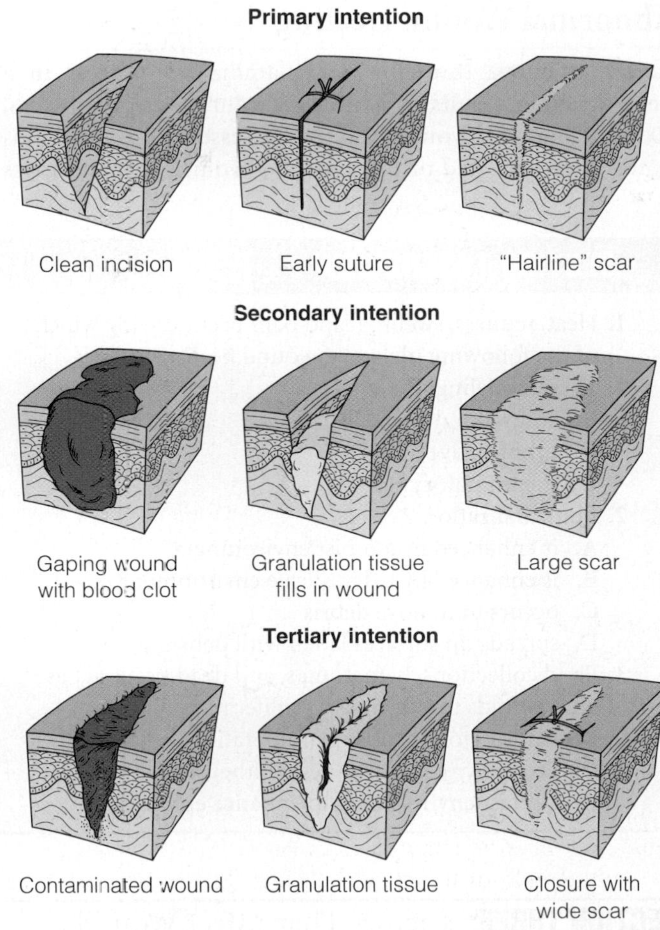

Figure 35–4 ■ Wound healing by primary, secondary, and tertiary intention.

Wounds that repair by primary intention progress through the normal phases of wound healing in an efficient fashion. However, the open tissue defect is rather small which decreases the distance new blood vessels and epithelial cells must migrate. Proliferation consists mainly of reepithelialization across the incision and begins within 24 hours of approximation (Myers, 2008b).

Wounds that heal by **secondary intention** usually are large wounds in which there is significant tissue loss, damage, or bacterial contamination. These wound cavities heal gradually and use the biological phases of wound healing to fill in the cavity or defect. Wounds healing by secondary intention include open abdominal wounds, dehisced sternal wounds, and stages III and IV pressure ulcers. These wounds require significantly more time to heal than do wounds healing by primary intention. The time to wound closure is determined by the rate of wound contraction and depth of tissue loss (Myers, 2008b).

Tertiary intention is a method of wound closure that uses a combination of primary and secondary intention. The wound is left open for a short period of time, usually a few days, to allow edema and exudate to resolve. The wound is packed with dressings that are changed to remove any debris and is closed later by primary intention. If the wound is contaminated, this technique may be used to decrease the bacterial load in the wound.

Abnormal Wound Healing

Failure to move through the inflammatory process in a timely fashion results in abnormal wound healing (Myers, 2008b). Abnormal wound healing is assessed if progression is slower than expected or by observing wound characteristics for atypical characteristics of each phase of wound healing (Myers, 2008b). Wounds with signs of abnormal healing should be inspected for underlying local or systemic factors that interfere with wound healing. These factors are discussed in Section Three.

SECTION TWO REVIEW

1. Heat, redness, swelling, and pain occur during which of the following phases of wound healing?
   A. remodeling
   B. contraction
   C. proliferative
   D. inflammatory
2. Epithelialization
   A. is enhanced by a moist environment
   B. is enhanced by a dry, sterile environment
   C. occurs to remove debris
   D. spreads on surfaces laden with debris
3. Fluid collections, hematomas, and dead tissue act as
   A. scaffolds for fibroblast proliferation
   B. barriers for fibroblast proliferation
   C. protective covers for new epithelial cells
   D. a moist environment to enhance epithelialization
4. An incision for a cholecystectomy usually would be allowed to heal by
   A. tertiary intention
   B. secondary intention
   C. primary intention
   D. delayed secondary intention
5. Delayed primary (tertiary) intention allows
   A. immediate resolution of the inflammatory phase
   B. edema and exudate to resolve
   C. gradual healing of the wound
   D. reorganization and cell differentiation for remodeling

Answers: 1. D, 2. A, 3. B, 4. C, 5. B

SECTION THREE: Factors That Affect Wound Healing

At the completion of this section, the learner will be able to state physiologic and environmental factors that affect wound healing.

Acutely ill patients experience many risk factors that increase their risk for impaired wound healing. These include impaired oxygenation, compromised nutritional status, age, preexisting disease, medications, and obesity. These risk factors increase the risk of delayed wound healing, development of wound infections, and wound dehiscence. It is a nursing challenge to provide the optimal environment that supports the wound healing process.

Oxygenation/Tissue Perfusion

Many drugs and treatments have been investigated to accelerate healing. However, perfusion of injured tissue with well-oxygenated blood may be most important. Adequate oxygen supply to wounds is required by immune and inflammatory cells to produce proteins, reestablish vascular structure and epithelium, and provide resistance to bacterial invasion of the wound space (Whitney, 2003). Adequate oxygenation promotes neovascularization and optimizes collagen deposition, which increases the tensile strength of wound beds (Gordillo & Sen, 2003). Adequate levels of oxygen in wound beds also act as a major determinant of susceptibility to infection (Gordillo & Sen, 2003). Furthermore, wounds in ischemic tissue become infected more frequently than wounds in well-oxygenated tissue (Porth & Sommer, 2009).

Availability of oxygen to tissue and wound beds depends on vascular supply, vasomotor tone, arterial oxygen tension, and the diffusion distance for oxygen to cross the capillary membrane. Edema and necrotic debris increase the diffusion distance for oxygen to reach cells in the wound. For optimal wound perfusion and oxygenation, patients must be warm, have adequate intravascular volume, and have adequate control of pain and anxiety. Stress associated with cold, pain, and fear cause peripheral vasoconstriction and can decrease oxygen delivery to wounds. Additionally, the nurse should ensure a warm environment for the patient with a wound, not only in his/her room, but also during invasive procedures and during transport.

Many conditions interfere with the delivery of oxygen to the wound (e.g., thrombosis, radiation, obesity, diabetes, cardiovascular disease, cigarette smoking, hypotension, hypothermia, and administration of vasoactive drugs). Significant blood loss, as frequently occurs in traumatically injured patients, results in hypovolemia, hypotension, and decreased tissue perfusion. Poor glycemic control and diabetic neuropathy place the diabetic patient at increased risk for traumatic injury, particularly to the feet, and subsequent poor healing. Smoking adversely affects wound healing. Toxins of greatest concern include nicotine and carbon monoxide. Nicotine causes vasoconstriction and decreased tissue perfusion. Carbon monoxide combines with hemoglobin, inhibits the binding with oxygen, and decreases the oxygen-carrying capacity of hemoglobin; all contribute to decreased oxygen delivery to wound beds. Smoking also increases platelet adhesiveness, making them more "sticky," setting up a situation of microclots in small vessels that decrease oxygen delivery.

Hyperbaric oxygen therapy (HBOT) is a treatment to improve oxygen delivery to wounds and promote wound healing. It is used in conjunction with standard wound care. HBOT delivers 100 percent oxygen at two to three atmospheres of pressure. This exposes tissues to greater concentrations of oxygen than would otherwise be possible and essentially "hypersaturates" the bloodstream with oxygen. HBOT can increase arterial oxygen tension to 1,200 mm Hg (Gordillo & Sen, 2003). This increase in oxygen tension encourages wound healing, enhances neutrophil actions to kill bacteria, impairs growth of anaerobic bacteria and promotes angiogenesis and fibroblast activity (Porth & Sommer, 2009). Patients typically require mulitple treatments, each lasting an hour or more, performed in specialized chambers at facilities equipped with a hyperbaric oxygen chamber. HBOT is useful for resolution of hypoxic conditions, such as gas gangrene, necrotizing fasciitis, traumatic crush injuries, and carbon monoxide poisoning.

Nutrition

Adequate nutrition is a critical factor predisposing the acutely ill patient to immunocompetence and poor wound healing. It is essential to ensure that patients with wounds receive adequate nutritional support.

Metabolic processes involved in wound healing rely heavily on adequate nutritional substances. Physiologic and psychological stress, traumatic injury, and fever further increase the basal metabolic rate, demanding adequate nutritional reserves. Because of these demands, malnutrition in the acutely ill patient is common. During the wound healing process, the main components of energy requirements emanate from collagen synthesis. Large, complicated wounds or thermal injuries require a significant amount of energy to heal the wound. Active cells require energy to function, with carbohydrates being the preferred fuel source (Myers, 2008c). A sufficient amount of protein is another important nutritional substance for wound healing. Protein is required for collagen synthesis, immune responses, formation of granulation tissue, and fibroblast proliferation. It is desirable for patients to maintain a positive nitrogen balance to enhance wound healing. Protein deficiencies prolong the inflammatory phase of wound healing and impair fibroblast proliferation, collagen and protein matrix synthesis, angiogenesis and wound remodeling (Porth & Sommer, 2009). Patients with draining wounds lose vital nutrients and protein. Every reasonable effort is made to quantify the loss so that correctional measures are instituted. Frequently, amino acid supplementation is prescribed to enhance the functioning of growth factors and immune cells, and to support the collagen deposition. Serum albumin levels reflect the level of visceral protein stores. Because the half-life of albumin is 18 to 21 days, a prealbumin is ordered in a high-acuity setting. The half-life of prealbumin is only one to two days. This allows for a more accurate prescription of protein replacement. Glycolysis contributes the majority of the energy needed for restoring tissue integrity and fighting infection. Fats serve as building blocks for prostaglandins, which regulate cell metabolism, inflammation, and circulation. Vitamins and trace elements are necessary for numerous events in the tissue healing and rebuilding process.

TABLE 35–1 The Roles of Vitamins in Wound Healing

Vitamin A	Collagen synthesis Promotes tissue formation Facilitates epithelialization Enhances macrophage function Reverses inhibitory effects of long-term corticosteroid therapy Increases wound tensile strength Decreases risk of wound dehiscence
Vitamin C	Helps the body absorb iron Required for collagen synthesis Activates WBCs and enhances their migration into wounds Limits damage from oxygen free radicals
Vitamin K	Essential for blood clotting Deficiencies can lengthen the inflammatory phase
B Complex	Aids in WBC function, antibody formation, resistance to infection Facilitates fibroblast function and collagen synthesis Improves wound tensile strength
Vitamin E	Prevents oxygen free-radical related cellular damage Decreases platelet adhesion

Vitamins are needed to build new tissues and aide in normal immune funtion. Vitamins A, C, E, K and B complex vitamins are especially important for wound healing. The roles of these vitamins in wound healing, as summarized by Myers (2008d), are listed in Table 35–1.

Age

Aging affects almost every stage of wound healing; the wound healing process is markedly slower as patients age. Patients with advanced age have reduced collagen and fibroblast synthesis, impaired wound contraction, and slower reepithelialization of open wounds (Porth & Sommer, 2009). In addition to the physiologic effects of aging, people with advancing age are more likely to have nutritional deficiencies and pulmonary or cardiovascular diseases that further diminish local oxygenation to wounds and immunologic resistance.

Diabetes

Wound healing in the patient with diabetes is compromised as a result of macrovascular and microvascular changes, poor glycemic control, and loss of sensation. These disease-associated changes result in impaired oxygenation and perfusion, slowed epithelialization and wound contraction, and impaired phagocytosis. Glucose levels have direct effects on several phases of wound healing, and the importance of glycemic control cannot be overstated. The nurse caring for the acutely ill diabetic patient with a wound can achieve a significant, positive impact on wound healing through scrupulous glucose monitoring and maximizing glycemic control.

Medications

Steroid therapy, used to block the inflammatory component of many diseases, has a well-known inhibitory effect on wound healing.

Decreased protein synthesis, delayed development of granulation tissue, inhibition of fibroblast proliferation, and reduced epithelialization are effects of steroid administration. In addition, inhibition of the inflammatory response and the immunosuppressive actions of steroids make the patient more susceptible to developing a wound infection. There is some disagreement as to whether nonsteroidal anti-inflammatory medications impact wound healing. While these medications are given to decrease inflammation, there is little evidence that they directly affect the inflammatory phase of wound healing. Other medications that interfere with wound healing include chemotherapeutic agents, immunosuppressive drugs, and anticoagulants.

Obesity

The obese patient (weight greater than 20 percent ideal body weight) experiences an increased incidence of dehiscence, herniation, and infection. Adipose tissue is poorly vascularized, which increases the risk of ischemia. Adipose tissue is difficult to suture, which makes the obese patient at risk to develop a wound dehiscence. A binder or splint (pillow) to the incision provides support during straining or coughing and takes excess tension off the incision.

Blood Chemistries

Normal serum electrolytes enhance wound repair. Potassium is necessary for building proteins for wound repair. Phagocytosis is inhibited by elevated sodium and glucose levels. Oxygen is released more rapidly from oxyhemoglobin in slightly acidic environments. Wounds may heal more effectively in this type of local environment.

Moisture

Water is absolutely vital to wound healing. Dehydration results in impaired wound healing. Patients with severe pressure ulcers who are on air-fluidized beds or specialty beds require up to 40 to 60 mL of water per kilogram of body weight to counteract the dehydrating effect of the bed (Myers, 2008d). The rate of epithelialization is enhanced in a moist, not dry, local wound environment. A wound bed is kept moist through the use of appropriate dressings. Ideally, the dressing will keep the wound surface moist without accumulation of excessive fluids that macerate the skin and allow bacterial proliferation.

Emerging Evidence

- Hyperspectral imaging is a new noninvasive technology that provides an assessment of oxygenation and microcirculation status and provides information predictive of wound healing potential. This technology measures the amount of oxyghemoglobin in wound tissues. Preliminary analysis demonstrates a positive predictive value for wound healing when oxyhemoglobin levels are greater than 65 percent. Further research will give more information about the usefulness and accuracy of this technology *(Nouvong, 2008)*.
- Wound assessment pH measured with litmus paper strips may be a useful assessment tool for wound healing. As wound condition improved and exudate levels decreased, the pH of wound reduced to less than 8.0. This change in pH may help predict the likelihood of wound healing *(Shukla, Shukla, Tiwany et al., 2007)*.
- Patients undergoing cardiac surgery are at significant risk for developing pressure ulcers postoperatively as a result of comorbidities and perioperative factors (extracorporeal circulation, hypothermia, use of vasopressors). The use of a fluid, pressure-reducing mattress in the operating room reduced the incidence of development of postoperative pressure ulcers in cardiac surgery patients *(Sewchuk, Padula, & Osborne, 2006)*.

SECTION THREE REVIEW

1. Small-vessel changes occur that impair tissue perfusion/oxygenation with
   A. malnutrition
   B. elevated sodium levels
   C. diabetes
   D. steroid therapy
2. The most important nutritional substance for wound healing is
   A. glucose
   B. fat
   C. vitamins
   D. protein
3. Which of the following is NOT an effect of steroid therapy on wound healing?
   A. decreased protein synthesis
   B. proliferation of fibroblasts
   C. delayed development of granulation tissue
   D. reduced epithelialization
4. The most important factor that affects wound healing is
   A. preventing infection
   B. total parenteral nutrition
   C. perfusion of injured tissues with well-oxygenated blood
   D. potassium replacements
5. A moist wound environment
   A. enhances epithelialization
   B. macerates the skin
   C. promotes bacterial proliferation
   D. impedes epithelialization

Answers: 1. C, 2. D, 3. B, 4. C, 5. A

SECTION FOUR: Clinical Assessment of Wound Healing

At the completion of this section, the learner will be able to identify the common clinical assessments to evaluate wound healing.

In assessing wound healing, it is important to assess the patient's preexisting health problems; perform a physical assessment of the wound using inspection and palpation; and collect and evaluate objective data to assess the patient's tissue perfusion/oxygenation, immunologic, and nutritional status. Systematic assessment and comprehensive evaluation of both patient and wound provide a consistent method for assessing wound healing.

Preexisting Health Problems

In collecting the initial nursing database, it is important to assess the patient for diseases, conditions, and medications or treatments that may impair the healing process, as discussed in Section Three. This will assist in identifying patients at risk for impaired wound healing. It is important to assess for conditions that alter tissue perfusion/oxygenation and impair the body's resistance to infection.

Inspection

Wounds, suture lines, casts, pins, and surrounding skin integrity are inspected for signs of infection, breakdown, and irritation. Inspect wounds to assess and evaluate the healing process and the effectiveness of wound care. Inspection includes at least the following components.

Measurement of the Wound

Wound size is a major indicator of improvement or decline in wound status. Measure and record the length, width, and depth of the wound. Measure the wound from the widest width perpendicular to its length (see Fig. 35–5). The amount and depth of tissue loss are assessed because these greatly influence the choice of treatment for wound management. Depth can be determined by inserting a sterile, cotton-tipped applicator into the deepest part of the wound and grasping the applicator where it meets the wound's edge (as shown in Fig. 35–6). Irregular wound beds are difficult to measure accurately, so it is important to take measurements of depth and length from the same point each time.

Wound tracings can also be used to measure wound size. A clean tranparency and permanent marker are required. There are several commercially available wound tracing sheets. Plastic wrap can also be used. The transparency or plastic wrap are placed on the wound and the wound is traced (see Fig. 35–7). The entire wound bed should be probed for the presence of **tunneling.** Tunneling is a narrow passageway created by the separation of, or destruction to, facial planes. It is measured by inserting a probe (or cotton tip swab) into the passageway until resistance is met, as shown in figures 35–8 and 35–9.

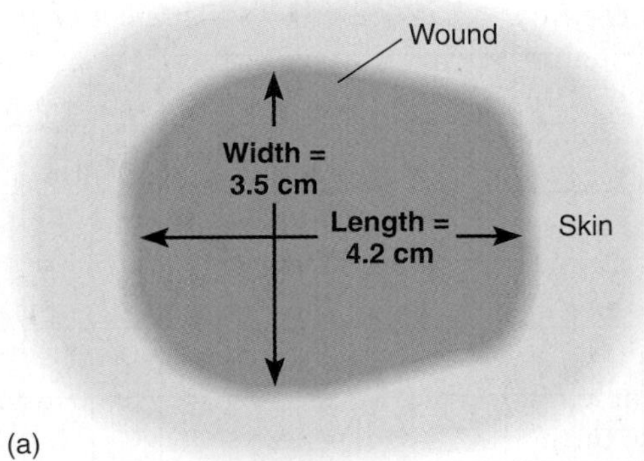

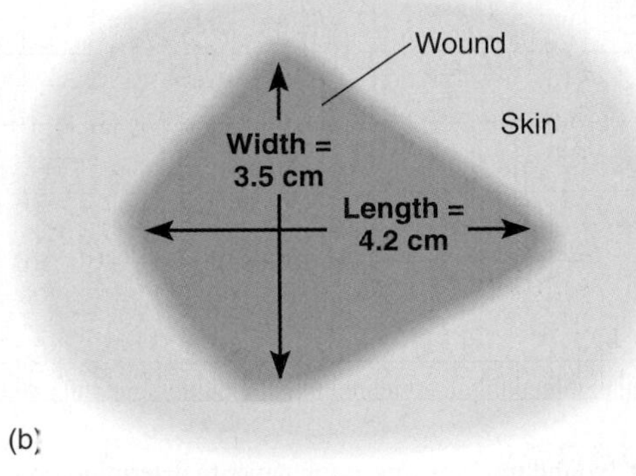

Figure 35–5 ■ Measurement of wound size.

Presence of Exudate or Drainage

Estimating the amount of blood and fluid loss allows for appropriate fluid and electrolyte replacement. The fluid produced by wounds is called **exudate;** it can consist of blood, serum, serosanguineous fluid, and leukocytes. Exudate bathes the wound continuously, keeping it moist, supplying nutrients and providing the best conditions for migration and mitosis of epithelial cells and control of bacteria at the wound surface. Documentation of all wound drainage includes color, amount, consistency, and odor. The amount of drainage is estimated as "mild," "moderate," or "heavy," and the presence or absence of odor is documented. In some cases, wound drainage can be

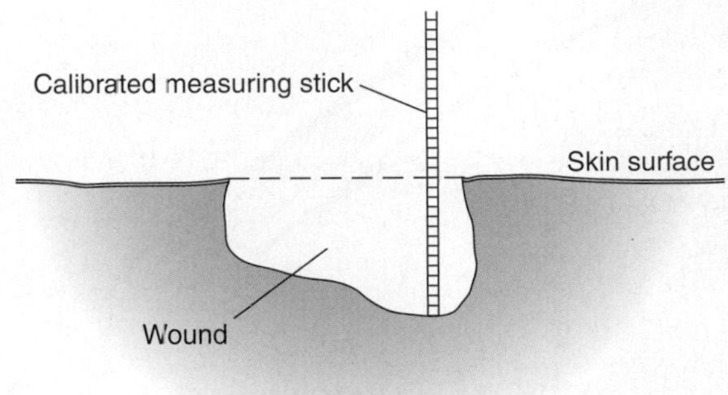

Figure 35–6 ■ Measurement of wound depth. It is documented as level of wound depth (e.g. wound depth 1.4 cm).

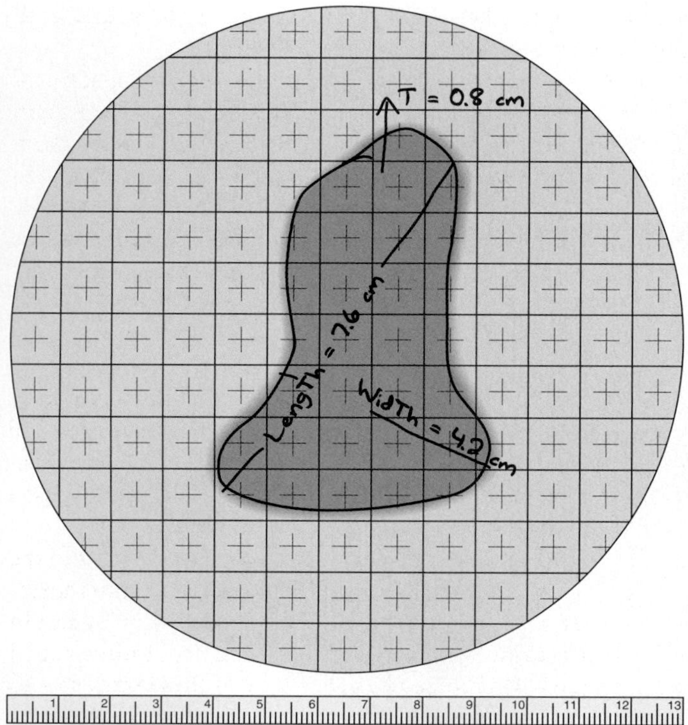

Figure 35–7 ■ Wound tracing using graph paper to determine wound area.

measured more accurately if a wound manager is used with a canister to collect the drainage.

Appearance of Wound Tissue

Wound color depends on the balance between granulation and necrotic tissue. Healing wounds are pink or "beefy" red, characteristic of granulation tissue. Granulation tissue that is pale or dusky has poor blood supply. In the presence of moisture and bacteria, exudate and devitalized tissue are yellow or cream-colored and puslike in consistency. This is **slough.** Black or dark-brown color indicates the presence of **eschar,** which is thick, nonpliable necrotic tissue. Slough and necrotic tissue have a negative effect on wound healing because they prevent granulation and epithelialization. The ideal local wound environment should be free from slough and eschar and be moist with red-pink budding granulation tissue.

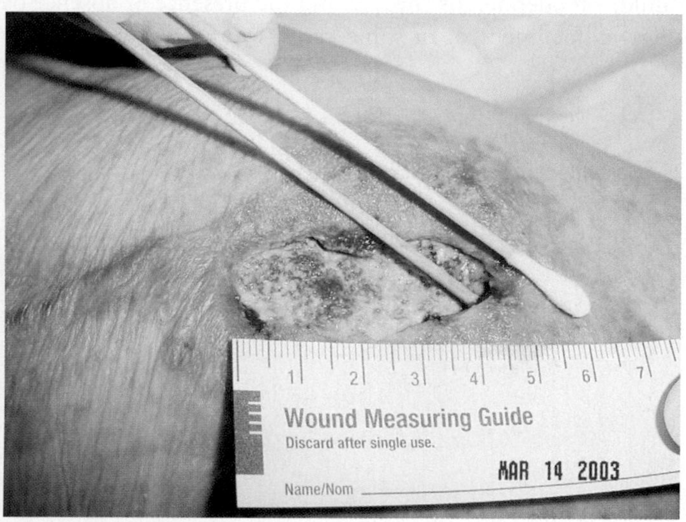

Figure 35–8 ■ Tunneling wound.

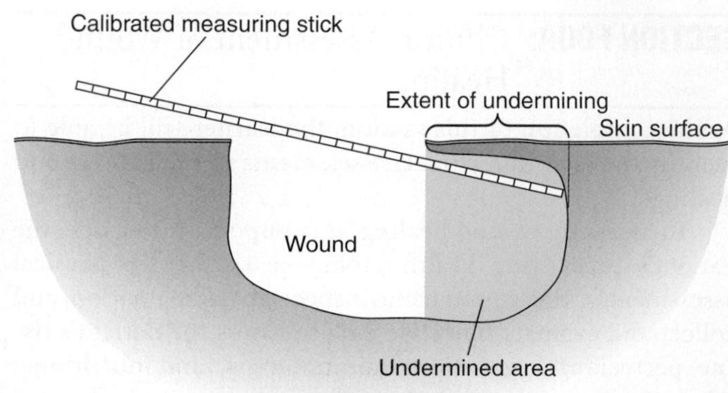

Figure 35–9 ■ Cross-sectional schematic of a wound with tunneling. Documentation must include the tunnel's depth and position within the wound bed, most commonly using clock terms: "wound tunnels at 3 o'clock position."

Inspection of Wound Edges

Impaired periwound skin integrity compromises and complicates wound healing and contracture. Inspect the wound for contraction (gradual healing from the edges to the center of the wound), and assess for gradual healing from the interior to the surfaces of deep wounds. Wound margins should not be erythematous or tender; nor should the wound margins have evidence of **maceration.** Maceration is evident when the periwound skin is white or pale. This occurs when drainage from the wound has prolonged contact with healthy skin tissue around the wound. If not stopped, macerated skin leads to altered skin integrity and further wound compromise. The periwound skin integrity can also be altered by frequent tape removal. Simple measures to protect the periwound area include the use of skin barriers before application of tape or other adhesives or the use of other protectant agents prior to covering the wound.

Palpation

Palpation of the wound and surrounding areas assists in recognizing changes in size, consistency, moisture, and texture. If bone is visible or palpable, it is highly probable that osteomyelitis exists and needs to be reported to the health care provider. To assess circulation into and from the wound, assess the proximal and distal pulses by palpation or by doppler. Proximal pulses demonstrate adequate circulation to the area. Capillary refill time is assessed. Compare the skin temperature bilaterally. Sensorimotor assessment distal to the wound is done by testing for discrimination between sharp and dull pressures.

Assessment of Tissue Perfusion/ Oxygenation Status

Adequate tissue perfusion/oxygenation is the most important factor to assess for in wound healing. Local and systemic factors that alter tissue perfusion and oxygenation are assessed. Necrotic areas, debris, and foreign materials in the wound do not allow adequate local tissue perfusion/oxygenation. Adequate systemic tissue perfusion/oxygenation depends on a full blood volume, adequate arterial oxygen content, and an adequate cardiac output. The nurse should assess capillary refill, skin temperature, and the presence of proximal and distal pulses around the wound. However, caution should be exercised because the presence of palpable pulses is not necessarily an accurate indicator of sufficient circulation to the wound (Myers, 2008c).

Assessment of Immunologic Status

An intact immunologic response to injury, regardless of the cause of injury, is a key factor in proper wound healing. The patient is assessed for the three elements that predispose the patient to a wound infection: susceptible host, compromised wound, and infectious organism. Factors that cause local and systemic resistance of infection are assessed. Compromised wounds containing devitalized tissue, hematomas, and debris are debrided to prevent an environment conducive to bacterial proliferation. The patient is assessed for sources of pathogenic organisms.

Assessment of immunologic status includes WBC, fibrinogen, body temperature, wound cultures, and serum antimicrobial levels. The inflammatory phase of wound healing releases WBCs. It is not uncommon for patients with wounds to have elevated WBC counts during the initial phase of wound healing. Elevated WBCs in later phases of wound healing are more indicative of an infectious process.

Neutrophils are the primary cells involved in phagocytosis. Elevated neutrophil counts are indicative of an acute infection as mature and immature neutrophils are released in response to an increased need for phagocytosis. Neutrophils are essential in the presence of infection if wound healing is to occur. Adequate amounts of fibrinogen are needed to convert to fibrin. This aids in localizing the infectious process by providing a matrix for phagocytosis.

Increased body temperature is triggered by microorganisms, bacterial toxins and antigens, and the inflammatory process. Because fever is a manifestation of the inflammatory process and the infectious process, it is important to assess the patient's overall clinical picture for etiologic factors of the fever. Patients in a hypothermic state experience decreased tissue perfusion/oxygenation and decreased leukocyte activity.

Monitoring concentrations of antimicrobial agents in the blood confirms therapeutic drug levels and determines toxicity. The best assessment of this can be made by drawing serum peak and trough samples, depending on the antimicrobial administered. The nurse must be aware of these protocols so that accurate therapeutic concentrations and toxicity can be assessed.

Assessment of Nutritional Status

The metabolic processes involved in wound healing rely on an adequate nutritional supply. Malnutrition affects the patient's ability to defend against pathogenic microorganisms. A complete and thorough nutritional assessment for all patients with altered skin and tissue integrity is made. Nutritional assessment is discussed in detail in Module 32, Determinants and Assessment of Nutrition and Metabolic Function.

SECTION FOUR REVIEW

1. In assessing wound healing, it is important to assess the patient's
   A. medical history
   B. renal status
   C. mental status
   D. fluid and electrolyte balance
2. Assessment of a wound bed reveals yellow-colored tissue that is stringy and puslike. What term would you use to describe this assessment in your documentation?
   A. infection
   B. eschar
   C. slough
   D. macerated tissue
3. If a wound is suspected as being infected
   A. the WBC and core temperature will be high
   B. there will be exudate in the wound
   C. antimicrobial levels should be drawn
   D. wound cultures should be taken
4. Which of the following techniques can be used to assess size of the wound? (choose all that apply)
   A. measure from widest width perpendicular to its length
   B. clean, transparency tracing
   C. plastic wrap
   D. relate to a common object, such as size of a quarter
5. In assessing a wound, the nurse notes that the wound contains granulation tissue that is pale and dusky. What is the cause of this?
   A. drainage in the wound
   B. maceration
   C. infection
   D. poor blood supply

Answers: 1. A, 2. C, 3. D, 4. (A, B, C) 5. D

POSTTEST

1. Dark grey adipose tissue may be a sign of
   A. infection
   B. fluid volume excess
   C. fluid volume deficit
   D. lack of vitamin B
2. Which of the following wounds is an example of a full thickness skin loss?
   A. abrasion
   B. contusion
   C. stage II pressure ulcer
   D. avulsion
3. Epithelialization
   A. occurs even in the presence of debris
   B. spreads on surfaces laden with bacteria
   C. is enhanced by a moist environment
   D. provides a barrier against the external environment
4. A patient has undergone an open appendectomy. Most likely, his incision would be allowed to heal by
   A. primary intention
   B. secondary intention
   C. delayed primary (tertiary) intention
   D. delayed secondary intention
5. Which of the following are signs of inflammation?
   A. heat
   B. redness
   C. edema
   D. pain
6. Which of the following wounds would heal the slowest?
   A. linear wound
   B. square wound
   C. circular wound
   D. all the above
7. Of the factors that affect wound healing, which of the following has been found to be the most important?
   A. age
   B. normal serum potassium levels
   C. moisture
   D. adequate tissue perfusion
8. Which of the following vitamins improve wound tensile strength? (choose all that apply)
   A. vitamin A
   B. vitamin B
   C. vitamin C
   D. vitamin E
9. Patients on air-fluidized beds are at risk for impaired wound healing as a result of
   A. immobility
   B. dehydration
   C. moist wound environment
   D. pain
10. The nurse assesses a wound and notes the wound bed has pale granulation tissue. What assessment should the nurse do next? (choose all that apply)
    A. Assess for local and systemic factors that impair tissue perfusion.
    B. Assess for elements that predispose the patient to a wound infection.
    C. Assess for the presence of tunneling.
    D. Assess for the presence of eschar.
11. The nurse assesses the wound margins and notes the periwound skin is white and pale. What could cause this?
    A. infection
    B. prolonged contact with wound drainage
    C. this is a normal part of the healing process.
    D. frequent tape removal
12. Why is it important to remove devitalized tissue and debris in a wound? (choose all that apply)
    A. They improve the appearance of the wound.
    B. They impair epithelialization.
    C. They provide an environment conducive to bacterial proliferation.
    D. It is not important to remove these substances.

Posttest answers with rationale are found on MyNursingKit.

REFERENCES

Brown, P. (2009). Normal healing process. In P. Brown (ed.), *Quick reference to wound care* (3rd ed.). Sudbury, Mass: Jones and Bartlett Publishers, 17–21

Gordillo, G. M., & Sen, C. K. (2003). Revisiting the essential role of oxygen in wound healing. *American Journal of Surgery, 186,* 259–263.

Nouvong, A. (2008). Hyperspectral imaging for evaluating tissue oxygenation. *Podiatry Management,* August, 111–115.

Myers, B. A. (2008a). Integumentary anatomy. In B. A. Myers (ed.), *Wound management: principles and practice* (2d ed.). Upper Saddle River, NJ: Pearson Education, 3–10.

Myers, B. A. (2008b). Wound healing, In B. A. Myers (ed.), *Wound management: principles and practice* (2d ed.). Upper Saddle River, NJ: Pearson Education, 11–24.

Myers, B. A. (2008c). Factors affecting wound healing. In B. A. Myers (ed.), *Wound management: principles and practice* (2d ed.). Upper Saddle River, NJ: Pearson Education, 25–37.

Myers, B. A. (2008d). Holistic management of patients with wounds. In B. A. Myers (ed.), *Wound management: principles and practice* (2d ed.). Upper Saddle River, NJ: Pearson Education, 196–213.

Porth, C. M. & Sommer, C. (2009). Inflammation, tissue repair, and wound healing. In C. M. Porth & Matfin, G. (eds.), *Pathophysiology: concepts of altered health states* (5th ed.). Philadelphia, PA: Wolters Luwer Health/Lippincott, Williams, & Wilkins, 377–399.

Sewchuk, D., Padula, C., Osborne, E. (2006). Prevention and early detection of pressure ulcers in patients undergoing cardiac surgery. *AORN Journal 84*(1), 75–96.

Skukla, V. K., Shukla, D., Tiwary, S. K., et al. (2007). Evaluation of pH measurements as a method of wound assessment. *J Wound Care 16*(7), 291–294.

Whitney, J. D. (2003). Supplemental perioperative oxygen and fluids to improve surgical wound outcomes: translating research into practice. *Wound Repair and Regeneration, 11,* 462–467.

MODULE

36 Alterations in Skin Integrity: Complex Wound Management

Karen L. Johnson

OBJECTIVES

Following completion of this module, the learner will be able to

1. Discuss the rationale for various treatment modalities used in wound management.
2. Identify conditions that predispose a patient to developing a wound infection.
3. Identify criteria used to diagnose a wound infection.
4. State interventions that can be used to treat wound infections.
5. Identify risk factors and causes of necrotizing fasciitis and Fournier's gangrene.
6. Describe the clinical presentation of necrotizing fasciitis and Fournier's gangrene.
7. Discuss the treatment options and nursing care for patients with necrotizing fasciitis and Fournier's gangrene.
8. Identify the risk factors for the development of an enterocutaneous fistula.
9. Recognize the signs of symptoms of an enterocutaneous fistula.
10. Discuss the treatment strategies for enterocutaneous fistulas including fluid and electrolyte replacement, nutritional support and complex wound management.

This self-study module focuses on complex wound management and the unique needs of the high-acuity patient population with infections, necrosis and fistulas. For nursing care of patients with simple wound management needs and for patients with pressure ulcers, the reader is referred to a general medical-surgical nursing textbook. The module is composed of four sections. Section One reviews the principles of wound management including the rationale for wound cleansing, wound debridement and dressing changes. Section Two reviews the etiology, diagnosis and treatment of wound infections, with an emphasis on resistant organisms. Section Three discusses the risk factors, clinical presentation, treatment options, and nursing care for high-acuity patients with necrotizing soft-tissue infections. This section focuses on patients with necrotizing fasciitis and Fournier's gangrene, otherwise known as "flesh-eating bacteria" and emphasizes the importance of treatment with broad-spectrum antibiotic administration. Section Four describes the risk factors, signs and symptoms, treatment strategies, and nursing care for the patient with an enterocutaneous fistula. Each section includes a set of review questions to help the learner evaluate his or her understanding of the section's content before moving on to the next section. All Section Reviews include answers. It is suggested that the learner review those concepts answered incorrectly in the review questions before proceeding to the next section.

PRETEST

1. Which of the following does NOT promote local wound healing?
   A. application of a heat lamp
   B. debridement with scissors
   C. irrigation with normal saline
   D. application of dressings
2. A solution used for wound irrigation that aids in mechanical debridement but does not damage granulation tissue is
   A. betadine (povidone–iodine)
   B. normal saline
   C. acetic acid
   D. hydrogen peroxide
3. A patient has an abdominal wound that is healing by secondary intention. On assessment of this wound, seropurulent drainage is noted from granulating tissue, with some necrotic tissue present. Which type of dressing would you select to remove the debris and necrotic tissue without causing harm to the granulation tissue?
   A. dry sterile dressing
   B. alginate dressing

C. synthetic dressing
D. hydrocolloid dressing

4. Necrotizing fasciitis is an infection that commonly involves the
A. lung parenchyma
B. heart
C. abdomen
D. scrotum

5. The most common organism that causes necrotizing fasciitis is
A. *staphyloccus aureus*
B. VRE
C. streptococcus
D. acinobacter

6. Which of the following assessments are associated with necrotizing fasciitis? (choose all that apply)
A. crepitus around the wound bed
B. bullae
C. blisters
D. frank purulent drainage

7. An enterocutaneous fistula is defined as
A. a fistula that drains more than 500 mL/day
B. a passageway between two segments of the bowel
C. a passageway between the colon and the perineum
D. a passageway between the bowel and the skin

8. Which of the following are important to consider when developing the plan of care for a patient with an ECF? (choose all that apply)
A. skin protection
B. drainage containment
C. drainage quantification
D. location of the ECF

9. Somatostatin is administered to patients with ECF to
A. decrease bowel motility
B. lower gastric pH content
C. decrease ECF drainage
D. protect the periwound skin integrity

Pretest answers are found on MyNursingKit.

SECTION ONE: Principles of Wound Management

At the completion of this section, the learner will be able to discuss the rationale for wound cleansing, wound debridement, and dressing changes.

The outcome of wound management is wound healing, as evidenced by a wound bed that is completely resurfaced with epithelial cells and the tissue is remodeled so that its strength approaches normal (Myers, 2008a). Nursing has a major influence on the outcome of wound healing. Nurses have the opportunity to favorably manipulate certain environmental factors that promote wound healing. This includes local wound care, which includes cleansing, debridement, and selection of appropriate wound dressing materials. The short-term goal of wound management is to obtain a clean, moist, warm, granular wound bed while protecting the periwound and intact skin (Myers, 2008a).

Wound Cleansing

Wound cleansing involves the use of nontoxic fluids to remove debris, microorganisms, contaminants, exudate, and devitalized tissue, usually by flushing the surface of the wound with an irrigating solution. The size and condition of the wound determines the method of wound cleansing. A large wound with a significant amount of necrosis requires high-pressure (8 to 15 pounds per square inch [psi]) irrigation, using enough solution to adequately remove the debris. Several devices can be used to accomplish a high-pressure irrigation, and there are numerous commercially available irrigation kits. Conversely, a 30 mL syringe used with a 19-gauge angiocath delivers about 8 psi to the wound. The fluid should be warmed to body temperature because cool fluid inhibits phagocytic and cellular growth in the wound. The goal of cleansing proliferative, granulating wounds is to remove inorganic debris from the wound using a gentle flushing technique. Wounds are not scrubbed, as this can cause trauma to healthy tissue. The use of pressures higher than 15 psi actually forces bacteria deeper into the tissue (Myers, 2008b). Whirlpool, as a method of wound cleansing, has significant limitations, including infection control, patient comfort, and the number of staff needed to perform the procedure. Pulsatile lavage with suction effectively irrigates the wound and removes fluid and debris with suction.

Sterile normal saline is the solution of choice (Myers, 2008b). Frequently used as an irrigant, saline can also be soaked in gauze and gently swiped around the wound, working from the least contaminated to the most contaminated portion of the wound. Tap water is a safe and effective alternative to sterile saline as a cleansing solution for chronic wounds without increased incidence of infection. Skin disinfectants (povidine–iodine, hydrogen peroxide, acetic acid, etc.) are not used because of toxicity to cells and potential systemic absorption of these chemicals. In particular, iodine absorbs through tissues and elevates serum levels. Diluted solutions of acetic acid and sodium hypochloride may be used. However, the concentrations needed to eliminate bacteria are often toxic to granulating cells.

Debridement

Debridement, the removal of necrotic tissue, foreign material, and debris from the wound bed, is important to healing because the presence of foreign material fosters bacterial growth and inhibits formation of granulation tissue. Wound healing cannot take place until nonviable tissue is removed. The four methods of debridement are sharp, mechanical, chemical, and autolytic. **Sharp debridement** is the removal of necrotic areas using a scapel or scissors. Sharp debridement selectively removes devitalized tissue, foreign material, and debris. **Mechanical debridement** is accomplished with moist dressing changes, irrigation, or whirlpool. **Chemical (or enzymatic) debridement** involves the use of topical enzymes that are applied to necrotic areas. This form of debridement requires an order by a health care provider. Commonly used enzymatic debriding agents include accuzyme, Gladase, Granulex spray, Panafil, and Travase. **Autolytic debridement** involves the use of dressing materials (hydrocolloid wafer, Carrington gel gauze, etc.). When applied, these dressings allow endogenous enzymes in the wound to selectively liquefy necrotic tissue. In addition, the growth factors and inflammatory cells within the wound fluid may hasten the inflammatory and proliferative phases of wound healing (Meyers, 2008a). It is vital that clinicians do not mistake the wound fluid for an infectious process. It is normal to have a fluid collection under the dressing. After removal of the dressing, the nurse should irrigate the wound with normal saline prior to assessing the wound. (Note: these dressings are to be left in place for several days and should not be removed.)

Dressings

Dressings are placed over wounds for multiple purposes, including debridement; protection from the external environment; provision of a physiological environment conducive to wound healing; and to provide immobilization, support, comfort, information regarding quality and quantity of drainage, pressure, and absorption. The goal of using dressings in wound management is to provide a moist environment at the wound surface to optimize wound healing, prevent infection, control wound drainage, and minimize scarring.

The purpose of the dressing and condition of the wound bed determine the type of dressing used. As a wound changes, the dressing care is modified. It is essential that the nurse continues to assess the patient's wound throughout the wound healing process to evaluate the effectiveness of the wound management plan.

TABLE 36–1 Wound Dressings

TYPE	INDICATIONS	CONSIDERATIONS
Wet-to-dry gauze: apply wet; remove dry	Use with wounds healing by secondary intention Removes debris and necrotic materials from wounds; use as a debriding alternative for yellow wounds	No solution should be visibly dripping from the dressing as it is placed into the wound; this retards wound closure, increases bacteria, and macerates periwound skin Gauze touching wound surfaces should be a single layer Wounds with large amounts of exudate should be dressed using gauze with large interstices; as exudate decreases, gauze with small interstices should be used
Wet-to-damp gauze: apply moist; remove moist	Use with wounds healing by secondary intention Use for mechanical debridement of red or yellow wounds Provides moist wound environment	As above Packing material is soaked in a solution, wrung out until moist, and packed into the wound If packing sticks to tissue as it is removed, remoisten it with normal saline before removing it; this will preserve regenerating tissue Continuous moist dressings can be used for protection of red wounds, for delivery of topical medications, or for autolytic debridement of yellow or black wounds May macerate periwound skin if drainage or moisture is allowed to remain in contact
Dry dressings: apply dry; remove dry	Use with wounds healing by primary intention Protects the wound during epithelialization Can be used with heavily exudating red wounds	Carefully remove dressing to avoid reopening of incision
Polyurethane films	Cutaneous wounds Minor burns Abrasions Donor sites Protects partial-thickness red wounds Protects granulation and epithelial tissue Occlusive Autolytic debridement of small, noninfected yellow wounds	Do not use with draining or infected wounds Change only if dressing leaks
Hydrocolloid	Use on moderate to heavily exudating wounds; normally used as a wound filler; most require secondary dressing	Gel-like substance becomes puslike in appearance and may even become odiferous; this should not become confused with the development of a wound infection Is water resistant and can adhere to uneven surfaces Do not use on documented or suspected infected wounds Change when leakage or dislodgment becomes apparent
Alginates	Highly absorbant secondary cover for wounds with packing	Alginates absorb secretions to form a gel that provides humidity and temperature conducive to wound healing Use gentle irrigation with normal saline to remove the dressing
Foams	Pressure ulcers Skin graft donor sites Skin tears and abrasions	Some foams have adherent border, provide thermal insulation, and absorb light to heavy amounts of exudates Effective for wounds with dry eschar May not be used around tubes

Specific types of dressings and their care are summarized in Table 36–1. Wounds healing by primary intention require dressings that absorb exudate and protect the wound from trauma and contamination. Dry, sterile gauze dressings remain the gold standard for wounds healing by primary intention. The length of time a dressing is required for wounds healing by primary intention varies greatly (usually less than three days).

Wounds healing by secondary or tertiary intention require dressing materials that provide a warm, moist, local wound environment conducive to wound healing; debride necrotic tissue; absorb exudate; and protect the wound from further trauma and contamination. As noted in Table 36–1, a variety of dressings can be used, including alginates, hydrocolloids, and traditional moist gauze dressings. Solutions frequently used when dressing wounds are listed in Table 36–2.

TABLE 36–2 Solutions for Dressings

Normal saline	Most commonly used solution Aids in mechanical debridement Does not damage granulation tissue
0.5% acetic acid	Used to treat *Pseudomonas* infections Toxic to fibroblasts
0.25% Dakin's solution	Chlorine bleach compound; use in a weak solution Antiseptic that slightly dissolves necrotic tissue Can be used in dirty, malodorous wounds Can inhibit growth of granulation tissue
Antibiotic solutions	Antibiotics in a solution that are applied topically Commonly used solutions include neomycin or bacitracin

Negative Pressure Wound Therapy

There is increasing evidence to support the use of negative pressure wound therapy (NPWT) to enhance wound healing. Commercial systems include Vacuum-Assisted Closure® (VAC) (Kinetic Concepts Inc., San Antonio, Texas) and Blue Sky Medical Verstaile-1 Wound Management System™. These systems use a polyurethane foam that is placed into the wound, then the dressing and the suction tubing is sealed to the skin with transparent film dressing and connected to a canister that collects the wound exudate (Fig. 36–1). NPWT provides subatmospheric pressure to the wound bed (-125 mm Hg). In some wounds the pressures may be lower, such as in split-thickness skin grafts. Once the amount of drainage has decreased, NPWT may be changed to intermittent suction, which further improves granulation rates. NPWT improves local wound perfusion by decreasing edema and bacterial contamination and improves neovascularization, granulation, and wound contraction (Venturi et al., 2005). NPWT allows for accurate measurement of wound drainage and decreases the time spent doing dressing changes.

NPWT can be used in a variety of complex wounds, especially those that are deep in appearance. NPWT has been effective in treating Stage III and IV pressure ulcers, leg ulcers, diabetic foot ulcers, and dehisced incisions. Prior to application of NPWT, the wound must be debrided of necrotic tissue and the wound must be well vascularized. The sponge is changed every 48 to 72 hours (Venturi et al., 2005). Changing the sponge can be painful, especially if granulation tissue has grown into the sponge. This can be addressed by wetting the sponge with normal saline or with topical xylocaine (without epinephrine) or changing the sponge more frequently if rapid tissue growth continues to be a problem (Venturi et al., 2005).

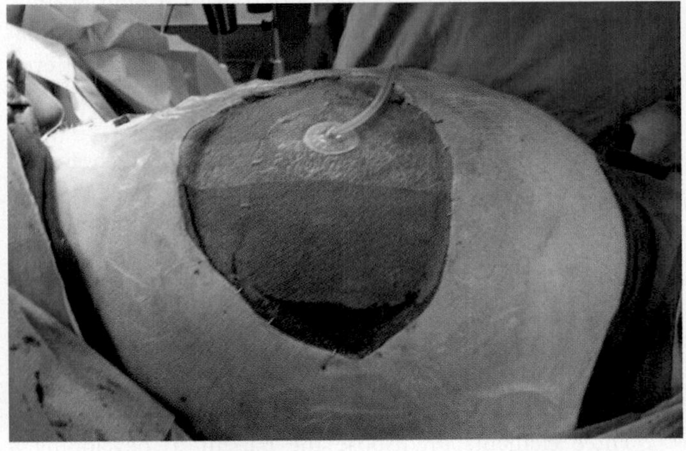

Figure 36–1 ■ Negative Pressure Wound Therapy. From Trish Martin.

SECTION ONE REVIEW

1. What size syringe would you select to irrigate a wound?
   A. 30-mL
   B. 50-mL
   C. 60-mL
   D. 100-mL
2. What type of dressing would be indicated to cover a wound healing by primary intention?
   A. dry
   B. wet-to-wet
   C. wet-to-dry
   D. polyurethane
3. The layer next to the wound in wet-to-dry dressings
   A. should adhere to the wound to prevent disruption of epithelial layers
   B. provides protection and strength in immobilizing the wound
   C. debrides the wound
   D. should be put on wet so the wound remains soupy
4. A solution used to treat *Pseudomonas* wound infections is
   A. Dakin's solution
   B. acetic acid
   C. Betadine (povidone–iodine)
   D. half-strength hydrogen peroxide

(continued)

(continued)

5. NPWT systems should be set to achieve pressure of
   A. +125 mm Hg
   B. −125 mm Hg
   C. + 5 mm Hg
   D. − 200 mm Hg

Answers: 1. A, 2. A, 3. C, 4. B, 5. B

SECTION TWO: Etiology, Diagnosis, and Treatment of Wound Infections

At the completion of this section, the learner will be able to identify conditions that predispose a patient to developing a wound infection, identify criteria used to diagnose a wound infection, and state interventions that can be used to treat wound infections.

The presence of nonreplicating microbes is called **contamination.** The skin is normally contaminated with microflora such as *Acinetobacter, Streptococcus,* and *Staphylococcus.* Wound **colonization** occurs if these microflora replicate but do not adversely affect wound healing. Contamination and colonization is normal. Wound **infection** occurs when microorganisms multiply and invade body tissues. A wound is considered to be infected when it contains 1×10^5 microorganisms per gram (Conner-Kerr & Sullivan, 2003). However, the mere presence of certain types of bacteria can interfere with wound healing. Beta-hemolytic *Streptococcus* is a potent strain of bacteria that produces toxins that allow this bacteria to cause infections even at very low concentrations (Myers, 2008c). Adverse effects of microbes in wounds are summarized in Table 36–3.

A wound infection occurs when microorganisms overcome host defenses and invade healthy tissue. Cardinal signs of a wound infection include purulent drainage, erythema, induration, warmth, edema, increased pain, and sometimes fever. Unfortunately, it is not possible to diagnose a wound infection based on these symptoms alone because these are also signs of the inflammatory process. However, if the wound is infected, these signs are typically excessive or disproportionate to the size and extent of integumentary damage due to the increasing wound bioburden (Myers, 2008c).

Three elements predispose the patient to developing a wound infection: (1) a susceptible host, (2) a compromised wound, and (3) an infectious organism.

Susceptible Host

One of the major determinants of a subsequent infection after surgery or trauma is the patient's own ability to use defense mechanisms to resist the threat of infection. The patient who is a **susceptible host** has some degree of local or systemic impairment of resistance to bacterial invasion. Local impairment may be the result of dead, foreign material or hematomas directly in the wound or some interference in blood supply to the area as a result of vascular disease. Systemic impairment of the patient's resistance may include diabetes, acute or chronic use of steroids, renal disease, malnutrition, cardiovascular disease, extremes of age, obesity, cancer, or the use of immunosuppressive therapies. These patients usually have some impairment in the acute inflammatory response or phagocytic mechanisms. Any patient with altered skin integrity has lost the major mechanical barrier blocking invasion by pathologic organisms and, thus, is a susceptible host.

TABLE 36–3 Adverse Effects of Microbes on Wound Healing

- Microbes compete with host cells for nutrients and oxygen
- Bacteria release exotoxins that are cytoxic
- Bacteria endotoxins within their cell walls activate host inflammatory response
- Wound infections delay wound healing

Compromised Wound

A **compromised wound** is one that contains devitalized tissue. Devitalized tissue is tissue that has been separated from the circulation and the body's antimicrobial defenses. Bacteria proliferate on wounds that contain dead tissue, hematomas, or foreign material. Debridement of these materials is essential to prevent an environment conducive to bacterial growth.

Infectious Organism

Many different organisms are capable of initiating a wound infection. Organisms come from endogenous or exogenous sources. Endogenous sources arise from within the patient. Many organisms exist on and in the human body—on the skin, in the respiratory tract, and in the gastrointestinal and genitourinary tracts. Organisms in these areas are not pathogenic until they are released from their normal inhabitant sites and allowed to proliferate in a sterile area of the body. Exogenous organisms enter the body from the external environment when the skin barrier has been broken. The external environment may be the accident scene (for trauma patients) or the health care setting.

Infection

A differentiation in wound bacterial colonization and infection is necessary. Colonization of wounds refers to a large number of organisms loosely attached to the wound surface, but there is no movement of bacteria into viable tissue and no host immune response. Infection is defined as the process by which organisms bind to tissue, multiply, invade viable tissue, and elicit a host immune response. Wound infection alters all three phases of wound healing.

Diagnosis of Wound Infections

Wound infections range from superficial cases of cellulitis to deep-seated abscesses. The cardinal signs of inflammation are present in a wound infection (redness, warmth, pain, and edema). The nurse may note a change in the drainage from serosanguinous in consistency to purulent and often malodorous. Wounds that have signs of inflammation that last longer than five days may be infected.

Fever and elevated WBCs indicate a more invasive infection. Wound cultures are needed to confirm the presence of an infection. There are two types of wound cultures: anaerobic and aerobic. Aerobic cultures are the standard culture taken from wounds because oxygen-metabolizing microbes are more likely to be present in superficial wound beds (Myers, 2008c). Anaerobic organisms are more likely to be found in deep wounds because of the oxygen-depleted environment of these wound beds. Tissue or pus, or both, should be collected whenever possible because these samples are more representative of the pathogenic flora (Healy & Freedman, 2006). The results guide the appropriate administration of systemic antibiotics.

Bacteria contaminating wounds must be sensitive to the antibiotic administered. However, as previously stated, it may take up to three days to obtain bacterial information. Thus, a knowledge of the likely wound contaminants and their established sensitivities is helpful in instituting prompt treatment. For example, organisms in the colon that have leaked into the peritoneum and are likely to cause infections in wounds in the abdomen are anaerobic organisms (*Bacteroides, Clostridium, Escherichia coli*), which respond to aminoglycosides.

Bacteria that continue to multiply in the presence of antimicrobials agents are considered **resistant.** Bacterial resistance occurs when bacteria produce enzymes that inactivate the antimicrobial, alter cell metabolism, or alter cell permeability to prevent antimicrobial entry into the bacterial cell (Myers, 2008c). The two most prevalent strains of resistant bacteria are methicillin-resistant *Staphylococcus aureus* (MRSA) and vancomycin-resistant *Enterococci* (VRE). A high percentage of MRSA infections occur in high-acuity patients. Risk factors for MRSA infections include diabetes, immunosuppression, malnutrition, recent surgery, immobility or significant debility (Myers, 2008c). VRE infections are common in surgical wounds and in urinary tract infections. Risk factors for VRE infections include high-acuity patients who have received multiple antimicrobial therapies, have had a prolonged hospitalization and have immunosuppression (Myers, 2008c).

Treatment of locally infected wounds with topical antiseptics may be sufficient. However, antiseptic agents should not be used in the treatment of open wounds and are not recommended (Myers, 2008c). Reasons for this include inadequate penetration for deep skin infections, development of antibiotic resistance, hypersensitivity reactions, systemic absorption when applied to large wounds, and local irritant effects leading to further delay in wound healing. The one major exception is burn wounds, as topical agents are applied (see Module 37, Alterations in Skin Integrity: Acute Burn Injury).

Prevention of Wound Infections

One of the greatest priorities in wound care is prevention of infection. Prevention of wound infections begins with recognition of the three elements that predispose the patient to a wound infection: susceptible host, compromised wound, and infectious organism.

For elective surgical procedures, prevention begins preoperatively through skin preparation, mechanical and antibiotic bowel preparations, prophylactic administration of antibiotics, and sterile operative site draping. Intraoperatively, careful surgical technique minimizes injury, and aseptic technique prevents endogenous and exogenous sources of bacterial contamination.

For patients with traumatically injured wounds, resuscitation and lifesaving measures often take priority over immediate treatment of wounds. After the resuscitative phase is completed, prompt and proper management of the wounds decreases the likelihood of subsequent infection. It is not uncommon for traumatically incurred wounds to be contaminated with dirt, grass, glass, twigs, leaves, stool, schrapnel, or bullet or knife fragments. Management of these wounds begins with cleansing of the wounds using high-pressure irrigation and debridement to remove bacteria and foreign debris.

The importance of hand washing to prevent the transmission of infectious organisms was determined more than a century ago. Hand washing is still considered one of the most important methods of preventing wound infections. This is especially important in high-acuity settings where susceptible hosts, compromised wounds, and infectious organisms are in close proximity to each other.

SECTION TWO REVIEW

1. Which of the following would NOT predispose the development of a wound infection?
   A. susceptible host
   B. exogenous organisms
   C. compromised wound
   D. infectious organisms
2. Local impairment of resistance to bacterial invasion may be the result of
   A. foreign material
   B. malnutrition
   C. cancer
   D. immunosuppressive drugs
3. Organisms from endogenous sources may come from
   A. debris in the wound
   B. the accident scene
   C. the gastrointestinal tract
   D. the hospital setting
4. Which of the following conditions is NOT a criterion for the diagnosis of a wound infection?
   A. purulent drainage from a wound
   B. culture and sensitivity testing
   C. the four cardinal signs of inflammation
   D. elevated temperature
5. Large open wounds with deep tunnels are more likely to be infected with ______ organisms.
   A. resistant
   B. aerobic
   C. anaerobic
   D. gram negative

Answers: 1. B, 2. A, 3. C, 4. B, 5. C

SECTION THREE: Necrotizing Soft Tissue Infections

At the completion of this section, the learner will be able to identify risk factors and causes of necrotizing fasciitis and Fournier's gangrene, describe the clinical presentation of necrotizing fasciitis and Fournier's gangrene, and discuss the treatment options and nursing care for the patient with necrotizing fasciitis or Fournier's gangrene.

Necrotic tissue is dead, devitalized in the wound bed. It is an impediment to wound healing and promotes infection. Necrotizing soft tissue infections (NSTIs) involve necrosis of the skin, subcutaneous fat, superficial fascia, deep muscular fascia, or any combination of these structures. This section reviews two types of life-threatening NSTIs that may occur in high-acuity patients: necrotizing fasciitis and Fournier's gangrene.

Necrotizing Fasciitis

Necrotizing fasciitis (NF) is necrosis of the fascia and subcutaneous tissue without involvement of the underlying muscle. This complex wound is potentially fatal as it can rapidly progress to systemic toxicity if not promptly diagnosed and treated. The etiology of NF is not well understood but appears to be multi-factorial. In many cases there is prior trauma to the area (infection, surgery, burn, muscle injury). It tends to develop in a susceptible host with preexisting risk factors, as summarized in Table 36–4.

Signs and Symptoms

NF can affect any part of the body, but most commonly involves the extremities, perineum, or abdomen. The extent of involvement in these tissues can range from simple contamination to an unpredictable clinical course and finally to septic shock, multisystem organ dysfunction, and death (Angoules, 2007). Early signs include those associated with the inflammatory process: erythema, edema, and pain in the affected area (see Fig. 36–2). Frank purulence is rare (Manaham et al., 2008). As the infection continues, the skin may change color from red-purple to dusky blue before progressing to necrosis and the formation of bullae (Hasham et al., 2005). The development of bullae, or blisters, is important in the differential diagnosis of NF because they are rarely associated with other skin infections such as cellulitis or phlebitis (see Fig. 36–3). They are caused by ischemia in the vessels supplying the skin as a result of vessel necrolysis and thrombosis (Salcido, 2007). The serous or hemorrhagic fluid inside them can turn into a grey foul-smelling fluid that is commonly described as "dishwater pus." Hemorrhage from the bullae can cause significant blood loss (Hasham, 2005). Crepitus may be palpated in the affected area or may be seen radiographically. Crepitus results from hydrogen, methane, and nitrogen gas produced by anaerobes and coliforms (Manahan et al., 2008). Symptoms can develop over several hours or days. Necrosis of soft tissue can progress as fast as one inch per hour, which may not be easily recognizable because the necrosis of subcutaneous

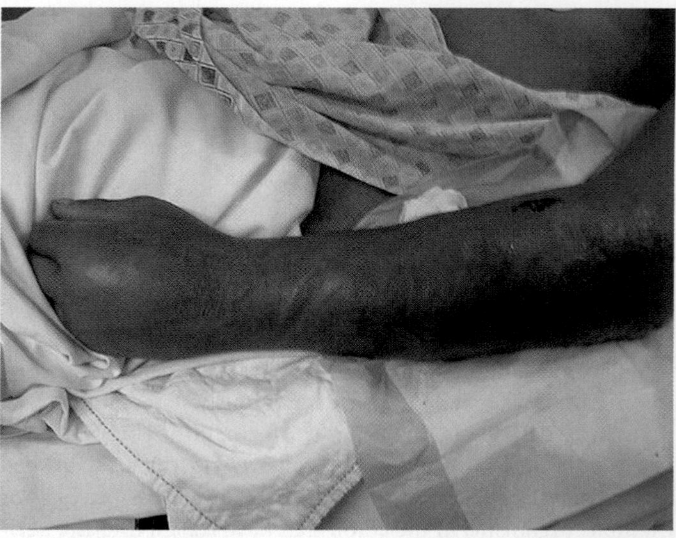

Figure 36–2 ■ Signs of Inflammation. Note erythema and edema. Skin appears very taught. From Trish Martin.

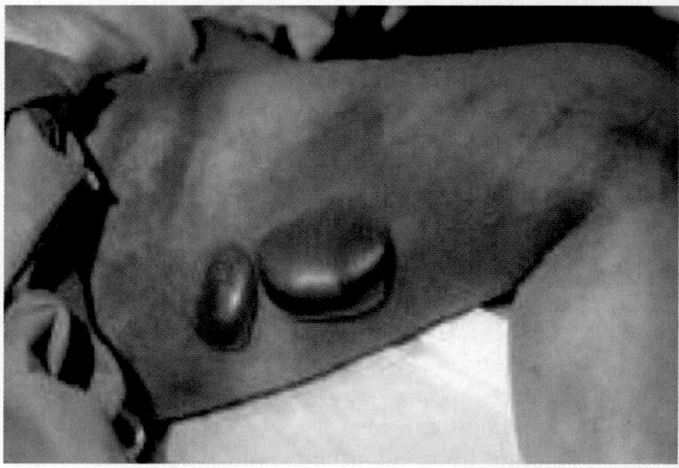

Figure 36–3 ■ Bullae. Note skin color changes with areas of red-purple with other areas of dusky blue. Note the bullae are filled with serous and hemorrhagic fluid. From Trish Martin.

TABLE 36–4 Predisposing Risk Factors for Necrotizing Fasciitis

Chronic Disease Heart disease Diabetes mellitus Renal failure Underlying malignancy Peripheral vascular disease
Drugs Steroids Intravenous drug abuse
Immunosuppression Steroids Cancer chemotherapy
Malnutrition
Advancing age
Obesity

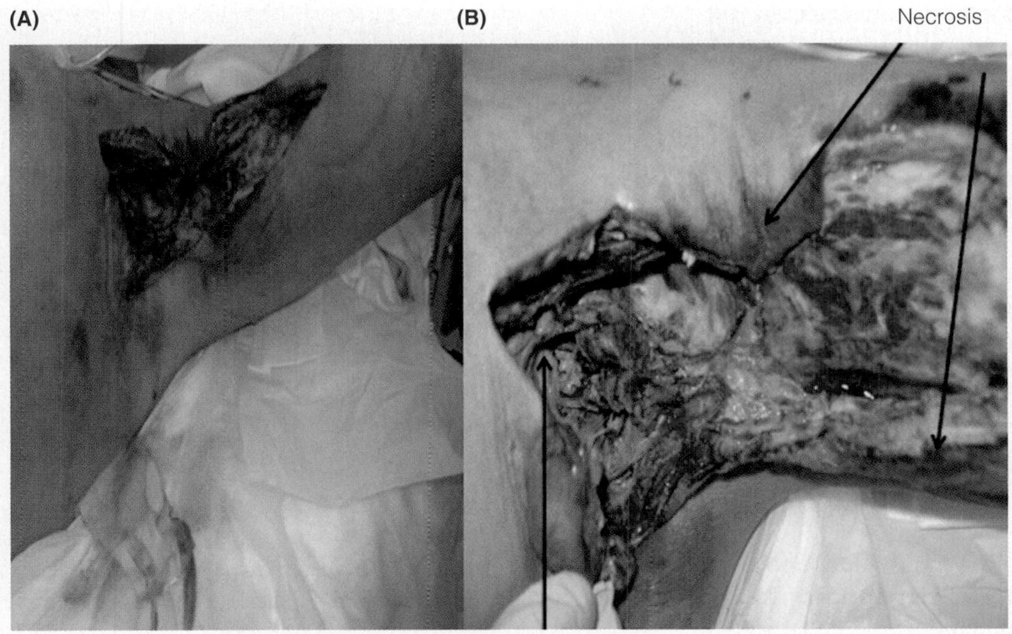

Figure 36–4 ■ Note how necrosis of the subcutaneous tissue and fascia is far more extensive than that of the skin (A). Note the dusky blue discoloration of the skin around the wound (B). When the wound is further opened and debrided, note the devitalized tissue and necrosis. Also note the absence of frank purulence. From Trish Martin.

tissue and fascia is far more extensive than that of the skin (Salcido, 2007) (see Figures 36–4A and 36–4B).

Laboratory findings may include elevated WBC (greater than 15,000 cells/mm^3), hyponatremia (less than 135 mEq/L), and elevated blood urea nitrogen (greater than 15 mg/dL) (Cainzos & Rodriquez, 2007). Increased serum creatine kinase levels indicate muscle involvement.

Wound cultures may reveal a mixture of aerobic and anaerobic organisms, although the most common causative organism is *Streptococcus* (Manahan et al., 2008). There has been a lot of attention in the media about "flesh-eating bacteria" which is caused by a strain of *Streptococcus,* group A beta-hemolytic streptococci; however, this organism is isolated in less than 15 percent of cases of NF (Eke, 2000). This type of NF often occurs in young healthy patients who may not have protective antibodies due to a lack of exposure to these strains of streptococci (Salcido, 2007).

Depending on the causative organism, NF is categorized as Type I, II or III. Type I is a mixed infection of aerobic and anaerobic bacteria; Type II is caused by anaerobic group A streptococci; and Type III is caused by marine vibrios (Angoules et al., 2007).

Pathogenesis of NF

The pathogens invade the subcutaneous tissue and rapidly proliferate. They then invade and block blood vessels and the lymphatic system, causing vasoconstriction and thrombosis (Salcido, 2007). Hypoxic conditions in the subcutaneous tissue impair neutrophil actions. Furthermore, decreased blood flow to the area impairs the delivery of oxygen, nutrients and antibiotics and results in necrosis of the skin, fascia and muscles. Some bacteria release cytokines that increase the synthesis of oxygen free-radicals that further contribute to necrosis of affected tissue (Salcido, 2007).

Emerging Evidence

- In patients with NSTI, the appearance of hemorrhagic bullae is an independent risk factor for mortality. Despite aggressive treatment, most patients in this study died within 48 hours of the emergence of hemorrhagic bullae *(Ming, Kun-Jung, Chien-Hung et al., 2008).*
- In the United States, emergency department visits for NSTIs increased threefold from 1993-2005 as a result of the emergence of MRSA. Potential confounding variables include diabetes and obesity *(Pallin, Egan, Pelletier et al., 2008).*
- In patients admitted to high-acuity units with NSTI, factors associated with increased mortality include admission serum lactate levels greater than 6 mmol/L *(Yaghoubian, de Virgilio, Dauphine et al., 2007).*
- Diabetes is a prognostic factor for mortality in patients with FG. Infection in diabetic patients spreads easily leading to systemic sepsis in a shorter period of time. Patients with diabetes mellitus who develop FG have a higher rate of sepsis. The existence of sepsis on admission is also a prognostic factor for mortality in patients with FG *(Unalp, Kamer, Derici et al, 2008).*

Treatment

Treatment includes intravenous administration of broad-spectrum antibiotics and wound management including aggressive surgical debridement and dressing changes. Antibiotic therapy typically consists of intravenous administration of penicillin for gram-positive cocci, an aminoglycoside for gram-negative aerobes, and metronidazole for anaerobes. Because of the lack of antibiotic penetration, surgical debridement is the only effective treatment. Antibiotics alone may suppress the systemic sequela of the infection, but will not address the underlying source leading to the demise of the patient (Cainzos & Rodriquez, 2007).

RELATED PHARMACOTHERAPY: Combination Antimicrobials for NSTIs

Penicillin G
Magacillan

Action and Uses
Beta-lactam antibiotic. Acts by interfering with synthesis of mucopeptides essential to formation and integrity of bacterial cell wall. Highly active against gram-positive cocci and gram-negative cocci.

Major Side Effects
Systemic anaphylaxis
Uticaria, delayed skin reactions

Nursing Implications
Treatment may be started before wound cultures are known.
Administer intravenous solutions over at least an hour to avoid electrolyte imbalance from potassium or sodium content.

Aminoglycosides
Gentamycin

Action and Uses
Active against a wide variety of aerobic gram negative bacteria, and certain gram positive organisms, such as MRSA.

Major Side Effects
Nephrotoxicity
Decreased creatinine clearance

Nursing Implications
Monitor renal function particularly for patients with impaired renal function, advancing age, or therapy beyond ten days.
Draw blood specimens for peak concentrations 30 to 60 minutes after completion of IV administration. Draw blood specimens for trough concentrations just before administration of IV dose. Use nonheparinized tubes to collect blood samples.

Antitrichomonal
Metronidazole (Flagyl)

Action and Uses
Synthetic compound that has antitrichomonacidal and amebicidal activity as well as antibacterial activity against anaerobic bacteria and some gram negative bacteria.

Major Side Effects
Overgrowth of candida
Nausea

Nursing Implications
Administer IV slowly over an hour.
Assess for signs of central nervous system toxicity.

All nonviable tissues, including fascia, must be surgically debrided. The patient may require debridement in the operating room every couple of days. NPWT, as discussed in Section One, may be used (see Figures 36–5A and 36–5B). More aggressive surgery, such as amputation of an extremity, may be required if the patient does not heal or develops septic shock. Given the high rate of systemic toxicity, these patients often require intensive monitoring, hemodynamic resuscitation, and nutritional support; all of which have been shown to decrease mortality (Manahan et al., 2008). Patients with NF are at high risk for developing multiple-system organ dysfunction. Judicious control of glucose and other therapeutic approaches

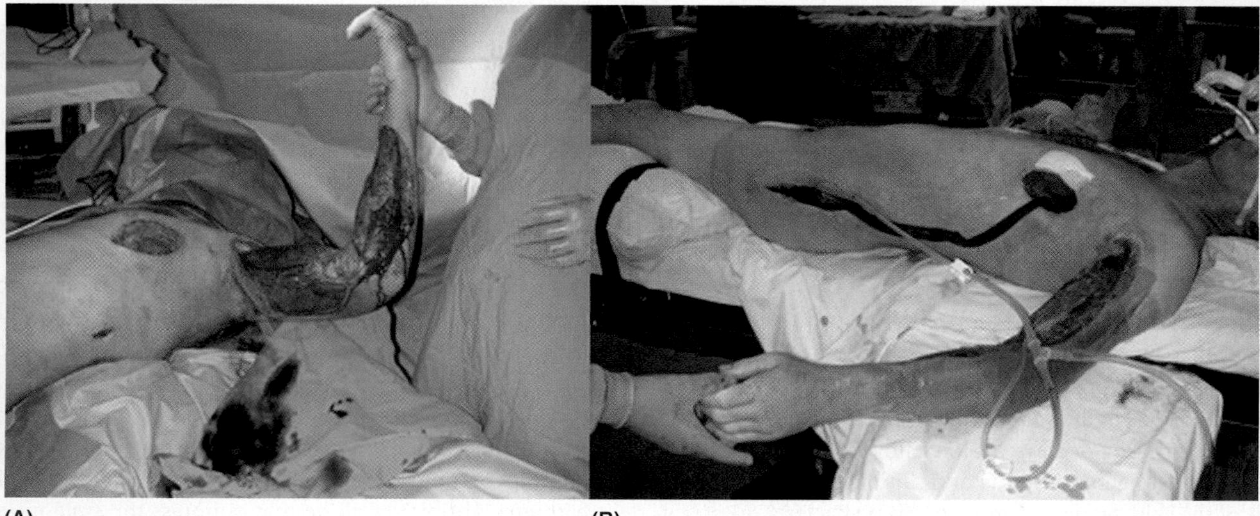

Figure 36–5 ■ After wide surgical debridement of NF of the arm (A), a NPWT system is placed (B). From Trish Martin.

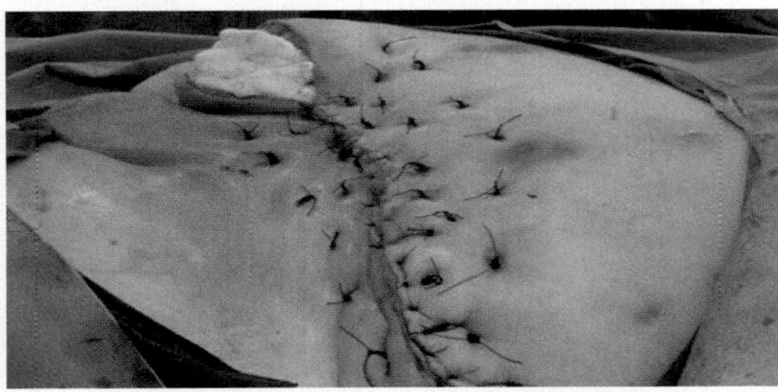

Figure 36–6 ■ Delayed primary closure of the abdomen after NF has cleared. From Trish Martin.

for septic shock are used to optimize the host response to infection (see Module 18, Alterations in Oxygen Delivery and Oxygen Consumption: Shock States). Hyperbaric oxygen therapy and intravenous immunoglobulins are possible adjunct therapies, but their efficacy has not been proven (Cainzos & Rodriquez, 2007).

Once systemic manifestations of an infectious process disappear, organisms appear to be reduced or eradicated, and transudate decreases in volume, healthy granulation tissue appears. The next phase is to restore dermal and fascial integrity. This can be accomplished in several ways. Delayed primary closure is often used for NF of the abdomen (see Fig. 36–6). The best way to achieve wound closure rapidly and safely is with split thickness skin grafts. Skin is taken from a donor site and placed on healthy granulation tissue to cover the defect (see Fig. 36–7).

Fournier's Gangrene

Fournier's gangrene (FG) is a form of necrotizing fasciitis that occurs in the genital or perineal area and progresses towards the thighs and abdominal wall (Unalp et al., 2008). It is more common in males than females. The risk factors and mechanisms of tissue destruction are the same as that described for NF. FG can arise spontaneously or from a perineal abscess, an infection of a Bartholin's gland or the scrotum, or a genitourinary procedure, such as a urinary catheter (Salcido, 2007). The onset of symptoms after injury to the perineum is typically between two to seven days (Champion, 2007). Pain out of proportion to visible signs of injury is typically the first symptom noted. Edema and erythema of the surrounding tissues follows. Skin color changes and crepitus, similar to those with NF, can occur (see Fig. 36–8).

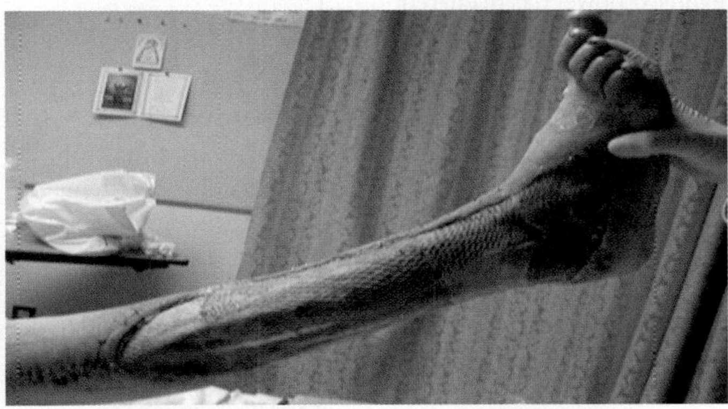

Figure 36–7 ■ Split thickness skin graft. From Trish Martin.

Treatment is similar to that for patients with NF: wound management, aggressive surgical debridement, and administration of broad-spectrum antibiotics. Along with antibiotic therapy, tetanus prophylaxis is recommended (Champion, 2007). Wound management may include dressing changes with saline or NPWT. Adequate pain management is essential as dressing changes are usually very painful. A temporary colostomy or urinary diversion may be required to control elimination into the wound area. Complications following treatment may include sexual dysfunction related to penile deviation, loss of sensitivity, and pain during erections (Champion, 2007).

Nursing Care

Patients with NSTIs require complex, specific wound management. Dressing changes are usually done several times a day and are often complex and time-consuming. Administration of antibiotics in a timely fashion is imperative. Peak and trough levels should be drawn accurately so that antibiotic doses can be adjusted for maximal effect. Aggressive pain management is essential as dressing changes can be extremely painful. Some patients may require anesthesia for dressing changes. Because of the rapidity of progressiveness of NSTIs, patients must be monitored for signs of septic shock and multisystem organ dysfunction. Psychological support is integral because patients are often disfigured and experience depression, anxiety, and anger (Salcido, 2007).

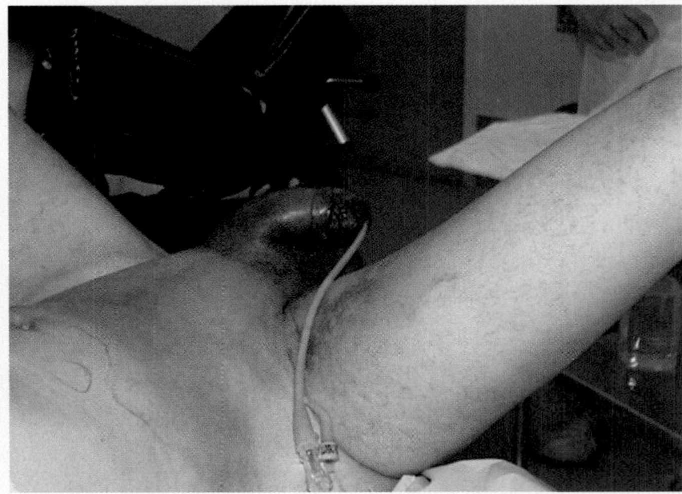

Figure 36–8 ■ Fournier's gangrene. Note the dusky blue discoloration moving from the penis and extending proximally in the abdomen. Soft tissue necrosis extends from the penis through the muscle planes in the abdomen. From Trish Martin.

SECTION THREE REVIEW

1. Which of the following are predisposing risk factors for NF? (choose all that apply)
   A. heart disease
   B. immunosuppression
   C. diabetes mellitus
   D. obesity
2. Which of the following assessments is associated with NF?
   A. crepitus
   B. enlarged lymph nodes
   C. frank purulence
   D. pitting edema
3. "Flesh eating bacteria" is a lay term for which organism?
   A. *Staphylococcus aureus*
   B. group A beta-hemolytic *streptococci*
   C. marine vibrios
   D. *Streptococcus aureus*
4. Which of the following antibiotics is likely to be prescribed for the treatment of NF? (choose all that apply)
   A. penicillin
   B. gentamycin
   C. metronidazole
   D. erythromycin
5. The onset of FG occurs within ______ of injury to the perineum.
   A. one to six hours
   B. 24 hours
   C. two to seven days
   D. one month

Answers: 1. (A, B, C, D) 2. A, 3. B, 4. (A, B, C) 5. C

SECTION FOUR: Enterocutaneous Fistulas

At the completion of this section, the learner will be able to identify the risk factors for the development of an enterocutaneous fistula, recognize the signs of symptoms of an enterocutaneous fistula, and discuss the treatment strategies including fluid and electrolyte replacement, nutritional support, and complex wound management.

A **fistula** is a tubelike passage that forms a connection between different sites (e.g., a cavity and a tube or a cavity and a free surface). An **enterocutaneous fistula (ECF)** is a passageway that develops between a segment of the GI tract and the skin. The vast majority of ECFs occur as a complication of abdominal surgery, usually involving a bowel anastomosis, repair of an enterotomy, or unrecognized bowel injury (Kassis & Makary, 2008). Management of ECFs is complex and challenging and often requires a multidisciplinary team of surgeons, enterostomal therapy nurses, nutritionists, and physical therapists and occupational therapists. Patients with ECFs have fluid and electrolyte imbalances, malnutrition, and altered skin integrity requiring complex wound management.

Risk Factors

Certain risk factors, as summarized in Table 36–5, are known to increase the chance of developing an ECF. Hypoalbuminemia (albumin less than 3 mg/dL) is a known risk factor for the development of ECF (Visschers et al., 2008). In malnourished states, tissue repair and regeneration is compromised and bowel anastamoses are more likely to fail, which allows GI contents to leak into the peritoneum. Patients who have been on long-term and/or high-dose steroids are at risk for developing ECF as a result of poor wound healing (see Module 35, Determinants and Assessment of Altered Skin Integrity). Chemotherapy and radiation therapy to the abdomen cause decreased tissue integrity and interfere with wound healing after abdominal surgery. ECFs can occur in patients who had abdominal surgery for trauma, especially if a bowel injury is missed at the initial operation or if the patient developed abdominal compartment syndrome and required damage control surgery in which the abdomen was left open to heal by secondary intention (see Module 38, Alterations in Multisystem Function: Multiple Trauma). Exposed bowel, as in the case of the abdomen left open to close by secondary intention, receives mechanical debridement from dressing changes. Epithelial cells are removed with the dressing changes, causing a thinning of the bowel wall, which eventually breaks open. It is important for the nurse to prevent these situations by protecting the bowel with Vaseline gauze until sufficient epithelialization over the exposed bowel has occurred.

TABLE 36–5 Conditions That Increase the Risk of Development of Enterocutaneous Fistulas

Malnutrition at the time of surgery
History of steroid use
History of chemotherapy or radiation therapy to the abdomen
Inflammatory bowel disease
Trauma to the abdomen, abdominal compartment syndrome

Clinical Presentation

The first sign of an ECF appears as a local wound infection. If the abdominal incision is healing by primary intention, the skin around the sutures or staples may become erythematous and the skin becomes shiny and tight. Within a couple of days, the appearance and odor of GI contents may be noted. A small amount of drainage may seep out of the sutures and appear on the patient's gown or bed linens. For patients with open abdomens healing by secondary intention, the drainage may not be visible in the wound bed, but may only be apparent on the dressings as they are removed from the wound (Fig. 36–9). Drainage on dressings may change from serosanguinous to

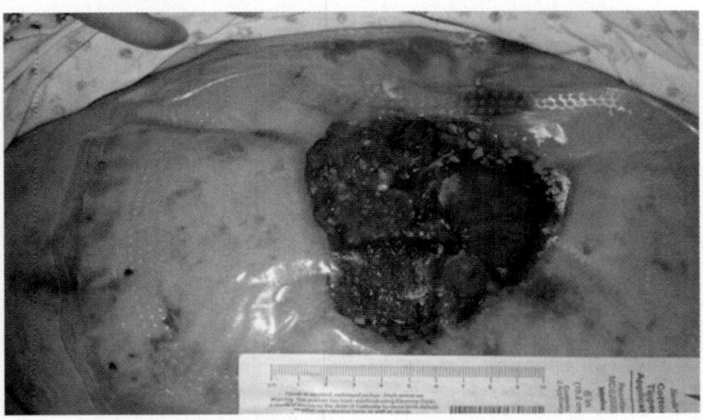

Figure 36–9 ▪ Enterocutaneous fistula. Note the green stool drainage in the wound bed. From Trish Martin.

green or brown and may have a fecal odor. In these situations, it is imperative that the nurse notifies the health care provider immediately. Early recognition is crucial to prevent life-threatening metabolic, septic, and nutritional complications (Kassis & Makary, 2008). An upper GI contrast study or CT scan may be ordered to determine the exact anatomic location of the ECF. Location is an important prognostic factor. ECFs that form in the proximal GI tract (small bowel) are associated with worse outcomes (Martinez et al., 2008). These ECFs have a higher output of GI drainage that results in severe fluid and electrolyte imbalances and malnutrition because nutrients and water are not absorbed. High-output drainage is generally defined as ECF drainage greater than 500 mL/day (Lloyd et al., 2006). ECFs that form in the distal GI tract (colon) do not have as much drainage and the stool from the ECF will be more formed. Small bowel ECFs tend to take longer to heal and require longer courses of treatment and hospitalization than ECFs that develop in the colon (Martinez et al., 2008).

Treatment

Treatment of patients with ECFs includes correction of fluid and electrolyte imbalances, nutritional support, and complex wound management. With high-output ECFs, the nurse should monitor the patient for signs of hypovolemia. Serum electrolytes should be monitored for the development of hypokalemia, hypocholoremia, and acidosis, depending on the location of the ECF in the GI tract (Lloyd et al., 2006). The nurse should ensure accurate measurement of ECF drainage so that fluids and electrolytes can be replaced accordingly.

Nutritional support may include enteral or parenteral nutrition; however, there is increasing evidence that enteral nutrition is associated with maintenance of GI mucosal integrity and improved immunologic host response (Kassis & Makary, 2008). Patients with a small bowel ECF with high-output drainage may not tolerate enteral nutrition. Parenteral nutrition may be required to allow administration of full nutritional requirements and to aide in wound healing by decreasing ECF drainage (Visshers et al., 2008). Nutritional support decisions are individualized based on the location of the ECF, the output from the ECF, and the patient's overall metabolic and nutritional requirements.

Management of skin integrity in patients with an ECF is extremely complex and challenging for the high-acuity nurse. If available, a wound ostomy nurse should be consulted to help manage these complex wounds. Skin protection, drainage quantification, and drainage containment must be considered when developing the plan of care for these patients (Davis et al., 2000). The enzyme content of the ECF drainage coupled with the prolonged exposure of the perifistula skin to moisture leads to alteration in skin integrity around the fistula. This prevents spontaneous closure of the ECF and predisposes the patient to infection (Lloyd et al., 2006). Skin care may include application of ostomy appliances to help protect skin and contain drainage. As noted, periwound barrier products can be used to protect the skin from ECF drainage.

Decreasing ECF output is important in reducing fluid and electrolyte imbalances and promoting wound healing. ECF drainage may be reduced by reducing GI secretions by administration of H_2 receptor antagonists or proton pump inhibitors. Bowel transit may be slowed with antimotility agents. The use of antisecretory agents, such as somatostatin and octreotide, is controversial. These agents reduce secretion of GI hormones (gastrin and cholecystokinin), which in turn decreases gastric and pancreatic secretions. There is evidence that these agents reduce fistula drainage and decrease time to closure of ECFs; however, there is insufficient evidence that they increase the overall likelihood of spontaneous closure of ECFs (Lloyd et al., 2006).

SECTION FOUR REVIEW

1. Risk factors for the development of an ECF after abdominal surgery include (choose all that apply)
   A. hypoalbuminemia
   B. long-term use of steroids
   C. radiation therapy to the abdomen
   D. abdominal compartment syndrome
2. High-output ECF drainage is defined as
   A. 100 mL/hour
   B. 200 mL/day
   C. 500 mL/hour
   D. 500 mL/day
3. ECFs that develop in the large bowel would tend to produce what type of drainage?
   A. high-output liquid stool
   B. high-output green drainage
   C. semiformed or formed stool
   D. highly acidic fluid

(continued)

(continued)

4. The patient with a high-output ECF is at risk for developing which of the following? (choose all that apply)
   A. alkalosis
   B. hypokalemia
   C. hypochloremia
   D. hypomagnesemia
5. Skin protection, drainage quantification, and drainage containment of an ECF may be obtained by using
   A. wet to dry dressings
   B. ostomy appliances
   C. hydrocolloid wafers
   D. skin barrier protection products

Answers: 1. (A, B, C, D), 2. D, 3. C, 4. (B,C), 5. B

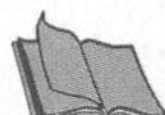

POSTTEST

1. A patient is receiving autolytic debridement with a hydrocolloid wafer dressing. The nurse notes the wound has a collection of yellow fluid under the dressing. Which action should the nurse take?
   A. Remove the dressing as the wound may be infected.
   B. Irrigate the wound with normal saline.
   C. Leave the dressing intact.
   D. Call the health care provider.
2. A patient is receiving NPWT. Upon removal of the sponge, the nurse notes granulation tissue has grown into the sponge and the patient complains of pain. What action(s) should the nurse take? (choose all that apply)
   A. Stop the procedure, call the health care provider immediately.
   B. Wet the sponge with normal saline.
   C. Discuss with the health care provider the need to change the sponge more frequently.
   D. Wet sponge with hydrogen peroxide.
3. Which of the following are risk factors for the development of a VRE infection? (choose all that apply)
   A. multiple antimicrobial therapy
   B. malnutrition
   C. recent surgery
   D. immunosuppression
4. Which of the following must be present to diagnose a wound as being infected?
   A. pus
   B. foul odor
   C. fever
   D. positive wound culture
5. Bullae are associated with NF. The bullae are typically filled with what type of fluid? (choose all that apply)
   A. blood
   B. "dishwater pus"
   C. protein
   D. chyme
6. Frequent surgical debridement of wounds with NF is required because (choose all that apply)
   A. Necrotic tissue is an impediment to wound healing.
   B. Antibiotics can not penetrate the wound bed.
   C. Nonviable tissue must be removed.
   D. Dressing changes alone can not reduce the infection.
7. A wound culture reveals gram-negative aerobes. Which of the following antibiotics would be effective against this organism?
   A. penicillin
   B. gentamycin
   C. metronidazole
   D. ampicillin
8. Which of the following are risk factors for the development of an ECF?
   A. hypoalbuminemia
   B. previous radiation therapy to the abdomen
   C. gallbladder disease
   D. alcohol abuse
9. When changing a patient's abdominal dressing, the nurse notes drainage on the dressing. During the previous dressing change, the drainage was serosanguinous. It is now green-brown in color and has a foul odor. What could be the cause of the change in drainage?
   A. Fournier's gangrene
   B. necrotizing fasciitis
   C. enterocutaneous fistula
   D. wound infection
10. Which of the following nursing diagnoses are appropriate for the patient with ECF?
    A. alteration in nutrition (less than body requirements)
    B. alteration in fluid volume (deficit)
    C. body image disturbance
    D. altered bowel elimination

Posttest answers with rationale are found on MyNursingKit.

REFERENCES

Angoules, A. G., Kontakis, G., Drakoulakis, E. (2007). Necrotizing fasciitis of upper and lower limbs: a systematic review. *Injury 38* (Suppl), S18–S25.

Cainzos, M. & Rodriquez, J. F .(2007). Necrotizing soft tissue infections. *Curr Opinion in Crit Care 13,* 433–439.

Champion, S. E. (2007). A case of Fournier's gangrene. *Urologic Nursing 27,* 296–299.

Davis, M., Dere, K., Hadley, G. (2000). Options for managing an open wound with draining enterocutaneous fistula. *J Wound Ostomy Care Nursing 27,* 118–123.

Eke, N. (2000). Fournier's gangrene: a review of 1726 cases. *Br J Surg 87,* 718–728.

Hasham S., Matteucci, P., Stanley P. R., et al. (2005). Necrotizing fasciitis. *Brit Med J 330,* 830–833.

Kassis, E. S. & Makary, M. A. (2008). Enterocutaneous fistula. In J. L. Cameron (ed.), *Current Surgical Therapy* (9th ed.). Philadelphia: Mosby Elsevier, 143–145.

Lloyd, D. A., Gabe, S. M., & Windsor A. C. (2006). Nutrition and management of enterocutaneous fistulas. *Brit J Surg 93,* 1045–1055.

Manahan, M. A., Milner, S. M., Freeswick P., et al. (2008). Necrotizing skin and soft tissue infections. In J. L. Cameron (ed.), *Current surgical therapy* (9th ed.). Philadelphia: Mosby Elsevier, 1128–1131.

Martinez, J. L., Luque-de-Leon, E., Mier, J., et al. (2008). Systematic management of postoperative enterocutaneous fistulas: Factors related to outcomes. *World J Surg 32,* 436–443.

Ming, L., Kun-Jung, C., Chien-Hung, C., et al. (2008). Risk factors for the outcome of cirrhotic patients with soft tissue infections. *J Clin Gastroenterol 42,* 312–316.

Myers, B. A. (2008a). Debridement. In B. A. Myers (wd.), *Wound management: principles and practice* (2d ed.). Upper Saddle River, NJ: Prentice Hall, 70–93.

Myers, B. A. (2008b). Electrotherapeutic modalities, physical agents, and mechanical modalities. In B. A. Myers (ed.), *Wound management: principles and practice* (2d ed.). Upper Saddle River, NJ: Prentice Hall, 160–195.

Myers, B. A. (2008c). Management of infection. In B. A. Myers (ed.), *Wound management: principles and practice* (2d ed.). Upper Saddle River, NJ: Prentice Hall, 94–122.

Pallin, D. J., Egan, D. J., & Pelletier, A. J. (2008). Increased US emergency department visits for skin and soft tissue infections, and changes in antibiotic choices during the emergence of community associated methicillan-resistant staphyloccus aureus. *Annals of Emerg Med 51,* 291–298.

Porth, C. M. (2009). Disorders of gastrointestinal function. In C. M. Porth & Matfin G. (eds.). *Pathophysiology: concepts of altered health states* (8th ed.). Philadelphia: Lippincott Williams & Wilkens, 916–948.

Salcido, R. (2007). Necrotizing fasciitis: reviewing the causes and treatment strategies. *Adv in Skin Wound Care 20,* 288–293.

Unalp, H. R., Kramer, E., Derici, H., et al. (2008). Fournier's gangrene: evaluation of 68 patients and analysis of prognostic values. *J Postgrad Med 54,* 102–105.

Venturi, M. L., Attinger, C. E., Mesbahi, A. N., et al. (2005). Mechanisms and clinical applications of the vacuum-assisted closure device. *Am J Clin Dermatol 6*(3), 185–194.

Visschers R. J., Damink S. W., Winkens, B., et al. (2008). Treatment strategies in 135 consecutive patients with enterocutaneous fistulas. *World J Surg 32,* 445–453.

Yagoubian, A., de Virgilio, C., Dauphine C., et al. (2007). Use of admission serum lactate levels and sodium levels to predict mortality in necrotizing soft tissue infections. *Arch Surg 142,* 840–846.

MODULE

37 Alterations in Skin Integrity: Acute Burn Injury

Karen L. Johnson

OBJECTIVES Following completion of this module, the learner will be able to

1. List the risk factors that place people at a greater risk for burn injury and have greater morbidity and mortality as a result of burn injury.
2. Discuss five mechanisms of burn injury.
3. Differentiate burn wound descriptors based on level of dermis and tissue involved in the injury.
4. Calculate the extent of total body surface area involved.
5. Discuss criteria for transfer of a patient to a burn center.
6. Describe the unique structures, processes, and personnel that make up a burn center.
7. Discuss priority cardiovascular and pulmonary assessments and interventions during the resuscitative phase for the patient with a burn injury.
8. Discuss priority neurological assessments and interventions during the resuscitative phase for the patient with a burn injury.
9. Discuss pain management strategies for the patient with a burn injury.
10. Discuss priority nursing assessments and interventions during the resuscitative phase for gastrointestinal, metabolic, and renal effects of burn injury.
11. Compare burn wound healing with wound healing from other injuries.
12. State the wound care priorities during the resuscitative phase.
13. Describe burn wound management in the acute rehabilitative phase.
14. Describe expected behaviors, emotional status, and levels of pain for burn patients during the acute rehabilitative phase as well as related nursing actions.
15. Describe the goals, interventions, and health professionals involved with promoting physical mobility during the acute rehabilitative phase of burn care.
16. Discuss nursing interventions related to physical conditioning, protection of new skin, scar management, and psychosocial adjustment during the long-term rehabilitative phase of burn care.

This self-study module focuses on the three phases of burn injury: the resuscitative phase, acute rehabilitative phase, and the long-term rehabilitative phase. The module is composed of 11 sections. Sections One through Three discuss the mechanisms of burn injury, assessment and classification of burns, and burn centers. Sections Four through Six describe the cardiovascular, pulmonary, neurologic, metabolic, and renal effects of burn injury during the resuscitative phase. Section Seven provides an overview of burn wound healing and describes initial wound care during the resuscitative phase. Section Eight describes burn wound management in the acute rehabilitative phase. Sections Nine and Ten describe the acute rehabilitative phase of burn injury. Section Eleven discusses the long-term rehabilitative phase of burn care. All Section Reviews include answers. It is suggested that the learner review those concepts answered incorrectly in the review questions before proceeding to the next section.

PRETEST

1. Of the following demographic groups, which is at highest risk for burn injury/death?
   A. Caucasians
   B. suburbanites
   C. women
   D. children

2. Which of the following mechanisms of burn injury causes protein liquification producing a soupy wound that allows for continued tissue damage into deeper structures?
   A. acid burn
   B. alkali burn

C. electrical burn
D. radiation burn

3. A sunburn is an example of a
A. superficial burn
B. superficial partial-thickness burn
C. deep partial-thickness burn
D. subdermal burn

4. A patient arrives at the emergency department with burns to bilateral anterior lower limbs and perineum. Calculate the extent of total body surface area (TBSA) of this injury using the rule of nines.
A. 10 percent
B. 18 percent
C. 19 percent
D. 36 percent

5. Single rooms with positive airflow are ideal in a burn unit because this arrangement promotes
A. privacy
B. noise reduction
C. infection control
D. adequate ventilation

6. Current guidelines recommend that an escharotomy should be performed when compartment pressures are
A. greater than 20 mm Hg
B. 25 to 40 mm Hg
C. greater than 40 mm Hg
D. greater than 75 mm Hg

7. Upper airway edema usually peaks during which time period postinhalation injury?
A. 24 to 48 hours
B. one to two hours
C. four to eight hours
D. 12 to 24 hours

8. Fluid resuscitation should be calculated for patients with ______ total body surface area burned.
A. 10 percent
B. 15 percent
C. 20 percent
D. 30 percent

9. The most effective method for delivering pain medication during the resuscitative phase is
A. orally
B. subcutaneously
C. intramuscularly
D. intravenously

10. During the initial stage of psychological adaptation after burn injury (survival anxiety) the nurse should
A. praise attempts for autonomous functioning
B. give reality-based responses
C. acknowledge reality-based responses
D. force the staff's expectations on the patient

11. Enteral nutrition should be initiated
A. within 24 hours postburn injury
B. when bowel sounds return
C. at 72 hours postburn
D. after parenteral nutrition is completed

12. A red-brown color in the urine that appears after an electrical burn may indicate
A. a urinary tract infection
B. renal tubular acidosis
C. renal hypoperfusion
D. myoglobinuria

13. The major consequence of hypertrophic scar formation is
A. contractures
B. muscle atrophy
C. that epithelialization cannot occur
D. wound healing is delayed

14. Ointments and creams should not be applied during initial care of burn wounds because they
A. induce the inflammatory process
B. make wounds soupy and susceptible to infection
C. interfere with burn wound evaluation
D. interfere with an escharotomy

15. Bullae larger than 2 cm may be
A. left intact
B. drained by aspiration
C. opened with the loose skin removed
D. all of the above

16. Monitoring the patient after a tangential excision includes monitoring the patient for
A. infection
B. bleeding
C. bullae
D. soupy drainage

17. Which of the following organizations or groups might be MOST helpful in helping the patient with burn injuries through psychosocial issues in the acute rehabilitative phase?
A. Tuscon Society
B. Phoenix Society
C. American Burn Association
D. The patient's visitors

18. Failure to apply compression wraps to recently grafted lower extremities prior to ambulation could result in
A. extreme pain
B. contracture formation
C. graft loss
D. bullae formation

19. Pressure garments are worn
A. only at night
B. continuously
C. to help regain muscle stability
D. until hospital discharge

Pretest answers are found on MyNursingKit.

SECTION ONE: Mechanisms of Burn Injury

At the completion of this section, the learner will be able to list the risk factors that place people at a greater risk for burn injury and discuss five mechanisms of burn injury.

Incidence and Risk Factors

More than 500,000 people are burned each year, resulting in approximately 3,500 deaths annually (American Burn Association [ABA], 2007a). Each year in the United States, burn injuries account for approximately 40,000 to 50,000 admissions to acute-care hospitals (Holmes, 2008). The economic costs from burn injury recovery rise into the billions of dollars per year as do the costs from days lost from work and for physical and vocational rehabilitation. Most burn injuries occur in the home (ABA, 2007a). Children and people with advancing age are most prone to burn injuries. People with advancing age have impaired senses and reaction times, and tend to incorrectly assess risk. They have thinner skin, with decreased microcirculation and an increased susceptibility to infection. All of these factors not only put them at a greater risk for burn injuries but also lead to greater morbidity and mortality.

Mechanisms of Injury

Burn injury may occur from exposure to heat (flames, hot objects), caustic chemicals, electrical current, radiation, or extreme cold. The severity of the injury depends on the length of exposure, temperature of the offending substance, and tissue conductance.

Thermal burns caused by exposure to flame or a hot object produce microvascular and inflammatory responses within minutes of the injury (Fig. 37–1). The effects from these two responses can last from two to three days. Substances released by damaged cells increase vascular permeability, causing fluid, electrolytes, and proteins to leak into the interstitial space. The various inflammatory mediators also contribute to cell wall changes that permit intravascular fluid and proteins to leak into the interstitial spaces. Both of these responses contribute to burn edema formation. Burn edema is usually limited to the injured tissues with smaller size burns. In larger size burns edema occurs in noninjured tissues also. The fluid shift from intravascular to interstitial spaces may cause a hypovolemic shock state. Fluid loss by evaporation from the burn wound also contributes to the volume deficit. This hypovolemic shock state is frequently referred to as **burn shock.**

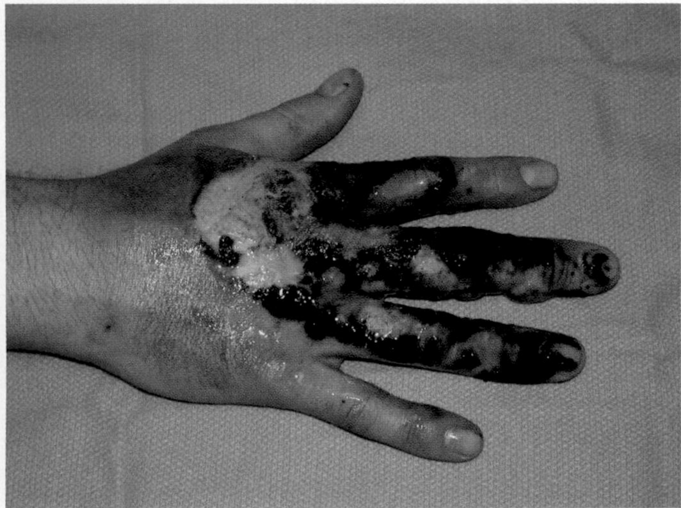

Figure 37–1 ■ Thermal burn.

Chemical burns are the result of exposure to acid, alkali, or organic substances. The extent of injury depends on the concentration of the substance, the amount, the length of exposure, and the mechanism of chemical action. An acid substance will cause an eschar type of wound resulting from a coagulation necrosis. The eschar prevents continued tissue damage beneath the layer of eschar. An alkali substance usually causes more tissue damage than an acid substance (given the same volume) because an alkali causes protein liquefaction producing a soupy wound, which allows continued tissue damage into deeper structures. Damage occurs rapidly and will continue until the pH level returns to a normal physiologic level. Organic substances produce a thermal component and may be absorbed systemically, producing renal and hepatic toxicity. Inhalation of chemical substances can cause direct parenchymal lung injury. Absorption of a chemical through either the pulmonary system or through direct skin contact can cause systemic effects involving the pulmonary, cardiovascular, renal, or hepatic systems.

Electrical burns result from the conversion of electrical energy into heat. The extent of thermal injury depends on the type of current, the pathway of current flow, local tissue resistance, and the duration of contact. All tissues are conductive to some extent but there are differences in the resistance to the current flow. Externally, the skin is the primary resistor to electrical current. The ability to resist electrical current depends on its thickness and amount of moisture. Internally, nerves and blood vessels are the best electrical conductors (Spence, 2008). Because of the internal damage that can be caused by electrical injuries, the severity of an electrical burn is difficult to determine on initial exam.

Electrical contact injuries can be caused by low-voltage lines. These lines, most commonly found in homes and offices, are usually in the form of alternating current (AC). Because AC produces a current that flows back and forth in a cyclical manner, the former terminology of describing an entrance and exit wound is incorrect. AC, as opposed to direct current (DC), causes a more severe injury because it produces tetanic muscle contractions that do not allow disengagement from the current source. DC causes the person to be cast away from the current source. These differences between AC and DC are only significant with low voltages. Electrical burns can be caused by high-voltage lines. High-voltage injuries are caused by a current that is sent from the electrical source in an arc, either into or over the person. The arc can generate temperatures up to 5,000° Celsius, causing thermal injuries (Spence, 2008). Another type of electrical burn is electrical flash burn where the injury involves no electrical contact and it is a true thermal injury. Delineating among the different types of electrical burns is important because it will lead the health care practitioner to determine depth of injury as well as other possible associated injuries.

Radiation burns result from radiant energy being transferred to the body resulting in production of cellular toxins. The effect is most rapidly evident on those cells that reproduce rapidly, such as skin, blood vessels, intestinal lining, and bone marrow. The greater the exposure, the more significant the damage and the more types of cells are affected. A radiation victim's injury usually results from radiation therapy or from an industrial or laboratory incident.

Exposure to severe cold temperatures can cause frostbite injuries (see Fig. 37–2). Conditions that increase a person's susceptibility to this type of injury include amount of muscle and fat to provide insulation, nutrition status, amount of exertion required to generate heat, and alcohol and drugs affecting judgment, as well as the ability to shiver. The elderly are at greater risk for this type of injury because of their decreased ability for heat generation and vasoconstriction. Frostbite injuries are treated conservatively because it may take weeks before there is a clear demarcation between viable and nonviable tissue.

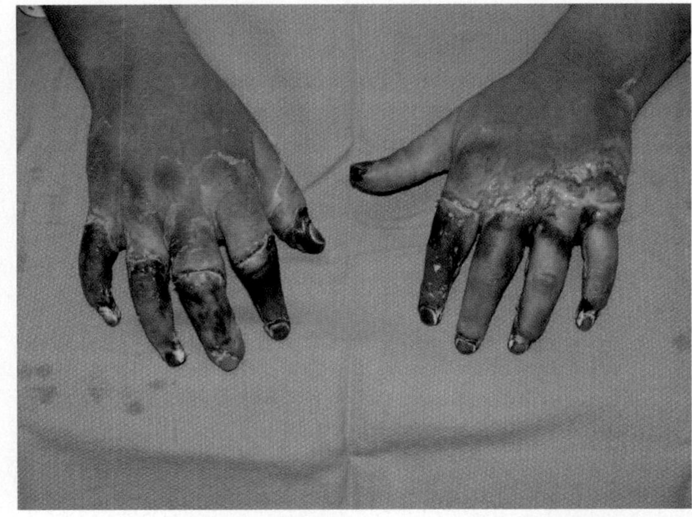

Figure 37–2 ■ Frostbite injury.

SECTION ONE REVIEW

1. Which of the following patient groups are NOT at an increased risk for burn injuries?
   A. African Americans
   B. people with advancing age
   C. children
   D. diabetics
2. The type of burn where tissues are deeply penetrated and necrosis may continue to occur for several hours after injury is MOST likely a(n)
   A. acidic burn
   B. alkaline burn
   C. electrical burn
   D. flash burn
3. Electrical contact injuries can be caused by low-voltage lines in the form of
   A. alternating current
   B. direct current
   C. current source
   D. a reflex arc
4. Which of the following areas are most prone to injury as a result of radiation? (choose all that apply)
   A. skin
   B. blood vessels
   C. intestinal lining
   D. bone marrow
5. Which of the following burn injuries are treated conservatively because it takes weeks before there is a demarcation of viable and nonviable tissue?
   A. thermal burns
   B. electrical burns
   C. radiation burns
   D. frostbite

Answers: 1. A, 2. B, 3. A, 4. (A, B, C, D) 5. D

SECTION TWO: Burn Wound Assessment

At the completion of this section, the learner will be able to differentiate burn wound descriptors based on level of dermis and tissue involved in the injury and calculate the extent of total body surface area involved.

After necessary life-saving measures have been taken, the goal is to preserve remaining functional integrity of the burn injured tissue.

Burns are classified according to depth of injury and extent of body surface area involved. Burn depth has been traditionally described as first-, second-, or third-degree (see Fig. 37–3). Currently, burn wounds are more specifically differentiated, depending on the level of dermis and subcutaneous tissue involved. Descriptors of burn depths include superficial, superficial partial-thickness, deep partial-thickness, full-thickness,

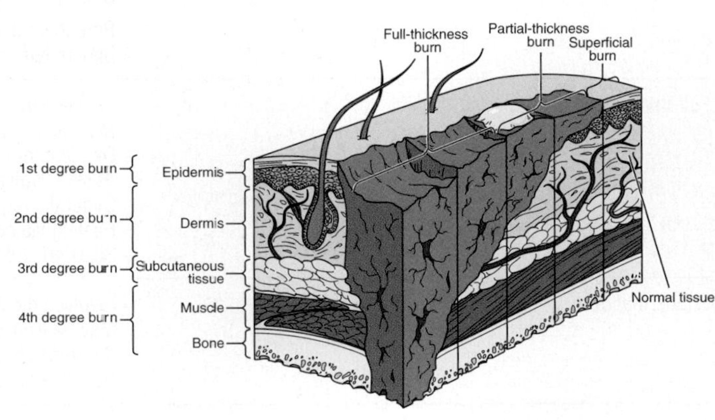

Figure 37–3 ■ Burn injury classification according to the depth of burn.

and subdermal burns (Table 37–1). **Superficial burns** involve the epidermis only. A sunburn is an example of a superficial burn. **Superficial partial-thickness burns** involve the epidermis and superficial layer of the dermis. These burns may occur with brief contact with hot objects. **Deep partial-thickness burns** involve the epidermis and deep layer of the dermis. An example is a tar burn. **Full-thickness burns** involve the epidermis, dermis, and subcutaneous layer. Exposure to flames, electricity, or chemicals can cause these severe burns. **Subdermal burns** usually involve all layers of skin and may include injury to muscle, tendons, or bone as a result of prolonged contact with flames, hot objects, or electricity.

The depth of the burn is often difficult to assess initially. Calculation of the extent of injury should be reevaluated after the initial wound debridement and over the course of the ensuing 72 hours to accurately describe the wound. Wound conversion sometimes occurs when viable tissue becomes nonviable, thereby increasing the depth of the wound. Thermal burns consist of three zones. The outermost area is termed the zone of hyperemia*;* it blanches with pressure and will heal in seven to ten days. The innermost area is termed the zone of coagulation*;* it is an area of immediately nonviable tissue. Surrounding this central zone is the *zone of stasis.* This area can easily convert to nonviable tissue if the restoration of blood flow is not adequately achieved. Proper fluid resuscitation is essential in preventing this from occurring. Other causes of wound conversion include infection, hypothermia, and external pressure.

The extent of injury is expressed by the percentage of total body surface area (TBSA) burned. When determining TBSA, superficial burns are not involved in the calculation. The most accurate guide in determining the extent of injury is the Lund and Browder Chart, which adjusts TBSA for age (shown in Fig. 37–4). This is important because various pediatric patients' body parts are disproportionate to adults'. For example, a child's head is allowed a greater TBSA percentage than an adult's. To use the guide, one assesses all partial- and full-thickness burns and shades the figure accordingly. The percentage of each anatomic area involved is calculated, then all are totaled. For example, if an adult were to sustain a scald injury to the right lower arm and hand, his or her TBSA burned wound would be 5.5 percent.

Another guide used to calculate TBSA is the rule of nines (see Fig. 37–5). This estimation divides the body into areas of 9 percent or multiples of 9 percent. The head is 9 percent, each upper extremity is 9 percent, each lower extremity is 18 percent, the back is 18 percent, the trunk (front) is 18 percent, and the genitalia is 1 percent, with the sum total equaling 100 percent.

TABLE 37–1 Descriptions of Burn Depths

DEPTH OF BURN	DESCRIPTION
Superficial burn	Involves epidermis only May be caused by the sun, or brief exposure to hot liquids Erythema, pain, minimal edema No blisters, dry skin Heals in three to five days via sloughing of the epidermal layer, no scarring
Superficial partial-thickness burn	Involves the epidermis and the papillary layer of the dermis (superficial layer) May be caused by hot liquids, brief contact with hot objects, or flash flame Erythema, brisk capillary refill, blisters, moist Moderate edema, very painful Heals in 10 to 14 days via reepithelialization No scarring; potential for hypo/hyperpigmentation
Deep partial-thickness burn	Involves the epidermis and the reticular layer of the dermis (deep layer) May be caused by flame, hot liquids, radiation, tar, or hot objects Erythematous or pale, sluggish or absent capillary refill Moist or dry, no blisters Significant edema and altered sensation Heals in two to three weeks or longer Potential for scarring and hypo/hyperpigmentation May require skin grafting for optimal function or appearance
Full-thickness burn	Involves the epidermis, dermis, and subcutaneous layer May be caused by flame, electricity, or chemicals Dry, leathery, white Absent capillary refill Generally requires skin grafting Healing via contraction and granulation tissue formation Scarring and hypo/hyperpigmentation
Subdermal burn	Involves the epidermis, dermis, subcutaneous layer, and muscle, tendon, or bone May be from electricity, prolonged contact with flame, or a hot object Charred, dry appearance Requires skin grafting, flap, or amputation

Area	Age (years)					% 1	% 2	% 3	% Total
	0–1	1–4	5–9	10–15	Adult				
Head	19	17	13	10	7				
Neck	2	2	2	2	2				
Ant. trunk	13	13	13	13	13				
Post. trunk	13	13	13	13	13				
R. buttock	2½	2½	2½	2½	2½				
L. buttock	2½	2½	2½	2½	2½				
Genitalia	1	1	1	1	1				
R.U. arm	4	4	4	4	4				
L.U. arm	4	4	4	4	4				
R.L. arm	3	3	3	3	3				
L.L. arm	3	3	3	3	3				
R. hand	2½	2½	2½	2½	2½				
L. hand	2½	2½	2½	2½	2½				
R. thigh	5½	6½	8½	8½	9½				
L. thigh	5½	6½	8½	8½	9½				
R. leg	5	5	5½	6	7				
L. leg	5	5	5½	6	7				
R. foot	3½	3½	3½	3½	3½				
L. foot	3½	3½	3½	3½	3½				
					Total				

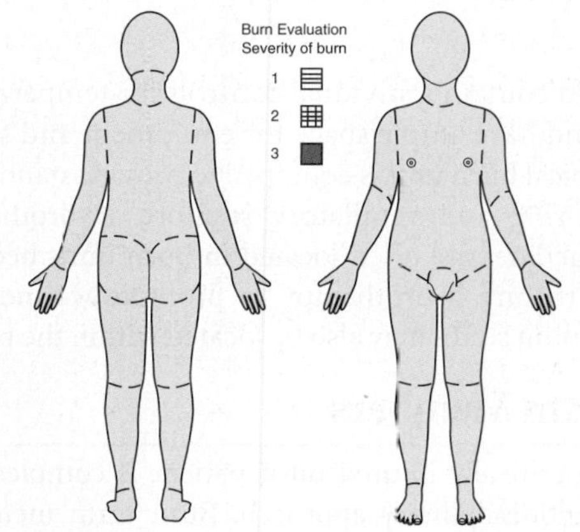

Figure 37–4 ■ The Lund and Browder chart.

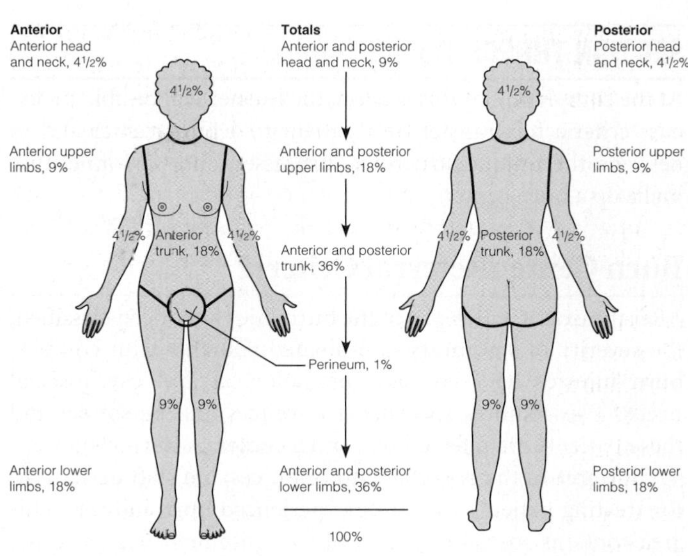

Figure 37–5 ■ The rule of nine's.

This method is quick and easy, but less accurate than the Lund and Browder method. This is especially true for children.

Another method of evaluating burn injuries, especially those that are irregularly shaped or occur in patches, is to use the palmar surface of the patient's hand which represents approximately 1 percent of the patient's body surface area. Just the palm accounts for 0.5 percent TBSA. For example, if a patchy burn to the torso includes four burned areas, each approximately the size of the patient's palm, the TBSA involved would be 2 percent.

SECTION TWO REVIEW

1. An adult patient received partial-thickness flash burns to his head and neck. The estimated extent of his injury according to the Lund and Browder Chart would be
   A. 21 percent
   B. 19 percent
   C. 9 percent
   D. 7 percent
2. Using the rule of nines, calculate the extent of burn for a patient with burns to the posterior head and posterior trunk.
   A. 22.5 percent
   B. 18 percent
   C. 20 percent
   D. 13 percent
3. White, charred, leathery-textured wounds are the result of
   A. full-thickness burns
   B. superficial burns
   C. deep partial-thickness burns
   D. superficial partial-thickness burns
4. Which of the following terms describes a burn that involves the epidermis and deep layer of the dermis and has sluggish or absent capillary refill?
   A. superficial partial-thickness burn
   B. deep partial-thickness burn
   C. full-thickness burn
   D. subdermal burns
5. Which of the following zones is an area of immediately nonviable tissue?
   A. hyperemia
   B. ischemia
   C. coagulation
   D. stasis

Answers: 1. C, 2. A, 3. A, 4. B, 5. C

SECTION THREE: Burn Centers

At the completion of this section, the learner will be able to discuss criteria for transfer of a patient to a burn center and to describe the unique structures, processes, and personnel that make up a burn center.

Burn Center Referral Criteria

After the extent and depth of the burn injury has been classified, the severity of the injury is evaluated. Patients with complex burn injuries have complex physiological and psychosocial needs. This requires specialized resources and personnel and these patients are referred to a **burn center.** A burn center is a specific area in the hospital with resources and staff designated for treating patients who have experienced burn injuries. This area contains special beds and other equipment related to the care of patients with burn injury (ABA, 2007b) and nurses who work in these areas receive special training and continuing education. The American Burn Association (2006) has established criteria that, when present, indicate the need to transfer a patient to a burn center (Table 37–2). As a general rule, if more than 5 to 10 percent of the TBSA is covered with burns, the patient should be transferred to a burn center (Holmes, 2008).

TABLE 37–2 Burn Center Referral Criteria

- Partial-thickness burns greater than 10% TBSA
- Burns involving face, hands, feet, genitalia, perineum, or over major joints
- Third degree burns in any age group
- Electrical burns, including lightning injuries
- Chemical burns
- Inhalation injuries
- Burn injury in patients with preexisting medical disorders that complicate management, prolong recovery, or affect mortality
- Any patient with burns and concomitant trauma in which the burn places the greatest risk of morbidity or mortality
- Burned children in hospitals without qualified personnel or equipment to take care of this type of patient
- Burn injury in patients that may require special social, emotional, or rehabilitation interventions

Structure of the Burn Unit

Patients in the burn unit are susceptible to infection because of altered resistance to microorganisms as a result of the presence of open wounds and immunosuppression. A model burn unit provides an environment that promotes isolation from pathogens and prevents infection. In the ideal unit each patient occupies a single room that provides positive airflow and the unit is access restricted. Techniques such as strict hand washing and the proper use of masks, gowns, gloves, and caps during dressing changes are strictly followed. These techniques decrease the patient's risk for infection. Each patient's room should contain individual controls for temperature and humidity and have ample space for equipment and supplies.

The typical burn unit is equipped to provide standard invasive monitoring and ventilatory support. Hydrotherapy or whirlpool facilities are often located in burn units because patients may require hydrotherapy to promote wound healing. Operating room suites may also be located within the burn unit.

Burn Team Members

Care of the critically injured burn patient is complex and requires a multidisciplinary approach. Burn team members include nurses, physicians (plastic and general surgeons), physical therapists (PTs), occupational therapists (OTs), pharmacists, dietitians, discharge planners, social workers, chaplains, and psychologists. Additional services may be needed. Nurses who work in burn centers must have an orientation program that documents nursing competencies specific to the care and treatment of burn patients, including critical care, wound care, and rehabilitation that are age-appropriate. Nurses must also attend a minimum of two burn-related continuing education opportunities annually (ABA, 2007).

SECTION THREE REVIEW

1. Which of the following criteria indicate a burn center referral should be made?
   A. partial-thickness burn greater than 10 percent
   B. chemical burns
   C. any patient with burns and trauma
   D. all of the above

2. In the ideal burn unit
   A. patients are in semiprivate rooms with positive airflow
   B. patients are in private rooms with positive airflow
   C. patients are in private rooms with negative airflow
   D. access is not restricted

Answers: 1. D, 2. B

SECTION FOUR: Resuscitative Phase: Cardiovascular and Pulmonary Effects

At the completion of this section, the learner will be able to discuss priority cardiovascular and pulmonary assessments and interventions during the resuscitation phase for the patient with a burn injury.

The **resuscitative phase** lasts from the time of burn injury to 48 to 72 hours postinjury. Burn shock with cardiovascular collapse can occur during this time period. Traumatic injuries, such as head trauma, internal injuries, and fractures that may occur concurrently with burn injuries, are identified and treated early in this phase. Primary and secondary assessments for traumatic injury are completed on all burn patients (see Module 38, Alterations in Multisystem Function: Multiple Trauma, for these assessments).

Cardiovascular

Severe burn injuries cause massive fluid shifts from the intravascular space to the interstitium in both burned and nonburned tissues, creating a hypovolemic state. Fluid resuscitation is challenging. Under-resuscitation can lead to ischemia of pulmonary, renal, and mesenteric vascular beds and can worsen injury. Over-resuscitation can lead to upper airway obstruction, pulmonary and cerebral edema, as well as extremity compartment and abdominal compartment syndromes (White, 2008).

Adults with large burns are frequently tachycardic (heart rate between 110 and 125 beats per minute). Burns covering more than 40 percent of the total body surface area produce significant myocardial dysfunction. A decrease in myocardial contractility occurs and cardiac output falls within the first few minutes of injury, even prior to a decreased plasma volume. During the initial few hours, plasma volume drops, contributing to the decreased cardiac output. An increased peripheral vascular resistance accompanies decreased cardiac output. The causes of myocardial dysfunction in burn patients are not well understood; however, there are several theories as to the causes including those that propound the release of a substance from the burn wound itself called myocardial depressant factor and the release of oxygen free-radicals from the ischemic myocardial tissues.

Administration of fluids dramatically improves the outcome of the burn patient. Fluid resuscitation will usually be initiated in adult patients with greater than 20 percent TBSA involvement, in the elderly with greater than 5 to 15 percent TBSA involvement, and in children with greater than 10 to 15 percent TBSA involvement. Children and the elderly are less able to tolerate the stress of injury. Volume replacement must be implemented very carefully in children and the elderly because they are very sensitive to volume. Children usually require more fluid than adults, averaging about 5.8 mL/kg percent TBSA burn (American Burn Association, 2001a). A pulmonary artery catheter may be used to monitor fluid status in the elderly.

Patients with thermal burns covering more than 40 percent of the body may experience burn shock, a state of hypovolemic shock that develops secondary to the fluid shifts that occur after burn injury. Chemical and vasoactive mediators produced as a result of burn injury cause arterial constriction initially, followed by vasodilation and increased capillary permeability. Vasodilation in combination with increased capillary permeability is referred to as a loss of capillary seal. The loss of capillary seal leads to massive fluid and electrolyte shifts from intravascular spaces to the interstitium. Hypovolemic shock is a complication of loss of capillary seal and other factors. Although the exact mechanisms for vascular and fluid changes are not well understood, the capillary seal is usually restored within 36 hours postinjury.

Restoration of intravascular volume by fluid resuscitation is a critical intervention for burn shock. The goal is to maintain vital organ perfusion without exacerbating tissue edema. A minimal mean arterial pressure (MAP) for the adult is 70 mm Hg (Arlati et al., 2007). The routine use of hemodynamic monitoring is not used to guide fluid resuscitation in patients with burn injury because of the risk of infections (Arlati et al., 2007). The patient's physiologic responses, such as urine output, adequate vital signs, appropriate mentation, capillary refill, and peripheral pulses, will guide fluid administration efforts. Although controversial, currently the best determinant of adequate fluid resuscitation (in the first 24 to 48 hours postburn injury) is urine output (Blumetti et al., 2008). However, urine output may not be an accurate measure of fluid resuscitation when the patient is receiving a medication that causes diuresis (e.g., diuretics) or in the presence of glucosuria (glucose in the urine causes an osmotic diuresis). After the initial resuscitation, urine output is not the best predictor of fluid status. Generally, in adults, a urine output of 30 to 50 mL/hour must be maintained (White, 2008). For children, a urine output of 1 to 2 mL/kg per hour for children weighing less than 30 kg should be maintained (Blumetti et al., 2008). Laboratory values such as serum sodium concentration, serum and urine glucose concentrations, as well as body weight changes, clinical examination, and intake and output records are followed to best determine fluid replacement (American Burn Association, 2001a).

Fluids are infused at a steady rate by two large-bore (14 to 16 gauge) intravenous (IV) catheters placed through unburned skin if possible. If an IV catheter must be inserted into a burned area, the cannula is threaded in a long vein so that edema does not push the hub out and cause an infiltration.

There are a number of formulas used to guide crystalloid fluid administration during the first 24 hours. Each formula will have to be modified according to the patient's response. One of the most frequent formulas used is the Parkland formula:

4 mL Ringer's lactate × TBSA % burned × patient weight (kg)

With the Parkland formula, one half of the amount is infused during the first eight hours postinjury. This is followed by the last half during the next 16 hours. For example, using the Parkland formula, a patient weighing 68 kilograms who experiences a 50 percent TBSA burn would require 6,800 mL of IV fluids during the first eight hours postinjury with a subsequent infusion of 6,800 mL during the next 16 hours. Urinary output trends are monitored to determine the adequacy of fluid replacement.

Fluid administration requirements are altered under certain circumstances. Patients with inhalation injuries in conjunction with thermal burns require increased amounts of fluid initially (up to 40 to 50 percent more). Patients with electrical burns and associated trauma, extensive deep thermal burns, alcohol intoxication, those receiving delayed resuscitation (greater than two hours after the time of injury), or those with preexisting medical conditions (e.g., patients receiving diuretic therapy) may require increased amounts of fluid according to their physiological responses.

Isotonic crystalloid fluids are used for patients with less than 40 percent TBSA and no pulmonary injury (American Burn Association, 2001a). For patients with greater than 40 percent TBSA or pulmonary injuries, hypertonic saline can be used in the initial eight hours, followed by lactated Ringer's (LR) solution. Although hypertonic saline is currently recommended (American

Burn Association, 2001a), considerable controversy exists over its efficacy. For pediatric and elderly patients, a lower hypertonic concentration is used to prevent excessive sodium retention and hypernatremia. A combination of fluids is used for patients with major burns, young children, and those with burns combined with a severe inhalation injury. Dextrose solutions are not to be given because these can cause osmotic diuresis, complicating fluid resuscitation. All resuscitative formulas should be considered guidelines and should be individualized according to patient assessments. Burn resuscitation fluids should be used until the volume infused is maintaining proper urine output and is equal to the maintenance rate, which consists of the normal maintenance volume plus considerations for evaporative water loss.

Patients who have been exposed to electrical currents may have necrosis of the myocardium and may be predisposed to cardiac dysrhythmias, including sinus tachycardia, nonspecific *ST* or *T* wave changes, *QT* segment prolongation, ventricular ectopy, atrial fibrillation, a bundle branch block, ventricular fibrillation, varying degrees of heart blocks, supraventricular tachycardia, and asystole. Patients who experience lethal dysrhythmias (ventricular fibrillation or asystole) from electrical or lightning contact receive aggressive resuscitation because of the frequency with which these patients can be successfully resuscitated. Cardiac monitoring continues for at least 24 hours postinjury, even for patients having electrical contact who do not seem to have any obvious injury.

Peripheral Vascular

Peripheral vascular assessment of each extremity occurs in the initial assessment and is repeated every hour thereafter throughout the resuscitative phase. Each extremity is evaluated for color, temperature, pulses, capillary refill, sensation, pain, and motor movement. A doppler may be required to make a better assessment of peripheral pulses because edema can interfere with palpation. Increased pressure within the limb from edema can cause tissue ischemia. Elevating burned extremities above the level of the heart helps decrease edema. Jewelry and constricting clothing are removed as soon as possible. **Compartment syndrome** occurs when the tissue pressure within a muscle compartment exceeds microvascular pressure causing an interruption in perfusion at the cellular level.

Signs and symptoms of compartment syndrome include pain on passive stretching of the muscle, decreased sensation, weakness, swelling, and pain beyond that expected for the injury sustained. Current guidelines recommend that escharotomies be performed (1) when compartmental pressures are greater than 40 mm Hg (however, pressures between 25 and 40 mm Hg may cause muscle and nerve ischemia leading to consideration of escharotomies at lower pressures) and (2) if doppler pulses are absent in the major distal arteries or in the palmar or plantar arches (however, the presence of doppler pulses does not confirm adequate perfusion of the underlying structures) (American Burn Association, 2001b). Escharotomies are performed in a longitudinal fashion midlateral or midmedial in the supinated extremity through the entire involved area as shown in Figure 37–6 (American Burn Association, 2001b). Continued close monitoring is necessary to ensure that the area was adequately released and that elevated pressures have not recurred.

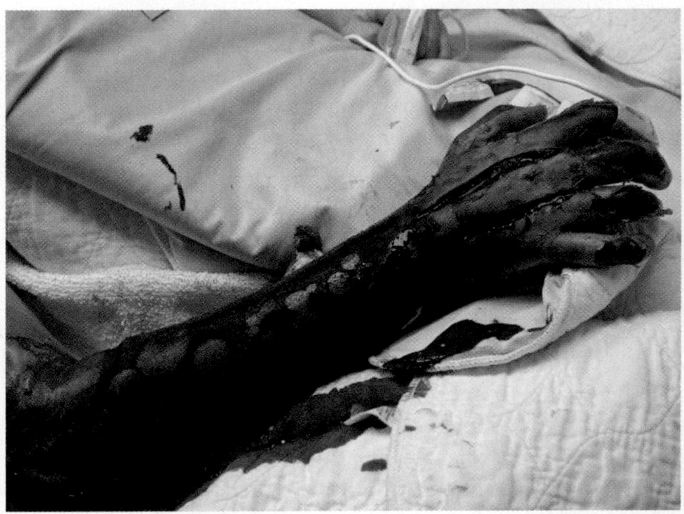

Figure 37–6 ■ Escharotomy of the hand.

Pulmonary

Alterations in pulmonary function can occur as part of the systemic response to burn injury or from direct inhalation injury. The systemic response to burn injury results in an increased systemic vascular resistance with a corresponding increase in pulmonary vascular resistance. This results in pulmonary edema from the increased capillary pressure and vasoconstriction of microcirculation. A decrease in pulmonary perfusion results in decreased diffusion of oxygen at the capillary level. Respiratory insufficiency can occur at two points postinjury: immediately during the resuscitation phase and ten days to two weeks postinjury during the acute rehabilitation phase. Respiratory failure during the resuscitative phase is usually a result of inhalation injury, and failure in the acute rehabilitation phase is usually a result of infection.

Circumferential (or near circumferential) full-thickness burns to the chest can also cause alterations in pulmonary function. Full-thickness burns result in **eschar** formation, a tough, dry, inelastic wound that does not allow for adequate expansion of the chest. If these eschar chest wounds are circumferential, the patient cannot adequately expand the chest to ventilate effectively and respiratory distress will develop. **Escharotomy** incisions may be performed at the bedside to allow movement of the chest wall and to restore adequate ventilation.

Upper-Airway Injury

Upper-airway injury refers to an injury that is supraglottic, resulting from either heat or chemicals dissolved in water. Heat causes an immediate injury to the mucosa. Thermal burns from hot air are usually isolated to the supraglottic (as opposed to the infraglottic) area because of the ability of the nasopharynx to absorb the heat and a reflex closure of the glottic opening when exposed to heat. Evaluation of patients with upper-airway burns may reveal facial burns, singed nasal hairs, erythema, swelling, tachypnea, dyspnea, hoarseness, a brassy cough or stridor, and ulceration, especially of the nasopharynx. Initial treatment for upper-airway injury is humidified 100 percent oxygen by a snugly fitting nonrebreather mask. Careful observation is necessary to identify impending airway obstruction. Once the tissues start to swell, patients can rapidly experience an airway occlusion. Patients with hoarseness, stridor, or pharyngeal burns are intubated and transferred to a burn center. Upper-airway edema peaks within 48 hours postinjury. If it is not contraindicated by concurrent trauma, the head of the bed is elevated to help reduce edema. Circumferential burns to the neck can also cause airway obstruction as a result of edema. These patients also require intubation.

An **inhalation injury** is suspected in the patient who presents with an altered level of consciousness or one from within a confined space in a burning environment. Inhalation injury is restricted to injury below the glottis caused by products of combustion (American Burn Association, 2007c). The diagnosis is made if there is evidence of history of exposure to products of combustion and by bronchoscopy that reveals evidence of carbonaceous material or signs of edema or ulceration below the glottis (American Burn Association, 2007c). Clinical indicators of inhalation injury are listed in Table 37–3. The composition and amount of the inhaled substance correlates with the severity of the injury.

Lower-Airway Injury

Lower-airway injury (infraglottic) is usually the result of toxic gases and chemicals contained in inhaled smoke. The inhaled smoke contains gaseous and chemical byproducts of combustion. When these products come into contact with the pulmonary mucosa, a variety of things happen, such as irritation, an inflammatory reaction, or alkali or acid burns. The result is an ulceration of mucous membranes, edema, excessive secretions, decreased ciliary action, bronchospasms, inactivation of surfactant, and atelectasis, among other things. The end result is an airflow obstruction causing hypoxemia and pulmonary dysfunction. These patients develop respiratory failure and are prone to the development of pulmonary infections.

The onset of symptoms of lower-airway injury is unpredictable. Patients with lower-airway injury may present without symptoms to the emergency department. However, they also may present with the signs and symptoms for upper-airway injury, in addition to a cough, carbonaceous (sooty) sputum, signs of hypoxemia (agitation, anxiety, cyanosis, impaired mental status), chest tightness, flaring nostrils, grunting, crackles, rhonchi, or wheezing. If the potential for inhalation injury exists, the patient is monitored closely for at least 24 hours postinjury. Parenchymal lung injuries may take longer to evolve. Diagnostic tests for determining the effects and extent of inhalation injury include physical examination, arterial blood gases (partial pressure of oxygen may be normal initially), serial chest radiographs, fiber-optic bronchoscopy (to visualize tracheobronchial injuries), ventilation–perfusion scan (to identify small airway and parenchymal injuries), carboxyhemoglobin levels, and cyanide levels (American Burn Association, 2001c).

Treatment for lower-airway injury is supportive. Any patient with the potential for inhalation injury must receive high-flow humidified oxygen (100 percent by nonrebreather mask). Patients with severe inhalation injuries or impending respiratory failure must receive high-flow humidified oxygen while preparations for endotracheal intubation are made. Intubation is not performed prophylactically; however, there must be a low threshold for intubation if there is concern about progressive edema (American Burn Association, 2001d). Mechanical ventilation provides positive pressure ventilation, peak inspiratory pressures to below 40 cm H_2O, and allows for permissive hypercapnia (although this is contraindicated in the presence of closed-head injury) (American Burn Association, 2001d).

One of the major goals of nursing care is meticulous pulmonary hygiene. Ensuring that the patient does the coughing and deep breathing exercises, turning the patient, suctioning, chest physiotherapy, and pharmacologic interventions will help achieve this goal. Repeated assessments of respiratory status and accurate documentation for other caregivers is necessary. Ventilatory support is tailored to each patient's needs, with the ultimate goal of improvement to a point such that support is no longer needed. Ensuring that the endotracheal tube is secured appropriately is very important, especially in children under the age of eight because the endotracheal tube may not have a cuff, although the routine use of uncuffed endotracheal tubes in children has recently been challenged (Namias, 2007). Accidental displacement of an endotracheal tube in a patient with airway edema can have catastrophic results. A fine balance must be made between tightly securing the airway and preventing pressure ulcers from the straps, which are especially difficult with facial burns and the resulting edema.

TABLE 37–3 Clinical Indicators of Inhalation Injury

- Facial burns with charred lips and tongue
- Carbonaceous sputum
- Wheezing or rhonchi on auscultation
- Stridor
- Cough
- Tachypnea
- Singed nasal hair
- Altered level of consciousness
- Injury in enclosed space
- History of flash burn
- Elevated carboxyhemoglobin levels
- Abnormal arterial blood gases

Carbon Monoxide Poisoning

Carbon monoxide (CO) poisoning is a chemical inhalation injury that has an action different from other inhaled chemicals. Carbon monoxide is a colorless, odorless gas that is a byproduct of the combustion of organic material. CO is more than 200 times more likely to bind to hemoglobin than oxygen. In the presence of CO, hemoglobin becomes saturated with CO rather than oxygen. This results in hypoxemia. The diagnosis of CO poisoning is made by obtaining a history of exposure to byproducts of combustion, especially in an enclosed space, and by drawing a serum **carboxyhemoglobin** level (percentage of CO bound to hemoglobin). CO poisoning represents a transport shock state (refer to Module 18, Alterations in Oxygen Delivery and Consumption: Shock States).

Symptoms caused by CO poisoning are the result of exposure to low levels of CO for prolonged periods or from exposure to higher levels for a shorter duration. The severity of poisoning depends on several factors, including underlying health. The most common symptoms of carbon monoxide poisoning are headache, malaise, nausea, difficulties with memory, and personality changes, as well as gross neurologic dysfunction. An elevated carboxyhemoglobin level confirms CO poisoning. Whereas carboxyhemoglobin levels may be greater than 70 percent, the carboxyhemoglobin level is not indicative of the level of neurological injury.

The treatment for CO poisoning consists of the administration of high fractional concentrations of supplemental oxygen. Data indicate that early, aggressive hyperbaric oxygen therapy may decrease the negative sequelae of CO poisoning. Serial carboxyhemoglobin levels are monitored to evaluate patient response to treatment. Pulse oximetry does not differentiate between hemoglobin saturated with oxygen and hemoglobin saturated with CO, so readings may be misleading.

SECTION FOUR REVIEW

1. The resuscitative phase of burn injury occurs from the time of injury to
   A. 24 to 48 hours after injury
   B. 36 to 60 hours after injury
   C. 48 to 72 hours after injury
   D. 60 to 84 hours after injury
2. Critically burned patients are at high risk for which of the following complications during the resuscitative phase?
   A. burn shock
   B. neurogenic shock
   C. contractures
   D. myocardial infarction
3. Calculate the fluid resuscitation requirements for Mr. C. using the Parkland formula. Mr. C. has a 55 percent TBSA burn and weighs 75 kilograms. His requirements for the first eight hours are
   A. 8,250 mL
   B. 16,500 mL
   C. 4,125 mL
   D. 12,375 mL
4. Patients exposed to electrical injuries are at risk for developing
   A. nonspecific *ST* wave changes
   B. *QT* segment prolongation
   C. ventricular ectopy
   D. all of the above
5. To detect compartmental syndrome in those with critical burns, assess for
   A. pain in extremity with exercise
   B. pain in extremity with passive movement
   C. contractures
   D. pallor in extremity
6. Treatment for carbon monoxide poisoning includes
   A. 100 percent O_2
   B. hypertonic saline
   C. keeping peak inspiratory pressure less than 40 cm H_2O
   D. pulmonary hygiene

Answers: 1. C, 2. A, 3. A, 4. D, 5. B, 6. A

SECTION FIVE: Resuscitative Phase: Pain and Neurologic Disorders

At the completion of this section, the learner will be able to discuss priority neurological and pain assessments and interventions during the resuscitative phase for the patient with a burn injury.

Neurological

Neurological effects are common with electrical and lightning injuries. Since neurological tissue offers low resistance to electrical current it is easily damaged. The skull is a common entry site for electrical current. While it is usually transient, respiratory paralysis can occur and loss of consciousness is frequent, especially with high-voltage injury. Patients may experience confusion, exhibit a flat affect, lose the ability to concentrate, or have short-term memory problems. Seizures, headaches, peripheral nerve damage, and loss of muscle strength may also be observed. Long-term or permanent numbness, prickling, tingling, heightened sensitivity, or paralysis may also occur. Spinal cord injuries can occur with high-voltage injuries. The onset of clinical manifestations may be acute or delayed.

Pain

Pain expressed by patients with burn injuries is extremely variable. Full-thickness burns are usually insensate, except for the edge of the wound where partial-thickness injury exists. Partial-thickness burns are exceptionally sensitive and painful even to an air current passing over them. The patient should be asked to rate pain as either procedural or nonprocedural pain (Meyer et al., 2007). Procedural pain is pain related to wound care or stretching of the patient's scar tissue. Nonprocedural (or background) pain is the discomfort experienced at rest.

Analgesics are most effective in burn survivors when they are given on a regularly scheduled basis (rather than intermittent, or as needed). There are a variety of treatments for background and procedural pain during the stages of burn treatment. According to Meyer et al., (2007) the three stages are

- Emergency or resuscitative phase (0-72 hours after injury)
- Acute phase (72 hours to three to five weeks, until wounds are closed)
- Rehabilitative phase (from time of wound closure to scar maturity; phase may last months to years)

For patients with greater than 10 percent TBSA, during the emergency phase the preferred route for most medications is IV because of potential problems with absorption from the intramuscular route secondary to decreased perfusion (Meyer et al., 2007). Morphine is the most widely used analgesic. Fentanyl may be used during procedures, however it should be administered 15 to 30 minutes prior to the procedure (Gordon & Marvin, 2007). During the acute phase, oral opioid analgesics may be given for procedural pain. Background pain is best controlled by patient-controlled analgesia. During the rehabilitative phase, most patients complain of an aching pain. Mild opioid analgesics, acetaminophen, or nonsteroidal anti-inflammatory drugs may be given. Nonpharmacologic therapies play an important role in addressing the psychological factors that exacerbate pain as well as directly affect the pain itself (Meyer et al., 2007). These therapies include classical conditioning, relaxation therapy, cognitive interventions, distraction (music therapy), hypnosis, and massage therapy.

Anxiety

Patients with burn injuries have increased levels of anxiety, especially related to treatment and outcome. Anticipatory anxiety related to treatments can lead to perceptions of increased pain; the increased pain leads to further increasing anxiety (Meyer et al., 2007). Anxiolytics may be given. However, anxiolytics should be considered only after the patient's pain has been aggressively treated. Benzodiazepam agents may be given IV during procedures. Otherwise, they may be given orally.

Itching

Pruritis is one of the most common subjective symptoms in patients after burn injury. The mechanism is not well understood. Scratching can further injure the skin, leading to graft loss and skin breakdown and can impede exercise or sleeping. Moisturizing body shampoos and lotions can be used to alleviate itching associated with dry skin. Topical steroids may be used once the skin is well healed. Other agents may include antihistamines (orally or topically) and colloid and oatmeal baths.

Psychiatric Symptoms

Common psychiatric symptoms during the emergency and acute-care phase may include delirium, acute stress and posttraumatic stress disorder symptoms, sleep disturbances, and depression. Causes of these symptoms are often multifactorial. Delirium may be caused by disturbances in fluid and electrolytes, glucose, altered cerebral perfusion, and history of substance abuse. Antipsychotic phenothiazines in the acute-burn phase are commonly used to address delirium and/or combative uncooperative behavior such as pulling off dressings, attempting to get out of bed, or striking out at caregivers (Thomas et al., 2007). During the acute phase, a significant number of burn survivors will experience posttraumatic stress disorder symptoms, including intrusive memories of injury, hypervigilance, or disturbed sleep patterns (Thomas et al., 2007). Antidepressants may be administered.

SECTION FIVE REVIEW

1. In general, full-thickness burns are
   A. not painful
   B. mildly painful
   C. moderately painful
   D. extremely painful
2. The patient should be asked to rate pain as ______ or ______.
3. Which of the following burn injuries are associated with pain that is exceptionally sensitive and painful even to an air current passing over them?
   A. full-thickness
   B. partial-thickness
   C. third-degree
   D. electrical
4. The acute-care phase for background and procedural pain treatment is (choose all that apply)
   A. 0 to 72 hours after injury
   B. 72 hours to three to five weeks
   C. from time wound closure to scar maturity
   D. until wounds are closed
5. Burned patients have increased levels of anxiety related to (choose all that apply)
   A. treatments
   B. outcomes
   C. anticipatory anxiety related to dressing changes
   D. pain

Answers: 1. A, 2. procedural or nonprocedural (background), 3. D, 4. (B, D) 5. (A, B, C, D)

SECTION SIX: Resuscitative Phase: Metabolic and Renal Effects

At the completion of this section, the learner will be able to discuss priority nursing assessments and interventions during the resuscitative phase for gastrointestinal (GI), metabolic, and renal effects of burn injury.

Metabolic Effects

The metabolic changes that occur in the burn patient are related to the extent of injury. Severe burns covering more than 40 percent of the body are typically associated with a period of physiologic stress, hypermetabolism, and inflammation; this results in glycolysis, proteolysis, lipolysis and hypermetabolism (Gauglitz et al., 2008). The hypermetabolic response to burn injury occurs in two distinct patterns. The "ebb phase" occurs in the first 48 hours of injury and is characterized by decreases in cardiac output, oxygen consumption and metabolic rate (Gauglitz et al., 2008). The "flow phase" occurs within five days postinjury. This phase is associated with a hypermetabolic hyperdynamic state with persistent elevation of cortisol, cytokines, catecholamines, and glucose (Gauglitz et al., 2008). Patients experience an increase in cardiac output, oxygen consumption, carbon dioxide production, caloric requirements, energy consumption, heart rate, respiratory rate, and body temperature. This hypermetabolic response has been shown to last up to a year, impacting both acute recovery and rehabilitation (Tam et al., 2008). Although adequate fluid resuscitation, prompt surgical excision, and grafting of burn wounds remain the cornerstones of burn care, recent evidence suggests modulation of the hypermetabolic response may improve outcomes. In patients with burn injuries covering more than 40 percent of the body, the resting metabolic rate is 180 percent of basal rate during acute admission, 150 percent at full healing of the burn wound, 140 percent at six months, 120 percent at nine months and 110 percent at 12 months after the burn injury.

Emerging Evidence

- Resuscitation volume can be safely reduced below the Parkland Formula estimate, provided that reduction of administered fluids is guided by close non-invasive hemodynamic monitoring with intrathoracic blood volume and cardiac output by PiCCO© (Pulsion Medical Systems, Munich, Germany). Permissive hypovolemia (3.2 ± 0.75 mL/kg/percent TBSA) seems to be effective in reducing both organ and system dysfunction induced by edema formation. This hemodynamic resuscitative approach allows for better refinement of fluid volume administered during early postburn period and minimizes unnecessary fluid volume overload *(Arlati, Storti, Pradella et al., 2007).*
- Oxandrolone is a testosterone analog that improves net protein balance, lean body mass, and liver protein synthesis. Early administration of oxandrolone (initiated within seven days of admission and continuing treatment for a mean of 43 days) is associated with higher survival and shortened length of hospitalization *(Pham, Klein, Gibran et al., 2008).*

Nutritional requirements are strongly influenced by the metabolic response to stress. Adequate caloric intake is imperative for wound healing and maintaining the immune system. Multiple formulas exist for estimating caloric needs of burn patients. Energy requirements are assessed and formulas that calculate both energy and protein needs are used. Increased protein intake is needed to counteract the use of lean body mass and viscera as sources of protein in this hypermetabolic state. Skeletal muscle is the major fuel source in the burned patient and leads to significant wasting of lean body mass within days of injury (Saffle & Graves, 2007). Stress induced hyperglycemia occurs in patients with burn injury as it does in patients with critical illness or injury. Administration of insulin in severely burned patients has been shown to improve muscle protein synthesis, accelerate healing time, attenuate loss of lean body mass, and decrease the acute phase response (Gauglitz et al., 2008).

Enteral nutrition is initiated early—within 24 hours postinjury (American Burn Association, 2001e). Early nutrition reduces cumulative caloric deficits, stimulates insulin secretion, and conserves lean body mass. Enteral nutrition should provide a calorie-to-nitrogen ratio of 110:1 for burns 20 percent or greater TBSA (American Burn Association, 2001e). Enteral nutrition is preferred over parenteral nutrition because enteral nutrition maintains gastrointestinal motility and reduces translocation of bacteria (Pereira, 2005). Parenteral nutrition is reserved for patients with prolonged ileus or intolerance to enteral feedings. Adequate protein intake is crucial because burn patients oxidize amino acids at rates 50 percent higher than healthy individuals (Pereira, 2005). Nutritional status is closely monitored via clinical examination of wound healing, serial weights, prealbumin levels, and indirect calorimetry.

Renal Effects

During the hypermetabolic phase, cardiac output and therefore renal blood flow and glomerular filtration rate are increased. As a result, the dose of many of the drugs given will be adjusted. With antibiotics eliminated by glomerular filtration, some patients will eliminate drugs extremely rapidly, leading to poor efficacy (Conil et al., 2006). During this hypermetabolic state, serum creatinine may be less reliable as a tool to detect changes in renal function (Conil et al., 2006).

Acute renal failure is a major complication associated with burn injury that can be caused by prerenal conditions or intrarenal parenchymal damage (see Module 27, Alterations in Renal Function: Acute Renal Failure). Etiologic factors include fluid shifts, stress related hormones, myocardial depression, inflammatory mediators, denatured proteins and nephrotoxic agents (Sun et al., 2007). Continuous renal replacement therapy may be used for supportive treatment of acute renal failure.

If a patient has experienced muscle damage from exposure to an electrical current or a crush-type injury, the urine may be red to reddish-brown in color. This discoloration results from **myoglobin** in the urine. Myoglobin is released from damaged muscle tissue and can clog the renal tubules, causing renal failure, especially in the face of inadequate fluid resuscitation, shock, or acidosis (refer to Module 27, Alterations in Renal Function:

Acute Renal Failure). If myoglobin is present in the urine (**myoglobinuria**), adequate urine output (75 to 100 mL/hour in an adult) must be maintained (through IV fluid administration) to prevent myoglobinuric renal failure (White, 2008). This rate of urine output is maintained as long as pigment in the urine is present. In addition to increasing the amount of fluids administered, alkalinization of the urine also prevents myoglobin from crystallizing in the tubules and causing an obstruction. The solubility of myoglobin increases in an alkaline environment, so maintaining alkaline urine will increase the rate of myoglobin clearance. By adding 50 mEq of sodium bicarbonate to each liter of intravenous fluids, a slight alkalinization of the blood is maintained (pH 7.45), ensuring that the urine is also alkaline. However, this treatment can worsen hypocalcemia (White, 2008). An osmotic diuretic, such as mannitol, may be used to increase diuresis and promote the clearance of myoglobin.

In addition to myoglobin causing discoloration of the urine, hemoglobin released from damaged red blood cells can also cause red to reddish-brown urine. It is difficult to distinguish myoglobin from hemoglobin by looking at the urine, so until laboratory tests confirm the presence of one or both of these substances, treat all red to reddish-brown discoloration of the urine as if it were myoglobin. Both myoglobin and hemoglobin are excreted more readily if the urine pH is alkaline.

SECTION SIX REVIEW

1. Which of the following statements reflect current recommendations for meeting the hypermetabolic needs of a burn patient?
   A. Total parenteral nutrition should be started within 24 hours after injury.
   B. Enteral nutrition should be started within 24 hours after injury.
   C. The patient should not be fed until bowel sounds are present.
   D. Enteral nutrition should be started after 48 hours of admission.
2. Which of the following routes is the preferred method of nutrition for patients with burn injury?
   A. IV
   B. oral
   C. parenteral
   D. enteral
3. Which of the following injuries places the burn patient at risk for developing renal failure?
   A. full-thickness burn to the perineum
   B. full-thickness burn to the flank
   C. electrical or crush-type injury
   D. traumatic brain injury
4. Diagnosis of myoglobinuria can be made by
   A. assessing the color of urine
   B. assessment of arterial blood gases
   C. urinalysis
   D. blood sample
5. In the presence of myoglobin in the urine, alkalinization of the urine will
   A. promote renal clearance of myoglobin
   B. promote hepatic clearance of myoglobin
   C. increase urine output
   D. concentrate the myoglobin so it can be removed more easily

Answers: 1. B, 2. D, 3. C, 4. C, 5. A

SECTION SEVEN: Overview of Burn Wound Healing and Initial Wound Care

At the completion of this section, the learner will be able to compare burn wound healing and wound healing from other injuries, and state the wound care priorities during the resuscitative phase. Before reading this section, it may be helpful to review normal wound healing as discussed in Module 35, Determinants and Assessment of Skin Integrity.

Wound Healing

The cellular and biochemical events that occur during the healing of burn injuries are similar to those that occur in the healing of other wounds. The major difference is that the phases of wound healing in the burn occur more slowly and last longer. Wound healing begins immediately after the injury occurs with the inflammatory response. The inflammatory phase lasts approximately two weeks, extending into the acute rehabilitative phase; thus, overall wound repair is delayed. After the inflammatory phase is finished, the proliferative phase of healing begins. This phase lasts up to one month, during which time collagen synthesis, revascularization, and reepithelialization occur, although at a slower rate than in wounds from other injuries. Collagen layers are not as organized as they are in other wounds; this contributes to excessive scar tissue (Fig. 37–7). The maturation phase of wound healing follows the proliferative phase and can last six to 18 months or longer, depending on the wound. New collagen layers are placed, strengthening the wound, whereas old collagen layers are broken down. Excessive deposits of collagen during this time will produce hypertrophic scars that are characteristic of deep partial- and full-thickness burns. Hypertrophic scars contract while maturing, which can lead to contractures. Wound contraction can produce both cosmetic and functional deformities.

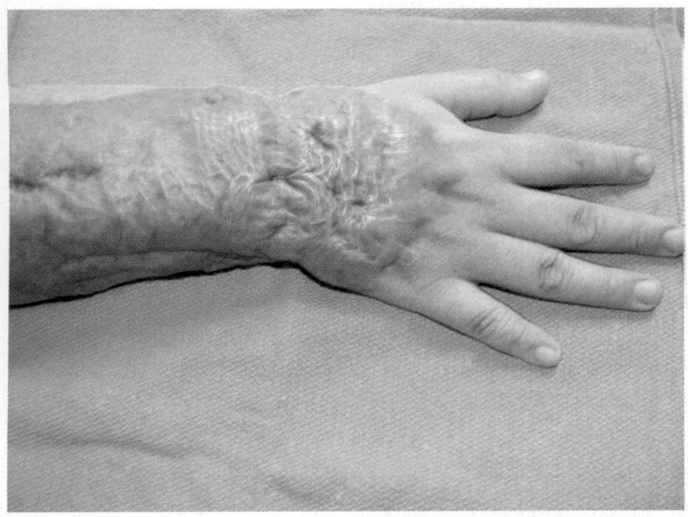

Figure 37–7 ■ Disorganized collagen layers lead to excessive scar tissue.

Initial Wound Care During the Resuscitative Phase

The first step in caring for the burn wound is to ensure the burning process has stopped. The longer the patient's skin is in contact with the burning agent and the higher the temperature, the deeper the cellular damage. Clothing, jewelry, belts, or anything containing heat is removed from the patient (adhered clothing or tar is left in place and cooled with water because removing it will cause further damage to the skin). Dry chemicals are brushed from the patient (taking care not to contaminate the caregiver) and continuous water lavage is initiated.

The initial assessment of the burn wound takes place in the secondary assessment after the head-to-toe evaluation has been completed. Burned extremities are elevated above the level of the heart to decrease edema formation. The head of the bed is also elevated to reduce upper body and head edema if not contraindicated by trauma. Tetanus prophylaxis is administered.

Initial care of the burn wound depends on the severity of the burn. If the patient meets criteria for transfer to a burn center, the patient is covered with a clean, dry sheet. Care is taken to avoid hypothermia. If time permits, the wound is gently cleansed with sterile saline or a mild soap. Creams or ointments are not applied as removal of the substance is necessary on arrival to the burn center to evaluate the wound (White, 2008). This is a painful procedure, so unless directed to do so by the receiving physician, leave the wound clean and cover with a sheet. An escharotomy may be required for a circumferential burn. Definitive care of the wound begins once the patient has been admitted to the hospital, whether that is a burn center or a hospital with the ability to care for the burn injury effectively.

SECTION SEVEN REVIEW

1. Initial evaluation of burn wounds takes place
   - **A.** immediately on arrival
   - **B.** at the end of the primary assessment
   - **C.** at the end of the head-to-toe evaluation during the secondary assessment
   - **D.** on admission to the burn center
2. You are the nurse in the emergency department caring for a patient with 60 percent TBSA burns. The helicopter is 20 minutes away, and the patient is to be transferred to a regional burn center. What is the appropriate initial wound care management at this time?
   - **A.** Cleanse the wounds and cover the patient with a sheet.
   - **B.** Place Neosporin ointment on all open burn wounds.
   - **C.** Put antibiotic cream on all wounds.
   - **D.** Cleanse the wounds and leave them open to air to dry out.
3. The maturation phase of burn wound injury can last
   - **A.** six weeks to 18 weeks
   - **B.** six months to 18 months
   - **C.** two weeks
   - **D.** one month
4. Wound contraction in burn wounds produces (choose all that apply)
   - **A.** infection
   - **B.** inflammation
   - **C.** cosmetic deformities
   - **D.** functional deformities
5. The first step in caring for the burn wound is to
   - **A.** clean the wound
   - **B.** administer pain medications
   - **C.** ensure the burning process has stopped
   - **D.** prevent infection

Answers: 1. C, 2. A, 3. B, 4. (C, D) 5. C

SECTION EIGHT: Acute Rehabilitative Phase: Burn Wound Management

At the completion of this section, the learner will be able to describe burn wound management in the acute rehabilitative phase.

The acute rehabilitative phase of burn care occurs after the resuscitative phase, beginning two to three days postinjury and lasting until wound closure. The goals of burn wound management include prevention and control of infection, preservation of viable tissue, and promotion of wound closure with minimal side effects. Interventions aimed at supporting these goals include wound cleansing, debridement, topical antimicrobial therapy, and wound closure.

Early excision and closure of burn wounds has greatly advanced in treating patients with thermal burn injuries in the past 20 years and has lead to substantial reduction in resting energy requirements and subsequent improvement in mortality rates (Gauglitz et al., 2008).

Wound Cleansing

Inpatient burn care begins with wounds being initially cleansed with water, known as hydrotherapy, and a mild soap to remove exudate and devitalized tissue. This can be accomplished (1) by showering if the patient is able, (2) by immersion in a tub if the burn is moderate in size, (3) by placing the patient on a table where the wounds are washed and rinsed with running water from spray hoses or, if these methods are contraindicated, (4) wounds can be cleaned while the patient is in bed. Once the wound has been cleaned, it must be debrided.

Wound Debridement

Wound **debridement** is the removal of debris and nonviable tissue from a wound. Wound debridement can be achieved mechanically, biologically, chemically, or surgically (refer to Module 35, Determinants and Assessment of Skin Integrity). Mechanical debridement includes hydrotherapy, or wound irrigation. With all methods of mechanical debridement, care is taken to avoid disrupting newly formed granulation tissue or epithelial buds in the healing wound. Wound irrigation and pulse lavage are easier to control than hydrotherapy, but all can cause disruption of newly formed tissue. The use of wet-to-dry dressings is no longer recommended because this is a nonselective form of debridement and causes harm to newly formed tissue and is also very painful. Biological debridement is the use of maggot therapy. This type of debridement is very beneficial because it only affects dead tissue.

Treatment of burn blisters, or **bullae,** is controversial. Fluid-filled blisters less than 2 cm in diameter are usually left intact (White, 2008). Blisters larger than 2 cm in diameter may be left intact, drained by aspiration using sterile technique, or opened and the loose skin removed.

Chemical debridement involves the application of an enzymatic or fibrinolytic preparation to the burn wound to digest necrotic tissue and hasten eschar separation. Eschar is tough, dry nonelastic tissue associated with full-thickness burns. Removal of eschar prevents bacterial colonization of dead tissue.

Surgical debridement is accomplished under anesthesia in the operating room and usually takes place within the resuscitative phase or within the first week postburn. There are two methods of burn wound excision: tangential excision and fascial excision. The method used depends on the depth and extent of burn. Tangential excision involves the shaving away of thin layers of eschar until viable tissue is exposed (Fig. 37–8). This method gives a better cosmetic result than fascial excision; however, significant blood loss may occur, causing hypovolemia. Fascial excision involves removing nonviable tissue down to the fascial or subcutaneous planes. This method is often used for patients with a large component of full-thickness burns because it is less stressful. Fascial excision does not produce as good a cosmetic result as tangential excision; however, if the injury is such that the patient will not survive the stress of tangential excision, fascial excision is used.

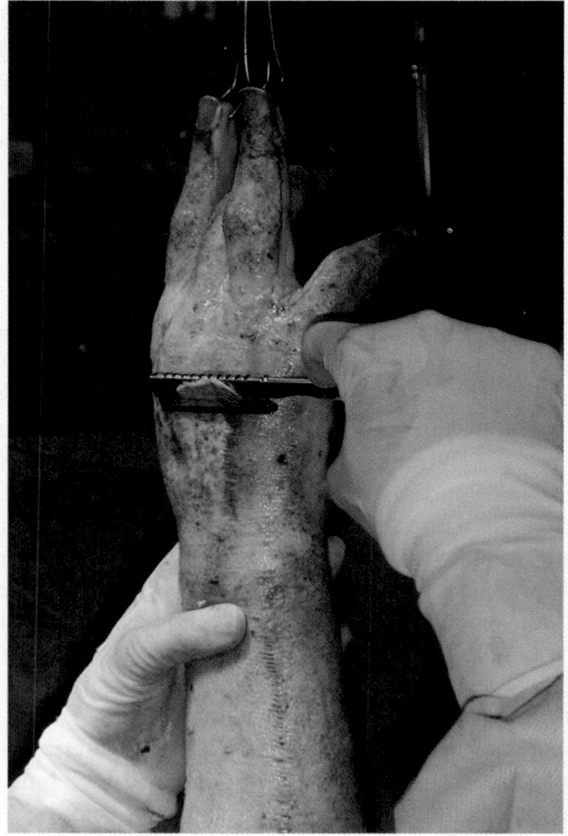

Figure 37–8 ■ Tangential excision.

Infection

All burn wounds have bacteria present; however, the presence of bacteria alone does not indicate an infection. The nurse must perform diligent surveillance of burn wounds to identify any changes in appearance. The wound may change color, have increased exudate, have increased pain, or appear to increase in depth. A classic sign of an infectious process in a burn is early separation of burn eschar (American Burn Association, 2007c). Early separation indicates an **invasive infection,** defined as the presence of pathogens in a burn wound at sufficient concentrations in conjunction with depth, surface area involved, and age of the patient, causing supportive separation of eschar or graft loss, invasion of adjacent unburned tissue, or causing the systemic response of sepsis syndrome (American Burn Association, 2007c).

Topical Antimicrobial Therapy

Initially, the burn wound surface is colonized by gram-positive bacteria. After the first week, the surface becomes colonized by gram-negative bacteria. Burn wounds are typically treated with a topical antimicrobial to control bacterial proliferation. Systemic antibiotics are not used prophylactically, but are initiated when there is clinical evidence of an infection and culture confirmation. To prevent the formation of antibiotic-resistant strains of bacteria, the health care provider chooses an antibiotic based on sensitivity results. See the RELATED PHARMACOTHERAPY box: Topical Antimicrobials for additional information.

Application of the topical agent is performed using aseptic technique once or twice daily. Table 37–4 lists the topical agents most frequently used, and the advantages and disadvantages of each. Dressing the wound in a silver nylon dressing (Silverlon, Argentum Medical LLL, Willowbrook, IL; SilverSeal, Noble Biomaterials, Scranton, PA) covered by a layer of gauze provides a clean protective environment. The silver ions act as antimicrobial agents. These dressings are effective for many hours to several days without need for reapplication of the topical agents such as silvadene (White, 2008).

Once the antimicrobial has been applied, an open- or closed dressing technique is used. The open method leaves the antimicrobial-covered wound open to air. This method is primarily used for burns to the face and ears. The closed method involves the application of gauze dressings over the antimicrobial agent. Proponents of this method argue its superiority because it assists with debridement and protects granulation tissue and fragile epithelial buds, while also decreasing the evaporative fluid loss from the wounds. It is crucial that the dressings are applied with function in mind. The dressings should not be so tight as to restrict motion but tight enough to stay in place with motion. Disadvantages to the closed method include fewer opportunities to evaluate the wound.

Biological, synthetic, and biosynthetic materials act as skin substitutes and are used to temporarily cover a burn. The type used depends on the depth of the wound and the goal of therapy. Biological dressings obtained from animals (frequently pigs) are referred to as **xenografts** or **heterografts.** Biological dressings obtained from humans are called **allografts** or **homografts.** These grafts are used to cover clean, superficial partial-thickness burns; maintain a moist wound environment; protect the ungrafted wound; and test the receptivity of a wound to autografting. If an infection or necrotic tissue is present in the wound, the biological dressing will not adhere to the wound. If the biological dressing will not adhere, it is termed a failure. It is preferable to have failure of a biological dressing than failure of a valuable donor site autograft. Biological dressings are occlusive, so they also help to reduce pain. The functions of temporary wound coverings are listed in Table 37–5.

Synthetic materials such as thin film dressings are used to cover donor sites and to protect clean, small superficial wounds. These dressings are waterproof and transparent, reduce pain, and maintain moisture in the wound to promote healing. Examples include Opsite and Tegaderm (from 3M Medical Surgical Division, St. Paul, Minnesota).

Biosynthetic dressings may be used to cover clean, superficial partial-thickness burns, meshed autografts, donor sites, and exudative wounds. An example is Biobrane (from Dow Hickam Pharmaceuticals, Inc., Sugar Land, Texas). TransCyte (Smith & Nephew, Largo, Florida) is a human fibroblast-derived temporary skin. This product can be used on

TABLE 37–4 Topical Antimicrobials

MEDICATIONS	ADVANTAGES	DISADVANTAGES
1% silver sulfadiazine (Silvadene, SSD)	Bacteriostatic Broad spectrum Soothing Painless on application	Poor penetration through eschar Transient leukopenia Poor cartilage penetration Questionable use with sulfa allergy Delays partial-thickness wound healing
Mafenide acetate cream (Sulfamylon cream)	Bacteriostatic Broad spectrum Effective against *Pseudomonas* species Penetrates eschar Penetrates cartilage	Limited fungal coverage Painful on partial-thickness burns Metabolic acidosis
Mafenide acetate solution (5% Sulfamylon solution)	Same properties as above Used as an irrigant after debridement and postgraft Less painful on application than Sulfamylon cream Less incidence of metabolic acidosis than Sulfamylon cream	Same as above
0.5% silver nitrate solution	Broad spectrum, yeast and fungus No known bacterial resistance No pain	Poor penetration of eschar Staining Messy Leeching of electrolytes
Antimicrobial ointments (e.g., Bacitracin, Bactroban)	Bactericidal for a variety of gram-positive and gram-negative organisms (exact coverage depends on type of ointment)	Poor eschar penetration Rash
Acticoat (Smith & Nephew)	Broad spectrum, fungus Can be left on wound up to seven days When used over mesh grafts, found to increase reepithelialization	May be difficult to remove If minimal wound exudate, must be moistened with water to release silver Unable to visualize wound daily
Aquacel Ag (Convatec)	Broad spectrum Can be left on wound up to 14 days Absorbent	Unable to visualize wound daily Shrinks and may expose burn

RELATED PHARMACOTHERAPY: Topical Antimicrobials

Sulfonamide
Silver Sulfadiazine (Silvadene)

Action and Uses
Silver salt is slowly released and exerts its bactericidal effect only on the bacterial cell membrane and wall; has broad antimicrobial activity including many gram-negative and gram-positive bacteria and yeast.

Major Side Effects
Potential for toxicity if applied to extensive areas of the body surface.

Nursing Implications
Apply with sterile, gloved hands to cleansed, debrided burned areas. Reapply cream to areas where it has been removed by patient activity; cover burn wounds with medication at all times.
Reapply after bathing.
Dressings not required but may be used if necessary. Drug does not stain clothing.
Store at room temperature, away from heat.
Pain may be experienced upon application; intensity and duration depend on depth of burn.

Sulfonamide Derivative
Mafenide Acetate (Sulfamylon)

Action and Uses
Produces marked reduction of bacterial growth in vascular tissue; active in presence of purulent matter; bacteriostatic against may gram-positive and gram-negative organisms.

Major Side Effects
Intense pain, burning, or stinging at application sites

Nursing Implications
Apply to burn areas to a thickness of approximately 15 mm (1/16 inch) one or two times daily with sterile, gloved hands to cleansed, debrided burned areas. Reapply cream to areas where it has been removed by patient activity; cover burn wounds with medication at all times.
Reapply after bathing.
Dressings not required but may be used if necessary. Drug does not stain clothing.
Store in light-resistant container, avoid extremes of heat.
Pain may be experienced upon application; intensity and duration depend on depth of burn.

TABLE 37–5 Functions of Temporary Wound Coverings

- Decrease bacterial proliferation
- Prevent desiccation
- Control heat loss
- Decrease protein loss in wound exudate
- Increase patient comfort
- Protect underlying structures
- Stimulate healing
- Prepare and test wound bed for autografting

middermal to indeterminate-depth partial-thickness burns as well as middermal burns after debridement.

Nonbiologic dressings can be used on superficial and superficial partial-thickness burns to provide a moist wound healing environment. Examples of nonbiologic dressings include Mepitel (from Molnlycke Health Care, Newton, Pennsylvania) and Xeroform (from Kendall Healthcare, Mansfield, Massachusetts).

Vacuum Assisted Closure (VAC, Kinetic Concepts, San Antonio, TX) provides negative-pressure wound therapy to promote wound healing. The VAC promotes the formation of granulation tissue, decreases wound size, removes exudate, and provides an environment for moist wound healing. This treatment device is typically used postdebridement and the goals are to decrease the wound size prior to grafting or to promote graft take by placing it on top of skin grafts. These dressings easily conform to the wound beds, facilitate removal of exudate, and expedite granulation (White, 2008).

The use of growth factors is another type of topical wound covering that can be used on burn injuries to stimulate wound healing. This is a current area of great interest, but few studies have been performed to determine its efficacy.

Nursing care related to temporary wound coverings include the periodic application and removal of the dressing material. It is imperative that dressings and the surrounding tissues be inspected for dislodgment, suppuration, fluid accumulation, and cellulitis. Most of these complications can be prevented by stabilizing the temporary covering with gauze, keeping it dry, keeping out contamination, and preventing wound shearing. It is important to note that wounds are dynamic and the wound management choices should be based on the state of the wound at a particular time. Wounds are evaluated at regular intervals, and wound dressings are changed as indicated by the wound state.

Wound Closure

Superficial partial-thickness burns heal by spontaneous reepithelialization within seven to ten days. Small full-thickness burns may be allowed to heal on their own by granulation tissue formation and contraction. Full-thickness burns are typically grafted for several reasons, including better cosmetic appearance, improved function, decreased risk of infection, and for a faster return to preinjury lifestyle. A large TBSA or a deep partial-thickness burn will also be grafted because healing usually takes more than 14 days and because otherwise, significant scarring will usually occur.

Early excision and closure of burn wounds have several advantages, including improved survival rates, reduction in the incidence of infection, reduced in-hospital stays, decrease in amount of grafting required, improved cosmetic results, and better functional outcome. Once the wound has been excised, steps are taken to close the wound. Small wounds are closed via primary wound closure. Larger wounds are closed via skin grafts, flaps, or skin substitutes. **Autografting** is the process of transplanting skin from one part of the body to fill in another part that has been injured. It is a method of permanent burn wound closure and uses either full-thickness or split-thickness skin grafts.

When the skin is removed down to the subcutaneous layer for grafting, it is termed a full-thickness skin graft (Fig. 37–9). Full-thickness skin grafts are used to cover areas that need the extra thickness and the durability it provides, such as the palm of the hand, or to cover a point that will be exposed to pressure, such as the elbow or the scapula. When removing skin for a full-thickness graft, the donor site becomes a full-thickness skin defect. This defect is closed by either suturing or by using a split-thickness skin graft. Full-thickness grafting is used for small areas only.

Split-thickness skin grafts (0.2 to 0.3 mm thick) are not as thick as full-thickness grafts (0.64 to 0.76 mm thick). The donor site is a partial-thickness skin defect that will heal within 10 to 14 days. A split-thickness skin graft can be used as a sheet graft or as a meshed graft. Skin is harvested from a donor site using an instrument called a dermatome. The sheet graft is taken from the donor site and placed on the recipient wound (Fig. 37–10). To make a meshed graft, the skin is taken from the donor site, then expanded using a mesh dermatome (Fig. 37–11). The mesh dermatome makes multiple small slits in the skin, giving it a netting type of appearance. A meshed graft is expanded to cover a larger area; however, the wider the mesh is spread, the longer it takes for wound closure which causes an increase in scar formation (Fig. 37–12). Sheet grafts usually provide a better cosmetic appearance than meshed grafts, so they are usually used for conspicuous sites such as the face and hands and are the most optimal coverage for burns less than 40 percent TBSA.

Skin grafts adhere to the recipient site by the presence of serum between the two layers. Soon, a fibrin matrix forms, which better secures the graft to the donor site. Within 48 hours, the wound will take on a pink or red color, indicating graft vascularization has taken place.

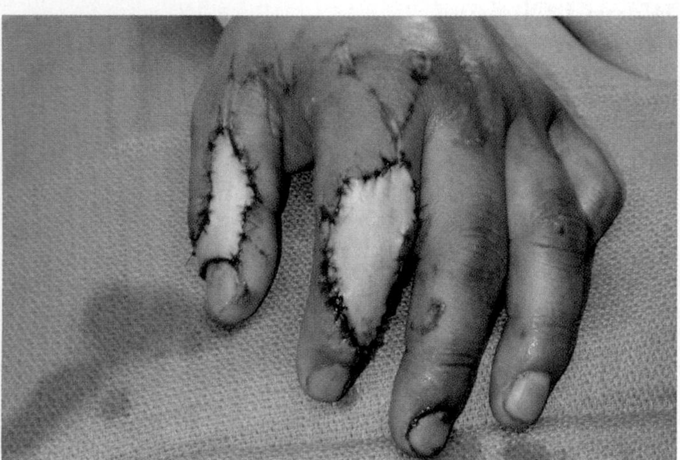

Figure 37–9 ■ Full thickness skin grafts on fingers.

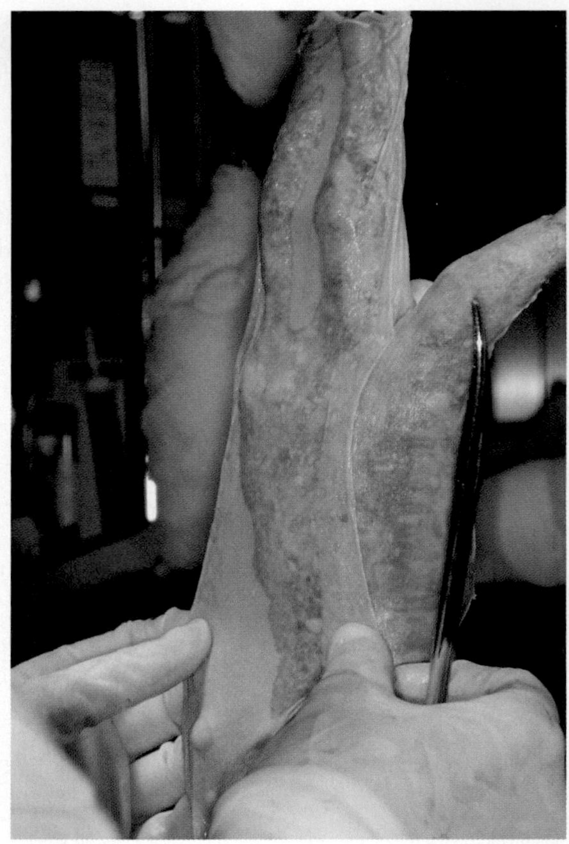

Figure 37–10 ■ Sheet graft taken from donor site and placed on recipient's wound.

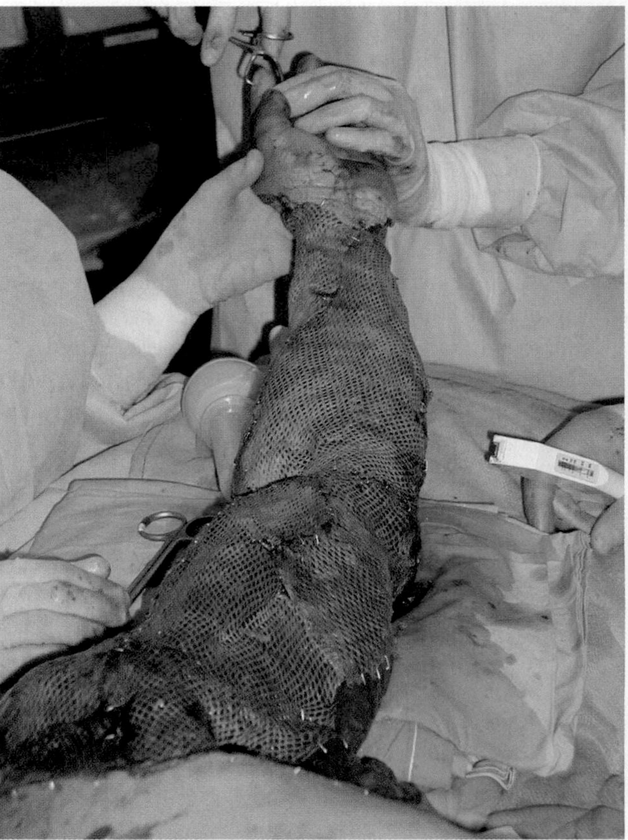

Figure 37–11 ■ Placement of mesh graft on arm.

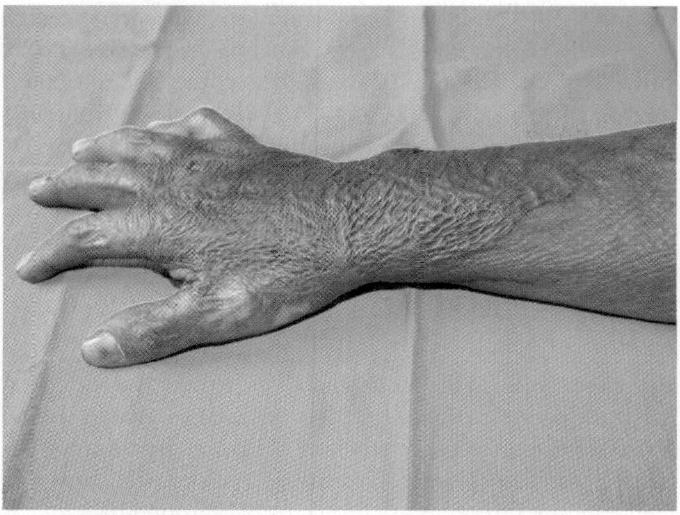

Figure 37–12 ■ Mature mesh graft on hand.

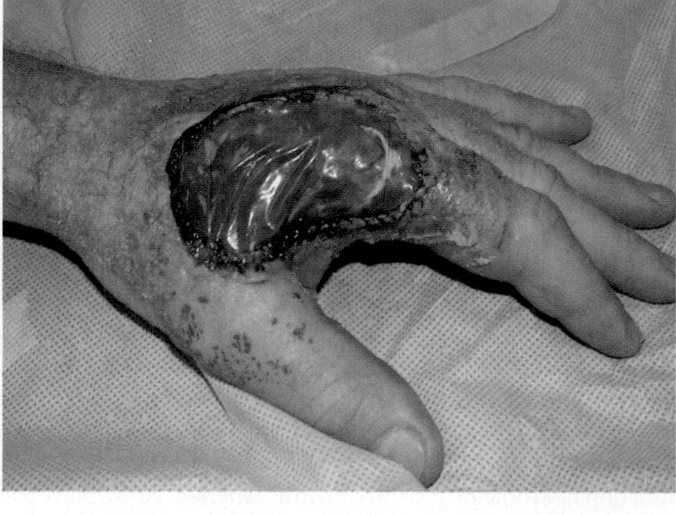

Figure 37–13 ■ Integra artificial skin.

Flaps are another choice for burn wound coverage. Flaps are typically chosen for full-thickness burns over tendons and subdermal burns where the wound either will not support skin graft coverage or would benefit from a thicker and more stable covering.

Integra Artificial Skin (from Integra Lifesciences, Plainsboro, New Jersey) is composed of a dermal replacement layer consisting of cross-linked bovine tendon collagen and chondroitin-6-sulfate covered with a silicone layer. Typically, Integra is applied to an excised full-thickness burn wound and provides a structure for a more organized neodermis to form (Fig. 37–13). Approximately two to three weeks after placement, the silicone layer is removed and a thin epidermal autograft is placed. This product allows for early coverage of extensive full-thickness burns. Integra also has been used in conjunction with cultured skin substitutes. Further applications include the use of Integra for burn wound reconstruction.

Nursing care of the burn wound includes monitoring for infection. Signs of noninvasive wound infection include reddened wound edges, generalized wound discoloration, change in the color of the wound exudate, foul-smelling exudate, loss of a healed skin graft, and an increase in wound pain. Signs of more severe invasive infection include conversion of a partial-thickness injury to a full-thickness injury, early separation of eschar, small necrotic subcutaneous vessels, tenderness at the wound edges, and edema. Burn wounds are not always easy to evaluate, so surface wound culture and sensitivity tests are frequently done. A burn wound biopsy will be done if an infection is suspected.

SECTION EIGHT REVIEW

1. Which of the following harms newly formed tissue and is, therefore, not recommended for burn wound care?
   A. sharp debridement
   B. biological debridement
   C. chemical debridement
   D. wet-to-dry dressings
2. Which topical antimicrobial is the most frequently used?
   A. Neomycin ointment
   B. silver nitrate
   C. silver sulfadiazine (Silvadene)
   D. mafenide acetate (Sulfamylon)
3. Biological dressings (allografts, homografts) are used to
   A. determine if the wound bed is adequate to accept an autograft
   B. maintain a moist environment
   C. protect the ungrafted wound
   D. all of the above
4. The process of transplanting skin from one part of the body to fill in another part that has been injured is known as
   A. xenograft
   B. autograft
   C. heterograft
   D. allograft
5. Nursing care related to temporary wound coverings includes inspection for
   A. dislodgement
   B. suppuration
   C. cellulitis
   D. all of the above

Answers: 1. D, 2. C, 3. D, 4. B, 5. D

SECTION NINE: Acute Rehabilitative Phase: Psychosocial Needs

At the completion of this section, the learner will be able to describe expected behaviors, emotional status, and levels of pain for burn patients during the acute rehabilitative phase, as well as their related nursing actions.

Behavioral Changes

In addition to the physical recovery during the rehabilitative phase, emotional recovery also must continue. The ramifications of the injury begin to be apparent to the patient and patient response is varied. The ability to cope with the injury will, in part, depend on past coping mechanisms the patient has learned. These mechanisms may be healthy or they may be dysfunctional. Problems most frequently experienced by burn patients include anxiety, fear, grief, depression, sleep problems, acute stress disorder, and aggressive or regressive behavior.

Personally meaningful rehabilitation and recovery from burn injuries can be greatly facilitated by learning behavioral and image enhancement strategies (Kammerer-Quayle, 2006). Psychological and emotional problems can be minimized by involving the patient in self-care activities soon after the injury is sustained. Patients should participate in wound care, feeding, exercising, and administering medications as soon as they are physically and emotionally able to improve their self-concept. Fear and anxiety as a result of burn injury can be reduced with repeated and consistent explanations in appropriate terms. Nurses play an important role in facilitating the presence and involvement of family and friends in the recovery and rehabilitation of burn survivors (Moi et al., 2008). Visits by recovered burn patients allow patients to discuss their concerns with nonmedical personnel who can offer practical advice on coping with burns. This can be arranged by contacting the national office of the Phoenix Society, a support group for burn survivors (www.phoenix-society.org).

Pain

Pain experienced in the acute rehabilitative phase may be different from pain experienced in the resuscitative phase (Section Five). During the acute rehabilitative phase of burn injury, patients generally experience decreasing levels of pain. However, pain continues to occur as chronic or background pain and as procedural pain. Procedures, surgery, or infection delay the easement of pain. Interventions vary depending on the duration and severity of the pain. Patients achieve better pain control when they are given opportunities to choose interventions that work best for them. As the patient stabilizes and pain levels begin to decrease, oral analgesics are used with greater frequency. Nonpharmacologic interventions for pain control include, but are not limited to, biofeedback, hypnosis, relaxation therapy, and guided imagery. Thorough pain assessments are conducted on a regular basis throughout the patient's recovery and the plan of care is adjusted accordingly.

SECTION NINE REVIEW

1. Members of the Phoenix Society are
   A. burn nurses
   B. safety educators
   C. social workers
   D. burn survivors
2. Which of the following statements is true?
   A. Burn wounds are ischemic so burn patients do not experience pain.
   B. Pain generally increases during the acute rehabilitative phase.
   C. Patients achieve better pain control when they can choose the interventions that work best for them.
   D. Nonpharmacologic interventions have been tried in burn patients, but they do not work.
3. Psychological and emotional problems can be minimized by involving the patient in (choose all that apply)
   A. wound care
   B. feeding themselves
   C. exercise programs
   D. taking their own medications

Answers: 1. D, 2. C, 3. (A, B, C, D)

SECTION TEN: Acute Rehabilitative Phase: Physical Mobility

At the completion of this section, the learner will be able to describe the goals, interventions, and health care professionals involved with promoting physical mobility during the acute rehabilitative phase of burn care.

Physical mobility problems during the acute rehabilitative phase of burn care are directly related to the healing wound itself and the therapeutic interventions necessary to maintain life and close the wound. During the resuscitative phase, excessive edema develops in the extremities, and mobility is restricted by edema and pain. Later, this problem is compounded by the limitations placed on mobility in an effort to protect healing grafts from shearing. As the wound heals, mobility is restricted by scar formation and contraction, and the desire to assume a position of comfort, which is typically flexed. Therefore, the treatment goals related to physical mobility during the acute rehabilitative phase include

- Returning to preinjury level of functioning
- Maintaining musculoskeletal, cardiopulmonary, and respiratory function
- Promoting wound healing
- Protecting healing skin grafts
- Preventing contractures and soft tissue deformity

- Preserving and strengthening extremity function
- Scar management
- Achieving maximum functional recovery
- Patient and family education

The burn team members involved in this process include the physical therapist (PT), occupational therapist (OT), and nursing staff. The OT and PT develop a treatment plan, fashion appliances, and perform daily treatments. The role of the nursing staff is to integrate the treatment plan into their delivery of care and to provide assessment feedback to the OT and PT. In addition, nurses play a pivotal role in gaining patient compliance because they have continuous contact with the patient and many opportunities to support the patient toward these rehabilitation goals.

Interventions to promote physical mobility during the acute phase of burn care employ many techniques and devices. Antideformity positioning begins at the time of admission unless contraindicated by a complicating condition. Its use is imperative during the acute phase because it decreases scar contracture across flexor surfaces, which often compromises joint mobility and functional capacity.

Joint function is also preserved by active and passive range of motion exercises. Mobility outcomes may actually be improved by the administration of analgesics prior to therapy and is discussed with the patient.

Early total body mobilization is important because of the impact that upright positioning has on cardiopulmonary functioning. Patients are assisted out of bed and ambulated early in the acute phase after hemodynamic stabilization. It is important to apply compression wraps on lower extremities before getting the patient out of bed, in order to prevent venous stasis. If extremities are not wrapped, the patient is at risk for capillary bed bleeding, which could cause autograft failure or delay donor-site healing. Venous pooling coupled with prolonged immobility also predisposes the patient to deep-vein thromboses. Wrapping the extremities continues until all wounds are healed and pressure garments are applied.

SECTION TEN REVIEW

1. Antideformity positioning should begin
   - **A.** after skin grafting
   - **B.** after the patient can walk again
   - **C.** at the time of admission
   - **D.** on discharge from the high-acuity area
2. Which nursing action is MOST important in the prevention of autograft failure secondary to capillary bed bleeding?
   - **A.** applying compression wraps to extremities
   - **B.** encouraging high vitamin K intake
   - **C.** monitoring prothrombin time/partial thromboplastin time (PT/PTT) and INR lab values
   - **D.** maintaining the patient on bedrest
3. Treatment goals related to physical mobility during the acute rehabilitative phase include
   - **A.** return to preinjury functioning
   - **B.** promotion of wound healing
   - **C.** scar management
   - **D.** all of the above
4. Which of the following statements is TRUE regarding mobility after a burn injury? (choose all that apply)
   - **A.** During the acute resuscitation phase, patients have decreased mobility due to treatments to maintain life.
   - **B.** During the resuscitation phase, edema restricts mobility.
   - **C.** Patients have limited mobility in an effort to protect healing grafts from shearing.
   - **D.** As wounds heal, mobility is restricted by scar formation.
5. Joint function is preserved by (choose all that apply)
   - **A.** active range of motion
   - **B.** passive range of motion
   - **C.** restrictive training
   - **D.** aerobic exercise

Answers: 1. C, 2. A, 3. D, 4. (A, B, C, D), 5. (A, B)

SECTION ELEVEN: Long-Term Rehabilitative Phase

At the completion of this section, the learner will be able to discuss nursing interventions related to physical conditioning, protection of new skin, scar management, and psychosocial adjustment during the long-term rehabilitative phase of burn care.

Traditionally, the rehabilitative phase of burn care was thought to begin at the time that all wounds were healed and continue throughout the patient's life span. From this paradigm it would seem that the rehabilitative phase would not fall into the realm of high-acuity nursing. However, it is important to recognize that preventive rehabilitative interventions actually begin during the resuscitative phase—which directly involves high-acuity nurses.

Physical Conditioning

Interventions during the rehabilitative phase are focused on physical conditioning, care of healing skin, and support of psychosocial adjustment. Physical conditioning during the rehabilitative phase moves beyond range of motion exercises and begins to address aerobic endurance and muscle strength. This process begins in the burn unit but is mainly accomplished after discharge.

Care of Healing Skin

Interventions related to the care of healing skin include protection of newly formed epithelium, scar management, and prevention of joint contractures. The epithelium over healing burn wounds is extremely fragile. Daily skin care includes cleansing with a mild soap and generous application of a high-quality emollient. Patients are instructed to apply this emollient several times a day because their sebaceous glands have been destroyed in the burning and grafting process. The skin is protected from mechanical traumas, such as shearing and pressure. Finally, patients are instructed to protect their scar from sun exposure for one year or until the scar turns silvery-white. Otherwise, the scar will "tan" and remain permanently pigmented, leaving the patient with a less satisfactory cosmetic result.

Scar management is achieved by wearing compression garments (Fig. 37–14). These garments are custom made and costly. The constant pressure from the garment assists in the remodeling of irregular collagen into a more parallel pattern to improve both function and appearance. Because hypertrophic scars are also hypervascular, pressure therapy also may help to reduce local blood supply, thereby improving the scars' appearance. Patient compliance is difficult to obtain because the garments are hot, difficult to put on, and require continuous wearing (except when bathing). Compression garments are worn until scars are mature as evidenced by a flat, white, and avascular appearance, which is usually achieved in 12 to 18 months.

Patients with burn wounds over a joint are at risk for future joint contracture. Preventive measures include compression garments, night splinting, silicone, serial splinting/casting, and range of motion exercises. Should a contracture and functional deficit occur, surgical intervention may be necessary to regain full mobility.

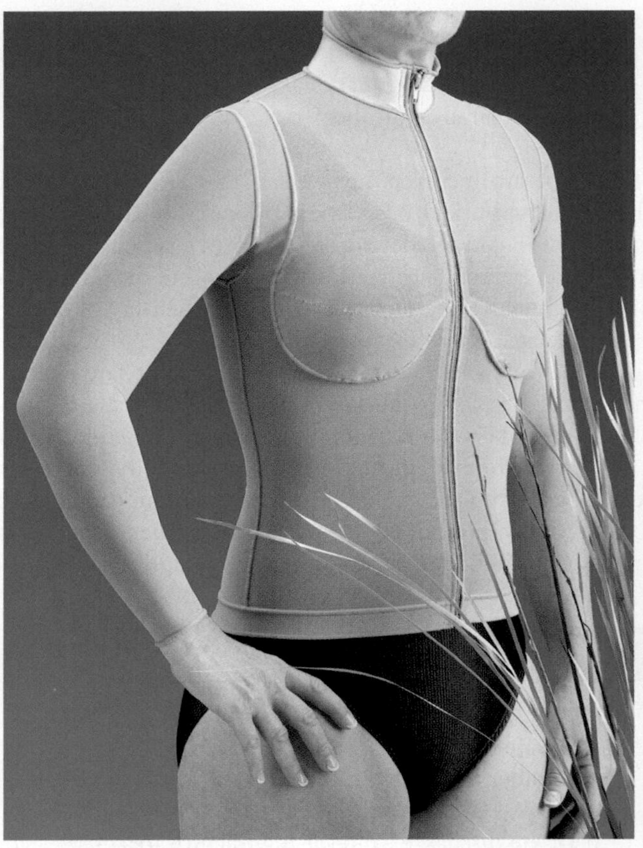

Figure 37–14 ■ Jobst compression garments. From © Gottfried Medical, Inc., used with permission

Psychosocial Adjustment

Social and psychological rehabilitation is, for the vast majority of burn survivors, profoundly more important than the recovery of physical functioning (Kammerer-Quayle, 2006). Psychosocial adjustment is a major task of the rehabilitative phase. During this time, patients begin to renew their interests in the outside world, invest in their rehabilitation, and reintegrate their identities. Burn-unit nurses may witness some of these behaviors, but the majority of the behaviors occur after discharge. The burn team is challenged to find appropriate community resources for discharged patients as they adapt to postburn alterations in appearance, level of physical functioning, and role concept. For example, patients with facial burns often struggle with their altered body image and have difficulty resuming their preburn lifestyle. Therefore, it may be helpful to refer these patients to a licensed aesthetician familiar with scar therapy and camouflage makeup techniques. The Phoenix Society maintains a registry of these professionals and can assist with appropriate referrals.

There is a growing body of evidence that demonstrates a high prevalence of psychological distress syndromes following burn injury. Acute stress disorder and posttraumatic stress disorder are common. Acute stress disorder is reported in 11 to 32 percent of patients with burn injury and posttraumatic stress disorder is observed in approximately 23 percent to 33 percent of patients between three and six months after burn, and 15 to 45 percent one year after burn (McKibben et al., 2008).

SECTION ELEVEN REVIEW

1. Rehabilitative interventions begin during which phase of burn care?
   A. resuscitative
   B. acute rehabilitative
   C. long-term rehabilitative
   D. transitional
2. Interventions during the rehabilitation phase are focused on
   A. physical conditioning
   B. care of healing skin
   C. support of psychosocial adjustment
   D. all of the above
3. Pressure garments improve immature scars by
   A. thinning hypertrophic epithelium
   B. remodeling irregular collagen
   C. reducing skin friction
   D. increasing arterial blood flow
4. Preventive measures for contractures include (choose all that apply)
   A. compression garments
   B. night splinting
   C. silicone
   D. range of motion exercises

5. In relation to psychological adjustment, which behavior is MOST likely to occur in the long-term rehabilitative phase?
   A. survival anxiety
   B. searching for meaning
   C. adaptation to severe pain
   D. reintegration of identity

Answers: 1. A, 2. D, 3. B, 4. (A, B, C, D) 5. D

POSTTEST

1. People with advancing age are prone to burn injuries because they (choose all that apply)
   A. have impaired senses
   B. have decreased reaction times
   C. tend to incorrectly assess risk
   D. participate in risk taking activities
2. Which of the following structures is the primary resistor to electrical current?
   A. skin
   B. nerves
   C. blood vessels
   D. none of the above
3. Using the Lund and Browder chart, what is the TBSA to an adult patient with burns to his head, neck, and anterior trunk?
   A. 13 percent
   B. 22 percent
   C. 15.5 percent
   D. 18.5 percent
4. Which of the following terms describe a burn injury that is painful, erythematous, has blisters and brisk capillary refill?
   A. full-thickness burns
   B. superficial partial-thickness burns
   C. deep partial-thickness burns
   D. first-degree burns
5. Using the American Burn Association's criteria, which of the following conditions would warrant admission to a burn center?
   A. first-degree burn, less than 5 percent TBSA
   B. first-degree burn, 90 percent TBSA
   C. deep partial-thickness burn, entire face
   D. superficial partial-thickness burn, 10 percent
6. Which pulmonary tests are indicated to assess inhalation injury?
   A. electrocardiogram, thallium
   B. arterial blood gases, bronchoscopy
   C. serum potassium, sodium levels
   D. pulmonary angiograms, hemoglobin levels
7. Patients experiencing full-thickness burns involving the entire circumference of an extremity require frequent peripheral vascular checks to detect
   A. ischemia
   B. adequate wound healing
   C. arteriosclerotic changes
   D. hypothermia
8. Which of the following is the most important to monitor during initial fluid resuscitation?
   A. hemoglobin
   B. blood pressure
   C. thirst
   D. urine output
9. Which of the following medications would provide the best pain relief to patients with partial-thickness burn injury?
   A. oxycodone by mouth
   B. meperidine intramuscular
   C. methadone by mouth
   D. morphine sulfate intravenous
10. Which of the following may be present in the burn survivor? (choose all that apply)
    A. posttraumatic stress disorder
    B. acute stress disorder
    C. depression
    D. anxiety
11. The hypermetabolic state of burn injury is characterized by
    A. decreased cardiac output, tachycardia
    B. increased cardiac output, increased oxygen consumption
    C. decreased caloric requirement, tachycardia
    D. increased heart rate, decreased carbon dioxide production
12. Myoglobinuria can be treated with
    A. increasing amount of IV fluids
    B. slight alkalinization of the blood
    C. osmotic diuresis
    D. all of the above
13. The major difference between burn wound healing and wound healing from other injuries is that burn wounds
    A. do not go through an inflammatory phase
    B. do not go through a proliferative phase
    C. do not mature
    D. have the same phases, but occur more slowly and last longer
14. Until a transfer to a burn center, the nurse should
    A. debride all wounds as soon as possible
    B. place ointment on the wounds as soon as possible
    C. clean all wounds with sterile saline
    D. prepare for an escharotomy

15. The surgical procedure used to shave thin layers of eschar until viable tissue is exposed is called
    A. tangential excision
    B. fascial excision
    C. eschar excision
    D. escharotomy
16. Which of the following topical antimicrobials have poor penetration through eschar?
    A. Silvadene
    B. 0.5 percent silver nitrate
    C. Bacitracin
    D. all of the above
17. Psychological and emotional problems that occur during the acute rehabilitative phase can be minimized by
    A. involving the patient in self-care activities soon after injury
    B. giving the patient sedatives
    C. keeping the patient from negative interactions
    D. not letting the patient see himself or herself in a mirror
18. Antideformity positioning
    A. decreases deep vein thrombosis formation
    B. decreases scar contractures across flexor surfaces
    C. increases deep vein thrombosis formation
    D. increases scar contractures across flexor surfaces
19. Patients require emollient application several times a day to
    A. prevent wound infection
    B. keep skin moist because sebaceous glands are destroyed
    C. protect the skin from shearing injuries when moving in bed
    D. protect the skin from sun exposure

Posttest answers with rationale are found on MyNursingKit.

REFERENCES

American Burn Association. (2001a). Burn shock resuscitation: initial management and overview. *Journal of Burn Care & Rehabilitation, 22* (suppl), 27S–37S.

American Burn Association. (2001b). Escharotomy. *Journal of Burn Care & Rehabilitation, 22* (suppl), 53S–58S.

American Burn Association. (2001c). Inhalation injury: diagnosis. *Journal of Burn Care & Rehabilitation, 22* (suppl), 19S–22S.

American Burn Association. (2001d). Inhalation injury: initial management. *Journal of Burn Care & Rehabilitation, 22* (suppl), 23S–26S.

American Burn Association. (2001e). Initial nutritional support of burn patients. *Journal of Burn Care & Rehabilitation, 22* (suppl), 59S–66S.

American Burn Association. (2007a). Burn incidence and treatment in the US: 2007 fact aheet. Retrieved November 21, 2008 from http://www.ameriburn.org/resources_factsheet.php.

American Burn Association. (2007b). Guidelines for the operation of burn centers. Retrieved November 20, 2008 from http://www.ameriburn.org/chapter14.pdf.

American Burn Association. (2007c). Consensus conference on burn sepsis and infection. *J Burn Care and Research, 28*(6), 776–790.

Arlati, S., Storti, E., Pradella, V., et al. (2007). Decreased fluid volume to reduce organ damage: a new approach to burn shock resuscitation. *Resuscitation, 72,* 371–378.

Blumetti, J., Hunt, J. L., Arnoldo, B. D., et al. (2008). The Parkland Formula under fire: is the criticism justified? *J Burn Care and Research, 29*(1), 180–186.

Concil, J. M., Georges, B., Fourcade, O., et al. (2006). Assessment of renal function in clinical practice at the bedside of burn patients. *Brit J Clinical Pharm, 63*(5), 583–594.

Fauerbach, J. A., Pruzinkey, T., Saxe, G. N. (2007). Psychological health and function after burn injury: setting research priorities. *J Burn Care and Research, 28*(4), 587–592.

Gauglitz, G. C., Herndon, D. N., & Jeschke, M. G. (2008). Insulin resistance postburn: underlying mechanisms and current therapeutic strategies. *J Burn Care and Research, 29*(5), 683–694.

Gordon, M. & Marvin, J. (2007). Burn nursing. In Herndon, D. N. (ed). *Total burn care* (3rd ed.). Philadelphia, PA: Saunders Elsevier, 477–484.

Holmes, J. H. (2008). Critical issues in burn care. *J Burn Care and Research 29*(6), Suppl 2, S180-S187.

McKibben, J. B., Bresnick, M. G., Wiechman, A., et al. (2008). Acute stress disorder and posttraumatic stress disorders: a prospective study of prevalence, course and predictors in a sample with major burn injuries. *J Burn Care and Research, 29(1), 22–35.*

Meyer, W. J., Patterson, D. R., & Jaco, M. (2007). Management of pain and other discomforts in burned patients. In Herndon, D. N. (ed). *Total burn care* (3rd ed.). Philadelphia, PA: Saunders Elsevier, 797–818.

Moi, A. L., Vindenes, H. A., & Gjengedal, E. (2008). The experience of life after burn injury: a new bodily awareness. *J Adv Nursing, 64*(3), 278–286.

Perceira, C. T., Murphy, K. D., & Herndon, D. N. (2005). Altering metabolism. *J Burn Care and Research, 26*(1), 194–199.

Phan, T. N., Klein, M., & Gibran, N. S. (2008). Impact of oxandrolone treatment on acute outcomes after severe burn injury. *J Burn Care and Research, 29*(6), 902–906.

Saffle, J. R. & Graves, C. (2007). Nutritional support of the burned patient. In Herndon, D. N. (ed.). *Total burn care* (3rd ed.). London: Saunders Elsevier, 398–419.

Spence, R. J. (2008). Electrical and lightning injuries. In Cameron, J. L. (ed.). *Current surgical therapy* (9th ed.). Philadelphia, PA: Mosby Elsevier, 1079–1083.

Sun, J. F., Les, S. S., Lin, S. D., et al. (2006). Continuous arteriovenous hemodialysis and continuous venovenous hemofiltration in burn patients with acute renal failure. *Kaotisiung J Med Sci, 23,* 344–351.

Thomas, C. R., Meyer, W. J., Blakeney, P. E. (2007). Psychiatric disorders associated with burn injury. In Herndon, D. N. (ed.). *Total burn care* (3rd ed.). Philadelphia, PA: Saunders Elsevier, 819–828.

White, C. E., Renz, E. M. (2008). Advances in surgical care: management of severe burn injury. *Crit Care Med, 36*[Suppl], S318–S324.

MODULE

38 Alterations in Multisystem Function: Multiple Trauma

Paul Thurman

OBJECTIVES Following completion of this module, the learner will be able to

1. Define injury, potential mechanisms of injury, and risk factors that influence injury patterns.
2. Define the forces associated with blunt trauma and apply these concepts to the clinical assessment of a patient with blunt trauma.
3. Define the forces associated with penetrating trauma and apply these concepts to the clinical assessment of a patient with penetrating trauma.
4. Translate the mechanism of injury into potential injury patterns manifested by the patient for both blunt and penetrating injuries.
5. State clinical conditions that mediate a patient's response to injury, including underlying medical conditions, substance abuse, and physiological alterations, including pregnancy and advancing age.
6. Identify the clinical assessment format used to identify life-threatening injuries during the primary survey.
7. Discuss the components of the secondary survey and the suggested format for conducting the secondary survey.
8. Describe the trimodal distribution of trauma-related mortalities and how this is integrated into clinical assessment.
9. Discuss nursing responsibilities during the trauma resuscitation phase.
10. Compare and contrast various end points of traumatic shock resuscitation.
11. Describe basic principles of collaborative management for injuries to the chest, abdomen, and pelvis.
12. Cluster patient symptoms and provide nursing diagnoses appropriate for the patient with traumatic injuries.
13. Link posttrauma complications with the physiology of a traumatic injury and preexisting risk factors.
14. Discuss interventions to prevent complications of traumatic injury.

This self-study module is intended to facilitate the learner's understanding of trauma. Particular focus is given to mechanism of injury for both blunt and penetrating trauma as an assessment factor to raise the learner's index of suspicion for certain injuries. The module is composed of 11 sections. Sections One through Four focus on mechanism of injury and kinematics of trauma. Section Five presents specific clinical and age-related variances that may mediate injury response. Sections Six and Seven focus on the trauma assessment and resuscitation principles based on primary and secondary assessments. Section Eight summarizes key points in the mediation of life-threatening injury related to trauma with a brief discussion on traumatic shock. Section Nine discusses the management of the patient with traumatic injuries to the chest, abdomen, and pelvis. Section Ten examines nursing care of the trauma patient, and Section Eleven addresses trauma sequelae. Each section includes a set of review questions to help the learner evaluate his or her understanding of the section's content before moving on to the next section. All Section Reviews include answers. It is suggested that the learner review those concepts answered incorrectly in the review questions before proceeding to the next section.

PRETEST

1. Which of the following are TRUE about blunt trauma? (choose all that apply)
   A. It interrupts skin integrity.
   B. The extent of the injury may be covert.
   C. It may be difficult to diagnose.
   D. Surrounding tissue deformation occurs.

2. Which of the following is the leading cause of death in all Americans ages 1 to 44 years of age?
   A. cancer
   B. heart disease
   C. injury
   D. Acquired Immune Deficiency Syndrome

3. The most common forces associated with blunt trauma are (choose all that apply)
   A. acceleration
   B. compression
   C. shearing
   D. axial loading
4. An improperly placed seat belt can cause ______injury to the small bowel.
   A. deceleration
   B. shearing
   C. acceleration
   D. compression
5. Damage from low to medium energy missiles (knives, arrows) usually result in
   A. damage located to structures directly in the missile's path
   B. cavitation
   C. injury up to 30 times the diameter of the missile
   D. blast effect to surrounding tissue
6. Secondary missiles often are created with penetrating trauma involving
   A. teeth and bone
   B. brain and soft tissue
   C. abdominal organs and vessels
   D. great vessels and brain
7. The most frequently seen pattern of injury for a pedestrian child hit by an automobile is
   A. fractures of femur, tibia, and fibula on side of impact
   B. fracture of femur, chest injury, and injury to contralateral skull
   C. contralateral head injury
   D. spleen, liver injuries
8. An unrestrained driver is likely to have injuries to the (choose all that apply)
   A. head
   B. ribs
   C. small bowel
   D. hip
9. Alcohol interferes with assessment of the trauma patient because it
   A. increases heart rate and blood pressure
   B. interferes with the neurologic assessment
   C. dilates pupils
   D. can cause chest pain
10. Which of the following statements is/are TRUE about the pregnant patient with traumatic injury? (choose all that apply)
   A. Heart rate is increased.
   B. Blood pressure is decreased.
   C. Mild blood loss is not well tolerated.
   D. Elevated hematocrits are common.
11. Ordered priorities in the primary survey are
   A. disability, airway, breathing
   B. cervical spine immobilization, circulation, breathing
   C. hemorrhage, fractures, chest trauma
   D. airway, breathing, circulation, disability, and exposure
12. During the primary survey, when assessing the "D" component, which of the following would you assess?
   A. ability to move extremities
   B. neurologic status
   C. breath sounds
   D. dyspnea
13. Key assessment techniques used in the secondary survey include (choose all that apply)
   A. palpation
   B. inspection
   C. X-rays
   D. auscultation
14. When should the secondary survey begin?
   A. before the primary survey is completed
   B. before life-threatening injuries are identified
   C. after the primary survey is completed
   D. upon arrival to the ER
15. The distribution of trauma-related mortalities is
   A. modal
   B. bimodal
   C. trimodal
   D. quasimodal
16. After a loss of up to 15 percent of circulating blood volume, a patient would most likely demonstrate
   A. hypotension
   B. tachycardia
   C. tachypnea
   D. none of the above
17. The most frequently injured organ in the abdomen is the
   A. liver
   B. spleen
   C. pelvis
   D. small intestine
18. Perianal ecchymosis, pain with palpation to the iliac crests, and hematuria are signs of
   A. bladder rupture
   B. liver laceration
   C. splenic laceration
   D. pelvic fracture
19. Which of the following data suggests the presence of life-threatening injury?
   A. absent breath sounds
   B. paradoxical chest wall movement
   C. deviated trachea
   D. all of the above

20. Which of the following is a key assessment finding that helps to differentiate spinal shock from hypovolemia?
A. bradycardia
B. tachycardia
C. hypotension
D. pulmonary edema

21. Which of the following contributes the greatest to the development of posttrauma complications?
A. hypoperfusion
B. delay in supporting nutrition
C. infection
D. vasoconstriction

Pretest answers are found on MyNursingKit.

SECTION ONE: Overview of the Injured Patient

At the completion of this section, the learner will be able to define injury, potential mechanisms of injury, and personal and environmental factors that influence injury patterns.

Injury

Understanding trauma enables the nurse to approach a patient in crisis with a level-headed, systematic plan based on a solid body of nursing knowledge. Historically, injuries or accidents were viewed as the result of random chance beyond human control. Now, injury is viewed as an event with an identifiable cause via the interaction of energy and force with a recipient. The recipient may be an inanimate object, such as a car or human being.

Injury results from acute exposure to energy, such as kinetic (for example, a motor vehicle crash [MVC], fall, or bullet), chemical, thermal, electrical, and ionizing radiation, or from a lack of essential agents, such as oxygen (drowning) and heat (frostbite). The injury occurs because of the body's inability to tolerate excessive exposure to the energy source. Effects of injury on the human body vary depending on the injuring agent. For the purposes of this module, the focus will be on two major categories of injury—blunt and penetrating.

Mechanism of Injury

Blunt trauma is considered injury without interruption of skin integrity. Blunt trauma may be life-threatening because the extent of the injury may be covert, making diagnosis difficult. Blunt forces transfer energy causing tissue deformation. The nature of the injury is related to both the transfer of energy and the anatomic structure involved.

Penetrating trauma refers to injury sustained by the transmission of energy to body tissues from a moving object that interrupts skin integrity. Penetrating trauma produces actual tissue penetration and may also cause surrounding tissue deformation based on the energy transferred by the penetrating object.

Because the transfer of energy occurs with both blunt and penetrating injury, deformation and displacement of body tissue and organs occur with both forms of injury. Injury takes place as the structural limits of the organ are exceeded. Damage may be localized, such as hematoma formation, or systemic, as in shock states. The local response of the patient varies according to the organ involved. Additional examples are bone fractures, bleeding vessels, or tissue edema.

Injuries, like other diseases, do not occur at random. Identifiable risk factors are present that predispose individuals to certain injury patterns. These risk factors include age, gender, and alcohol use as well as race, income, and geography.

Age

Injury continues to be the leading cause of death in all Americans ages 1 through 44 (Bergen et al., 2008). The death rate from injury is highest for patients more than 75-years-old. The highest injury rate is for patients ages 15 through 24 because of their exposure to high-risk activities (including poor judgment with the use of alcohol, drugs, and driving practices). The highest homicide rate occurs among people between 20 and 29 years of age.

The elderly are predisposed to trauma because of age-related changes in reaction time, balance and coordination, and sensory motor function. Trauma in the elderly is associated with higher mortality and morbidity with less severe injury. A 79-year-old with multiple rib fractures will have a very different clinical course than

Emerging Evidence

- An estimated 1.85 million adults aged 65 years and older were treated in the United States emergency rooms for fall-related injuries at a mean cost of $17,000 per admission (*Roudsari, Ebel, Corso et al., 2005*).
- Patients with advancing age are at an increased risk for falls while hospitalized. For hospitalized patients, fall risk is greatest during the first week of hospitalization (*McCarter-Bayer, Bayer & Hall, 2005*).
- Older adult pedestrians are frequently injured by automobiles due to problems with vision, reflexes, and increased time needed to cross intersections. Their injuries are more severe than younger pedestrians involved in similar accidents and they are four times more likely to die if injured than younger patients (*Simms & O'Neill, 2005*).
- Driving skills and abilities should be assessed and encouraged to promote independence in adults with advancing age. However, no tools exist that aid clinicians in quickly screening patients for safe driving ability. A neurologist experienced with detecting Alzheimer's disease was shown to accurately predict driving ability in elders with mild cognitive impairment (*Brown, Ott, Papandonatos et al., 2005*).
- Traumatic injury places a patient at risk for depression. Traumatically injured adults over age 55 met criteria for depressive symptoms immediately following their injury, but showed improvement by three months postinjury in contrast to posttraumatic stress disorders, which remained elevated at three months. This indicates that the immediate postinjury period is a time of increased vulnerability for the trauma patient with advancing age (*Richmond, Thompson, Kauder et al., 2006*).

an 18-year-old with multiple rib fractures. This is attributed to the elderly patients' decreased ability to compensate for severe injury (or a "limited physiological reserve") and preexisting medical conditions (Lewis et al., 2007). Limited physiological reserve is a concept of limited organ function in the face of a physiologic challenge. Organ dysfunction may not appear in the resting state, but in a physiological stress situation (such as traumatic injury), the ability of the organs to augment function is compromised (Lewis, 2007).

Gender

Injury rates are highest for 15- to 24-year-old males. The risk for males is 2.5 times that of females, possibly because of male involvement in hazardous activities.

Alcohol

Alcohol use and abuse influences the likelihood of virtually all types of injury, even among young teenagers. An alcohol-related MVC kills someone every 31 minutes, and every two minutes a nonfatal crash occurs (NHTSA, 2006). Alcohol-related trauma is a major public health problem. Communities have enacted programs to decrease alcohol-related MVCs, including reducing legal blood alcohol levels to 0.08 percent and initiating sobriety checkpoints.

Race, Income, and Geography

Native Americans have the highest death rates from unintentional injury; African Americans have the highest homicide rates; and Caucasians and Native Americans have the highest suicide rates (Bergen et al., 2008). An inverse relationship between income levels and death rates exists for African Americans and Caucasians. There is a higher unintentional injury rate in rural areas and a higher intentional injury rate in urban areas (Bergen et al., 2008). Behaviors associated with rural unintentional injuries may include increased use of recreational vehicles and employment in high-risk occupations such as farming (Tiesman et al., 2007). Urban intentional injuries are usually related to homicide attempts.

SECTION ONE REVIEW

1. The two major categories of injury are
   A. chemical and thermal
   B. fractures and burns
   C. blunt and penetrating
   D. MVCs and gunshot wounds
2. The death rate from injury is highest for patients
   A. 24 to 42 years old
   B. 15 to 24 years old
   C. 5 to 14 years old
   D. more than 75 years old
3. The elderly have higher mortality and morbidity with traumatic injury because they
   A. have limited physiological reserve
   B. are exposed to high-risk activities
   C. drink more alcohol
   D. have poor judgment
4. The risk for males versus females for injury is
   A. 2.5 times lower
   B. 2.5 times higher
   C. 5 times higher
   D. equal
5. Reducing blood alcohol levels to ______ has been shown to decrease alcohol-related MVCs.
   A. 0.10 percent
   B. 0.05 percent
   C. 0.08 percent
   D. 0.04 percent

Answers: 1. C, 2. D, 3. A, 4. B, 5. C

SECTION TWO: Mechanism of Injury: Blunt Trauma

At the completion of this section, the learner will be able to define the forces associated with blunt trauma and apply these concepts to the clinical assessment of a patient with blunt trauma.

Blunt trauma is most commonly seen with MVCs, motor vehicles striking pedestrians, and falls from significant heights. One of the most basic principles of physics is used to explain trauma: the law of conservation of energy. Energy can neither be created nor destroyed; it is only changed from one form to another. Blunt trauma is this translation of energy from one form to another, through force.

Forces Associated with Blunt Trauma

Force is a physical factor—the push or pull that changes the state of an object that is either at rest or already in motion. Injury resulting from force is related to the amount and speed (velocity) of energy transmission, the surface area to which the energy is applied, and the elasticity of the tissues affected. The more slowly the force is applied, the more slowly energy is released, with less subsequent tissue deformation. The forces most often applied are acceleration, deceleration, shearing, and compression (ACSCT, 2004).

Acceleration is an increase in the rate of velocity or speed of a moving body. The most significant determinant of the amount of injury sustained is velocity. As velocity increases, so does tissue damage due to a greater amount of energy present. The concept of acceleration can be illustrated with a simple example. Upon impact with a solid object (e.g., another car, a brick wall, or a telephone pole), the driver of a car is suddenly propelled forward. He experiences a sudden acceleration of body mass determined by the rate of speed at which he was traveling and his body mass. This relationship is reflected in the following formula.

$$\text{Body weight} \times \text{mph} = \text{pounds per square inch of impact}$$

A person weighing 100 pounds, traveling at 35 miles per hour (mph), will hit at 3,500 pounds per square inch. This is equivalent to jumping head-first from a three-story building!

Deceleration is a decrease in the rate of velocity of a moving object. The same driver in the preceding example who is moving forward after hitting a solid object will experience a sudden deceleration after he comes into contact with the mass that impedes his forward (or backward) progression (e.g., the steering wheel, a tree, the road, or another passenger).

Shearing refers to injury resulting from two structures or two parts of the same structure, sliding in opposite directions causing a tearing or degloving type of injury. For example, shearing forces are frequently the cause of spinal injury at the C7–T1 juncture because the mobile cervical spine attaches at that point to the relatively immobile thoracic spine. Shearing forces are often the cause of aortic tears; splenic and renal injuries; and liver, brain, or heart injuries. These structures have a relatively immobile section connected to a relatively mobile section and, therefore, are subject to shearing forces.

Compression is the process of being pressed or squeezed together with a resulting reduction in volume or size. For example, sudden acceleration or deceleration during an MVC can cause compression of the heart and lung parenchyma between the posterior and anterior chest wall. The small bowel may be compressed between the vertebral column and the lower part of the steering wheel or an improperly placed seat belt. The bowel may rupture. The same mechanism can cause compression of the liver, causing it to burst.

Acceleration and deceleration injuries are most common with blunt trauma—for example, those involving the thoracic aorta. MVCs and falls from 20 feet or higher precipitate stretching, bowing, and shearing in major vessels. Damage may occur to any or all layers of the vessel wall. The vessel wall can tear, dissect, rupture, or form an aneurysm immediately or at any time postinjury. Shearing damage occurs in the vessels when deceleration occurs at a different rate than that occurring in other internal structures. For example, the relatively mobile ascending aorta continues to move after the relatively stationary descending aorta has stopped moving, resulting in a shearing injury.

Injuries Associated with Blunt Trauma

Injuries associated with blunt traumatic forces include head injuries (the movement of the brain inside the skull with acceleration, deceleration, and shearing coup injury), spinal cord injuries (the instability and poor support of the cervical spine predisposes it to shearing and acceleration/deceleration injury), fractures (from shearing and compression), and abdominal injuries (especially to the spleen and liver).

Tissue responsiveness to applied forces varies, creating characteristic limits of the tissues' abilities to withstand the forces of acceleration, deceleration, compression, and shearing. Tissue deformation is generally the result of tensile forces or shear forces. **Tensile forces** cause tissues to stretch and extend. Tensile strength of a specific tissue is the greatest longitudinal stretch or stress it can withstand without tearing apart. Joint dislocations, muscle sprains, and strains are frequently the result of tensile forces. Tensile forces are also the cause of contrecoup brain injuries. Brain tissue is pulled away from the skull with the initial alteration in motion as a result of acceleration or deceleration.

SECTION TWO REVIEW

1. Acceleration is a change in the rate of velocity or speed of a moving body. As velocity increases, tissue damage
   - A. decreases
   - B. increases
   - C. remains constant
   - D. cannot be determined
2. A decrease in the velocity of a moving object is
   - A. acceleration
   - B. deceleration
   - C. compression
   - D. shearing
3. Structures slipping in opposite directions to each other is a force known as
   - A. acceleration
   - B. deceleration
   - C. compression
   - D. shearing
4. The process of being pressed or squeezed is known as
   - A. acceleration
   - B. deceleration
   - C. compression
   - D. shearing
5. Forces that cause tissues to stretch are known as
   - A. tensile
   - B. shearing
   - C. mass
   - D. compression

Answers: 1. B, 2. B, 3. D, 4. C, 5. A

SECTION THREE: Mechanism of Injury: Penetrating Trauma

At the completion of this section, the learner will be able to define the forces associated with penetrating trauma and apply these concepts to the clinical assessment of a patient with penetrating trauma.

Forces Associated with Penetrating Trauma

Penetrating trauma is the result of the transmission of energy from a moving object into body tissues as the object disrupts the integrity of the skin and the underlying structures. The amount of kinetic energy transmitted by the object has a direct relationship to the degree of tissue damage. With tissue or organ penetration, the severity of the injury depends on the structures damaged by the transmission of the energy. A penetrating object can be almost anything—a knife, a bullet, shrapnel, an arrow, a stick, a metal rod, a fork, a gear shift, and so on.

The amount of kinetic energy available to be transmitted to tissues depends on the surface area of the point of impact, the density of the tissue, and the velocity of the projectile at the time of impact (ACSCT, 2004). Weapons are usually classified by the amount of energy they are capable of producing: Low-energy weapons include knives, arrows, or any type of hand missile; medium-energy weapons include handguns and some rifles; and high-energy weapons include hunting rifles and shotguns.

Low- to Medium-Energy Missiles

Low- to medium-energy missiles travel less than 2,000 feet per second. The injury sustained usually results from the missile contacting the tissue. Typically, damage is localized to those structures directly in the missile's path. However, special consideration must be given when injury occurs where body cavities lie in close proximity to one another. This principle is of critical importance when considering the close proximity of the thoracic and abdominal cavities, especially with injuries occurring near the diaphragm, which offers very little resistance to the penetrating agent. Penetrating injuries to the chest below the nipple line, the sixth rib, or the scapula may involve both thoracic and abdominal structures.

If the offending weapon is impaled in the body, it is critical that the object be left in place and protected from further movement until definitive surgical intervention is available. Protective padding can be placed around the object, such as gauze rolls or abdominal pads. A protective device, such as a plastic cup, may be used to secure the protruding handle of objects such as knives or the end of a stick or metal rod. Impaled objects may actually be controlling hemorrhage from damaged structures and removal may precipitate exsanguination.

High-Energy Missiles

High-energy missiles are those traveling more than 2,000 feet per second. At higher velocities, a tremendous amount of tissue destruction can occur as a result of forces transmitted to the tissues by the missile. High-energy missiles (also referred to as high-velocity missiles) transmit more kinetic energy, creating an intense blast result within the tissues. As the missile penetrates the tissue, the transmission of kinetic energy displaces tissues forward and laterally to form a temporary cavity, a process of cavity formation known as **cavitation** (Fig. 38–1). The degree of cavitation is directly related to the amount of kinetic energy transmitted to the tissues, which in turn is determined by the velocity of the missile. The size of the cavity may be up to 30 times the diameter of the missile (ACSCT, 2004). Tissue surrounding the missile tract is exposed to tensile (stretching), compressing, and shearing forces, which produce damage outside the direct path of the missile. Vessels, nerves, and other structures that are not directly damaged by the missile may be affected. The phenomenon of structure injury outside the direct missile path is referred to as "blast effect." Higher-velocity missiles produce more serious injury because of the destructive process of cavitation and blast effect to surrounding tissue and organs.

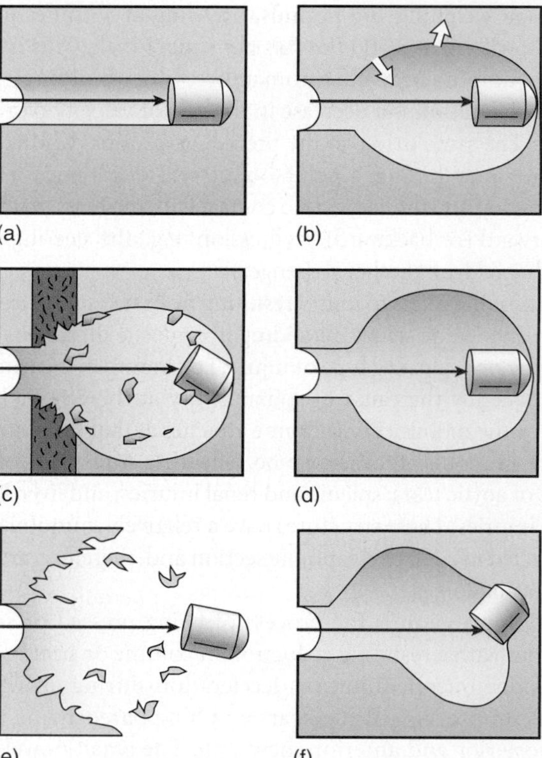

Figure 38–1 ■ Patterns of tissue injury secondary to gunshot wounds. (a) Low velocity, small entrance, and exit wounds. (b) Higher velocity, cavitation present with energy dispersion outward from missile path (blast effect). (c) Same velocity as in *B* but with penetration of bone and greater blast effect because of projections of bone being spread through tissue. (d) Higher velocity than in *B* or *C* with greater cavitation effect, small entrance and exit wounds. (e) same velocity as in *D*, but person or extremity hit is thinner resulting in large exit wound. (f) Asymmetrical cavitation as bullet begins to yaw and tumble.

Another contributing factor is the missile's trajectory. Consider a missile moving in stable flight toward the host (for our purposes, the patient). The missile passes from air into human tissue, which is several hundred times denser than air. As the missile passes into the tissue, the surrounding environment changes, precipitating instability of the missile. The unstable missile may yaw, tumble, deform, fragment, or any combination of these actions.

Yaw is the deviation of a missile either horizontally or vertically about its axis. *Tumble* is the action of forward rotation around the center of a mass (somersaulting) (Fig. 38–1F). The action of yawing or tumbling increases the surface area of the missile as it impacts the body (side of the missile versus the point of the missile). This creates a larger entrance wound. It also allows for increased energy transfer to the surrounding tissues, creating a larger area of tissue destruction. Higher-velocity missiles have a greater propensity for yaw and tumble.

Secondary Missiles

Another principle to consider when analyzing the effects of penetrating injury is the creation of secondary missiles by the penetrating object. A missile or its fragments may impart sufficient kinetic injury to dense tissue, such as bone or teeth, to create highly destructive secondary missiles. These secondary missiles may take erratic, unpredictable courses, resulting in additional injury. Secondary missiles also may be created by fragmentation of the primary missile. Thus, the anticipated missile path may be compounded, complicated, or enhanced by tissue damage precipitated by a secondary missile.

Injuries Associated with Penetrating Trauma

An evaluation of the wounds caused by the missile is necessary, noting the location, size, and shape. It is also important to determine if there is any foreign substance on the surrounding tissue, such as a black powder; and if the wound is actively bleeding. If there are two wounds, noting the location of each gives the clinician a hint of the trajectory the missile may have taken if the same missile caused both wounds. Missiles usually take the path of least resistance, so the path the missile followed may not be a straight line between the two wounds. Entrance wounds are usually smaller than exit wounds. However, the characteristics of a wound depend on the forces causing the injury, such as velocity, cavitation, and blast effect. Identifying the entrance wound and the exit wound is not necessary and should be left to experienced personnel. Simply identifying the wounds as wound 1 and wound 2 will suffice. The presence of two wounds does not necessarily mean one is an entrance and one is an exit wound, as there may be two entrance wounds from two separate missiles. Not all medium- and high-energy penetrating injuries have a resulting exit wound because the missile may remain inside the body.

SECTION THREE REVIEW

1. As a missile penetrates, the tissue is temporarily displaced forward and laterally, creating a tract. This process is known as
   A. velocity
   B. yaw
   C. tumbling
   D. cavitation
2. Cavitation demonstrates a(n) ______ relationship with the amount of kinetic energy transmitted to tissue.
   A. inverse
   B. direct
   C. insignificant
   D. diagonal
3. The phenomenon of structure injury outside the direct missile path is referred to as
   A. cavitation
   B. blast effect
   C. yaw
   D. tumbling
4. Yaw and tumble will ______ the area of tissue destruction precipitated by a missile.
   A. decrease
   B. increase
   C. minimize
   D. not affect
5. A patient has an impaled knife in the upper abdomen. You should immediately
   A. remove the knife and apply pressure
   B. manipulate the knife to facilitate assessment of injured organs
   C. stabilize the knife without removal and minimal manipulation
   D. leave the knife alone

Answers: 1. D, 2. B, 3. B, 4. B, 5. C

SECTION FOUR: Mechanism of Injury Patterns

At the completion of this section, the learner will be able to translate mechanism of injury into potential injury patterns manifested by the patient for both blunt and penetrating injuries.

Certain mechanisms result in predictable injury patterns (Table 38–1). Thus, the history of the event preceding the injury, such as pedestrian/motor vehicle injuries, motor vehicle driver and passenger injuries, fall injuries, and missile injuries, should elicit an increased index of suspicion for certain combinations of injured structures.

TABLE 38–1 Commonly Seen Injuries

MECHANISM OF INJURY	POTENTIAL STRUCTURE INJURY
Pedestrian hit by automobile	
Adult	Fractures of femur, tibia, and fibula on side of impact; ligamental damage to impacted knee; mild contralateral head injury
Child	Fractures of femur, chest injury, contralateral head injury
Unrestrained driver	Head and/or facial injury, rib fractures, sternum with underlying myocardial or pulmonary contusion, cervical spine fractures, laryngotracheal injuries, spleen injuries, liver injuries, small bowel injuries, posterior fracture–dislocation of hip, femur fractures
Unrestrained front seat passenger	Head and/or facial injuries, laryngotracheal injuries, posterior fracture–dislocation of femoral head, femur/patellar fractures

(continued)

TABLE 38–1 (*continued*)

MECHANISM OF INJURY	POTENTIAL STRUCTURE INJURY
Restrained driver (lap and shoulder harness)	Contusions of structures underlying harness (i.e., pulmonary contusion, contusion of small bowel)
Restrained passenger (lap belt only)	Flexion/distraction fractures, especially lumbar vertebrae (L1–L4), duodenal injuries, cervical spine injuries
Fall injuries	Compression fractures of lumbosacral spine and calcaneous fractures; fractures of radius/ulna, patella if victim falls forward
Vehicular ejection	Multiple injuries, especially head and cervical spine injuries; injury risk increases by 300% when ejection occurs
Low-velocity impalement	Local tissue/organ disruption, little or no cavitation
High-velocity missile, short missile path	Entrance wound larger than missile caliber; large ragged exit wound with cavitation
High-velocity missile, long missile path	Entrance wound larger than missile caliber; exit wound slightly larger than or equal to missile caliber; extensive cavitation (blast effect to deep structures absorbing lost kinetic energy)
High-velocity missile hitting bone or teeth	Entry wound larger than missile caliber; possibly no exit wound with missile fragmentation; secondary missile injury in unpredictable, erratic pattern

The following situation demonstrates the importance of the application of mechanism of injury. A 21-year-old male, unrestrained driver hits another vehicle head-on (Fig. 38–2).

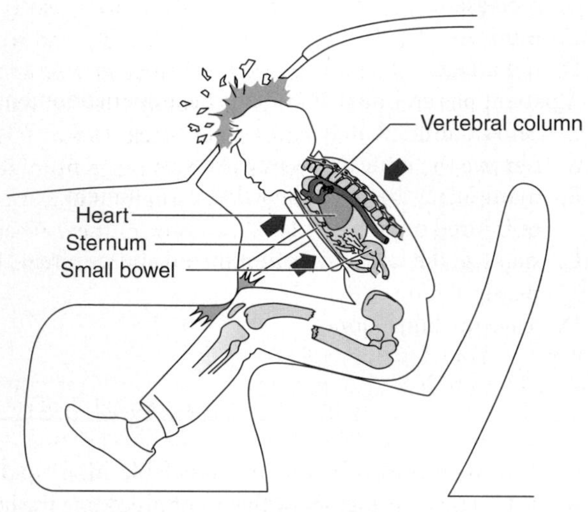

Figure 38–2 ■ Typical injuries of an unrestrained driver.

Traveling speed was in excess of 95 mph. Both the steering wheel and windshield were broken. A high index of suspicion must be maintained for the following injuries:

1. Potential intracranial injury because of the high rate of speed and shattered windshield
2. Potential cervical vertebrae injury because of suspected acceleration/deceleration at a high rate of speed and the broken windshield
3. Potential intrathoracic injuries because of the broken steering wheel—suspect rib fractures, myocardial and pulmonary contusions, and great vessel injury
4. Potential intraabdominal injuries because of the broken steering wheel and acceleration/deceleration mechanism; injuries could include splenic/liver lacerations, small bowel injuries, and great vessel injuries
5. Potential long-bone fractures, especially femur fractures or posterior hip fracture–dislocation, because of impact of knees with dashboard
6. Potential multiple skin lacerations, avulsions, punctures from the patient impacting various parts of the vehicle interior

SECTION FOUR REVIEW

1. A restrained passenger (lap belt only) may exhibit flexion/distraction fractures in which area of the vertebral column?
   A. cervical
   B. lumbar
   C. thoracic
   D. sacral
2. A restrained (lap and shoulder harness) occupant involved in an MVC can receive what types of injuries from the restraints?
   A. pulmonary contusions
   B. lumbar fractures
   C. femur fractures
   D. facial injuries
3. Which of the following is true?
   A. Vehicular ejection increases the risk for potential injury.
   B. Vehicular ejection decreases the risk for potential injury.
   C. Vehicular ejection is not related to the risk for potential injury.
   D. Vehicular ejection is associated with seat belt use.

4. An unrestrained front seat passenger involved in an MVC can receive what types of injuries? (choose all that apply)
   A. head or facial injuries
   B. laryngotracheal injuries
   C. posterior fracture-dislocation
   D. femur, patellar fractures

5. A broken steering wheel should induce a high suspicion of injury to the
   A. head
   B. neck
   C. abdomen
   D. long bones of the legs

Answers: 1. B, 2. A, 3. A, 4. (A, B, C, D) 5. C

SECTION FIVE: Mediators of Injury Response

At the completion of this section, the learner will be able to state clinical conditions that mediate a patient's response to injury, including underlying medical conditions, substance abuse, and physiological alterations such as pregnancy and advancing age.

Comorbidities

It is extremely important to identify comorbidities or underlying medical conditions when considering the patient's physiological and hemodynamic response to trauma. The most commonly encountered conditions include chronic obstructive pulmonary disease (COPD), heart disease, and underlying cerebral insufficiency, as with brain attacks (stroke). These conditions or the medications used to control their effects may alter the physiological response to trauma. The patient with COPD who sustains a minor pulmonary contusion related to blunt trauma may require prompt, life-saving intubation because of the alteration in the ventilation–perfusion ratio and effects on the resilience of affected lung tissue. Beta blockade used for coronary artery disease to minimize oxygen demands by the heart could prevent a normal response to hypovolemia (i.e., tachycardia). The patient with a head injury who has a history of stroke may experience an altered level of consciousness, difficulty in communication, or sensory/motor dysfunction from the prior stroke and not the acute head injury. Eliciting a complete medical history is crucial during the initial assessment.

Substance Abuse

Substance abuse is characterized by recurrent and clinically significant adverse consequences related to the repeated use of substances. Adverse consequences include failing to meet major role obligations, use of drugs in physically hazardous situations, substance-abuse related legal problems, and persistent or recurrent social or interpersonal problems as a result of continued drug use.

The high incidence of alcohol as a contributing factor to injury has been demonstrated. The most common effect is the inability to establish a baseline level of consciousness. As a central nervous system (CNS) depressant, the effects of alcohol on the brain are concentration dependent. The most sensitive tool for evaluation of brain injury is level of consciousness. Therefore, alcohol involvement is a critical consideration.

Blood alcohol concentration (BAC) is a measurement of intoxication. Measurement is conducted in milligrams per deciliter (mg/dL) or grams per deciliter (g/dL), varying from institution to institution. Legal intoxication in most states is 80 mg/dL or 0.08 g/dL. However, impaired judgment occurs at a level of 50 mg/dL or 0.05 g/dL. A history of alcohol use should be obtained because a degree of tolerance ensues with frequent alcohol ingestion. As plasma levels increase, sedation, lack of motor coordination, ataxia, and impaired psychomotor performance become apparent. The concomitant use of alcohol and other CNS depressants (e.g., barbiturates, opiates, sedative–hypnotics) potentiates each drug's effects, creating a synergistic effect. CNS stimulants, such as cocaine, also can alter the level of consciousness in the injured patient. Cocaine use mimics and intensifies a sympathetic stimulation or the fight-or-flight response in the patient. Notably, an increase in heart rate and blood pressure occur along with vasoconstriction, dilated pupils, tremors, excitability, and restlessness. Cocaine can induce myocardial ischemia as well as many dysrhythmias, including heart block, tachydysrhythmias, ventricular fibrillation, asystole, and bundle branch block (Devlin & Henry, 2008). Neurologically, mental status changes range from anxiety to acute paranoid psychosis. For the high-acuity nurse, it is very difficult to obtain a baseline level of consciousness when the patient is intoxicated with alcohol or other drugs that cloud his or her sensorium.

The Pregnant Patient

The pregnant trauma patient presents unique aspects of care that must be carefully considered. Major trauma affects 6 to 7 percent of pregnant patients (Hill & Pickinpaugh, 2008). Familiarity with trauma assessment and management during pregnancy is important for the nurse in the high-acuity setting.

Anatomic Changes

Anatomic rearrangement as pregnancy progresses is inevitable and may cause confusion in physical diagnosis. Depending on the gestational size of the uterus, different patterns of injury may occur to the mother as well as to the fetus. Blunt abdominal trauma in the pregnant patient is associated with different injuries from those in the nonpregnant patient.

Hemodynamic Changes

After the tenth week of pregnancy, cardiac output is increased by up to 50 percent. A high-output, low-resistance hemodynamic state is characteristic in pregnancy. Maternal heart rate increases by 10 to 15 beats per minute throughout pregnancy, with a slight increase in stroke volume. Blood pressure decreases during pregnancy by 5 to 15 mm Hg (Hill & Pickinpaugh, 2008). It is important to remember that some women experience profound hypotension when placed in the supine position (especially during the third trimester). This is known as the *vena cava syndrome* and is caused by the enlarged uterus compressing the inferior vena cava against the spinal column, decreasing venous return and preload. The hypotension can be relieved by turning the patient to the left lateral decubitus position.

Blood Volume and Composition

During pregnancy, maternal blood volume increases by 50 percent by the end of the third trimester, with maximal volume expansion by 28 to 32 weeks gestation (Hill & Pickinpaugh, 2008). Therefore, mild blood loss as a result of traumatic injury is usually well tolerated. Pregnant and nonpregnant trauma patients respond very differently to physiological stress. Because of the hypervolemic state associated with pregnancy, a 30 to 40 percent (up to 2,000 mL) blood loss may occur in a pregnant patient before signs and symptoms of hypovolemia occur; however, the patient may deteriorate rapidly once 2,500 mL blood loss has occurred. During pregnancy, a physiological anemia results as plasma volume increases by 50 percent and red blood cell volume increases by only 30 percent. Late in pregnancy, the hemoglobin may have fallen to 10.5 to 11 g and the hematocrit to 31 to 35 percent. The white blood cell count increases during pregnancy (15,000 to 18,000/mm^3) and during labor may be as high as 25,000/mm^3.

Advancing Age

Physiological changes associated with aging (individuals ages 65 and older), such as delayed reaction times, disturbances of gait and balance, diminished visual acuity, and hearing loss predispose older adults to traumatic injury. Also, age-related deterioration in body systems alters the elderly trauma victim's response to injury and increases the susceptibility to complications. The four most common mechanisms of injury in this age group are falls, motor vehicle crashes, pedestrian versus automobile crashes, and penetrating trauma, respectively.

Chronic Disease States

Chronic disease states exacerbate or compound traumatic injury. Common underlying medical conditions include COPD, coronary artery disease, diabetes mellitus, congestive heart failure, hypertension, and conditions leading to diminished neurological acuity (e.g., stroke and carotid insufficiency). The patient not only may have a chronic medical condition but also could be treated with a polypharmaceutical regimen that may affect the response to a traumatic injury.

Limited Physiologic Reserve

The higher morbidity and mortality rates associated with trauma and advancing age can be attributed to limited physiological reserve (as discussed in Section One). The limited physiological reserve is most often in the cardiorespiratory, neurological, and musculoskeletal systems. Cardiorespiratory effects include decreased distensibility of blood vessels, increased systolic blood pressure and systemic vascular resistance, increased vascular resistance, decreased coronary blood flow, decreased cardiac output, decreased respiratory muscle strength, limited chest expansion, and decreased number of functioning alveoli. These alterations combine to reduce greatly the ability to sustain adequate tissue perfusion and oxygenation. Mild anemia is also common in this age group and potentiates alterations in oxygenation by limiting oxygen transport capabilities.

Neurological changes associated with advancing age include short-term memory loss and reduced cerebral blood flow. Preexisting neurological conditions, such as senility, dementia, and Alzheimer's disease, may significantly affect evaluation of the patient's neurological status. Head injuries are common in the elderly. A high index of suspicion, awareness of the patient's preexisting neurological status, and frequent, thorough neurological assessments are necessary to avoid detrimental delays in diagnosis and intervention.

Osteoporosis and decreasing muscle mass contribute to the high incidence of fractures. The incidence of rib fractures with blunt chest trauma is 39 to 71 percent (Sharma et al., 2008). Patients with advancing age have twice the mortality and morbidity of younger patients. Mortality increases with the number of rib fractures. Normal aging processes diminish blood supply to the skin and result in delayed healing of soft tissue injuries. This reduction of blood supply also predisposes the elderly trauma patient to the development of pressure ulcers.

Difficulties during the initial assessment related to normal aging may present themselves to the clinician. Shock is difficult to diagnose secondary to age-related changes that affect the patient's response to trauma, including decreased cardiac output, decreased maximal heart rate, and increased peripheral vascular resistance (Calloway & Wolfe, 2007). Because of the decline in gag and cough reflexes, airway integrity may be difficult to maintain. Detection of shock may be difficult because of the propensity toward hypertension. Thus, normal blood pressures actually may indicate low perfusion states. Aggressive care and resuscitation have a dramatic effect in improving outcome; therefore, they require a more aggressive approach than younger patients who have similar mechanism during their initial emergency management (Calloway & Wolfe, 2007).

SECTION FIVE REVIEW

1. Eliciting a medical history is crucial during the initial assessment because (choose all that apply)
   A. comorbidities alter the physiologic response to trauma
   B. medications alter the physiologic response to trauma
   C. a medical history helps to identify the cause of injury
   D. the patient may be comatose later

2. Cocaine use in the trauma patient acts as a CNS
   A. stimulant
   B. depressant
   C. vasodilator
   D. vasoconstrictor

3. After the tenth week of pregnancy, cardiac output is increased by ______.
   A. 10 percent
   B. 25 percent
   C. 50 percent
   D. 100 percent
4. Patients with advanced age are at a high risk of rib fractures because of (choose all that apply):
   A. limited chest expansion
   B. lack of wearing seat belts
   C. decreased muscle mass
   D. osteoporosis
5. Shock is difficult to assess in elderly trauma patients, secondary to which of the following age-related changes?
   A. decrease in cardiac output
   B. decrease in heart rate
   C. increase in peripheral vascular rate
   D. all of the above

Answers: 1. (A, B) 2. A, 3. C, 4. (C, D) 5. D

SECTION SIX: Primary Survey

At the completion of this section, the learner will be able to identify the clinical assessment format used to identify life-threatening injuries during the primary survey.

Because of the unpredictable effects of trauma-related injury on the patient, the nurse must develop a rapid, systematic approach to assessing each patient to ensure no effects of injury are overlooked. Trauma should always be approached as a multisystem disease. Thus, a rapid systematic approach to assessment with establishment of management priorities is essential.

Trauma presents myriad of potentially life-threatening injuries. The life-threatening injuries must be evaluated quickly, with immediate interventions. The trauma assessment is divided into three phases: primary survey, resuscitation, and secondary survey.

The primary survey is the focus of this section. The purpose of the primary survey is to identify and treat life-threatening conditions and intervene appropriately. Primary survey is done using the A, B, C, D, and E approach, as outlined here

- **A—Airway (with cervical spine immobilization).** Ensure that the patient has an open airway.
- **B—Breathing.** Is the patient breathing? Are respirations effective? Does the patient need assistance via bag-valve-mask or mechanical ventilation?
- **C—Circulation.** The trauma patient is at very high risk of hypovolemic shock from acute blood loss and third spacing of fluid with soft tissue damage. Identify hypovolemia quickly and search for the etiology.
- **D—Disability.** Perform a quick neurological examination of the patient's level of consciousness and motor function.
- **E—Exposure and evacuation.** Completely undress the patient to provide for visualization of external causes of injury. If the severity of the patient's injury exceeds the capability of the hospital, consider transport of the patient to a definitive care facility.

Each of the components of the primary survey is explored in detail here, providing the learner with information needed to approach the multiple-injured patient using critical thinking and problem-solving strategies.

Airway and Cervical Spine

The goal of airway management is optimization of ventilation and oxygenation, with cervical spine protection. The first step in the primary survey is assessment of patency of the patient's airway. An injury to the cervical spine should always be assumed in the patient with multisystem trauma, especially in the patient with an injury above the clavicle. Excessive manipulation of the head, face, or neck, such as hyperextension or hyperflexion of the cervical spine, may convert a fracture without neurological manifestations into a fracture–dislocation with spinal cord contusion, laceration, compression, or transection. Therefore, cervical immobilization is imperative during airway assessment.

Potential causes of airway obstruction include the tongue falling back into the oropharynx; blood, vomitus, secretions, or foreign objects in the airway; and fractures of the facial bony structures or crushing injuries of the laryngotracheal tree. Actual or potential airway obstruction may be present with the following symptoms:

- Dyspnea
- Diminished breath sounds despite respiratory effort
- Dysphonia (hoarseness, stridor)
- Dysphagia
- Drooling

Airway management techniques range from simple positional maneuvers to complex surgical procedures. During all maneuvers, it is critical that the cervical spine be maintained by in-line immobilization with the head in the neutral position. Cervical spine immobilization is best achieved by manual in-line axial traction either by a caregiver or hard cervical collar. Disposable head blocks or towel rolls may be placed on both sides of the patient's head with tape across the patient's forehead to immobilize the cervical spine. These actions prevent forward flexion, hyperextension, and lateral rotation of the cervical spine. Sandbags are no longer an acceptable means of lateral cervical immobilization because of the increased lateral pressure to the cervical spine that occurs with turning or tilting of the backboard.

The first, and most simple, maneuver used to open the airway is a chin lift or modified jaw thrust. This maneuver may open the airway adequately and allow ventilation to take place. The airway can be suctioned for debris, secretions, blood, or vomitus. An oropharyngeal or nasopharyngeal airway may be used to facilitate airway maintenance. The oropharyngeal airway should be used in patients who are unconscious and have no gag reflex. Using this airway in a conscious patient may precipitate gagging, vomiting, and potential aspiration. Improper placement of the oropharyngeal airway may cause airway obstruction. The nasopharyngeal airway can be used to facilitate airway integrity in the conscious victim with an intact gag reflex; however, it should be avoided if a basal skull fracture is suspected.

If the aforementioned procedures are inadequate in establishing an airway, more aggressive measures must be taken. The patient is preoxygenated with a bag-valve-mask using 100 percent oxygen. A frequent complication of ventilation with this technique is gastric distention. Increased risks secondary to the distention include vomiting, aspiration, and diaphragmatic impingement. To minimize gastric distention avoid using too large a volume or too many breaths. After a definitive airway has been secured, placement of a gastric tube decompresses the stomach.

Endotracheal intubation is achieved either orally or nasally. Nasotracheal intubation may be performed in the injured patient because hyperextension of the neck is minimized. With the nasotracheal method, the tube is advanced during the inspiratory effort when the epiglottis is open. Orotracheal intubation is necessary when the patient is apneic or a cribriform plate fracture is suspected, as with basilar skull fractures. With fractures of the cribriform plate, the nasally inserted endotracheal tube could pass into the cranial vault, injuring brain tissue. If orotracheal intubation is necessary, absolute and vigilant care must be taken to avoid hyperextension of the cervical spine. The most important determinant when choosing either method is the experience of the provider.

After intubation is achieved, breath sounds are auscultated to confirm tracheal intubation. The clinician also should first ausculate over the epigastrium for gurgling sounds to help rule out an esophageal intubation. Repeated assessment of breath sounds in any intubated patient is a critical nursing action.

The indication for a surgical airway is the inability to intubate the trachea. Inability to intubate the trachea may result from edema of the glottis, laryngeal fracture, severe oropharyngeal hemorrhage, or gross instability of the midface. A surgical airway can be achieved by a needle cricothyroidotomy, surgical cricothyroidotomy, or tracheostomy. Surgical cricothyroidotomy is performed by making an incision through the cricothyroid membrane and passing an endotracheal or tracheostomy tube into the trachea. Tracheostomy must be considered in the patient with suspected laryngeal trauma. Symptoms of laryngeal injury include tenderness, hoarseness, subcutaneous emphysema, and intolerance of the supine position. The supine position is poorly tolerated by these patients because, on assuming the position, the airway will collapse where the laryngeal injury has occurred. With the patient sitting upright, an open airway is maintained even though the larynx is injured.

Assurance of airway integrity is the priority in the primary survey. Airway integrity does not ensure adequate ventilation, but the airway must be opened and secured before ventilation is assessed.

Breathing

The next step in the primary survey is to assess adequacy of ventilation. The primary goal of ventilation is to achieve maximum cellular oxygenation by providing an oxygen-rich environment. Thus, all trauma patients should receive high-flow oxygen during the initial evaluation.

Breathing is evaluated by the look, listen, and feel parameters. Look to detect the presence of respiratory excursion, listen for breath sounds, and feel for breathing. Positive pressure ventilation may be required in some patients and is provided in a number of ways: mouth-to-mask, bag-valve-mask, or a mechanical ventilator.

Confirmation of the adequacy of ventilation is best achieved by evaluating the $Pa{O_2}$ and $Pa{CO_2}$ obtained from an arterial blood gas (ABG) or by continuous monitoring of end-tidal carbon dioxide and arterial oxygen saturation using noninvasive measures. If arterial blood gases are inadequate, the airway is reevaluated, and the patient is evaluated for the presence of pneumothorax, hemothorax, hemopneumothorax, or tension pneumothorax. Tube thoracostomy is indicated for any of these conditions because they are all life-threatening injuries.

Circulation

The third step in the primary survey is assessment of circulation. Inadequate circulation is manifested as shock, a clinical state characterized by inadequate organ perfusion and tissue oxygenation, discussed further in Module 18, Alterations in Oxygen Delivery and Consumption: Shock States.

Assessment for adequate circulation includes palpating for strength, rate, rhythm, and symmetry of carotid, radial, femoral, and pedal pulses. Skin temperature is evaluated, as is capillary refill. Adequacy of tissue perfusion is reflected by the patient's level of consciousness.

Successful treatment of shock depends on early recognition, controlling obvious hemorrhage, and aggressive fluid resuscitation to prevent the development of hypotension. Intravenous (IV) access is critical for volume infusion. Two large-bore IVs are established (16 gauge or larger in adults), and crystalloids are administered. Warm lactated Ringer's solution is the solution of choice. Lactated Ringer's solution can be infused at a wide-open rate. If there are no signs of improvement after 2 liters, crystalloid infusion continues along with administration of blood products. Failure to respond to crystalloid and blood infusions indicates a rapid surgical intervention is required (ACSCT, 2004).

Recognition of the source of blood loss is critical. Blood volume loss in quantities large enough to produce a shock state can occur in one or more of the following five areas

1. **Chest.** In the adult, 2.5 L of blood can be lost in each hemothorax. Thus, a total of 5 L can be lost inside the chest, which would be the total blood volume of a 70-kg person.
2. **Abdomen.** As much as 6 L of blood can be lost via intraperitoneal bleeding from damaged organs or vessels.

3. **Pelvis and retroperitoneum.** Unstable pelvic fractures, especially those involving the posterior elements of the pelvis, can precipitate liters of blood loss. A patient actually may exsanguinate from an unstable pelvic fracture involving posterior bony elements.
4. **Femur fractures.** For each femur fracture, 500 to 1,000 mL of blood can be lost.
5. **External hemorrhage.** Bleeding wounds are a consideration. A scalp laceration, particularly, requires proper hemostasis because a significant amount of blood can be lost with this injury.

Of the causes of early postinjury deaths in the hospital that are amenable to effective treatment, hemorrhage is predominant. The most common cause of shock in the injured patient is hypovolemia, resulting from acute blood loss. Fluid resuscitation is the fundamental treatment for hypovolemic shock until definitive surgical intervention is available to treat the site (or sites) of injury.

Disability

After airway, breathing, and circulation are assessed and adequately managed, the fourth step in the primary survey is assessment of neurological disability. The purpose of the neurological examination in the primary survey is to establish quickly the patient's level of consciousness and pupillary size and reaction.

The patient's level of consciousness is quickly determined using the AVPU method.

- A—Alert
- V—Responds to verbal stimulation
- P—Responds to painful stimulation
- U—Unresponsive

A more detailed neurological examination is included in the secondary survey.

Exposure

At this point in the primary survey, the patient is completely disrobed in preparation for the secondary survey. Exposure to cold ambient temperatures of resuscitation areas, large volumes of room temperature IV fluids and cold blood products, and wet clothing all predispose the trauma patient to hypothermia. Careful attention to heat conservation measures cannot be overemphasized.

SECTION SIX REVIEW

1. Life-threatening injuries are detected during
   A. the primary survey
   B. resuscitation
   C. the secondary survey
   D. the tertiary survey
2. The primary survey is done using the A, B, C, D, E approach. The D stands for assessment of
   A. dyspnea
   B. diminished breath sounds
   C. dysphagia
   D. disability
3. Assessment of ventilation can be made using
   A. ABG determination
   B. continuous end-tidal CO_2
   C. listening to all breath sounds
   D. all of the above
4. Assessment for circulation should include
   A. palpation of all pulses
   B. capillary refill
   C. level of consciousness
   D. all of the above
5. Which of the following assessments is done during the "E" component of the primary survey?
   A. Expel all gastric contents.
   B. Extricate the patient from harm.
   C. Apply external pressure to hemorrhage.
   D. Disrobe patient in preparation for secondary survey.

Answers: 1. A, 2. D, 3. D, 4. D, 5. D

SECTION SEVEN: Secondary Survey

This section outlines the components of the secondary assessment during the initial trauma evaluation. At the completion of this section, the learner will be able to discuss the components and the suggested format for conducting the secondary survey.

The secondary survey begins after the primary survey is completed and all immediately life-threatening injuries have been addressed. A head-to-toe approach is used, with a thorough examination of each body system. A critical point to remember is that if the patient becomes hemodynamically unstable at any point during the secondary survey, immediately return to the primary survey format (A, B, C, D, and E) to troubleshoot the problem. A summary of key points in the secondary survey has been adapted in Table 38–2 from the American College of Surgeons Committee on Trauma's *Advanced Trauma Life Support Course Manual* (ACSCT, 2004).

During the completion of the secondary survey, the trauma patient demands repeated reevaluation so that any new signs or symptoms are not overlooked. Other life-threatening problems may appear, or exacerbation of previously treated injuries may occur (such as tension pneumothorax, pericardial tamponade, or intracranial bleeding). Continuous monitoring of vital signs is critical.

TABLE 38–2 Key Points in the Secondary Survey

SURVEYED SYSTEM	EVALUATED CRITERIA
Head	Complete neurological examination using a tool such as the Glasgow Coma Scale (GCS); reevaluation of pupillary size and reactivity; inspection and palpation of cranium for lacerations, fractures, contusions, hemotympanium, cerebrospinal fluid leakage, and edema
Maxillofacial	Assessment for facial fractures via inspection, palpation for open fractures, lacerations, and mobility or instability of facial structures
Cervical spine/neck	Inspection and palpation of neck anteriorly (maintaining cervical spine immobilization) and palpation anteriorly and posteriorly for pain, crepitus, bony stepoffs indicating fracture–dislocation, neck vein distention, and tracheal deviation
Chest	Inspection for paradoxical movement, flail segments, open chest wounds, and ecchymosis; palpation for rib fractures, subcutaneous emphysema, respiratory excursion, and sternal fractures; auscultation for quality, equality of breath sounds, and presence of adventitious sounds; auscultation of heart sounds for quality, extra heart sounds, murmurs, or pericardial friction rubs possibly indicating pericardial effusion
Abdomen	Inspection and auscultation before palpation to prevent precipitation of misleading bowel sounds by manual manipulation; abdomen inspection for abrasions, contusions, lacerations, and distention; auscultation for bowel sounds in four quadrants, bruits, and breath sounds; light and deep palpation precipitating a painful response may indicate intraperitoneal bleeding and should be quickly attended
Pelvis, perineum, genitalia	Pelvis inspection for deformation and palpation for stability; perineum and genitalia inspection for bleeding at the meatus, hematoma, vaginal bleeding, and lacerations; rectal examination to evaluate rectal wall integrity, presence of blood, position of prostate, presence of palpable pelvic fractures, and quality of sphincter tone
Musculoskeletal	Visual evaluation of extremities for contusions or deformities; palpation of all extremities for tenderness, crepitation, or abnormal range of motion, which may raise index of suspicion for fracture; all peripheral pulses should be evaluated, and capillary refill, skin color, temperature rechecked
Back	All patients should be log rolled with careful attention to spinal immobilization to afford the clinician a full view of the patient's posterior surfaces, including neck, back, buttocks, and lower extremities; these areas should be carefully inspected and palpated to detect any area of injury
Complete neurologic examination	Motor and sensory evaluation of the extremities and reevaluation of the patient's GCS score and pupils; any evidence of paralysis or paresis should prompt immediate immobilization of the entire patient if not already done

SECTION SEVEN REVIEW

1. During the secondary assessment, the patient becomes hemodynamically unstable. You should immediately
   A. stop the secondary survey and reinstitute the primary assessment
   B. finish the secondary survey, looking for potential etiologies of instability
   C. start at the beginning of the secondary survey
   D. reevaluate patency and flow rates of IVs
2. The purpose of the secondary survey is to
   A. identify and intervene with life-threatening injuries
   B. identify the existence of all injuries
   C. facilitate treatment of airway and breathing
   D. assess response of resuscitative interventions
3. The complete and immediate immobilization of the entire patient should take place with the following findings during secondary survey
   A. inability to establish airway
   B. tense, distended abdomen
   C. Glasgow Coma Scale score less than eight
   D. evidence of paralysis or paresis
4. Presence of abdominal pain on light or deep palpation in the injured patient usually indicates
   A. gastritis
   B. presence of intraperitoneal blood
   C. pelvic fracture
   D. intracerebral pathology
5. Rectal examination should be done to evaluate which of the following? (choose all that apply)
   A. rectal wall integrity
   B. presence of blood
   C. bladder injury
   D. palpable pelvic fractures

Answers: 1. A, 2. B, 3. D, 4. B, 5. (A, B, D)

SECTION EIGHT: Trauma Resuscitation

At the completion of this section, the learner will be able to describe the trimodal distribution of trauma-related mortalities and how this is integrated into clinical assessment. The learner will also be able to discuss important nursing responsibilities during the trauma resuscitation phase, and compare and contrast various end points of traumatic shock resuscitation.

The primary survey and resuscitation occur simultaneously. As this happens, other therapies are also initiated. For example, a Foley catheter is inserted during resuscitation (unless contraindicated). A nasogastric tube is placed to prevent aspiration.

Trauma Deaths

When plotted on a graph, trauma-related mortalities exhibit a trimodal distribution; that is, death from trauma has three peak periods of occurrence. The first peak occurs within minutes of the injury. These deaths usually result from injuries to the brain, upper spinal cord, heart, aorta, or other major blood vessel. The second peak occurs within two hours of injury, and death usually is related to subdural or epidural hematomas, hemopneumothorax, ruptured spleen, lacerated liver, fractured femurs, or other injuries resulting in significant blood loss. The third peak occurs days to weeks after the injury and usually results from complications of sepsis or MODS (ACSCT, 2004).

How does the knowledge of this distribution affect clinical practice? It can empower the nurse to anticipate the needs of the patient based on time from injury and physiological manifestation of the injury. If a patient is received within minutes of injury, what are the life-threatening injuries that may cause death in this time frame? Has the patient experienced brainstem compression or laceration resulting in respiratory center dysfunction? What assessments and interventions must be performed to mediate these injuries?

If an unstable patient arrives within 30 minutes of injury, certain conditions must be appreciated clinically to anticipate a life-threatening situation. Conditions might include hemopneumothorax (assess respiratory effort, lung sounds and necessity of a chest tube), ruptured spleen or lacerated liver (assess for a tense and painful abdomen, hypotension with no signs of obvious blood loss), or fractured femur (assess for a painful leg, with an obvious fracture).

The high-acuity nurse caring for a patient three days postinjury anticipates a much different scenario. The nurse identifies precipitating or contributing factors in a patient experiencing sepsis or multiple organ dysfunction syndrome, such as overhydration during the first 24 to 48 hours with development of acute respiratory distress syndrome (ARDS) or a missed intraabdominal injury predisposing the patient to sepsis.

Shock from Trauma

Mortality from trauma may result from what is considered a preventable cause. One of the most frequently encountered clinical states in the injured patient is traumatic shock. Because of the frequency of traumatic shock, a brief discussion of hemorrhagic shock ensues. Refer to Module 18, Alterations in Oxygen Delivery and Consumption: Shock States, for an in-depth examination of the cellular tissue, organ, and system response to shock.

Shock has been defined as the consequence of insufficient tissue perfusion that results in inadequate cellular oxygenation and accumulation of metabolic wastes (ACSCT, 2004). The most common cause of shock in the injured patient is hypovolemia resulting from acute blood loss. Acute blood loss can occur externally, as with lacerations, open fractures, avulsion injuries, or amputations, or internally within a body cavity, as with bleeding into the chest cavity, abdominal cavity, retroperitoneum, or soft tissue.

Exsanguination is the most extreme form of hemorrhage. There is an initial loss of 40 percent of the patient's blood volume, with a rate of blood loss, or a rate of hemorrhage, exceeding 250 mL per minute. If uncontrolled, the patient may lose 50 percent of the entire blood volume within a very few minutes. Loss of up to 15 percent of circulating volume (700 to 750 mL for a 70-kg patient) may produce little in terms of obvious symptoms, whereas loss of up to 30 percent of circulating volume (1.5 mL) may result in mild tachycardia, tachypnea, and anxiety. Hypotension, marked tachycardia (pulse 110 to 120 beats per minute) and confusion may not be evident until more than 30 percent of blood volume has been lost. Loss of 40 percent of circulating volume (2 L) is immediately life-threatening. Most injuries precipitating exsanguination are from penetrating trauma. Regardless of the mechanism, exsanguinations will lead to hypovolemic shock.

Resuscitation of the patient who is exsanguinating rests on the intensified basic principles of circulation management. IV access is established quickly with adequate, large-bore catheters. Because the underlying source of the hypotension is hypovolemic shock, administering fluids is crucial in shock management. Vasopressors are not given to treat hypotension until fluid volume has been restored. Blood and blood products may be given in addition to IV fluids. Type specific blood should be given, but in an emergency situation low-titer O-positive blood may be given to men and O-negative to women of childbearing age.

Other adjuncts are available in the acute phase of resuscitation of the patient with exsanguination. Rapid infusion devices are available that can deliver large amounts of crystalloid and colloid quickly. The use of autotransfusion devices facilitates resuscitative efforts. Emergency department open resuscitative thoracotomy also may be used to manage the exsanguinating patient, especially if exsanguination is suspected to be related to injury to the great vessels (i.e., aorta) or the heart.

Critical analysis during the primary assessment and quick recognition of traumatic shock are essential skills in the resuscitative phase of trauma. Twenty percent of preventable trauma-related mortalities can be mediated with improved prehospital and hospital care under the provision of highly skilled clinicians trained to evaluate the injured patient rapidly and effectively.

End Points of Resuscitation

How is it determined that the patient has been adequately resuscitated? The goal of the resuscitation is to treat shock so it does not progress to an irreversible state.

Recall that shock has been defined as the consequence of insufficient tissue perfusion that results in inadequate cellular oxygenation and accumulation of metabolic wastes (ACSCT, 2004). The patient who is in shock, therefore, would have signs and symptoms of inadequate tissue perfusion and cellular oxygenation and accumulation of metabolic wastes. The patient who is not in shock would have signs of adequate tissue perfusion that results in adequate cellular oxygenation and no evidence of accumulation of metabolic wastes. Determining when tissue perfusion has been restored is a challenge. Unfortunately, traditional signs of sufficient tissue perfusion (normal blood pressure, heart rate, and urine output) cannot be used in shock states because normal vital signs and urine output may be the result of compensatory mechanisms (renin–angiotensin–aldosterone and the sympathetic nervous system; see Module 18, Alterations in Oxygen Delivery and Consumption: Shock States. The best clinical indicator of sufficient tissue perfusion is not currently available. Current indicators include traditional hemodynamic parameters, global parameters, and organ specific parameters (Table 38–3).

The high-acuity nurse should not be lured into a false sense of security when vital signs and basic hemodynamic parameters have been restored to normal values during resuscitation. During resuscitation from traumatic hemorrhagic shock, normalization of blood pressure, heart rate, and urine output are not adequate, as occult hypoperfusion and ongoing tissue acidosis (compensated shock) may be present, which may lead to organ dysfunction and death (Tisherman et al., 2004). Optimizing hemodynamic variables to improve cardiac output/index, oxygen delivery, and oxygen consumption may be beneficial. Numerous parameters, including hemodynamic profiles, acid-base status, gastric tonometry, and regional measures of tissue O_2 and CO_2 levels, have been studied and found to be useful for predicting risk of organ failure and death; however, use as parameters for endpoints of resuscitation have failed to show clear benefit in terms of patient outcomes (Tisherman et al., 2004). Using one of these parameters as an endpoint seems sensible as traditional clinical parameters are inadequate.

TABLE 38–3 End Points in Trauma Resuscitation

Parameter	End-Point Value
Traditional Hemodynamic Parameters	
Blood pressure	Systolic blood pressure greater than 90 mm Hg; mean arterial pressure (MAP) greater than 70 mm Hg
Heart rate	Less than 100 beats per minute
Urine output	Greater than 30 mL per hour
Skin	Warm, dry
Global Parameters	
Oxygen delivery index	Greater than 500 mL/min/m^2
Oxygen consumption index	125 mL/min/m^2
Systemic mixed venous oxygen saturation	65 to 80%
Lactate	Less than 2.2 mMol/L
Base deficit	± 3.0 mMol/L
Tissue arteriovenous carbon dioxide gradient	Less than 11 mm Hg
Sublingual capnography	Less than 70
Gastric pH$_i$	pH$_i$ greater than 7.35

SECTION EIGHT REVIEW

1. Trauma-related mortalities exhibit a ______ distribution.
   A. modal
   B. bimodal
   C. trimodal
   D. bell-shaped
2. The most common shock state in the injured patient is
   A. hypovolemic
   B. cardiogenic
   C. neurogenic
   D. septic
3. Hypotension, marked tachycardia, and confusion may not be evident until ______ of blood volume is lost.
   A. 15 percent
   B. 30 percent
   C. 50 percent
   D. 75 percent
4. Which of the following parameters is the BEST reflection that resuscitation efforts have improved the shock state?
   A. MAP greater than 70 mm Hg
   B. heart rate 80 beats per minute
   C. urine output 30 mL per hour
   D. lactate less than 2.2 mmol
5. Current guidelines recommend which of the following parameters should be corrected within 24 hours of injury?
   A. base deficit
   B. lactate
   C. gastric pH$_i$
   D. all of the above

Answers: 1. C, 2. A, 3. B, 4. D, 5. D

SECTION NINE: Management of Selected Injuries

At the completion of this section, the learner will be able to describe basic principles of collaborative management for injuries to the chest, abdomen, and pelvis. Care of the patient with traumatic brain injury is discussed in Module 22, Alteration in Sensory Perceptual Disorders: Acute Head Injury and care of the patient with spinal cord injury is reviewed in Module 23, Alteration in Sensory Perceptual Function: Acute Spinal Cord Injury. The focus of this section is on management of chest, abdominal, and pelvic injuries because these injuries are commonly seen in high-acuity units. As with any emergent condition, these systems are not addressed until the airway, breathing, and circulation are stabilized as described in Section Six.

Chest Injuries

Injuries to the chest are usually a result of an MVC or a violent crime. Chest injuries cause one in every four deaths in North America. Injuries to the chest involve trauma to the chest wall, lungs, and heart.

Rib Fractures

Rib fractures are typically caused by blunt trauma. Multiple ribs can be fractured. Rib fractures are very painful; the pain is aggravated by any movement of the chest wall, even breathing. Therefore, the patient with rib fractures often takes shallow breaths. Atelectasis can develop and the patient is at risk for developing pneumonia. Pain management, including nonsteroidal anti-inflammatory agents, intercostal nerve block, thoracic epidural analgesia, and narcotics may be used to optimize pain management. There is no treatment for rib fractures other than to let the fractures heal naturally over time; however, the use of the incentive spirometer has been found to decrease the incidence of pneumonia, intensive care unit and hospital length of stay, as well as mortality (Keel & Meier, 2007)

Flail Chest

Flail chest occurs when two or more rib fractures occur in two or more places (Fig. 38–3). The chest wall does not have bony support and normal chest wall movement is disrupted. Complications ensue as a result of extreme pain with inspiration and expiration, and hypoxemia often results from inadequate respiratory effort. Signs of a flail chest include uncoordinated, asymmetrical movement of the chest wall, crepitus, and hypoxemia on blood gas. Treatment goals are directed at preventing and treating hypoxemia. Mechanical ventilation may be required.

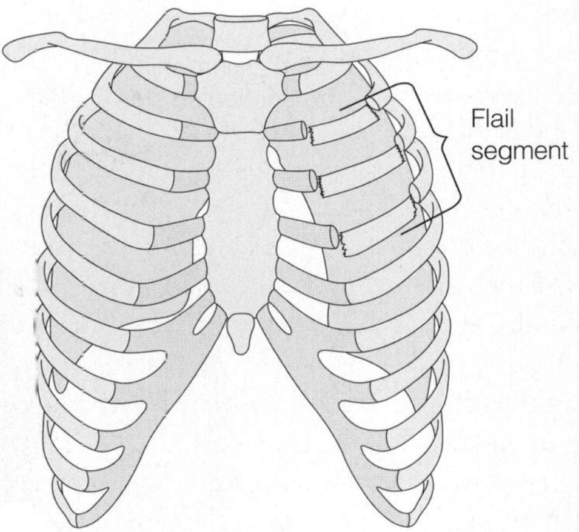

A Fracture pattern of flail chest

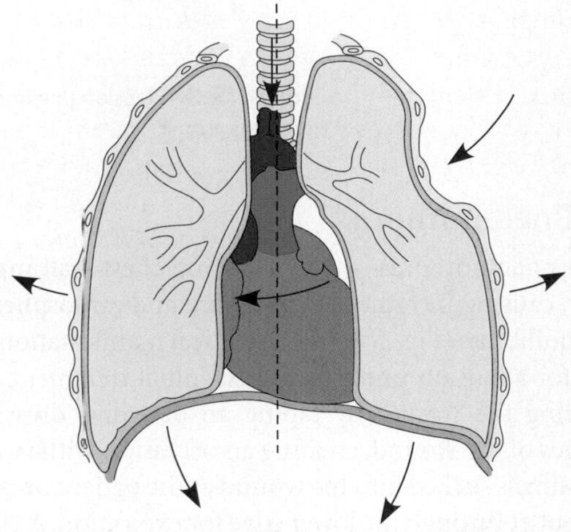

B Inspiration

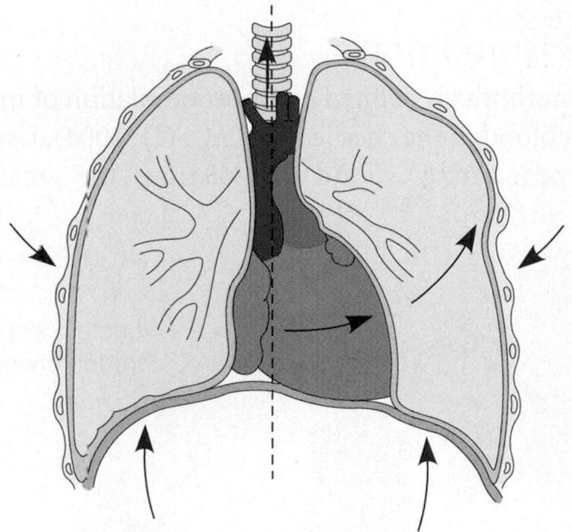

C Expiration

Figure 38–3 ■ Flail chest. Physiologic function of the chest wall is impaired as the flail segment (*A*) is sucked inward during inspiration (*B*) and moves outward with expiration (*C*).

Pulmonary Injuries

Pulmonary Contusions

Blunt trauma to lung parenchyma can result in a unilateral or bilateral pulmonary contusion (a bruising of lung parenchyma). These injuries can be quite serious because the bruising can lead to alveolar hemorrhage, edema, and inflammation within the lung. A large pulmonary contusion can result in respiratory failure. Clinical manifestations of pulmonary contusion may not be present for several days. A chest X-ray may reveal pulmonary infiltrates. Crackles may be auscultated. The patient is at risk for impaired gas exchange. Therefore, nursing care must focus on improving gas exchange through deep breathing exercises, ambulation, and removal of secretions. As with rib fractures, pain management is paramount. The patient is monitored for worsening respiratory status. Intubation and mechanical ventilation may be required if signs of respiratory failure are present. The major complications of pulmonary contusions include pneumonia and ARDS (refer to Module 10, Alterations in Pulmonary Gas Exchange).

Tension Pneumothorax

A tension pneumothorax occurs when air leaks from the lung or through the chest wall. The air trapped in the thoracic cavity without means of escape collapses the affected lung (Fig. 38–4). As intrathoracic pressure continues to increase, this pressure is transmitted to the heart, causing decreased venous return and cardiac output. Tension pneumothorax is characterized by chest pain, air hunger, respiratory distress, tachycardia, neck vein distention, trachea displaced from midline, and absent breath sounds on the affected side. In an emergent situation, the increased intrathoracic pressure is relieved by a large-bore (14-gauge) needle or immediate placement of a chest tube.

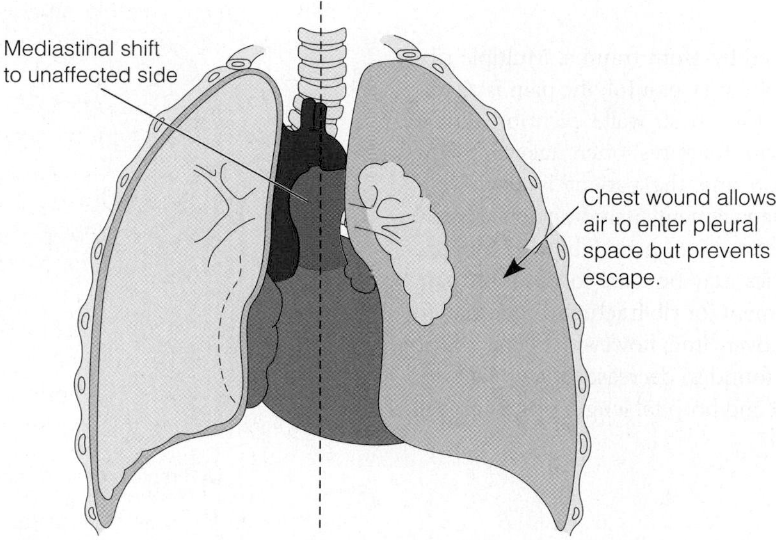

Figure 38–4 ■ Tension pneumothorax. Chest wound allows air to enter pleural space but prevents escape.

Open Pneumothorax

An open pneumothorax is a penetrating chest wall injury that sucks air, causing intrathoracic pressure and atmospheric pressure to equilibrate (Fig. 38–5). The clinical manifestations are the same as for a tension pneumothorax. Initial treatment includes temporizing the wound by taping an occlusive dressing over three edges of the wound, creating an occlusion with inspiration (the dressing is sucked into the wound as the patient breathes in), with an outlet through the lower edge for expiration. A chest tube is placed as soon as possible and surgery may be required.

Massive Hemothorax

Massive hemothorax is defined as the accumulation of more than 1,500 mL of blood in the chest cavity (ACSCT, 2004). Usually, the cause is a penetrating wound that disrupts the great vessels.

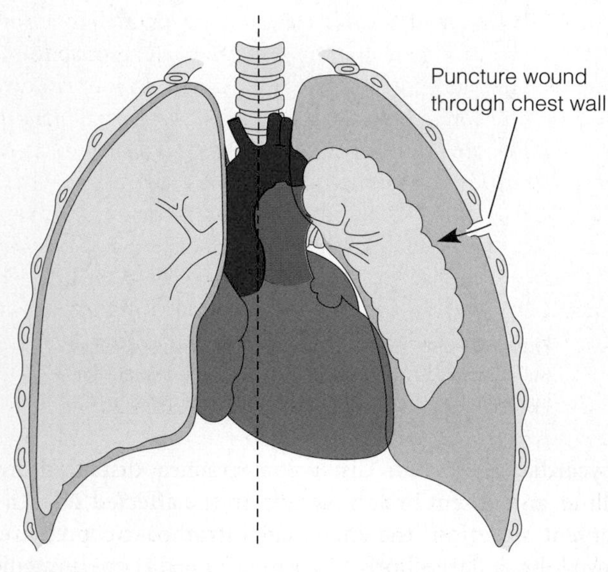

Figure 38–5 ■ Open pneumothorax.

Assessment findings may include decreased breath sounds or dullness to percussion on the affected side and hypotension. Management is aimed at restoring blood volume and decompression of the chest cavity with a chest tube. An autotransfusion device may be attached to the chest tube collection chamber. Surgery may be required for patients who have continued bleeding requiring persistent transfusions and changes in physiologic status (ACSCT, 2004).

Cardiac Injuries

Cardiac Tamponade

Whether from penetrating or blunt trauma, cardiac tamponade causes the pericardium (the sac around the heart) to fill with blood. This restricts the heart's ability to pump and also impedes venous return. Signs and symptoms include Beck's triad (elevated right atrial pressure with neck vein distention, hypotension, and muffled heart sounds). Pulsus paradoxus (decrease of greater than 10 mm Hg systolic blood pressure on inspiration) is also a classic sign of cardiac tamponade. Pulseless electrical activity (PEA) may be present (refer to Module 14, Assessment of Cardiac Rhythm: Basic Electrocardiographic Rhythm Interpretation). Treatment is initially directed at volume resuscitation until pericardiocentesis can be performed (Fig. 38–6).

Blunt Cardiac Injury

Blunt cardiac injury, formerly called cardiac contusion, is a bruising of the myocardium. Chest discomfort, sinus tachycardia, and hypotension are suggestive of this injury. Electrocardiogram (ECG) changes may also be present and may include *ST* changes, dysrhythmias, or heart block. If the admission ECG is abnormal on admission, the patient is admitted to the high-acuity unit for continuous ECG monitoring for 24 to 48 hours (McGillicuddy & Rosen, 2007). An echocardiogram may be done to evaluate cardiac function.

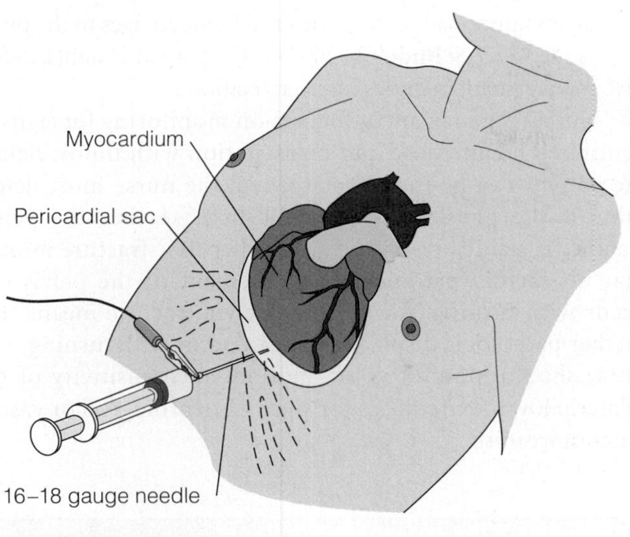

Figure 38–6 ■ Pericardiocentesis.

Abdominal Injuries

Blunt trauma creates devastating injury to the abdomen. In a motor vehicle crash, a compression injury from a steering wheel may rupture solid organs. Shearing injury from a seat belt can result in similar injuries. Deceleration may cause lacerations to the spleen and liver because these organs are movable from the fixed structures surrounding them. The incidence of injury to the spleen is the highest (40 to 55 percent) followed by injury to the liver (35 to 45 percent) (ACSCT, 2004). Penetrating trauma from stab wounds most commonly involve the liver, small bowel, diaphragm, or colon. Gunshot wounds have a greater kinetic energy and more often involve the small bowel, colon, liver, and abdominal vascular structures.

Spleen Injuries

The spleen is located in the left upper quadrant of the abdomen and is the most common organ injured in blunt trauma to the abdomen. The spleen has important immunologic functions; therefore, steps are taken to let the spleen wound heal after injury instead of removing it. Diagnosis of injury to the spleen is made by CT scan. Patients with splenic injury are admitted to a high-acuity unit for serial monitoring of vital signs and hematocrit. It is crucial to monitor vital signs for evidence of continued bleeding in or around the spleen. Continued hemodynamic instability may indicate the need for surgical intervention (Galvan & Peitzman, 2006). Patients who do have a splenectomy will be at risk for infections, and will require vaccinations prior to discharge from the hospital.

Liver Injuries

Though anterior and lateral portions of the liver are protected by the lower rib cage, the liver remains vulnerable to injury in blunt or penetrating trauma. The majority of liver injuries are minor and do not require surgery. However, the mortality may be greater than 50 percent in a complex liver injury, and death is usually the result of hemorrhage. Diagnosis of liver injury is made by CT scan. Liver injuries are graded using a liver injury scale. A grade of one to six is given, with six being a complete hepatic avulsion and the worst injury possible. Medical management may include hepatic arteriography to embolize any bleeding in the liver, or surgery may be required stop the bleeding. That said, most liver injuries up to grade four are successfully managed nonoperatively (EAST, 2003c). Bleeding is the most common complication associated with liver injury, and patients must be monitored for changes in vital signs and continued decline in hematocrit values.

Patients with liver injuries are usually admitted to a high-acuity unit for serial monitoring of vital signs and hematocrit. In the event the patient becomes hemodynamically unstable from continued bleeding and develops hypovolemic shock, the high-acuity nurse must be prepared to implement volume resuscitation as ordered. This may include crystalloids and blood or blood products. Coagulopathies may be corrected with fresh-frozen plasma, platelets, or cryoprecipitate. It is crucial that the nurse monitors the patient's response to these interventions. Continued hemodynamic instability may require surgical interventions to find and control the source of hemorrhage within the liver.

Damage Control Surgery. Patients with abdominal injuries that need an operative procedure may require a technique referred to as *damage control surgery.* There are three phases to this surgical technique: initial operation, resuscitation, and definitive restoration. During the *initial operation,* time in the operating room (OR) is kept to a minimum. The goal is to quickly locate and control sources of hemorrhage. The longer this takes, the greater the risk of three conditions: hypothermia, continued bleeding, and systemic acidosis. The triad of hypothermia, coagulopathy, and acidosis creates a self-propagating cycle that can eventually lead to an irreversible physiological insult (McArthur, 2006). Therefore, the goal of this initial operation is to quickly control hemorrhage, which may be done by simply packing the abdomen with sterile dressing to control the bleeding.

After this initial phase, the patient is taken to the ICU for *resuscitation.* The goal is to correct hypothermia, acidosis, and coagulopathies. Serial measurements of lactate and base deficit are assessed for signs of improving metabolic acidosis. Coagulopathies are corrected with blood and blood products. During this time, the patient is assessed for abdominal compartment syndrome. Abdominal compartment syndrome is essentially intraabdominal hypertension, or too much pressure within the abdominal cavity. It is caused by continued bleeding or visceral edema. Signs and symptoms include a taut distended abdomen, decreased cardiac output, increased peak pulmonary pressures, and decreased urine output (An & West, 2008). Intraabdominal pressures may be directly measured via a Foley catheter. Fluid is instilled to create a fluid filled column used to transmit pressure from the bladder to the transducer. The transducer should be leveled and zeroed to the mid-axillary line with the patient in the supine position. The measurement is obtained at end expiration (An & West, 2008). These pressures can be monitored intermittently or continuously as ordered. Abdominal pressures greater than 20 to 25 mm Hg are considered high and may indicate that the patient's abdomen needs to be opened to relieve the pressure (An & West, 2008).

Once the hypothermia, acidosis, and coagulopathies are corrected (usually within 72 hours of the initial operation), the patient is returned to the OR for definitive repair of injuries.

Pelvic Injuries

Pelvic fractures can be life-threatening injuries. They are associated with blunt trauma—an MVC or a crushing injury to the pelvic region. Because the pelvis protects major blood vessels, patients with pelvic fractures are at high risk for hemorrhage. Signs of a pelvic fracture include perianal ecchymosis, pain on palpation or "rocking" of the iliac crests, hematuria, and lower extremity rotation or paresis (ACSCT, 2004). Confirmation of pelvic fractures is made by CT scan.

Initial management includes the prevention or treatment of life-threatening hemorrhage. Stabilization may be temporary with a pelvic binder or external fixation device for patients who are unstable. The patient may have embolization of bleeding vessels in the interventional radiology suite or may require pelvic packing to tamponade retroperitoneal hemorrhages in the operating suite. (Rice & Rudolph, 2007) If the patient is stable, definitive management includes internal fixation.

Nursing management focuses on monitoring for signs of continued hemorrhage and resuscitation with fluids. Before the patient can be moved or turned, the nurse must determine if the physician has established whether the pelvic fracture is stable or unstable. A stable pelvic fracture implies that no further pathologic displacement of the pelvis can occur with turning. An unstable pelvic fracture means that further pathologic displacement can occur with turning. The nurse should monitor color, motion, and sensitivity of the bilateral lower extremities for signs of neurological or vascular compromise.

SECTION NINE REVIEW

1. A major complication of pulmonary contusions is
   A. ARDS
   B. pneumothorax
   C. hemothorax
   D. tension pneumothorax
2. Which of the following are important interventions for the patient with multiple rib fractures?
   A. chest tube placement
   B. needle aspiration
   C. pain management and pulmonary hygiene
   D. placing a gauze dressing over the wound
3. Patients with injuries to the spleen or liver may require operative repair if
   A. their abdominal girths increase
   B. they have a change in level of consciousness
   C. the hematocrit increases
   D. they become hemodynamically unstable
4. During damage control surgery, the initial operation time is restricted to prevent
   A. hypothermia
   B. coagulopathy
   C. metabolic acidosis
   D. all of the above
5. You are the nurse caring for a patient with a pelvic fracture. Before turning the patient you must first
   A. medicate the patient
   B. ask the physician if the fracture is stable or unstable
   C. remove the fixation device
   D. assess color, motion, and sensitivity of the legs

Answers: 1. A, 2. C, 3. D, 4. D, 5. B

SECTION TEN: Nursing Diagnoses Associated with Traumatic Injury

At the completion of this section, the learner will be able to cluster patient symptoms and derive appropriate nursing diagnoses for the patient with traumatic injuries.

If a traumatic injury is suspected, the nurse focuses on assessing the symptoms most commonly associated with life-threatening conditions. These symptoms include ineffective breathing, altered blood pH, hypotension, distended neck veins, decreased urine output, and a change in level of consciousness. The nursing diagnoses associated with these symptoms include *altered airway clearance, ineffective breathing patterns, impaired gas exchange, fluid volume deficit, altered urinary elimination,* and *altered cerebral tissue perfusion.*

Ineffective Airway Clearance, Ineffective Breathing Patterns, and Impaired Gas Exchange

In the trauma patient, the airway is always assessed first and necessary interventions completed. The airway may be compromised if the patient has a depressed mental status. The gag reflex may be absent, and foreign bodies may be present in the oropharynx. A partially obstructed airway will be noisy, and snoring, gargling, or wheezing may be present. If the airway is obstructed, it is reopened using a manual maneuver (chin lift maneuver if cervical spine injury has not been ruled out), immediately suctioned, and an oral or nasopharyngeal artificial airway placed. Oral or nasotracheal intubation is another method of securing a patent airway. Facial trauma may produce copious amounts of bleeding, and skeletal integrity of the face may be disrupted. The performance of a **cricothyroidotomy** (surgical airway) is preferred to obtain a patent airway in a patient with massive facial injuries. Direct trauma to the airway may occur from blunt injuries to the larynx or pharynx. These patients are hoarse, unable to tolerate a supine position, have subcutaneous emphysema, and are tender over the tracheal area. A **tracheostomy** is the best method of securing an airway in these patients.

Ineffective breathing patterns are associated with tracheobronchial and thoracic injuries. The chest is observed for bruising, open wounds, and symmetry of chest wall movement. Open wounds are evaluated further by log rolling the patient and inspecting the posterior surface. No chest wall movement and the presence of abdominal breathing may indicate a cervical cord lesion. The patient's respiratory rate is noted, as is the degree of breathing effort. Paradoxical movement of the chest (inward motion of a segment of the chest during inhalation and outward motion of the same segment with expiration) indicates multiple rib fractures and a flail segment. The patient with a large flail segment may require intubation and mechanical ventilation or pain control therapy to prevent respiratory compromise and to promote tissue oxygenation. The chest area is palpated to detect the presence of subcutaneous emphysema, rib/sternum tenderness, or defects. Auscultation detects the presence of breath sounds bilaterally in the primary survey. Gross differences in breath sounds are an important finding; this usually indicates a pneumothorax or hemothorax. A more detailed pulmonary assessment is performed during the secondary assessment. High-flow oxygen is administered to trauma patients before obtaining arterial blood gas results. A nonrebreathing mask or a bag-valve-mask device with an oxygen reservoir may be used depending on the patient's responsiveness level. Pulse oximetry and end-tidal carbon dioxide measurement (if the patient is intubated) provide additional data regarding oxygenation.

Fluid Volume Deficit

Peripheral vasoconstriction, a compensatory mechanism, may artificially elevate blood pressure readings even though central arterial pressures are low. The value of clustering assessment data is to prevent misdiagnosis by focusing on one symptom while ignoring others. It is important to monitor the trauma patient's blood pressure and at the same time assess neck veins, level of consciousness, and urine output.

Hypotension in the trauma patient usually is related to hypovolemia. Hypovolemia may result from internal bleeding or uncontrolled external bleeding. Fractures and lacerations of abdominal organs are frequent sources of bleeding in the trauma patient. However, hypotension may be related to factors that inhibit cardiac output (CO) or cause the loss of peripheral vascular resistance. The two most frequently encountered conditions associated with restriction of CO are cardiac tamponade and tension pneumothorax. In cardiac tamponade, hypotension occurs in response to decreased CO. A tear in the pericardium produces bleeding into the pericardial sac. The increased pressure prohibits filling of the ventricles and decreases stroke volume. The increased pericardium pressure also impedes coronary blood flow. Myocardial ischemia results and further decreases CO. Lung parenchymal injury from chest trauma may produce a tension pneumothorax. As atmospheric air enters the pleural cavity through the injury site, the lung on the affected side collapses while mediastinal contents and the trachea are pushed away from the injury site. The pressure placed on the great vessels inhibits venous return. Thus, the neck veins become distended.

Both cardiac tamponade and tension pneumothorax are life-threatening conditions that require immediate treatment. Blood in the pericardial sac is removed by pericardiocentesis. Insertion of a chest tube and covering the open chest wound (if present) with an impermeable dressing are appropriate interventions for the patient with a tension pneumothorax.

Hypotension also may occur in patients with spinal cord injuries who develop spinal shock. In spinal shock, the patient's blood pressure may be less than 70 mm Hg as a result of a loss of sympathetic tone that occurs secondary to transection of the spinal cord. The parasympathetic nervous system is unopposed, resulting in peripheral vasodilation and bradycardia. Bradycardia is the key assessment finding that helps to differentiate spinal shock from hypovolemic shock. The patient also may be hemorrhaging but unable to compensate by increasing the heart rate. Atropine or intravenous fluids are administered to increase the heart rate enough to perfuse core organs. Fluid resuscitation is appropriate for a patient with spinal cord injury who is hypotensive because internal trauma cannot be ruled out initially. However, caution must be taken to avoid causing pulmonary edema. For the patient with an isolated spinal cord injury, if a fluid challenge does not resolve the hypotension, careful administration of a vasopressor may be considered (ACSCT, 2004).

The nurse can discriminate hypotension resulting from hypovolemia from that associated with increased pericardial pressure by assessing for the presence of a paradoxical pulse. The systolic blood pressure will fall more during inspiration if tension pneumothorax or cardiac tamponade exists. In these conditions, the increased thoracic pressure from inspiration further decreases left ventricle filling and results in blood backing up into the right heart, compromising CO. If a right atrial pressure (RAP) catheter or pulmonary arterial catheter is in place, the RAP reading is elevated because of increased right atrial filling with decreased emptying. A RAP reading greater than 15 cm H_2O is significant. Jugular venous distention will be present. Hypotension resulting from hypovolemia is associated with flat neck veins. Decreased pedal pulses and pale or mottled skin also may be present.

Altered Urinary Elimination

The kidneys receive 25 percent of the CO, and may reflect decreased CO earlier than other organs. In most circumstances, decreased or absent urine output in the trauma patient indicates decreased core perfusion from an extrarenal cause. The adult trauma patient should maintain an hourly urine output of at least 0.5 mL/kg/hr to ensure adequate core circulation.

Altered Cerebral Tissue Perfusion

A change in consciousness in the trauma patient may be related to numerous factors. In the presence of hypovolemia, cerebral blood flow decreases, resulting in stupor, unconsciousness, and eventually failure of subconscious mental processes, including vasomotor control and respiration. The more highly specialized the tissue, the more vulnerable it is to hypoxemia. Cortical functions are lost first with cerebral hypoxia. Cerebral hypoperfusion is present when the systolic blood pressure is below 60 mm Hg. Hypoxia, hypoglycemia, and drug use also may impair responsiveness. Because a change in responsiveness may be present from cerebral injury or from systemic causes, clustering of assessment data is helpful. Responsiveness generally is evaluated at the same time that pupillary size and reaction and motor responses are assessed. If a spinal cord injury is present, patients may not be able to respond to commands even if they comprehend what is being said. It is important to document the stimulus used to elicit a motor response, the exact response, and bilateral differences. The use of a standardized scale, such as the Glasgow Coma Scale (refer to Module 20, Determinants and Assessment of Cerebral Tissue Perfusion), can facilitate monitoring of neurological status and improve communication among multiple health care providers.

Airway protection is of major concern in a patient with decreased responsiveness. An oral or nasopharyngeal airway is inserted to maintain airway patency. Unconscious patients should be intubated endotracheally. Oxygen administration is necessary in a patient with decreased responsiveness to promote cerebral oxygenation.

Focused Assessment Findings and Nursing Diagnoses

Life-threatening conditions produce characteristic symptoms that the nurse can identify. The following cluster of data strongly suggests the presence of a life-threatening injury

- Noisy airway
- Absent breath sounds
- Deviated trachea
- Flat or distended neck veins
- Paradoxical chest movement
- Open chest wound
- Subcutaneous emphysema
- Hypotension
- Decreased responsiveness
- Decreased urine output

Nursing diagnoses that pertain to the trauma patient can be clustered in the same manner as the assessment data. Clustering around the ABCs of airway, breathing, and circulation will assist the nurse in prioritizing nursing care.

- *Ineffective airway clearance* related to obstruction or cognitive impairment
- *Ineffective breathing pattern* related to tracheobronchial or chest wall injury, decreased area for gas exchange, or pain
- *Impaired gas exchange* related to ventilation–perfusion imbalance or decreased hemoglobin
- *Decreased cardiac output* related to impairment of venous return or myocardial injury
- *Altered tissue perfusion* related to an imbalance between cellular oxygen demands and supply
- *Fluid volume deficit* related to hemorrhage or extravasation (i.e., burns)

SECTION TEN REVIEW

Mary arrives at the ER following an assault where she was beaten in the face and head. She has a large amount of facial edema, and both eyes are swollen shut. She has broken teeth and blood in her mouth. Mary follows commands but does not verbalize a response to questions. Breathing pattern is rapid and noisy.

1. Based on Mary's history, which of the following interventions should be performed first?
   A. Open the airway and clear the oral pharynx.
   B. Apply 100 percent oxygen by mask.
   C. Obtain arterial blood gases.
   D. Insert an intravenous catheter.
2. Mary's arterial blood gases reflect respiratory acidosis. The acidosis is most likely related to
   A. ineffective breathing pattern
   B. pain
   C. partially obstructed airway
   D. head injury
3. Mary loses consciousness. The nurse should prepare for which of the following first?
   A. CT scan of the head
   B. endotracheal intubation or surgical airway placement
   C. placement of a second IV line
   D. placement of a nasogastric tube
4. Which of the following signs and symptoms are potentially life-threatening? (choose all that apply)
   A. rapid and noisy breathing
   B. decreased consciousness
   C. eyes swollen shut
   D. facial edema
5. Which of the following nursing diagnoses pertain to Mary?
   A. impaired gas exchange
   B. decreased cardiac output
   C. ineffective breathing patterns
   D. impaired gas exchange

Answers: 1. A, 2. C, 3. B, 4. (A, B) 5. C

SECTION ELEVEN: Complications of Traumatic Injury

At the completion of this section, the learner will be able to link posttrauma complications with the physiology of a traumatic injury and preexisting risk factors, and discuss interventions to prevent complications of traumatic injury.

As discussed in Section Eight, trauma deaths occur in three peaks. The first peak is within the first hour postinjury, and the major causes of death are massive bleeding secondary to great vessel tears and head injuries. The second peak occurs during the initial hours postinjury during the resuscitation phase. Deaths in this phase generally are attributed to internal bleeding. The final peak of trauma-related deaths occurs days to weeks after the injury event.

The primary responsibilities of the nurse caring for a trauma patient in the final phase are prevention and surveillance. Treatment of trauma sequelae is controversial and primitive because research in this area is still in its infancy as compared with trauma resuscitation research. Therefore, the goal of nursing care is to prevent complications. Patients with traumatic injuries are at a greater risk of complications than patients with other injuries for a variety of reasons. Patients with traumatic injuries are at risk for venous thromboembolism (VTE), undernutrition, ARDS, disseminated intravascular coagulation (DIC), acute kidney injury (AKI), and multiple organ dysfunction syndrome (MODS). Many of these complications have been discussed in detail throughout this book, but they will be reviewed here briefly, as they relate to the patient with traumatic injuries. The reader is referred to the following modules for additional information: undernutrition (Module 32, Determinants and Assessment of Nutrition and Metabolic Function), ARDS (Module 10, Alterations in Pulmonary Gas Exchange), acute kidney injury (Module 27, Alteration in Renal Function: Acute Renal Failure), and MODS (Module 19, Alterations in Tissue Perfusion: Multiple Organ Dysfunction Syndrome).

Risks for Complications

Several types of injuries predispose the trauma patient to complications. Table 38–4 summarizes traumatic injuries and their associated sequelae. Thoracic trauma may produce massive hemorrhage in addition to disruption in the lung parenchyma. Thus, the thoracic trauma patient is at high risk for DIC and ARDS. Abdominal trauma increases the likelihood of hemorrhage, abdominal compartment syndrome, and infection. Orthopedic trauma predisposes the patient to VTE and prolonged immobility, which may compound the effect on gas exchange. The physiological complications of trauma are intimately related. It is common for a patient to have a combination of these disorders. Although the etiologies of these conditions may differ slightly, the result is the same: inadequate oxygen delivery to the tissue. For this reason, it is important to keep in mind that the patient may be at higher risk for one of these disorders because of the initial injury but, in reality, any one of and more than one of these conditions may occur.

TABLE 38–4 Traumatic Injuries and Associated Sequelae

CONDITION	PATHOPHYSIOLOGY	COMPLICATION
Thoracic Trauma		
Great vessel tears	Hemorrhage	DIC, ARF
Hemothorax	Decreased gas exchange	ARDS
Tension pneumothorax	Decreased gas exchange	ARDS
Open pneumothorax	Disruption in skin integrity	Sepsis
Abdominal Trauma		
Perforation of intestine	Extravasation of GI contents into peritoneum	Sepsis
Liver/splenic laceration	Hemorrhage	DIC, ACS, ARF
Orthopedic Trauma		
Femur/pelvis fracture	Hemorrhage	DIC, ARF
Long-bone fractures	Disruption of fat-containing tissue, increased flow of fat globules in microcirculation	ARDS, ARF

DIC = disseminated intravascular coagulation; ARF = acute renal failure; ARDS = acute respiratory distress syndrome; ACS = abdominal compartment syndrome

Metabolic Response to Injury: Risk for Undernutrition

Two phases occur in the metabolic response after injury: ebb phase and flow phase. The ebb phase occurs in the first three days during acute resuscitation. Characteristics of the ebb phase are summarized in Table 38–5. The body requires a large amount of glucose during this time, which is achieved by breakdown of glycogen stores through gluconeogenesis. Prolonged gluconeogenesis depletes skeletal muscle protein and can lead to wasting. This phase typically ends after the resuscitative phase, about 72 hours after injury.

The next phase is the flow phase, which is characterized by a hypermetabolic response. This hypermetabolic phase results in catabolism of lean body mass, negative nitrogen balance, and altered glucose metabolism.

Nutritional support is required for amino acids and adequate energy for protein synthesis as new tissues are synthesized and wounds are repaired. Patients with an open abdomen may be at a higher risk for negative nitrogen balance due to protein loss in the abdominal fluid (Cheatam et al., 2007). Starting nutritional support as early as possible is essential in the trauma patient as malnutrition is associated with increased morbidity and mortality, while those patients whose nutritional requirements are properly met experience reduced time on a ventilator, fewer complications and shorter time in rehabilitation (Woien & Bjork, 2006). Following nutritional guidelines helps ensure patients receive adequate nutritional support. The use of algorithms encourage early initiation and rapid increment of nutritional support thus increasing the amount of nutrition delivered to the patient (Woien & Bjork, 2006).

TABLE 38–5 Metabolic Response to Trauma

METABOLIC PHASE	CHARACTERISTICS PRESENT
Ebb phase (first 72 hours after injury)	Hypometabolism Decreased body temperature Decreased energy expenditure Normal glucose production with insulin resistance Mild protein catabolism Increased catecholamines Increased glucocorticoids Decreased cardiac output Decreased oxygen consumption Vasoconstriction
Flow phase (72 hours after injury)	Hypermetabolism Increased energy expenditure Increased glucose production Increased oxygen consumption Profound protein catabolism Increased glucocorticoids Increased catecholamines Increased potassium and sodium losses Loss of serum proteins through wounds, exudates, drains, and hemorrhage

Venous Thromboembolism

Venous thromboembolism encompasses both deep vein thrombosis (DVT) and pulmonary embolism (PE), both of which constitute a major health problem with significant morbidity and mortality (Sharma et al., 2007). The trauma patient has one of the highest incidences of VTE among hospitalized patients for myriad reasons including stasis from immobility and increased coagulability from the inflammatory process of injury. Prophylaxis in the trauma patient may be difficult because high bleeding risk injuries preclude anticoagulant use and lower extremity injuries hinder the use of pneumatic sequential compression devices, or SCDs (Sharma et al., 2007). The high-acuity nurse must be ever vigilant in ensuring the use of SCDs when able and monitoring for complications of VTE.

Sepsis

Sepsis is the inflammatory response to microorganisms in the blood. Septic shock is the physiologic response to an infection that results in hemodynamic instability (refer to Module 18, Alterations in Oxygen Delivery and Consumption: Shock States). A pathogen is identified in the body from cultures. The pathogens may be part of the patient's normal flora or may be present in the external environment. Gram-negative and gram-positive bacteria, viruses, and fungi can produce sepsis. There are several portals of entry for these microorganisms.

The patient with traumatic injuries is at particular risk for infection and sepsis because of so many potential ports of entry, including urinary catheters, endotracheal tubes, surgical wounds, invasive hemodynamic monitoring catheters, and IV catheters. Foreign devices in the nose represent a major risk factor for the development of nosocomial sinusitis, which itself is a risk factor for the development of pneumonia. Additional risk factors for infection are summarized in Table 38–6.

Acute Respiratory Distress Syndrome

ARDS is characterized by the presence of bilateral pulmonary infiltrates, a pulmonary capillary wedge pressure of 18 mm Hg (in the absence of left ventricular dysfunction), and a PaO_2/FiO_2 ratio less than 200, regardless of the amount of positive end-expiratory pressure, or PEEP (Bernard et al., 1994). The trauma patient is at risk for ARDS as a result of direct and indirect lung injury. Primary lung injury includes direct blunt or penetrating injury to the lungs, aspiration, or inhalation. Indirect injuries include sepsis, fat embolism, ischemia/reperfusion, and missed injuries.

TABLE 38–6 Risk Factors for Infection in the Patient with Traumatic Injury

- High injury severity
- Shock on admission
- Prolonged ICU length of stay
- Age greater than 60 years
- Size of ICU (more than 10 beds)
- Parenteral nutrition
- Days with arterial catheter
- Days with mechanical ventilation
- Days with central venous catheters
- Tracheostomy
- Neurological failure at day three
- ICP monitor

Disseminated Intravascular Coagulation

DIC is an exaggeration of a normal response. Normal clotting is a localized reaction to injury, whereas DIC is a systemic response. The healthy individual maintains a balance between clot formation and lysis. In trauma, both the extrinsic and intrinsic pathways of coagulation may be stimulated. Head injury can precipitate the release of tissue thromboplastin (extrinsic pathway). Hypoxia and acidosis also stimulate the extrinsic pathway. Crush injuries, burns, and sepsis result in blood cell injury as well as platelet aggregation (intrinsic pathway).

Acute Kidney Injury

In the trauma patient, renal failure rarely occurs as a result of direct trauma to the kidneys. Often AKI is the result of acute tubular necrosis from renal hypoperfusion or toxin-mediated damage to the tubules. Toxin-mediated kidney injury may be caused by many of the drugs trauma patients frequently receive, including aminoglycosides, nonsteroidal anti-inflammatory agents, and radiologic contrast dyes used for CT scanning. Myoglobin from crushed skeletal muscle can accumulate in the tubules and cause obstruction and renal failure.

Assessment and Nursing Diagnosis

Complications may occur at any time in the postinjury phase. It should be clear from this discussion why baseline laboratory and diagnostic data are so important in the trauma patient. With these data, the nurse is able to monitor for subtle changes that indicate that a complication is occurring. The following

RELATED PHARMACOTHERAPY: Anticoagulants

Low Molecular Weight Heparin
Enoxaparin (Lovanox)

Action and Uses
Antithrombotic properties are due to its antifactor Xa and antithrombin in the coagulation activities. An effective anticoagulation agent, it is used for prophylactic treatment as an antithrombotic agent after trauma and surgery. Used for venous thromboembolism prevention.

Major Side Effects
Angioedema, hemorrhage

Nursing Implications
Does not affect prothrombin time. Does affect thrombin time and activated thromboplastin time up to 1.8 times the control value
Monitor for and report immediately any sign or symptom of bleeding

assessment data would indicate the presence of a posttrauma complication

- Elevation of white blood cell count
- Fever
- Change in characteristics of wound drainage (foul odor, thick, and colored)
- Inability to tolerate movement or nursing procedures (e.g., decreasing Spo_2, Pao_2)
- Decreasing level of responsiveness (related to decreased oxygenation or increased serum ammonia levels)
- Decreased urine output
- Diaphoresis
- Cool, mottled skin
- Presence of bleeding (melena, hemoptysis, hematemesis, petechiae, or hematuria)
- Changing trends in vital signs/hemodynamic readings (e.g., elevated CO, decreased systemic vascular resistance, SVR)

Nursing diagnoses that pertain to the trauma patient can be clustered mainly into the two broad areas of ventilation and perfusion.

Ventilation

- *Impaired gas exchange* related to increased capillary permeability and decreased surface area for gas exchange, or obstruction in pulmonary capillary perfusion
- *Ineffective breathing patterns* related to decreased skeletal muscle mass and denervation
- *Ineffective airway clearance* related to fatigue and artificial airway placement with mechanical ventilation

Perfusion

- *Fluid volume deficit* related to vasodilation, bleeding, or interstitial fluid shift
- *Decreased tissue perfusion* related to capillary obstruction and vasodilation
- *Increased cardiac output* related to catecholamine excretion and decreased systemic vascular resistance
- *Decreased cardiac output* related to decreased vascular volume

Additional nursing diagnoses would include

- *Altered urinary elimination patterns* related to obstruction (microemboli and myoglobin) of renal blood flow and tissue necrosis
- *Altered nutrition:* less than body requirements related to catecholamine release, activation of inflammatory response resulting in a hypermetabolic state, and decreased or absent oral intake
- *Risk of infection* related to open wounds, invasive procedures, surgical incisions, debilitated state, and altered nutrition

While the emphasis here has been on physical manifestations of posttrauma complications, psychosocial aspects should not be ignored. Patients who have complications posttrauma remain in the high-acuity unit for prolonged periods and are susceptible to sensory disturbances. Quality-of-life issues need to be considered by the patient and the family. Extensive rehabilitation may be necessary to regain skeletal muscle mass and neurological function. The family's standard of living may decrease because of financial factors related to change in the role of the patient, and health care costs may become a financial burden.

SECTION ELEVEN REVIEW

Consider the following: S.W. was pinned underneath his tractor for one hour before being extricated and transported to the hospital for treatment. He has open fractures of both legs and abdominal tenderness. Questions one through three pertain to S.W.

1. What risk is associated with this delay in treatment?
   - **A.** He will not be able to produce the same number of immunoglobulins.
   - **B.** He will have a higher microorganism count because of delay in wound debridement.
   - **C.** He is at higher risk for antibiotic resistance.
   - **D.** He will be unable to mount a local inflammatory response.
2. Because of his crush injury, DIC may occur as a result of
   - **A.** activation of the intrinsic pathway via platelet aggregation
   - **B.** activation of the extrinsic pathway via thromboplastic release
   - **C.** a high microorganism count
   - **D.** long-bone injury
3. Which of the following nursing diagnoses would be appropriate for S.W.? (choose all that apply)
   - **A.** risk for infection
   - **B.** decreased peripheral tissue perfusion
   - **C.** risk for fluid volume deficit
   - **D.** risk for trauma
4. Which of the following statements best describes the relationship between ARDS and MODS?
   - **A.** Decreased ventilation leads to decreased tissue oxygenation and cellular death.
   - **B.** Pulmonary edema produces a fluid volume deficit and hypoperfusion of tissues.
   - **C.** Organ death releases endotoxins that kill pulmonary epithelial cells.
   - **D.** Increased carbon dioxide retention stimulates peripheral vasodilation and hypoperfusion of tissue.
5. Nutritional support in the trauma patient is instituted (choose all that apply)
   - **A.** when the patient has bowel function
   - **B.** using algorithms with rapid increment
   - **C.** as early as possible
   - **D.** as soon as the patient is removed from mechanical ventilation

Answers: 1. B, 2. A, 3. (A, B, C) 4. A, 5. (B, C)

POSTTEST

1. Typically, a trauma patient has which demographic profile?
   A. 15 to 24 years, male, using alcohol
   B. 24 to 32 years, male, using alcohol
   C. 15 to 24 years, female, using alcohol
   D. 15 to 24 years, male, no alcohol involvement
2. Diminished physiological reserve occurs in response to trauma in
   A. Native Americans
   B. the elderly
   C. women
   D. African Americans
3. What are the four forces that must be considered in assessment of injury?
   A. acceleration, mass, axial loading, deceleration
   B. shearing, compression, impact, axial loading
   C. acceleration, deceleration, shearing, synergistic
   D. acceleration, deceleration, shearing, compression
4. The coup and contrecoup injury is an example of application of______ and ______ forces, respectively.
   A. shear, tensile
   B. tensile, shear
   C. compression, axial loading
   D. acceleration, tensile
5. The extent of cavitation and tissue deformation is most determined by
   A. yaw
   B. velocity
   C. blast effect
   D. tissue density
6. A patient is admitted to the ER with two gunshot wounds. What can the clinician determine from these two wounds? (choose all that apply)
   A. One is an entrance wound and one is an exit wound.
   B. The patient was shot twice.
   C. A hint of the trajectory the missile might have taken if the same missile caused both wounds.
   D. The path the missile followed may not be a straight line between two wounds.
7. Which of the following statements is true about high-velocity missiles and potential structural injury?
   A. The entrance wound is smaller than missile caliber.
   B. There is little or no cavitation.
   C. There is no exit wound.
   D. The exit wound is usually large.
8. Fall injuries are typically associated with
   A. cervical spine fractures
   B. multiple injuries to long bones
   C. compression fractures of lumbosacral spine
   D. contusions to underlying structures
9. Trauma victims who have ingested cocaine may exhibit
   A. tachycardia, dilated pupils, tremors, elevated blood pressure
   B. tachycardia, constricted pupils, tremors, elevated blood pressure
   C. bradycardia, hypotension
   D. dilated pupils, hypotension, bradycardia
10. Which of the following age-related changes significantly impacts recovery from trauma in elderly patients? (choose all that apply)
    A. decreased distensibility of blood vessels
    B. increased systemic vascular resistance
    C. decreased cardiac output
    D. decreased respiratory muscle strength
11. The first three components of the primary assessment are
    A. airway, circulation, cervical spine control
    B. airway, breathing, circulation
    C. circulation, cervical spine control, breathing
    D. breathing, disability, circulation
12. Actual or potential airway obstruction may be evidenced by (choose all that apply)
    A. dyspnea
    B. diminished breath sounds
    C. dysphonia
    D. drooling
13. IV access and administration of fluids is achieved during the "C" component of the primary survey. Which of the following scenarios is recommended for this intervention?
    A. two 19-gauge IVs with lactated Ringer's solution
    B. two 22-gauge IVs with lactated Ringer's solution
    C. an 18-gauge IV with normal saline
    D. a 22-gauge IV with normal saline
14. Any injured patient in a shock state should be evaluated for the most common etiology of traumatic shock, which is
    A. hypovolemic
    B. cardiogenic
    C. neurogenic
    D. sepsis
15. The third peak of death after trauma occurs
    A. within minutes of the injury
    B. within two hours of injury
    C. days to weeks after the injury
    D. at the injury scene
16. An occlusive dressing should be placed over a(n)
    A. open pneumothorax
    B. tension pneumothorax
    C. flail chest
    D. pulmonary contusion
17. Which of the following bladder pressures is consistent with intraabdominal hypertension and abdominal compartment syndrome?
    A. 100 mm Hg
    B. 75 mm Hg
    C. 50 mm Hg
    D. 25 mm Hg
18. Which of the following assessments is important for the nurse to perform for a patient with an unstable pelvic fracture? (choose all that apply)
    A. assess color and motion of extremities
    B. assess for signs of bleeding

C. assess urine for hematuria
D. lower extremity paresis

19. Which of the following are signs of cardiac tamponade? (Choose all that apply)
A. pulsus paradoxus
B. neck vein distention
C. hypertension
D. muffled heart sounds

20. In damage control surgery, certain conditions can lead to an irreversible physiological insult. These conditions include (choose all that apply)
A. hypothermia
B. coagulopathy
C. acidosis
D. hyperthermia

21. The initial metabolic response in the first 24 hours postinjury is associated with
A. hypermetabolism
B. hypometabolism
C. increased O_2 consumption
D. increased energy expenditure

22. Which of the following is a risk factor for the development of acute renal injury in the trauma patient? (choose all that apply)
A. hypoperfusion
B. radiologic contrast dye
C. myoglobinuria
D. aminoglycoside antibiotics

Posttest answers with rationale are found on MyNursingKit.

PEARSON
EXPLORE mynursingkit™

MyNursingKit is your one stop for online chapter review materials and resources. Prepare for success with additional NCLEX®-style practice questions, interactive assignments and activities, web links, animations and videos, and more!

Register your access code from the front of your book at **www.mynursingkit.com.**

REFERENCES

ACSCT [American College of Surgeons Committee on Trauma]. (2004). *Advanced trauma life support for doctors student course manual.* (7th ed.). Chicago: American College of Surgeons.

An, G. & West, M. (2008). Abdominal compartment syndrome: a concise clinical review. *Critical Care Medicine*, 36,1304–1310.

Bergen G , Chen, L. H., Warner, M., Fingerhut, L. A. (2008) *Injury in the United States: 2007 chartbook.* Hyattsville, MD: National Center for Health Statistics.

Bernard, G. R., Artigas, A., Brigham, K. L., et al. (1994). The American European Consensus Conference on ARDS: definitions, mechanisms, relevant outcomes and clinical trial coordination. *American Journal of Respiratory and Critical Care Medicine, 149*, 818–824.

Brown, L. B., Ott, B. R. and Papandonatos, G. D., et al. (2005). Prediction of on-road driving performance in patients with early Alzheimer's disease. *J Am Geriatr Soc, 53* (1), 94–98.

Callaway, D. & Wolfe, R. (2007). Geriatric trauma. *Emergency Medical Clinics of North America, 25*, 837-860.

Cheatham, M., Safcsak, K., Brzenzinski, S. & Lube, M. (2007). Nitrogen balance, protein loss, and the open abdomen. *Critical Care Medicine, 35*, 127–131.

Dept of Transportation (US), National Highway Traffic Safety Administration (NHTSA).(2006) *Traffic safety facts 2005 data: alcohol.* Washington (DC): NHTSA.

Devlin, R., & Henry, J. (2008). Clinical review: major consequences of illicit drug consumption. *Critical Care*, 12, 202–209.

Galvan, D. & Peitzman A. (2006). Failure of non-operative management of abdominal solid organ injuries. *Current Opinions in Critical Care, 12*, 590-594.

Hill, C. & Pickinpaugh, J. (2008). Trauma and surgical emergencies in the obstetric patient. *Surgical Clinics of North America, 88*, 421–440.

Keel, M. & Meier, C. (2007). Chest injuries - what is new? *Current Opinions in Critical Care,13*, 674-679.

Lewis, M. C., Abouelenin, K., & Paniagua, M. (2007). Geriatric trauma: special considerations in the anesthetic management of the injured elderly patient. *Anesthesiology Clinics, 25*: 75–90.

McArthur, B. (2006). Damage control surgery for the patient who has experienced multiple traumatic injuries. *AORN Journal, 84*(6), 992–1000.

McCarter-Bayer, A., Bayer, F. and Hall, K. (2005). Preventing falls in acute care: an innovative approach. *J Gerontol Nurs, 31*(3), 25–33.

McGillicuddy, D. & Rosen, P. (2007). Diagnostic dilemmas and current controversies in blunt chest trauma. *Emergency Medical Clinics of North America, 25*, 595–711.

Rice, P. & Rudolph, M. (2007). Pelvic fractures. *Emergency Medical Clinics of North America, 25*, 795–802.

Richmond, T. S., Thompson, H. J., and Kauder, D., et al. (2006). A feasibility study of methodological issues and short-term outcomes in seriously-injured older adults. *Am J Crit Care, 15*(2),158–165.

Roudsari, B. S., Ebel, B. E. Corso, P. S., et al. (2005). Acute medical care costs of fall-related injuries among US older adults. *Injury, 36* (11), 1316–1322.

Sharma, O., Oswanski, M., Jolly S., Lauer, S., Dressel, R., & Stombaugh, H. (2008). Perils of rib fractures. *The American Surgeon*, 74, 310–314.

Sharma, O., Oswanski, M., Joseph, R., Tonui, P., Westrick, L., Raj, S., Tatchell, T., Waite, P., Ches, F., & Gandaio, A. (2007). Venous thromboembolism in trauma patients. *The American Surgeon, 73*, 1173-1180.

Simms, C. and O'Neill, D. (2005). Sports utility vehicles and older pedestrians. *BMJ, 331*(7520), 787–788.

Tiesman, H., Zwerling, C., Peek-Asa, C., Sprince, N., Cavanaugh, J. (2007). Non-fatal injuries among urban and rural residents: The National Health Interview Survey, 1997-2001. *Injury Prevention,13*, 115–119.

Tisherman, S., Barie, P., Bokhari, F., Bonadies, J., Daley, B., Diebel, L., Eachempati, S., Kurek, S., Luchette, F., Puyana, J., Schreiber, M., & Simon, R. (2004). Clinical practice guidelines: endpoints of resuscitation. The *Journal of Trauma® Injury, Infection, and Critical Care*, 57; 898–912.

Woien, H. & Bjork, I. (2006). Nutrition of the critically ill patient and effects of implementing a nutritional support algorithm in ICU. *Journal of Clinical Nursing, 15*, 168–177.

Glossary

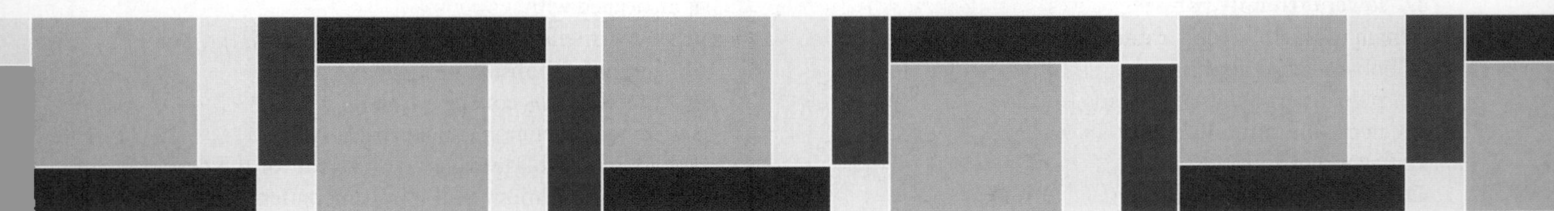

$\dot{V}/\dot{Q}$ ratio A ratio expressing the relationship of ventilation to perfusion.

β-hydroxybutyric acid One component of ketone bodies.

abdominal compartment syndrome (ACS) Occurs when the intra-abdominal pressure increases to a point where vascular tissue is compromised with subsequent loss of tissue viability and function.

abrasion Partial-thickness denudation of skin caused by friction or scraping. Top layer of the skin has been removed, revealing the top layer of the dermis.

absolute refractory period The period after an action potential when a stimulus cannot produce a second action potential no matter how strong the stimulus.

absolute shunt The sum of anatomic shunt and capillary shunt. It is refractory to oxygen therapy.

acceleration An increase in the rate of velocity or speed of a moving body.

accessory muscles Muscles not normally used during quiet breathing that are available for assisting either inspiration or expiration during times of increased work of breathing.

acetoacetic acid Produced by fat catabolism, it is one component of ketone bodies.

acetone (dimethyl ketone) Produced by fat catabolism, it is a component of ketone bodies.

acetyl-CoA (acetylcoenzyme A) A product of the reaction between acetic acid and coenzyme A.

acids Substances that dissociate or lose ions.

acinus The exocrine functional unit of the pancreas; composed of acinar cells that produce, store, and secrete digestive enzymes and ductal cells that secrete bicarbonate and water (plural: acini).

action potential A change in cell polarity. Signal produced from rapid change in membrane permeability that is transmitted from one part of the nerve or muscle cell to another.

active acquired immunity A type of immunity that results from exposure to a specific antigen and subsequent formation and programming of antibodies.

acute coronary syndrome (ACS) Coronary artery insufficiency typically resulting from disruption of intracoronary plaque, resulting in partial or total occlusion of the artery with subsequent ECG changes and cardiac biomarker release.

acute disseminated intravascular coagulation (DIC) A type of coagulopathy associated with systemic activation of the coagulation cascade.

acute hepatic failure A rapidly developing (less than eight weeks) dysfunction of the liver that is characterized by sudden onset and a brief course.

acute hepatitis An inflammatory liver disease, usually of viral origin, that results in liver injury and necrosis.

acute kidney injury Abruptly diminished renal function with many possible causes and typically having the presenting characteristics of oliguria, and elevations of serum BUN and creatinine.

acute lung injury (ALI)/acute respiratory distress syndrome (ARDS) ALI and ARDS are "syndromes with a spectrum of increasing severity of lung injury defined by physiologic and radiographic criteria in which widespread damage to cells and structures of the alveolar capillary membrane occurs within hours to days of a predisposing insult" (Matthay et al., 2003, p. 1027).

acute lymphocytic leukemia (ALL) A type of acute leukemia characterized by the proliferation of immature lymphoblasts that cannot carry on normal immune functions.

acute myelogenous leukemia (AML) A type of acute leukemia characterized by the proliferation of malignant blast cells from myeloid stem cells.

acute pain Pain that is continually changing and transient; onset is rapid and pain is of brief duration (less than six months).

acute rejection A cell-mediated immune response in which the T lymphocytes and macrophages of the host suddenly attack and destroy the graft tissue; it occurs within days, months, or even years following the transplant.

acute respiratory distress syndrome (ARDS) A type of respiratory failure caused by diffuse injury to the alveolar–capillary membrane, resulting in noncardiogenic pulmonary edema.

acute ventilatory failure (AVF) A state of respiratory decompensation in which the lungs are unable to maintain adequate alveolar ventilation, losing the ability to eliminate carbon dioxide.

addiction (psychological dependence) See psychological dependence.

adenosine triphosphate (ATP) A nucleotide that contains large amounts of chemical energy stored in high-energy phosphate bonds; when it is broken down by a process called hydrolysis, energy is released and utilized for metabolic processes.

aerobic metabolism The mechanism used by the body for energy generation in the presence of oxygen.

affinity The degree to which hemoglobin releases oxygen.

afterload The resistance against which the ventricle pumps blood.

agnosia A perceptual impairment resulting in the failure to recognize familiar objects by the senses even though sensation is intact; types include tactile, visual, or auditory.

agranulocytosis An absolute neutrophil count (ANC) of less than 100 cells/mcL; a potentially life-threatening degree of neutropenia

air trapping The abnormal retention of air in the lungs on exhalation.

airway resistance (R_{aw}) The amount of opposition to airway flow through the conducting system.

akinesis Lack of myocardial wall movement.

alanine aminotransferase (ALT, SGPT) An enzyme primarily found in the cells of the liver, kidneys, heart, and skeletal muscles.

alkaline phosphatase (Alk Phos, ALP) An enzyme primarily found in the cells of the liver and kidneys.

allergic response A hypersensitivity reaction of antigen–antibody activity in response to a specific substance that in nonsensitive people in similar amounts produces no effect.

allograft Tissue that is transplanted between members of the same species; also referred to as a *xenograft.*

alveolar ventilation ($\dot{V}_A$) The air that fills the alveoli and is available for gas exchange.

aminoacidemia Amino acids in the blood.

ampulla of Vater Formed by the junction at the duodenum of the main pancreatic duct and the common bile duct.

amylase A pancreatic enzyme that breaks down starch; when found in the blood may be indicative of acute pancreatitis.

amylolytic Facilitating the breakdown of carbohydrates.

anabolism A constructive metabolic process whereby simple molecules are converted into more complex molecules.

anaerobic metabolism The mechanism used by the body for energy generation in the absence of oxygen.

anaphylactic shock A form of hypovolemic shock; the extreme result of type I hypersensitivity response with mediator-induced generalized vasodilatation and increased vascular permeability causing rapid loss of plasma into interstitial spaces.

anaphylaxis A severe type I hypersensitivity response caused by the massive release of chemical mediators and other substances from mast cells.

anastomosis Site at which a graft is sutured into a recipient.

anatomic shunt Movement of blood from the right heart and back into the left heart without coming into contact with alveoli.

anemia A condition marked by decreased numbers of RBCs, decreased hemoglobin, or decreased hematocrit.

anergy Lack of immune response.

aneurysm Thin-walled balloon-like outpouching of the arterial intima.

angina pectoris Chest pain that is usually precipitated by exercise and relieved by rest.

anginal equivalents Symptoms suggestive of coronary artery disease but that do not include angina (examples include dyspnea, fatigue, dizziness).

angiogenesis Formation of new blood vessels in order to reestablish perfusion to the wound bed.

anicteric hepatitis Hepatitis with no jaundice present.

anion gap A measurement of excessive unmeasurable anions.

anions Negatively charged ions.

anosognosia A severe form of neglect in which the patient fails to recognize his or her illness or paralysis.

antigen A substance capable of triggering an immune response.

antigen-presenting cells (APC) Special cells that process antigen and present a fragment for recognition by the T and B lymphocytes.

antrum The terminal portion of the stomach, located between the gastric body and the pyloric sphincter.

anuria Cessation of urine production.

anxiety Both a symptom and a disorder ranging from mild unease to severe panic.

aortic regurgitation (AR) Aortic valve insufficiency that allows blood to flow back into the left ventricle from the aorta during diastole.

aortic stenosis (AS) A narrowing of the aortic valve orifice so that blood flow is obstructed from the left ventricle into the aorta during systole.

aphasia The inability to understand language, use language, or both.

apheresis A therapeutic procedure in which blood is removed from the body and run through a special cell-separating apparatus to remove specific blood components, such as platelets, plasma, or hematopoietic stem cells.

apical–radial pulse deficit The difference between the apical and radial pulse rates, which reflects the number of heartbeats too weak to be transmitted to the periphery.

apoptosis Programmed cell death.

apraxia A perceptual and cognitive impairment resulting in an inability to perform movements voluntarily in the presence of intact motor power, sensation, or coordination; may move automatically but not purposefully; types of apraxia include dressing, ideational, ideomotor, motor, and constructional.

aromatherapy Use of oils to reduce stress and anxiety.

arousal The component of consciousness concerned with the ability of an individual simply to respond to environmental stimuli, such as opening the eyes to speech or turning the head toward a noise; degree of alertness or responsiveness to stimuli.

ascites An abnormal accumulation of fluid in the peritoneal cavity; often occurs with renal or liver failure.

aspartate aminotransferase (AST, SGOT) An enzyme primarily found in the cells of the liver, kidneys, heart, pancreas, and brain.

assist-control mode (AC or ACMV) A mechanical ventilation mode that combines two single modes: assist, a patient-sensitive mode; and control, a time-triggered mode.

asystole Complete myocardial electrical standstill or "without" systole.

ataxia Impaired gait characterized by unsteadiness, poor balance, and lack of coordination (lesion site: cerebellum).

atheroma Complicated atherosclerotic lesion that is calcified and contains hemorrhage, ulceration, and scar tissue deposits.

atherosclerosis A form of arteriosclerosis characterized by plaque deposits in the intimal lining of medium and large arteries.

atrial gallop Abnormal S4 heart sound caused by atrial contraction.

Auer rods Abnormal, large granule-containing, needle-like rods in the cytoplasm; most commonly found in blast cells of the bone marrow and blood in patients with AML (Acute myelogenous [myelocytic] leukemia).

autodigestion Breakdown of pancreatic tissues by its own enzymes.

autograft Transplantation of tissue from one part of a person's body to another part.

autografting Transplanting tissue from one part of the patient's body to another part of the patient's body.

autoimmunity A destructive response in which the immune system recognizes self as foreign and begins to destroy the body's own cells and tissues.

autolytic debridement Use of dressing materials that allow endogenous enzymes to liquefy necrotic tissue.

automaticity Ability to initiate an impulse.

autonomic dysreflexia Potentially life-threatening complication following spinal cord injury; caused by excessive sympathetic nervous system stimulation that produces extreme vasoconstriction and hypertension.

auto-PEEP The unintentional buildup of positive end-expiratory pressure caused by airtrapping.

autoregulation Mechanism used by tissues to regulate their own blood supply by dilating or constricting local blood vessels; the localized matching of cerebral blood flow with cerebral metabolism.

avulsion Full-thickness skin loss; wound edges cannot be approximated.

awareness Having or showing realization, perception, or knowledge of surroundings, situation, circumstances.

azotemia Accumulation of abnormally large amounts of nitrogenous waste products in the blood.

B lymphocytes (B cells) Lymphocytes primarily responsible for antibody production on exposure to a specific antigen; the primary cells of humoral immunity.

bacteremia The presence of bacteria in the blood.

band (stab) An immature neutrophil.

bandemia Elevated serum band (immature neutrophil) level.

baroreceptors Pressure receptors located in the arch of the aorta and carotid sinus that detect arterial pressure changes.

barotrauma Injury to pulmonary tissues as a result of excessive pressures.

base deficit The amount of base required to titrate 1 liter of arterial blood to a normal pH. It is calculated from an arterial blood gas.

base excess A measure of the amount of buffer required to return the blood to a normal pH state. It is used in reference to metabolic acid–base states. A person can develop a base excess (metabolic alkalosis) or a base deficit (metabolic acidosis).

bases Substances capable of accepting ions.

Beck's triad Classic signs of cardiac tamponade that include elevated right atrial pressure, hypotension, and muffled heart sounds.

bigeminy A cardiac dysrhythmia of one SA node–generated beat followed by one premature ventricular contraction.

bile A substance produced by the hepatocytes that is essential to normal digestion, particularly for fats.

bilirubin The end product of hemoglobin degradation.

blast cells Immature, undifferentiated blood cells.

bleb A type of cyst (or blister) of gas that develops in the visceral pleura of the lung.

blood–brain barrier A network of cells and membranes that control brain volume and contents by controlling permeability.

blunt trauma Injury without interruption of skin integrity.

body surface area (BSA) A measure of overall body size using both height and weight in its calculation.

body, gastric The largest portion of the stomach located between the fundus and the antrum.

bradycardia Heart rate less than 60 bpm.

brain death Irreversible cessation of all brain function, including brainstem function.

brain herniation A catastrophic complication of traumatic brain injury caused by increased intracranial pressure.

B-type natriuretic peptide (BNP) Hormone released from the ventricles in response to increased preload; causes urinary excretion of sodium and diuresis. Its action results in reduced preload.

buffer A substance that reacts with acids and bases to maintain a neutral environment of stable pH.

bulla A large blister or skin vesicle filled with fluid (plural, bullae).

burn center A specific area in the hospital with resources and staff designated for treating patients who have experienced burn injuries.

burn shock Hypovolemic shock that develops secondary to fluid shifts occurring with burn injury.

burnout A syndrome of emotional exhaustion, depersonalization, and reduced personal accomplishments that occurs among individuals who work with people on a daily basis.

bursa equivalent Tissue thought to be located in the bone marrow that is primarily responsible for differentiating lymphocytes into B cells for humoral immunity.

cachetic Relating to having cachexia.

cachexia Observable wasting of body mass caused by malnutrition.

cadaver donor A donor from whom tissue or an organ is recovered after death.

canaliculi Small channels or canals that branch out and connect to lacunae.

capillary shunt Normal flow of pulmonary blood past completely unventilated alveoli.

capnogram Graphic representation of carbon dioxide levels during respiration.

capnometry Measurement of carbon dioxide in expired gas.

carbohydrates Nutritional substances composed of complex and simple sugars.

carboxyhemoglobin A compound formed by carbon monoxide and hemoglobin.

cardiac index (CI) Cardiac output divided by body surface area.

cardiac markers Proteins that necrotic myocytes release into the blood; when present in the serum, they signal myocardial damage.

cardiac output (CO) The amount of blood pumped by the heart each minute.

cardiac tamponade A life-threatening postoperative complication of coronary artery bypass surgery caused by bleeding into the pericardial sac.

cardiogenic shock Impaired oxygenation because the heart fails to function as a pump to deliver oxygenated blood.

cardiomyopathy End-stage heart failure (class IV); the patient has symptoms of HF at rest and cannot perform activities of daily living.

cardioversion A synchronized direct current electrical countershock that depolarizes all the cells simultaneously, allowing the SA node to resume the pacemaker role.

carina The junction of the Y formed by the right and left mainstem bronchi in the lungs.

catabolism Process by which complex nutrients are converted into more basic elements, such as glucose, fatty acids, and amino acids; breakdown of a substance.

catheter-related sepsis (CRS) A potentially lethal complication of total parenteral nutrition (TPN); microorganisms are introduced through the TPN catheter, eventually causing a systemic infection (sepsis).

cations Positively charged ions.

cavitation Creation of a temporary cavity as tissues are stretched, compressed, and displaced forward and laterally, creating a tract from a penetrating missile.

CD markers Refers to "clusters of differentiation" cell surface antigens markings on lymphocytes.

cell differentiation Development of specific cell functions through a maturation process.

cell-mediated immunity A type of protection against invading antigens characterized by surveillance and direct attack of foreign material; the primary effector cell is the T lymphocyte.

central stimulation Involves the trunk or central portion of the body and produces an overall body response; should be used for initial introduction of pain; refers to stimulation of the cerebral hemispheres rather than spinal cord.

cerebral blood flow (CBF) Blood flow to the brain is maintained at a constant rate by vasodilation of the vessels to increase the flow or vasoconstriction to decrease the flow.

cerebral blood volume The amount of blood in the cranial vault at any given point in time; occupies about 10 percent of the total intracranial volume.

cerebral hematoma A group of focal cerebral injuries associated with the accumulation of blood in the cranial vault.

cerebral perfusion pressure (CPP) An estimate of the adequacy of cerebral circulation; perfusion pressure to the brain that is the difference between the mean systemic arterial pressure and the mean intracranial pressure. It is calculated as follows: **CPP = MAP – ICP.**

cerebral salt wasting A state of fluid overload of which the end result is the loss of sodium into the urine causing water to follow.

chemical debridement Use of topical enzymes applied to a wound to remove necrotic tissue; also known as *enzymatic debridement.*

chemotaxis The movement of leukocytes along an increasing concentration of chemical stimulus (chemotactic factors) towards an area of inflammation.

chief cells The particular cells of gastric glands that secrete pepsinogen, a precursor of pepsin for protein digestion.

cholecystokinin (CCK) Hormone that stimulates pancreatic enzymes, increases contractility of the gallbladder, and inhibits gastric motility.

cholestatic hepatitis Hepatitis with retention of bile as a result of biliary obstruction.

chronic lymphocytic leukemia (CLL) A condition marked by smaller than normal mature lymphocytes; the second most commonly diagnosed leukemia in adults.

chronic myelogenous leukemia (CML) A condition characterized by a chromosomal abnormality that causes accelerated cell growth and decreased cell death, resulting in the proliferation of both mature and immature myelocytic cells.

chronic obstructive pulmonary disease (COPD) (chronic airflow limitation disease). A group of pulmonary diseases that cause obstruction to expiratory airflow.

chronic rejection A humoral immune response in which antibodies slowly attack and destroy a graft.

chronic renal failure A slow and progressive destruction of kidney function.

chyme The mixture of partially digested food and secretions of digestion found in the stomach and small bowel.

chymotrypsin A proteolytic pancreatic enzyme.

circle of Willis An area in the brain where carotid arteries and vertebral arteries unite to provide collateral blood flow to either side of the brain.

CO_2 narcosis A state of hypercapnic encephalopathy caused by toxic levels of Pa_{CO_2} that produces drowsiness, stupor, or coma.

Cognition Thinking skills that include language use, calculation, perception, memory, awareness, reasoning, judgment, learning, intellect, social skills, and imagination.

collagen Major component of new connective tissue that gives tensile strength to the wound.

colonization The replication of microflora that do not adversely affect wound healing.

coma A state of unconsciousness from which one cannot be aroused and is the most severe of the alterations of consciousness.

committed stem cell A pluripotential stem cell that has committed its development to either the myeloid or lymphoid cell line.

common bile duct The duct formed by the union of the hepatic and cystic ducts and opening into the duodenum.

compartment syndrome Pressure within a muscle compartment rises and exceeds microvascular pressure, thereby interfering with cellular perfusion.

compensated A state in which the pH is within normal limits with the acid–base imbalance being neutralized but not corrected.

complement system A progressive, sequential cascade of events produced by substances found naturally in the circulating sera; components of the system must be triggered individually and cause cellular lysis of antigens.

complementary and alternative therapies Therapies used in lieu of, or along with, standard medical treatment.

complete spinal cord injury A traumatic injury that results in the loss of motor and sensory function below the level of injury, extending to the lowest sacral segment.

compliance (C_L) Measurement of the relative ease with which an organ can expand; reflects relative stiffness of the organ; in the lungs, it is the amount of force required to expand the lungs; measured in mL/cm H_2O; normal is 50 to 100 mL/cm H_2O.

compression The process of being pressed or squeezed together, resulting in reduction in size or volume.

compromised wound Wound that contains devitalized tissue.

concussion Mild traumatic brain injury caused by blunt trauma to the head.

conductivity The ability of the cardiac stimulus to transmit throughout the myocardium.

conjugated bilirubin Bilirubin that has been joined with glucuronic acid to make it water soluble.

conscious sedation Moderate (level two) sedation primarily used to induce relaxation while minimally disturbing the vital signs when cooperation is needed for a procedure.

consciousness State of general awareness of oneself and the environment; made up of the components of arousal and content.

constrictive cardiomyopathy Condition associated with normal left ventricular size and a slightly depressed ejection fraction with a marked decrease in cardiac muscle compliance.

contamination The presence of nonreplicating microbes.

content The component of consciousness concerned with interpreting environmental stimuli; includes thinking, memory, problem solving, orientation, and speech.

continuous positive airway pressure (CPAP) The application of positive pressure to the airway of a spontaneously breathing person (see positive end-expiratory pressure [PEEP]).

contractility The ability of a muscle to shorten when stimulated; in particular, the force of myocardial contraction.

contraction, wound Wound margins begin to pull toward the center of the wound to decrease the wound surface area.

contusion Injury to superficial tissues, with disruption of blood vessels (bruising) with extravasation into the skin; in brain injury it is a moderate-to-severe injury with bruising of brain tissue.

cor pulmonale Right ventricular hypertrophy and dilation secondary to pulmonary disease, resulting in pulmonary hypertension.

corrected A state in which all acid–base parameters have returned to normal ranges after a state of acid–base imbalance.

crackles (rales) Adventitious breath sounds associated with fluid or secretions or both in small airways or alveoli.

C-reactive protein (CRP) Peptide released by the liver in response to inflammation, infection, and tissue damage; downstream marker for inflammation now considered a major risk factor for heart disease.

cricothyroidotomy A surgical airway created by division and cannulation of the trachea between the cricoid and thyroid cartilage.

Cullen's sign A bluish discoloration around the umbilicus seen in hemorrhagic pancreatitis.

cultural competence An awareness of one's own thoughts and feelings without letting them influence caring for patients with different backgrounds.

Cushing's triad Vital sign changes that occur where the pulse pressure widens until ICP equals MAP and includes (1) increased systolic blood pressure, (2) decreased diastolic blood pressure, and (3) bradycardia.

cytokine-release syndrome (CRS) A group of clinical manifestations associated with the initial dose of monoclonal antibody therapy.

cytokines Special secreted cellular proteins that serve as messengers for activation of components of the immune system and other hematopoietic functions.

cytopathic hypoxia A pathologic state in which tissue hypoxia results from derangements in the cellular use of oxygen in the face of adequate oxygen delivery.

cytotoxic agents Drugs that have the capability of destroying target cells.

D-dimer A protein that is released into the circulation during the breakdown of fibrin blood clots.

debridement Removal of necrotic tissue, devitalized tissue, or debris from the wound bed.

deceleration A decrease in the rate of velocity or speed of a moving body.

decerebrate posturing Abnormal extension; neck is extended with jaw clenched; arms pronate and extend straight out; feet are plantar flexed.

decorticate posturing Abnormal flexion; upper arms move upward to the chest; elbows, wrists, and fingers flex; legs extend with internal rotation; feet flex.

deep partial-thickness burn Burn that involves the epidermis and deep layers of the dermis.

defibrillation An unsynchronized direct current electrical countershock that depolarizes all the cells simultaneously, allowing the SA node to resume the pacemaker role.

delirium Acute onset of fluctuating awareness, impaired ability to attend to environmental stimuli, and disorganized thinking. May include hallucinations or delusions, difficulty in focusing attention and sleeping; and emotional, physical and autonomic overactivity.

dementia A progressive, often irreversible decline in mental functioning that involves increasing deficits of reasoning, judgment, abstract thought, comprehension, learning, task execution, and speech.

depolarization A wave of electrical current that causes cardiac cells to become positively charged; should result in cardiac muscle contraction.

dermatome A cutaneous section of the body innervated by a spinal or cranial nerve.

dermis Middle layer of skin, referred to as true skin.

diabetes insipidus A condition associated with improper water balance and characterized by the decrease or absence of antidiuretic hormone (ADH) secreted by the posterior pituitary gland; this loss of ADH secretion results in diuresis.

diabetes mellitus A complex metabolic disorder in which the person has either an absolute or a relative insulin deficiency; this insulin deficiency results in impaired carbohydrate, protein, and fat metabolism.

diabetic ketoacidosis (DKA) A potentially devastating form of metabolic acidosis, characterized by a clinical syndrome of symptoms associated with elevated blood glucose, blood ketone levels and metabolic acidosis.

diapedesis The movement of WBCs through an intact vessel wall using ameboid movement.

diastolic dysfunction Heart failure characterized by impairment of ventricular relaxation.

diffuse axonal injury (DAI) Injury that occurs when shearing forces disrupt the structure of neurons and their nearby blood vessels.

diffusion Movement of gases across a pressure gradient from an area of high concentration to one of low concentration.

dilated cardiomyopathy Condition associated with left ventricular dilation and decreased ejection fraction.

dilutional effect Net gain of water in the extracellular spaces.

direct calorimetry Measurement of the body's heat production while the individual is isolated in a chamber or room specifically equipped for this purpose.

doll's eye movements Oculocephalic reflex; reflexive movements of the eyes in the opposite direction of head rotation.

donor One who donates an organ or tissue.

drug allergy Refers to an immune-based hypersensitivity reaction (for example, rash, or hypotension).

drug side effect Refers to a predictable or expected undesirable effect of a drug.

duct of Santorini An accessory duct of the pancreas that exists in approximately 70 percent of the population.

duct of Wirsung The main pancreatic duct.

dysarthria Impairment of the muscles that control speech.

dyskinesis Myocardial wall movement in the opposite direction.

dysoxia Condition characterized by an inability of the cells to use oxygen properly despite adequate levels of oxygen delivery.

dysphagia Dysfunction of one or more parts of the swallowing process.

dysphasia Impaired capacity to interpret, formulate, or express meaningful language by speaking, writing, or gesturing (expressive or Broca's dysphasia); the inability to understand the written or spoken language (receptive or Wernicke's dysphasia).

dyspnea Subjective sensation of difficulty breathing.

dysrhythmia Abnormal heart rhythm.

ebb phase The first phase of the metabolic stress response, characterized by reduced systemic circulation, decreased metabolic rate (reduced temperature and oxygen consumption), gluconeogenesis, glycogenolysis, hyperglycemia, lactic acidosis, and persisting for 24 to 48 hours.

echocardiogram Noninvasive technology that allows visualization of the valves; their movement; as well as the size, thickness, and function of the aorta and ventricles.

echocardiography Imaging technique used to assess functional structures of the heart using ultrasound waves.

ectopic pacemaker Premature heartbeats that originate from an excitable focus outside of the normal SA node.

edema Excess accumulation of fluid in interstitial spaces.

ejection fraction (EF) The amount of blood ejected from the left ventricle per each heartbeat; normal is above 50 percent.

elastase A proteolytic pancreatic enzyme; its proenzyme, proelastase, requires trypsin to become activated; responsible for erosion of blood vessels contributing to hemorrhage in severe acute pancreatitis.

electrodes Small adhesive patches with conducting gel placed on the skin for ECG monitoring.

electrodiagnostic testing The use of electrical and electronic devices for diagnostic purposes of the heart, nerves, and muscles.

electrolytes Electrically charged microsolutes found in body fluids.

electromyograms The graphic record of resting and voluntary muscle activity as a result of electrical stimulation.

emphysema A pathologic pulmonary process characterized by enlargement of alveoli and destruction of alveoli and surrounding capillary beds.

empyema Abnormal accumulation of purulent fluid in the intrapleural space as a result of inflammation or infection.

end stage renal disease Decline in renal function to less than 10 percent of normal.

endoscopic retrograde cholangiopancreatography (ERCP) An invasive endoscopic test that allows cannulation and direct viewing of the ampulla of Vater, and the pancreatic and bile ducts.

endothelium Thin inner layer of blood vessels composed of endothelial cells.

end-tidal carbon dioxide (P_{ETCO_2} or $ETCO_2$) Concentration of carbon dioxide at the end of exhalation.

energy The ability to do work; synonymous with calories; most common sources are carbohydrates and fats.

enteral nutrition Nutrition delivered into the gastrointestinal tract through a feeding tube; it is a lactose-free, nutritionally complete formula composed of protein, carbohydrates, fats, electrolytes, vitamins, and minerals.

enterocutaneous fistula A passageway that develops between a segment of the gastrointestinal tract and the skin.

enzymes Catalyst substances found in cells that assist in cellular activities.

epidermis Outermost layer of skin.

epidural hematoma (EDH) Bleeding in the space between the dura mater and the skull.

epithelialization Migration of epithelial cells along the wound surface.

erythrocytes Red blood cells; part of the hematopoietic stem cell line; produced in the bone marrow.

erythropoiesis Refers to production of erythrocytes.

erythropoietin A circulating hormone, produced by the kidneys that regulates production of erythrocytes.

eschar A tough, dry inelastic wound indicative of a full-thickness burn.

escharotomy Surgical incision of the eschar and superficial fascia of a circumferentially burned limb or trunk in order to restore blood flow distal to the affected area.

ethnicity A set of social, cultural, and political beliefs held by a group of individuals.

expressive aphasia The inability to write or use language appropriately.

exsanguination The most extreme form of hemorrhage, with an initial loss of blood volume of 40 percent and a rate of hemorrhage exceeding 250 mL per minute.

external respiration Movement of gases across the alveolar-capillary membrane.

extracellular Fluid compartment within the body composed of plasma and interstitial fluid.

extravasation The escape of fluid from its physiologic contained space into the surrounding tissues.

extrinsic pathway A coagulation cascade of events triggered by blood being exposed to extravascular tissue that results in clot formation.

extubation Removal of an endotracheal or tracheostomy tube from the patient's airway.

exudate Fluid produced by wounds.

failure to capture Term used to describe the situation in which the pacemaker initiates an impulse but the stimulus is not strong enough to produce depolarization.

failure to sense Term used to describe when the pacemaker competes with the patient's own impulse generation.

fatty streaks Type II atherosclerotic skin lesions characterized by macrophage migration across the endothelium and smooth muscle cells that contain lipid droplets.

fibrous atheromatous plaque Basic lesion associated with atherosclerosis; lesion filled with lipids, collagen, scar tissue, and vascular smooth muscle cells.

fistula Tubelike passages that form connections between different sites of the gastrointestinal tract.

flaccid paralysis Damage to lower motor neurons, producing loss of both voluntary and involuntary movement.

flaccidity Absence of muscle tone resulting in floppy, limp, flabby, hyporeflexic, nonfunctional limbs.

flow phase The second phase of the metabolic stress response, characterized by a neuroendocrine response of hypermetabolism (increased temperature and oxygen consumption), hypercatabolism, increased nitrogen losses, gluconeogenesis, and hyperglycemia.

focal injury One of the two types of traumatic brain injury; typically occurs in a well-defined area of the brain and may be the result of a hematoma.

forced expiratory volume (FEV) Measure of how rapidly a person can forcefully exhale air after a maximal inhalation; a measurement of dynamic lung function.

fraction of inspired oxygen (FIO_2) That portion of the total gas being inspired that is composed of oxygen; expressed in decimals from 0.21 to 1.0.

full-thickness wound Injury to the epidermis and dermis with exposure of subcutaneous tissue.

full-thickness burn A burn that destroys epidermis, dermis, and portions of subcutaneous tissues (formerly known as third- and fourth-degree burns).

fulminant hepatic failure (FHF) A rapidly developing (less than eight weeks) acute failure of the liver, characterized by severe encephalopathy (stage III or IV), that develops in a person with no preexisting liver dysfunction.

functional decline The loss of ability to carry out daily self-care activities common in older adults during acute illness and hospitalization.

fundus The anatomic area of the stomach located above the lower esophageal sphincter, appearing as a bulge at the top of the stomach.

GALT A term that stands for gut associated lymphoid tissue, used for all lymphoid tissue associated with the gastrointestinal tract, including the tonsils, appendix, and Peyer's patches.

gastric inhibitory peptide (GIP) Hormone that helps digest carbohydrates and fats.

gastric tonometry A technique to assess gut perfusion by using a gastric balloon to measure the mucosal CO_2 level.

gastrin A hormonal regulator produced by cells located in the pyloric region of the stomach; stimulates gastric glands to produce hydrochloric acid and pepsinogen.

gastrocolic reflex A mass movement of the contents of the colon, frequently preceded by a similar movement in the small intestine, which sometimes occurs immediately following the entrance of food into the stomach.

G-cell Gastrin secreting cells located in the mucosa of the pyloric area of the stomach and duodenum.

global aphasia The inability to use or understand language.

glucagon A hormone produced by the alpha cells of the islets of Langerhans of the pancreas.

gluconeogenesis Formation of glucose from protein and fat stores in the body; seen in the ebb phase and flow phase; formation of glycogen in the liver from a noncarbohydrate substance.

glycogen The stored form of carbohydrate for conversion into glucose.

glycogenolysis Conversion of glycogen to glucose in the liver and muscles; seen in the ebb phase of the metabolic stress response.

glycosuria Excretion of glucose in the urine.

glycosylated hemoglobin (Hb A_1c) Hemoglobin with glucose attached to it.

graft The transfer of tissue or organ from one part of the body to a different part, or from another donor source.

Graft-vs-host disease (GVHD) A complication of hematopoeitic stem cell transplantation in which donor T-cells, after being implanted in the recipient, recognize the recipeient's tissues as being foreign and muster an attack.

granulation tissue Tissue in a wound with a characteristic pink-red color.

granulocyte A type of blood cell with granules located in the cytoplasm.

granulocyte monocyte-colony stimulating factors (GM-CSF) A group of cytokines involved in the division and differentiation of neutrophils and monocytes and other chemical mediator activities.

Grey Turner's sign A bluish discoloration of the flank region seen in hemorrhagic pancreatitis.

guided imagery A complementary alternative therapy that uses patients' past experiences to promote a vision or fantasy that encourages relaxation.

Guillain-Barré syndrome A rare neurological illness marked by an ascending paralysis.

gut Refers to the bowel or intestine.

Harris–Benedict equation Estimates caloric requirements of a resting, fasting, unstressed individual based on the individual's height, weight, age, and sex; expressed in kilocalories.

haustral churning Movement of the large intestine.

healthy work environment. A work environment that supports quality patient care and high levels of nurse satisfaction.

heart failure (HF) Clinical syndrome that can result from structural or functional cardiac disorders that decrease the ability of the ventricle to fill or eject.

hematemesis Vomiting of bright red blood or blood that resembles "coffee grounds."

hematochezia Bright red blood or maroon colored stool secondary to bleeding.

hemianopsia Loss of a visual field of one or both eyes; the person with left hemianopsia cannot see objects in the left visual field.

hemiparesis Weakness of one side of the body.

hemiplegia Paralysis or loss of voluntary movement of one side of the body.

hemoglobin The oxygen-carrying protein found on erythrocytes.

hemolytic anemia Breakdown (pathologic destruction) of red blood cells.

hemopneumothorax Abnormal accumulation of air and blood in the intrapleural space.

hemoptysis Expectoration of bloody sputum.

hemostasis Stoppage of bleeding; stagnation of blood flow.

hemothorax Abnormal accumulation of blood in the intrapleural space.

hepatic encephalopathy An altered neurologic status that is caused by a buildup of circulating toxins of hepatic origin.

hepatic failure The inability of the liver to perform its normal functions.

hepatorenal syndrome (HRS) Acute renal failure associated with advanced liver dysfunction.

herniation A catastrophic shifting or displacement of brain tissue, which causes pressure and traction on cerebral structures and produces clinical symptoms.

heterograft Transplantation of tissue between two different species; (e.g., animals and humans); can be used as a temporary biological dressing; also referred to as xenograft.

high-density lipoprotein (HDL) Lipoprotein molecule that has a high density (amount) of protein and a small amount of cholesterol; commonly known as the "good" cholesterol.

histocompatibility antigens (human leukocyte antigen [HLA]) Genetically determined surface antigens found in all nucleated cells in the body; one's own HLA antigens are substances that the body recognizes as self.

histocompatibility The ability of cells and tissues to live without interference from the immune system.

homograft Tissue transplanted from another individual to be used as a biological dressing.

hormone-sensitive lipase A fat-splitting enzyme.

humoral immunity The type of protection against foreign antigens provided by antibody formation from B lymphocytes.

hyalinization A degenerative cell process affecting the basement membrane of arteries and arterioles; hyalinized cells take on a glassy appearance.

hydrocephalus A clinical syndrome caused by an increased production of cerebrospinal fluid that exceeds the absorption rate.

hydrochloric acid Secreted by the parietal cells to lower gastrointestinal pH and to regulate bacterial growth.

hyperacute rejection A humoral immune response in which the B lymphocytes are activated to produce antibodies against the donor organ; it occurs within minutes to hours following transplantation.

hypercapnia Abnormally high level of carbon dioxide in the blood.

hypercatabolism Breakdown of total body protein; skeletal muscle protein is used initially for conversion to glucose through gluconeogenesis; visceral (organ) protein is used after skeletal muscle protein; occurs in the flow phase of the metabolic stress response.

hypercholesterolemia High levels of serum cholesterol.

hyperemia A state in which cerebral blood flow is higher than cerebral metabolic needs; also known as *luxury perfusion.*

hyperglycemia Abnormally high level of glucose in the blood.

hyperglycemic hyperosmolar state (HHS) A hyperglycemic complication of diabetes mellitus that results from insulin deficiency or insulin resistance; previously referred to as hyperglycemic hyperosmolar nonketotic syndrome (HHNS).

hyperlipidemia A condition manifested by high levels of lipids in the blood.

hypermetabolism An increased metabolic rate in response to a major bodily insult requiring increased quantities of oxygen and nutrients to meet the increased metabolic needs; occurs in the flow phase of the metabolic stress response.

hypersensitivity An exaggerated response of the immune system to an antigen or antigens otherwise considered nonpathogenic; an allergy to a certain substance is an example of a hypersensitivity reaction.

hypertonic A high-osmolarity state in which the concentration of particles is greater on one side of a membrane than on the other side; in the body, the solution has a higher osmolarity than exists inside of the cells.

hypertrophic cardiomyopathy Condition associated with left ventricular hypertrophy that decreases the ability of the chamber to relax (diastolic dysfunction).

hypervolemia Excess volume of circulating fluids.

hypochromic The abnormal pale coloring of RBCs, indicating reduced hemoglobin content.

hypogammaglobulinemia Abnormally low serum levels of gamma globulin.

hypoglycemia Abnormally low level of glucose in the blood.

hypokinesis Decreased myocardial wall movement resulting from myocardial ischemia or injury.

hypotonic A low-osmolarity state in which the concentration of particles in a solution is greater on one side of a membrane than on the other side; in the body, the solution has a lower osmolarity than exists inside of the cells.

hypovolemia Decreased volume of circulating fluids.

hypovolemic shock Impaired oxygenation because of inadequate cardiac output as a result of decreased intravascular volume.

hypoxemia Condition characterized by an inadequate amount of oxygen in the blood as a result of impaired gas exchange, frequently quantified as a PaO_2 of less than 60 mm Hg.

hypoxia An inadequate amount of oxygen available at the cellular level.

idiopathic thrombocytopenia purpura (ITP) Abnormally low platelet count of unknown origin; platelet antibodies are present in the patient's serum.

immunity A normal adaptive response to the external environment; it functions to protect the body from disease by means of both resistance to offending organisms and attack on offending organisms.

immunodeficiency A deficiency of T cells or B cells or both resulting from illnesses, chemotherapy, radiation therapy, or a direct pathogenic attack on the immune system.

immunodeficiency state A general term referring to a state of deficient immune activity.

immunogenicity/immunogenic Capable of evoking an immune response; in varying degrees, antigens are immunogenic; some antigens do not evoke an immune response (e.g., CEA, AFP).

immunoglobulin (Ig) The product of plasma cells in the humoral immune response following exposure to a specific antigen; the five classes of immunoglobulins are IgA, IgD, IgE, IgG, and IgM; antibodies.

immunosuppressant A drug that suppresses the immune response.

incomplete spinal cord injury Trauma to the spinal cord that leads to partial loss of sensory or motor function below the neurological level of injury; includes the lower sacral segment.

indirect calorimetry A technique of estimating an individual's metabolic or energy expenditure through the measurement of oxygen consumed ($\dot{V}O_2$) and carbon dioxide produced (VCO_2); can also calculate respiratory quotient (RQ).

infarction Death of tissue.

infection The multiplication of microorganisms that invade body tissues.

infective endocarditis (IE) A disease caused by microbial infection of the endothelial lining of the heart, usually presenting with vegetations on a heart valve.

inhalation injury Burn-associated injury caused by inhaling products of combustion.

innate (natural) immunity Species-specific protection composed of natural resistance and the activities of certain leukocytes.

inotrope Factor that influences myocardial contractility; a positive inotrope increases myocardial contractility; a negative inotrope decreased myocardial contractility.

insomnia Prolonged or abnormal inability to sleep.

insulin An anabolic hormone produced by the beta cells of the islets of Langerhans of the pancreas.

insulin-dependent cells Cells that require insulin to facilitate diffusion of glucose through the cell membrane.

interferon A cytokine involved in the signaling between cells of the immune system and in protection against viral infections; see cytokines.

interleukin A cytokine involved in signaling between cells of the immune system; see cytokines.

intermediate-care unit High-acuity nursing unit that provides an efficient distribution of resources for the patient whose acute illness requires less use of monitoring equipment and staffing than an intensive care unit.

internal respiration Movement of gases across the systemic capillary–cell membrane in the tissues.

intestinal strangulation Intestine twists to such an extent that circulation to the twisted area is impaired.

intracellular Fluid compartment within the body's cells; composes approximately two thirds of the total body water.

intracerebral hematoma (ICH) Accumulation of blood in the parenchyma of brain tissue.

intracranial hypertension Increased intracranial pressure.

intracranial pressure Pressure exerted by the cerebrospinal fluid within the ventricles of the brain; normal pressure is 0 to 15 mm Hg.

intrathecal Within a sheath (e.g., cerebrospinal fluid that is contained within the dura mater) (AHCPR, 1992).

intravascular Fluid compartment in the blood vessels; fluid is available for exchange of nutrients and oxygen.

intrinsic factor Secreted by the parietal cells; necessary for vitamin B_{12} absorption.

intrinsic pathway A coagulation cascade of events triggered by direct exposure of blood to subendothelial vascular tissue that results in clot formation.

intrinsic renal failure Kidney dysfunction caused by damage to the renal parenchyma.

isoelectric Consistent with baseline on an ECG tracing.

isoenzymes A subgrouping of parent enzymes that are more specific to a particular cell type.

isograft Transplantation of tissues between identical twins; also referred to as a *syngraft.*

isotonic The concentration of particles in a solution on one side of a membrane is the same as it is on the other side of the membrane; in the body, it closely approximates normal serum plasma osmolality.

jaundice A yellow cast of the skin, sclera, and mucous membranes caused by elevated bilirubin, a yellow pigment.

kallikrein An enzyme found in plasma, body tissues, and urine that forms kinin; it normally circulates in the plasma in its inactive state, as the proenzyme kallikreinogen; when activated by trypsin, it is an extremely potent vasodilator.

ketonuria The presence of ketones in the urine.

ketosis The presence of ketones in the blood.

Kupffer's cells Fixed tissue macrophages found in the liver.

kwashiorkor A state of malnutrition in which there is a prolonged deficiency for absence of protein in the presence of adequate carbohydrate intake.

lead Electrographic picture of the heart.

leukostasis (or leukostasis syndrome) A complication of extreme elevations (greater than 100,000 cells/mcL) in circulating leukocytes (usually blast cells); most commonly associated with AML.

lipase A lipolytic pancreatic enzyme; its action contributes to necrosis of fatty tissue surrounding the pancreas in the presence of pancreatitis.

lipogenesis The liver's production of lipids from glucose or amino acid.

lipolysis Breakdown or splitting of fat.

lipolytic Facilitating the breakdown of fats.

lipoproteins Cholesterol bound to protein and carried in the blood.

living donor A person who volunteers to have an organ, part of an organ, or hematopoietic stem cells removed for transplantation into another person while still alive.

lobectomy Surgical procedure that removes one or more lobes of the lung.

lobule The functional unit of the liver.

low-density lipoprotein (LDL) Lipoprotein molecule that has a low density (amount) of protein and a large amount of cholesterol; commonly known as the "bad" cholesterol.

lower esophageal sphincter (cardiac sphincter) Separates the esophagus from the stomach.

lymphocytosis Higher than normal levels of lymphocytes.

lymphokine A type of cytokine (chemical messenger) produced by lymphocytes; see cytokines.

maceration Situation in which drainage from the wound has prolonged contact with healthy skin tissue around the wound; periwound skin is white or pale.

macroangiopathy Disease of the large and medium-sized blood vessels; essentially atherosclerosis.

macrocytic Abnormally large RBC.

macronutrients Carbohydrates, lipids (fats), and proteins.

macrophages Activated, mature monocytes that ingest and digest antigens, then carry the antigen to the T cells and B cells; the link between the immune response and the inflammatory response.

magnetic resonance cholangiopancreatography (MRCP) A test using magnetic resonance imaging to produce images of the hepatobiliary tree.

major histocompatibility complex (MHC) A group of genes located on the sixth chromosome responsible for coding histocompatibility antigens for discrimination of self from nonself.

malnutrition A state of poor nutrition that arises from a lack of meeting the body's minimum nutritional requirements of carbohydrates, proteins, lipids, and other essential nutrients; may be caused by anorexia, poor diet, or malabsorption of nutrients in the gastrointestinal tract.

marasmus A state of malnutrition in which there is inadequate intake of protein and calories and generalized wasting is evident.

margination The movement and adhering of circulating WBCs to the capillary wall in preparation for shifting out of the vessel to move to the site of injury.

mast cells Large granule-containing tissue cells that are located in connective tissue throughout the body.

maximum inspiratory pressure (MIP, PImax) The amount of negative pressure a person can exert during maximal inspiration; normal is –50 to –100 cm H_2O. Also referred to negative inspiratory pressure (NIF).

mean arterial pressure (MAP) Average pressure within the arterial system throughout the cardiac cycle.

mean corpuscular volume (MCV) A measurement of the size (volume) of RBCs.

mechanical debridement Use of moist dressings, irrigation, or whirlpool to remove foreign material from a wound.

mediators A broad category of bioactive substances that stimulate physiologic change in cells.

melena Black, tarry, foul-smelling stools containing blood.

mentation Refers to mental activity.

mesenteric circulation Blood flow to the intestines.

mesentery Part of the peritoneum that suspends the small intestine to the abdominal wall.

metabolic acidosis An alteration in acid–base balance characterized by an arterial blood gas pH of less than 7.35 (normal is 7.35 to 7.45) with a bicarbonate level of less than 22 mEq/L (normal is 22 to 28 mEq/L).

metabolic stress response A well-defined pattern of metabolic and physiologic responses that occur as the result of injured tissue in the body.

microangiopathy Small blood vessel disease.

microcytic Abnormally small RBC.

micronutrients Electrolytes, vitamins, minerals, and trace elements.

microvascular disease Disease of the capillaries.

microvilli Fingerlike projections covering the villi.

minute ventilation ($\dot{V}_E$) The total volume of expired air in one minute.

mitral regurgitation (MR) Incompetent mitral valve allows blood to flow back into the left atrium during systole because the mitral valve does not fully close.

mitral stenosis (MS) A narrowing of the mitral valve orifice so that blood flow is obstructed from the left atrium into the left ventricle during diastole.

mitral valve prolapse A type of mitral valve insufficiency that occurs when one or both of the mitral valve cusps flow into the atria during ventricular systole.

magnet designation Accreditation awarded to hospitals that create working environments that are successful in recruiting and retaining professional nurses.

modifiable risk factors Risk factors that can be altered through either lifestyle modification or medications (examples include obesity and smoking).

monoclonal antibodies (mAb) Antibodies that are pure clones of specific B lymphocytes.

monocyte-macrophages Large phagocytic cells that are found in circulation and in tissues. They are crucial cells of the innate immune system.

Monro–Kellie hypothesis A principle that states that the skull is a rigid vault filled with noncompressible contents: brain, blood, and cerebrospinal fluid; if any one component increases in volume, one or both remaining components must decrease in volume for overall volume to remain constant.

mucosa Innermost layer of the GI wall.

multifocal Premature contractions originating from more than one ectopic pacemaker.

multimodal or balanced analgesia A balanced approach to pain treatment that targets several pain signaling pathways and matches the treatment to the type of pain.

multiple organ dysfunction syndrome (MODS) The presence of altered organ function in an acutely ill patient such that homeostasis cannot be maintained without intervention.

muscularis Muscular layer of the GI wall.

myelin sheath An insulating layer that is produced by Schwann cells and covers axons, providing protection and increasing the velocity of information transmission.

myocardial depressant factor (MDF) A small peptide produced when proteolytic enzymes autodigest the pancreas. MDF has a negative inotropic (decreases cardiac output) effect.

myocardial infarction (MI) The complete occlusion of one or more coronary arteries leading to cell and tissue death.

myocardial ischemia A state where oxygen demand exceeds supply causing chest pain (angina pectoris).

myoglobin An oxygen binding protein similar to hemoglobin and primarily found in muscle; substance released from damaged muscle tissue.

myoglobinuria The presence of myoglobin in the urine.

myopathy Any muscle disease that is marked by focal or diffuse muscular weakness.

natural killer lymphocyte (NK cell) A large granulated lymphocyte with strong phagocytic properties; a part of the innate immune system.

neurogenic shock Condition that occurs with an injury above T6; manifested by hypotension, bradycardia, decreased cardiac output, and inability to sweat below the level of the injury.

neuroplasticity Changes in the structure and function of the spinal segment of the nervous system.

neutropenia Abnormally low number of neutrophils.

neutrophils Segmented granulocytes of the myeloid cell line.

nitrogen A basic unit of protein (amino acid) breakdown; excreted primarily in urine in the form of urea; a 24-hour urinary urea nitrogen (UUN) measures nitrogen losses for a 24-hour period.

nociception The activation of pain receptors and the pain pathway by a noxious stimulus of sufficient strength to threaten tissue integrity.

nociceptors Refers to pain receptors; sensory receptors that, when stimulated, cause the sensation of pain.

nocturnal myoclonus Involuntary limb movements during the night.

noninvasive intermittent positive pressure ventilation (NIPPV) The application of positive pressure ventilation using a mechanical ventilator and a mask in place of an artificial airway.

nonmodifiable risk factors Risk factors that, regardless of therapy, cannot be altered (examples include genetics and age).

nonvolatile acids Metabolic acids that cannot be converted to a gas, requiring excretion through the kidneys.

normochromic The normal coloring of RBCs, indicating normal hemoglobin content.

normocytic Normal-sized cells.

nuchal rigidity Neck pain or stiffness.

nutrients Elements and compounds required for growth and maintenance of life; consist of macro- and micronutrients.

nutrition A complex process by which an organism takes in and uses food substrates for the purpose of providing energy for growth, maintenance, and repair; nutrition involves ingestion, digestion, absorption, and metabolism.

nystagmus Lateral tonic deviation of the eyes toward a stimulus.

obstructive pulmonary disorders Pulmonary disorders that are associated with decreased or delayed airflow during expiration.

obstructive shock Impaired oxygenation because of a mechanical barrier to blood flow.

occult blood Blood present in the GI tract but not really visible.

oligoanalgesia Treating pain with minimal drug use.

oliguria Production of an abnormally small amount (less than 400 mL) of urine per 24 hours; can be a symptom of kidney disease or obstruction of the urinary tract.

opioid pseudoaddiction A term that has been applied to patient behaviors that mimic those associated with addiction; the behaviors result from inadequate pain management rather than psychological dependence.

opiophobia The fear of prescribing (or consuming) adequate amounts of opiates for therapeutic results.

opsonins Factors that provide binding sites for attachment of macrophages or neutrophils to the antigens; composed of IgG and C3b, a fragment of the complement system.

opsonization A process by which antigen is modified, making it more susceptible to phagocytosis.

orthopnea Difficulty breathing while laying down, relieved in the upright position.

orthostatic hypotension A drop in blood pressure greater than 20 mm Hg or an increase in heart rate greater than 20 bpm when going from sitting to standing or lying to sitting position.

osmolality The solute concentration per volume of a solution (refers to body fluids).

osmolarity The solute concentration per volume of a solution (refers to outside of body).

osmosis The net diffusion of water from an area of greater concentration to an area of lesser concentration across the cell membrane; occurs as the result of osmotic pressure.

osmotic diuresis Excessive urinary excretion caused by osmotic shifting of fluids.

otorrhea The drainage of cerebral spinal fluid through the ear; indicates possible tear in the meninges.

oxygen consumption (VO_2) The amount of oxygen used by the body; described as a product of cardiac output and the difference between arterial oxygen content and venous oxygen content.

oxygen delivery (DO_2) The process of transportation of oxygen to cells, dependent on cardiac output, hemoglobin saturation with oxygen, and the partial pressure of oxygen in arterial blood.

oxygen extraction The process by which cells take oxygen from the blood.

oxygenation failure A respiratory crisis in which the primary problem is one of hypoxemia; clinically, it is defined as a PaO_2 of less than 60 mm Hg.

oxyhemoglobin dissociation curve A graphic representation of the relationship between oxygen saturation of hemoglobin (SaO_2) and the partial pressure of oxygen (PaO_2) in the plasma.

pacemaker Specialized cardiac nervous tissue that is able to initiate an electrical impulse, resulting in contraction of the heart; an artificial pulse generator used to provide electrical stimulus to the heart when the heart fails to conduct or generate impulses on its own at a rate that maintains cardiac output.

$PaCO_2$ The partial pressure of carbon dioxide as it exists in the arterial blood; normal range is 35 to 45 mm Hg.

pain behavior A person's physical reaction to the conscious perception of pain.

pain receptor See nociceptor.

pain (1) An unpleasant sensory and emotional experience associated with actual or potential tissue damage or described in terms of such damage (AHCPR, 1992, p. 95). (2) An unpleasant but protective phenomenon that is uniquely experienced by each individual and cannot be adequately defined, identified, or measured by an observer (Defriez and Huether, 2008, p. 305). (3) Whatever the experiencing person says it is, existing whenever the experiencing person says it does (McCaffery & Pasero, 1999, p. 17). (4) "the perception of a noxious stimulus dependent upon events in the neurons of the spinal cord and brain stem" (Loeser & Cousins, 1990, p. 179).

palliative care An interdisciplinary approach to patient care to relieve suffering and improve quality of life.

palpitations Subjective feeling of heart rhythm abnormalities; perceived as a "skipping" or "thumping"; related to premature cardiac beats.

pancreatitis Inflammation of the pancreas; it may occur as an acute or chronic condition.

pancytopenia Deficiency of all three cell lines of the blood: white blood cells, red blood cells, and platelets.

PaO_2 The partial pressure of oxygen as it exists in the arterial blood; normal range is 75 to 100 mm Hg.

paraplegia Injury to the thoracolumbar region of the spine, causing loss of motor function in the lower extremities.

paresthesias Abnormal sensations, such as burning or tingling of the skin, often occurring during stroke recovery.

parietal cells A fundic gland that secretes hydrochloric acid for pH regulation and intrinsic factor for vitamin B_{12} absorption.

parietal pleura The moist membrane that adheres to the thoracic walls, diaphragm, and mediastinum.

paroxysmal nocturnal dyspnea (PND) A symptom usually associated with transient pulmonary edema secondary to heart failure; patient awakens from sleep with severe orthopnea.

partial pressure Pressure each gas exerts in a total volume of gases.

partial-thickness wound Injury to the epidermis and part of the dermis.

partial thromboplastin time (PTT) Measures the intrinsic coagulation pathway.

partially compensated A state in which the pH is abnormal but the body buffers and regulatory mechanisms have started to respond to the imbalance.

passive acquired immunity A temporary immunity acquired through transfer of antibodies from one individual to another or from some other source to an individual. Examples include breast feeding (antibodies transferred to baby through milk) and gamma globulin (antibodies transferred through injection).

pathogens Disease-producing microorganisms.

peak airway pressure (PAP) Amount of pressure required to deliver a volume of gas.

penetrating trauma The result of the transmission of energy from a moving object into the body tissue as the object disrupts the integrity of the skin and the underlying structures.

penumbra An ischemic zone of viable, threatened tissue surrounding the brain infarct.

pepsin A gastric enzyme that breaks down protein.

pepsinogen An enzyme secreted by chief cells; converts to its active form of pepsin for protein digestion.

percutaneous coronary intervention (PCI) The use of angioplasty balloons and coronary stents to alleviate stenoses of arteries and reestablish blood flow to ischemic myocardium.

perfusion The pumping or flow of blood into tissues and organs.

perfusionist A specially trained technician who controls the cardiopulmonary bypass machine during coronary artery bypass surgery.

pericarditis Accumulation of fluid in the pericardial sac.

peripheral nerve block A pain management procedure that involves injecting a local anesthetic at the origin of the pain.

peripheral stimulation Pain stimulus that is delivered more distally in extremities and is important in the differentiation between hemispheric conditions and spinal cord injury.

peritoneum Serous membrane that lines the abdominal cavity and abdominal organs.

Peyer's patches Lymph tissue on the outer wall of the intestine.

pH Represents free hydrogen ion concentration.

phagocytosis An important innate immune response whereby invading foreign materials or injured cells are ingested and destroyed by phagocytic cells, such as neutrophils, macrophages, or NK cells.

phlebostatic axis An imaginary point determined by the intersection of two lines; 4th intercostal space midpoint between the anterior and posterior diameter; this is the correct level for positioning transducers used for hemodynamic monitoring.

phospholipase A A lipolytic pancreatic enzyme, activated by either bile salts or trypsin; contributes to the development of pulmonary complications (acute respiratory distress syndrome [ARDS]) by decreasing surfactant in the lungs.

physical dependence A physical adaptation of the body to the presence of opioids, existing when rapid drug withdrawal produces signs and symptoms.

plasma cells The result of the transformation of mature B cells in response to exposure to a specific antigen; primary cells for antibody production.

plateau phase Part of the repolarization when the calcium channels open to allow movement of calcium into the cell to help maintain the cell in a depolarized state.

platelet activating factor (PAF) A potent proinflammatory phospholipid mediator whose inappropriate activation results in inflammatory disease states.

platelet factor 4 A protein located in the platelet alpha granules.

platelet plug A rapid onset hemostatic function of platelets in which the platelets aggregate and adhere to each other at the site of a vessel injury to form a temporary seal and facilitate clot formation.

pleural effusion Abnormal accumulation of fluid in the intrapleural space.

pleural infusion A pain management route in which a catheter is inserted between the parietal and visceral pleura; often used when the patient has fractured ribs.

pleural rub Adventitious breath sound caused by inflammation of the pleural membrane.

pleurisy (pleuritis) Pain caused by inflammation of the parietal pleura.

pluripotential hematopoietic stem cells (PHSC) Stem cells produced in the bone marrow that have the potential to become erythrocytes, leukocytes, or thrombocytes.

pneumonectomy Surgical procedure that removes one entire lung.

pneumothorax Abnormal accumulation of air in the intrapleural space.

poikilothermia Loss of internal temperature control whereby the patient assumes the temperature of the environment.

polarized Negatively charged.

polyclonal antibodies Antibodies produced by immunizing animals with human lymphocytes.

polycythemia Abnormally elevated red blood cell mass.

polydipsia Excessive thirst.

polymorphonuclear The presence of multiple nuclei in a cell (e.g., segmented neutrophils).

polyneuropathy Disease that affects multiple peripheral nerves resulting in weakness.

polyuria Excessive urination.

portal hypertension Elevated portal vein pressure that is sustained at above-normal levels.

positive end-expiratory pressure (PEEP) The application of positive pressure to the airway at the end of expiration such that the airway pressure never returns to ambient.

postrenal injury Kidney dysfunction caused by bilateral obstruction distal to the kidney parenchyma.

prerenal injury Kidney dysfunction caused by inadequate renal blood flow.

renal insufficiency Decline in renal function to approximately 25 percent of normal.

precursor lesions Types II and III atherosclerotic lesions that form during the teenage years.

prehypertension Defined as systolic blood pressure of 139 to 150 mm Hg and diastolic blood pressure of 80 to 89 mm Hg.

preload The degree of stretch in myocardial fibers at the end of diastole.

pressure gradient Difference between the partial pressures of a gas; influences rate of diffusion.

pressure support ventilation (PSV) A type of mechanical ventilatory support in which a preset level of positive pressure augments the inspiratory effort required to attain a tidal volume, thereby decreasing the work of breathing.

pressure-regulated volume-controlled (PRVC) A dual mode of mechanical ventilation where the pressure support is adjusted breath to breath to deliver a set tidal volume.

priapism Persistent penile erection produced by reflex activity.

primary injury Neurons sustain direct injury at the moment of impact.

primary intention Method of wound closure using sutures or tape.

primary MODS Organ dysfunction directly related to an organ insult.

primary response The initial humoral response to antigen exposure.

primary immunodeficiency Failure of either T cell or B cell function or both, resulting from embryonic or congenital lack of development of such organs as the thymus.

Prinzmetal's angina See variant angina.

proliferative phase Phase of wound healing that lasts for several weeks after injury; wound is restored with a functional barrier.

proprioception The ability to determine spatial position; knowing where the body or a body part is positioned in space.

proteolytic Facilitating the breakdown of proteins.

prothrombin time (PT) Measures the coagulation extrinsic pathway.

pseudocyst A combination of pancreatic enzymes, necrotic tissue and possible blood which is enclosed by pancreatic or adjacent tissues.

pseudopods Fingerlike projections.

psychological dependence (addiction) A pattern of compulsive drug use characterized by a continued craving for an opioid and the need to use the opioid for effects other than pain relief (or other medical indications) (AHCPR, 1994).

pulmonary artery diastolic (PAD) pressure Reflects diastolic filling pressure in the left ventricle.

pulmonary artery systolic (PAS) pressure Pressure generated by the right ventricle during systole.

pulmonary artery wedge pressure (PAWP) Pressure obtained when the inflated balloon wedges in a small branch of the pulmonary artery, reflecting pressures from the left heart.

pulmonary embolism Blockage of a pulmonary vessel caused by lodging of a thromboembolism or other blood-borne material.

pulmonary gas exchange The process that involves the intake of oxygen from the external environment into the internal environment and is carried out by ventilation, diffusion, and perfusion.

pulmonary shunt The percentage of cardiac output that flows from the right heart and back into the left heart without undergoing pulmonary gas exchange or not achieving normal levels of PaO_2 because of abnormal alveolar functioning.

pulmonary vascular resistance (PVR) Afterload of the right ventricle; the resistance the right ventricle must overcome to open the pulmonic valve and eject the stroke volume into the pulmonary artery.

pulse oximetry Noninvasive technique for monitoring arterial capillary hemoglobin saturation.

pulse pressure Difference between diastolic and systolic pulse pressure.

pulsus alternans Alternating weak and strong pulses.

pulsus paradoxus Exaggerated decrease (greater than 10 mm Hg) in systolic blood pressure during inspiration.

pus A thin liquid residue that is an important indicator of inflammation.

quadriplegia Injury to cervical or thoracic regions of the spinal cord that may result in impaired function of the arms, trunk, legs, and pelvic organs; also known as tetraplegia.

race Human biological variation.

receptive aphasia The inability to understand written or spoken words.

recipient One who receives an organ or tissue.

refeeding syndrome (RFS) A nutritional complication associated with reinitiating nutritional support in a significantly malnourished person, characterized by electrolyte imbalances.

regurgitation Backward blood flow through the chambers of the heart.

rejection The activation of the immune response against a transplanted tissue or organ.

relative refractory period The period after an action potential when a stimulus can produce a second action potential if the stimulus is greater than the threshold level.

remodeling/maturation phase Final wound repair process; lasts up to two years; final product is the scar.

renal insufficiency Decline in renal function to approximately 25 percent of normal.

repolarization Return of the cellular membrane to its resting membrane potential. Should result in cardiac muscle relaxation.

resistant bacteria Bacteria that continue to multiply in the presence of antimicrobial agents.

respiration The process by which the body's cells are supplied with oxygen and carbon dioxide is eliminated from the body; also refers to breathing, the movement of air in and out of the lungs.

respiratory failure A state of pulmonary decompensation in which the body is no longer able to maintain normal gas exchange; it can be expressed as PaO_2 less than 60 mm Hg or $PaCO_2$ greater than 50 mm Hg at pH less than 7.30.

respiratory insufficiency A state of pulmonary compensation in which a normal blood pH is maintained only at the expense of the cardiopulmonary system.

respiratory quotient (RQ) A ratio of carbon dioxide ($\dot{V}CO_2$) to oxygen consumed ($\dot{V}O_2$); provides information about fuel composition used by the body; $\dot{V}CO_2$ and $\dot{V}O_2$ are obtained from an indirect calorimetry study.

resting membrane potential Point at the end of repolarization when the membrane is relatively permeable to potassium but is almost impermeable to sodium; thus, intracellular concentration of potassium is greater than extracellular concentration.

restrictive disorders Pulmonary disorders associated with a decrease in lung volume.

resuscitative phase The period of 48 to 72 hours immediately following a burn injury.

reticular activating system (RAS) A pathway of neurons and neuronal connections for transmission of sensory stimuli from the lower brainstem to the cerebral cortex; the anatomic basis of the arousal component of consciousness.

reticulocytes Immature RBCs.

reticuloendothelial system A group of cells found throughout the body that are capable of ingesting particles; cells include macrophages, reticular cells, and other tissue macrophages.

Rh incompatibility A type of hemolytic disease of the newborn in which the baby has a different Rh blood type than the mother (for example, the baby has Rh positive blood and the mother has Rh negative blood).

rhinorrhea The drainage of cerebral spinal fluid through the nose; indicates possible tear in the meninges.

rhonchi Adventitious breath sounds associated with an accumulation of fluid or secretions in the larger airways.

right atrial pressure (RAP) A measure of the pressure in the right ventricle at end diastole; represents right ventricular preload.

secondary (acquired) injury Injury that occurs in response to a primary (direct) injury; involves complex biochemical processes that occur within minutes of a primary injury and can last for days to weeks.

secondary intention Method of wound closure in which the wound is allowed to heal gradually, using the biological phases of wound healing to fill in a cavity or defect.

secondary MODS An abnormal and excessive inflammatory response as a consequence of the patient's response to a secondary insult.

secondary response The humoral response to subsequent exposures to the same antigen; immune response is heightened, and antibody formation is triggered more quickly than in the primary response.

secretin A hormone present in the small bowel mucosa that stimulates sodium bicarbonate secretion by the pancreas and bile secretion by the liver; it decreases gastrointestinal peristalsis and motility.

sedation A state of drowsiness and clouding of mental activity that may be accompanied by impaired reasoning ability (Way et al., 2001).

segmentectomy Surgical procedure that removes a portion of a lobe of the lung.

segmented cells (segs) Mature neutrophils.

seizure activity A complication of traumatic brain injury.

seizure A convulsion or other clinically detectable event caused by a sudden discharge of electrical activity in the brain.

sensory perceptual alterations The amount, character, or intensity of stimuli that exceeds the person's minimum or maximum threshold of tolerance for sensory input; accompanied by a diminished, exaggerated, distorted, or impaired response.

sepsis A pathologic state in which microorganisms, or their toxins, are present in the bloodstream; syndrome of systemic inflammation in response to infection; a subcategory of systemic inflammatory response syndrome (SIRS).

septic encephalopathy Generalized brain dysfunction marked by varying degrees of impairment of speech, cognition, orientation, and arousal that is associated with systemic inflammatory response syndrome or septicemia.

septic shock Severe sepsis plus hypotension not reversed with fluid resuscitation.

serosa Outermost layer of the GI wall.

severe abdominal compartment syndrome IAP greater than 25 mm Hg.

severe acute respiratory syndrome (SARS) An atypical pneumonia caused by a novel form of coronavirus called SARS-CoV.

severe sepsis Acute organ dysfunction secondary to infection.

sharp debridement Removal of necrotic areas in wounds using scissors or a scalpel.

shearing Structures sliding in opposite directions causing a tearing or degloving type of injury.

shock A syndrome; a complex of signs and symptoms that describe a sequence of changes that occur when tissue oxygen supply does not meet oxygen demand.

shunting The state in which pulmonary capillary perfusion is normal but alveolar ventilation is lacking.

shuntlike effect Effect created by an excess of perfusion in relation to alveolar ventilation.

sigh Intermittent hyperinflation of the lungs.

slough Moist, stringy, thick, yellow tissue that is dying.

sodium-potassium pump (also known as Na^+/K^+ pump) An active transport ion gradient mechanism that maintains intracellular sodium and potassium homeostasis.

somatosensory-evoked potentials (SEPs) Stimulation of pain and touch to peripheral nerves to determine whether a response is elicited by the cerebral cortex.

Somogyi effect A nocturnal hypoglycemia rebound phenomenon characterized by wide swings in serum glucose levels.

spastic paralysis Damage to upper motor neurons resulting in the inability to carry out a skilled movement.

spasticity A state of increased tone of a muscle resulting in a stiff muscle and continuous resistance to stretching.

sphincter of Oddi A circular muscle that surrounds the ampulla of Vater; it helps control the rate of pancreatic enzyme and bile flow into the duodenum.

spinal shock A condition that occurs within 60 minutes after spinal cord injury. Manifested by hypotension, bradycardia, flaccid paralysis, absence of muscle contractions, and bowel and bladder dysfunction.

spiral CT scan A specialized computerized axial tomography scan (CT scan) that continuously moves the patient through the scan quickly; provides greater visualization of blood vessels.

spirituality A sense of faith and transcendence.

splanchnic circulation The combination of the portal venous and arterial circulatory systems of the viscera; blood flow through the gut, spleen, pancreas, and liver.

spontaneous breaths Breaths that use the patient's own respiratory effort and mechanics.

stable angina Chest pain that is predictable and relieved with rest or nitrates.

stabs (bands) A commonly used alternative name for immature neutrophils.

status asthmaticus A life-threatening emergency of acute airway obstruction that does not respond to usual therapy.

status epilepticus Continuous seizure activity without a pause, that is, without an intervening period of normal brain function. A life-threatening emergency.

stenosis Valve leaflets fuse together and cannot fully open or close.

stomatitis Inflammation of any or all of the oral mucous membranes (i.e., tongue, gums, pharynx, lips, and cheeks).

stridor A type of wheeze heard loudest over the neck suggesting obstruction of the trachea or larynx.

stroke A brain attack; an acute neurologic deficit that occurs when impaired blood flow to a localized area of the brain results in injury to brain tissue.

stroke volume (SV) The volume of blood pumped with each heartbeat.

stroke volume index The volume of blood pumped with each beat, indexed to body size.

subarachnoid hemorrhage (SAH) Accumulation of blood between the arachnoid layer of the meninges and the brain.

subdermal burn Burn that destroys all layers of the skin and may include injury to muscle, tendons, or bone.

subdural hematoma (SDH) Accumulation of blood between dura and arachnoid layers of the meninges.

subluxation Incomplete dislocation, most often seen in the shoulder joint following stroke.

submucosa Layer of the GI wall that contains blood and lymphatic vessels.

summation gallop S3 and S4 heart sounds are present; indicative of severe heart failure.

superficial burn Burn that destroys the epidermis only.

superficial partial-thickness burn Burn that destroys the epidermis and superficial layer of the dermis.

superficial wound Injury to the epidermis.

supranormal period The period after an action potential during which a stimulus that is slightly less than normal can precipitate another action potential.

surfactant A lipoprotein produced by type II alveolar cells that reduces the surface tension of the alveolar fluid lining.

synchronous intermittent mandatory ventilation (SIMV) A mechanical ventilator mode that allows the patient to breathe spontaneously through ventilator circuitry while interspersing mandatory mechanical breaths at even intervals via a preset rate. The mandatory breaths are synchronized to the patient's own breathing cycle.

syncope A temporary loss of consciousness, followed by a spontaneous and complete recovery.

syndrome of inappropriate antidiuretic hormone (SIADH) The retention of water due to the excessive secretion of antidiuretic hormone (ADH); characterized by the production of small amounts of concentrated urine with an associated decrease in serum sodium.

syngraft See isograft.

synthesis Formation of a substance.

systemic inflammatory response syndrome (SIRS) A term used to describe a condition in which there is a systemic (rather than local) inflammatory process.

systemic vascular resistance (SVR) Afterload of left ventricle; the resistance the left ventricle must overcome to open the aortic valve and eject the stroke volume into the aorta.

systolic dysfunction. Heart failure characterized by ejection fraction less than 40 percent.

T lymphocytes (T cells) Lymphocytes primarily responsible for direct attack and destruction of invading antigens and for primary cell-mediated immunity

tachycardia Heart rate greater than 100 bpm.

target organ damage Dysfunction that occurs in organs affected by high blood pressure.

tensile forces Forces that cause tissues to stretch or extend.

tertiary intention Method of wound closure in which a combination of primary and secondary intention is used.

tetraplegia Injury to cervical or thoracic regions of the spinal cord that may result in impaired function of the arms, trunk, legs, and pelvic organs; also known as quadriplegia.

thermodilution Method used to obtain cardiac output with a pulmonary artery catheter; uses theory of a known amount of volume infused at a known temperature and change in blood temperature over time as a result of that infusion.

third spacing Shift of fluid from the intravascular compartment to a third (transcellular) space, usually a serous cavity.

thirst The awareness of the desire to drink.

thrombosis Intravascular aggregation of cells creating a blood clot.

thymus Organ in the mediastinum primarily responsible for differentiating lymphocytes into various types of T cells for cell-mediated immunity.

tidal volume (TV or V_T) The volume of air moved in and out of the lungs during one normal breath. It is also an important setting on a mechanical ventilator – if set too high the patient is hyperventilated and if set too low the patient is hypoventilated.

tissue typing Identification of the HLA antigens of both the donor and the recipient.

tolerance A common physiologic result of chronic opioid use; it means that a larger dose of opioid is required to maintain the same level of analgesia.

tonicity Osmolarity of an intravenous fluid.

total lung capacity (TLC) The amount of gas present in the lungs after maximal inspiration.

total parenteral nutrition (TPN) A nutritionally complete, IV-delivered solution composed of protein, carbohydrate, fat, electrolytes, vitamins, and trace elements; TPN with a glucose concentration of greater than 10 percent is administered through a central vein.

tracheostomy A surgical airway created by cutting into the trachea below the cricothyroid membrane.

transfer anxiety Anxiety experienced by the individual who is moved from a familiar, somewhat secure environment to an environment that is unfamiliar.

transient ischemic attacks (TIAs) Episodes of focal neurologic deficits that usually resolve in a few minutes or hours.

transport shock Impaired oxygenation because of a diminished supply of hemoglobin in which to carry oxygen to tissues.

traumatic brain injury (TBI) Injury that results from any mechanical disruption of brain tissue from an impact or injury to the head.

trigeminy A cardiac dysrhythmia of two normal *QRS* complexes followed by one premature ventricular contraction.

troponin A protein found in cardiac muscle; when present in the blood, it is used as a marker of myocardial cell death.

true shunt Flow of blood from the right heart, through the lungs, and on into the left heart without taking part in alveolar–capillary diffusion or oxygen exchange.

trypsin A proteolytic pancreatic enzyme; it exists in the pancreas in its proenzyme (inactive) state as trypsinogen. Most of the other pancreatic enzymes require trypsin for activation.

tunneling Narrow passageway created by the separation of, or destruction to, fascial planes.

type I (allergic) hypersensitivity response A hypersensitivity immune response that involves an interaction between IgE and mast cells; its systemic form is anaphylaxis.

type II (cytotoxic) hypersensitivity response A hypersensitivity immune response; IgM and IgG react directly with cell surface antigens, injuring or destroying targeted cells.

type III (immune complex) hypersensitivity response A hypersensitivity immune response involving antigen-antibody complexes with IgG and IgM; complexes are deposited vessel walls or tissues causing an inflammatory response.

type IV (cell-mediated) hypersensitivity response A delayed hypersensitivity immune response involving tissue injury by direct T cell attack in the absence of antibody activity.

uncompensated An acid–base state in which the pH is abnormal because other buffer and regulatory mechanisms have not begun to correct the imbalance.

unconjugated bilirubin Fat-soluble bilirubin that has not yet joined with glucuronic acid.

unifocal Premature contractions originating from one ectopic pacemaker.

unstable angina Chest pain that is not predictable, and that occurs with rest or with minimal activity.

unstable spinal injury An injury to two or more of the spinal columns; vertebral and ligamentous structures are unable to support and protect the injured area.

uptake To take a substance into a cell.

urea A nitrogen substance produced by the liver from ammonia.

uremia Clinical symptoms of azotemia.

urobilinogen Bilirubin in the urine.

variant angina Chest pain that is not predictable, may occur at night, and is caused by coronary artery spasm; also known as Prinzmetal's angina.

varices Dilated veins (singular form: varix).

vascular thrombosis A blood clot in the vasculature of the graft.

venous admixture The effect that a physiologic shunt has on the oxygen content of the blood as it drains into the left heart.

ventilation The gross movement of air in and out of the lungs; airflow between the atmosphere and alveoli.

ventilation–perfusion ratio ($\dot{V}/\dot{Q}$) The relationship of pulmonary ventilation to pulmonary perfusion expressed as a ratio in L/min; normal is 4:5.

ventilatory failure A condition caused by alveolar hypoventilation; clinically, it is called acute respiratory acidosis.

ventricular gallop S3 heart sound caused by decreased ventricular compliance.

ventricular stroke work index The work involved in moving blood in the ventricle with each heartbeat against afterload.

villi Fingerlike projections covering intestinal folds.

visceral pleura The moist membrane that adheres to the lung parenchyma and is adjacent to the parietal pleura.

vital capacity (VC) The volume of air that can be exhaled after maximum inhalation; an indication of respiratory muscle strength; normal is 65 to 75 mL/kg.

volatile acids Acids that can convert to a gas form for excretion.

volutrauma Injury to pulmonary tissues as a result of excessive volumes.

weaning Withdrawal of mechanical ventilation.

wedge resection Surgical procedure that removes a wedge-shaped section of the peripheral portion of the lung.

wheeze Adventitious breath sound caused by air passing through constricted airways.

xanthoma A cholesterol-filled skin lesion.

xenograft Biological dressings or grafts obtained from animals; also referred to as heterografts.

Abbreviations

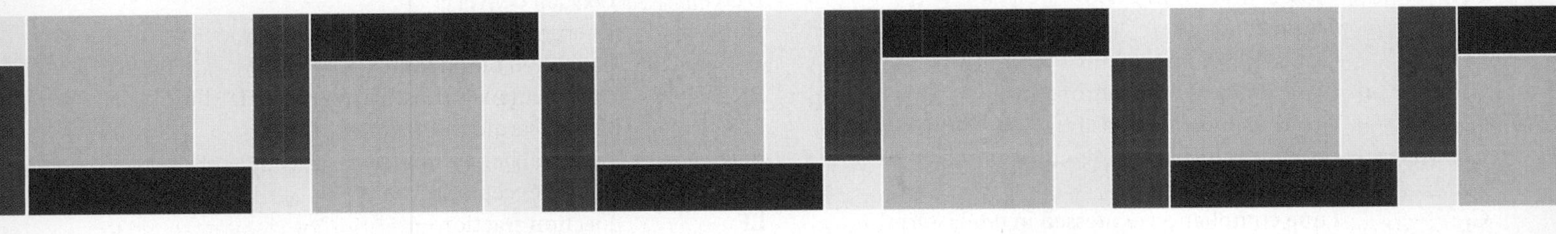

2,3 DPG	Diphosphoglycerate
5'-N	5'-nucleotidase
$A\dot{V}$	Alveolar ventilation
AAA	Aromatic amino acid
AACN	American Association of Critical Care Nurses
ABG	Arterial blood gas
ABO	Refers to the A, B, and O blood types
AC	Assist-control mode; alternating current
ACC	American College of Cardiology
ACCM	American College of Critical Care Medicine
ACE	Angiotensin-converting enzyme
ACS	Acute coronary syndromes; abdominal compartment syndrome
ACTH	Adrenocorticotropic hormone
ADH	Antidiuretic hormone
ADL	Activities of daily living
ADP	Adenosine diphosphate
ADR	Adverse drug reaction
AED	Automatic external defibrillator
AFib	Atrial fibrillation
Aflutter	Atrial flutter
AFP	Alpha-fetoprotein
AHA	American Heart Association
AHCPR	Agency for Health Care Policy and Research
AHF	Acute hepatic failure
AI	Anemia of inflammation
AICD	Automatic implantable cardioverter/defibrillator
AIDS	Acquired immune deficiency syndrome
AKI	Acute kidney injury
ALG	Antilymphocyte globulin
ALI/ARDS	Acute lung injury/acute respiratory distress syndrome
Alk phos	(ALP) Alkaline phosphatase; previously SGOT
ALL	Acute lymphocytic leukemia
ALT	Alanine aminotransferase (SGPT)
AMI	Acute myocardial infarction
AML	Acute myelogenous (myelocytic) leukemia
AMSN	Academy of Medical Surgical Nurses
ANA	American Nurses Association
AND	Allow natural death
ANP	Atrial natriuretic peptide
APC	Activated protein C; antigen-presenting cells
APS	American Pain Society
aPTT	Activated partial thromboplastin time
AR	Aortic regurgitation
ARB	Angiotensin receptor blocker
ARDS	Acute respiratory distress syndrome
ARS	Adjective Rating Scale
AS	Aortic stenosis
ASA	Acetylsalicylic acid (aspirin)
ASPM	American Society for Pain Management Nursing
AST	Aspartate aminotransferase (SGOT)
ATG	Antithymocyte globulin
ATN	Acute tubular necrosis
ATP	Adenosine triphosphate
AV	Atrioventricular
AV Block	Atrioventricular block
AVF	Acute ventilatory failure
AVM	Arteriovenous malformation
AZT	Azidothymidine
B cells	Bursa cells
BAC	Blood alcohol concentration
BB	Beta blocker
BBB	Bundle branch block
BCAA	Branched-chain amino acid
BCR-ABL	Breakpoint cluster region-Abelson (oncogene)
BE	Base excess
BMI	Body mass index
BNP	Brain natriuretic peptide
BPM	Beats per minute; breaths per minute
BPOC	Barcode point-of-care
BSA	Body surface area
BUN	Blood urea nitrogen
C	Cervical vertebrae (C1–C7)
Ca	Calcium
CABG	Coronary artery bypass graft
CAD	Coronary artery disease
CAM	Confusion Assessment Method
CAM-ICU	Confusion assessment method for the ICU
CaO_2	Oxygen content of arterial blood
CAP	Community-acquired pneumonia
CAPM	Continuous airway pressure monitoring
CARS	Compensatory anti-inflammatory response syndrome
CAT	Complementary and alternative therapies
CAVH	Continuous arterial venous hemofiltration
CBC	Complete blood count
CBF	Cerebral blood flow
CCB	Calcium channel blocker
CCK	Cholecystokinin
CCSC	Canadian Cardiology Society Classification
CD	Clusters of differentiation
CEA	Carcinoembryonic antigen
CEO_2	Cerebral oxygen extraction

CHD	Coronary heart disease
CHI	Closed-head injury
CI	Cardiac index
CIM	Critical illness myopathy
CIP	Critical illness polyneuropathy
CK	Creatine phosphokinase
CK-MB	Creatine phosphokinase–myocardial bands
Cl	Chloride
C_L	Lung compliance, expressed in cm H_2O/mL
CLL	Chronic lymphocytic leukemia
cm H_2O	Centimeters of water pressure
CML	Chronic myelogenous (myelocytic) leukemia
CMO	Comfort measures only
CMV	Cytomegalovirus
CNS	Central nervous system
CO	Cardiac output; carbon monoxide
CO_2	Carbon dioxide
COPD	Chronic obstructive pulmonary disease
CPAP	Continuous positive airway pressure
CPB	Cardiopulmonary bypass
CPOE	Computerized provider order entry
CPP	Coronary perfusion pressure; cerebral perfusion pressure
CPR	Cardiopulmonary resuscitation
Cr	Creatinine
CrCl	Creatinine clearance
CRF	Chronic renal failure
CRP	C-reactive protein
CRRT	Continuous renal replacement therapy
CRS	Catheter-related sepsis, cytokine-release syndrome
CRT	Cardiac resynchronization therapy
CSF	Cerebrospinal fluid
CSW	Cerebral salt wasting
CT	Computed tomography
cTn	Troponin
cTnI	Troponin-I
cTnT	Troponin-T
CVD	Cardiovascular disease
Cvo_2	Oxygen content of venous blood
CVP	Central venous pressure
CVVH	Continuous veno-venous hemofiltration
CVVHD	Continuous veno-venous hemofiltration dialysis
CyA	Cyclosporine (or CsA)
DAI	Diffuse axonal injury
DASH	Dietary approaches to stop hypertension
dBA	Decibel
DBP	Diastolic blood pressure
DC	Direct current
DCD	Donation after cardiac death
DDAVP	Desmopressin
DES	Drug-eluting stents
DI	Diabetes insipidus
DIC	Disseminated intravascular coagulation
DKA	Diabetic ketoacidosis
DNA	Deoxyribonucleic acid
DNI	Do not intubate
DNR	Do not resuscitate
DO_2	Oxygen delivery
DVT	Deep vein thrombosis
EBL	Estimated blood loss
ECF	Enterocutaneous fistula', extracellular fluid
ECG	Electrocardiogram
EDH	Epidural hematoma
EEG	Electroencephalography
EF	Ejection fraction
EGD	Esophagogastroduodenoscopy
ELISA	Enzyme-linked immunosorbent assay
EPAP	Expiratory positive airway pressure
EBP	Evidence-based practice
EPS	Electrophysiology studies
ERCP	Endoscopic retrograde cholangiopancreatography
ERV	Expiratory reserve volume of lungs
ESR	Erythrocyte sedimentation rate
ESRD	End stage renal disease
EST	Exercise stress test
ET tube	Endotracheal tube
ETOH	Ethanol (alcohol)
EUS	Endoscopic ultrasound
f	Frequency, rate of breathing, expressed in breaths per minute
FeNa	Fractional excretion of sodium
FEV	Forced expiratory volume
FFA	Free fatty acid
FG	Fournier's gangrene
FHF	Fulminant hepatic failure
Fio_2	Fraction of inspired oxygen
FRC	Functional residual capacity
ft	Foot (measurement)
FVD	Fluid volume deficit
GALT	Gut-associated lymphoid tissue
GCS	Glasgow Coma Scale
G-CSF	Granulocyte-colony stimulating factor
GDS	Geriatric Depression Scale
GFR	Glomerular filtration rate
GGT	Gamma glutamyl transferase
GH	growth hormone
GI	Gastrointestinal
GIP	Gastric inhibitory peptide
GM-CSF	Granulocyte macrophage-colony stimulating factor
GP	Glycoprotein
H^+	Hydrogen ion
H_2CO_3	Carbonic acid
H_2O	Water
H_2RA	Histamine-2 receptor antagonist
HAP	Hospital-acquired pneumonia
HAV	Hepatitis A virus
Hb (Hgb)	Hemoglobin
Hb A	Hemoglobin A
Hb A_1c	Glycosylated hemoglobin
HbO_2	Oxyhemoglobin
HBOT	Hyperbaric oxygen therapy
HBsAg	Hepatitis B surface antigen

HBV	Hepatitis B virus
HCAP	Healthcare-associated pneumonia
HCO_3	Bicarbonate
HCP	Health care provider
Hct	Hematocrit
HCV	Hepatitis C virus
HDL	High-density lipoprotein
HDV	Hepatitis D virus
HEV	Hepatitis E virus
HF	Heart failure
Hgb (Hb)	Hemoglobin
HHS	Hyperglycemic hyperosmolar state (previously referred to as HHNS, hyperglycemic hyperosmolar nonketotic syndrome)
HIPAA	Health Insurance Portability and Accountability Act
HIV	Human immunodeficiency virus
HLA DR	Human leukocyte antigen genotype
HLA	Human leukocyte antigen
HOB	Head of bed
HR	Heart rate
HRS	Hepatorenal syndrome
HTLV	Human T cell lymphotropic virus
HTLV-1	Human T cell leukemia virus type I
IABP	Intraaortic balloon pump
IAH	Intraabdominal hypertension
IAP	Intraabdominal pressure
IBW	ideal body weight
ICD	Implantable cardioverter defibrillator
ICF	Intracellular fluid
ICG	Impedance cardiography
ICH	Intracerebral hematoma
ICP	Intracranial pressure
ICU	Intensive care unit
IE	Infective endocarditis
IF	Intrinsic factor
Ig	Immunoglobulin
IgG	Immunoglobulin G
IgM	Immunoglobulin M
IHD	Intermittent hemodialysis
IL	Interleukin
IM	Intramuscular route
IMC	Intermediate-care unit
INF	Interferon
INR	International normalized ratio
IOM	Institute of Medicine
IPAP	Inspiratory positive airway pressure
IPPB	Intermittent positive pressure breathing
IRV	Inspiratory reserve volume
ITP	Idiopathic thrombocytopenia purpura
IV	Intravenous
IVC	Intraventricular catheter
J	Joules
JVD	Jugular venous distention
K	Potassium
kcal	Kilocalorie
kg	Kilogram
KODA	Kentucky Organ Donor Affiliates
L	Lumbar vertebrae (L1–L5)
L/min	Liters per minute
LA	Left atrium
LAD	Left anterior descending artery
LCX	Left circumflex artery
LDH	Lactic dehydrogenase
LDL	Low-density lipoprotein
LES	Lower esophageal sphincter
LGL	Large granulated lymphocytes (NK cells)
LIMA	Left internal mammary artery
LMCA	Left main coronary artery
LMWH	Low molecular weight heparin
LOC	Level of consciousness
LP	Lumbar puncture
LV	Left ventricle
LVAD	Left ventricular assist device
LVEDP	Left ventricular end-diastolic pressure
LVSWI	Left ventricular stroke work index
$M\dot{V}$	Minute ventilation; also $\dot{V}E$
mAb	Monoclonal antibody
MABP	Mean arterial blood pressure
MALT	Mucosa associated lymphoid tissue
MAP	Mean arterial pressure
MARS	Mixed antagonistic response syndrome
mcg	Micrograms
MCH	Mean corpuscular hemoglobin
MCHC	Mean corpuscular hemoglobin concentration
mcL	Microliters
mcm	Micrometers
MCV	Mean corpuscular volume
MDF	Myocardial depressant factor
mEq/L	Milliequivalents per liter
Mg	Magnesium
MHC	Major histocompatibility complex
MI	Myocardial infarction
mL	Milliliter
mm Hg	Millimeters of mercury
MMV	Mandatory minute ventilation
MODS	Multiple organ dysfunction syndrome
mOsm	Milliosmole
MOsm/L	Milliosmoles per liter
MPI	Myocardial perfusion imaging
MPQ	McGill Pain Questionnaire
MPV	Microprocessor ventilator
MR	Mitral regurgitation
MRA	Magnetic resonance angiography
MRI	Magnetic resonance imaging
MRSA	Methicillin-resistant *Staphylococcus aureus*
MS	Mitral stenosis
MTBI	Mild traumatic brain injury
MUGA	Multigated angiographic scan
MVC	Motor vehicle crash
Na	Sodium
Na^+/K^+	sodium/potassium ions
NAD^+	nicotinic acid dehydrogenase

NANDA North American Nursing Diagnosis Association
NF Necrotizing fasciitis
NG Nasogastric
NIPPV Noninvasive intermittent positive pressure ventilation
NK cells Natural killer cells
NMB Neuromuscular blockade
NPO Nothing by mouth
NPWT Negative pressure wound therapy
NRS Numeric Rating Scale
NSAID Nonsteroidal anti-inflammatory drug
NSR Normal sinus rhythm
NSTEMI Non-*ST* elevation myocardial infarction
NSTI Necrotizing soft tissue infection
NYHA New York Heart Association
O_2 Oxygen
OCT Ornithine carbamoyl transferase
OPO Organ procurement organization
OPTN National Organ Procurement and Transplantation Network
OT Occupational therapist
OTC Over-the-counter (nonprescription)
PA Pulmonary artery
$\overline{PA}$ Mean airway pressure
PAC Premature atrial contraction
$PACO_2$ Partial pressure of alveolar carbon dioxide in the alveoli
$PaCO_2$ Partial pressure of dissolved carbon dioxide in the plasma of arterial blood
PAD Peripheral artery disease; pulmonary artery diastolic
PAF Platelet activating factor
PAG Periaqueductal gray
PAO_2 Partial pressure of oxygen in the alveoli
PaO_2 Partial pressure of oxygen in the arterial blood
PAP Peak airway pressure; proximal airway pressure; pulmonary artery pressure
PAR Pressure adjusted heart rate
PAS Pulmonary artery systolic
PAWP Pulmonary artery wedge pressure
$Pbto_2$ Brain tissue oxygen partial pressure
PCA Patient-controlled analgesia; posterior cerebral artery
PCEA Patient-controlled epidural analgesia
PCI Percutaneous coronary intervention
PCO_2 Partial pressure of carbon dioxide
PCP *Pneumocystis jiroveci* pneumonia
PCR Polymerase chain reaction
PD Peritoneal dialysis
PDA Posterior descending artery; personal digital assistant
PE Pulmonary embolism
PEEP Positive end-expiratory pressure
PET Positron emission tomography
$PETCO_2$ Partial pressure of end-tidal carbon dioxide
PFT Pulmonary function tests
pH Free hydrogen ion concentration
Ph^1 Philadelphia chromosome
pHi Intramucosal pH
PHSC Pluripotential hematopoietic stem cell
PIM Potentially inappropriate medication
PImax Maximum inspiratory pressure
PIP Peak inspiratory pressure
PMI Point of maximal impulse
PMN Polymorphonuclear neutrophil
PND Paroxysmal nocturnal dyspnea
PO Oral route
PO_2 Partial pressure of oxygen or oxygen tension, expressed in mm Hg
PO_4 Phosphate
PPI Proton pump inhibitor
PPV Positive pressure ventilation
PRN As needed
PRVC Pressure-regulated volume-controlled
PSA Prostate-specific antigen
psi Pounds per square inch
PSV Pressure support ventilation
PT Prothrombin time; physical therapist
PTCA Percutaneous transluminal coronary angioplasty
PTH Parathyroid hormone
PTT Partial thromboplastin time
PUD Peptic ulcer disease
PVC Premature ventricular contraction
$PvCO_2$ Partial pressure of carbon dioxide in the venous blood
PVD Peripheral vascular disease
PvO_2 Partial pressure of oxygen in the venous blood
PVR Pulmonary vascular resistance
PVRI Pulmonary vascular resistance index
$\dot{Q}$ Perfusion
Qs/Qt Intrapulmonary shunt
RA Right atrium
RAP Right atrial pressure
RBC Red blood cell
RCA Right coronary artery
RDW Red blood cell (R) distribution width
REE Resting energy expenditure
REM Rapid eye movement
RFS Refeeding syndrome
RIMA Right internal mammary artery
RLE Right lower extremity
RN Registered nurse
ROM Range of motion
RQ Respiratory quotient
RR Respiratory rate
RRT Renal replacement therapy
RV Residual volume of lungs; right ventricle
RVEDP Right ventricular end-diastolic pressure
RVSWI Right ventricular stroke work index
SA node Sinoatrial node
SAH Subarachnoid hemorrhage
SaO_2 Oxygen saturation of arterial blood
SARS Severe acute respiratory syndrome
SB Sinus bradycardia
SBP Systolic blood pressure
SCCM Society of Critical Care Medicine

SCD	Sequential compression devices
SCI	Spinal cord injury
SCID	Severe combined immune deficiencies
SCUF	Slow continuous ultrafiltration
SDH	Subdural hematoma
SEPs	Somatosensory-evoked potentials
SF-MPQ	Short-form McGill Pain Questionnaire
SG	Specific gravity
SGA	Subjective Global Assessment of Nutritional Status
SGOT	Serum glutamic oxaloacetic transaminase (AST)
SGPT	Serum glutamic pyruvic transaminase (ALT)
SIADH	Syndrome of inappropriate antidiuretic hormone
SIMV	Synchronous intermittent mandatory ventilation
SIRS	Systemic inflammatory response syndrome
SLE	Systemic lupus erythematosus
SOFA	Sequential Organ Failure Assessment
SPA	Sensory perceptual alterations
SPECT	Single photon emission computed tomography
SpO_2	Saturation of arterial capillary hemoglobin determined by pulse oximetry
ST	Sinus tachycardia
STD	Sexually transmitted disease
STEMI	*ST* segment elevation myocardial infarction
SV	Spontaneous ventilation; stroke volume
SVG	Saphenous vein graft
SVI	Stroke volume index
SvO_2	Mixed venous oxygen saturation
SVR	Systemic vascular resistance
SVRI	Systemic vascular resistance index
SVT	Supraventricular tachycardia
T	Thoracic vertebrae (T1–T12)
TBGH	Traumatic basal ganglia hemorrhage
TBI	Traumatic brain injury
TBSA	Total body surface area
TCD	Transcranial Doppler
TE	Tracheoesophageal
TEE	Transesophageal echocardiogram
TIA	Transient ischemic attack
TJC	The Joint Commission
TLC	Total lymphocyte count; total lung capacity
TNF	Tumor necrosis factor
tPA	Tissue plasminogen activator
TPN	Total parenteral nutrition
TRALI	Transfusion-related acute lung injury
UA	Unstable angina
UAGA	Uniform Anatomical Gift Act
UAP	Unlicensed assistive personnel
UH	Unfractionated heparin
UNOS	United Network for Organ Sharing
UUN	Urine urea nitrogen
$\dot{V}$	Ventilation
$\dot{V}_A$	Alveolar ventilation
$\dot{V}/\dot{Q}$	Ventilation–perfusion ratio
$\dot{V}CO_2$	Carbon dioxide produced
$\dot{V}O_2$	Oxygen consumption
VAC	Vacuum-assisted closure®
VAD	Ventricular assist device
VAE	Venous air embolism
VAP	Ventilator-associated pneumonia
VAS	Visual Analog Scale
VATS	Video-assisted thoracoscopic surgery
VC	Vital capacity
$\dot{V}_E$	Minute ventilation
VFib	Ventricular fibrillation
VO_2	Oxygen consumption
VRE	Vancomycin-resistant *Enterococci*
VT	Tidal volume; ventricular tachycardia
VTE	Venous thromboembolism
WBC	White blood cell count
WHO	World Health Organization

Index

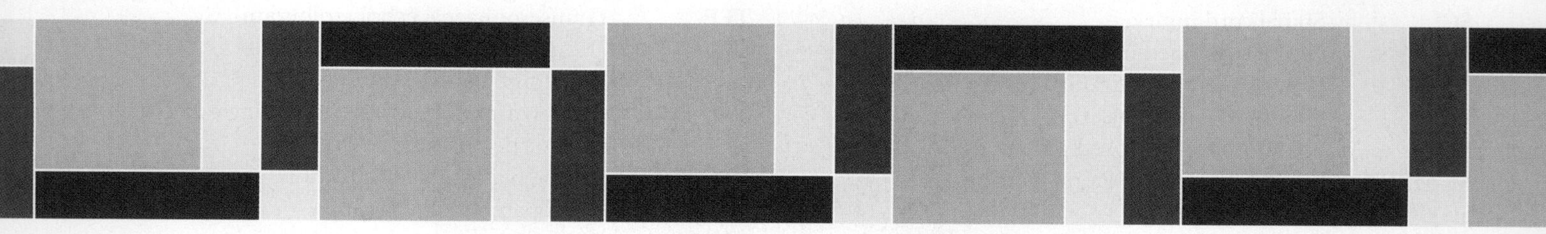

E

F

G

H

I

N

O

P

Q

R

S

T

X

Y

Z

Appendix

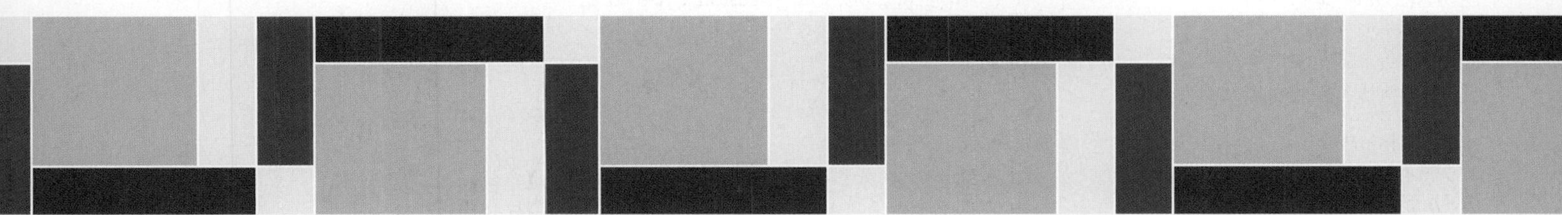

SUPPLEMENTAL ABG EXERCISES ANSWERS IN CHAPTER NINE

1. pH 7.58 (alkaline) and HCO_3 30 mEq/L (alkaline) match. $PaCO_2$ 38 mm Hg (normal). Interpretation: metabolic alkalosis. Compensation: uncompensated.
2. pH 7.20 (acid) and $PaCO_2$ 60 mm Hg (acid) match. HCO_3 26 mEq/L (normal). Interpretation: respiratory acidosis. Compensation: uncompensated.
3. pH 7.39 (normal, slightly to acid side of 7.4) and $PaCO_2$ 43 mm Hg (normal). HCO_3 24 (normal). Interpretation: normal. Compensation: none required.
4. pH 7.32 (acid) and $PaCO_2$ 60 mm Hg (acid) match. HCO_3 30 mEq/L (alkaline). Interpretation: respiratory acidosis. Compensation: partial compensation.
5. pH 7.5 (alkaline) and HCO_3 38 mEq/L (alkaline) match. $PaCO_2$ 50 mm Hg (acid). Interpretation: metabolic alkalosis. Compensation: partial compensation.
6. pH 7.45 (normal, alkaline side) and $PaCO_2$ 30 mm Hg (alkaline) match. HCO_3 20 mEq/L (acid). Interpretation: respiratory alkalosis. Compensation: full compensation.
7. pH, $PaCO_2$, and HCO_3 are all normal. Interpretation: normal. Compensation: none required.
8. pH 7.37 (normal range, acid) and $PaCO_2$ 48 mm Hg (acid) match. HCO_3 29 mEq/L (alkaline) is opposite. PaO_2 80 mm Hg and SaO_2 95 percent both are low normal. Acid–base state: compensated respiratory acidosis (pH normal). Oxygenation status: adequate. The Hgb is not known, but the relationship between PaO_2 and SaO_2 appears normal. Assessing trends is important. Is the $PaCO_2$ continuing to increase and PaO_2 continuing to decrease? Continue to monitor.
9. pH 7.48 (alkaline) and $PaCO_2$ 30 mm Hg (alkaline) match, HCO_3 24 mEq/L, PaO_2 90 mm Hg, and SaO_2 98 percent are all normal. Acid–base state: acute respiratory alkalosis (uncompensated). Oxygenation status: within normal limits and seems adequate. Look at your patient.
10. pH 7.48 (alkaline) and $PaCO_2$ 33 mm Hg (alkaline) match. HCO_3 25 mEq/L is normal. PaO_2 68 mm Hg (low) and SaO_2 98 percent (normal). Acid–base state: acute respiratory alkalosis. Oxygenation status: low oxygen with high saturation. Hemoglobin is carrying a full load but needs more carriers. What is this patient's hemoglobin? Nursing interventions may focus on decreasing oxygen demand. Is this patient tachypneic? Is supplemental oxygen available? Is a transfusion ordered?
11. pH 7.38, $PaCO_2$ 38 mm Hg, HCO_3 24 mEq/L are all normal. PaO_2 269 mm Hg is high, and SaO_2 100 percent is high normal. Acid–base state: normal. Oxygenation status: too high! What oxygen percentage is this patient on? Oxygenation supplement needs to be decreased.
12. pH 7.17 (acid) and HCO_3 7 mEq/L (acid) match. $PaCO_2$ 18 mm Hg (alkaline) is opposite. PaO_2 100 mm Hg is high, and SaO_2 99 percent is high normal. Acid–base state: severe metabolic acidosis with partial compensation. Oxygenation status: adequate oxygen provided, but it is doubtful that the patient can use what is available efficiently because of the state of severe acidosis. Cellular metabolism is compromised and cannot function efficiently in the acid environment. Cardiovascular status is very likely compromised. The reactivity and effectiveness of many drugs are altered severely in an acidic environment such as this.